D0206408

VOLUME 2

Section 8
Problems of Ingestion, Digestion, Absorption, and Elimination

38 Assessment of Gastrointestinal System, 833
39 Nutritional Problems, 854
40 Obesity, 874
41 Upper Gastrointestinal Problems, 893
42 Lower Gastrointestinal Problems, 929
43 Liver, Pancreas, and Biliary Tract Problems, 974

Section 9
Problems of Urinary Function

44 Assessment of Urinary System, 1015
45 Renal and Urologic Problems, 1033
46 Acute Kidney Injury and Chronic Kidney Disease, 1069

Section 10
Problems Related to Regulatory and Reproductive Mechanisms

47 Assessment of Endocrine System, 1102
48 Diabetes Mellitus, 1120
49 Endocrine Problems, 1156
50 Assessment of Reproductive System, 1184
51 Breast Disorders, 1204
52 Sexually Transmitted Infections, 1227
53 Female Reproductive and Genital Problems, 1242
54 Male Reproductive and Genital Problems, 1268

Section 11
Problems Related to Movement and Coordination

55 Assessment of Nervous System, 1294
56 Acute Intracranial Problems, 1314
57 Stroke, 1345
58 Chronic Neurologic Problems, 1368
59 Dementia and Delirium, 1399
60 Spinal Cord and Peripheral Nerve Problems, 1419
61 Assessment of Musculoskeletal System, 1446
62 Musculoskeletal Trauma and Orthopedic Surgery, 1462
63 Musculoskeletal Problems, 1496
64 Arthritis and Connective Tissue Diseases, 1517

Section 12
Nursing Care in Critical Care Settings

65 Critical Care, 1554
66 Shock, Sepsis, and Multiple Organ Dysfunction Syndrome, 1587
67 Acute Respiratory Failure and Acute Respiratory Distress Syndrome, 1609
68 Emergency and Disaster Nursing, 1628

Appendixes

A Basic Life Support for Health Care Professionals, 1650
B Nursing Diagnoses, 1653
C Laboratory Reference Intervals, 1655

Glossary, 1663
Index, I-1

evolve

ELSEVIER

YOU'VE JUST PURCHASED MORE THAN A TEXTBOOK!

Evolve Student Resources for *Medical-Surgical Nursing* include the following:

- Review Questions
- Key Points
- Answer Keys for Questions
  - Rationales for Bridge to NCLEX Examination Questions
  - Answer Guidelines for Case Studies
  - Answer Guidelines for Managing Care of Multiple Patients Case Studies
- Student Case Studies
- Nursing Care Plans
- Conceptual Care Map Creator
- Conceptual Care Maps
- Audio Glossary
- Stress-Busting Kit for Nursing Students
- Supporting Media
  - Animations
  - Audio
- Fluids and Electrolytes Tutorial
- Content Updates

Activate the complete learning experience that comes with each textbook purchase by registering at

http://evolve.elsevier.com/Lewis/

REGISTER TODAY!

You can now purchase Elsevier products on Evolve!
Go to evolve.elsevier.com/html/shop-promo.html to search and browse for products.

2015v1.0

10th Edition

MEDICAL-SURGICAL NURSING

Assessment and Management of Clinical Problems

Volume 1

Sharon L. Lewis, RN, PhD, FAAN
Professor Emerita, University of New Mexico, Albuquerque, New Mexico
Former Castella Distinguished Professor, School of Nursing, University of Texas Health Science Center at San Antonio, San Antonio, Texas
Developer and Consultant, Stress-Busting Program for Family Caregivers

Linda Bucher, RN, PhD, CEN, CNE
Emerita Professor, School of Nursing, University of Delaware, Newark, Delaware
Per Diem Staff Nurse, Emergency Department, Virtua Memorial Hospital, Mt. Holly, New Jersey

Margaret McLean Heitkemper, RN, PhD, FAAN
Professor and Chairperson, Biobehavioral Nursing and Health Systems, Elizabeth Sterling Soule Endowed Chair in Nursing, School of Nursing
Adjunct Professor, Division of Gastroenterology, School of Medicine, University of Washington, Seattle, Washington

Mariann M. Harding, RN, PhD, CNE
Associate Professor of Nursing, Kent State University at Tuscarawas, New Philadelphia, Ohio

Section Editors

Jeffrey Kwong, DNP, MPH, ANP-BC, FAANP
Associate Professor of Nursing at CUMC
Program Director, Adult-Gerontology Nurse Practitioner Program
Program Director, HIV Sub-Specialty
Program Director, Elder LGBT Interprofessional Collaborative Care Program (ELINC)
Program Director, Collaborative Access for LGBT Adults (CALA)
Columbia University School of Nursing
New York, New York

Dottie Roberts, RN, EdD, MSN, MACI, OCNS-C, CMSRN, CNE
Executive Director,
Orthopaedic Nurses Certification Board,
Chicago, Illinois;
Editor, "MEDSURG Nursing,"
Official Journal of the Academy
of Medical-Surgical Nurses
Pitman, New Jersey

ELSEVIER

ELSEVIER

3251 Riverport Lane
St. Louis, Missouri 63043

MEDICAL-SURGICAL NURSING; ASSESSMENT AND MANAGEMENT OF CLINICAL PROBLEMS, 10TH EDITION

ISBN (two-volume set): 978-0-323-35593-3
ISBN (Volume 1): 978-0-323-49759-6

Copyright © 2017 by Elsevier, Inc. All rights reserved.

No part of this publication may be reproduced or transmitted in any form or by any means, electronic or mechanical, including photocopying, recording, or any information storage and retrieval system, without permission in writing from the publisher. Details on how to seek permission, further information about the Publisher's permissions policies and our arrangements with organizations such as the Copyright Clearance Center and the Copyright Licensing Agency, can be found at our website: www.elsevier.com/permissions.

This book and the individual contributions contained in it are protected under copyright by the Publisher (other than as may be noted herein).

Notices

Knowledge and best practice in this field are constantly changing. As new research and experience broaden our understanding, changes in research methods, professional practices, or medical treatment may become necessary.

Practitioners and researchers must always rely on their own experience and knowledge in evaluating and using any information, methods, compounds, or experiments described herein. In using such information or methods they should be mindful of their own safety and the safety of others, including parties for whom they have a professional responsibility.

With respect to any drug or pharmaceutical products identified, readers are advised to check the most current information provided (i) on procedures featured or (ii) by the manufacturer of each product to be administered, to verify the recommended dose or formula, the method and duration of administration, and contraindications. It is the responsibility of practitioners, relying on their own experience and knowledge of their patients, to make diagnoses, to determine dosages and the best treatment for each individual patient, and to take all appropriate safety precautions.

To the fullest extent of the law, neither the Publisher nor the authors, contributors, or editors, assume any liability for any injury and/or damage to persons or property as a matter of products liability, negligence or otherwise, or from any use or operation of any methods, products, instructions, or ideas contained in the material herein.

Herdman, T.H. & Kamitsuru, S. (Eds.). (2014). *NANDA International Nursing Diagnoses: Definitions & Classification, 2015-2017.* Oxford: Wiley Blackwell.

Previous editions copyrighted 2014, 2011, 2007, 2004, 2000, 1996, 1992, 1987, and 1983 by Mosby, Inc., an affiliate of Elsevier Inc.

Library of Congress Cataloging-in-Publication Data

Names: Lewis, Sharon Mantik, author.
Title: Medical-surgical nursing : assessment and management of clinical problems / Sharon L. Lewis [and five others].
Description: Tenth edition. | St. Louis, Missouri : Elsevier, Inc, [2017] | Includes bibliographical references and index.
Identifiers: LCCN 2016018182| ISBN 9780323328524 (v. 1 : hardcover : alk. paper) | ISBN 9780323355933 (v. 2 : hardcover : alk. paper)
Subjects: | MESH: Nursing Care | Nursing Assessment | Perioperative Nursing
Classification: LCC RT41 | NLM WY 100 | DDC 617/.0231—dc23 LC record available at https://lccn.loc.gov/2016018182

Senior Content Strategist: Jamie Blum
Content Development Manager: Jean Sims Fornango
Content Development Specialist: Jennifer Hermes, Melissa Rawe
Publishing Services Manager: Julie Eddy
Senior Project Manager: Mary G. Stueck
Design Direction: Ashley Miner, Renée Duenow

Printed in the United States of America

Last digit is the print number: 9 8 7 6 5 4 3 2 1

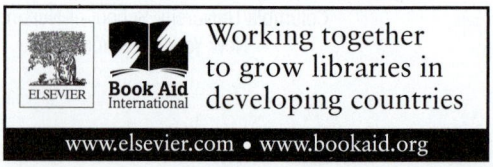

ABOUT THE AUTHORS

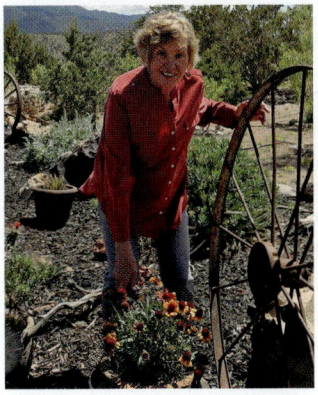

SHARON L. LEWIS, RN, PhD, FAAN

Sharon Lewis received her Bachelor of Science in nursing from the University of Wisconsin–Madison, Master of Science in nursing with a minor in biological sciences from the University of Colorado–Denver, and PhD in immunology from the Department of Pathology at the University of New Mexico School of Medicine. She had a 2-year postdoctoral fellowship from the National Kidney Foundation. Her more than 45 years of teaching experience include inservice education and teaching in associate degree, baccalaureate, master's degree, and doctoral programs in Maryland, Illinois, Wisconsin, New Mexico, and Texas. Favorite teaching areas are pathophysiology, immunology, and family caregiving. She has been actively involved in clinical research for the past 35 years, investigating altered immune responses in various disorders and developing a stress management program for family caregivers. Her current primary professional responsibility is disseminating the Stress-Busting for Family Caregivers Program that she developed. Her free time is spent biking, landscaping, gardening, and being a grandmother.

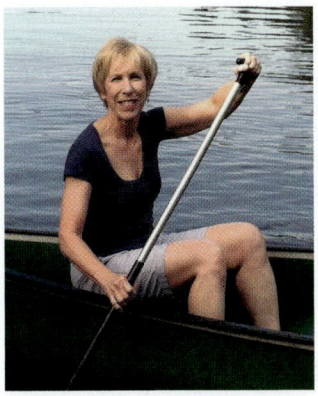

LINDA BUCHER, RN, PhD, CEN, CNE

Linda Bucher is an Emerita Professor in the School of Nursing at the University of Delaware in Newark, Delaware. She received her Bachelor of Science in nursing from Thomas Jefferson University in Philadelphia, her Master of Science in adult health and illness from the University of Pennsylvania in Philadelphia, and her doctorate in nursing from Widener University in Chester, Pennsylvania. Her 40 years of nursing experience have spanned staff and patient education, acute and critical care nursing, and teaching in associate, baccalaureate, and graduate nursing programs in New Jersey, Pennsylvania, and Delaware. Her preferred teaching areas include emergency and cardiac nursing and evidence-based practice. She maintains her clinical practice by working as an emergency nurse, actively participates in the American Association of Critical Care Nurses, and volunteers as a postoperative nurse for Operation Smile. In her free time, she enjoys traveling and skiing with her family.

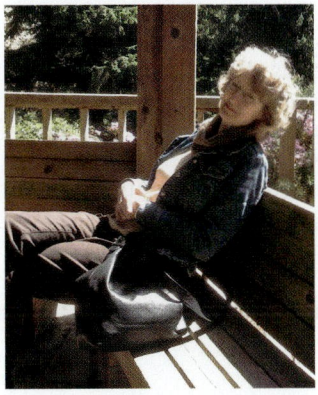

MARGARET MCLEAN HEITKEMPER, RN, PhD, FAAN

Margaret Heitkemper is Professor and Chairperson, Department of Biobehavioral Nursing and Health Systems at the School of Nursing, and Adjunct Professor, Division of Gastroenterology at the School of Medicine at the University of Washington. She is also Director of the National Institutes of Health-National Institute for Nursing Research–funded Center for Research on Management of Sleep Disturbances at the University of Washington. In the fall of 2006, Dr. Heitkemper was appointed the Elizabeth Sterling Soule Endowed Chair in Nursing. Dr. Heitkemper received her Bachelor of Science in nursing from Seattle University, a Master of Nursing in gerontologic nursing from the University of Washington, and a doctorate in Physiology and Biophysics from the University of Illinois–Chicago. She has been on faculty at the University of Washington since 1981 and has been the recipient of three School of Nursing Excellence in Teaching awards and the University of Washington Distinguished Teaching Award. In addition, in 2002 she received the Distinguished Nutrition Support Nurse Award from the American Society for Parenteral and Enteral Nutrition (ASPEN), in 2003 the American Gastroenterological Association and Janssen Award for Clinical Research in Gastroenterology, and in 2005 she was the first recipient of the Pfizer and Friends of the National Institutes for Nursing Research Award for Research in Women's Health.

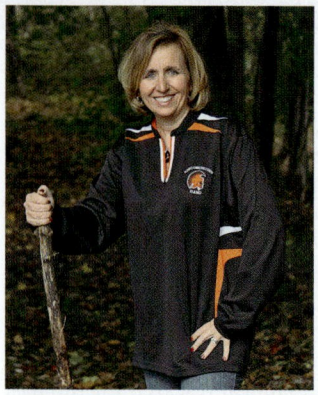

MARIANN M. HARDING, RN, PhD, CNE

Mariann Harding is an Associate Professor of Nursing at Kent State University Tuscarawas, New Philadelphia, Ohio, where she has been on the faculty since 2005. She received her diploma in nursing from Mt. Carmel School of Nursing in Columbus, Ohio, her Bachelor of Science in nursing from Ohio University in Athens, Ohio, her Master of Science in Nursing as an adult nurse practitioner from the Catholic University of America in Washington D.C., and her doctorate in nursing from West Virginia University in Morgantown, West Virginia. Her 29 years of nursing experience has primarily been in critical care nursing, and teaching in licensed practical, associate, and baccalaureate nursing programs. She currently teaches medical-surgical nursing, health care policy, and evidence-based practice. Her research has focused on promoting student success and health promotion among individuals with gout and facing cancer. Free time is spent with her family or traveling, walking, and reading.

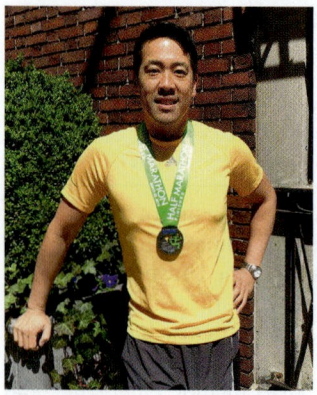

JEFFREY KWONG, DNP, MPH, ANP-BC, FAANP

Jeffrey Kwong is an Associate Professor of Nursing at Columbia University School of Nursing where he also serves as Director of the Adult-Gerontology Nurse Practitioner Program. He has worked in the area of adult primary care with a special focus on HIV for over 20 years. He received his undergraduate degree from the University of California–Berkeley, his nurse practitioner degree from the University of California–San Francisco, and completed his doctoral training at the University of Colorado–Denver. He also has a Master's Degree in Public Health with a focus on Health Education and Behavioral Sciences from the University of California–Los Angeles and was appointed a Hartford Geriatric Interprofessional Scholar while completing his gerontology education at NYU. In addition to teaching, Dr. Kwong maintains a clinical practice at Gotham Medical Group in New York City. In 2015 he was inducted as a Fellow in the American Association of Nurse Practitioners.

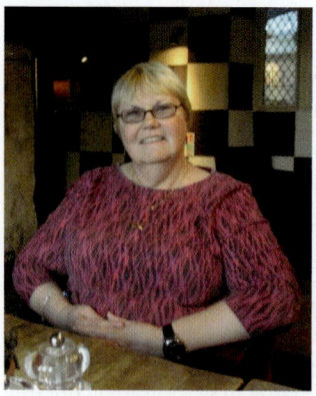

DOTTIE ROBERTS, RN, EdD, MSN, MACI, OCNS-C, CMSRN, CNE

Dottie Roberts received her Bachelor of Science in nursing from Beth-El College of Nursing, Colorado Springs, Colorado, Master of Science in adult health nursing from Beth-El College of Nursing and Health Sciences, Master of Arts in curriculum and instruction from Colorado Christian University, Colorado Springs, Colorado, and EdD in healthcare education from Nova Southeastern University, Ft. Lauderdale, Florida. She has over 25 years of experience in medical-surgical and orthopaedic nursing, and holds certifications in both specialties. She has also taught in two baccalaureate programs in the Southeast and is certified as a nurse educator. For her dissertation, Dottie completed a phenomenological study on facilitation of critical-thinking skills by clinical faculty in a baccalaureate nursing program. She has been Executive Director of the Orthopaedic Nurses Certification Board since 2005 and editor of "MEDSURG Nursing," the official journal of the Academy of Medical-Surgical Nurses, since 2003. Her free time is spent traveling, reading, and cross-stitching.

CONTRIBUTORS

Richard B. Arbour, RN, MSN, CCRN, CNRN, CCNS, FAAN
Clinical Faculty
School of Nursing
LaSalle University
Philadelphia, Pennsylvania

Adena Bargad, RN, PhD, CNM
Assistant Professor, Columbia University Medical Center
Director, Sub-Specialty Program in Women's Health
Columbia University School of Nursing
New York, New York

Diana Taibi Buchanan, RN, PhD
Associate Professor
Biobehavioral Nursing and Health Systems
University of Washington
Seattle, Washington

Darcy Burbage, RN, MSN, AOCN, CBCN
Survivorship Nurse Navigator
Helen F. Graham Cancer Center and Research Institute
Newark, Delaware

Kim K. Choma, RN, DNP, WHNP
Women's Health Nurse Practitioner–Training Consultant
NY/NJ AIDS Education and Training Centers (AETC)
New York, New York

Susan Collazo, MSN, APN-CNP
Thoracic Surgery
Northwestern Memorial Hospital
Chicago, Illinois

Paula P. Cox-North, PhD, ARNP
Clinical Assistant Professor
School of Nursing
University of Washington School of Nursing
Seattle, Washington

Hazel A. Dennison, RN, DNP, APNc, CPHQ, CNE
Director of Education Services
American Nephrology Nurses Association
Anthony J. Jannetti, Pub.
Pitman, New Jersey

Jane K. Dickinson, RN, PhD, CDE
Program Coordinator/Faculty
Diabetes Education and Management
Teachers College
Columbia University
New York, New York

Rose Ann DiMaria-Ghalili, RN, PhD, CNSC
Associate Professor of Nursing
College of Nursing and Health Professions
Drexel University
Philadelphia, Pennsylvania

Mechele Fillman, RN, MSN
Nursing Practitioner
Pain Management
Stanford Healthcare
Palo Alto, California

Diana L. Gallagher, RN, MS, CWOCN, CFCN
Clinical Nursing and Education
HealthMatters Consulting
Fayetteville, Arkansas

Sherry A. Greenberg, RN, PhD, GNP-BC
Coordinator, Advanced Practice Nursing: Geriatrics Program
Hartford Institute for Geriatric Nursing
New York University College of Nursing
New York, New York

Angela DiSabatino Herman, RN, MS
Manager, Cardiovascular Clinical Trials
Christiana Care Health Services
Newark, Delaware

Christine R. Hoch, RN, MSN
Nursing Instructor
University of Delaware
Newark, Delaware

David M. Horner, CRNA, MS, APN
CRNA Anesthesia
Marlton Hospital
Marlton, New Jersey

Melissa L. Hutchinson, RN, MN, CCNS, CCRN
Clinical Nurse Specialist
MICU/CCU
VA Puget Sound Health Care System
Seattle, Washington

Katherine A. Kelly, RN, DNP, FNP-C, CEN
Assistant Professor of Nursing
California State University
Sacramento, California

Judy Knighton, RN, MScN
Clinical Nurse Specialist—Burns
Ross Tilley Burn Centre
Sunnybrook Health Sciences Centre
Toronto, Ontario, Canada

Nancy Kupper, RN, MSN
Associate Professor of Nursing
Tarrant County College
Fort Worth, Texas

Janet Lenart, RN, MN, MPH
Senior Lecturer and Director for Online Education
University of Washington School of Nursing
Seattle, Washington

Linda Littlejohns, RN, MSN, CNRN, FAAN
Neuroscience Clinical Nursing Consultant
San Juan Capistrano, California

Amy McKeever, PhD, CRNP, WHNP-BC
Assistant Professor
College of Nursing
Villanova University
Villanova, Pennsylvania

De Ann F. Mitchell, RN, PhD
Director of Nursing
Tarrant County College
Fort Worth, Texas

Carolyn Moffa, RN, MSN, FNP-C, CHFN
Clinical Leader, Heart Failure Program
Christiana Care Health System
Newark, Delaware

Eugene E. Mondor, RN, MN, CNCC(C)
Clinical Nurse Educator—Adult Critical Care
Royal Alexandra Hospital
Edmonton, Alberta, Canada

Janice A. Neil, RN, PhD
Associate Professor and Chair
Undergraduate Nursing Science Junior Division
College of Nursing
East Carolina University
Greenville, North Carolina

Suzanne Teresa Parsell, MSN, ANP-BC, CUNP
Division of Endourology
University of Michigan
Ann Arbor, Michigan

Madona Dawn Plueger, RN, MSN, ACNS-BC, CNRN
Neuroscience Clinical Nurse Specialist
Barrow Neurological Institute
St. Joseph's Hospital and Medical Center
Phoenix, Arizona

Carolee Polek, RN, PhD, AOCNS, BMTCN
Associate Professor
School of Nursing
University of Delaware
Newark, Delaware

Rosemary C. Polomano, RN, PhD, FAAN
Professor of Pain Practice
Department of Biobehavioral Health Sciences
University of Pennsylvania School of Nursing;
Professor of Anesthesiology and Critical Care (Secondary)
University of Pennsylvania Perelman School of Medicine
Philadelphia, Pennsylvania

Matthew C. Price, RN, MS, CNP, ONP-C, RNFA
Manager, Orthopedic Advanced Practice Providers
Orthopedics
Riverside Methodist Hospital
Columbus, Ohio

Susanne A. Quallich, RN, MSN, ANP-BC, NP-C, CUNP
Andrology Nurse Practitioner
Urology
University of Michigan Health System
Ann Arbor, Michigan

Kathleen A. Rich, RN, PhD, CCNS, CCRN-CSC, CNN
Cardiovascular Clinical Specialist
Patient Care Services
IU Health La Porte Hospital
La Porte, Indiana

Sandra Irene Rome, RN, MN, AOCN, CNS
Clinical Nurse Specialist
Blood and Marrow Transplant Program
Cedars-Sinai Medical Center
Los Angeles, California

Jennifer Saylor, RN, PhD, ACNS-BC
Assistant Professor
School of Nursing
University of Delaware
Newark, Delaware

Maureen A. Seckel, RN, MSN, APN, ACNS-BC, CCNS, CCRN
Clinical Nurse Specialist
Medical Pulmonary Critical Care
Christiana Care Health System
Newark, Delaware

Rose Shaffer, RN, MSN, ACNP-CS, CCRN
Cardiology Nurse Practitioner
Thomas Jefferson University Hospital
Philadelphia, Pennsylvania

Anita Jo Shoup, RN, MSN, CNOR
Perioperative Clinical Nurse Specialist
Swedish Edmonds
Edmonds, Washington

Cindy M. Sullivan, MN, ANP-C, CNRN
Nurse Practitioner
Neurosurgery
Barrow Neurological Institute
Phoenix, Arizona

Linda A. L. Upchurch, DNP, ANP-BC
Assistant Professor
School of Nursing
Georgia Southern University
Statesboro, Georgia

Deidre D. Wipke-Tevis, RN, PhD
Associate Professor
PhD Program Director
MU Sinclair School of Nursing
University of Missouri
Columbia, Missouri

Mary K. Wollan, RN, BAN, ONC
Orthopaedic Nurse Educator
Excelen
Minneapolis, Minnesota

Kathy H. Wu, MSN, ANP-BC
Nurse Practitioner
Liver Transplant Center
New York Columbia Presbyterian Hospital
New York, New York

Meg Zomorodi, RN, PhD, CNL
Clinical Associate Professor
School of Nursing
University of North Carolina at Chapel Hill
Chapel Hill, North Carolina

Michael E. Zychowicz, RN, DNP, ANP, ONP, FAAN, FAANP
Associate Professor and Director, MSN Program
School of Nursing
Duke University
Durham, North Carolina

REVIEWERS

Karen S. Abate, PhD, FNP-BC
Trenton, New Jersey

Marian Altman, RN, MS, CNS-BC, ANP
Richmond, Virginia

Carol Annesser, RN, MSN, BC, CNE
Toledo, Ohio

Tara Back, RN, MSN
St. Louis, Missouri

Carolyn Baird, DNP, MBA, RN-BC, CARN-AP, CCDPD, FIAAN
Canonsburg, Pennsylvania

Adena Bargad, PhD, CNM
New York, New York

Janica Barnett, JD, AGPCNP-BC
New York, New York

Margaret Barton-Burke, RN, PhD, FAAN
St. Louis, Missouri

Vera Barton-Caro, RN, PhD, FNP-BC, CHFN
Wheeling, West Virginia

Cecilia M. Bidigare, RN, MSN, CNS-BC, CNE
Dayton, Ohio

Sonya H. Blevins, RN, DNP, CMSRN, CNE
Greenville, South Carolina

Donna C. Bond, RN, DNP, CCNS, AE-C, CTTS
Roanoke, Virginia

Marilyn Borkgren, APN, MS, CCNS
Elk Grove Village, Illinois

Elisabeth G. Bradley, MS, APN, ACNS-BC, AGPCNP-BC
Newark, Delaware

Marylee Bressie, RN, DNP, CCRN, CCNS, CEN
Minneapolis, Minnesota

Barbara Brunow, RN, MSN, MEd, CNS, CNE
Sandusky, Ohio

Diana Taibi Buchanan, RN, PhD
Seattle, Washington

Geraldine M. Budd, RN, PhD, FNP-BC, FAANP
Harrisburg, Pennsylvania

Darcy Burbage, RN, MSN, AOCN, CBCN
Newark, Delaware

Patricia Gable Burke, RN, BSN, CWOCN
Cincinnati, Ohio

Hope Bussenius, DNP, APRN, FNP-BC
Atlanta, Georgia

Judy Carlyle, RN, MNSc
Nashville, Arkansas

Kim K. Choma, RN, DNP, WHNP
New York, New York

Kim Clevenger, RN, EdD, BC
Morehead, Kentucky

Deborah Cline, RN, MS
Reno, Nevada

Susan Collazo, MSN, APN-CNP
Chicago, Illinois

Janie Corbitt, RN, MLS
Milledgeville, Georgia

Hazel A. Dennison, RN, DNP, APNc, CPHQ, CNE
Pitman, New Jersey

Jane K. Dickinson, RN, PhD, CDE
New York, New York

Vickie Lee Doscher, MSN, FNP-C, APRN
Chesapeake, Virginia

Deborah Ehlers, RN, MSN
Yakima, Washington

Susan J. Eisel, RN, MSEd
Toledo, Ohio

Rowena W. Elliott, RN, PhD, CNN, CNE, AGNP-C, FAAN
Hattiesburg, Mississippi

Dana R. Epstein, RN, PhD
Tempe, Arizona

Deborah Erickson, RN, PhD
Peoria, Illinois

Christine Espina, RN, DNP
Seattle, Washington

Cora Espina, RN, MN, ARNP, CWN
Seattle, Washington

Abimbola Farinde, PharmD, MS
Orange Beach, Alabama

Brian J. Fasolka, RN, MSN, CEN
Philadelphia, Pennsylvania

Marianne Ferrin, MSN, ACNP-BC
Philadelphia, Pennyslvania

Diana L. Gallagher, RN, MS, CWOCN, CFCN
Fayetteville, Arkansas

Karen Gilbert, RN, MSN, CNSC, CRNP
Riverton, New Jersey

Nelda S. Godfrey, RN, PhD, ACNS-BC, FAAN
Kansas City, Kansas

Roberta Goff, MSN Ed, RN-BC, ACNS-BC, ONC
Traverse City, Michigan

Regina Gonzalez-Lama, RN, MS
Staten Island, New York

Debra B. Gordon, RN-BC, DNP, ACNS-BC, FAAN
Seattle, Washington

Shari Gould, RN, MSN
Victoria, Texas

Sherry A. Greenberg, RN, PhD, GNP-BC
New York, New York

Kelly S. Grimshaw, RN, MSN, APRN, CCRN, CCTN
New Haven, Connecticut

Sharon Haas, RN, MSN, CDN
Milwaukee, Wisconsin

Debra Hagler, RN, PhD, ACNS-BC, CNE, CHSE, ANEF, FAAN
Phoenix, Arizona

Cynthia Hambach, RN, MSN, CCRN
Philadelphia, Pennsylvania

Janet L. Hannah, RN, CGRN
Leesburg, Virginia

Carla V. Hannon, MS, APRN, CCRN, CCNS
New Haven, Connecticut

Helene Harris, RN, MSN
Temple, Texas

Misty Hobart, RN, MSN, CNE
Spokane, Washington

Deena Hollingsworth, MSN, FNP-BC, CORLN
Arlington, Virginia

Michele M. Hughes, RN, MSN, ACNP, ONP-C
Mechanicvsille, Virginia

Melissa Hutchinson, RN, MN, CCNS, CCRN
Seattle, Washington

Stephanie Jackson, RN, MSN, AOCNS
Los Angeles, California

Suzanne Jed, MSN, FNP-BC
Pretoria, South Africa

Monica L. Johnson, RN, MSN, MBA-HCM, CMSRN, ONC, LNC
New Orleans, Louisiana

Jane Kaufman, MS, CRNP, ANP-BC
Philadelphia, Pennsylvania

Christina D. Keller, RN, MSN-Ed
Radford, Virginia

Lauren Kemph, RN, DNP, AGPCNP
New York, New York

Tracy H. Knoll, RN, MSN
St. Louis, Missouri

Regina Kukulski, RN, MSN, ACNS, BC, CNE
Trenton, New Jersey

Jane E. Lacovara, RN, MSN, CMSRN
Tucson, Arizona

Katherine A. Ladetto, RN, MSN, APRN, ANP-BC, GNP-BC
Peabody, Massachusetts

Susan C. Landis, RN, MN
Seattle, Washington

Marci Langenkamp, RN, MS
Piqua, Ohio

Patricia Lea, RN, DNP, CCRN
Galveston, Texas

Judith M. Lewis, DNP, APRN, CRNA
Akron, Ohio

Linda R. Lewis, MSN, RN-BC
Scranton, Pennsylvania

Rebecca Liebert, RN, MSN, FNP-C, ONP-C
Tomah, Wisconsin

Linda Littlejohns, RN, MSN, CNRN, FAAN
San Juan Capistrano, California

Anthony R. Lutz, RN, MSN, A-GNP-C
Charlotte, North Carolina

Carolyn Lyon, RN, MSN
Roanoke, Virginia

Angela M. Martinelli, RN, PhD, CNOR
Fairfield, Connecticut

Donna E. McCabe, DNP, APRN-BC, GNP
New York, New York

Molly McClelland, RN, PhD, ACNS-BC, CMSRN
Detroit, Michigan

Tara McMillan-Queen, RN, MSN, ANP, GNP
Charlotte, North Carolina

Molly McNett, RN, PhD, CNRN
Cleveland, Ohio

Karen Meneses, RN, PhD, FAAN
Birmingham, Alabama

Eugene E. Mondor, RN, MN, CNCC(C)
Edmonton, Alberta, Canada

Heidi E. Monroe, MSN, RN-BC, CPAN, CAPA
Green Bay, Wisconsin

Anna P. Moore, RN, MS
Richmond, Virginia

Kathy Morrison, RN, MSN, CNRN, SCRN
Hershey, Pennsylvania

Pamela K. Newland, RN, PhD, CMSRN
St. Louis, Missouri

Lorraine Nowakowski-Grier, MSN, APRN-BC, CDE
Newark, Delaware

Ellen Odell, DNP, ACNS-BC, CNE, APRN
Siloam Springs, Arkansas

Suzanne Teresa Parsell, MSN, ANP-BC, CUNP
Ann Arbor, Michigan

Jessica Pastor, MSN, DNP(c), ACNP-BC, SANE-A, TNCC
Detroit and Troy, Michigan

Rebecca Personett, RN, PhD, NEA-BC
Gainesville and Dallas, Texas

Madona Dawn Plueger, RN, MSN, ACNS-BC, CNRN
Phoenix, Arizona

Carolee Polek, RN, PhD, AOCNS, BMTCN
Newark, Delaware

Julia R. Popp, RN, MSN
Toledo, Ohio

Sarah Byram Poppe, MSN, ANP-BC
Olympia, Washington

Matthew C. Price, RN, MS, CNP, ONP-C, RNFA
Columbus, Ohio

Susanne A. Quallich, RN, MSN, ANP-BC, NP-C, CUNP
Ann Arbor, Michigan

Margaret R. Rateau, RN, PhD, CNE
East Liverpool, Ohio

Patricia S. Regojo, RN, MSN
Philadelphia, Pennsylvania

Courtney Reinisch, RN, DNP, APN-BC, DCC
Newark, New Jersey

Janet M. Riggs, RN, DrNP
Philadelphia, Pennsylvania

Julie Rogan, RN, MSN, ACCNS-AG, AOCNS, CCRN
Philadelphia, Pennsylvania

Diane Marie Rudolphi, RN, MS
Newark, Delaware

Diane Ryzner, MSN, APN, CNS, OCNS-C
Arlington Heights, Illinois

Susan A. Sandstrom, RN, MSN, BC, CNE
Omaha, Nebraska

Christine L. Savage, RN, PhD, CARN, FAAN
Baltimore, Maryland

Jennifer Saylor, RN, PhD, ACNS-BC
Newark, Delaware

Mary Scheid, RN, MSN, OCN, CBCN
Greeley, Colorado

Teresa J. Seright, RN, PhD, CCRN
Bozeman, Montana

Crystal Sheaves, RN, MSN, APRN, FNP-BC
Charleston, West Virginia

Crystal R. Sherman, DNP, CNP, FNP-BC, APHN-BC
Portsmouth, Ohio

Michelle Smeltzer, RN, MSN, DNPc, CEN
East Norriton, Pennsylvania

Matthew Soos, RN, BSN, BA, EMT
Atlantic City, New Jersey

Lisa Spruce, DNP, ACNS, ACNP, ANP, CNOR, CNS-CP
Denver, Colorado

Whitney Starr, MSN, FNP-BC
Denver, Colorado

Cynthia M. Steinwedel, RN, PhD, CNE
Peoria, Illinois

Laura A. Stokowski, RNC, MS
Falls Church, Virginia

Beth D. Strauss, RN, DNP, ACNS-BC
Madison, Wisconsin

Cindy M. Sullivan, MN, ANP-C, CNRN
Phoenix, Arizona

Joseph Tariman, RN, PhD, ANP-BC
Chicago, Illinois

Allison J. Terry, RN, PhD
Montgomery, Alabama

Tamekia L. Thomas, MSN, APN, PCCN, ACNS-BC
Newark, Delaware

Andrea H. Thurler, RN, DNP, FNP-BC
Boston, Massachusetts

Bonnie Tong, MSN, ACNP-BC
New York, New York

Mary Ellen Tresgallo, DNP, MPH, FNP-BC
New York, New York

Kathryn J. Trotter, DNP, CNM, FNP-C
Durham, North Carolina

Linda A. L. Upchurch, DNP, ANP-BC
Statesboro, Georgia

Olga Van Dyke, RN, MSN, CAGS
Boston, Massachusetts

Dawn M. Vanderhoef, PhD, DNP, PMHNP/CS-BC
Nashville, Tennessee

Deborah Kirk Walker, DNP, FNP-BC, NP-C, AOCN
Birmingham, Alabama

Colleen R. Walsh, RN, DNP, ONC, ONP-C, CNS, ACNP-BC
Evansville, Indiana

Daryle Wane, PhD, ARNP, FNP-BC
New Port Richey, Florida

Robert M. Welch, RN, MSN, FNP, CRNO
Reno, Nevada

Laura C. Williams, RN, MSN, CNS, ONC, CCNS
Orlando, Florida

Daniel Worrall, MSN, ANP-BC
Boston, Massachusetts

Kathy H. Wu, MSN, ANP-BC
New York, New York

Elsa Wuhrman, DNP, RN-BC, FNP, BC, DCC
New York, New York

Kenneth Wysocki, PhD, FNP-BC, FAANP
Scottsdale, Arizona

Linda H. Yoder, RN, PhD, AOCN, FAAN
Austin, Texas

Meg Zomorodi, RN, PhD, CNL
Chapel Hill, North Carolina

To the Profession of Nursing
and to the Important People in Our Lives

Sharon
My husband Peter and our grandchildren
Malia, Halle, Aidan, Cian, Layla, Ryker, and Archer

Linda
My nieces, Stefany and Jayme,
who so admirably reflect the ideals of the nursing profession
and my godchild, Liz, for her love of written words.

Margaret
My husband David, our daughters Elizabeth and Ellen,
and our grandsons Jaxon James and Axel

Mariann
My husband Jeff and our daughters Kate and Sarah

Jeff
To my mother, Virginia, whose dedication to the field of nursing
led me on this wonderful journey.

Dottie
My husband Steve and my children Megan, E.J., Jessica, and Matthew,
who have supported me through four college degrees and countless writing projects,
and to our grandsons Oscar and Stephen.

PREFACE

The tenth edition of *Medical-Surgical Nursing: Assessment and Management of Clinical Problems* has been thoroughly revised to incorporate the most current medical-surgical nursing information in an easy-to-use format. More than just a textbook, this is a comprehensive resource containing essential information that students need to prepare for lectures, classroom activities, examinations, clinical assignments, and the safe, comprehensive care of patients. In addition to the readable writing style and full-color illustrations, the text and accompanying resources include many special features to help students learn key medical-surgical nursing content, including patient and caregiver teaching, gerontology, interprofessional care, cultural and ethnic considerations, patient safety, genetics, nutrition and drug therapy, evidence-based practice, and much more.

The comprehensive and timely content, special features, attractive layout, and student-friendly writing style combine to make this the number one medical-surgical nursing textbook used in more nursing schools than any other medical-surgical nursing textbook.

The strengths of the first nine editions have been retained, including the use of the nursing process as an organizational theme for nursing management. Numerous new features have been added to address some of the rapid changes in practice. Contributors have been selected for their expertise in specific content areas; one or more specialists in the subject area have thoroughly reviewed each chapter to increase accuracy. The editors have undertaken final rewriting and editing to achieve internal consistency. All efforts have been directed toward building on the strengths of the previous edition while preparing an even more effective new edition.

ORGANIZATION

Content is organized into two major divisions. The first division, Section 1 (Chapters 1 through 10), discusses general concepts related to adult patients. The second division, Sections 2 through 12 (Chapters 11 through 68), presents nursing assessment and nursing management of medical-surgical problems.

The various body systems are grouped to reflect their interrelated functions. Each section is organized around two central themes: assessment and management. Chapters dealing with assessment of a body system include a discussion of the following:

1. A brief review of anatomy and physiology, focusing on information that will promote understanding of nursing care
2. Health history and noninvasive physical assessment skills to expand the knowledge base on which treatment decisions are made
3. Common diagnostic studies, expected results, and related nursing responsibilities to provide easily accessible information

Management chapters focus on the pathophysiology, clinical manifestations, diagnostic studies, interprofessional care, and nursing management of various diseases and disorders. The nursing management sections are organized into assessment, nursing diagnoses, planning, implementation, and evaluation. To emphasize the importance of patient care in various clinical settings, nursing implementation of all major health problems is organized by the following levels of care:

1. Health Promotion
2. Acute Care
3. Ambulatory Care

CLASSIC FEATURES

- **Nursing management** is presented in a consistent and comprehensive format, with headings for Health Promotion, Acute Care, and Ambulatory Care. Over 60 nursing care plans on the Evolve website incorporate Nursing Interventions Classification (NIC) and Nursing Outcomes Classification (NOC) in a way that clearly shows the linkages among NIC, NOC, and nursing diagnoses, and applies them to nursing practice.
- **Cultural and ethnic health disparities** content and boxes in the text highlight risk factors and important issues related to the nursing care of various ethnic groups. A special Culturally Competent Care heading denotes cultural and ethnic content related to diseases and disorders. Chapter 2: Health Disparities and Culturally Competent Care discusses health status differences among groups of people related to access to care, economic aspects of health care, gender and cultural issues, and disease risk.
- **Interprofessional care** is highlighted in special Interprofessional Care sections in all management chapters and Interprofessional Care tables throughout the text.
- **Coverage on delegation and prioritization** includes the following:
  - Teamwork & Collaboration boxes highlight the nurse's role in working with members of the interprofessional team and also cover specific topics and skills related to delegation
  - Delegation and prioritization questions in case studies and Bridge to NCLEX Examination Questions
  - Nursing interventions throughout the text are listed in order of priority
  - Nursing diagnoses in the nursing care plans are listed in order of priority
- **Focused Assessment boxes** in all assessment chapters provide brief checklists that help students do a more practical "assessment on the run" or bedside approach to assessment. They can be used to evaluate the status of previously identified health problems and monitor for signs of new problems.
- **Safety Alert boxes** highlight important patient safety issues and focus on the National Patient Safety Goals.
- **Pathophysiology Maps** outline complex concepts related to diseases in flowchart format, making them easier to understand.
- **Patient and caregiver teaching** is an ongoing theme throughout the text. Chapter 4: Patient and Caregiver Teaching emphasizes the increasing importance and prevalence of patient management of chronic illnesses and conditions and the role of the caregiver in patient care.
- **Gerontology and chronic illness** are discussed in Chapter 5: Chronic Illness and Older Adults, and included throughout

the text under Gerontologic Considerations headings and in Gerontologic Differences in Assessment tables.

- **Nutrition** is highlighted throughout the book. Nutritional Therapy tables summarize nutritional interventions and promote healthy lifestyles in patients with various health problems.
- ***Healthy People* boxes** present health care goals as they relate to specific disorders such as diabetes and cancer.
- **Extensive drug therapy** content includes Drug Therapy tables and concise Drug Alerts highlighting important safety considerations for key drugs.
- **Genetics content** includes:
  - Genetics in Clinical Practice boxes that summarize the genetic basis, genetic testing, and clinical implications for genetic disorders that affect adults
  - A genetics chapter that focuses on practical application of nursing care as it relates to this important topic
  - Genetic Risk Alerts in the assessment chapters call attention to important genetic risks
  - Genetic Link headings in the management chapters highlight the specific genetic bases of many disorders
- **Gender Differences** boxes discuss how women and men are affected differently by conditions such as pain and hypertension.
- **Complementary & Alternative Therapies boxes** expand on this information and summarize what nurses need to know about therapies such as herbal remedies, acupuncture, and biofeedback.
- **Ethical/Legal Dilemmas boxes** promote critical thinking for timely and sensitive issues that nursing students may deal with in clinical practice—topics such as informed consent, advance directives, and confidentiality.
- **Emergency Management tables** outline the emergency treatment of health problems most likely to require emergency intervention.
- **Assessment Abnormalities tables** in assessment chapters alert the nurse to frequently encountered abnormalities and their possible etiologies.
- **Nursing Assessment tables** summarize the key subjective and objective data related to common diseases. Subjective data are organized by functional health patterns.
- **Health History tables** in assessment chapters present key questions to ask patients related to a specific disease or disorder.
- **Evidence-based practice** is covered throughout the book in Applying the Evidence boxes, Translating Research Into Practice boxes, and evidence-based practice-focused questions in the case studies.
- **Student-friendly pedagogy** includes the following:
  - Learning Outcomes and Key Terms at the beginning of each chapter help students identify the key content for that chapter.
  - Evolve website boxes at the end of each chapter alert students to supplemental online content and exercises, making it easy for students to facilitate online learning.
  - Bridge to NCLEX® Examination Questions at the end of each chapter are matched to the learning outcomes and help students learn the important points in the chapter. Answers are provided just below the questions for immediate feedback, and rationales are provided on the Evolve website.
  - Case Studies with photos bring patients to life. Management chapters have case studies at the end of the chapters. These cases help students learn how to prioritize care and manage patients in the clinical setting. Unfolding case studies are included in each assessment chapter and case studies that focus on managing care of multiple patients are included at the end of each section. Discussion questions with a focus on prioritization, delegation, and evidence-based practice are included in all case studies. Answer guidelines are provided on the Evolve website.
- A **glossary** of key terms and definitions is provided at the back of the text. An expanded version of the glossary with audio pronunciations is included on the Evolve website.

NEW FEATURES

- **Check Your Practice boxes** challenge students to think critically, analyze patient assessment data, and implement the appropriate intervention. Scenarios and discussion questions are provided to promote active learning.
- **Becoming a Nurse Leader boxes** introduce students to concepts related to being a responsible team member and leader. They cover topics such as how nurses can build supportive relationships in the work environment, how to manage a team when providing care, dealing with a changing environment, and more.
- **Informatics boxes and content** in the Patient and Caregiver Teaching chapter reflect the current use and importance of technology as it relates to patient self-management.
- **Increased focus on developing critical thinking skills** is apparent in the Evidence-Based Practice boxes where students are engaged in discussing the implications of EBP findings for nursing practice. The unfolding case studies in assessment chapters also include additional discussion questions to facilitate critical thinking.
- **Increased focus on ambulatory and chronic care** addresses the increasing management of patients on an outpatient basis.
- **QSEN competencies** are highlighted in the core content, case studies, and nursing care plans.

LEARNING SUPPLEMENTS FOR STUDENTS

- The handy **Clinical Companion** presents approximately 200 common medical-surgical conditions and procedures in a concise, alphabetical format for quick clinical reference. Designed for portability, this popular reference includes the essential, need-to-know information for treatments and procedures in which nurses play a major role. An attractive and functional four-color design highlights key information for quick, easy reference.
- An exceptionally thorough **Study Guide** contains over 500 pages of review material that reflect the content found in the book. It features a wide variety of clinically relevant exercises and activities, including NCLEX-format multiple choice and alternate format questions, case studies, anatomy review, critical thinking activities, and much more. It features an attractive four-color design and many alternate-item format questions to better prepare students for the NCLEX examination. An answer key is included to provide students with immediate feedback as they study.

- The **Evolve Student Resources** are available online at http://evolve.elsevier.com/Lewis/medsurg and include the following valuable learning aids organized by chapter:
  - Printable **Key Points** summaries for each chapter
  - 1000 NCLEX Examination **Review Questions**
  - **Answer Guidelines** to the case studies in the textbook
  - **Rationales for the Bridge to NCLEX® Examination Questions** in the textbook
  - 55 **Interactive Case Studies** with state-of-the-art animations and a variety of learning activities, which provide students with immediate feedback. Ten of the case studies are enhanced with photos and narration of the clinical scenarios.
  - Customizable **Nursing Care Plans**
  - **Conceptual Care Map Creator** and conceptual care maps for selected case studies in the textbook
  - **Audio glossary** of key terms, available as comprehensive alphabetical glossary and organized by chapter
  - **Stress-Busting Kit**
  - **Supporting Media**, including animations and audio clips
  - **Fluids and Electrolytes Tutorial**
  - **Content Updates**
- **Virtual Clinical Excursions (VCE)** is an exciting learning tool that brings learning to life in a "virtual" hospital setting. VCE simulates a realistic, yet safe, nursing environment where the routine and rigors of the average clinical rotation abound. Students can conduct a complete assessment of a patient and set priorities for care, collect data, analyze and interpret data, prepare and administer medications, and reach conclusions about complex problems. Each lesson has a textbook reading assignment and online activities based on "visiting" patients in the hospital. Instructors receive an implementation manual with directions for using VCE as a teaching tool.
- More than just words on a screen, **Elsevier eBooks** come with a wealth of built-in study tools and interactive functionality to help students better connect with the course material and their instructors. Plus, with the ability to fit an entire library of books on one portable device, students have the ability to study when, where, and how they want.

TEACHING SUPPLEMENTS FOR INSTRUCTORS

- The **Evolve Instructor Resources** (available online at http://evolve.elsevier.com/Lewis/medsurg) remain the most comprehensive set of instructor's materials available, containing the following:
  - **TEACH for Nurses Lesson Plans** with electronic resources organized by chapter to help instructors develop and manage the course curriculum. This exciting resource includes:
    - Objectives
    - Teaching focus
    - Key terms
    - Nursing curriculum standards
    - Student and instructor chapter resource listings
    - Teaching strategies with learning activities and assessment methods tied to learning outcomes
    - **Case studies** with answer guidelines
  - The **Test Bank** features over 2000 NCLEX Examination test questions with text page references and answers coded for NCLEX Client Needs category, nursing process, and cognitive level. The test bank includes hundreds of prioritization, delegation, and multiple patient questions. All alternate item format questions are included. The ExamView software allows instructors to create new tests; edit, add, and delete test questions; sort questions by NCLEX category, cognitive level, nursing process step, and question type; and administer and grade online tests.
  - The **Image Collection** contains more than 800 full-color images from the text for use in lectures.
  - An extensive collection of **PowerPoint Presentations** includes over 125 different presentations focused on the most common diseases and disorders. The presentations have been thoroughly revised to include helpful instructor notes/teaching tips, unfolding case studies, new illustrations and photos not found in the book, new animations, and updated audience response questions for use with iClicker and other audience response systems.
  - Course management system.
  - Access to all student resources listed above.
- The **Simulation Learning System (SLS)** is an online toolkit that helps instructors and facilitators effectively incorporate medium- to high-fidelity simulation into their nursing curriculum. Detailed patient scenarios promote and enhance the clinical decision-making skills of students at all levels. The SLS provides detailed instructions for preparation and implementation of the simulation experience, debriefing questions that encourage critical thinking, and learning resources to reinforce student comprehension. Each scenario in the SLS complements the textbook content and helps bridge the gap between lecture and clinical. The SLS provides the perfect environment for students to practice what they are learning in the text for a true-to-life, hands-on learning experience.

ACKNOWLEDGMENTS

The editors are especially grateful to many people at Elsevier who assisted with this major revision effort. In particular, we wish to thank the team of Jamie Blum, Jennifer Hermes, Mary Stueck, Julie Eddy, and Ashley Miner. In addition, we want to thank Becky Ramsaroop in marketing.

Special thanks and appreciation go to Peter Bonner who assisted with many details of manuscript preparation and review and photography for the book and interactive case studies.

We are particularly indebted to the faculty, nurses, and student nurses who have put their faith in our book to assist them on their path to excellence. The increasing use of this book throughout the United States, Canada, Australia, and other parts of the world has been gratifying. We appreciate the many users who have shared their comments and suggestions on the previous editions. All feedback is welcome.

We also wish to thank our contributors and reviewers for their assistance with the revision process. We sincerely hope that this book will assist both students and clinicians in practicing truly professional nursing.

Sharon L. Lewis
Linda Bucher
Margaret McLean Heitkemper
Mariann M. Harding
Jeffrey Kwong
Dottie Roberts

AUTHORS OF TEACHING AND LEARNING RESOURCES

TEST BANK

Debra Hagler, RN, PhD, ACNS-BC, CNE, CHSE, ANEF, FAAN
Clinical Professor
College of Nursing and Healthcare Innovation
Arizona State University
Phoenix, Arizona

CASE STUDIES

Interactive and Managing Care of Multiple Patients Case Studies

Katherine A. Kelly, RN, DNP, FNP-C, CEN
Assistant Professor of Nursing
California State University
Sacramento, California

Sarah Barnes, RN, DNP
Assistant Professor of Nursing
California State University
Sacramento, California

POWERPOINT PRESENTATIONS

Jane E. Oehme, RN, MS
Associate Professor of Nursing
Pennsylvania College of Technology
Williamsport, Pennsylvania

Michele A. Walczak, RN, MSN
Associate Professor of Nursing
Pennsylvania College of Technology
Williamsport, Pennsylvania

TEACH FOR NURSES

Margaret R. Rateau, RN, PhD, CNE
Associate Professor of Nursing
Kent State University–Columbiana at East Liverpool
East Liverpool, Ohio

AUDIENCE RESPONSE QUESTIONS

Jane E. Oehme, RN, MS
Associate Professor of Nursing
Pennsylvania College of Technology
Williamsport, Pennsylvania

Michele A. Walczak, RN, MSN
Associate Professor of Nursing
Pennsylvania College of Technology
Williamsport, Pennsylvania

NCLEX EXAMINATION REVIEW QUESTIONS

Mary Boyce, RN, MSN, CCRN, CNE
Mesa Community College
Mesa, Arizona

Sarah Barnes, RN, DNP
Assistant Professor of Nursing
California State University
Sacramento, California

Leigh W. Moore, RN, MSN, CNOR, CNE
Associate Professor of Nursing–ADN
Southside Virginia Community College
Alberta, Virginia

STUDY GUIDE

Susan A. Sandstrom, RN, MSN, BC, CNE
Associate Professor in Nursing, Retired
College of Saint Mary
Omaha, Nebraska

CLINICAL COMPANION

Debra Hagler, RN, PhD, ACNS-BC, CNE, CHSE, ANEF, FAAN
Clinical Professor
College of Nursing and Healthcare Innovation
Arizona State University
Phoenix, Arizona

ETHICAL/LEGAL DILEMMAS BOXES

Katherine K. Anselmi, JD, PhD, WHNP-BC
Associate Clinical Professor
Assistant Dean of Accreditation/Regulatory Affairs and Online Innovation
College of Nursing and Health Professions
Drexel University
Philadelphia, Pennsylvania

Vicki D. Lachman, RN, PhD, APRN, FAAN, NEA-BC
President
V.L. Associates
Avalon, New Jersey

EVIDENCE-BASED PRACTICE BOXES

Shannon Ruff Dirksen, RN, PhD, FAAN
Associate Professor
College of Nursing and Health Innovation
Arizona State University
Phoenix, Arizona

NURSING CARE PLANS

Collin Bowman-Woodall, RN, MS
Assistant Professor
Samuel Merritt University
San Francisco Peninsula Learning Center
San Mateo, California

BECOMING A NURSE LEADER BOXES

Donna Jean Middaugh, RN, PhD
Associate Dean for Academic Programs
College of Nursing
University of Arkansas for Medical Sciences
Little Rock, Arkansas

GLOSSARY

Cory Retherford, MSOM
Former Research Assistant
University of Texas Health Science Center at San Antonio
San Antonio, Texas

SPECIAL PROJECTS

Peter Bonner, MS
Former Professor and Research Statistician
New Mexico Highlands University
Las Vegas, New Mexico;
DSI
Placitas, New Mexico

CONTENTS

VOLUME 1

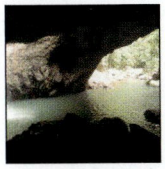

Section 1
Concepts in Nursing Practice

1 Professional Nursing Practice, 2
2 Health Disparities and Culturally Competent Care, 18
3 Health History and Physical Examination, 34
4 Patient and Caregiver Teaching, 46
5 Chronic Illness and Older Adults, 60
6 Stress and Stress Management, 77
7 Sleep and Sleep Disorders, 89
8 Pain, 102
9 Palliative Care at End of Life, 129
10 Substance Use Disorders, 145

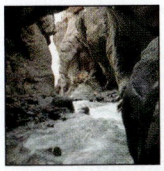

Section 2
Pathophysiologic Mechanisms of Disease

11 Inflammation and Wound Healing, 160
12 Genetics and Genomics, 178
13 Altered Immune Responses and Transplantation, 191
14 Infection and Human Immunodeficiency Virus Infection, 213
15 Cancer, 234
16 Fluid, Electrolyte, and Acid-Base Imbalances, 270

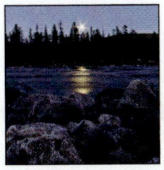

Section 3
Perioperative Care

17 Preoperative Care, 301
18 Intraoperative Care, 315
19 Postoperative Care, 330

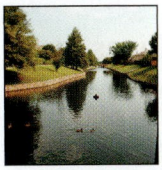

Section 4
Problems Related to Altered Sensory Input

20 Assessment of Visual and Auditory Systems, 350
21 Visual and Auditory Problems, 367
22 Assessment of Integumentary System, 394
23 Integumentary Problems, 407
24 Burns, 429

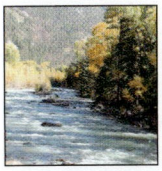

Section 5
Problems of Oxygenation: Ventilation

25 Assessment of Respiratory System, 453
26 Upper Respiratory Problems, 475
27 Lower Respiratory Problems, 499
28 Obstructive Pulmonary Diseases, 538

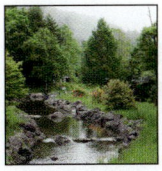

Section 6
Problems of Oxygenation: Transport

29 Assessment of Hematologic System, 587
30 Hematologic Problems, 606

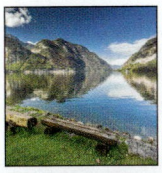

Section 7
Problems of Oxygenation: Perfusion

31 Assessment of Cardiovascular System, 658
32 Hypertension, 681
33 Coronary Artery Disease and Acute Coronary Syndrome, 702
34 Heart Failure, 737
35 Dysrhythmias, 757
36 Inflammatory and Structural Heart Disorders, 780
37 Vascular Disorders, 802

VOLUME 2

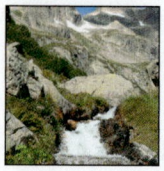

Section 8
Problems of Ingestion, Digestion, Absorption, and Elimination

38 Assessment of Gastrointestinal System, 833
39 Nutritional Problems, 854
40 Obesity, 874
41 Upper Gastrointestinal Problems, 893
42 Lower Gastrointestinal Problems, 929
43 Liver, Pancreas, and Biliary Tract Problems, 974

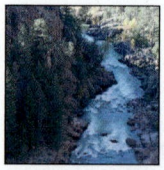

Section 9
Problems of Urinary Function

44 Assessment of Urinary System, 1015
45 Renal and Urologic Problems, 1033
46 Acute Kidney Injury and Chronic Kidney Disease, 1069

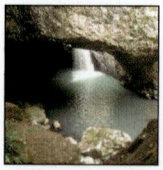

Section 10
Problems Related to Regulatory and Reproductive Mechanisms

47 Assessment of Endocrine System, 1102
48 Diabetes Mellitus, 1120
49 Endocrine Problems, 1156
50 Assessment of Reproductive System, 1184
51 Breast Disorders, 1204
52 Sexually Transmitted Infections, 1227
53 Female Reproductive and Genital Problems, 1242
54 Male Reproductive and Genital Problems, 1268

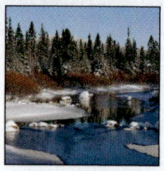

Section 11
Problems Related to Movement and Coordination

55 Assessment of Nervous System, 1294
56 Acute Intracranial Problems, 1314
57 Stroke, 1345
58 Chronic Neurologic Problems, 1368
59 Dementia and Delirium, 1399
60 Spinal Cord and Peripheral Nerve Problems, 1419
61 Assessment of Musculoskeletal System, 1446
62 Musculoskeletal Trauma and Orthopedic Surgery, 1462
63 Musculoskeletal Problems, 1496
64 Arthritis and Connective Tissue Diseases, 1517

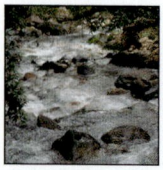

Section 12
Nursing Care in Critical Care Settings

65 Critical Care, 1554
66 Shock, Sepsis, and Multiple Organ Dysfunction Syndrome, 1587
67 Acute Respiratory Failure and Acute Respiratory Distress Syndrome, 1609
68 Emergency and Disaster Nursing, 1628

Appendixes

A Basic Life Support for Health Care Professionals, 1650
B Nursing Diagnoses, 1653
C Laboratory Reference Intervals, 1655

Glossary, 1663
Index, I-1

SPECIAL FEATURES

ASSESSMENT ABNORMALITIES TABLES

Auditory System, 20, p. 365
Breast, 50, p. 1197
Cardiovascular System, 31, p. 668
Endocrine System, 47, p. 1113
Female Reproductive System, 50, p. 1197
Fluid and Electrolyte Imbalances, 16, p. 292
Gastrointestinal System, 38, p. 846
Hematologic System, 29, p. 597
Integumentary System, 22, p. 403
Male Reproductive System, 50, p. 1198
Musculoskeletal System, 61, p. 1456
Nervous System, 55, p. 1308
Respiratory System, 25, p. 467
Urinary System, 44, p. 1025
Visual System, 20, p. 357

BECOMING A NURSE LEADER BOXES

Bullying in the Workplace, 33, p. 730
Coaching in Nursing, 28, p. 581
Dealing With a Changing Environment, 57, p. 1365
Dealing With Conflict in the Workplace, 49, p. 1159
Elder Abuse, 59, p. 1414
Impaired Nurse, 8, p. 125
Importance of Being a Leader, 30, p. 646
Leadership vs. Management, 46, p. 1090
Patient and Visitor Violence/Abuse, 68, p. 1644
Practicing Safe Delegation, 39, p. 868
Protecting Patient Privacy, 51, p. 1222
Self-Care in Nursing, 6, p. 86

CASE STUDIES

End-of-Chapter Case Studies

Acute Respiratory Distress Syndrome, 67, p. 1626
Alzheimer's Disease, 59, p. 1417
Benign Prostatic Hyperplasia With Acute Urinary Retention, 54, p. 1289
Breast Cancer, 51, p. 1225
Burn Injury, 24, p. 449
Chronic Kidney Disease, 46, p. 1097
Chronic Obstructive Pulmonary Disease, 28, p. 582
Cirrhosis of the Liver, 43, p. 1010
Colorectal Cancer, 42, p. 971
Critical Care and Mechanical Ventilation, 65, p. 1584
Diabetic Ketoacidosis, 48, p. 1154
Dysrhythmia and Cardiac Arrest, 35, p. 778
Epilepsy With Headache, 58, p. 1396
Fluid and Electrolyte Imbalance, 16, p. 297
Glaucoma and Diabetic Retinopathy, 21, p. 392
Gonococcal and Chlamydial Infection, 52, p. 1240
Graves' Disease, 49, p. 1182
Health Disparities, 2, p. 32
Heart Failure, 34, p. 755
HIV Infection, 14, p. 231
Inflammation and Infection, 11, p. 176
Insomnia, 7, p. 100
Intraoperative Patient, 18, p. 328
Laryngeal Cancer, 26, p. 496
Leukemia, 30, p. 652
Malignant Melanoma and Dysplastic Nevi, 23, p. 427
Metastatic Bone Tumor/Pathologic Fracture, 63, p. 1514
Myocardial Infarction, 33, p. 734
Obesity, 40, p. 891
Older Adults, 5, p. 75
Pain, 8, p. 127
Painful Bladder and Frequent Urination, 45, p. 1067
Patient and Caregiver Teaching, 4, p. 57
Peptic Ulcer Disease, 41, p. 926
Peripheral Artery Disease, 37, p. 828
Periprosthetic Hip Fracture and Revision Arthroplasty, 62, p. 1493
Pneumonia and Lung Cancer, 27, p. 535
Postoperative Patient, 19, p. 346
Preoperative Patient, 17, p. 313
Primary Hypertension, 32, p. 700
Rheumatoid Arthritis, 64, p. 1549
Shock, 66, p. 1607
Spinal Cord Injury, 60, p. 1443
Spiritual Distress at End of Life, 9, p. 142
Stress-Induced Complaints, 6, p. 87
Stroke, 57, p. 1366
Substance Use Disorder, 10, p. 156
Trauma, 68, p. 1647
Traumatic Brain Injury, 56, p. 1342
Undernutrition, 39, p. 872
Uterine Fibroids and Endometrial Cancer, 53, p. 1265
Valvular Heart Disease, 36, p. 800

Managing Care of Multiple Patients Case Studies

Concepts in Nursing Practice, Section 1, p. 158
Nursing Care in Critical Care Settings, Section 12, p. 1649
Pathophysiologic Mechanisms of Disease, Section 2, p. 299
Perioperative Care, Section 3, p. 348
Problems of Ingestion, Digestion, Absorption, and Elimination, Section 8, p. 1013
Problems of Oxygenation: Perfusion, Section 7, p. 831
Problems of Oxygenation: Transport, Section 6, p. 656
Problems of Oxygenation: Ventilation, Section 5, p. 585
Problems of Urinary Function, Section 9, p. 1100
Problems Related to Altered Sensory Input, Section 4, p. 451
Problems Related to Movement and Coordination, Section 11, p. 1552
Problems Related to Regulatory and Reproductive Mechanisms, Section 10, p. 1292

Assessment Case Studies

Cardiovascular System, 31, p. 663
Endocrine System, 47, p. 1109
Gastrointestinal System, 38, p. 839
Hematologic System, 29, p. 593
Integumentary System, 22, p. 398
Musculoskeletal System, 61, p. 1451

Nervous System, 55, p. 1302
Reproductive System, 50, p. 1191
Respiratory System, 25, p. 460
Urinary System, 44, p. 1020
Visual and Auditory Systems, 20, p. 353

COMPLEMENTARY & ALTERNATIVE THERAPIES BOXES

Acupuncture, 64, p. 1523
Assessment of Use of Herbs and Dietary Supplements, 3, p. 38
Biofeedback, 45, p. 1057
Echinacea, 26, p. 480
Fish Oil and Omega-3 Fatty Acids, 32, p. 689
Ginger, 41, p. 895
Glucosamine and Chondroitin, 64, p. 1523
Hawthorn, 34, p. 749
Herbal and Dietary Supplements That May Affect Clotting, 37, p. 820
Herbal Products and Surgery, 17, p. 304
Herbs and Supplements for Menopause, 53, p. 1249
Herbs and Supplements That May Affect Blood Glucose, 48, p. 1141
Imagery, 51, p. 1221
Lipid-Lowering Agents, 33, p. 710
Melatonin, 7, p. 95
Milk Thistle (Silymarin), 43, p. 980
Music Therapy, 18, p. 319
Yoga, 6, p. 83
Zinc, 26, p. 482

CULTURAL & ETHNIC HEALTH DISPARITIES BOXES

Alzheimer's Disease and Dementia, 59, p. 1402
Arthritis and Connective Tissue Disorders, 64, p. 1525
Brain Tumors, 56, p. 1333
Breast Cancer, 51, p. 1218
Cancer, 15, p. 267
Cancers of the Female Reproductive System, 53, p. 1256
Cancers of the Male Reproductive System, 54, p. 1276
Chronic Kidney Disease, 46, p. 1076
Colorectal Cancer, 42, p. 954
Coronary Artery Disease, 33, p. 704
Cultural & Ethnic Health Disparities Boxes Throughout Book, 2, p. 20
Diabetes Mellitus, 48, p. 1137
Heart Failure, 34, p. 738
Hematologic Problems, 30, p. 607
Hypertension, 32, p. 682
Integumentary Problems, 23, p. 410
Liver, Pancreas, and Gallbladder Disorders, 43, p. 986
Lung Cancer, 27, p. 514
Obesity, 40, p. 878
Obstructive Pulmonary Diseases, 28, p. 539
Oral, Pharyngeal, and Esophageal Problems, 41, p. 898
Osteoporosis, 63, p. 1511
Sexually Transmitted Infections, 52, p. 1228
Stroke, 57, p. 1347
Tuberculosis, 27, p. 506
Urologic Disorders, 45, p. 1034
Visual and Auditory Problems, 21, p. 368

DIAGNOSTIC STUDIES TABLES

Auditory System, 20, p. 365
Cardiovascular System, 31, p. 673
Clotting Studies, 29, p. 601
Common Preoperative Diagnostic Studies, 17, p. 308
Complete Blood Count Studies, 29, p. 600
Endocrine System, 47, p. 1115
Gastrointestinal System, 38, p. 847
Headaches, 58, p. 1370
Hematologic System, 29, p. 603
Integumentary System, 22, p. 405
Liver Function Tests, 38, p. 852
Male and Female Reproductive Systems, 50, p. 1198
Miscellaneous Blood Studies, 29, p. 602
Musculoskeletal System, 61, p. 1457
Nervous System, 55, p. 1310
Respiratory System, 25, p. 469
Shock, 66, p. 1590
Stroke, 57, p. 1352
Urinalysis, 44, p. 1030
Urinary System, 44, p. 1025
Venous Thromboembolism, 37, p. 819
Viral Hepatitis, 43, p. 979
Visual System, 20, p. 359

DRUG THERAPY TABLES

Acute and Chronic Glaucoma, 21, p. 381
Acute and Chronic Pancreatitis, 43, p. 1001
Adjuncts to General Anesthesia, 18, p. 326
Adjuvant Drugs Used for Pain, 8, p. 116
Alzheimer's Disease, 59, p. 1408
Androgen Deprivation Therapy for Prostate Cancer, 54, p. 1280
Anticoagulant Therapy, 37, p. 820
Antidiarrheal Drugs, 42, p. 931
Antidysrhythmia Drugs, 35, p. 771
Antithrombotic Therapy for Atrial Fibrillation, 35, p. 766
Arthritis and Connective Tissue Diseases, 64, p. 1521
Asthma and Chronic Obstructive Pulmonary Disease (COPD), 28, p. 548
Bacterial Community-Acquired Pneumonia, 27, p. 504
Breast Cancer, 51, p. 1217
Burns, 24, p. 441
Causes of Medication Errors by Older Adults, 5, p. 73
Chemotherapy, 15, p. 247
Chronic Stable Angina and Acute Coronary Syndrome, 33, p. 715
Cirrhosis, 43, p. 993
Combination Therapy for Hypertension, 32, p. 694
Common Bases for Topical Medications, 23, p. 423
Commonly Used Preoperative Medications, 17, p. 311
Constipation, 42, p. 936
Diseases/Disorders Treated With Corticosteroids, 49, p. 1180
Drugs That May Cause Photosensitivity, 23, p. 408
Effects and Side Effects of Corticosteroids, 49, p. 1180
Gastroesophageal Reflux Disease (GERD) and Peptic Ulcer Disease (PUD), 41, p. 903
General Anesthesia, 18, p. 325
Heart Failure, 34, p. 745
Helicobacter pylori Infection, 41, p. 910
Hematopoietic Growth Factors Used in Cancer Treatment, 15, p. 260

HIV Infection, 14, p. 224
Hormone Therapy, 15, p. 259
Hyperlipidemia, 33, p. 711
Hypertension, 32, p. 691
Immunosuppressive Therapy, 13, p. 211
Immunotherapy and Targeted Therapy, 15, p. 258
Infertility, 53, p. 1243
Inflammation and Healing, 11, p. 164
Inflammatory Bowel Disease, 42, p. 947
Insomnia, 7, p. 94
Insulin Regimens, 48, p. 1127
Latent Tuberculosis Infection Regimens, 27, p. 510
Leukemia, 30, p. 639
Long-Term Control versus Quick Relief of Asthma, 28, p. 546
Managing Side Effects of Pain Medications, 8, p. 111
Medication Guidelines for Stable COPD, 28, p. 563
Medication Use by Older Adults, 5, p. 74
Methods of Chemotherapy Administration, 15, p. 248
Multiple Sclerosis, 58, p. 1385
Nausea and Vomiting, 41, p. 895
Obesity, 40, p. 884
Opioid Analgesics, 8, p. 113
Oral Agents and Noninsulin Injectable Agents, 48, p. 1131
Parkinson's Disease, 58, p. 1391
Pulmonary Hypertension, 27, p. 532
Replacement Factors for Hemophilia, 30, p. 628
Rhinitis and Sinusitis, 26, p. 479
Seizure Disorders, 58, p. 1378
Selected Nonopioid Analgesics, 8, p. 111
Shock, 66, p. 1599
Smoking Cessation, 10, p. 150
Tuberculosis (TB), 27, p. 509
Tuberculosis Disease Regimens, 27, p. 509
Types of Insulin, 48, p. 1125
Viral Hepatitis B and C, 43, p. 981
Voiding Dysfunction, 45, p. 1059

EMERGENCY MANAGEMENT TABLES

Abdominal Trauma, 42, p. 942
Acute Abdominal Pain, 42, p. 939
Acute Gastrointestinal Bleeding, 41, p. 924
Acute Soft Tissue Injury, 62, p. 1464
Anaphylactic Shock, 13, p. 202
Chemical Burns, 24, p. 436
Chest Pain, 33, p. 723
Chest Trauma, 27, p. 519
Depressant Toxicity, 10, p. 152
Diabetic Ketoacidosis, 48, p. 1144
Dysrhythmias, 35, p. 763
Electrical Burns, 24, p. 435
Emergency Management Tables, 68, p. 1629
Eye Injury, 21, p. 371
Fractured Extremity, 62, p. 1474
Head Injury, 56, p. 1330
Hyperthermia, 68, p. 1636
Hypothermia, 68, p. 1639
Inhalation Injury, 24, p. 435
Sexual Assault, 53, p. 1264
Shock, 66, p. 1597
Spinal Cord Injury, 60, p. 1425
Stimulant Toxicity, 10, p. 151
Stroke, 57, p. 1354
Submersion Injuries, 68, p. 1641
Thermal Burns, 24, p. 434
Thoracic Injuries, 27, p. 520
Tonic-Clonic Seizures, 58, p. 1378

ETHICAL/LEGAL DILEMMAS BOXES

Advance Directives, 28, p. 575
Allocation of Resources, 46, p. 1093
Board of Nursing Disciplinary Action, 59, p. 1416
Brain Death, 56, p. 1331
Competence, 34, p. 754
Confidentiality and HIPAA, 52, p. 1239
Do Not Resuscitate, 36, p. 794
Durable Power of Attorney for Health Care, 48, p. 1153
End-of-Life Care, 9, p. 137
Entitlement to Treatment, 62, p. 1482
Family Presence and Visitation in the Adult ICU, 65, p. 1558
Genetic Testing, 12, p. 185
Good Samaritan, 68, p. 1646
Health Disparities, 2, p. 19
Individual vs. Public Health Protection, 14, p. 226
Informed Consent, 17, p. 310
Medical Futility, 15, p. 266
Pain Management, 30, p. 619
Patient Adherence, 27, p. 510
Rationing, 43, p. 995
Religious Beliefs, 30, p. 649
Right to Refuse Treatment, 60, p. 1424
Scope and Standards of Practice, 35, p. 770
Social Networking: HIPAA Violation, 1, p. 14
Withdrawing Treatment, 46, p. 1097
Withholding Treatment, 56, p. 1338

EVIDENCE-BASED PRACTICE BOXES

Applying the Evidence Boxes

Adherence to Tuberculosis Treatment Program, 27, p. 510
Condom Use and HIV, 14, p. 228
Dancing and Parkinson's Disease, 58, p. 1390
Education: Text Messaging and Diabetes, 48, p. 1135
Exercise and Hematologic Cancer, 30, p. 643
Falls and Osteoarthritis, 64, p. 1520
Home Care and Heart Failure, 34, p. 752
HPV Vaccine and Young Men, 52, p. 1235
Lifestyle Changes and Uncontrolled Hypertension, 32, p. 688
Modifying Risk Factors for Dementia, 59, p. 1410
Music and Preoperative Anxiety, 17, p. 303
Obesity Interventions in Faith-Based Organizations, 40, p. 889
Pap Test and Cervical Cancer, 53, p. 1256
Physical Activity and COPD, 28, p. 574
Prevention of Recurrent Kidney Stones, 45, p. 1048
Probiotics and Constipation, 42, p. 935
Repositioning and Pressure Ulcers, 10, p. 174
Screening and Testing for Hepatitis C, 43, p. 977
Tanning Booths and Skin Cancer, 23, p. 408
Treatment for Breast Cancer, 51, p. 1220
Virtual Reality and Stroke, 57, p. 1363
Walking and Stroke, 57, p. 1364

Translating Research Into Practice Boxes

Are Integrative Therapies Helpful During Breast Cancer Treatment?, 51, p. 1221
Can Exercise Improve Blood Pressure Levels in Patients With Diabetes?, 48, p. 1142
Can Home-Based Blood Pressure Monitoring Improve Hypertension Screening?, 32, p. 694
Can Tai Chi Help Cognitive Function in Older Adults?, 5, p. 72
Do Behavioral Interventions Reduce Cardiovascular Risk Factors?, 33, p. 730
Do Cardiac Rehabilitation Programs Improve Outcomes?, 33, p. 707
Do Nonpharmacologic Interventions Improve Sleep in Dialysis Patients?, 46, p. 1080
Do Physical Activity Exercises Decrease Sport Injuries?, 62, p. 1476
Do Proton Pump Inhibitors Increase Gastric Cancer Risk?, 41, p. 902
Do Tobacco Cessation Programs Affect Smoking Behavior?, 10, p. 148
Does Culturally Appropriate Education Improve Diabetic Glycemic Control and Knowledge?, 4, p. 53
Does Exercise Reduce Fatigue in Chronic Fatigue Syndrome?, 64, p. 1549
Does Home Palliative Care Affect Odds of Dying at Home?, 9, p. 131
Does Prehospital Therapeutic Hypothermia Improve Outcomes in Cardiac Arrest?, 68, p. 1635
Is Home-Based STI Testing Effective?, 52, p. 1229
Is Sleep Disturbance Associated With Menopausal Stage?, 53, p. 1249
What Is the Effect of Capsaicin on Chronic Neuropathic Pain?, 8, p. 119
What Is the Effect of Internet-Based Interventions on Eating Disorders?, 39, p. 871
What Types of Diet Programs Result in Weight Loss?, 40, p. 882

FOCUSED ASSESSMENT BOXES

Auditory System, 20, p. 364
Cardiovascular System, 31, p. 669
Clotting Studies, 29, p. 601
Endocrine System, 47, p. 1114
Gastrointestinal System, 38, p. 846
Hematologic System, 29, p. 599
Integumentary System, 22, p. 402
Musculoskeletal System, 61, p. 1457
Nervous System, 55, p. 1308
Reproductive System, 50, p. 1196
Respiratory System, 25, p. 466
Urinary System, 44, p. 1024
Visual System, 20, p. 356

GENDER DIFFERENCES BOXES

Alzheimer's Disease and Dementia, 59, p. 1402
Asthma, 28, p. 539
Cancer, 15, p. 235
Cholelithiasis, 43, p. 1006
Chronic Obstructive Pulmonary Disease (COPD), 28, p. 558
Coronary Artery Disease and Acute Coronary Syndrome, 33, p. 705
Effects of Aging on Sexual Function, 50, p. 1191
Endocrine Problems, 49, p. 1163
Gout, 64, p. 1533
Headaches, 58, p. 1370
Heart Failure, 34, p. 739
Hernia, 42, p. 965
Hypertension, 32, p. 682
Irritable Bowel Syndrome (IBS), 42, p. 940
Lung Cancer, 27, p. 514
Older Adults, 5, p. 63
Osteoarthritis (OA), 64, p. 1518
Osteoporosis, 63, p. 1511
Pain, 8, p. 103
Sexually Transmitted Infections, 52, p. 1231
Urinary Incontinence, 45, p. 1055
Urinary Tract Calculi, 45, p. 1045
Vascular Disorders, 37, p. 803

GENETICS IN CLINICAL PRACTICE BOXES

α_1-Antitrypsin (AAT) Deficiency, 28, p. 559
Alzheimer's Disease (AD), 59, p. 1402
Ankylosing Spondylitis, 64, p. 1536
Breast Cancer, 51, p. 1210
Cystic Fibrosis (CF), 28, p. 576
Duchenne and Becker Muscular Dystrophy (MD), 63, p. 1502
Familial Adenomatous Polyposis (FAP), 42, p. 953
Familial Hypercholesterolemia, 33, p. 704
Genetic Information Nondiscrimination Act (GINA), 12, p. 184
Genetics in Clinical Practice Boxes Throughout Book, 12, p. 183
Hemochromatosis, 30, p. 620
Hemophilia A and B, 30, p. 627
Hereditary Nonpolyposis Colorectal Cancer (HNPCC) or Lynch Syndrome, 42, p. 954
Huntington's Disease (HD), 58, p. 1396
Ovarian Cancer, 53, p. 1258
Polycystic Kidney Disease (PKD), 45, p. 1051
Sickle Cell Disease, 30, p. 616
Types 1 and 2 Diabetes Mellitus and MODY, 48, p. 1122

GERONTOLOGIC ASSESSMENT DIFFERENCES TABLES

Adaptations in Physical Assessment Techniques, 3, p. 42
Auditory System, 20, p. 361
Cardiovascular System, 31, p. 663
Cognitive Function, 5, p. 64
Effects of Aging on Hematologic Studies, 29, p. 593
Effects of Aging on the Immune System, 13, p. 196
Endocrine System, 47, p. 1108
Gastrointestinal System, 38, p. 840
Integumentary System, 22, p. 397
Musculoskeletal System, 61, p. 1451
Nervous System, 55, p. 1302
Reproductive Systems, 50, p. 1191
Respiratory System, 25, p. 459
Summary of Tables, 5, p. 64
Urinary System, 44, p. 1020
Visual System, 20, p. 353

HEALTH HISTORY TABLES

Auditory System, 20, p. 362
Cardiovascular System, 31, p. 665
Endocrine System, 47, p. 1110
Functional Health Pattern Format, 3, p. 37
Gastrointestinal System, 38, p. 841
Hematologic System, 29, p. 595
Integumentary System, 22, p. 398
Musculoskeletal System, 61, p. 1452
Nervous System, 55, p. 1303
Reproductive System, 50, p. 1193
Respiratory System, 25, p. 461
Urinary System, 44, p. 1021
Visual System, 20, p. 354

HEALTHY PEOPLE BOXES

Health Impact of a Well-Balanced Diet, 39, p. 855
Health Impact of Good Oral Hygiene, 41, p. 900
Health Impact of Maintaining a Healthy Weight, 40, p. 878
Health Impact of Regular Physical Activity, 62, p. 1464
Health Impact of Responsible Eye Care, 21, p. 370
Health Impact of Wearing Ear Protection, 21, p. 388
Lesbian, Gay, Bisexual, and Transgender (LGBT) Individuals, 2, p. 21
Prevention and Detection of Chronic Kidney Disease, 46, p. 1084
Prevention and Early Detection of Cancer, 15, p. 242
Prevention and Early Detection of Diabetes Mellitus, 48, p. 1138
Prevention and Early Detection of HIV, 14, p. 226
Prevention of Osteoarthritis, 64, p. 1523
Prevention of Respiratory Diseases, 27, p. 500
Prevention of Stroke, 57, p. 1353

INFORMATICS IN PRACTICE BOXES

Chest Drainage System, 27, p. 523
Communication Devices for Patient With Laryngectomy, 26, p. 494
Computer Monitoring of Antibiotic Safety, 46, p. 1075
Computer-Based Timing for Antibiotic Administration, 17, p. 311
Digital Images, 11, p. 175
Discharge Teaching, 19, p. 345
Heart Surgery DVD/TV, 36, p. 795
Home Monitoring of Asthma, 28, p. 551
Importing Monitor and Ventilator Data, 65, p. 1578
Managing Cancer Patients' Symptoms, 15, p. 248
Monitoring Blood Pressure, 32, p. 697
Older Adults and Internet Use, 5, p. 65
Patient Teaching Using Smart Phone Apps, 48, p. 1141
Respiratory Monitoring, 19, p. 336
Sleep Apnea Diagnosis and Monitoring, 7, p. 97
Smart Infusion Pumps, 65, p. 1556
Social Media Use for Patients With Migraine Headaches, 58, p. 1371
Staff Training Using Gaming, 24, p. 438
Texting for Chronic Obstructive Pulmonary Disease (COPD) Patients, 28, p. 573
Use of Cell Phone for Weight Loss, 40, p. 889
Use of Internet and Mobile Devices to Manage HIV, 14, p. 229
Use of Internet to Access Information on Unfamiliar Diseases, 30, p. 635
Use of Translation Applications, 2, p. 31
Video Games for Stroke Recovery, 57, p. 1363
Voice Banking Applications in Amyotrophic Lateral Sclerosis, 58, p. 1395
Web-Based Knee and Hip Replacement Community, 62, p. 1477
Wireless ECG Monitoring, 35, p. 760

INTERPROFESSIONAL CARE TABLES

Abnormal Uterine Bleeding, 53, p. 1246
Acute Kidney Injury, 46, p. 1073
Acute Pancreatitis, 43, p. 1001
Acute Pericarditis, 36, p. 786
Acute Pulmonary Embolism, 27, p. 530
Acute Pyelonephritis, 45, p. 1039
Acute Respiratory Distress Syndrome, 67, p. 1624
Acute Respiratory Failure, 67, p. 1616
Addison's Disease, 49, p. 1179
Alzheimer's Disease, 59, p. 1407
Amputation, 62, p. 1487
Aortic Dissection, 37, p. 815
Asthma, 28, p. 544
Bacterial Meningitis, 56, p. 1340
Benign Prostatic Hyperplasia, 54, p. 1270
Bladder Cancer, 45, p. 1054
Breast Cancer, 51, p. 1213
Burn Injury, 24, p. 438
Cardiomyopathy, 36, p. 797
Cataract, 21, p. 374
Cervical Cord Injury, 60, p. 1426
Chlamydial Infections, 52, p. 1229
Cholelithiasis and Acute Cholecystitis, 43, p. 1007
Chronic Kidney Disease, 46, p. 1080
Chronic Obstructive Pulmonary Disease (COPD), 28, p. 562
Chronic Otitis Media, 21, p. 385
Cirrhosis of the Liver, 43, p. 991
Colorectal Cancer, 42, p. 955
Cor Pulmonale, 27, p. 533
Cushing Syndrome, 49, p. 1176
Diabetes Mellitus, 48, p. 1125
Diabetic Ketoacidosis (DKA) and Hyperosmolar Hyperglycemic Syndrome (HHS), 48, p. 1144
Diverticulosis and Diverticulitis, 42, p. 964
Endometriosis, 53, p. 1253
Epilepsy and Seizure Disorders, 58, p. 1377
Erectile Dysfunction, 54, p. 1287
Esophageal Cancer, 41, p. 905
Fractures, 62, p. 1470
Gastroesophageal Reflux Disease (GERD) and Hiatal Hernia, 41, p. 901
Genital Herpes, 52, p. 1233
Glaucoma, 21, p. 380
Gonococcal Infections, 52, p. 1231
Gout, 64, p. 1533
Head and Neck Cancer, 26, p. 491
Headaches, 58, p. 1369
Heart Failure, 34, p. 744
Hypertension, 32, p. 687
Hyperthyroidism, 49, p. 1165
Hypoglycemia, 48, p. 1146
Hypothyroidism, 49, p. 1169

Increased Intracranial Pressure, 56, p. 1319
Infertility, 53, p. 1243
Inflammatory Bowel Disease, 42, p. 946
Insomnia, 7, p. 93
Intervertebral Disc Disease, 63, p. 1506
Iron-Deficiency Anemia, 30, p. 611
Lung Cancer, 27, p. 516
Ménière's Disease, 21, p. 386
Multiple Sclerosis, 58, p. 1385
Myasthenia Gravis, 58, p. 1394
Neurogenic Bladder, 60, p. 1433
Neutropenia, 30, p. 633
Obesity, 40, p. 882
Oral Cancer, 41, p. 898
Osteoarthritis, 64, p. 1520
Osteoporosis, 63, p. 1512
Otosclerosis, 21, p. 385
Ovarian Cancer, 53, p. 1259
Parkinson's Disease, 58, p. 1389
Peptic Ulcer Disease, 41, p. 914
Peripheral Artery Disease, 37, p. 804
Peritonitis, 42, p. 943
Pneumonia, 27, p. 503
Premenstrual Syndrome (PMS), 53, p. 1245
Prostate Cancer, 54, p. 1278
Pulmonary Tuberculosis, 27, p. 508
Renal Cancer, 45, p. 1053
Retinal Detachment, 21, p. 377
Rheumatic Fever, 36, p. 789
Rheumatoid Arthritis, 64, p. 1528
Scleroderma, 64, p. 1544
Shock, 66, p. 1600
Stomach Cancer, 41, p. 920
Stroke, 57, p. 1353
Syphilis, 52, p. 1237
Systemic Lupus Erythematosus, 64, p. 1540
Thrombocytopenia, 30, p. 625
Trigeminal Neuralgia, 60, p. 1438
Urinary Tract Infection, 45, p. 1036
Valvular Heart Disease, 36, p. 793
Viral Hepatitis, 43, p. 980

NURSING ASSESSMENT TABLES

Acute Coronary Syndrome, 33, p. 726
Acute Pancreatitis, 43, p. 1002
Acute Respiratory Failure, 67, p. 1615
Allergies, 13, p. 201
Alzheimer's Disease, 59, p. 1409
Anemia, 30, p. 609
Assessment Techniques: Visual System, 20, p. 356
Assessment Variations in Light- and Dark-Skinned Persons, 22, p. 404
Asthma, 28, p. 553
Benign Prostatic Hyperplasia, 54, p. 1273
Breast Cancer, 51, p. 1219
Care of Patient on Admission to Clinical Unit, 19, p. 345
Cholecystitis or Cholelithiasis, 43, p. 1009
Chronic Obstructive Pulmonary Disease, 28, p. 572
Cirrhosis, 43, p. 993
Colorectal Cancer, 42, p. 957
Constipation, 42, p. 937
Cushing Syndrome, 49, p. 1176
Cystic Fibrosis, 28, p. 580
Diabetes Mellitus, 48, p. 1138
Diarrhea, 42, p. 932
Elder Mistreatment, 5, p. 67
Epilepsy and Seizure Disorders, 58, p. 1380
Fracture, 62, p. 1475
Head and Neck Cancer, 26, p. 494
Head Injury, 56, p. 1331
Headaches, 58, p. 1373
Heart Failure, 34, p. 750
Hepatitis, 43, p. 982
HIV-Infected Patient, 14, p. 225
Hypertension, 32, p. 695
Hyperthyroidism, 49, p. 1167
Infective Endocarditis, 36, p. 783
Inflammatory Bowel Disease, 42, p. 949
Leukemia, 30, p. 639
Low Back Pain, 63, p. 1503
Lung Cancer, 27, p. 518
Malnutrition, 39, p. 860
Multiple Sclerosis, 58, p. 1386
Nausea and Vomiting, 41, p. 896
Obese Patient, 40, p. 880
Oral Cancer, 41, p. 899
Osteomyelitis, 63, p. 1499
Pain, 8, p. 108
Parkinson's Disease, 58, p. 1392
Pelvic Inflammatory Disease, 53, p. 1252
Peptic Ulcer Disease, 41, p. 915
Peripheral Artery Disease, 37, p. 807
Pneumonia, 27, p. 505
Pressure Ulcers, 11, p. 174
Prostate Cancer, 54, p. 1281
Rheumatic Fever and Rheumatic Heart Disease, 36, p. 789
Rheumatoid Arthritis, 64, p. 1530
Sexually Transmitted Infections, 52, p. 1237
Sleep, 7, p. 95
Spinal Cord Injury, 60, p. 1427
Stroke, 57, p. 1357
Systemic Lupus Erythematosus, 64, p. 1541
Thrombocytopenia, 30, p. 624
Upper Gastrointestinal Bleeding, 41, p. 923
Urinary Tract Calculi, 45, p. 1049
Urinary Tract Infection, 45, p. 1037
Valvular Heart Disease, 36, p. 795
Venous Thromboembolism, 37, p. 822

NURSING MANAGEMENT TABLES

Physical Care at End of Life, 9, p. 140
Psychosocial Care at End of Life, 9, p. 138

NUTRITIONAL THERAPY TABLES

1200-Calorie–Restricted Weight-Reduction Diet, 40, p. 882
Celiac Disease, 42, p. 967
Chronic Kidney Disease, 46, p. 1082
Diabetes Mellitus, 48, p. 1133
Effects of Food on Stoma Output, 42, p. 961
Foods High in Iron, 39, p. 856
Foods High in Protein, 39, p. 855

High-Calorie Foods, 15, p. 262
High-Calorie, High-Protein Diet, 39, p. 863
High-Fiber Foods, 42, p. 937
High-Potassium Foods, 46, p. 1083
Low-Sodium Diets, 34, p. 749
Maximizing Food Intake in COPD, 28, p. 571
MyPlate Tips for a Healthy Lifestyle, 39, p. 862
Nutrients for Erythropoiesis, 30, p. 610
Postgastrectomy Dumping Syndrome, 41, p. 918
Protein Foods With High Biologic Value, 15, p. 262
Sources of Calcium, 63, p. 1513
Therapeutic Lifestyle Changes Diet, 33, p. 709
Tips to Make Diet and Lifestyle Changes, 33, p. 709
Urinary Tract Calculi, 45, p. 1049

PATIENT & CAREGIVER TEACHING TABLES

Acute Coronary Syndrome, 33, p. 731
Acute or Chronic Sinusitis, 26, p. 483
Addison's Disease, 49, p. 1179
After Eye Surgery, 21, p. 376
Anticoagulant Therapy, 37, p. 824
Antiretroviral Drugs, 14, p. 228
Asthma, 28, p. 557
Autonomic Hyperreflexia, 60, p. 1431
Avoiding Allergens in Allergic Rhinitis, 26, p. 478
Bowel Management After Spinal Cord Injury, 60, p. 1433
Cancer Survivors, 15, p. 267
Cardiomyopathy, 36, p. 800
Cast Care, 62, p. 1477
Characteristics of Menstruation, 50, p. 1190
Chronic Kidney Disease, 46, p. 1084
Chronic Obstructive Pulmonary Disease, 28, p. 573
Cirrhosis, 43, p. 995
Constipation, 42, p. 937
Corticosteroid Therapy, 49, p. 1181
Decrease Risk for Antibiotic-Resistant Infection, 14, p. 217
Early Warning Signs of Alzheimer's Disease, 59, p. 1405
Effective Huff Coughing, 28, p. 569
Exercise for Patients With Diabetes Mellitus, 48, p. 1134
FAST for Warning Signs of Stroke, 57, p. 1346
FITT Activity Guidelines After Acute Coronary Syndrome, 33, p. 732
Following Lower Extremity Amputation, 62, p. 1490
Foot Care, 48, p. 1151
Gastroesophageal Reflux Disease (GERD), 41, p. 902
Genetic Testing, 12, p. 185
Halo Vest Care, 60, p. 1428
Head Injury, 56, p. 1332
Headaches, 58, p. 1374
Heart Failure, 34, p. 751
Heat and Cold Therapy, 8, p. 122
Hip Replacement, 62, p. 1483
Home Oxygen Use, 28, p. 569
How to Use a Dry Powder Inhaler (DPI), 28, p. 552
How to Use Your Peak Flow Meter, 28, p. 556
Hypertension, 32, p. 697
Hypothyroidism, 49, p. 1170
Ileal Conduit Appliances, 45, p. 1066
Implantable Cardioverter-Defibrillator (ICD), 35, p. 773
Improving Adherence to Antiretroviral Therapy, 14, p. 229
Instructions for Patients With Diabetes Mellitus, 48, p. 1142
Insulin Therapy, 48, p. 1128
Joint Protection and Energy Conservation, 64, p. 1524
Low Back Problems, 63, p. 1504
Management of Diabetes Mellitus, 48, p. 1141
Mitral Valve Prolapse, 36, p. 792
Neck Exercises, 63, p. 1508
Neutropenia, 30, p. 634
Ostomy Self-Care, 42, p. 961
Pacemaker, 35, p. 776
Pain Management, 8, p. 123
Pelvic Floor Muscle (Kegel) Exercises, 45, p. 1058
Peptic Ulcer Disease (PUD), 41, p. 916
Peripheral Artery Bypass Surgery, 37, p. 808
Postoperative Laparoscopic Cholecystectomy, 43, p. 1010
Preoperative Preparation, 17, p. 309
Pressure Ulcer, 11, p. 175
Prevention and Early Treatment of Lyme Disease, 64, p. 1535
Prevention of External Otitis, 21, p. 384
Prevention of Food Poisoning, 41, p. 926
Prevention of Hypokalemia, 16, p. 283
Prevention of Musculoskeletal Problems in Older Adults, 62, p. 1463
Protection of Small Joints, 64, p. 1531
Pursed Lip Breathing (PLB), 28, p. 554
Radiation Skin Reactions, 15, p. 255
Reducing Barriers to Pain Management, 8, p. 124
Reducing Risk Factors for Coronary Artery Disease, 33, p. 708
Seizure Disorders, 58, p. 1381
Self-Monitoring of Blood Glucose (SMBG), 48, p. 1136
Sexual Assault Prevention, 53, p. 1265
Sexually Transmitted Infections, 52, p. 1239
Signs and Symptoms HIV-Infected Patients Need to Report, 14, p. 229
Skin Care After Spinal Cord Injury, 60, p. 1434
Sleep Hygiene, 7, p. 93
Smoking and Tobacco Use Cessation, 10, p. 149
Systemic Lupus Erythematosus, 64, p. 1542
Thrombocytopenia, 30, p. 626
Urinary Tract Infection, 45, p. 1037

TEAMWORK & COLLABORATION BOXES

Assessment and Data Collection, 3, p. 36
Blood Transfusions, 30, p. 649
Cardiac Catheterization and Percutaneous Coronary Intervention (PCI), 33, p. 729
Care of Postoperative Patient, 19, p. 334
Caring for Patients With Alzheimer's Disease, 59, p. 1412
Caring for the Incontinent Patient, 45, p. 1059
Caring for the Patient Requiring Mechanical Ventilation, 65, p. 1581
Caring for the Patient With a Cast or Traction, 62, p. 1471
Caring for the Patient With a Seizure Disorder, 58, p. 1381
Caring for the Patient With an Acute Stroke, 57, p. 1359
Caring for the Patient With Chronic Venous Insufficiency, 37, p. 827
Caring for the Patient With Diabetes Mellitus, 48, p. 1152
Caring for the Patient With Hypertension, 32, p. 696
Caring for the Patient With Neutropenia, 30, p. 632
Caring for the Patient With Osteomyelitis, 63, p. 1498
Caring for the Patient With Rheumatoid Arthritis, 64, p. 1529

Caring for the Patient With Venous Thromboembolism (VTE), 37, p. 824
Corrective Lenses and Hearing Aids, 21, p. 392
IV Therapy, 16, p. 294
Nasogastric and Gastric Tubes and Enteral Feedings, 39, p. 867
Ostomy Care, 42, p. 960
Oxygen Administration, 28, p. 568
Pain, 8, p. 123
Patient Receiving Bladder Irrigation, 54, p. 1274
Skin Care, 23, p. 425
Suctioning and Tracheostomy Care, 26, p. 490
Teamwork & Collaboration Boxes Throughout Book, 1, p. 10
Urinary Catheters, 45, p. 1061
Wound Care, 11, p. 170

MEDICAL-SURGICAL NURSING

Assessment and Management of Clinical Problems

SECTION 1

Concepts in Nursing Practice

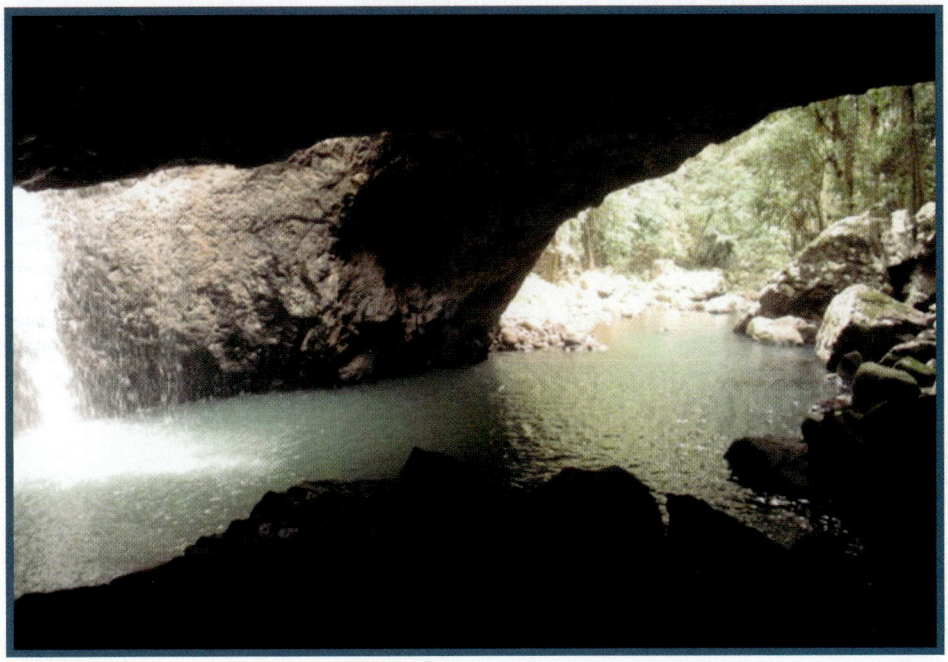

Peter Bonner

Life is like the river, sometimes it sweeps you gently along and sometimes the rapids come out of nowhere.
Emma Smith

Chapter 1 Professional Nursing Practice, 2

Chapter 2 Health Disparities and Culturally Competent Care, 18

Chapter 3 Health History and Physical Examination, 34

Chapter 4 Patient and Caregiver Teaching, 46

Chapter 5 Chronic Illness and Older Adults, 60

Chapter 6 Stress and Stress Management, 77

Chapter 7 Sleep and Sleep Disorders, 89

Chapter 8 Pain, 102

Chapter 9 Palliative Care at End of Life, 129

Chapter 10 Substance Use Disorders, 145

1

Professional Nursing Practice

Mariann M. Harding

Knowledge has to be improved, challenged, and increased constantly, or it vanishes.

Peter Drucker

http://evolve.elsevier.com/Lewis/medsurg/

LEARNING OUTCOMES

1. Describe professional nursing practice in terms of domain, definitions, and recipients of care.
2. Compare the different scopes of practice available to professional nurses.
3. Analyze the effect of external influences on professional nursing practice.
4. Describe the role of critical thinking skills and use of the nursing process to provide patient-centered care.
5. Explain how standardized nursing terminologies for nursing diagnoses, patient outcomes, and nursing interventions can be used and linked.
6. Explore the role of the professional nurse in delegating care to licensed practical/vocational nurses and unlicensed assistive personnel.
7. Discuss the role of integrating safety and quality improvement processes into nursing practice.
8. Evaluate the role of informatics and technology in nursing practice.
9. Apply concepts of evidence-based practice to nursing practice.

KEY TERMS

advanced practice registered nurse (APRN), p. 3
case management, p. 9
clinical pathways, p. 10
clinical reasoning, p. 9
critical thinking, p. 9
delegation, p. 11
electronic health records (EHRs), p. 14
evidence-based practice (EBP), p. 15
interprofessional team, p. 9
nursing, p. 3
nursing process, p. 5
nursing-sensitive patient outcome, p. 7
SBAR (Situation-Background-Assessment-Recommendation), p. 10
serious reportable event (SRE), p. 12
telehealth, p. 9

This chapter presents an overview of professional nursing practice, discussing the wide variety of roles and responsibilities that nurses fulfill to meet the health care needs of society.

PROFESSIONAL NURSING PRACTICE

Domain of Nursing Practice

Nursing practice today consists of a wide variety of roles and responsibilities necessary to meet society's health care needs. As a nurse, you are the frontline professional of health care (Fig. 1-1). You can practice in virtually all health care settings and communities. You have never been more important to health care than you are today. As a nurse, you (1) offer skilled care to those recuperating from illness or injury, (2) advocate for patients' rights, (3) teach patients to manage their health, (4) support patients and their caregivers at critical times, and (5) help them navigate the complex health care system. Although the majority of nurses work in acute care facilities, many nurses practice in long-term care, home care, primary and preventive care, ambulatory or outpatient clinics, and community health. Wherever you practice, recipients of your care include individuals, families, groups, or communities.

The American Nurses Association (ANA) states that the authority for the practice of nursing is based on a contract with society that acknowledges professional rights and responsibilities, as well as mechanisms for public accountability.[1] The knowledge and skills that make up nursing practice are derived from society's expectations and needs. Nursing practice continues to evolve according to society's health care needs and as knowledge and technology expand. This chapter introduces concepts and factors that affect professional nursing practice.

Definitions of Nursing

Several well-known definitions of nursing indicate that the basic themes of health, illness, and caring have existed since Florence Nightingale described nursing. Following are two such examples:

- Nursing is putting the patient in the best condition for nature to act (Nightingale).[2]
- The nurse's unique function is to assist patients, sick or well, in the performance of those activities contributing to health or its recovery (or to peaceful death) that they would perform unaided if they had the necessary strength, will, or

Reviewed by Nelda S. Godfrey, PhD, RN, ACNS-BC, FAAN, Associate Dean and Clinical Professor, University of Kansas School of Nursing, Kansas City, Kansas; Laura A. Stokowski, RNC, MS, Inova Fairfax Hospital for Children, Falls Church, Virginia; and Dawn M. Vanderhoef, PhD, DNP, PMHNP/CS-BC, Assistant Professor, Vanderbilt University School of Nursing, Nashville, Tennessee.

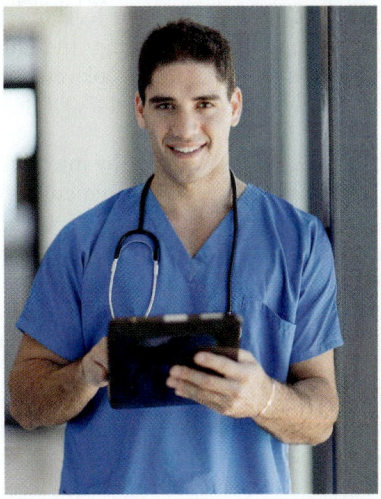

FIG. 1-1 Nurses are frontline professionals of health care. (©Michael Jung/iStock/Thinkstock)

knowledge—and to do this in such a way as to help them gain independence as rapidly as possible (Henderson).[3]

In 1980 the ANA defined **nursing** as "the diagnosis and treatment of human responses to actual and potential health problems."[1] In this context, your care of a person with a fractured hip would focus on the patient's possible responses to impaired mobility, pain, and loss of independence.

The widely accepted ANA definition of nursing was reaffirmed in the 2010 edition of the ANA's *Nursing: A Social Policy Statement* to reflect the continuing evolution of nursing practice:

> ***Nursing*** *is the protection, promotion, and optimization of health and abilities, prevention of illness and injury, alleviation of suffering through the diagnosis and treatment of human response, and advocacy in the care of individuals, families, communities, and populations.*[1]

This definition reflects nurses' increasing role in promoting health and wellness and advocating for the recipients of their care.

Nursing's View of Humanity

An individual has physiologic (or biophysical), psychologic (or emotional), sociocultural (or interpersonal), spiritual, and environmental components or dimensions. In this book, the individual is considered "a biopsychosocial spiritual being in constant interaction with a changing environment."[4] The individual is composed of dimensions that are interrelated and not separate entities. Thus a problem in one dimension may affect one or more of the other dimensions. A person's behavior is meaningful and oriented toward fulfilling needs, coping with stress, and developing one's self. However, at times a person requires help to meet these needs, cope successfully, or develop his or her unique potential.

Scope of Nursing Practice

The essential core of nursing practice is to deliver holistic, patient-centered care. It includes assessment and evaluation, administering a variety of interventions, patient and family teaching, and being a member of the interprofessional health care team.

The extent that nurses engage in the scope of practice depends on their educational preparation, experience, and role and is guided by individual state laws. To enter into practice, a nurse must complete an accredited program and pass an examination verifying that the nurse has the knowledge necessary to provide safe care. Entry-level nurses with associate or baccalaureate degrees are prepared to function as generalists. At this level, nurses provide direct health care and focus on ensuring coordinated and comprehensive care to patients in a variety of settings. Nurses work collaboratively with other health care providers to manage the needs of individuals and groups.[5]

With experience and continued study, nurses may specialize in an area of practice. Certification is a formal way for nurses to obtain professional recognition for having expertise in a specialty area. A variety of nursing organizations offer certification in a number of nursing specialties.[6] Certification usually requires a certain amount of clinical experience and successful completion of an examination. Recertification usually requires ongoing clinical experience and continuing education. Common nursing specialties include cardiovascular care; critical care; women's health; nursing informatics; and geriatric, medical-surgical, perinatal, emergency, psychiatric/mental health, and community health nursing.

Additional formal education and experience can prepare nurses for advanced practice. An **advanced practice registered nurse (APRN)** is a nurse educated at the master's or doctoral level, with advanced education in pathophysiology, pharmacology, and health assessment and expertise in a specialized area of practice. APRNs include clinical nurse specialists, nurse practitioners, nurse midwives, and nurse anesthetists. APRNs play a vital role in the health care delivery system. In addition to managing and delivering direct patient care, APRNs have roles in leadership, quality improvement, evidence-based practice, and informatics.[5]

The doctor of nursing practice (DNP) degree is a practice-focused terminal nursing degree. By raising the educational preparation for APRNs to the doctoral level, nursing is moving in the same direction as other health professions that offer practice doctorates (e.g., pharmacy [PharmD], physical therapy [DPT]). Nurses with a research-focused doctorate (PhD) typically serve as faculty in schools of nursing, policy analysts, and researchers. However, they are being increasingly used in health care settings as clinical experts, researchers, and health care system executives.

INFLUENCES ON PROFESSIONAL NURSING PRACTICE

Complex Health Care Environments

Expanding Knowledge and Technology. Rapidly changing technology and dramatically expanding knowledge are adding to the complexity of health care environments. Advances in patient care technologies are transforming care delivery and extending patients' lives. Discoveries in genetics are changing the way we think about a number of diseases, such as cancer and heart disease. For example, genetic information guides breast cancer screening. If cancer is diagnosed, this information then allows for treatment and drug therapy based on the patient's genetic makeup. With advances in knowledge, ethical dilemmas and controversies arise regarding the use of new scientific knowledge and the disparities that exist in patients' access to technologically advanced health care. Throughout this book, expanding knowledge and technology's impact on nursing

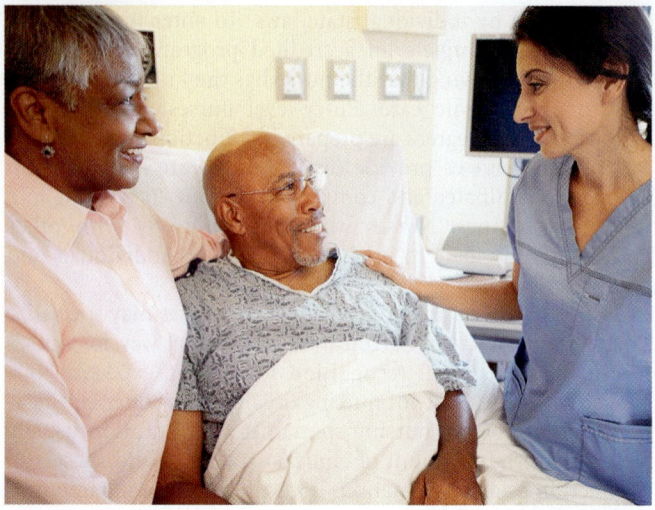

FIG. 1-2 The patient, family, and nurse collaborate as part of coordinating high-quality care. (©monkebusinessimages/iStock/Thinkstock)

practice are highlighted in genetics, informatics, and ethical/legal boxes.

Diverse Populations. Patient populations are more diverse than ever. Americans are living longer, with the number of people with chronic illnesses and multiple comorbidities increasing. Unlike those who receive acute, episodic care, patients with chronic illnesses have complex needs. They see a variety of health care providers in various settings over an extended period. With care shifting from hospitals and nursing homes to managed care in the community, you need to be able to manage and coordinate care when patients are transitioning among different settings.

At the same time, you will be caring for a more culturally and ethnically diverse population. When delivering care, you must consider the patient's and caregiver's cultural beliefs and values. Immigrants, particularly undocumented immigrants, often lack the resources necessary to access health care. Inability to pay for health care is associated with a tendency to delay seeking care, resulting in illnesses that are more serious at the time of diagnosis. Boxes throughout this book emphasize the influence of such factors as gender, culture, and ethnicity on nursing practice.

Consumerism. Health care is a consumer-focused business, and patients today are more involved in their health care. They want more control over their health care and expect high-quality, coordinated, and financially reasonable care. Health information is readily available. Many patients are very knowledgeable about their health and seek information about health problems and health care from media and Internet sources. They gather information so that they can have a voice in making decisions about their health care. As a nurse, you must be able to help patients access, interpret, and use appropriate and valid health care information (Fig. 1-2).

Health Care Systems

Health Care Financing. Many changes in health care systems that influence nursing care delivery are initiated by the government, employers, insurance companies, and regulating agencies in efforts to provide more cost-effective health care. Historically, the most notable event related to reimbursement was the establishment of prospective payment systems in the Medicare program. With this system, payment for hospital services for Medicare patients are based on flat fees determined by the diseases and problems treated during the admission. For example, if a patient had a total knee replacement, the hospital receives a set sum of money, such as $45,000 for the patient's care.

Other health care systems followed by introducing managed care systems that use prospective payment as a means of offering cost-effective health care delivery. In health maintenance organizations (HMOs) and preferred provider organizations (PPOs), charges are negotiated in advance of the delivery of care using predetermined reimbursement rates or capitation fees for medical care, hospitalization, and other health care services.

Now, quality and performance initiatives are driving further changes in health care financing. Value-based purchasing programs base reimbursement to health care providers on their performance on certain quality measures. These quality measures include clinical outcomes, patient safety, patient satisfaction, and the provider's adherence to evidence-based practice. Those who provide quality care at a lower cost may receive additional payments.

As part of value-based purchasing, payment for care can be withheld if a patient experiences events such as developing a pressure ulcer during a hospital stay or having something happen that is considered preventable (e.g., acquiring an injury after falling or having wrong site surgery).[7] This type of event is considered a *serious reportable event (SRE)*. SREs are discussed later in this chapter on p. 12.

Health Policy. Legislation has serious implications for health care delivery and nursing practice. The 2010 Patient Protection and Affordable Care Act (ACA) is the most important health care legislation since the creation of Medicare in 1965. The ACA's main goal is to increase access to health care. Other provisions affect how health care is delivered, expand wellness and preventive care, and promote quality and efficiency in the health care system.

The ACA encourages the creation of Accountable Care Organizations (ACOs). ACOs are groups of physicians, hospitals, and other health care providers who unite to coordinate care for Medicare patients. The goal of an ACO is to ensure that patients, especially the chronically ill, get the right care at the right time, while avoiding duplicate services and preventing errors.

The ACA supports nursing through funding for education and nurse-based clinics. The ACA has triggered changes throughout the health care system. As a nurse, you must take a leadership role in creating health care systems that provide safe, quality, patient-centered care. Becoming a Nurse Leader boxes throughout this book focus on developing leadership skills needed to fulfill this role.

Healthy People Initiative

The U.S. government is active in establishing goals and objectives for improving health through the *Healthy People* initiative.[8] The vision of *Healthy People* is a society in which all people live long, healthy lives. The overarching goals of the *Healthy People 2020* initiative are presented in Table 1-1. You will play a significant role in the *Healthy People* agenda by emphasizing health promotion, health maintenance, and cost-effective care that is responsive to the needs of older adults, culturally diverse groups, and underserved populations. *Healthy People* boxes related to these goals are integrated throughout this book.

TABLE 1-1 *Healthy People 2020*

Overarching Goals

- Attain high-quality, longer lives free of preventable disease, disability, injury, and premature death.
- Achieve health equity, eliminate disparities, and improve the health of all groups.
- Create social and physical environments that promote good health for all.
- Promote quality of life, healthy development, and healthy behaviors across all life stages.

Source: U.S. Department of Health and Human Services: *Healthy People 2020.* Retrieved from *www.healthypeople.gov.*

Organizational Influences

Professional Nursing Organizations. The American Nurses Association is the primary professional nursing organization. There are numerous professional specialty organizations, such as the American Association of Critical-Care Nurses (AACN), Association of periOperative Registered Nurses (AORN), and Oncology Nursing Society (ONS). Professional organizations have numerous roles in promoting quality patient care and professional nursing practice. These roles include developing standards of practice and codes of ethics, supporting research, and lobbying for legislation and regulations. Major nursing organizations promote research into the causes of errors, develop strategies to prevent future errors, and address nursing issues that affect the nurse's ability to deliver patient care safely. Nurses join a professional organization to keep current in their practice and network with others who are interested in a particular practice area.

A program that supports nurses is the American Nurses Credentialing Center's Magnet Recognition Program. The Magnet program "recognizes health care organizations for quality patient care, nursing excellence and innovations in professional nursing practice."[9] Magnet designation demonstrates a high quality of nursing care and achievement of a positive practice environment for nurses. Nurses who work in Magnet facilities have low turnover and burnout rates and more opportunities for professional and personal growth. This leads to better patient outcomes and greater career satisfaction.

Quality and Safety Education for Nurses (QSEN). A number of high-profile reports over the past 15 years have highlighted problems with the quality of health care. One of these reports, *The Future of Nursing: Leading Change, Advancing Health* from the Health and Medicine Division (HMD) of the National Academy of Medicine (formerly called the Institute of Medicine), acknowledges the link between professional nursing practice and health care delivery. The report discusses how health care providers, including nurses, are not being adequately prepared to provide the highest quality care possible. It recommends making changes so that nurses will have the skills to advance health care and play leadership roles in a reformed health care system[10] (Table 1-2).

To address nursing's role in solving these problems, the Robert Wood Johnson Foundation funded the *Quality and Safety Education for Nurses (QSEN) Institute.* QSEN has made a major contribution to nursing by defining specific competencies that nurses need to have to practice safely and effectively in today's complex health care system. The remainder of this chapter describes each of the QSEN competencies and the knowledge, skills, and attitudes (KSAs) necessary in each of the six areas: (1) patient-centered care, (2) teamwork and collaboration, (3) safety, (4) quality improvement, (5) informatics, and (6) evidence-based practice[11] (Table 1-3).

TABLE 1-2 Key Messages for the Future of Nursing

- Nurses should practice to the full extent of their education and training.
- Nurses should achieve high education and training through an improved education system that promotes seamless academic progression.
- Nurses should be full partners with physicians and other health professionals in redesigning health care.
- Effective workforce planning and policy making require better data collection and information infrastructure.

Source: IOM (now HMD) Recommendations. Retrieved from *www.thefutureofnursing.org/recommendations.*

PATIENT-CENTERED CARE

Nurses have long demonstrated that they truly deliver patient-centered care based on each patient's unique needs and understanding of the patient's preferences, values, and beliefs. Patient-centered care is interrelated with quality and safety. In the patient-centered care model, patients and caregivers seek and receive care from competent and knowledgeable health care professionals. In addition, patients and caregivers are involved in making decisions and coordinating care.

Nursing Process

Nurses provide patient-centered care using an organizing framework called the *nursing process*. The **nursing process** is a problem-solving approach to the identification and treatment of patient problems that is the foundation of nursing practice. The nursing process framework provides a structure for the delivery of nursing care and the knowledge, judgments, and actions that nurses use to achieve best patient outcomes. Once started, the nursing process is continuous and cyclic.

The nursing process consists of five phases: assessment, diagnosis, planning, implementation, and evaluation (Fig. 1-3). There is a basic order to the nursing process, beginning with assessment. *Assessment* is the collection of subjective and objective patient information on which you will base your plan of care. *Nursing diagnosis* is the act of analyzing the assessment data and making a judgment about the nature of the data. It includes identifying and labeling human responses to actual or potential health problems or life processes. During *planning* the nursing diagnosis directs developing patient outcomes or goals and identifying nursing interventions to accomplish the outcomes. *Implementation* is the activation of the plan with the use of nursing interventions. *Evaluation* is a continual activity in the nursing process. Evaluation determines whether the patient outcomes have been met as a result of nursing interventions. If the outcomes were not met, a review of the steps of the process is necessary to determine why not. Revision may be needed in assessment (data collection), nursing diagnoses, planning (determining patient outcomes), or implementation (nursing interventions).

Standardized Nursing Terminologies

The demands of the health care system challenge nursing to define its contribution to health care. The nursing profession can describe its unique role by answering questions such as: What do nurses do? How do they do it? How does it make a measurable difference in the health of those for whom they

TABLE 1-3 QSEN Competencies

Competency	Knowledge, Skills, and Attitudes
Patient-Centered Care Recognize the patient and caregiver as full partners in providing compassionate and coordinated care based on respect for patient's preferences, values, and needs	• Provide care with sensitivity and respect, taking into consideration the patient's perspectives, beliefs, and cultural background • Assess level of comfort and treat appropriately • Engage the patient in an active partnership that promotes health, well-being, and self-care management • Facilitate patient's informed consent for care
Teamwork and Collaboration Function effectively within nursing and interprofessional teams	• Value the expertise of each interprofessional member • Initiate referrals when appropriate • Follow communication practices that minimize risks associated with handoffs and transitions in care • Participate in interprofessional rounds
Safety Minimize risk of harm to patients and providers	• Follow recommendations from national safety campaigns • Appropriately communicate observations or concerns related to hazards and errors • Contribute to designing systems to improve safety
Quality Improvement Use data to monitor the outcomes of care and to improve the quality and safety of health care systems	• Use quality measures to understand performance • Identify gaps between local and best practices • Participate in investigating the circumstances surrounding a sentinel event (never event) or serious reportable event (SRE)
Informatics Use information and technology to communicate, manage knowledge, reduce errors, and support decision making	• Protect confidentiality of patient's protected health information • Document appropriately in electronic health records • Use communication technologies to coordinate patient care • Respond correctly to clinical decision-making alerts
Evidence-Based Practice Integrate best current evidence with clinical expertise and the patient/family preferences and values for delivery of optimal health care	• Read research, clinical practice guidelines, and evidence reports related to area of practice • Base individual patient care plan on patient's values, clinical expertise, and evidence • Continuously improve clinical practice based on new knowledge

Source: QSEN Competencies. Retrieved from *http://qsen.org/competencies.*

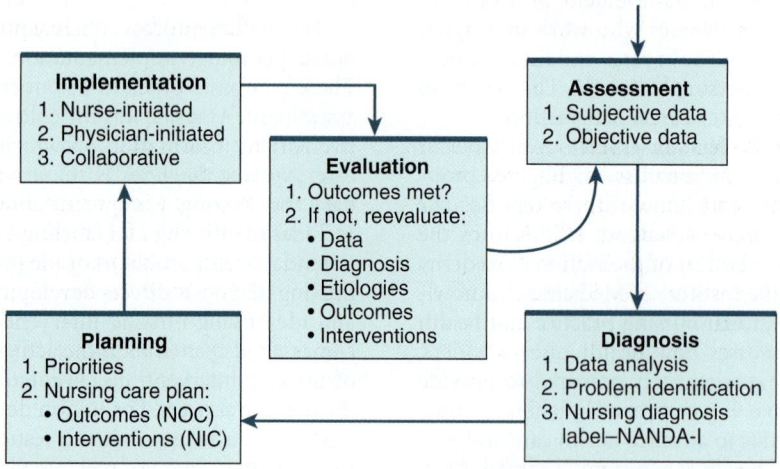

FIG. 1-3 Nursing process.

care? How are nursing's contributions different from those of medicine?

In response to these questions, nursing uses standardized terminologies (also called *nomenclatures, classification systems,* and *taxonomies*) to clearly define and evaluate nursing care. This promotes continuity of patient care and provides data showing nursing's impact on patient outcomes. Instead of using a variety of words to describe the same patient problems and nursing interventions, nurses use a readily understood common language to improve communication.

Standardized terminologies help identify new knowledge and practice guidelines and are essential in exchanging information between different electronic records systems. For example, do the patient problems of pressure ulcer and skin breakdown mean the same thing? What nursing interventions prevent these problems? Does turning the patient every 2 hours mean the same thing as repositioning the patient every 2 hours? If the patient is turned or repositioned every 2 hours, what happens as a result? Does placing the patient on a pressure-relieving mattress or a standard mattress change the results? How are the results described? How do you know what works best?

Three of the most widely used nursing terminologies focus on specific phases of the nursing process: (1) NANDA International (NANDA-I): Nursing Diagnoses, Definitions, and Classification; (2) the Nursing Outcomes Classification (NOC); and (3) the Nursing Interventions Classification (NIC). Patients' responses or problems can be labeled using the nursing diagnoses classified and defined by NANDA-I.[12] Nursing-sensitive patient outcomes can be identified and evaluated by selecting appropriate NOC outcomes and nursing interventions, or treatments, can be selected and implemented from NIC.[13,14]

NANDA-I Nursing Diagnoses. NANDA-I is the nursing organization that develops and maintains the standard classification system for nursing diagnoses.[12] Nursing diagnoses provide the basis for selecting nursing interventions to achieve patient outcomes for which nursing is accountable. Delivering care based on accurately identified nursing diagnoses results in more effective and safer patient care. The NANDA-I list is continually evolving as new research results are available and nurses identify new human responses.

Nursing Outcomes Classification (NOC). Nursing Outcomes Classification (NOC) is a list of patient outcomes developed to evaluate the effects of interventions provided by nurses. A **nursing-sensitive patient outcome** is defined as an individual, family, or community state, behavior, or perception that is measured along a continuum in response to a nursing intervention(s).[13] The impact of your nursing practice on patient outcomes can be identified and measured when you choose a NOC outcome. Currently there are more than 490 outcomes. Each outcome has a designated code, definition, a set of indicators to use to evaluate patient status, and a five-point Likert scale for rating the outcome and indicators. A rating of a "5" is always the best possible score and "1" is always the worst possible score.

Nursing Interventions Classification (NIC). Nursing Interventions Classification (NIC) includes independent and collaborative interventions that you carry out, or direct others to carry out, on behalf of patients. An intervention is "any treatment, based upon clinical judgment and knowledge, which a nurse performs to enhance patient/client outcomes."[14] It includes treatments that you perform in all settings and includes direct and indirect care. NIC includes more than 550 interventions with a label name, a definition, and a set of activities for you to choose from to carry out the intervention.

A list of more than 550 interventions may seem overwhelming. You will soon discover those interventions that are often used in your particular specialty or with your patient population. When planning care for a patient, choose specific interventions that are appropriate for the patient based on the nursing diagnosis and desired patient outcomes. Each intervention has a list of activities, and you select the appropriate activities from the list to implement the intervention. NIC does not prescribe interventions for specific situations. You are responsible for making the important decision of when and which interventions to use for a specific patient and situation based on your knowledge of the patient and the patient's condition.

NANDA-NOC-NIC Linkages. NANDA, NOC, and NIC (NNN) linkages show how the three distinct nursing terminologies can be connected and used together when planning care for patients. Linkages may assist in determining a nursing diagnosis, projecting a desired outcome, and selecting interventions to achieve the desired outcome. Because each outcome or intervention has a coded number, the use of NNN facilitates electronic collection of standardized nursing data to evaluate the effectiveness of nursing care. Table 1-4 shows an example of an NNN linkage.

TABLE 1-4 Example of NANDA-I–NOC–NIC Linkage

NANDA-I Nursing Diagnosis: *Impaired skin integrity:* A state in which the individual has altered epidermis and/or dermis

NANDA-I–Related Factors	NOC Outcomes	NIC Interventions
Pressure	Tissue integrity: skin and mucous membranes	Pressure management Skin surveillance
Nutritional deficit	Nutritional status: food and fluid intake	Nutrition monitoring Nutrition therapy
Knowledge deficit	Knowledge: illness care	Teaching: disease

Source: *Nursing Diagnoses—Definitions and Classification 2015-2017.* © 2014, 1994-2014 by NANDA International. Used by arrangement with Blackwell Publishing Limited, a company of John Wiley & Sons, Inc.
NANDA-I, NANDA International; *NIC,* Nursing Interventions Classification; *NOC,* Nursing Outcomes Classification.

Nursing Care Plans

In any clinical setting, you are responsible for providing an individualized plan of care that includes nursing diagnoses, outcomes, and interventions. In clinical practice, electronic care plans often follow a standard format that has been adapted to the specific setting. These plans are guides for routine nursing care. You individualize each to your patient's unique needs and problems.

In nursing education, the nursing process is often documented differently from clinical practice. The nursing process is frequently recorded in nursing care plans similar to those located on the website for this book *(http://evolve.elsevier.com/Lewis/medsurg)*. These nursing care plans are teaching and learning tools. You practice and learn the nursing process by collecting assessment data, identifying nursing diagnoses, and selecting patient outcomes and nursing interventions. You usually have to identify rationales for the selected interventions.

The nursing care plans associated with this book use NANDA-I–approved nursing diagnoses, listed in order of priority, with NOC outcomes and NIC interventions (NCP 1-1). When any of these care plans are used, you should individualize the plan for your specific patient. You must use critical thinking to continually evaluate the situation and revise the nursing diagnoses, outcomes, and interventions to fit each patient's unique care needs.

With *collaborative problems,* the nurse must monitor the patient to detect the onset or change in status of actual or potential complications.[15] Nurses use physician and nurse prescribed interventions to manage collaborative problems and prevent morbidity and mortality. During the diagnosis phase of the nursing process, you identify these risks in addition to nursing diagnoses. Identifying collaborative problems requires knowledge of pathophysiology and possible complications of medical treatment. Collaborative problem statements are usually written as "potential complication: _____" or "PC:

NURSING CARE PLAN 1-1

*Patient With Heart Failure**

Nursing Diagnosis

Impaired gas exchange *related to* increased preload and alveolar-capillary membrane changes *as evidenced by* abnormal O_2 saturation,, hypoxemia, dyspnea, tachypnea, tachycardia, restlessness, and patient's statement, "I am so short of breath"

Patient Goal

Maintains adequate O_2/CO_2 exchange at the alveolar-capillary membrane to meet O_2 needs of the body

Outcomes (NOC)	Interventions (NIC) and *Rationales*
Respiratory Status: Gas Exchange • O_2 saturation ____ • Arterial pH ____ • PaO_2 ____ • $PaCO_2$ ____ • Chest x-ray findings ____ **Measurement Scale** 1 = Severe deviation from normal range 2 = Substantial deviation from normal range 3 = Moderate deviation from normal ranage 4 = Mild deviation from normal range 5 = No deviation from normal range • Dyspnea with exertion ____ • Dyspnea at rest ____ • Restlessness ____ • Impaired cognition ____ **Measurement Scale** 1 = Severe 2 = Substantial 3 = Moderate 4 = Mild 5 = None	**Respiratory Monitoring** • Monitor pulse oximetry, respiratory rate, rhythm, depth, and effort of respirations *to evaluate changes in respiratory status.* • Auscultate breath sounds, noting areas of decreased or absent ventilation and presence of adventitious sounds *to detect presence of pulmonary edema.* • Monitor for increased restlessness, anxiety, and work of breathing *to detect increasing hypoxemia.* **Oxygen Therapy** • Administer supplemental O_2 or other noninvasive ventilator support (e.g., bilevel positive airway pressure [BiPAP]) as needed *to maintain adequate O_2 levels.* • Monitor the O_2 liter flow rate and placement of O_2 delivery device *to ensure O_2 is adequately delivered.* • Change O_2 delivery device from mask to nasal prongs during meals as tolerated *to sustain O_2 levels while eating.* • Monitor the effectiveness of O_2 therapy *to identify hypoxemia and establish range of O_2 saturation.* **Positioning** • Position patient to alleviate dyspnea (e.g., semi-Fowler's position), as appropriate, *to improve ventilation by decreasing venous return to the heart and increasing thoracic capacity.*

*This example presents one nursing diagnosis for heart failure. The complete nursing care plan for heart failure is available on *http://evolve.elsevier.com/Lewis/medsurg.*

_____" without a *"related to"* statement. An example is PC: pulmonary embolism.

A *concept map* is another method of recording a nursing care plan. In a concept map the nursing process is recorded in a visual diagram of patient problems and interventions that illustrates the relationships among clinical data. Nurse educators use concept mapping to teach nursing process and care planning. There are various formats for concept maps.

Conceptual care maps blend a concept map and a nursing care plan. On a conceptual care map, assessment data used to identify the patient's primary health concern are centrally positioned. Diagnostic testing data, treatments, and medications surround the assessment data. Positioned below are nursing diagnoses that represent the patient's responses to the health state. Listed with each nursing diagnosis are the assessment data that support the nursing diagnosis, outcomes, nursing interventions with rationales, and evaluation. After completing the map, you draw connections between identified relationships and concepts. A conceptual care map creator is available online on the website for this book. For selected case studies at the end of the management chapters, related concept maps are available on the website at *http://evolve.elsevier.com/Lewis/medsurg.*

Continuum of Patient Care

Nursing is a part of health care at all points along the patient care continuum. Depending on their health status, patients often move among a multitude of different health care settings. For example, a young man is in a trauma unit of an acute care hospital following a motor vehicle crash. After he is stabilized, he may be transferred to a general medical-surgical unit and then to an acute rehabilitation facility. After rehabilitation is complete, he is discharged home to continue with outpatient rehabilitation, with follow-up by home health care nurses and care in an ambulatory clinic.

Decisions regarding the most appropriate setting for obtaining health care frequently depend on the cost of care and the patient's health care insurance plan and personal finances. Although the hospital remains the mainstay for acute care interventions, community-based settings offer patients the opportunity to live or recover in settings that maximize their independence and preserve human dignity.

Community-based health care settings include ambulatory care, transitional care, and long-term care. *Transitional care* settings provide care in between the acute care and the home or long-term care setting. Patients may receive transitional care at an acute rehabilitation facility after head trauma or a spinal cord injury. *Long-term care* refers to the care of patients for a period greater than 30 days. It may be required for those who are severely developmentally disabled, who are mentally impaired, or who have physical deficits requiring continuous medical and nursing management (e.g., patients who are ventilator dependent or have Alzheimer's disease). Long-term care facilities include skilled nursing facilities, assisted living facilities, and residential care facilities.

With the Affordable Care Act, there is a new emphasis on care coordination when patients transition between care settings. *Transitions of care* refer to patients moving among health care practitioners, settings, and home as their condition and care needs change.[16] As a nurse, you are an essential part of care coordination by stressing actions that meet patient's needs and facilitate safe, quality care. Collaborating with other members of the interprofessional team is critical. A lack of communication can result in an ineffective care transition, leading to medication errors and higher hospital readmission rates. For example, you are a nurse in acute care admitting a long-term care patient who has been receiving propranolol 20 mg/5 mL twice a day. The admitting orders read "propranolol 20 mg/mL, give 5 mL twice a day."

Delivery of Nursing Care

Nurses deliver patient-centered care in collaboration with the interprofessional health care team and within the framework of a care delivery model. A care delivery model outlines how responsibilities and authority are structured to accomplish patient care.[17] More positive care outcomes occur when the number and type of care providers match patient needs and there is a designated care coordinator.

In acute care settings, two basic models are used, team care and total patient care. *Team care* models involve a group of providers who work together to deliver care. A professional nurse is usually the team leader. As team leader, you manage and coordinate care with others, such as licensed practical/vocational nurses (LPNs/LVNs) and unlicensed assistive personnel (UAP). You have accountability for the quality of care delivered by team members during a work period. In total patient care models, you are responsible for planning and providing all care.

Other care models include case management and telehealth. **Case management** is "a collaborative process of assessment, planning, facilitation, care coordination, evaluation, and advocacy for options and services to meet an individual's and family's comprehensive health needs through communication and available resources to promote quality, cost-effective outcomes."[18] Although health care agencies implement case management in various ways, it involves managing the patient's care with other interprofessional team members across multiple care settings and levels of care.

A professional nurse often serves as the case manager. In this role, the nurse assesses the needs of patients and/or caregivers, coordinates services for them, makes referrals as appropriate, and evaluates the progress towards meeting care goals.

For example, a nurse case manager in an outpatient clinic has been working for 3 months with an older male patient who has multiple co-morbidities, including severe coronary artery disease, diabetes, and osteoarthritis. After he is scheduled for a coronary artery bypass, the nurse manager coordinates his care with other members of the interprofessional team. She arranges his preoperative appointments and informs the other team members so that all health care providers understand the patient's unique needs. After the patient has surgery, he develops a deep venous thrombosis in his leg. The case manager then works with the interprofessional team to evaluate the patient's discharge needs and determine whether rehabilitation or home health care are necessary for the patient. With the patient and caregiver, the team decides to discharge the patient to a rehabilitation facility. The case manager assists with the transition, again coordinating care so that the providers at the rehabilitation facility are aware of the patient's needs.

Telehealth nursing is using the nursing process to provide nursing care to patients through telecommunication technologies, including high-speed Internet, wireless, satellite, and video communications.[17] Among the many uses of telehealth are triaging patients, monitoring patients with chronic or critical conditions, helping patients manage symptoms, providing patient and caregiver education and emotional support, and providing follow-up care. Telehealth increases access to care. The nurse engaged in telehealth can assess the patient's health status, deliver interventions, and evaluate the outcomes of nursing care while separated geographically from the patient (Fig. 1-4).

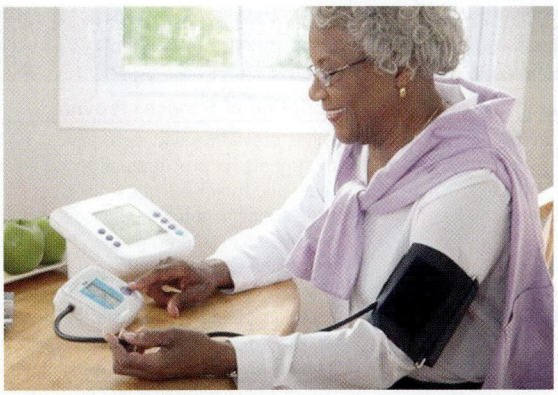

FIG. 1-4 An older adult performing remote blood pressure monitoring. (From Cooper K, Gosnell K: *Foundations of nursing*, St Louis, 2015, Elsevier.)

Critical Thinking

Complex health care environments require that you use critical thinking and clinical reasoning skills to make decisions that lead to the best patient outcomes. **Critical thinking**, your ability to focus your thinking to get the results you need in various situations, has been described as knowing how to learn, be creative, generate ideas, make decisions, and solve problems.[19]

Critical thinking is not memorizing a list of facts or the steps of a procedure. Instead, it is the ability to make judgments and solve problems by making sense of information. Learning and using critical thinking is a continual process that occurs inside and outside of the clinical setting.

Clinical reasoning is using critical thinking to examine and analyze patient care issues.[19] It involves understanding the medical and nursing implications of a patient's situation when making decisions regarding patient care. You use clinical reasoning when you identify a change in a patient's status, take into account the context and concerns of the patient and caregiver, and decide what to do about it.

Given the complexity of patient care today, nurses are required to learn and implement critical thinking and clinical reasoning skills long before they gain those skills through the experience of professional practice. Clinical experiences during nursing education provide opportunities for you to learn and make decisions about patient care. Various education models and techniques, including interactive case studies and simulation exercises, promote practice in critical thinking and clinical reasoning. Throughout this book, select boxes, case studies, and review questions promote your use of critical thinking and clinical reasoning skills.

TEAMWORK AND COLLABORATION

Interprofessional Team

To deliver high-quality care, you need to establish effective working relationships with members of the health care team. The **interprofessional team** is composed of providers from various disciplines, working together and sharing their expertise to provide individualized care. It may consist of physicians, nurses, pharmacists, occupational and physical therapists, social workers, and others (Table 1-5). To be competent in interprofessional practice, you must collaborate in many ways by exchanging knowledge, sharing responsibility for problem

TABLE 1-5 Interprofessional Team Members

Team Member	Description of Services Provided
Dentist	Provides preventive and restorative treatments for problems affecting the teeth and mouth
Dietitian	Provides general nutrition services, including dietary consultation regarding health promotion or specialized diets
Occupational therapist (OT)	May assist patient with fine motor coordination, performance of activities of daily living, cognitive-perceptual skills, sensory testing, and the construction or use of assistive or adaptive equipment
Pastoral care	Offers spiritual support and guidance to patients and caregivers
Pharmacist	Prepares medications and infusion products
Physical therapist (PT)	Works with patients on improving strength and endurance, gait training, transfer training, and developing a patient education program
Physician (medical doctor [MD])	Practices medicine and treats illness and injury by prescribing medication, performing diagnostic tests and evaluations, performing surgery, and providing other medical services and advice
Physician assistant	Conducts physical exams, diagnoses and treats illnesses, and counsels on preventive health care in collaboration with a physician
Respiratory therapist	May assist with oxygen therapy in the home, provide specialized respiratory treatments, and instruct patient or caregiver regarding the proper use of respiratory equipment
Social worker	Assists patients with developing coping skills, meeting caregiver concerns, securing adequate financial resources or housing assistance, or making referrals to social service or volunteer agencies
Speech pathologist	Focuses on treatment of speech defects and disorders, especially through the use of physical exercises to strengthen muscles used in speech, speech drills, and audiovisual aids that develop new speech habits

solving, and making patient care decisions. You may be responsible for coordinating care among the team members, participating in interprofessional team meetings or rounds, and initiating appropriate referrals when you need expertise in specialized areas to help the patient. To do so, you must be aware of the knowledge and skills of other team members and be able to communicate effectively with them.

To assist you in developing the competencies necessary to practice within an interprofessional clinical environment, you may participate in education activities with students from other disciplines. Throughout this book, teamwork and collaboration boxes, case studies, and review questions discuss the roles other professionals have in managing clinical problems.

Coordinating Care

Communication. Effective communication is a key component of fostering teamwork and coordinating care. To provide safe, effective care, everyone involved in a patient's care should understand the patient's condition and his or her needs.

TEAMWORK & COLLABORATION

Teamwork & Collaboration Boxes Throughout Book

Title	Chapter	Page
Assessment and Data Collection	3	36
Blood Transfusions	30	649
Cardiac Catheterization and Percutaneous Coronary Intervention (PCI)	33	729
Corrective Lenses and Hearing Aids	21	392
Incontinent Patient	45	1059
IV Therapy	16	294
Nasogastric and Gastric Tubes and Enteral Feedings	39	867
Ostomy Care	42	960
Oxygen Administration	28	568
Pain	8	123
Patient Receiving Bladder Irrigation	54	1274
Patient Requiring Mechanical Ventilation	65	1581
Patient With a Cast or Traction	62	1471
Patient With a Seizure Disorder	58	1381
Patient With Alzheimer's Disease	59	1412
Patient With an Acute Stroke	57	1359
Patient With Chronic Venous Insufficiency	37	827
Patient With Diabetes Mellitus	48	1152
Patient With Hypertension	32	696
Patient With Neutropenia	30	632
Patient With Osteomyelitis	63	1498
Patient With Rheumatoid Arthritis	64	1529
Patient With Venous Thromboembolism (VTE)	37	824
Postoperative Patient	19	334
Skin Care	23	425
Suctioning and Tracheostomy Care	26	490
Urinary Catheters	45	1061
Wound Care	11	170

Unfortunately many issues result from a breakdown in communication. Miscommunication often occurs during transitions of care. One structured model used to improve communication is the **SBAR (Situation-Background-Assessment-Recommendation)** technique (Table 1-6). This technique provides a way to talk about a patient's condition among members of the health care team in a predictable, structured manner. Other ways to enhance communication during transitions include performing surgical time-outs, using a standard change-of-shift process, and conducting interprofessional rounds to identify risks and develop a plan for delivering care.

Clinical Pathways. **Clinical pathways** (critical paths, patient care protocols, care maps) are interprofessional care plans that specify care and desired outcomes during a specific time period for patients with a particular diagnosis or health condition. Think of a clinical pathway as a road map the patient and health care team should follow. As the patient progresses along the road, the patient should receive specific care and accomplish specific goals. If a patient's progress differs from the planned path, a variance has occurred. A negative variance occurs when specific goals are not met. The nurse usually identifies when a negative variance is present and works with the interprofessional team to create a plan to address the issue.[16]

The exact content and format of clinical pathways vary among agencies and settings. Each agency usually develops its own pathways based on evidence-based practice guidelines. Common components include assessment guidelines, laboratory and diagnostic testing, medications, activity, diet, and teaching. In

TABLE 1-6 Guidelines for Communicating Using SBAR

Purpose: SBAR is a model for effective transfer of information by providing a standardized structure for concise factual communications from nurse-to-nurse, nurse-to-physician, or nurse-to–other health professionals.

Steps to Use: Before speaking with a physician or other health care professional about a patient problem, assess the patient yourself, read the most recent physician progress and nursing notes, and have the patient's chart available.

S **Situation**	• What is the situation you want to discuss? What is happening at the present time? • Identify self, unit. State: I am calling about: *patient, room number.* • Briefly state the problem: what it is, when it happened or started, and how severe it is. State: I have just assessed the patient and I am concerned about: *identify why you are concerned.*
B **Background**	• What is the background or circumstances leading up to the situation? State pertinent background information related to the situation that may include • Admitting diagnosis and date of admission • List of current medications, allergies, IV fluids • Most recent vital signs • Date and time of any laboratory testing and results of previous tests for comparison • Synopsis of treatment to date • Code status
A **Assessment**	• What do you think the problem is? What is your assessment of the situation? State what you think the problem is: • Changes from prior assessments • Patient condition unstable or worsening
R **Recommendation/ Request**	• What should we do to correct the problem? What is your recommendation or request? State your request. • Specific treatments • Tests needed • Patient needs to be seen now

Source: Institute for Health Care Improvement: SBAR technique for communication: a situational briefing model. Retrieved from *www.ihi.org/resources/Pages/Tools/SBARTechniqueforCommunicationASituationalBriefingModel.aspx.*

acute care, clinical pathways often describe which patient care components are required at specific times for each day of hospitalization. The case types selected for this type of pathway are usually those that are high volume or high risk and predictable, such as myocardial infarction and surgical procedures (e.g., joint replacements, cholecystectomies, cataract surgery).

Delegation and Assignment. As a registered nurse (RN), you will delegate nursing care and supervise others who are qualified to deliver care. **Delegation** is transferring authority to a competent individual for completing selected nursing tasks in a selected situation.[20] The delegation and assignment of nursing activities is a process that, when used appropriately, can result in safe, effective, and efficient patient care. Delegating can allow you more time to focus on complex patient care needs. Delegating care and supervising others will be one of your fundamental roles as a professional nurse.

Delegation typically involves tasks and procedures that licensed practical/vocational nurses (LPNs/LVNs) and unlicensed assistive personnel (UAP) perform. Nursing interventions that require independent nursing knowledge, skill, or judgment (e.g., initial assessment, determining nursing diagnoses, patient teaching, evaluating care) are your responsibility and cannot be delegated. State boards of nursing and agency policies identify activities that you can delegate to LPNs/LVNs and UAP. You need to use professional judgment to determine appropriate activities to delegate based on the patient's needs, the LPN/LVN's and UAP's education and training, and extent of supervision required. The most common delegated nursing actions occur during the implementation phase of the nursing process. For example, the nurse can delegate measuring oral intake and urine output to UAP, but the RN uses nursing judgment to decide if the intake and output are adequate.

The general guideline for LPN/LVN practice is that they can function independently in a stable, routine situation. However, they must work under the direct supervision of a professional nurse in acute, unstable situations when a patient's condition can rapidly change. In most states, LPNs/LVNs may administer medications, perform sterile procedures, and provide a wide variety of interventions planned by the RN. The procedure itself is not the issue in determining what can be delegated. Rather, the stability of the patient determines whether it is appropriate for an RN to delegate a procedure to an LPN/LVN. For example, the LPN/LVN can change a dressing on an abdominal surgical wound, but the RN should perform the initial dressing change and wound assessment.

UAPs hold many titles, including nurse aides, orderlies, nursing assistants, patient care assistants, or technicians. The activities UAPs perform typically include obtaining routine vital signs on stable patients, feeding and assisting patients at mealtimes, ambulating stable patients, and helping patients with bathing and hygiene.

Delegation can also occur among professional nurses. For example, if one RN has accountability for an outcome and asks another RN to perform a specific intervention related to that outcome, that is delegation. This type of delegation typically occurs when one RN leaves the unit/work area for a meal break.

Assignment is different from delegation in that assignment is the work each staff member is to accomplish during a given work period.[20] Staff members can only be assigned activities that are within their scope of practice. Therefore the term *assign* is used when you direct a person to do something that he or she is authorized to do. For example, you can assign an LPN/LVN to administer medications to a patient, because this is within the LPN/LVN's scope of practice. You cannot assign an LPN/LVN to a patient who needs an admission assessment, because an RN must perform the initial patient assessment.

Whether you delegate or are working with staff to whom you assign tasks, you are responsible for the patient's total care during your work period. You need to determine what patient care tasks must be accomplished during the given time period, identify who will accomplish them, and prioritize the order in which the tasks must be completed. You are responsible for supervising UAP or LPNs/LVNs. Clearly communicate what tasks must be done and provide necessary guidance. Since you are accountable for ensuring that delegated tasks are completed in a competent manner, evaluate the care given, follow-up as needed, and make sure no care was missed.

Delegation is a skill that is learned and you must practice to be proficient in managing patient care. You need to use critical thinking and professional judgment to ensure that the Five Rights of Nursing Delegation are implemented (Table 1-7). To

TABLE 1-7 Five Rights of Delegation

The Five Rights of Delegation

The registered nurse uses critical thinking and professional judgment to be sure that the delegation or assignment is:

1. The right task
2. Under the right circumstances
3. To the right person
4. With the right directions and communication
5. Under the right supervision and evaluation

Rights of Delegation	Description	Questions to Ask
Right Task	One that can be delegated for a specific patient	Is it appropriate to delegate based on legal and agency factors? Has the person been trained and evaluated in performing the task? Is the person able and willing to do this specific task?
Right Circumstances	Appropriate patient setting, available resources, and considering relevant factors, including patient stability	What are the patient's needs right now? Is staffing such that the circumstances support delegation strategies?
Right Person	Right person is delegating the right task to the right person to be performed on right person	Is the prospective delegatee a willing and able employee? Are the patient needs a "fit" with the delegatee?
Right Directions and Communication	Clear, concise description of task, including its objective, limits, and expectations	Have you clearly communicated the task? With directions, limits, and expected outcomes? Does the delegatee know what and when to report? Does the delegatee understand what needs to be done?
Right Supervision and Evaluation	Appropriate monitoring, evaluation, intervention, and feedback	Do you know how and when you will interact about patient care with the delegatee? How often will you need to provide direct observation? Will you be able to give feedback to the staff member if needed?

Source: Delegation Joint Statement NCSBN-ANA. Retrieved from *www.ncsbn.org/1625.htm.*

assist you, information on delegation is presented in teamwork and collaboration boxes and questions in case studies at the end of the management chapters.

SAFETY

As the complexity of health care environments increases, patient safety is affected. It is estimated that between 210,000 and 440,000 patients each year suffer some type of harm that contributes to their death because of preventable medical errors.[21] A number of organizations are addressing this issue by providing safety goals for health care organizations and identifying safety competencies for health professionals. By implementing various procedures and systems to improve health care delivery to meet safety goals, health care systems are working to attain a culture of safety that minimizes the risk of harm to the patient.

Serious Reportable Events

The National Quality Forum (NQF) uses the term **serious reportable event (SRE)**, also called a *"never" event,* to describe adverse events that are serious, largely preventable, and of concern to the public and health care providers.[22] These events include such things as a patient acquiring a stage III or greater pressure ulcer while hospitalized and death or disability from a fall or hypoglycemia.

To reduce the occurrence of these events, the NQF provides a list of effective *Safe Practices* that should be used in health care settings to improve the safety of care. You are implementing NQF practices when you perform a time-out prior to a surgical procedure, complete accurate medication records, and implement interventions to prevent catheter-associated urinary tract infections, pressure ulcers, and falls.

National Patient Safety Goals

The Joint Commission (TJC), the accrediting agency for health care organizations, gathers and reports data on serious errors they call sentinel events. A *sentinel event* is a patient safety event not related to the patient's illness or underlying condition that reaches a patient and results in death, permanent harm, or severe temporary harm.[23] Events are "sentinel" because they signal the need for immediate investigation and response. Many sentinel events are also serious reportable events. If the patient undergoes a wrong-site or wrong-procedure surgery, experiences an assault in the health care setting or receives an incompatible blood product, the occurrence is both a sentinel event, reportable to TJC, and a serious reportable event, reportable to NQF.

To address specific patient safety concerns, TJC issues National Patient Safety Goals (NPSGs).[23] NPSGs promote patient safety by providing evidence-based solutions to common safety problems. The 2016 NPSGs are listed in Table 1-8.

The latest safety goal, focusing on improving the safety of clinical alarm systems, will greatly affect nursing. Patient monitoring systems provide important information. Alarms that work well improve patient safety and care by telling you when a patient requires your attention. However, so many alarms can go off that *alarm fatigue* occurs, and nurses can become desensitized to the sounds. By better managing alarms, alarm fatigue will be reduced and patient safety improved.

Because you have the greatest amount of interaction with patients, you play a key role in promoting safety. Many describe nurses as the patient's last line of defense. Every nurse has the responsibility to ensure the patient receives care in a manner that prevents errors and promotes patient safety. Throughout this book, safety alerts highlighting patient care issues and NPSGs will assist you in learning to apply safety principles.

QUALITY IMPROVEMENT

Quality care is related to safety: the higher the culture of safety, the better the quality of care. Health care systems focused on

TABLE 1-8 National Patient Safety Goals

Safety Goal	Examples
Goal 1: Identify patients correctly.	• Use at least two ways to identify patients (e.g., have them state full name and date of birth). • Give the correct patient the correct blood with every blood transfusion.
Goal 2: Improve communication among the health care team.	• Quickly get critical test results to the right staff person.
Goal 3: Use medications safely.	• Label all medicines that are not already labeled. Discard any found unlabeled. • Use appropriate precautions with patients who take anticoagulants. • Find out what medications each patient is taking. Make certain that it is safe for the patient to take any new medicines with his or her current medicines. • Give a list of the patient's medicines to the patient and his or her caregiver before they go home. Explain the list.
Goal 6: Use clinical alarm systems safely.	• Respond to alarms in a timely manner. • Do not turn alarms off.
Goal 7: Prevent health care–associated infections.	• Use soap, water, and hand sanitizer before and after every patient contact. • Use evidence-based practices to prevent infections related to central lines, indwelling urinary catheters, and multidrug-resistant organisms.
Goal 15: Identify the safety risks inherent in the agency's patient population.	• Assess patients at risk for suicide. • Assess any risks for patients who are getting home oxygen therapy, such as fires.
Universal Protocol (UP) Preprocedure verification Mark procedure site Performance of time-out	• Conduct a time-out before the start of any invasive or surgical procedure. • Confirm correct patient, procedure, and site.

Adapted from The Joint Commission (TJC): *2016 National patient safety goals*, Oakbrook Terrace, Ill. Retrieved from *www.jointcommission.org/assets/1/6/2016_NPSG_HAP_ER.pdf/*.

quality outcomes use practice standards and protocols based on best evidence while considering the patient's unique preferences and needs. Your role is to coordinate the complex aspects of patient care, including the care delivered by others, and identify and correct issues associated with poor quality and unsafe care.

Quality improvement (QI) programs involve systematic actions that monitor, assess, and improve health care quality. QI is an interprofessional team effort that is required by accrediting agencies. As part of professional nursing practice, you need to be able to collect data using QI tools, implement interventions to improve quality of care, and monitor patient outcomes. Several public and private groups focusing on improving health care quality have developed standard QI measures. These performance measures assess how well the health care team cares for a patient with a certain condition or receives a specific treatment. They describe what data must be collected and monitored. Fig 1-5 shows an example of a QI system for adult patients with asthma. In this example, you would monitor

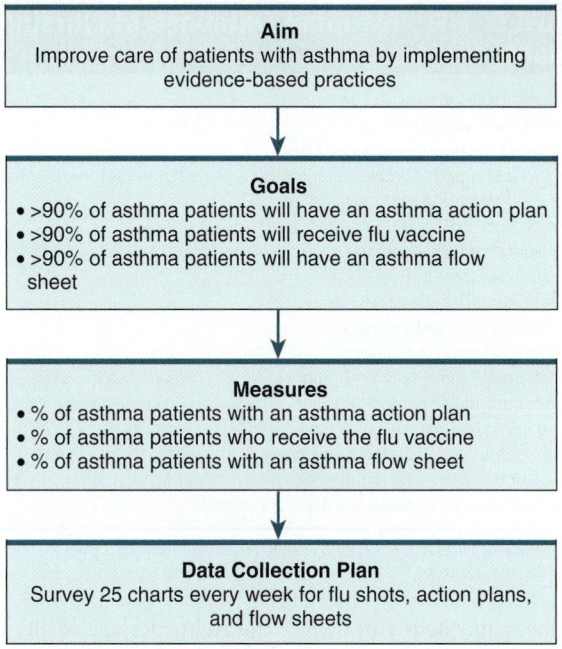

FIG. 1-5 Quality improvement system. (Adapted from Courtlandt CD, Noonan L, Leonard GF: Model for improvement—part 1: A framework for health care quality, *Ped Clin North Am* 56:757, 2009.)

patient medical records to determine if the rate of flu vaccine administration exceeds 90%. You would share the results with the interprofessional team and, if the identified proficiency was not met, work as a team to implement measures to correct the deficiency.

National Database of Nursing Quality Indicators

The National Database of Nursing Quality Indicators (NDNQI) provides data on nursing-sensitive measures to evaluate the impact of nursing care on patient outcomes. Patient outcomes are nursing sensitive if they improve with a greater quantity or quality of nursing care. NDNQI outcomes are unique because they identify how nursing workforce factors, including nurse staffing and skill mix, directly influence patient outcomes. NDNQI data show the incidence of falls and health care–associated pressure ulcers and infections decreases with adequate staffing and increased nurse education and satisfaction with the work environment. Table 1-9 lists the current NDNQI.

INFORMATICS

Nursing is an information-intense profession. Advances in informatics and technology have changed the way nurses plan, deliver, document, and evaluate care. All nurses, regardless of their setting or role, use informatics and technology every day in practice. Informatics has changed how you obtain and review diagnostic information, make clinical decisions, communicate with patients and health care team members, document, and provide care.

Technology advances have increased the efficiency of nursing care, improving the work environment and the care nurses provide. Computers and mobile devices allow you to document at the time you deliver care and give you quick and easy access to information, including clinical decision-making tools, patient education materials, and references. Texting, video chat, and e-mail enhance communication among health care team

TABLE 1-9 National Database of Nursing Quality Indicators

- Workforce factors
  - Nurse turnover
  - Nursing hours per patient day
  - RN surveys on job satisfaction and practice environment scale
  - RN education and certification
  - Skill mix: RNs, LPNs/LVNs, UAP
- Hospital readmission rates
- Pain assessment cycle
- Peripheral IV infiltration rate
- Physical restraint prevalence
- Physical/sexual assault rate
- Patient falls and falls with injury
- Pressure ulcer incidence
- Health care–associated infections (HAI)
  - Ventilator-associated pneumonia and events
  - Central line-associated bloodstream infection
  - Catheter-associated urinary tract infection

Source: National Database of Nursing Quality Indicators. Retrieved from *www.nursingquality.org.*

members and help you deliver the right message to the right person at the right time.

Technology plays a key role in providing safe, quality patient care. Medication administration applications improve patient safety by flagging potential errors, such as look-alike and sound-alike medications and adverse drug interactions, before they can occur. Computerized provider order entry (CPOE) systems can eliminate errors caused by misreading or misinterpreting handwritten orders. Sensor technology can decrease the number of falls in high-risk patients. Care reminder systems provide cues that decrease the amount of missed nursing care.

Being able to use technology skills to communicate and access information is now an essential component of your professional nursing practice. You must be able to use word processing software, communicate by e-mail and book messaging, access appropriate information, and follow security and confidentiality rules. You need to demonstrate the skills to safely use patient care technologies and navigate electronic documentation systems.

Protected health information (PHI) is highly sensitive. *The Health Insurance Portability and Accountability Act (HIPAA)* is part of federal legislation that addresses actions for how PHI is used and disclosed. With the increased use of informatics and technology come new concerns on how to comply with HIPAA regulations and maintain a patient's privacy. New wireless technologies, increased use of e-mail and computer networking, and the ongoing threat of computer viruses increase the need for properly protecting a patient's privacy.

As a nurse, you have an obligation to ensure the privacy of your patient's health information. To do so, you need to understand your agency's policies regarding the use of technology. You need to know the rules regarding accessing patient records and releasing PHI, what to do if information is accidentally or intentionally released, and how to protect any passwords you use. If you are using social networking, you must be careful not to place any individually identifiable PHI online. Throughout this book, Informatics in Practice boxes offer suggestions on how to use informatics in your practice.

Electronic Health Records

The largest use of informatics is **electronic health records (EHRs)**, also called *electronic medical records.* An EHR is a computerized record of patient information. It is shared among all health care team members involved in a patient's care and moves with the patient—to other providers and across care settings. The ideal EHR provides a single place for team members to review and update a patient's health record, document care given, and enter patient care orders, including medications, procedures, diets, and diagnostic and laboratory tests (Fig. 1-6). The EHR should contain a patient's medical history, diagnoses, medications, treatment plans, immunization dates, allergies, and test results.[24]

With the ACA, an increase in EHR use is under way. EHRs have the potential to reduce medical errors associated with traditional paper records and improve clinical decision making, patient safety, and quality of care. Unfortunately, several obstacles remain in the way of fully implementing EHRs. Systems are expensive and technologically complex, requiring a number of resources to implement and maintain. In addition, communication is still lacking among computer systems and software

ETHICAL/LEGAL DILEMMAS

Social Networking: HIPAA Violation

Situation

You log into a closed group on a social networking site and read a posting from a fellow nursing student. The posting describes in detail the complex care the student provided to an older patient in a local hospital the previous day. The student comments on how stressful the day was and asks for advice on how to deal with similar patients in the future.

Ethical/Legal Points for Consideration

- Protecting and maintaining patient privacy and confidentiality are basic obligations defined in the Code of Ethics for Nurses, which nurses and nursing students should uphold.[1]
- As outlined in the Health Insurance Portability and Accountability Act (HIPAA), a patient's private health information is any information that relates to the person's past, present, or future physical or mental health. This includes not only specific details such as a patient's name or picture but also information that gives enough details that someone may be able to identify that person.
- You may unintentionally breach privacy or confidentiality by posting patient information (diagnosis, condition, or situation) on a social networking site. Using privacy settings or being in a closed group does not guarantee the secrecy of posted information. Others can copy and share any post without your knowledge.
- Potential consequences for improperly using social networking vary based on the situation. These may include (1) disciplinary action by the state board of nursing, (2) being disciplined, suspended, or fired by an employer, (3) dismissal from a nursing program, and (4) civil and/or criminal charges.
- A student nurse who experienced a stressful day and is looking for advice and support from peers (e.g., "Today my patient died. I wanted to cry.") could share the experience by clearly limiting the posts to the student's personal perspective and not sharing any identifying information. This is one area in which it is safest to err on the side of caution to avoid the appearance of impropriety.

Discussion Questions

1. How would you deal with the situation involving the fellow nursing student or a nursing colleague?
2. How would you handle a situation in which you observed a staff member who violated HIPAA?

Reference

1. Code of Ethics for Nurses: Retrieved from *www.nursingworld.org/MainMenuCategories/EthicsStandards/Ethics-Position-Statements.*

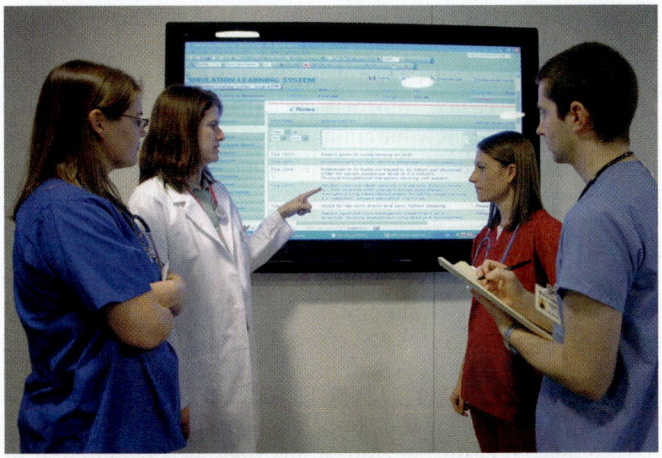

FIG. 1-6 Members of the interprofessional team review a patient's electronic health record. (From Arnold EC, Boggs KU: *Interpersonal relationships*, St Louis, 2011, Mosby.)

applications in use. Finally, patients must be assured of their privacy and that information is only accessed by those with a right to know.

EVIDENCE-BASED PRACTICE

Evidence-based practice (EBP) is a problem-solving approach to clinical decision making. Using the best available evidence (e.g., research findings, QI data), combined with your expertise and the patient's unique circumstances and preferences, leads to better clinical decisions and improved patient outcomes. EBP closes the gap between research and practice, providing more reliable and predictable care than that based on tradition, opinion, and trial and error.

EBP does not mean that you have to conduct a research study. Instead, EBP depends on you to take an active role in using the best available evidence when delivering care. You need to have an ongoing curiosity about what are the best nursing practices and routinely ask questions about your patient's care. Recognize when you need more information. When you base your practice on valid evidence, you are solving problems and supporting best patient outcomes.

Steps of EBP Process

The EBP process has six steps (Table 1-10).

Step 1. Step 1 is asking a clinical question in the PICOT format. Developing the clinical question is the most important step in the EBP process.[25] A good clinical question sets the context for integrating evidence, clinical judgment, and patient preferences. In addition, the question guides the literature search for the best evidence to influence practice.

An example of a clinical question in PICOT format is, "In adult abdominal surgery patients (**P** = patients/population) is splinting with an elasticized abdominal binder (**I** = intervention) or a pillow (**C** = comparison) more effective in reducing pain associated with ambulation (**O** = outcome) on the first postoperative day (**T** = time period)?" A properly stated clinical question may not have all components of PICOT. Some only include four components. The (T) timing or (C) comparison components are not appropriate for every question. The (C) component of PICOT may include a comparison with a specific intervention, the usual standard of care, or no intervention at all.

TABLE 1-10 Steps of Evidence-Based Practice (EBP) Process

1. Ask the clinical question using the **PICOT** format:
   Patients/population
   Intervention
   Comparison or comparison group
   Outcome(s)
   Time (as applicable)
2. Search for the best evidence based on the clinical question.
3. Critically appraise and synthesize the evidence.
4. Implement the evidence in practice.
5. Evaluate the practice decision or change.
6. Share the outcomes of the decision or change.

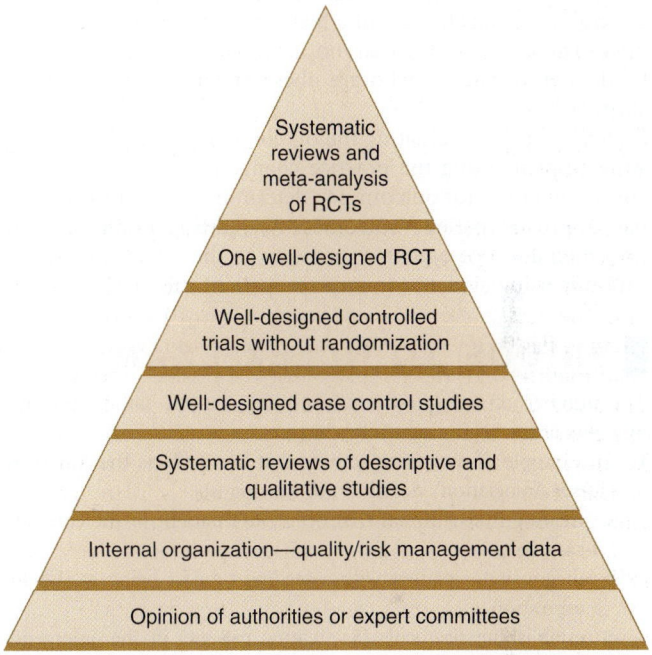

FIG. 1-7 Hierarchy of evidence. (Modified from Guyatt G, Rennie D: *User's guide to the medical literature*, Chicago, 2002, American Medical Association; Harris RP, et al: Current methods of the U.S. Prevention Services Task Force: a review of the process. *Am J Prevent Med* 20:21, 2001; Melnyk BM, Fineout-Overholt E: *Evidence-based practice in nursing and healthcare: a guide to best practice*, ed 3, Philadelphia, 2014, Lippincott Williams & Wilkins.)

Step 2. Step 2 is searching for the best evidence that applies to the clinical question. Technology provides you with ready access to data. You can easily search a number of online resources and collect large amounts of clinical information and evidence. It is important to evaluate all data sources for their credibility and reliability. Not all evidence is equal. Figure 1-7 presents the hierarchy of evidence. As you go down the pyramid, the strength of the evidence becomes weaker. Systematic reviews and evidence-based clinical practice guidelines save time and effort in the EBP process. However, they are available for only a limited number of clinical topics and may not suit all types of clinical questions. When insufficient research exists to guide practice, recommendations from expert panels and authority figures may be the best evidence available.

Step 3. Step 3 is critically appraising and synthesizing evidence found in the search. A successful critical appraisal process focuses on three essential questions: (1) What are the results? (2) Are the results reliable and valid? and (3) Will the results help me in caring for my patients? You must determine the strength of the evidence and synthesize the findings related to the clinical question to conclude what is the best practice. For example, you find strong evidence supporting effectiveness of elasticized binders and pillows in reducing pain associated with ambulation. However, the binder appears to be more effective if the patient is obese or has had prior abdominal surgery.

Step 4. Step 4 involves implementing the evidence in practice. The decision to implement change is made by combining the evidence, clinical judgment, and the preferences and values of patients and caregivers. You may be part of an interprofessional team charged with implementing a practice change or applying evidence in a specific patient care situation. This may include developing clinical practice guidelines; policies and procedures; or new assessment, teaching, or documentation tools. For example, you may be part of a team implementing a new postoperative protocol focused on using elasticized abdominal binders with patients who are obese or had prior abdominal surgery.

Step 5. Step 5 is evaluating the outcome in the clinical setting. After implementing the practice change for a specific period, you should monitor outcomes to determine whether the change has improved patient outcomes. Accrediting bodies require documentation of outcome measures to show that the organization is using evidence to improve patient care.[25]

Step 6. Step 6 is sharing the results of the EBP change. If you do not share the outcomes of EBP, then other health care providers and patients cannot benefit from what you learned from your experience. Information is shared locally using unit- or hospital-based newsletters and posters and regionally and nationally through journal publications and presentations at conferences.

Implementing EBP

To implement EBP, you must develop the skills to be able to seek and incorporate into practice scientific evidence that supports best patient outcomes. Throughout this book, two different types of EBP boxes are used to show how EBP is used in nursing practice. The Translating Research into Practice boxes provide initial answers to specific clinical questions. These boxes contain the clinical question, critical appraisal of the supportive evidence, implications for nursing practice, and the source of the evidence. Applying the Evidence boxes provide an opportunity for you to practice your critical thinking skills in applying EBP to patient scenarios. To assist you in identifying the use of evidence incorporated throughout this book, an asterisk (*) is used in the reference list at the end of each chapter to indicate evidence-based information for clinical practice.

BRIDGE TO NCLEX EXAMINATION

The number of the question corresponds to the same-numbered outcome at the beginning of the chapter.

1. An example of a nursing activity that best reflects the American Nurses Association's definition of nursing is
   a. treating dysrhythmias that occur in a patient in the coronary care unit.
   b. diagnosing a patient with a feeding tube as being at risk for aspiration.
   c. establishing protocols for treating patients in the emergency department.
   d. providing antianxiety drugs for a patient who has disturbed sleep patterns.
2. A nurse working on the medical-surgical unit at an urban hospital would like to become certified in medical-surgical nursing. The nurse knows that this process would most likely require
   a. a bachelor's degree in nursing.
   b. formal education in advanced nursing practice.
   c. experience for a specific period in medical-surgical nursing.
   d. membership in a medical-surgical nursing specialty organization.
3. A nurse is providing care to a patient after right hip surgery. Within a pay-for-performance system, a critical role of the nurse is to
   a. ensure that care is provided using a minimal amount of supplies.
   b. discharge the patient at completion of the number of approved days of care.
   c. implement measures to decrease the risk of the patient acquiring an infection.
   d. assess the patient's ability to pay for health care services at the time of admission.
4. The nurse is assigned to care for a newly admitted patient. Number in order the steps for using the nursing process to prioritize care. (Number 1 is the first step, and number 5 is the last step.)
   ___ Evaluate whether the plan was effective.
   ___ Identify any health problems.
   ___ Collect patient information.
   ___ Carry out the plan.
   ___ Determine a plan of action.
5. The linkages among NANDA-I nursing diagnoses, NOC patient outcomes, and NIC nursing interventions can be used to
   a. evaluate patient outcomes.
   b. provide guides for planning care.
   c. predict the results of nursing care.
   d. shorten written care plans for individual patients.
6. The nurse is caring for a diabetic patient in the ambulatory surgical unit who has undergone debridement of an infected toe. Which task is appropriate for the nurse to delegate to unlicensed assistive personnel (UAP)?
   a. Check the patient's vital signs.
   b. Monitor the patient's pain level.
   c. Assess the patient's IV catheter site.
   d. Evaluate the patient's tibial and pedal pulses.
7. The nurse's role in addressing the National Patient Safety Goals established by The Joint Commission includes *(select all that apply)*
   a. answering monitoring alarms in a timely manner.
   b. using side rails and alarm systems as necessary to prevent patient falls.
   c. obtaining a complete, accurate list of the patient's medications on admission.
   d. memorizing and implementing all the rules published by The Joint Commission.
   e. encouraging patients to be actively involved in and question their own health care.

8. Advantages of using informatics in health care delivery are *(select all that apply)*
   a. reduced need for nurses in acute care.
   b. increased patient anonymity and confidentiality.
   c. the ability to achieve and maintain high standards of care.
   d. access to standard plans of care for many health problems.
   e. improved communication of the patient's health status to the health care team.
9. When using evidence-based practice, the nurse
   a. must use clinical practice guidelines developed by national health agencies.
   b. should use findings from randomized controlled trials to plan care for all patient problems.
   c. uses clinical decision making and judgment to determine what evidence is appropriate for a specific clinical situation.
   d. statistically analyzes the relationship of nursing interventions to patient outcomes to establish evidence for the most appropriate patient interventions.

1. b, 2. c, 3. c, 4. 5, 2, 1, 4, 3, 5. b, 6. a, 7. a, b, c, 8. c, d, e, 9. c.

For rationales to these answers and even more NCLEX review questions, visit *evolve.elsevier.com/Lewis/medsurg*

EVOLVE WEBSITE

http://evolve.elsevier.com/Lewis/medsurg

Review Questions (Online Only)
Key Points
Answer Key for Questions
- Rationales for Bridge to NCLEX Examination Questions

Conceptual Care Map Creator
Audio Glossary
Content Updates

REFERENCES

1. American Nurses Association: *Nursing: a social policy statement,* ed 3, Washington DC, 2010, The Association. (Classic)
2. Nightingale F: *Notes on nursing: what it is and what it is not* (facsimile edition), Philadelphia, 1946, Lippincott. (Classic)
3. Henderson V: *The nature of nursing,* New York, 1966, Macmillan. (Classic)
4. Roy S, Andrews H: *The Roy adaptation model,* ed 2, Stamford, Conn, 1999, Appleton & Lange. (Classic)
5. American Association of Colleges of Nursing: Essentials of baccalaureate education for professional nursing practice. Retrieved from *www.aacn.nche.edu.*
6. American Nurses Credentialing Center: Certification. Retrieved from *www.nursecredentialing.org/certification.aspx.*
7. Robert Wood Johnson Foundation: Achieving the potential of health care performance measures. Retrieved from *www.rwjf.org.*
8. US Department of Health and Human Services: *Healthy People 2020.* Retrieved from *www.healthypeople.gov.*
9. ANCC Magnet Recognition Program. Retrieved from *www.nursecredentialing.org/magnet.aspx.*
10. Committee on the Robert Wood Johnson Foundation Initiative on the Future of Nursing at the Institute of Medicine: *The future of nursing: leading change, advancing health,* Washington, DC, 2011, National Academies Press.
11. QSEN Institute. Retrieved from *http://qsen.org.*
12. NANDA International: Defining the knowledge of nursing. Retrieved from *www.nanda.org.*
13. Overview: Nursing Outcomes Classification (NOC). Retrieved from *www.nursing.uiowa.edu/cncce/nursing-outcomes-classification-overview.*
14. Overview: Nursing Interventions Classification (NIC). Retrieved from *www.nursing.uiowa.edu/cncce/nursing-interventions-classification-overview.*
15. Carpenito LJ: *Nursing care plans: transitional patient and family-centered care,* ed 6, Philadelphia, 2014, Lippincott Williams & Wilkins.
16. Transitions of care portal. Retrieved from *www.jointcommission.org/toc.aspx.*
17. Cherry B, Jacob SR: *Contemporary nursing practice,* ed 6, St Louis, 2013, Elsevier.
18. What is a case manager? Retrieved from *www.cmsa.org.*
19. Alfaro-LeFevre R: *Critical thinking, clinical reasoning, and clinical judgment,* ed 5, St Louis, 2013, Saunders.
20. Delegation. Retrieved from *www.ncsbn.org/1625.htm.*
21. James J: A new, evidence-based estimate of patient harms associated with hospital care, *Journal of Patient Safety* 9:122, 2013.
22. Safe practices for better healthcare. Retrieved from *www.qualityforum.org/Projects/Safe_Practices_2010.aspx.*
23. National Patient Safety Goals. Retrieved from *www.jointcommission.org/standards_information/npsgs.aspx.*
24. Benefits of EHRs. Retrieved from *www.healthit.gov/providers-professionals.*
25. Echevarria IM, Walker S: To make your case, start with a PICOT question, *Nursing* 44:18, 2014.

2

Health Disparities and Culturally Competent Care

Janet Lenart

No culture can live if it attempts to be exclusive.

Mahatma Gandhi

http://evolve.elsevier.com/Lewis/medsurg/

LEARNING OUTCOMES

1. Identify the key determinants of health and equity.
2. Describe the factors that contribute to health disparities and health equity.
3. Define the terms *culture, values, acculturation, ethnicity, race, stereotyping, ethnocentrism, cultural imposition, cultural competency,* and *culture-bound syndrome.*
4. Explain how culture and ethnicity may affect a person's physical and psychologic health.
5. Describe strategies for successfully communicating with a person who speaks a language that you do not understand.
6. Apply strategies for incorporating cultural information in the nursing process with all patients.
7. Describe the role of nursing in reducing health disparities.
8. Examine ways that your own cultural background may influence nursing care.

KEY TERMS

acculturation, p. 22
cultural competence, p. 23
culture, p. 21
culture-bound syndromes, p. 29
determinants of health, p. 18
ethnicity, p. 19
ethnocentrism, p. 23
folk healers, p. 24
health disparities, p. 19
health equity, p. 19
health status, p. 18
lesbian, gay, bisexual, and transgender (LGBT), p. 21
place, p. 20
race, p. 19
sexuality, p. 21
stereotyping, p. 23
transcultural nursing, p. 23
values, p. 21

This chapter discusses health disparities and culture. Nurses play a key role in recognizing and reducing health disparities and providing culturally competent care.

DETERMINANTS OF HEALTH

Why are there differences in the health status of people in America? How do these differences occur? The **determinants of health** are factors that (1) influence the health of individuals and groups and (2) help explain why some people experience poorer health than others.[1] Where people are born, grow up, live, work, and age helps determine their health status, behaviors, and care.

Health status describes the health of a person or a community.[2] Many measures make up the concept of health status. For individuals, this means the sum of their current health problems plus their coping resources (e.g., family, financial resources). For a community, health status is the combination of health measures for all individuals living in the community. Community health measures include birth and death rates, life expectancy, access to care, and morbidity and mortality rates related to disease and injury.

Factors in a person's social and physical environment, including personal relationships, workplace, housing, transportation, and neighborhood violence, contribute to health status.[1] For example, the risk of youth homicide is much higher in neighborhoods with gang activity and high crime rates. The physical environment in which one lives, works, and plays may expose a person to such risks as environmental hazards (workplace injuries), toxic agents (chemical spills, industrial pollution), unsafe traffic patterns (lack of sidewalks), or absence of fresh and healthy food choices.

An individual's behavior is influenced by his or her environment, education, and economic status. Behaviors such as tobacco and illicit drug use are strongly linked to a number of health conditions (e.g., lung cancer, liver disease). An individual's biologic makeup, such as genetics and family history of disease (e.g., heart disease), can increase the risk for specific diseases.

Reviewed by Christine Espina, RN, DNP, Nurse Planner and Continuing Education Specialist, University of Washington Continuing Nursing Education, Seattle, Washington; Shari Gould, RN, MSN, Associate Professor of Nursing, Victoria College, Victoria, Texas; and Ellen Odell, DNP, ACNS-BC, CNE, APRN, Director of Nursing, Associate Professor, Department of Nursing, John Brown University, Siloam Springs, Arkansas.

The availability of health care also contributes to an individual's health. The Affordable Care Act (ACA) reduced the number of uninsured Americans by 5.4 million in the first year of implementation. However, millions remain uninsured and have limited access to care, which will affect both individual and community health.[3]

HEALTH DISPARITIES AND HEALTH EQUITY

Health disparities are differences in the incidence, prevalence, mortality rate, and burden of diseases that exist among specific population groups in the United States because of social, economic, or environmental disadvantages. Health disparities can affect population groups based on gender, age, ethnicity, socioeconomic status, education, geography, sexual orientation, disability, or special health care needs.[4] **Health equity** is achieved when every person has the opportunity to attain his or her health potential, and no one is disadvantaged.

Factors and Conditions Leading to Health Disparities

Many factors and conditions can lead to the development of health disparities (Table 2-1). Awareness of these factors will assist you in providing optimal care for your patients.

ETHICAL/LEGAL DILEMMAS

Health Disparities

Situation

E.M., a 47-year-old Mexican American woman with type 2 diabetes mellitus, comes to the clinic to have her blood glucose measured. It has been 12 months since her last visit. At that time the nurse requested that she bring along her glucometer and strips to demonstrate how she checks her blood glucose because her glucose values were high at her previous visits.

When you check E.M.'s equipment and glucose strips, it is clear that the strips are for a different machine and they expired more than 2 years ago. When you inquire about the situation, E.M. explains that she cannot afford to come to the clinic or to buy new equipment and supplies to check her blood glucose level. During the day E.M. cares for her three grandchildren so her daughter can work. E.M. spends most of her income on food for her family, so little money is left over for her own health care.

Ethical/Legal Points for Consideration

- Ethnic minorities and other vulnerable or disadvantaged groups experience certain chronic illnesses at higher rates. Limited access to high-quality, accessible, and affordable health care services is clearly associated with an increased incidence of illness and complications, as well as a reduced life span.
- People with certain health problems such as diabetes may have difficulty obtaining health care insurance. These issues must be considered in the broader context of social justice.
- In many states the legal definition of the role of the professional nurse includes patient advocacy. Advocacy includes the obligation to provide adequate follow-up care for all patients, especially those who are experiencing health care disparities.
- When disparities are observed in an individual patient and family, as a nurse you must consider the possibilities of discrimination and abuse. Professional nurses are legally and ethically responsible for patient advocacy. When failure to fulfill this obligation results in harm to the patient, the nurse may incur legal liability.

Discussion Questions

1. How would you work with E.M. to help her obtain the necessary resources and knowledge to care for her diabetes?
2. What can you do to begin working on the problems of health disparities in your community?

TABLE 2-1 Factors and Conditions Leading to Health Disparities

- Ethnicity and race
- Place
- Income status
- Education
- Occupation or unemployment
- Health literacy
- Gender
- Age
- Sexual orientation
- Disability status
- Health care provider attitudes
- Lack of health care services access
- Language barrier

Ethnicity and Race. The terms **ethnicity** and **race** are subjective and based on self-report. These terms are used interchangeably in conversation and cannot be defined by genetic markers. Social context and lived experiences influence people's decision about the ethnic and race category to which they identify or are assigned. For example, ethnic and race categories may differ on a person's birth certificate and death certificate.

People are asked to identify their own ethnicity and race for the purpose of health data collection (e.g., for birth and death certificates). Collection of health data based on self-reported ethnic and race categories is important for research, to inform policy, and to understand and eliminate disparities. For example, federal agencies are required to list a minimum of two ethnicities for people who self-identify as either *Hispanic or Latino* and *Not Hispanic or Latino.* A Hispanic or Latino is typically a person of Cuban, Mexican, Puerto Rican, South or Central American, or other Spanish descent, regardless of race.

In addition, federal agencies are required to list a minimum of five race categories: white, black or African American, American Indian or Alaska Native, Asian, and Native Hawaiian or other Pacific Islander. People are asked to identify their race using one or more categories. In this book the terms *ethnicity* and *race* are used interchangeably or together.

Despite dramatic improvements in treatments to prolong life and improve quality of life for most individuals, racial and ethnic minorities have benefited far less from these advances. Disparities are generally determined by comparing population groups. In the United States minority groups include Hispanics/Latinos 16.3%, African Americans 12.6%, Asian Americans 4.8%, Native Hawaiians and other Pacific Islanders 0.2%, Native Americans and Native Alaskans 0.9%, and two or more races 2.9% of the U.S. population.[5] The percentages for most of these groups are expected to increase in the coming decades.

Obesity and chronic illness rates for diabetes, hypertension, chronic obstructive pulmonary diseases, cancer, and stroke are higher among minority people. Racial, ethnic, and cultural differences exist in health services, treatments provided, and access to health care providers (HCPs). For example, African American men are less likely to be offered intervention procedures for cardiovascular disease and stroke. African American and Hispanic women are less likely to have mammography for breast cancer screening. Differences in access to screening and treatment exist even when minority groups are insured at the same level as whites. When patient groups are given the same care, the treatment outcomes are similar across racial and ethnic groups.[6]

Disease risk and outcomes are also influenced by race and ethnicity. For example, compared with U.S. white and African American populations, Native Americans have a higher incidence of stroke and are more likely to die as a consequence.[7] Cervical cancer mortality rates are higher in Hispanic and

CULTURAL & ETHNIC HEALTH DISPARITIES

Cultural & Ethnic Health Disparities Boxes Throughout Book

Title	Chapter	Page
Alzheimer's Disease and Dementia	59	1402
Arthritis and Connective Tissue Disorders	64	1525
Brain Tumors	56	1333
Breast Cancer	51	1218
Cancer	15	267
Cancers of the Female Reproductive System	53	1256
Cancers of the Male Reproductive System	54	1276
Chronic Kidney Disease	46	1076
Colorectal Cancer	42	954
Coronary Artery Disease	33	704
Diabetes Mellitus	48	1137
Heart Failure	34	738
Hematologic Problems	30	607
Hypertension	32	682
Integumentary Problems	23	410
Liver, Pancreas, and Gallbladder Disorders	43	986
Lung Cancer	27	514
Obesity	40	878
Obstructive Pulmonary Diseases	28	539
Oral, Pharyngeal, and Esophageal Problems	41	898
Osteoporosis	63	1511
Sexually Transmitted Infections	52	1228
Stroke	57	1347
Tuberculosis	27	506
Urologic Disorders	45	1034
Visual and Auditory Problems	21	368

African American women than in other American women. Numerous strategies are being developed to promote health equity and reduce disparities.

Place. Place refers to the geographic and environmental location where a person is born, grows, lives, works, and ages. Place affects the use of health services, health status, and health behaviors.

Approximately 25% of Americans live in nonurban or rural areas.[5] Three percent of Americans live in designated frontier counties. Differences in access to health care services among frontier, rural, and urban settings can create geographic health disparities. For example, rural populations and Native Americans living on reservations may need to travel long distances to receive health care. This can result in inadequate or less-frequent access to health care services. Some parts of the rural United States are considered "medically underserved" because of decreased numbers of health care providers per population.

People living in rural areas have higher rates of cancer, heart disease, diabetes, depression, and injury-related deaths than people living in urban areas. For example, in rural Appalachia the rates of lung, colon, cervical, and colorectal cancer are higher than the national average. Rural populations tend to be older than urban populations. Many rural areas have higher rates of obesity and chronic disease. The impact of social and physical environment on health choices can be illustrated by the problem of intimate partner violence in rural communities.[8] The decision to seek help is affected by geographic isolation, traditional gender roles, patriarchal attitudes, fear of lack of confidentiality, and economic factors that exist in some small rural communities.

Living in urban centers may also predispose a person to health disparities. Concerns about personal safety (e.g., clinics located in high-crime neighborhoods) can make patients reluctant to visit HCPs. At the same time, providers, such as home health nurses, working in high-risk areas may experience distress when they witness crime, drug use, or other illegal activities.

Among the most obvious health behaviors affected by place are physical activity and nutrition. Safe, walkable neighborhoods with playgrounds and sources of healthy foods promote physical activity and healthy eating. Social support and networks are related to health and coping with illness. Social networks are more likely to be found in communities where neighbors interact and rely on one another.

Income, Education, and Occupation. People of lower income, education, or occupational status experience worse health. In addition, they die at a younger age than those who are more affluent. Adults without a high school diploma or equivalent are three times more likely to die before age 65 than those with a college degree. Health care costs are one of the important factors that contribute to health disparities. Individuals who have no insurance, are underinsured, or lack financial resources to pay for treatment of diseases may forgo health care visits, screenings, and treatments. Patients who lack the knowledge and/or access to apply for government assistance programs (e.g., Medicaid) are also at risk. Hazardous work environments and high-risk occupations of laborers also increase health risk and contribute to higher rates of illness, injury, and death.

Health Literacy. *Health literacy* is defined as the degree to which individuals have the capacity to obtain, process, and understand basic health information and services needed to make appropriate health decisions. This includes the ability to (1) read, comprehend, and analyze information; (2) understand instructions; (3) weigh risks and benefits; and (4) ultimately make decisions and take action. The most recent national literacy survey reported that more than 40% and two thirds of people over age 60 have basic to below basic literacy skills, and another 5% are nonliterate in English.[9] Low health literacy is associated with more hospitalizations, greater use of emergency department care, decreased use of cancer screening and influenza vaccine, decreased ability to use medications correctly, and higher mortality rates among older adults.

On a daily basis, patients need to self-manage conditions such as diabetes and asthma. For example, patients with diabetes may not be able to maintain adequate blood glucose levels if they cannot read or understand the numbers on the home glucose monitoring system. The inability to read and understand medication labels can result in taking medications at the wrong time or in the wrong dose. Health literacy is discussed further in Chapter 4.

Gender. Health disparities exist between men and women. Adult women use health care services more than men. Women may not receive the same quality of care (Fig. 2-1). For example, women are less likely than men to receive procedures (e.g., coronary angiography) for cardiovascular disease.[10] When gender is combined with racial and ethnic differences, the disparities are even greater. (Gender Differences boxes are presented throughout this book, which highlight gender differences in disease risk, manifestations, and treatment.)

Age. Older adults are at risk for experiencing health disparities in the number of diagnostic tests performed and aggressiveness of treatments used. Biases toward older adults that affect their care, or ageism, are discussed in Chapter 5. Older women are less likely to be offered mammograms. Older people of low

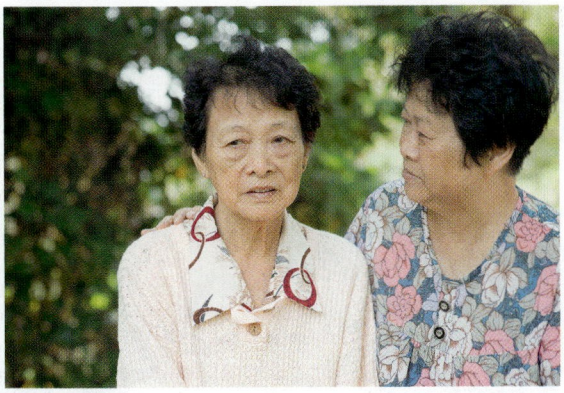

FIG. 2-1 Older Asian women are especially at risk for health disparities. (©szefei/iStock/Thinkstock)

socioeconomic status experience greater disability, more limitations in activities of daily living, and more frequent and rapid cognitive decline. Older adults who belong to minority groups are less likely than their white counterparts to receive screening for prostate and colorectal cancer.

Sexual Orientation. Sexuality is defined as a person's romantic, emotional, or sexual attraction to another person.

Lesbian, Gay, Bisexual, and Transgender (LGBT). Lesbian, gay, bisexual, and transgender (LGBT) is a term that refers to the sexual orientation of these groups of people. LGBT individuals encompass all races and ethnicities, religions, and social classes. Being LGBT places an individual at risk for health disparities resulting from social, economic, or environmental disadvantages. Personal, family, and social acceptance of sexual orientation and gender identity affects the mental health and personal safety of LGBT individuals. Discrimination against LGBT people has been associated with high rates of psychiatric disorders, substance abuse, and suicide.[2]

Lesbian women are more likely to be obese when compared with their heterosexual counterparts. Lesbian and bisexual women have increased risk factors for cardiovascular disease.[11] Gay men have higher rates of human immunodeficiency virus and hepatitis infections than other groups. Gay men and lesbian women have higher smoking rates than heterosexuals.

Older LGBT individuals may face additional barriers to health because of isolation and a lack of social services and culturally competent providers.[2]

Understanding the cause of these disparities among LGBT individuals is essential to providing safe and high-quality care. One of the barriers to accessing high-quality health care by LGBT adults is the current lack of HCPs who are knowledgeable about their health needs. LGBT people may also experience fear of discrimination in health care settings.

Some health care settings are addressing the negative stereotypes that health care professionals may have, but of which they may not be aware. The Joint Commission (TJC) requires that patients be allowed the presence of a support individual of their choice. In addition, hospitals must adopt policies that bar discrimination based on factors such as sexual orientation and gender identification and expression.

Health Care Provider Attitudes. Certain behaviors and biases of the HCP can contribute to health disparities. Factors such as bias and prejudice can affect health care–seeking behavior in minority populations.[12] The health care system may also contribute to the problem of health disparities. For example, a clinic located in an area with a large population of Vietnamese immigrants that does not provide interpreters or educational materials and financial forms in Vietnamese may limit these families' ability to understand how to access health care.

Discrimination and *bias* based on a patient's race, ethnicity, gender, age, body size, sexual orientation, or ability to pay are likely to result in less aggressive or negative treatment practices. Discrimination can result in the delay of a proper diagnosis due to assumptions made about the patient. Sometimes discrimination is difficult to identify, especially when it occurs at the institutional level.

Because an HCP's overt discriminatory behavior may not be immediately evident to the patient or yourself, it may be difficult to confront. Even well-intentioned providers who try to eliminate bias in their care can demonstrate their prior beliefs or prejudices through nonverbal communication. Many policies are in place to eliminate discrimination, but it still exists.[12]

HEALTHY PEOPLE

Lesbian, Gay, Bisexual, and Transgender (LGBT) Individuals

A *Healthy People 2020* goal is to improve the health, safety, and well-being of LGBT individuals.

- Efforts to improve LGBT health include the following:
  - Decreasing human immunodeficiency virus (HIV)/sexually transmitted infections (STI) with effective interventions
  - Implementing antibullying policies in schools
  - Creating advisory groups consisting of community representatives
  - Providing supportive social services to reduce suicide and homelessness risk among young people
  - Appropriately inquiring about and being supportive of a patient's sexual orientation to enhance the patient-provider interaction and patient's regular use of care
  - Providing health care professional students with access to LGBT patients to increase their knowledge of the health care needs of LGBT patients and ability to provide care to them
- Efforts to address health disparities among LGBT people include the following:
  - Expansion of domestic partner health insurance coverage
  - Establishment of LGBT health centers
  - Dissemination of effective HIV/STI interventions
  - Guarantee of appropriate health care screening

CULTURE

Culture is a way of life for a group of people. It includes the behaviors, beliefs, values, traditions, and symbols that the group accepts, generally without thinking about them. This way of life is passed along by communication and imitation from one generation to the next. You can also think of culture as cultivated behavior that is acquired through social learning. It is the totality of a person's learned, accumulated experience that is socially transmitted. The four classic characteristics of culture are described in Table 2-2.

Values are the sets of rules by which individuals, families, groups, and communities live. They are the principles and standards that serve as the basis for beliefs, attitudes, and behaviors. Although all cultures have values, the types and expressions of those values differ from one culture to another. These cultural values develop over time, guide decision making and actions, and may affect a person's self-esteem. Cultural values are often unconsciously developed early in life as a child learns about acceptable and unacceptable behaviors. The extent to which a person's cultural values are internalized influences that person's

TABLE 2-2 Basic Characteristics of Culture

- *Dynamic* and ever-changing
- *Not always shared* by all members of a cultural group
- *Adapted* to specific conditions such as environmental factors
- *Learned* through oral and written histories, as well as socialization

TABLE 2-3 Cultural Characteristics of Different Ethnic Groups

Native American
- Doing the honorable thing
- Folk healing
- Living in harmony with people and nature
- Respect for tribal elders and children
- Respect for all things living
- Returning what is taken from nature
- Spiritual guidance

Hispanic/Latino
- Cultural foods
- Folk healing
- Extended family valued
- Interdependence and collectivism
- Involvement of family in social activities
- Religion and spirituality highly valued
- Respect for elders and authority

African American
- Cultural foods
- Family networks
- Folk healing
- Importance of religion
- Interdependence within ethnic group
- Music and physical activities valued

European American
- Equal rights of genders
- Independence and freedom
- Individualistic and competitive
- Materialistic
- Self-reliance valued
- Youth and beauty valued

Asian American
- Cultural foods
- Family loyalty
- Folk healing
- Harmonious relationships
- Harmony and balance within body vital for preservation of life energy
- Respect for elders
- Respect for one's parents and ancestors

Pacific Islander American
- Collective concern and involvement
- Kinship alliance among nuclear and extended family
- Knowledge is collective; belongs to group, not individual
- Natural order and balanced relationships

Adapted from Andrews MM, Boyle JS: *Transcultural concepts in nursing care*, ed 6, Philadelphia, 2012, Lippincott Williams & Wilkins; and Giger JN, Davidhizar RE: *Transcultural nursing: assessment and intervention*, ed 6, St Louis, 2012, Mosby.

tendency toward judging other cultures, while usually using his or her own culture as the accepted standard. Table 2-3 provides some examples of cultural characteristics of different ethnic groups in the United States.[13]

Although individuals within a cultural group may have many similarities through their shared values, beliefs, and practices, there is also diversity within groups (Fig. 2-2). Each person is culturally unique. Such diversity may result from different perspectives and interpretations of situations. These differences may be based on age, gender, marital status, family structure, income, education level, religious views, and life experiences. Within any cultural group, there are smaller groups that may not hold all of the values of the dominant culture. These smaller cultural groups have experiences that differ from those of the dominant group. These differences may be related to ethnic background, residence, religion, occupation, health, age, gender, education, or other factors that unite the group. Members of a subculture share certain aspects of culture that are different from those of the overall cultural group. For example, among

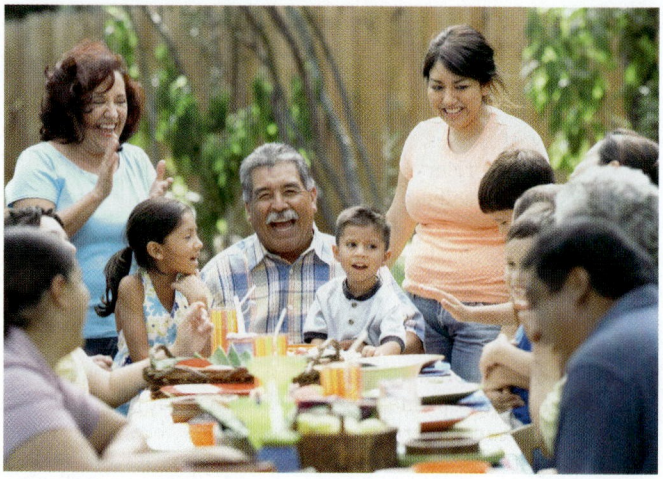

FIG. 2-2 Members of this family share a common heritage. (©Jack Hollingsworth/Photodisc/Thinkstock)

Hispanics some seek professional health care immediately when symptoms appear, whereas other Hispanics rely first on folk healers. Other Hispanics first seek the opinion of family and friends before seeking formal health care.

Cultural beliefs about symptom tolerance and health care–seeking behavior can contribute to health disparities. Some cultures consider pain something to be endured or ignored, and as a result, the patient does not seek help. Some cultures may view diseases or problems fatalistically; that is, people see no reason to seek treatment because they believe it is unlikely to have any benefit. Some cultures view the signs and symptoms of an illness as "God's will" or as a punishment for some prior behavior.

Fatalism is higher in individuals with lower socioeconomic status. Fatalistic beliefs are associated with reduced cancer prevention activities such as exercising, not smoking, and following a healthy diet.[14] In some cultures it may not be acceptable to see an HCP who is not of the same gender or ethnic group. Such beliefs can result in delays in seeking health care or inadequate treatment.

Acculturation is the lifelong process of incorporating cultural aspects of the contexts in which a person grows, lives, works, and ages.[15] Acculturation is often bidirectional. In other words, the context also changes as it is influenced by a person's culture. Change may be in attitudes, behaviors, and values. For example, a sedentary person who loves to cook may change his or her attitude toward exercise when living with athletic roommates, who in turn also change as they begin to appreciate cooking. Behaviors change when an immigrant child learns the local language while also influencing the conduct of classmates. Last, a deeply held value such as self-sufficiency may change for a person exposed to a culture in which reliance on others dominates.

Newcomers may adopt both the strengths and limitations of the dominant culture. This is relevant when considering health behaviors of individuals and the quality of health care delivered by professionals. For example, an immigrant may be negatively influenced by a dominant cultural context in which unhealthy eating habits prevail.[16] As a new nurse, you may be negatively or positively influenced by the culture of care that is most prevalent in your workplace.

The result of acculturation for the individual may be new cultural variations in attitudes, behaviors, and values. All people participate in this process over their lives. People who move to a new cultural context are more aware of the acculturation experience than people who are not exposed to new experiences. Exposure to new cultural contexts increases the cultural competency of nurses.

Stereotyping refers to an overgeneralized viewpoint that members of a specific culture, race, or ethnic group are alike and share the same values and beliefs. This oversimplified approach does not take into account the individual differences that exist within a culture. Being a member of a particular cultural, ethnic, or racial group does not make the person an expert on other members of that same group. Such stereotyping can lead to false assumptions and affect a patient's care. For example, it would be inappropriate for you to assume that just because a nurse is Mexican American, he would know how a Mexican American patient's beliefs may affect that patient's health care practices. As another example, a young Mexican American nurse born and raised in a large city has experienced a different culture than the older patient who was born and raised in a rural area of Mexico.

Ethnocentrism refers to the belief that one's own culture and worldview are superior to those of others from different cultural, ethnic, or racial backgrounds. Comparing others' ways to your own can lead to seeing others as different or inferior. HCPs' ethnocentrism can result in poor communication, patient alienation, and potentially inadequate treatment. To avoid ethnocentrism, you need to remain open to a variety of perspectives and maintain a nonjudgmental view of the values, beliefs, and practices of others. Failure to do this can result in ethnic stereotyping or cultural imposition.

Cultural imposition occurs when one's own cultural beliefs and practices are imposed on another person or group of people. In health care it can result in disregarding or trivializing a patient's health care beliefs or practices. Cultural imposition may happen when an HCP is unaware of the patient's cultural beliefs and plans and implements care without taking them into account.[17]

Cultural safety describes care and advocacy for a person of another culture determined by that person or family. Care that is culturally safe prevents cultural imposition. Culturally safe practice requires cultural competency and action to ensure that cultural histories, experiences, and traditions of patients, their families, and communities are valued and shape health care approaches and policies.[18]

The term **transcultural nursing** was coined by Madeleine Leininger in the 1950s. Transcultural nursing is a specialty that focuses on the comparative study and analysis of cultures and subcultures. The goal of transcultural nursing is the discovery of culturally relevant facts that can guide the nurse in providing culturally appropriate care.[19]

CULTURAL COMPETENCE

Cultural competence is the ability to understand, appreciate, and work with individuals from cultures other than your own. It involves an awareness and acceptance of cultural differences, self-awareness, knowledge of the patient's culture, and adaptation of skills to meet the patient's needs. The four components of cultural competence are (1) cultural awareness, (2) cultural knowledge, (3) cultural skill, and (4) cultural encounter[20] (Table 2-4).

Specific information is presented throughout this book to assist you in developing an awareness of cultural differences and learning assessment skills for different cultural groups. Table 2-7 (later in this chapter) presents a cultural assessment guide. It may be helpful to review general cultural characteristics associated with a cultural group when preparing to interview a patient. However, recognize that the patient may not identify with the assumed cultural group, and the provider's own biases and stereotypes may impact the patient and result in more patient-provider barriers.

Providing culturally competent care may increase patient satisfaction, reduce health disparities, increase patient safety,

TABLE 2-4 How to Develop Cultural Competence

Description	Role of Nurse
Cultural Awareness	
• Ability to understand patients' unique cultural needs	• Identify your own cultural background, values, and beliefs, especially as related to health and health care. • Examine your own cultural biases toward people whose cultures differ from your own culture.
Cultural Knowledge	
• Process of learning key aspects of a group's culture, especially as it relates to health and health care practices • Patients are best source of information about their culture	• Learn basic general information about predominant cultural groups in your geographic area. Cultural pocket guides can be a good resource. • Assess patients for presence or absence of cultural traits based on an understanding of generalizations about a cultural group. • Do not make assumptions based on cultural background because the degree of acculturation varies among individuals. • Read research studies that describe cultural differences. • Read ethnic newspaper articles and books. • View documentaries about cultural groups.
Cultural Skill	
• Ability to collect relevant cultural data • Performance of a cultural assessment	• Be alert for unexpected responses with patients, especially as related to cultural issues. • Become aware of cultural differences in predominant ethnic groups. • Develop assessment skills to do a competent cultural assessment for any patient.* • Learn assessment skills for different cultural groups, including cultural beliefs and practices.
Cultural Encounter	
• Direct cross-cultural interactions between people from culturally diverse backgrounds • Extended contact with a cultural group to enhance understanding of its values and beliefs	• Create opportunities to interact with predominant cultural groups. • Attend cultural events, such as religious ceremonies, significant life passage rituals, social events, and demonstrations of cultural practices. • Visit markets and restaurants in ethnic neighborhoods. • Explore ethnic neighborhoods, listen to different types of ethnic music, and learn games of various ethnic groups. • Visit or volunteer at health fairs in local ethnic neighborhoods. • Learn about prominent cultural beliefs and practices, and incorporate this knowledge into planning nursing care.

*See Table 2-7 later in the chapter.

and prevent misunderstandings between you and your patients. It also involves integrating cultural practices into Western medicine. For example, before some diagnostic procedures and interventions, it is typical to have patients remove personal objects that are worn on the body. Ask patients whether they wear personal objects and the significance of their removal, since they may have cultural or spiritual significance. You also should know whether wearing these objects will compromise patient safety, test results, or outcomes of the intervention.

CULTURAL DIVERSITY IN THE HEALTH CARE WORKPLACE

Poorer health outcomes for minorities are linked to the shortage of culturally and ethnically diverse HCPs, who have historically been underrepresented in the health professions. A diversity gap exists between the ethnic composition of the interprofessional health care team and the overall population in the United States (Fig. 2-3). For example, the diversity of nurses in the United States is increasing but still lags behind that of the overall population. African Americans, Hispanic/Latino Americans, and Native Americans make up more than 35% of the population but only 17% of the nation's nurses. Biased behaviors against nurses of diverse cultural and ethnic backgrounds by patients and health care professionals may contribute to their underrepresentation.

Cultural differences exist in how well patients believe they can communicate with their HCP. Communication issues include not understanding the HCP, feeling that they are not listened to, and having questions but not asking them. In the United States approximately 25% to 33% of minority patients have difficulty communicating with their HCP, compared with 16% of white patients. As increasing numbers of internationally educated nurses join the workforce, sufficient training and transitional support must be in place to ensure communication and quality of care.[21]

When HCPs from different cultures work together as members of the health care team, opportunities for miscommunication and conflict can occur. This is termed *cultural conflict.* The cultural origins of miscommunication and conflict in the workplace are often interconnected with cultural beliefs, values, and etiquette. Seeking clarification about misperceptions and misunderstandings is a communication strategy to foster effective teamwork among a multicultural health care team. To ensure the recruitment and retention of nurses from minority populations, all members of the health care team and leadership must create an environment that promotes effective cross-cultural communication and reduces bias and discrimination.

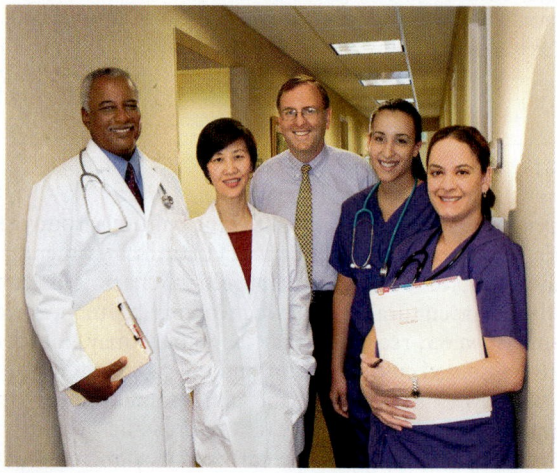

FIG. 2-3 Interprofessional team working together in a multicultural health care environment. (©Thinkstock/Stockbyte/Thinkstock)

CULTURAL FACTORS AFFECTING HEALTH AND HEALTH CARE

Many cultural factors affect the patient's health and health care. Several potential factors are presented in Table 2-5.

Folk Healers and Traditions

Many cultures have **folk healers**, who are also known as *traditional healers.* Most folk healers speak the person's native language and cost less than conventional HCPs. Among the many folk healers found worldwide, Hispanics, particularly from regions in Mexico and Central and South America, may choose to use a *curandero* (or *curandera*), African Americans may visit a *hougan,* Native Americans may seek help from a medicine man or *shaman,* and Asian Americans may use folk healers such as a Chinese herbal therapist. In addition to folk healers, some cultures involve lay midwives (e.g., *parteras* for Hispanic women) in the care of pregnant women.

Folk medicine and traditions are forms of prevention and treatment that are culturally based and traditionally rely on oral transmission of healing techniques from one generation to the next. The patient may not use the term *folk medicine* but thinks of these as cultural home remedies or treatment practices. Folk medicine may be practiced in the home without the guidance of a folk healer. It is important to assess whether the patient is practicing traditional or folk healing.

Some traditions that are practiced as a rite of passage in some cultures can be considered harmful in the dominant culture in the United States. For example, female genital cutting is a tradition that is illegal in most countries yet still practiced in many countries in Africa and the Middle East. It results in physical and emotional trauma and may affect childbirth. Nurses have the opportunity to advocate for immigrant women who have experienced this trauma and to prevent return of young girls to their country of origin for the procedure.

Spirituality and Religion

Spirituality and religion are aspects of culture that may affect a person's beliefs about health, illness, and end-of-life care. They may also play a role in nutrition and decisions related to health, wellness, and how to respond to or treat an illness.

Spirituality refers to a person's effort to find purpose and meaning in life. It is influenced by a person's unique life experiences and reflects one's personal understanding of life's mysteries. Spirituality relates to the soul or spirit more than to the body, and it may provide hope and strength for an individual during an illness.

Religion is a more formal and organized system of beliefs, including belief in or worship of God or gods. Religious beliefs include the cause, nature, and purpose of the universe and involve prayer and rituals. Religion is based on beliefs about life, death, good, and evil. You can use several interventions to meet a patient's religious and spiritual needs, including prayer, scripture reading, listening, and referral to a chaplain, rabbi, or priest.

Many patients find that rituals help them during times of illness. Rituals help a person make sense of life experiences and may take the form of prayer, meditation, or other rituals that

TABLE 2-5 Cultural Factors Affecting Health and Health Care

Time Orientation

- For some cultures it is more important to attend to a social role than to arrive on time for an appointment with HCP.
- Some cultures are future oriented; others are past or present oriented.

Language and Communication

- Patients may not speak English and may not be able to communicate with HCP.
- Even with interpreters, communication may be difficult.

Economic Factors

- Patients may not get health care because they cannot pay for it or because of the costs associated with travel for health care.
- Refugee or undocumented immigrant status may deter some patients from using the health care system.
- Immigrant women who are heads of households or single mothers may not seek health care for themselves because of child care costs.
- Patients may lack health insurance.

Health Care System

- Patients may not make or keep appointments because of the time lag between the onset of an illness and an available appointment.
- Hours of operation of health care facilities may not accommodate patients' need to work or use public transportation.
- Requirements to access some types of care may discourage some patients from taking the steps to qualify for health care or health care payment assistance.
- Some patients have a general distrust of HCPs and health care systems.
- Lack of ethnic-specific health care programs may deter some individuals from seeking health care.
- Transportation may be a problem for patients who have to travel long distances for health care.
- Adequate interpreter services may be unavailable.
- Patients may not have a primary HCP and may use emergency departments or urgent care centers for health care.
- Shortages of HCPs from specific ethnic groups may deter some people from seeking health care.
- Patients may lack knowledge about the availability of existing health care resources.
- Facility policies may not be culturally competent (e.g., hospital policy may limit the number of visitors, which is problematic for cultures that value having many family members present).

Beliefs and Practices

- Care provided in established health care programs may not be perceived as culturally relevant.
- Religious reasons, beliefs, or practices may affect a person's decision to seek (or not seek) health care.
- Patients may delay seeking health care because of fear or dependence on folk medicine and herbal remedies.
- Patients may stop treatment or discontinue visits for health care because the symptoms are no longer present, and they believe that further care is not required.
- Some patients associate hospitals and extended care facilities with death.
- The patient may have had a previous negative experience with culturally incompetent HCPs or discriminatory practices.
- Some people mistrust the majority population and institutions dominated by them.
- Some patients may feel apprehensive about unfamiliar diagnostic procedures and treatment options.

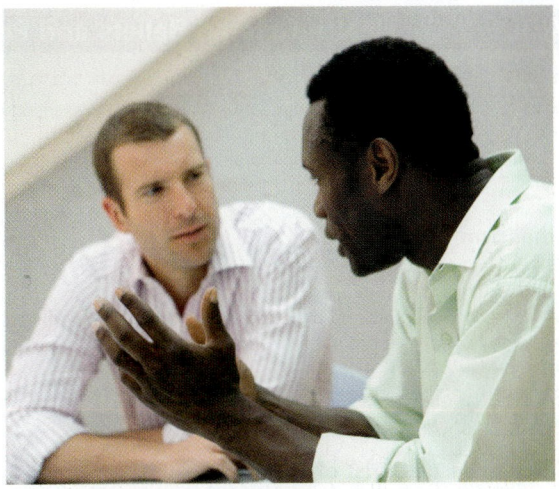

FIG. 2-4 Co-workers from different cultures communicate with verbal and nonverbal cues. (©BananaStock/Thinkstock)

the patient may create. With appropriate training, you may include spiritual questions in the complete assessment of the patient and plan care based accordingly. (Table 9-5 has a spiritual assessment guide that may be used with patients.) Table 2-6 summarizes health-related beliefs and practices of selected religious groups.[19]

Cross-Cultural Communication

Communication refers to an organized, patterned system of behavior that may be verbal or nonverbal (Fig. 2-4). *Verbal communication* includes not only one's language or dialect, but also voice tone, volume, timing, and ability to share thoughts and feelings. More than 45 million people in the United States speak a language other than English in their home, with Spanish being the most common. Hispanic people who do not speak English at home are less likely to receive a variety of health care services regardless of whether or not they are comfortable speaking English.

Nonverbal communication may take the form of writing, gestures, body movements, posture, facial expressions, and personal dress in some cultures. Nonverbal communication also includes eye contact, use of touch, body language, style of greeting, and spatial distancing. Eye contact varies greatly among cultural groups. Patients who are Asian, Arab, or Native American may avoid direct eye contact and consider it disrespectful or aggressive. Hispanic patients may expect you to look directly at them but may not return that direct gaze. Other variables to consider include the role of gender, age, acculturation, status, or position on what is considered appropriate eye contact. For example, Muslim-Arab women exhibit modesty when avoiding eye contact with men other than their husbands and when in public situations.

Silence has many meanings, and it is important to understand the meaning of silence for different cultural groups. Some people are comfortable with silence, whereas others become uncomfortable and may speak to decrease the amount of silent time. It is important to clarify what silence means in an interaction with a patient. Patients sometimes nod their head or say "yes" as if agreeing with you or to indicate they understand. Actually, they may be doing this because it is a culturally acceptable manner of showing respect, not because they understand or agree.

Many Native Americans are comfortable with silence and interpret silence as essential for thinking and carefully considering a response. In these interactions, silence shows respect

TABLE 2-6 Health-Related Beliefs and Practices of Selected Religious Groups

Amish
- Alcoholic beverages and drugs are prohibited unless prescribed by HCPs.
- Abortion, artificial insemination, and stem cell use are prohibited.
- Amish seldom purchase commercial health insurance.

Catholicism
- Many fast and abstain from meat and meat products on Ash Wednesday and the Fridays of Lent.
- Artificial contraception and direct abortion are prohibited. Indirect abortion (e.g., treatment of uterine cancer in a pregnant woman) may be morally justified.
- Sacrament of the Sick includes anointing of sick with oil, blessing by a priest, and communion (unleavened wafer made of flour and water).

Church of Jesus Christ of Latter-Day Saints (Mormons)
- Strict dietary code called Word of Wisdom prohibits all alcoholic beverages, hot drinks (nonherbal teas and coffee), tobacco, and illegal or recreational drugs.
- Fasting for 24-hour period occurs monthly on "Fast Sunday."
- During hospitalization or serious illness, an elder anoints the ill person with oil while a second elder seals the anointing with a prayer and blessing (laying on of hands).
- Abortion is prohibited except when the mother's life is in danger.

Hinduism
- Eating meat is prohibited because it involves harming a living creature.
- Cremation is most common form of body disposal, but fetuses or newborns are sometimes buried.

Islam
- Fasting during daytime hours occurs during a month-long period called Ramadan.
- Ritual cleansing with water before eating and before prayer is practiced.
- Eating pork or taking medicines with pork derivatives is prohibited.
- Drinking alcoholic beverages is prohibited.
- Artificial insemination is permissible only if from the husband to his own wife.

Jehovah's Witness
- Transfusions of blood in any form or agents in which blood is an ingredient are not acceptable. Blood volume expanders are acceptable if they are not derivatives of blood.
- Transplants that involve bodily mutilation are prohibited.
- Therapeutic and on-demand abortions are prohibited.
- Artificial insemination is prohibited for both donors and recipients.

Judaism
- Strictly observant Jews never eat pork, shellfish, or predatory fowl and never mix milk dishes and meat dishes in preparing foods. Fish with fins and scales are permissible.
- Certain foods and drink are designated as kosher, which means "proper." All animals must be ritually slaughtered.
- On the eighth day after birth, boys are circumcised in a ritual called Brit Milah, and girls are given a dedication ceremony involving prayers and blessings.
- Abortion is morally unacceptable except when the mother's life is in danger.
- Organized support system for the sick includes a visit from the rabbi. The rabbi may pray with the sick person alone or in a minyan, a group of 10 adults over age 13.
- If an autopsy is performed, all body parts must be returned for burial.

Seventh-Day Adventism
- Vegetarian diet encouraged.
- Nonvegetarian members refrain from eating foods derived from any animal having a cloven hoof that chews its cud (e.g., pigs, goats). Eating fish with fins and scales is acceptable, but consuming shellfish is prohibited.
- Consumption of alcoholic beverages is prohibited.
- Fasting is practiced and involves abstaining from food or liquids by healthy members of the church.

Buddhism
- Consumption of alcoholic beverages and illicit drugs is prohibited.
- Moderation in diet and avoidance of extremes are practiced.
- Central tenets are maintaining right views, intentions, speech, actions, livelihood, effort, mindfulness, and concentration.

Data from Andrews MM, Boyle JS: *Transcultural concepts in nursing care*, ed 6, Philadelphia, 2012, Lippincott Williams & Wilkins.

for the other person and demonstrates the importance of the remarks. In traditional Japanese and Chinese cultures, the speaker may stop talking and leave a period of silence for the listener to think about what has been said before continuing. Silence may be intended to show respect for the speaker's privacy, whereas in some cultures (e.g., French, Spanish, Russian) the person may interpret silence as meaning agreement. Asian Americans may use silence to demonstrate respect for elders, whereas African Americans may use silence as a response to what is perceived to be an inappropriate question.

Racism and microaggression affect communication. *Racism* is a belief that differences among the various racial/ethnic groups determine cultural or individual achievement. It usually involves the idea that one's own race/ethnicity is superior and has the right to dominate others or that a particular racial/ethnic group is inferior to the others.

Microaggression is social exchanges in which a person says or does something than can either intentionally or unintentionally belittle or alienate a person, especially someone of a different racial/ethnic group. It is imperative that nurses seek to understand racism and microaggression through education, self-awareness, and open dialogue with peers.[22]

Family Roles and Relationships

Family roles differ from one culture to another (Fig. 2-5). It is important for you to determine who should be involved in communication and decision making related to health care. Some cultural groups emphasize interdependence rather than independence. In the United States many in the mainstream culture have strong beliefs related to autonomy. An individual is expected to sign consent forms when receiving health care. In other cultural groups a family member may be expected to make health care decisions. When you encounter a family that values interdependence over independence, the health care system may have difficulty adapting to how decisions are made. Treatment may have to be delayed while the patient waits for significant family members to arrive before giving consent for a procedure or treatment. In other instances the patient may make a decision that is best for the family despite adverse outcomes for the patient. Being aware of such values will better prepare you to advocate for the patient.

Some cultural differences relate to expectations of family members in providing care. In some cultures, family members expect to provide care for the patient even in the hospital. The patient may expect that the family, along with the HCPs, will provide all care. This view is the opposite of the predominant Western expectation that the patient will assume self-care as quickly as possible.

Ask about culturally relevant gender relationships. For example, in some cultures, such as many Arab groups, it is not appropriate for a man to be alone with a woman other than his wife. Nor is it appropriate for a woman other than a man's wife to provide physical care for him. The clinical implication of this cultural belief is that for many patients from Arab cultures, nurses cannot provide direct physical care for patients of the opposite gender. In some instances, procedures or treatments may be carried out for patients from the opposite gender but only if a third party is present.

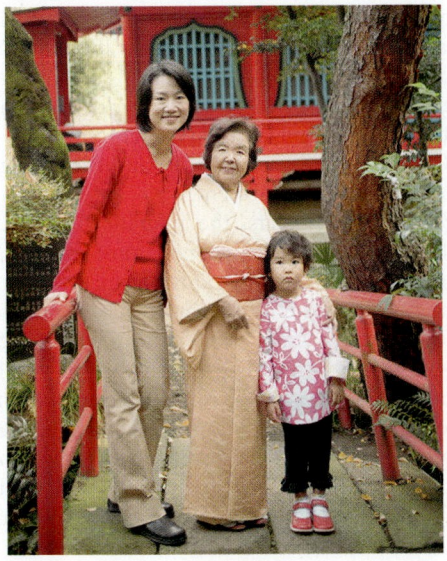

FIG. 2-5 Family roles and relationships differ from one culture to another. (©Jupiterimages/Photos.com/Thinkstock)

Personal Space

Personal space zones are the variable and subjective distance at which one person feels comfortable talking to another. A representative example of personal space zones for European Americans is shown in Fig. 2-6. Personal space distances vary from culture to culture, as well as within a culture. As a nurse, you often interact with patients in the intimate or personal distance, which may be uncomfortable for the patient.

Cultural groups have wide variations in their perception of appropriate distances. Whereas an American nurse of European descent may be comfortable with a certain distance, a person from a Hispanic or Middle Eastern background may believe that the distance is too far and will move closer, perhaps causing you to feel uncomfortable. If you then move away to a more comfortable distance, this may cause the other person to think that you are unfriendly, or the person may be offended. Personal space distance also varies within cultures.

Touch

Physical contact with patients conveys various meanings depending on the culture. Performing a comprehensive assessment requires touching a patient. Many people of Asian and Hispanic heritage believe that touching a person's head is a sign of disrespect, especially because the head is believed to be the source of one's strength and/or soul. Numerous people in the world believe in the evil eye, or *mal ojo.* In this culture-bound syndrome, the illness—usually in a child or a woman—is believed to result from excessive admiration by another person. In some cultures the proper way to ward off the evil eye is to touch the area of admiration. For example, if the person admires

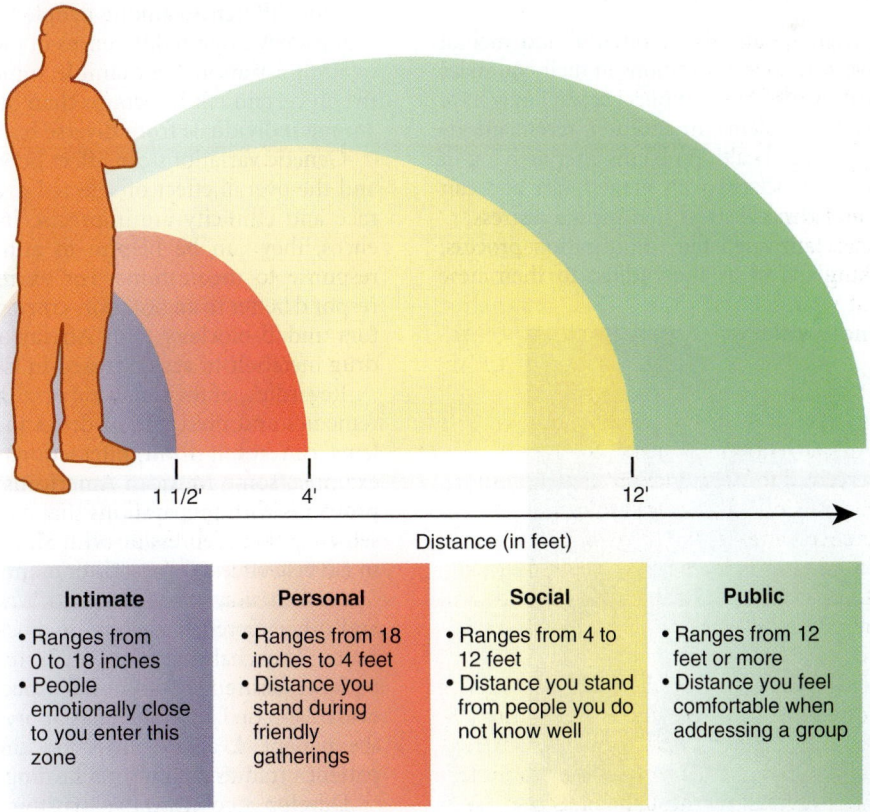

FIG. 2-6 Personal space zones.

the hair, the top of the head may be touched. It is important for you to ask permission before touching anyone, particularly if it is necessary to touch the person's head.

Nutrition

An important part of cultural practices is food, including both the foods that are eaten and rituals and practices associated with food. Muslims fast during the daytime during the Islamic month of Ramadan. Such practices may affect when and how medications are taken. Patients may be asked to make major changes in their diets because of health problems, or alternatively food may be used to cope with life changes such as homesickness. Specific foods may be considered essential to good health during pregnancy or other life stages. The HCP should take into account food-related cultural beliefs, practices, and habits when discussing nutrition with patients and planning their diets.

When individuals and families immigrate to an area that is very different from their country of origin, they may experience unfamiliar foods, food-storage systems, and food-buying habits. They also may come from countries that have limited food supplies because of poverty, wars, and poor sanitation. They may arrive with conditions such as malnutrition, diarrhea, and dental caries. Other problems may develop after the person arrives in the new country. For example, second-generation Hispanic immigrants have a greater chance of becoming overweight than their first-generation counterparts. The increase in weight is related to the degree of acculturation experienced by the immigrant.

Immigrants and Immigration

Migration is driven by a number of conditions, such as overcrowding, natural disasters, geopolitical conflict, persecution, and economic forces. Because of these migrations, a rich diversity of cultures exists in many communities and countries today (Fig. 2-7).

Recent immigrants may be at risk for physical and mental health problems for many reasons. Conditions in their countries of origin (e.g., malnutrition, poor sanitation, civil war) may have resulted in chronic health problems. In addition, recent immigrants are at increased risk for health problems after arriving in a new area. Relocation is associated with many losses and can cause economic hardship, physical stress, and mental distress.

As new immigrants go through the acculturation process, many experience cultural stress as they adjust to their new environment, especially if they have left relatives behind or are unable to return to their home country. Older immigrants are especially affected by changes in role and social position. This may result in depression. Posttraumatic stress disorder is seen in immigrants who have survived wars and violence. Immigrants may face barriers to social acceptance, such as prejudice or discrimination, and experience a lack of ethnic and cultural resources. For some, it may mean loss of the social status that they experienced in their countries of origin.

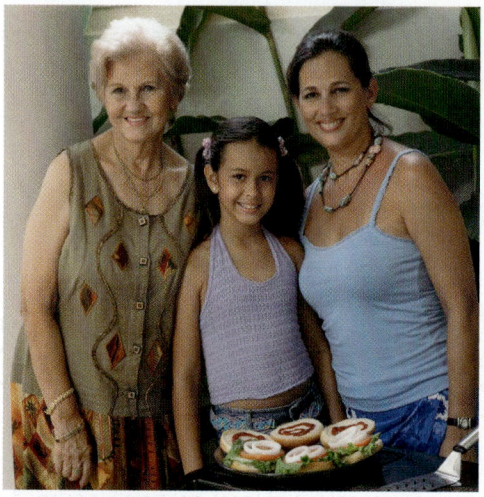

FIG. 2-7 Recently arrived immigrants join a neighbor for a barbecue, a common American tradition. (©Jack Hollingsworth/Photodisc/Thinkstock)

Another potential problem is tuberculosis (TB). More than half of the TB cases in the United States occur in individuals born outside the country. Individuals who have recently immigrated from areas that have a high endemic rate of TB are more likely to have TB. Foreign-born Hispanics and Asians combined account for 48% of the nation's TB cases. The top five countries of the origin of foreign-born people with TB are Mexico, Philippines, Vietnam, India, and China. The *Refugee Health Guidelines* from the Centers for Disease Control and Prevention supports early identification and treatment.[23]

During the past 45 years, the migration pattern of North America has shifted. Whereas once most immigrants came from Europe, now most immigrants originate from Asia, Latin America, and Africa. Additionally, an increased number of first- and second-generation immigrants enter the United States after visiting friends and relatives. These individuals have a higher risk for malaria, typhoid fever, cholera, and hepatitis A than people born in the United States. Many immigrants lack health insurance and may primarily obtain their health care in emergency departments and urgent care clinics. Therefore nurses in all settings need to be aware of refugee health screening, treatment recommendations, and resources for access to health care and social services.

Medications

Genetic differences among people from diverse ethnic or racial groups may explain differences in medication selection, dosage, or administration. For example, some medicines are more effective in certain ethnic groups than others. Side effects may vary among individuals from diverse backgrounds.

Genetic variations can affect how the body processes a drug and the overall effect of selected drugs on the body. Although race and ethnicity are imprecise indicators of genetic differences, they can be helpful in anticipating variations in the response to medications. For example, European Americans respond better to angiotensin-converting enzyme (ACE) inhibitors and β-blockers than African Americans. (Genetics and drug metabolism are discussed in Chapter 12.)

Regardless of their cultural origins, many people use cultural remedies and prescription drugs to treat their illnesses. Problems can result from interactions of these substances. For example, some Mexican Americans may treat gastrointestinal problems with preparations that contain lead. Individuals may self-treat their depression with St. John's wort, which can result in adverse effects if prescription antidepressants are also taken.

Patients may avoid standard Western medicine until herbs and other remedies become ineffective or the illness becomes acute. The challenge for you is to try to accommodate the patient's desire for traditional aspects of care while also using evidence-based approaches as appropriate and as acceptable to the patient. Evaluate the safety and appropriateness of the patient's traditional cultural healing therapies.

Develop a collaborative, trusting relationship with patients and encourage them to discuss their traditional approaches to healing. Seek out information on potential drug and herbal

TABLE 2-7 Cultural Assessment

A cultural assessment should include the following:

- Brief history of the cultural group with which person identifies
- Values orientation
- Cultural sanctions and restrictions
- Communication
- Health-related beliefs and practices
- Nutrition
- Socioeconomic considerations
- Organizations providing cultural support
- Educational background
- Religious affiliation
- Spiritual considerations

Adapted from Jarvis C: *Physical examination and health assessment*, ed 6, Philadelphia, 2012, Saunders.

product interaction from the pharmacist. Honor the patient's choices, if safe and effective, since this will enhance collaboration and may have a positive impact on health outcomes.

Psychologic Factors

Symptoms are interpreted through a person's cultural norms and may vary from the recognized interpretations of Western medicine. All symptoms have meaning, and the meanings may vary from one culture to another. For example, the degree of depression following a cardiac diagnosis is mediated by cultural views. It is important to ask patients what their illness means to them, what they believe is the cause, and what they think is the best treatment (Table 2-7).

Culture-bound syndromes are illnesses or afflictions that are recognized only within a cultural group (Table 2-8). The symptoms, course of the illness, and people's reactions to the illness are limited to specific cultures. Culture-bound syndromes are expressed through psychologic or physical symptoms.

TABLE 2-8 Culture-Bound Syndromes

Syndrome	Description
Hispanics/Latinos	
Bilis or Colera	Caused by strong anger or rage. Many Hispanic/Latino groups believe that anger results in excess bile that gets into the systemic circulation. Symptoms include acute nervous tension, headache, trembling, screaming, stomach disturbances, and, in severe cases, loss of consciousness.
Ataque de Nervios	Brought on by a stressful family event (e.g., death, divorce). Symptoms may include uncontrollable shouting, crying and trembling, and verbal or physical aggression.
Empacho	Condition described as food forming into a ball that clings to the stomach or intestines, causing pain and cramping.
Susto	Sometimes referred to as "fright sickness" or "soul loss." A traumatic anxiety-depressive state that may result from a frightening experience, such as a loud sound or some threat. Can cause anxiety, insomnia, listlessness, loss of appetite, and social withdrawal. One treatment is to have the affected person lie on the floor. The healer then sweeps indigenous herbs over the person's body while praying to release the evil wind.
Native Americans	
Ghost Sickness	Condition sometimes associated with witchcraft and a preoccupation with death. Symptoms include general weakness, loss of appetite, a feeling of suffocation, recurring nightmares, and a pervasive feeling of terror.
Chinese	
Shenjing Shuairuo	Characterized by physical and mental fatigue, headaches and other pains, dizziness, sleep disturbances, and concentration difficulties.
African Americans	
Brain Fag	Term describing brain "fatigue" caused by the challenges of school. Symptoms include difficulties concentrating, remembering, and thinking.
Thin Blood	Affects older adults, women, and children. Generally weakens an individual and increases susceptibility to illness.
Caribbean and Southern United States	
Falling Out	Characterized by a sudden collapse, which may sometimes be preceded by dizziness or "swimming" in the head. The person can hear but is unable to move.
Cambodians	
Koucharang or Kit Chroeun	Translates as "thinking too much," brought about by having witnessed or experienced a horrific trauma. Characterized by physical and emotional exhaustion, immobilization, and constant preoccupation with past suffering and loss.
Koreans	
Hwa-Byung	Ailment characterized by resentment that is brought about by bitterness and discontent.

❖ NURSING MANAGEMENT: REDUCING HEALTH DISPARITIES AND INCREASING CULTURAL COMPETENCY

Nurse's Self-Assessment

The first step in reducing health disparities and providing culturally competent care is for you to assess your own cultural background, values, and beliefs, especially those that are related to health and health care. Many tools are available to assist you with this process *(http://nccc.georgetown.edu)*.

Table 2-4 suggests ways for you to improve your cultural competence. This information can help you better understand patients and provide culturally competent care. It is important to understand that cultures evolve and change over time. Culturally competent care requires continual learning and self-reflection.[24] Many other important aspects of culture related to health care are included in the Culturally Competent Care sections throughout this book.

In today's increasingly multicultural environment, you will meet patients, families, significant others, and members of the health care team from many different cultures. You will find yourself in patient care situations that require an understanding of the patient's cultural beliefs and practices. Even when you provide care for patients from your own cultural background, you may be from a different subculture than the patient. For example, there are more than 550 federally recognized Native American tribes in the United States, so it would be inappropriate for you to assume that a Native American nurse can give culturally appropriate care to a Native American patient when they may be from different tribes. A white nurse from an urban upbringing may find cultural differences with a white patient from a rural community. Cultural competence is a lifelong process that involves self-reflection and continual learning.[24]

Patient Assessment

HCPs play an important role in reducing health disparities. However, the causes of health disparities are not always easy to identify. Assess patients for their risk for reduced health care services because of limited access, inadequate resources, age, or low health literacy.

A cultural assessment should be included in the nursing process.[25] Table 2-7 lists important components of the assessment. Determine the patient's (1) health beliefs and health care practices; and (2) perspective of the meaning, cause, and preferred treatment of illness. Ask questions that you are comfortable with based on your own culture.

How can you be aware of the differences among ethnic groups? Using guides for cultural assessment will facilitate the nursing process when working with patients, families, or other groups who are from different cultures. Although guides can assist in this process, you need to be careful not to stereotype or assume that common cultural characteristics pertain to each individual patient. Use guides to explore the degree to which patients share commonalities with the traits generally attributed to their cultural group. You must be informed about traditional characteristics of cultural groups while recognizing that culture is constantly evolving and unique for each individual.

Nursing Implementation

Although the issues associated with health disparities can seem overwhelming, a number of strategies are available to reduce and ultimately eliminate health disparities. Table 2-9 presents nursing interventions to reduce health disparities.

Advocacy. The solutions to reduce health disparities often rest with the policymakers. Economic issues often determine health care delivery. Access and public policy decisions determine who is eligible for federal and state health insurance coverage. You, along with the social worker, can help by identifying key resources in the community, including transportation services, reduced-fee screening programs, and appropriate federal and state offices for Medicaid and Medicare.

You can be an advocate in your health care setting by helping to create a community advisory group. Such a group can be very helpful when establishing health programs within a community. This can also increase the distribution of culturally sensitive information. Another powerful strategy is to increase the number of underrepresented populations in the health care professions (Fig. 2-8).

Standardized Guidelines. The use of standardized, evidence-based care guidelines can reduce disparities in diagnosis and treatments. For example, guidelines for the management of hypertension should be based on the patient's BP, symptoms, history, and laboratory values rather than other characteristics such as gender, age, or culture. Racial or cultural differences in outcomes are reduced when the guidelines are followed. In addition, recommendations related to cultural competency will guide you in your learning and practice.

The National Standards for Culturally and Linguistically Appropriate Services in Health Care (CLAS standards) are guidelines that improve the quality of health care. The CLAS standards provide practical guidance for care of people with limited English proficiency and of diverse cultural backgrounds.

Communication. Improving interpersonal skills is an important first step in reducing health disparities and providing culturally competent care. To show respect for the patient, take into account the patient's usual communication style. For instance, conduct a health history in an unhurried manner and in a way that is appropriate for the culture. In some cultures it is best to start with general rather than direct questions. For some cultures it is most effective to engage in "small talk," with the discussion including answers that may seem to be unrelated to the questions. If you appear to be "too busy," communication may be impaired.

When meeting patients or family members, introduce yourself and indicate how you would like them to address you—whether they should use first names; Mr., Ms., or Mrs.; or a title, such as nurse. Also ask the patient how he or she prefers to be addressed. This shows respect and will help you begin the relationship in a culturally appropriate manner.

If you need to gather personal information, it is important to understand the most effective approach to use. For instance,

TABLE 2-9 Nursing Interventions to Reduce Health Disparities

- Treat all patients equally.
- Be aware of your own biases or prejudices and work toward eliminating them.
- Learn about services and programs that focus on specific cultural/ethnic groups.
- Inform patients about health care services available for their specific cultural/ethnic group.
- Make sure the same standards of care are followed for all patients regardless of culture or ethnicity.
- Identify health care practices and cultural practices that are important to cultural and ethnic identity.
- Participate in research focused on understanding and improving care to culturally and ethnically diverse populations.
- Identify stereotypic attitudes toward a culture/ethnic group that may interfere with getting appropriate health care.
- Support patients of specific cultural/ethnic groups who are fearful about traveling outside the accepted neighborhood for health care services.
- Advocate for patients of specific cultural/ethnic groups to receive health care services that pay special attention to English-language limitations and cultural health practices.
- Learn advocacy and interpersonal strategies from leaders of specific cultural/ethnic groups. For example, African Americans may respond to themes such as "do it for your loved ones." Asian Americans may respond to fear of dependency themes.
- Ensure availability of culturally appropriate patient educational resources.

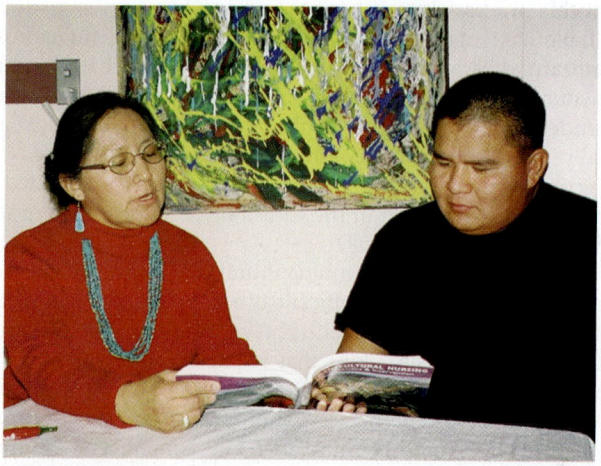

FIG. 2-8 A Navajo nurse teaching a Navajo patient. (From Giger JN: *Transcultural nursing*, ed 6, St Louis, 2013, Mosby.)

TABLE 2-10 Using a Medical Interpreter

Choosing an Interpreter

- Use an agency interpreter if possible.
- Use a trained medical interpreter who knows how to interpret, has a health care background, understands patients' rights, and can help with advice about the cultural relevance or appropriateness of the health care plan and instructions.
- Use a family member only if necessary. Be aware of limitations if the family member does not understand medical terms, is younger or a different gender than the patient, or is not aware of the health care procedures or medical ethics.
- Interpreter should be able to do the following:
  - Interpret the patient's nonverbal as well as verbal communication.
  - Translate the message into understandable terms.
  - Act as a patient advocate to represent the patient's needs to the health care team.
  - Be culturally competent and understand how to provide teaching instructions.

Strategies for Working With an Interpreter

- If possible, have the interpreter meet with the patient ahead of time to establish rapport before the interpreting begins.
- Speak slowly.
- Maintain eye contact with the patient.
- Talk to the patient, not the interpreter.
- Use simple language with as few medical terms as possible.
- Speak one or two sentences at a time to allow for easier interpretation.
- Avoid raising your voice during the interaction.
- Obtain feedback to be certain the patient understands.
- Plan on taking twice as long to complete the interaction.

when talking with people from some cultural groups, it is imperative that you take time to establish trust and listen to the patient's responses to questions. There may be long silences as the person thinks about the question, showing respect by giving the question appropriate consideration before answering. Take time to listen and help establish trust.

Consider how the patient's age may impact his or her views and communication. For example, African American older adults with mental health concerns may struggle with shame, uncertainty, and lack of trust in the system.

Do not try to serve as an interpreter if your patient does not understand English, because this could lead to misunderstandings. Get the assistance of a person who is qualified to do medical interpretation when you cannot speak the patient's primary language (Table 2-10). Interpreters are available by phone anywhere in the United States through a fee-based service and should be used rather than a family member. Table 2-11 provides guidelines for communicating when no interpreter is available.

TABLE 2-11 Communicating When No Interpreter Is Available

1. Be polite and formal.
2. Pronounce name correctly. If unsure, ask about the correct pronunciation of the name. Use proper titles of respect, such as "Mr.," "Mrs.," "Ms.," "Dr." Greet the person using the last or complete name.
3. Gesture to yourself and say your name.
4. Offer a handshake or nod. Smile.
5. Proceed in an unhurried manner. Pay attention to any effort by the patient or family to communicate.
6. Speak in a low, moderate voice and avoid excessive hand gestures. Remember that there is a tendency to raise the volume and pitch of your voice when the listener appears not to understand. The listener may perceive that you are shouting or angry.
7. Use any words that you might know in the person's language. This indicates that you are aware of and respect his or her culture.
8. Use simple words such as "pain" instead of "discomfort." Avoid medical jargon, idioms, and slang. Avoid using contractions (e.g., don't, can't, won't). Use nouns repeatedly instead of pronouns. *Example:*
   Do not say: "He has been taking his medicine, hasn't he?"
   Do say: "Does Juan take medicine?"
9. Pantomime words and simple actions while you verbalize them.
10. Give instructions in the proper sequence. *Example:*
    Do not say: "Before you rinse the bottle, sterilize it."
    Do say: "First, wash the bottle. Second, rinse the bottle."
11. Discuss one topic at a time. Avoid using conjunctions. *Example:*
    Do not say: "Are you cold and in pain?"
    Do say: "Are you cold [while pantomiming]? Are you in pain?"
12. Validate whether the person understands by having him or her repeat instructions, demonstrate the procedure, or act out the meaning.
13. Write out several short sentences in English and determine the person's ability to read them.
14. Try a third language. Many Indochinese people speak French. Europeans often know two or more languages. Try Latin words or phrases. Use English words that have Latin roots (e.g., use precipitation instead of rain).
15. Ask the person's family and friends who could serve as an interpreter.
16. Use websites that translate words from one language to another. Some of them also have audio to help you know how to say the word correctly.
17. Obtain phrase books from a library or bookstore, make or purchase flash cards, contact hospitals for a list of interpreters, and use both a formal and an informal network to locate a suitable interpreter.

Source: Jarvis C: *Physical examination and health assessment*, ed 6, Philadelphia, 2012, Saunders.

A dictionary that translates from both your language and the patient's language (e.g., Spanish-English/English-Spanish dictionary) is useful. Patients may find it helpful if you have a list of questions and potential answers in several languages prepared by using these types of dictionaries. Many websites translate words and documents from one language into another (see Informatics in Practice box).

It is helpful to have resources for those cultural groups who frequently use the health care facility. This is especially beneficial when a qualified medical interpreter is not readily available and you need to learn important phrases in another language.

INFORMATICS IN PRACTICE

Use of Translation Applications

- Communication barriers can negatively affect the type of care received by non–English-speaking patients.
- Use a language translation app to help you translate one language into another language.
- Some apps allow you to speak critical phrases and have the translation immediately spoken back to you or the patient in a natural human voice with the proper accent.
- Check the policy of the health care institution on the use of medical interpreters or translators, including the use of apps for translation.

CASE STUDY

Health Disparities

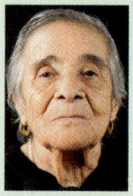

(©Luevanos/ iStock/ Thinkstock)

Patient Profile

M.S. is an 81-year-old woman who came to the United States from India 4 years ago with her son and daughter-in-law and their four children. She has a number of health problems, including coronary artery disease, hypertension, osteoarthritis in her right hip, and diabetes. Her daughter-in-law is the primary caregiver and frequently brings her to the urban community health clinic for a variety of health-related complaints. Recently M.S. has been experiencing memory problems.

The entire family comes to the health clinic with M.S. Because English is a second language (Hindustani is their first language) for all of the adult family members, the staff relies on the oldest granddaughter to interpret.

At this clinic visit, M.S. is complaining of shortness of breath. Through her granddaughter's interpretation, she tells the nurse that she is having trouble walking up the stairs in the apartment building. The nurse does the history and assessment, checks her blood glucose (which is within normal limits), and advises that she get more exercise. Given M.S.'s memory problems and limited English, the nurse does not complete a 24-hour dietary recall or counsel her or the family about diabetes management. M.S. is scheduled for an appointment with the cardiologist for an evaluation of her hypertension and heart disease. Two weeks later, when she is seen by the cardiologist, her shortness of breath is much worse and she is complaining of chest pain. She is hospitalized immediately.

Meanwhile, the clinic supervisor is completing a chart audit for the clinic's quality review program. She is reviewing M.S.'s chart and notices that, although she has been a patient in the clinic for 3 years, she has never received instructions on blood glucose monitoring or general diabetes management. The clinic has a nurse diabetes educator who teaches individual patients and groups of patients with diabetes. The clinic manager reviews these findings with the nurse and asks why she has not recommended that M.S. see the diabetes educator. The nurse states that with M.S.'s memory problems and the language barrier, she just assumed that M.S. and her family would not benefit from the consultation.

Discussion Questions

1. What type of health disparity has M.S. experienced?
2. What factors led to her not receiving the standard of care?
3. What additional assessment should have been done at the initial visit?

Patient-Centered Care

4. What strategies may have worked to enhance patient education?
5. How would you assess M.S.'s religious and spiritual needs?

Quality Improvement

6. If you were the clinic manager, how would you recommend that the nurse improve her practice?

Answers available at *http://evolve.elsevier.com/Lewis/medsurg.*

BRIDGE TO NCLEX EXAMINATION

The number of the question corresponds to the same-numbered outcome at the beginning of the chapter.

1. What are the *leading* determinants of a patient's health (*select all that apply*)?
   a. Genetics
   b. Health behaviors
   c. Family history of disease
   d. Social and physical environment
   e. Type and quality of medical care received
2. In identifying patients at the *greatest* risk for health disparities, the nurse would note that
   a. patients who live in urban areas have readily available access to health care services.
   b. cultural differences exist in patients' ability to communicate with their health care provider.
   c. a patient receiving care from a health care provider of a different culture would have decreased quality of care.
   d. men are more likely than women to have their cardiovascular disease symptoms ignored by their health care provider.
3. Forcing one's own cultural beliefs and practices on another person is an example of
   a. stereotyping.
   b. ethnocentrism.
   c. cultural relativity.
   d. cultural imposition.
4. Which statement *most* accurately describes cultural factors that may affect health?
   a. Diabetes and cancer rates differ by cultural/ethnic groups.
   b. Most patients find that religious rituals help them during times of illness.
   c. There are limited ethnic variations in physiologic responses to medications.
   d. Silence during a nurse-patient interaction usually means that the patient understands the instructions.
5. When communicating with a patient who speaks a language that the nurse does not understand, it is important to *first* attempt to
   a. have a family member interpret.
   b. use a trained medical interpreter.
   c. use specific medical terminology so there will be no mistakes.
   d. focus on the translation rather than nonverbal communication.
6. As part of the nursing process, cultural assessment is *best* accomplished by
   a. judging the patient's cultural values based on observations.
   b. using a cultural assessment guide as part of the nursing process.
   c. seeking guidance from a nurse from the patient's cultural background.
   d. relying on the nurse's previous experience with patients from that cultural group.

7. Nurses play an important role in reducing health disparities. An important mechanism to do this is to
   a. discourage use of evidence-based practice guidelines.
   b. insist that patients adhere to the *Healthy People 2020* guidelines.
   c. teach patients to use the Internet to find resources related to their health.
   d. engage in active listening and establish relationships with patients and families.

8. What is the *first* step in developing cultural competence?
   a. Create opportunities to interact with a variety of cultural groups.
   b. Examine the nurse's own cultural background, values, and beliefs about health and health care.
   c. Learn about a multitude of folk medicines and herbal substances that different cultures use for self-care.
   d. Learn assessment skills for different cultural groups, including cultural beliefs and practices and physical assessments.

1. a, b, d, 2. b, 3. d, 4. a, 5. b, 6. b, 7. d, 8. b.

For rationales to these answers and even more NCLEX review questions, visit *http://evolve.elsevier.com/Lewis/medsurg.*

EVOLVE WEBSITE

http://evolve.elsevier.com/Lewis/medsurg

Review Questions (Online Only)
Key Points
Answer Keys for Questions
- Rationales for Bridge to NCLEX Examination Questions
- Answer Guidelines for Case Study on p. 32

Conceptual Care Map Creator
Audio Glossary
Content Updates

REFERENCES

1. World Health Organization: Health impact assessment. Retrieved from *www.who.int.hia.en.*
2. Healthy People 2020: Social determinants of health. Retrieved from *www.healthypeople.gov/2020/topicsobjectives2020/overview.spx?topicid=39.*
3. Health Reform Monitoring Survey: Number of uninsured adults falls by 5.4 million since 2013. Retrieved from *http://hrms.urban.org/quicktakes/changeInUninsurance.html.*
4. Centers for Disease Control and Prevention: Chronic disease prevention and health promotion. Retrieved from *www.cdc.gov/chronicdisease/healthequity.*
5. US Census Bureau: Population estimates. Retrieved from *www.census.gov/prod/cen2010/briefs/c2010br-02.pdf.*
6. Cancer Facts & Figures for African Americans 2013-2014. Retrieved from *www.cancer.org/acs/groups/content/@epidemiologysurveilance/documents/document/acspc-036921.pdf.*

*7. Schieb LJ, Ayala C, Valderrama AL, et al: Trends and disparities in stroke mortality by region for American Indians and Alaska Natives, *Am J Public Health* 104(suppl 3):s359, 2014.

8. Edwards KM: Intimate partner violence and the rural-urban-suburban divide: myth or reality? A critical review of the literature, *Trauma Violence Abuse* 16:359, 2015.
9. The Joint Commission: What did the doctor say? Improving health literacy to protect patient safety. Retrieved from *www.jointcommission.org/assets/1/18/improving_health_literacy.pdf.*
10. Fabreau GI, Leung AA, Southern DA, et al: Sex, socioeconomic status, access to cardiac catheterization, and outcomes for acute coronary syndromes in the context of universal healthcare coverage, *Circ Cardiovasc Qual Outcomes* 7:540, 2014.
11. Farmer GW, Jabson JM, Bucholz KK, Bowen DJ: A population-based study of cardiovascular disease risk in sexual-minority women, *Am J Public Health* 103(10):1845, 2013.

*12. Blair I, Havranek E, Price D, et al: Assessment of biases against Latinos and African Americans among primary care providers and community members, *Am J Public Health* 103:92, 2013.

13. Giger JN, Davidhizar RE: *Transcultural nursing: assessment and intervention,* ed 6, St Louis, 2012, Mosby.
14. Harper FW, Nevedal A, Eggly S, et al: "It's up to you and God": understanding health behavior change in older African American survivors of colorectal cancer, *Transl Behav Med* 3:94, 2013.
15. Lopez-Class M, Castro FG, Ramirez AG: Conceptions of acculturation: a review and statement of critical issues, *Soc Sci Med* 72:1555, 2011.

*16. Ramírez A, Rutten L, Oh A, et al: Perceptions of cancer controllability and cancer risk knowledge: the moderating role of race, ethnicity, and acculturation, *J Cancer Educ* 28:254, 2013.

17. Melluish S: Globalization, culture and psychology, *Int Rev Psychiatry* 26:538, 2014.
18. Doutrich D, Arcus K, Dekker L, et al: Cultural safety in New Zealand and the United States. Looking at a way forward together, *J Transcult Nurs* 23:143, 2012.
19. Andrews MM, Boyle JS: *Transcultural concepts in nursing care,* ed 6, Philadelphia, 2012, Lippincott Williams & Wilkins.
20. Douglas MK, Pierce JU, Rosenkoetter M, et al: Standards of practice for culturally competent nursing care: 2011 update, *J Transcult Nurs* 22:317, 2011.
21. Sherwood G, Shaffer F: The role of internationally educated nurses in a quality, safe workforce, *Nurs Outlook* 62:46, 2014.
22. Hall J, Fields B: Continuing the conversation in nursing on race and racism, *Nurs Outlook* 61:164, 2013.
23. CDC: Implementation of new TB screening requirements for U.S.-bound immigrants and refugees—2007-2014. Retrieved from *www.cdc.gov/mmwr/preview/mmwrhtml/mm6311a3.htm.*
24. American Association of Colleges in Nursing: Cultural competency in baccalaureate nursing education. Retrieved from *www.aacn.nche.edu/education-resources/cultural-competency.*
25. Jarvis C: *Physical examination and health assessment,* ed 6, Philadelphia, 2012, Saunders.

*Evidence-based information for clinical practice.

3

Health History and Physical Examination

Jennifer Saylor

Believe in yourself and all that you are. Know that there is something inside you greater than any obstacle.

Christian D. Larson

http://evolve.elsevier.com/Lewis/medsurg/

LEARNING OUTCOMES

1. Explain the purpose, components, and techniques of a patient's health history and physical examination.
2. Obtain a nursing history using a functional health pattern format.
3. Select appropriate techniques of inspection, palpation, percussion, and auscultation for physical examination of a patient.
4. Differentiate among emergency, comprehensive, and focused types of assessment in terms of indications, purposes, and components.

KEY TERMS

auscultation, p. 40
database, p. 34
functional health patterns, p. 35
inspection, p. 39
nursing history, p. 34
objective data, p. 35
palpation, p. 39
percussion, p. 39
subjective data, p. 35

During the assessment phase of the nursing process, you will obtain a patient's health history and perform a physical examination. The findings of your assessment (1) contribute to a database that identifies the patient's current and past health status and (2) provide a baseline against which future changes can be evaluated. The purpose of the nursing assessment is to enable you to make clinical judgments or nursing diagnoses about your patient's health status.[1] Assessment is the first step of the nursing process, but it is performed continually throughout the nursing process to validate nursing diagnoses, evaluate nursing interventions, and determine whether patient outcomes and goals have been met.

The language of assessment is complex, with many overlapping and confusing terms. In this text, *assessment* describes a hands-on data collection process, whereas a database identifies a specific list of information (data) to be collected.

DATA COLLECTION

In the broadest sense, the **database** is all the health information about a patient. This includes the nursing history and physical examination, the medical history and physical examination, results of laboratory and diagnostic tests, and information contributed by other health care providers (HCPs). As a nurse, you and HCPs perform a patient history and a physical examination but use different formats and analyze the data based on each discipline's focus.

Medical Focus

A *medical history* is designed to collect data to be used primarily by the HCP to determine risk for disease and diagnose medical conditions. The medical history is usually collected by a member of the health care team (e.g., physician, advanced practice nurse [APN], resident, physician's assistant, medical student). The HCP's physical examination and diagnostic tests aid in establishing medical diagnoses, effectiveness of previous treatments, and new treatment plan (if indicated). The information collected and reported by the HCP is also used by nurses and other members of the health care team (e.g., pharmacist, physical therapist, dietitian, social worker) based on the focus of their care. For example, the abnormal results of a neurologic examination by an APN may assist in the diagnosis of a stroke. You may use the same results of the neurologic examination to identify a nursing diagnosis of risk for falls. A physical therapist may also use this information to plan therapy involving range-of-motion exercises.

Nursing Focus

The focus of nursing care is the diagnosis and treatment of human responses to actual or potential health problems or life processes. The information obtained from the **nursing history** and physical examination is used to determine the patient's strengths and responses to a health problem. For example, for the patient with a diagnosis of diabetes, the patient's responses

Reviewed by Karen S. Abate, PhD, FNP-BC, Family Nurse Practitioner/Nurse Educator, W. Cary School of Nursing, Thomas Edison State College, Trenton, New Jersey; Janie Corbitt, RN, MLS, Retired Instructor of Nursing, Milledgeville, Georgia; and Misty Hobart, RN, MSN, CNE, Department Chair, Nursing, Spokane Community College, Spokane, Washington.

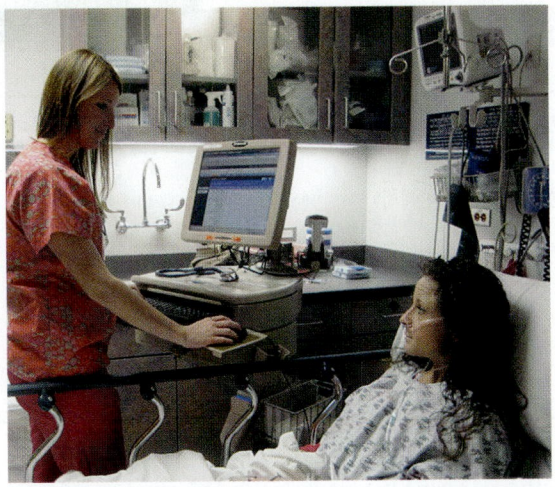

FIG. 3-1 Obtaining and recording data from a nursing history and physical examination using a computer. (Courtesy Linda Bucher, RN, PhD, CEN, CNE, Staff Nurse, Virtua Memorial Hospital, Mt. Holly, N.J.)

may include anxiety or a lack of knowledge about self-management of the condition. This patient may also experience the physical response of fluid volume deficit because of the abnormal fluid loss caused by hyperglycemia. These human responses to the condition of diabetes are diagnosed and treated by nurses. During the nursing history interview and physical examination, you will obtain and record the data to support the identification of nursing diagnoses (Fig. 3-1).

Types of Data

The database includes subjective and objective data. **Subjective data**, also known as *symptoms,* are collected by interviewing the patient and/or caregiver during the nursing history. This type of data includes information that can be described or verified only by the patient or caregiver. It is what the person tells you either spontaneously or in response to a direct question.

Objective data, also known as *signs,* are data that can be observed or measured. You obtain this type of data using inspection, palpation, percussion, and auscultation during the physical examination. Objective data are also acquired by diagnostic testing. Patients will often provide subjective data while you are performing the physical examination. You will also observe objective signs while interviewing the patient. All of the findings related to a specific problem, whether subjective or objective, are known as *clinical manifestations* of that problem.

Interview Considerations

The purpose of the patient interview is to obtain a health history (i.e., subjective data) about the patient's past and present health state. Effective communication is a key factor in the interview process. Creating a climate of trust and respect is critical to establishing a therapeutic relationship.[2] You need to communicate acceptance of the patient as an individual by using an open, responsive, nonjudgmental approach. You communicate not only through language but also in your manner of dress, gestures, and body language. Modes of communication are learned through one's culture and influence: not only the words, gestures, and postures one uses but also the information that is shared with others (see discussion on culture in Chapter 2).

In addition to understanding the principles of effective communication, you have to develop a personal style of relating to patients. Although no single style fits all people, your wording of questions can increase the probability of eliciting the needed information. The ease of asking questions, particularly those related to sensitive areas such as sexual functioning, comes with training and experience.

The amount of time you need to complete a nursing history varies with the format used and your experience. The nursing history may be completed in one or several sessions, depending on the setting and patient. For example, you may have to plan several short sessions for an older adult patient with a low energy level to allow time for the patient to provide the needed information. You must also make a judgment about the amount of information collected on initial contact with the patient. In interviews with patients with chronic disease, patients in pain, and patients in emergency situations, ask only those questions that are pertinent to a specific problem. You can complete the health history interview at a more appropriate time.

Judge the reliability of the patient as a historian. An older adult may give a false impression about his or her mental status because of a prolonged response time or visual and hearing impairments. The complexity and long duration of health problems may make it hard for an older adult or a chronically ill younger patient to be an accurate historian.

It is important for you to determine the patient's priority concerns and expectations, since your priorities may be different from the patient's. For example, your priority may be to complete the health history, whereas the patient is interested only in relief from symptoms. Until the patient's priority need is met, you will probably be unsuccessful in obtaining complete and accurate data.

Symptom Investigation

At any time during the assessment the patient may report a symptom such as pain, fatigue, or weakness. Symptoms experienced by the patient are not observed, so the symptom must be explored. Table 3-1 shows a mnemonic (PQRST) to help you remember the areas to explore if a symptom is reported. The information you receive may help determine the cause of the symptom. A common symptom that you will assess is pain (see Chapter 8). For example, if a patient states that he has "pain in his leg," you would assess and record the data using PQRST.

> Has right midcalf pain that usually occurs at work when climbing stairs after lunch (P). Pain is alleviated by stopping and resting for 2 to 3 minutes. Patient states he has been "eating a banana every day for extra potassium" but "it hasn't helped" (P). Pain is described as "stabbing" and is non-radiating (Q, R). Pain is so severe (rating 9 on 0-10 scale) that patient cannot continue activity (S). Onset is abrupt, occurring once or twice daily. It last occurred yesterday while cutting the lawn (T).

Data Organization

Assessment data must be systematically obtained and organized so that you can readily analyze and make judgments about the patient's health status and any health problems. Some assessment forms are organized using body systems. Although helpful, these types of forms may be incomplete because they omit areas such as health promotion behaviors, sleep, coping, and values.

Functional health patterns, developed by Gordon,[3] provide the framework used throughout this book for obtaining a nursing history. This format includes an initial collection of important health information followed by assessment of 11

TABLE 3-1 Investigation of Patient-Reported Symptom

	Factor	Questions for Patient and Caregiver	Record
P	Precipitating and Palliative	Were there any events that came before the symptom? What makes it better? Worse? What have you done for the symptom? Did this help?	Influence of physical and emotional activities. Patient's attempts to alleviate (or treat) the symptom.
Q	Quality	Tell me what the symptom feels like (e.g., aching, dull, pressure, burning, stabbing).	Patient's own words (e.g., "Like a pinch or stabbing feeling").
R	Radiation	Where do you feel the symptom? Does it move to other areas?	Region of body. Local or radiating, superficial or deep.
S	Severity	On a scale of 0-10, with 0 meaning no pain and 10 being the worst pain you could imagine, what number would you give your symptom?	Pain rating number (e.g., 5/10).
T	Timing	When did the symptom start? Any particular time of day, week, month, or year? Has the symptom changed over time? Where are you and what are you doing when the symptom occurs?	Time of onset, duration, periodicity, and frequency. Course of symptoms. Where patient is and what patient is doing when the symptom occurs.

TEAMWORK & COLLABORATION

Assessment and Data Collection

Ongoing data collection is expected of all members of the health care team. In acute care the initial (admission) nursing assessment must be completed by a registered nurse (RN) and within the timeframe determined by the agency.

Role of Nursing Personnel

Role of Registered Nurse (RN)

- On admission, complete a comprehensive assessment (Table 3-4).
- Obtain patient's health history by interviewing patient and/or caregiver.
- Perform physical examination using inspection, palpation, percussion, and auscultation as appropriate.
- Document findings from the health history and physical examination in the patient's record.
- Organize patient data into functional health patterns, if appropriate (Table 3-2).
- Develop and prioritize nursing diagnoses and collaborative problems for the patient.
- Throughout hospitalization, perform focused assessments based on patient's history or clinical manifestations (Table 3-7).

Role of Licensed Practical/Vocational Nurse (LPN/LVN)

- Collect and document specific patient data as delegated by the RN (after the RN has developed the plan of care based on the admission assessment).
- Perform focused assessment based on patient's history, clinical manifestations, or as instructed by the RN (Table 3-7).

Role of Unlicensed Assistive Personnel (UAP)

- Take and record vital signs, including oxygen saturation.
- Report abnormal findings to RN.
- Measure and document patient's height and weight, oral intake and output.
- Report patient's subjective complaints to RN.
- Per agency policy, perform point-of-care testing (e.g., glucose) and report findings to RN.

areas of health status or function (Table 3-2). Data organized in this format allow for the identification of areas of wellness (or positive function) as well as health problems.[2]

Culturally Competent Care: Assessment

The process of obtaining a health history and performing a physical examination is an intimate experience for you and the patient. As noted earlier in the chapter, one's culture influences patterns of communication and what information is shared with others. During the interview and physical examination, be sensitive to issues of eye contact, space, modesty, and touching, as discussed in Chapter 2. Knowing the cultural norms related to male-female relationships is especially important during the physical examination. To avoid violating any culturally based practices, ask the patient about cultural values. Determine if the patient would like to have someone present during the history or physical examination or someone of the same gender to perform the history and physical examination.[1]

NURSING HISTORY: SUBJECTIVE DATA

Important Health Information

Important health information provides an overview of past and present medical conditions and treatments. Past health history, medications, allergies, and surgery or other treatments are included in this part of the history.

Past Health History. The past health history provides information about the patient's prior state of health. Ask the patient about major childhood and adult illnesses, injuries, hospitalizations, and surgeries. Specific questions are more effective than simply asking whether the patient has had any illness or health problems in the past. For example, asking "Do you have a history of diabetes?" elicits better information than asking "Do you have any chronic health problems?"

Medications. Ask the patient for specific details related to past and current medications, including prescription and illicit drugs, over-the-counter drugs, vitamins, herbs, and dietary supplements. Patients frequently do not consider herbs and dietary supplements as drugs. It is important to specifically ask about their use because they can interact adversely with existing or newly prescribed medications (Complementary & Alternative Therapies box).

Question older adult and chronically ill patients about medication routines. Polypharmacy, including medication costs and changes in absorption, metabolism, and elimination of drugs can pose serious potential problems for these patients.[4]

Allergies. Fully explore the patient's history of allergies to drugs, latex, contrast media, food, and the environment (e.g., pollen). Include a detailed description of any allergic reaction(s) reported by the patient.

Surgery or Other Treatments. Record all surgeries, along with the date of the event, reason for the surgery, and outcome. The outcome includes whether the problem was completely resolved or has residual effects. Be sure to ask about and record any blood products that the patient has received.

TABLE 3-2 Health History

Functional Health Pattern Format

Demographic Data

Name, address, age, occupation, gender
Race, ethnicity, culture, spirituality

Important Health Information

Past health history
Medications, supplements
Allergies
Surgery or other treatments

Health Perception–Health Management Pattern

1. Reason for visit?
2. General state of health?
3. Most important things done to keep healthy? Testicular self-examination? Colorectal cancer, hypertension, and cardiac disease risk screening? Papanicolaou (Pap) test? Immunizations such as tetanus, pneumonia, hepatitis, and flu vaccines?
4. Who is your primary health care provider?
5. Health adherence problems?
6. Cause of illness? Action taken? Results?
7. Things important to you while here?
8. Family health history (e.g., cardiovascular disease, hypertension, cancer, diabetes, psychiatric illness, genetic disorders)?
9. Illness and injury risk factors (e.g., sexual abuse, intimate partner abuse, violence, use of tobacco or alcohol, substance abuse)?

Nutritional-Metabolic Pattern

1. Typical daily food intake (describe)? Supplements?
2. Typical daily fluid intake (describe)?
3. Weight loss or gain (amount, time span, intentional)?
4. Desired weight?
5. Appetite?
6. Food or eating: Discomfort? Diet restrictions?
7. Change in appetite with anxiety?
8. Heal well or poorly?
9. Skin problems: Lesions? Dryness?
10. Dentition: Dental problems? Well-fitting dentures?
11. Food preferences?
12. Food allergies?

Elimination Pattern

1. Bowel elimination pattern (describe): Frequency? Character? Discomfort? Laxatives? Enemas?
2. Urinary elimination pattern (describe): Frequency? Problem in control? Diuretics?
3. Any external devices?
4. Excess perspiration? Odor problems? Itching?

Activity-Exercise Pattern

1. Sufficient energy for desired or required activities?
2. Exercise pattern? Type? Regularity?
3. Spare time (leisure) activities?
4. Dyspnea? Chest pain? Palpitations? Stiffness? Aching? At rest? With activity?
5. Perceived ability for (rate Functional Level 0-III for each):
   Eating __ Cooking __ Grooming __
   Transfer (e.g., bed to chair) __ Toileting __
   Bathing __Dressing __ Shopping __ General mobility __

   Functional Levels
   Level 0: Full self-care
   Level I: Requires use of equipment or device
   Level II: Requires assistance or supervision from another person
   Level III: Is dependent and does not participate

Sleep-Rest Pattern

1. Generally rested and ready for daily activities after sleep?
2. Sleep onset problems? Aids (e.g., drugs, CPAP)? Dreams (nightmares)? Early awakening?
3. Usual sleep rituals?
4. Usual sleep pattern?

Cognitive-Perceptual Pattern

1. Hearing impairment? Hearing aids?
2. Vision? Wear glasses? Wear contact lens? Last checked?
3. Any change in taste? Any change in smell?
4. Any recent change in memory?
5. Easiest way to learn things?
6. Any discomfort? Pain (rating on scale of 0-10)? How managed?
7. Ability to communicate (e.g., primary language)?
8. Understanding of illness?
9. Understanding of treatments?

Self-Perception–Self-Concept Pattern

1. Self-description? Self-perception?
2. Effect of illness on self-image?

Role-Relationship Pattern

1. Live alone? Family/caregiver? Family structure?
2. Family problems?
3. Family problem solving?
4. Family dependence on you for things? How managing?
5. Family's and others' feelings about illness or hospitalization?*
6. Problems with children? Difficulty handling?*
7. Belong to social groups? Have close friends? Feel lonely (frequency)?
8. Work (school) satisfaction? Income sufficient for needs?*
9. Feel part of or isolated from neighborhood where living?

Sexuality-Reproductive Pattern

1. Any changes or problems in sexual relations?*
2. Effect of illness?
3. Use of contraceptives? Problems?
4. When menstruation started? Last menstrual period? Menstrual problems? Gravida? Para?†
5. Effect of present condition or treatment on sexuality?
6. Sexually transmitted infections?

Coping–Stress Tolerance Pattern

1. Tense a lot of the time? What helps? Use any drugs, alcohol?
2. Have someone to confide in? Available to you now?
3. Recent life changes?
4. Problem-solving techniques? Effective?

Value-Belief Pattern

1. Satisfied with life?
2. Religion important in your life?
3. Conflict between treatment and beliefs?

Modified from Gordon M: *Manual of nursing diagnosis*, ed 13, Boston, 2014, Jones & Bartlett.
CPAP, Continuous positive airway pressure.
*If appropriate.
†For women.

COMPLEMENTARY & ALTERNATIVE THERAPIES

Assessment of Use of Herbs and Dietary Supplements

Why Assessment Is Important

- Herbs and dietary supplements may have side effects or may interact adversely with prescription or OTC drugs.
- Patients at high risk for drug-herb interactions include those taking anticoagulant, antihypertensive, antidepressant, or immune-regulating therapy and patients undergoing anesthesia. Most herbs must be discontinued 2 to 3 weeks before surgery.
- Many patients do not tell health care providers (HCPs) that they are using herbs and dietary supplements. They may fear HCPs will disapprove of their use.
- Many herbal preparations contain a variety of ingredients. Ask the patient or caregiver to bring labeled containers to the health care site to determine the composition of the products.

Nurse's Role

- Patients typically share information about the use of herbs and dietary supplements with you if they are specifically asked.
- Create an accepting and nonjudgmental attitude when assessing use or interest in herbs or dietary supplements.
- Use open-ended questions such as, "What types of herbs, vitamins, or supplements do you take?" and "What effects have you noticed from using them?"
- Document the use of any herb(s) or dietary supplements in the patient record, including the name, amount, frequency of use, and any side effects.
- Inform patients of the following:
  - Risks and benefits associated with herbal use, including drug-herb interactions
  - Employees of health food stores are not licensed HCPs
  - Importance of carefully reading the labels of herbal therapies and dietary supplements and only taking the recommended amount
  - Moisture, sunlight, and heat may change the components of herbs
  - Many herbal therapies have side effects and these should be reported immediately to the HCP

Functional Health Patterns

Assess the patient's functional health patterns to identify positive, dysfunctional, and potential dysfunctional health patterns. *Dysfunctional health patterns* result in nursing diagnoses, and *potential dysfunctional patterns* identify risk conditions for problems. In addition, you may identify patients with effective health function who express a desire for a higher level of wellness. Examples of possible questions to ask the patient related to the functional health patterns are presented in Table 3-2.

Health Perception–Health Management Pattern. Assessment of the health perception–health management functional health pattern focuses on the patient's perceived level of health and well-being and on personal practices for maintaining health. Ask the patient to describe his or her personal health and any concerns about it. Explore the patient's feelings of effectiveness at staying healthy by asking what helps and what hinders his or her well-being. Ask the patient to rate his or her health as excellent, good, fair, or poor. When possible, record this information in the patient's own words.

Next, ask about the type of HCP the patient uses. For example, if the patient is Native American, a medicine man may be considered the primary HCP. If the patient is of Hispanic origin, a *curandero* (Hispanic healer who uses folk medicine and herbs to treat patients) may be the primary HCP (see Chapter 2).

The questions for this pattern also seek to identify risk factors by obtaining a thorough family history (e.g., cardiac disease, cancer, genetic disorders), history of personal health habits (e.g., tobacco, alcohol, drug use), and history of exposure to environmental hazards (e.g., asbestos). If the patient is hospitalized, ask about the expectations for this experience. Have the patient describe his or her understanding of the current health problem, including its onset, course, and treatment. These questions obtain information about a patient's knowledge of the health problem and ability to use appropriate resources to manage the problem.

Nutritional-Metabolic Pattern. The processes of ingestion, digestion, absorption, and metabolism are assessed in this pattern. Obtain a 24-hour diet recall from the patient to evaluate the quantity and quality of foods and fluids consumed. If a problem is identified, ask the patient to keep a 3-day food diary for a more careful analysis of dietary intake. Assess the impact of psychologic factors such as depression, anxiety, stress, and self-concept on nutrition. Additionally, determine socioeconomic and cultural factors such as food budget, who prepares the meals, and food preferences. Determine whether the patient's present condition has interfered with eating and appetite by exploring any symptoms of nausea, intestinal gas, or pain. Food allergies should be differentiated from food intolerances, such as lactose or gluten intolerance.

Elimination Pattern. Assess bowel, bladder, and skin function in this pattern. Ask the patient about the frequency of bowel and bladder activity, including laxative and diuretic use. The skin is assessed in the elimination pattern in terms of its excretory function.

Activity-Exercise Pattern. Assess the patient's usual pattern of exercise, work activity, leisure, and recreation. Question the patient about his or her ability to perform activities of daily living and note any specific problems. Table 3-2 includes a scale for rating the functional levels of common activities.

Sleep-Rest Pattern. This pattern describes the patient's perception of his or her pattern of sleep, rest, and relaxation in a 24-hour period. This information can be elicited by asking, "Do you feel rested when you wake up?"

Cognitive-Perceptual Pattern. Assessing this pattern involves a description of all of the senses and cognitive functions. In addition, assess pain as a sensory perception in this pattern. (See Chapter 8 for details on pain assessment.) Ask the patient about any sensory deficits that affect the ability to perform activities of daily living. Record ways in which the patient compensates for any sensory-perceptual problems. To plan for patient teaching, ask the patient how he or she communicates best and what he or she understands about the illness and treatment plan. (See Chapter 4 for details on patient teaching.)

Self-Perception–Self-Concept Pattern. This pattern describes the patient's self-concept, which is critical in determining the way the person interacts with others. Included are attitudes about self, perception of personal abilities, body image, and general sense of worth. Ask the patient for a self-description and about how his or her health condition affects self-concept. Patients' expressions of hopelessness or loss of control frequently reflect an inability to care for oneself.

Role-Relationship Pattern. This pattern reveals the patient's roles and relationships, including major responsibilities. Ask the patient to describe family, social, and work roles and relationships and to rate his or her performance of the expected behaviors related to these. Determine whether patterns in these roles and relationships are satisfactory or whether strain is evident. Note the patient's feelings about how the present condition affects his or her roles and relationships.

Sexuality-Reproductive Pattern. This pattern describes satisfaction or dissatisfaction with personal sexuality and describes reproductive issues. Assessing this pattern is important because many illnesses, surgical procedures, and drugs affect sexual function. A patient's sexual and reproductive concerns may be expressed and teaching needs may be identified through information obtained in this pattern.

Obtaining information related to sexuality may be difficult for you. However, it is important to take a health history and screen for sexual function and dysfunction in a nonjudgmental way and provide information as appropriate, or refer the patient to a more experienced HCP.

Coping–Stress Tolerance Pattern. This pattern describes the patient's general coping pattern and the effectiveness of the coping mechanisms. Assessment of this pattern involves analyzing the specific stressors or problems that confront the patient, the patient's perception of the stressors, and the patient's response to the stressors. Document any major losses or stressors experienced by the patient in the previous year. Note strategies used by the patient to deal with stressors and relieve tension. Ask about individuals and groups that make up the patient's social support networks.

Value-Belief Pattern. This pattern describes the values, goals, and beliefs (including spiritual) that guide health-related choices. Document the patient's ethnic background and effects of culture and beliefs on health practices. Note and respect the patient's wishes about continuation of religious or spiritual practices and the use of religious articles.

PHYSICAL EXAMINATION: OBJECTIVE DATA

General Survey

After the nursing history, make a *general survey statement.* This is your general impression of a patient, including behavioral observations. This initial survey begins with your first encounter with the patient and continues during the health history interview.

Although you may include other data that seem pertinent, the major areas included in the general survey statement are (1) body features, (2) mental state, (3) speech, (4) body movements, (5) obvious physical signs, (6) nutritional status, and (7) behavior. Vital signs and body mass index (BMI) (calculated from height and weight [kg/m^2]) may be included. The following is a sample of a general survey statement:

> A.H. is a 34-year-old Hispanic woman, BP 130/84, P 88, R 18. No distinguishing body features. Alert but anxious. Speech rapid with trailing thoughts. Wringing hands and shuffling feet during interview. Skin flushed, hands clammy. Overweight relative to height (BMI = 28.3 kg/m^2). Sits with eyes downcast and shoulders slumped and avoids eye contact.

Physical Examination

The *physical examination* is the systematic assessment of a patient's physical status. Throughout the physical examination, explore any positive findings using the same criteria used during the investigation of a symptom in the nursing history (Table 3-1). A *positive finding* indicates that the patient has or has had the particular problem or sign under discussion (e.g., if the patient with jaundice has an enlarged liver, it is a positive finding). Relevant information about this problem should then be gathered.

Negative findings may also be significant. A pertinent *negative finding* is the absence of a sign or symptom usually associated with a problem. For example, peripheral edema is common with advanced liver disease. If edema is not present in a patient with advanced liver disease, specifically note this as "no peripheral edema."

Techniques. Four major techniques are used in performing the physical examination: inspection, palpation, percussion, and auscultation. The techniques are usually performed in this sequence, except for the abdominal examination (inspection, auscultation, percussion, and palpation). Performing percussion and palpation of the abdomen before auscultation can alter bowel sounds and produce false findings. Not every assessment area requires the use of all four assessment techniques (e.g., musculoskeletal system requires only inspection and palpation).

Inspection. **Inspection** is the visual examination of a part or region of the body to assess normal conditions or deviations. Inspection is more than just looking. This technique is deliberate, systematic, and focused. Compare what is seen with the known, generally visible characteristics of the body part that you are inspecting. For example, most 30-year-old men have hair on their legs. Absence of hair may indicate a vascular problem and the need for further investigation, or it may be normal for a patient of a particular ethnicity (e.g., Filipino men have little body hair). Always compare one side of the patient's body to the other to assess bilaterally for any abnormal findings.

Palpation. **Palpation** is the examination of the body using touch. Using light and deep palpation can yield information related to masses, pulsations, organ enlargement, tenderness or pain, swelling, muscular spasm or rigidity, elasticity, vibration of voice sounds, crepitus, moisture, and texture. Different parts of the hand are more sensitive for specific assessments. For example, use the palmar surface (base of fingers) to feel vibrations, the dorsa (backs) of your hands and fingers to assess skin temperature, and tips of your fingers to palpate the abdomen[1] (Fig. 3-2).

Percussion. **Percussion** is a technique that produces a sound and vibration to obtain information about the underlying

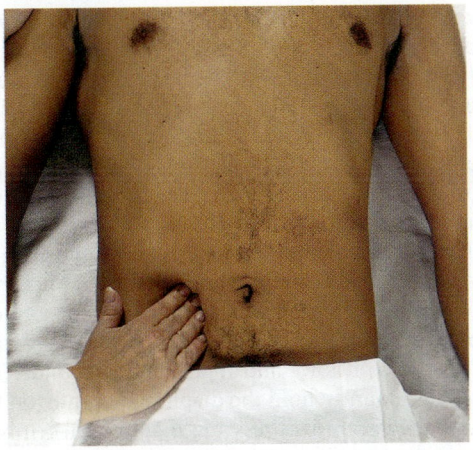

FIG. 3-2 Palpation is the examination of the body using touch. (From Jarvis C: *Physical examination and health assessment,* ed 6, St Louis, 2012, Saunders.)

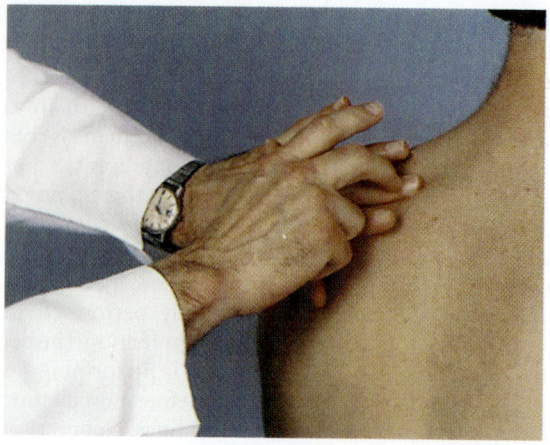

FIG. 3-3 Percussion technique. Tapping the interphalangeal joint. Only the middle finger of the nondominant hand should be in contact with the skin surface. Normal percussion sounds: *resonant*—lung tissue; *tympany*—air-filled viscus (e.g., intestines); *dull*—dense organs (e.g., liver); *flat*—no air present (e.g., bone, muscle). (Modified from Seidel HM, Ball JW, Dains JE, et al: *Mosby's guide to physical examination*, ed 7, St Louis, 2011, Saunders.)

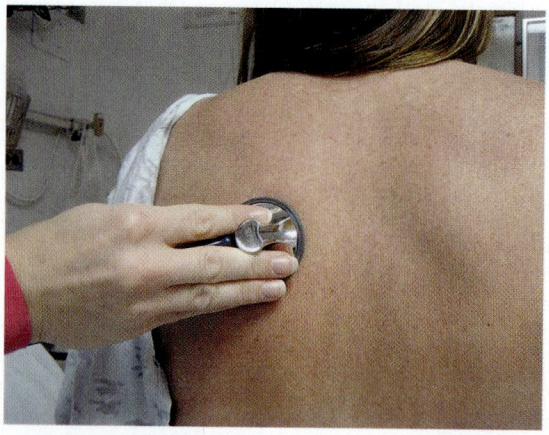

FIG. 3-4 Auscultation is listening to sounds produced by the body to assess normal conditions and deviations from normal. (Courtesy Linda Bucher, RN, PhD, CEN, CNE, Staff Nurse, Virtua Memorial Hospital, Mt. Holly, N.J.)

area (Fig. 3-3). The sounds and vibrations are relative to the underlying structures. A change from an expected sound may indicate a problem (Fig. 3-3). For example, dullness in the right lower quadrant instead of the normal sound of tympany should be explored. (Specific percussion sounds of various body parts and regions are discussed in the appropriate assessment chapters.)

Auscultation. **Auscultation** is listening to sounds produced by the body with a stethoscope to assess normal conditions and deviations from normal. This technique is particularly useful in evaluating sounds from the heart, lungs, abdomen, and vascular system. The bell of the stethoscope is more sensitive to low-pitched sounds (e.g., heart murmurs). The diaphragm of the stethoscope is more sensitive to high-pitched sounds (e.g., bowel sounds). Some stethoscopes have only a diaphragm, designed to transmit low- and high-pitched sounds. To listen for low-pitched sounds, hold the diaphragm lightly on the skin. For high-pitched sounds, press the diaphragm firmly on the skin[1] (Fig. 3-4). (Specific auscultatory sounds and techniques are discussed in the appropriate assessment chapters.)

TABLE 3-3 Equipment for Physical Examination*

- Alcohol swabs
- Blood pressure cuff
- Cotton balls
- Examining table or bed
- Eye chart (e.g., Snellen eye chart)
- Paper cup with water
- Patient gown
- Pocket flashlight
- Reflex hammer
- Stethoscope (with bell and diaphragm or a dual-purpose diaphragm; tubing 15-18 inches [38-46 cm])
- Tongue blades
- Watch (with second hand or digital)

*These are examples of commonly used equipment; other equipment may be used depending on the situation.

Equipment. Collect the equipment needed for the physical examination before you begin (Table 3-3). This saves time and energy for you and the patient. (The uses of specific equipment are discussed in the appropriate assessment chapters.)

Organization of Examination. Perform the physical examination systematically and efficiently. Provide explanations to the patient as the examination proceeds and consider the patient's comfort, safety, and privacy. If you follow the same sequence every time, you are less likely to forget a procedure, a step in the sequence, or a portion of the body. Table 3-4 presents a comprehensive and organized physical examination outline.

Adaptations of the physical examination are often useful for the older adult patient, who may have age-related problems such as decreased mobility, limited energy, and perceptual changes.[5] An outline listing some of the useful adaptations is found in Table 3-5.

Recording Physical Examination. At the conclusion of the examination, record the normal and abnormal findings in the patient's record. See Table 3-6 for an example of how to record findings of a normal physical examination of a healthy adult. See Table 5-5 to locate age-related assessment findings in the book.

TYPES OF ASSESSMENT

Various types of assessment are used to obtain information about a patient. These approaches can be divided into three types: emergency, comprehensive, and focused (Table 3-7). You need to decide what type of assessment to perform based on the clinical situation. Sometimes the health care agency provides guidelines, and other times it is a nursing judgment.

Emergency Assessment

In an emergency or life-threatening situation an *emergency assessment* may be done. This involves a rapid history and examination of a patient while maintaining vital functions.

Comprehensive Assessment

A *comprehensive assessment* includes a detailed health history and physical examination of all body systems. This is typically done on admission to the hospital or onset of care in a primary care setting.

Focused Assessment

A *focused assessment* is an abbreviated health history and examination. It is used to evaluate the status of previously

TABLE 3-4 Outline for Physical Examination

1. General Survey

Observe general state of health (patient is seated).

- Body features
- Mental state and level of orientation
- Speech
- Body movements
- Physical appearance
- Nutritional status
- Behavior

2. Vital Signs

Record vital signs.

- Blood pressure—both arms for comparison
- Apical/radial pulse
- Respiration
- Temperature
- Oxygen saturation

Record height and weight; calculate body mass index (BMI).

3. Integument

Inspect and palpate skin for the following:

- Color
- Integrity (e.g., lacerations, lesions, breakdown)
- Scars, tattoos, piercings
- Bruises, rash
- Edema
- Moisture
- Texture
- Temperature
- Turgor
- Vascularity

Inspect and palpate nails for the following:

- Color
- Lesions
- Size
- Shape
- Angle
- Capillary refill time

4. Head and Neck

Inspect and palpate head for the following:

- Shape and symmetry of skull
- Masses
- Tenderness
- Condition of hair and scalp
- Temporal arteries
- Temporomandibular joint
- Sensory (CN V, light touch, pain)
- Motor (CN VII, shows teeth, purses lips, raises eyebrows)
- Looks up, wrinkles forehead (CN VII)
- Raises shoulders against resistance (CN XI)

Inspect and palpate (occasionally auscultate) neck for the following:

- Skin (vascularity and visible pulsations)
- Symmetry
- Range of motion
- Pulses and bruits (carotid)
- Midline structure (trachea, thyroid gland, cartilage)
- Lymph nodes (preauricular, postauricular, occipital, mandibular, tonsillar, submental, anterior and posterior cervical, infraclavicular, supraclavicular)

Test visual acuity.

Inspect and lightly palpate eyes/eyebrows for the following:

- Position and movement of eyelids (CN VII)
- Visual fields (CN II)
- Extraocular movements (CN III, IV, VI)
- Cornea, sclera, conjunctiva
- Pupillary response (CN III)
- Red reflex*

Inspect and palpate nose and sinuses for the following:

- External nose: shape, blockage
- Internal nose: patency of nasal passages, shape, turbinates or polyps, discharge
- Frontal and maxillary sinuses

Inspect and palpate ears for the following:

- Placement
- Pinna
- Auditory acuity (whispered voice, ticking watch) (CN VIII)
- Mastoid process
- Auditory canal
- Tympanic membrane

Inspect and palpate mouth for the following:

- Lips (symmetry, lesions, color)
- Buccal mucosa (Stensen's and Wharton's ducts)
- Teeth (absence, state of repair, color)
- Gums (color, receding from teeth)
- Tongue for strength (asymmetry, ability to stick out tongue, side to side, fasciculations) (CN XII)
- Palates
- Tonsils and pillars
- Uvular elevation (CN IX)
- Posterior pharynx
- Gag reflex (CN IX and X)
- Jaw strength (CN V)
- Moisture
- Color
- Floor of mouth

5. Extremities

Observe size and shape, symmetry and deformity, involuntary movements. Inspect and palpate arms, fingers, wrists, elbows, shoulders for the following:

- Strength
- Range of motion
- Joint pain
- Swelling
- Pulses (radial, brachial)
- Sensation (light touch, pain, temperature)
- Test reflexes: triceps, biceps, brachioradialis

Inspect and palpate legs for the following:

- Strength
- Range of motion
- Joint pain
- Swelling, edema
- Hair distribution
- Sensation (light touch, pain, temperature)
- Pulses (dorsalis pedis, posterior tibialis)
- Test reflexes: patellar, Achilles, plantar

6. Posterior Thorax

Inspect for muscular development, scoliosis, respiratory movement, approximation of AP diameter.

- Palpate for symmetry of respiratory movement, tenderness of CVA, spinous processes, tumors or swelling, tactile fremitus
- Percuss for pulmonary resonance
- Auscultate for breath sounds
- Auscultate for egophony, bronchophony, and whispered pectoriloquy

7. Anterior Thorax

- Assess breasts for configuration, symmetry, dimpling of skin
- Assess nipples for rash, direction, inversion, retraction
- Inspect for apical impulse, other precordial pulsations
- Palpate the apical impulse and the precordium for thrills, lifts, heaves, tenderness
- Inspect neck for venous distention, pulsations, waves
- Palpate lymph nodes in the subclavian, axillary, and brachial areas
- Palpate breasts
- Auscultate for rate and rhythm; character of S_1 and S_2 in the aortic, pulmonic, Erb's point, tricuspid, mitral areas; bruits at carotid, epigastrium

Continued

TABLE 3-4 Outline for Physical Examination—cont'd

8. Abdomen

- Inspect for scars, shape, symmetry, bulging, muscular position and condition of umbilicus, movements (respiratory, pulsations, presence of peristaltic waves)
- Auscultate for peristalsis (i.e., bowel sounds), bruits
- Percuss then palpate to confirm positive findings; check liver (size, tenderness), spleen, kidney (size, tenderness), urinary bladder (distention)
- Palpate femoral pulses, inguinofemoral nodes, and abdominal aorta

9. Neurologic

Observe motor status.

- Gait
- Toe walk
- Heel walk
- Drift

Observe coordination:

- Finger to nose
- Romberg sign
- Heel to opposite shin

Observe the following:

- Proprioception (position sense of great toe)

10. Genitalia*

Male External Genitalia

- Inspect penis, noting hair distribution, prepuce, glans, urethral meatus, scars, ulcers, eruptions, structural alterations, discharge
- Inspect epidermis of perineum, rectum
- Inspect skin of scrotum; palpate for descended testes, masses, pain

Female External Genitalia

- Inspect hair distribution; mons pubis, labia (minora and majora); urethral meatus; Bartholin's, urethral, Skene's glands (may also be palpated, if indicated); introitus; any discharge
- Assess for presence of cystocele, prolapse
- Inspect perineum, rectum

AP, Anteroposterior; *CN,* cranial nerve; *CVA,* costovertebral angle.
*If the nurse has the appropriate education, additional techniques can be performed. A retinal reflex examination (red reflex) would be performed with the eye examination. Speculum and bimanual examination of women and the prostate gland examination of men would be performed after inspection of genitalia. Examination of the genitalia may require a second person to be present in the room.

TABLE 3-5 Gerontologic Assessment Differences

Adaptations in Physical Assessment Techniques

General Approach

Keep patient warm and comfortable because loss of subcutaneous fat decreases ability to stay warm. Adapt positioning to physical limitations. Avoid unnecessary changes in position. Perform as many activities as possible in the position of comfort for the patient.

Skin

Handle with care because of fragility and loss of subcutaneous fat.

Head and Neck

Provide a quiet environment free from distraction because of possible sensory impairments (e.g., decreased vision, hearing).

Extremities

Use gentle movements and reinforcement techniques. Avoid having patient hop on one foot or perform deep knee bends if patient has limited range of motion of the extremities, decreased reflexes, or diminished sense of balance.

Thorax

Adapt examination for changes related to decreased force of expiration, weakened cough reflex, and shortness of breath.

Abdomen

Use caution in palpating patient's liver because it is readily accessible because of a thinner, softer abdominal wall. The older adult patient may have diminished pain perception in the abdominal wall.

identified problems and monitor for signs and symptoms of new problems. It can be done when a specific problem (e.g., pneumonia) is identified. The patient's clinical manifestations should alert you to the appropriate focused assessment. For example, abdominal pain indicates the need for a focused assessment of the abdomen. Some problems require a focused assessment of more than one body system. A complaint of headache may indicate the need to do musculoskeletal, neurologic, and head and neck examinations. Examples of focused assessments for the various body systems can be found in each assessment chapter of this book.

Using Assessment Approaches

Assessment in a hospital inpatient setting, particularly in acute care, is markedly different from assessment in other settings. Focused assessment of the hospitalized patient is frequent and performed by many different people. Such a team approach demands a high degree of consistency among different HCPs.

As you provide ongoing care for a patient, you will be constantly refining your mental image of the patient. As you gain experience, you will form a mental image of a patient's status from a few basic details, such as "85-year-old African American woman admitted for COPD exacerbation." Your picture of her becomes clearer as you receive a more complete verbal report, such as length of stay, laboratory results, physical findings, and vital signs. Next, perform your own assessment using a focused approach. During your assessment, you will confirm or revise the findings that you read in the medical record and what you heard from other HCPs.

Keep in mind that the process does not end once you have done your first assessment on a patient during your rounds. You will continue to gather information about all your patients throughout your shift. Everything that you learned previously about each patient is considered in the light of new information. For example, when you are doing a respiratory assessment on your patient with COPD, you hear crackles in her lungs. This finding should lead you to do a cardiovascular assessment because cardiac problems (e.g., heart failure) can also cause crackles. As you gain experience, the importance of new findings will be more obvious to you. Assessment case studies are integrated into all of the assessment chapters for this book to help you develop your assessment skills and knowledge.

Table 3-8 shows how you can perform different types of assessments based on a patient's progress through a given hospitalization. When a patient arrives at the emergency

TABLE 3-6 Findings From a Physical Examination of a Healthy Adult

Example

General Status
Well-nourished, well-hydrated, well-developed white (woman) or (man) in NAD, appears stated age, speech clear and evenly paced; is alert and oriented ×3; cooperative, calm; BMI 23.8

Skin
Clear s̄ lesions, warm and dry, trunk warmer than extremities, normal skin turgor, no ↑ vascularity, no varicose veins

Nails
Well-groomed, round 160-degree angle s̄ lesions, nail beds pink, capillary refill <2 sec

Hair
Thick, brown, shiny, normal (male, female) distribution

Head
Normocephalic, nontender

Eyes
Visual fields intact on gross confrontation
Visual acuity: Right eye 20/20
Left eye 20/20
Both eyes 20/20
s̄ glasses
EOM: Intact on all gazes s̄ ptosis, nystagmus
Pupils: PERRLA, negative cover and uncover tests

Ears
Pinna intact, in proper alignment; external canal patent; small amount of cerumen present bilaterally; TMs intact; pearly gray LM, LR visible, not bulging; whisper heard at 3 ft bilaterally

Nose
Patent bilaterally; turbinates pink, no swelling
Sinuses nontender

Mouth
Moist and pink, soft and hard palates intact, uvula rises midline on "ahh," 24 teeth present and in good repair

Throat
Tonsils surgically removed, no redness

Tongue
Moist, pink, size appropriate for mouth, no lesions

Neck
Supple, s̄ masses, s̄ bruits, lymph nodes nonpalpable and nontender
Thyroid: Palpable, smooth, not enlarged
ROM: Full, intact strong
Trachea: Midline, nontender

Breasts
Soft, nonpendulous, s̄ venous pattern, s̄ dimpling, puckering
Nipples: s̄ inversion, point in same direction, areola dark and symmetric, no discharge, no masses, nontender

Axilla
Hair present, no lesions, no palpable lymph nodes

Thorax and Lungs
Respiratory rate 18, regular rhythm, oxygen saturation 98% on room air; AP < transverse diameter, no ↑ in tactile fremitus, no tenderness, lungs resonant throughout, diaphragmatic excursion 4 cm bilaterally, chest expansion symmetric, lung fields clear throughout

Heart
Rate 82, regular rate and rhythm; blood pressure: RA: 122/76, LA: 120/78; no lifts, heaves
Apical impulse: 5th ICS at MCL; no palpable thrills; S_1, S_2 louder, softer in appropriate locations; no S_3, S_4; no murmurs, rubs, clicks
Carotid, femoral, pedal, and radial pulses present; equal, 2+ bilaterally

Abdomen
No pulsations visible, rounded, positive bowel sounds in four quadrants, no bruits or CVA tenderness, no palpable masses

Liver
Lower border percussed at costal margin, smooth, nontender; approx. 9-cm span

Spleen
Nonpalpable, nontender

Neurologic System
Cranial nerves I-XII intact
Motor (drift, toe stand) intact
Coordination (FN, Romberg) intact
Reflexes: *See diagram*

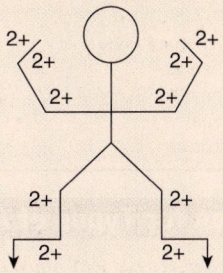

Grading Scale
0 No response
1+ Diminished
2+ Normal
3+ Increased
4+ Hyperactive
Sensation (touch, vibration, proprioception) normal bilaterally, upper and lower extremities

Musculoskeletal System
Well developed, no muscle wasting; s̄ crepitus, nodules, swelling; no scoliosis
ROM: Full and equal bilaterally, upper and lower extremities
Strength: Equal, strong 5/5 bilaterally, upper and lower extremities
Gait: Walks erect 2-foot steps, arms swinging at side s̄ staggering

Continued

TABLE 3-6 Findings From a Physical Examination of a Healthy Adult

Example—cont'd

Female Genitalia*	Male Genitalia*
External genitalia: No swelling, redness, tenderness in BUS; normal hair distribution, no cysts Vagina: No lesions, discharge; bulging, pink Cervix: Os closed; pink, no lesions, erosions, nontender Uterus: Small, firm, nontender Adnexa: No enlargement; nontender Rectovaginal: Sphincter intact; confirms above findings	Normal male hair distribution, negative inguinal hernia Penis: Urethral opening patent; no redness, swelling, discharge; no lesions, structural alterations Scrotum: Testes descended; no redness, masses, tenderness Rectal: No lesions, redness; sphincter intact; prostate small, nontender

AP, Anterior-posterior; *BMI,* body mass index; *BUS,* Bartholin's gland, urethral meatus, Skene's duct; *CVA,* costovertebral angle; *EOM,* extraocular movements; *FN,* finger to nose; *ICS,* intercostal space; *LA,* left arm; *LM,* landmarks; *LR,* light reflex; *MCL,* midclavicular line; *NAD,* no acute distress; *PERRLA,* pupils equal, round, reactive to light and accommodation; *RA,* right arm; *ROM,* range of motion; $\bar{s}$, without; S_1, S_2, S_3, and S_4, heart sounds; *TM,* tympanic membrane.
*These data would be obtained from an examination of the genitalia if the nurse has the appropriate education.

TABLE 3-7 Types of Assessment

The following describes types of assessment that you may use in various situations.

Description	When and Where Performed	Where to Find in Book
Emergency • Limited to assessing life-threatening conditions (e.g., inhalation injuries, anaphylaxis, myocardial infarction, shock, stroke) • Conducted to ensure survival. Focuses on elements in primary survey (e.g., airway, breathing, circulation, disability) • After life-saving interventions are initiated, perform brief systematic assessment to identify any and all other injuries or problems	• Performed in any setting when signs or symptoms of a life-threatening condition appear (e.g., emergency department, critical care unit, surgical setting)	• Chapter 68, Table 68-3 and Table 68-5 • Emergency management tables throughout the book and listed in Table 68-1
Comprehensive • Detailed assessment of all body systems (head-to-toe assessment)	• Onset of care in primary or ambulatory care setting • On admission to hospital, rehabilitation, or long-term care setting • On initial home care visit	• Assessment chapters for each body system • Outline for physical examination (Table 3-4) • Findings for normal physical examination (Table 3-6)
Focused • Abbreviated assessment that focuses on one or more body systems that are the focus of care • Includes an assessment related to a specific problem (e.g., pneumonia, specific abnormal laboratory findings) • Monitors for signs and symptoms of new problems	• Throughout hospital admission—at beginning of a shift and as needed throughout shift • Revisit in ambulatory care setting or home care setting	• Focused assessment boxes in each assessment chapter • Tables on nursing assessment of specific diseases throughout book

TABLE 3-8 Clinical Application for Types of Assessment

The following is an example of how various types of assessment would be used for a patient progressing from the emergency department to a clinical unit of a hospital.

Timeline	Type of Assessment
Emergency Department Patient arrives in acute respiratory distress. Problem is identified and critical interventions are performed. Patient stabilizes.	• Perform emergency assessment (see Table 68-3). • Conduct a focused assessment of the respiratory and related body systems (e.g., cardiovascular). • May begin comprehensive assessment of all body systems.
Clinical Unit Patient is admitted to a monitored clinical unit. Beginning of each shift: reassess per orders and more frequently as determined by the nurse.	• Complete comprehensive assessment of all body systems within proper timeframe. • Perform focused assessment of respiratory system and other related body systems per agency protocol. • Perform focused assessment of appropriate body system(s) if new symptoms are reported.

department with a life-threatening condition, you will perform an emergency assessment based on the elements of a primary survey (e.g., airway, breathing, circulation, disability) (see Table 68-3). Once the patient is stabilized, you can begin a focused assessment of the respiratory and related body systems. Once the patient is admitted, a comprehensive assessment of all body systems, whether or not they are involved in the current clinical problem, is obtained.

PROBLEM IDENTIFICATION AND NURSING DIAGNOSES

After completing the history and physical examination, analyze the data to develop a list of nursing diagnoses and collaborative problems. See Chapter 1 for a description of the nursing process, including the identification of nursing diagnoses and collaborative problems.

BRIDGE TO NCLEX EXAMINATION

The number of the question corresponds to the same-numbered outcome at the beginning of the chapter.

1. The patient health history and physical examination provide the nurse with information to primarily
   a. diagnose a medical problem.
   b. investigate a patient's signs and symptoms.
   c. classify subjective and objective patient data.
   d. identify nursing diagnoses and collaborative problems.
2. The nurse would place information about the patient's concern that his illness is threatening his job security in which functional health pattern?
   a. Role-relationship
   b. Cognitive-perceptual
   c. Coping–stress tolerance
   d. Health perception–health management
3. The nurse is preparing to examine a patient's abdomen. Identify the proper order of the steps in the assessment of the abdomen, using the numbers 1-4, with 1 = the first technique and 4 = the last technique:
   ___ Inspection
   ___ Palpation
   ___ Percussion
   ___ Auscultation
4. Which situation would require the nurse to obtain a focused assessment *(select all that apply)*?
   a. A patient denies a current health problem.
   b. A patient reports a new symptom during rounds.
   c. A previously identified problem needs reassessment.
   d. A baseline health maintenance examination is required.
   e. An emergency problem is identified during physical examination.

1. d, 2. a, 3. 1, 4, 3, 2, 4. b, c.

For rationales to these answers and even more NCLEX review questions, visit *http://evolve.elsevier.com/Lewis/medsurg.*

EVOLVE WEBSITE

http://evolve.elsevier.com/Lewis/medsurg

Review Questions (Online Only)
Key Points
Answer Key for Questions
- Rationales for Bridge to NCLEX Examination Questions

Conceptual Care Map Creator
Audio Glossary
Content Updates

REFERENCES

1. Jarvis C: *Physical examination and health assessment*, ed 6, St Louis, 2012, Saunders.
2. Wilson S, Giddens J: *Health assessment for nursing practice*, ed 5, St Louis, 2013, Mosby.
3. Gordon M: *Manual of nursing diagnosis*, ed 13, Boston, 2014, Jones & Bartlett.
4. Lehne R: *Pharmacology for nursing care*, ed 8, St Louis, 2013, Mosby.
5. Eliopoulos C: *Gerontological nursing*, ed 8, Philadelphia, 2013, Lippincott Williams & Wilkins.

4

Patient and Caregiver Teaching

Linda Bucher

Tell me and I'll forget; show me and I may remember; involve me and I'll understand.

Chinese Proverb

http://evolve.elsevier.com/Lewis/medsurg/

LEARNING OUTCOMES

1. Apply the teaching-learning process to diverse patient populations.
2. Apply strategies to manage challenges to nurse-teacher effectiveness.
3. Evaluate the role of the caregiver in patient teaching.
4. Relate the physical, psychologic, and sociocultural characteristics of the patient and caregiver to the teaching-learning process.
5. Prioritize patient teaching goals for diverse patients and caregivers.
6. Select appropriate teaching strategies for diverse patient populations and their caregivers.
7. Select appropriate methods to evaluate patient and caregiver teaching.

KEY TERMS

caregivers, p. 49
health literacy, p. 52
learning, p. 47
learning needs, p. 53
motivational interviewing, p. 47
positive reinforcement, p. 53
self-efficacy, p. 48
teaching, p. 46
teaching plan, p. 46
teaching process, p. 51

This chapter describes the process of patient and caregiver teaching. In addition, it discusses the strategies and methods that contribute to successful teaching and learning experiences.

ROLE OF PATIENT AND CAREGIVER TEACHING

Patient and caregiver (family member or significant other) teaching is an interactive and dynamic process that involves a change in a patient's knowledge, behavior, and/or attitude to maintain or improve health. You will find that teaching is one of your most challenging and rewarding roles. Teaching patients and caregivers is a key nursing intervention that makes a difference in their lives.

General goals of patient teaching include health promotion, disease prevention, management of illness, and appropriate selection and use of treatment options. In patients with acute and chronic health problems, teaching can prevent complications and promote recovery, self-care, and independence. The leading causes of death and disability in the United States are chronic diseases.[1] Whether patients adequately manage their health problems and maintain quality of life depends on what they learn about their conditions and what they choose to do with this knowledge. Patients who have the knowledge, skills, and desire to take responsibility for managing their health are less likely to be readmitted or visit the emergency department than patients who do not have this information or motivation.[2]

Teaching may occur wherever you work. Although agencies may employ advanced practice nurses and patient educators to establish and oversee patient teaching programs, you are always responsible for patient and caregiver teaching.[3] It is a responsibility that cannot be delegated to unlicensed assistive personnel (UAP).

Every interaction with a patient and a caregiver is a potential *teachable moment.* On any given day, more informal opportunities to teach will occur than formal opportunities. Take advantage of and document all of these moments. For example, when you teach a patient with asthma how to use a peak flow meter, you do not need a formal teaching plan. However, when your patient has a specific learning need about health promotion or management of a health problem, you should develop a teaching plan. A **teaching plan** includes (1) assessment of the patient's ability and readiness to learn, (2) identification of teaching needs, (3) development of learning goals with the patient, (4) implementation of the teaching, and (5) evaluation of the patient's learning.

TEACHING-LEARNING PROCESS

Teaching is not just imparting information. **Teaching** is a process of deliberately arranging conditions to promote learning that results in a change in behavior.[4] Teaching can be a planned or informal experience. It uses a combination of methods such as instruction, counseling, and behavior modification.

Reviewed by Debra Hagler, RN, PhD, ACNS-BC, CNE, CHSE, ANEF, FAAN, Clinical Professor, Arizona State University, College of Nursing and Health Innovation, Phoenix, Arizona; Regina Kukulski, RN, MSN, ACNS, BC, CNE, Clinical Nurse Specialist Renal Services, Capital Health Regional Medical Center, Trenton, New Jersey; and Laura A. Stokowski, RNC, MS, Inova Fairfax Hospital for Children, Falls Church, Virginia.

Learning is acquiring knowledge and/or skills. It can result in a permanent change in a person.[4] Observation of this change is an indication that learning has occurred. Learning may also result in the potential or capability to change behavior. This is seen in a patient who understands the instruction and is fully informed but chooses not to change behavior. In this case, teaching gives the patient the capability to change behavior, but the decision to change is the patient's.

Although learning may occur without teaching, teaching helps to organize information and skills to make learning more efficient. In patient teaching the teaching-learning process involves the patient, the patient's caregiver(s), and you.

Adult Learner

Adult Learning Principles. Understanding how and why adults learn is important for you to effectively teach patients and their caregivers. Many theories of adult learning have evolved from the work of Malcolm Knowles. He identified six principles of *andragogy* (adult learning) that are important for you to consider when teaching adults[5] (Table 4-1).

Models to Promote Health. When a change in health behaviors is recommended, patients and their caregivers may progress through a series of steps before they are willing or able to accept the change. Prochaska and Velicer proposed six stages of change in their *Transtheoretical Model of Health Behavior Change*[6] (Table 4-2). This model is frequently used to help patients stop smoking, manage diabetes, and lose weight.

Motivational interviewing *(www.motivationalinterview.org)* uses nonconfrontational interpersonal communication techniques to motivate patients to change behavior.[7] This strategy includes the use of any intervention that enhances the patient's motivation for change (Table 4-3). The techniques used in motivational interviewing are linked to the stages of change as identified by Prochaska and Velicer.

During the process of change, relapse and recycling through the stages are expected. Sometimes patients do not change behaviors or return to previous behaviors after a period of change. This may indicate that the interventions used did not consider the patient's stage of change.[8] Identify the patient's current stage of readiness for change and the stage to which the patient is moving. Patients who are in the early stages of change need and use different kinds of motivational support than patients at later stages of change.

For example, a patient who smokes cigarettes who is hospitalized is often in the *precontemplation* or *contemplation* stage of change. In the precontemplation stage, patients are not concerned about their substance use and are not considering changing their behavior. During this stage, help the patient increase awareness of risks and problems related to smoking and create doubt about the use of cigarettes. Ask the patient what he or she thinks could happen if the behavior is continued, provide evidence of the problem (e.g., x-ray changes), and share facts about the risks of smoking. Although patients may not be ready to change behavior while experiencing an acute health problem, the seeds of doubt are sown. In other cases, such as when a patient experiences a life-threatening condition (e.g., heart attack), there may be an immediate awareness of the problem and motivation to change.

TABLE 4-1 Adult Learning Principles Applied to Patient and Caregiver Teaching

Principles	Teaching Implications for Nurse	Examples
Need to know	• Patients need to know why they should learn something, what they need to learn, and how it will benefit them. • Ask the patient questions such as, "What do you think you need to learn about this topic?"	Your patient and his caregiver ask what they need to know about exercise guidelines after a heart attack.
Readiness to learn	• Readiness and motivation to learn are high when facing new tasks. • Health crises provide opportunities for patients to learn and change behavior. • Stress and anxiety may interfere with learning, thus requiring frequent reinforcement of content.	While recovering from a transient ischemic attack, your patient tells you that she is ready to learn about the changes she needs to take to reduce her risk for stroke.
Prior experiences	• Motivation is increased when patients already know something about the subject from past experiences. • Identification of past knowledge and experiences can help find familiar ground to increase patients' confidence.	Your patient needs to begin injections of enoxaparin (Lovenox). She tells you that she gives her father insulin injections and is ready to learn how to administer this medication.
Motivation to learn	• Patients prefer to apply learning immediately. • Long-term goals may have less appeal than short-term goals. • Focus teaching on information that the patient views as being needed right now.	Your patient is scheduled to be discharged in the morning. Both she and her caregiver have received instruction on wound care and have watched the procedure. The caregiver tells you that he wants to perform the wound care today.
Orientation to learning	• Patients seek out various resources for specific learning and prefer to have choices. • When the patient does not recognize the relevancy of the teaching, offer explanations of the value of the learning. • Teaching should target the specific problem or circumstance.	Your patient, who is newly diagnosed with diabetes mellitus, tells you that he is worried about the diet changes he will need to make. Share several options with him to learn about diet changes (e.g., cooking classes, Web-based tutorials, mobile applications, individual sessions with the dietitian, brochures).
Self-concept	• Patients need control and self-direction (sense of autonomy) to maintain their sense of self-worth. • Patients do not learn when they are treated like children and told what they must do.	Your patient has a temporary colostomy. She says she is not ready to look at the stoma. Work out a schedule with her for learning colostomy care that meets her need for control and prepares her for self-care.

TABLE 4-2 Stages of Change in Transtheoretical Model

Stage	Patient Behavior	Nursing Implications
1. Precontemplation	Is not considering a change. Is not ready to learn.	Provide support, increase awareness of condition. Describe benefits of change and risks of not changing.
2. Contemplation	Thinks about a change. May verbalize recognition of need to change. Says "I know I should," but identifies barriers.	Introduce what is involved in changing the behavior. Reinforce the stated need to change.
3. Preparation	Starts planning the change, gathers information, sets a date to initiate change, shares decision to change with others.	Reinforce the positive outcomes of change, provide information and encouragement, develop a plan, help set priorities, and identify sources of support.
4. Action	Begins to change behavior through practice. Tentative and may experience relapses.	Reinforce behavior with reward, encourage self-reward, discuss choices to help minimize relapses and regain focus. Help patient plan to deal with potential relapses.
5. Maintenance	Practices the behavior regularly. Able to sustain the change.	Continue to reinforce behavior. Provide additional teaching on the need to maintain change.
6. Termination	Change has become part of lifestyle. Behavior no longer considered a change.	Evaluate effectiveness of the new behavior. No further intervention needed.

Adapted from Prochaska J, Velicer W: The transtheoretical model of health behavior change, *Am J Health Promot* 12:38, 1997. (Classic)

TABLE 4-3 Key Aspects of Motivational Interviewing

- Listen rather than tell.
- Adjust to, rather than oppose, patient resistance.
- Express empathy through reflective listening.
- Focus on the positive. Do not criticize the patient.
- Gently persuade with the understanding that change is up to the patient.
- Focus on the patient's strengths to support the hope needed to make changes.
- Avoid argument and direct confrontation, which can cause defensiveness and a power struggle.
- Help the patient recognize the "gap" between where he or she is and where he or she hopes to be.

A patient in the *contemplation* stage of change often experiences ambivalence. The patient understands that the behavior is a problem and that change is necessary. However, he or she believes that change is too difficult or that the pleasures of the behavior are worth the risks. This is seen in the patient who says, "I know that I have to stop smoking. This heart attack really scared me. I know I need to lose weight and start exercising, but I can't change everything all at once. Smoking helps me control my eating—I can't stop until I lose some weight." During this stage of change, help the patient consider the positive and negative aspects of his or her behavior (e.g., tobacco use), gently trying to tip the balance in favor of positive behavior. Helping the patient discover internal motivators in addition to those external motivators (e.g., second heart attack, lung disease) that push the patient toward change can move the patient from contemplating change to preparation and action. Throughout this process, emphasize the patient's personal choices and responsibilities for change.

As the patient moves from contemplation to *preparation*, a commitment to change is strengthened by helping the patient develop **self-efficacy**, which is the belief that one can succeed in a given situation. In this case it is the patient's belief that tobacco-use behaviors can be changed. Support even the smallest effort to change. Movement through action and maintenance stages of change requires continued support to increase the patient's involvement and participation in treatment. A comprehensive discussion of motivational interviewing is presented in the Treatment Improvement Protocols available at *www.ncbi.nlm.nih.gov/books/NBK14856.*

The resolution of acute health problems or discharge from the hospital often occurs before the patient moves to the preparation and action stages of change. As the patient develops readiness to change in the contemplative stage of change, continue to support him or her with referral to appropriate community and outpatient resources.

Nurse as Teacher

Required Competencies

Knowledge of Subject Matter. Although it is impossible to be an expert in all subject areas, develop confidence as a teacher by becoming knowledgeable about the topic to be taught. For example, if you are teaching patients about the management of hypertension, you must be able to explain what hypertension is and why it is important to treat it. Also teach patients what they need to know about exercise, diet, and side effects of medications. Teach the patient and caregiver how to use BP equipment to monitor BP and to describe situations that must be reported to the HCP. Finally, provide the patient with additional resources, such as valid websites, brochures, and information about support organizations (e.g., American Heart Association).

Sometimes you will not be able to answer patients' or caregivers' questions. Clarify their questions to be sure of what they are asking. When you do not have the knowledge to answer the question, tell this to the patient and caregiver and seek help from co-workers, patient educators, and other reliable sources.

Communication Skills. Patient teaching depends on effective communication between you and the patient or caregiver. Medical jargon is intimidating and frightening to most patients and their caregivers. Introduce medical words and define their meanings. Limit the use of acronyms (e.g., CABG for coronary artery bypass graft) and abbreviations (e.g., IV) when talking with patients. Have the patient and caregiver clarify their understanding of the disease process. Ask them to explain what they know in their own words. For example, if a patient is told that he has leukopenia, define this term in words that mean something to him. Explain that *leuko-* refers to a leukocyte, a white blood cell that fights infections; and that

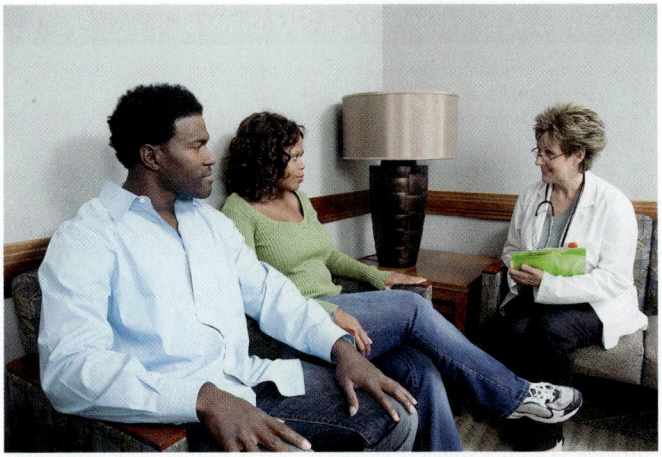

FIG. 4-1 Open, relaxed positioning of patient, spouse, and nurse at eye level promotes communication in teaching and learning. (©Jupiterimages/Photos.com/Thinkstock.)

penia refers to a shortage. To enhance learning, use a brief explanation such as, "You have a shortage of white blood cells, the cells that fight infection."

Nonverbal communication is critical when teaching. Nonverbal communication is often guided by cultural practices. For example, in Western culture, sitting in an open, relaxed position facing the patient with eyes at the same level delivers a positive nonverbal message (Fig. 4-1). In a hospital setting this may require raising the patient's bed or sitting in a chair at the bedside. Open body gestures communicate interest and a willingness to share. With patients from Eastern cultures, you may need to avoid direct eye contact and provide health information to a family spokesperson rather than directly to the patient.

Also develop the art of *active listening* by paying attention to what is said, observing the patient's nonverbal cues, and not interrupting. Nod in response to the patient's statements and restate what the patient is saying to help clarify communication.

Empathy is the courage to enter into the world of another in a manner that does not judge or correct but attempts to understand. Empathy means putting aside your own self and stepping into the patient's shoes. Active listening, combined with empathy, is a powerful way to communicate caring and prepare the patient to learn.

Challenges to Nurse-Teacher Effectiveness. Teaching patients and caregivers has many challenges, including (1) lack of time, (2) your own feelings as a teacher, (3) nurse-patient differences in learning goals, and (4) early discharge from the health care system.

Lack of time can be a barrier to effective teaching. For example, the patient's physical needs may compete for time that could be used for teaching. To make the most of limited time, it is critical to set learning priorities with the patient. Tell the patient at the beginning of the interaction how much time you can devote to the session. Some teaching should be delivered or reinforced during every contact with the patient or caregiver. For example, when giving medications, explain the purpose and side effects of each drug. Reinforcing small pieces of information over time is an effective teaching strategy, especially if information is new or complex.

Additional barriers are your *own feelings as a teacher* and insecurity about your own knowledge and skill. Teaching is a skill that takes time to master. Become familiar with the various resources for patient teaching that are available at your agency.

TABLE 4-4 Assessment of Caregiver Needs

Ask caregivers the following questions:

1. How are you coping with your caregiver role?
2. Do you have any difficulties performing your caregiver responsibilities?
3. How much support do you get from outside sources (e.g., other family members, friends)?
4. Are you aware of and do you use community resources (e.g., disease-specific professional organizations [such as Alzheimer's Association, American Heart Association], adult day care centers, church, synagogue)?
5. Do you know about resources that are available for respite (someone caring for your loved one while you have time to yourself)?
6. What kind of help or services do you need now and in the near future?
7. How can I or other health care providers help you in your caregiving role?

Consult with nurse educators or experienced co-workers for further help with developing your teaching skills.

Also, disagreements can arise among the patient, the caregiver, and you regarding the expectations or outcomes of teaching. Having realistic discussions about discharge plans, identifying timelines, and exploring home care options can emphasize the need for learning. For example, after a diagnosis of heart failure due to aortic valve insufficiency and subsequent emergent valve surgery, the patient and caregiver may reject teaching efforts until they realize and accept the seriousness of the patient's health problem.

Last, another important challenge to patient teaching relates to patients having early and quick discharges from the health care system. Shortened lengths of hospital stays have resulted in patients only having basic teaching plans implemented.

Caregiver Support in the Teaching-Learning Process

The teaching and learning process is applicable to the caregiver as well as the patient. **Caregivers** are people who care for those who cannot care for themselves. Most common, caregivers are family members or significant others who (1) give or assist with direct patient care; (2) provide emotional, social, spiritual, and possibly financial support for the patient; and (3) manage and coordinate health care services.

Approximately one in four American adults provides care to someone on a daily basis. Caregivers are often categorized by their relationship to the patient. The most common types of caregivers are spouses, adult children, parents, grandparents, and life partners. Although older adult women are the most common family caregivers, other examples include husbands who care for wives with Alzheimer's disease, adult children who care for a parent with a stroke, grandparents who care for a grandchild with a developmental disorder, parents who care for an adult child with a spinal cord injury, and life partners who care for loved ones with a chronic illness.[9]

Identify the key caregiver(s) for the patient. Assess the caregiver's roles and relationships to the patient. The patient's health problem affects family roles and functions. Identify the needs of caregivers, whether it is in the acute care setting, during the transition to home, or in a home setting[10] (Table 4-4).

Consider cultural differences when assessing the caregiver. In some cultures a male family member may be the designated spokesperson. This person would receive and communicate information among family members and the patient. In planning for discharge to home, it is important to include caregivers who will actually provide the care for the patient, along with the family spokesperson (see Chapter 2 for more information on culturally competent care).

As much as possible, teach the caregiver along with the patient. Explain the goals of the teaching plan to both of them. Caregivers may need help to learn the physical and technical requirements of care, find resources for home care, locate equipment and supplies, and rearrange the home to accommodate the patient. Sources of support for the transition from hospital to home include community-based agencies, Medicare and Medicaid offices, and case managers at the hospital and insurance companies.

Patients and caregivers may have different teaching needs. For example, the first priority of an older patient with a diabetic leg ulcer may be to learn how to transfer from a bed to a chair in the least painful manner. On the other hand, the caregiver may be most concerned about learning the technique for dressing changes. Both the patient's and caregiver's learning needs are important. The patient and caregiver may also have differing or conflicting views of the illness and treatment options. Developing a successful teaching plan requires you to view the patient's needs within the context of the caregiver's needs. For instance, you may teach a patient with right-sided *paresis* (weakness) self-feeding techniques with special tools, but at a home visit you find the patient being fed by the caregiver. On questioning, the caregiver reveals that it is too hard to watch the patient struggle with feeding, it takes too long, and it is messy. As a result, the caregiver decides that it is easier to feed the patient. This is an example of a situation in which the patient and caregiver need additional discussion about the goals for self-care.

Finally, discuss the potential that support groups, family and friends, and community resources have for providing ongoing support. Support groups help by people sharing experiences and information, offering understanding and acceptance, and suggesting solutions to common problems and concerns. Encourage the caregiver to seek help from the social support system on matters such as housing, health coverage, finances, and respite care. *Respite care,* which is planned temporary care for the patient, includes adult day care, in-home care, and assisted living services.

Caregiver Stress. Caregiver responsibilities are usually taken on gradually with the progression of the patient's illness. As the caregiving responsibilities become more demanding, caregivers often realize that their lives have changed because of this experience. Overwhelmingly, caregivers want to continue their usual activities (e.g., work) despite the hardships they face in caring for acute and chronically ill patients.[11]

Prolonged periods of caregiving coupled with a patient's life-limiting illness can contribute to stress and burnout. Some common caregiver stressors are listed in Table 4-5. As caregiving progresses, stressors may change. For example, a caregiver may initially need only to adjust work schedules to accommodate a patient's health care appointments. Later, as the patient's condition worsens, the caregiver may have to reduce work hours, incurring financial hardships.

Caregiving is an experience for which most people are not prepared. It is common for caregivers to become physically, emotionally, and economically overwhelmed by the responsibilities and demands of caring for a loved one. The stress of caregiving may lead to emotional problems such as depression, anger, and resentment. Signs of caregiver stress include irritability, inability to concentrate, fatigue, and sleeplessness. The caregiver often experiences decreased social interactions and may be at risk for social isolation. Multiple commitments, fatigue, and, at times, the patient's socially inappropriate behaviors contribute to the caregiver's social isolation. Stress can progress to burnout and result in negligence and abuse of the patient by the caregiver. See Chapter 5 for information on elder mistreatment and abuse.

TABLE 4-5 Caregiver Stressors

- Change in roles and relationships within family unit
- Lack of respite or relief from caregiving responsibilities
- Need to juggle day-to-day activities, decisions, and caregiving
- Change in living conditions to accommodate family member
- Conflict in the family unit related to decisions about caregiving
- Other people's lack of understanding of the time and energy needed for caregiving
- Inability to meet personal self-care needs, such as socialization, sleep, eating, exercise, and rest
- Financial depletion of resources as a result of patient's or caregiver's inability to work
- Inadequate information or skills related to specific caregiving tasks such as bathing, drug administration, wound care

In the family system an illness experienced by one family member affects the entire family and alters family interactions. Often family members do not communicate with each other about the patient's needs, and this results in tension. Family conflicts regarding how patient care should be given can lead to disagreements and conflict within the family.

At the same time, many family members involved in caregiver activities also share rewards associated with this role. Positive aspects of caregiving include (1) knowing that their loved one is receiving good care (often in a home environment), (2) learning and mastering new skills, and (3) finding opportunities for intimacy. The tasks involved in caregiving often provide opportunities for family members to gain greater insights into each other and strengthen their relationships.

Encourage caregivers to take care of themselves. Suggest journaling or joining a support group to help them share feelings that may be difficult to express. Remind caregivers that getting regular exercise and sleep and eating balanced meals enhance their well-being. Encourage contact with others to provide emotional support. Finally, humor is important, and sometimes its use by caregivers can provide distraction and relieve stress-filled situations. See the Caregiving Resource Center at *www.aarp.org/home-family/caregiving* for additional information.

Regulatory Mandates for Patient Teaching

Several important agencies have provided specific mandates related to teaching hospitalized patients. The Joint Commission's (TJC's) accreditation standards, National Patient Safety Goals,[12] and the American Hospital Association's Patient Care Partnership[13] clearly state that patients have a fundamental right to receive information about their care. This information includes their diagnosis, treatment, and prognosis in terms that they can reasonably be expected to understand. For example, this means that written materials must be appropriate for the patient's reading level. One program initiated by TJC, called Speak Up, was developed to encourage patients to become more involved and informed about their plan of care[14] (Table 4-6). Another program proposed by the National Patient Safety Foundation is called Ask Me 3.[15] A variety of resources that

TABLE 4-6 The Joint Commission's Speak Up Initiative

Speak up if you have questions or concerns. If you still do not understand, ask again. It is your body and you have a right to know.
Pay attention to the care you get. Always make sure you are getting the right treatments and medicines by the right health care professionals. Do not assume anything.
Educate yourself about your illness. Learn about the medical tests you get and your treatment plan.
Ask a trusted family member or friend to be your advocate (advisor or supporter).
Know what medicines you take and why you take them. Medicine errors are the most common health care mistakes.
Use a hospital, clinic, surgery center, or other type of health care organization that has been carefully checked out.
Participate in all decisions about your treatment. You are the center of the health care team.

Source: The Joint Commission: To prevent health care errors, patients are urged to Speak Up (poster). Retrieved from *www.jointcommission.org/assets/1/18/SpeakUp_Poster.pdf.*

prompt patients to ask specific questions about their care are available as a part of these initiatives *(www.jointcommission.org/topics/speakup_brochures.aspx)*.

PROCESS OF PATIENT TEACHING

Many different approaches are used in the process of patient teaching. However, the approach used most frequently by nurses parallels the nursing process. The **teaching process** and the nursing process involve the development of a plan that includes assessment, setting of patient goals, implementation, and evaluation. The teaching process, like the nursing process, may not always flow in linear order, but the steps serve as checkpoints.

Assessment

During the general nursing assessment, gather data to determine if the patient has learning needs. For example, what does the patient know about the health problem? How does he or she perceive the problem? If a learning need is identified, a more detailed assessment is needed, and that problem is addressed with the teaching plan. Assessment also includes the caregivers to determine their role and ability to care for the patient at home.[10] Key questions to use in the assessment are included in Table 4-7.

Physical Factors. The patient's age is a factor to consider in the teaching plan. Age affects the patient's experiences and rate of learning.[16] Some effects of increased age on learning may be obvious, but the inexperience of younger people can also affect learning. For example, a man in his twenties who has never thought about his own mortality may be unable to accept the long-term health implications of diabetes mellitus.

Sensory impairments (e.g., hearing or vision loss) decrease sensory input and can alter learning. Magnifying glasses, bright lighting, and materials printed in a large font may help the patient with impaired vision read teaching materials. People with hearing loss can be helped with hearing aids and teaching techniques that use more visual stimuli. Cognition may be affected by disorders of the nervous system (e.g., stroke, head trauma), and by other diseases (e.g., liver impairment, heart failure). Patients with alterations in cognition may have difficulty learning and may require greater caregiver involvement in the teaching process. Manual dexterity is needed to perform skills such as administration of injections or BP monitoring.

TABLE 4-7 Assessment of Factors Affecting Patient Teaching

Key Factors and Questions

Physical
- What is the patient's age?
- Is the patient acutely ill?
- Is the patient fatigued or in pain?
- What is the primary diagnosis?
- Are there additional medical problems?
- What is the patient's current mental status?
- What is the patient's hearing ability? Visual ability? Motor ability?
- What drugs does the patient take that may affect learning?

Psychologic
- Does the patient appear anxious, afraid, depressed, defensive?
- Is the patient in a state of denial?
- What is the patient's level of motivation? Self-efficacy?

Sociocultural
- What are the patient's beliefs regarding his or her illness or treatment?
- Is proposed teaching consistent with the patient's cultural values?
- What is the patient's educational experience, reading ability, primary language?
- What is the patient's present or past occupation?
- How does the patient describe his or her financial status?
- What is the patient's living arrangement?
- Does the patient have family or close friends?

Learner
- What does the patient already know about his or her health problem?
- What does the patient think is most important to learn?
- What prior learning experiences could act as a frame of reference for current learning needs?
- Is the patient ready to learn? Change behavior?
- How does the patient learn best (e.g., reading, listening, looking at pictures, doing, playing games)?
- In what kind of environment does the patient learn best? Formal classroom? Computer/Web-based setting? Informal setting, such as home? Alone or in a group?
- In what way should the caregiver(s) be involved in patient teaching?

Problems performing manual skills may be resolved by using adaptive equipment.

Pain, fatigue, and certain drugs also influence the patient's ability to learn. No one can learn effectively when in pain. Provide teaching only after the patient's pain is controlled. A fatigued and weakened patient cannot learn effectively because of the inability to concentrate. Sleep disruption is common during hospitalization, and patients are frequently sleep deprived at the time of discharge. Drugs that cause central nervous system depression, such as opioids and sedatives, cause a general decrease in mental alertness and can affect the patient's ability to learn new information. Adjust the teaching plan to accommodate these factors by setting high-priority goals based on need-to-know information and realistic expectations. Patients often need a referral for follow-up so that teaching continues and learning is confirmed after discharge.

Psychologic Factors. Psychologic factors have a major influence on the patient's ability to learn. Anxiety and depression are common reactions to illness. Although mild anxiety increases the learner's perceptual and learning abilities, moderate or severe anxiety limits learning. Anxiety and depression can negatively affect the patient's motivation and readiness to learn. For instance, the patient newly diagnosed with diabetes mellitus who is depressed about the diagnosis may not listen or respond to instructions about glucose testing. Discussions with the patient about these concerns or referrals to an appropriate support group may help the patient to learn that management of diabetes is possible.

Patients also respond to the stress of illness with a variety of defense mechanisms, such as denial, rationalization, or even humor. A patient who denies having cancer will not be receptive to information related to treatment options. Similarly, a caregiver may have difficulty accepting a terminal diagnosis. A patient using rationalization will imagine any number of reasons for avoiding change or for rejecting teaching. For example, a patient with heart disease who does not want to change dietary habits will relate stories of people who have eaten bacon and eggs every day and lived to be 100. Some patients also use humor to filter reality or decrease anxiety. They may use laughter to escape from the experience of facing threatening situations. Humor in the teaching process is important and useful, but determine when humor is used excessively or inappropriately to avoid reality.

One important determinant of successful adoption of new behaviors is the patient's sense of self-efficacy. There is a strong relationship between self-efficacy and outcomes of illness management.[17] Self-efficacy increases when a person gains new skills in managing a threatening situation but decreases when the individual experiences repeated failure, especially early in the course of events. Plan easily achievable goals early in the teaching sessions. Proceed from simple to more complex content to create a feeling of success.

Sociocultural Factors

Health Literacy. *Literacy* is the ability to use printed and written information to function in society. The recent focus on the literacy rates of the U.S. population and their effects on health and health care have major implications for patient and caregiver teaching. The most recent national literacy survey reported that 43% of the general population and 66% of people older than 60 have basic to below basic literacy skills and another 5% are not literate in English.[18] Assessment of literacy is challenging, since patients rarely admit they have difficulty reading because of feelings of inadequacy and low self-esteem.[19]

Health literacy is the degree to which individuals have the capacity to obtain and understand basic health information needed to make appropriate health decisions.[12] Patients with limited literacy have trouble understanding and acting on health information, leading to *health illiteracy*. Even patients with higher general literacy can have low health literacy when trying to understand complex health information. Health illiteracy results in poor patient outcomes, nonadherence to treatment plans, limited self-management skills, and increased health disparities.[20]

Easy-to-use assessment tools are available to determine a patient's health literacy. The Single-Item Literacy Screener (SILS) uses one question to identify adults who need help with reading.[21] The question is, "How often do you need to have someone help you when you read instructions, pamphlets, or other written material from your doctor or pharmacy?"

Patient teaching materials should be written at the fifth-grade or lower reading level.[21] TJC has established that patient teaching should be tailored to the patient's literacy needs. For example, patients should be taught in their primary language.

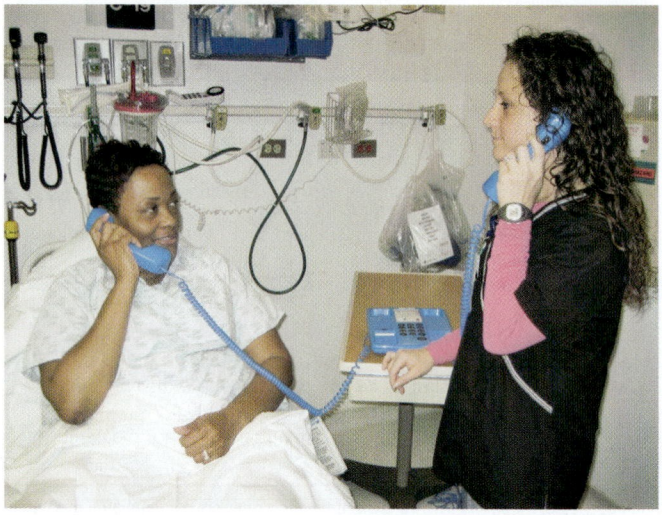

FIG. 4-2 Nurse communicating with a non-English-speaking patient using a translation phone service. (Courtesy Linda Bucher, RN, PhD, CEN, CNE, Staff Nurse, Virtua Memorial Hospital, Mt. Holly, N.J.)

This is accomplished using medical interpreters (e.g., translators, sign language interpreters)[22] (Fig. 4-2). (Medical interpreters are discussed in Chapter 2 on p. 31.) Many patient teaching materials are currently available in languages other than English. Ideally, written materials should always be available in the patient's primary language.

Cultural Considerations. Learning is influenced by the wider culture to which a patient belongs. Health practices, beliefs, and behavior are influenced by one's cultural traditions. These traditions, which can affect patient teaching, can be identified in a cultural assessment (see Table 2-7). TJC requires that patient teaching be tailored to the patient's cultural needs.[22] To prevent stereotyping patients, it is important to simply ask if there is a cultural group with which the patient identifies. Ask patients to describe their beliefs regarding health and illness.

One cultural element that specifically affects the teaching-learning process is a conflict between the patient's cultural beliefs and values and the behaviors promoted by the health care team. For example, a patient who values a trim figure can be taught to use diet and exercise to retain that figure while at the same time improving BP control. However, in another patient's culture, being heavier may be valued as a sign of financial success and sexuality. This patient may have more difficulty accepting the need for diet and exercise unless the importance of BP control is understood.

Assess the patient's use of cultural remedies and folk healers (see the Complementary & Alternative Therapies Box: Assessment of Use of Herbs & Dietary Supplements in Chapter 3, p. 38). Also consider the cultural remedies that may interfere with or are contraindicated by the treatment plan.

Last, it is important to know who has authority in the patient's culture. The patient may defer to the authority, such as an elder or a spiritual leader, for decisions. In this case, identify and work with the decision makers in the patient's cultural group. (See Chapter 2 for more information on cultural competence.)

Socioeconomic Considerations. A variety of socioeconomic factors are considered when preparing to teach patients. Knowing the patient's present or past occupation may assist you in determining the vocabulary to use during teaching. For example, an auto mechanic may understand the volume

EVIDENCE-BASED PRACTICE

Translating Research Into Practice

Does Culturally Appropriate Education Improve Diabetic Glycemic Control and Knowledge?

Clinical Question

For adults with diabetes mellitus (P), what is the effect of culturally appropriate health education (I) versus usual care (C) on glycemic control and diabetes knowledge (O) in the short- and long-term (T)?

Synthesis of Best Available Evidence

- Systematic review of randomized controlled trials (RCTs) and quasi RCTs.
- 33 trials of patients (n = 7453) from ethnic minority groups with type 2 diabetes. Culturally appropriate interventions were any type of health education tailored for cultural needs of a minority group with type 2 diabetes. Glycemic control was measured by glycosylated hemoglobin A1C (A1C). Knowledge assessment varied across studies.
- A1C levels improved at 3, 6, 12, and 24 months after the intervention.
- Knowledge scores increased at 6 and 12 months after the intervention.

Conclusion

- Culturally appropriate education improved glycemic control and diabetes knowledge on a short- and long-term basis.

Implications for Nursing Practice

1. How would you modify diabetes education for someone from an ethnic minority group?
2. Why is it important for health care providers to provide culturally appropriate diabetes education?

Reference for Evidence

Attridge M, Creamer J, Ramsden M, et al: Culturally appropriate health education for people in ethnic minority groups with type 2 diabetes mellitus. Cochrane Database Syst Rev (9):CD006424, 2014.

P, Patient population of interest; *I*, intervention or area of interest; *C*, comparison of interest or comparison group; *O*, outcomes of interest; *T*, timing (see p. 15).

overload associated with heart failure as flooding an engine. An engineer may understand the principles of physics associated with gravity and pressures when discussing vascular problems.

Ask the patient about living arrangements. Whether the patient lives alone, with friends, or with family influences who is included in the teaching process. You may need to modify the teaching plan if the patient does not have access to electricity or phones. If the patient has unmet learning needs by the time of discharge, arrange for ongoing teaching after discharge.

Learner Factors. Finally, assess learner factors, including the patient's learning needs, readiness to learn, and learning style.

Learning Needs. **Learning needs** are the new knowledge and skills that an individual must have to meet a goal. The assessment of learning needs determines what the patient already knows and any past experiences with health problems. Patients with long-standing health problems may have different learning needs from those patients with newly diagnosed health problems.

What patients should learn about managing an illness or what behaviors have to be changed to promote health may seem obvious to you. However, what you think is important may be different from what patients want to know. Remember that adults learn best when the teaching provides information that they view as being immediately needed (Table 4-1). Ask patients to prioritize what they see as the most critical information. Start by giving the patient a list of the recommended topics and then ask the patient to identify other topics not on the list. Having patients prioritize their own learning needs lets you begin with the patient's most important needs. If critical information needs to be taught, explain why the information is "need to know."

Readiness to Learn. Readiness to learn and motivation depend on multiple factors, such as perceived need, attitudes, and beliefs. When teaching adults, identify what information the person values. Readiness to learn is increased if the patient perceives a need for information, has a belief that a behavior change has value, or perceives the learning activities as new and stimulating.[5]

Before implementing the teaching plan, determine where the patient is in the stages of change (Table 4-2). If the patient is in the precontemplation stage, provide support and increase the patient's awareness of the problem until the patient is ready to consider a change in behavior. Nurses in outpatient settings and home health care can continue to evaluate the patient's readiness to learn and implement the teaching plan as the patient moves through the stages of change. Reinforcement is a strong motivational factor for achieving a desired behavior and must be incorporated throughout the change process. **Positive reinforcement** involves rewarding the target behavior with positive feedback or other rewards to maintain the behavior.[6]

Learning Style. Each person has a distinct style of learning. The three general learning styles are (1) *visual* (reading, pictures), (2) *auditory* (listening), and (3) *physical* (doing things). People often use more than one learning style to gain new knowledge or skills. To assess a patient's learning style, ask how the patient likes to learn and has learned in the past.[23] During assessment of the patient's learning style, identify the patient who does not read or who has limited health literacy. For example, the patient may tell you that he or she does not read much but likes to learn from television. In addition, assess the patient's *ehealth literacy*. This refers to the degree that patients use digital information (e.g., webinars, online health management tools) and communication technologies (e.g., online communication with HCP, online support groups) to improve their health[24] (Fig. 4-3). If possible, always use the patient's or caregiver's preferred learning style.

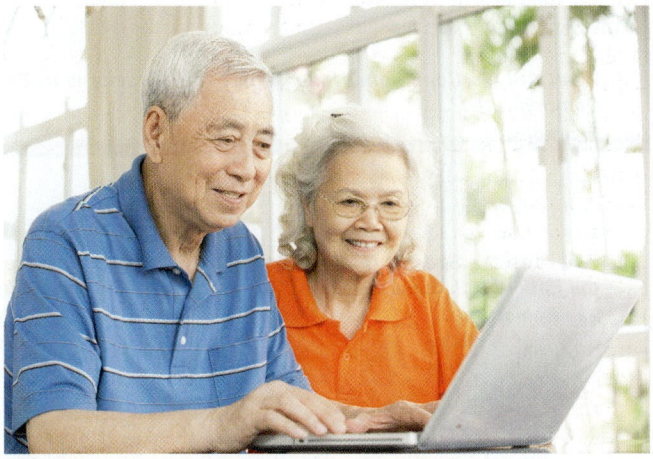

FIG. 4-3 Older couple accessing the Web for health information. (©monkebusinessimages/iStock/Thinkstock.)

Planning

Prioritize the patient's learning needs and agree on learning goals. If the patient's physical or psychologic condition interferes with his or her participation, involve the patient's caregiver(s) in the planning phase.

Setting Goals. It is important to have clear and measurable learning goals or outcomes (Table 4-8). Learning goals relate to the intended outcome of the learning process, guide the selection of teaching strategies, and help evaluate the patient's progress. Learning goals are parallel to patient outcomes in the nursing care plan (NCP). Most settings have standardized NCPs that contain preset goals and interventions for specific learning needs. You will modify these NCPs based on the patient's unique sociocultural and learner characteristics.

Selecting Teaching Strategies. Three factors that influence the selection of teaching strategies are (1) patient characteristics (e.g., learning style, educational background, culture, language skills), (2) subject matter, and (3) available resources. Table 4-9 provides a summary of the learner characteristics and recommended teaching approaches based on the generation of the patient or caregiver.[25,26]

Consider various teaching strategies (Table 4-10) when developing a teaching plan. Often, multiple strategies are used to improve learning (Fig. 4-4). Discussion is the most common type of interaction used in teaching patients and caregivers. Another type of group teaching involves *peer teaching*, as occurs in support groups. Patients dealing with common problems such as cancer, alcoholism, and eating disorders can benefit from peer teaching.

Learning Materials. Use learning materials that are provided in multiple formats. Learn what resources are available in your agency and from support services and professional groups. The use of CDs/DVDs is helpful, particularly when teaching content

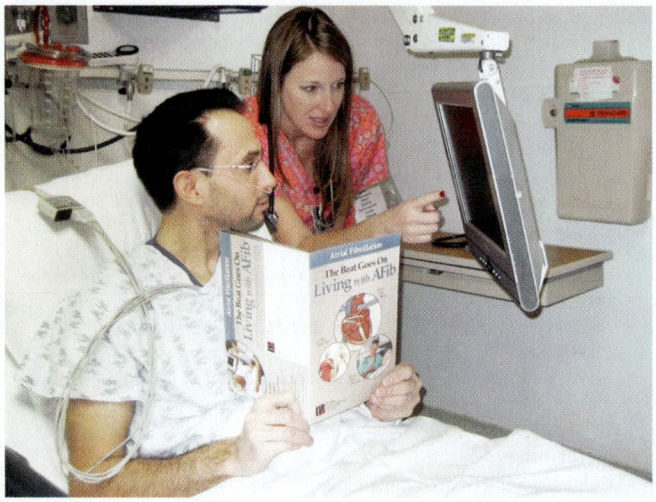

FIG. 4-4 Effective teaching using a variety of strategies (written materials, computer-based patient education programs). (Courtesy Linda Bucher, RN, PhD, CEN, CNE, Staff Nurse, Virtua Memorial Hospital, Mt. Holly, N.J.)

TABLE 4-8 Writing Learning Goals

Elements of Learning Goals

Learning goals (also called outcomes or objectives) are written statements that define exactly how patients demonstrate their mastery of the content. Goals address the following four questions:

1. ***Who Will Perform the Activity or Acquire the Desired Behavior?***
   Examples:
   I (the patient) will
   I (the caregiver) will
   We (patient's family/caregivers) will

2. ***What Is the Actual Behavior That the Learner Will Exhibit to Demonstrate Mastery of the Goal?***
   Examples:
   List the symptoms.
   Self-administer an insulin injection.
   Select from a hospital menu.

3. ***What Are the Conditions Under Which the Behavior Is to Be Demonstrated?***
   Examples:
   In front of the nurse
   From a random list
   Using sterile technique

4. ***What Are the Specific Criteria That Will Be Used to Measure the Patient's Success, Such as Time and Degree of Accuracy?***
   Examples:
   With 100% accuracy
   Over the next week
   Before discharge

Verbs in Learning Goals

Avoid vague, ambiguous verbs that are difficult to measure:
- Appreciate
- Learn
- Understand
- Enjoy
- Feel
- Value

Use verbs that have precise descriptions with few interpretations:
- Identify
- List
- Describe
- Demonstrate
- Perform
- Select

Poorly and Well-Written Learning Goals

Example of Poorly Written Learning Goal	Examples of Well-Written Learning Goals
• The patient will understand the importance of managing his own colostomy. *Analysis*: It is not clear how the patient will demonstrate that he "understands" the importance of managing his colostomy, when and to whom he will demonstrate this behavior, or what criteria will be used to determine whether the objective has been met.	• The patient will describe to the nurse the basic steps for changing the colostomy pouch and skin barrier by 2/14/17. • Using correct technique, the patient will empty his colostomy pouch when one-third full. • The patient's caregiver will perform colostomy care including changing the pouch and skin barrier. • Given a list of signs and symptoms related to complications of a colostomy, the patient and caregiver will identify signs and symptoms to report to a health care provider before discharge. *Analysis*: When learning goals are clear and specific and when they are documented in the patient's record, all members of the health care team can work together to accomplish the same outcomes.

TABLE 4-9 Learner Characteristics and Teaching Strategies by Generation

Birth Year	Learner Characteristics	Recommended Teaching Strategies
Millennials (Generation Y, Yers, Nexters, Digital Natives)		
1981-2000	• Multitaskers • Prefer interactive and virtual environments • Technologically focused • Require flexibility • Short attention span • Team players • Prefer more structured learning compared to Xers • Demand 24/7 access to learning	• Integrate technology and media in teaching (e.g., webinars, social networking sites, Avatars, Podcasts, Wii Fit). • Discuss reliable websites. • Consider health-related mobile applications. • Download health information to smart phones, tablets, or similar devices. • Consider group teaching.
Generation X (Xers, Digital Natives)		
1965-1980	• Self-directed or self-paced learning • Self-reliant • Consumers of education • Short attention span	• Integrate technology and media in teaching. • Discuss reliable websites. • Consider health-related mobile applications. • Provide Web-based education materials. • Provide education materials that are brief and easy to read. • Encourage questions.
Baby Boomers (Digital Immigrants)		
1946-1964	• Emphasis on self-knowledge • Solve problems by action • Acquisition of knowledge from authoritative sources • Receptive to feedback • Prefer text over graphics • Process (step-by-step) oriented	• Assess ehealth literacy and consider strategies as appropriate. • Consider lecture or lecture-discussion (e.g., PowerPoint presentation). • Use patient education TV channels. • Provide printed materials.
Veterans (Traditionalists, Digital Immigrants)		
Born before 1946	• Emphasis on rote learning • Memorization of knowledge • Follow rules	• Assess ehealth literacy and consider strategies as appropriate. • Consider lecture or lecture-discussion. • Use pictures and printed materials such as books.

Compiled from Bradshaw M, Lowenstein A: *Innovative teaching strategies in nursing*, ed 6, Burlington, MA, 2014, Jones & Bartlett Learning; and United Nations Joint Staff Pension Fund: Traditionalists, baby boomers, generation X, generation Y (and generation Z) working together. Retrieved from *www.un.org/staffdevelopment/pdf/Designing%20Recruitment,%20Selection%20&%20Talent%20Management%20Model%20tailored%20to%20meet%20UNJSPF's%20Business%20Development%20Needs.pdf.*

that is mostly visual, such as the steps of a procedure (e.g., suctioning a tracheostomy). The health care agency's television system may also provide patient teaching programs (Fig. 4-4). A dedicated channel may be available and contain high-quality, professionally produced programs provided on demand or on a rotating schedule.

Printed materials continue to be used for teaching patients and caregivers and especially for those whose preferred learning style is reading. Many of these can be printed as needed for teaching (e.g., *www.kramesstaywell.com/home*). These materials are often used in combination with previously discussed teaching strategies. For instance, after a discussion on the effects of smoking on health, you may use material from the American Cancer Society to reinforce the information.

When writing teaching materials, use several techniques to keep the reading level at a fifth-grade level. These include the following: (1) place key information first using bold or italics; (2) use short, common words of one or two syllables; (3) define medical words in simple language if used; (4) keep sentences under 10 words if possible, and 15 at the most; (5) use pictures or drawings; and (6) use an active voice in the manner you would normally say something.[27] Whenever possible, evaluate written materials for readability level using word processing (e.g., Microsoft Word) or Web-based (e.g., *www.wordscount.info*) programs.

Using Technology. Patients' use of the Internet and other digital technology (e.g., smart phones) to obtain health information and manage their health has steadily increased.[28] Patients can quickly do a Web search or open an application and have access to information about their disease, drugs, treatments, and surgeries (e.g., *www.hhs.gov/digitalstrategy/mobile/mobile-apps.html*). Your job is to help patients sift through the wide variety of information to decide if it is valid, reliable, and usable.[29] Understanding the principles of Web searching for health information and instructing patients in finding valid information are critical skills. The presence of Internet connections in many patient rooms (e.g., *www.getwellnetwork.com*) provides an opportunity for you to teach patients about their illness and how to use the Web to find related information.

Explore the use of digital technology by young and older patients and their caregivers. Factors that predict the use of the Web for health information (ehealth literacy) include access to high-speed connections, younger age, some college education, and confidence in using technology.[28] Patients who are chronically ill are more likely to seek health information on the Web.[30,31] Encourage patients to use websites established by the government, universities, or reputable health-related organizations (e.g., American Diabetes Association, American Heart Association, National Institutes of Health, U.S. Food and Drug Administration).

Although older adults are accessing the Web in greater numbers, many may not have the mental capacity, patience, or technical skills to successfully find health information.[32] Organizations dedicated to improving the quality of life for older adults promote the development of user-friendly websites (e.g., *www.nlm.nih.gov/pubs/checklist.pdf*) and publish guides to help older adults evaluate Web-based health information (e.g., *www.mlanet.org/resources/userguide.html*).

The quantity and complexity of digital health care technology available to patients and you will continue to increase.[33] *Telehealth,* a broad term that refers to the delivery of health-related services and information via telecommunications technologies, allows for (1) remote HCP-patient consultations *(telemedicine);* (2) monitoring of vital signs, weight, heart rhythm, blood glucose, etc.; and (3) ongoing patient teaching[34] (see Fig. 34-7). Always educate yourself about these technologies and determine if any will be used when teaching patients.

Implementation

During the implementation phase, use the planned teaching strategies to present information and teach new skills

TABLE 4-10 Comparison of Teaching Strategies

Description	Advantages	Limitations
Discussion ("Teach Back") • Purpose is to exchange points of view about a topic or to arrive at a decision or conclusion • Can be done with patient, with patient and caregiver, or with group • *Example:* Weight loss	• Allows for an active exchange of information and previous experiences among participants • Good choice when patients have previous experience with subject and have information to share • Nonthreatening format • Can use peers (patients with common problems) to teach	• May require additional time depending on topic and number of participants
Lecture-Discussion • Commonly used when group of patients and caregivers can benefit from basic information • Lecture portion is short (i.e., 15-20 min) • Discussion ("teach back") follows lecture • *Example:* Basic principles of cardiac rehabilitation (e.g., exercise, nutrition)	• Combines short lecture to present basic information with time for discussion • Provision of printed material related to lecture content is useful and recommended	• Need to limit number of lecture topics to three to five • May require additional time depending on topic and number of participants
Demonstration/Return Demonstration ("Show Back") • Purpose is to teach patient and caregiver to perform a skill • Through return demonstration ("show back") can evaluate patient's ability to perform skill (Fig. 4-5) • *Examples:* Dressing change, injection	• Provides for learning and practice of physical skills • Dividing skill into series of smaller steps facilitates mastery and provides reinforcement	• May require additional time for practice needed to master skill • Patients with limited manual dexterity may have difficulty
Use of Teaching Resources • Audiovisual aids to supplement teaching • Printed materials (e.g., brochures) • CDs/DVDs • Hospital-based TV (Fig. 4-4) • Digital and communication technologies (e.g., mobile applications, Web-based patient education programs, game-based education, online support groups) • Telehealth (see Fig. 34-7)	• Enhance the presentation through visual and/or auditory stimulation • Best used in combination with other teaching strategies • Use of digital and communication technologies for health information is the preferred choice for many • Web access in patient rooms is standard in most health care agencies • Health information can be provided and reinforced to patients remotely	• Materials must be previewed and evaluated (e.g., accuracy, completeness, reading level) before using • Websites, games, applications, programs, etc. must be evaluated for validity of information • May not be appropriate for all learners (e.g., lack of interest, decreased mental capacity) • Finances (e.g., equipment purchase, Internet service) may be a limiting factor to using digital technology

(Table 4-10). Incorporate verbal and nonverbal communication skills, active listening, and empathy into the process. Based on the assessment of the patient's physical, psychologic, sociocultural, and learner characteristics, determine how much the patient can participate. Whenever possible and appropriate, involve the patient's caregiver(s) in the teaching-learning process.

In implementing the teaching plan, remember the principles and characteristics of the adult learner. Reinforcement and reward are important, but be aware that phrases such as, "Aren't you doing well!" in a tone one would use with a child can be condescending to adult learners.

Evaluation

Evaluation, the final step in the learning process, is a measure of the degree to which the patient has achieved the learning goals. Various evaluation techniques can be used (Table 4-11). Use techniques such as "teach back" and "show back" to determine the knowledge and skill levels of the patient and/or caregiver throughout the teaching and learning process[35] (Fig. 4-5). If certain goals are not reached, reassess the patient and revise the teaching plan accordingly.

The patient most likely had been administering insufficient insulin to himself for some time. The patient's vision had declined over the 20 years, and special equipment was now necessary for him to safely and correctly administer the insulin. The lesson here is that assumptions regarding a patient's

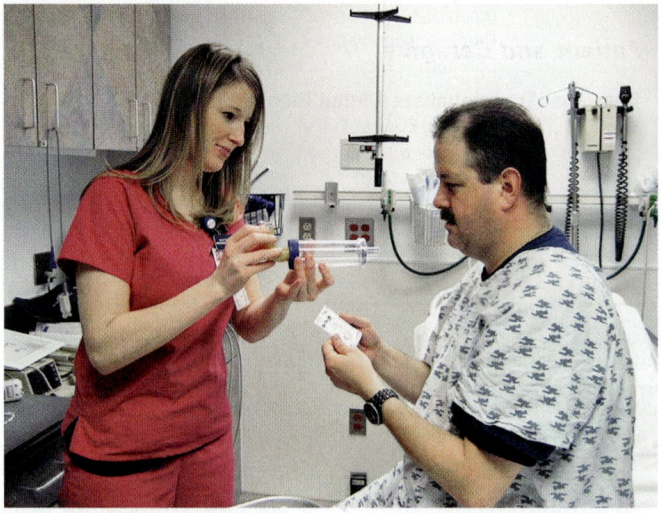

FIG. 4-5 Teaching using discussion ("teach back") and demonstration/return demonstration ("show back") increases successful learning by the patient. (Courtesy Linda Bucher, RN, PhD, CEN, CNE, Staff Nurse, Virtua Memorial Hospital, Mt. Holly, N.J.)

TABLE 4-11 Evaluation of Patient and Caregiver Learning

Technique	Strategy and Examples

Observe patient or caregiver directly.	• Ask person to show you how to change the dressing.
	• Return demonstration ("show back") determines whether
	  • Skill has been mastered
	  • Further instruction is needed
	  • Patient and caregiver are ready for new or additional content

Observe verbal and nonverbal cues.	• Teaching may have to be delayed, further teaching is needed, or different strategy should be used if patient or caregiver
	  • Asks you to repeat instructions
	  • Loses eye contact
	  • Begins to doze in chair or bed
	  • Becomes restless or fidgety
	  • Does not speak English

Ask open-ended questions ("teach back").	• Open-ended questions provide more information about understanding than close-ended questions, which require only a "yes" or "no."
	• Ask questions such as
	  • "How often do you need to change the dressing?"
	  • "What will you do if you develop chest pain at home?"

Talk with caregiver ("teach back").	• Involve caregiver in the evaluation process.
	• Ask questions such as
	  • "What medications is she taking?"
	  • "When does he use his oxygen?"

Seek the patient's self-evaluation of progress.	• Ask patient's opinion about his or her progress.
	  • What evidence does the patient have that the goals are being met?
	  • Is the patient ready to go forward with learning new material?

CHECK YOUR PRACTICE

Your patient is a 53-yr-old male with type 1 diabetes mellitus who entered the hospital with a blood glucose level of 550 mg/dL (30.53 mmol/L). He is now stable and soon will be discharged.

You prepare his insulin and plan to give him the syringe to let him do his own injection. Before you go to his room, your preceptor suggests that you observe his technique of preparing the insulin as well as the injection. You are puzzled by this comment because he has had diabetes for 32 years and should know how to do it.

When you go to his room, you ask him to prepare the insulin injection ("show back"). You notice that he filled the syringe with 30 units of insulin and 10 units of air, instead of 40 units of insulin. After correcting the dose and questioning the patient more fully ("teach back"), you wonder what happened because you thought he knew the correct dosage of insulin.

- What are possible reasons that he did not draw up the correct amount of insulin?

knowledge and skills are dangerous. Always evaluate past and new knowledge and skills.

Long-term evaluation of learning goals often requires follow-up after discharge. Provide a written schedule of visits and other appropriate referrals for the patient before he or she leaves the hospital or clinic. The patient's caregiver(s) also must be familiar with the follow-up plan so that everyone involved in the patient's long-term progress is on the same page.[36]

Documentation is an essential and required component throughout the entire teaching-learning process. Record everything from the assessment through plans for evaluation and follow-up. Because various members of the health care team use these records in different settings and for different reasons, the teaching goals, strategies, and evaluation results need to be clear, complete, and available to all members of the health care team.

CASE STUDY

Patient and Caregiver Teaching

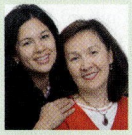

(©Thomas M Perkins/ Shutterstock)

Patient Profile

M.L., a 60-year-old Asian woman, is admitted to the hospital with a diagnosis of exacerbation of chronic obstructive pulmonary disease (COPD).

Subjective Data

- History of COPD for 10 years. Reports a chronic cough but denies any recent change in color of sputum. States "I stopped smoking last year, but my son-in-law smokes."
- Past medical history: gastroesophageal reflux disease; macular degeneration in right eye.
- Social history: widowed 5 years ago and since then has lived with daughter and son-in-law who work full time. Cares for two young grandchildren after school. English is M.L.'s second language.

Objective Data

Physical Examination

- Alert, cognitively intact, anxious, thin woman with dyspnea on minimal exertion. Speaking in short phases or sentences. States "I have no energy."
- Using oxygen via nasal cannula at 2 L/min
- Weight 100 lb, height 5 ft 2 in

Diagnostic Studies

- Chest x-ray negative for acute infection
- Arterial blood gases on room air: pH 7.35, $PaCO_2$ 47 mm Hg, PaO_2 75 mm Hg, HCO_3^- 30 mEq/L
- O_2 saturation (via pulse oximetry) during 6-minute walk test on room air = 83%
- Forced expiratory volume in 1 second of expiration (FEV_1) = 60% of predicted

Interprofessional Care

- Medications: bronchodilator therapy (inpatient nebulizer therapy, inhalers on discharge), oral corticosteroids
- Continuous home O_2 therapy: O_2 at 2 L/min via nasal cannula
- Pulmonary rehabilitation: inpatient and outpatient

Discussion Questions

1. ***Priority Decision:*** Given M.L.'s history, what are the priority learning needs?
2. ***Patient-Centered Care:*** What factors (e.g., sociocultural, physical, psychologic) may influence M.L.'s response to teaching?
3. ***Patient-Centered Care:*** What potential challenges might you expect when planning to teach M.L.? How would you manage them?
4. ***Priority Decision:*** Identify two priority nursing diagnoses. Develop a teaching plan for M.L. based on these nursing diagnoses.

Answers available at *http://evolve.elsevier.com/Lewis/medsurg.*

BRIDGE TO NCLEX EXAMINATION

The number of the question corresponds to the same-numbered outcome at the beginning of the chapter.

1. Which technique is *most* appropriate when using motivational interviewing with a patient who tells you that he is ready to start a weight-loss program?
   a. Confirm that the patient is serious about losing weight.
   b. Insist that the patient consider an organized group weight-loss program.
   c. Focus on the patient's strengths to support his optimism that he can successfully lose weight.
   d. Ask a prescribed set of questions to increase the patient's awareness of his dietary behaviors.
2. Which is the *priority* patient teaching strategy when limited time is available?
   a. Setting realistic goals that have high priority for the patient
   b. Referring the patient to a nurse educator in private practice for teaching
   c. Observing more experienced nurse-teachers to learn how to teach faster and more efficiently
   d. Providing reading materials for the patient instead of discussing information the patient needs to learn
3. The nurse needs to include caregivers in patient teaching primarily because *(select all that apply)*
   a. they provide all of the care for patients after discharge.
   b. they might feel rejected if they are not included in the teaching.
   c. patients have better outcomes when their caregivers are involved.
   d. the patient may be too ill or too stressed to fully understand the teaching.
   e. caregivers are responsible for the overall management of the patient's care.
4. Which patient characteristic enhances the teaching-learning process?
   a. Moderate anxiety
   b. High self-efficacy
   c. Being in the precontemplative stage of change
   d. Being able to laugh about the current health problem
5. What would be the *priority* teaching goal for a middle-aged Hispanic woman regarding methods to relieve symptoms of menopause?
   a. Prevent the development of future disease.
   b. Maintain the patient's current state of health.
   c. Provide information on possible treatment options.
   d. Change the patient's beliefs about herbal supplements.
6. A patient tells the nurse that she enjoys talking with others and sharing experiences but often falls asleep when reading. Which teaching strategy would be *most* effective with this patient?
   a. Role playing
   b. Group teaching
   c. Lecture-discussion
   d. Web-based programs
7. The nurse has taught a patient's wife (his primary caregiver) how to administer insulin to her husband. Evaluation of the nurse's teaching effectiveness before discharge would include
   a. arranging for follow-up with a home care nurse.
   b. monitoring the patient's glucose readings before discharge.
   c. asking the caregiver to "show back" her ability to administer insulin.
   d. asking the caregiver what she found helpful about the teaching experience.

1. c, 2. a, 3. c, d, 4. b, 5. c, 6. b, 7. c.

For rationales to these answers and even more NCLEX review questions, visit *http://evolve.elsevier.com/Lewis/medsurg.*

EVOLVE WEBSITE

http://evolve.elsevier.com/Lewis/medsurg

Review Questions (Online Only)
Key Points
Answer Keys for Questions
- Rationales for Bridge to NCLEX Examination Questions
- Answer Guidelines for Case Study on p. 57

Conceptual Care Map Creator
Audio Glossary
Content Updates

REFERENCES

1. Centers for Disease Control and Prevention: Chronic disease prevention and health promotion, Washington, DC, 2014. Retrieved from *www.cdc.gov/chronicdisease/overview/#sec1.*

*2. Mitchell S, Gardiner P, Sadikova E, et al: Patient activation and 30-day post-discharge hospital utilization, *J Gen Int Med* 29:349, 2014.

3. American Nurses Credentialing Center: Forces of magnetism: force 11: nurses as teachers, 2014. Retrieved from *www.nursecredentialing.org/ForcesofMagnetism.aspx#11.*

4. Redman BK: *The practice of patient education*, ed 10, St Louis, 2007, Mosby.

5. Knowles MS, Holton EF, Swanson RA: *The adult learner: the definitive classic in adult education and human resource development*, ed 7, St Louis, 2011, Mosby.

*6. Prochaska J, Velicer W: The transtheoretical model of health behavior change, *Am J Health Promot* 12:38, 1997. (Classic)

7. Rollnick S, Miller WR, Yahne CE: *Motivational interviewing in health care: helping patients change behavior*, New York, 2008, Guilford Press. (Classic)

*8. Miller WR: *Enhancing motivation for change in substance abuse treatment: Treatment Improvement Protocol (TIP) series 35, DHHS pub no (SMA) 99-3354*, Rockville, Md, 1999, US Department of Health and Human Services. Retrieved from *www.ncbi.nlm.nih.gov/books/NBK64967.* (Classic)

9. Feinberg L, Reinhard SC, Houser A, et al: Valuing the invaluable: 2011 update—the growing contributions and costs of family caregiving, AARP Public Policy Institute. Retrieved from *http://assets.aarp.org/rgcenter/ppi/ltc/i51-caregiving.pdf.*

10. Levine C: Supporting family caregivers: the hospital nurse's assessment of family caregiver needs, *Am J Nurs* 111:47, 2011.

11. Fowler C: Caring for the caregiver, *Nursing* 44:60, 2014.

12. The Joint Commission: 2014 Hospital national patient safety goals. Retrieved from *www.jointcommission.org/standards_information/npsgs.aspx.*

13. American Hospital Association: The patient care partnership. Retrieved from *www.aha.org/advocacy-issues/communicatingpts/pt-care-partnership.shtml.*

14. The Joint Commission: Speak up initiatives, 2014. Retrieved from *www.jointcommission.org/speakup.aspx.*

15. National Patient Safety Foundation: Ask me 3. Retrieved from *https://npsf.site-ym.com/default.asp?page=askme3.*

16. Geriatric Mental Health Foundation: Consumer/patient information. Retrieved from *www.gmhfonline.org/gmhf/consumer/factsheets/hlthage_mental.html.*
*17. Farrell K, Wicks MN, Martin JC: Chronic disease self-management improved with enhanced self-efficacy, *Clin Nurs Res* 13(4):289, 2004. (Classic)
18. The Joint Commission: What did the doctor say? Improving health literacy to protect patient safety, 2007. Retrieved from *www.jointcommission.org/assets/1/18/improving_health_literacy.pdf.*
19. Barclay L: Screening questions may help predict limited health literacy, *Ann Fam Med* 7:24, 2009.
20. U.S. Department of Health and Human Services, Office of Disease Prevention and Health Promotion: Quick guide to health literacy, fact sheet, health literacy and health outcomes. Retrieved from *www.health.gov/communication/literacy/quickguide/factsliteracy.htm.*
*21. Morris NS, MacLean CD, Chew LD, et al: The single item literacy screener: evaluation of a brief instrument to identify limited reading ability, *BMC Fam Pract* 7:21, 2006. (Classic)
22. Wilson-Stronks A, Lee KK, Cordero CL, et al: One size does not fit all: meeting the health care needs of diverse populations, Oakland Terrace, Ill, The Joint Commission. Retrieved from *www.jointcommission.org/assets/1/6/HLCOneSizeFinal.pdf.*
23. Inott T, Kennedy BB: Assessing learning styles: practical tips for patient education, *Nurs Clin North Am* 46:313, 2011.
24. Office of Disease Prevention and Health Promotion: What is e-health? Retrieved from *www.health.gov/communication/ehealth.*
25. Bradshaw M, Lowenstein A: *Innovative teaching strategies in nursing*, ed 6, Burlington, Mass, 2014, Jones & Bartlett Learning.
26. United Nations Joint Staff Pension Fund: Traditionalists, baby boomers, generation X, generation Y (and generation Z) working together. Retrieved from *www.un.org/staffdevelopment/pdf/Designing%20Recruitment,%20Selection%20&%20Talent%20Management%20Model%20tailored%20to%20meet%20UNJSPF's%20Business%20Development%20Needs.pdf.*
27. Medline Plus: How to write easy-to-read health materials, 2013. Retrieved from *www.nlm.nih.gov/medlineplus/etr.html.*
28. Pew Research Internet Project: Trends to watch. Retrieved from *www.pewinternet.org/2009/06/11/trends-to-watch.*
29. Wood F, Robson M, Thompson M, et al: Selecting the best type of mobile application for chronic disease self-management, *Comput Inform Nurs* 31:208, 2013.
*30. Stellefson M, Chaney B, Ochipa K, et al: YouTube as a source of chronic obstructive pulmonary disease patient education: a social media content analysis, *Chronic Resp Dis* 11:61, 2014.
*31. Lee S, Shin S: Effectiveness of virtual reality using video gaming technology in elderly adults with diabetes mellitus, *Diabetes Technol Ther* 15:489, 2013.
*32. Levy H, Janke AT, Langa KM: Health literacy and the digital divide among older Americans, *J Gen Intern Med* 30:384, 2015.
33. Trossman S: Back to the future? Telehealth services, tele-nursing are on the rise, *American Nurse* Sept/Oct:1, 2014.
34. GlobalMed: Telehealth, telecare, telemedicine…what's the difference? Retrieved from *www.globalmed.com/additional-resources/telehealth-telecare-and-telemedicine-whats-the-difference.php.*
35. Minnesota Health Literacy Partnership: Teach-back: what does your patient really understand? Retrieved from *healthliteracymn.org/sites/default/files/images/files/Teach-Back_program_guide_updated_011212.pdf.*
*36. Agency for Healthcare Research and Quality: Implementing re-engineered hospital discharges (Project RED): frequently asked questions, 2009. Retrieved from *www.ahrq.gov/news/kt/red/redfaq.htm.*

*Evidence-based information for clinical practice.

5

Chronic Illness and Older Adults

Sherry A. Greenberg

You don't stop laughing when you grow old, you grow old when you stop laughing.

George Bernard Shaw

http://evolve.elsevier.com/Lewis/medsurg/

LEARNING OUTCOMES

1. Describe the prevention and major causes of chronic illness.
2. Explain the characteristics of a chronic illness.
3. Describe the demographics of aging.
4. Define *ageism.*
5. Explain the needs of special populations of older adults.
6. Describe nursing interventions to assist older adults with chronic illnesses.
7. Describe common problems of older adults related to hospitalization and acute illness and the nurse's role in assisting them.
8. Differentiate among care alternatives to meet needs of older adults.
9. Describe the nurse's role in health promotion, disease prevention, and managing the special needs of older adults.

KEY TERMS

ageism, p. 63
chronic illness, Table 5-1, p. 61
elder mistreatment (EM), p. 66
ethnogeriatric, p. 66
frail older adult, p. 63
gerontologic nursing, p. 69
Medicaid, p. 68
Medicare, p. 68
old-old adult, p. 63
young-old adult, p. 63

This chapter discusses issues related to chronic illness and aging. The population of older adults is growing rapidly. You need to consider their multiple, complex health care conditions and needs.

CHRONIC ILLNESS

Illness can be categorized as either acute or chronic (Table 5-1). The U.S. health care system faces a growing burden of chronic illness as the population ages. Chronic illnesses account for 70% of all deaths in the United States. Chronic illness results in limitations in physical functioning, work productivity, and quality of life for nearly 1 out of 10 Americans. Older adults often live with more than one chronic illness, frequently up to six or more. A significant portion of U.S. health care dollars go toward the treatment of chronic illnesses.[1] The management of a chronic illness can greatly affect the lives of the patient, family, and caregiver. Table 5-2 presents the impact of some chronic illnesses.

In addition to people living longer, other societal changes have contributed to the increase in chronic illnesses. These include insufficient physical activity, lack of access to fresh fruits and vegetables, tobacco use, and alcohol consumption.[1]

Trajectory of Chronic Illness

The individual with a chronic illness can move from a level of optimum functioning, with the illness well controlled, to a period of physical instability. Corbin and Strauss proposed a view of chronic illness as a trajectory (Fig. 5-1) with overlapping phases[2] (Table 5-3). This trajectory characterizes the common course of most chronic conditions. In addition, Corbin and Strauss identified the seven tasks of those who are chronically ill (Table 5-4). These tasks are discussed in the following sections.

Preventing and Managing a Crisis. Most chronic illnesses have the potential for an acute exacerbation of symptoms, which may result in further disability or death. Examples include the patient with heart disease who has another myocardial infarction or the patient with asthma who has a severe attack. A major task for the patient and caregiver is to learn to prevent or manage the crisis. First, the patient and caregiver need to understand the potential for the crisis to occur. Second, they need to know ways to prevent or modify the threat. This often involves adherence to a prescribed medical regimen. Patients also need to know the signs and symptoms of the onset of a crisis. Depending on the chronic illness, signs and symptoms may occur suddenly (e.g., bleeding in a patient with inflammatory bowel disease) or

Reviewed by Donna E. McCabe, DNP, APRN-BC, GNP, New York University, College of Nursing, New York, New York; and Lorraine Nowakowski-Grier, MSN, APRN, BC, CDE, Diabetes Nurse Practitioner, Christiana Care Health Services, Nursing Development & Education, Newark, Delaware.

TABLE 5-1 Characteristics of Acute and Chronic Illness

Description	Characteristics
Acute Illness Diseases that have a rapid onset and short duration *Examples:* colds, influenza, acute gastroenteritis	• Usually self-limiting • Responds readily to treatment • Complications infrequent • After illness, return to previous level of functioning
Chronic Illness Diseases that are prolonged, do not resolve spontaneously, and are rarely cured completely *Examples:* see Table 5-2	• Permanent impairments or deviations from normal • Irreversible pathologic changes • Residual disability • Special rehabilitation required • Need for long-term medical and/or nursing management

slowly (e.g., heart failure in a patient with untreated hypertension). It is important for the patient and caregiver to develop a plan to manage a crisis that is likely to occur.

Carrying Out Prescribed Treatment Regimen. Treatment regimens vary in degree of difficulty and the impact they have on the person's lifestyle. Treatment regimens may appear challenging or time consuming, such as changing a dressing multiple times a day or instituting a toileting program. However, they generally save time and prevent complications.

Controlling Symptoms. An important task for those with chronic illnesses is to learn to control symptoms so that desired activities may be continued. Some individuals redesign their lifestyle by learning to plan ahead, such as individuals with heart failure adjusting the time they take diuretics to avoid needing to rush to a bathroom if going out for the day. Independence in decision making is encouraged, but changes in treatment regimens should be done in collaboration with their health care provider (HCP) to avoid an exacerbation of the illness. Others may redesign their living space. Patients and their families and/or caregivers need to learn about the pattern of symptoms, such as typical onset, duration, and severity, so that lifestyle may be changed accordingly, while maintaining safety.

Reordering Time. People with chronic illness often report having too much or too little time. Treatment plans that require large amounts of time for the person, as well as caregivers, may necessitate changing schedules or eliminating other activities. For example, the patient with a new ileostomy needs to plan for increased time in the bathroom to change the drainage bag.

Adjusting to Changes in the Course of Disease. Some diseases, such as multiple sclerosis, have unpredictable courses that make planning activities difficult. Part of the individual's task is to develop a personal identity that includes the chronic illness and adjust to the lifestyle changes it necessitates. For example, an individual taking warfarin (Coumadin) due to a mechanical heart valve may need to avoid extreme physical sports that have a high potential for injury.

Preventing Social Isolation. Social isolation may occur with chronic illness because the individual chooses to withdraw from previous activities or because others withdraw from the chronically ill person. For example, a woman who has aphasia secondary to a stroke may be unwilling to go out in public because of embarrassment related to communication issues.

TABLE 5-2 Impact of Chronic Illnesses

Chronic Illness	Impact	CONTENT IN BOOK Chapter	Page
Alzheimer's disease	• Affects 5.4 million people • Sixth leading cause of death	59	1401
Arthritis	• Affects 1 in 5 people • One of most common chronic illnesses	64	1517
Cancer	• Second leading cause of death	15	234
Chronic obstructive pulmonary disease	• Affects many older adults • Third leading cause of death	28	557
Coronary artery disease	• Affects about 17 million adults • Leading cause of death	33	702
Diabetes	• Affects >29 million Americans • 8.1 million do not know they have the disease • Seventh leading cause of death	48	1120
Heart failure	• Most common reason older adults are hospitalized	34	737
Obesity	• Affects about 34% of adults • Major contributor to other health problems	40	874
Stroke	• Affects about 7 million adults, 15%-30% disabled • Leading cause of serious disability • Fifth leading cause of death	57	1345
HIV/AIDS	• 50,000 new cases each year • Affects >1 million Americans	14	213

Data from Centers for Disease Control and Prevention: CDC's Chronic Disease Press Releases. Retrieved from *www.cdc.gov/chronicdisease/resources/press*, 2014.
AIDS, Acquired immunodeficiency syndrome; *HIV*, human immunodeficiency virus.

Attempting to Normalize Interactions With Others. Most individuals with chronic illness attempt to manage symptoms so that they can hide their disabilities or disfigurement. This may involve wearing a prosthesis or demonstrating that they can function the same as a person without a disability or chronic illness. An example of this is the woman with heart failure who stops walking to catch her breath but appears to be inspecting a plant or looking in a store window.

Prevention of Chronic Illness

Chronic illnesses are often preventable. *Primary prevention* refers to measures such as nutritious diet, proper exercise, and immunizations that prevent the occurrence of a specific disease. Appropriate immunizations for older adults include influenza, pneumococcal, herpes zoster, tetanus/diphtheria/pertussis (Td/Tdap), and hepatitis A and B. *Secondary prevention* refers to actions aimed at early detection of disease that can lead

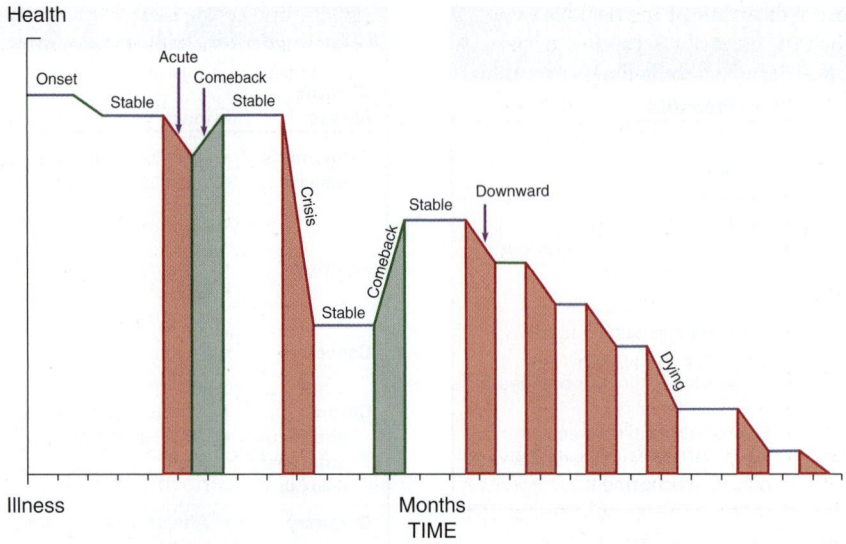

FIG. 5-1 The Chronic Illness Trajectory is a theoretical model of chronic illness. The trajectory model of chronic illness recognizes that chronic illness will have many phases (Table 5-3). (From Woog P: *The chronic illness trajectory framework: the Corbin and Strauss nursing model,* New York, 1992, Springer.)

TABLE 5-3 Chronic Illness Trajectory

Phases	Description
Onset	• Signs and symptoms are present. • Disease diagnosed.
Stable	• Illness course and symptoms controlled by treatment regimen. • Person maintains everyday activities.
Acute	• Active illness with severe and unrelieved symptoms or complications. • Hospitalization may be required for management.
Comeback	• Gradual return to an acceptable way of life.
Crisis	• Life-threatening situation occurs. • Emergency services are necessary.
Unstable	• Unable to keep symptoms or disease course under control. • Life becomes disrupted while patient works to regain stability. • Hospitalization not required.
Downward	• Gradual and progressive deterioration in physical or mental status. • Accompanied by increasing disability and symptoms. • Continuous alterations in everyday life activities.
Dying	• Patient has to relinquish everyday life interests and activities, let go, and die peacefully. • Immediate weeks, days, hours preceding death.

Source: Woog P: *The chronic illness trajectory framework: the Corbin and Strauss nursing model,* New York, 1992, Springer.

to interventions to prevent disease progression. *Tertiary prevention* refers to activities that limit disease progression such as rehabilitation.

❖ NURSING MANAGEMENT: CHRONIC ILLNESS

Diagnosis and treatment of the acute phase or acute exacerbations of a chronic illness sometimes take place in a hospital. Other phases of a chronic illness are regularly assessed and managed in an ambulatory care setting, at home, in an assisted living facility, or in a skilled nursing facility.

TABLE 5-4 Seven Tasks of People With Chronic Illness

1. Prevent and manage a crisis.
2. Carry out prescribed treatment regimen.
3. Control symptoms.
4. Reorder time.
5. Adjust to changes in course of disease.
6. Prevent social isolation.
7. Attempt to normalize interactions with others.

Source: Corbin JM, Strauss A: A nursing model for chronic illness management based upon the trajectory framework, *Sch Inq Nurs Pract* 5:155, 1991.

An assessment of health status, at least annually, includes an individual's level of daily functioning and his or her perception of relative health, function, and/or illness. Health assessment includes activities of daily living (ADLs), such as bathing, dressing, eating, toileting, and transferring. It also includes instrumental ADLs (IADLs), such as using a phone, shopping, preparing food, housekeeping, doing laundry, arranging transportation, taking medications, and handling finances.[3]

Because the majority of chronic illnesses are treated in an ambulatory care setting, it is increasingly important for patients and caregivers to understand and manage their own health. The term *self-management* refers to the individual's ability to manage his or her health, especially in response to living with a chronic illness. It refers to the ability to manage symptoms, medications and treatment regimen, physical and psychosocial consequences, and lifestyle changes.[4] Self-management is in conjunction with family and HCP.

You play an important role in the management of individuals with chronic illness. This includes conducting a comprehensive history and physical assessment, participating in interventions and plan of care, teaching the patient and caregiver regarding the treatment plan, implementing strategies for symptom management, and evaluating patient outcomes.

Family caregivers (e.g., spouses, partners, adult children) often have important roles in the life of the chronically ill person. The ideal situation is one in which family caregivers work together with the patient to manage the chronic condition(s). This collaboration begins under the direction of the health care team at the time of diagnosis. When the caregiver is a spouse or partner who is also older, he or she may have a chronic illness or multiple chronic conditions as well, which may complicate the coordination of care.[5] The stresses and needs of family caregivers are discussed in Chapter 4.

OLDER ADULTS

DEMOGRAPHICS OF AGING

The older adult population (those 65 years of age and older) continues to outpace the rest of the population. More than 41 million people, or 13% of the population, are age 65 or older.[6] Nearly one in five U.S. residents is expected to be 65 or older by 2030. The U.S. Census Bureau predicts life expectancy to continue to increase for both men and women. Those reaching 65 years have an average life expectancy of an additional 19.2 years, specifically 20.4 years for females and 17.8 years for males.[7] Whether this gender difference is due to differences in health behaviors (e.g., smoking, alcohol use) or occupation is not known.

GENDER DIFFERENCES

Older Adults

Men

- More likely to be married and living with spouse or partner
- More likely to have health insurance
- Higher income after retirement
- Less likely to be involved in caregiving activities
- Generally have fewer chronic health conditions than women

Women

- More likely to live alone
- More likely to be widowed
- Less likely to have health insurance
- More likely to live in poverty
- Poverty rates highest among minority women
- More likely to lack formal work experience leading to lower income
- More likely to rely on Social Security as major source of income
- More likely to be caregiver of ill spouse or partner
- Have a higher incidence of chronic health conditions such as arthritis, hypertension, stroke, and diabetes

The fastest-growing segment of older Americans is people ages 85 or older. The increase in life span is due to declining infant mortality, new drug therapies, mechanical devices, and improved surgical interventions. In addition, greater emphasis on health promotion, disease prevention, and earlier detection as well as better care management has led to more Americans living past 85 years.

In the United States 13% of people over age 65 are of racial or ethnic minority populations, including 9% African Americans; 4% Asian/Pacific Islanders; and less than 1% American Indians, Eskimos, and Aleuts. People of Hispanic/Latino ethnicity (who may be of any race) represent 7% of the older population.[7] By 2030 the proportion of older adults who are people of racial or ethnic minority will increase 125% (Latinos 155%; African Americans 104%; American Indians, Eskimos, and Aleuts 116%; and Asian/Pacific Islanders 119%), while growth in the European-American population will increase by only 54%.[7]

Upcoming cohorts of older adults will likely have increased access to higher education, employment, technology, and resources than previous cohorts. According to the U.S. Census Bureau, the majority of the population 65 and older completed high school or higher education. Additionally, a quarter of the population 65 and older earned a bachelor's degree or higher.[8]

The terms **young-old adult** (65 to 74 years of age) and **old-old adult** (85 years of age and older) describe two groups of older adults with different characteristics and needs. Nearly 6% of individuals age 65 to 74 and 25% of those 85 and older live in nursing homes. The old-old adult is often a widowed, divorced, or single woman dependent on family for support or care. Many old-old adults have outlived children, spouses or partners, and siblings.

The **frail older adult** is usually over age 75 and has physical, cognitive, and/or mental conditions that may interfere with independently performing ADLs. (Frail older adults are discussed later in this chapter.)

ATTITUDES TOWARD AGING

Who is old? The answer to this question often depends on the respondent's age and attitude. It is important to understand that aging is normal and is not related to pathology or disease. Age is established by a date in time and is influenced by many factors, including emotional and physical health, developmental stage, socioeconomic status, culture, and ethnicity.

As people age, they are exposed to new and different life experiences. The accumulation of these differences makes older adults more diverse than any other age group. As you assess older adults, consider and value their diversity and life history. Also assess their own perceptions of what it means to be an older adult. The majority of older adults report having good-to-excellent health despite having a chronic condition. However, older adults with poor health often report a higher perceived age and lower sense of well-being when compared with healthy older adults. Age is important, but it may not be the most relevant factor in determining appropriate care of an individual older adult.

Myths and stereotypes about aging are often supported by media reports of older adults who are "problematic." These commonly held misconceptions may lead to omissions or errors in assessment and unnecessary limitations or interventions. For example, if you think that all older people are rigid in their thinking, you may not present new ideas to a patient.[9]

Ageism is a negative attitude based on age. Ageism leads to discrimination and disparities in the care given to older adults. If you demonstrate negative attitudes, it may be because you fear your own aging process or you are not knowledgeable about aging and the health care needs of the older adult.

BIOLOGIC AGING

From a biologic view, *aging* reflects the changes that occur over time. Biologic aging is a multifactorial process involving genetics, diet, and environment.[10] In part, biologic aging can be viewed as a balance of positive and negative factors (Fig. 5-2). Current research is directed at increasing the average life span and the quality of life of older adults. The hope is that new antiaging therapies will be developed to slow down or reverse age-related changes that result in chronic illness and disability.

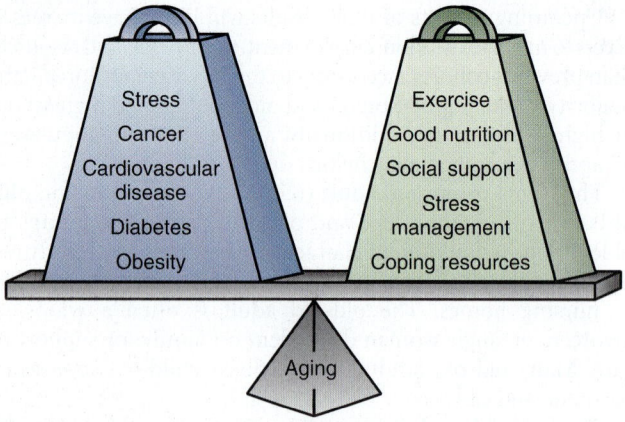

FIG. 5-2 The aging process can be viewed as a balance between negative and positive factors.

AGE-RELATED PHYSIOLOGIC CHANGES

Age-related changes affect every body system. These changes are normal and occur as people age. However, the age at which specific changes occur differs from person to person and within the same person. For instance, a person may have gray hair at age 45 but have relatively unwrinkled skin at age 80. In your role as a nurse, assess for age-related changes. Table 5-5 presents a list of tables in which specific age-related assessment findings can be found throughout the book.

SPECIAL OLDER ADULT POPULATIONS

Chronically Ill Older Adults

Daily living with chronic illness is a reality for many older adults. The incidence of chronic illness triples after age 45. Most people 65 years of age and older have at least one chronic condition, and many have multiple conditions.[1] The most common chronic conditions in older adults are hypertension, heart failure, coronary artery disease, chronic obstructive pulmonary disease, cancer, diabetes, and osteoarthritis. Other common chronic conditions include Alzheimer's disease, vision and hearing deficits, osteoporosis, stroke, Parkinson's disease, and depression.

Cognitively Impaired Older Adults

Most healthy older adults have no noticeable decline in cognitive abilities (Table 5-6). Older adults may have a mild decline in memory and may require more time to recall events or new information. This differs from cognitive impairment. New learning may be slower. Encourage older adults with memory loss to be evaluated by their HCP and to use memory aids, attempt recall in a calm and quiet environment, and actively engage in enhancing memory. Memory aids include clocks, calendars, notes, marked pillboxes, safety alarms on stoves, and identification necklaces or bracelets. Memory techniques include word association, mental imaging, and mnemonics.

Dementia, delirium, and depression are common and may co-exist in older adults. Declining physical health and acute illness are important factors that may influence cognition. For example, an older adult who undergoes surgery may demonstrate an acute change in mental status known as *delirium.*[11] Delirium superimposed on dementia may signify an acute or emergent condition such as heart failure. Hence, it is important to differentiate signs and symptoms of each. Cognitive impairment, delirium, dementia, and differentiation of each are discussed in Chapter 59.

TABLE 5-5 Gerontologic Assessment Differences

Summary of Tables

Body System	Table Number	Page
Visual	20-1	353
Auditory	20-7	361
Integumentary	22-1	397
Respiratory	25-4	459
Hematologic	29-3	593
Cardiovascular	31-1	663
Gastrointestinal	38-5	840
Urinary	44-2	1020
Endocrine	47-3	1108
Reproductive	50-3	1191
Nervous	55-2	1302
Musculoskeletal	61-1	1451

TABLE 5-6 Gerontologic Assessment Differences

Cognitive Function

Effect of Aging	Cognitive Function
Improves with aging	• Vocabulary and verbal reasoning • Crystallized intelligence (ability to use skills, knowledge, and experience)
Declines during middle age	• Mental performance speed • Synthesis of new information • Fluid intelligence (ability to think logically and solve problems in new situations)
Declines during old age	• Short-term recall memory
Constant (no changes with aging)	• Long-term recall memory

Rural Older Adults

Five barriers to health care access for rural older adults are transportation, limited supply of health care workers and facilities, lack of quality health care, social isolation, and financial limitations. Particularly vulnerable are older adults of racial or ethnic minority living in rural areas, who have even less access to HCPs. In addition, older adults who live in rural areas may be less likely to engage in health-promoting activities.

When you work with older adults in rural areas, recognize lifestyle values and practices of rural life (Fig. 5-3). In planning care, be aware that transportation is the number one barrier to health care for rural older adults. Alternative service approaches such as computer-based Internet sources and chat rooms, DVDs, radio, community centers, and church social events may be used to promote healthy practices or to conduct health screening (Fig. 5-4).

The use of telehealth devices for monitoring patients in their home environments has enhanced the ability to provide care, including to those more isolated.[12] Innovative models of nursing practice must continue to be developed to assist the rural older adult. Older adults are increasingly using technology in their daily lives. Most older adults use the Internet and own a cell phone.[12]

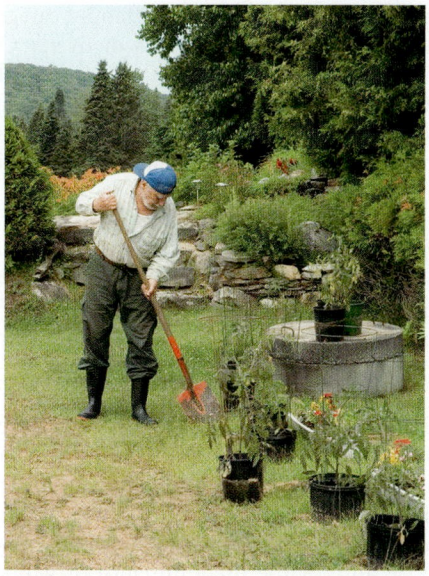

FIG. 5-3 Older adults living in rural areas often enjoy outside activities, such as gardening. (©iStockphoto/Thinkstock.)

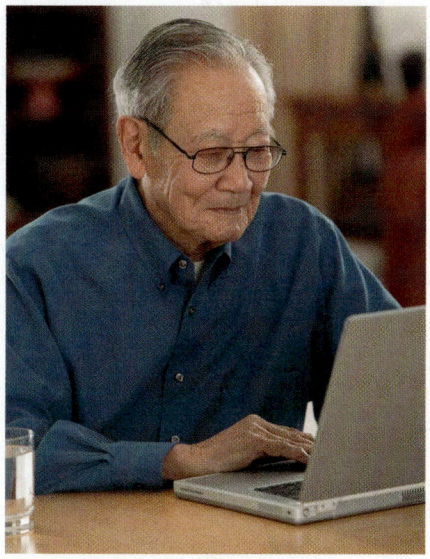

FIG. 5-4 Older adults are using computers more frequently and accessing health care information on the Internet. (©iStockphoto/Thinkstock.)

INFORMATICS IN PRACTICE

Older Adults and Internet Use

- Thirty percent of older adults use the Internet to look for health information.
- Many adults over age 65 track their weight, diet, and exercise using apps.
- Older adults are more likely to accept as true what they read on the Internet. This is related to limited Internet experience and confusion from the large amounts of available information.
- Teach patients who use the Internet as a source of information how to assess the credibility of a website.
- Suggest the use of websites and apps that include senior-friendly design elements.

Source: *http://nihseniorhealth.gov/#.U4T10ruX3IA.emai.*

Homeless Older Adults

The number of older adults who are homeless is increasing. Key factors associated with homelessness include (1) having a low income, (2) having reduced cognitive capacity, (3) living alone, and (4) living in a community that lacks affordable housing. Homeless older adults may be chronically homeless or recently homeless because of a crisis in either health, economic, or social status.

Mortality rates for homeless older adults are higher than for older adults who have housing. Older homeless adults are at higher risk for more health problems because many aging network services are not designed to reach out to homeless people. Older people who are homeless are less likely to use shelters or meal site services than younger homeless people. This may be due to fear of institutionalization. Care for homeless older adults requires an interprofessional approach (including nurses, physicians, social workers, clerical workers, and transporters) that links shelters with outreach, primary care clinics, Medicare and Medicaid offices, pharmacies, senior centers, and Area Agencies on Aging. Long-term care placement is often an alternative to homelessness, especially when the person is cognitively impaired.

Frail Older Adults

Frailty is a common clinical syndrome seen in older adults. Clinical manifestations of frailty include older adults with three or more of the following criteria: (1) unintentional weight loss (greater than or equal to 10 pounds in a year); (2) self-reported exhaustion; (3) weakness (measured by grip strength); (4) slow walking speed; (5) low level of physical activity.[13] Risk factors include disability, multiple chronic conditions, and dementia. People are more likely to become frail if they smoke, have a history of depression or long-term medical health problems, or are underweight. The old-old population (85 years of age or older) is most at risk for frailty, although many in this age group remain healthy and robust.

Older frail adults experience declining function and decreasing daily energy. When stressful life events (e.g., death of a close friend) and daily strain (e.g., caring for an ill spouse) occur, frail older adults often show ineffective coping mechanisms and, as a result, may become ill. Common health problems of frail older adults include mobility limitations, sensory impairment, cognitive decline, and falls.

Frail older adults may tire easily; have little physical reserve; and are at risk for physical dependence and institutionalization. Frail older adults are especially at risk for malnutrition and dehydration, which are related to factors such as living alone, depression, and low income. Other factors, such as dementia, inadequate dental care, sensory deficits, fatigue, and limited mobility increase the risk of malnutrition and dehydration. Monitor frail older adults for adequate calorie, protein, iron, calcium, vitamin D, and fluid intake. A tool to assess the risk factors for poor nutritional status in older adults with or without evidence of frailty is presented in Table 5-7. Once an older adult's nutritional needs are identified, common interventions include home-delivered meals, dietary supplements, Supplemental Nutrition Assistance Program (SNAP),[14] dental referrals, and vitamin supplements. Because medications may affect appetite or interact with nutrients, perform a thorough medication review, including prescription drugs, over-the-counter (OTC) drugs, vitamins, minerals, supplements, as well as herbs and cultural remedies. Nutrition is discussed in Chapter 39.

TABLE 5-7 SCALES: Nutritional Assessment of Older Adults

The acronym SCALES can remind you to assess important nutritional indicators:

Sadness, or mood change
Cholesterol, high
Albumin, low
Loss or gain of weight
Eating problems (e.g., mechanical problems such as impaired swallowing, poor dentition)
Shopping and food preparation problems

Culturally Competent Care: Older Adults

The term **ethnogeriatric** describes the specialty area of providing culturally competent care to older adults.[15] As American society changes, ethnic institutions and neighborhoods may also change. For the older adult with strong ethnic and cultural roots, there may be a loss of friends who speak the "mother tongue," a loss of the religious institution that supports social ethnic activities, and a loss of stores that carry desired ethnic foods. This sense of loss is increased when children and others deny or ignore ethnic and cultural practices. Support for older adults of racial or ethnic minority is most frequently found in the family, religious practices, and isolated geographic or community ethnic clusters.

Ethnic populations of older adults face unique problems. Older adults may live in neighborhoods where physical security and personal safety related to crime may be a concern. Individuals who identify with particular ethnic groups often have disproportionately lower incomes and may not be able to afford Medicare deductibles or drugs needed to treat chronic illnesses. Older individuals from minority populations such as Hispanics use health care services less often when compared to nonminority groups.[15]

Assess each older adult's ethnic and cultural background. Assume that ethnicity and culture are important and of value to older adults and their families unless they tell you otherwise during an assessment. For you to be effective with the ethnic older adult, a sense of respect and clear communication are critical. Nursing interventions to assist in meeting the needs of ethnic populations[16] are described in Table 2-9. (Culturally competent care is discussed in Chapter 2.)

SOCIAL SUPPORT FOR OLDER ADULTS

Social support for older adults occurs at three levels. First, family members are the primary and preferred providers of social support. Second, a semiformal level of support is found in clubs, religious (faith-based) organizations, neighborhoods, adult day care, and senior citizen centers. Third, older adults may be linked to formal systems of social welfare agencies, health facilities, and government support. Generally, you, as a nurse, are part of the formal support system.

Family Caregivers

Many older adults require caregiving by family members. This includes those with multiple chronic conditions, those needing assistance with ADLs and IADLs, and older adults with dementia. Many family caregivers are caring for themselves, their aging parents, as well as their children and grandchildren. Caregiving contributes to stress or burden. Many family caregivers caring for older adults are themselves age 65 or over.[17] Older adults may take on the role of caregiver for someone in their family, usually their spouse or partner. Consider collaborating with a social worker if caregiver stress or strain is present and caregivers are in need of respite. The challenges of caregiving are discussed in Chapter 4 on p. 50.

Elder Mistreatment

Elder mistreatment (EM) describes intentional acts of omission or commission by a caregiver or "trusted other" that cause harm or serious risk of harm to a vulnerable older adult. EM may occur in community (home or assisted living facility) or long-term care (institutional) settings.

Approximately 2% to 10% of community-dwelling older adults in the United States are abused, neglected, or exploited by trusted others.[18] The prevalence of EM in institutional settings is unknown, but it is thought to be widespread. Although EM rates are similar in women and men, the majority of victims are women because of the predominance of women in older age cohorts. Victims of EM have a mortality risk that is three times higher than that of non-mistreated peers. The higher mortality risk is not due to the abuse or neglect itself but rather may be due to stress-related illnesses associated with prolonged mistreatment.[18]

EM is a hidden problem. For every reported case in the community setting, more than five cases go unreported. Underreporting may be higher based on immigration status, ethnic background, or sexual orientation. Victims are unlikely to report mistreatment by "trusted others" because of isolation; impaired cognitive or physical function; feelings of shame, guilt, or self-blame; fear of reprisal; pressure from family members; fear of long-term care; or cultural norms. HCPs also underreport EM, possibly because of failure to suspect or recognize EM, perceived inability to successfully intervene, desire to avoid responsibility for further action, or ageism.

Family members are responsible for up to 90% of domestic EM.[18] Adult children who abuse, neglect, or exploit their parents are usually dependent on their parent(s) for housing and financial support, have a history of violence, are unemployed, and/or are disabled from substance abuse or mental illness. Abusive spouses or partners may either initiate intimate partner violence in older age or continue a lifelong pattern of abuse.

Many factors put community-dwelling older adults at risk for domestic EM. These include (1) physical or cognitive dysfunction that leads to an inability to perform ADLs (and therefore produces dependence on others for care), (2) any psychiatric diagnoses (especially dementia and depression), (3) alcohol abuse, and (4) decreased social support.[19] In long-term care settings the same factors that lead to institutionalization are risk factors for mistreatment by staff, visitors, and others. These include dependence on others for care because of physical or cognitive limitations.

Types of EM, characteristics, and manifestations are shown in Table 5-8. In institutional settings EM includes the types described in Table 5-8 but also includes failure to follow the plan of care, unauthorized use of physical or chemical restraints, overuse or underuse of medication, or isolation as punishment.

Follow your organization's protocols for EM screening and interventions. Perform a thorough history and physical examination that includes screening for mistreatment. It is important that you interview people alone because, if

TABLE 5-8 Types of Elder Mistreatment

Characteristics	Manifestations
Physical Abuse	
Slapping, striking, restraining, incorrect positioning. Oversedation with medications.	Bruises, bilateral injuries (upper arms, ankles, wrists), repeated injuries in various stages of healing, burn marks, oversedation. Use of several emergency departments.
Neglect	
Failure or refusal to provide basic life needs, including food, water, medications, clothing, hygiene. Failure to provide physical aids such as dentures, eyeglasses, hearing aid. Failure to ensure safety.	Older adult's report of being neglected. Untreated or infected pressure ulcers on sacral area, heels. Loss of body weight. Laboratory values showing dehydration (e.g., ↑ Hct, ↑ serum sodium), malnutrition (↓ serum protein). Poor personal hygiene. Lack of adherence with medical treatment.
Failure to provide social stimulation. Leaving alone for long periods. Failure to provide companionship.	Depression, withdrawn behavior, agitation. Ambivalent attitude toward caregiver or family member.
Psychologic Abuse	
Berating verbally, harassment, intimidation, threats of punishment, or deprivation. Childlike treatment, isolation.	Depression, withdrawn behavior, agitation. Ambivalent attitude toward caregiver or family member.
Sexual Abuse	
Nonconsensual sexual contact, including touching inappropriately. Forced sexual contact.	Older adult's report of sexual abuse. Unexplained vaginal or anal bleeding, bruised breasts, unexplained STIs or genital infections.
Financial Abuse	
Denying access to personal resources, stealing money or possessions. Coercing to sign contracts or durable power of attorney. Making changes in will or trust.	Living situation below level of personal resources. Sudden change in personal finances, sudden transfer of assets.
Violation of Personal Rights	
Denying right to privacy or right to make decisions regarding health care or living environment. Forcible eviction.	Sudden inexplicable changes in living situation, confusion.
Abandonment	
Desertion of an older person by an individual who has assumed responsibility for providing care or by a person with physical custody.	Older adult's reports of being abandoned; desertion of an older adult at a hospital or skilled nursing facility, shopping center, or other public place.

Hct, Hematocrit; *STIs,* sexually transmitted infections.

mistreatment is occurring, they may not disclose it in the presence of the person who accompanied them, especially if that person is the abuser. Be especially attentive to explanations about injuries that are not consistent with what you observe, contradictory explanations between the patient and the caregiver, or behavioral clues that suggest the patient is being threatened or intimidated. Additional nursing assessments and interventions are listed in Table 5-9. In most states, health care workers and others are mandated to report suspected or actual EM to Adult Protective Services (APS) and/or law enforcement. Know your legal responsibilities by checking the laws in your state.

Self-Neglect

The majority of referrals made to APS are for self-neglect. Older adults who self-neglect are often unable to meet their basic needs and refuse help; have multiple, untreated medical or psychiatric conditions; and live alone and often in squalor. Older community-dwelling adults who self-neglect face a higher risk of mortality than peers who do not self-neglect.[20] Nursing interventions include assessment for possible self-neglect, referrals for long-term interprofessional case management, and referral to APS.

SOCIAL SERVICES FOR OLDER ADULTS

A network of services supports older adults in the community and health care facilities. In the United States, most older adults are the beneficiaries of at least one social or governmental service. To understand the older adult's situation, learn about government structures that fund and regulate programs for older adults. The Administration on Aging (AoA), which is part of the Department of Health and Human Services, is the federal agency responsible for many older adult programs. Funding from the AoA is given to state and local Area Agencies on Aging (AAAs).

TABLE 5-9 Nursing Assessment and Intervention

Elder Mistreatment

When elder mistreatment is suspected, it is important to do the following:

- Screen for possible elder mistreatment, including domestic violence.
- Conduct a thorough history and head-to-toe physical assessment. Document your findings, including any statements made by the older adult or accompanying adult.
- If the older adult appears to be in immediate danger, develop and implement a safety plan in collaboration with the interprofessional team involved in the person's care.
- Identify, collect, and preserve physical evidence (e.g., dirty or bloody clothing, dressings, sheets).
- After obtaining consent, take photographs to document physical findings of suspected abuse or neglect. If possible and appropriate, do this before treating or bathing the alleged victim.
- If you suspect that mistreatment is occurring, report your findings to the appropriate state agency and/or law enforcement as mandated by the laws in your state.
- Initiate social work, forensic nursing, adult protective services, and other consultations as appropriate.

MEDICARE AND MEDICAID

Medicare is a federally funded health insurance program for people ages 65 years or older, as well as for people under age 65 with certain disabilities and people of any age with end-stage renal disease (ESRD) requiring dialysis or a kidney transplant.

Medicare has four options for coverage: A, B, C, and D. Part A covers inpatient hospital care and partially covers skilled nursing facility care, hospice, and home health care. Part A coverage is "free" because workers support Medicare through payroll taxes. Medicare Part B partially covers outpatient care, physicians' or primary care providers' services, and home health care. It also covers some preventive services, such as mammograms. Medicare Part B is voluntary and has a monthly premium and an annual deductible before payment begins. Medicare Advantage Plans, sometimes called "Part C" or "MA Plans," are offered by private companies approved by Medicare to provide Part A and Part B benefits. Part D is available to Medicare enrollees and provides a prescription drug benefit. Members pay a yearly deductible, monthly premium, and copayment. People with lower incomes and limited assets may qualify for extra help to pay for prescriptions.

Medicare does not cover long-term care, custodial ADLs or IADLs care, dental care or dentures, hearing aids, or eyeglasses. (More information is available at *www.medicare.gov.*) Out-of-pocket expenditures for people on Medicare continue to rise. The costs increase with age, functional disabilities, number of chronic conditions, and number of hospitalizations.[21]

Medicaid is a state-administered, needs-based program to assist eligible low-income people, including Medicare beneficiaries, with certain medical expenses. Individuals who qualify for both Medicare and Medicaid are referred to as *dual-eligible.* Eligibility and coverage vary by state. For qualified Medicare beneficiaries, Medicaid pays Medicare premiums, deductibles, and co-insurance, as well as long-term care and home health expenses. In the United States the majority of long-term care is paid for by Medicaid or private pay. (More information is available at *www.medicaid.gov.*)

CARE ALTERNATIVES FOR OLDER ADULTS

Older adults with special care needs include people who are homeless, in need of assistance with ADLs, cognitively impaired, homebound, or no longer able to live at home. Older adults may be served by adult day care, adult day health care, home health care, and long-term care. Continuing care retirement communities, congregate housing, and assisted living facilities are housing options for older adults.

Adult Day Care and Adult Day Health Care

Adult day care centers provide social, recreational, and health-related services to individuals in a safe, community-based environment (Fig. 5-5). This includes daily supervision, social activities, opportunities for social interaction, and ADLs assistance for two major groups of adults: (1) those who are cognitively impaired and (2) those who have problems independently performing ADLs. Services offered in adult day care programs are individualized based on need. Programs designed for adults who are cognitively impaired offer therapeutic recreation, support for family, family counseling, and social involvement.

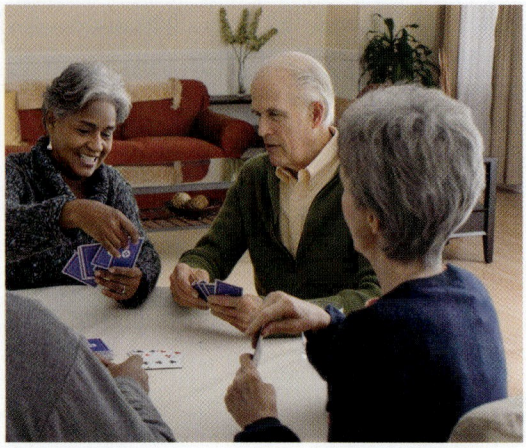

FIG. 5-5 Senior centers offer places for older adults who live independently to meet and gather with friends. (©Jupiterimages/Comstock/Thinkstock.)

Adult day health care centers are similar to adult day care but are designed to meet the needs of older adults and people with disabilities who need a higher level of care. This might include health monitoring, therapeutic activities, one-on-one ADLs training, and personal services.

Adult day care centers and adult day health care centers may provide respite to allow continued employment for the caregiver and delay institutionalization of older adults. Centers are regulated, and standards are set by the state. Medicare does not cover costs. Adult day health care is tax deductible as dependent care. Appropriate placement in adult care programs that match participants' needs is important. You can assist caregivers and adults with self-care deficits by knowing the available centers in your area and assessing the needs of older adults and their families. You will then be in a position to assist older adults and their families in making good decisions about their care.

Home Health Care

Home health care (HHC) can be a cost-effective care alternative for older adults who are homebound, have health needs that are intermittent or acute, and have supportive caregiver involvement. HHC is not an alternative for adults in need of 24-hour assistance with ADLs or continuous safety supervision. (Private duty care may be an alternative in these situations.) HHC services require physician orders and skilled nursing care for Medicare reimbursement. Unless these requirements are met, assistance by home health aides for ADLs management or assistance by a homemaker for IADLs management will not be paid by Medicare.

In addition to HHC, respite, and personal care, homemaker services are often sought by caregivers through organizations that provide nonmedical assistance. These services help older adults stay at home.

Long-Term Care Facilities

Three factors appear to precipitate placement in a long-term care facility: (1) rapid patient deterioration, (2) caregiver inability to continue care because of stress and burnout, and (3) an alteration in or loss of the family support system. Progressive dementia, incontinence, or a major health event (e.g., stroke) can accelerate long-term care placement.

The conflicts and fears faced by older adults and their families make placement a difficult transition. Common caregiver

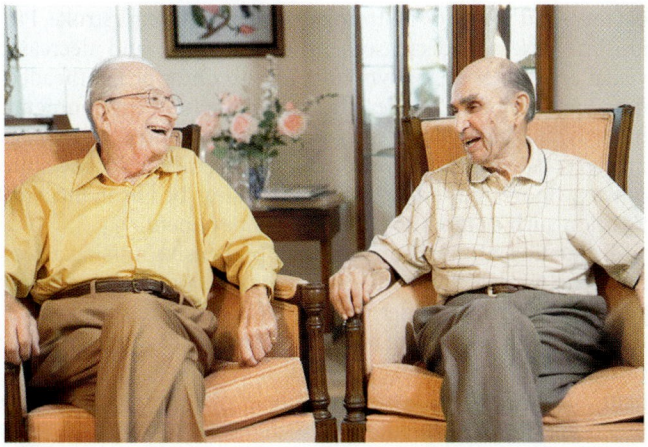

FIG. 5-6 Social interaction and acceptance are important for older adults. (©Hemera/Thinkstock.)

concerns include: (1) Will the older adult resist the admission process? (2) Will the level of care given by staff be insufficient? (3) Will the resident be lonely? and (4) Will nursing care be affordable?

The physical relocation of the older adult may lead to adverse health effects. *Relocation stress syndrome* is a nursing diagnosis that is associated with the disruption, confusion, and challenges that older adults face when moving from one environment to a new environment. Older adults may experience anxiety, depression, and disorientation. Appropriate interventions can reduce the effects of relocation. Whenever possible, involve older adults in the decision to move and fully inform them about the location. Caregivers can share information, pictures, or a video recording of the new location. Personnel at the institution can send a welcome message. On arrival, new residents can be greeted by staff members to provide orientation. To bridge the relocation, new residents can be "buddied" with seasoned residents (Fig. 5-6).

Programs for All-Inclusive Care for the Elderly (PACE)

Programs for All-Inclusive Care for the Elderly (PACE) provide care for adults age 55 and older. PACE services include primary care including prescription medications and wound care; physical, occupational, recreational, and speech therapy; adult day care; dental; podiatry; social services; and home health care. Respite care, hospitalization, short-term rehabilitation, and long-term care are provided as needed.[22]

A person who has Medicaid will not have to pay a monthly premium for the long-term portion of the PACE benefit. A person who does not qualify for Medicaid but has Medicare will be charged a monthly premium to cover the long-term care portion.

LEGAL AND ETHICAL ISSUES

Legal guidance and assistance is needed by many older adults. Legal issues include advance directives, estate planning, taxation issues, appeals for denied services (e.g., disability), financial decisions, or exploitation by strangers or "trusted others."

Advance directives are written statements of a person's wishes regarding medical care. A health care proxy may be appointed to make medical decisions in the event that a person is unable to make his or her own medical decisions. These documents allow individuals to more specifically direct their own care at end of life. Advance directives are discussed in detail in Chapter 9 and Table 9-6.

When working with older adults, you may find several ethical issues that influence practice, such as the assessment of older adults' ability to make decisions. Other ethical issues related to end-of-life care include decisions about resuscitation, treatment of infections, nutrition and hydration, and transfer to more intensive treatment units. These situations are often complex, especially during emotionally difficult times. You can assist the older adult, family, and other health care workers by (1) keeping current on the ethical issues, (2) acknowledging when an ethical dilemma is present, and (3) advocating for an institutional ethics committee to help provide guidance in the decision-making process and assist when differences of opinion occur.

❖ NURSING MANAGEMENT: OLDER ADULTS

Gerontologic nursing is the care of older adults based on the specialty body of knowledge of gerontology and nursing. These specialty nurses provide care for older adults using a whole-person (physical, psychologic, functional, developmental, socioeconomic, cultural) perspective. Care of older adults is complex and presents challenges that require skilled assessment and creative nursing interventions tailored to this population.

Diseases and conditions in older adults may be difficult to accurately assess and diagnose. Older adults may underreport symptoms and "treat" these symptoms by altering their functional status. For example, a woman having loss of feeling in her feet because of neuropathy may start using a walker to get around, while not reporting the symptom to her HCP. The older adult may attribute a new symptom to "aging" and ignore it. The older adult may eat less, sleep more, or "wait it out."

In older adults, disease symptoms are often atypical. For example, confusion may be a sign of an infection. Asymptomatic cardiac disease may be diagnosed when the patient is being treated for a urinary tract infection. Pathologic conditions with similar symptoms are often confused. For example, depression may be misdiagnosed and treated as dementia. The most common atypical illness presentations are "delirium" or "acute change in mental status" and change in functional status. A caregiver may say that their relative "is acting differently," "doesn't appear as him/herself," or is no longer participating in usual activities or self-care.

In older adults a *cascade disease pattern* may occur. For example, a person who experiences insomnia treats the condition with a sleeping medication, becomes lethargic and confused, falls, sustains a hip fracture, decreases activity and mobility, and subsequently develops pneumonia. You play a vital role in preventing this downward trajectory.

For older adults, the stress of an illness may lead to fear and anxiety. They may view health care personnel as helpful but perceive institutions as negative and potentially harmful places. Communicate a sense of concern and care by use of direct and simple statements, appropriate eye contact, direct touch, and gentle humor. These actions help the older adult relax in this stressful situation.

◆ Nursing Assessment

Prior to assessment, attend to the person's primary needs. For example, ensure that older adults are comfortable and ask if they need to use the bathroom. If older adults normally use eyeglasses and hearing aids, ask them to use these during the assessment. Place all assistive devices, such as walkers, within reach. Assess your patient's level of fatigue and pause the interview if necessary. Allow adequate time to offer information and time for the person to respond to questions. Interview both the older adult and his or her family or caregivers. This can be done separately, unless the patient is cognitively impaired or specifically requests the caregiver's presence. Although the health history may be lengthy, it is important to obtain. Review medical records and determine what information is most relevant or needs more detail.

The focus of a comprehensive geriatric assessment is to determine appropriate interventions to maintain and enhance the health, quality of life, function, and independence of older adults. Comprehensive geriatric assessment is interprofessional and, at a minimum, includes the medical history, functional assessment, medication review, cognitive and mood evaluation, social resources, physical examination, followed by recommended diagnostic tests. Comprehensive geriatric assessment is often conducted by an interprofessional geriatric assessment team. The interprofessional team minimally includes a staff nurse, an HCP such as a physician or adult-geriatric nurse practitioner, and a social worker. It may also include a physical and/or occupational therapist, dietitian, podiatrist, ophthalmologist, dentist, and pastoral care representative. After the assessment is complete, the interprofessional team meets with the patient and family to present the team's findings and recommendations.

Specific elements in a comprehensive nursing assessment include a thorough history, mood assessment, functional assessment including ADLs and IADLs, mental status evaluation, social-environmental assessment, and physical assessment. Evaluation of mental status is particularly important for older adults because these results often determine the potential for independent living. *SPICES,* an effective tool for obtaining assessment data in older adults, may be used as an initial nursing assessment when working in any setting (Fig. 5-7). Multiple evidence-based geriatric assessment tools and best practice approaches to nursing care for older adults are available from the *Try This* Series at the Hartford Institute for Geriatric Nursing (available at: *www.ConsultGeriRN.org/resources*).

A comprehensive geriatric assessment includes a fall risk (including fear of falling) and cause(s) of past falls. Individuals are at increased risk for falls if they have a history of falls or have a fear of falling. Many factors increase the risk of falls, including medications (including OTC ones), infection, electrolyte imbalance or other laboratory abnormalities, arthritis, changes in gait, balance, and mobility, neurologic impairment (e.g., stroke, Parkinson's disease), decreased muscle strength, and decreased visual acuity. Assess for symptoms of dizziness or lightheadedness upon standing. Other risk factors include environmental hazards, feet abnormalities, poor footwear, clutter, throw rugs, incorrect use of an assistive device such as a walker or cane, shiny or waxy floors, slippery floors, poor lighting, bed in an incorrect position such as too high, and uneven pavement.

Evaluation of the results of a comprehensive nursing assessment helps determine the service and potential long-term placement needs of older adults. Collect data regarding community resources that are needed to assist older adults and their caregivers in maintaining maximal functioning. The goal is to plan and implement actions that help older adults remain as functionally independent as possible and to promote their quality of life.

Patient name:	Date:	
	EVIDENCE	
SPICES	Yes	No
Sleep disorders		
Problems with eating or feeding		
Incontinence		
Confusion		
Evidence of falls		
Skin breakdown		

FIG. 5-7 SPICES. (Adapted from Fulmer T: The geriatric nurse specialist role: a new model. *Nursing Management* 22:91, 1991. © Copyright Lippincott Williams & Wilkins, *http://lww.com.*)

◆ Planning

When setting goals with older adults, identify their strengths and abilities. Include caregivers in planning. Priority goals for older adults may include gaining a sense of control, feeling safe, and reducing stress.

◆ Nursing Implementation

When carrying out a plan of action for older adults, modify your approach and actions based on their physical, functional, and mental status. Small body size (common in older adults who meet frailty criteria) may necessitate the use of pediatric equipment (e.g., BP cuff). As with all patient groups, safety is a primary concern when caring for an older adult. Bone and joint changes often require transfer assistance, altered positioning, and use of gait belts and lift devices. Older adults with declining energy reserves may require additional time to complete tasks. A slower approach and the use of other adaptive equipment may be necessary. Cognitive impairment, if present, requires that you offer careful explanations and a calm approach to avoid producing anxiety and resistance in the older adult. Depression can result in apathy and poor cooperation with the treatment plan.

◆ **Health Promotion.** Health promotion and prevention of health problems for older adults focus on three areas: (1) increased participation in health promotion and disease prevention activities (Fig. 5-8), (2) reduction in diseases and health-related

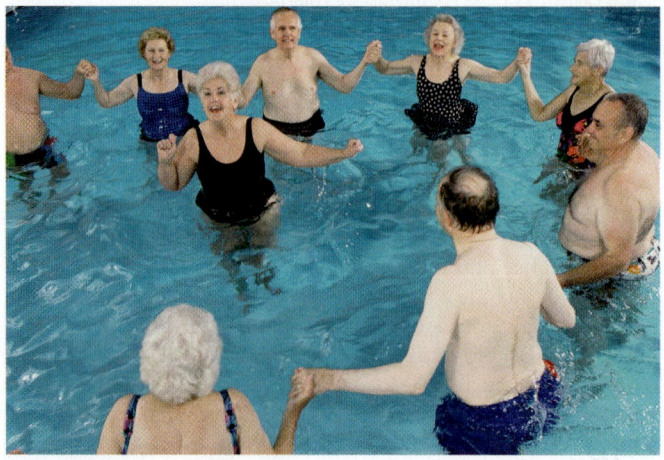

FIG. 5-8 Water aerobics is an example of a health promotion activity for older adults. (©Purestock/Thinkstock.)

issues, and (3) increased use of services that reduce health hazards. Programs have been successfully developed for screening for chronic health conditions, tobacco cessation, geriatric foot care, vision and hearing screening, stress reduction, exercise programs, fall prevention programs, drug usage, crime prevention, elder mistreatment, and home safety assessment.[3,23] Teach older adults about the need for specific preventive services and available programs.

Health promotion and disease prevention should be included in nursing interventions and plans at any setting or level of care where nurses and older adults interact. You can use health promotion activities to increase personal responsibility for health and independent functioning. Teaching and reinforcement are important tools for you to use to enhance self-care practices by older adults. (Patient teaching is discussed in Chapter 4.)

◆ **Acute and Ambulatory Care.** The hospital may be the first point of contact for older adults with the health care system. Conditions that most commonly result in hospitalization include falls, dysrhythmias, heart failure, stroke, fluid and electrolyte imbalances (e.g., hyponatremia, dehydration), pneumonia, urosepsis, and hip fractures. Older adults are often hospitalized with multiple problems.

When older adults are being cared for in the acute care setting, both patients and caregivers need assistance with a variety of functions (Table 5-10). The outcome of hospitalization for older adults varies. Of particular concern are patients undergoing high-risk surgical procedures (e.g., hip replacement) and those who experience delirium while hospitalized.

◆ ***Care Transitions.*** The time of a care transition to another setting (e.g., acute care hospital to rehabilitation) is challenging for many older adults. While in the hospital, patients and caregivers are counseled on how to prepare for posthospital care. Those with multiple health conditions are particularly at high risk for rehospitalization.

Medicare regulations require a registered nurse, social worker, or qualified person to develop a care transition plan for patient discharge. Safe and effective care transitions are most likely to occur when interprofessional team members work together with the patient and family to coordinate care.

The Transitional Care Model (TCM) is an evidence-based, innovative approach to care coordination and management of the complex needs of older adults.[24] In this model a transitional care nurse delivers and coordinates care by nurses and other team members throughout potential and acute episodes of illness. Those most likely to benefit from transitional care nursing include those of older age and those with functional deficits, behavioral or psychiatric issues, multiple chronic conditions, a need for polypharmacy, a recent hospitalization, lack of a support system, low health literacy, and history of nonadherence to treatment.[24]

◆ ***Rehabilitation.*** The goal of rehabilitation is to help older adults adapt to or recover from disability or an acute functional decline. Rehabilitation may occur in acute inpatient rehabilitation, subacute rehabilitation, or long-term care settings. With proper training, assistive equipment, and attendant personal care, people with functional deficits may live independently. Older adults, primarily through Medicare reimbursement, can receive rehabilitative assistance through acute inpatient rehabilitation (limited days) and home health care programs (Fig. 5-9).

Older adults with chronic conditions, such as arthritis, have increased risk of functional decline. Decreased function or disabilities lead to increased self-care deficits, increased rates of institutionalization, decreased quality of life, and higher mortality rates.

Rehabilitation of older adults is influenced by several factors. First, preexisting conditions associated with decreased reaction time, visual acuity, fine motor ability, physical strength, and cognitive function affect the short- and long-term rehabilitation potential of older adults. Older adults may have anxiety, fear, or concern about falling. They may also be limited in the rehabilitation process by poor nutrition and financial issues. Encouragement, support, and acceptance from the interdisciplinary team members as well as their caregivers can assist older adults in remaining motivated for potentially physically challenging rehabilitation.

Second, older adults often lose function because of inactivity and immobility. This deconditioning can occur as a result of unstable acute medical conditions, lack of assistive devices, and a lack of motivation to stay fit. The effect of inactivity leads to "use it or lose it" consequences. Older adults can improve flexibility, strength, and aerobic capacity even into very old age. Passive and active range-of-motion exercises are used with all older adults to preserve muscle tone and strength and prevent deconditioning and subsequent functional decline.

TABLE 5-10 Care of the Hospitalized Older Adult

When an older adult is hospitalized, give special consideration to the following nursing interventions.

- Identify older adults at risk for iatrogenesis (consequences of medical and/or surgical treatments).
- Consider discharge needs early in the hospital stay, especially assistance with ADLs, IADLs, and medications.
- Encourage the development and use of interprofessional teams, special care units, and individuals who focus on the special needs of older patients.
- Implement standard protocols to screen for at-risk conditions commonly present in the hospitalized older adult, such as urinary tract infection, falls, and delirium.
- Implement mobility programs to prevent functional decline such as *"The bed is not your friend."*
- Monitor for and prevent skin integrity changes.
- Focus on safety (e.g., prevention of falls).
- Advocate for referral of the patient to appropriate community-based services.

ADLs, Activities of daily living; *IADLs,* instrumental activities of daily living.

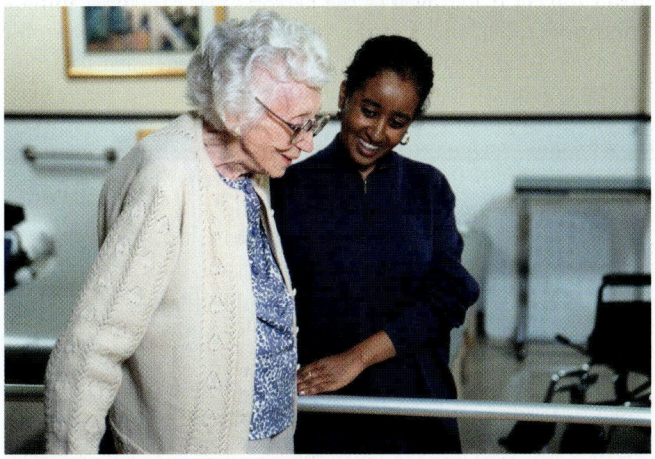

FIG. 5-9 The nurse assists a patient in a geriatric rehabilitation facility. (©KeithBrofsky/Photodisc/Thinkstock.)

EVIDENCE-BASED PRACTICE

Translating Research Into Practice

Can Tai Chi Help Cognitive Function in Older Adults?

Clinical Question

In older adults (P), what is the effect of Tai Chi (I) on cognitive functioning (O)?

Synthesis of Best Available Evidence

- Systematic review of randomized controlled trials (RCTs), cross-sectional studies, and prospective randomized controlled and noncontrolled observational studies
- 20 studies of adults aged 60 years and older ($n = 2553$) in residential and community care settings with and without cognitive impairment. Intervention was Tai Chi lasting 20 to 60 minutes, 1 to 4 times per week, for up to 1 year. Most RCT control groups were stretching and toning, resistance and nonresistance exercise, and education. Outcomes of cognitive functioning were global cognition (dementia assessment), executive function (e.g., attention, memory), language, and learning.
- In cognitively healthy adults, Tai Chi had a positive effect on executive function with improvement maintained at 1 year. Global cognition, memory, learning, and fluency also improved.
- In cognitively impaired adults, Tai Chi had positive effects on global cognition and executive function.

Conclusion

- Tai Chi improved cognitive function, particularly in adults without significant cognitive impairment.

Implications for Nursing Practice

- How would you advise older adults who want information on activities that will help to maintain memory and ability to learn?
- How may the caregiver of a spouse or partner with dementia also benefit from engaging in Tai Chi?

Reference for Evidence

Wayne PM, Walsh JN, Taylor-Piliae RE, et al: Effect of Tai Chi on cognitive performance in older adults: systematic review and meta-analysis, *J Am Geriatr Soc* 62:25, 2014.

P, Patient population of interest; *I*, intervention or area of interest; *O*, outcomes of interest (see p. 15)

Last, the goal of rehabilitation is to strive for maximal function and physical capabilities considering the individual's current health and functional status. For example, on admission to an acute or long-term care facility and home health services, assess for fall risk as well as the person's fear of falling. Initiate appropriate fall prevention interventions and evaluate for ongoing risk. Conduct accurate and comprehensive foot and peripheral vascular assessments for all older adults, especially those with diabetes, and arrange appropriate follow-up care.

◆ ***Assistive Devices.*** Consider the use of assistive devices as interventions for older adults. Using appropriate assistive devices such as dentures, glasses, hearing aids, walkers, wheelchairs, adaptive utensils, elevated toilet seats, and skin protective devices can increase function. Include these tools and devices in the older adult's care plan when appropriate and provide instruction in the proper use of the devices. For example, using a cane appropriately may decrease fall risk.

Technology can assist with rehabilitation and living with functional impairments. For example, electronic monitoring equipment can be used to monitor heart rhythm and BP. Monitoring can also locate a person with dementia who has wandered away from home or a long-term care facility. Computerized assistive devices may help patients with speech difficulties following stroke, and small electronic devices can serve as memory aids.

◆ ***Safety.*** Safety is crucial in the health maintenance of older adults. When compared to younger adults, older adults are at higher risk for accidents due to normal sensory changes, slowed reaction time, decreased thermal and pain sensitivity, changes in gait and balance, and medication effects. Most accidents occur in or around the home. Falls, motor vehicle accidents, and fires are common causes of accidental death in older adults. Declining thermoregulation impairs the older person's ability to adapt to extremes in environmental temperatures. The bodies of older adults can neither conserve nor dissipate heat as efficiently as younger adults. Therefore both hypothermia and hyperthermia occur more readily. The older adult age-group accounts for the majority of deaths during severe cold spells and heat waves.

You can provide counsel regarding environmental changes, which may improve safety for older adults. Measures such as colored step strips, tub and toilet grab bars, and stairway handrails can be effective in "safety-proofing" the living spaces of older adults. Uncluttered floor space (e.g., removal of throw rugs), railings, and increased lighting and night-lights are some of the easiest and most practical adaptations. Social workers may help older adults implement these environmental changes. You can also advocate for home fire and security alarms.

Other interventions to decrease the risk of falling include exercise, physical therapy, and management of foot and footwear issues. Prevention of falls also includes encouraging the patient's use of glasses and hearing aid as ordered. Fear of falling can affect the older adults' decisions about the activities that they engage in and how active they remain.

Older adults who are new to inpatient or long-term care settings need a thorough orientation to the environment. Reassure the older adult that he or she is safe, and answer all questions and refer to interprofessional team members and specialists as needed. Foster orientation by displaying large-print clocks, avoiding complex or visually confusing wall designs, clearly designating doors and exits, and using simple bed and nurse or family-call controls. Provide diffuse lighting while avoiding glare.

◆ ***Medication Use.*** Medication use in older adults requires thorough and regular assessment, care planning, and evaluation. Nonadherence to medication regimens by older adults is common. Many older adults are unable to read prescription drug labels, and many are unable to understand the health information that is provided to them.

Age-related changes alter the pharmacodynamics and pharmacokinetics of drugs. Drug-drug, drug-nutrient, and drug-disease interactions influence the absorption, distribution, metabolism, and excretion of drugs. The most dramatic changes with aging are related to drug metabolism (Fig. 5-10). Hepatic blood flow decreases markedly with aging, and the enzymes largely responsible for drug metabolism are decreased as well. As a result, drug half-life is increased in older adults as compared with younger adults. This can lead to greater risk for drug toxicity and adverse drug events. Overall, by age 75 to 80, there is a 50% decline in the renal clearance of drugs. Older adults with altered renal function may need a lower dose and/or decreased frequency of administration of a drug excreted by the kidney. When drug level monitoring is available (e.g., digoxin [Lanoxin]), identify toxic levels by serum monitoring at regular

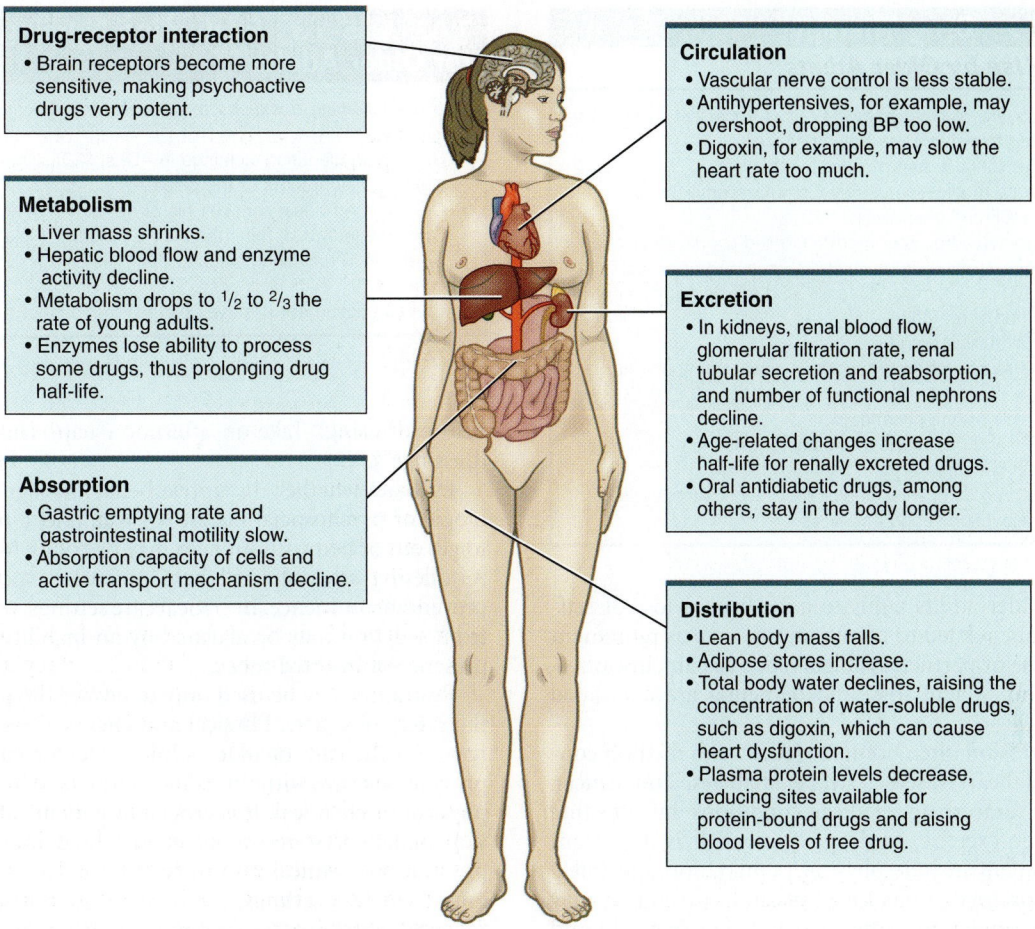

FIG. 5-10 The effects of aging on drug metabolism.

TABLE 5-11 Drug Therapy

Causes of Medication Errors by Older Adults

- Decreased vision
- Forgetting to take drugs
- Use of nonprescription over-the-counter drugs
- Use of medications prescribed for someone else
- Lack of financial resources to obtain prescribed medication
- Failure to understand instructions or importance of drug treatment
- Refusal to take medication because of undesirable side effects

intervals, especially at change of dose and/or frequency of administration.

In addition to changes in the pharmacodynamics and pharmacokinetics of drugs, older adults may have difficulty managing medication regimens due to cognitive impairment, altered sensory perceptions, limited hand mobility or dexterity, and the high cost of many drugs. Common reasons for drug errors made by older adults are listed in Table 5-11.

Polypharmacy (the use of multiple medications by a person who has more than one health problem), overdose, and addiction to prescription drugs are major causes of illness in older adults.[25] Potential medication errors include the (1) administration of both brand and generic medications, (2) refilling medications too soon or too late (resulting in taking the medication incorrectly), and (3) drug-drug interactions. These errors can be prevented by having a pharmacist review the medication regimen regularly. Suggest the use of one pharmacy for filling all prescription medications.

The effects of medications in older adults with multiple health problems are particularly challenging to assess and manage. As one disease is treated, another may be affected. For example, the use of a drug such as oxybutynin (Ditropan), which is prescribed for overactive bladder, may cause confusion. To accurately assess medication knowledge and use, ask older adults to bring all medications (OTC drugs, prescription drugs, vitamins and supplements, laxatives, sleep aids, and herbal remedies) that they take regularly or occasionally to their health care appointment. You will then be able to accurately assess all medications that the patient is taking, including drugs that the person may have omitted or thought unimportant. The American Geriatrics Society (AGS) Beers Criteria are designed to reduce problems with medications in older adults.[25] Additional nursing interventions to assist older adults in following a safe medication routine are listed in Table 5-12.

◆ ***Depression.*** Depression is not a normal part of aging. However, it is often an underrecognized problem in older adults. Approximately 15% of older adults living in their homes have manifestations of depression. Rates of depressive symptoms in older adults in institutional settings are higher. The second highest rate of suicide occurs in those over 75.

Depression is associated with female gender, divorced or separated marital status, low socioeconomic status, poor social support, and a recent adverse and unexpected event.

TABLE 5-12 Drug Therapy

Medication Use by Older Adults

When older adults are using medications, it is important to take the following measures to prevent medication errors.

- Assess cognitive function and monitor for changes.
- Attempt to reduce medication use that is not essential by consulting the HCP and pharmacist.
- Assess ability to self-administer medication and overall medication use, including prescription drugs; over-the-counter drugs; antihistamines; cough syrups; vitamins, minerals, and supplements; sleep remedies; and herbal remedies.
- Assess alcohol and illicit drug use.
- Encourage the use of written or electronic medication-reminder systems.
- Encourage the use of one pharmacy.
- Work with HCPs and pharmacists to establish routine drug profiles on all older adult patients.
- Advocate, with drug companies and/or social work services, for low-income prescription support services.

Depression in older adults tends to arise from a loss of self-esteem and may be related to life situations, such as retirement or loss of a spouse or partner. Problems such as pain, insomnia, lethargy, agitation, weight loss, and dementia are associated with depression.

Late-life depression often occurs together with medical conditions, such as heart disease, stroke, diabetes, and cancer. Depression can exacerbate medical conditions by affecting adherence to diet, exercise, or drug regimens. It is important that your assessment include physical examination and interpretation of laboratory results for physical disorders that may have symptoms similar to those of depression (e.g., thyroid disorders, vitamin deficiencies).

Encourage older adults who exhibit depressive symptoms to seek treatment. Because older adults with depression may feel unworthy, withdrawn, and isolated, the support of the family or others in encouraging older adults to seek treatment is important. Assist older adult caregivers who exhibit depressive symptoms to seek medical attention, and assist them in securing respite services and support for their caregiving role. (Family caregiving is discussed in Chapter 4 on pp. 49 to 50.)

◆ ***Use of Restraints.*** *Physical restraints* are devices, materials, and equipment that physically prevent individuals from moving freely, such as walking, standing, lying, transferring, or sitting. *Chemical restraints* are drugs used to restrict the freedom or movement of a patient or in some cases to sedate a patient.

Before considering the use of any restraint, completely assess the perceived need for the restraint and document the assessment. Behavioral symptoms, such as crying and shouting, may arise from co-morbidities, pain, medication effects, unmet needs, and/or environmental factors. When behavioral manifestations are evident, ask the following questions to better understand the patient's behavior: Is the person able to verbalize what she or he needs and wants? People with dementia may respond by speaking, gesturing, nodding, or making eye contact. Questions that use "yes" or "no" answers are better than open-ended questions for gathering assessment information. Ask family, friends, or staff members from previous care settings about the patient's (1) history; (2) usual communication style and cues to indicate pain, fatigue, hunger, or a need to urinate or defecate; (3) abilities in ADLs; and (4) daily routines (e.g., "Is he often awake at night or an early riser?" "Does she prefer breakfast before dressing? Take an afternoon nap? Have a routine for dressing?").

TABLE 5-13 Evaluating Nursing Care for Older Adults

Use the following questions to evaluate the effectiveness of care for older adults.

- Is there an identifiable change in ADLs, IADLs, mental status, or signs and symptoms of the disease?
- Does the individual consider his or her health state to be improved?
- Does the individual think the plan is helpful?
- Do the individual and caregiver think the care is worth the time and cost?
- Can you document positive changes that support the interventions?

ADLs, Activities of daily living; *IADLs,* instrumental activities of daily living.

Evaluate whether disruptive behaviors signal unmet physiologic or psychosocial needs. For example, a patient who tries to get out of bed without help may be trying to reach the toilet. A toileting schedule will help to curtail such attempts and prevent incontinence. In critical care settings, patients emerging from sedation may be alarmed by an inability to speak or the presence of inserted tubes.

Restraints may be used only to ensure the person's safety or the safety of others. Physical and chemical restraints are a last resort in the care of older adults. The current standard is to provide safe care without using restraints of any form, whether physical or chemical. It is crucial to patient safety and prevention of falls that restraints not be used for this purpose. If physical or chemical restraints are used in acute, subacute, or long-term care settings, use of the least restrictive restraint is required. Restraints require an order from an HCP.

Carefully document restraint use and the behaviors that necessitate its perceived need. It is not appropriate to use restraints based on fall risk, avoidance of interference with medical devices, or perceived irritating behaviors, such as calling out. Frequent scheduled reviews of the ongoing necessity of the restraint are needed with consideration of discontinuation of the restraint. Long-term care regulations and The Joint Commission set standards for restraint usage. These include time limit, observation and care, use of least restrictive measures (e.g., mittens), and alternatives to the use of restraints. Restraint alternatives include low beds, body props, and electronic devices (such as bed and chair alarm signaling). Such approaches support the development of a "restraint-free," safe environment. Alternatives to restraints require vigilant, creative, and sensitive nursing care.

◆ ***Sleep.*** Adequacy of sleep is often a concern for older adults because of altered sleep patterns. Older people experience a marked decrease in deep sleep and are easily aroused. Many older adults report difficulty initiating sleep and maintaining prolonged sleep. They may state they feel "unrefreshed" after sleep. (Sleep problems of older adults are discussed in Chapter 7.)

◆ Evaluation

The evaluation phase of the nursing process is similar for all patients. The results of evaluation direct you to continue the plan of care or revise as indicated. When evaluating nursing care with older adults, focus on functional improvement and quality of life. Useful questions to consider when evaluating the plan of care for older adults are included in Table 5-13.

CASE STUDY

Older Adults

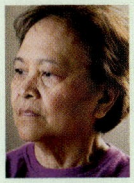

(©azndc/iStock/Thinkstock)

Patient Profile

C.L., a 73-year-old Taiwanese woman, was admitted through the emergency department with shortness of breath. She was diagnosed with community-acquired pneumonia. Her history also indicates she has chronic obstructive pulmonary disease (COPD), hypertension, diabetes, mild cognitive impairment, depression, macular degeneration, and significant hearing loss.

Subjective Data

- A stroke 5 years ago and has right-sided weakness
- A 100 pack-year history of tobacco use but quit smoking after her stroke
- Not seen primary care physician in 1 year
- In past year has had an unplanned weight loss of 15 pounds
- Spends her days either in bed or in a recliner watching television
- Shortness of breath for past 5 days

Psychosocial Data

- Came to the United States 15 years ago from Taiwan.
- Speaks Mandarin Chinese with limited English proficiency.
- Lives with her unemployed adult son who provides assistance with ADLs and IADLs.
- Has three daughters who live within a 2-hour drive.
- Limited financial resources but has Medicare and Medicaid benefits.
- Daughters raise concerns about their mother's care and safety at home, given their brother's history of anger issues and a gambling addiction.
- When daughters ask their brother about how he is caring for his mother, he says, "I'm doing the best I can. She refuses help. She refuses to go to the doctor. What do you want me to do? She's old. She's crazy. She's going to die anyway!"
- Daughters state their mother does not want to go to a nursing home.

Objective Data

Physical Examination

- Unwashed, matted hair, poor oral hygiene, overgrown toenails
- Two stage III sacral ulcers
- Unstageable right heel ulcer
- Multiple small bruises on her forearms and shins
- 5 x 10–cm bruise in the middle of her back

Diagnostic Tests

- Serum albumin 2.4 g/dL
- X-ray reveals consolidation in lower left and right lung lobes

Discussion Questions

1. What other information do you need to assess C.L.'s condition? How should questions regarding potential elder mistreatment be addressed?
2. Identify the stage(s) of Corbin and Strauss chronic illness trajectory that describe C.L.'s current status. Which stage(s) is the goal of your nursing care?
3. ***Patient-Centered Care:*** What is your assessment of C.L.'s ability to successfully complete these tasks? What will you include in your care planning to optimize her ability to complete these tasks?
4. ***Priority Decision:*** Based on your assessment of C.L., what are the priority nursing diagnoses? Are there collaborative problems?
5. ***Safety:*** To ensure C.L.'s safety, what nursing interventions are necessary during her hospitalization?
6. ***Teamwork and Collaboration:*** How would you use unlicensed assistive personnel (UAP) on the hospital unit to carry out the priorities that you identified in question 4?
7. ***Teamwork and Collaboration:*** What referrals may be indicated?
8. Define ageism, and explain how it may be manifested in this case.
9. What risk factors does C.L. have for development of frailty? Which of these factors are modifiable?
10. Based on your knowledge of care alternatives for older adults, what setting or settings may be appropriate for C.L. upon hospital discharge?
11. What risk factors does C.L. have for becoming a victim of elder mistreatment? List and provide the rationale for nursing interventions and legal and ethical responsibilities in this case.

Answers available at *http://evolve.elsevier.com/Lewis/medsurg.*

BRIDGE TO NCLEX EXAMINATION

The number of the question corresponds to the same-numbered outcome at the beginning of the chapter.

1. Examples of primary prevention strategies include
   a. colonoscopy at age 50.
   b. avoidance of tobacco products.
   c. teaching the importance of exercise to a patient with hypertension.
   d. intake of a diet low in saturated fat in a patient with high cholesterol.
2. A characteristic of a chronic illness is that it *(select all that apply)*
   a. has reversible pathologic changes.
   b. has a consistent, predictable clinical course.
   c. results in permanent deviation from normal.
   d. is associated with many stable and unstable phases.
   e. always starts with an acute illness and then progresses slowly.
3. Ageism is characterized by
   a. denial of negative stereotypes regarding aging.
   b. positive attitudes toward the elderly based on age.
   c. negative attitudes toward the elderly based on age.
   d. negative attitudes toward the elderly based on physical disability.
4. An ethnic older adult may feel a loss of self-worth when the nurse *(select all that apply)*
   a. prohibits visits from a faith healer.
   b. informs the patient about ethnic support services.
   c. allows a patient to rely on ethnic health beliefs and practices.
   d. emphasizes that a therapeutic diet does not allow ethnic foods.
   e. uses a medical interpreter to provide explanations and teaching.
5. An important nursing action to help a chronically ill older adult is to
   a. avoid discussing future lifestyle changes.
   b. ensure the patient that the condition is stable.
   c. treat the patient as a competent manager of the disease.
   d. encourage the patient to "fight" the disease as long as possible.

6. Older adults who become ill are more likely than younger adults to
   a. complain about the symptoms of their problems.
   b. refuse to carry out lifestyle changes to promote recovery.
   c. seek medical attention because of limitations on their lifestyle.
   d. alter their daily living activities to accommodate new symptoms.
7. An appropriate care choice for an older adult who lives with an employed daughter but needs help with activities of daily living is
   a. adult day care.
   b. long-term care.
   c. a retirement center.
   d. an assisted living facility.
8. Nursing interventions directed at health promotion in the older adult are primarily focused on
   a. disease management.
   b. controlling symptoms of illness.
   c. teaching positive health behaviors.
   d. teaching regarding nutrition to enhance longevity.

1. b, 2. c, d, 3. c, 4. a, d, 5. c, 6. d, 7. a, 8. c.

For rationales to these answers and even more NCLEX review questions, visit *http://evolve.elsevier.com/Lewis/medsurg.*

EVOLVE WEBSITE

http://evolve.elsevier.com/Lewis/medsurg

Review Questions (Online Only)
Key Points
Answer Keys for Questions
- Rationales for Bridge to NCLEX Examination Questions
- Answer Guidelines for Case Study on p. 75

Conceptual Care Map Creator
Audio Glossary
Content Updates

REFERENCES

1. Centers for Disease Control and Prevention: Chronic diseases and health promotion, Retrieved from *www.cdc.gov/chronicdisease.*
2. Corbin JM, Strauss A: A nursing model for chronic illness management based upon the Trajectory Framework, *Sch Inq Nurs Pract* 5:155, 1991. (Classic)
3. Hartford Institute for Geriatric Nursing: Try This Series. Retrieved from *www.ConsultGeriRN.org/resources.*
4. Department of Health and Human Services. Self-management for health in chronic conditions. Retrieved from *www.grants.nih.gov/grants/guide/pa-files/PA-14-344.html.*

*5. Martinez-Marcos M, De la Cuesta-Benjumea C: Women's self management of chronic illnesses in the context of caregiving: a grounded theory study, *J Clin Nurs* 24:1557, 2015.

6. U.S. Census Bureau: Facts for features: Older Americans month: May 2014. Retrieved from *www.census.gov/newsroom/facts-for-features/2014/cb14-ff07.html.*
7. Administration on Aging: A profile of older Americans. Retrieved from *www.aoa.gov/Aging_Statistics/Profile/2012/docs/2012profile.pdf.*
8. Administration on Aging: Projected future growth of the older population. Retrieved from *www.aoa.acl.gov/Aging_Statistics/future_growth/future_growth.aspx.*
9. Scott G: Ageism is rife in health care, *Nurs Stan* 25:1, 2011.
10. Daniel M, Tollefsbol TO: Epigenetic linkage of aging, cancer and nutrition, *J Exp Biol* 218: 59, 2015.
11. Kim S, Brooks AK, Groban L: Preoperative assessment of the older surgical patient: honing in on geriatric syndromes, *Clin Interv Aging* 10:13, 2014.
12. Pew Research Internet Project. Older adults and technology use. Retrieved from *www.pewinternet.org/2014/04/03/older-adults-and-technology-use.*

*13. Xue QL: The frailty syndrome: definition and natural history, *Clin Geriatr Med* 27:1, 2011.

14. USDA Food and Nutrition Service. Supplemental Nutrition Assistance Program (SNAP). Retrieved from *www.fns.usda.gov/snap/snap-special-rules-elderly-or-disabled.*
15. Hardin SR: Ethnogeriatric in critical care, *Crit Care Nurs Clin North Am* 16:21, 2014.
16. Stanford Medicine, Geriatric Education Center. A national resource center in ethnogeriatrics. Retrieved from *http://sgec.stanford.edu.*
17. Administration on Aging Family Caregiver Alliance: Selected caregiver statistics. Retrieved from *www.caregiver.org/selected-caregiver-statistics.*
18. National Center for Elder Abuse. Retrieved from *www.ncea.aoa.gov/Library/Data.*
19. Preventing elder abuse and neglect in older adults: tools and tips. Retrieved from *www.ncea.aoa.gov/Library/Data.*

*20. Dong X: Self-neglect in an elderly community-dwelling U.S. Chinese population: findings from the population study of Chinese elderly in Chicago study, *J Am Geriatr Soc* 62:2391, 2014.

21. How much is enough? Out-of-pocket spending among Medicare beneficiaries: a chartbook. Retrieved from *www.kff.org/out+of+pocket.*
22. National PACE Association. Retrieved from *www.npaonline.org/website/article.asp.*
23. American Geriatrics Society. AGS/BGS Clinical practice guideline: prevention of falls in older persons. Retrieved from *www.americangeriatrics.org/health_care_professionals/clinical_practice/clinical_guidelines_recommendations/prevention_of_falls_summary_of_recommendations.*
24. Transitional care model: Essential elements. Retrieved from *www.transitionalcare.info/essential-elements.*
25. The American Geriatrics Society 2012 Beers criteria update expert panel for potentially inappropriate medication use in older adults, *J Am Geriatr Soc* 60:616, 2012.

*Evidence-based information for clinical practice.

6

Stress and Stress Management

Sharon L. Lewis, Peter N. Bonner

What is the triumph of the human spirit? It is the ability to rise above our problems and not only survive, but thrive in the face of adversity.

Brian Luke Seaward

http://evolve.elsevier.com/Lewis/medsurg/

LEARNING OUTCOMES

1. Differentiate between the terms *stressor* and *stress*.
2. Describe the role of the nervous and endocrine systems in the stress process.
3. Describe the effects of stress on the immune system.
4. Describe how stress affects the mind-body-spirit connection.
5. Discuss the effects of stress on health.
6. Explain the role of coping in managing stress.
7. Describe the coping and relaxation strategies that can be used by you, a patient, or caregiver experiencing stress.
8. Describe the nursing assessment and management of a patient experiencing stress.

KEY TERMS

coping, p. 82
emotion-focused coping, p. 82
imagery, p. 84
massage, p. 85
meditation, p. 84
mind-body-spirit connection, p. 81
problem-focused coping, p. 82
psychoneuroimmunology (PNI), p. 80
relaxation breathing, p. 83
stress, p. 77
stressors, p. 77

High levels of stress are common among patients and their caregivers. How they deal with their stress is critical to their well-being. As a nurse, you have an important role in helping them manage stressful events.

Stress has a powerful effect on the mind and therefore a significant effect on one's health and well-being. This chapter focuses on how stress can affect the mind, body, and spirit and how a person can effectively cope with stress.

WHAT IS STRESS?

Stress is the inability to cope with perceived (real or imagined) demands or threats to one's mental, emotional, or spiritual well-being.[1] What is perceived as stressful to one person may not be perceived as stressful to another. Individual responses to the same stressor vary greatly. *Perception* of the potential stressor influences the way an individual responds to that stressor (Fig. 6-1). This is demonstrated in the following examples.

- B.J., a 43-year-old woman, becomes depressed after a laparoscopic hysterectomy for fibroids. She is unwilling to participate in normal self-care activities. You are surprised by her response and think that this is fairly simple surgery and she should get on with her life. After further assessment, you discover that the removal of her uterus is a great psychologic stressor because she perceives it as a loss of her womanhood and femininity.
- K.R., a 52-year-old woman, has just been told by her physician of her new diagnosis of type 2 diabetes. After the physician's visit with her, you are prepared to provide emotional support. However, you are puzzled when she is smiling and breathing a sigh of relief. You think that this diagnosis should be stressful. However, K.R. tells you that she is so relieved because for weeks she has worried that her symptoms were related to cancer.

Many different events or factors can be **stressors**. They can be physiologic or emotional/psychologic (Fig. 6-1). The emotional/psychologic stressors can be positive or negative. For example, the birth of a baby is a positive stressor. Marital discord is a negative stressor.

Is Stress Bad or Good?

We tend to think of stress as bad or a threat. Actually any event or situation that is out of the ordinary can be considered a stressor. Events that are normally considered happy or enjoyable (e.g., getting married, going on a vacation) are also stressors.

Stress can be helpful. A little stress can motivate you. Stress can actually inspire you to achieve a goal and become more confident or stronger physically.

Reviewed by Ellen Odell, DNP, ACNS-BC, CNE, APRN, Director of Nursing, Associate Professor, Department of Nursing, John Brown University, Siloam Springs, Arkansas; and Teresa J. Seright, RN, PhD, CCRN, Associate Teaching Professor, College of Nursing, Montana State University, Bozeman, Montana.

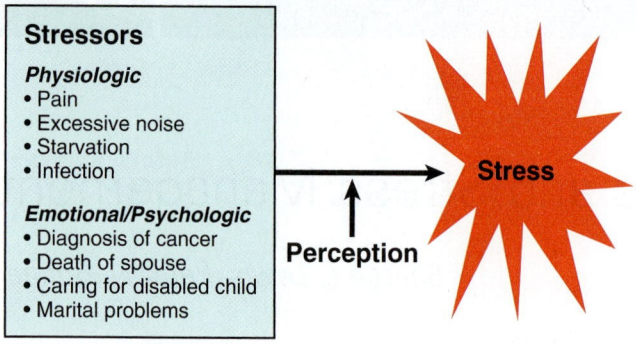

FIG. 6-1 Stressors can be physiologic or emotional/psychologic. Your perception of these stressors will determine whether they cause stress. Events or circumstances become stressful when you perceive them to be.

The body does not differentiate between bad stress and good stress, or real or imaginary stress. It responds to the stressor with the same stress response. This stress response is the way our bodies react both physically and emotionally to any change, be it good, bad, real, or imagined.

For you as a nursing student, a test can be a stressful situation. A little bit of stress related to the upcoming test makes you study and become better prepared. If you are mildly stressed during the test, it may help your test performance as a little stress heightens your awareness and increases your mental acuity. However, if you are overly stressed, it causes mental blocks, lack of concentration, and inability to remember things.

Stress is a key for survival, but too much stress can be detrimental. That is why it is important for you and your patients to learn to cope more effectively with the stressors in life.

Factors Affecting Response to Stress

Why do people respond so differently to stress? Why do some people cope better with stress than others? Interestingly, some individuals experience significant adverse life events but do not succumb to the effects of stress.

Differences in the responses to a stressor can be based on the duration of a stressor (acute or chronic) and intensity of a stressor (mild, moderate, or severe). For example, an individual dealing with the chronic stress of caring for a loved one may also be exposed to many acute stressors (e.g., car accident, influenza). Therefore the type, duration, and intensity of a stressor are important variables that can influence an individual's response (Fig. 6-2).

Factors that affect an individual's response to stress include internal and external influences (Table 6-1). These factors indicate the importance of using a holistic approach when assessing the impact of stress on a person. Four key personal characteristics that buffer the effects of stress are resilience, hardiness, attitude, and being optimistic.

Resilience is being resourceful and flexible and having good problem-solving skills. Individuals who possess a high degree of resilience are not as likely to perceive an event as stressful.

Hardiness is a combination of three characteristics: commitment, control, and openness to change. Together they provide the courage and motivation needed to turn stressful circumstances from potential calamities into opportunities for personal growth.[2]

Attitude can also influence the effect of stress on a person. People with positive attitudes view situations differently from those with negative attitudes. A person's attitude also influences how he or she manages stress. To some extent, positive emotional attitudes can prevent disease and prolong life.[3]

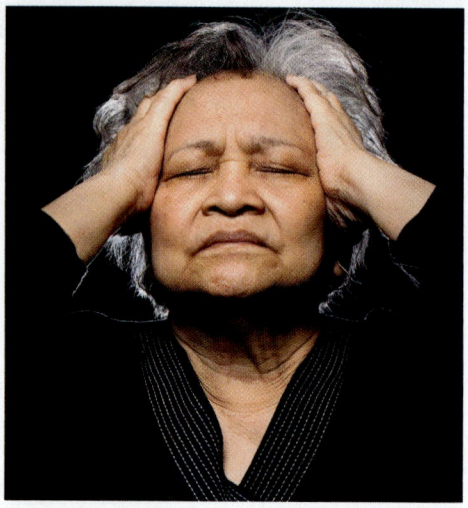

FIG. 6-2 During stressful situations, the demands seem to exceed the resources. (©azndc/iStock/Thinkstock)

TABLE 6-1 Factors Affecting Response to Stress

Internal	External
• Age	• Cultural and ethnic influences
• Health status	• Socioeconomic status
• Personality characteristics	• Social support
• Previous experience with stressors	• Religious or spiritual influences
• Genetic background	• Timing of stressors
• Resilience	• Number of stressors already experiencing
• Hardiness	
• Attitude	
• Optimistic outlook	
• Nutritional status	
• Sleep status	

Being optimistic can help you cope more effectively with stress. Optimism also reduces a person's chances of developing stress-related illnesses. When optimistic people do become ill, they tend to recover more quickly. Pessimists are likely to deny the problem, distance themselves from the stressful event, focus on stressful feelings, or allow the stressor to interfere with achieving a goal. People with a more pessimistic attitude tend to report poorer health than people with optimistic attitudes.[3]

In addition to personal characteristics, external factors play an important role in one's ability to cope with stress. Being surrounded by a strong social support system and receiving positive support from friends and family have a large impact on an individual's ability to cope with stressors.

PHYSIOLOGIC RESPONSE TO STRESS

The following section discusses the roles of the nervous, endocrine, and immune systems. These systems are interrelated, and that interrelationship is reflected in a person's physiologic response to stress (Fig. 6-3). Further, stress activation of these systems affects other body systems, such as the cardiovascular, respiratory, gastrointestinal, renal, and reproductive systems. A person's response to a stressor (real or imagined, and

PATHOPHYSIOLOGY MAP

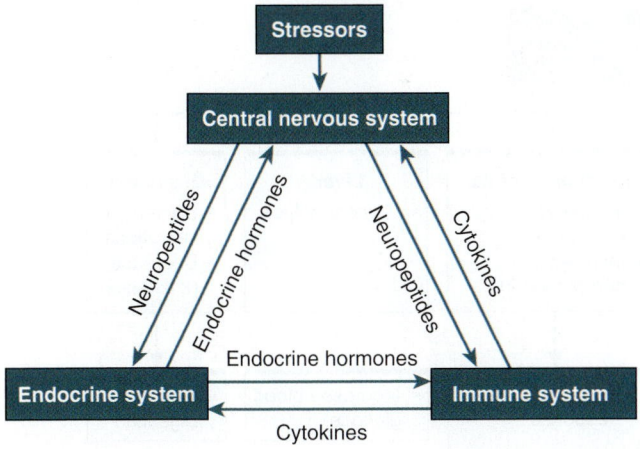

FIG. 6-3 Neurochemical links among the nervous, endocrine, and immune systems. The communication among these three systems is bidirectional.

physiologic or emotional/psychologic) determines the impact that stress will have on the body.

Nervous System

Cerebral Cortex. The cerebral cortex evaluates the stressor in light of past experiences and future consequences. These functions are involved in the perception of a stressor.

Limbic System. The *limbic system* lies in the inner midportion of the brain near the base of the brain. The limbic system is an important mediator of emotions and behavior. When the limbic system is stimulated, emotions, feelings, and behaviors can occur that ensure survival and self-preservation.

Reticular Formation. The *reticular formation* is located between the lower end of the brainstem and thalamus. It contains the *reticular activating system* (RAS), which sends impulses contributing to alertness to the limbic system and cerebral cortex. When the RAS is stimulated, it increases its output of impulses, leading to wakefulness. Stress usually increases the degree of wakefulness and can lead to sleep disturbances.

Hypothalamus. The hypothalamus, which lies at the base of the brain just above the pituitary gland, has many functions that assist in adaptation to stress. Stress activates the limbic system, which in turn stimulates the hypothalamus. Because the hypothalamus secretes neuropeptides that regulate the release of hormones by the anterior pituitary, it is central to the connection between the nervous and endocrine systems in responding to stress (Fig. 6-4).

The hypothalamus plays a primary role in the stress response by regulating the function of both the sympathetic and parasympathetic branches of the autonomic nervous system. When an individual perceives a stressor, the hypothalamus sends signals that initiate both the nervous and endocrine responses to the stressor. It does this primarily by sending signals via nerve fibers to stimulate the sympathetic nervous system (SNS) and by releasing corticotropin-releasing hormone (CRH), which stimulates the pituitary to release adrenocorticotropic hormone (ACTH) (see Chapter 47).

Endocrine System

Once the hypothalamus is activated in response to stress, the endocrine system becomes involved. The SNS stimulates the

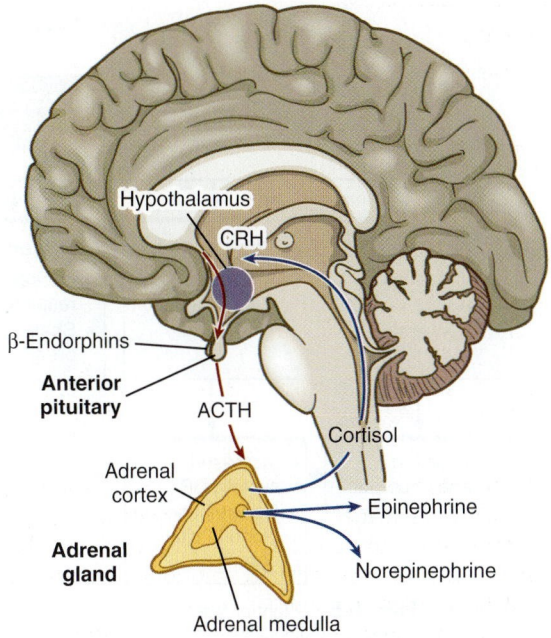

FIG. 6-4 Hypothalamic-pituitary-adrenal axis. *ACTH,* Adrenocorticotropic hormone; *CRH,* corticotropin-releasing hormone.

adrenal medulla to release epinephrine and norepinephrine (catecholamines). The effect of catecholamines and the activation of the SNS, including the response of the adrenal medulla, is referred to as the *sympathoadrenal response.* Epinephrine and norepinephrine prepare the body for the *fight-or-flight response* (Fig. 6-5).

Stress activates the hypothalamic-pituitary-adrenal (HPA) axis. In response to stress, the hypothalamus releases CRH, which stimulates the anterior pituitary to release proopiomelanocortin (POMC). Both ACTH (a hormone) and β-endorphin (a neuropeptide) are derived from POMC. Endorphins have analgesic-like effects and blunt pain perception during stress situations involving pain stimuli. ACTH, in turn, stimulates the adrenal cortex to synthesize and secrete corticosteroids (e.g., cortisol) and, to a lesser degree, aldosterone.

Corticosteroids are essential for the stress response. Cortisol produces a number of physiologic effects, such as increasing blood glucose levels, potentiating the action of catecholamines on blood vessels, and inhibiting the inflammatory response. Corticosteroids play an important role in "turning off" or blunting the stress response, which, if uncontrolled, can become self-destructive. This is shown by corticosteroids' ability to suppress the release of proinflammatory mediators, such as the cytokines tumor necrosis factor (TNF) and interleukin-1 (IL-1). The persistent release of such mediators is believed to initiate organ dysfunction in conditions such as sepsis. Thus corticosteroids act not only to support the body's adaptive response to a stressor but also to suppress an overzealous and potentially self-destructive response.

The stress response involves increases in (1) cardiac output (resulting from the increased heart rate and increased stroke volume), (2) blood glucose levels, (3) oxygen consumption, and (4) metabolic rate (Fig. 6-5). In addition, dilation of skeletal muscle blood vessels increases blood supply to the large muscles and provides for quick movement. Increased cerebral blood flow increases mental alertness. For example, in the case of stressful situations (e.g., blood loss from trauma), the increased

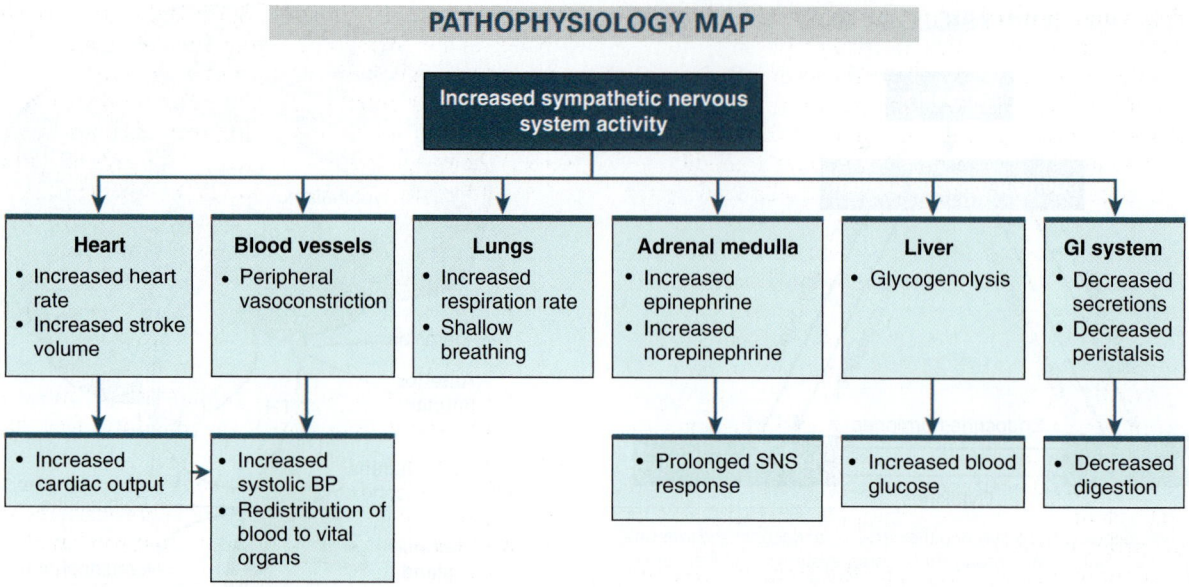

FIG. 6-5 "Fight-or-flight" reaction. Alarm reaction responses resulting from increased sympathetic nervous system *(SNS)* activity.

blood volume (from increased extracellular fluid and the shunting of blood away from the gastrointestinal system) helps to maintain adequate circulation to vital organs.

Summary of Stress Response

In summary, the fight-or-flight response is an important and necessary adaptive mechanism of the body to acute stress. This response to stressors is activated regardless of whether they are physiologic (e.g., acute pain) or emotional/psychologic (e.g., death of a child, loss of a home through fire, fear).

Acute stress leads to physiologic changes that are important to a person's survival. This is your "alarm system." It puts you on high alert. The acute stress response is a state of physiologic and psychologic arousal characterized by increased SNS activity that leads to increased heart and respiratory rate, increased BP, increased muscle tension, increased brain activity, and decreased skin temperature.

Immune System

Stress also has an impact on the immune system. **Psychoneuroimmunology (PNI)** is an interdisciplinary science that studies the interactions among psychologic, neurologic, and immune responses.[4] Because the brain is connected to the immune system by neuroanatomic and neuroendocrine pathways, stressors have the potential to lead to alterations in immune function (Fig. 6-6).

Nerve fibers extend from the nervous system and synapse on cells and tissues of the immune system (i.e., spleen, lymph nodes). In turn, the cells of the immune system have receptors for many neuropeptides and hormones, which permit them to respond to nervous and neuroendocrine signals. As a result, the mediation of stress by the central nervous system leads to corresponding changes in immune cell activity.

Both acute and chronic stress can cause immunosuppression. Stress affects immune function by (1) decreasing the number and function of natural killer cells; (2) decreasing lymphocyte proliferation; (3) altering production of *cytokines* (soluble factors secreted by white blood cells and other cells, e.g., interferon, interleukins); and (4) decreasing phagocytosis

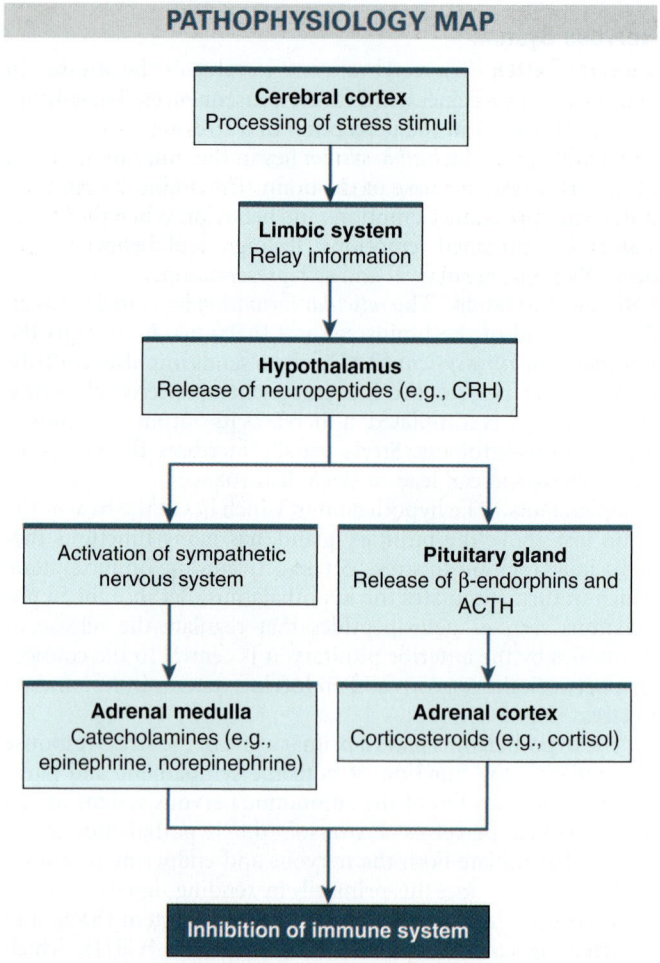

FIG. 6-6 The cerebral cortex processes stressful stimuli and relays the information via the limbic system to the hypothalamus. Corticotropin-releasing hormone *(CRH)* stimulates the release of adrenocorticotropic hormone *(ACTH)* from the pituitary gland. ACTH stimulates the adrenal cortex to release corticosteroids. The sympathetic nervous system is also stimulated, resulting in the release of epinephrine and norepinephrine from the adrenal medulla. The end result is the inhibition of the immune system.

by neutrophils and monocytes.[4] (Natural killer cells, lymphocytes, and cytokines are discussed in Chapter 13.)

Importantly, the network that links the brain and immune system is bidirectional (Fig. 6-3). Signals from these systems travel back and forth, allowing for communication among these systems. Consequently, not only do emotions modify the immune response, but products of immune cells send signals back to the brain and alter its activity. Many of the communication signals sent from the immune system to the brain are mediated by cytokines, which are central to the coordination of the immune response. For example, IL-1 (a cytokine made by monocytes) acts on the temperature regulatory center of the hypothalamus and initiates the febrile response to infectious pathogens (see Fig. 11-4).

The central nervous system is capable of influencing the function of the immune system. Stress-induced immunosuppression may exacerbate or increase the risk of progression of immune-related diseases such as multiple sclerosis, asthma, rheumatoid arthritis, and cancer.[5]

Many questions about stress and the immune response remain unanswered. For example, it is not known how much stress (intensity or chronicity) is needed to cause changes or how much of an alteration in the immune system is necessary before disease susceptibility occurs.

MIND-BODY-SPIRIT CONNECTION

The **mind-body-spirit connection** demonstrates the relationship and interconnectedness among the various parts that a person is made of: mind, body, and spirit (Fig. 6-7). All three parts are important in your life and in determining who you are. What goes on in your mind influences every part of the body. Your body and your mind are affected by how connected you feel to your spirit (soul). Spirit is the life force within you that gives life, energy, and power. You are a spiritual being with a mind that affects every aspect of your body.

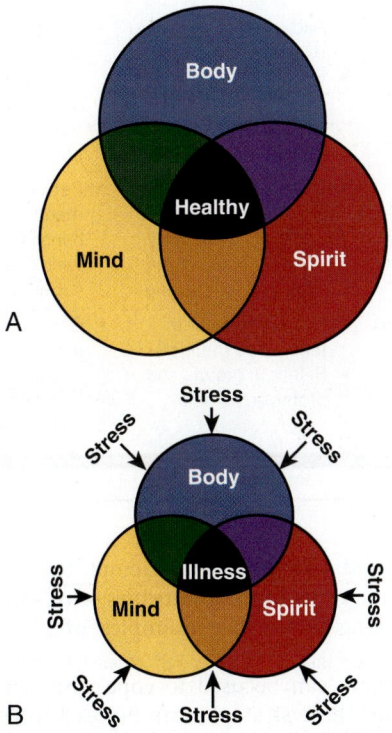

FIG. 6-7 The connections among the mind, body, and spirit can lead to a person being healthy **(A)** or the effects of stress on the mind, body, and spirit connections can lead to illness **(B)**.

When your mind is healthy, your body can resist illness better. When your body is healthy, your feelings are more positive. When your spirit is renewed and energized, your mind is alert and your body feels good. The well-being of your spirit is linked to your mental, emotional, and physical health.

Stress has a powerful effect on your mind, body, and spirit. Therefore it has a significant effect on your health and well-being. Emotional thoughts and feelings can affect the body and spirit. Negative thoughts such as, "I am a terrible nurse … I cannot handle this one more day" can cause a physical response in your body (e.g., headaches, stomachaches), and it will make you feel down in your spirits; your life force feels sucked out. You can become physically ill.

Since the mind can affect the body and spirit, conscious use of the mind can effect positive changes in your body. Your mind is one of the most powerful weapons that you have to deal with and conquer stress.

How you deal with difficult situations or stressful times can greatly influence your overall well-being: your mind, body, and spirit. You have a choice in how you respond to a crisis or a difficult time. Even if the outcome of the situation is not what a person desired, one can emerge with a winning attitude. Sometimes you may feel that the world is against you and life is not fair. Or you can say, "This is rough, but I'm not going to let this get me down."

EFFECTS OF STRESS ON HEALTH

As previously mentioned, the acute stress response is your alarm system and puts you on alert. However, your body was not meant to be on high alert all of the time. If stress is excessive or prolonged, these same "helpful" physiologic responses can lead to harm and disease. When a person sustains chronic, unrelieved stress, the body's defenses can no longer keep up with the demands. Therefore stress plays a role in the development and/or progression of diseases of adaptation, or stress-related illnesses (Table 6-2).

Stress is linked to leading causes of death, including cancer, accidents, and suicides. Stress can have effects on cognitive function, including poor concentration, memory problems, distressing dreams, sleep disturbances, and impaired decision making. Stress can also cause a wide variety of changes in behavior. These include people withdrawing from others, becoming quiet or unusually talkative, changing eating habits, drinking alcohol excessively, or becoming irritable.[5,6]

Long-term exposure to catecholamines resulting from excessive activation of the SNS may increase the risk of cardiovas-

TABLE 6-2 Disorders With a Stress Component*

• Depression	• Hypertension
• Dyspepsia	• Insomnia
• Eating disorders	• Irritable bowel syndrome
• Erectile dysfunction	• Low back pain
• Fatigue	• Menstrual irregularities
• Fibromyalgia	• Peptic ulcer disease
• Headaches	• Sexual dysfunction

*List is not all inclusive.

cular diseases such as atherosclerosis and hypertension.[7] Other conditions that are precipitated or aggravated by stress include migraine headaches, irritable bowel syndrome, and peptic ulcers.[8,9] Control of metabolic conditions, such as diabetes mellitus, is also affected by stress. Behavioral interventions aimed at stress reduction and relaxation have helped manage these diseases in conjunction with standard medical therapy.[10]

Stressful life events can make a person more susceptible to infection. For example, psychologic stress may increase one's risk for developing the common cold. In a landmark study, healthy volunteers were inoculated intranasally with low doses of upper respiratory tract viruses. The subjects underwent psychologic testing to determine the occurrence of stressful events in their lives and their reactions to such stresses. The results showed that the rates of both viral infection and clinical colds increased with the degree of psychologic stress. In this study, social support buffered the harmful effects of stress.[11]

At the cellular level, stress may promote earlier onset of age-related diseases. There is a link between stress and telomere length. Telomeres are the protective end caps on chromosomes, and their diminishing size is an indication of age. Telomeres are highly susceptible to stress and depression. Telomeres are shorter in people who are stressed and depressed than in healthy people. Thus chronic stress can have a long-term effect on our overall health by changing our DNA and accelerating the rate at which our cells age.[12,13]

Chronic stress is a major contributor to chronic illness, which in turn is a major driver of escalating health care costs. It is critical that the entire health care community recognize the role of stress and unhealthy behaviors in causing and exacerbating chronic health conditions.

COPING STRATEGIES

Coping is a person's efforts to manage stressors.[14] *Coping strategies* are what you do (your behaviors and actions) to help deal with stress. Coping can be either positive or negative. Positive coping includes activities such as exercise and spending time with friends and family. Healthy coping helps you handle your stressors so that they do not overwhelm you. Negative coping may include substance abuse and denial.

Unfortunately, some coping strategies actually make the stress worse. Sometimes coping strategies temporarily relieve the stress, but in the long run they actually increase the stress. For example, a person may really enjoy watching a favorite TV show as a form of coping. However, then it soon becomes a fixation on many soap operas and TV becomes an addiction and escape from dealing with the real stressors.

> You cannot always choose your destiny in life, but you can choose how you cope with it.
>
> **Norman Vincent Peale**

A variety of coping strategies can be used to cope with stress. Table 6-3 has examples of coping strategies that you can use in your life and teach to patients and caregivers. Coping strategies can be divided into two broad categories: emotion-focused coping and problem-focused coping. **Emotion-focused coping** involves managing the emotions that an individual feels when a stressful event occurs. Examples of emotion-focused coping include discussing feelings with a friend or taking a hot bath.

TABLE 6-3 Coping Strategies

Strategy	Description	How to Implement
Aromatherapy	• Use of essential oils (fragrant molecules from plants) for inhalation or topical application • Variety of essential oils including lavender, peppermint, rosemary, eucalyptus, sandalwood, etc.	• Place 5-8 drops in a full bath and agitate water before bathing. • Place a few drops on a tissue or in diffuser or vaporizer.
Art therapy	• Allows a person to nonverbally express and communicate feelings, emotions, and thoughts • Can reduce stress, promote relaxation, and help process experiences • Based on the belief that the creative process is healing and life enhancing	• Close your eyes and draw a line on a piece of paper. Open your eyes. Continue to build on that line and draw whatever comes to mind. • Get a piece of paper and doodle. Do not edit. • Get a coloring book and crayons and just start coloring.
Exercise	• Any form of movement, especially aerobic movement • Can be viewed as meditation in motion	• Walk, swim, garden, bicycle, dance, climb stairs, participate in group exercises.
Humor	• Can take the form of laughter, cartoons, funny movies, videos, riddles, comic books, and joke books	• Keep a "tickler" scrapbook with funny photos, cartoons, etc. • Humor carts can be set up in many clinical settings to be used by patients and families.
Journaling	• Allows an individual to express self in writing • Enhances personal development and awareness through self-reflection	• Use a journaling notebook or computer to write down thoughts, feelings, memories, and perceptions.
Pet therapy (animal-assisted therapy) (Fig. 6-8)	• Use of animals as a form of treatment • Improves a patient's social, emotional, or cognitive functioning	• Pet therapist or family member or friend brings a pet with which patient can socialize.
Social support	• Relationships with family and friends • Self-help groups and professional help	• Get together with family and friends on a regular basis. • Join a support group that specifically helps to meet needs (e.g., grief support group).

Problem-focused coping involves attempts to resolve the problems causing the stress. Setting priorities or collecting information and seeking advice are examples of problem-focused coping.

Both strategies can be used to cope with stressors, and a combination of these strategies can be used to cope with the same stressor. Table 6-4 provides examples of emotion- and problem-focused coping when applied to the same stressful situation. When a situation is unchangeable or uncontrollable,

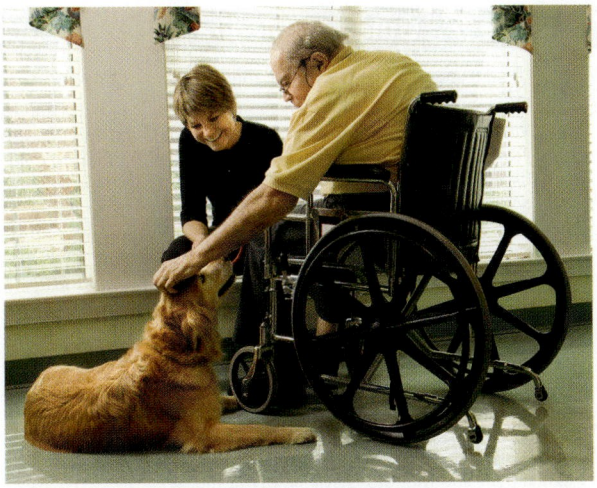

FIG. 6-8 Pet therapy can be used in a variety of settings including rehabilitation. (©RonChappleStudios/Hemera/Thinkstock)

TABLE 6-4 Problem- and Emotion-Focused Coping

Stressor	Problem-Focused Coping	Emotion-Focused Coping
Failing an examination	Obtaining a tutor	Going for a run
Being diagnosed with diabetes	Attending education classes about diabetes	Getting a massage
Receiving questionable mammogram results	Scheduling follow-up testing for ultrasound	Expressing feelings of anxiety to friends and nurse

emotion-focused coping may predominate. The primary purpose of emotion-focused coping is to help decrease negative emotions and create a feeling of well-being. Although it may not seem to be working toward a solution, emotion-focused coping is a valid and appropriate way to deal with stressful situations.

If a problem can be changed or controlled, problem-focused coping is the most helpful coping strategy. Problem-focused coping strategies allow an individual to look at a challenge objectively, take action to address the problem, and thereby reduce the stress.

RELAXATION STRATEGIES

The *relaxation response* is a state of physiologic and psychologic rest. It is the opposite of the stress response. The relaxation response is characterized by decreased SNS activity, which leads to decreased heart and respiratory rate, decreased BP, decreased muscle tension, decreased brain activity, and increased skin temperature.[15]

The relaxation response can be elicited through a variety of relaxation strategies (Table 6-5). Regular elicitation of the relaxation response has been proven to be an effective treatment for a wide range of stress-related disorders, including chronic pain, insomnia, and hypertension. Individuals who regularly engage in relaxation strategies are able to deal better with their stressors, increase their sense of control over stressors, and reduce their tension.[16]

TABLE 6-5 Relaxation Strategies*

- Imagery
- Massage
- Meditation
- Muscle relaxation
- Music
- Qigong
- Relaxing breathing
- Tai Chi
- Yoga

*This list is not all inclusive. Further description of the most common ones are discussed in the text.

COMPLEMENTARY & ALTERNATIVE THERAPIES

Yoga

Yoga is an ancient system of relaxation, exercise, and healing with origins in Indian philosophy. The goal of yoga is physical and mental well-being achieved through the use of stretching, postures, breathing practices, and meditation.

Scientific Evidence

Yoga can be used to treat hypertension and reduce stress and anxiety.

Nursing Implications

- Regardless of the type of yoga, deep abdominal relaxation breathing is a main component and helps one to focus on the inner self and promote the relaxation response.
- Yoga is often used to promote relaxation, decrease stress, improve flexibility, and enhance overall health.
- Yoga is generally considered safe. Some postures should not be used by patients with certain medical conditions or illnesses.

Relaxation Breathing

The way one breathes affects every aspect of one's life. When a person is stressed, muscles tense and breathing becomes shallow and rapid. Therefore one of the simplest and most effective ways to stop the stress response is to breathe deeply and slowly. It is difficult to maintain tension when breathing in a slow, deep, and relaxed pattern.

Relaxation (abdominal) **breathing** can be performed while sitting, standing, or lying down. It is especially useful during a stressful or anxious situation to reduce stress. Relaxation breathing forms the basis for most relaxation strategies.

Before practicing relaxation breathing, it is important to assess one's normal breathing pattern (Table 6-6). Relaxation breathing, which involves the diaphragm, is natural for newborns and sleeping adults. It is a more efficient type of breathing. Chest breathing, which involves the upper chest and shoulders, is inefficient. This type of breathing is often used during times of anxiety and distress.

Relaxation breathing involves the primary use of the diaphragm and less use of the upper chest and shoulders to assist in each breath. In this type of breathing, the abdomen gently moves in and out during exhalation and inhalation. The breaths should be slow, steady, and deep.

One basic technique for relaxation breathing is as follows: (1) Inhale slowly and deeply, pushing the abdomen out. Think about breathing in peace. (2) Exhale slowly, letting the abdomen come in and all the muscles relax. Think about breathing out tension. (3) Repeat these deep breaths 10 times without interruption. As with any breathing exercise, if a light-headed feeling arises, stop for 30 seconds and then start again.

Other methods used to teach relaxation breathing are the 4 × 4 technique and relaxation sigh (Table 6-6). Breathing

TABLE 6-6 Relaxation Breathing Techniques*

Breathing Assessment

1. Begin by placing one hand gently on your abdomen below your waistline.
2. Place the other hand on the center of your chest on the sternum.
3. Without changing the normal breathing pattern, take several breaths. During inhalation notice which hand rises the most.
4. When relaxation breathing is performed properly, the hand on the abdomen should rise more than the hand on the chest.

4 × 4 Technique

1. Sit up straight with your back flush to the support of the chair and your feet flat on the floor.
2. Rest your arms on your lap, thighs, or arms of the chair.
3. Take in a deep breath through your nose to a count of four (1 ... 2 ... 3 ... 4).
4. Hold your breath to a count of four (1 ... 2 ... 3 ... 4).
5. Release your breath through your mouth to a count of four (1 ... 2 ... 3 ... 4).
6. Rest for a count of four (1 ... 2 ... 3 ... 4).
7. Repeat the cycle four times.

Relaxing Sigh

1. Sit up straight with your back against the support of the chair and your feet flat on floor.
2. Inhale a natural breath and then sigh deeply. Let out a sound of relief as the air rushes out of your lungs.
3. Do not think about inhaling at the end of the sigh; just let the air come in naturally as you breathe deeply.
4. Repeat this sigh about 4 to 6 times very slowly.
5. You can repeat this exercise whenever you need it.

*Video demonstrations of these techniques are available in the Stress-Busting Kit for Nursing Students on the website for this book.

techniques are discussed in the Stress-Busting Kit for Nursing Students available on the website for this book.

Initially, relaxation breathing may feel unusual. With practice it becomes easier, and its relaxing benefits are soon obvious. You should personally learn to use relaxation breathing before teaching it to patients and their caregivers. Once learned, relaxation breathing can be easily taught to patients in a variety of settings, particularly when they are undergoing stressful and painful procedures.

Meditation

Meditation is a practice of concentrated focus on a sound, object, visualization, the breath, or movement. The purpose of meditation is to increase awareness, reduce stress, promote relaxation, and enhance personal and spiritual growth.

Although meditation can be performed anywhere, it is best to practice meditation in a quiet place, free of distractions. Table 6-7 provides some basic guidelines on how to meditate. Meditation is often practiced while seated, and it is important to maintain a comfortable posture. Meditation can also be performed while walking and focusing on a single action such as the movement of the feet. In the beginning, individuals typically start with just 5 to 10 minutes of meditation at a time and often increase the time as the practice becomes more comfortable.

Prayer. Prayer can be a form of meditation. It is a spiritual communion with God or an object of worship. Many people find deep comfort in their faith. Religious services, conversations with clergy, and individual worship and prayer may help to alleviate a person's stress and give one a greater perspective, strength, and inspiration.

TABLE 6-7 Guide to Meditation*

You can teach yourself the basics of meditation by following a few simple steps:

1. Find a quiet place.
2. Make sure there are no distractions.
3. Sit in a comfortable position.
4. Close your eyes.
5. Shut out the world so that your brain can stop processing information coming from your senses.
6. Pick a focus word, short phrase, song verse (melody), or prayer that is firmly rooted in your belief system, such as *one, peace, The Lord is my shepherd, Hail Mary full of grace,* or *shalom.*
7. Breathe slowly and practice relaxation breathing. Say your focus word, short phrase, song verse, or prayer silently to yourself as you exhale.
8. Say the word or phrase again and again.
9. Try saying the word or phrase silently to yourself with every exhalation. The monotony will help you focus.
10. Relax your muscles, progressing from your feet to your calves, thighs, abdomen, shoulders, head, and neck.
11. Do not be concerned when other thoughts come to mind. Just acknowledge them and return calmly to your word or phrase.
12. Continue for 10 to 20 minutes, but even 5 minutes can leave you feeling calm and refreshed. Rise slowly.
13. Practice once or twice daily.

*Meditation exercises are available in the Stress-Busting Kit for Nursing Students on the website for this book.

Imagery

Imagery is the use of one's mind to generate images that have a calming effect on the body. It involves focusing the mind and incorporates all the senses to create physiologic and emotional changes. It is a simple relaxation technique that requires no equipment other than an active imagination. *Guided imagery* is a variation of imagery in which images are suggested by another person (either live or on a CD or in an MP3 file).

Imagery can be used in many clinical settings for stress reduction and pain relief. Benefits of imagery include anxiety reduction, decreased muscle tension, improved comfort during medical procedures, enhanced immune function, decreased recovery time after surgery, and reduction in sleeping problems.

You can use imagery in your own life or use guided imagery with your patients. One of the uses of imagery is to create a special place for a mental retreat. Table 6-8 describes the steps involved in creating a special place.

When imagery is performed, it is best to find a comfortable position. Take slow, deep breaths. Focus should involve all senses (sight, hearing, touch, smell). For example, one can use an image such as Fig. 6-9, engaging all the senses as one focuses on the image.

Imagery can also be used to specifically target a disease, problem, or stressor. Table 6-9 describes some suggestions for using imagery in specific diseases or disorders.

Imagery can also be used to enhance performance or process stressful or difficult tasks. For example, an athlete or musician can use imagery to achieve greater success. Imagery allows one to mentally rehearse the difficult or challenging situation. Imagery can help a fearful nurse start an IV line or perform a difficult procedure. It can also be used with a patient who is afraid to have a stressful or painful procedure performed (e.g., bone marrow biopsy).

TABLE 6-8 Imagery: Creating Your Special Place*

1. Begin by closing your eyes and taking several slow, deep breaths.
2. Imagine a place where you feel completely comfortable and peaceful. It may be a real place or one you imagine: one from your past or some place you have always wanted to go.
3. Allow this special place to take form, slowly. As it takes form, look around to your left, to your right. Enjoy the scenery: the colors, the texture, the shapes.
4. Listen carefully to the sounds of your place. What do you hear?
5. Is there a gentle breeze or sunshine warming your face? Pick up or touch some favorite objects from your special place.
6. Take in a deep breath through your nose, and notice the rich smells around you. Perhaps your favorite flower is in bloom, or you smell the scents of the ocean.
7. Take another deep breath and relax. Enjoy the peace, comfort, and safety of your special place.
8. This is your special place. You relax and feel thankful that you are here, in your special place.
9. You can return to this place any time that you wish.

*Imagery exercises are available in the Stress-Busting Kit for Nursing Students on the website for this book.

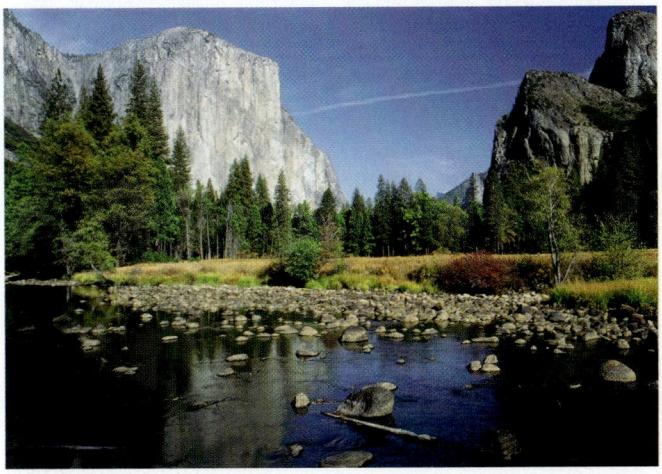

FIG. 6-9 In imagery, special places are created involving all the senses, such as a place where one can hear rustling water, smell flowers, feel the wind, and see a colorful landscape. (©iStockphoto/Thinkstock)

Music

Music can help achieve relaxation and bring about healthy changes in emotional or physical states. Listening to relaxing music can divert one's focus from a stressful situation.

Music has been used in many clinical settings. Music decreases anxiety and elicits the relaxation response. Music helps people with insomnia go to sleep. It can decrease muscle tension, pain sensation, and emotional stress.[17]

Music that contains approximately 60 to 80 beats/min is considered soothing. Low-pitched tones and music without words is recommended for relaxation. Mozart's music is a popular form of music used for relaxation. On the other hand, fast-tempo music can stimulate and uplift a person. Each person considers different types of music to be relaxing, so it is important to find music that best matches the person's needs and circumstance. To achieve optimal relaxation while listening to music, minimize all interruptions and assume a comfortable posture.

Music can be incorporated into clinical practice. It is noninvasive, safe, inexpensive, and easy to use. First, it is important to establish the purpose and benefit of using music with patients in a given clinical setting. Then assess each patient's interest and preference in music. Create a listening environment, encouraging the patient to find a comfortable position. Headphones or earphones and an MP3 or CD player can be used. Evaluate patients' response to the music, asking them how it sounds and how it makes them feel.

TABLE 6-9 Examples of Imagery

Imagery can be used to relieve stress and promote health and healing in conjunction with regular medical care. Special images can be created to alleviate symptoms or treat diseases or disorders. The image should be strong and vivid for the person, using many senses to create the image. Below are some examples that some people have found useful.

Disease or Disorder	Images
Infection	• White blood cells with flashing red sirens arrest and imprison harmful germs.
Cancer	• Shark gobbles up cancer cells. • Radiation or chemotherapy treatments enter the body like healing rays of light; they destroy cancer cells.
Coronary artery disease	• Water flows freely through a wide, open river.
Weakened immune system	• White blood cells rapidly multiply like millions of seeds bursting from a ripe seed pod.
Asthma	• Tiny elastic rubber bands that constrict the airways pop open.
Depression	• Troubles and feelings of sadness are attached to big colorful helium balloons and are floating off into a clear blue sky.
Pain	• Pain is washed away by a cool calm river flowing through the entire body.

Adapted from Sobel DS, Ornstein R: *Healthy mind, healthy body,* New York, 1996, Patient Education Materials, Time Life.

Massage

Massage includes a range of techniques that manipulate the soft tissues and joints of the body. Involving touch and movement, massage is typically delivered with the hands. It reduces muscle tension and positively affects mental and emotional states.

Massage is an important form of touch. It is also a form of caring, communication, and comfort. Your role related to massage differs from that of the registered massage therapist. Whereas massage therapists can provide more comprehensive massage therapies, as a nurse, you can use specific massage techniques as part of nursing care. For example, you can give a back massage to help promote sleep. For a bedridden patient, gentle massage can stimulate circulation and help prevent skin breakdown. A simple hand massage can be used to have a calming and relaxing effect, especially for patients who are anxious or agitated. During end-of-life care, hospice nurses may incorporate massage into their nursing care as the massaging touch can lessen pain and restlessness.

When you identify that massage may be useful, first assess the patient's preference regarding touch and massage. Consider cultural and social beliefs and discuss potential benefits with the patient. Family members can be taught to massage their loved one, providing a way for family members to participate in patient care. This can be therapeutic for the patient and family, even when the loved one is cognitively impaired or unresponsive.

> You may not be able to change the stressors in your life, but you can change your reaction or response to them.
>
> **Florence Nightingale**

❖ NURSING MANAGEMENT: STRESS

◆ Nursing Assessment

Patients and caregivers face many potential stressors that can have health consequences. Be aware of situations that are likely to result in stress and determine the patient's and caregiver's perception of these situations. In addition to the stressor itself, specific coping strategies have health consequences and therefore must be included in the assessment.

As a nurse, you are in a key position to (1) assess stress in patients and their caregivers, (2) assist them in identifying high-risk periods for stress, and (3) implement stress management strategies that can prevent the negative consequences of stress on their health (Fig. 6-10). Assess the number of stressors, duration of these stressors, and previous experience with similar demands. Assess the personal meaning attached to the stressful situation to provide useful insight for planning stress management strategies with the patient. Also consider the caregivers' responses to the stressors.

Be specific with your questions: Have you experienced this stressor before? How did you handle it? What worked well and what did not? Although the manifestations of stress may vary from person to person, assess the patient for the signs and symptoms of the stress response, including an increased heart rate and BP, hyperventilation, sweating, headache, musculoskeletal pain, gastrointestinal upset, loss of appetite, insomnia, and fatigue. In addition, the patient may exhibit some of the stress-related illnesses or diseases of adaptation (Table 6-2).

Behavioral manifestations may include an inability to concentrate, accident proneness, impaired speech, anxiety, crying, frustration, and irritability. Work-related responses to stress may include absenteeism or tardiness at work, decreased productivity, and job dissatisfaction. Cognitive responses include self-reports of an inability to make decisions and forgetfulness. Some of these responses may also be apparent to significant others.

Another major source of stress relates to the patient's illness, which often also causes stress for the caregiver and other family members. Assess what aspects of the illness are the most stressful for the patient and caregiver. These may include the patient's physical health, job responsibilities, finances, and children. This information is valuable because it helps you to understand the patient's perspective of the stressors. Knowledge of stressors, the feelings these stressors evoke, and the psychologic sequelae they can produce will assist you in identifying potential and actual sources of stress and their effect on the patient.

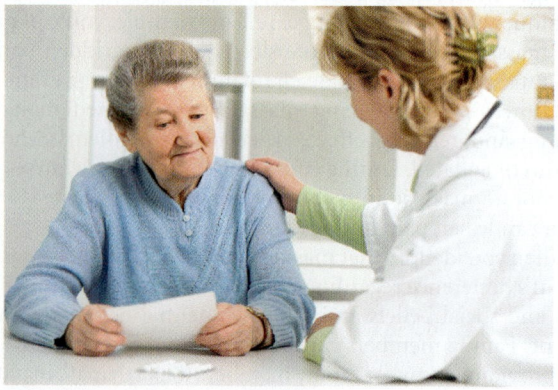

FIG. 6-10 As a nurse, you have an important role in helping patients deal with stress. (©AlexRaths/iStock/Thinkstock)

◆ Nursing Implementation

The first step in managing stress is to become aware of its presence. This includes identifying what the stressors are and the person's response to them. Your role is to facilitate and enhance the patient's coping and adaptation. Nursing interventions depend on the severity of the stress experience. For example, a patient with multiple trauma expends energy in an attempt

BECOMING A NURSE LEADER

Self-Care in Nursing

Situation

You are a nursing student and becoming more anxious every day. You are constantly fatigued, have trouble sleeping, and are prone to muscle tension, headaches, and frequent gastrointestinal problems. In addition, you cannot concentrate or study, and you dread going to class and clinical. Seeing the pain and suffering of patients and family members is very stressful for you and causes you to feel hopeless. You are increasingly worried about being asked a question you cannot answer by physicians, nurses, and your instructors.

Points for Consideration

- Being an effective leader begins with taking care of yourself.
- Effective nurses remain honest with themselves and keep an open mind to getting help when they need it.
- Although nurses are taught to care for others, they often express reluctance to take the time required to care for themselves. Self-care can help practicing and student nurses cope with stressors and alleviate symptoms such as exhaustion, tension, and fatigue/burnout.[1]
- *Compassion fatigue* is identified as a unique form of burnout that affects individuals in caregiving roles. This may affect nurses when they personally experience the pain of their patients and families.[2]
- Be open to help. Don't feel ashamed or alone. Reach out for help by talking to your faculty, co-workers, or supervisor. Take advantage of student/employee health counseling.
- Keep work and home life separate. Easier said than done, but one of the key causes of compassion fatigue is losing sight of the boundaries between personal and work life.
- Some nursing school programs are incorporating self-care activities in their curriculums. These include discussions about self-care and stress management techniques (e.g., relaxation breathing, yoga, meditation, exercise, journaling) and seeing life as a blend and balance of teacher, healer, leader, and visionary.[2]

Discussion Questions

1. What are the first steps that you can take to decrease your stress and anxiety?
2. What self-care measures can you include in your daily life?
3. How can dealing with your own stressors help you to be a better nurse leader?

References

1. Blum CA: Practicing self-care for nurses: a nursing program initiative, *Online J Issues Nurs* 19(3), 2014. doi: 10.3912/OJIN.Vol19No03Man03.
2. Lombardo B, Eyre C: Compassion fatigue: a nurse's primer, *Online J Issues Nurs* 16(1):3, 2011. doi:10.3912/OJIN.Vol16No01Man03.

TABLE 6-10 Personal Tips for Handling Stress

- Do not try to be superhuman.
- Learn to "let go" of things that are outside of your control.
- Learn acceptance of yourself.
- Exercise regularly.
- Share your feelings.
- Keep a sense of humor; laugh often.
- Learn relaxation breathing.
- Use imagery.
- Meditate or pray.
- Get adequate sleep.
- Live a healthy lifestyle.
- Try to look at change as a positive challenge, not as a threat.
- Solve the little problems, since this can help you gain a feeling of control.
- Work to resolve conflicts with other people.
- If needed, get professional counseling.

to physically survive. As a nurse, your efforts are directed to life-supporting interventions and approaches aimed at reducing additional stressors for the patient. The patient with multiple trauma is much less likely to adapt or recover if faced with additional stressors such as sleep deprivation or an infection.

Coping strategies that are used should be helpful and not a source of additional stress for the patient. Coping strategies were previously discussed in this chapter.

You can assume a primary role in implementing stress management strategies. Some personal tips for handling stress are presented in Table 6-10. These tips will benefit you personally and enhance your own level of health and wellness. It is essential that you first care for yourself before you can help the patients who need your care. Once you have incorporated these strategies into your life, you can share them with patients and caregivers.

Ideas for how to incorporate stress management strategies into nursing practice are presented in Table 6-11. Although some may require additional training, many stress management strategies are within the scope of nursing practice. These include relaxation breathing, imagery, music, exercise, massage, meditation, art therapy, and journaling. (Additional resources are in the Stress-Busting Kit for Nursing Students on the website for this book.)

TABLE 6-11 How to Implement Stress Management in Practice

1. Learn relaxation breathing. It is the easiest method of relaxation to use.
2. Practice teaching relaxation breathing with peers, then patients.
3. Pick coping strategies (Table 6-4) and relaxation strategies that are appropriate for your clinical area.
4. Practice using the strategy yourself. It becomes easier with time.
5. Take advantage of opportunities to teach coping and relaxation strategies to patients.
6. If you have setbacks, think about what went wrong. Do NOT quit!
7. Attend seminars and workshops on stress management to learn more.

Most coping and relaxation strategies can be taught to patients in 10 to 15 minutes. Choose a coping or relaxation strategy to best suit the patient and situation. Give directions calmly and slowly in short, simple sentences.

Effective stress management provides an individual a sense of control of the stressful situation. As stress management practices are incorporated into daily activities, the individual is able to increase his or her confidence and self-reliance and limit the emotional response to the stressful circumstances. Having a sense of control can prevent the harmful effects of a stress response.

As a nurse, you are in an ideal situation to integrate stress management in clinical practice. You are also well equipped to develop and test the effectiveness of new approaches to manage stress and promote positive health outcomes. However, it is very important to recognize when the patient or caregiver needs to be referred to a professional with advanced training in counseling.

CASE STUDY

Stress-Induced Complaints

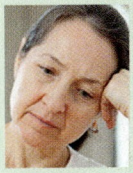

(©JackF/iStock/Thinkstock)

Patient Profile

K.F., a 48-year-old woman, recently moved to the United States from Romania with her two teenage children. She has no family in the country and was recently divorced. She has taken a job as a waitress in a hectic restaurant and works as a seamstress out of her home in the evenings.

She has developed some unusual symptoms and comes to see the nurse practitioner at a community clinic. Although she states that she was in good health when she left Romania, she now complains of fatigue, inability to sleep, and aches all over her body. Even when she is able to get some extra sleep, she still feels exhausted. Her co-worker told her she has fibromyalgia.

Discussion Questions

1. Consider K.F.'s situation and describe the stressors with which she is dealing. Describe the possible effects of these stressors on her health.
2. ***Priority Decision:*** What are the priority coping strategies that you should include in K.F.'s plan of care?
3. What limitations should be considered when discussing specific coping strategies?
4. ***Patient-Centered Care***: What cultural considerations should be included in the plan of care?

Answers available at *http://evolve.elsevier.com/Lewis/medsurg.*

BRIDGE TO NCLEX EXAMINATION

The number of the question corresponds to the same-numbered outcome at the beginning of the chapter.

1. Determination of whether an event is a stressor is based on a person's
   a. tolerance.
   b. perception.
   c. adaptation.
   d. stubbornness.
2. The nurse would expect which finding in a patient as a result of the physiologic effect of stress on the reticular formation?
   a. An episode of diarrhea while awaiting painful dressing changes
   b. Refusal to communicate with nurses while awaiting a cardiac catheterization
   c. Inability to sleep the night before beginning to self-administer insulin injections
   d. Increased blood pressure, decreased urine output, and hyperglycemia after a car accident
3. The nurse uses knowledge of the effects of stress on the immune system by encouraging patients to
   a. sleep for 10 to 12 hours per day.
   b. avoid exposure to upper respiratory tract infections.
   c. receive regular immunizations when they are stressed.
   d. use emotion-focused rather than problem-focused coping strategies.
4. Which of the following examples reflects the relationship among the mind-body-spirit (*select all that apply*)?
   a. A 75-year-old man who enjoys doing crossword puzzles every day
   b. A 25-year-old man who has been successfully treated for testicular cancer
   c. A 55-year-old man who is impotent because of his prostate cancer surgery
   d. A 34-year-old woman who is angry because of her recent diagnosis of breast cancer
   e. A 65-year-old woman struggling with rehabilitation after having hip replacement surgery
5. The nurse recognizes that a person who experiences chronic stress could be at higher risk for (*select all that apply*)
   a. osteoporosis.
   b. fibromyalgia.
   c. colds and flu.
   d. high blood pressure.
   e. high serum cholesterol.
6. The nurse recognizes that a patient with newly diagnosed breast cancer is using an emotion-focused coping process when she
   a. joins a support group for women with breast cancer.
   b. considers the pros and cons of the various treatment options.
   c. delays treatment until her family can take a weekend trip together.
   d. tells the nurse that she has a good prognosis because the tumor is small.
7. During a stressful circumstance that is unchangeable, which type of coping strategy is the *most* effective?
   a. Avoidance
   b. Coping flexibility
   c. Emotion-focused coping
   d. Problem-focused coping
8. An appropriate nursing intervention for a hospitalized patient who states she cannot cope with her illness is
   a. controlling the environment to prevent sensory overload and promote sleep.
   b. encouraging the patient's family to offer emotional support by frequent visiting.
   c. arranging for the patient to phone family and friends to maintain emotional bonds.
   d. asking the patient to describe previous stressful situations and how she managed to resolve them.

1. b, 2. c, 3. b, 4. a, b, c, d, e, 5. b, c, d, 6. a, 7. c, 8. d.

For rationales to these answers and even more NCLEX review questions, visit *http://evolve.elsevier.com/Lewis/medsurg.*

EVOLVE WEBSITE

http://evolve.elsevier.com/Lewis/medsurg

Review Questions (Online Only)
Key Points
Answer Keys for Questions
- Rationales for Bridge to NCLEX Examination Questions
- Answer Guidelines for Case Study on p. 87

Conceptual Care Map Creator
Stress-Busting Kit for Nursing Students
Audio Glossary
Content Updates

REFERENCES

1. Seward BL: *Managing stress: principles and strategies for health and well-being*, ed 8, Burlington, Mass, 2014, Jones & Bartlett.
*2. Maddi SR: Hardiness: the courage to grow from stresses, *J Pos Psych* 1(3):160, 2006. (Classic)
3. Positive thinking: Stop negative self-talk to reduce stress. Retrieved from *www.mayoclinic.org/healthy-living/stress-management/in-depth/positive-thinking/art-20043950.*
4. Segerstrom S, editor: *The Oxford handbook of psychoneuroimmunology*, 2012.
5. American Institute of Stress. Retrieved from *http://www.stress.org.*
6. Chronic stress can damage brain structure and connectivity. Retrieved from *www.psychologytoday.com/blog/the-athletes-way/201402/chronic-stress-can-damage-brain-structure-and-connectivity.*
7. Stress and heart health. Retrieved from *www.heart.org/HEARTORG/Conditions/More/MyHeartandStrokeNews/Stress-and-Heart-Health_UCM_437370_Article.jsp.*
8. Feeling 'worn out'? Your heart may pay the price. Retrieved from *www.medicinenet.com/script/main/art.asp?articlekey=185327.*
9. Stress and migraines. Retrieved from *http://womenshealth.gov/publications/our-publications/fact-sheet/migraine.html.*
10. Feeling stressed? Stress relief might help your health. Retrieved from *http://newsinhealth.nih.gov/issue/Dec2014/Feature1.*
*11. Cohen S, Tyrrell DA, Smith AP: Psychological stress and susceptibility to the common cold, *N Engl J Med* 325:606, 1991. (Classic)
12. Mitchell C: Social disadvantage, genetic sensitivity and children's telomere length, *PNAS* 111:5944, 2014.
13. American Psychological Association: Stress in America: our health at risk. Retrieved from *www.apa.org/news/press/releases/stress.*
14. Lazarus R, Folkman S: *Stress, appraisal, and coping*, New York, 1984, Springer. (Classic)
15. Benson H: *The relaxation response*, New York, 1975, Avon. (Classic)
16. National Center for Complementary and Integrative Health. *https://nccih.nih.gov/health/stress/relaxation.htm.*
17. The power of music to reduce stress. Retrieved from *http://psychcentral.com/lib/the-power-of-music-to-reduce-stress/000930.*

*Evidence-based information for clinical practice.

7

Sleep and Sleep Disorders

Diana Taibi Buchanan

When you have a dream, you've got to grab it and never let go.

Carol Burnett

http://evolve.elsevier.com/Lewis/medsurg/

LEARNING OUTCOMES

1. Define sleep.
2. Describe the stages of sleep.
3. Explain the relationship of various diseases/disorders and sleep disorders.
4. Describe the etiology, clinical manifestations, and interprofessional and nursing management of insomnia.
5. Describe the etiology, clinical manifestations, interprofessional care, and nursing management of obstructive sleep apnea.
6. Describe the etiology, clinical manifestations, and interprofessional and nursing management of periodic limb movement disorder.
7. Describe clinical manifestations and interprofessional management of narcolepsy, parasomnias (including sleepwalking, sleep terrors, and nightmares), and circadian rhythm disorders.
8. Select appropriate strategies for managing sleep problems associated with shift work sleep disorder.

KEY TERMS

circadian rhythms, p. 90
insomnia, p. 91
jet lag disorder, p. 98
narcolepsy, p. 98
obstructive sleep apnea (OSA), p. 96
parasomnias, p. 99
periodic limb movement disorder (PLMD), p. 98
shift work sleep disorder, p. 100
sleep, p. 89
sleep-disordered breathing (SDB), p. 96
sleep disorders, p. 89
sleep disturbance, p. 89
sleep hygiene, p. 93
wake behavior, p. 90

SLEEP

Sleep is a state in which an individual lacks conscious awareness of environmental surroundings but can be easily aroused. Sleep is distinct from unconscious states such as coma, in which the individual cannot be aroused. Sleep is a basic, dynamic, highly organized, and complex behavior that is essential for healthy functioning and survival. Over a life span of 80 years, an individual who sleeps 7 hours each night will spend approximately 24 years sleeping. Sleep influences both behavioral and physiologic functions, including memory, mood, hormone secretion, glucose metabolism, immune function, and body temperature.

Most adults require 7 to 8 hours of sleep within a 24-hour period.[1] Adequate sleep is defined as the amount of sleep one needs to be fully awake and alert the next day. *Insufficient sleep* refers to obtaining less than the recommended amount of sleep. *Fragmented sleep* refers to frequent arousals or actual awakenings that interrupt sleep continuity. *Nonrestorative sleep* refers to sleep that is of adequate duration but does not result in the individual feeling refreshed and alert the next day.

Sleep disturbance is a term used broadly to indicate conditions of poor sleep quality. Sleep disturbance may be related to external factors (e.g., noise, light), health-related factors (e.g., pain), or sleep disorders.

Sleep disorders refer to abnormalities unique to sleep. Sleep disorders discussed in this chapter include insomnia, obstructive sleep apnea syndrome, periodic limb movement disorder, circadian sleep disorders, narcolepsy, and parasomnias.

General sleep disturbances and sleep disorders can result in insufficient sleep. Many people get insufficient sleep because they simply do not allot enough time in bed to get adequate sleep. About 30% of Americans report getting less than 6 hours of sleep per night. An estimated 50 to 70 million people in the United States have a sleep disorder, and many are unaware that they have a problem[2] (Fig. 7-1).

Reviewed by Marylee Bressie, RN, DNP, CCRN, CCNS, CEN, Core Faculty/Nurse Planner, Department of Nursing, School of Public Service Leadership, Capella University, Minneapolis, Minnesota; Dana R. Epstein, RN, PhD, Chief, Nursing Research and Evidence-Based Practice Phoenix VA Health Care System, Phoenix, Arizona; and Teresa J. Seright, RN, PhD, CCRN, Associate Teaching Professor, College of Nursing, Montana State University, Bozeman, Montana.

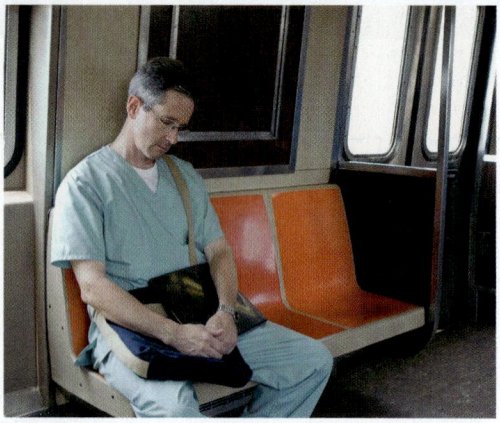

FIG. 7-1 Sleep disorders are common in our society. (©Jupiterimages/Creatas/Thinkstock)

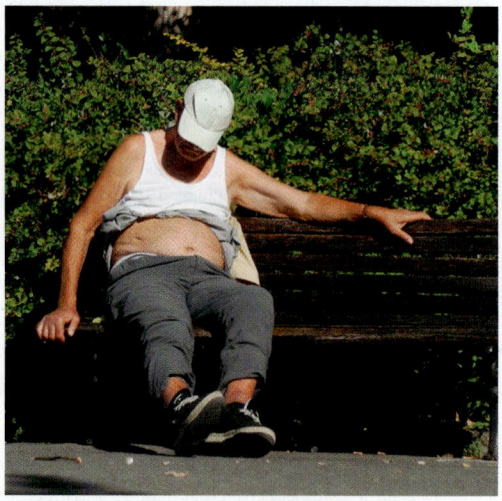

FIG. 7-2 Excessive daytime sleepiness can occur in people with sleep disorders. (©iStockphoto/Thinkstock)

Untreated sleep disorders cause considerable health, safety, and economic consequences. Daytime sleepiness can be so severe that it interferes with work and social functioning (Fig. 7-2). People with chronic illnesses are at the greatest risk for sleep disturbances. Driving while drowsy is related to 100,000 accidents and 1500 traffic fatalities per year.[3] Each year, sleep disorders, sleep loss, and excessive daytime sleepiness cost the United States billions of dollars from the cost of health care, work-related accidents, and lost productivity.[2] Opportunities to address sleep problems are often missed because health care providers (HCPs) do not ask, and patients do not readily talk about them.

PHYSIOLOGIC SLEEP MECHANISMS

Sleep-Wake Cycle

The brain controls the cyclic changes between sleep and waking. Complex networks in the brainstem, hypothalamus, and thalamus interact to regulate the sleep and wake cycle.

Wake Behavior. **Wake behavior** is maintained by an integrated network of arousal systems from the brainstem and forebrain. A cluster of neuronal structures in the middle of the brainstem, called the *reticular activating system (RAS)*, is associated with generalized cortical activation and behavioral arousal. Various neurotransmitters (glutamate, acetylcholine, norepinephrine, dopamine, histamine, serotonin) promote wake behavior.[4]

People with Alzheimer's disease have a loss of cholinergic neurons in the forebrain, which results in sleep disturbances. People with Parkinson's disease have degeneration of dopamine neurons in the substantia nigra, leading to excessive daytime sleepiness. Histamine neurons in the hypothalamus stimulate cortical activation and wake behavior. The sedating properties of many over-the-counter (OTC) medications (e.g., diphenhydramine [Benadryl]) result from inhibiting histamine-related arousal systems.

Orexin (also called hypocretin) is a neuropeptide found in the hypothalamus. Orexin is involved in regulating the sleep-wake cycle and plays a role in keeping people awake.[5,6] Decreased levels of orexin or its receptors lead to difficulties staying awake, which is a syndrome called *narcolepsy*. (Narcolepsy is discussed later in this chapter on pp. 98-99.)

Sleep Behavior. An area in the hypothalamus just above the optic chiasm contains many sleep-promoting neurons. These neurons act to inhibit the RAS and promote sleep.[7] Sleep is stimulated by a variety of sleep-promoting neurotransmitters and peptides, including γ-aminobutyric acid (GABA), galanin, melatonin, adenosine, somatostatin, growth hormone–releasing hormone (GHRH), delta-sleep–inducing peptide, prostaglandins, and proinflammatory cytokines. When a person has an infection, proinflammatory cytokines (interleukin-1, tumor necrosis factor, interleukin-6) mediate symptoms such as sleepiness and lethargy. Peptides, such as cholecystokinin, released by the gastrointestinal tract after food ingestion, may mediate *postprandial sleepiness* (sleepiness after eating).

Melatonin is an endogenous hormone (from the amino acid tryptophan) produced by the pineal gland in the brain. Melatonin secretion is linked to the environmental light-dark cycle and its release signals the time for sleep. Under normal day-night conditions, melatonin is released in the evening as it gets dark. Light exposure at night can suppress melatonin secretion.[7]

Circadian Rhythms. Many biologic rhythms of behavior and physiology fluctuate within a 24-hour period. Because the **circadian** (*circa dian,* about a day) **rhythms** are controlled by internal clock mechanisms, they persist when people are placed in environments free of external time cues. The suprachiasmatic nucleus (SCN) in the hypothalamus is the master clock of the body. The 24-hour cycle of sleep and wake is synchronized to the environmental light and dark periods through specific light detectors in the retina. Pathways from the retina reach the SCN, and pathways from the SCN innervate brain regions controlling wake and sleep behavior.[7]

Light is the strongest time cue for the sleep-wake rhythm. Thus light can be used as a therapy to shift the timing of the sleep-wake rhythm. For example, bright light used early in the morning will cause the sleep-wake rhythm to move to an earlier time; bright light used in the evening will cause the sleep-wake rhythm to move to a later time.

Sleep Architecture

Sleep architecture refers to the pattern of nighttime sleep recorded from physiologic measures of brain waves, eye movements, and muscle tone called *polysomnography* (PSG). Sleep consists of two basic states: *rapid eye movement (REM) sleep* and *non–rapid eye movement (NREM) sleep*. During sleep, the body cycles between NREM and REM sleep. Once asleep, a person goes through four to six NREM and REM sleep cycles, each cycle lasting 60 to 110 minutes.

NREM Sleep. In healthy adults the largest percentage of total sleep time, approximately 75% to 80%, is spent in NREM sleep. NREM sleep is subdivided into three stages:[8]

Stage 1 occurs in the beginning of sleep, with slow eye movements, and is a transition phase from wakefulness to sleep. During this period the person can be easily awakened.

Stage 2 encompasses most of the night's sleep. The heart rate slows down and body temperature drops. This stage is associated with specific electroencephalographic (EEG) wave forms that represent sleep-maintaining neural activity.

Stage 3 is deep sleep or slow-wave sleep (SWS). This stage is associated with large EEG wave forms, called delta waves, which are used as a measure of sleep intensity. SWS sleep declines as people age such that most adults over 60 years of age have little NREM stage 3 sleep.

REM Sleep. REM sleep accounts for 20% to 25% of sleep. REM sleep follows NREM sleep in a sleep cycle. In this stage, brain waves resemble wakefulness and postural muscles are inhibited, leading to greatly reduced skeletal muscle tone. During REM sleep an individual cannot initiate muscle movement (e.g., cannot stand up). REM sleep is the period when the most vivid dreaming occurs.

INSUFFICIENT SLEEP AND SLEEP DISTURBANCES

Insufficient sleep is associated with changes in body function (Fig. 7-3) and health problems (Table 7-1). Impaired cognitive function and impaired performance on simple behavioral tasks occur within 24 hours of sleep loss. The effects of sleep loss are cumulative.

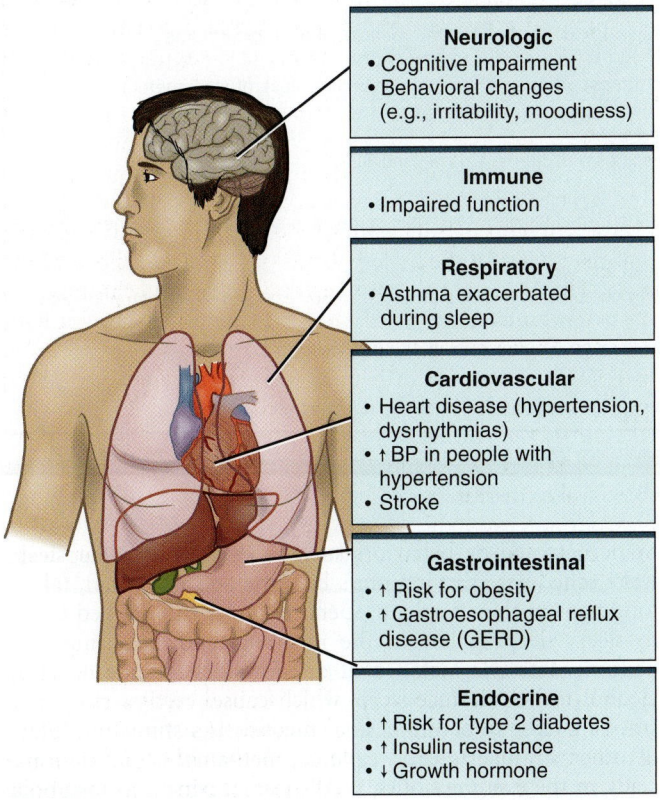

FIG. 7-3 Effects of sleep deprivation and sleep disorders on the body.

Individuals who report less than 6 hours of sleep a night have a higher body mass index (BMI) and are more likely to be obese. The risk for developing glucose intolerance and diabetes is increased in individuals with a history of insufficient sleep. Chronic loss of sleep places older adults at risk for depression, impaired daytime functioning, social isolation, and overall reduction in quality of life. In patients with chronic illnesses, especially cardiovascular disease and stroke, insomnia and sleep-disordered breathing are associated with increased morbidity and mortality.[9]

SLEEP DISTURBANCES IN THE HOSPITAL

Hospitalization, especially in the intensive care unit (ICU), is associated with decreased total sleep time and decreased SWS and REM sleep.[10] Because of the nature of a critical illness and its treatment, some degree of sleep loss may be inevitable for patients in ICUs. Preexisting sleep disorders may be aggravated or triggered in patients who are hospitalized.

In the hospital, environmental sleep-disruptive factors, psychoactive medications, and acute and critical illness all contribute to poor sleep. Patient symptoms, including pain, dyspnea, and nausea, can also contribute to sleep loss in the acutely ill patient. Medications commonly used in acutely and critically ill patients can further contribute to sleep loss. Hospitalized patients are also at risk for poor sleep because of circadian rhythm disruptions.

Hospital and ICU noise (e.g., staff paging system, ventilator alarms, bedside monitors, infusion alarms) and especially staff conversations near patients (e.g., in hallways) during both the day and night disturb sleep. Bright lights during the night also disrupt sleep and reduce melatonin levels. Patient care activities (e.g., dressing changes, blood draws, vital sign monitoring) disrupt sleep. Inactivity, boredom, and certain medications lead to napping during the day and evening that can affect nighttime sleep.

Decreased sleep duration and sleep loss increase the sensitivity and lower the tolerance to pain.[11] Adequate pain management may improve total sleep time, but medications commonly used to relieve pain, especially opioids, alter sleep and place an individual at risk for sleep-disordered breathing.

You have an important role in creating an environment conducive to sleep. This includes the scheduling of medications and procedures, including those performed by unlicensed assistive personnel (UAP). Reducing light and noise levels can promote opportunities for sleep. Hypnotic medications are often available on an as-needed basis.

SLEEP DISORDERS

INSOMNIA

The most common sleep disorder is insomnia, affecting one in three adults. **Insomnia** is characterized by difficulty falling asleep, difficulty staying asleep, waking up too early, or complaints of waking up feeling unrefreshed. The main complaint of people with insomnia is overall dissatisfaction with sleep quality and quantity.

Acute insomnia refers to difficulties falling or remaining asleep at least 3 nights per week for less than a month. *Chronic insomnia* is defined by the same symptoms and a daytime complaint (e.g., fatigue, poor concentration, interference with social

TABLE 7-1 Relationship of Sleep Disturbances to Diseases and Disorders

Disease or Disorder	Sleep Disturbance
Respiratory	
Asthma	• Exacerbated during sleep
Chronic obstructive pulmonary disease (COPD)	• Associated with poor sleep quality, nocturnal oxygen desaturation, and coexisting sleep apnea
Obstructive sleep apnea (OSA)	• Linked with heart disease (hypertension, stroke, heart failure, coronary artery disease, dysrhythmias) • Results in impaired glucose control similar to that which occurs in type 2 diabetes
Renal	
End-stage renal disease (ESRD)	• Disrupted nocturnal sleep with excessive daytime sleepiness • Patients on dialysis have a high incidence of SDB and RLS, which are both significant predictors of mortality in these patients.
Immune Disorders	
Human immunodeficiency virus (HIV)	• Sleep disturbances and fatigue highly prevalent and associated with increased morbidity and mortality
Endocrine	
Diabetes	• Insufficient sleep linked to increased risk for type 2 diabetes • Sleep deprivation in healthy people increases insulin resistance. • Sleep duration and quality are predictors of HbA1C (A1C) levels, an important marker of blood glucose control.
Musculoskeletal	
Arthritis	• Increased rates of RLS and SDB • Disease activity linked to sleep complaints
Fibromyalgia	• Co-morbid insomnia, especially complaint of nonrestorative sleep • Increased rates of PLMD and RLS • Lower levels of sleep-dependent hormones (growth hormone, prolactin)
Systemic exertion intolerance disease (chronic fatigue syndrome)	• Co-morbid insomnia • Increased rates of SDB
Cardiovascular (CV)	
	• People with sleep apnea or sleep disorders are at increased risk for CV disorders, including hypertension, dysrhythmias, and coronary artery disease.
Heart failure (HF)	• Sleep disturbances (insomnia, PLMD, SDB) are common. • Cheyne-Stokes breathing and central apnea are signs of HF exacerbation related to fluid overload.
Hypertension	• Inadequate sleep in people with hypertension can lead to further elevations in BP.
Gastrointestinal	
Obesity	• Association between short sleep duration and excess body weight. Short sleep duration may result in metabolic changes that are linked to obesity. • Higher BMI in people who sleep <6 hours compared with people who sleep >8 hours • Risk factor for SDB
Gastroesophageal reflux disease (GERD)	• Reflux of gastric contents into the esophagus occurs during sleep because of incompetent lower esophageal sphincter. • Swallowing is depressed during sleep.
Chronic liver disease	• Associated with excessive sleepiness, nocturnal arousal, and RLS
Neurologic	
Parkinson's disease	• Associated with difficulty initiating or maintaining sleep, parasomnias, and excessive daytime sleepiness
Alzheimer's disease	• Many have SDB (frequently sleep apnea). • Circadian rhythm alterations with nocturnal wandering, daytime sleepiness, and sleep disruption and awakening
Pain (acute and chronic)	• Decreased quantity and quality of sleep. Poor sleep can intensify pain.
Cancer	• Higher rates of insomnia • Chemotherapy for cancer treatment associated with fragmented sleep and fatigue

Source: National Center on Sleep Disorders and National Heart, Lung, and Blood Institute: National Sleep Disorders Research Plan: section 4, sleep and health. Retrieved from *www.cdc.gov/sleep/about_sleep/chronic_disease.htm.*
BMI, Body mass index; *PLMD,* periodic limb movement disorder; *RLS,* restless legs syndrome; *SDB,* sleep-disordered breathing.

or family activities) that persist for 3 months or longer. Chronic insomnia occurs in 10% to 15% of Americans and is more common in women than men. Insomnia is more common in people who are divorced, widowed, and separated than in those who are married. Insomnia is more prevalent in individuals with low socioeconomic status and less education.[3]

Etiology and Pathophysiology

Behaviors, lifestyle, diet, physical and mental conditions, and medications contribute to insomnia. Insomnia is exacerbated or perpetuated by behaviors such as keeping irregular sleep-wake schedules (varying one's bedtime and rise time), taking long naps in the afternoon, spending more time in bed trying to sleep, sleeping late in the morning, and exercising near bedtime. Lifestyle factors that disrupt sleep include drinking alcohol to help induce sleep, which causes restless sleep, and smoking close to bedtime, since nicotine is a stimulant. Intake of other stimulants (e.g., caffeine, methamphetamine), especially in the evening hours, predisposes a person to insomnia. Insomnia is a common side effect of many medications (e.g., antidepressants, antihypertensives, corticosteroids, psychostimulants, analgesics).

Chronic insomnia often has no known medical or psychologic cause. Often individuals report that the onset occurred after a stressful life event (e.g., loss of loved one). In other cases, the onset of insomnia may be precipitated by psychiatric illnesses, medical conditions, medications, or substance abuse. Patients with psychiatric or medical conditions are more likely to have insomnia than individuals without these conditions. Once chronic insomnia manifests, symptoms are likely to persist over time.

Clinical Manifestations

Manifestations of insomnia include one or more of the following symptoms: (1) difficulty falling asleep *(long sleep latency)*, (2) frequent awakenings *(fragmented sleep)*, (3) prolonged nighttime awakenings or awakening too early and not being able to fall back to sleep *(difficulty maintaining sleep)*, and (4) awakening feeling unrefreshed *(nonrestorative sleep)*. Daytime or functional consequences of insomnia include fatigue, having trouble concentrating at work or school, and having an altered mood. Behavioral manifestations of poor sleep include irritability, sleepiness during the day, forgetfulness, and attention and concentration problems.

Diagnostic Studies

Self-Report. The diagnosis of insomnia is made based on subjective complaints and on an evaluation of a 1- or 2-week sleep diary completed by the patient. A diary or log usually includes the number and times of naps, times of going to bed, awakening and getting up, number of awakenings, as well as overall sleep quality.

In ambulatory care settings the evaluation of insomnia requires a comprehensive sleep history to establish the type of insomnia and to screen for possible psychiatric, medical, or other sleep disorders that would require specific treatment. Questionnaires, such as Pittsburgh Quality Sleep Index, Insomnia Severity Index, and Epworth Daytime Sleepiness, are commonly used to assess sleep quality and negative daytime symptoms related to insomnia.

Actigraphy. *Actigraphy* is a relatively noninvasive method of monitoring rest and activity cycles. An actigraph is a device that measures gross motor activity. It is worn on the wrist like a watch and is about the same size and shape. The unit continuously records the patient's movements, producing data that are downloaded to a computer and analyzed. Activity corresponds to time spent awake, and continuous inactivity corresponds to time spent asleep. Actigraphy is not necessary for diagnosing insomnia, but it is useful for confirming patient's sleep self-reports and monitoring the effects of treatments.

Polysomnography. A polysomnography (PSG) study is not required to establish a diagnosis of insomnia. A PSG study is done only if there are symptoms or signs of another sleep disorder, such as sleep-disordered breathing (discussed later in the chapter). In a PSG study, electrodes simultaneously record physiologic measures that define the main stages of sleep and wakefulness. These measures include (1) muscle tone recorded using an electromyogram (EMG), (2) eye movements recorded with an electro-oculogram (EOG), and (3) brain activity recorded through EEG. To determine additional characteristics of specific sleep disorders, other measures made during PSG include airflow at the nose and mouth, respiratory effort around the chest and abdomen, heart rate, noninvasive oxygen saturation, and EMG of the anterior tibialis muscles (used to detect periodic leg movements). Finally, a patient's gross body movements are monitored continuously by cameras and microphones.

Interprofessional Care

Insomnia treatments are oriented toward symptom management (Table 7-2). A key to management is to change behaviors that perpetuate insomnia. The goal is to (1) prevent acute insomnia from becoming chronic and (2) treat chronic insomnia. An important first step is to provide teaching about sleep along with behavioral strategies. **Sleep hygiene** is a variety of different practices that are important to have normal, quality nighttime sleep and daytime alertness (Table 7-3). Patients often have some familiarity with sleep hygiene principles, but they may still benefit from coaching on how to use these principles effectively.

Cognitive-Behavioral Therapy for Insomnia. Although teaching about sleep hygiene practices is useful, individuals with chronic insomnia require more in-depth *cognitive-behavioral therapy for insomnia (CBT-I)*.[12] CBT-I is based on structured treatment plans that include cognitive and behavioral components.

TABLE 7-2 Interprofessional Care

Insomnia

Diagnostic Assessment

History
- Self-report sleep log or diary
- Sleep assessment (Table 7-5)
- Pittsburgh Sleep Quality Index
- Insomnia Severity Index
- Epworth Sleepiness Scale

Management

Nondrug Therapy
- Sleep hygiene (Table 7-3)
- Cognitive behavioral therapies for insomnia (CBT-I)

Drug Therapy (Table 7-4)
- Benzodiazepines
- Benzodiazepine-receptor–like agents
- Orexin-receptor antagonist
- Melatonin-receptor agonist
- Antidepressants
- Antihistamines

Complementary and Alternative Therapy
- Melatonin

TABLE 7-3 Patient Teaching

Sleep Hygiene

Include the following instructions when teaching a patient who has a sleep disturbance or disorder.
- Do not go to bed unless you are sleepy.
- If you are not asleep after 20 minutes, get out of bed.
- Adopt a regular pattern in terms of bedtime and awakening.
- Begin rituals (e.g., warm bath, light snack, reading) that help you relax each night before bed.
- Get a full night's sleep on a regular basis.
- Make your bedroom quiet, dark, and a little bit cool.
- Do not read, write, eat, watch TV, talk on the phone, or use technologies such as smart phones and tablet computers in bed.
- Avoid caffeine, nicotine, and alcohol at least 4 to 6 hours before bedtime.
- Do not go to bed hungry, but don't eat a big meal near bedtime either.
- Avoid strenuous exercise within 6 hours of your bedtime.
- Avoid sleeping pills, or use them cautiously.
- Practice relaxation techniques (e.g., relaxation breathing) to help you cope with stress in your life (see Chapter 6).

Adapted from American Academy of Sleep Medicine: Healthy sleep habits, 2014. Retrieved from *www.sleepeducation.com/essentials-in-sleep/healthy-sleep-habits.*

The cognitive part of CBT-I may include stress management techniques (e.g., relaxation breathing, imagery) or cognitive strategies to address misconceptions about sleep. The specific approach used varies based on the patient's need. The behavioral part of CBT-I includes instructions to (1) limit the amount of time an individual can stay in bed, (2) maintain a scheduled time to get up in the morning, (3) go to bed only when feeling sleepy, and (4) get out of bed when unable to sleep. CBT-I also includes teaching about sleep hygiene practices (Table 7-3). CBT-I requires individuals to change behavior, which sometimes is difficult.

Although full CBT-I treatment should be delivered by qualified providers with training in this treatment, you can apply many of the principles to help patients. Encourage individuals with insomnia not to watch television or read in bed. Time in bed is limited to the actual time that the individual can sleep. Teach the person with insomnia to avoid naps and consumption of large meals, alcohol, and stimulants, especially a few hours before bedtime. Naps are less likely to affect nighttime sleep if they are limited to 15 to 20 minutes, once per day, and scheduled 7 to 9 hours after morning awakening. Regular exercise may enhance sleep quality but should not be performed within several hours of bedtime.

Drug Therapy. Most medications for insomnia work by producing sleepiness to promote the onset or maintenance of sleep. Medications are generally recommended for short-term treatment of insomnia. Medications that treat insomnia can cause next-day drowsiness and impair driving and other activities that require alertness. People can be impaired even when they feel fully awake. Hypnotic and anxiolytic medications are effective for improving sleep, but the benefits for improving daytime functioning are less certain.

Few studies have evaluated the use of hypnotics for chronic insomnia, and their use in older adults is controversial due to side effects and safety concerns, such as fall risk.[13] Many individuals with insomnia become accustomed to taking OTC or prescription medications to treat insomnia and risk becoming dependent on them, psychologically and physically. *Rebound insomnia* is common with abrupt withdrawal of some hypnotic medications. The daytime fatigue resulting from some medications can negatively influence the patient's efforts to use nondrug approaches.

Classes of medications used to treat insomnia include benzodiazepines, benzodiazepine-receptor agonists, orexin-receptor antagonist, melatonin-receptor agonist, antidepressants, and antihistamines (Table 7-4).

Benzodiazepine Hypnotics. Benzodiazepines such as diazepam (Valium) activate the γ-aminobutyric acid (GABA) receptors to promote sleep. The prolonged half-life of some of these agents (e.g., flurazepam) can result in daytime sleepiness, amnesia, dizziness, and rebound insomnia. Tolerance to these agents develops, and there is a risk for dependence. The use of benzodiazepines should be limited to 2 to 3 weeks. All benzodiazepines have the potential for abuse. In addition, benzodiazepines interact with alcohol and other central nervous system (CNS) depressants. These agents are no longer recommended as first-line therapy for insomnia.

Non-Benzodiazepine Hypnotics. Zolpidem (Ambien), zaleplon (Sonata), and eszopiclone (Lunesta) are the drugs of first choice for insomnia. Because they are benzodiazepine-receptor agonists, they work similarly to benzodiazepines. These drugs are effective and safe for use from 6 months to a year. Food has the potential to delay onset of action and should not be taken with these agents. These agents have short half-lives, making their duration of action short and reducing the risk of daytime sedation. The extended-release formulation of zolpidem (Ambien CR) is used for problems of sleep onset and sleep maintenance. A dissolvable tablet form of zolpidem (Edluar) and an oral spray formulation (ZolpiMist) may be useful for individuals who have difficulty swallowing pills or are on restricted oral fluid intake. Zolpidem tartrate (Intermezzo), a sublingual tablet, is used for patients with insomnia characterized by middle-of-the-night waking followed by difficulty returning to sleep.

TABLE 7-4 Drug Therapy

Insomnia

Benzodiazepines
- Diazepam (Valium)
- Flurazepam
- Lorazepam (Ativan)
- Quazepam
- Triazolam (Halcion)

Benzodiazepine-Receptor–Like Agents
- Zolpidem (Ambien, Ambien CR, Intermezzo, Edluar, ZolpiMist)
- Zaleplon (Sonata)
- Eszopiclone (Lunesta)

Orexin-Receptor Antagonist
- Suvorexant (Belsomra)

Melatonin-Receptor Agonist
- Ramelteon (Rozerem)

Antidepressants
- Amitriptyline
- Doxepin
- Trazodone

Antihistamines
- Diphenhydramine
- Doxylamine (Unisom)

Orexin-Receptor Antagonist. Suvorexant (Belsomra) is the first approved orexin-receptor antagonist. It promotes sleep by blocking the effects of orexin. (Orexin is discussed on p. 90 earlier in this chapter.) Suvorexant should be taken no more than once per night, within 30 minutes of going to bed, with at least 7 hours remaining before the planned time of waking. The most common side effect is drowsiness.

Melatonin-Receptor Agonist. Ramelteon (Rozerem) is a melatonin-receptor agonist. It has a rapid onset that is effective for sleep onset but a short duration of action. Ramelteon does not cause tolerance, but the drug is not always effective in improving sleep quality. Ramelteon is used for insomnia with sleep onset difficulty, not for sleep maintenance problems.

Antidepressants. Certain atypical and tricyclic antidepressants are used as sleep aids due to their side effects of sedation. Trazodone, an atypical antidepressant, is one of the most common agents prescribed to treat insomnia, especially in older adults. The insomnia dose of antidepressants such as trazodone is much lower than the antidepressant dose. The administration of this drug to older adults is controversial. Daytime sleepiness is a common side effect. Tolerance can develop within a few weeks. Doxepin and amitriptyline are tricyclic antidepressants that may be used to treat insomnia. Doxepin improves sleep without next-day drowsiness in older and middle-aged adults with chronic primary insomnia.[14]

Antihistamines. Many individuals with insomnia self-medicate with OTC sleep aids. Most OTC agents include diphenhydramine or doxylamine (Unisom). These drugs may also be constituents of "nighttime" pain medicines. Antihistamine agents are less effective than benzodiazepines, and tolerance develops quickly. In addition, antihistamines have anticholinergic side effects, including daytime sleepiness, impaired cognitive function, blurred vision, urinary retention, constipation, and risk of increased intraocular pressure. Agents with diphenhydramine are not intended for long-term use and should not be used by older adults.[15]

Complementary and Alternative Therapy. Many types of complementary and alternative therapies are used as sleep aids. As noted earlier in the chapter, melatonin is a hormone produced by the pineal gland (Complementary & Alternative Therapies box on below). Melatonin is effective for improving sleep disturbance associated with jet lag. It also helps night shift workers sleep during the daytime.[16] However, melatonin is not considered effective for improving nighttime sleep. Valerian is a herb that has been used for many years as a sleep aid and to relieve anxiety. Although valerian is safe, it is not effective in treating insomnia.[17] Additional sleep aids include white noise devices or relaxation strategies.

COMPLEMENTARY & ALTERNATIVE THERAPIES

Melatonin

Scientific Evidence

Overall, the scientific evidence suggests the benefits of melatonin in people who take it for jet lag. The majority of scientific evidence suggests that it may decrease the time it takes to fall asleep (sleep latency).

Nursing Implications

- Regarded as safe in recommended doses for short-term use
- Avoid in patients using warfarin (Coumadin).
- Avoid in patients using central nervous system depressants.
- May cause a drop in BP. Caution is advised in patients taking drugs that may also lower BP.

Source: Based on a systematic review of scientific literature. Retrieved from *www.naturalstandard.com.*

NURSING MANAGEMENT: INSOMNIA

Nursing Assessment

As a nurse, you are in a key position to assess sleep problems in patients and their caregivers. Sleep assessment is important in helping patients identify personal habits and environmental factors that contribute to poor sleep. Family caregivers may experience sleep disruptions due to the necessity of providing care to patients in the home. These sleep disruptions can increase the burden of caregiving.

Self-report and objective data are used to assess sleep duration and quality. Many patients do not tell their HCP about their sleep problems. Make sure to ask patients about their sleep and problems with sleep. A sleep history includes characteristics of sleep such as sleep duration, the pattern of sleep, and daytime alertness (Table 7-5). Before using any questionnaire, assess the patient's cognitive function, reading level (if a paper form is used), and language ability. Also assess the diet. Question the patient about the intake of caffeine. Ask about alcohol consumption and whether it is used as a sleep aid. Although the sedative effects of alcohol hasten sleep onset, it suppresses REM sleep and increases awakenings later in the night.

Ask the patient about sleep aids. This includes OTC and prescription medications. Note the drug dose, frequency of use, and any side effects (e.g., daytime drowsiness, dry mouth). Many individuals also consume herbal or dietary supplements that they believe will improve sleep. Common supplements include valerian, melatonin, hops, lavender, passion flower, kava, and skullcap. Inform the patient that many of these products are sold as dietary supplements and do not have U.S. Food and Drug Administration (FDA) approval or regulatory oversight. The exact components and concentrations of herbs and supplements often are unknown, and patients may experience adverse effects. Certain agents such as kava are associated with liver toxicity.

TABLE 7-5 Nursing Assessment

Sleep

Use the following questions to do an initial assessment regarding sleep.

1. What time do you normally go to bed at night? What time do you normally wake up in the morning?
2. Do you often have trouble falling asleep at night?
3. About how many times do you wake up at night?
4. If you do wake up during the night, do you usually have trouble falling back asleep?
5. Does your bed partner say or are you aware that you frequently snore, gasp for air, or stop breathing?
6. Does your bed partner say or are you aware that you kick or thrash about while asleep?
7. Are you aware that you ever walk, eat, punch, kick, or scream during sleep?
8. Are you sleepy or tired during much of the day?
9. Do you usually take one or more naps during the day?
10. Do you usually doze off without planning to during the day?
11. How much sleep do you need to feel alert and function well?
12. Are you currently taking any type of medication or other preparation to help you sleep?

Source: Bloom HG, Ahmed I, Alessi CA, et al: Evidence-based recommendations for the assessment and management of sleep disorders in older people, *J Am Geriatr Soc* 57:761, 2009.

Encourage individuals to keep a sleep diary for 1 to 2 weeks. In the diary have them record when they go to sleep, when they wake up, and how long they were awake during the night. The number and duration of naps should also be recorded.

The patient's medical history can also provide important information about factors that contribute to poor sleep. For example, a man with benign prostatic hyperplasia may report frequent awakenings during the night for voiding. Psychiatric problems (e.g., depression, anxiety, posttraumatic stress disorder [PTSD], drug abuse) are associated with sleep disturbances. Sleep disturbances often develop as a consequence or complication of a chronic or terminal condition (e.g., heart disease, dementia, cancer). Painful conditions such as arthritis may also contribute to nighttime awakenings.

Ask about work schedules and cross-country and international travel. Shift work contributes to reduced or poor-quality sleep. Work-related behaviors resulting from poor sleep may include poor performance, decreased productivity, and job absenteeism.

Nursing Diagnoses

Nursing diagnoses related to sleep include insomnia, sleep deprivation, disturbed sleep pattern, and readiness for enhanced sleep.

Nursing Implementation

Nursing interventions depend on the severity and duration of the sleep problem, as well as individual characteristics. Optimally, healthy adults should have 7 to 8 hours of sleep a night. Occasional difficulty getting to sleep or awakening during the night is not unusual. However, sleep disturbances longer than 1 month are problematic.

Although teaching about sleep hygiene practices (Table 7-3) is beneficial, individuals with chronic insomnia require more in-depth intervention using CBT-I strategies. An important component of sleep hygiene is reducing dietary intake of substances containing caffeine (Table 7-6). Caffeine has a half-life of about 6 hours, and possibly as long as 9 hours in older adults. Consuming caffeinated beverages after 12 noon should be avoided.

Suggest and implement changes in home and institutional environments to enhance sleep. Reducing light and noise levels enhances sleep. Awareness of time passing and watching the clock adds to anxieties about not falling asleep or returning to sleep. Keeping the bedroom dark and cool is conducive to good sleep.

Teach patients about sleeping medications. With the benzodiazepines, non-benzodiazepine hypnotics, and melatonin-receptor agonists, teach the patient to take the drug right before bedtime, be prepared to get a full night's sleep of at least 6 to 8 hours, and do not plan activities the next morning that require highly skilled psychomotor coordination. Advise patients not to take these medications with high-fat food (delays absorption), alcohol, or other CNS depressants. Patient follow-up regarding medications is important. Ask about daytime sleepiness, nightmares, and any difficulties in activities of daily living.

TABLE 7-6 Caffeine Content of Foods and Beverages*

Food or Beverage	Caffeine (mg)
Coffee, brewed (8 oz)	95-200
Coffee, instant (8 oz)	27-173
Coffee, decaffeinated	2-12
Tea, leaf or bag (8 oz)	14-70
Celestial Seasoning herbal tea, all varieties	0
Diet Coke (12 oz)	23-47
Coca-Cola (12 oz)	23-35
Dr. Pepper (12 oz)	36-42
Pepsi-Cola (12 oz)	32-39
Diet Pepsi-Cola (12 oz)	27-37
7-Up, Sprite, or Diet 7-Up (12 oz)	0
A&W Root Beer (12 oz)	0
Red Bull (12 oz)	75-80
Mountain Dew (12 oz)	42-55
Ben & Jerry's no-fat coffee fudge frozen yogurt (1 cup)	85
Dannon coffee yogurt (8 oz)	45
Hershey's special dark chocolate bar (1.5 oz)	31
Hershey bar (milk chocolate)	10
Hot chocolate (8 oz)	5

*List only includes selected foods and beverages.

OBSTRUCTIVE SLEEP APNEA

The term **sleep-disordered breathing (SDB)** indicates abnormal respiratory patterns associated with sleep. These include snoring, apnea (temporary cessation of respiration), and hypopnea (temporary restriction of respiration without full cessation) with increased respiratory effort leading to frequent arousals. SDB results in frequent sleep disruptions and alterations in sleep architecture. Obstructive sleep apnea is the most commonly diagnosed SDB problem.

Obstructive sleep apnea (OSA), also called *obstructive sleep apnea–hypopnea syndrome* (OSAHS), is characterized by partial or complete upper airway obstruction during sleep. *Apnea* is the cessation of respiratory airflow (90% or greater reduction) lasting longer than 10 seconds. *Hypopnea* is a condition characterized by shallow respirations (30% to 90% reduction in airflow).[8] Airflow obstruction in OSA occurs because of (1) narrowing of the air passages with relaxation of muscle tone during sleep and/or (2) the tongue and soft palate falling backward to partially or completely obstruct the pharynx (Fig. 7-4). Each obstruction may last from 10 to 90 seconds. During the apneic period the patient can experience *hypoxemia* (decreased PaO_2 or SpO_2) and *hypercapnia* (increased $PaCO_2$). These changes are ventilatory stimulants and cause brief arousals, but the patient may not fully awaken.

The patient has a generalized startle response, snorts, and gasps, which cause the tongue and soft palate to move forward and the airway to open. Apnea and arousal cycles occur repeatedly throughout the night. Apneic episodes occur most often during REM sleep, when airway muscle tone is lowest.

There is no single cause for OSA, but rather the condition is related to multiple factors that influence airway patency and the tone of airway musculature. Risk factors include obesity (BMI greater than 30 kg/m^2), age greater than 65 years, neck circumference greater than 17 inches, craniofacial abnormalities that affect the upper airway, and acromegaly (a pituitary disorder discussed in Chapter 49). Smokers are more likely to have OSA. OSA is more common in men than in women until after menopause, when the prevalence of the disorder is equal.[18] Women with OSA have higher mortality rates than men with OSA. OSA patients with excessive daytime sleepiness have increased mortality.

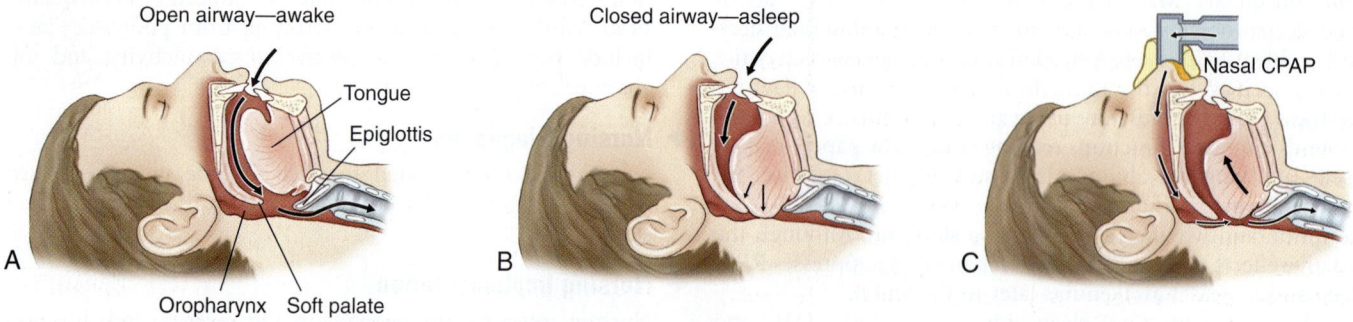

FIG. 7-4 How sleep apnea occurs. **A,** The patient predisposed to obstructive sleep apnea (OSA) has a small pharyngeal airway. **B,** During sleep, the pharyngeal muscles relax, allowing the airway to close. Lack of airflow results in repeated apneic episodes. **C,** Continuous positive airway pressure *(CPAP)* splints the airway open, preventing airflow obstruction. (Modified from LaFleur Brooks M: *Exploring medical language: a student-directed approach,* ed 8, St Louis, 2012, Mosby.)

INFORMATICS IN PRACTICE

Sleep Apnea Diagnosis and Monitoring

- Home respiratory monitoring is a cost-effective alternative for diagnosing sleep-related breathing disorders that allows patients the convenience of sleeping in their own home.
- Home respiratory monitoring is used as part of a comprehensive sleep evaluation and in patients likely to have moderate to severe obstructive sleep apnea but without heart failure, obstructive lung disease, or neuromuscular disease.
- Home respiratory monitoring is used to monitor the effectiveness of non-CPAP therapies for patients with sleep-related breathing disorders.
- Wireless monitors can detect changes in vital signs and pulse oximetry, raising an alarm if values fall outside of set parameters.
- Your patient may benefit from telehealth to diagnose and monitor for sleep apnea in the home.

CPAP, Continuous positive airway pressure.

Clinical Manifestations

Clinical manifestations of sleep apnea include frequent arousals during sleep, insomnia, excessive daytime sleepiness, and witnessed apneic episodes. The patient's bed partner may complain about the patient's loud snoring. Other symptoms include morning headaches (from hypercapnia or increased BP that causes vasodilation of cerebral blood vessels), personality changes, and irritability.

A major risk of OSA is cardiovascular complications. Apnea during sleep causes hypoxia, nocturnal arousals, and increased pressure in the thoracic cavity. These events can lead to negative physiologic consequences, including overactivation of the sympathetic nervous system, increased vascular resistance, and reduced oxygenation of the cardiac muscle. Long-term effects include hypertension, cardiac dysrhythmias, arteriosclerosis, heart failure, and cardiovascular-related mortality.[9]

Chronic sleep loss predisposes the person to diminished ability to concentrate, impaired memory, failure to accomplish daily tasks, and interpersonal difficulties. Men may experience impotence. Hypercapnia and arousals contribute to daytime sleepiness in people with OSA. Driving accidents may occur due to excessive daytime sleepiness. Family life and the patient's ability to maintain employment are often compromised. As a result, the patient may experience depression. Cessation of breathing reported by the bed partner is usually a source of great anxiety because of the fear that breathing may not resume.

Diagnostic Studies

Assessment of the patient with OSA includes a thorough sleep and medical history. A common questionnaire used to screen for OSA is the STOP-BANG questionnaire,[18] which assesses for clinical manifestations highly suspicious of OSA.

Typically, OSA is diagnosed by PSG done in a clinical sleep laboratory. The patient's chest and abdominal movement, oral and nasal airflow, SpO_2, ocular movement, and heart rate and rhythm are monitored. In some instances, portable sleep studies are conducted in the home setting. Overnight pulse oximetry assessment may be done to determine whether nocturnal oxygen supplementation is indicated.

A diagnosis of sleep apnea requires documentation of apneic events or hypopneas of at least 10 seconds' duration. OSA is defined as more than 5 apnea/hypopnea events per hour accompanied by a 3% to 4% decrease in oxygen saturation. Severe apnea can be associated with apneic events of more than 30 to 50 per hour of sleep.[8]

❖ NURSING AND INTERPROFESSIONAL MANAGEMENT: SLEEP APNEA

◆ Conservative Treatment

Mild sleep apnea (5 to 10 apnea/hypopnea events per hour) may respond to simple measures. Conservative treatment at home begins with sleeping on one's side rather than on the back (called *positional therapy*), which reduces the effects of gravity on the airway. Elevating the head of the bed may eliminate OSA in some patients.

Medications that relax airway muscle tone often make OSA worse. Instruct the patient to avoid taking sedatives or consuming alcoholic beverages for 3 to 4 hours before sleep. Sleep medications often make OSA worse. Excessive weight worsens sleep apnea as the pressure of adipose tissue in the neck and on the chest restricts ventilation. Referral to a weight loss program may be indicated. Bariatric surgery may also reduce OSA.[19] Instruct the patient on the dangers of driving or using heavy equipment due to the profound sleepiness that is common in people with OSA. Insomnia is common in people with OSA, and they may need additional specific treatment for the insomnia (such as CBT-I).

Symptoms may resolve in up to half of patients with OSA who use a special mouth guard, also called an oral appliance, during sleep to prevent airflow obstruction. Oral appliances bring the mandible and tongue forward to enlarge the airway space, thereby preventing airway occlusion.[19] Some individuals find a support group beneficial, where they can express concerns and feelings and discuss strategies for resolving problems.

In patients with more severe symptoms (>15 apnea/hypopnea events/hour), *continuous positive airway pressure (CPAP)* by mask is the treatment of choice. With CPAP, the patient applies a nasal mask that is attached to a high-flow blower (Fig. 7-5). The blower is adjusted to maintain sufficient positive pressure (5 to 25 cm H_2O) in the airway during inspiration and expiration to prevent airway collapse.

Some patients cannot adjust to wearing a mask over the nose or mouth or to exhaling against the high pressure. A technologically more sophisticated therapy, bilevel positive airway pressure (BiPAP), can deliver a higher inspiration pressure and a lower

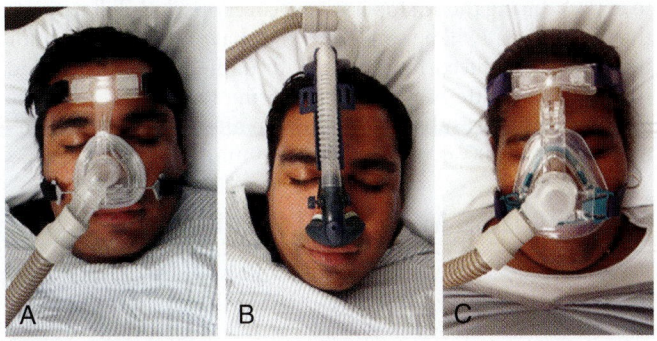

FIG. 7-5 Examples of positive airway pressure devices for sleep apnea. **A,** Patient wearing a nasal mask and headgear (positive pressure only through nose). **B,** Patient wearing nasal pillows (positive pressure only through nose). **C,** Patient wearing a full face mask (positive pressure to nose and mouth). (From Goldman L, Schafer AI: *Goldman's Cecil medicine,* ed 24, Philadelphia, 2012, Saunders.)

pressure during expiration. With BiPAP, the apnea can be relieved with a lower mean pressure and may be better tolerated.

CPAP reduces apnea episodes, daytime sleepiness, and fatigue. It improves quality of life ratings and returns cognitive functioning to normal. Although CPAP is a highly effective treatment, patients have problems with adherence to using it on a daily basis.[19] Approximately two thirds of patients using CPAP report side effects such as nasal stuffiness.

First assess the patient's knowledge about OSA and CPAP, and involve the bed partner in teaching. Evaluate the patient for nasal resistance. To ensure successful adherence to CPAP treatment, patients need to be involved in the selection of the mask and device before the start of therapy.

When patients with a history of OSA are hospitalized, be aware that the administration of opioid analgesics and sedating medications (benzodiazepines, barbiturates, hypnotics) may worsen OSA symptoms by depressing respiration.[20] This will necessitate that the patient wear the CPAP or BiPAP when resting or sleeping. Many patients are able to use their own CPAP equipment, but hospital policy should be checked to be certain it can be used. Check with the HCP in charge of the patient's care to determine if a patient who uses home CPAP should continue this therapy in the hospital. If CPAP is ordered, you can encourage and assist with the patient's use of this therapy.

◆ Surgical Treatment

If other measures fail, OSA can be managed surgically. The goal of OSA surgery is to reduce collapsibility and increase patency of the upper airway, including oral, nasal, and pharyngeal passages. The two most common procedures are uvulopalatopharyngoplasty (UPPP or UP3) and genioglossal advancement and hyoid myotomy (GAHM). UPPP involves excision of the tonsillar pillars, uvula, and posterior soft palate to remove the obstructing tissue. GAHM involves advancing the attachment of the muscular part of the tongue on the mandible. When GAHM is performed, UPPP is generally done as well. Depending on the site of the obstruction, symptoms are relieved in up to 80% of patients. Radiofrequency ablation (RFA) of obstructive tissues alone or in combination with other surgical techniques is also used. RFA is the least invasive surgical intervention.

After surgery, complications of airway obstruction or hemorrhage occur most often in the immediate postoperative period. Patients can usually be discharged home within 1 day after the procedure. Before going home, teach the patient what to expect during the postoperative recovery period. Tell patients that their throat will be sore. They may have a foul breath odor that may be reduced by rinsing with diluted mouthwash and then salt water after several days. Snoring may persist until the inflammation has subsided. Follow-up after surgery is important. A repeat PSG is performed 3 to 4 months after surgery.

PERIODIC LIMB MOVEMENT DISORDER

Periodic limb movement disorder (PLMD) is characterized by *periodic limb movements in sleep* (PLMS): involuntary, repetitive movement of the limbs that affects people only during sleep.[21] PLMD usually involves the legs and rarely involves the arms. Sometimes abdominal, oral, and nasal movement accompanies PLMD. Movements typically occur for 0.5 to 10 seconds, in intervals separated by 5 to 90 seconds. PLMD causes poor-quality sleep and excessive daytime sleepiness. The causes of PLMD are not fully understood, but iron deficiency and dopamine dysfunction in the CNS have been implicated.[21]

PLMS can occur with medical disorders (e.g., sleep apnea, narcolepsy) and certain medications. For a diagnosis of PLMD, the occurrence of PLMS must not be due to another disorder. PLMS affects many individuals with restless legs syndrome (RLS). (RLS is a disorder that is discussed in Chapter 58.)

PLMD is diagnosed using a detailed history from the patient and/or bed partner and doing PSG. PLMD is treated by medications aimed at reducing or eliminating the limb movements or the arousals. Clonazepam (Klonopin) (a benzodiazepine) is used to treat PLMD, although it likely helps patients by improving sleep quality rather than reducing limb movements. Other medications shown to be effective are valproic acid (Depakene), an antiseizure drug that reduces muscle activity, and selegiline (Eldepryl), a dopaminergic agent. Dopamine agonists (pramipexole [Mirapex] and ropinirole [Requip]) are recommended for RLS, but there is little research on their efficacy for PLMD. However, in common practice these drugs are prescribed to treat PLMD.

CIRCADIAN RHYTHM DISORDERS

Circadian rhythm disorders can occur when the circadian time-keeping system loses synchrony with the environment. Lack of synchrony between the circadian time-keeping system and environment disrupts the sleep-wake cycle and affects the patient's ability to have quality sleep. The two common symptoms are insomnia and excessive sleepiness. Jet lag disorder and shift work sleep disorder (see Special Sleep Needs of Nurses section on p. 100) are the most common types of circadian rhythm disorders.[16]

Jet lag disorder occurs when a person travels across multiple time zones. One's body time is not synchronized with environmental time. Most individuals crossing at least three time zones experience jet lag. The number of time zones crossed affects the severity of symptoms and the time it takes to recover. Resynchronization of the body's clock occurs at a rate of about 1 hr/day when traveling eastward and 1.5 hr/day when traveling westward. Melatonin and exposure to daylight help to synchronize the body's rhythm.

Several strategies may help to reduce the risk of developing jet lag. Before travel the individual can start to get in harmony with the time schedule of the destination. When time at destination is brief (i.e., 2 days or less), keeping home-based sleep hours rather than adopting destination sleep hours may reduce sleepiness and jet lag symptoms.

NARCOLEPSY

Narcolepsy is a chronic neurologic disorder caused by the brain's inability to regulate sleep-wake cycles normally. At various times throughout the day, people with narcolepsy experience uncontrollable urges to sleep. Patients with narcolepsy often go directly into REM sleep from wakefulness.[21] This does not occur in normal sleep and is a unique feature of narcolepsy. Patients with narcolepsy also experience fragmented and disturbed nighttime sleep. There are two types of narcolepsy: with cataplexy (type 1) and without cataplexy (type 2).[21] Cataplexy is a brief and sudden loss of skeletal muscle tone. It can manifest as a brief episode of muscle weakness or complete postural collapse and falling. Laughter, anger, or surprise often triggers episodes.

In both genders the onset of narcolepsy typically occurs in adolescence or early in the third decade. Head trauma, a sudden change in sleep-wake habits, and infection may trigger the onset of narcolepsy symptoms. The cause of narcolepsy remains unknown. It is associated with destruction of neurons that produce orexin. The resulting deficiency of orexin causes instability of wake and transitions from wake to sleep that occur unpredictably. The loss of neurons may be due to an autoimmune process.

Narcolepsy is diagnosed based on a history of sleepiness, PSG, and daytime *multiple sleep latency tests* (MSLTs).[21] For the MSLT, patients undergo an overnight PSG evaluation followed by four or five naps scheduled every 2 hours during the next day. Short sleep latencies and onset of REM sleep in more than two MSLTs are diagnostic signs of narcolepsy.

Narcolepsy cannot be cured. Management of narcolepsy is focused on symptom management (Table 7-3). Provide teaching about sleep and sleep hygiene. Advise the patient with narcolepsy to take three or more short (15-minute) naps throughout the day and to avoid large or heavy meals and alcohol. You can play a key role in ensuring patient safety by teaching safety behaviors and encouraging adherence to the prescribed medication regimen. Safety precautions, especially when driving, are critically important for patients with narcolepsy. The behavioral therapies for insomnia (discussed earlier in this chapter) are also used to address the sleep disturbances. Stimulants are used to counter daytime sleepiness.

Modafinil (Provigil), a nonamphetamine wake-promotion drug, is considered a first-line drug therapy. Sodium oxybate (Xyrem), a metabolite of GABA, is another wake-promoting medication that is used. High doses of selective serotonin reuptake inhibitors (SSRIs) (e.g., fluoxetine [Prozac], venlafaxine) may be prescribed for the management of cataplexy.

PARASOMNIAS

Parasomnias are unusual and often undesirable behaviors that occur while falling asleep, transitioning between sleep stages, or arousing from sleep.[21] They are due to CNS activation and often involve complex behaviors. The parasomnia is generally goal directed, although the person is not aware or conscious of the act. Parasomnias may result in fragmented sleep and fatigue.

Sleepwalking and sleep terrors are arousal parasomnias that occur during NREM sleep. *Sleepwalking* behaviors can range from sitting up in bed, moving objects, and walking around the room to driving a car. During a sleepwalking event the individual may not speak and may have limited or no awareness of the event. On awakening, the individual does not remember the event. In the ICU, a parasomnia may be misinterpreted as ICU psychosis. Sedated ICU patients can exhibit manifestations of a parasomnia.

Sleep terrors (night terrors) are characterized by a sudden awakening from sleep along with a loud cry and signs of panic. The person has marked increases in heart rate and respiration and diaphoresis. Factors in the ICU such as sleep disruption and deprivation, fever, stress, and exposure to noise and light can contribute to sleep terrors.

Nightmares are a parasomnia characterized by recurrent awakening with recall of a frightful or disturbing dream. These normally occur during REM sleep during the final third of sleep. In critically ill patients nightmares are common and are most likely due to medications. Drug classes most likely to cause nightmares are sedative-hypnotics, β-adrenergic antagonists, dopamine agonists, and amphetamines.

Gerontologic Considerations: Sleep

Older age is associated with overall shorter total sleep time, decreased sleep efficiency, and more awakenings (Fig. 7-6). A common misconception is that older people need less sleep than younger people. In fact, the amount of sleep needed as a person ages remains relatively constant. Other sleep disorders (e.g., sleep-disordered breathing) also increase with age and may manifest with symptoms of insomnia.[22]

Multiple factors impair older adults' ability to obtain quality sleep. Insomnia symptoms in older adults frequently occur with depression, cardiovascular disease, pain, and cognitive problems. Chronic conditions that are more common in older adults (COPD, diabetes, dementia, chronic pain, cancer) can affect sleep quality.[22] Medications used to treat these conditions can contribute to sleep problems. OTC medications also can lead to sleep disturbance. Cough and cold medications, especially those containing pseudoephedrine; caffeine-containing drugs; and drugs containing nicotine (e.g., nicotine gum, transdermal patches), are stimulants.

Awakening and getting out of bed during the night (e.g., to use the bathroom) increase the risk for falls. Older adults may use OTC medications or alcohol as a sleep aid. This practice can further increase the risk of falls at night. Chronic disturbed sleep in older adults can result in disorientation, delirium, impaired intellect, disturbed cognition, and increased risk of accidents and injury.

Because older adults may attribute their disturbed sleep to normal aging, they may fail to report symptoms of sleep disorders to their HCPs.[22] Use a sleeping assessment (Table 7-5) to detect sleep disturbances in older adults.

Sleep medications should be used with great caution in older adults. Diphenhydramine, alone or in combination with other drugs, is sedating with anticholinergic effects. Any OTC medication labeled "PM" probably has diphenhydramine and should be used cautiously by older adults. Metabolism of most hypnotic drugs decreases with aging. Older adults have increased sensitivity to hypnotic and sedative medications. Thus drug therapies for sleep disturbances are started at lower doses and monitored carefully. Whenever possible, long-acting benzodiazepines should be avoided. Older adults receiving

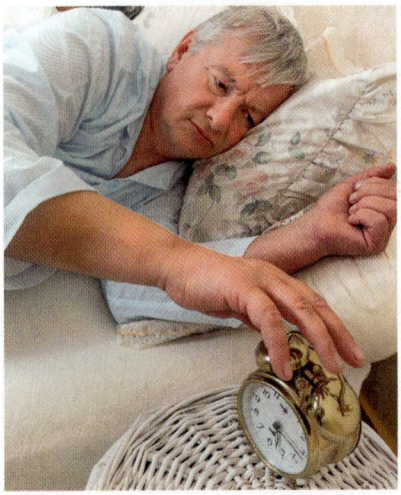

FIG. 7-6 Many older people have sleep problems. (©Studio-Annika/iStock/Thinkstock)

benzodiazepines are at increased risk of daytime sedation, falls, and cognitive and psychomotor impairment.

❖ SPECIAL SLEEP NEEDS OF NURSES

Nursing is one of several professions that necessitates night shift and rotating shift schedules. In many settings, nurses are asked to or volunteer to work a variety of day and night shifts, often alternating and rotating them. Unfortunately, nurses who do shift work often report less job satisfaction and more job-related stress.[23] There is a higher incidence of driving errors in nurses doing shift work, especially those who work rotating shifts.[24]

Nurses on permanent night or rapidly rotating shifts are at increased risk of experiencing **shift work sleep disorder**, which is characterized by insomnia, sleepiness, and fatigue. Nurses on rotating shifts get the least amount of sleep. With repeated periods of inadequate sleep, the sleep debt grows. Chronic fatigue in nurses doing shift work poses challenges for the individual nurse's health and for patient safety.[23]

Shift work alters the synchrony between circadian rhythms and the environment, leading to sleep disruption. Nurses working the night shift are often too sleepy to be fully alert at work and too alert to sleep soundly the next day. Sustained alterations in circadian rhythms such as those imposed by rotating shift work have been linked to increased morbidity and mortality risks associated with cardiovascular problems. In addition, mood disorders such as anxiety are higher in nurses who work rotating shifts.

From a safety perspective, disturbed sleep and subsequent fatigue can result in errors and accidents for nurses as well as for their patients. Fatigue diminishes or distorts perceptual skills, judgment, and decision-making capabilities. Lack of sleep reduces the ability to cope and handle stress and may result in physical, mental, and emotional exhaustion.

The problem of sleep disruption is critically important to nursing. Several strategies may help reduce the distress associated with rotating shift work. These include brief periods of on-site napping. Maintaining a consistent sleep-wake schedule even on days off is optimum but perhaps unrealistic. For night shift work, scheduling the sleep period just before going to work increases alertness and vigilance, improves reaction times, and decreases accidents during night shift work. Nurses who have control over their work schedules appear to experience less sleep disruption than those whose schedule is imposed. As a nurse, you need to manage the impact of sleep disruption through the use of sleep hygiene practices.

CASE STUDY

Insomnia

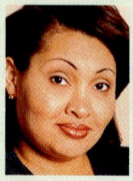

(©JackF/ iStock/ Thinkstock)

Patient Profile

G.P., a 49-year-old African American woman, is seen in the primary care clinic for complaints of chronic fatigue and disturbed sleep. She is postmenopausal based on self-report. In the past year, since the end of her periods, she has experienced daily hot flashes and sleep problems. She denies any other health problems. On a usual workday she drinks two cups of hot tea in the morning and one can of diet cola in the late afternoon. Currently she is taking OTC diphenhydramine for sleep. Her partner, who has accompanied her to the clinic, states that her snoring has gotten worse, and it is interfering with his sleep.

Subjective Data

- Reports hot flashes and nighttime sweating
- Reports daytime tiredness and fatigue
- States she has trouble getting to sleep and staying asleep

Objective Data

Physical Examination

- Laboratory evaluations within normal limits
- Height 5′6″
- Weight 180 lb

Diagnostic Studies

- Nighttime PSG study reveals episodes of obstructive sleep apnea

Interprofessional Care

- CPAP nightly
- Referred for weight reduction counseling
- Education about sleep hygiene

Discussion Questions

1. What are G.P.'s risk factors for sleep apnea?
2. How does CPAP work?
3. Based on the data above, what are the major health risks for G.P. from sleep apnea?
4. ***Patient-Centered Care:*** What specific sleep hygiene practices could G.P. use to improve the quality of her sleep?
5. ***Priority Decision:*** Based on your assessment of G.P., what are the priority nursing interventions for her?
6. ***Teamwork and Collaboration:*** For the interventions that you identified in the above question, which of the following personnel could be responsible for implementing them: RN, LPN, unlicensed assistive personnel (UAP)?
7. ***Priority Decision:*** Based on the assessment data provided, what are the priority nursing diagnoses?
8. ***Teamwork and Collaboration:*** What referrals may be indicated for G.P.?

Answers available at *http://evolve.elsevier.com/Lewis/medsurg.*

BRIDGE TO NCLEX EXAMINATION

The number of the question corresponds to the same-numbered outcome at the beginning of the chapter.

1. Sleep is *best* described as a
   - **a.** loosely organized state similar to coma.
   - **b.** state in which pain sensitivity decreases.
   - **c.** quiet state in which there is little brain activity.
   - **d.** state in which an individual lacks conscious awareness of the environment.
2. Which statement(s) is/are true regarding rapid eye movement (REM) sleep (*select all that apply*)?
   - **a.** The EEG pattern is quiescent.
   - **b.** Muscle tone is greatly reduced.
   - **c.** It occurs only once in the night.
   - **d.** It is separated by distinct physiologic stages.
   - **e.** The most vivid dreaming occurs during this phase.

3. Insufficient sleep is associated with *(select all that apply)*
   a. increased body mass index.
   b. increased insulin resistance.
   c. impaired cognitive functioning.
   d. increased immune responsiveness.
   e. increased daytime body temperature.
4. When teaching the patient with primary insomnia about sleep hygiene, the nurse should emphasize
   a. the importance of daytime naps.
   b. the need to exercise before bedtime.
   c. the need for long-term use of hypnotics.
   d. avoiding caffeine-containing beverages 6-9 hours before bedtime.
5. While caring for a patient with a history of narcolepsy with cataplexy, the nurse can delegate which activity to the unlicensed assistive personnel (UAP)?
   a. Teaching about the timing of medications
   b. Walking the patient to and from the bathroom
   c. Developing a plan of care with a family member
   d. Planning an appropriate diet that avoids caffeine-containing foods
6. An overweight patient with sleep apnea would like to avoid using a nasal CPAP device if possible. To help him reach this goal, the nurse suggests that the patient
   a. lose excess weight.
   b. take a nap during the day.
   c. eat a high-protein snack at bedtime.
   d. use mild sedatives or alcohol at bedtime.
7. A patient on the surgical unit has a history of parasomnia (sleepwalking). What statement describes parasomnia?
   a. Hypnotic medications reduce the risk of sleepwalking.
   b. The patient is often unaware of the activity on awakening.
   c. The patient should be restrained at night to prevent personal harm.
   d. The potential for sleepwalking is reduced by exercise before sleep.
8. Strategies to reduce sleepiness during nighttime working include
   a. exercising before work.
   b. taking melatonin before working the night shift.
   c. sleeping for at least 2 hours immediately before work time.
   d. walking for 10 minutes every 4 hours during the night shift.

1. d, 2. b, e, 3. a, b, c, 4. d, 5. b, 6. a, 7. b, 8. c.

For rationales to these answers and even more NCLEX review questions, visit *http://evolve.elsevier.com/Lewis/medsurg.*

EVOLVE WEBSITE

http://evolve.elsevier.com/Lewis/medsurg

Review Questions (Online Only)
Key Points
Answer Keys for Questions
- Rationales for Bridge to NCLEX Examination Questions
- Answer Guidelines for Case Study on p. 100

Conceptual Care Map Creator
Audio Glossary
Content Updates

REFERENCES

1. National Heart, Lung, and Blood Institute: *How much sleep is enough?* Retrieved from *www.nhlbi.nih.gov/health/health-topics/topics/sdd/howmuch.html.*
2. Centers for Disease Control and Prevention: *Insufficient sleep is a public health epidemic.* Retrieved from *www.cdc.gov/features/dssleep/index.html#References.*
3. National Sleep Foundation: *Facts and stats.* Retrieved from *http://drowsydriving.org/about/facts-and-stats.*
4. Monti JM: The neurotransmitters of sleep and wake, a physiological reviews series, *Sleep Med Rev* 17:313, 2013.
5. de Lecea L, Huerta R: Hypocretin (orexin) regulation of sleep-to-wake transitions, *Front Pharmacol* 5:1, 2014.
6. National Sleep Foundation: *Orexin receptor antagonists: a new class of sleeping pill.* Retrieved from *http://sleepfoundation.org/sleep-news/orexin-receptor-antagonists-new-class-sleeping-pill.*
7. LeGates TA, Fernandez DC, Hattar S: Light as a central modulator of circadian rhythms, sleep and affect, *Nat Rev Neurosci* 15:443, 2014.
8. Iber C, Ancoli-Israel S, Chesson A, et al: *The American Academy of Sleep Medicine: The AASM manual for the scoring of sleep and associated events: rules, terminology and technical specifications*, 2007, Westchester, Ill.
9. Stopford E, Ravi K, Nayar V: The association of sleep disordered breathing with heart failure and other cardiovascular conditions, *Cardiol Res Pract* 2013:356280 (ISSN: 2090-8016), 2013.
10. Nesbitt L, Goode D: Nurses perceptions of sleep in the intensive care unit environment: a literature review, *Intensive Crit Care Nurs* 30:231, 2014.
11. Finan PH, Goodin BR, Smith MT: The association of sleep and pain: an update and a path forward, *J Pain* 14:1539, 2013.
12. Williams J, Roth A, Vatthauer K, et al: Cognitive behavioral treatment of insomnia, *Chest* 143:554, 2013.

*13. Tannenbaum C, Paquette A, Hilmer S, et al: A systematic review of amnestic and non-amnestic mild cognitive impairment induced by anticholinergic, antihistamine, GABAergic and opioid drugs, *Drugs Aging* 29:639, 2012.

*14. Yeung WF, Chung KF, Yung KP, et al: Doxepin for insomnia: a systematic review of randomized placebo-controlled trials, *Sleep Med Rev* 19:75, 2015.

15. Zisapel N: Drugs for insomnia, *Expert Opin Emerg Drugs* 17:299, 2012.
16. Zee PC, Attarian H, Videnovic A: Circadian rhythm abnormalities, *Continuum (Minneap Minn)* 19:132, 2013.

*17. Taibi DM, Landis CA, Petry H, et al: A systematic review of valerian as a sleep aid: safe but not effective, *Sleep Med Rev* 11:209, 2007.

*18. Chung F, Subramanyam R, Liao P, et al: High STOP-BANG score indicates a high probability of obstructive sleep apnoea, *Br J Anaesth* 108:768, 2012.

19. Freedman N: Improvements in current treatments and emerging therapies for adult obstructive sleep apnea, *F1000 Prime Rep* 6:1, 2014.
20. Ward CW: Safe use of opioids in individuals with obstructive sleep apnea, *Pain Manag Nurs* 16 (3):411, 2015.
21. American Academy of Sleep Medicine: *International classification of sleep disorders*, Darien, Ill, 2014, American Academy of Sleep Medicine.
22. Gooneratne NS, Vitiello MV: Sleep in older adults: normative changes, sleep disorders, and treatment options, *Clin Geriatr Med* 30:591, 2014.

*23. Matheson A, O'Brien L, Reid JA: The impact of shiftwork on health: a literature review, *J Clin Nurs* 23:3309, 2014.

*24. Ftouni S, Sletten TL, Howard M, et al: Objective and subjective measures of sleepiness, and their associations with on-road driving events in shift workers, *J Sleep Res* 22:58, 2013.

*Evidence-based information for clinical practice.

8

Pain

Rosemary C. Polomano, Mechele Fillman

It's not the load that breaks you down, it's the way you carry it.

Lou Holtz

http://evolve.elsevier.com/Lewis/medsurg/

LEARNING OUTCOMES

1. Define pain.
2. Describe the neural mechanisms of pain and pain modulation.
3. Differentiate between nociceptive and neuropathic types of pain.
4. Explain the physical and psychologic effects of unrelieved pain.
5. Interpret the subjective and objective data that are obtained from a comprehensive pain assessment.
6. Describe effective interprofessional pain management techniques.
7. Describe drug and nondrug methods of pain relief.
8. Explain your role and responsibility in pain management.
9. Discuss ethical and legal issues related to pain and pain management.
10. Evaluate the influence of one's own knowledge, beliefs, and attitudes about pain assessment and management.

KEY TERMS

analgesic ceiling, p. 111
breakthrough pain (BTP), p. 108
central sensitization, p. 105
complex regional pain syndrome (CRPS), p. 107
equianalgesic dose, p. 117
modulation, p. 106
multimodal analgesia, p. 110
neuropathic pain, p. 106
nociception, p. 103
nociceptive pain, p. 104
pain, p. 102
patient-controlled analgesia (PCA), p. 120
patient-controlled epidural analgesia (PCEA), p. 120
peripheral sensitization, p. 104
transduction, p. 103
transmission, p. 104
trigger point, p. 121

Pain is a complex, multidimensional experience that can cause suffering and decreased quality of life. Pain is one of the major reasons that people seek health care. To effectively assess and manage patients with pain, you need to understand the physiologic and psychosocial dimensions of pain. This chapter presents evidence-based information to help you assess and safely manage pain in collaboration with other interprofessional team members.

MAGNITUDE OF PAIN PROBLEM

Millions of people suffer from pain. Annually in the United States, at least 25 million people experience acute pain as a result of injury or surgery. Common chronic pain conditions such as arthritis, migraine headache, and back pain affect more than 1 million American adults.[1] Of the approximately 1.7 million people diagnosed with cancer each year, about 60% experience pain during treatment.[2] Despite the high prevalence and costs of acute and chronic pain, inadequate pain management occurs. Consequences of unrelieved acute pain are presented in Table 8-1.

DEFINITIONS AND DIMENSIONS OF PAIN

In 1968 Margo McCaffery, a nurse and pioneer in pain management, defined **pain** as "whatever the person experiencing the pain says it is, existing whenever the person says it does."[3] The International Association for the Study of Pain (IASP) defines *pain* as "an unpleasant sensory and emotional experience associated with actual or potential tissue damage, or described in terms of such damage."[1]

These definitions emphasize the subjective nature of pain, in which the patient's self-report is the most valid means of assessment. Although understanding the patient's experience and relying on his or her self-report is essential, this view is problematic for many patients. For example, patients who are comatose or who suffer from dementia, patients who are mentally disabled or challenged, and patients with expressive aphasia

Reviewed by Marylee Bressie, RN, DNP, CCRN, CCNS, CEN, Core Faculty/Nurse Planner, Department of Nursing, School of Public Service Leadership, Capella University, Minneapolis, Minnesota; Debra B. Gordon, RN-BC, DNP, ACNS-BC, FAAN, Co-Director, Harborview Integrated Pain Care Program, Department of Anesthesiology and Pain Medicine, University of Washington, Seattle, Washington; and Elsa Wuhrman, DNP, RN-BC, FNP, BC, DCC, Nurse Practitioner and Assistant Professor of Nursing, Department of Anesthesiology/Acute Pain Services, Columbia University Medical Center, New York, New York.

TABLE 8-1 Negative Consequences of Unrelieved Acute Pain

Response	Possible Consequences
Endocrine and Metabolic	
↑ Adrenocorticotropic hormone (ACTH)	Weight loss (from ↑ catabolism)
↑ Cortisol	↑ Respiratory rate
↑ Antidiuretic hormone (ADH)	↑ Heart rate
↑ Epinephrine and norepinephrine	Shock
↑ Renin, ↑ aldosterone	Glucose intolerance
↓ Insulin	Hyperglycemia
Gluconeogenesis	Fluid overload
Glycogenolysis	Hypertension
Muscle protein catabolism	Urinary retention, ↓ urine output
Cardiovascular	
↑ Heart rate	Hypertension
↑ Cardiac output	Unstable angina
↑ Peripheral vascular resistance	Myocardial infarction
↑ Myocardial oxygen consumption	Deep vein thrombosis
↑ Coagulation	
Respiratory	
↓ Tidal volume	Atelectasis
Hypoxemia	Pneumonia
↓ Cough, sputum retention	
Renal and Urologic	
↓ Urine output	Fluid imbalance
Urinary retention	Electrolyte disturbance
Gastrointestinal	
↓ Gastric and intestinal motility	Constipation
	Anorexia
	Paralytic ileus
Musculoskeletal	
Muscle spasm	Immobility
Impaired muscle function	Weakness and fatigue
Neurologic	
Impaired cognitive function	Confusion
	Impaired ability to think, reason, and make decisions
Immunologic	
↓ Immune response	Infection

TABLE 8-2 Dimensions of Pain

Dimension	Description
Physiologic	• Genetic, anatomic, and physical determinants of pain influence how painful stimuli are processed, recognized, and described.
Affective	• Emotional responses to pain include anger, fear, depression, and anxiety. • Negative emotions impair patient's quality of life.
Cognitive	• Beliefs, attitudes, memories, and meaning attributed to pain influence the ways in which a person responds to pain.
Behavioral	• Observable actions (e.g., grimacing, irritability, coping skills) are used to express or control pain. • People unable to communicate may have behavioral changes (e.g., agitation, combativeness).
Sociocultural	• Age and gender influence nociceptive processes and responses to opioids. • Families and caregivers influence patient's response to pain through their beliefs, behaviors, and support. • Culture affects pain expression, medication use, and pain-related beliefs and coping methods.

GENDER DIFFERENCES

Pain

Men

- Men are less likely to report pain than women.
- Men report more control over pain.
- Men are less likely than women to use alternative treatments for pain.

Women

- Women more frequently experience migraine headache, back pain, arthritis, fibromyalgia, irritable bowel syndrome, neuropathic pain, abdominal pain, and foot ache.
- Women are more likely to be diagnosed with a nonspecific, somatic disorder and less likely to receive analgesics for symptoms of chest and abdominal pain.

have varying abilities to report pain. In these instances, you must incorporate nonverbal information such as observed behaviors into your pain assessment.

The emotional distress of pain can cause *suffering*, which is the state of distress associated with loss. Suffering can result in a sense of insecurity, lack of control, and spiritual distress. It is important to assess the ways in which a person's spirituality influences and is influenced by pain.[4]

The meaning of the pain to the person is important. For example, a woman in labor may experience severe pain but can manage it without analgesics because for her it is associated with a joyful event. Moreover, she may feel control over her pain because of the training she received in prenatal classes and the knowledge that the pain is time-limited. In contrast, a woman with chronic, undefined musculoskeletal pain may be stressed by thoughts that her pain is "not real," is uncontrollable, or is caused by her own actions. Perceptions influence the ways in which a person responds to pain and must be incorporated into a comprehensive treatment plan.

Some people cope with pain by distracting themselves, whereas others convince themselves that the pain is permanent, untreatable, and overwhelming. People who believe that their pain is uncontrollable and overwhelming are more likely to have poor outcomes.[5] The biopsychosocial model of pain includes the physiologic, affective, cognitive, behavioral, and sociocultural dimensions of pain (Table 8-2).

Families and caregivers influence the patient's response to pain through their beliefs and behaviors. For example, families may discourage the patient from taking opioids because they have preconceived notions and fears that the patient may become addicted. Understanding these beliefs helps you address them through patient and family teaching.

Pain Mechanisms

Nociception is the physiologic process by which information about tissue damage is communicated to the central nervous system (CNS). It involves four processes: (1) transduction, (2) transmission, (3) perception, and (4) modulation (Fig. 8-1).

Transduction. **Transduction** involves the conversion of a noxious mechanical, thermal, or chemical stimulus into an electrical signal called an action potential. Noxious (tissue-damaging) stimuli, including thermal (e.g., sunburn), mechanical (e.g.,

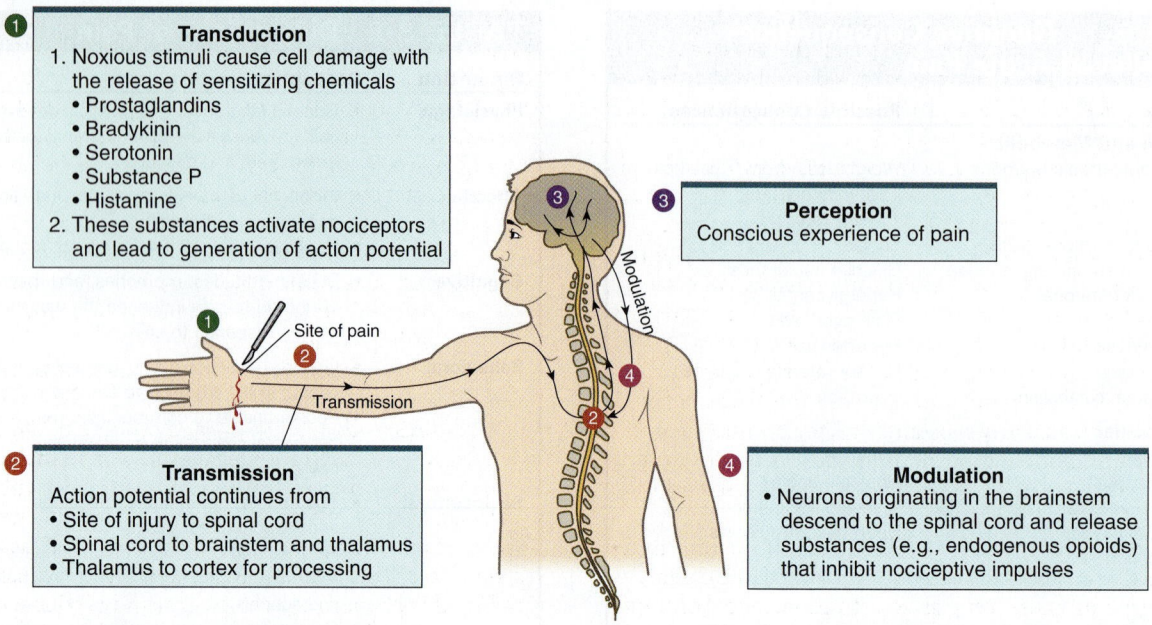

FIG. 8-1 Nociceptive pain originates when the tissue is injured. *1,* Transduction occurs when there is release of chemical mediators. *2,* Transmission involves the conduct of the action potential from the periphery (injury site) to the spinal cord and then to the brainstem, thalamus, and cerebral cortex. *3,* Perception is the conscious awareness of pain. *4,* Modulation involves signals from the brain going back down the spinal cord to modify incoming impulses. (Developed by McCaffery M, Pasero C, Paice JA. Modified from McCaffery M, Pasero C: *Pain: clinical manual,* ed 2, St Louis, 1999, Mosby.)

surgical incision), or chemical (e.g., toxic substances) stimuli, cause the release of numerous chemicals such as substance P and adenosine triphosphate (ATP) into the damaged tissues. Other chemicals are released from mast cells (e.g., serotonin, histamine, prostaglandins) and macrophages (e.g., cytokines). These chemicals activate nociceptors, which are specialized receptors, or free nerve endings, that respond to painful stimuli. Activation of nociceptors results in an action potential that is carried from the nociceptors to the spinal cord primarily via small, rapidly conducting, myelinated A-delta fibers and slowly conducting unmyelinated C fibers.

In addition to stimulating nociceptors, inflammation and the subsequent release of chemical mediators lower nociceptor thresholds. As a result, nociceptors may fire in response to stimuli that previously were insufficient to elicit a response. They may also fire in response to non-noxious stimuli, such as light touch. This increased susceptibility to nociceptor activation is called **peripheral sensitization**. Leukotrienes, prostaglandins, cytokines, and substance P are involved in peripheral sensitization. Cyclooxygenase (COX), produced in the inflammatory response, also plays an important role in peripheral sensitization. A clinical example of this process is sunburn. This thermal injury causes inflammation that results in a sensation of pain when the affected skin is lightly touched. Peripheral sensitization amplifies signal transmission, which in turn contributes to central sensitization (discussed under Dorsal Horn Processing). The pain produced from activation of peripheral nociceptors is called **nociceptive pain** (described later in the chapter on p. 106).

Therapies that alter either the local environment or sensitivity of the peripheral nociceptors can prevent transduction and initiation of an action potential. Decreasing the effects of chemicals released at the periphery is the basis of several drug approaches to pain relief. For example, nonsteroidal antiinflammatory drugs (NSAIDs), such as ibuprofen (Advil), exert their analgesic effects by blocking the action of COX (see Fig. 11-2).

Transmission. **Transmission** is the process by which pain signals are relayed from the periphery to the spinal cord and then to the brain. Nerves that carry pain impulses from the periphery to the spinal cord are called *primary afferent fibers.* These include A-delta and C fibers, each of which is responsible for a different pain sensation. As previously mentioned, A-delta fibers conduct pain rapidly and are responsible for the initial, sharp pain that accompanies tissue injury. C fibers transmit painful stimuli more slowly and produce pain that is typically aching or throbbing. Primary afferent fibers terminate in the dorsal horn of the spinal cord. Activity in the dorsal horn integrates and modulates pain inputs from the periphery.

The propagation of pain impulses from the site of transduction to the brain is shown in Fig. 8-1. Three segments are involved in nociceptive signal transmission: (1) transmission along the peripheral nerve fibers to the spinal cord, (2) dorsal horn processing, and (3) transmission to the thalamus and cerebral cortex.

Drugs that stabilize the neuronal membrane act on peripheral sodium channels to inhibit propagation of nerve impulses. These medications include local anesthetics (e.g., injectable or topical lidocaine, bupivacaine [Sensorcaine]) and antiseizure drugs (e.g., gabapentin [Neurontin]).

Transmission to Spinal Cord. The *first-order neuron* extends the entire distance from the periphery to the dorsal horn with no synapses. For example, an afferent fiber from the great toe travels from the toe through the fifth lumbar nerve root into the spinal cord; it is one cell. Once generated, an action potential travels all the way to the spinal cord unless it is blocked by a sodium channel inhibitor (e.g., local anesthetic) or disrupted by a lesion such as a dorsal root entry zone lesion.

The manner in which nerve fibers enter the spinal cord is central to the notion of spinal dermatomes. *Dermatomes* are areas on the skin that are innervated primarily by a single spinal cord segment. The distinctive pattern of the rash caused by herpes zoster (shingles) across the back and trunk is determined by dermatomes (see Fig. 23-7). Different dermatomes and their innervations are illustrated in Fig. 55-7.

Dorsal Horn Processing. Once a nociceptive signal arrives in the spinal cord, it is processed within the dorsal horn. Neurotransmitters released from the afferent fiber bind to receptors on nearby cells. Some of these neurotransmitters (e.g., glutamate, substance P) produce activation, whereas others (e.g., γ-aminobutyric acid [GABA], serotonin) inhibit activation of nearby cells. In this area, exogenous and endogenous opioids (e.g., encephalin, β-endorphin) also play an important role by binding to opioid receptors and blocking the release of neurotransmitters, particularly substance P. They produce analgesic effects similar to those of exogenous opioids such as morphine. The neurons that project to the thalamus are called *second-order neurons.*

Increased sensitivity and hyperexcitability of neurons in the CNS is called **central sensitization**. Peripheral tissue damage or nerve injury can cause central sensitization, and continued nociceptive input from the periphery maintains it (Fig. 8-2). As a result of the increased excitability of CNS neurons, normal sensory inputs cause abnormal sensing and responses to painful and other stimuli. This explains why some people experience significant pain from touch or tactile stimulation in and around the areas of tissue or nerve injury. This is called *allodynia,* pain from a stimulus that is not typically painful. It also explains why some people experience *hyperalgesia,* an exaggerated or increased pain response to noxious stimuli.

With central sensitization, the central processing circuits are altered. In some cases, central sensitization can be long lasting due to multiple changes that occur in the periphery and CNS.[6]

With ongoing stimulation of slowly conducting unmyelinated C-fiber nociceptors, firing of specialized dorsal horn neurons gradually increases. These inputs can lead to the sprouting of wide dynamic range (WDR) neuron dendrites and the induction of glutamate-dependent *N*-methyl-D-aspartate (NMDA) receptors. This results in an increased capacity to transmit a broader range of stimuli-producing signals, which are then passed up the spinal cord and to the brain. This process is known as *windup.*[7]

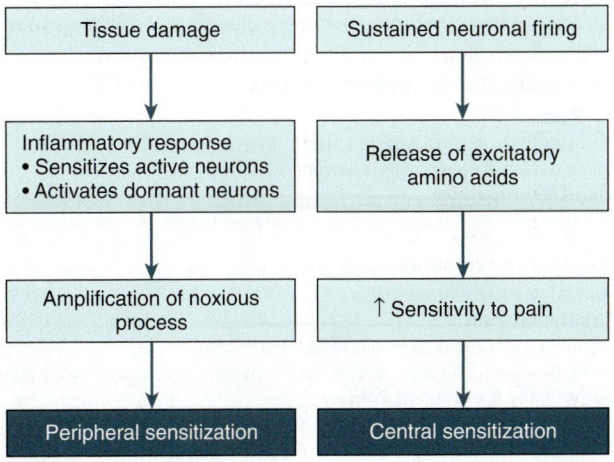

FIG. 8-2 Sequence of mechanisms leading to peripheral and central sensitization. Increased susceptibility to nociceptor activation is called *peripheral sensitization.* Increased sensitivity and hyperexcitability of neurons in the CNS is called *central sensitization.*

Activation of NMDA receptors also plays a role in windup. NMDA receptor antagonists, such as ketamine (Ketalar), potentially interrupt or block mechanisms that lead to or sustain central sensitization. Windup is like central sensitization and hyperalgesia in that it occurs in response to C-fiber inputs. Windup is different, however, in that it can be short lasting, whereas central sensitization and hyperalgesia persist over time.

It is important for you to understand that acute, unrelieved pain leads to chronic pain through central sensitization. Even brief intervals of acute pain are capable of inducing long-term neuronal remodeling and sensitization *(plasticity),* chronic pain, and lasting psychologic distress.

Neuroplasticity refers to processes that allow neurons in the brain to compensate for injury and adjust their responses to new situations or changes in their environment.[8] Neuroplasticity contributes to adaptive mechanisms for reducing pain but also can result in maladaptive mechanisms that enhance pain sensitivity. Genetic variability among individuals may play an important role in changes that occur in the CNS as well as the response to different analgesic therapies to treat pain.[9] Understanding this phenomenon helps explain individual differences in response to pain and why some patients develop chronic pain conditions, whereas others do not.[10]

Referred pain must be considered when interpreting the location of pain reported by the person with an injury or a disease involving visceral organs. The location of a stimulus may be distant from the pain location reported by the patient (Fig. 8-3). For example, pain from liver disease is frequently located in the right upper abdominal quadrant but can also be referred to the anterior and posterior neck region, shoulder area, and posterior flank area. If referred pain is not considered when evaluating a pain location report, diagnostic tests and therapy could be misdirected.

Transmission to Thalamus and Cortex. From the dorsal horn, nociceptive stimuli are communicated to the *third-order neuron,* primarily in the thalamus. Fibers of dorsal horn projection cells enter the brain through several pathways, including the spinothalamic tract and spinoreticular tract. Distinct thalamic nuclei

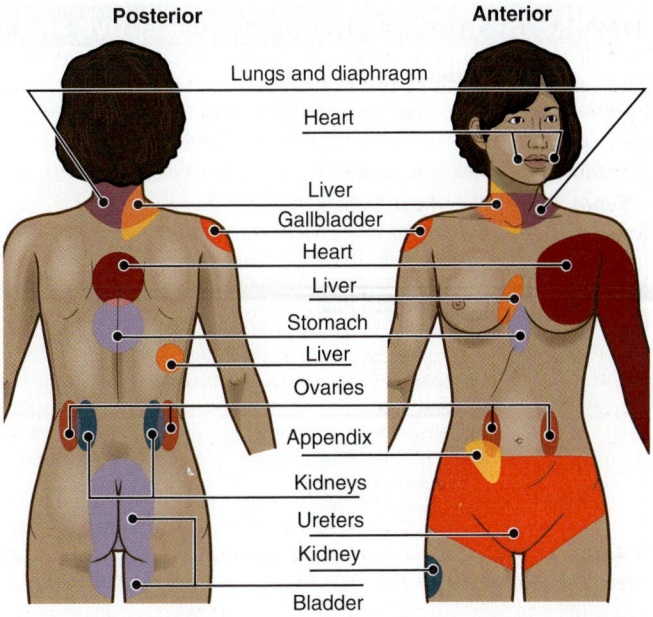

FIG. 8-3 Typical areas of referred pain.

receive nociceptive input from the spinal cord and have projections to several regions in the cerebral cortex, where the perception of pain is presumed to occur.

Therapeutic approaches that target pain transmission include opioid analgesics that bind to opioid receptors on primary afferent and dorsal horn neurons. These agents mimic the inhibitory effects of endogenous opioids. Another medication, baclofen (Lioresal), inhibits pain transmission by binding to GABA receptors, thus mimicking the inhibitory effects of GABA.

Perception. *Perception* occurs when pain is recognized, defined, and assigned meaning by the individual experiencing the pain. In the brain, nociceptive input is perceived as pain. There is no single, precise location where pain perception occurs. Instead, pain perception involves several brain structures. For example, it is believed that the reticular activating system is responsible for warning the individual to attend to the pain stimulus; the somatosensory system is responsible for localization and characterization of pain; and the limbic system is responsible for the emotional and behavioral responses to pain. Cortical structures also are crucial to constructing the meaning of the pain.

Therefore behavioral strategies such as distraction and relaxation are effective pain-reducing therapies for many people. Meditation and imagery also affect pain perception. By directing attention away from the pain sensation, patients can reduce the sensory and affective components of pain.

Modulation. Modulation involves the activation of descending pathways that exert inhibitory or facilitatory effects on the transmission of pain (Fig. 8-1). Depending on the type and degree of modulation, nociceptive stimuli may or may not be perceived as pain. Modulation of pain signals can occur at the level of the periphery, spinal cord, brainstem, and cerebral cortex. Descending modulatory fibers release chemicals such as serotonin, norepinephrine, GABA, and endogenous opioids that can inhibit pain transmission.

Several antidepressants exert their effects through the modulatory systems. For example, tricyclic antidepressants (e.g., amitriptyline [Elavil]) and serotonin norepinephrine reuptake inhibitors (SNRIs) (e.g., venlafaxine [Effexor]) are used in the management of chronic noncancer and cancer pain. These agents interfere with the reuptake of serotonin and norepinephrine, thereby increasing their availability to inhibit noxious stimuli.

CLASSIFICATION OF PAIN

Pain can be categorized in several ways. Most commonly, pain is categorized as nociceptive or neuropathic based on underlying pathology (Table 8-3). Another useful scheme is to classify pain as acute or chronic (Table 8-4).

Nociceptive Pain

Nociceptive pain is caused by damage to somatic or visceral tissue. *Somatic pain* often is further categorized as superficial or deep. *Superficial pain* arises from skin, mucous membranes, and subcutaneous tissues. It is often described as sharp, burning, or prickly. *Deep pain* is often characterized as aching or throbbing and originates in bone, joint, muscle, skin, or connective tissue.

Visceral pain comes from the activation of nociceptors in the internal organs and lining of the body cavities such as the thoracic and abdominal cavities. Visceral nociceptors respond to inflammation, stretching, and ischemia. Stretching of hollow viscera in the intestines and bladder that occurs from tumor involvement or obstruction can produce intense cramping pain. Examples of visceral nociceptive pain include pain from a surgical incision, pancreatitis, and inflammatory bowel disease.

Neuropathic Pain

Neuropathic pain is caused by damage to peripheral nerves or structures in the CNS. While neuropathic pain is commonly associated with diabetic neuropathy and other neuropathic pain syndromes, approximately 8% of the general population has pain with neuropathic characteristics.[10] Typically described as numbing, hot, burning, shooting, stabbing, sharp, or electric shock–like, neuropathic pain can be sudden, intense, short lived, or lingering. Paroxysmal firing of injured nerves is

TABLE 8-3 Comparison of Nociceptive and Neuropathic Pain

	Nociceptive Pain	Neuropathic Pain*
Definition	Normal processing of stimulus that damages normal tissue or has the potential to do so if prolonged	Abnormal processing of sensory input by the peripheral or central nervous system
Treatment	Usually responsive to nonopioid and/or opioid drugs	Treatment usually includes adjuvant analgesics.
Types	**Superficial Somatic Pain** Pain arising from skin, mucous membranes, subcutaneous tissue. Tends to be well localized *Examples:* sunburn, skin contusions **Deep Somatic Pain** Pain arising from muscles, fasciae, bones, tendons. Localized or diffuse and radiating *Examples:* arthritis, tendonitis, myofascial pain **Visceral Pain** Pain arising from visceral organs, such as the GI tract and bladder. Well or poorly localized. Often referred to cutaneous sites *Examples:* appendicitis, pancreatitis, cancer affecting internal organs, irritable bowel and bladder syndromes	**Central Pain** Caused by primary lesion or dysfunction in the CNS *Examples:* poststroke pain, pain associated with multiple sclerosis **Peripheral Neuropathies** Pain felt along the distribution of one or many peripheral nerves caused by damage to the nerve *Examples:* diabetic neuropathy, alcohol-nutritional neuropathy, trigeminal neuralgia, postherpetic neuralgia **Deafferentation Pain** Pain resulting from a loss of or altered afferent input *Examples:* phantom limb pain, postmastectomy pain, spinal cord injury pain **Sympathetically Maintained Pain** Pain that persists secondary to sympathetic nervous system activity *Examples:* phantom limb pain, complex regional pain syndrome

Adapted from National Institute of Neurological Disorders and Stroke: Complex regional pain syndrome fact sheet. Retrieved from *www.ninds.nih.gov/disorders/reflex_sympathetic_dystrophy/detail_reflex_sympathetic_dystrophy.htm.*

CNS, Central nervous system; *GI,* gastrointestinal.

*Note: Some types of neuropathic pain (e.g., postherpetic neuralgia) are caused by more than one neuropathologic mechanism.

TABLE 8-4 Differences Between Acute and Chronic Pain

	Acute Pain	Chronic Pain
Onset	Sudden	Gradual or sudden
Duration	<3 mo or as long as it takes for normal healing to occur	>3 mo. May start as acute injury or event but continues past the normal time for recovery
Severity	Mild to severe	Mild to severe
Cause of pain	Generally can identify a precipitating event (e.g., illness, surgery)	May not be known. Original cause of pain may differ from mechanisms that maintain the pain.
Course of pain	Decreases over time and goes away as recovery occurs	Typically pain does not go away. Characterized by periods of increasing and decreasing pain
Typical physical and behavioral manifestations	Manifestations vary but can reflect sympathetic nervous system activation: • ↑ Heart rate, respiratory rate, BP • Diaphoresis, pallor • Anxiety, agitation, confusion • Urine retention	Predominantly behavioral manifestations: • Flat affect • ↓ Physical activity • Fatigue • Withdrawal from social interaction
Usual goals of treatment	Pain control with ability to participate in recovery activities Minimize side effects of treatment	Pain control to the extent possible. Focus on enhancing function and quality of life.

responsible for shooting and electric shock–like sensations. Common causes of neuropathic pain include trauma, inflammation, metabolic diseases (e.g., diabetes mellitus), alcoholism, infections of the nervous system (e.g., herpes zoster, human immunodeficiency virus), tumors, toxins, and neurologic diseases (e.g., multiple sclerosis). Examples of neuropathic pain conditions include phantom limb sensation, diabetic neuropathy, and trigeminal neuralgia. No single sign or symptom is diagnostic for neuropathic pain.

Deafferentation pain results from loss of or altered afferent input secondary to either peripheral nerve injury (e.g., amputation) or CNS damage, including a spinal cord injury. *Sympathetically maintained pain* is associated with dysregulation of the autonomic nervous system, and *central pain* is caused by CNS lesions or dysfunction. Painful peripheral polyneuropathies (pain felt along the distribution of multiple peripheral nerves) and painful mononeuropathies (pain felt along the distribution of a damaged nerve) arise from damage to peripheral nerves and generate pain that may be described as burning, paroxysmal, or shock-like. The patient may have associated positive or negative motor and sensory signs, including numbness, allodynia, or change in reflexes and motor strength.

One particularly debilitating type of neuropathic pain is **complex regional pain syndrome (CRPS)**. Typical features include dramatic changes in the color and temperature of the skin over the affected limb or body part, accompanied by intense burning pain, skin sensitivity, sweating, and swelling. CRPS type I is frequently triggered by tissue injury, surgery, or a vascular event such as stroke.[11] CRPS type II includes all these features in addition to a peripheral nerve lesion.

Neuropathic pain often is not well controlled by opioid analgesics alone. Treatment frequently necessitates a multimodal approach combining various adjuvant analgesics from different drug classes, including tricyclic antidepressants (e.g., amitriptyline [Elavil]), SNRIs (e.g., bupropion [Wellbutrin, Zyban]), antiseizure drugs (e.g., pregabalin [Lyrica]), transdermal lidocaine, and α_2-adrenergic agonists (e.g., clonidine [Catapres]). NMDA receptor antagonists such as ketamine have shown promise in alleviating neuropathic pain refractory to other drugs.

Acute and Chronic Pain

Acute pain and chronic pain differ in their cause, course, manifestations, and treatment (Table 8-4). Examples of *acute pain* include postoperative pain, labor pain, pain from trauma (e.g., lacerations, fractures, sprains), pain from infection (e.g., dysuria from cystitis), and pain from acute ischemia. For acute pain, treatment includes analgesics for symptom control and treatment of the underlying cause (e.g., splinting for a fracture, antibiotic therapy for an infection). Normally, acute pain diminishes over time as healing occurs. However, acute pain that persists can ultimately lead to disabling chronic pain states. For example, pain associated with herpes zoster subsides as the acute infection resolves, usually within a month. However, sometimes the pain persists and develops into a chronic pain state called *postherpetic neuralgia.* Because of the connection between inadequately treated acute pain and chronic pain, it is important to treat acute pain aggressively.

Chronic pain, or *persistent pain,* lasts for longer periods, often defined as longer than 3 months or past the time when an expected acute pain or acute injury should subside. The severity and functional impact of chronic pain often are disproportionate to objective findings because of changes in the nervous system not detectable with standard tests. Whereas acute pain functions as a signal, warning the person of potential or actual tissue damage, chronic pain does not appear to have an adaptive role. Chronic pain can be disabling and often is accompanied by anxiety and depression.

PAIN ASSESSMENT

Assessment is an essential, although often overlooked, step in pain management. Regularly screen all patients for pain and, when present, perform a more thorough pain assessment. The key to accurate and effective pain assessment is to consider the principles of pain assessment (Table 8-5).

The goals of a nursing pain assessment are to (1) describe the patient's pain experience to identify and implement appropriate pain management techniques and (2) identify the patient's goal for therapy and resources for self-management.

Elements of a Pain Assessment

Most components of a pain assessment involve direct interview or observation of the patient. Diagnostic studies and physical examination findings complete the initial assessment. Although the assessment differs according to the clinical setting, patient

TABLE 8-5 Principles of Pain Assessment

Principles	Nursing Implications
1. Patients have the right to appropriate assessment and management of pain.	• Assess pain in *all* patients.
2. Pain is always subjective.	• Patient's self-report of pain is the single most reliable indicator of pain. • Accept and respect this self-report unless there are clear reasons for doubt.
3. Physiologic and behavioral signs of pain (e.g., tachycardia, grimacing) are not reliable or specific for pain.	• Do not rely primarily on observations and objective signs of pain unless the patient is unable to self-report pain.
4. Pain is an unpleasant sensory and emotional experience.	• Address physical and psychologic aspects of pain when assessing pain.
5. Assessment approaches, including tools, must be appropriate for the patient population.	• Special considerations are needed for assessing pain in patients with difficulty communicating. • Include family members in the assessment process (when appropriate).
6. Pain can exist even when no physical cause can be found.	• Do not attribute pain that does not have an identifiable cause to psychologic causes.
7. Different patients experience different levels of pain in response to comparable stimuli.	• A uniform pain threshold does not exist.
8. Patients with chronic pain may be more sensitive to pain and other stimuli.	• Pain tolerance varies among and within individuals depending on various factors (e.g., genetics, energy level, coping skills, prior experience with pain).
9. Unrelieved pain has adverse consequences. Acute pain that is not adequately controlled can result in physiologic changes that increase the likelihood of developing persistent pain.	• Encourage patients to report pain, especially patients who are reluctant to discuss pain, deny pain when it is probably present, or fail to follow through on prescribed treatments.

population, and point of care (i.e., whether the assessment is part of an initial workup or a reassessment of pain following therapy), the evaluation of pain should always be multidimensional (Table 8-6).

Before beginning any assessment, recognize that patients may use words other than "pain." For example, older adults may deny that they have pain but respond positively when asked if they have soreness or aching. Document the specific words that the patient uses to describe pain. Then consistently ask the patient about pain using those words.

Pain Pattern. Assessing pain *onset* involves determining when the pain started. Patients with acute pain resulting from injury, acute illness, or treatment (e.g., surgery) typically know exactly when their pain began. Those with chronic pain may be less able to identify when the pain started. Establish the *duration* of the pain (how long it has lasted). This information helps to determine whether the pain is acute or chronic and assists in identifying the cause of the pain. For example, a patient with advanced cancer who also has chronic low back pain from spinal stenosis reports a sudden, severe pain in the back that began 2 days ago. Knowing the onset and duration can lead to a diagnostic workup that may reveal new metastatic disease in the spine.

Pain pattern also provides clues about the cause of the pain and directs its treatment. Many types of chronic pain (e.g., arthritis pain) can increase and decrease over time. A patient may have pain all the time (around-the-clock pain), as well as discrete periods of intermittent pain.

Breakthrough pain (BTP) is transient, moderate to severe pain that occurs in patients whose baseline persistent pain is otherwise mild to moderate and fairly well controlled. The average peak of BTP can be 3 to 5 minutes and can last up to 30 minutes or even longer. BTP can be either predictable or unpredictable, and patients can have one to many episodes per day. Several transmucosal fentanyl products are used specifically to treat BTP.

TABLE 8-6 Nursing Assessment

Pain

Subjective Data

Important Health Information

Health history: Pain history includes onset, location, intensity, quality, patterns, aggravating and alleviating factors, and expression of pain. Coping strategies. Past treatments and their effectiveness. Review of health care utilization related to the pain problem (e.g., emergency department visits, treatment at pain clinics, visits to primary HCPs and specialists)

Medications: Use of any prescription or over-the-counter, illicit, or herbal products for pain relief. Alcohol use

Nondrug measures: Use of therapies such as, but not limited to, massage, heat or ice, Reiki, aromatherapy, acupuncture, hypnosis, yoga, or meditation

Functional Health Patterns

Health perception–health management: Social and work history, mental health history, smoking history. Effects of pain on emotions, relationships, sleep, and activities. Interviews with family members. Records from psychologic/psychiatric treatment related to the pain

Elimination: Constipation related to opioid drug use, other medication use, or pain related to elimination

Activity-exercise: Fatigue, limitations in ability to perform ADLs (activities of daily living), IADLs (instrumental activities of daily living), and pain related to use of muscles

Sexuality-reproductive: Decreased libido

Coping–stress tolerance: Psychologic evaluation using standardized measures to examine coping style, depression, anxiety

Objective Data

Physical examination, including evaluation of functional limitations

Psychosocial evaluation, including mood

End-of-dose failure is pain that occurs before the expected duration of a specific analgesic. It should not be confused with BTP. Pain that occurs at the end of the duration of an analgesic often leads to a prolonged increase in the baseline persistent pain. For example, in a patient on transdermal fentanyl (Duragesic patches) the typical duration of action is 72 hours. An increase in pain after 48 hours on the drug would be characterized as end-of-dose failure. End-of-dose failure signals the need for changes in the dose or scheduling of the analgesic. Episodic, procedural, or *incident pain* is a transient increase in pain that is caused by a specific activity or event that precipitates pain. Examples include dressing changes, movement, position changes, and procedures such as catheterization.

Location. Determining the *location* of pain assists in identifying possible causes and treatment. Some patients may be able to specify the precise location(s) of their pain, whereas others may describe general areas or comment that they "hurt all over." The location of the pain may also be referred from its origin to another site (Fig. 8-3). For example, myocardial infarction can result in pain in the left shoulder. Pain may also radiate from its origin to another site. For example, angina pectoris can radiate from the chest to the jaw or down the left arm. This is referred to as radiating pain. *Sciatica* is pain that follows the course of the sciatic nerve. It may originate from joints or muscles around the back or from compression or damage to the sciatic nerve. The pain is projected along the course of the peripheral nerve, causing painful shooting sensations down the back of the thigh and inside of the leg to the foot.

Obtain information about the location of pain by asking the patient to (1) describe the site(s) of pain, (2) point to painful areas on the body, or (3) mark painful areas on a pain map. Because many patients have more than one site of pain, make certain that the patient describes every location.

Intensity. Assessing the severity, or *intensity*, of pain provides a reliable measure to determine the type of treatment and its effectiveness. Pain scales help the patient communicate pain intensity. Base your choice of a scale on the patient's developmental needs and cognitive status. Most adults can rate the intensity of their pain using a numeric rating scale (e.g., 0 = no pain, 10 = the worst pain), which is commonly used. A verbal descriptor scale (e.g., none, mild, moderate, severe) may be preferred for patients who wish to have word choices to quantify pain. For those oriented to vertical representations, the Pain Thermometer Scale is an option[12] (Fig. 8-4). Other visual pain measures such as the Wong-Baker FACES pain tool (*http://wongbakerfaces.org*) are useful for patients with cognitive or language barriers to describe their pain.[13] Pain assessment measures for cognitively impaired adults and nonverbal adults are addressed later in this chapter.

Although intensity is an important factor in determining analgesic approaches, do not dose patients with opioids solely based on reported pain scores.[14] Opioid "dosing by numbers" without taking into account a patient's sedation level and respiratory status can lead to unsafe practices and serious adverse events. Safer analgesic administration can be achieved by balancing an amount of pain relief with analgesic side effects and using a multimodal approach. (Multimodal approach is described later in this chapter.) Adjustments in therapy can be made to promote better pain control and minimize adverse outcomes.

Quality. The pain *quality* refers to the nature or characteristics of the pain. For example, patients often describe neuropathic pain as burning, numbing, shooting, stabbing, electric shock–like, or itchy. Nociceptive pain may be described as sharp, aching, throbbing, dull, and cramping. Since the quality of pain relates to some degree to the classification of pain (e.g., neuropathic, nociceptive), these descriptors can help to guide treatment options that best address the specific mechanism of pain.

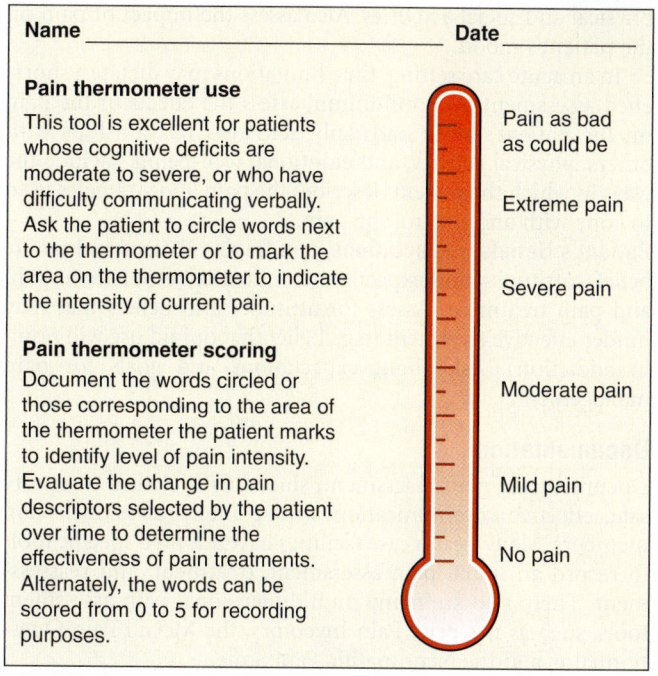

FIG. 8-4 Pain thermometer scale. Ask the patient to circle words or point next to the thermometer or to mark or point to the area on the thermometer to indicate the intensity of pain. (Used with permission of Keela Herr, RN, PhD, AGSF, FAAN, University of Iowa.)

Associated Symptoms. *Associated symptoms* such as anxiety, fatigue, and depression may exacerbate or be exacerbated by pain. Patients with pain often report poor sleep and subsequent daytime sleepiness. Poor sleep can further increase pain perception. Ask about aggravating factors that increase pain as well as activities and situations that alleviate pain. For example, musculoskeletal pain may be increased or decreased with movement and ambulation. Resting or immobilizing a painful body part can decrease pain. Knowing what makes pain better or worse can help characterize the type of pain and be helpful in selecting treatments.

Management Strategies. As people experience and live with pain, they may cope differently and be more or less willing to try different strategies to manage it. Some strategies are successful, whereas others are not. To maximize the effectiveness of the pain treatment plan, ask patients what they are using now to control pain, what they have used in the past, and the outcomes of these methods. Strategies include prescription and nonprescription drugs and nondrug therapies, such as hot and cold applications, complementary and alternative therapies (e.g., acupuncture), and relaxation strategies (e.g., imagery). It is important to document both those that work and those that are ineffective.

Impact of Pain. Pain can have a profound influence on a patient's quality of life and functioning. Assess the effect of the pain on the patient's ability to sleep, enjoy life, interact with others, perform work and household duties, and engage in physical and social activities. Also assess the impact of pain on the patient's mood.

In an acute care setting, time limitations may dictate a shortened assessment. At a minimum, assess the effects of the pain on the patient's sleep and daily activities, relationships with others, physical activity, and emotional well-being. Include the ways in which the patient describes the pain and strategies used to cope with and control the pain.

Patient's Beliefs, Expectations, and Goals. Patient and family beliefs, attitudes, and expectations influence responses to pain and pain treatment. Assess for attitudes and beliefs that may hinder effective treatment (e.g., belief that opioid use will result in addiction). Ask about expectations and goals for pain management.

Documentation

Document the pain assessment, since this is critical to ensure safe, effective communication among interprofessional team members. Many health care facilities have adopted specific tools to record an initial pain assessment, treatment, and reassessment. There also are many multidimensional pain assessment tools, such as the Brief Pain Inventory, the McGill Pain Questionnaire, and the Neuropathic Pain Scale.

Reassessment

It is critical for you to reassess pain at appropriate intervals. The frequency and scope of reassessment are guided by factors such as pain severity, physical and psychosocial condition, type of intervention and risks of adverse effects, and institutional policy. For example, reassessment of a postoperative patient may be done frequently, such as at the time of peak effect for each analgesic dose. In a long-term care facility, residents with chronic pain are reassessed at least quarterly or with a change in condition or functional status.

PAIN TREATMENT

Basic Principles

All pain treatment plans are based on the following 10 principles and practice standards:

1. *Follow the principles of pain assessment* (Table 8-5). Remember that pain is a subjective experience. The patient is not only the best judge of his or her own pain but also the expert on the effectiveness of each pain treatment.
2. *Use a holistic approach to pain management.* The experience of pain affects all aspects of a person's life. Thus a holistic approach to assessment, treatment, and evaluation is required.
3. *Every patient deserves adequate pain management.* Many patient populations, including ethnic minorities, cognitively impaired adults, and people with past or current substance abuse, are at risk for inadequate pain management. Be aware of your own biases and ensure that all patients are treated respectfully.
4. *Base the treatment plan on the patient's goals.* Discuss with the patient realistic goals for pain relief during the initial pain assessment. Although goals can be described in terms of pain intensity (e.g., the desire for average pain to decrease from "8/10" to "3/10"), with chronic pain conditions functional goal setting should be encouraged (e.g., a goal of performing certain daily activities, such as socializing and recreational activities). Encourage functional activities for the patient with acute pain as well. For example, the pain must be at a level that allows the patient to use the incentive spirometer, get out of bed, and ambulate. Over time, reassess these goals and progress made toward meeting them. The patient, in collaboration with the interprofessional team, determines new goals. If the patient has unrealistic goals for therapy, such as wanting to be completely rid of all chronic arthritis pain or be completely pain free after a major surgery, work with the patient to establish a more realistic goal.
5. *Use both drug and nondrug therapies.* Although drugs are often considered the mainstay of therapy, incorporate self-care activities and nondrug therapies to increase the overall effectiveness of therapy and to allow for the reduction of drug dosages to minimize adverse drug effects.
6. *When appropriate, use a multimodal approach to analgesic therapy.* **Multimodal analgesia** employs the use of two or more classes of analgesic agents to take advantage of the various mechanisms of action. For acute, postoperative pain, a multimodal approach may include the use of an opioid (morphine), nonopioid (nonsteroidal antiinflammatory drug), and/or an antiseizure drug (e.g., gabapentin). Regional anesthesia and continuous peripheral neural blockade can be used with local anesthetics as part of multimodal regimens.[15] Factors such as age, type of surgery, risk for developing chronic pain, and co-existing conditions are all taken into account when designing a multimodal analgesic regimen. Multimodal analgesia is also used to treat chronic or persistent pain. Similar to the strategies for acute postoperative pain, the goal is to combine classes of analgesics for the maximum benefit of relieving pain with minimum doses to achieve relief and reduce adverse events from analgesics. Multimodal regimens achieve superior pain relief, enhance patient satisfaction, and decrease adverse effects of individual drugs.[16]
7. *Address pain using an interprofessional approach.* The expertise and perspectives of an interprofessional team are often necessary to provide effective assessment and therapies for patients with both acute and chronic pain. For hospitalized patients or those with complex acute or chronic pain issues, anesthesiology-based pain services may be available to manage patients with technology-supported pain care (e.g., patient-controlled analgesia or regional analgesia). Team members for these services can include pain management nurses, nurse practitioners, clinical nurse specialists, anesthesiologists, and clinical pharmacists. These teams also help to establish realistic goals with patients and families to facilitate recovery and discharge. Many outpatient pain management centers or clinics are available. Some provide comprehensive pain care and employ multiple providers including anesthesiologists, rehabilitation physicians, nurses, psychologists, physical and occupational therapists, and social workers. Services may focus on medication management, pain interventional therapies, psychologic counseling, cognitive and behavioral therapies, rehabilitative therapies (physical and occupational therapy), and social services. Specialized pain treatment centers may also offer more holistic therapies such as massage, music and art therapy, and acupuncture. Advise patients seeking specialized pain care from outpatient treatment centers to check about services that are provided.

TABLE 8-7 Drug Therapy

Managing Side Effects of Pain Medications

Side effects can be managed in one or more of the following methods.
- Decreasing the dose of analgesic by 10% to 15%
- Changing to a different medication in the same class
- Adding a drug to counteract the adverse effect of the analgesic (e.g., using a stool softener for patients experiencing opioid-induced constipation)
- Using an administration route that minimizes drug concentrations (e.g., intraspinal administration of opioids used to minimize high drug levels that produce sedation, nausea, and vomiting)

8. *Evaluate the effectiveness of all therapies to ensure that they are meeting the patient's goals.* Achievement of an effective treatment plan often requires trial and error. Adjustments in drug, dosage, or route are common to achieve maximal benefit while minimizing adverse effects. This trial-and-error process can become frustrating for the patient and caregivers. Reassure them that pain relief, if not pain cessation, is possible and that the interprofessional team will continue to work with them to achieve adequate pain relief.
9. *Prevent and/or manage medication side effects.* Side effects or adverse events are a major reason for treatment failure and nonadherence. Side effects are managed in one of several ways, as described in Table 8-7. You play a key role in monitoring for and treating side effects and in teaching patients and caregivers how to minimize these effects.
10. *Incorporate patient and caregiver teaching throughout assessment and treatment.* Content should include information about the causes of the pain, pain assessment methods, treatment goals and options, expectations of pain management, proper use of drugs, side effect management, and nondrug and self-help pain relief measures. Document the teaching and include evaluation of patient and caregiver comprehension.

Drug Therapy for Pain

Pain medications generally are divided into three categories: nonopioids, opioids, and adjuvant drugs. Patient-centered treatment regimens may include medications from one or more of these groups. Mild pain often can be relieved using nonopioids alone. Moderate to severe pain usually requires an opioid. Certain types of pain, such as neuropathic pain, typically require adjuvant drug therapy alone or in combination with an opioid or another class of analgesics. Pain caused by cancer may be treated with chemotherapy or radiation therapy as well as pain medications.

Nonopioids. Nonopioid analgesics include acetaminophen, aspirin and other salicylates, and NSAIDs (Table 8-8). These agents are characterized by the following: (1) their analgesic properties have an **analgesic ceiling**; that is, increasing the dose beyond an upper limit provides no greater analgesia; (2) they do not produce tolerance or physical dependence; and (3) many are available without a prescription. To provide safe care, monitor over-the-counter (OTC) analgesic use to avoid serious problems related to drug interactions, side effects, and overdose.

Nonopioids are effective for mild to moderate pain. They are often used in conjunction with opioids because they allow for effective pain relief using lower opioid doses (thereby causing fewer opioid side effects). This phenomenon is called the *opioid-sparing effect.*

Aspirin is effective for mild pain, but its use is limited by its common side effects, including increased risk for bleeding, especially gastrointestinal (GI) bleeding. Other salicylates such as choline magnesium trisalicylate (Trilisate) cause fewer GI disturbances and bleeding abnormalities. Similar to aspirin, acetaminophen (Tylenol) has analgesic and antipyretic effects, but

TABLE 8-8 Drug Therapy

Selected Nonopioid Analgesics

Drug	Nursing Considerations
Nonsalicylate	
acetaminophen (Tylenol)	• Chronic overdose: liver toxicity • Rectal suppository and injectable form (OFIRMEV) available. Sustained-release preparations available. Maximum daily dose of 3 g • Oral doses of >3 g may cause hepatotoxicity. • Acute overdose: acute liver failure • Chronic overdose: liver toxicity • Maximum daily IV dose should not exceed 4 g/day for adults ≥50 kg.
Salicylates	
aspirin	• Rectal suppository and sustained-release preparations available. • Possibility of upper GI bleeding • Used more commonly in low doses as a cardioprotective measure than for its analgesic properties
choline magnesium trisalicylate (Trilisate)	• Unlike aspirin and NSAIDs, does not increase bleeding time
Nonsteroidal Antiinflammatory Drugs (NSAIDs)	
ibuprofen (Advil)	• Use lowest effective dose for shortest possible duration. • Increased risk of serious GI adverse events (bleeding, ulceration, perforation), especially in older adults • May increase risk of serious cardiovascular thrombotic events, myocardial infarction, and stroke • May increase risk of hypertension and renal insufficiency
naproxen (Naprosyn, Aleve)	• Use lowest effective dose for shortest possible duration. • Increased risk of serious GI adverse events (bleeding, ulceration, perforation), especially in older adults • Contraindicated for the treatment of perioperative pain in setting of coronary artery bypass graft (CABG) surgery
ketorolac	• Limit treatment to 5 days. • May precipitate renal failure in dehydrated patients
diclofenac K (Cataflam)	• Use lowest effective dose for shortest possible duration. • Available in oral, ophthalmic, topical preparations
celecoxib (Celebrex)	• Causes fewer GI side effects (e.g., bleeding) than other NSAIDs but risk still present. Is more costly than other NSAIDs • May increase risk of serious cardiovascular thrombotic events, myocardial infarction, and stroke • Risks may increase with duration of use, preexisting cardiovascular disease, or risk factors for cardiovascular disease.

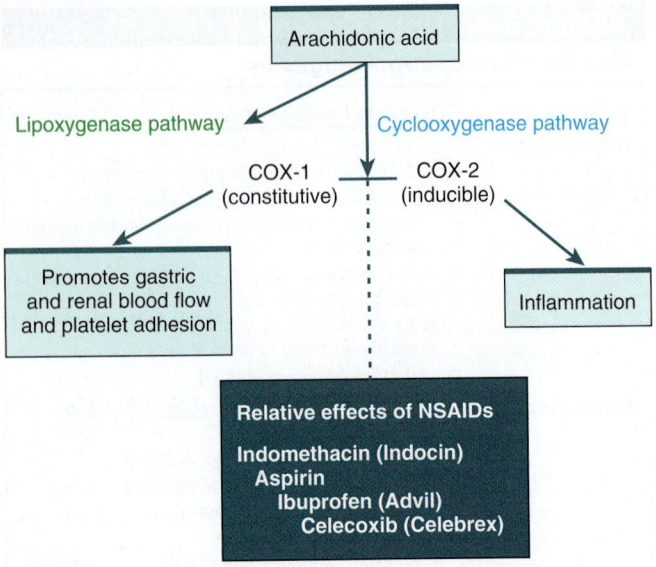

FIG. 8-5 Arachidonic acid is oxidized by two different pathways: lipoxygenase and cyclooxygenase. The cyclooxygenase pathway leads to two forms of the enzyme cyclooxygenase: COX-1 and COX-2. COX-1 is known as *constitutive* (always present), and COX-2 is known as *inducible* (its expression varies markedly depending on the stimulus). Nonsteroidal anti-inflammatory drugs (NSAIDs) differ in their actions, with some having more effects on COX-1 and others more on COX-2. Indomethacin acts primarily on COX-1, whereas ibuprofen is equipotent on COX-1 and COX-2. Celecoxib primarily inhibits COX-2.

unlike aspirin, it has no antiplatelet or antiinflammatory effects. Although acetaminophen is well tolerated, it is metabolized by the liver. Hepatotoxicity may result from chronic dosing of more than 3 g/day, acute overdose, or use by patients with severe preexisting liver disease.[17] The addition of acetaminophen to opioid therapy produces an opioid-sparing effect, lower pain scores, and fewer side effects, which is the reason for opioid-acetaminophen combinations such as Percocet. Acetaminophen is available for administration by parenteral route (OFIRMEV) administered over 15 minutes. IV acetaminophen is used for the treatment of acute mild to moderate pain and moderate to severe pain as an adjunct to opioid analgesics or part of a multimodal analgesic regimen. It has a short duration of action. The daily dose should not exceed 4 g/day.

NSAIDs represent a broad class of drugs with varying efficacy and side effects. All NSAIDs inhibit cyclooxygenase (COX), the enzyme that converts arachidonic acid into prostaglandins and related compounds. The enzyme has two forms: COX-1 and COX-2. COX-1 is found in almost all tissues and is responsible for several protective physiologic functions. In contrast, COX-2 is produced mainly at the sites of tissue injury, where it mediates inflammation (Fig. 8-5). Inhibition of COX-1 causes many of the untoward effects of NSAIDs, such as impairment of renal function, bleeding tendencies, GI irritation, and ulceration. Inhibition of COX-2 is associated with the therapeutic, antiinflammatory effects of NSAIDs. (Celecoxib [Celebrex] is a COX-2 inhibitor.) Older NSAIDs, such as ibuprofen, inhibit both forms of COX and are referred to as nonselective NSAIDs.

Patients vary greatly in their responses to a specific NSAID, so when one NSAID does not provide relief, another should be tried. NSAIDs are associated with many side effects, including GI problems ranging from dyspepsia to life-threatening ulceration and hemorrhage. NSAIDs can also cause cognitive impairment and hypersensitivity reactions with asthma-like symptoms.

Individuals at risk for NSAID-associated GI toxicity include those who have a recent history of peptic ulcer disease, patients who are older than 65, and those concurrently using corticosteroids or anticoagulants. If NSAIDs are used in patients at risk for GI bleeding, they should have concomitant therapy with misoprostol (Cytotec) or a proton pump inhibitor such as omeprazole (Prilosec). NSAIDs should not be administered concurrently with aspirin, since this increases the risk for GI bleeding.

DRUG ALERT Nonsteroidal Antiinflammatory Drugs (NSAIDs)

- NSAIDs (except aspirin) have been linked to a higher risk for cardiovascular events such as myocardial infarction, stroke, and heart failure.
- Patients who have just had heart surgery should not take NSAIDs.

Opioids. Opioids (Table 8-9) produce their effects by binding to receptors in the CNS. This results in (1) inhibition of the transmission of nociceptive input from the periphery to the spinal cord, (2) altered limbic system activity, and (3) activation of the descending inhibitory pathways that modulate transmission in the spinal cord. Thus opioids act on several nociceptive processes.

Types of Opioids. Opioids are categorized according to their physiologic action (i.e., agonist, antagonist) and binding at specific opioid receptors (e.g., mu, kappa, delta). The most commonly administered subclass of opioids is the pure opioid agonists, or morphine-like opioids, which bind to mu receptors.

Opioid agonists are used for acute and chronic pain. Although nociceptive pain appears to be more responsive to opioids than neuropathic pain, opioids may be used to treat both types of pain. In the treatment of neuropathic pain, antineuropathic pain drugs such as antidepressants and antiseizure drugs are recommended as first-line agents. Pure opioid agonists include morphine, oxycodone (OxyContin), hydrocodone, codeine, methadone, hydromorphone (Dilaudid), oxymorphone (Opana), and levorphanol (Levo-Dromoran) (Table 8-9). These drugs are effective for moderate to severe pain because they are potent, theoretically have no analgesic ceiling, and can be administered via several routes. When opioids are prescribed for moderate pain, they are usually combined with a nonopioid analgesic such as acetaminophen (e.g., codeine plus acetaminophen [Tylenol #3], or hydrocodone plus acetaminophen or ibuprofen [Vicoprofen]). Addition of acetaminophen or NSAIDs limits the total daily dose that can be given.

DRUG ALERT Morphine

- Morphine may cause respiratory depression.
- If respirations are 12 or less breaths per minute, withhold medication and contact the HCP.

Methadone is a unique mu opioid receptor agonist, which is used primarily in the treatment of chronic pain but can be used for acute pain. It has a unique mechanism of action as an NMDA receptor antagonist, which is believed to produce analgesic effects independent of its action as an opioid.[18]

DRUG ALERT Methadone (Dolophine)

- Methadone may cause respiratory depression.
- Methadone can cause cardiac toxicity, specifically QT prolongation.

TABLE 8-9 Drug Therapy

Opioid Analgesics

Drug	Routes of Administration	Nursing Considerations
Mu Agonists		
morphine (MS Contin, Avinza, Kadian, Epimorph, Oramorph SR)	PO (short-acting and sustained-release forms), rectal, IV, subcutaneous, epidural, intrathecal, sublingual, intranasal	• Standard of comparison for opioid analgesics (Table 8-12 [later in chapter]) • Indicated for moderate to severe pain • Can stimulate histamine release, leading to pruritus, with systemic administration • Tablets for sustained-release preparations are to be swallowed whole, and must not be broken, chewed, dissolved, or crushed. • Preparations for neuraxial* administration must be preservative free.
hydromorphone (Dilaudid)	PO (short-acting and long-acting forms), rectal, IV, subcutaneous, epidural, intrathecal	• Slightly shorter duration than morphine • Indicated for moderate to severe pain • Tablets for sustained-release preparations are to be swallowed whole, and must not be broken, chewed, dissolved, or crushed. • Preparations for neuraxial* administration must be preservative free.
methadone (Dolophine)	PO, IV, IM	• High oral and rectal bioavailability • Accumulates with repeated dosing • Use with caution in older adults. • Risk of QT interval prolongation
levorphanol (Levo-Dromoran)	PO, IV, IM, subcutaneous	• Accumulates with repeated dosing
fentanyl (Sublimaze [IV], Duragesic [transdermal], Actiq [transmucosal]), buccal tablet (Fentora), sublingual (Abstral), buccal soluble film (Onsolis), nasal spray (Lazanda)	IV, epidural, intrathecal, transmucosal, transdermal	• Immediate onset after IV route, 7-8 min after IM route, 5-15 min after transmucosal route, up to 6 hr after transdermal route • For procedures, IV fentanyl often combined with benzodiazepines for analgesia and sedation • Very potent; dosage is in micrograms (mcg). • Transdermal fentanyl indicated only for chronic pain and should not be administered to opioid-naive patients.
oxymorphone (Opana, Opana ER, Numorphan)	IV, PO (short-acting and extended-release forms)	• Tablets for extended-release forms are to be swallowed whole and must not be broken, chewed, dissolved, or crushed. • Use with caution in older and debilitated patients and patients with hepatic and renal impairment.
oxycodone (Roxicodone) oxycodone extended-release (OxyContin) oxycodone plus acetaminophen (Percocet) oxycodone plus aspirin (Percodan) oxycodone plus ibuprofen (Combunox) oxycodone extended-release plus acetaminophen (Xartemis)	PO (short-acting and extended-release forms)	• Available as single entity and in combination with a nonopioid • Can be used similarly to oral morphine for moderate to severe pain • Often combined with a nonopioid for acute, moderate pain • Extended-release indicated for chronic pain
oxycodone and naloxone extended release (Targiniq ER)	PO (extended release)	• Used for severe pain needing treatment around the clock • Naloxone in drug blocks euphoric effects of oxycodone when crushed and snorted or crushed, dissolved, and injected. • Makes it less liked by abusers than oxycodone alone
hydrocodone (with acetaminophen [Norco]) (with bitartrate [Hysingla, Zohydro])	PO (short acting and long-acting)	• Used for moderate or moderately severe pain • Generally indicated for short-term management of acute pain (e.g., trauma, musculoskeletal)
codeine oral (with acetaminophen [Tylenol #3]), codeine injectable	PO, subcutaneous	• Associated with higher incidence of nausea and constipation than other mu agonists • Many codeine preparations are combined with acetaminophen. • 5%-10% of European Americans lack the enzyme to metabolize codeine to morphine.
tramadol (Ultram)	PO (short-acting and extended release)	• Dual mechanism of action: mu opioid agonist and blocks reuptake of norepinephrine and serotonin • Used for moderate pain
tapentadol (Nucynta)	PO (short-acting and extended release)	• Dual mechanism of action: mu opioid agonist and blocks reuptake of norepinephrine and serotonin

*Neuraxial anesthesia pertains to local anesthetics placed around the nerves of the central nervous system such as spinal and epidural anesthesia.

Continued

TABLE 8-9 Drug Therapy

Opioid Analgesics—cont'd

Drug	Routes of Administration	Nursing Considerations
Mixed Agonist-Antagonists		
pentazocine (Talwin) pentazocine plus naloxone (Talwin NX)	Formulated in combination with acetaminophen, aspirin, ibuprofen Abuse-deterrent preparation includes naloxone to discourage parenteral abuse	• May cause psychotomimetic effects (e.g., hallucinations) and may precipitate withdrawal in opioid-dependent patients • Not recommended for treatment of chronic pain and rarely for acute pain
butorphanol	Available in a nasal spray and injectable form Not available orally	• Psychotomimetic effects lower than with pentazocine • May precipitate withdrawal in opioid-dependent patients • Injectable used for acute pain • Nasal spray indicated for migraine headaches
Partial Agonists		
buprenorphine buprenorphine plus naloxone sublingual (Suboxone)	Sublingual, injectable, implant	• Sublingual form should not be chewed or swallowed • Lower abuse potential than morphine. Does not produce psychotomimetic effects • May precipitate withdrawal in opioid-dependent patients. Not readily reversed by naloxone • Buprenorphine plus naloxone used as a sublingual preparation to treat opioid dependence for easier withdrawal when necessary to taper from opioids

Mixed agonist-antagonists (e.g., pentazocine [Talwin], butorphanol) bind as agonists on kappa receptors and as weak antagonists or partial agonists on mu receptors. Because of this difference in binding, mixed agonist-antagonists produce less respiratory depression than drugs that act only at mu receptors. These drugs cause more dysphoria and agitation. In addition, opioid agonist-antagonists have an analgesic ceiling and can precipitate withdrawal if used by a patient who is physically dependent on mu agonist drugs. Partial opioid agonists (e.g., buprenorphine [Buprenex]) can produce some pain relief but bind tightly to mu receptors and can block the effect of other drugs. Agonist-antagonists and partial agonists currently have limited clinical application in pain management.

Dual-Mechanism Agents. Some analgesics have two distinct actions, or dual mechanisms. Tramadol (Ultram) is a weak mu agonist and inhibits the reuptake of norepinephrine and serotonin. It is effective in low back pain, osteoarthritis, fibromyalgia, diabetic peripheral neuropathic pain, polyneuropathy, and postherpetic neuralgia. The most common side effects are similar to those of other opioids, including nausea, constipation, dizziness, and sedation. As with other medications that increase serotonin and norepinephrine, avoid this drug in patients with a history of seizures because it lowers seizure threshold.

Tapentadol (Nucynta) is a centrally acting analgesic that works at mu receptors and inhibits norepinephrine reuptake. It is approved for management of moderate to severe acute pain. For chronic moderate to severe pain, an extended-release formula is available. The side effects are similar to those of conventional opioids, except that this drug is associated with less nausea and constipation.

Opioids to Avoid. Some opioids should be avoided for pain relief because of limited efficacy and/or toxicities. Meperidine (Demerol) or pethidine is associated with neurotoxicity (e.g., seizures) caused by accumulation of its metabolite, normeperidine. Its use is limited for very short-term (i.e., less than 48 hours) treatment of acute pain when other opioid agonists are contraindicated.

DRUG ALERT Meperidine (Demerol)
The American Pain Society does not recommend the use of meperidine as an analgesic.

Side Effects of Opioids. Common side effects of opioids include constipation, nausea and vomiting, sedation, respiratory depression, and pruritus. With continued use, many side effects diminish; the exception is constipation. Less common side effects include urinary retention, myoclonus, dizziness, confusion, and hallucinations. *Constipation* is the most common side effect of opioids. Left untreated, constipation may increase the individual's pain and can lead to fecal impaction and paralytic ileus.

Because tolerance to opioid-induced constipation does not develop, a bowel regimen should be initiated at the beginning of opioid therapy and continued for as long as the person takes opioids. Although dietary fiber, fluids, and exercise should be encouraged, these measures alone may not be sufficient. Most patients should use a gentle stimulant laxative (e.g., senna) plus a stool softener (e.g., docusate sodium [Colace]). Other agents (e.g., milk of magnesia, bisacodyl [Dulcolax], polyethylene glycol [MiraLAX], or lactulose [Constulose]) can be added if necessary. Methylnaltrexone (Relistor) and naloxegol (Movantik) are peripheral opioid receptor antagonists used for opioid-induced constipation when the response to traditional laxative and stool softener therapy is insufficient.

Nausea is often a problem in opioid-naive patients. The use of an antiemetic such as ondansetron (Zofran), metoclopramide (Reglan), transdermal scopolamine (Transderm Scōp), hydroxyzine (Vistaril), or a phenothiazine (e.g., prochlorperazine) can prevent or minimize nausea and vomiting until tolerance develops, usually within 1 week. Opioids delay gastric emptying (patient complains of gastric fullness), and this effect can be reduced by metoclopramide. If nausea and vomiting are severe and persistent, changing to a different opioid may be necessary.

Sedation is usually seen in opioid-naive patients being treated for acute pain. Regularly monitor patients receiving opioid analgesics for acute pain, especially in the first few days (e.g., after surgery). Be aware that the risk for unintended sedation in postoperative patients is greatest within 4 hours after leaving the postanesthesia care unit. Opioid-induced sedation resolves with the development of tolerance. Persistent sedation with chronic opioid use can be effectively treated with psychostimulants such as caffeine, dextroamphetamine (Dexedrine), methylphenidate (Ritalin), or the anticataleptic drug modafinil (Provigil).

The risk of *respiratory depression* is also higher in opioid-naive, hospitalized patients who are treated for acute pain. Clinically significant respiratory depression is rare in opioid-tolerant patients and when opioids are titrated to analgesic effect. Patients most at risk for respiratory depression include those who are age 65 or older, have a history of snoring or witnessed apneic episodes, report excessive daytime sleepiness, have underlying cardiac or lung disease, are obese (body mass index greater than 30 kg/m^2), have a history of smoking (more than 20 pack-years), or are receiving other CNS depressants (e.g., sedatives, benzodiazepines, antihistamines). For postoperative patients the greatest risk for opioid-related respiratory adverse events is within the first 24 hours after surgery. Clinically significant respiratory depression cannot occur in patients who are fully awake.

CHECK YOUR PRACTICE

A 74-yr-old male patient returned to the clinical unit following surgery for a hip replacement. You are having difficulty arousing him with either verbal or physical stimulation. His wife tells you to just let him sleep. His respiratory rate ranges from 8-10 breaths/min.

- What should you do?

Frequently monitor both the sedation level and respiratory rate in patients receiving opioid analgesics.[19] A sedation scale can be used for monitoring and providing appropriate interventions based on the level of sedation (Table 8-10).

SAFETY ALERT Sedation and Respiratory Depression

- If the number of patient's respirations falls below 8 or 10 breaths/minute and the sedation level is 3 or greater, you should vigorously stimulate the patient and try to keep the patient awake.
- If the patient becomes oversedated, administer oxygen.
- In this situation, the opioid dose should be reduced.

For patients who are excessively sedated or unresponsive, naloxone, an opioid antagonist that rapidly reverses the effects of opioids, can be administered. Naloxone can be given IV, subcutaneously, or intranasally. Evzio (handheld autoinjector containing naloxone) can be used by a caregiver or family member to treat a person known or suspected to have had an opioid overdose.

If the patient has been taking opioids regularly for more than a few days, use naloxone carefully because it can precipitate severe, agonizing pain; profound withdrawal symptoms; hypertension; and pulmonary edema. Because naloxone's half-life is shorter than that of most opioids, frequently monitor the patient.

Pruritus (itching) is another common side effect of opioids and occurs most frequently when opioids are administered via neuraxial (i.e., epidural, intrathecal) routes. Management of opioid-induced pruritus in non-cancer patients may include low-dose infusions of naloxone.

TABLE 8-10 Pasero Opioid-Induced Sedation Scale (POSS) With Interventions

Level of Sedation	Nursing Intervention
S = Sleep, easy to arouse	• Acceptable • No action necessary • May increase opioid dose if needed
1 Awake and alert	• Acceptable • No action necessary • May increase opioid dose if needed
2 Slightly drowsy, easily aroused	• Acceptable • No action necessary • May increase opioid dose if needed
3 Frequently drowsy, arousable, drifts off to sleep during conversation	• Unacceptable • Monitor respiratory status and sedation level closely until sedation level is stable at less than 3 and respiratory status is satisfactory. • Decrease opioid dose 25%-50% or notify HCP or anesthesiologist for orders. • Consider administering a nonsedating, opioid-sparing nonopioid, such as acetaminophen or an NSAID, if not contraindicated.
4 Somnolent, minimal or no response to verbal or physical stimulation	• Unacceptable • Stop opioid • Consider administering naloxone. • Notify HCP or anesthesiologist. • Monitor respiratory status and sedation level closely until sedation level is stable at less than 3 and respiratory status is satisfactory.

Adapted from Pasero C: Assessment of sedation during opioid administration for pain management, *J PeriAnesthesia Nurs* 24:186, 2009.

A rare but concerning problem with long-term and even short-term use of high-dose opioids is *opioid-induced hyperalgesia* (OIH). OIH is a state of nociceptive sensitization caused by exposure to opioids. It is characterized by a paradoxic response in which patients actually become more sensitive to certain painful stimuli and report increased pain with opioid use. The exact mechanism is not clearly understood, but it may be due to neuroplasticity changes. This may explain why opioids tend to lose their effectiveness in certain patients over time.

Adjuvant Analgesic Therapy. Analgesic adjuvants are drugs that can be used alone or in conjunction with opioid and nonopioid analgesics (Table 8-11). Generally, these agents were developed for other purposes (e.g., antiseizure drugs, antidepressants) and found to be effective for treating pain.

Corticosteroids. Corticosteroids include dexamethasone, prednisone, and methylprednisolone (Medrol). They are used for management of acute and chronic cancer pain, pain secondary to spinal cord compression, and inflammatory joint pain syndromes. Mechanisms of action may be related to the ability of corticosteroids to decrease edema and inflammation.

Corticosteroids have many side effects, especially when given chronically in high doses. These include hyperglycemia, fluid retention, dyspepsia and GI bleeding, impaired healing, muscle wasting, osteoporosis, adrenal suppression, and susceptibility to infection. Because they act through the same final pathway as NSAIDs, do not give corticosteroids at the same time as NSAIDs.

TABLE 8-11 Drug Therapy

Adjuvant Drugs Used for Pain

Drug	Specific Indication	Nursing Considerations
Corticosteroids	Inflammation	• Avoid high doses for long-term use.
Antidepressants		
Tricyclic Antidepressants		
amitriptyline doxepin imipramine (Tofranil) nortriptyline (Pamelor) desipramine (Norpramin)	Neuropathic pain	• Side-effect profile differs for each agent and is often dose dependent. • Common side effects include anticholinergic effects (e.g., dry mouth) and sedation. • Monitor for anticholinergic side effects. • Titrate slowly over days to weeks to reach optimal therapeutic doses.
Serotonin Norepinephrine Reuptake Inhibitor (SNRI) Antidepressants		
venlafaxine duloxetine (Cymbalta) milnacipran (Savella)	Neuropathic pain Multimodal therapy for acute pain (venlafaxine) Fibromyalgia (duloxetine, milnacipran)	• Side effects vary with each agent. • Decrease arousal and desire for sex
Other Antidepressants		
bupropion (Wellbutrin)	Neuropathic pain Headaches Distinguished from TCAs and SNRIs as an inhibitor of norepinephrine and dopamine uptake	• Low risk of sexual dysfunction and sedation
Antiseizure Drugs		
First generation: carbamazepine (Tegretol) phenytoin (Dilantin) *Second generation:* gabapentin (Neurontin) pregabalin (Lyrica) lamotrigine (Lamictal)	Neuropathic pain Multimodal therapy for acute pain (gabapentin, pregabalin) Fibromyalgia (pregabalin)	• Start with low doses, increase slowly. • Side effects vary with each agent.
GABA Receptor Agonist		
baclofen (Lioresal)	Neuropathic pain Muscle spasms	• Monitor for weakness, urinary dysfunction. • Avoid abrupt discontinuation because of CNS irritability.
α_2-Adrenergic Agonist		
clonidine (Duraclon) tizanidine (Zanaflex)	Particularly useful for neuropathic pain when administered intrathecally	• Side effects include sedation, orthostatic hypotension, dry mouth. • Often combined with anesthetics (e.g., bupivacaine [Sensorcaine])
Anesthetics: Oral or Systemic		
mexiletine	Diabetic neuropathy Neuropathic pain	• Monitor for side effects: high incidence of nausea, dizziness, perioral numbness, paresthesias, tremor, seizures (at high doses), dysrhythmias, and myocardial depression. • Avoid in patients with preexisting cardiac disease.
5% lidocaine-impregnated transdermal patch (Lidoderm patch)	Postherpetic neuralgia	• Local skin reactions (e.g., change in color, colored spots, irritation, itching, rash, burning) occur at the site of application; typically mild.
Anesthetics: Local		
lidocaine (L-M-X)	Topical local anesthetic cream applied to intact skin before venipuncture or lumbar puncture. Possibly effective for postherpetic neuralgia	• Apply bubble layer to intact skin, wait at least 20-30 min before wiping and performing painful procedure. • Duration is approximately 60 min after wiped from skin. • Available without prescription
lidocaine 2.5% + prilocaine 2.5% (topical EMLA [eutectic mixture of local anesthetics])	Longer time to take effect than L-M-X	• Apply under an occlusive dressing (e.g., Tegaderm, DuoDerm) or on an anesthetic disk. • Side effects include mild erythema, edema, skin blanching.
5% lidocaine-impregnated transdermal patch (Lidoderm patch)	Postherpetic neuralgia	• Local skin reactions (e.g., change in color, colored spots, irritation, itching, rash, burning) occur at the site of application—typically mild.
capsaicin (active compound of chili peppers)	Pain associated with arthritis, postherpetic neuralgia, diabetic neuropathy	• Apply very sparingly onto affected area. Use gloves or wash hands with soap and water after application. • Monitor for side effects: skin irritation (burning, stinging) at application site and cough when inhaled.

Adapted from Pasero C, Polomano RC, McCaffery M, et al: Adjuvant analgesics. In Pasero C, McCaffery M, editors: *Pain: assessment and pharmacological management,* New York, 2011, Elsevier.
CNS, Central nervous system.

Antidepressants. Tricyclic antidepressants (TCAs) enhance the descending inhibitory system by preventing the cellular reuptake of serotonin and norepinephrine. Higher levels of serotonin and norepinephrine in the synapse inhibit the transmission of nociceptive signals in the CNS. Other potential beneficial actions of TCAs include sodium channel modulation, α_1-adrenergic antagonist effects, and a weak NMDA receptor modulation. They are effective for a variety of pain syndromes, especially neuropathic pain syndromes. However, side effects such as sedation, dry mouth, blurred vision, and weight gain limit their usefulness. Antidepressants that selectively inhibit reuptake of serotonin and norepinephrine (SNRIs) are effective for many neuropathic pain syndromes and have fewer side effects than the TCAs. These agents include venlafaxine, desvenlafaxine (Pristiq), milnacipran (Savella), and bupropion.

Antiseizure Drugs. Antiseizure drugs affect peripheral nerves and the CNS in several ways, including sodium channel modulation, central calcium channel modulation, and changes in excitatory amino acids and other receptors. Agents such as gabapentin, lamotrigine, and pregabalin are valuable adjuvant agents in chronic pain therapy and are being used increasingly in the treatment of acute pain.

GABA-Receptor Agonist. Baclofen, an agonist at GABA receptors, can interfere with the transmission of nociceptive impulses and is used for muscle spasms and neuropathic pain. It crosses the blood-brain barrier poorly and is much more effective for spasticity when delivered intrathecally.

α_2-Adrenergic Agonists. Clonidine and tizanidine (Zanaflex), the most widely used α_2-adrenergic agonists, are thought to work on the central inhibitory α-adrenergic receptors. These agents may also decrease norepinephrine release peripherally. They are used for chronic headache and neuropathic pain.

Local Anesthetics. For acute pain from surgery or trauma, local anesthetics such as bupivacaine and ropivacaine can be administered epidurally by continuous infusion but also by intermittent or continuous infusion with regional nerve blocks. Topical applications of local anesthetics are used to interrupt transmission of pain signals to the brain. For example, 5% lidocaine patch (Lidoderm) is recommended as a first-line agent for the treatment of several types of neuropathic pain. In the treatment of chronic severe neuropathic pain that is refractory to other analgesics, oral therapy with mexiletine (Mexitil) may be tried. Systemic lidocaine administered in the form of an IV infusion is also sometimes used for neuropathic and postoperative visceral pain.

Cannabinoids. Cannabinoid-derived medications show promise in the treatment of certain pain syndromes and symptoms. However, these preparations have sparked considerable controversy and confusion, mostly because cannabinoids are related to the cannabis plant, also known as marijuana. Synthetic cannabinoids (e.g., dronabinol [Marinol]) have been approved for medical use. Smoking marijuana or cannabis rapidly increases plasma levels of tetrahydrocannabinol (THC). The increase is dependent on composition of the marijuana cigarette and inhalation technique. As a result, this form of use is associated with variable pain relief. With commercially available oral preparations, the absorption and bioavailability are more reliable and predictable.

Cannabinoids exert their analgesic effects primarily through the cannabinoid-l (CB1) and CB2 receptors. Activation of cannabinoid receptors modulates neurotransmission in the serotoninergic, dopaminergic, and glutamatergic systems, as well as other systems. Cannabinoids also enhance the endogenous opioid system. Other beneficial effects include alleviation of nausea and increased appetite. They may also have opioid-sparing effects, possibly reduce opioid tolerance, and even ameliorate symptoms of opioid withdrawal.[20]

Administration

Scheduling. Appropriate analgesic scheduling focuses on preventing or controlling pain, rather than providing analgesics only after the patient's pain has become severe. Premedicate a patient before procedures and activities that are expected to produce pain. Similarly, a patient with constant pain should receive analgesics around the clock rather than on an "as needed" (PRN) basis. These strategies control pain before it starts and usually result in lower analgesic requirements. Use fast-acting drugs for incident or breakthrough pain, whereas long-acting analgesics are more effective for constant pain. Examples of fast-acting and sustained-release analgesics are described later in this section.

Titration. *Analgesic titration* is dose adjustment based on assessment of the adequacy of analgesic effect versus the side effects produced. The amount of analgesic needed to manage pain varies widely, and titration is an important strategy in addressing this variability. An analgesic can be titrated upward or downward, depending on the situation. For example, in a postoperative patient the dose of analgesic generally decreases over time as the acute pain resolves. On the other hand, opioids for chronic, severe cancer pain may be titrated upward many times over the course of therapy to maintain adequate pain control. The goal of titration is to use the smallest dose of analgesic that provides effective pain control with the fewest side effects.

Equianalgesic Dosing. The term **equianalgesic dose** refers to a dose of one analgesic that is approximately equivalent in pain-relieving effects to a given dose of another analgesic (Table 8-12). This equivalence helps guide opioid dosing when changing routes or opioids when a particular drug is ineffective or causes intolerable side effects. Equianalgesic charts and conversion programs are widely available in clinical guidelines, in health care facility pain protocols, and on the Internet. They are useful tools, but you need to understand their limitations, since equianalgesic doses are estimates. To ensure safety, all changes

TABLE 8-12 Opioid Equianalgesic Doses*

	DOSE EQUAL TO PARENTERAL MORPHINE 10 MG	
Drug	**Oral (mg)**	**Parenteral (IM, IV, Subcutaneous) (mg)**
Morphine	30	10
Codeine	200	120-130
Fentanyl	NA	0.1 (100 mcg)
Hydrocodone	30	NA
Hydromorphone	7.5	1.5
Levorphanol	4	2
Meperidine	300	75
Methadone†		
Oxycodone	15-30	NA
Oxymorphone	NA	1

NA, Not available.
*All equivalencies should be considered approximations. These amounts can be affected by many factors, including interpatient variability, type of pain, and tolerance. Monitor patients for effectiveness and adverse reactions and adjust the dose accordingly.
†The equianalgesic dose of methadone compared with other opioids varies widely in patients on chronic opioids (*www.aafp.org/afp/20050401/1353.html*).

in opioid therapy must be carefully monitored and adjusted for the individual patient.

Administration Routes. Opioids and other analgesic agents can be delivered via many routes. This flexibility allows the HCP to (1) target a particular anatomic source of the pain, (2) achieve therapeutic blood levels rapidly when necessary, (3) avoid certain side effects through localized administration, and (4) provide analgesia when patients are unable to swallow. The following discussion highlights the uses and nursing considerations for analgesic agents delivered through a variety of routes.

Oral. Generally, oral administration is the route of choice for the person with a functioning GI system. Most pain medications are available in oral preparations, such as liquid and tablet. For opioids, larger oral doses are needed to achieve the equivalent analgesia of doses administered intramuscularly (IM) or IV (Table 8-12). For example, 10 mg of parenteral morphine is equivalent to approximately 30 mg of oral morphine. The reason larger doses are required is related to the *first-pass effect* of hepatic metabolism. This means that oral opioids are absorbed from the GI tract into the portal circulation and shunted to the liver. Partial metabolism in the liver occurs before the drug enters the systemic circulation and becomes available to peripheral receptors or can cross the blood-brain barrier and access CNS opioid receptors, which is necessary to produce analgesia. Oral opioids are as effective as parenteral opioids if the dose administered is large enough to compensate for the first-pass metabolism.

Many opioids are available in short-acting (immediate-release) and long-acting (sustained-release or extended-release) oral preparations. Immediate-release products are effective in providing rapid, short-term pain relief. Sustained- or extended-release preparations generally are administered every 8 to 12 hours, although some preparations (e.g., Kadian, Avinza, Exalgo) may be dosed every 24 hours.

SAFETY ALERT Sustained- or Extended-Release Preparations

- These should not be crushed, broken, dissolved, or chewed. These drugs are meant to be swallowed whole.
- If all of the medicine is released into a person at once, very serious side effects can occur, including death from overdose.

Transmucosal and buccal routes. Although morphine has historically been administered sublingually to people with cancer pain who have difficulty swallowing, little of the drug is actually absorbed from the sublingual tissue. Instead, most of the drug is dissolved in saliva and swallowed, making its absorption similar to oral morphine.

Several transmucosal fentanyl products are used for the treatment of breakthrough pain. These include (1) oral transmucosal fentanyl citrate (OTFC) (Actiq) with the fentanyl embedded in a flavored lozenge on a stick, which is absorbed by the buccal mucosa after being rubbed actively over it when administered as the lozenge (not sucked as a lollipop), (2) fentanyl buccal tablet (FBT) (Fentora) in the form of a buccal tablet that disintegrates, (3) fentanyl sublingual (Abstral), and (4) fentanyl buccal soluble film (Onsolis) for application to the buccal membrane. Transmucosal absorption allows the drug to enter the bloodstream and travel directly to the CNS. Pain relief typically occurs 5 to 7 minutes after administration. These formulations of fentanyl should only be used for patients who are already receiving and are tolerant to opioid therapy.[21]

An oromucosal spray delivery of cannabinoid extract (Sativex) is an adjunctive treatment for neuropathic pain and spasticity in patients with multiple sclerosis. It is not currently available in the United States.

Intranasal route. Intranasal administration allows delivery of medication to highly vascular mucosa and avoids the first-pass effect. Butorphanol is indicated for acute headache and other intense, recurrent types of pain. A transmucosal fentanyl nasal spray (Lazanda) is available for the treatment of breakthrough pain.

Rectal. The rectal route is often overlooked but is particularly useful when the patient cannot take an analgesic by mouth, such as those patients with severe nausea and vomiting. Analgesics that are available as rectal suppositories include hydromorphone, oxymorphone, morphine, and acetaminophen. If rectal preparations are not available, many oral formulations can be given rectally if the patient is unable to take medications by mouth.

Transdermal route. Fentanyl (Duragesic) is available as a transdermal patch system for application to intact, nonhairy skin. This delivery system is useful for the patient who cannot tolerate oral analgesic drugs. Absorption from the patch is slow, and it takes 12 to 17 hours to reach full effect with the first application. Therefore transdermal fentanyl is not suitable for rapid dose titration but can be effective if the patient's pain is stable, and the dose required to control it is known. Patches may have to be changed every 48 hours rather than the recommended 72 hours based on individual patient responses. Rashes caused by the adhesive of the patch may be reduced by preparing the skin 1 hour before placement with a weak corticosteroid cream. Bioocclusive dressings are available if the patch keeps falling off because of sweating. A transdermal patient-controlled analgesia (PCA) system (iontophoretic transdermal system [ITS]) is available.

DRUG ALERT Fentanyl Patches

- Fentanyl patches (Duragesic) may cause death from overdose.
- Signs of overdose include trouble breathing or shallow respirations; tiredness, extreme sleepiness, or sedation; inability to think, talk, or walk normally; and faintness, dizziness, or confusion.

An important distinction should be made between transdermal patches designed for systemic drug delivery (e.g., Duragesic) and those for topical or local delivery (e.g., Lidoderm).

A 5% lidocaine-impregnated transdermal patch (Lidoderm patch) is used for postherpetic neuralgia. The patch is placed directly on the intact, nonhairy skin in the area of postherpetic pain and left in place for up to 12 hours. Topical local anesthetics are generally well tolerated and cause few systemic side effects, even with chronic use.

Creams and lotions containing 10% trolamine salicylate (Aspercreme, Myoflex Creme) are available for joint and muscle pain. This aspirin-like substance is absorbed locally. This route of administration avoids GI irritation but not the other side effects of high-dose salicylates. Topical diclofenac solution and a diclofenac patch (Flector) are effective for osteoarthritic pain of the knee.

Other topical analgesic agents, such as capsaicin (e.g., Zostrix) and lidocaine (L-M-X cream), also provide analgesia. Derived from red chili pepper, capsaicin acts on C-fiber heat receptors. If used three or four times a day for 4 to 6 weeks, it will cause the C nociceptor fibers to become inactive. The result is neuronal resistance to painful stimuli. Capsaicin is used to control pain associated with diabetic neuropathy, arthritis, and postherpetic neuralgia. L-M-X cream is useful for

EVIDENCE-BASED PRACTICE

Translating Research Into Practice

What Is the Effect of Capsaicin on Chronic Neuropathic Pain?

Clinical Question

For adults with chronic neuropathic pain (P), what is the effect of high-concentration capsaicin (I) versus placebo or usual care (C) on pain relief (O) for up to 12 weeks (T)?

Synthesis of Best Available Evidence

- Systematic review of randomized controlled trials (RCTs)
- Six trials (n = 2073) of participants with moderately intense postherpetic neuralgia or painful HIV-neuropathy lasting at least 3 months. Intervention was single application of high-concentration capsaicin patches to affected areas under carefully controlled conditions. The concentration of capsaicin (8%) was almost 100 times greater than conventional creams. Pain relief was expected to occur for approximately 12 weeks.
- About 1 in 8 patients with high-concentration capsaicin patch had significant pain relief. People with high pain relief reported improved sleep, fatigue, depression, and quality of life. Short-term local skin effects were erythema, burning, and pain at application site.

Conclusion

- High-concentration capsaicin patches may relieve chronic neuropathic pain.

Implications for Nursing Practice

1. What information would you provide a patient with intense chronic shingles pain who seeks your help when other therapies have failed?
2. What is your role as a member of the interprofessional pain management team for patients with constant, severe chronic pain?

Reference for Evidence

Derry S, Rice ASC, Cole P, et al: Topical capsaicin (high concentration) for chronic neuropathic pain in adults, *Cochrane Database Syst Rev* (2):CD007393, 2013.

P, Patient population of interest; *I*, intervention or area of interest; *C*, comparison of interest or comparison group; *O*, outcomes of interest; *T*, timing (see p. 15).

control of pain associated with venipunctures. Cover the targeted area of intact skin with a layer of L-M-X for at least 20 to 30 minutes before it is wiped off prior to beginning a painful procedure.

Parenteral routes. The parenteral routes include IV and subcutaneous administration. Single, repeated, or continuous dosing (IV or subcutaneous) is possible via parenteral routes. IV administration is the best route when immediate analgesia and rapid titration are necessary. Continuous IV infusions provide excellent steady-state analgesia through stable blood levels.

Onset of analgesia after subcutaneous administration is slow, and thus the subcutaneous route is rarely used for acute pain management. However, continuous subcutaneous infusions are effective for pain management at the end of life. This route is especially helpful for people with abnormal GI function and limited venous access.

The IM route is not recommended because injections cause significant pain and result in unreliable absorption. With chronic use, IM injections can result in abscesses and fibrosis.

Intraspinal delivery. Intraspinal or neuraxial opioid therapy involves inserting a catheter into the subarachnoid space

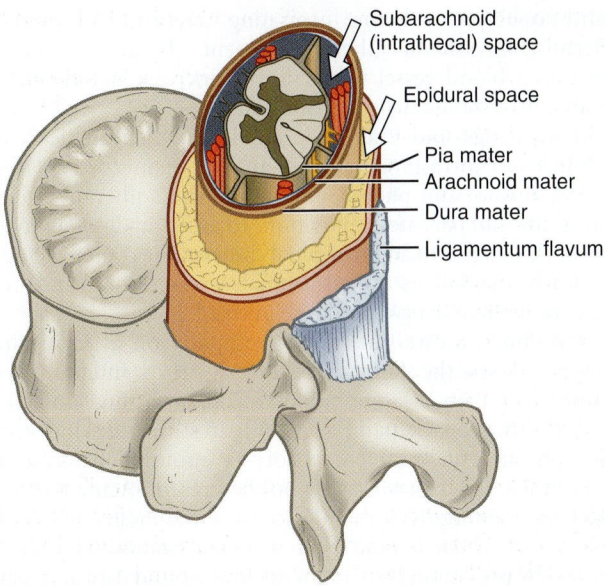

FIG. 8-6 Spinal anatomy. The spinal cord extends from the foramen magnum to the first or second lumbar vertebral space. The subarachnoid space (intrathecal space) is filled with cerebrospinal fluid that continuously circulates and bathes the spinal cord. The epidural space is a potential space filled with blood vessels, fat, and a network of nerve extensions.

(intrathecal delivery) or the epidural space *(epidural delivery)* (Fig. 8-6). Analgesics are injected either by intermittent bolus doses or continuous infusion.

Percutaneously placed temporary catheters are used for short-term therapy (2 to 4 days), and surgically implanted catheters are used for long-term therapy. Although the lumbar region is the most common site of placement, epidural catheters may be placed at any point along the spinal column (cervical, thoracic, lumbar, or caudal). The tip of the epidural catheter is placed as close to the nerve supplying the painful dermatome as possible. For example, a thoracic catheter is placed for upper abdominal surgery, and a high lumbar catheter is used for lower abdominal surgery. Fluoroscopy is used to ensure correct placement of the catheter.

Intraspinally administered analgesics are highly potent because they are delivered close to the receptors in the spinal cord dorsal horn. Smaller doses of analgesics are needed than with other routes, including IV. For example, 1 mg of intrathecal morphine is approximately equivalent to 10 mg of epidural morphine, 100 mg of IV morphine, and 300 mg of oral morphine. Drugs that are delivered intraspinally include morphine, fentanyl, sufentanil (Sufenta), alfentanil (Alfenta), hydromorphone, ziconotide (Prialt) (a calcium channel receptor modulator for use in neuropathic pain syndromes), and clonidine. Nausea, itching, and urinary retention are common side effects of intraspinal opioids.

Complications of intraspinal analgesia include catheter displacement and migration, accidental infusions of neurotoxic agents, epidural hematomas, and infection. Clinical manifestations of catheter displacement or migration depend on catheter location and the drug being infused. A catheter that migrates out of the intrathecal or epidural space causes a decrease in pain relief with no improvement with additional boluses or increases in the infusion rate. If an epidural catheter migrates into the subarachnoid space, increased side effects become quickly apparent. Somnolence, confusion, and increased anesthesia (if the infusate contains an anesthetic) occur. Check with institutional policy before aspirating cerebrospinal fluid to determine intrathecal catheter placement. Migration of a catheter into a blood vessel may cause an increase in side effects because of systemic drug distribution.

Many drugs and chemicals are highly neurotoxic when administered intraspinally. These include many preservatives such as alcohol and phenol, antibiotics, chemotherapy agents, potassium, and parenteral nutrition. To avoid inadvertent injection of IV drugs into an intraspinal catheter, the catheter should be clearly marked as an intraspinal access device, and only preservative-free drugs should be injected.

Infection is a rare but serious complication of intraspinal analgesia. Assess the skin around the exit site for inflammation, drainage, or pain. Manifestations of an intraspinal infection include diffuse back pain, pain or paresthesia during bolus injection, and unexplained sensory or motor deficits in the lower limbs. Fever may or may not be present. Acute bacterial infection (meningitis) is manifested by photophobia, neck stiffness, fever, headache, and altered mental status. Infection is avoided by providing regular, meticulous wound care and using sterile technique when caring for the catheter and injecting drugs.

Long-term epidural catheters may be placed for terminal cancer patients or patients with certain pain syndromes that are unresponsive to other treatments. If a long-term indwelling epidural catheter is used, bacterial filters are recommended.

Implantable pumps. Intraspinal catheters can be surgically implanted for long-term pain relief. The surgical placement of an intrathecal catheter to a subcutaneously placed pump and reservoir allows for the delivery of drugs directly into the intrathecal space. The pump, which is normally placed in a pocket made in the subcutaneous tissue of the abdomen, may be programmable or fixed.

Changes are made by either reprogramming the pump or changing the mixture or concentration of drug in the reservoir. The pump is refilled every 30 to 90 days depending on flow rate, mixture, and reservoir size.

Patient-controlled analgesia. **Patient-controlled analgesia (PCA)** (demand analgesia) is a method that allows the patient to self-administer preset doses of an analgesic within a prescribed time period by activating an infusion pump. Routes of administration include oral, IV, epidural, inhaled, nasal, and transcutaneous. In acute care, PCA often refers to an electronically controlled infusion pump that delivers the medication by an IV or epidural route (**patient-controlled epidural analgesia [PCEA]**). PCEA often combines an opioid and local anesthetic. PCA can also be adapted for oral administration. With PCA/PCEA, a dose of opioid is delivered when the patient decides a dose is needed. PCA/PCEA uses an infusion system in which the patient pushes a button to receive a bolus infusion of an analgesic. PCA/PCEA is used widely for the management of acute pain, including postoperative pain and cancer pain.

Opioids, such as morphine and hydromorphone, are commonly administered via PCA therapy for acute and chronic pain. Sometimes IV PCA is administered with a continuous or background infusion called a *basal rate,* depending on the patient's opioid requirement. The addition of a basal rate in opioid-naive patients and those at risk for adverse respiratory outcomes (e.g., older age, obstructive sleep apnea, pulmonary disease) may lead to serious respiratory events. Basal rates are often used with epidural catheter pain management. Because the medication is delivered directly into the epidural space, the amount of opioid is 10 times less than is needed by IV route. This lessens the risk of respiratory depression but does not totally eliminate it.

Patient teaching is very important with the use of PCA/PCEA. Help the patient understand the mechanics of getting a drug dose and how to titrate the drug to achieve good pain relief. Teach the patient to self-administer the analgesic before pain is severe. Assure the patient that he or she cannot "overdose" because the pump is programmed to deliver a maximum number of doses per hour. Pressing the button after the maximum dose is administered will not result in additional analgesic. If the maximum doses are inadequate to relieve pain, the pump can be reprogrammed to increase the amount or frequency of dosing. In addition, you can give bolus doses if they are included in the HCP's orders. To make a smooth transition from infusion PCA to oral drugs, the patient should receive increasing doses of oral drug as the PCA analgesic is tapered.

Patient-controlled delivery systems are intended for use by the patient. An *authorized agent controlled analgesia (AACA)* is a method of delivery performed by a consistently available and competent individual for patients who are unable to independently activate PCA devices.[22] This authorized agent must be carefully selected, educated on the principles of PCA, and be capable of recognizing pain and the appropriate times to administer medication via the PCA device. Understand your institution's policies regarding PCA and AACA.

Interventional Therapy

Therapeutic Nerve Blocks. Nerve blocks generally involve one-time or continuous infusion of local anesthetics into a particular area to produce pain relief. These techniques are also called *regional anesthesia.* Nerve blocks interrupt all afferent and efferent transmission to the area and thus are not specific to nociceptive pathways. They include local infiltration of anesthetics into a surgical area (e.g., chest incisions, inguinal hernia) and injection of anesthetic into a specific nerve (e.g., occipital or pudendal nerve) or nerve plexus (e.g., brachial or celiac plexus). Nerve blocks often are used during and after surgery to manage pain. For longer-term relief of chronic pain syndromes, local anesthetics can be administered via a continuous infusion.

Adverse effects of nerve blocks are similar to those for local anesthetics delivered via other systemic routes and include systemic toxicity resulting in dysrhythmias, confusion, nausea and vomiting, blurred vision, tinnitus, and metallic taste. Temporary nerve blocks affect motor function and sensation and typically last 2 to 24 hours, depending on the agent and the site of injection. Motor ability generally returns before sensation.

Neuroablative Techniques. *Neuroablative interventions* are performed for severe pain that is unresponsive to all other therapies. Neuroablative techniques destroy nerves, thereby interrupting pain transmission. Destruction is by surgical resection or thermocoagulation, including radiofrequency coagulation. Neuroablative interventions that destroy the sensory division of a peripheral or spinal nerve are classified as *neurectomies, rhizotomies,* and *sympathectomies.* Neurosurgical procedures that ablate the lateral spinothalamic tract are classified as *cordotomies* if the tract is interrupted in the spinal cord, or *tractotomies* if the interruption is in the medulla or midbrain of the brainstem (Fig. 8-7). Cordotomy and tractotomy can be performed with the aid of local anesthesia by a percutaneous technique under fluoroscopy.

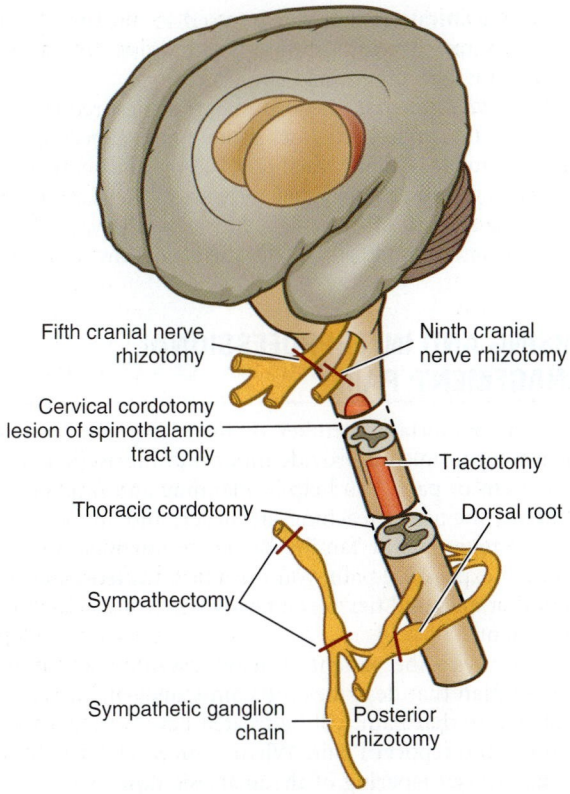

FIG. 8-7 Sites of neurosurgical procedures for pain relief.

TABLE 8-13 Nondrug Therapies for Pain

Physical Therapies	Cognitive Therapies

• Acupuncture
• Application of heat and cold (Table 8-14)
• Exercise
• Massage
• Transcutaneous electrical nerve stimulation (TENS)
	• Distraction
	• Hypnosis
	• Imagery
	• Relaxation strategies (see Chapter 6)
	  • Relaxation breathing
	  • Imagery
	  • Meditation
	  • Art therapy
	  • Music therapy

Neuroaugmentation. *Neuroaugmentation* involves electrical stimulation of the brain and spinal cord. Spinal cord stimulation (SCS) is performed much more often than brain stimulation. The most common use of SCS is for chronic back pain secondary to nerve damage that is unresponsive to other therapies. Other uses include complex regional pain syndrome (CRPS), spinal cord injury pain, and interstitial cystitis. Potential complications include those related to the surgery (bleeding and infection), migration of the generator (which usually is implanted in the subcutaneous tissues of the upper gluteal or pectoralis area), and nerve damage.

Nondrug Therapies for Pain

Nondrug strategies play an important role in pain management (Table 8-13). They can reduce the dose of an analgesic required to relieve pain and thereby minimize side effects of drug therapy. Moreover, they increase the patient's sense of personal control about managing pain and increase coping skills. Some strategies are believed to alter ascending nociceptive input or stimulate descending pain modulation mechanisms (see the section on Perception on p. 106). These nondrug therapies are useful for both acute and chronic pain.

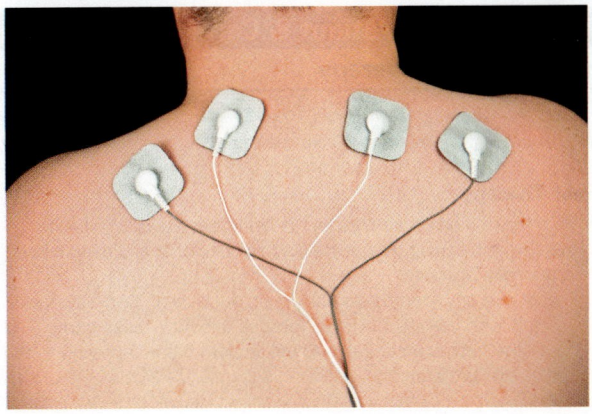

FIG. 8-8 Transcutaneous electrical nerve stimulation (TENS) treatment being given for treatment of pain after shoulder surgery. (©Noel Moore/Hemera/Thinkstock)

Physical Pain Relief Strategies

Massage. Massage is useful for acute and chronic pain. Many different massage techniques exist, including moving the hands or fingers over the skin slowly or briskly with long strokes or in circles (superficial massage) or applying firm pressure to the skin to maintain contact while massaging the underlying tissues (deep massage). Another type is trigger point massage. A **trigger point** is a circumscribed hypersensitive area within a tight band of muscle. It is caused by acute or chronic muscle strain. It feels like a tight knot under the skin. Trigger point massage is performed by applying either strong, sustained digital pressure; deep massage; or gentler massage with ice followed by muscle heating. (Massage is discussed in Chapter 6.)

Exercise. Exercise is an essential part of the treatment plan for patients with chronic pain, particularly those with musculoskeletal pain. Many patients become physically deconditioned as a result of their pain, which in turn leads to more pain. Exercise acts via many mechanisms to relieve pain. It enhances circulation and cardiovascular fitness, reduces edema, increases muscle strength and flexibility, and enhances physical and psychosocial functioning. Tailor an exercise program to the patient's physical needs and lifestyle. It may include aerobic exercise, stretching, and strengthening exercises. The program should be supervised by trained personnel (e.g., physical therapist).

Transcutaneous Electrical Nerve Stimulation. *Transcutaneous electrical nerve stimulation* (TENS) involves the delivery of an electric current through electrodes applied to the skin surface over the painful region, at trigger points, or over a peripheral nerve. A TENS system consists of two or more electrodes connected by lead wires to a small, battery-operated stimulator (Fig. 8-8). Usually a physical therapist is responsible for administering TENS therapy, although nurses can be trained in the technique.

TENS may be used for acute pain, including postoperative pain and pain associated with physical trauma. The effects of TENS on chronic pain are less clear, but it may be effective in these cases.[23]

Acupuncture. Acupuncture is a technique of Traditional Chinese Medicine in which very thin needles are inserted into the body at designated points. Acupuncture is used for many different kinds of pain.

TABLE 8-14 Patient & Caregiver Teaching

Heat and Cold Therapy

Include the following instructions when teaching the patient and caregiver about superficial heat or cold techniques.

Heat Therapy

- Do not use heat on an area that is being treated with radiation therapy, is bleeding, has decreased sensation, or has been injured in the past 24 hours.
- Do not use any menthol-containing products (e.g., Ben-Gay, Vicks, Icy Hot) with heat applications because this may cause burns.
- Cover the heat source with a towel or cloth before applying to the skin to prevent burns.

Cold Therapy

- Cover the cold source with a cloth or towel before applying to the skin to prevent tissue damage.
- Do not apply cold to areas that are being treated with radiation therapy, have open wounds, or have poor circulation.
- If it is not possible to apply the cold directly to the painful site, try applying it right above or below the painful site or on the opposite side of the body on the corresponding site (e.g., left elbow if the right elbow hurts).

Heat Therapy. Heat therapy is the application of either moist or dry heat to the skin. Heat therapy can be either superficial or deep. Superficial heat can be applied using an electric heating pad (dry or moist), a hot pack, hot moist compresses, warm wax (paraffin), or a hot water bottle. To expose large areas of the body, patients can immerse themselves in a hot bath, shower, or whirlpool. Physical therapy departments provide deep-heat therapy through such techniques as short-wave diathermy, microwave diathermy, and ultrasound therapy. Patient and caregiver teaching regarding heat therapy is described in Table 8-14.

Cold Therapy. Cold therapy involves the application of either moist or dry cold to the skin. Dry cold can be applied by means of an ice bag, moist cold by means of towels soaked in ice water, cold hydrocollator packs, or immersion in a bath or under running cold water. Icing with ice cubes or blocks of ice made to resemble Popsicles is another technique used for pain relief. Cold therapy is believed to be more effective than heat for a variety of painful conditions, including acute pain from trauma or surgery, acute flare-ups of arthritis, muscle spasms, and headache. Patient and caregiver teaching regarding cold therapy is described in Table 8-14.

Cognitive Therapies. Techniques to alter the affective, cognitive, and behavioral components of pain include a variety of cognitive strategies and behavioral approaches. For example, patients can identify and challenge negative pain-related thoughts and replace them with more positive coping thoughts. Some of these techniques require little training and often are adopted independently by the patient. For others, a trained therapist is necessary.

Distraction. Distraction involves redirection of attention away from the pain and onto something else. It is a simple but powerful strategy to relieve pain. Distraction can be achieved by engaging the patient in any activity that can hold his or her attention (e.g., watching TV or a movie, conversing, listening to music). It is important to match the activity with the patient's energy level and ability to concentrate.

Hypnosis. Hypnotherapy is a structured technique that enables a patient to achieve a state of heightened awareness and focused concentration that can be used to alter the patient's pain perception. Hypnosis should be administered and monitored only by specially trained clinicians.

Relaxation Strategies. Relaxation strategies reduce stress, decrease acute anxiety, distract from pain, alleviate muscle tension, combat fatigue, facilitate sleep, and enhance the effectiveness of other pain relief measures.[24] Relaxation strategies include relaxation breathing, music, imagery, meditation, muscle relaxation, and art.[25] (These strategies are described in Chapter 6.)

❖ NURSING AND INTERPROFESSIONAL MANAGEMENT: PAIN

You are an important member of the interprofessional pain management team. You provide input into the assessment and reassessment of pain. You help in planning and implementing treatments, including teaching, advocacy, and support of the patient, caregiver, and family. Because patients in any care setting can experience pain, you must be knowledgeable about current therapies and flexible in trying new approaches to pain management.

Together with the patient, develop a written agreement or treatment plan that describes the pain management. The plan should ensure that pain will be treated based on the patient's perception and report of pain. When appropriate, the plan outlines the gradual tapering of the analgesic dose, with eventual substitution of parenteral analgesics with long-acting oral preparations, and possibly cessation of opioids.

Many nursing roles are described earlier in this chapter, including assessing pain, administering treatment, monitoring for side effects, and teaching patients and caregivers. However, the success of these actions depends on your ability to establish a trusting relationship with the patient and caregiver and to address their concerns regarding pain and its treatment.

◆ Effective Communication

Because pain is a subjective experience, patients need to feel confident that their reporting of pain will be believed and will not be perceived as "complaining." The patient and caregiver also need to know that you consider the pain significant and understand that pain may profoundly disrupt a person's life. Communicate concern and commit to helping the patient obtain pain relief and cope with any unrelieved pain. Support the patient and caregiver through the period of trial and error that may be necessary to implement an effective therapeutic plan. It also is important to clarify responsibilities in pain relief. Help the patient understand the role of the interprofessional team members, as well as the patient's roles and expectations.

In addition to addressing specific aspects of pain assessment and treatment, evaluate the impact that the pain has on the lives of the patient and caregiver. Table 8-15 addresses teaching needs of patients and caregivers related to pain management.

◆ Challenges to Effective Pain Management

Common challenges to effective pain management include misunderstandings about tolerance, physical dependence, and addiction. It is important for you to understand and be able to explain these concepts. Table 8-16 lists barriers to pain management and strategies to address them.

◆ **Tolerance.** *Tolerance* occurs with chronic exposure to a variety of drugs. In the case of opioids, tolerance to analgesia is

TABLE 8-15 Patient & Caregiver Teaching

Pain Management

Include the following information in the teaching plan for the patient with pain and caregiver.

- Self-management techniques
- Realistic goals for pain control
- Negative consequences of unrelieved pain
- Need to maintain a record of pain level and effectiveness of treatment
- Treat pain with drugs and/or nondrug therapies before it becomes severe.
- Medication may stop working after it is taken for a period of time, and dosages may have to be adjusted.
- Potential side effects and complications associated with pain therapies can include nausea and vomiting, constipation, sedation and drowsiness, itching, urinary retention, and sweating.
- Need to report when pain is not relieved to tolerable levels

TEAMWORK & COLLABORATION

Pain

Effective pain management should be a focus for all members of the nursing team.

Role of Nursing Personnel

Registered Nurse (RN)

- Assess pain characteristics (pattern and onset, area or location, intensity, quality, associated symptoms, and management strategies).
- Develop treatment plan for patient's pain (including drug and nondrug therapies).
- Evaluate whether current treatment plan is effective.
- Teach patient and caregiver about treatment plan.
- Implement discharge teaching about pain management.

Licensed Practical/Vocational Nurse (LPN/LVN)

- Administer ordered pain medications (consider the state nurse practice act and agency policy, since LPNs may not be able to give medications by all routes).
- Assess patient's pain.

Unlicensed Assistive Personnel (UAP)

- Assist with screening for pain and notify RN if patient expresses pain.
- Take and report vital signs before and after pain medications are given.
- Note and report if patient is refusing to participate in ordered activities such as ambulation (since this may indicate inadequate pain management).

characterized by the need for an increased opioid dose to maintain the same degree of analgesia. Although the development of tolerance to side effects (except constipation) is more predictable, the incidence of clinically significant analgesic opioid tolerance in chronic pain patients is unknown, since dosage needs may increase as the disease (e.g., cancer) progresses. It is essential to assess for increased analgesic needs in patients on long-term therapy. The interprofessional team must evaluate and rule out other causes of increased analgesic needs, such as disease progression or infection.

If significant tolerance to opioids develops and it is believed that an opioid is losing its effectiveness, or intolerable side effects are associated with escalation of doses, the practice of *opioid rotation* may be considered. This involves switching from one opioid to another, assuming that the new opioid will be more effective at lower equianalgesic doses. However, very high opioid doses can result in opioid-induced hyperalgesia (OIH) rather than pain relief. This means that increases in the dose can lead to higher pain levels. (OIH is discussed on p. 115.)

- **Physical Dependence.** Like tolerance, physical dependence is a normal physiologic response to ongoing exposure to drugs. It is manifested by a withdrawal syndrome when the drug is abruptly decreased. Manifestations of opioid withdrawal are listed in Table 8-17. When opioids are no longer needed to provide pain relief, a tapering schedule should be used in conjunction with careful monitoring. A typical tapering schedule may involve reducing the dose by 20% to 50% per day. The goal is to reduce the amount of medication and at the same time minimize adverse and withdrawal effects.
- **Pseudoaddiction.** Inadequate treatment of pain can lead to a phenomenon called *pseudoaddiction*. This occurs when patients exhibit behaviors commonly associated with addiction (e.g., frequent requests for analgesic refills or higher dosages), but the behaviors resolve with adequate treatment of the patient's pain. These patients are often labeled as drug seeking, which can result in mistrust between the patient and HCP. This problem can be avoided by effective communication strategies and optimal pain management.
- **Addiction.** *Addiction* is a complex neurobiologic condition characterized by aberrant behaviors arising from a drive to obtain and take substances for reasons other than the prescribed therapeutic value (see Chapter 10). Tolerance and physical dependence are not indicators of addiction. Rather they are normal physiologic responses to chronic exposure to certain drugs, including opioids. Addiction rarely occurs in patients who receive opioids for pain control. If addiction is suspected, it must be investigated and diagnosed, if appropriate, but it should not be implied without evidence because this interferes with pain management. The hallmarks of addiction include (1) compulsive use, (2) loss of control of use, and (3) continued use despite risk of harm.
- **Risk Monitoring.** Several opioid risk assessments are available to help clinicians assess patient for abuse, misuse, and addiction. A controlled substance agreement for those at risk of addiction may be used. Addiction risk assessment tools such as the Opioid Risk Tool (*www.painmed.org/SOPResources/ClinicalTools*) and the Screener and Opioid Assessment for Patient Pain (*http://nhms.org/sites/default/files/Pdfs/SOAPP-14.pdf*) are available. Patient monitoring with urine drug screens and access to state prescription monitoring programs to track prescriptions are effective in detecting misuse of drugs. The risk of addiction should not prevent HCPs from using opioids to effectively treat moderate to severe acute and chronic pain.

INSTITUTIONALIZING PAIN EDUCATION AND MANAGEMENT

Besides patient and caregiver barriers, other barriers to effective and safe pain management include inadequate HCP education and lack of institutional support. Traditionally, medical and nursing school curricula have spent little time teaching future physicians and nurses about pain and symptom management. The lack of emphasis on pain has contributed to inadequate training of HCPs.

Progress has been made in overcoming these barriers. Medical and nursing schools now devote more time to

TABLE 8-16 Patient & Caregiver Teaching

Reducing Barriers to Pain Management

When teaching the patient and caregiver about pain management, discuss the following barriers.

Barrier	Nursing Considerations
Fear of addiction	• Explain that addiction is uncommon in patients taking opioids for pain.
Fear of tolerance	• Teach that tolerance is a normal physiologic response to chronic opioid therapy. If tolerance does develop, the drug may have to be changed (e.g., morphine in place of oxycodone). • Teach that there is no absolute upper limit to pure opioid agonists (e.g., morphine). Dosages can be increased, and patient should not save drugs for when the pain is worse. • Teach that tolerance develops more slowly to analgesic effects of opioids than to side effects (e.g., sedation, respiratory depression). Tolerance does not develop to constipation. Thus a regular bowel program should be started early.
Concern about side effects	• Teach methods to prevent and to treat common side effects. • Emphasize that side effects such as sedation and nausea decrease with time. • Explain that different drugs have unique side effects, and other pain drugs can be tried to reduce the specific side effect.
Fear of injections	• Explain that oral medicines are preferred. • Emphasize that even if oral route becomes unusable, transdermal or indwelling parenteral routes can be used rather than injections.
Desire to be "good" patient	• Explain that patients are partners in their care and that partnership requires open communication by both patient and nurse. • Emphasize to patients that they have a responsibility to keep you informed about their pain.
Desire to be stoic	• Explain that although stoicism is a valued behavior in many cultures, failure to report pain can result in undertreatment and severe, unrelieved pain.
Forgetting to take analgesic	• Provide and teach use of pill containers. • Provide methods of record keeping for drug use. • Recruit caregivers to assist with the analgesic regimen.
Concern that pain indicates disease progression	• Explain that increased pain or the need for analgesics may reflect tolerance. • Emphasize that new pain may come from a non–life-threatening source (e.g., muscle spasm, urinary tract infection). • Institute drug and nondrug strategies to reduce anxiety. • Ensure that patient and caregivers have current, accurate, comprehensive information about the disease and prognosis. • Provide psychologic support.
Sense of fatalism	• Explain that pain can be managed in most patients. • Explain that most therapies require a period of trial and error. • Emphasize that side effects can be managed.
Ineffective medication	• Teach that there are multiple options within each category of medication (e.g., opioids, NSAIDs), and another medication from the same category may provide better relief. • Emphasize that finding the best treatment regimen often requires trial and error. • Incorporate nondrug approaches in treatment plan.

Adapted from Ersek M: Enhancing effective pain management by addressing patient barriers to analgesic use, *J Hospice Palliat Nurs* 1:87, 1999.
NSAIDs, Nonsteroidal antiinflammatory drugs.

TABLE 8-17 Manifestations of Opioid Withdrawal Syndrome

	Early Response (6-12 Hr)	Late Response (48-72 Hr)
Psychosocial	• Anxiety	• Excitation
Secretions	• Lacrimation • Rhinorrhea • Diaphoresis	• Diarrhea
Other	• Yawning • Piloerection • Shaking, chills • Dilated pupils • Anorexia • Tremor	• Restlessness • Fever • Nausea and vomiting • Abdominal cramping pain • Hypertension • Tachycardia • Insomnia

addressing pain. Numerous professional organizations have published evidence-based guidelines for assessing and managing pain in many patient populations and clinical settings.

Institutional commitment and practices are changing clinical practice. One major step in institutionalizing pain management is the development and adoption of The Joint Commission (TJC) guideline on pain.[26] TJC is the accrediting body for most health care facilities (hospitals, nursing homes, and health care clinics). Under these standards, health care facilities are required to (1) recognize the patient's right to appropriate assessment and management of pain; (2) identify pain in patients during their initial assessment and as needed, during ongoing, periodic reassessments; (3) educate HCPs about pain assessment and management and ensure competency; and (4) educate patients and their families about pain management.

ETHICAL ISSUES IN PAIN MANAGEMENT

Fear of Hastening Death by Administering Analgesics

A common concern of health care professionals and caregivers is that providing a sufficient amount of drug to relieve pain will

BECOMING A NURSE LEADER

Impaired Nurse

Situation

You are a nurse on a very busy postsurgical cardiac care unit. Although Mr. Zeller is not your patient, you answer his call light while his nurse Bill is off the unit. Mr. Zeller is complaining of severe pain from his surgical site, stating he is not receiving relief from his pain medication. You check the medication administration record and notice that it is charted that he received morphine IV 30 minutes ago. You find this very strange and ask Bill about it when he returns from his break. Bill dismisses you and says that Mr. Zeller has a low pain tolerance. After you return from your break, Bill tells you that your patient Mrs. Zink is still complaining of severe pain, although he gave her morphine IV 15 minutes ago. While packing up to leave for the day, you notice Bill taking two syringes out of his pocket and throwing them in the hazardous waste container.

Points for Consideration

- As an advocate for the patient, nurses must be alert to and take appropriate action regarding any instances of incompetent, unethical, illegal, or impaired practice by any member of the health care team.[1]
- When nurses are aware of inappropriate or questionable practice in the provision or denial of health care, express your concern to the person carrying out the questionable practice.
- When the welfare of the patient is threatened, similar action should be directed to the responsible administrator and/or higher authority within the institution, or to an appropriate external authority.[1]
- About 1 in 10 nurses may be impaired or in recovery from alcohol or drug addiction. Nurses' overall pattern of dependency is unique because they have greater access to drugs in the workplace.[2]
- Nurses must educate themselves about the signs, symptoms, and behaviors that characterize substance abuse. It may be difficult to suspect a co-worker, and the fear of retaliation may keep some nurses from action. It is important to take steps to confront or notify the nurse manager of your suspicions.
- Do not allow yourself to be manipulated or fear confronting a nurse if patient safety is in jeopardy.[2]
- Substance-abusing nurses most likely will not seek treatment until confronted by peers, family, or nursing management, or if their job is in jeopardy. Those who do enter and complete structured treatment programs can be successful and reenter the profession of nursing.

Discussion Questions

1. Based on your suspicions of Bill, what action will you take first?
2. Do you have enough evidence to report Bill to your supervisor?
3. What responsibility do you have to Bill's patients?

References

1. American Nurses Association (ANA): Code of ethics for nurses with interpretive statements: Provision 3. Retrieved from *www.nursingworld.org/provision-3.*
2. Thomas CM, Siela D: The impaired nurse: would you know what to do if you suspected substance abuse? Retrieved from *www.americannursetoday.com/the-impaired-nurse-would-you-know-what-to-do-if-you-suspected-substance-abuse.*

hasten or precipitate death of a terminally ill person. However, there is no scientific evidence that opioids can hasten death, even among patients at the very end of life. Moreover, you have a moral obligation to provide comfort and pain relief at the end of life. Even if there is a concern about the possibility of hastening death, the rule of double effect provides ethical justification. This rule states that if an unwanted consequence (i.e., hastened death) occurs as a result of an action taken to achieve a moral good (i.e., pain relief), the action is justified if the nurse's intent is to relieve pain and not to hasten death.

Requests for Assisted Suicide

Unrelieved pain is one of the reasons that patients make requests for assisted suicide. Aggressive and adequate pain management may decrease the number of such requests. Assisted suicide is a complex issue that extends beyond pain and pain management. Physician-assisted suicide is legal in some states (e.g., Oregon, Washington). To address the legal and ethical issues confronting nurses in this unique situation, the Oregon Nurses Association prepared a position paper on this topic.[27]

Use of Placebos in Pain Assessment and Treatment

Placebos are still sometimes used to assess and treat pain. Using a placebo involves deceiving patients by making them believe that they are receiving an analgesic when in fact they are typically receiving an inert substance such as saline. The use of placebos to assess or treat pain is condemned by several professional organizations.

Gerontologic Considerations: Pain

Persistent pain is a common problem in older adults and is often associated with physical disability and psychosocial problems. The prevalence of chronic pain among community-dwelling older adults exceeds 50%, and among older nursing home patients, it is approximately 80%. The most common painful conditions among older adults are musculoskeletal conditions such as osteoarthritis and low back pain. Chronic pain often results in depression, sleep disturbance, decreased mobility, increased health care utilization, and physical and social role dysfunction. Despite its high prevalence, pain in older adults is often inadequately assessed and treated.

Several barriers to pain assessment in the older patient exist. Older adults and their HCPs often believe that pain is a normal, inevitable part of aging and that nothing can be done to relieve the pain. Older adults may not report pain for fear of being a "burden" or a "complainer." They may fear taking opioids. In addition, older patients are more likely to use words such as "aching," "soreness," or "discomfort" rather than "pain." Be persistent in asking older adults about pain. Carry out the assessment in an unhurried, supportive manner.

Another barrier is the increased prevalence of cognitive, sensory-perceptual, and motor problems that interfere with a person's ability to process information and communicate. Examples include dementia and delirium, poststroke aphasia, and other communication barriers. Hearing and vision deficits may complicate assessment. Therefore pain assessment tools may have to be adapted for older adults. For example, it may be necessary to use a large-print pain intensity scale. Most older adults, even those with mild to moderate cognitive impairment, can use quantitative scales accurately and reliably.

In older patients with chronic pain, perform a thorough physical examination and history to identify causes of pain, possible therapies, and potential problems. Also assess for depression and functional impairments, because they are also common among older adults with pain.

Treatment of pain in older adults is complicated by several factors. First, older adults metabolize drugs more slowly than younger people and thus are at greater risk for higher blood levels and adverse effects. The adage "start low and go slow" must be applied to analgesic therapy in this age group. Second, the use of NSAIDs in older adults is associated with a high frequency of GI bleeding. Third, older adults often are taking many drugs for one or more chronic conditions. The addition of analgesics can result in dangerous drug interactions and increased side effects. Fourth, cognitive impairment and ataxia can be exacerbated by analgesics such as opioids, antidepressants, and antiseizure drugs. This requires that HCPs titrate drugs slowly and monitor carefully for side effects.

Treatment regimens for older adults must incorporate nondrug modalities. Exercise and patient teaching are important nondrug interventions for older adults with chronic pain. Also include family and caregivers in the treatment plan (Tables 8-15 and 8-16).

MANAGING PAIN IN SPECIAL POPULATIONS

Patients Unable to Self-Report Pain

Although the patient's self-report is the gold standard of pain assessment, many illnesses and conditions affect a patient's ability to report pain. These diagnoses and conditions include dementia and delirium. For these people, behavioral and physiologic changes may be the only indicators of pain. You must be astute at recognizing behavioral symptoms of pain.

A guide for assessing pain in nonverbal patients is presented in Table 8-18. Several scales have been developed to assess pain-related behaviors in nonverbal patients, particularly those with advanced dementia and the critically ill. Several pain assessment tools for people with dementia are available at the City of Hope Pain and Palliative Care Resource Center website *(http://prc.coh.org)*.

Patients With Substance Abuse Problems

HCPs are often reluctant to administer opioids to patients at risk for addiction or those with substance-abuse disorders for fear of promoting or worsening addictions. However, there is no evidence that providing opioid analgesia to these patients in any way worsens their addictive disease. In fact, the stress of unrelieved pain may contribute to relapse in the recovering patient or increased drug use in the patient who is actively abusing drugs.

TABLE 8-18 Assessing Pain in Nonverbal Patients

The following assessment techniques are recommended.

- Obtain a self-report when possible.
- Never assume a nonverbal person is unable to communicate pain in some manner as blinking, writing, hand gestures, or nodding can be ways to express pain or the absence of pain.
- Investigate potential causes of pain.
- Observe patient behaviors that indicate pain (e.g., grimacing, frowning, rubbing a painful area, groaning, restlessness).
- Obtain surrogate reports of pain from professional and family caregivers.
- Try to use analgesics and reassess the patient to observe for a decrease in pain-related behaviors.

Modified from Herr K, Coyne PJ, McCaffery M, et al: Position statement from the American Society for Pain Management Nursing (ASPMN). Pain assessment in the patient unable to self-report: position statement with clinical practice recommendations, *Pain Manag Nurs* 12:230, 2011.

CHECK YOUR PRACTICE

A 36-yr-old male patient is recovering from abdominal surgery to remove his spleen after an automobile accident. He is a known drug user. You are taking care of him and he is very irritable because he is not getting enough pain medication. You are reluctant to give him his PRN morphine as you are afraid you will contribute to his addiction problem.

- What should you do?

Guidelines for pain management in patients with addictive disease have been established by the American Society for Pain Management Nursing (ASPMN). These guidelines reflect your role in a team approach in which patients with addictive disease and pain have the right to be treated with dignity, respect, and the same quality of pain assessment and management as all other patients.

If the patient acknowledges substance abuse, determine the types and amounts of drugs used. Avoid exposing the patient to the drug of abuse, and effective equianalgesic doses of other opioids may be determined if daily drug doses are known. If a history of drug abuse is unknown or if the patient does not acknowledge substance abuse, suspect abuse when normal doses of analgesics do not relieve the patient's pain.

Aggressive behavior patterns and signs of withdrawal may also occur. Withdrawal symptoms can exacerbate pain and lead to drug-seeking behavior or illicit drug use. Toxicology screens may be helpful in determining recently used drugs. Discussing these findings with the patient may help gain the patient's cooperation in pain control.

Severe pain should be treated with opioids and at much higher doses than those used with drug-naive patients. The use of a single opioid is preferred. Avoid using a mixed opioid agonist-antagonist such as butorphanol or a partial agonist such as buprenorphine because these drugs may precipitate withdrawal symptoms. Nonopioid and adjuvant analgesics and nondrug pain relief measures may also be used as appropriate. To maintain opioid blood levels and prevent withdrawal symptoms, provide analgesics around the clock. Use supplemental doses to treat breakthrough pain. IV or PCA infusions may be considered for acute pain management.

Pain management for people with addiction is challenging and requires an interprofessional team approach. When possible, the team includes pain management and addiction specialists. Team members need to be aware of their own attitudes about people with substance abuse problems, which may result in undertreatment of pain.

CASE STUDY

Pain

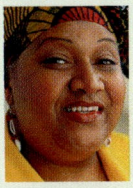

(©Ryan McVey/ Photodisc/ Thinkstock)

Patient Profile

K.C. is a 280-lb (127-kg) 68-year-old African American woman with diabetes who was admitted for an incision and drainage of a right abdominal abscess. She is being discharged on her second postoperative day. Her daughter will assist with dressing changes at home.

Subjective Data

- Lives alone
- Desires 0 pain but will accept 1 or 2 on a scale of 0 to 10
- Reports incision area pain as a 2 or 3 between dressing changes and as a 6 during dressing changes
- States sharp pain persists 1 to 2 hours after dressing change
- Reports pain between dressing changes controlled by two Percocet tablets
- Has history of fibromyalgia and is complaining of pain "everywhere"

Objective Data

- Requires qid dressing changes after discharge
- For discharge, Percocet (two tablets q4hr for pain PRN) is prescribed.

Discussion Questions

1. Describe the assessment data that are important for determining whether K.C. has adequate pain management.
2. How long should the daughter wait after the Percocet is given to begin the dressing change?
3. ***Patient-Centered Care:*** What additional pain therapies might you plan to help K.C. through the dressing change?
4. ***Priority Decision:*** What are the priority nursing interventions for K.C.?
5. ***Safety:*** What side effects might she experience because of her pain medication? How can these be safely managed?
6. ***Teamwork and Collaboration:*** To whom can you delegate teaching K.C. and her daughter the plan of care at home?
7. ***Priority Decision:*** Based on the data presented, what are the priority nursing diagnoses? Are there any collaborative problems?
8. ***Evidence-Based Practice:*** K.C.'s daughter asks you if any other strategies could be used to help decrease her mother's incisional pain and her overall fibromyalgia pain.

Answers available at *http://evolve.elsevier.com/Lewis/medsurg.*

BRIDGE TO NCLEX EXAMINATION

The number of the question corresponds to the same-numbered outcome at the beginning of the chapter.

1. Pain is *best* described as
   a. a creation of a person's imagination.
   b. an unpleasant, subjective experience.
   c. a maladaptive response to a stimulus.
   d. a neurologic event resulting from activation of nociceptors.
2. A patient is receiving a PCA infusion after surgery to repair a hip fracture. She is sleeping soundly but awakens when the nurse speaks to her in a normal tone of voice. Her respirations are 8 breaths/minute. The *most* appropriate nursing action in this situation is to
   a. stop the PCA infusion.
   b. obtain an oxygen saturation level.
   c. continue to closely monitor the patient.
   d. administer naloxone and contact the physician.
3. Which words are *most* likely to be used to describe neuropathic pain *(select all that apply)*?
   a. Dull
   b. Mild
   c. Burning
   d. Shooting
   e. Shock-like
4. Unrelieved pain is
   a. expected after major surgery.
   b. expected in a person with cancer.
   c. dangerous and can lead to many physical and psychologic complications.
   d. an annoying sensation, but it is not as important as other physical care needs.
5. A cancer patient who reports ongoing, constant moderate pain with short periods of severe pain during dressing changes is
   a. probably exaggerating his pain.
   b. best treated by referral for surgical treatment of his pain.
   c. best treated by receiving a long-acting and a short-acting opioid.
   d. best treated by regularly scheduled short-acting opioids plus acetaminophen.
6. An example of distraction to provide pain relief is
   a. TENS.
   b. music.
   c. exercise.
   d. biofeedback.
7. Appropriate nonopioid analgesics for mild pain include *(select all that apply)*
   a. oxycodone.
   b. ibuprofen (Advil).
   c. lorazepam (Ativan).
   d. acetaminophen (Tylenol).
   e. codeine with acetaminophen (Tylenol #3).
8. An *important* nursing responsibility related to pain is to
   a. leave the patient alone to rest.
   b. help the patient appear to not be in pain.
   c. believe what the patient says about the pain.
   d. assume responsibility for eliminating the patient's pain.
9. Providing opioids to a dying patient who is experiencing moderate to severe pain
   a. may cause addiction.
   b. will probably be ineffective.
   c. is an appropriate nursing action.
   d. will likely hasten the person's death.

10. A nurse believes that patients with the same type of tissue injury should have the same amount of pain. This statement reflects
- **a.** a belief that will contribute to appropriate pain management.
- **b.** an accurate statement about pain mechanisms and an expected goal of pain therapy.
- **c.** a belief that will have no effect on the type of care provided to people in pain.
- **d.** a lack of knowledge about pain mechanisms, which is likely to contribute to poor pain management.

1. b, 2. c, 3. c, d, e, 4. c, 5. c, 6. b, 7. b, d, 8. c, 9. c, 10. d.

For rationales to these answers and even more NCLEX review questions, visit *http://evolve.elsevier.com/Lewis/medsurg.*

EVOLVE WEBSITE

http://evolve.elsevier.com/Lewis/medsurg

Review Questions (Online Only)

Key Points

Answer Keys for Questions

- Rationales for Bridge to NCLEX Examination Questions
- Answer Guidelines for Case Study on p. 127

Student Case Study

- Patient With Pain

Conceptual Care Map Creator

Audio Glossary

Content Updates

REFERENCES

1. Institute of Medicine Report from the Committee on Advancing Pain Research, Care, and Education: *Relieving pain in America: a blueprint for transforming prevention, care, education, and research*, Washington, DC, 2011, National Academies Press.
2. American Cancer Society. Retrieved from *http://www.cancer.org/research/survivaltreatmentresearch/palliative-care-research.*
3. McCaffery M: *Nursing practice theories related to cognition, bodily pain and man-environmental interactions*, Los Angeles, 1968, UCLA Students Store. (Classic)
4. Richardson P: Spirituality, religion and palliative care, *Ann Palliat Med* 3:150, 2014.
5. Sturgeon JA, Zautra AJ: Psychological resilience, pain catastrophizing, and positive emotions: perspectives on comprehensive modeling of individual pain adaptation, *Curr Pain Headache Rep* 17:317, 2013.
6. Mifflin KA, Kerr BJ: The transition from acute to chronic pain: understanding how different biological systems interact, *Can J Anaesth* 61:112, 2014.
7. Kerstman E, Ahn S, Battu S, et al: Neuropathic pain, *Handb Clin Neurol* 110:175, 2013.
8. Pelletier R, Higgins J, Bourbonnais D: Is neuroplasticity in the central nervous system the missing link to our understanding of chronic musculoskeletal disorders? *BMC Musculoskelet Disord* 12:25, 2015.
9. Mogil JS: Pain genetics: past, present and future, *Trends Genet* 28:258, 2012.

*10. van Hecke O, Austin SK, Khan RA, et al: Neuropathic pain in the general population: a systematic review of epidemiological studies, *Pain* 155:654, 2014.

*11. Bean DJ, Johnson MH, Kydd RR: The outcome of complex regional pain syndrome type 1: a systematic review, *J Pain* 15:677, 2014.

12. Herr K, Bjoro K, Decker S: Tools for assessment of pain in nonverbal older adults with dementia: a state-of-the-science review, *J Pain Symptom Manage* 31:170, 2006. (Classic)
13. Bashir MS, Khade A, Borkar P, et al: A comparative study between different pain rating scales in patients with osteoarthritis, *Indian J Physiol Pharmacol* 57:205, 2013.

*14. Gordon DB, Dahl J, Phillips P, et al: The use of "as-needed" range orders for opioid analgesic in the management of acute pain: a consensus statement of the American Society of Pain Management Nurses and the American Pain Society, *Pain Manag Nurs* 5:53, 2004. (Classic)

*15. de Leon-Casasola O: A review of the literature on multiple factors involved in postoperative pain course and duration, *Postgrad Med* 126:42, 2014.

16. Prabhakar A, Mancuso KF, Owen CP, et al: Perioperative analgesia outcomes and strategies, *Best Pract Res Clin Anesthesiol* 28:105, 2014.

*17. dela Cruz Ubaldo C, Hall NS, Le B: Postmarketing review of intravenous acetaminophen dosing based on Food and Drug Administration prescribing guidelines, *Pharmacotherapy* 34(Suppl 1):34S, 2014.

*18. Weimer MB, Chou R: Research gaps on methadone harms and comparative harms: findings from a review of the evidence for an American Pain Society and College on Problems of Drug Dependence clinical practice guideline, *J Pain* 15:366, 2014.

*19. Jungquist CR, Pasero C, Tripoli NM, et al: Instituting best practice for monitoring for opioid-induced advancing sedation in hospitalized patients, *Worldviews Evid Based Nurs* 11:350, 2014.

*20. Maguire DR, France CP: Impact of efficacy at the μ-opioid receptor on antinociceptive effects of combinations of μ-opioid receptor agonists and cannabinoid receptor agonists, *J Pharmacol Exp Ther* 35:383, 2014.

21. Simon SM, Schwartzberg LS: A review of rapid-onset opioids for breakthrough pain in patients with cancer, *J Opioid Manag* 10:207, 2014.

*22. Cooney MF, Czarnecki M, Dunwoody C, et al: American Society for Pain Management Nursing position statement with clinical practice guidelines: authorized agent controlled analgesia, *Pain Manag Nurs* 14:176, 2013.

23. Song JJ, Popescu A, Bell RL: Present and potential use of spinal cord stimulation to control chronic pain, *Pain Physician* 17:235, 2014.

*24. Shengelia R, Parker SJ, Ballin M, et al: Complementary therapies for osteoarthritis: are they effective? *Pain Manag Nurs* 14:e274, 2013.

*25. Crawford C, Lee C, Bingham J: Active Self-Care Therapies for Pain (PACT) Working Group: Sensory art therapies for the self-management of chronic pain symptoms, *Pain Med* 15(Suppl 1):S66, 2014.

26. The Joint Commission: Standard on pain assessment and management. Retrieved from *www.jointcommission.org.*
27. Oregon Nurses Association: ONA provides guidance on nurses' dilemma. Retrieved from *http://c.ymcdn.com/sites/www.oregonrn.org/resource/resmgr/imported/Assisted%20Suicide%20Adjusted.pdf.*

*Evidence-based information for clinical practice.

9

Palliative Care at End of Life

Linda A. L. Upchurch

You matter because you are you. You matter to the last moment of your life, and we will do all we can, not only to help you die peacefully, but also to live until you die.

Dame Cicely Saunders

http://evolve.elsevier.com/Lewis/medsurg/

LEARNING OUTCOMES

1. Discuss the purpose of palliative care.
2. Describe the purpose of and services provided by hospice.
3. Describe the physical and psychologic manifestations at the end of life.
4. Explain the process of grief and bereavement at the end of life.
5. Describe the nursing management of the dying patient.
6. Examine the cultural and spiritual issues related to end-of-life care.
7. Discuss vulnerable populations in end-of-life care.
8. Discuss ethical and legal issues in end-of-life care.
9. Explore the special needs of family caregivers in end-of-life care.
10. Discuss the special needs of the nurse who cares for dying patients and their families.

KEY TERMS

advance directives, p. 135
bereavement, p. 133
brain death, p. 131
Cheyne-Stokes respiration, p. 132
death, p. 131
death rattle, p. 132
end of life, p. 132
grief, p. 133
hospice, p. 130
palliative care, p. 129
spirituality, p. 134

PALLIATIVE CARE

Palliative care is any form of care or treatment that focuses on reducing the severity of disease symptoms. The overall goals of palliative care are to (1) prevent and relieve suffering and (2) improve quality of life for patients with serious life-limiting illnesses[1] (Fig. 9-1). Specific goals of palliative care are listed in Table 9-1.

Ideally all patients receiving curative or restorative health care should receive palliative care at the same time. Palliative care extends into the period of end-of-life (EOL) care. Bereavement care follows the patient's death (Fig. 9-2).

Palliative care originated as EOL care in the 1960s. Initially this care focused on providing the relief of symptoms and emotional support to the patient, family, and significant others during the terminal phases of a serious life-limiting disease. Now that phase of palliative care is called palliative care at the end of life, which is the focus of this chapter.

The role of palliative care at the end of life is increasing in our current health care environment. Demographic changes in the population are increasing the demand for palliative care. For example, there are growing numbers of Baby Boomers turning 65. At the same time improvements in health care technology have led to longer life expectancies and an increased number of older adults. Older adults often have multiple chronic illnesses resulting in increased health care utilization.[2] Palliative care has been shown to (1) improve quality of life for those with chronic illness, (2) decrease the associated economic costs for their health care, and (3) alleviate the burden of caregivers for those with chronic and terminal illnesses.[3]

To optimize the benefits of palliative care, it should be initiated after a person receives a diagnosis of a life-limiting illness,

TABLE 9-1 Goals of Palliative Care

- Regard dying as a normal process.
- Provide relief from symptoms, including pain.
- Affirm life and neither hasten nor postpone death.
- Support holistic patient care and enhance quality of life.
- Offer support to patients to live as actively as possible until death.
- Offer support to the family during the patient's illness and in their own bereavement.

Adapted from World Health Organization: WHO definition of palliative care. Retrieved from *www.who.int/cancer/palliative/definition/en.*

Reviewed by Ellen Odell, DNP, ACNS-BC, CNE, APRN, Director of Nursing, Associate Professor, Department of Nursing, John Brown University, Siloam Springs, Arkansas; and Mary Ellen Tresgallo, DNP, MPH, FNP-BC, Assistant Professor of Nursing, Columbia University School of Nursing, New York, New York.

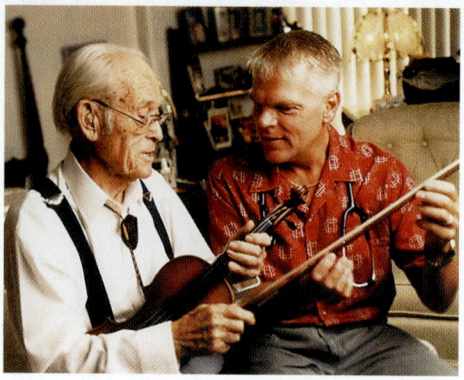

FIG. 9-1 One goal of palliative care is to improve the quality of the patient's remaining life. (Courtesy Kathleen A. Pollard, RN, MSN, CHPN, Phoenix, Ariz.)

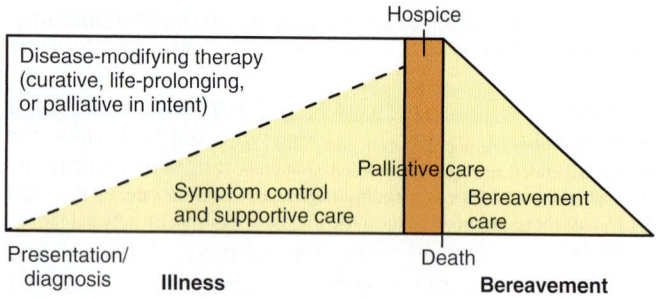

FIG. 9-2 Continuum of care model showing integration of curative care, palliative and end-of-life/hospice care, and bereavement care. (Redrawn from Robert Wood Johnson Foundation: *The EPEC Project: Elements and models of end-of-life care*, 1999.)

such as cancer, heart failure, chronic obstructive pulmonary disease, dementia, or end-stage kidney disease. The palliative care team is an interprofessional collaboration involving physicians, nurses, social workers, pharmacists, chaplains, and other health care professionals. Communication among the patient, family, and interprofessional palliative team is important to provide optimal care. Patients may receive palliative care services in multiple settings, including the home, long-term and acute care, mental health facilities, rehabilitation centers, and prisons. Many institutions have established interprofessional palliative and hospice care teams.[1]

HOSPICE CARE

Palliative care often includes hospice care before or at the end of life (Fig. 9-3). **Hospice** is not a place but a concept of care that provides compassion, concern, and support for persons in the last phases of a terminal disease (Fig. 9-4). The main goals of hospice care are to assist the patient to live fully as comfortable as possible and to die pain free and with dignity.[4] Hospice programs provide care with an emphasis on symptom management, advance care planning, spiritual care, and family support.

The major difference between palliative care and hospice care is that palliative care allows a person to simultaneously receive curative and palliative treatments. Hospice care is provided when the physician determines a person has 6 months or less to live, and that person or health care proxy decides to forgo curative treatments. Hospice is often underutilized, as many assume the person must be actively dying before hospice is necessary. On the contrary, it is important that the person be

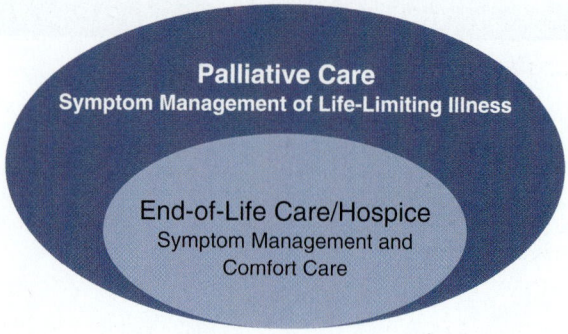

FIG. 9-3 Relationship of palliative care and end-of-life care/hospice. (From Rosenberg M, Lamba S, Misra S: Palliative medicine and geriatric emergency care: challenges, opportunities, and basic principles, *Clin Geriatr Med* 29[1]:1, 2013.)

referred to hospice as soon as possible to facilitate palliation of physical, emotional, and spiritual distress so common at the end of life.

Approximately 1.5 million patients every year receive services through hospice programs. Almost half of the patients who die in the United States are under the care of a hospice program. More than three quarters of persons in hospice programs are over the age of 65 years, and the majority are white. The most common diagnoses are cancer and heart disease. Currently the median length of stay in a hospice program is 21 days.[4]

Hospice programs are organized under a variety of models. Some are hospital-based programs, others are part of existing home health care agencies, and others are freestanding or community-based programs. However, regardless of their organization, all hospice programs emphasize palliative rather than curative care, and quality rather than quantity of life.

Like palliative care, hospice care is provided in a variety of locations, including the home, inpatient settings, acute and long-term care facilities, and rehabilitation centers. Hospice services are available 24 hours a day, 7 days a week to provide help to patients and families in their homes. Inpatient hospice settings often have a relaxed and homelike atmosphere as much as possible (Fig. 9-5). Staff and volunteers are available for the patient and family.

A medically supervised interprofessional team and volunteers provide holistic hospice services. The hospice nurse plays a pivotal role in coordination of the hospice team.[5] Hospice nurses work with other interprofessional team members to provide care and support to the patient and family. Hospice

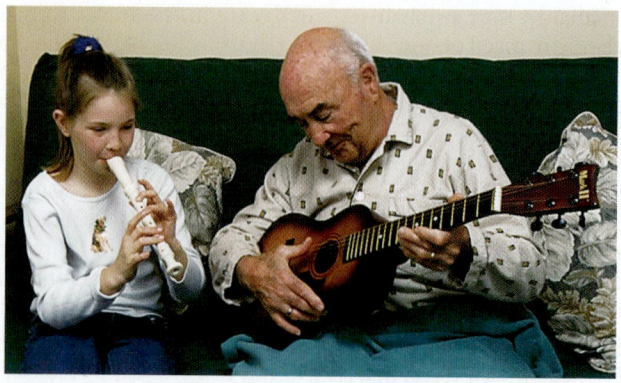

FIG. 9-4 Hospice care is designed to provide compassion, concern, and support for the dying. (From Rick Brady, Riva, Md.)

EVIDENCE-BASED PRACTICE

Translating Research Into Practice

Does Home Palliative Care Affect Odds of Dying at Home?

Clinical Question

In adults with advanced disease (P) what is the effect of home palliative care (I) versus usual care (C) on odds of dying at home, caregiver outcomes, and cost-effectiveness (O)?

Synthesis of Best Available Evidence

- Systematic review of randomized controlled trials (RCTs), controlled clinical trials (CCTs), controlled before and after studies (CBAs), and interrupted time series (ITSs)
- 23 studies of family caregivers (n = 4042) and patients (n = 37,561) mainly with advanced cancer. Palliative care was specialized with home-based care teams for patients and/or family caregivers. Usual care included community, hospital, home health, and hospice care. Caregiver outcomes were (1) burden in last weeks of care and (2) grief after the patient's death.
- Although >50% of people worldwide prefer to die at home, less than 33% of all deaths take place at home.
- Specialized palliative home care almost doubled the odds of the patient's death occurring at home. There was no difference in caregiver grief when specialized care was compared to usual care from the time the patient died to 13 months later.
- Conflicting evidence exists if palliative home care reduces caregiver burden or is cost effective.

Conclusions

- Home palliative team care increases the likelihood of the patient dying at home compared to usual care.
- It is inconclusive if palliative home care is cost effective or affects caregiver outcomes.

Implications for Nursing Practice

1. How would you help patients who are undecided about palliative home care and yet desire to die at home?
2. What information would you provide caregivers who are concerned that palliative home care will result in greater grief related to the patient's death?

Reference for Evidence

Gomes B, Calanzani N, Curiale V, et al: Effectiveness and cost-effectiveness of home palliative care services for adults with advanced illness and their caregivers, *Cochrane Database Syst Rev* 6:CD007760, 2013.

P, Patient population of interest; *I*, intervention or area of interest; *C*, comparison of interest or comparison group; *O*, outcomes of interest; *T*, timing (see p. 15).

nurses are educated in pain control and symptom management, spiritual assessment, and assessment and management of family needs. To meet patient and family needs, the hospice nurse needs excellent teaching skills, compassion, flexibility, cultural competence, and adaptability.

The decision to begin hospice care is difficult for several reasons. Frequently patients, families, physicians, and other HCPs lack information about hospice care. Some cultural/ethnic groups may underutilize hospice because of lack of awareness of hospice services, desire to continue with potentially curative therapies, and concerns about lack of minority hospice workers.[6] Physicians may be reluctant to give referrals because they sometimes view a patient's decline as their personal failure. Some patients or family members see it as giving up.

It is important for you to consider potential barriers to hospice care in vulnerable populations. These may include

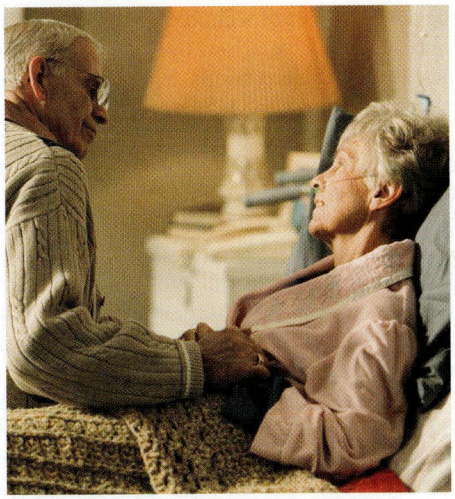

FIG. 9-5 Inpatient hospice settings have been deinstitutionalized to make the atmosphere as relaxed and homelike as possible. (©Photodisc/Thinkstock)

veterans, homeless, immigrants, impoverished, disabled, or institutionalized persons. In these populations, besides the hospice team, you may need to collaborate with community partners to facilitate supportive services to meet everyday needs of the patient and family.[7]

Hospice services are covered by Medicare, Medicaid, and many private insurance agencies. Admission to a hospice program has two criteria. The first criterion is that the patient must desire the services and agree in writing that only hospice care (and not curative care) can be used to treat the terminal illness. Patients in hospice programs can withdraw from the program at any time (e.g., if their condition unexpectedly improves). Patients can receive care for other health problems that are not related to the terminal illness. However, those services may not be covered by the hospice, Medicare, Medicaid, or by the patient's insurance company.[8]

The second criterion is that the patient must be considered eligible for hospice. Medicare, Medicaid, and other insurers require that two physicians certify that the patient's prognosis is terminal, with less than 6 months to live. After this initial certification, only one physician (e.g., the hospice medical director) is needed to recertify the patient. It is important to realize that the physician who certified that a hospice patient is terminal does not "guarantee" death within 6 months. If a patient in hospice survives beyond 6 months, Medicare and other reimbursement organizations will continue to reimburse for more extended periods of treatment if the patient still meets enrollment criteria.

Occasionally, a patient's condition stabilizes, at which time the patient may be discharged from hospice care. This decision is made after review of the current treatment plan and input from members of the interprofessional hospice team.

DEATH

Death occurs when all vital organs and body systems cease to function. It is the irreversible cessation of cardiovascular, respiratory, and brain function.

Brain death is an irreversible loss of all brain functions, including those of the brainstem. Brain death is a clinical diagnosis, and it occurs when the cerebral cortex stops functioning or is irreversibly destroyed.[9]

Since the development of technology that assists in supporting life, controversies have arisen over the exact definition of death. Questions and discussions have focused on whether brain death occurs when the whole brain (cortex and brainstem) ceases activity or when function of the cortex alone stops. The American Academy of Neurology developed the diagnostic criteria guidelines for clinical diagnosis of brain death. These criteria for brain death include coma or unresponsiveness, absence of brainstem reflexes, and apnea. Specific assessments by a physician are required to validate each of the criteria.[9]

Currently, legal and medical standards require that all brain function must cease for brain death to be pronounced and life support to be disconnected. Diagnosis of brain death is of particular importance when organ donation is an option. In some states and under specific circumstances, registered nurses are legally permitted to pronounce death. Policies and procedures may vary from state to state and among health care institutions.

END-OF-LIFE CARE

End of life generally refers to the final phase of a patient's illness when death is imminent. The time from diagnosis of a terminal illness to death varies considerably, depending on the patient's diagnosis and extent of disease.

The Institute of Medicine defines *end of life* as the period during which an individual copes with declining health from a terminal illness or from the frailties associated with advanced age, even if death is not clearly imminent.[10] In some cases it is obvious to HCPs that the patient is at the end of life, but in other cases they may be uncertain if the end is close at hand. This uncertainty adds to the challenge of answering common questions the patient and family may ask, such as, "How much time is left?"

End-of-life care (EOL care) is the term used for issues and services related to death and dying. EOL care focuses on physical and psychosocial needs for the patient and family. The goals for EOL care are to (1) provide comfort and supportive care during the dying process, (2) improve the quality of the patient's remaining life, (3) help ensure a dignified death, and (4) provide emotional support to the family.

Physical Manifestations at End of Life

As death approaches, metabolism is reduced and the body gradually slows down until all functions end. Respiratory changes are common at the end of life. Respirations may be rapid or slow, shallow, and irregular. Breath sounds may become wet and noisy, both audibly and on auscultation. Noisy, wet-sounding respirations, termed the **death rattle** or terminal secretions, are caused by mouth breathing and accumulation of mucus in the airways. **Cheyne-Stokes respiration** is a pattern of breathing characterized by alternating periods of apnea and deep, rapid breathing. When respirations cease, the heart stops beating within a few minutes. The physical manifestations of approaching death are listed in Table 9-2.

Psychosocial Manifestations at End of Life

A variety of feelings and emotions can affect the dying patient and family at the end of life (Table 9-3). Most patients and families struggle with a terminal diagnosis and the realization that there is no cure. The patient and family may feel overwhelmed, fearful, powerless, and fatigued. The family's response

TABLE 9-2 Physical Manifestations at End of Life

System	Manifestations
Sensory system	
Hearing	• Usually last sense to disappear
Touch	• Decreased sensation • Decreased perception of pain and touch
Taste and smell	• Decreased with disease progression
Sight	• Blurring of vision • Sinking and glazing of eyes • Blink reflex absent • Eyelids remain half-open
Cardiovascular system	• Increased heart rate; later slowing and weakening of pulse • Irregular rhythm • Decreased BP • Delayed absorption of drugs administered IM or subcutaneously
Respiratory system	• Increased respiratory rate • Cheyne-Stokes respiration (pattern of respiration characterized by alternating periods of apnea and deep, rapid breathing) • Inability to cough or clear secretions resulting in grunting, gurgling, or noisy congested breathing (death rattle or terminal secretions) • Irregular breathing, gradually slowing down to terminal gasps (may be described as guppy breathing)
Urinary system	• Gradual decrease in urine output • Incontinence of urine • Inability to urinate
Gastrointestinal system	• Slowing or cessation of GI function (may be enhanced by pain-relieving drugs) • Accumulation of gas • Distention and nausea • Loss of sphincter control, producing incontinence • Bowel movement before imminent death or at time of death
Musculoskeletal system	• Gradual loss of ability to move • Sagging of jaw resulting from loss of facial muscle tone • Difficulty speaking • Swallowing becoming more difficult • Difficulty maintaining body posture and alignment • Loss of gag reflex • Jerking seen in patients on high doses of opioids
Integumentary system	• Mottling on hands, feet, arms, and legs • Cold, clammy skin • Cyanosis of nose, nail beds, knees • "Waxlike" skin when very near death

TABLE 9-3 Psychosocial Manifestations at End of Life

- Altered decision making
- Anxiety about unfinished business
- Decreased socialization
- Fear of loneliness
- Fear of meaninglessness of one's life
- Fear of pain
- Helplessness
- Life review
- Peacefulness
- Restlessness
- Saying goodbyes
- Unusual communication
- Vision-like experiences
- Withdrawal

TABLE 9-4 Kübler-Ross Model of Grief

Stage	What Person May Say	Characteristics
Denial	No, not me. It cannot be true.	Denies the loss has taken place and may withdraw. This response may last minutes to months.
Anger	Why me?	May be angry at the person who inflicted the hurt (even after death) or at the world for letting it happen. May be angry with self for letting an event (e.g., car accident) take place, even if nothing could have stopped it.
Bargaining	Yes me, but ...	May make bargains with God, asking, "If I do this, will you take away the loss?"
Depression	Yes me, and I am sad.	Feels numb, although anger and sadness may remain underneath
Acceptance	Yes me, but it is okay.	Anger, sadness, and mourning have tapered off. Accepts the reality of the loss

Adapted from Kübler-Ross E: *On death and dying*, New York, 1969, Macmillan. (Classic)

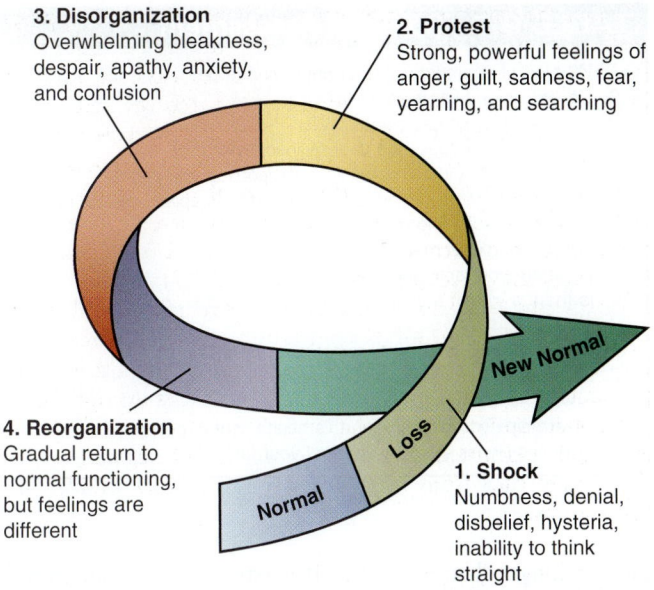

FIG. 9-6 The grief wheel model begins with the normal state at the bottom. After a person goes through the grief process, eventually the grief will resolve. However, because of the loss, the normal state is not the same as before. The challenge is to accept the "new normal." (Adapted from Stress Free Living by Trevor Powell with permission from DK, a division of Penguin Random House LLC. Copyright © 2000 Dorling Kindersley Limited.)

depends in part on the type and length of the illness and their relationship with the person.

The patient's needs and wishes must be respected. Patients need time to think and express their feelings. Response time to questions may be sluggish because of fatigue, weakness, and confusion.

Bereavement and Grief

Although the terms are often used interchangeably, *bereavement* refers to the state of loss, and *grief* refers to the reaction to loss. **Bereavement** is the period following the death of a loved one during which grief is experienced and mourning occurs. The time spent in bereavement depends on a number of factors, including how attached one was to the person who died and how much time was spent anticipating the loss.

Grief is a normal reaction to loss. Grief occurs in response to the real loss of a loved one and the loss of what might have been. Grief is dynamic and includes both psychologic and physiologic responses following a loss. Psychologic responses include anger, guilt, anxiety, sadness, depression, and despair. Physiologic reactions include sleeping problems, changes in appetite, physical problems, and illness.

Grief is a powerful emotional state that affects all aspects of a person's life. It is a complex and intense emotional experience. In the Kübler-Ross model of grief, there are five stages[11] (Table 9-4). Not every person experiences all the stages of grieving, and they are not always progressive. It is common to reach a stage and then go backward. For example, a person may have reached the stage of bargaining and then revert to the denial or anger stage.

Another model of grief is the grief wheel (Fig. 9-6). After a person experiences the loss, he or she feels *shock* (numbness, denial, inability to think straight). Next is the *protest* stage, in which a person experiences anger, guilt, sadness, fear, and searching. Then comes the *disorganization* stage, in which a person feels despair, apathy, anxiety, and confusion. The next stage is *reorganization*, in which a person gradually returns to normal functioning, but he or she feels different. The final stage is the *new normal*. Eventually the destabilization experienced in grief resolves and a normal state can begin. However, because of the loss, the normal state is not the same as before. The challenge is to accept the new normal. Trying to go back to the "old" normal (which is not there anymore) is what causes a great deal of anxiety and stress.

The manner in which a person grieves depends on factors such as the relationship with the person who has died (e.g., spouse, parent), physical and emotional coping resources, concurrent life stresses, cultural beliefs, and personality. Additional factors that affect the grief response include mental and physical health, economic resources, religious influences or spiritual beliefs, family relationships, social support, and time spent preparing for the death. Issues that occurred before the death (e.g., marital problems) may affect the grief response.[12]

The grief experience for the caregiver of the patient with a chronic illness often begins long before the actual death event. This is called *anticipatory grief*. Patients at the end of life can also experience anticipatory grief.

Working in a positive way through the grief process helps to adapt to the loss.[12] Grief that assists the person in accepting the reality of death is called *adaptive grief*, which is a healthy response. It may be associated with grieving before a death actually occurs or when the inevitability of the death is known. Indicators of adaptive grief include the ability to see some good resulting from the death and positive memories of the deceased person.

Dysfunctional reactions to loss can occur, and the physical and psychologic impact of the loved one's death may persist for years. *Prolonged grief disorder*, formerly called *complicated grief*, is a term used to describe prolonged and intense mourning. Prolonged grief disorder can include symptoms such as recurrent and severe distressing emotions and intrusive thoughts related to the loss of a loved one, self-neglect, and denial of the

TABLE 9-5 Spiritual Assessment

1. Who or what provides you strength and hope?
2. Do you use prayer in your life?
3. How do you express spirituality?
4. How would you describe your philosophy of life?
5. What type of spiritual or religious support do you desire?
6. What is the name of your clergy, minister, chaplain, pastor, rabbi?
7. What does suffering mean to you?
8. What does dying mean to you?
9. What are your spiritual goals?
10. Is there a role of a church, synagogue, mosque, or temple in your life?
11. Has belief in God been important in your life?
12. How does your faith help you cope with illness?
13. How do you keep going day after day?
14. What helps you get through this health care experience?
15. How has illness affected you and your family?

Copyright The Joint Commission. Adapted with permission.

loss for longer than 6 months. It is estimated that one in five bereaved individuals experiences prolonged grief disorder. Those who experience prolonged grief disorder are at great risk for illness and may have work and social impairments.[13]

Bereavement and grief counseling are core components of patient- and family-centered palliative care. The goal of a bereavement program is to provide support and to assist survivors in the transition to a life without the deceased person. Incorporate grief support into the plan of care for the family and significant others during the patient's illness and after the death.

Priority interventions for grief must focus on providing an environment that allows the patient and family to express their feelings, such as anger, fear, and guilt. Discussion of feelings helps the patient and family work toward resolution of the grief process. Respect for the patient's privacy and need or desire to talk (or not to talk) is important. Honesty in answering questions and giving information is essential.

Spiritual Needs

Assessment of spiritual needs in EOL care is a key consideration (Table 9-5). Spiritual needs do not necessarily equate to religion. **Spirituality** is defined as those beliefs, values, and practices that relate to the search for existential meaning and purpose. It may or may not include a belief in a higher power.[14] A person may not be part of a particular religion but have a deep spirituality. Many times at the end of life, patients question their beliefs about a higher power, their journey through life, religion, and an afterlife (Fig. 9-7). Some patients may choose to pursue a spiritual path. Some may not. Respect an individual's choice. Assess the patient's and family's preferences related to spiritual guidance or pastoral care services and make appropriate referrals.

Deep-seated spiritual beliefs may surface for some patients when they deal with their terminal diagnosis and related issues. Spiritual distress may occur.[15] Characteristics of spiritual distress include anger toward God or a higher being, change in behavior and mood, desire for spiritual assistance, or displaced anger toward clergy.

Spirituality has been associated with decreased despair in patients at the end of life. Some dying patients are secure in their faith about the future. It is common to observe patients relinquishing material possessions of life and focusing on values

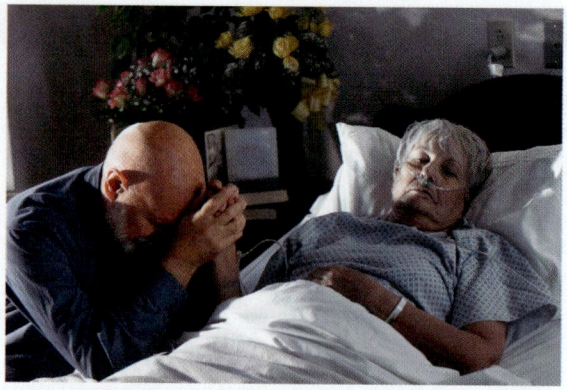

FIG. 9-7 Spiritual needs are an important consideration in end-of-life care. (©Photodisc/Thinkstock)

that they believe will lead them on to another place. Many turn to religion because it may provide order to the world even in the presence of physical decline, social losses, suffering, and impending death. Religion may offer an existential meaning that offers a sense of peace and recognition of one's place in the broader cosmic context.[15]

Culturally Competent Care: End of Life

Culture and ethnicity are important considerations for patients who are receiving palliative and EOL care and their families. Cultural beliefs affect a person's understanding of and reaction to death or loss. In some cultural/ethnic groups, death and dying are private matters shared only with significant others. Often feelings are repressed or internalized. People who believe in "toughing it out" or "being strong" may not express themselves when they are experiencing a loss. Some cultural groups, such as African Americans and Hispanic/Latinos, may easily express their feelings and emotions. Kinship tends to be strong in the Hispanic culture, and immediate and extended family provide support for one another. Expressing feelings of loss is encouraged and accepted easily.[16]

If palliative or hospice care is recommended, some cultural/ethnic groups are less likely to use these resources. For example, African Americans use hospice care less often because they value "toughness" in times of hardship. For Hispanics, often spouses and daughters are involved in decisions regarding palliative care and hospice.[16]

Consider patient attitudes toward death and suffering and preferences for information. The decision to use palliative care or hospice services may be perceived as "giving up" or receiving second-rate care. Such attitudes are best approached through clear, open discussions with the patient and family about the philosophy and services of palliative and hospice organizations. Culture and ethnicity affect decision making with regard to life support and withholding and withdrawing of treatments.[17] In some cultures, such as the Filipino American culture, it may be appropriate to first discuss a terminal diagnosis with the family before informing the patient.

Rituals associated with dying are part of all cultures.[16] In certain cultures the family may want to keep constant vigil in the room of a dying patient or in the waiting area. For example, some Jewish Americans believe that the spirit should not be alone when it leaves the body at the time of death. Therefore someone who is terminally ill should never be left alone. The

Jewish culture believes all body tissues must be buried with the individual. Once a death has occurred, some cultures, such as the Puerto Rican American culture, may want to kiss and touch the body to say goodbye. In the Islamic cultures the traditional rites of washing, shrouding, funeral prayers, and burial are done as soon as possible.

Families with non–English-speaking members are at risk for receiving less information about their family member's critical illness and prognosis.[18] Cultural variations also exist in symptom expression (e.g., pain expression) and use of health care services. Providing culturally competent care requires assessment of nonverbal cues such as grimaces, body position, and decreased or guarded movements. Issues related to pain assessment and management are discussed in Chapter 8.

Many differences exist among cultural beliefs and values in relation to death and dying. Your assessment of beliefs and preferences should be made on an individual basis to avoid stereotyping individuals with different cultural belief systems. This includes assessing and documenting the patient's cultural background, concerns, health practices, and attitudes about suffering. Early in the assessment, ask the patient and family to describe their desires for care before death and care of the body after death. Use open-ended questions related to the patient's perspectives on his or her illness and the patient's expectations of care. Use this assessment to guide the patient's plan of care and evaluation. You can also suggest or plan grief and bereavement counseling for the family. Accommodations must be made related to the patient's language, diet, and cultural beliefs and practices. When appropriate, access medical interpreter services so that the patient's wishes are known. (Culturally competent care is discussed in Chapter 2.)

LEGAL AND ETHICAL ISSUES AFFECTING END-OF-LIFE CARE

Patients and families struggle with many decisions during the terminal illness and dying experience. Many people decide that the outcomes related to their care should be based on their own wishes and values. It is important to provide information to assist patients with these decisions. The decisions may involve the choice for (1) organ and tissue donations, (2) advance directives (e.g., medical power of attorney, living wills), (3) resuscitation, (4) mechanical ventilation, and (5) feeding tube placement.

Decisional capacity refers to the ability to consent or refuse care. It means that the individual has an understanding and appreciation of the information that is shared and has the capacity to engage in the reasoning process.

Organ and Tissue Donation

Persons who are legally competent may choose organ donation. Any body part or the entire body may be donated. The decision to donate organs or to provide anatomic gifts may be made by a person before death or by immediate family after death. Family permission must be obtained at the time of donation.[19]

Some people carry donor cards. Some states allow organ donation to be marked on drivers' licenses. The names of agencies that handle organ donation vary by state and community. Common names for such an agency may be the organ bank, organ-sharing network, and organ-sharing alliance. Organ and tissue donations follow specific legal guidelines. Legal requirements and facility policies for organ or tissue donation must be followed. The physician must be notified immediately when organ donation is intended, because some tissues must be used within hours after death.

Advance Care Planning and Advance Directives

Advance care planning is a process that involves having patients (1) think through their values and goals for treatment, (2) talk about their values and goals with others, and (3) document them. **Advance directives** are the written documents that provide information about the patient's wishes and his or her designated spokesperson (Table 9-6).

The first advance directive was known by laypersons as a *living will.* Most states have replaced the idea of living wills with *natural death acts,* which may include *directive to physicians* (DTPs), *durable power of attorney for health care* (DPAHC), *medical power of attorney* (MPOA), and *power of attorney for health care* (POAH). Under the natural death acts, an individual can tell the physician exactly what treatment is or is not desired. Each state has its own unique requirements. Keep in mind that patients often change their minds about desired treatments as their disease state progresses. Therefore it is important to reassess a patient's advance directives. For cognitively impaired older adults, consider the person's values and manner of life to make health care decisions consistent with decisions they made when they were cognitively intact.

Copies of state-specific forms can be obtained from local medical associations and on the Internet. However, a person may write his or her wishes without special forms. Verbal directives may be given to physicians with specific instructions in the presence of two witnesses. Based on this directive, the physician may use a Physician Order for Life-Sustaining Treatment (POLST) or Medical Order for Life-Sustaining Treatment (MOLST) to outline current treatment options that honor the person's desire for treatment (Table 9-6).

The person retains a copy of the order to be used in the case of any emergency in which the primary physician is not readily available for consultation. Attorneys and notaries may not be required in the development of these directives. If the person is not capable of communicating his or her wishes, the surrogate decision maker (most often family or significant other) determines the measures that will or will not be taken. In this case, the physician and nurse can discuss the options that are available with the family. Then it is important to document the family's decision. This is important because often nurses and other medical professionals do not know who can legally make EOL decisions for patients when they no longer have decisional capacity.

Resuscitation

Cardiopulmonary resuscitation (CPR) has become common practice in health care. Patients who have respiratory or cardiac arrest are given CPR unless a *do-not-resuscitate (DNR) order* is given by the physician. A DNR order is a written medical order that documents a patient's wishes regarding resuscitation and, more important, the patient's desire to avoid CPR.[20]

The patient or family has the right to decide whether CPR will be used. It is no longer the sole decision of the physician. The American Nurses Association (ANA) supports the patient's right to self-determination and believes that nurses have a primary role in supporting the patient and family's decisions.[21]

TABLE 9-6 Common Documents Used in End-of-Life Care

Document	Description	Special Considerations
Advance directive	General term used to describe documents that give instructions about future medical care and treatments and who should make the decisions in the event the person is unable to communicate	• Should comply with guidelines established by state of residence
Allow Natural Death (AND)	Written order acknowledging that comfort measures only are being provided to patient. Used in many palliative care and hospice settings to indicate that patient wants to die naturally with dignity and comfort	• In many settings may be used in conjunction with DNR terminology to ensure patient/family wishes for advance directives are followed (DNR/AND)
Directive to physicians (DTP)	Written document specifying the patient's wish to be allowed to die without heroic or extraordinary measures	• Indicates specific measures to be used or withheld
Do not resuscitate (DNR)	Written physician's order instructing HCPs not to attempt CPR. DNR order often requested by family	• Must indicate any specific measures to be used or withheld. Must be signed by a physician to be valid
Power of attorney for health care (POAH)	Term used by some states to describe a document used for listing the person(s) to make health care decisions should a patient become unable to make informed decisions for self	• May be the same as medical power of attorney • Indicates specific measures to be used or withheld
Living will	Lay term used to describe any documents that give instructions about future medical care and treatments or the wish to be allowed to die without heroic or extraordinary measures should the patient be unable to communicate for self	• Must identify specific treatments that a person wants or does not want at end of life
Medical power of attorney (MPOA)	Term used by some states to describe a document used for listing the person(s) to make health care decisions should a patient become unable to make informed decisions for self	• May be the same as durable power of attorney for health care, health care proxy, or appointment of a health care agent or surrogate. Specifies measures to be used or withheld • Person appointed may be called a health care agent, surrogate, attorney-in-fact, or proxy.
Physician Order for Life-Sustaining Treatment (POLST) or Medical Order for Life-Sustaining Treatment (MOLST)	A standardized physician order guided by the patient's medical condition and based upon personal preferences verbalized by patient or expressed in advance directive	• Only for those whose illness may limit life to less than 12 months • Guides current treatments. Differs from advance directive, which guides future treatments • Physician completes form based on discussion with patient or authorized representative, or in review of advance directive. Signed by physician, patient, or patient representative • Printed on bright pink paper

CPR, Cardiopulmonary resuscitation.

A physician's order should be written concerning the patient's or family's wishes for the use of CPR. Several different types of CPR decisions can be made. Complete and total heroic measures, which may include CPR, drugs, and mechanical ventilation, can be referred to as a *full code.* Some people choose variations of the full code. A *chemical code* involves the use of drugs for resuscitation without the use of CPR. A "no code," or a DNR order, allows the person to die with comfort measures only and without the interference of technology. Some states have implemented a form called *out-of-hospital DNR* for use by terminally ill patients who wish to have no heroic measures used to prolong life after they leave an acute care facility.[22]

Allow Natural Death (AND) is a term being used to replace "no code" or DNR. This term more accurately conveys what actually happens. It is also sometimes referred to as *"comfort measures only"* status, meaning that all comfort measures associated with pain control and symptom management are carried out, but the natural physiologic progression to death is not delayed or interrupted. The use of this type of language means that care is not withheld, but rather is supportive while allowing nature to take its course. It is meant to promote comfort and dignity at the end of life.

Withholding or withdrawing treatments must be included in an advance directive. The directive must clearly state what is to be done and what is not to be done. The ANA position statement states that the decision to withhold artificial nutrition and hydration should be made by the patient or surrogate together with the interprofessional team.[21] For patients who are no longer receiving artificial nutrition and hydration, it is important to continue to provide expert nursing care.

You need to be aware of legal issues and the patient's wishes. Advance directives and organ donor information should be located in the medical record and identified on the patient's record and/or the nursing care plan. All caregivers responsible for the patient need to know the patient's wishes. Additionally, you are responsible for becoming familiar with state, local, and agency procedures in EOL care documentation.

Euthanasia is the deliberate act of hastening death. The ANA statement on active euthanasia states that the nurse should not participate in active euthanasia, because such an act is in direct violation of the Code for Nurses, ethical traditions and goals of the profession, and its covenant with society.

Physician-assisted suicide is legal in some states. In this case, the physician provides the means and/or information about how the patient can commit suicide. As a nurse, you have an obligation to provide timely, humane, comprehensive, and compassionate EOL care. Euthanasia should not be confused with *palliative sedation,* which is the use of medications to intentionally produce sedation to relieve intractable symptoms and distress in a patient who is imminently dying.[5] The intent of palliative sedation is to relieve pain and suffering and not to shorten life or to hasten death, as is the case with euthanasia.

The use of opioids for symptom management at the end of life is often misunderstood and feared by patients, families, and HCPs. For this reason, many patients refuse to take the medications, which leads to physical and emotional suffering due to uncontrolled pain and symptoms. Your ethical obligation is to relieve suffering, which includes giving medications that have the potential of producing harm, such as with opioids. The *principle of double effect* refers to a principle that regards it morally permissible to give a medication that has the potential for harm if it is given with the intent of relieving pain and suffering and not intended to hasten death.[5]

As a nurse, your role is to teach the patient and family about addiction and tolerance to and dependence on medications. The person with terminal illness should not be concerned with addiction when the goal of treatment is comfort. Pain management is discussed in Chapter 8.

❖ NURSING MANAGEMENT: END OF LIFE

Nurses spend more time with patients near the end of life than any other health care professionals. Nursing care of terminally ill and dying patients is holistic and encompasses all psychosocial and physical needs. Respect, dignity, and comfort are important for the patient and family. Although there is no cure for the person's disease, the treatment plan still consists of assessment, planning, implementation, and evaluation. The main difference is that the focus of care is on the management of the symptoms of the disease, not necessarily the disease itself. Additionally, nurses who care for the dying need to recognize their own needs when dealing with grief and dying.

◆ Nursing Assessment

Assessment of the terminally ill or dying patient varies with the patient's condition. Be sensitive and do not impose repeated, unnecessary assessments on the dying patient. When possible, use health history data that are available in the medical record rather than tiring the patient with an interview.

Document the specific event or change that brought the patient into the health care setting. Record the patient's medical diagnoses, medication profile, and allergies.

If the patient is alert, do a brief review of the body systems. Assess for discomfort, pain, nausea, and dyspnea so that prompt interventions can be implemented using evidence-based tools for symptom assessment. These include numeric scales or visual analog scales for pain rating. In addition, evaluate and manage co-morbidities or acute episodes of problems such as diabetes mellitus or headache. Elicit information about the patient's abilities, food and fluid intake, patterns of sleep and rest, and response to the stress of terminal illness. Assess the patient's ability to cope with the diagnosis and prognosis of the illness. Also determine the family's capacity to manage the needed care and to cope with the illness and its consequences.

The physical assessment is abbreviated and focuses on changes that accompany terminal illness and the specific disease process.[23] The frequency of assessment depends on the patient's stability, but assessment is performed at least every 8 hours in the institutional setting. For patients cared for in their homes by hospice programs, assessment may occur weekly. As changes occur, assessment and documentation may have to be completed more frequently. If the patient is in the final hours of life, the physical assessment may be limited to essential data.

Key elements of a social assessment include determining the relationships and patterns of communication among the family. If multiple family members are present, listen to concerns from different members. Differences in expectations and interpersonal conflict can produce disruptions during the dying process and after the death of the loved one. Social assessment also includes evaluating the goals of the patient and family.

As death approaches, monitor the patient for multiple systems that often are failing during the EOL period. This requires vigilance and attention to physical changes that are often subtle. Neurologic assessment is especially important and

ETHICAL/LEGAL DILEMMAS

End-of-Life Care

Situation

A.P. is a terminally ill 50-year-old woman with metastatic breast cancer who has been hospitalized with severe bone pain. She moans at rest and verbalizes severe pain from any movement to reposition her. The present dose of IV morphine is not adequately controlling her pain. At the team conference the nurses discuss the need for more effective pain control but are concerned that additional pain medicine could hasten her death.

Ethical/Legal Points for Consideration

- Adequate pain relief is an important outcome for all patients, especially patients who are terminally ill.
- The *Code of Ethics for Nurses* addresses the responsibility of the nurse to relieve suffering and have conversations with patients and families about pain and symptom management.[1]
- The *principle of beneficence* means that care is provided to benefit patients. The goal of adequate pain control in the terminally ill to alleviate suffering is based on the *principle of nonmaleficence* (preventing or reducing harm to the patient). The secondary effect of hastening the patient's death is ethically justified and known as the *double effect*.
- Legally, the *standard of care* is used to define the nursing acts that are required for safe and competent nursing practice. When the actual nursing care falls below the standard of care, it is considered negligent and unsafe, and the nurse is at risk for being found incompetent.
- In a court of law, the standard of care in nursing is determined by nursing experts and evidence-based practices. The increasing use of technology to access the latest scientific findings is changing the standard of nursing care to a national, if not global, standard defined by research findings and nationally recognized expert testimony. Standards for providing expert nursing care and counseling at end of life are available.[1]
- In A.P.'s situation the standard of care is that the patient will experience pain relief. Failure of the nurse to act assertively to achieve pain relief for the patient and failure to effectively use resources to obtain that pain relief will be considered below the standard of care and unsafe and incompetent practice.

Discussion Questions

1. What types of discussions need to occur among the health care team, patient, and family as the terminally ill patient approaches this phase of care?
2. Distinguish between promotion of comfort and relief of pain in dying patients, and between assisted suicide and euthanasia.

Reference

1. Code of Ethics for Nurses: *www.nursingworld.org/MainMenuCategories/EthicsStandards/Ethics-Position-Statements.*

includes level of consciousness, presence of reflexes, and pupil responses. Evaluation of vital signs, skin color, and temperature indicates changes in circulation. Monitor and describe respiratory status, character and pattern of respirations, and characteristics of breath sounds. Monitor nutritional and fluid intake, urine output, and bowel function, since this provides assessment data for renal and gastrointestinal functioning. Assess skin condition on an ongoing basis, because skin becomes fragile and may easily break down.

In the last hours of life, assessments should be limited to only those that are needed to determine patient comfort. Assessment of pain and respiratory status may be the most important during this time. It may be more peaceful and comforting to the patient and family to refrain from overstimulation that may occur from certain types of assessments, such as measuring BP or checking for pupillary response. As death approaches, your efforts may be better spent providing emotional support to the patient and family rather than performing tasks that will have no impact on the patient's physical care.

Planning

The patient and family need to be involved in planning and coordinating EOL care. In some cases, a family conference may be helpful to develop a coordinated plan of care.

Develop a comprehensive plan to support, teach, and evaluate patients and families. Nursing care goals during the last stages of life involve comfort and safety measures and care of the patient's emotional and physical needs. These goals may also include determining where the patient would like to die and whether this is possible. For example, the patient may want to die at home, but the family may object. Many factors contribute to the patient and family's decision. Interprofessional EOL care that includes the physician, social worker, chaplain, as well as other members of the palliative and/or hospice care team is important. Advocate for the patient so that his or her wishes are met as much as possible.

The last hours or days of the patient experiencing brain death (e.g., from trauma) are frequently spent in the ICU. Planning for EOL care may be particularly challenging in the ICU environment. At this time, some families are approached about organ donation. Consultation from palliative care specialists may help the family plan and cope with EOL issues.

Nursing Implementation

Psychosocial care and physical care are interrelated for both the dying patient and family. Teaching them is an important part of EOL care. Families need ongoing information on the disease, the dying process, and any care that will be provided. They need information on how to cope with the many issues during this period of their lives. Denial and grieving may be barriers to learning and understanding at the end of life for both the patient and family.

Psychosocial Care. As death approaches, respond appropriately to the patient's psychosocial manifestations at the end of life (Table 9-7).

Anxiety and Depression. Patients often exhibit signs of anxiety and depression during the EOL period. Anxiety is an uneasy feeling whose cause is not easily identified. Anxiety is frequently related to fear.

Causes of anxiety and depression may include uncontrolled pain and dyspnea, psychosocial factors related to the disease process or impending death, altered physiologic states, and drugs used in high dosages. Encouragement, support, and teaching decrease some of the anxiety and depression. Management of anxiety and depression may include both medications and nonpharmacologic interventions. Relaxation strategies such as relaxation breathing, muscle relaxation, music, and imagery may be useful (see Chapter 6).

Anger. Anger is a common and normal response to grief. A grieving person cannot be forced to accept the loss. The surviving family members may be angry with the dying loved one who is leaving them. Encourage the expression of feelings, but at the same time realize how difficult it is to come to terms with loss. As a nurse, you may be the target of the anger. You need to understand what is happening and not react on a personal level.

Hopelessness and Powerlessness. Feelings of hopelessness and powerlessness are common during the EOL period. Encourage realistic hope within the limits of the situation. Allow the patient and family to deal with what is within their control, and help them to recognize what is beyond their control. When

TABLE 9-7 Nursing Management

Psychosocial Care at End of Life

Characteristic	Nursing Management
Withdrawal	
Patient near death may seem withdrawn from the physical environment, maintaining the ability to hear but unable to respond.	Converse as though the patient were alert, using a soft voice and gentle touch.
Unusual Communication	
This may indicate that an unresolved issue is preventing the dying person from letting go. Patient may become restless and agitated or perform repetitive tasks (may also indicate terminal delirium).	Encourage the family to talk with and reassure the dying person.
Vision-Like Experiences	
Patient may talk to persons who are not there or see places and objects not visible. Vision-like experiences assist the dying person in coming to terms with meaning in life and transition from it.	Affirm the dying person's experience as a part of transition from this life.
Saying Goodbyes	
It is important for the patient and family to acknowledge their sadness, mutually forgive one another, and say goodbye.	Encourage the dying person and family to verbalize their feelings of sadness, loss, forgiveness and to touch, hug, cry. Allow the patient and family privacy to express their feelings and comfort one another.
Spiritual Needs	
Patient or family may request spiritual support, such as the presence of a chaplain.	Assess spiritual needs. Allow patient to express his or her spiritual needs. Encourage visit by appropriate spiritual care service provider, chaplain, or family member.

possible, support the patient's involvement in decision making about care to foster a sense of control and autonomy.

- ***Fear.*** Fear is a typical feeling associated with dying. Four specific fears associated with dying are fear of pain, fear of shortness of breath, fear of loneliness and abandonment, and fear of meaninglessness.
- **Fear of pain.** Many people assume that pain always accompanies death. Physiologically, there is no absolute indication that death is always painful. Psychologically, pain may occur based on the anxieties and separations related to dying. Terminally ill patients who do experience physical pain should have pain-relieving drugs available. Assure the patient and family that drugs will be given promptly when needed and that side effects of drugs can and will be managed. Reassessment of pain after medications are given is an important nursing action. Patients can participate in their own pain relief by discussing pain relief measures and their effects. Most patients want their pain relieved without the side effects of grogginess or sleepiness. Pain relief measures do not have to deprive the patient of the ability to interact with others.
- **Fear of shortness of breath.** Respiratory distress and dyspnea are common near the end of life. The sensation of air hunger results in anxiety for the patient and family. Current therapies include opioids, bronchodilators, and oxygen, depending on the cause of the dyspnea. Anxiety-reducing agents (e.g., anxiolytics) may help produce relaxation.
- **Fear of loneliness and abandonment.** Most terminally ill and dying people fear loneliness and do not want to be alone. Many dying patients are afraid that loved ones who are unable to cope with the patient's imminent death will abandon them. The simple presence of someone provides support and comfort (Fig. 9-8). Holding hands, touching, and listening are important nursing interventions. Providing companionship allows the dying person a sense of security.
- **Fear of meaninglessness.** Fear of meaninglessness leads people to review their lives. They review their intentions during life, examining actions and expressing regrets about what might have been. *Life review* helps patients recognize the value of their lives. Assist patients and their families in identifying the positive qualities of the patient's life. Practical ways of helping may include looking at photo albums or collections of important mementos. Sharing thoughts and feelings may enhance spirituality and provide comfort for the patient at this time. Respect and accept the practices and rituals associated with the patient's life review while remaining nonjudgmental.[24]

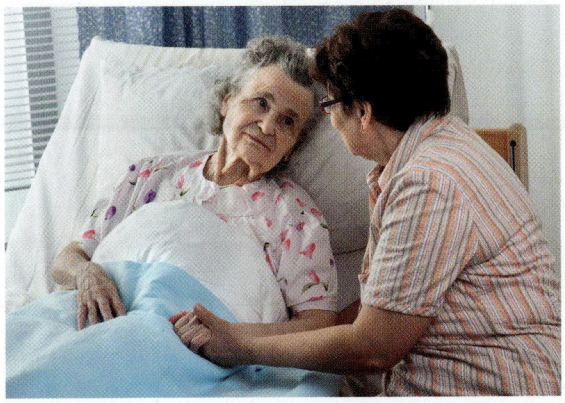

FIG. 9-8 Dying patients typically want someone whom they know and trust to stay with them. (©iStockphoto/Thinkstock)

- ***Communication.*** Communication among the interprofessional team, patient, and family is essential at the end of life. Empathy and active listening are essential components of communication in EOL care. *Empathy* is the identification with and understanding of another's situation, feelings, or motives. *Active listening* is paying attention to what is said, observing the patient's nonverbal cues, and not interrupting.

  There may be silence. Frequently silence is related to the overwhelming feelings experienced at the end of life. Silence can also allow time to gather thoughts. Listening to the silence sends a message of acceptance and comfort. Communication also must be respectful of the patient's ethnic, cultural, and religious backgrounds.

  Patients and family members may have difficulties expressing themselves emotionally. Allow time for them to express their feelings and thoughts. Make time to listen and interact in a sensitive way to enhance the relationship among you, the patient, and the family. A family conference is one way to create a more conducive environment for communication.

  Prepare family members for changes in emotional and cognitive function that occur at the end of life. Unusual communication by the patient may take place at the end of life. The patient's speech may become confused, disoriented, or garbled. Patients may speak to or about family members or others who have predeceased them, give instructions to those who will survive them, or speak of projects yet to be completed. Active, careful listening allows for the identification of specific patterns in the dying person's communication and decreases the risk for inappropriate labeling of behaviors.
- **Physical Care.** Nursing management related to physical care at the end of life focuses on symptom management and comfort rather than treatment for curing a disease or disorder (Table 9-8). The priority is meeting the patient's physiologic and safety needs. Physical care focuses on the needs for oxygen, nutrition, pain relief, mobility, elimination, and skin care. People who are dying deserve and require the same physical care as people who are expected to recover. If possible, it is important to discuss with the patient and family the goals of care before treatment begins. An advance directive should be completed so that the patient and family wishes are followed.
- ***Postmortem Care.*** After the patient is pronounced dead, prepare or delegate preparation of the patient's body for immediate viewing by the family with consideration for cultural customs and in accord with state law and agency policies and procedures. In some cultures and in some types of death, it may be important to allow the family to prepare or assist in caring for the patient's body. In general, close the patient's eyes, replace dentures, wash the body as needed (placing pads under the perineum to absorb urine and feces), and remove tubes and dressings (if appropriate). The patient's body is straightened, leaving the pillow to support the head and prevent pooling of blood and discoloration of the face.

  Allow the family privacy and as much time as they need with the deceased person. When the death is unexpected or unanticipated, preparation of the patient's body for viewing or release to a funeral home depends on state law and agency policies and procedures. Never refer to the deceased person as "the body." Care of and discussion related to the person should continue to be respectful even after death.

TABLE 9-8 Nursing Management

Physical Care at End of Life

Characteristic	Nursing Management
Pain • Pain may be a major symptom associated with terminal illness and the one most feared. • Pain can be acute or chronic. • Bone pain can be caused by metastases, fractures, arthritis, immobility. • Physical and emotional stressors can aggravate pain.	• Assess pain thoroughly and regularly to determine the quality, intensity, location, and contributing and alleviating factors. • Minimize possible irritants such as skin irritations from wetness, heat or cold, and pressure. • Administer medications around the clock in a timely manner and on a regular basis to provide constant relief rather than waiting until the pain is unbearable and then trying to relieve it. • Provide complementary and alternative therapies such as guided imagery, massage, and relaxation techniques as needed (see Chapter 6). • Evaluate effectiveness of pain relief measures frequently to ensure that the patient is on a correct, adequate drug regimen. • Do not delay or deny pain relief measures to a terminally ill patient.
Delirium • A state characterized by confusion, disorientation, restlessness, clouding of consciousness, incoherence, fear, anxiety, excitement, and often hallucinations • May be misidentified as depression, psychosis, anger, or anxiety • Use of opioids or corticosteroids as well as their withdrawal may cause delirium. • Underlying disease process may contribute to delirium. • Generally considered a reversible process	• Perform a thorough assessment for reversible causes of delirium, including pain, constipation, and urinary retention. • Provide a room that is quiet, well lit, and familiar to reduce the effects of delirium. • Reorient the dying person to person, place, and time with each encounter. • Administer ordered benzodiazepines and sedatives as needed. • Stay physically close to frightened patient. Reassure in a calm, soft voice with touch and slow strokes of the skin. • Provide family with emotional support and encouragement in their efforts to cope with the behaviors associated with delirium.
Anxiety/Restlessness • May occur as death approaches and cerebral metabolism slows • May occur with tachypnea, dyspnea, sweating	• Assess for previous anxiety disorder. • Assess for spiritual distress and/or concerns related to death as causes of restlessness and agitation. • Assess for urinary retention and stool impaction. • Do not restrain. • Use soothing music; slow, soft touch and voice. • Limit the number of persons at the bedside.
Dysphagia • May occur because of extreme weakness and changes in level of consciousness • Difficulty swallowing • Aspiration of liquids and/or solids • Drooling/inability to swallow secretions	• Identify the least invasive alternative routes of administration for drugs needed for symptom management. • Suction orally as needed. • Modify diet as tolerated/desired (soft, pureed, chopped meats). • Hand feed small meals. • Head elevated for meals and at least 30 minutes after • If necessary use alternative (rectal, buccal, transdermal) medication routes. • Discontinue nonessential medications. • Discuss risk of aspiration.
Weakness and Fatigue • Expected at the end of life • Metabolic demands related to disease process contribute to weakness and fatigue.	• Assess the patient's tolerance for activities. • Time nursing interventions to conserve energy. • Help the patient identify and complete valued or desired activities. • Provide support as needed to maintain positions in bed or chair. • Provide frequent rest periods.
Dehydration • May occur during the last days of life • Hunger and thirst are rare in the last days of life. • As the end of life approaches, patients tend to take in less food and fluid.	• Assess mucous membranes frequently for dryness, which can lead to discomfort. • Maintain complete, regular oral care to provide for comfort and hydration of mucous membranes. • Encourage consumption of ice chips and sips of fluids or use moist cloths to provide moisture to the mouth. • Use moist cloths and swabs for unconscious patients to avoid aspiration. • Apply lubricant to the lips and oral mucous membranes as needed. • Do not force the patient to eat or drink. • Teach family that hunger and thirst are rare in the last days of life. • Reassure family that cessation of food and fluid intake is a natural part of the process of dying.

TABLE 9-8 Nursing Management

Physical Care at End of Life—cont'd

Characteristic	Nursing Management
Dyspnea • Subjective symptom • Accompanied by fear of suffocation and anxiety • Underlying disease process can exacerbate dyspnea. • Coughing and expectorating secretions become difficult.	• Assess respiratory status regularly. • Elevate the head and/or position patient on side to improve chest expansion. • Use a fan or air conditioner to facilitate movement of cool air. • Teach and encourage the use of pursed-lip breathing. • Administer supplemental oxygen as ordered. • Suction PRN to remove accumulation of mucus from the airways. Suction cautiously in the terminal phase. • Administer expectorant as ordered.
Myoclonus • Mild to severe jerking or twitching sometimes associated with use of high dose of opioids. • Patient may complain of involuntary twitching of extremities.	• Assess for initial onset, duration, and any discomfort or distress experienced by patient. • If myoclonus is distressing or becoming more severe, discuss possible drug therapy modifications with the HCP. • Changes in opioid medication may alleviate or decrease myoclonus.
Skin Breakdown • Skin integrity is difficult to maintain at the end of life. • Immobility, urinary and bowel incontinence, dry skin, nutritional deficits, anemia, friction, and shearing forces lead to a high risk for skin breakdown. • Disease and other processes may impair skin integrity. • As death approaches, circulation to the extremities decreases and they become cool, mottled, and cyanotic.	• Assess skin for signs of breakdown. • Implement protocols to prevent skin breakdown by controlling drainage and odor and keeping the skin and any wound areas clean. • Perform wound assessments as needed. • Follow appropriate nursing management protocol for dressing wounds. • Follow appropriate nursing management protocol for a patient who is immobile, but consider realistic outcomes of skin integrity vs. maintenance of comfort. • Follow appropriate nursing management to prevent skin irritations and breakdown from urinary and bowel incontinence. • Use blankets to cover for warmth. Never apply heat. • Prevent the effects of shearing forces.
Bowel Patterns • Constipation can be caused by immobility, use of opioid medications, depression, lack of fiber in the diet, and dehydration. • Diarrhea may occur as muscles relax or from a fecal impaction related to the use of opioids and immobility.	• Assess bowel function. • Assess for and remove fecal impactions. • Encourage movement and physical activities as tolerated. • Encourage fiber in the diet if appropriate. • Encourage fluids if appropriate. • Use suppositories, stool softeners, laxatives, or enemas if ordered. • Assess for confusion, agitation, restlessness and pain, which may be signs of constipation.
Urinary Incontinence • May result from disease progression or changes in the level of consciousness. • As death becomes imminent, the perineal muscles relax.	• Assess urinary function. • Use absorbent pads for urinary incontinence. • Follow appropriate nursing protocol for the consideration and use of indwelling or external catheters. • Follow appropriate nursing management to prevent skin irritations and breakdown from urinary incontinence.
Anorexia, Nausea, and Vomiting • May be caused by complications of disease process • Drugs contribute to nausea. • Constipation, impaction, and bowel obstruction can cause anorexia, nausea, and vomiting.	• Assess the patient for complaints of nausea or vomiting. • Assess possible contributing causes of nausea or vomiting. • Have family provide the patient's favorite foods. • Discuss modifications to the drug regimen with the HCP. • Provide antiemetics before meals if ordered. • Offer and provide frequent meals with small portions of favorite foods. • Offer culturally appropriate foods. • Provide frequent mouth care, especially after vomiting. • Ensure uninterrupted mealtimes. • If ordered, administer medications (e.g., megestrol, corticosteroids) to increase appetite. • Teach family that appetite naturally decreases at end of life.
Candidiasis • White, cottage-cheese–like oral plaques • Fungal overgrowth in the mouth due to chemotherapy and/or immunosuppression	• If ordered, administer oral antifungal nystatin. • Clean dentures and other dental appliances to prevent reinfection. • Provide oral hygiene and use soft toothbrush.

SPECIAL NEEDS OF CAREGIVERS AND NURSES IN END-OF-LIFE CARE

Special Needs of Family Caregivers

Family caregivers are important in meeting the patient's physical and psychosocial needs. The role of caregivers includes working and communicating with the patient and other family members, supporting the patient's concerns, and helping the patient resolve any unfinished business. Families often face emotional, physical, and economic consequences as a result of caring for a family member who is dying. The caregiver's responsibilities do not end when the person is admitted to an acute care, inpatient hospice, or long-term care facility.

An understanding of the grieving process as it affects both the patient and family is important. Being present during a family member's dying process can be highly stressful. Recognize signs and behaviors among family members who may be at risk for abnormal grief reactions, and be prepared to intervene if necessary. Warning signs may include dependency and negative feelings about the dying person, inability to express feelings, sleep disturbances, a history of depression, difficult reactions to previous losses, perceived lack of social or family support, low self-esteem, multiple previous bereavements, alcoholism, or substance abuse. Caregivers with concurrent life crises (e.g., divorce) will be especially at risk.

Family caregivers and other family members need encouragement to continue their usual activities as much as possible. They need to discuss their activities and maintain some control over their lives. Inform caregivers about appropriate resources for support, including respite care. Resources such as community counseling and local support may assist some people in working through their grief.

Encourage caregivers to build a support system of extended family, friends, faith community, and clergy. The caregivers should have people to call on at any time to express any feelings they are experiencing. (The stressors and special needs of family caregivers are discussed in Chapter 4 on p. 50.)

Special Needs of Nurses

Many nurses who care for dying patients do so because they are passionate about providing high-quality EOL care. Caring for patients and their families at the end of life is challenging and rewarding but also intense and emotionally charged.[24] A bond or connection may develop between you and the patient or family. Be aware of how grief personally affects you. When you provide care for terminally ill or dying patients, you are not immune to feelings of loss. It is common to feel helpless and powerless when dealing with death. Express feelings of sorrow, guilt, and frustration. It is important to recognize your own values, attitudes, and feelings about death.

Interventions are available that may help ease your physical and emotional stress. Be aware of what you can and cannot control. Recognizing personal feelings allows openness in exchanging feelings with the patient and family. Realizing that it is okay to cry with the patient or family during the end of life may be important for your well-being.

To meet your personal needs, focus on interventions that will help decrease your stress. Get involved in hobbies or other interests, schedule time for yourself, ensure time for sleep, maintain a peer support system, and develop a support system beyond the workplace.[25] Hospice agencies can help you cope through professionally assisted groups, informal discussion sessions, and flexible time schedules.

CASE STUDY

Spiritual Distress at End of Life

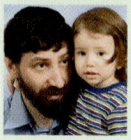

(©Mocker_bat/iStock/Thinkstock)

Patient Profile

G.M. is a 42-year-old Orthodox Jewish man. He is being visited by the hospice nurse for complaints of increasing abdominal pain, nausea, vomiting, lack of appetite, and constipation. He was diagnosed 6 months ago with pancreatic cancer that has metastasized to the liver and lungs. He quit work 1 month later. Two weeks ago he ended the drug trial he was on for 5 months and enrolled in hospice. Currently, he is taking oral opioids for pain, ondansetron (Zofran) PRN for nausea and vomiting, sertraline (Zoloft) for depression, and megestrol for appetite. His wife is worried that he will become addicted to the pain medication.

Subjective Data

- States that he is angry at God for giving him this illness
- Reports fatigue and lack of appetite
- Reports pain at 7 (0- to 10-point scale) not relieved by medication
- States he is worried about the loss of his health benefits and what will happen to his young family (including a son age 3) when he is gone

Objective Data

Physical Examination

- Underweight (20% less than ideal body weight for height)
- Skin is jaundiced
- Yellow sclera

Interprofessional Care

- Review pain medications for dosage adjustment.
- Hospice social worker to review medical benefits and disability application
- Ensure that advance directives are in place.
- Request a visit from his rabbi.

Discussion Questions

1. What are G.M.'s risk factors for spiritual distress?
2. Based on the data above, what are the major health problems for G.M.?
3. ***Patient-Centered Care:*** What specific palliative care needs does G.M. have?
4. ***Priority Decision:*** Based on the assessment data provided, what are the priority nursing diagnoses? Are there any collaborative problems?
5. ***Priority Decision:*** Based on your assessment of G.M., what are the priority nursing interventions for him?
6. ***Teamwork and Collaboration:*** For the interventions that you identified in the above question, which personnel could be responsible for implementing them: RN, LPN, unlicensed assistive personnel (UAP)?
7. ***Teamwork and Collaboration:*** What referrals may be indicated?

Answers available at *http://evolve.elsevier.com/Lewis/medsurg.*

BRIDGE TO NCLEX EXAMINATION

The number of the question corresponds to the same-numbered outcome at the beginning of the chapter.

1. An 80-year-old female patient is receiving palliative care for heart failure. The *primary* purpose(s) of her receiving palliative care is (are) to (*select all that apply*)
   a. improve her quality of life.
   b. assess her coping ability with disease.
   c. have time to teach patient and family about disease.
   d. focus on reducing the severity of disease symptoms.
   e. provide care that the family is unwilling or unable to give.
2. The *primary* purpose of hospice is to
   a. allow patients to die at home.
   b. provide better quality of care than the family can.
   c. coordinate care for dying patients and their families.
   d. provide comfort and support for dying patients and their families.
3. A 67-year-old woman was recently diagnosed with inoperable pancreatic cancer. Before the diagnosis she was very active in her neighborhood association. Her husband is concerned because his wife is staying at home and missing her usual community activities. Which common EOL psychologic manifestation is she *most* likely demonstrating?
   a. Peacefulness
   b. Decreased socialization
   c. Decreased decision making
   d. Anxiety about unfinished business
4. For the past 5 years Tom has repeatedly asked his mother to donate his deceased father's belongings to charity, but his mother has refused. She sits in the bedroom closet, crying and talking to her long-dead husband. What type of grief is Tom's mother experiencing?
   a. Adaptive grief
   b. Disruptive grief
   c. Anticipatory grief
   d. Prolonged grief disorder
5. The home health nurse visits a 40-year-old patient with metastatic breast cancer who is receiving palliative care. The patient is experiencing pain at a level of 7 (0-10 point scale). In prioritizing activities for the visit, what should the nurse do *first*?
   a. Auscultate for breath sounds.
   b. Administer PRN pain medication.
   c. Check pressure points for skin breakdown.
   d. Ask family about patient's food and fluid intake.
6. While caring for his dying wife, the husband states that his wife is a devout Roman Catholic but he is a Baptist. Who is considered the *most* reliable source for spiritual preferences concerning EOL care for the dying wife?
   a. A priest
   b. Dying wife
   c. Hospice staff
   d. Husband of dying wife
7. A tearful patient tells the nurse that her brother (who is in prison) just received a diagnosis of terminal metastatic lung cancer. She is worried that her brother will die in pain and alone. What is the nurse's *best* response?
   a. "It's too bad that they don't have hospice services in prison."
   b. "I'm sure the prison will let him out if they know he is dying."
   c. "Maybe if he had not committed a crime, he wouldn't be in this situation."
   d. "Many prisons offer health care services, including hospice and palliative care."
8. The family attorney informed a patient's adult children and wife that the patient did not have an advance directive after he suffered a serious stroke. Who is responsible for making the decision about EOL measures when the patient cannot communicate his or her specific wishes?
   a. Notary and attorney
   b. Physician and family
   c. Wife and adult children
   d. Physician and nursing staff
9. The children caregivers of an older patient whose death is imminent have not left the bedside for the past 36 hours. In the nurse's assessment of the family, what findings indicate the potential for an abnormal grief reaction to occur *(select all that apply)*?
   a. Family cannot express their feelings to one another.
   b. Dying patient is becoming more restless and agitated.
   c. A family member is going through a difficult divorce.
   d. Family talks with and reassures the patient at frequent intervals.
   e. Siblings who were estranged from each other have now reunited.
10. A nurse has been working full time with terminally ill patients for 3 years. He has been experiencing irritability and mixed emotions when expressing sadness since four of his patients died on the same day. To optimize the quality of his nursing care, he should examine his own
    a. full-time work schedule.
    b. past feelings toward death.
    c. patterns for dealing with grief.
    d. demands for involvement in patient care.

1. a, d, 2. d, 3. b, 4. d, 5. b, 6. b, 7. d, 8. c, 9. a, c, 10. c.

For rationales to these answers and even more NCLEX review questions, visit *http://evolve.elsevier.com/Lewis/medsurg.*

EVOLVE WEBSITE

http://evolve.elsevier.com/Lewis/medsurg

Review Questions (Online Only)
Key Points
Answer Keys for Questions

- Rationales for Bridge to NCLEX Examination Questions
- Answer Guidelines for Case Study on p. 142

Student Case Study

- Patient With Chronic Myelogenous Leukemia Including End-of-Life Care

Conceptual Care Map Creator
Audio Glossary
Content Updates

REFERENCES

1. National Consensus Project for Quality Palliative Care: Clinical practice guidelines for quality palliative care, ed 3. Retrieved from *www.hpna.org/multimedia/NCP_Clinical_Practice_Guidelines_3rd_Edition.pdf.*
2. Centers for Disease Control and Prevention, U.S. Dept of Health and Human Services: The state of aging and health in America 2013. Retrieved from *www.cdc.gov/aging.*
3. Kelley AS, Deb P, Du Q, et al: Hospice enrollment saves money for Medicare and improves care quality across a number of different lengths-of-stay, *Health Aff* 32:552, 2013.
4. National Hospice and Palliative Care Organization: NHPCO facts and figures: hospice care in America. Alexandria, Va. Retrieved from *www.nhpco.org/sites/default/files/public/Statistics_Research/2014_Facts_Figures.pdf.*
5. Hospice and Palliative Nurses Association: HPNA position statements. Retrieved from *http://hpna.advancingexpertcare.org/education/position-statements.*
6. Johnson KS: Racial and ethnic disparities in palliative care, *J Palliat Med* 16:1329, 2013.
7. Olmsted CL, Johnson AM, Kaboli P, et al: Use of palliative care and hospice among surgical and medical specialties in the Veterans Health Administration, *JAMA Surg* 149:1169, 2014.
8. National Hospice and Palliative Care Organization: Palliative care costs and benefits. Retrieved from *www.caringinfo.org/i4a/pages/index.cfm?pageid=3297.*
9. Jackson J, Willmarth-Stec M, Shutter L: Update of clinical practice guidelines for brain death determination in an academic health center, *J Neurosci Nurs* 47:44, 2015.
10. Field M, Cassel C: *Approaching death: improving care at the end of life*, Washington, DC, 1997, National Academy Press. (Classic)
11. Kübler-Ross E: *On death and dying*, New York, 1969, Macmillan. (Classic).
12. National Cancer Institute: PDQ Grief, bereavement, and coping with loss, Bethesda, Md, 2014, National Cancer Institute. Retrieved from *http://cancer.gov/cancertopics/pdq/supportivecare/bereavement/HealthProfessional.*
13. Bryant RA, Kenny L, Joscelyne A, et al: Treating prolonged grief disorder: a randomized clinical trial, *JAMA Psychiatry* 71:1332, 2014.

*14. Skalla K, Ferrell B: Challenges in assessing spiritual distress in survivors of cancer, *Clin J Oncol Nurs* 19:99, 2015.

*15. Wilson KS, Korrke TE, Schettle S: Honoring Choices Minnesota: preliminary data from a community-wide advance care planning model, *J Am Geriatric Soc* 62:2420, 2014.

16. Rubin SS, Malkinson R, Witztum E: *Working with the bereaved: multiple lenses on loss and mourning*, Routledge Taylor and French, 2012, New York.

*17. LoPresti MA, Dement F, Gold HT: End-of-life care for people from ethnic minority groups: a systematic review, *Am J Hosp Palliat Care* 33(3):291, 2016.

*18. Leung D, Blastorah M, Nusdorfer L, et al: Nursing patients with chronic critical illness and their families: a qualitative study, *Nurs Crit Care* Feb 18, 2015. DOI: 10.1111/nicc.12154.

19. Stahler PA, Weese SE, Nygaard RM: Honoring patients' organ donation decisions when family conflict is present: experience from a single organ procurement organization, *J Trauma Acute Care Surg* 77:555, 2014.
20. Marcus B: Communicating patient DNR status using color-coded wristbands, *Am J Nurs* 115:11, 2015.
21. American Nurses Association: ANA position statements. Retrieved from *www.nursingworld.org/MainMenuCategories/EthicsStandards/Ethics-Position-Statements/etpain14426.pdf.*
22. Iowa Department of Public Health: Out of hospital DNR. Retrieved from *www.idph.state.ia.us/ems/dnr.asp.*

*23. Hui D, Dos Santos R, Chisholm G: Bedside clinical sign associated with impending death in patients with advanced cancer: preliminary findings of a prospective, longitudinal cohort study, *Cancer* 15:121, 2015.

24. Sliter MT, Sinclaire RR, Yuan Z, et al: Don't fear the reaper: trait death anxiety, mortality salience, and occupational health, *J Appl Psychol* 99:759, 2014.

*25. Wittenberg-Lyles E, Goldsmith J, Reno J: Perceived benefits and challenges of an oncology nurse support group, *Clin J Oncol Nurs* 18:E71, 2014.

*Evidence-based information for clinical practice.

10

Substance Use Disorders

Mariann M. Harding

No one is immune from addiction. It afflicts people of all ages, races, classes, and professions.

Patrick J. Kennedy

http://evolve.elsevier.com/Lewis/medsurg/

LEARNING OUTCOMES

1. Relate the effects of substance use to its resulting major health complications.
2. Differentiate among the effects of the use of stimulants, depressants, and cannabis.
3. Explain your role in promoting the cessation of smoking and tobacco use.
4. Summarize the nursing management and interprofessional care of patients who experience toxicity or withdrawal from stimulants and depressants.
5. Apply the Screening, Brief Intervention, and Referral to Treatment approach in clinical situations.
6. Describe the incidence and effects of substance use in the older adult.

KEY TERMS

acute alcohol toxicity, p. 149
alcohol use disorder (AUD), p. 148
alcohol withdrawal syndrome (AWS), p. 150
binge drinking, p. 148
electronic cigarettes, p. 146
Screening, Brief Intervention, and Referral to Treatment (SBIRT), p. 153
substance use disorder (SUD), Table 10-1, p. 146
tobacco use disorder (TUD), p. 145

Substance use is a serious problem affecting society and the health care system. Substance-related disorders involve several types of substances, ranging from widely used and accepted tobacco and alcohol to illegal, brain-altering drugs such as heroin and cocaine. The *Diagnostic and Statistical Manual of Mental Disorders V (DSM-V)* outlines criteria used to identify the presence of substance use disorder (SUD)[1] (Table 10-1).

SUD is defined as mild, moderate, or severe based on the person's pattern of use and the functional impact of use on the person's daily life. Knowing the severity of substance use allows the health care team to tailor treatment according to a patient's needs. For example, a person who binge drinks may not have alcohol SUD but is at increased risk for it. On the other hand, a person who uses heroin or cocaine is likely to have severe SUD because these substances are highly addictive.

Many of the patients with substance use problems whom you will encounter are receiving care for problems associated with substance use. Almost every drug associated with SUD harms some tissue or organ. Substance use causes specific health problems, such as liver damage related to alcohol use or chronic obstructive pulmonary disease (COPD) related to smoking. Other health problems result from behaviors associated with substance use, such as malnutrition or trauma-related injuries from automobile accidents. Common health problems related to substance use are presented in Table 10-2.

This chapter focuses on the role of the medical-surgical nurse in identifying and managing the patient with SUD in the acute care setting. A hospitalized patient who uses substances can develop withdrawal when the use of the substance is abruptly stopped. You need to be able to recognize substance use and its effects on health problems and manage withdrawal. The health care setting provides an opportunity for screening and providing teaching regarding substance use and abuse. It is your responsibility to motivate the patient to change behavior and provide referrals to programs that provide treatment and rehabilitation. Failing to address a patient's substance use problem, thus enabling the behavior, is a breach of your professional responsibility.

DRUGS ASSOCIATED WITH SUBSTANCE USE DISORDER

NICOTINE

You are most likely to encounter people with **tobacco use disorder (TUD)**. People with TUD are dependent on the drug

Reviewed by Carolyn Baird, DNP, MBA, RN-BC, CARN-AP, CCDPD, FIAAN, Therapist, Counseling and Trauma Services, Canonsburg, Pennsylvania; Abimbola Farinde, PharmD, MS, Professor, Columbia Southern University, Orange Beach, Alabama; and Christine L. Savage, RN, PhD, CARN, FAAN, Professor and Chair, Community Public Health Johns Hopkins School of Nursing, Baltimore, Maryland.

TABLE 10-1 Criteria for Substance Use Disorder

The following criteria (clustered in four groups) can be used to identify substance use disorder (SUD). The severity of SUD can be classified as mild (2-3 criteria), moderate (4-5 criteria), or severe (6 or more criteria).

Impaired Control
- Taking more or for longer than intended
- Failing to quit using despite multiple times of trying to do so
- Spending a great deal of time obtaining, using, or recovering from use
- Craving the substance

Social Impairment
- Missing school, work, or other responsibilities due to use
- Continuing use despite problems caused or exacerbated by use
- Giving up or reducing important activities because of use

Risky Use
- Recurrent use in hazardous situations
- Continued use despite problems that are caused or worsened by use

Pharmacologic Dependence
- Physical tolerance to effects of the substance
- Presence of withdrawal symptoms when not using or using less

Source: American Psychiatric Association: *The diagnostic and statistical manual of mental disorders*, ed 5, Arlington, Va, 2013, The Association.

TABLE 10-2 Health Problems Related to Substance Use

	Health Problems*
Substance	
Cocaine	• Cardiac dysrhythmias, myocardial ischemia and infarction • Seizures, stroke • Psychosis
Amphetamines	• Cardiac dysrhythmias, myocardial ischemia and infarction • Liver, lung, kidney damage • Mood disturbances, violent behavior, psychoses
Sedative-hypnotics	• Memory impairment • Personality changes, depression
Opioids	• Sexual dysfunction • Gastric ulcers • Glomerulonephritis
Inhalants	• Cognitive and motor impairment • Acute and chronic kidney injury
Cannabis	• Bronchitis, chronic cough • Depression, anxiety, schizophrenia • Memory impairment
Behaviors	
Injecting drugs	• Blood clots, phlebitis, skin infections • Hepatitis B and C • HIV/AIDS • Other infections: endocarditis, tuberculosis, pneumonia, meningitis, tetanus, bone and joint infections, lung abscesses
Snorting drugs	• Nasal sores, septal necrosis or perforation • Chronic sinusitis
Risky sexual behavior	• HIV/AIDS • Hepatitis B and C • Sexually transmitted infections
Personal neglect	• Malnutrition, impaired immunity • Accidental injuries

Adapted from National Institute on Drug Abuse: Medical consequence of drug abuse. Retrieved from *www.drugabuse.gov/related-topics/medical-consequences-drug-abuse.*
*Health problems related to substance use are discussed in the appropriate chapters throughout the text where they are identified as risk factors for these problems.

nicotine due to using tobacco products. A number of products contain nicotine, including smoked tobacco (cigarettes, cigars, pipes), smokeless tobacco (chew, snuff, dip), and some electronic cigarettes. Cigarette smoking is the main form of tobacco use in the United States.

Effects of Use and Complications

Nicotine is a central nervous system stimulant. Within seconds of entering the body, nicotine reaches the brain, causing the release of adrenaline and creating feelings of a "high" or a "buzz." The effects last about 1 to 2 hours before withdrawal symptoms occur, leaving the person feeling tired, irritable, and anxious. The need to have the "high" or "buzz" feelings again makes the person crave more nicotine, leading to addiction.

Smoked tobacco is the most harmful method of nicotine use and injures nearly every organ in the body. Smoking alone accounts for 14 million major medical conditions affecting adults in the United States.[2] Smoking causes chronic lung disease, cardiovascular disease, and lung and other cancers and is a major factor in a variety of other conditions, including delayed wound healing and overall diminished health (Fig. 10-1).

Although those who use smokeless tobacco have less risk of lung disease, it is not without complications. Holding tobacco in the mouth is associated with periodontal disease and cancer of the mouth, cheek, tongue, throat, and esophagus. Smokeless tobacco produces the systemic effects of nicotine on the cardiovascular system, increasing the risk for cardiovascular disease.[3]

Electronic cigarettes, or e-cigs, have a similar look and feel as traditional cigarettes. These battery-operated devices turn nicotine and other chemicals, including propylene glycol and flavorings, into an aerosol. Emerging information indicates e-cigs are not harmless. This is a serious concern because the overall impact of their use on health remains uncertain. Potentially harmful chemicals have been found in some cartridges, including irritants, genotoxins, and carcinogens. E-cigs containing nicotine have the potential to increase the risk of cardiovascular and respiratory problems similar to traditional cigarettes.[4] Other problems, such as seizures and pneumonia, have been attributed to inhaling chemicals in the vapor. Although some believe substituting an e-cig for a traditional cigarette may aid in smoking cessation, no e-cigs are FDA approved. Do not recommend them as a smoking cessation aid.

❖ NURSING AND INTERPROFESSIONAL MANAGEMENT: TOBACCO USE DISORDER

◆ Tobacco Cessation

As a nurse, you have a professional responsibility to help people stop smoking or using tobacco. The Joint Commission mandates that every health professional is responsible for identifying tobacco users and providing them with information on ways to stop using tobacco. Patients who receive even brief advice and intervention from you are more likely to quit than those who receive no intervention.

With each patient encounter, encourage the patient to quit and offer specific smoking cessation interventions. The Agency for Healthcare Research and Quality has issued clinical practice guidelines for clinicians, including nurses, to use to motivate users to quit[5] (Tables 10-3 and 10-4). Use these brief clinical

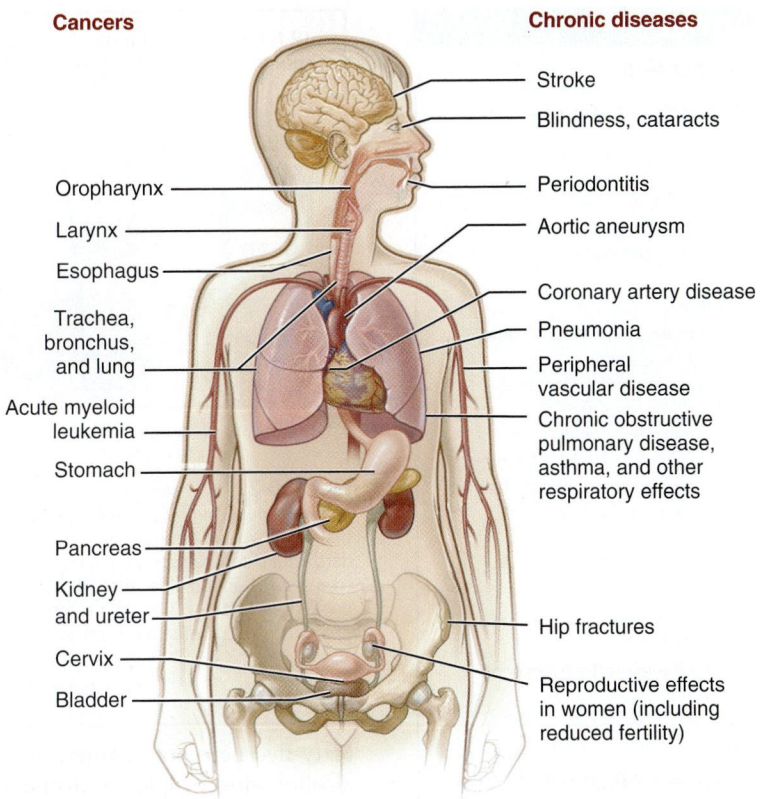

FIG. 10-1 Health effects of smoking. (From Samet JM: Tobacco smoking, *Thorac Surg Clin* 23(2):103, 2013.)

TABLE 10-3 Clinical Practice Guideline

Treating Tobacco Use Disorder

The Five *A*s for Users Who Desire to Quit	The Five *R*s for Users Unwilling to Quit
1. **Ask:** Identify all tobacco users at every contact.	1. **Relevance:** Ask the patient to indicate why quitting is personally relevant (e.g., health).
2. **Advise:** Strongly urge all tobacco users to quit.	2. **Risks:** Ask the patient to identify his or her potential risks/consequences of tobacco use.
3. **Assess:** Determine willingness to make a quit attempt.	3. **Rewards:** Ask the patient to identify potential benefits of stopping tobacco use.
4. **Assist:** Develop a plan with the patient to help the patient quit (e.g., counseling, medication).	4. **Roadblocks:** Ask patient to identify barriers or impediments to quitting.
5. **Arrange:** Schedule follow-up contact.	5. **Repetition:** Repeat process every clinic visit.

Source: Agency for Healthcare Research and Quality: *AHCPR supported clinical practice guideline: treating tobacco use and dependence: 2008 update,* Washington, DC, 2008, U.S. Public Health Service.

TABLE 10-4 Inpatient Tobacco Cessation Interventions

Take the following steps for every hospitalized patient.

- Ask each patient on admission if he or she uses tobacco and document tobacco use status.
- For current tobacco users, list tobacco use status on the admission problem list and as a discharge diagnosis.
- Use counseling and medication to help all tobacco users maintain abstinence and to treat withdrawal symptoms.
- Provide advice and assistance on how to quit during hospitalization and remain abstinent after discharge.
- Arrange for follow-up regarding smoking status. Supportive contact should be provided for at least a month after discharge.

Source: Agency for Healthcare Research and Quality: *AHCPR supported clinical practice guideline: treating tobacco use and dependence: 2008 update,* Washington, DC, 2008, U.S. Public Health Service.

interventions, called the "5 *A*s," with each patient encounter. These interventions will help you identify tobacco users, encourage them to quit, determine their willingness to quit, assist them in quitting, and arrange for follow-up. A patient teaching guide (Table 10-5) expands on the fourth strategy, *Assist,* to help you aid the user willing to quit. If a tobacco user is unwilling to quit, using the "5 *R*s" may motivate the user to quit in the future.

A variety of smoking cessation products are available to help support users in quitting. These include prescription medicines as well as over-the-counter (OTC) products such as skin patches, lozenges, and gum. Nicotine replacement products are one type of smoking cessation product. These products reduce the craving and withdrawal symptoms associated with cessation by supplying the body with smaller amounts of nicotine (Table 10-6).

Because most health care facilities are tobacco-free environments, admitted patients who are addicted to nicotine may experience withdrawal symptoms since they are unable to smoke. These symptoms are the same as for the person who stops using tobacco "cold turkey." Offering nicotine replacement therapy to those who desire it will assist in controlling withdrawal symptoms during hospitalization and promote continued cessation after discharge.

Non-nicotine products also play a role in helping users quit. Varenicline (Chantix) is a drug used to aid smoking cessation. Varenicline is unique in that it has both agonist and antagonist actions. Its agonist activity at one subtype of nicotinic receptors

EVIDENCE-BASED PRACTICE

Translating Research Into Practice

Do Tobacco Cessation Programs Affect Smoking Behavior?

Clinical Question

In adults who regularly smoke cigarettes (P), do mass media tobacco cessation programs (I) versus no intervention (C) reduce smoking prevalence, cigarette consumption, quit attempts, and quit rates (O)?

Synthesis of Best Available Evidence

- Systematic review of randomized controlled trials (RCTs), quasi-RCTs, controlled trials, and interrupted time series
- 11 studies of state and community-wide programs; smoking prevalence generally >15,000 individuals per program. Mass media interventions were cessation-related messages focusing on smokers and motivation to quit with dissemination of information through television, radio, print media, and billboards. Smoking behavior outcomes were prevalence, cigarette consumption, attempts to quit, and quit or abstinence rates.

Conclusions

- Most studies suggested mass media programs have positive effects on individual smoking behaviors.
- Intensity and length of program may influence effectiveness of intervention.

Implications for Nursing Practice

1. What community resources can you use to help individuals who want to quit smoking?
2. How could you assist with a statewide program that seeks to reduce tobacco use?

Reference for Evidence

Bala M, Strzeszynski L, Topor-Madry R, et al: Mass media interventions for smoking cessation in adults, *Cochrane Database of Syst Rev* 6:CD004704, 2013.

P, Patient population of interest; *I*, intervention or area of interest; *C*, comparison of interest or comparison group; *O*, outcomes of interest; *T*, timing (see p. 15).

provides some nicotine effects to ease withdrawal symptoms. If the person does resume smoking, its antagonist action blocks the effects of nicotine at another subtype of nicotinic receptor, making smoking less enjoyable. Bupropion (Zyban), an antidepressant drug, reduces the urge to smoke, reduces some symptoms of withdrawal, and helps prevent weight gain associated with smoking cessation.

DRUG ALERT Varenicline (Chantix) and Bupropion (Zyban)

- Serious neuropsychiatric symptoms such as changes in behavior, hostility, agitation, depressed mood, suicidal thoughts and behavior, and attempted suicide can occur.
- Advise patients to stop taking these drugs and contact the HCP immediately if they experience any of these manifestations.

Along with using a smoking cessation product, users who wish to quit are more likely to succeed if they participate in a tobacco cessation program. You should be aware of community resources that assist users who are motivated to quit. Cessation programs may involve hypnosis, acupuncture, behavioral interventions, aversion therapy, group support programs, individual therapy, and self-help options. Many of these programs teach users to avoid high-risk situations for smoking relapse (e.g., those that promote cue-induced craving) and help them develop coping skills, such as cigarette refusal skills, assertiveness, alternative activities, and peer support systems.

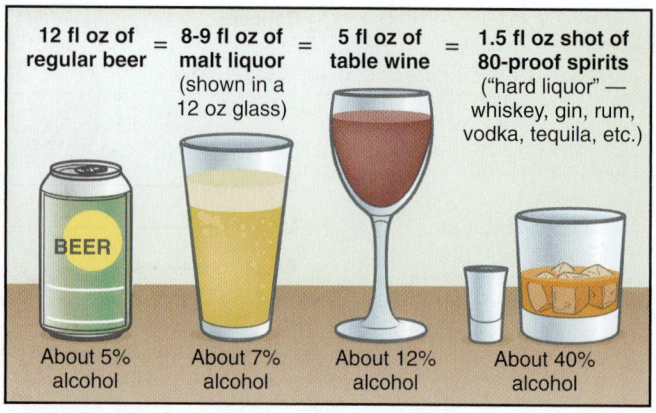

The percent of "pure" alcohol, expressed here as alcohol by volume (alc/vol), varies by beverage.

FIG. 10-2 U.S. standard drink equivalents. The National Institute on Alcohol Abuse and Alcoholism (NIAAA) guidelines for alcohol use indicate that healthy men younger than 65 should consume no more than 14 standard drinks per week or 4 drinks per drinking occasion. Healthy, nonpregnant women and adults older than 65 should consume no more than 7 standard drinks per week or 3 drinks per drinking occasion. (From NIAAA: *What's a standard drink?* Retrieved from *www.niaaa.nih.gov.*)

ALCOHOL

Sixty-five percent of Americans ages 18 and older consume alcohol. Most people use alcohol in moderation. *Risky drinking* is consuming alcohol in excess of established guidelines set forth by the National Institute on Alcohol Abuse and Alcoholism (Fig. 10-2). Risky drinking is associated with negative physical, emotional, and social consequences. **Alcohol use disorder (AUD)**, or alcoholism, affects about 7.2% of U.S. adults. A higher percent engage in periodic excess alcohol use. **Binge drinking** is alcohol use that brings blood alcohol concentration (BAC) levels over the legal limit for intoxication at least once per month.[6]

Effects of Use and Complications

Alcohol affects almost all cells of the body. It changes levels of neurotransmitters in the central nervous system (CNS), affecting all areas and functions of the CNS. These include centers that control our impulses, mood, and behavior; coordinate motor activity; and promote respiratory and cardiac function. The immediate effects of alcohol depend on a person's susceptibility to alcohol and their BAC.

For the person who is not dependent on alcohol, the BAC is generally predictable of alcohol's effects. The relationship between BAC and behavior is different in a person who has developed tolerance to alcohol and its effects. The *tolerant person* is usually able to drink large amounts without obvious impairment and perform complex tasks without problems at BAC levels much higher than levels that would produce obvious impairment in the *nontolerant drinker*. Women have higher blood alcohol levels than men do after the same amount of alcohol intake.

Alcohol use has been linked to many health problems (Table 10-7), which frequently are the reason that people seek health care. Long-term alcohol use can lead to the development of high BP, heart disease, stroke, liver disease, and digestive problems. Short-term, excess alcohol use increases the risk of injury from motor vehicle crashes, falls, firearms, assault, drowning, and burns. A patient with AUD undergoing surgery has increased

TABLE 10-5 Patient Teaching

Smoking and Tobacco Use Cessation

The following interventions are methods that work for quitting tobacco use. Tobacco users have the best chance of quitting if they use more than one method.

Develop a Quit Plan

- Set a quit date, ideally within 2 weeks.
- Talk to your HCP about getting help to quit.
- Tell family, friends, and co-workers about quitting and request understanding and support.
- Anticipate withdrawal symptoms and challenges when quitting.
- Before quitting, avoid smoking in places where you spend a lot of time (work, car, home).
- Throw away all tobacco products from your home, car, and work.
- Have support options in place by your quit date.

Use Approved Nicotine Replacement Systems

- Use a nicotine replacement agent unless you are a pregnant or nursing woman (Table 10-6).
- Do not use other forms of tobacco when using nicotine replacement systems.

Support and Encouragement

- Joining a quit-tobacco support group will increase your chances of stopping permanently.
- If you get the urge for tobacco, call someone to help talk you out of it—preferably an ex-user.
- Be proud every time you reach a quit milestone and reward yourself.
- Do not be afraid to talk about how you feel while quitting, especially fears of not being able to quit for good. Ask your spouse or partner, friends, and co-workers to support you. Self-help materials, mobile phone applications, and hot lines are available:
  - American Lung Association: 800-586-4872; *www.lung.org*
  - American Cancer Society: 800-227-2345; *www.cancer.org*
  - National Cancer Institute: 800-784-8669; *www.smokefree.gov*

Dealing With Urges to Use Tobacco

- Identify situations that may cause you to want to smoke or use other tobacco, such as being around other smokers, being under time pressure, feeling sad or frustrated, and drinking alcohol.
- Avoid difficult situations while you are trying to quit. Try to lower your stress level.
- Exercise can help, such as walking, jogging, or bicycling.
- Distract yourself from thoughts of smoking and the urge to use tobacco by talking to someone, going to a movie, getting busy with a task, or having a game night with friends.
- Drink a lot of water.
- Keep your hands busy with a pen or toothpick.

Avoiding Relapse

Most relapses occur within the first 3 months after quitting. Do not be discouraged if you start using tobacco again. Remember, most people try several times before they finally quit. Explore different ways to break habits. You may have to deal with some of the following triggers that cause relapse.

- *Change your environment.* Get rid of cigarettes, tobacco (in any form), and ashtrays in your home, car, and place of work. Get rid of the smell of cigarettes in your car and home.
- *Alcohol.* Consider limiting or stopping alcohol use while you are quitting tobacco.
- *Other smokers at home.* Encourage housemates to quit with you. Work out a plan to cope with others who smoke, and avoid being around them.
- *Weight gain.* Tackle one problem at a time. Work on quitting tobacco first. You will not necessarily gain weight, and increased appetite is often temporary. Eat healthy and exercise.
- *Negative mood or depression.* If these symptoms persist, talk to your HCP. You may need treatment for depression.
- *Withdrawal symptoms.* Your body will go through many changes when you quit tobacco. You may have a dry mouth, cough, or scratchy throat, and you may feel irritable. The nicotine patch or gum may help with cravings (Table 10-6).
- *Focus on the benefits of quitting:*
  - Your BP and heart rate will lower almost immediately.
  - Your risk of a heart attack declines within 24 hours and the blood will become less likely to clot, making dangerous blood clots less likely.
  - Within a few weeks, you will be less short of breath, cough less, and have more energy. Your ability to smell and taste should improve.
  - Your immune system will be stronger, so you will be less likely to be sick.
  - Quitting will improve your night vision and help preserve your overall vision.

Adapted from National Cancer Institute: 18 ways smoking affects your health. Retrieved from *http://smokefree.gov/health-effects.*

readmission rates, increased in-hospital death rates, and longer length of stay.[7]

Complications may arise from the interaction of alcohol with commonly prescribed or OTC drugs. Drugs that interact with alcohol in an additive manner include antihypertensives, antihistamines, and antianginals. Alcohol taken with aspirin may cause or exacerbate GI bleeding. Alcohol taken with acetaminophen may increase the risk of liver damage. Taking an additional CNS depressant with alcohol can increase, or potentiate, the effect of both. An alcohol-dependent person may have cross-tolerance, requiring an increased dose of CNS depressants to achieve the desired effect.

❖ NURSING AND INTERPROFESSIONAL MANAGEMENT: ALCOHOL USE DISORDER

◆ Alcohol Toxicity

Acute alcohol toxicity occurs when a person has a high level of alcohol in his or her blood, generally after the ingestion of a large amount of alcohol. This leads to behavior changes and alcohol-induced CNS depression, resulting in respiratory and circulatory failure. Unconsciousness, coma, and possibly death can occur. Other common effects include hypokalemia, hypomagnesemia, and hypoglycemia.

Obtain as accurate a health history as possible and assess for injuries, diseases, and hypoglycemia. No antidote for alcohol is available. Implement supportive care measures to maintain airway, breathing, and circulation (the ABCs) until the alcohol metabolizes. Frequently monitor vital signs and level of consciousness. Treat alcohol-induced hypotension with IV fluids.

Patients with hypoglycemia may receive glucose-containing IV solutions. IV thiamine may be given before or with IV glucose solutions to prevent *Wernicke-Korsakoff syndrome,* which can cause seizures and brain damage.[8] Many patients have low serum magnesium levels and other signs of malnutrition, so HCPs frequently add multivitamins and magnesium to the IV fluids.

Agitation and anxiety are common. Stay with the patient as much as possible, orienting as necessary. Assess the patient for increasing belligerence and a potential for violence. Since the

TABLE 10-6 Drug Therapy

Smoking Cessation*

Agents	Common Side Effects	Considerations
Nicotine Replacement Agents		
Nicotine Gum (OTC) Nicorette 2 mg, 4 mg • Use up to 12 wk • Use 1 piece q1-2hr for 6 wk then q2-4hr for 3 wk • Maximum dose: 24 pieces/day	Hiccups, mouth/jaw pain, mouth ulcers, indigestion, throat irritation, nausea	Specific 30-min chewing regimen with periods of holding the gum between cheek and teeth. Take only water 15 min before and during use. Difficult to use with dentures
Nicotine Lozenge (OTC) Commit 2 mg, 4 mg • Use 8-12 wk • Use 1 lozenge q1-2hr tapering to 1 lozenge q4-8hr in 12 wk	Insomnia, nausea, sore throat, hiccups, cough, heartburn, headache, flatulence	Dissolves in mouth in 20 to 30 min. Do not chew or swallow. Avoid food and drink during use. Occasionally rotate around the mouth.
Nicotine Patch (OTC) NicoDerm CQ, Habitrol, Nicotine transdermal system • 18- or 24-hr doses • Use ≥8 wk	Transient itching, burning, and redness at patch site. Insomnia, nausea, headache	Provides steady level of nicotine and is easy to use. Cannot be used by those with adhesive allergies. Rotate site to diminish skin irritation.
Nicotine Nasal Spray Nicotrol NS • 1-2 doses (2 sprays)/hr • Use 3-6 mo	Nose and throat irritation, sneezing, rhinitis, headache, cough	Requires a prescription. Provides fastest nicotine delivery. Do not sniff or inhale while dosing. Tilt head back slightly for best results.
Nicotine Inhaler Nicotrol nicotine inhalation system • Use 1 cartridge q1-2hr • Use 3-6 mo	Cough, mouth and throat irritation, headache, nausea, hiccups	Requires a prescription. Simulates smoking with mouthpiece and nicotine cartridge. May not be advisable for those with asthma or pulmonary disease
Non-Nicotine Agents		
bupropion (Zyban) • 150 mg/day for 3 days, then 150 mg bid • Use 12 wk; can use up to 6 mo	Insomnia, dry mouth, irritability, rash, tremors, anorexia	Contraindicated with history of seizures or eating disorders. Promotes weight loss. First choice for smokers with depression
varenicline (Chantix)† • 0.5 mg/day for 3 days, 0.5 mg bid for 4 days, then 1 mg bid • Use 12 wk; additional 12 wk may be used in select patients	Nausea, sleep disturbances, constipation, flatulence, vomiting, headache	If taken concurrently with nicotine replacement therapy, incidence of nausea, headache, vomiting, dizziness, dyspepsia, and fatigue is increased, but nicotine pharmacokinetics not affected.

*OTC nicotine replacement agents are also available in generic forms. Additional information and patient instructions are available from the American Lung Association at *www.lungusa.org*.
†See the Drug Alert for varenicline on p. 148.

patient is at risk for injury because of lack of coordination and impaired judgment, use protective measures.

Alcohol Withdrawal Syndrome

Alcohol withdrawal syndrome (AWS) can develop in a hospitalized patient when the use of alcohol abruptly stops. The onset of AWS is variable depending on the quantity, frequency, pattern, and duration of alcohol use. The early signs usually develop within a few hours after the last drink. They peak after 24 to 48 hours and then disappear unless the withdrawal progresses to alcohol withdrawal delirium.

Alcohol withdrawal delirium is a serious complication that can occur from 2 to 3 days after the last drink and last 2 to 3 days. The greater the patient's dependence on alcohol, the greater the risk of alcohol withdrawal delirium. Death may result from hyperthermia, sepsis, aspiration pneumonia, or peripheral vascular collapse.[8]

Management begins with identifying at-risk people. Use a symptom assessment tool, such as the Clinical Institute Withdrawal Assessment of Alcohol Scale, Revised (CIWA-Ar), to determine treatment[8] (Table 10-8). Table 10-9 presents the clinical manifestations and suggested treatment for alcohol withdrawal. A nursing care plan (eNursing Care Plan 10-1) for a patient with AWS is available on the website at *http://evolve.elsevier.com/Lewis/medsurg*.

CHECK YOUR PRACTICE

A 34-yr-old male patient was admitted for multiple trauma following a car accident. His girlfriend tells you that he always drinks too much and she knew he would get in trouble someday.

- What signs and symptoms would alert you to the presence of alcohol withdrawal syndrome?
- What measures would you use to protect his safety?
- How would you involve members of the interprofessional team in planning patient care?

USE OF OTHER SUBSTANCES

STIMULANTS

Amphetamine-related stimulants are highly addictive substances. While the use of crack cocaine and methamphetamine is illegal, amphetamines have a role in treating narcolepsy and attention deficit disorder. While most people responsibly use prescribed stimulants, prescription stimulants are frequently misused. All stimulants increase cardiac activity and excite the CNS by increasing levels of norepinephrine, serotonin, and dopamine. People use these drugs to produce feelings of euphoria, increase alertness, and boost their energy. Health problems associated with using stimulants are presented in Table 10-2.

TABLE 10-7 Effects of Chronic Alcohol Use

Body System	Effects
Neurologic	Alcoholic dementia, Wernicke-Korsakoff syndrome. Impaired cognitive function, psychomotor skills, abstract thinking, and memory. Depression, anxiety, attention deficit, labile moods, seizures, insomnia, peripheral neuropathy, chronic headache
Immunologic	Increased susceptibility to infections, depressed immune function
Hematologic	Bone marrow depression, anemia, leukopenia, thrombocytopenia, blood clotting abnormalities
Musculoskeletal	Myopathy, osteoporosis, gout
Cardiac	Hypertension, atrial fibrillation, cardiomyopathy, stroke, coronary artery disease, sudden cardiac death
Hepatic	Alcoholic hepatitis, cirrhosis, liver cancer
Gastrointestinal	Gastritis, gastroesophageal reflux disease (GERD), peptic ulcer, esophagitis, esophageal varices, gastrointestinal bleeding, pancreatitis, oropharyngeal cancer, colorectal cancer
Nutrition	Diabetes mellitus, anorexia, malnutrition, vitamin deficiencies (especially thiamine)
Urinary	Diuretic effect from inhibition of antidiuretic hormone
Reproductive	Breast cancer, testicular atrophy, decreased beard growth, decreased libido, decreased sperm count, gynecomastia
Integumentary	Palmar erythema, spider angiomas, rosacea, rhinophyma

TABLE 10-8 Clinical Institute Withdrawal Assessment of Alcohol Scale, Revised (CIWA-Ar)

CIWA-Ar categories, with the range of scores in each category, are as follows:

Agitation	0-7	Paroxysmal sweats	0-7
Anxiety	0-7	Tactile disturbances	0-7
Auditory disturbances	0-7	Tremor	0-7
Headache	0-7	Visual disturbances	0-7
Clouding of sensorium	0-4		

Source: University of Maryland School of Medicine. Available at *http://umem.org/files/uploads/1104212257_CIWA-Ar.pdf.*

NURSING AND INTERPROFESSIONAL MANAGEMENT: STIMULANT USE

Toxicity

Patients with stimulant toxicity present with *sympathetic overdrive* (increased stimulation of the sympathetic nervous system). The patient experiences restlessness, hypervigilance, agitated delirium, impaired judgment, and paranoia with psychotic symptoms. Physical effects include hypertension, tachycardia, fever, pupil dilation, seizures, confusion, and diaphoresis. Death may occur from stroke, dysrhythmias, or myocardial infarction.[1]

The emergency management depends on the clinical manifestations at the time of treatment (Table 10-10). A specific antidote for stimulant toxicity is not available. Supportive care measures include medications for agitation and cardiovascular symptoms.

TABLE 10-9 Manifestations and Treatment of Alcohol Withdrawal

Manifestations	Interprofessional Care
Alcohol Withdrawal Syndrome	
• Agitation • Anxiety • ↑ Heart rate • ↑ BP • Sweating • Nausea • Tremors • Insomnia • Hyperactivity	• Benzodiazepines (e.g., lorazepam [Ativan] or midazolam [Versed]) to prevent seizures and delirium • Thiamine to prevent Wernicke-Korsakoff syndrome • Multivitamins (e.g., folic acid, B vitamins) • Magnesium sulfate to treat low serum magnesium • IV glucose solution to treat hypoglycemia • β-blockers (e.g., propranolol) or α_2-agonists (e.g., clonidine) to stabilize VS • Respiratory support
Alcohol Withdrawal Delirium	
• Disorientation • Visual, tactile, or auditory hallucinations • Seizures	• Continued use of benzodiazepines • Carbamazepine (Tegretol) or valproate (Depakote) to treat seizures • Antipsychotic agents (e.g., chlorpromazine [Thorazine], haloperidol [Haldol]) • Chlordiazepoxide (Librium) if psychosis persists after benzodiazepine administration

TABLE 10-10 Emergency Management

Stimulant Toxicity

Assessment Findings	Interventions
Cardiovascular • Palpitations • Tachycardia • ↑ BP • Dysrhythmias • Myocardial ischemia or infarction **Central Nervous System** • Feeling of impending doom • Euphoria • Agitation • Combativeness • Seizures • Hallucinations • Confusion • Paranoia • Fever	• Ensure patent airway. • Establish IV access and initiate fluid replacement as appropriate. • Obtain a 12-lead ECG and initiate ECG monitoring. • Treat ventricular dysrhythmias as appropriate with lidocaine, bretylium (Bretylol), or procainamide (Pronestyl). • Hypertension and chest pain may require administration of nitroprusside (Nipride) or phentolamine (Regitine). • Aspirin may be administered to lower the risk of myocardial infarction. • Administer IV diazepam (Valium) or lorazepam (Ativan) for seizures. • Administer IV antipsychotic drugs for psychosis and hallucinations. • Monitor vital signs and level of consciousness. • Initiate cooling measures for hyperthermia.

Withdrawal

Stimulant withdrawal is usually not an emergency. Abrupt cessation can lead to a "crash." The patient may be depressed and experience fatigue, prolonged sleep, vivid dreams, irritability, increased appetite, and disorientation. Craving for the stimulant drug is intense during the first hours to days of drug cessation and may continue for weeks. Supportive care includes maintaining a quiet environment and allowing the patient to sleep and eat as desired. If a patient has severe depression, initiate suicide precautions and refer for further treatment.

DEPRESSANTS

Commonly used depressants include sedative-hypnotics and opioids. Depressants have a rapid development of tolerance and dependence. Their use is also associated with medical emergencies involving toxicity and withdrawal. Deaths related to overdose are frequently caused by depressants and often from multiple depressants (e.g., opioids and benzodiazepines).[9] Excessive alcohol consumption is also common among those reporting high rates of depressant drug use.[9] Common health problems resulting from depressant use are listed in Table 10-2.

Sedative-Hypnotics

Common sedative-hypnotic agents include barbiturates, benzodiazepines, and barbiturate-like drugs. Sedative-hypnotic drugs depress the CNS, causing sedation at low doses and sleep at high doses. Their use produces a euphoria and intoxication that resembles that of alcohol. Tolerance develops rapidly to the effects of these drugs, requiring higher doses to achieve euphoria. However, tolerance may not develop to the brainstem-depressant effects. As a result, an increased dose may trigger hypotension and respiratory depression, resulting in death.

Opioids

The term *opioid* refers to a group of substances including opium, opium derivatives, and synthetic compounds. Individuals dependent on opioids include those who use illegal drugs sold on the street and those who misuse prescription opioids. Opioids act on opiate receptors and neurotransmitter systems in the CNS, causing sedation and analgesia. The person taking an opioid experiences euphoria, mood changes, mental clouding, drowsiness, and pain reduction. While this makes prescription opioids useful in treating a number of medical conditions, their pleasurable effects promote misuse. Misusing oxycodone (OxyContin) or acetaminophen plus hydrocodone can result in the same harmful consequences as abusing heroin.

❖ NURSING AND INTERPROFESSIONAL MANAGEMENT: DEPRESSANT USE

◆ Toxicity

Unintentional overdose frequently occurs with misuse of depressants, especially when used with alcohol or other drugs. The first priority of care is always the patient's ABCs. Depressant toxicity can cause death from CNS and respiratory depression. Continuous monitoring of neurologic status and supporting respiratory and cardiovascular function is critical until the patient is stable. The emergency management depends on the substance used and the clinical manifestations (Table 10-11).

◆ **Sedative-Hypnotics.** On occasion, a patient with a benzodiazepine overdose may receive flumazenil, a specific benzodiazepine antagonist. Because flumazenil may have a shorter duration of action than some benzodiazepines, repeated doses may be needed until the benzodiazepine is metabolized. Place the patient on safety precautions, as flumazenil can cause seizures.

Since there are no antagonists for barbiturates or other sedative-hypnotic drugs, the patient who has overdosed on these agents receives treatment to promote drug elimination.[10]

✚ TABLE 10-11 Emergency Management

Depressant Toxicity

Assessment Findings	Interventions
• Aggressive behavior • Agitation • Confusion • Lethargy • Stupor • Hallucinations • Depression • Slurred speech • Pinpoint pupils • Nystagmus • Seizures • Cold, clammy skin • Rapid, weak pulse • Slow or rapid shallow respirations • Decreased O_2 saturation • Hypotension • Dysrhythmias • ECG changes • Cardiac or respiratory arrest	• Ensure patent airway. • Anticipate intubation if respiratory distress evident. • Establish IV access. • Obtain temperature. • Obtain 12-lead ECG and initiate continuous ECG monitoring. • Obtain information about substance (name, route, when taken, amount). • Obtain specific drug levels or comprehensive toxicology screen. • Obtain a health history, including drug use and allergies. • Administer antidotes as appropriate. • Perform gastric lavage if necessary. • Administer activated charcoal and cathartics as appropriate. • Monitor vital signs, level of consciousness, and O_2 saturation.

Dialysis is used to decrease the drug level and to prevent irreversible CNS effects and death. If the airway can be maintained, gastric lavage and activated charcoal are options.

◆ **Opioids.** Opioid overdose can occur when a person deliberately misuses an illegal or prescription opioid, takes an opioid prescribed for someone else, takes an opioid in combination with other depressants, or inadvertently receives an incorrect opioid dose.[11] First-line treatment includes administering an opioid antagonist such as naloxone. Naloxone reverses respiratory depression, coma, and other manifestations of toxicity. Monitor the patient closely because naloxone has a shorter duration of action than most opioids. Repeated doses of naloxone may be required until the opioid is metabolized.

In some states, laws are making naloxone more widely available. This allows police, first responders, family members, and friends to administer naloxone in emergencies, thus reversing the effects of an overdose sooner. As a result, you may see more patients requiring postreversal care.

◆ Withdrawal

◆ **Sedative-Hypnotics.** Withdrawal from sedative-hypnotics can be life threatening. The manifestations are nearly identical to those of alcohol withdrawal. Early, the patient may experience weakness, anxiety, insomnia, fever, orthostatic hypotension, and disorientation. Since the patient may experience delirium, seizures, and respiratory and cardiac arrest within 24 hours after the last dose, closely monitor the patient. Treatment consists of administering a long-acting benzodiazepine or phenobarbital in a tapered dose. IV diazepam is an option for severe manifestations. Supportive care includes implementing patient safety and comfort measures, frequently assessing neurologic status and vital signs, and providing reassurance and orientation.

◆ **Opioids.** Opioid withdrawal symptoms depend on the opioid used, route of administration, and duration of use. It is usually not life threatening but can be extremely uncomfortable. Manifestations include intense drug craving, diaphoresis, GI distress, restlessness, fever, insomnia, watery eyes, tremors, muscle aches, runny nose, and altered mood.[1] With shorter-acting drugs, withdrawal occurs 6 to 8 hours after the last dose and peaks within 1 to 3 days. With longer-acting drugs, manifestations may not appear until 1 to 3 days after the last dose and peak in 4 to 6 days.

Treatment focuses on relieving symptoms and often requires medications. Substituting a long-acting opioid (e.g., methadone, buprenorphine) at low doses or α_2-adrenergic agonists (e.g., clonidine [Catapres]) decreases withdrawal symptoms. Management includes GI medications (e.g., loperamide [Imodium], prochlorperazine [Compazine]), acetaminophen for muscle aches and fever, and benzodiazepines for acute anxiety and sleep disturbances.

INHALANTS

Many products found in the home or workplace, such as markers, glues, and cleaning fluid, contain chemicals with psychoactive properties when they are inhaled. Many people do not consider these products as drugs. However, they are sometimes misused. Inhalants are rapidly absorbed and reach the CNS quickly. Most are depressants, and their effects are similar to alcohol, including slurred speech, lack of coordination, euphoria, and dizziness. The effects are relatively brief, lasting only 60 to 90 minutes. Long-term use can result in neurologic problems, including damage to parts of the brain that control cognition, movement, vision, and hearing (Table 10-2).

The patient with inhalant toxicity may experience dizziness, euphoria, disinhibition, nystagmus, slurred speech, and lethargy. The effects usually resolve within minutes to a few hours. Managing inhalant toxicity usually consists of providing supportive care. However, in some cases, users need emergency treatment for dysrhythmias, heart failure, or CNS hyperactivity (e.g., seizures). Using some inhalants (i.e., toluene) can result in nephrotoxicity; therefore monitor renal function. Withdrawal is rare as the duration of most inhaled substances is relatively short. Any manifestations that may occur require supportive care.

CANNABIS

The use of cannabis, commonly referred to as marijuana or weed, continues to increase in the United States. The use patterns are similar to alcohol in that there is occasional use, misuse resulting in temporary problems, and the potential for SUD. The key ingredient in cannabis responsible for the psychoactive effects is tetrahydrocannabinol (THC). At low to moderate doses, THC produces effects similar to alcohol and other CNS depressants. These include euphoria, decreased inhibition, and impaired coordination. Long-term use is associated with a wide range of effects, particularly on cardiopulmonary and mental health[12] (Table 10-2).

The legalization of cannabis for medical and recreational use is controversial. While many states have legalized its use for specific medical reasons, legal sales for nonmedical use began for the first time in 2014.[12] THC-based medications, dronabinol (Marinol) and nabilone (Cesamet), are available to control nausea and vomiting resulting from cancer chemotherapy. Dronabinol is also used to stimulate the appetite in patients with acquired immunodeficiency syndrome (AIDS). Illegal synthetic THC derivatives (e.g., K2, Spice) contain varying amounts of different ingredients. The result is that these products have unpredictable effects and are more toxic. In some instances, death has occurred with a single use.

Patients with *acute marijuana toxicity* can present with acute psychotic episodes, especially if the patient used a synthetic derivative. Cannabis can induce tachycardia and hypertension, triggering dysrhythmias and myocardial infarction. Panic and flashbacks are managed by providing a quiet environment and reassuring the patient. Benzodiazepines provide symptom relief.

Withdrawal can occur in a hospitalized patient who heavily uses cannabis. The patient may experience irritability, anxiety, anorexia, chills, disturbed sleep, fever, and tremors.[1] These peak about 48 hours after cessation and last 3 to 4 days. No specific drug therapy is effective in treating withdrawal. Supportive care includes measures to ensure patient comfort, including analgesics and hydration.

CAFFEINE

Caffeine is the most widely used psychoactive substance in the world. It is very weak when compared with the other stimulants. Most people use it to promote wakefulness. Other uses include facilitating motor activity and treating headaches. Its use is safe in most people. Recently, problems from high doses of caffeine have occurred in association with specialized drinks. A large caffeine intake can cause cardiac dysrhythmias, hypertension, disturbed sleep, seizures, and anxiety. Treatment consists of seizure control with benzodiazepines or phenobarbital and supportive care until the effects wear off. In a hospitalized patient, caffeine dependence can result in muscle pain or stiffness, drowsiness, irritability, and headaches after general anesthesia or during restrictions on usual caffeine intake.[1]

❖ NURSING MANAGEMENT: SUBSTANCE USE

◆ Nursing Assessment

You need to be able to determine if the patient uses substances in a way that places them at risk or if a SUD is present. Screening is a simple effective way to identify patients who need further assessment. The **Screening, Brief Intervention, and Referral to Treatment (SBIRT)** approach can be used (Fig. 10-3). SBIRT consists of three components: (1) screening

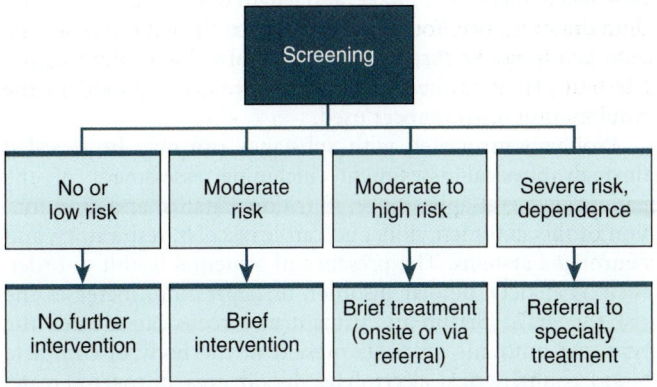

FIG. 10-3 Screening, Brief Intervention, and Referral to Treatment Approach. (From Substance Abuse and Mental Health Services Administration [SAMHSA]: Systems-level implementation of screening, brief intervention, and referral to treatment. Technical Assistance Publication [TAP] Series 33. HHS Publication No. 13-4741. Rockville, Md, 2013, SAMHSA. Retrieved from *http://www.integration.samhsa.gov/SBIRT/tap33.pdf.*)

TABLE 10-12 Brief Screening Tools for Substance Use

Single-Question Tests

Use one of the following questions to screen for the presence of alcohol, drug, or tobacco use.

- How often in the past year have you had 5 (men) or 4 (women) or more drinks in a day?
- How many times in the past year have you used illegal drugs or prescription medications for nonmedical reasons?
- In the past year, how often have you used tobacco products?

Two-Question Tests

Use the following two questions to screen for alcohol or drug use.

- In the past year, have you ever drunk or used drugs more than you meant to?
- Have you felt you wanted or needed to cut down on your drinking or drug use in the past year?

Adapted from Strobbe S: Prevention and screening, brief intervention, and referral to treatment for substance use in primary care, *Prim Care Clin Office Pract* 41:185, 2014.

or assessing for substance use problems using standardized screening tools, (2) brief intervention or teaching patients about the consequences of substance use and abuse, and (3) referring those who screen positive for further treatment.[13]

The first step of SBIRT is using screening tools to identify those who may have problems with substance use. As a baseline, ask every patient about the use of all substances, including prescribed medications, OTC drugs, caffeine, tobacco, and recreational drugs. Use simple one- or two-question screening tests to detect alcohol, tobacco, and/or other substance use problems (Table 10-12). If a patient has a positive screen, follow up with a detailed assessment to identify specific problems. A screening tool for AUDIT, the Alcohol Use Disorders Identification Test, is shown in Table 10-13. A score of 8 points or more in men or 7 or more in women is considered problematic. Another useful tool is the Drug Abuse Screening Test (DAST-10), shown in Table 10-14.

If there is any indication of substance use, determine when the patient last used the substance. Knowing this information will let you know when to expect the onset of withdrawal and help you anticipate drug interactions. Assess for factors that influence the onset of withdrawal including the substance used, dose taken, method of intake, and length of time the patient has used the substance. You may discover that the patient is dealing with *polysubstance use*, or the use of more than one substance. Alert the HCP as these patients require care tailored to the combination of substances used.

Problems associated with substance use may be revealed through physical assessment, including assessment of the patient's general appearance, nutritional status, and examination of the abdomen, skin, and cardiovascular, respiratory, and neurologic systems. The presence of a mental health disorder, such as anxiety, bipolar disorder, or depression, increases the risk for SUD.[14] Serum and urine drug screens can identify the type and amounts of drugs present in the body. A complete blood count, serum electrolytes, blood urea nitrogen, creatinine, and liver function tests evaluate for electrolyte imbalances and cardiac, kidney, or liver dysfunction.

During your assessment, observe for patient behaviors such as denial, avoidance, underreporting or minimizing substance use, or provision of inaccurate information. Possible behaviors and physical manifestations suggesting substance use are listed in Table 10-15. However, these behaviors are not all inclusive.

TABLE 10-13 Alcohol Use Disorders Identification Test (AUDIT)

Please answer each question by checking one of the circles in the second column.

		Score
1. How often do you have a drink containing alcohol?	○ Never	(0)
	○ Monthly or less	(1)
	○ 2 to 4 times per month	(2)
	○ 2 to 4 times per week	(3)
	○ 4+ times per week	(4)
2. How many drinks containing alcohol do you have on a typical day when you are drinking?	○ 1 or 2	(0)
	○ 3 or 4	(1)
	○ 5 or 6	(2)
	○ 7 to 9	(3)
	○ 10 or more	(4)
3. How often do you have six or more drinks on one occasion?	○ Never	(0)
	○ Less than monthly	(1)
	○ Monthly	(2)
	○ Weekly	(3)
	○ Daily or almost daily	(4)
4. How often during the last year have you found that you were not able to stop drinking once you had started?	○ Never	(0)
	○ Less than monthly	(1)
	○ Monthly	(2)
	○ Weekly	(3)
	○ Daily or almost daily	(4)
5. How often in the last year have you failed to do what was normally expected of you because you were drinking?	○ Never	(0)
	○ Less than monthly	(1)
	○ Monthly	(2)
	○ Weekly	(3)
	○ Daily or almost daily	(4)
6. How often during the last year have you needed a first drink in the morning to get yourself going after a heavy drinking session?	○ Never	(0)
	○ Less than monthly	(1)
	○ Monthly	(2)
	○ Weekly	(3)
	○ Daily or almost daily	(4)
7. How often during the last year have you had a feeling of guilt or remorse about drinking?	○ Never	(0)
	○ Less than monthly	(1)
	○ Monthly	(2)
	○ Weekly	(3)
	○ Daily or almost daily	(4)
8. How often during the last year have you been unable to remember what happened the night before because you had been drinking?	○ Never	(0)
	○ Less than monthly	(1)
	○ Monthly	(2)
	○ Weekly	(3)
	○ Daily or almost daily	(4)
9. Have you or someone else been injured as a result of your drinking?	○ No	(0)
	○ Yes, but not in the last year	(2)
	○ Yes, during the last year	(4)
10. Has a relative, friend, or other health worker been concerned about your drinking or suggested that you cut down?	○ No	(0)
	○ Yes, but not in the last year	(2)
	○ Yes, during the last year	(4)

Source: Babor TF, Higgins-Biddle JC, Saunders JB, Monteiro M: *The alcohol use disorders identification test*, ed 2, Geneva, Switzerland, 2001, WHO Press.
Scoring for AUDIT: Questions 1 through 8 are scored 0, 1, 2, 3, or 4. Questions 9 and 10 are scored 0, 2, or 4 only. The minimum score (nondrinkers) is 0 and the maximum possible score is 40. A score of 9 or more indicates hazardous or harmful alcohol consumption.

◆ Nursing Diagnoses

Nursing diagnoses for the patient with substance use disorder include, but are not limited to, the following:

TABLE 10-14 Drug Abuse Screening Test (DAST-10)

In the last 12 months:

1. Have you used drugs other than those required for medical reasons?	No	Yes
2. Do you abuse more than one drug at a time?	No	Yes
3. Are you always able to stop using drugs when you want to?	No	Yes
4. Have you had "blackouts" or "flashbacks" as a result of drug use?	No	Yes
5. Do you ever feel bad or guilty about your drug use?	No	Yes
6. Does your spouse (or parents) ever complain about your involvement with drugs?	No	Yes
7. Have you neglected your family because of your use of drugs?	No	Yes
8. Have you engaged in illicit activities in order to obtain drugs?	No	Yes
9. Have you ever experienced withdrawal symptoms or felt sick when you stopped taking drugs?	No	Yes
10. Have you had medical problems as a result of your drug use?	No	Yes

Copyright 1982 by Harvey A. Skinner, PhD, and the Centre for Addiction and Mental Health, Toronto, Canada. You may reproduce this instrument for noncommercial use (clinical, research, training purposes) as long as you credit the author, Dr. Harvey A. Skinner, Dean, Faculty of Health, York University, Toronto, Canada.

TABLE 10-15 Manifestations Suggesting Substance Use

- Fatigue
- Insomnia
- Headaches
- Seizure disorder
- Changes in mood
- Anorexia, weight loss
- Vague physical complaints
- Overuse of mouthwash or toiletries
- Appearing older than stated age, unkempt appearance
- Leisure activities that involve alcohol and/or other drugs
- Sexual dysfunction, decreased libido, erectile dysfunction
- Trauma secondary to falls, auto accidents, fights, or burns
- Driving while intoxicated (more than one citation suggests dependence)
- Failure of standard doses of sedatives to have a therapeutic effect
- Financial problems, including those related to spending for substances
- Defensive or evasive answers to questions about substance use and its importance in the person's life
- Problems in areas of life function (e.g., frequent job changes; marital conflict, separation, or divorce; work-related accidents, tardiness, absenteeism; legal problems; social isolation, estrangement from friends or family)

- Acute confusion *related to* toxicity or withdrawal
- Disturbed sensory perception *related to* toxicity or withdrawal
- Risk for injury *related to* altered mental status
- Ineffective health maintenance *related to* substance use

Planning

The overall goals are that the patient with a substance use problem will (1) have normal physiologic functioning, (2) acknowledge a substance use problem, (3) explain the psychologic and physiologic effects of substance use, (4) abstain from substance use, and (5) cooperate with a proposed treatment plan.

Nursing Implementation

Health Promotion. Your role in health promotion includes prevention and early detection of substance use. Prevention measures include abstinence from potentially harmful substances or limiting alcohol consumption. These measures decrease the risk of substance-related injury or illness.[14] You can help to prevent substance use problems by (1) teaching about the effects and negative outcomes of substance use and (2) providing support. Through early screening, you have the opportunity to prevent patients from becoming dependent on alcohol and other drugs. You can do this by initiating brief interventional techniques and helping them access appropriate care through referral to treatment if they exhibit risky behaviors or are already dependent.

Acute Intervention. The immediate result of overconsumption is acute toxicity or overdose. The patient may also present with trauma or injuries. The first priority of care is supporting the patient's ABCs, especially respiratory status. In addition to treating injuries, provide supportive care until detoxification can occur. Nursing care includes frequently assessing neurologic status and vital signs, administering IV fluids to prevent dehydration, orienting to time and place, and implementing patient safety measures.

Sometimes, uncertainty exists as to what substances are involved. If the patient used multiple substances, a complex clinical picture can result. For example, a patient presents with toxicity and the health care team does not know what substances are involved. Although blood and urine tests will help identify the substances, treatment is started while waiting for the test results. The patient in this situation would usually receive naloxone. If the substance used is a barbiturate or another CNS depressant, naloxone will not help the patient, but it will not hurt the patient either. If the patient does not respond to a total dose of 10 mg of naloxone, it is unlikely opioids are involved.

Once acute health issues are resolved, provide a brief intervention to teach patients about the consequences of substance use and support behavioral change. When patients have a substance use problem, it is critical to motivate the patient to engage in long-term treatment. You are in a unique position to facilitate behavior change. When a patient seeks care for health problems related to substance use or when hospitalization interferes with the usual pattern of use, the patient's awareness of a substance use problem is increased. Intervention at this time can promote behavior change. Take an active role in performing motivational interviewing and providing counseling aimed at cessation. (Motivational interviewing is discussed in Chapter 4.) Discuss the risks associated with substance use and provide feedback and advice. If the patient agrees, assist with referral to counseling or behavioral therapy.

Gerontologic Considerations: Substance Use

Substance use in older adults is often difficult to recognize. Older adults do not fit the image of users. For example, older users are less likely to be involved in drug-related criminal activity and less likely to binge drink. They use different substances than younger users. The effects of alcohol and drug use can be mistaken for medical conditions common among older adults (e.g., insomnia, depression, hypertension, dementia). Therefore substance use problems may be attributed to another cause and not adequately treated (Fig. 10-4).

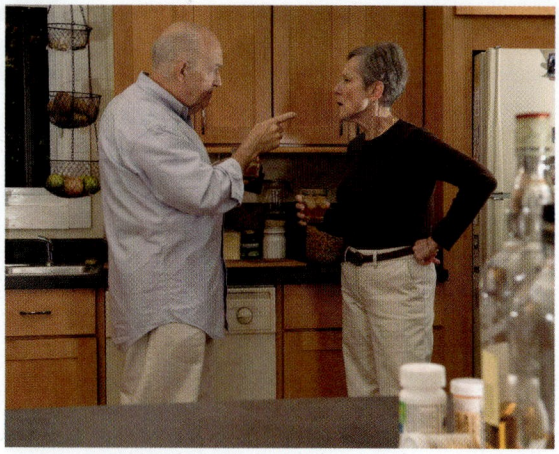

FIG. 10-4 Older adults are often unaware of their substance use problems. (©Ned White/iStock/Thinkstock)

Because of the higher rate of co-existing medical problems, older adults are at greater risk for medical problems associated with substance use. Common problems include liver damage and cardiovascular, GI, and endocrine problems. Substance use may cause confusion, delirium, memory loss, and neuromuscular impairment. Physiologic changes may lead to toxicity at levels that may not have been a problem at a younger age. Withdrawal symptoms may be more severe than in younger individuals.

It is important to screen older adults for substance use. Family members are important sources of information. Other potential sources include friends, home health aides, meal delivery personnel, and staff members at senior citizen centers and long-term care facilities. It is important for you to discuss all drug and alcohol use with older adult patients, including OTC, herbal, and homeopathic drug use. Assess the patient's knowledge of currently used medications. Common screening questionnaires may not identify an older adult with a substance use problem. The Short Michigan Alcoholism Screening Test–Geriatric version (SMAST-G) is available as a short-form alcoholism-screening instrument for older adults *(http://consultgerirn.org)* and can identify those with a potential AUD.

Smoking and other tobacco use is an issue in older adults. Those who have been chronic smokers for decades may feel unable to stop or believe there is no benefit to stopping at an advanced age. However, smoking contributes to and exacerbates many chronic illnesses found in the older adult population. Smoking cessation at any age is beneficial. The information about smoking cessation discussed earlier is appropriate for helping older adults with smoking cessation (Tables 10-3 to 10-6).

Patient teaching for the older adult includes teaching about the desired effects, possible side effects, and appropriate use of prescribed and OTC drugs. When you suspect alcohol or substance use, refer the patient for treatment. It is a mistaken belief that older people have little to gain from alcohol and drug dependence treatment. The rewards of treatment can lead to greater quality and quantity of life for older adults.

CASE STUDY

Substance Use Disorder

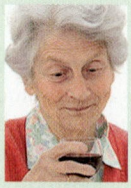

(©JPC-PROD/iStock/Thinkstock)

Patient Profile

C.M., a 78-year-old white woman, is admitted to the emergency department after falling and injuring her right hip. She has been widowed for 4 years and lives alone. Recently her best friend died. Her only family is a daughter who lives out of town. When contacted by phone, the daughter tells the nurse that her mother has appeared more disoriented and confused over the past few months when she has talked to her on the phone.

Subjective Data

- Is complaining of severe pain in her right hip
- Admits she had some wine in the late afternoon to stimulate her appetite
- Has experienced several falls in the past 2 months
- Reports that she fell after taking a sleeping pill prescribed by her physician because she does not sleep well
- Speech is hesitant and slurred
- Says she smokes about one-half pack of cigarettes a day

Objective Data

Physical Examination

- Oriented to person and place, but not time
- BP 162/94, pulse 92, respirations 24
- Severe pain and tenderness in the right hip region
- Tremors of hands

Diagnostic Tests

- X-ray reveals a subtrochanteric fracture of the right femur requiring surgical repair
- Blood alcohol concentration (BAC) 120 mg/dL (0.12 mg%)
- Complete blood count: hemoglobin 10.6 g/dL, hematocrit 33%

Discussion Questions

1. What other information is needed to assess C.M.'s condition?
2. How should you address questions regarding these areas?
3. What factors may contribute to C.M.'s substance use?
4. ***Priority Decision:*** Based on the assessment data presented, what are the priority nursing diagnoses? Are there any collaborative problems?
5. ***Priority Decision:*** What are the priority nursing interventions during C.M.'s preoperative period?
6. What possible complications and injury risks may become apparent during C.M.'s postoperative recovery?
7. ***Safety:*** To ensure C.M.'s safety, what nursing interventions are necessary after surgery?
8. ***Teamwork and Collaboration:*** How would you use the unlicensed assistive personnel (UAP) on the postoperative unit to carry out the interventions that you identified in question 5?
9. ***Teamwork and Collaboration:*** What referrals are indicated?

Answers available at *http://evolve.elsevier.com/Lewis/medsurg.*

BRIDGE TO NCLEX EXAMINATION

The number of the question corresponds to the same-numbered outcome at the beginning of the chapter.

1. When admitting a patient, the nurse must assess the patient for substance use based on the knowledge that long-term use of addictive substances leads to
   a. the development of coexisting psychiatric illnesses.
   b. a higher risk for complications from underlying health problems.
   c. potentiation of effects of similar drugs taken when the individual is drug free.
   d. increased availability of dopamine, resulting in decreased sleep requirements.
2. The nurse would suspect cocaine toxicity in the patient who is experiencing
   a. agitation, dysrhythmias, and seizures.
   b. blurred vision, restlessness, and irritability.
   c. diarrhea, nausea and vomiting, and confusion.
   d. slow, shallow respirations; bradycardia; and hypotension.
3. The *most* appropriate nursing intervention for a patient who is being treated for an acute exacerbation of chronic obstructive pulmonary disease who is not interested in quitting smoking is to
   a. accept the patient's decision and not intervene until the patient expresses a desire to quit.
   b. realize that some smokers never quit, and trying to assist them increases the patient's frustration.
   c. motivate the patient to quit by describing how continued smoking will worsen the breathing problems.
   d. ask the patient to identify the risks and benefits of quitting and what barriers to quitting are present.
4. While caring for a patient who is experiencing alcohol withdrawal, the nurse should *(select all that apply)*
   a. monitor neurologic status on a routine basis.
   b. provide a quiet, nonstimulating, dimly lit environment.
   c. pad the side rails and place suction equipment at the bedside.
   d. orient the patient to environment and person with each contact.
   e. administer antiseizure drugs and sedatives to relieve symptoms during withdrawal.
5. A patient admitted for scheduled surgery has a positive brief screening test result for an alcohol use disorder. Which initial action is *most* appropriate?
   a. notify the health care provider.
   b. complete a detailed alcohol use assessment.
   c. initiate a referral to a specialty treatment center.
   d. provide patient teaching on postoperative health risks.
6. Substance use problems in older adults are usually related to
   a. use of drugs and alcohol as a social activity.
   b. misuse of prescribed and over-the-counter drugs and alcohol.
   c. continuing the use of illegal drugs initiated during middle age.
   d. a pattern of binge drinking for weeks or months with periods of sobriety.

1. b, 2. a, 3. d, 4. a, c, d, e, 5. b, 6. b

For rationales to these answers and even more NCLEX review questions, visit *http://evolve.elsevier.com/Lewis/medsurg.*

EVOLVE WEBSITE

http://evolve.elsevier.com/Lewis/medsurg

Review Questions (Online Only)
Key Points
Answer Keys for Questions
- Rationales for Bridge to NCLEX Examination Questions
- Answer Guidelines for Case Study on p. 156
- Answer Guidelines for Managing Care of Multiple Patients Case Study (Section 1) on p. 158

Nursing Care Plan
- eNursing Care Plan 10-1: Patient in Alcohol Withdrawal

Conceptual Care Map Creator
Audio Glossary
Content Updates

REFERENCES

1. American Psychiatric Association: *The diagnostic and statistical manual of mental disorders*, ed 5, Arlington, Va, 2013, The Association.
2. CDC: Adult cigarette smoking in the U.S. Retrieved from *www.cdc.gov/tobacco/data_statistics/fact_sheets/adult_data/cig_smoking.*
3. CDC: Health effects of cigarette smoking. Retrieved from *www.cdc.gov/tobacco/data_statistics/fact_sheets/health_effects/effects_cig_smoking/#overview.*

*4. Hajek P, Etter J, Benowitz N, et al: Electronic cigarettes: review of use, content, safety, effects on smokers and potential for harm and benefit, *Addiction* 109:1801, 2014.

5. Agency for Healthcare Research and Quality: Treating tobacco use and dependence: 2008 update. Retrieved from *www.ahrq.gov/professionals/clinicians-providers/guidelines-recommendations/tobacco/index.html.*
6. Alcohol Facts and Statistics. Retrieved from *www.niaaa.nih.gov/alcohol-health/overview-alcohol-consumption/alcohol-facts-and-statistics.*
7. Miguel GM, Bejar-Prado L, Gili-Ortiz E, et al: Alcohol use disorders among surgical patients: Unplanned 30-days readmissions, length of hospital stay, excessive costs and mortality, *Drug Alc Dep* 137:55, 2014.
8. Patel G: The management of substance abuse in the critically ill, *Disease-a-Month* 60:429, 2014.
9. CDC: Prescription drug overdose in the United States. Retrieved from *www.cdc.gov/homeandrecreationalsafety/overdose/facts.html.*

*10. Mactier R, Laliberté M, Mardini J, et al: Extracorporeal treatment for barbiturate poisoning, *Am J of Kidney Dis* 64:347, 2014.

11. Substance Abuse and Mental Health Services Administration: *Opioid overdose prevention toolkit*, HHS Publication No. SMA 14-4742 2014, Rockville, Md, 2013, The Institute.
12. Durkin A: Legalization of marijuana for non-medical use, *J Psychosoc Nurs* 52:22, 2014.
13. SAMSA-HRSA Center for Integrated Health Solutions: SBIRT. Retrieved from *www.integration.samhsa.gov/clinical-practice/SBIRT.*
14. Strobbe S: Prevention and screening, brief intervention, and referral to treatment for substance use in primary care, *Prim Care Clin Office Pract* 41:185, 2014.

*Evidence-based information for clinical practice.

CASE STUDY

Managing Care of Multiple Patients

Introduction

You are assigned to care for the following five patients on a medical-surgical unit. Your team consists of yourself, a new LPN still on orientation, and a UAP (unlicensed assistive personnel).

Patients

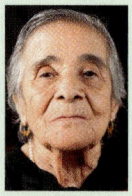

(©Luevanos/ iStock/ Thinkstock)

M.S. is an 81-yr-old woman who came to the United States from India 4 yr ago with her daughter, son-in-law, and their four children. She speaks minimal English, relying on her oldest granddaughter to translate. M.S., who has a history of diabetes mellitus, was admitted to the hospital yesterday with a diagnosis of heart failure.

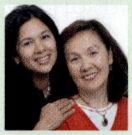

(©Thomas M Perkins/ Shutterstock)

M.L. is a 60-yr-old Asian woman who was admitted to the hospital with a diagnosis of exacerbation of chronic obstructive pulmonary disease (COPD). She is receiving O_2 at 2 L/min via nasal cannula and her condition is currently stable.

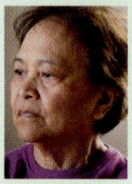

(©azndc/ iStock/ Thinkstock)

C.L. is a 73-yr-old Taiwanese woman who was brought to the ED by her son. Her chief complaint is shortness of breath. She has a history of COPD, hypertension, diabetes, and stroke. She was diagnosed with community-acquired pneumonia, which is being treated with IV antibiotics.

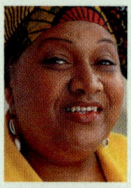

(©Ryan McVey/ Photodisc/ Thinkstock)

K.C. is a 280-lb (127-kg) 68-yr-old African American woman with diabetes who was admitted for an incision and drainage of a right abdominal abscess. She is being discharged on her second postoperative day. Her daughter will assist with dressing changes at home.

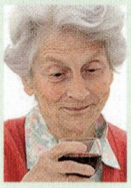

(©JPC-PROD/ iStock/ Thinkstock)

C.M. is a 78-yr-old white woman who was admitted from the ED after falling and fracturing her right hip. She is in Buck's traction and is scheduled to undergo surgical repair later this morning. She has a history of substance abuse and her blood alcohol content (BAC) was 120 mg/dL (0.12 mg%) on admission. The night nurse reports that she has been somewhat confused and restless overnight.

Discussion Questions

1. ***Priority Decision:*** After receiving report, which patient should you see first? Provide rationale.
2. **Teamwork and Collaboration:** Which morning task(s) could you delegate to the LPN *(select all that apply)*?
   a. Obtain a capillary blood glucose reading on K.C.
   b. Assess C.L.'s IV site for signs of phlebitis or infiltration.
   c. Access the hospital's available translation services for M.S.
   d. Provide discharge teaching on wound care for K.C. and her daughter.
   e. Titrate M.L.'s O_2 to obtain a pulse oximetry reading of 95% (as ordered by the health care provider).
3. ***Priority and Teamwork and Collaboration:*** When you and the LPN enter M.S.'s room, you find her sitting up in bed with labored respirations. Although you cannot understand what she is saying, you note that she is unable to say more than two words without stopping for a breath. Which *initial* action would be the *most* appropriate?
   a. Administer M.S.'s cardiac and respiratory medications and reassess her in 30 minutes.
   b. Ask the LPN to stay with M.S. while you go to the nurse's station to call her health care provider.
   c. Have the LPN find M.S.'s granddaughter so that she can translate what M.S. is trying to tell you.
   d. Ask the LPN to obtain an O_2 saturation and vital signs while you perform a respiratory assessment.

Case Study Progression

M.S.'s assessment reveals bibasilar crackles, 2+ dependent pitting edema, BP 175/84, pulse 116, RR 32, temp 36.8°C, and pulse oximetry 88% on room air. You administer O_2 at 4 L/min via nasal cannula and obtain an order from M.S.'s health care provider for furosemide 40 mg IV stat. After administering the diuretic, M.S.'s granddaughter arrives and you discuss her grandmother's condition. She tells you that her grandmother asked her to bring in potato chips and soda yesterday. She did not think her grandmother should be eating salt, but M.S. insisted that the dietitian said that she could eat them.

4. On further investigation, the dietitian tells you that an interpreter (translator) was not available when she saw M.S. yesterday. Because the dietitian did not understand what the patient was saying, she could not respond to any of her questions. She planned to visit M.S. today when the granddaughter is present. Being a culturally competent nurse, you realize that M.S. most likely interpreted the dietitian's silence as
   a. agreement with what A.Z. was asking.
   b. demonstrating a lack of respect for A.Z.'s wishes.
   c. a lack of understanding by the dietitian as to what she was asking.
   d. a need for the dietitian to get more information before answering her questions.
5. Which assessment findings may suggest elder mistreatment by C.L.'s son with whom she lives *(select all that apply)*?
   a. Two sacral ulcers
   b. Asking when her son is coming to visit
   c. Multiple small bruises on her forearms and shins
   d. Matted hair, poor oral hygiene, overgrown toenails
   e. C.L. becomes totally silent when her son comes to visit
6. Knowing that C.M.'s reported restlessness overnight may indicate acute alcohol withdrawal, you perform a more thorough assessment. Your assessment reveals a score of 11 on the Clinical Institute Withdrawal Assessment for Alcohol Scale. To prevent alcohol delirium, you plan to administer which medications per the health care provider's order *(select all that apply)*?
   a. IV thiamine
   b. morphine
   c. naloxone
   d. lorazepam (Ativan)
   e. haloperidol (Haldol)
7. ***Management Decision:*** The UAP informs you that the LPN is not following hospital protocol when caring for patients at risk for falling. What is your *most* appropriate action?
   a. Notify the unit manager as soon as possible.
   b. Ask the UAP to explain hospital protocol to the LPN.
   c. Write up the LPN's actions so they are included in her evaluation.
   d. Talk to the LPN about the importance of following hospital protocol to prevent injury in patients at risk for falling.

Answers available at *http://evolve.elsevier.com/Lewis/medsurg.*

SECTION 2

Pathophysiologic Mechanisms of Disease

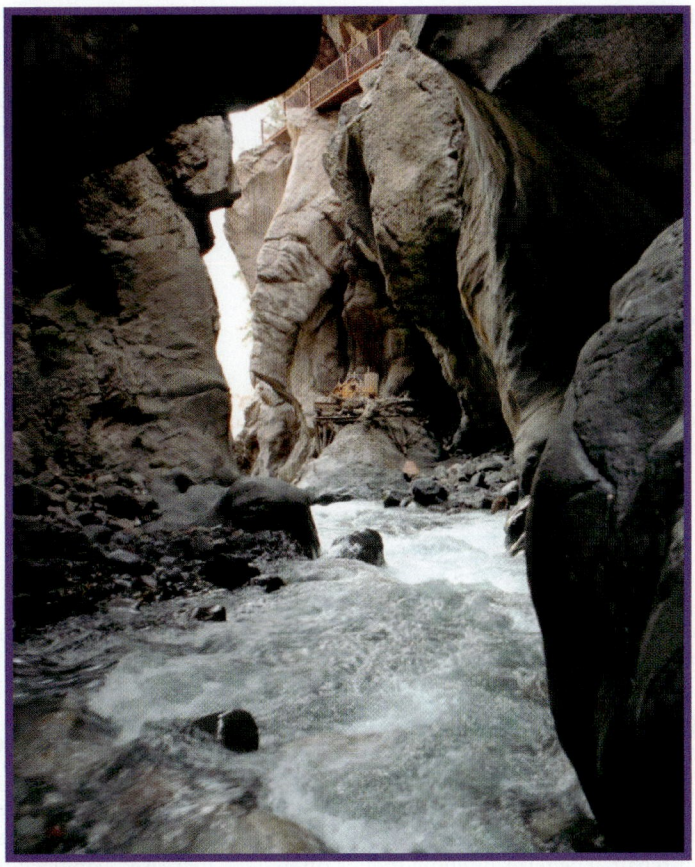

Peter Bonner

May what I do flow from me like a river,
no forcing and no holding back,
the way it is with children.

Rainer Maria Rilke

Chapter 11 Inflammation and Wound Healing, 160

Chapter 12 Genetics and Genomics, 178

Chapter 13 Altered Immune Responses and Transplantation, 191

Chapter 14 Infection and Human Immunodeficiency Virus Infection, 213

Chapter 15 Cancer, 234

Chapter 16 Fluid, Electrolyte, and Acid-Base Imbalances, 270

11

Inflammation and Wound Healing

Sharon L. Lewis

The most difficult thing is the decision to act, the rest is merely tenacity.

Amelia Earhart

http://evolve.elsevier.com/Lewis/medsurg/

LEARNING OUTCOMES

1. Describe the inflammatory response, including vascular and cellular responses and exudate formation.
2. Explain local and systemic manifestations of inflammation and their physiologic bases.
3. Describe the drug therapy, nutrition therapy, and nursing management of inflammation.
4. Differentiate among healing by primary, secondary, and tertiary intention.
5. Describe the factors that delay wound healing and common complications of wound healing.
6. Describe the nursing and interprofessional management of wound healing.
7. Explain the etiology and clinical manifestations of pressure ulcers.
8. Apply a patient risk assessment for pressure ulcers to measures used to prevent the development of pressure ulcers.
9. Discuss nursing and interprofessional management of a patient with pressure ulcers.

KEY TERMS

adhesions, Table 11-7, p. 167
dehiscence, Table 11-7, p. 167
evisceration, Table 11-7, p. 167
fibroblasts, p. 166
hypertrophic scars, Table 11-7, p. 167
inflammatory response, p. 160
pressure ulcer, p. 172
regeneration, p. 165
repair, p. 165
shearing force, p. 172

This chapter focuses on inflammation and wound healing. Pressure ulcer prevention and treatment are also described.

INFLAMMATORY RESPONSE

The **inflammatory response** is a sequential reaction to cell injury. It neutralizes and dilutes the inflammatory agent, removes necrotic materials, and establishes an environment suitable for healing and repair. The term *inflammation* is often but incorrectly used as a synonym for the term *infection*. Inflammation is always present with infection, but infection is not always present with inflammation. However, a person who is neutropenic may not be able to mount an inflammatory response. An infection involves invasion of tissues or cells by microorganisms such as bacteria, fungi, and viruses. In contrast, inflammation can also be caused by heat, radiation, trauma, chemicals, allergens, and an autoimmune reaction.

The mechanism of inflammation is basically the same regardless of the injuring agent. The intensity of the response depends on the extent and severity of injury and on the injured person's reactive capacity. The inflammatory response can be divided into a vascular response, cellular response, formation of exudate, and healing. Fig. 11-1 illustrates the vascular and cellular response to injury.

Vascular Response

After cell injury, local arterioles briefly undergo transient vasoconstriction. After release of histamine and other chemicals by the injured cells, the vessels dilate. Chemical mediators cause increased capillary permeability and facilitate fluid movement from capillaries into tissue spaces. Initially composed of serous fluid, this inflammatory exudate later contains plasma proteins, primarily albumin. These proteins exert oncotic pressure that further draws fluid from blood vessels. Both vasodilation and increased capillary permeability are responsible for redness, heat, and swelling at the site of injury and the surrounding area.

As the plasma protein fibrinogen leaves the blood, it is activated to fibrin by the products of the injured cells. Fibrin strengthens a blood clot formed by platelets. In tissues, the clot functions to trap bacteria, prevent their spread, and serve as a framework for the healing process. Platelets release growth factors that start the healing process.

Reviewed by Marylee Bressie, RN, DNP, CCRN, CCNS, CEN, Core Faculty/Nurse Planner, Department of Nursing, School of Public Service Leadership, Capella University, Minneapolis, Minnesota; Diana L. Gallagher, RN, MS, CWOCN, CFCN, Clinical Nursing and Education, HealthMatters Consulting, Fayetteville, Arkansas; and Christina D. Keller, RN, MSN-Ed, Instructor, Clinical Simulation Center, Radford University, Radford, Virginia.

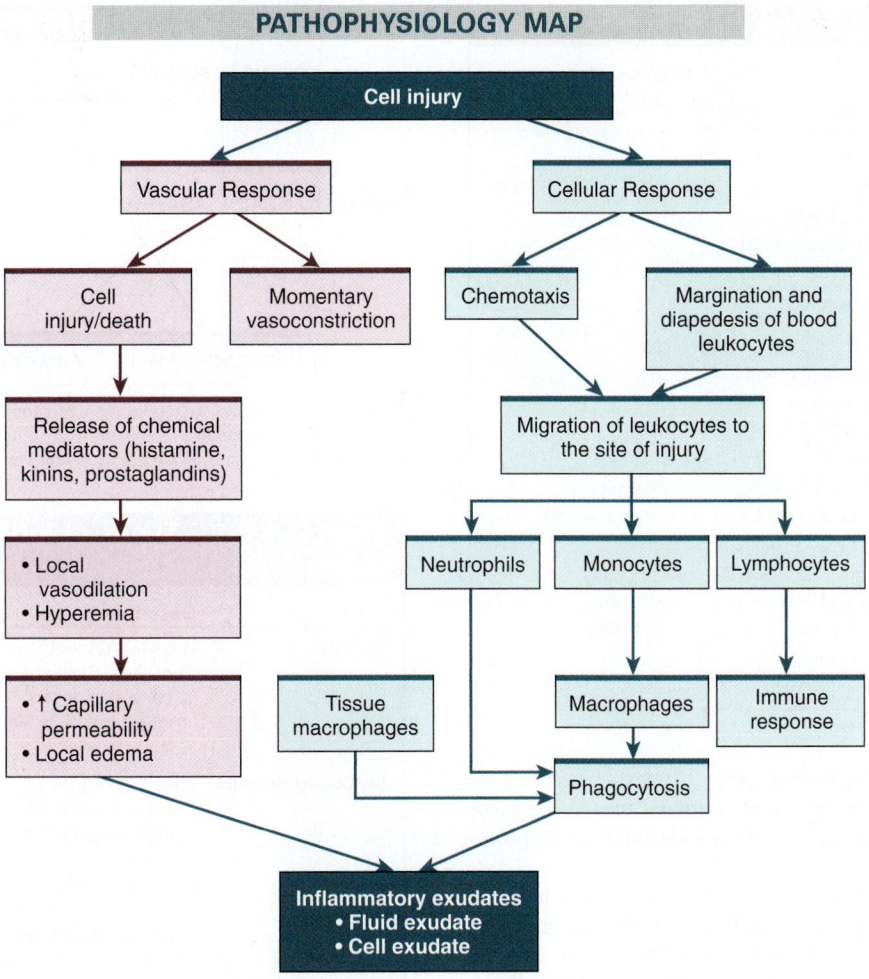

FIG. 11-1 Vascular and cellular responses to tissue injury.

Cellular Response

Neutrophils and monocytes move from circulation to the site of injury (Fig. 11-1). *Chemotaxis* is the directional migration of white blood cells (WBCs) to the site of injury, resulting in an accumulation of neutrophils and monocytes at the site.

Neutrophils. Neutrophils are the first leukocytes to arrive at the injury site (usually within 6 to 12 hours). They phagocytize (engulf) bacteria, other foreign material, and damaged cells. With their short life span (24 to 48 hours), dead neutrophils soon accumulate. In time a mixture of dead neutrophils, digested bacteria, and other cell debris accumulates as a creamy substance termed *pus.*

To keep up with the demand for neutrophils, the bone marrow releases more neutrophils into circulation. This results in an elevated WBC count, especially the neutrophil count. Sometimes the demand for neutrophils increases to the extent that the bone marrow releases immature forms of neutrophils *(bands)* into circulation. (Mature neutrophils are called *segmented neutrophils.*) The finding of increased numbers of band neutrophils in circulation is called a *shift to the left,* which is commonly found in patients with acute bacterial infections. (See Chapter 29 for a discussion of neutrophils.)

Monocytes. Monocytes are the second type of phagocytic cells that migrate from circulating blood. They usually arrive at the site within 3 to 7 days after the onset of inflammation. On entering the tissue spaces, monocytes transform into macrophages. Together with the tissue macrophages, these newly arrived macrophages assist in phagocytosis of the inflammatory debris. The macrophage role is important in cleaning the area before healing can occur. Macrophages have a long life span; they can multiply and may stay in the damaged tissues for weeks. These long-lived cells are important in orchestrating the healing process.

In cases in which particles are too large for a single macrophage, the macrophages accumulate and fuse to form a *multinucleated giant cell.* The giant cell is then encapsulated by collagen, leading to the formation of a granuloma. A classic example of this process occurs in tuberculosis of the lung. While the *Mycobacterium* bacillus is walled off, a chronic state of inflammation exists. The granuloma formed is a cavity of necrotic tissue.

Lymphocytes. Lymphocytes arrive later at the site of injury. Their primary role is related to humoral and cell-mediated immunity (see Chapter 13).

Chemical Mediators

Mediators of the inflammatory response are presented in Table 11-1.

Complement System. The complement system is an enzyme cascade (C1 to C9) consisting of pathways to mediate inflammation and destroy invading pathogens. Major functions of the

TABLE 11-1 Mediators of Inflammation

Mediator	Source	Mechanisms of Action
Histamine	Stored in granules of basophils, mast cells, platelets	Causes vasodilation and increased capillary permeability
Serotonin	Stored in platelets, mast cells, enterochromaffin cells of GI tract	Same as above. Stimulates smooth muscle contraction
Kinins (e.g., bradykinin)	Produced from precursor factor kininogen as a result of activation of Hageman factor (XII) of clotting system	Cause contraction of smooth muscle and vasodilation. Result in stimulation of pain
Complement components (C3a, C4a, C5a)	Anaphylatoxic agents generated from complement pathway activation	Stimulate histamine release and chemotaxis
Prostaglandins (PGs) **and leukotrienes** (LTs)	Produced from arachidonic acid (Fig. 11-2)	PGs cause vasodilation. LTs stimulate chemotaxis.
Cytokines	For information on cytokines, see Table 13-3	

complement system are enhanced phagocytosis, increased vascular permeability, chemotaxis, and cellular lysis. All of these activities are important mediators of the inflammatory response and healing.

Cell lysis occurs when the final components create holes in the cell membranes and cause targeted cell death by membrane rupture. In autoimmune disorders, healthy tissue can be damaged by complement activation and the resulting inflammatory response. Examples of this include rheumatoid arthritis and systemic lupus erythematosus.

Prostaglandins and Leukotrienes. When cells are activated by injury, the arachidonic acid in the cell membrane is rapidly converted to produce prostaglandins (PGs), thromboxane, and leukotrienes (Fig. 11-2). PGs are generally considered proinflammatory and are potent vasodilators contributing to increased blood flow and edema formation.

Some subtypes of PGs are formed when platelets are activated and can inhibit platelet and neutrophil aggregation. PGs also perform a significant role in sensitizing pain receptors to arousal by stimuli that would normally be painless. PGs have a pivotal role as pyrogens when stimulating the temperature-regulating area of the hypothalamus and producing a febrile response (see section on Fever on p. 163).

Thromboxane is a powerful vasoconstrictor and platelet-aggregating agent. It causes brief vasoconstriction and skin pallor at the injury site and promotes clot formation. It has a short half-life, and the pallor soon gives way to vasodilation and redness, which is caused by PGs and histamine.

Leukotrienes form the slow-reacting substance of anaphylaxis (SRS-A), which constricts smooth muscles of bronchi, causing narrowing of the airway, and increases capillary permeability, leading to airway edema.

Exudate Formation

Exudate consists of fluid and leukocytes that move from the circulation to the site of injury. The nature and quantity of exudate depend on the type and severity of the injury and tissues involved (Table 11-2).

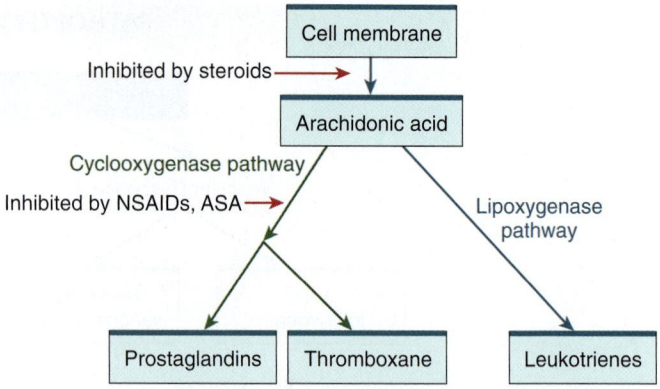

FIG. 11-2 Pathway of generation of prostaglandins, thromboxane, and leukotrienes. Corticosteroids, nonsteroidal antiinflammatory drugs *(NSAIDs)*, and acetylsalicylic acid *(ASA)* act to inhibit various steps in this pathway.

TABLE 11-2 Types of Inflammatory Exudate

Type	Description	Examples
Serous	Results from outpouring of fluid. Seen in early stages of inflammation or when injury is mild	Skin blisters, pleural effusion
Serosanguineous	Found during the midpoint in healing after surgery or tissue injury Composed of RBCs and serous fluid, which is semiclear pink and may have red streaks	Surgical drain fluid
Fibrinous	Occurs with increasing vascular permeability and fibrinogen leakage into interstitial spaces Excessive amounts of fibrin that coats tissue surfaces may cause them to adhere.	Adhesions, gelatinous ribbons seen in surgical drain tubing Frequently covers fluid-exuding wounds such as venous ulcers
Hemorrhagic	Results from rupture or necrosis of blood vessel walls	Hematoma, bleeding after surgery or tissue trauma
Purulent (pus)	Consists of WBCs, microorganisms (dead and alive), liquefied dead cells, and other debris	Furuncle (boil), abscess, cellulitis (diffuse inflammation in connective tissue)
Catarrhal	Found in tissues where cells produce mucus Mucus production is accelerated by inflammatory response	Runny nose associated with upper respiratory tract infection

Clinical Manifestations

The *local manifestations* of inflammation include redness, heat, pain, swelling, and loss of function (Table 11-3 and Fig. 11-3).

TABLE 11-3 Local Manifestations of Inflammation

Manifestations	Cause
Redness (rubor)	Hyperemia from vasodilation
Heat (calor)	Increased metabolism at inflammatory site
Pain (dolor)	Change in pH. Nerve stimulation by chemicals (e.g., histamine, prostaglandins). Pressure from fluid exudate
Swelling (tumor)	Fluid shift to interstitial spaces. Fluid exudate accumulation
Loss of function (functio laesa)	Swelling and pain

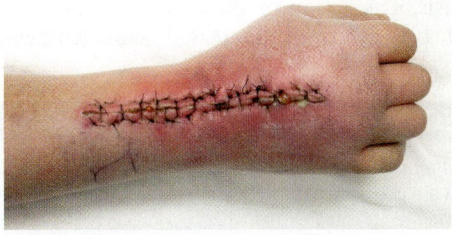

FIG. 11-3 Inflammation secondary to postoperative deep wound infection following wrist surgery. (From Hayden RJ, Jebson PJL: Wrist arthrodesis, *Hand Clinics* 21[4]:631, 2005.)

Systemic manifestations of inflammation include an increased WBC count with a shift to the left, malaise, nausea and anorexia, increased pulse and respiratory rate, and fever.

Leukocytosis results from the increased release of WBCs from the bone marrow. Although the causes of other systemic manifestations are poorly understood, they may be related to complement activation and the release of *cytokines* (soluble factors secreted by WBCs and other types of cells that act as intercellular and intracellular messengers). Some of these cytokines (e.g., interleukins [ILs], tumor necrosis factor [TNF]) are important in causing the systemic manifestations of inflammation, as well as inducing fever. An increase in pulse and respiration follows the rise in metabolism as a result of an increase in body temperature. (Cytokines are discussed in Chapter 13.)

Fever. The onset of fever is triggered by the release of cytokines, which cause fever by initiating metabolic changes in the temperature-regulating center in the hypothalamus (Fig. 11-4). The synthesis of PGs is the most critical metabolic change. PGs act directly to increase the thermostatic set point. The hypothalamus then activates the autonomic nervous system to stimulate increased muscle tone and shivering and decreased perspiration and blood flow to the periphery. Epinephrine released from the adrenal medulla increases the metabolic rate. The net result is fever.

With the physiologic thermostat fixed at a higher-than-normal temperature, the rate of heat production is increased until the body temperature reaches the new set point. As the set point is raised, the hypothalamus signals an increase in heat production and conservation to raise the body temperature to the new level. At this point the individual feels chilled and shivers. The shivering response is the body's method of raising the body's temperature until the new set point is attained.[1] This seeming paradox is dramatic: the body is hot, yet an individual piles on blankets and may go to bed to get warm. When the body temperature reaches the set point, the chills and warmth-seeking behavior cease.

PATHOPHYSIOLOGY MAP

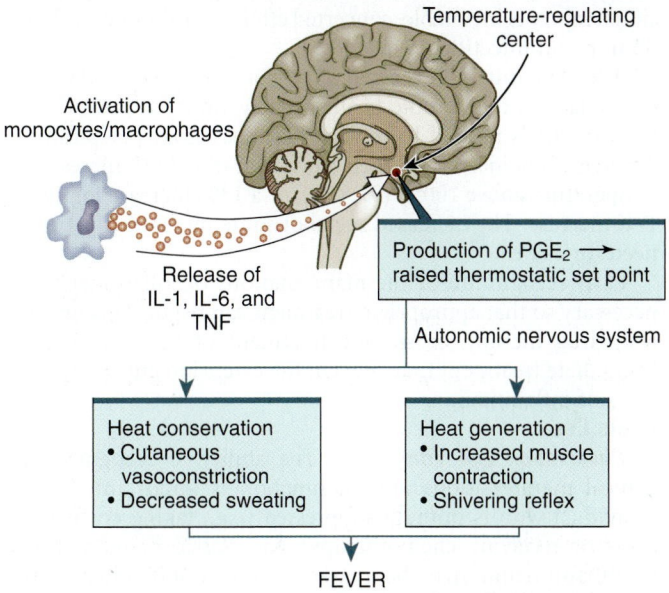

FIG. 11-4 Production of fever. When monocytes/macrophages are activated, they secrete cytokines such as interleukin-1 *(IL-1)*, interleukin-6 *(IL-6)*, and tumor necrosis factor *(TNF)*, which reach the hypothalamic temperature-regulating center. These cytokines promote the synthesis and secretion of prostaglandin E_2 *(PGE_2)* in the anterior hypothalamus. PGE_2 increases the thermostatic set point, and the autonomic nervous system is stimulated, resulting in shivering, muscle contraction, and peripheral vasoconstriction.

The released cytokines and the fever that they trigger activate the body's defense mechanisms. Beneficial aspects of fever include increased killing of microorganisms, increased phagocytosis by neutrophils, and increased proliferation of T cells. Higher body temperatures may also enhance the activity of interferon, the body's natural virus-fighting substance (see Chapter 13).

Types of Inflammation

The basic types of inflammation are acute, subacute, and chronic. In *acute inflammation*, the healing occurs in 2 to 3 weeks and usually leaves no residual damage. Neutrophils are the predominant cell type at the site of inflammation. A *subacute inflammation* has the features of the acute process but lasts longer. For example, infective endocarditis is a smoldering infection with acute inflammation, but it persists for weeks or months (see Chapter 36).

Chronic inflammation lasts for weeks, months, or even years. The injurious agent persists or repeatedly injures tissue. The predominant cell types present at the site of inflammation are lymphocytes and macrophages. Examples of chronic inflammation include rheumatoid arthritis and osteomyelitis. The prolongation and chronicity of any inflammation may be the result of an alteration in the immune response (e.g., autoimmune disease) and can lead to physical deterioration.

❖ NURSING AND INTERPROFESSIONAL MANAGEMENT: INFLAMMATION

◆ Nursing Implementation

◆ **Health Promotion.** The best management of inflammation is the prevention of infection, trauma, surgery, and contact with potentially harmful agents. This is not always possible. A simple mosquito bite causes an inflammatory response. Because occasional injury is inevitable, concerted efforts to minimize inflammation and infection are needed.

Adequate nutrition is essential so that the body has the necessary factors to promote healing when injury occurs. A high fluid intake is needed to replace fluid loss from perspiration. There is a 7% increase in metabolism for every 1°F increase in temperature above 100°F (37.8°C), or a 13% increase for every 1°C increase. The increased metabolic rate increases a patient's need for calories.

Early recognition of the manifestations of inflammation is necessary so that appropriate treatment can begin. This may be rest, drug therapy, or specific treatment of the injured site. Immediate treatment may prevent the extension and complications of inflammation.

Acute Care

Observation and Vital Signs. The ability to recognize the clinical manifestations of inflammation is important. In the individual who is immunosuppressed (e.g., taking corticosteroids or receiving chemotherapy), the classic manifestations of inflammation may be masked. In this individual, early symptoms of inflammation may be malaise or "just not feeling well."

Vital signs are important to note with any inflammation, especially when an infectious process is present. With infection, the temperature may rise, and pulse and respiration rates may increase.

Fever. An important aspect of fever management is determining its cause. Although fever is usually regarded as harmful, an increase in body temperature is an important host defense mechanism. In the seventeenth century, Thomas Sydenham noted that "fever is a mighty engine which nature brings into the world for the conquest of her enemies."[2]

Steps are frequently taken to lower body temperature to relieve the anxiety of the patient and health care professionals. Because mild to moderate fever usually does little harm, imposes no great discomfort, and may benefit host defense mechanisms, antipyretic drugs are rarely essential to patient welfare. Moderate fevers (up to 103°F [39.4°C]) usually produce few problems in most patients. However, if the patient is very young or very old, is extremely uncomfortable, or has a significant medical problem (e.g., severe cardiopulmonary disease, brain injury), the use of antipyretics should be considered. Fever in the immunosuppressed patient should be treated immediately with antibiotic therapy because infections can rapidly progress to septicemia. (Neutropenia is discussed in Chapter 30 on pp. 632-633.)

Fever (especially if greater than 104°F [40°C]) can damage body cells, and delirium and seizures can occur. At temperatures greater than 105.8°F (41°C), regulation by the hypothalamic temperature control center becomes impaired. Damage can occur to many cells, including those in the brain.

Older adults have a blunted febrile response to infection. The body temperature may not rise to the level expected for a younger adult, or the rise may be delayed in its onset. The blunted response can delay diagnosis and treatment. By the time fever (as defined for younger adults) is present, the illness may be more severe. Patients who are taking nonsteroidal anti-inflammatory drugs (NSAIDs) on a regular basis (e.g., for treatment of rheumatoid arthritis) may also have a blunted febrile response.

Although sponge baths increase evaporative heat loss, they may not decrease the body temperature unless antipyretic drugs have been given to lower the set point. Otherwise, the body will initiate compensatory mechanisms (e.g., shivering) to restore body heat. The same principle applies to the use of cooling blankets, which are most effective in lowering body temperature when the set point has also been lowered.

A nursing care plan for the patient with a fever (eNursing Care Plan 11-1) is available on the website for this chapter.

Drug Therapy. Drugs are used to decrease the inflammatory response and lower the body temperature (Table 11-4). Aspirin blocks PG synthesis in the hypothalamus and elsewhere in the body. Acetaminophen acts on the heat-regulating center in the hypothalamus. Some NSAIDs (e.g., ibuprofen [Motrin, Advil]) have antipyretic effects. Corticosteroids are antipyretic through the dual mechanisms of preventing cytokine production and PG synthesis. The action of these drugs results in dilation of superficial blood vessels, increased skin temperature, and sweating.

CHECK YOUR PRACTICE

A 76-yr-old female patient has acute osteomyelitis following a fractured femur. You are checking her temperature every 2 hours and giving acetaminophen when it is higher than 102°F. However, you notice that her temperature is greatly fluctuating from 96°F to 103°F.

- What should you do?

Antipyretics should be given around the clock to prevent acute swings in temperature. Chills may be evoked or perpetuated by the intermittent administration of antipyretics. These agents cause a sharp decrease in temperature. When the antipyretic wears off, the body may initiate a compensatory

TABLE 11-4 Drug Therapy
Inflammation and Healing

Drug	Mechanism of Action
Antipyretic Drugs	
Salicylates (aspirin)	Inhibit synthesis of PGs (Fig. 11-2). Lower temperature by action on heat-regulating center in hypothalamus, resulting in peripheral vasodilation and heat loss
Acetaminophen (Tylenol)	Inhibits synthesis of PGs. Lowers temperature by action on heat-regulating center in hypothalamus
NSAIDs (e.g., ibuprofen [Advil])	Inhibit synthesis of PGs
Antiinflammatory Drugs	
Salicylates (aspirin)	Inhibit synthesis of PGs, reduce capillary permeability
Corticosteroids (e.g., prednisone)	Interfere with tissue granulation, induce immunosuppressive effects (decreased synthesis of lymphocytes), prevent liberation of lysosomes
NSAIDs (e.g., ibuprofen, piroxicam [Feldene])	Inhibit synthesis of PGs
Vitamins	
Vitamin A	Accelerates epithelialization
Vitamin B complex	Acts as coenzymes
Vitamin C	Assists in synthesis of collagen and new capillaries
Vitamin D	Facilitates calcium absorption

PGs, Prostaglandins.

involuntary muscular contraction (i.e., chill) to raise the body temperature back up to its previous level. This unpleasant side effect of antipyretic drugs can be prevented by administering these agents regularly at 2- to 4-hour intervals.

Antihistamine drugs may also be used to inhibit the action of histamine. (Antihistamines are discussed in Chapters 13 and 26.)

- ***RICE.*** Rest, ice, compression, and elevation (RICE) is a key concept in treating soft tissue injuries and related inflammation.
- **Rest.** Rest helps the body use its nutrients and O_2 for the healing process. The repair process is facilitated by allowing fibrin and collagen to form across the wound edges with little disruption.
- **Cold and heat.** Cold application is usually appropriate at the time of the initial trauma to promote vasoconstriction and decrease swelling, pain, and congestion from increased metabolism in the area of inflammation. Heat may be used later (e.g., after 24 to 48 hours) to promote healing by increasing the circulation to the inflamed site and subsequent removal of debris. Heat is also used to localize the inflammatory agents. Warm, moist heat may help debride the wound site if necrotic material is present.
- **Compression and immobilization.** Compression counters the vasodilation effects and development of edema. Compression by direct pressure over a laceration occludes blood vessels and stops bleeding. Compression bandages provide support to injured joints that have tendons and muscles unable to provide support on their own. Assess distal pulses and capillary refill before and after application of compression to evaluate whether compression has compromised circulation (e.g., pale color of skin, loss of feeling).

  Immobilization of the inflamed or injured area promotes healing by decreasing the tissues' metabolic needs. Immobilization with a cast or splint supports fractured bones and prevents further tissue injury from sharp bone fragments that could sever nerves or blood vessels (causing hemorrhage). As with compression, evaluate the patient's circulation after application and at regular intervals. Swelling can occur within the closed space of a cast and compromise circulation.
- **Elevation.** Elevating the injured extremity above the level of the heart reduces the edema at the inflammatory site by increasing venous and lymphatic return. Elevation also helps reduce pain associated with blood engorgement at the injury site. Elevation may be contraindicated in patients with significantly reduced arterial circulation.

HEALING PROCESS

The final phase of the inflammatory response is healing. Healing includes two major components: regeneration and repair.

Regeneration

Regeneration is the replacement of lost cells and tissues with cells of the same type. The ability of cells to regenerate depends on the cell type (Table 11-5).

Repair

Repair is healing as a result of lost cells being replaced by connective tissue. Repair is the more common type of healing and usually results in scar formation. Repair is a more complex process than regeneration. Most injuries heal by connective tissue repair. Repair healing occurs by primary, secondary, or tertiary intention (Fig. 11-5).

TABLE 11-5 Regenerative Ability of Different Types of Tissues

Tissues	Cell Type	Description
Skin, lymphoid organs, bone marrow, and mucous membranes	Labile cells	Cells divide constantly. Injury to these organs is followed by rapid regeneration.
Liver, pancreas, kidney, and bone cells	Stable cells	Retain their ability to regenerate but do so only if the organ is injured. Regeneration is slow.
Neurons of the central nervous system (CNS) and skeletal and cardiac muscle cells	Permanent cells	Do not divide. Damage to CNS neurons or skeletal or heart muscle can lead to permanent loss. Healing of skeletal and cardiac muscle will occur by repair with scar tissue. If neurons in the CNS are destroyed, the tissue is generally replaced by glial cells. However, neurogenesis may occur from stem cells (see Chapter 55).

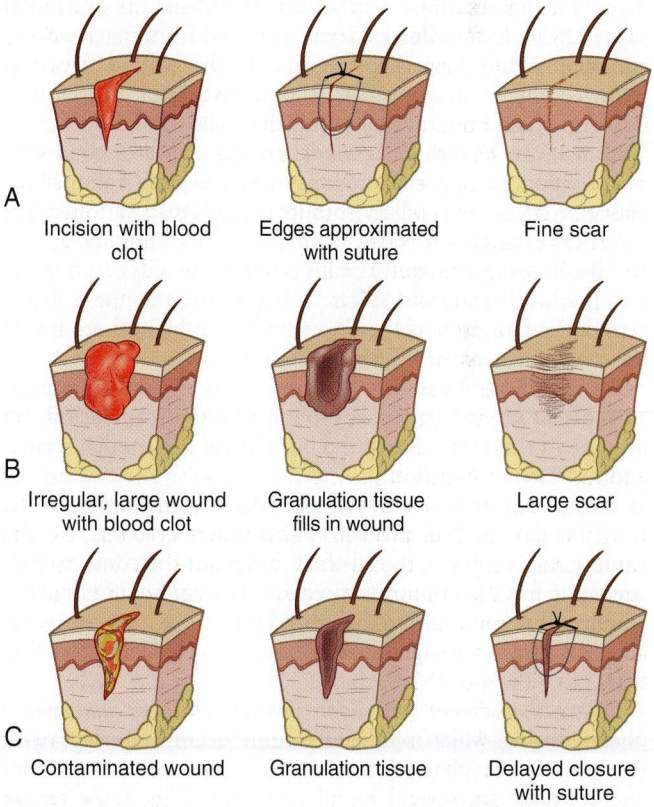

FIG. 11-5 Types of wound healing. **A,** Primary intention. **B,** Secondary intention. **C,** Tertiary intention.

Primary Intention. *Primary intention* healing takes place when wound margins are neatly approximated, as in a surgical incision or a paper cut. A continuum of processes is associated with primary healing (Table 11-6). These processes include three phases.

TABLE 11-6 Phases in Primary Intention Healing

Phase	Duration	Description
Initial	3 to 5 days	Approximation of incision edges. Migration of epithelial cells. Clot serving as meshwork for starting capillary growth
Granulation	5 days to 4 wk	Migration of fibroblasts. Secretion of collagen. Abundance of capillary buds. Wound fragile
Maturation and scar contraction	7 days to several months	Remodeling of collagen. Strengthening of scar

Initial Phase. In the *initial* (inflammatory) phase, the edges of the incision are first aligned and sutured (or stapled) in place. The incision area fills with blood from the cut blood vessels, blood clots form, and platelets release growth factors to begin the healing process. This forms a matrix for WBC migration. An acute inflammatory reaction occurs.

The area of injury is composed of fibrin clots, erythrocytes, neutrophils (dead and dying), and other debris. Macrophages ingest and digest cellular debris, fibrin fragments, and red blood cells (RBCs). Extracellular enzymes derived from macrophages and neutrophils help digest fibrin. As the wound debris is removed, the fibrin clot serves as a meshwork for future capillary growth and migration of epithelial cells.

Granulation Phase. The *granulation* phase is the second step. The components of granulation tissue include proliferating fibroblasts; proliferating capillary sprouts *(angioblasts);* various types of WBCs; exudate; and loose, semifluid, ground substance.

Fibroblasts are immature connective tissue cells that migrate into the healing site and secrete collagen. In time, the collagen is organized and restructured to strengthen the healing site. At this stage it is termed *fibrous* or *scar tissue.*

During the granulation phase, the wound is pink and vascular. Numerous red granules (young budding capillaries) are present. At this point the wound is friable, at risk for dehiscence, and resistant to infection.

Surface epithelium at the wound edges begins to regenerate. In a few days a thin layer of epithelium migrates across the wound surface in a one-cell-thick layer until it contacts cells spreading from the opposite direction. The epithelium thickens and begins to mature, and the wound now closely resembles the adjacent skin. In a superficial wound, re-epithelialization may take 3 to 5 days.

Maturation Phase and Scar Contraction. The *maturation* phase, during which scar contraction occurs, overlaps with the granulation phase. It may begin 7 days after the injury and continue for several months or years. This is the reason abdominal surgery discharge instructions limit lifting for up to 6 weeks.

Collagen fibers are further organized, and the remodeling process occurs. Fibroblasts disappear as the wound becomes stronger. The active movement of the myofibroblasts causes contraction of the healing area, helping to close the defect and bring the skin edges closer together. A mature scar is then formed. In contrast to granulation tissue, a mature scar is virtually avascular and pale. The scar may be more painful at this phase than in the granulation phase.

Secondary Intention. Wounds that occur from trauma, ulceration, and infection have large amounts of exudate and wide, irregular wound margins with extensive tissue loss. These wounds may have edges that cannot be *approximated* (brought together). The inflammatory reaction may be greater than in primary healing. This results in more debris, cells, and exudate. The debris may have to be cleaned away *(debrided)* before healing can take place.

The process of healing by secondary intention is essentially the same as healing by primary intention. The major differences are the greater defect and the gaping wound edges. Healing and granulation take place from the edges inward and from the bottom of the wound upward until the defect is filled. There is more granulation tissue, and the result is a much larger scar.

Tertiary Intention. *Tertiary intention* (delayed primary intention) healing occurs with delayed suturing of a wound in which two layers of granulation tissue are sutured together. This occurs when a contaminated wound is left open and sutured closed after the infection is controlled. It also occurs when a primary wound becomes infected, is opened, is allowed to granulate, and is then sutured. Tertiary intention usually results in a larger and deeper scar than primary or secondary intention.

Wound Classification

A *wound* is a break or opening into the skin. Wounds often occur because of accidents or injuries. Types of wounds can range from minor scrapes to deep wounds involving bones, blood vessels, and nerves.

Identifying the etiology of a wound is essential to classifying the wound properly. Wounds can be classified by their cause (surgical or nonsurgical; acute or chronic) or depth of tissue affected (superficial, partial thickness, or full thickness). A *superficial wound* involves only the epidermis. *Partial-thickness* wounds extend into the dermis. *Full-thickness* wounds have the deepest layer of tissue destruction because they involve the subcutaneous tissue and sometimes even extend into the fascia and underlying structures such as the muscle, tendon, or bone (see Fig. 24-3).

A *skin tear* is a wound caused by shear, friction, and/or blunt force resulting in separation of skin layers. A skin tear can be partial thickness or full thickness. This type of wound is common, especially in older adults and critically or chronically ill adults.[3]

Complications of Healing

Certain factors can interfere with wound healing and lead to complications (Table 11-7).

❖ NURSING AND INTERPROFESSIONAL MANAGEMENT: WOUND HEALING

◆ Nursing Assessment

The first step in wound care is to carefully assess and document the characteristics of the wound and surrounding area. This includes the location, size (longest length and widest width), depth, undermining and tunneling, wound margin (e.g., normal, macerated, erythema), and wound base (e.g., eschar, slough, exudate). Thoroughly assess the wound on admission (or first clinic visit) and on a regular basis thereafter. Deterioration in the wound requires you to assess and document changes more frequently.[4] Various methods exist for measuring wounds. One method is presented in Fig. 11-9.

TABLE 11-7 Complications of Wound Healing

Adhesions
- Bands of scar tissue that form between or around organs
- Adhesions may occur in the abdominal cavity or between the lungs and the pleura
- Adhesions in abdomen may cause an intestinal obstruction

Contractions
- Wound contraction is a normal part of healing
- Complications occur when excessive contraction results in deformity
- Shortening of muscle or scar tissue, especially over joints, results from excessive fibrous tissue formation (see Fig. 24-14)

Dehiscence
- Separation and disruption of previously joined wound edges (Fig. 11-6)
- Usually occurs when a primary healing site bursts open
- May be caused by the following:
  - Infection causing an inflammatory process
  - Granulation tissue not strong enough to withstand forces imposed on wound
  - Obesity placing individuals at high risk for dehiscence because adipose tissue has less blood supply and may slow healing
  - Pocket of fluid (seroma, hematoma) developing between tissue layers and preventing the edges of the wound from coming together

Evisceration
- Occurs when wound edges separate to the extent that intestines protrude through wound

Excess Granulation Tissue ("Proud Flesh")
- Excess granulation tissue may protrude above surface of healing wound
- If the granulation tissue is cauterized or cut off, healing continues in normal manner

Fistula Formation
- An abnormal passage between organs or a hollow organ and skin (abdominal or perianal fistula)

Infection (Fig. 11-3)
- ↑ Risk of infection when wound contains necrotic tissue or blood supply is ↓, patient's immune function is ↓ (e.g., from immunosuppressive drugs such as corticosteroids), undernutrition, multiple stressors, and hyperglycemia in diabetes

Hemorrhage
- Bleeding is normal immediately after tissue injury and ceases with clot formation
- Hemorrhage occurs as abnormal internal or external blood loss caused by suture failure, clotting abnormalities, dislodged clot, infection, or erosion of a blood vessel by a foreign object (tubing, drains) or infection process

Hypertrophic Scars
- Inappropriately large, raised red and hard scars (Fig. 11-7)
- Occur when an overabundance of collagen is produced during healing

Keloid Formation
- Great protrusion of scar tissue that extends beyond wound edges and may form tumor-like masses of scar tissue (Fig. 11-8)
- Permanent without any tendency to subside
- Patients often complain of tenderness, pain, and hyperparesthesia, especially in early stages
- Thought to be a hereditary condition occurring most often in dark-skinned people, particularly African Americans

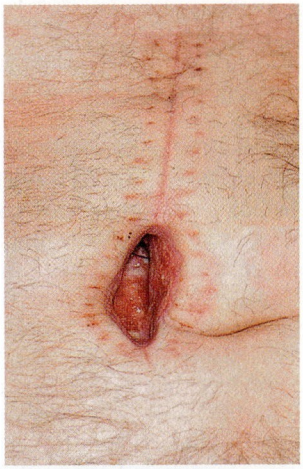

FIG. 11-6 Dehiscence following a cholecystectomy. (From Bale S, Jones V: *Wound care nursing: a patient-centered approach,* ed 2, St Louis, 2006, Mosby.)

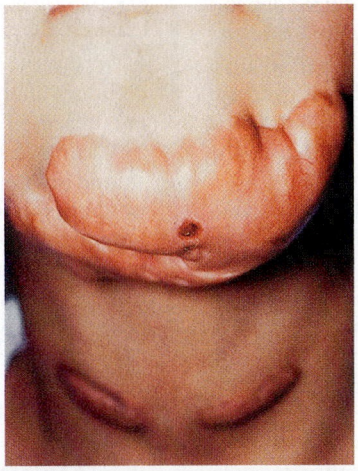

FIG. 11-7 Hypertrophic scarring. (Reproduced with kind permission from Dr. C. Lawrence, Wound Healing Research Unit, Cardiff. In S Bale, V Jones, editors: *Wound care nursing: a patient-centered approach,* ed 2, St Louis, 2006, Mosby.)

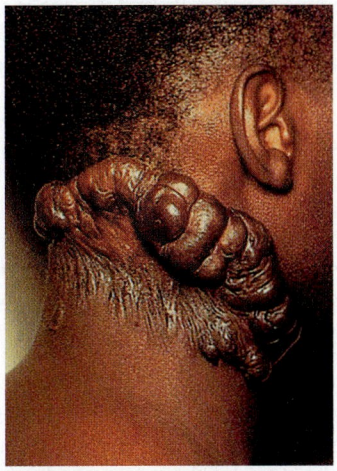

FIG. 11-8 Keloid scarring. (Reproduced with kind permission from Dr. C. Lawrence, Wound Healing Research Unit, Cardiff. In Bale S, Jones V, editors: *Wound care nursing: a patient-centered approach,* ed 2, St Louis, 2006, Mosby.)

Record the consistency, color, and odor of any drainage and report if abnormal for the situation. *Staphylococcus* and *Pseudomonas* are common organisms that cause purulent, draining wounds.

In healthy people, wounds heal at a normal, predictable rate. Identify factors that may delay wound healing and contribute to chronic nonhealing wounds (Table 11-8).

Chronic wounds are those that do not heal within the normal time (approximately 3 months). If a wound fails to heal in a timely manner, assess and identify factors that may delay healing. Refer the patient to an HCP specializing in wound management. Time does not heal all wounds. While caring for patients during the healing process, you need to continually assess for complications (e.g., infection) associated with healing (Table 11-7).

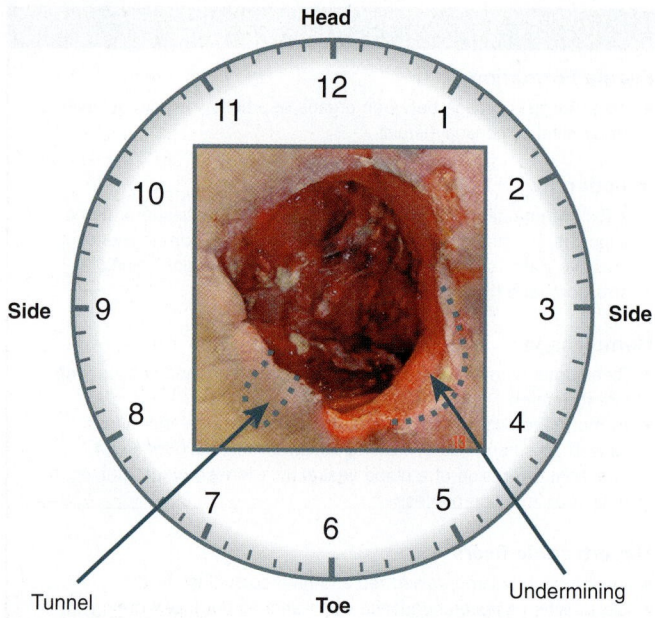

FIG. 11-9 Wound measurements are made in centimeters. The first measurement is oriented from head to toe, the second is from side to side, and the third is the depth (if any). If there is any tunneling (when cotton-tipped applicator is placed in wound, there is movement) or undermining (when cotton-tipped applicator is placed in wound, there is a "lip" around the wound), this is charted in respect to a clock, with 12 o'clock being toward the patient's head. This wound would be charted as a full-thickness, red wound, 7 × 5 × 3 cm, with a 3-cm tunnel at 7 o'clock and 2 cm undermining from 3 o'clock to 5 o'clock. (Courtesy Robert B. Babiak, RN, BSN, CWOCN, San Antonio, Tex.)

TABLE 11-8 Factors Delaying Wound Healing

Factor	Effect on Wound Healing
Nutritional deficiencies	
• Vitamin C	Delays formation of collagen fibers and capillary development
• Protein	Decreases supply of amino acids for tissue repair
• Zinc	Impairs epithelialization
Inadequate blood supply	Decreases supply of nutrients to injured area, decreases removal of exudative debris, inhibits inflammatory response
Corticosteroid drugs	Impair phagocytosis by WBCs, inhibit fibroblast proliferation and function, depress formation of granulation tissue, inhibit wound contraction
Infection	Increases inflammatory response and tissue destruction
Smoking	Nicotine, a potent vasoconstrictor, impedes blood flow to healing areas
Mechanical friction on wound	Destroys granulation tissue, prevents apposition of wound edges
Advanced age	Slows collagen synthesis by fibroblasts, impairs circulation, requires longer time for epithelialization of skin, alters phagocytic and immune responses
Obesity	Decreases blood supply in fatty tissue
Diabetes mellitus	Decreases collagen synthesis, delays capillary growth, impairs phagocytosis (result of hyperglycemia), reduces supply of O_2 and nutrients secondary to vascular disease
Poor general health	Causes generalized absence of factors necessary to promote wound healing
Anemia	Supplies less O_2 at tissue level

Nursing Implementation

The type of wound management and dressings required depend on the type, extent, and characteristics of the wound and the phase of healing. The purposes of wound management include (1) protecting a clean wound from trauma so that it can heal normally, (2) cleaning a wound to remove any dirt and debris from the wound bed, and (3) treating infection to prepare the wound for healing.

Clean Wounds. Superficial skin injuries may only need cleansing. Material used to close wounds include adhesive strips (e.g., Steri-Strips, butterflies), sutures (stitches), or tissue adhesives (fibrin sealants). Adhesive strips may be used instead of *sutures* in some injuries because they decrease *scarring,* and it is easier to care for them. Sutures are used to close wounds because suture material provides the mechanical support necessary to sustain closure. A wide variety of suturing materials are available. In contrast, tissue adhesives are a biologic adhesive that can be used by themselves or in conjunction with sutures or tape.

A dressing material that keeps the wound surface clean and slightly moist is optimal to promote epithelialization. For wounds that heal by primary intention, it is common to cover the wound or incision with a dry, sterile dressing that is removed as soon as the drainage stops or in 2 to 3 days. Medicated sprays that form a transparent film on the skin may be used for dressings on a clean incision or injury. Transparent film or adhesive semipermeable dressings (e.g., OpSite, Tegaderm) are occlusive dressings that are permeable to oxygen. The wound is then usually covered with a sterile dressing. Sometimes a surgeon will leave a surgical wound uncovered or remove the dressing within 48 hours after surgery.[5] (Examples of types of wound dressings are presented in Table 11-9.)

Clean wounds that are granulating and re-epithelializing should be kept slightly moist and protected from further trauma until they heal naturally.[6] Do not let a wound that has the potential to heal dry out. Dryness is an enemy of wound healing. "Airing out" a wound is a great mistake. Wounds need a moist environment to heal. Unnecessary manipulation during dressing changes may destroy new granulation tissue and break down fibrin formation.

Topical antimicrobials and antibactericidals (e.g., povidone-iodine [Betadine], Dakin's solution [sodium hypochlorite], hydrogen peroxide [H_2O_2], and chlorhexidine [Hibiclens]) should be used with caution in wound care because they can damage the new epithelium of healing tissue and delay healing. Therefore they should never be used in a clean granulating wound.

Sometimes drains are inserted into the wound to facilitate removal of fluid. The Jackson-Pratt drain is a suction drainage device consisting of a flexible plastic bulb connected to an internal plastic drainage tube (Fig. 11-10).

Contaminated Wounds. If the wound is contaminated, it must be converted into a clean wound before healing can occur normally. Debridement of a wound that has debris or dead tissue may be necessary. Absorption dressings can be used that absorb exudate and clean the wound surface. These dressings work by

TABLE 11-9 Types of Wound Dressings

Type of Dressing	Description	Uses	Examples
Gauze	Made of woven or nonwoven material. Provide absorption of exudates. Most often combined with another kind of dressing	Can be used on almost any kind of wound. Cleansing, packing, and covering a variety of wounds	Numerous products available (e.g., Curity, Kerlix)
Nonadherent	Woven or nonwoven dressings. May be impregnated with saline, petrolatum, or antimicrobials. Minimally absorbent	Minor wounds or as a second dressing	Adaptic, Vaseline gauze, Xeroform
Transparent films	Generally composed of polyurethane. Transparency allows visualization of the wound. Minimally absorbent. Use with caution over superficial wounds. In fragile wounds (e.g., skin tears) can result in further tissue loss. In other wounds, can draw in moisture, increasing risk for infection	Dry, uninfected wounds or wounds with minimal drainage	Bioclusive, OpSite, Suresite, Tegaderm, Transeal
Foams	Film-coated gel or polyurethane. Able to hold large amounts of exudate. Some come with adhesive backings; others require gauze wrapping	Wounds with moderate to heavy drainage. Often used on new wounds	Allevyn, Cutimed, Hydrocell, Lyofoam, Mepilex, PolyMem
Hydrocolloids	Gelatin, pectin, or carboxymethylcellulose bonded to a film or sheet. Produce a flat occlusive dressing that forms a gel on wound surface. Occlusion does not interfere with wound healing. Support debridement and prevent secondary infections	Wounds with light to moderate drainage	Bursamed, Comfeel, DuoDerm, Primacol
Hydrogels	Available in gels, gel-covered gauze, or sheets. Donate moisture to a dry wound and maintain a moist environment. Can rehydrate wound tissue. Debridement because of moisturizing effects. Require a secondary dressing	Dry wounds. Wounds with minimal drainage. Necrotic wounds	Aquasite, Curasol, IntraSite, Purilon, Solosite
Alginates	Derived from seaweed or kelp. Form a nonsticky gel on contact with draining wound. Easy to use over irregular-shaped wounds. Generally require a secondary dressing	Wounds with moderate to heavy exudates (e.g., pressure ulcers, infected wounds)	AlgiSite, Kalginate, Melgisorb, Sorbsan
Antimicrobials	Wound covers that deliver agents such as silver and iodine, and polyhexamethylene biguanide (PHMB), which have antibacterial properties. Bacteria are not able to develop resistance to metals. Available as sponges, impregnated woven gauzes, film dressings, absorptive products, nylon fabric, nonadherent barriers, or a combination of materials	Partial- and full-thickness wounds, over surgical incisions, or around tracheostomies	Acticoat, Curity AMD, Iodoflex, SilverSorb, Silvercel

For additional information, see *www.woundsource.com/product-category/dressings.*

drawing excess drainage from the wound surface. The amount of wound secretions determines the number of dressing changes.

In hydrocolloid dressings, such as DuoDerm, the inner part of these dressings interacts with the exudate, forming a hydrated gel over the wound. When the dressing is removed, the gel separates and stays over the wound. The wound must be cleansed gently to prevent damage to newly formed tissue. These types of dressings are designed to be left in place for up to 7 days or until leakage occurs around the dressing.

Dead tissue can be removed by debridement.[7] The debridement method used depends on the amount of debris and the condition of the wound tissue (Table 11-10).

◆ **Negative-Pressure Wound Therapy.** Negative-pressure wound therapy (NPWT) is used to treat acute and chronic wounds. A vacuum source creates continuous or intermittent negative pressure inside the wound to remove fluid, exudates, and infectious materials to prepare the wound for healing and closure. NPWT systems consist of a vacuum pump, drainage tubing, a foam or gauze wound dressing, and an adhesive film dressing that covers and seals the wound.[8]

In this therapy, the wound is cleaned and a gauze or foam dressing is cut to the dimensions of the wound. A large occlusive dressing is applied and a small hole is made over the gauze or foam dressing where the tubing is attached (Fig. 11-11). The tubing is connected to a pump, which creates a negative pressure in the wound bed.

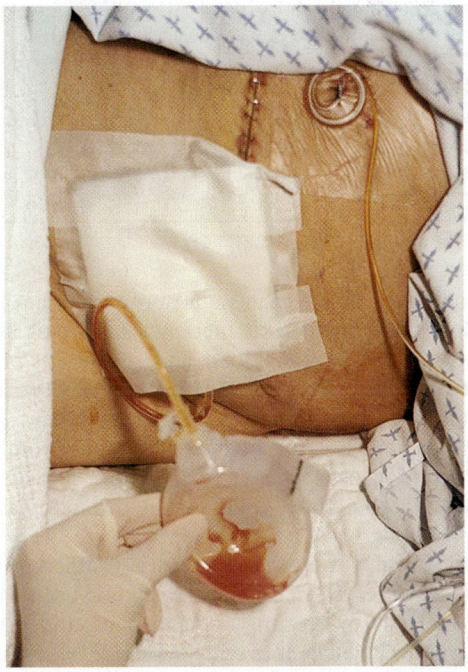

FIG. 11-10 Jackson-Pratt drainage device. (From Perry AG, Potter PA, Elkin MK: *Nursing interventions and clinical skills,* ed 5, St Louis, 2012, Mosby.)

TEAMWORK & COLLABORATION

Wound Care

In general, wound care for complex or nonhealing wounds should be managed by the registered nurse (RN). State nurse practice acts vary in the wound care actions allowed by licensed practical/vocational nurses (LPNs/LVNs) and unlicensed assistive personnel (UAP).

Role of Nursing Personnel

Registered Nurse (RN)

- Assess patients for pressure ulcer risk and develop a plan of care to prevent the development of pressure ulcers.
- Assess patients for factors that may delay wound healing and develop a plan of care to address these factors.
- Assess and document initial wound appearance, including wound size, depth, color, and drainage.
- Plan nursing actions to assist with wound healing, including wound care, positioning, and nutritional interventions.
- Choose dressings and therapies for wound treatment (in conjunction with the HCP and/or wound care specialist).
- Implement wound care for complex or new wounds, including negative-pressure wound therapy and hyperbaric O_2 therapy.
- Evaluate whether wound care is effective in promoting wound healing.
- Provide teaching to patient and caregivers about home wound care and pressure ulcer prevention.

Licensed Practical/Vocational Nurse (LPN/LVN)

- Perform sterile dressing changes on acute and chronic wounds.
- Apply ordered topical antimicrobials and antibactericidals to wounds.
- Apply prescribed dressings or medications for wound debridement.
- Collect and record data about wound appearance.
- Reinforce teaching that was provided by the RN.

Unlicensed Assistive Personnel (UAP)

- Perform dressing changes for chronic wounds using clean technique (must consider state nurse practice act and agency policy).
- Empty wound drainage containers and document drainage on intake and output record.
- Report changes in wound appearance or drainage to RN.

Role of Other Team Members

Dietitian

- Assess and monitor patient's nutritional status.
- Establish an intervention together with the interprofessional team.
- Monitor patient's progress toward achieving the goals of care.

Although the exact mechanism for promoting healing is not known, it is thought that this therapy pulls excess fluid from the wound, reduces bacterial load, and encourages blood flow into the wound base.

Monitor the patient's serum protein levels and fluid and electrolyte balance because of losses from the wound. Additionally, monitor the patient's coagulation studies (platelet count, prothrombin time [PT], partial thromboplastin time [PTT]).

◆ **Hyperbaric Oxygen Therapy.** Hyperbaric O_2 therapy (HBOT) is the delivery of O_2 at increased atmospheric pressures. It can be given topically by creating a chamber around the injured limb. Alternatively it can be given systemically with the patient placed in an enclosed chamber, where 100% O_2 is administered at 1.5 to 3 times the normal atmospheric pressure.

TABLE 11-10 Types of Debridement

Type	Description
Surgical debridement	• Quick method of debridement to prevent, control, or remove infection • Used when large amounts of nonviable tissue are present • Prepares wound bed for healing, skin grafting, or flaps
Mechanical debridement	• Two methods: • *Wet-to-dry dressings*, in which open-mesh gauze is moistened with normal saline, lightly packed into wound surface, and outer layer allowed to dry. Wound debris adheres to dressing and then dressing is removed • *Wound irrigation*. Make certain bacteria are not accidentally driven into wound with high irrigation pressure
Autolytic debridement	• Semiocclusive or occlusive dressings (Table 11-9) used to soften dry eschar by autolysis • Assess area around wound for maceration when using these dressings
Enzymatic debridement	• Drugs applied topically to dissolve necrotic tissue and then covered with moist dressing (e.g., saline-moistened gauze) • Examples of these drugs include collagenase (e.g., Santyl) • Process can be slow, and thick eschar may have to be scored with scalpel

HBOT allows O_2 to diffuse into the serum, rather than RBCs, and be transported to the tissues. By increasing the O_2 content in the serum, HBOT moves the O_2 past narrowed arteries and capillaries where RBCs cannot go.

In addition, elevated O_2 levels stimulate *angiogenesis* (production of new blood vessels), kill anaerobic bacteria, and increase the killing power of WBCs and certain antibiotics (e.g., fluoroquinolones, aminoglycosides). HBOT accelerates granulation tissue formation and wound healing.

The topical treatments can last 20 minutes twice daily or 4 to 6 hours daily. Most systemic treatments last from 90 to 120 minutes, and the number of treatments may vary from 10 to 60 depending on the condition being treated. The number of treatments is highly variable.

◆ **Drug Therapy.** Platelet-derived growth factor is released from the platelets and stimulates cell proliferation and migration. Becaplermin (Regranex), a recombinant human platelet–derived growth factor gel, actively stimulates wound healing. It is used to treat foot ulcers in patients with diabetes (see Chapter 48). Becaplermin should be used only when the wound is free of dead tissue and infection. It should not be used if cancer is suspected in the wound.

◆ **Nutritional Therapy.** Special nutritional measures facilitate wound healing. A high fluid intake is needed to replace fluid loss from perspiration and exudate formation. An increased metabolic rate intensifies water loss. Individuals at risk for wound healing problems are those with malabsorption problems (e.g., Crohn's disease, gastrointestinal [GI] surgery, liver disease), deficient intake or high energy demands (e.g., malignancy, major trauma or surgery, sepsis, fever), and diabetes.

Undernutrition puts a person at risk for poor healing. A diet high in protein, carbohydrate, and vitamins with moderate fat intake is necessary to promote healing. Protein is needed to

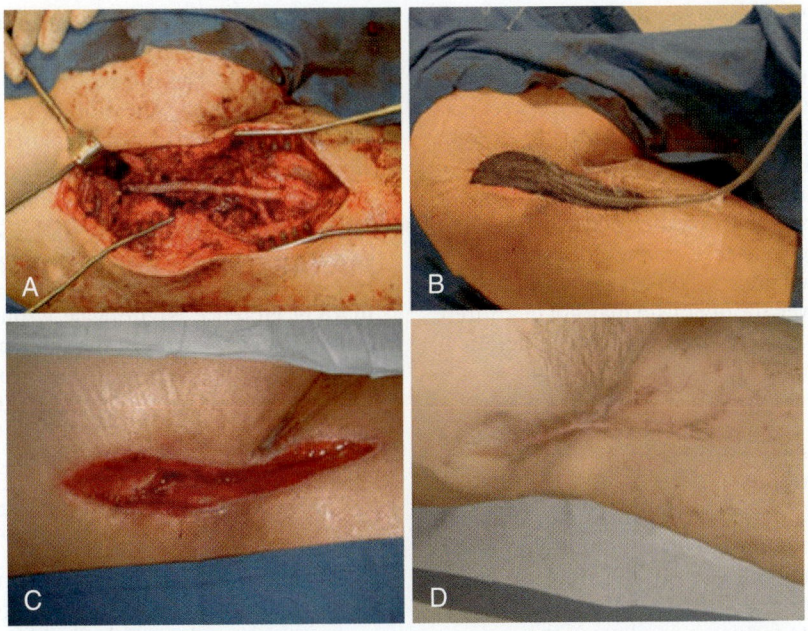

FIG. 11-11 Negative-pressure wound therapy in woman with history of IV drug abuse. **A,** The completely destroyed femoral artery was reconstructed with a homograft. **B,** A black open-pore polyurethane foam was directly applied to the vascular reconstruction and negative pressure applied to wound. **C,** Wound site 16 days after surgery. **D,** Healed wound at 28 months without reinfection. (Source: Reprinted from Mayer D, Hasse B, Koelliker J, et al: Long-term results of vascular graft and artery preserving treatment with negative pressure wound therapy in Szilagyi grade III infections justify a paradigm shift, *Ann Surg* 254:754, 2011. Copyright Southeastern Surgical Congress.)

correct the negative nitrogen balance resulting from the increased metabolic rate. Protein is also necessary for synthesis of immune factors, leukocytes, fibroblasts, and collagen, which are the building blocks for healing. Carbohydrate is needed for the increased metabolic energy required in inflammation and healing. If there is a carbohydrate deficit, the body will break down protein for the needed energy. Fats are also a necessary component in the diet to help in the synthesis of fatty acids and triglycerides, which are part of the cellular membrane.[9]

Vitamin C is needed for capillary synthesis and collagen production by fibroblasts. The B-complex vitamins are necessary as coenzymes for many metabolic reactions. If a vitamin B deficiency develops, a disruption of protein, fat, and carbohydrate metabolism will occur. Vitamin A is also needed in healing because it aids in the process of epithelialization. It increases collagen synthesis and tensile strength of the healing wound.

If the patient is unable to eat, enteral feedings and supplements should be the first choice if the GI tract is functional. Parenteral nutrition is indicated when enteral feedings are contraindicated or not tolerated. (Enteral and parenteral nutrition is discussed in Chapter 39.)

◆ **Infection Prevention and Control.** You and the patient must scrupulously follow aseptic procedures, including handwashing, for keeping the wound free from infection. Do not allow the patient to touch a recently injured area. The patient's environment should be as free as possible from contamination from items introduced by roommates and visitors. Antibiotics may be administered prophylactically to some patients.

If an infection develops, a culture and sensitivity test should be done to determine the organism and the most effective antibiotic for that specific organism. The culture should be taken before the first dose of antibiotic is given. Cultures can be obtained by needle aspiration, tissue culture, or swab technique. Physicians obtain needle and tissue punch biopsy samples. As a nurse, you can obtain cultures using the swab technique.

Swab specimens can be obtained from wounds using Levine's technique, which involves rotating a culture swab over a cleansed 1-cm^2 area near the center of the wound. Use sufficient pressure to extract wound fluid from deep tissue layers. (A culture must be taken of the clean tissue because exudate and necrotic tissue will not provide an accurate sample.) When collecting samples, do not use cotton-tipped applicators.[10] The sample must be sent to the laboratory within 1 hour.

◆ **Psychologic Implications.** The patient may be distressed at the thought or sight of an incision or wound because of fear of scarring or disfigurement. Drainage and odor from a wound often cause increased alarm. The patient needs to understand the healing process and normal changes that occur as the wound heals.

When changing a dressing, avoid inappropriate facial expressions that may alert the patient to problems with the wound or raise doubts about your ability to care for it. Wrinkling your nose may convey disgust to the patient. Be careful not to focus on the wound to the extent that the patient is not treated as a total person.

◆ **Patient Teaching.** Because patients are being discharged earlier after surgery and many have surgery as outpatients, it is important that the patient and caregiver know how to care for the wound and perform dressing changes. Wound healing may not be complete for 4 to 6 weeks or longer. Emphasize the importance of adequate rest and good nutrition throughout this time. Physical and emotional stress should be minimal. Observing the wound for complications such as contractures, adhesions, and secondary infection is important. Teach the patient and caregiver the signs and symptoms of infection. Have them note changes in the wound color and amount of drainage. Teach the patient to notify the HCP of any signs of abnormal wound healing.

Drugs are often taken for a time after recovery from the acute infection. Review drug-specific side effects and adverse effects with the patient and caregiver, as well as methods to prevent side effects (e.g., taking with food or not). Teach the patient to contact the HCP if any of these effects occur. Inform the patient of the need to continue the drugs for the specified time. For example, a patient is instructed to take an antibiotic for 10 days but may stop taking the drug after 5 days because of decreased or absent symptoms. However, the organism may not be entirely eliminated, and it may also become resistant to the antibiotic if the drug is not continued.

PRESSURE ULCERS

Etiology and Pathophysiology

A **pressure ulcer** is localized injury to the skin and/or underlying tissue (usually over a bony prominence) as a result of pressure or pressure in combination with shear.[11] Pressure ulcers generally fall under the category of healing by secondary intention. The most common site for pressure ulcers is the sacrum, with heels being second.

Factors that influence the development of pressure ulcers include the amount of pressure (intensity), length of time the pressure is exerted on the skin (duration), and ability of the patient's tissue to tolerate the externally applied pressure. Other factors that contribute to pressure ulcer formation include **shearing force** (pressure exerted on the skin when it adheres to the bed and the skin layers slide in the direction of body movement [e.g., when pulling patient up in bed]) and *excessive moisture* (increases risk for skin breakdown).

Factors that put a patient at risk for the development of pressure ulcers are presented in Table 11-11. Individuals at risk include those who are older, incontinent, unable to reposition or unaware of the need to reposition (e.g., spinal cord injury), and bed- or wheelchair-bound.

Clinical Manifestations

The clinical manifestations of pressure ulcers depend on the extent of the tissue involved. Pressure ulcers are staged or categorized based on the visible or palpable tissue in the ulcer bed. Table 11-12 illustrates the pressure ulcer stages based on the National Pressure Ulcer Advisory Panel (NPUAP) guidelines.[11]

If the pressure ulcer becomes infected, the patient may display signs of infection (e.g., leukocytosis, fever). In addition, the pressure ulcer may increase in size, odor, and drainage; have necrotic tissue; and be indurated, warm, and painful. Untreated ulcers may lead to *cellulitis* (spreading of inflammation to subcutaneous or connective tissue), chronic infection, sepsis, and possibly death. The most common complication of a pressure ulcer is recurrence. Therefore it is important to note the location of previously healed pressure ulcers on a patient's initial admission assessment.

TABLE 11-11 Risk Factors for Pressure Ulcers

- Advanced age
- Anemia
- Contractures
- Diabetes mellitus
- Elevated body temperature
- Friction (rubbing of surfaces together)
- Immobility
- Impaired circulation
- Incontinence
- Low diastolic blood pressure (<60 mm Hg)
- Mental deterioration
- Neurologic disorders
- Obesity
- Pain
- Prolonged surgery
- Vascular disease

NURSING AND INTERPROFESSIONAL MANAGEMENT: PRESSURE ULCERS

In 1859 Florence Nightingale wrote, "If he has a bedsore, it's generally not the fault of the disease, but of the nursing."[12] Her comment emphasizes the critical role that nurses have in prevention and treatment of pressure ulcers.

SAFETY ALERT Pressure Ulcers

- Stage III or IV (full skin–thickness injury) pressure ulcer acquired after admission to a health care setting is considered a serious reportable event (SRE) (never event).[13] (SREs are discussed in Chapter 1.)

Nursing and interprofessional management are discussed together because the activities are interrelated. In addition to the nurse, other members of the health team, such as the wound care specialist, plastic surgeon, dietitian, physical therapist, and occupational therapist, can provide valuable input into the complex treatment necessary to prevent and treat pressure ulcers.

Nursing Assessment

Assess patients for pressure ulcer risk initially on admission and at periodic intervals based on the patient's condition. Conduct a thorough head-to-toe assessment on admission to identify and document any pressure ulcers. Thereafter conduct periodic reassessment of the skin and wounds.

SAFETY ALERT Assessing for Pressure Ulcers

- In acute care, reassess patients for pressure ulcers every 24 hours.
- In long-term care, reassess residents weekly for the first 4 weeks after admission and then at least monthly or quarterly.
- In home care, reassess patients at every nurse visit.

To do a risk assessment, use a validated assessment tool such as the Braden Scale (available at *www.bradenscale.com*). Knowing the level of risk can help determine how aggressive preventive measures should be.

Identification of skin changes may be difficult in patients with dark skin. Table 11-13 presents techniques to help assess darker skin.

Subjective and objective data that should be obtained from a person with or at risk for a pressure ulcer are presented in Table 11-14.

Nursing Diagnoses

Nursing diagnoses for the patient with a pressure ulcer may include, but are not limited to, the following:

- Impaired skin integrity *related to* mechanical factors and physical immobilization
- Impaired tissue integrity *related to* impaired circulation and imbalanced nutritional state

Planning

The overall goals are that the patient with a pressure ulcer will (1) have no deterioration of the ulcer, (2) reduce or eliminate the factors that lead to pressure ulcers, (3) not develop an

TABLE 11-12 Pressure Ulcer Stages/Categories

Stage/Category I: Nonblanchable Erythema

Intact skin with nonblanchable redness of a localized area usually over a bony prominence. Darkly pigmented skin may not have visible blanching. Its color may differ from the surrounding area. The area may be painful, firm, soft, warmer, or cooler as compared to adjacent tissue.

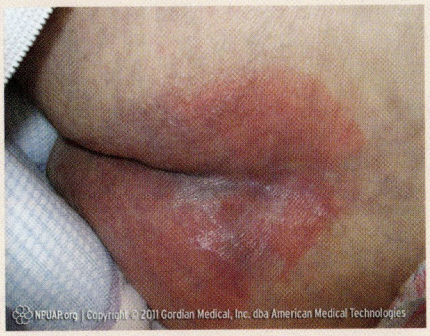

Stage/Category II: Partial Thickness

Partial-thickness loss of dermis presenting as a shallow open ulcer with a red-pink wound bed, without slough. May also present as an intact or open/ruptured serum-filled or serosanguineous-filled blister. Presents as a shiny or dry shallow ulcer without slough or bruising. (Bruising indicates deep tissue injury.)

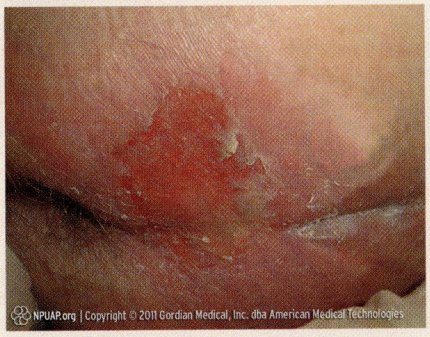

Stage/Category III: Full-Thickness Skin Loss

Full-thickness tissue loss. Subcutaneous fat may be visible but bone, tendon, or muscle are not exposed. Slough may be present but does not obscure depth of tissue loss. May include undermining and tunneling. The depth of a category/stage III pressure ulcer varies by anatomic location.

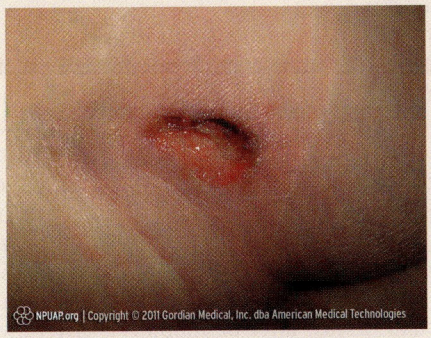

Stage/Category IV: Full-Thickness Tissue Loss

Full-thickness tissue loss with exposed bone, tendon, or muscle. Slough or eschar may be present. Often includes undermining and tunneling. Depth of pressure ulcer varies by anatomic location. Ulcers can extend into muscle and/or supporting structures (e.g., fascia, tendon, or joint capsule) making osteomyelitis or osteitis likely to occur. Exposed bone/muscle is visible or directly palpable.

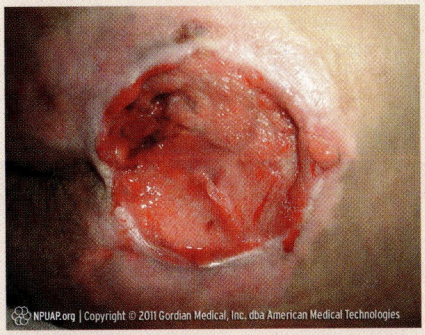

Unstageable/Unclassified: Full-Thickness Skin or Tissue Loss (Depth Unknown)

Full-thickness tissue loss in which actual depth of ulcer is completely obscured by slough (yellow, tan, gray, green, or brown) and/or eschar (tan, brown, or black) in wound bed. Until enough slough and/or eschar are removed to expose the base of wound, the true depth cannot be determined; but it will be either a stage III or stage IV. Stable (dry, adherent, intact without erythema, or fluctuance) eschar on the heels serves as "the body's natural (biologic) cover" and should not be removed.

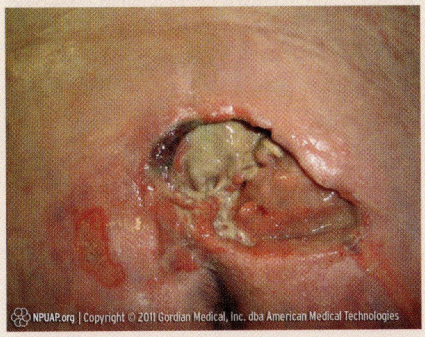

Suspected Deep Tissue Injury (Depth Unknown)

Purple or maroon localized area of discolored intact skin or blood-filled blister due to damage of underlying soft tissue from pressure and/or shear. The area may be preceded by tissue that is painful, firm, mushy, boggy, warmer, or cooler as compared to adjacent tissue. Deep tissue injury may be difficult to detect in individuals with dark skin tones. Evolution may include a thin blister over a dark wound bed. The wound may further evolve and become covered by thin eschar. Evolution may be rapid, exposing additional layers of tissue even with optimal treatment.

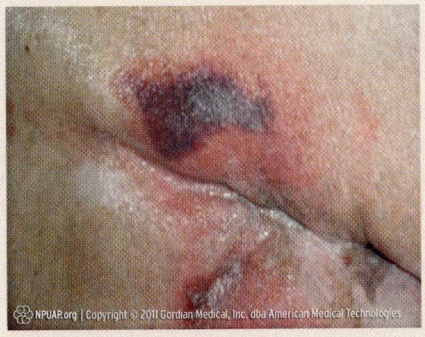

Photos used with permission of the National Pressure Ulcer Advisory Panel.

TABLE 11-13 Assessing Patients With Dark Skin

- Look for changes in skin color, such as skin that is darker (purplish, brownish, bluish) than surrounding skin.
- Use natural or halogen light source to accurately assess the skin color. Fluorescent light casts blue color, which can make skin assessment difficult.
- Assess the area for the skin temperature using your hand. The area may feel initially warm, then cooler.
- Touch the skin to feel its consistency. Boggy or edematous feel may indicate a stage I pressure ulcer.
- Ask the patient if he or she has any pain or itchy sensation.

TABLE 11-14 Nursing Assessment

Pressure Ulcers

Subjective Data

Important Health Information

Past health history: Stroke, spinal cord injury; prolonged bed rest or immobility; circulatory impairment; poor nutrition; altered level of consciousness; prior history of pressure ulcer; immunologic abnormalities; advanced age; diabetes; anemia; trauma

Medications: Use of opioids, hypnotics, systemic corticosteroids

Surgery or other treatments: Recent surgery

Functional Health Patterns

Nutritional-metabolic: Obesity, emaciation; decreased fluid, calorie, or protein intake; vitamin or mineral deficiencies; clinically significant malnutrition as indicated by low serum albumin, decreased total lymphocyte count, and decreased body weight (15% less than ideal body weight)

Elimination: Incontinence of urine, feces, or both

Activity-exercise: Weakness, debilitation, inability to turn and position body; contractures

Cognitive-perceptual: Pain or altered cutaneous sensation in pressure ulcer area; decreased awareness of pressure on body areas; capacity to follow treatment plan

Objective Data

General

Fever

Integumentary

Diaphoresis, edema, and discoloration, especially over bony areas such as sacrum, hips, elbows, heels, knees, ankles, shoulders, and ear rims, progressing to increased tissue damage characteristic of ulcer stages*

Possible Diagnostic Findings

Leukocytosis, positive cultures for microorganisms from pressure ulcer

*Table 11-12.

infection in the pressure ulcer, (4) have healing of pressure ulcers, and (5) have no recurrence.

Nursing Implementation

Health Promotion. A primary nursing responsibility is the (1) identification of patients at risk for developing pressure ulcers (Tables 11-11 and 11-14) and (2) implementation of pressure ulcer prevention strategies for those who are at risk. Prevention remains the best treatment for pressure ulcers. Implementing evidence-based pressure ulcer prevention programs can reduce the occurrence of health care–acquired pressure ulcers.[14,15]

EVIDENCE-BASED PRACTICE

Applying the Evidence

Repositioning and Pressure Ulcers

You are doing discharge planning with L.H., an obese 76-year-old woman with a history of diabetes, hypertension, and macular degeneration. L.H. has spent most of her time while hospitalized in a bed or wheelchair and now has a stage I pressure ulcer on her sacrum. You explain the importance of pressure ulcer care with her son, who is her primary caregiver.

Making Clinical Decisions

Best Available Evidence. Repositioning is the primary method of reducing the risk for pressure ulcers. Pressure-reducing devices (e.g., foam dressings, foam mattress, padded commode, wheelchair seats) may also be used but should not be a substitute for repositioning.

Clinician Expertise. You know that patients with pressure ulcers or at risk for pressure ulcers should be repositioned frequently. The frequency of repositioning is individualized based on patient need and risk. (It is no longer every 2 hours for every patient.)

Caregiver Preferences and Values. L.H.'s caregiver states he will reposition his mother during the day and instruct the home health care aide to reposition her frequently at night.

Implications for Nursing Practice

1. In addition to repositioning, what information is important to discuss with L.H.'s son to prevent further skin breakdown?
2. What are the risk factors for L.H. to develop new pressure ulcers?
3. What is important for the home health care nurse to monitor on her visits to L.H. related to pressure ulcers and healing?

Reference for Evidence

National Pressure Ulcer Advisory Panel. Retrieved from *www.npuap.org/wp-content/uploads/2014/08/Updated-10-16-14-Quick-Reference-Guide-DIGITAL-NPUAP-EPUAP-PPPIA-16Oct2014.pdf.*

SAFETY ALERT Preventing Pressure Ulcers

- Use devices to reduce pressure and shearing force (e.g., low-air-loss mattresses, foam mattresses, wheelchair cushions, padded commode seats, boots [foam, air], lift sheets) as appropriate. These devices do not replace the need for frequent repositioning.
- Reposition patients frequently to prevent pressure ulcers.

In the past, the "standard" was to turn and reposition patients every 2 hours. However, this "policy" is not evidence based. Time schedules and frequency should be individualized based on risk factors, patient's overall condition, and type of mattress and support surface. For example, some high-risk patients may need to be turned and repositioned every hour, whereas others at lower risk may need to be turned and repositioned only every 3 to 4 hours.[6,11]

Acute Care. Care of a patient with a pressure ulcer requires local care of the wound and support measures of the whole person, such as adequate nutrition, pain management, control of other medical conditions, and pressure relief. Both conservative and surgical strategies are used in the treatment of pressure ulcers, depending on the stage and condition of the ulcer.

Once a pressure ulcer has developed, initiate interventions based on the ulcer characteristics (e.g., stage, size, location, amount of exudate, type of wound, presence of infection or pain) and the patient's general status (e.g., nutritional state, age, cardiovascular status, level of mobility). Carefully document the size of the pressure ulcer. A wound-measuring card or tape can be used to note the ulcer's maximum length and width in centimeters. To find the depth of the ulcer, take a sterile cotton-tipped applicator and soak it with saline. Gently place it into the deepest part of the ulcer, and then measure the length of the portion of the applicator that probed the ulcer. Documentation of the healing wound can be done using several available pressure ulcer healing tools such as the NPUAP Pressure Ulcer Scale for Healing (PUSH) tool (available at *www.npuap.org/wp-content/uploads/2012/03/push3.pdf*).

Some agencies require that pictures of the pressure ulcer be taken initially and at regular intervals during the course of treatment. The Informatics box has suggestions for digital imaging.

INFORMATICS IN PRACTICE

Digital Images

To monitor wound progress, use digital photography. For the best images:

- Include a ruler with date, length, width, and depth of the wound in each photo.
- Position the patient the same way for each photo.
- Take the photo from the same angle each time. Pointing perpendicularly at the wound is best.
- Use natural light, without flash, whenever possible.
- Show the wound on a solid background, avoiding shiny underpads.
- Avoid patient identifiers such as jewelry, tattoos, or visible family members.

Local care of the pressure ulcer may involve debridement, wound cleaning, application of a dressing, and relief of pressure. It is important to select the appropriate pressure-relieving technique (e.g., pad, overlay, mattress, specialty bed) to relieve pressure and keep the patient off of the pressure ulcer. Whenever possible, do not turn the patient onto a body surface that is still reddened. Massage is contraindicated in the presence of acute inflammation and where there is the possibility of damaged blood vessels or fragile skin.

Sliding down in bed causes shear. Encourage patients to reposition themselves by lifting rather than sliding and to use a trapeze if indicated. Lift sheets may be used to move patients up in bed or to transfer them.

A pressure ulcer that has necrotic tissue or eschar (except for dry, stable necrotic feet or heels) must have the tissue removed by surgical, mechanical, enzymatic, or autolytic debridement methods. Once the pressure ulcer has been successfully debrided and has a clean granulating base, the goal is to provide an appropriate wound environment that supports moist wound healing and prevents disruption of the newly formed granulation tissue. Reconstruction of the pressure ulcer site by surgical repair, including skin grafting, skin flaps, musculocutaneous flaps, or free flaps, may be necessary.

Clean pressure ulcers with noncytotoxic solutions (e.g., normal saline) that do not kill or damage cells, especially fibroblasts. Solutions such as Dakin's solution (sodium hypochlorite solution), acetic acid, povidone-iodine, and hydrogen peroxide are cytotoxic. Therefore they should not be used to clean pressure ulcers. It is also important to use enough irrigation pressure to adequately clean the pressure ulcer (4 to 15 psi) without causing trauma or damage to the wound. To obtain this pressure, use a 30-mL syringe and a 19-gauge needle.

After the pressure ulcer has been cleansed, cover it with an appropriate dressing. Keep a pressure ulcer slightly moist, rather than dry, to enhance re-epithelialization. Some factors to consider when selecting a dressing are maintenance of a moist environment, prevention of the wound from drying out, ability to absorb the wound drainage, location of the wound, amount of caregiver time required to change the dressing, cost of the dressing, presence of infection, clean versus sterile dressings, and care delivery setting. Never use a wet-to-dry dressing on a clean granulating pressure ulcer. This type of dressing should be used only for mechanical debridement of a wound that has necrotic or sloughing tissue. (Dressings are discussed in Table 11-9.)

Stages II through IV pressure ulcers are considered contaminated or colonized with bacteria. Remember that in people who have chronic wounds or are immunocompromised, the clinical signs and symptoms of infection (purulent exudate, odor, erythema, warmth, tenderness, edema, pain, fever, and elevated WBC count) may not be present even though the pressure ulcer is infected.

The maintenance of adequate nutrition is an important nursing responsibility for the patient with a pressure ulcer. Often the patient is debilitated and has a poor appetite secondary to inactivity. Oral feedings must be adequate in calories, protein, fluids, vitamins, and minerals to meet the patient's nutritional requirements. The caloric intake needed to correct and maintain nutritional balance may be 30 to 35 calories/kg/day and 1.25 to 1.50 g of protein/kg/day.

Enteral feedings can be used to supplement the oral feedings. When oral and enteral feedings are inadequate, parenteral nutrition consisting of amino acid and glucose solutions is used. (Parenteral and enteral nutrition are discussed in Chapter 39.)

◆ **Ambulatory Care.** Pressure ulcers affect the quality of life of patients and their caregivers. Because pressure ulcers commonly recur, teaching prevention techniques to the patient and caregiver is extremely important (Table 11-15). A sixth-grade–level version of the patient guide to pressure ulcer prevention is available for use in patient teaching *(www.npuap.org/PU_Prev_Points.pdf)*.

The caregiver needs to know the etiology of pressure ulcers, prevention techniques, early signs, nutritional support, and

TABLE 11-15 Patient & Caregiver Teaching

Pressure Ulcer

When teaching the patient and caregiver to prevent and care for pressure ulcers, do the following.

1. Identify and explain risk factors and etiology of pressure ulcers to patient and caregiver.
2. Assess all at-risk patients at time of first hospital and/or home visit or whenever the patient's condition changes. Thereafter assess at regular intervals based on care setting (every 24 hours for acute care or every visit in home care).
3. Teach the caregiver techniques for incontinence. If incontinence occurs, cleanse skin at time of soiling and use absorbent pads or briefs.
4. Demonstrate correct positioning to decrease risk of skin breakdown. Instruct caregiver to reposition a bed-bound patient at least every 2 hours, a chair-bound patient every hour. NEVER position the patient directly on the pressure ulcer.
5. Assess resources (i.e., caregiver's availability and skill, finances, equipment) of patients requiring pressure ulcer care at home. When selecting ulcer care dressing, consider cost and amount of caregiver time required.
6. Teach patient and/or caregiver to place clean dressings over sterile dressings using "no touch" technique when changing dressings. Instruct caregiver on disposal of contaminated dressings.
7. Teach patient and caregiver to inspect skin daily. Tell them to report any significant changes to the HCP.
8. Teach patient and caregiver the importance of good nutrition to enhance ulcer healing.
9. Evaluate program effectiveness.

care techniques for actual pressure ulcers. Because the patient with a pressure ulcer often requires extensive care for other health problems, it is important that the nurse support the caregiver with the added responsibility for pressure ulcer treatment. eNursing Care Plan 11-2 (available on the website for this chapter) outlines the care for the patient with a pressure ulcer.

◆ Evaluation

The expected outcomes are that the patient with a pressure ulcer will have

- Healing of pressure ulcer(s)
- Intact skin with no further breakdown

CASE STUDY

Inflammation and Infection

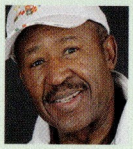

(©iStockphoto/Thinkstock)

Patient Profile

G.N., a 65-year-old African American man, was admitted to the hospital emergency department with partial-thickness burns that involved his face, neck, and upper trunk. He also had a lacerated right leg. His injuries occurred about 36 hours earlier when he fell out of a tree onto his gas grill (which was lit) while trimming tree branches.

Subjective Data

- Complains of slightly hoarse voice and irritated throat
- States that he tried to treat himself because he does not have health insurance
- Has been coughing up sooty sputum
- Complains of severe pain in left hip

Objective Data

Physical Examination

- Leg wound is gaping and has drainage: temperature 101.1°F (38.4°C)
- X-rays reveal a fractured right tibia and fractured left hip

Laboratory Studies

- WBC count 26,400/μL (26.4×10^9/L) with 80% neutrophils (10% bands)

Interprofessional Care

- Surgery is performed to repair the left hip.

Discussion Questions

1. What clinical manifestations of inflammation did G.N. exhibit, and what are their pathophysiologic mechanisms?
2. What type of exudate formation did he develop?
3. What is the basis for the development of the temperature?
4. What is the significance of his WBC count and differential?
5. Because his wound was gaping, primary tissue healing was not possible. How would you expect healing to take place? What complications could he develop?
6. What risk factors does G.N. have to develop a pressure ulcer?
7. ***Priority Decision:*** Based on the assessment data provided, what are the priority nursing diagnoses? Are there any collaborative problems?
8. ***Teamwork and Collaboration:*** What nursing activities related to wound care can be delegated to unlicensed assistive personnel (UAP)?
9. ***Quality Improvement:*** What outcomes would indicate that interprofessional care was effective?

Answers available at *http://evolve.elsevier.com/Lewis/medsurg.*

BRIDGE TO NCLEX EXAMINATION

The number of the question corresponds to the same-numbered outcome at the beginning of the chapter.

1. A patient 1 day postoperative after abdominal surgery has incisional pain, 99.5°F temperature, slight erythema at the incision margins, and 30 mL serosanguineous drainage in the Jackson-Pratt drain. Based on this assessment, what conclusion would the nurse make?
   a. The abdominal incision shows signs of an infection.
   b. The patient is having a normal inflammatory response.
   c. The abdominal incision shows signs of impending dehiscence.
   d. The patient's physician must be notified about her condition.
2. The nurse assessing a patient with a chronic leg wound finds local signs of erythema and the patient complains of pain at the wound site. What would the nurse anticipate being ordered to assess the patient's systemic response?
   a. Serum protein analysis
   b. WBC count and differential
   c. Punch biopsy of center of wound
   d. Culture and sensitivity of the wound
3. A patient in the unit has a 103.7°F temperature. Which intervention would be *most* effective in restoring normal body temperature?
   a. Use a cooling blanket while the patient is febrile.
   b. Administer antipyretics on an around-the-clock schedule.
   c. Provide increased fluids and have the UAP give sponge baths.
   d. Give prescribed antibiotics and provide warm blankets for comfort.
4. A nurse is caring for a patient who has a pressure ulcer that is treated with debridement, irrigations, and moist gauze dressings. How should the nurse anticipate healing to occur?
   a. Tertiary intention
   b. Secondary intention
   c. Regeneration of cells
   d. Remodeling of tissues
5. A nurse is caring for a patient with diabetes who is scheduled for amputation of his necrotic left great toe. The patient's WBC count is 15.0×10^6/μL, and he has coolness of the lower extremities, weighs 75 lb more than his ideal body weight, and smokes two packs of cigarettes per day. Which *priority* nursing diagnosis addresses the primary factor affecting the patient's ability to heal?
   a. Imbalanced nutrition: obesity *related to* high-fat foods
   b. Impaired tissue integrity *related to* decreased blood flow secondary to diabetes and smoking
   c. Ineffective peripheral tissue perfusion *related to* narrowed blood vessels secondary to diabetes and smoking
   d. Ineffective individual coping *related to* indifference and denial of the long-term effects of diabetes and smoking
6. Which one of the orders should a nurse question in the plan of care for an elderly immobile stroke patient with a stage III pressure ulcer?
   a. Pack the ulcer with foam dressing.
   b. Turn and position the patient every hour.
   c. Clean the ulcer every shift with Dakin's solution.
   d. Assess for pain and medicate before dressing change.

7. An 85-year-old patient is assessed to have a score of 16 on the Braden Scale. Based on this information, how should the nurse plan for this patient's care?
   a. Implement a 1-hr turning schedule with skin assessment.
   b. Place DuoDerm on the patient's sacrum to prevent breakdown.
   c. Elevate the head of bed to 90 degrees when the patient is supine.
   d. Continue with weekly skin assessments with no special precautions.
8. A 65-year-old stroke patient with limited mobility has a purple area of suspected deep tissue injury on the left greater trochanter. Which nursing diagnoses are *most* appropriate (*select all that apply*)?
   a. Acute pain *related to* tissue damage and inflammation
   b. Impaired skin integrity *related to* immobility and decreased sensation
   c. Impaired tissue integrity *related to* inadequate circulation secondary to pressure
   d. Risk for infection *related to* loss of tissue integrity and undernutrition secondary to stroke
   e. Ineffective peripheral tissue perfusion *related* to arteriosclerosis and loss of blood supply to affected area
9. An 82-year-old man is being cared for at home by his family. A pressure ulcer on his right buttock measures 1 × 2 × 0.8 cm in depth, and pink subcutaneous tissue is completely visible on the wound bed. Which stage would the nurse document on the wound assessment form?
   a. Stage I
   b. Stage II
   c. Stage III
   d. Stage IV

1. b, 2. b, 3. b, 4. b, 5. b, 6. c, 7. a, 8. b, c, 9. c

For rationales to these answers and even more NCLEX review questions, visit *http://evolve.elsevier.com/Lewis/medsurg.*

EVOLVE WEBSITE

http://evolve.elsevier.com/Lewis/medsurg

Review Questions (Online Only)
Key Points
Answer Keys for Questions
- Rationales for Bridge to NCLEX Examination Questions
- Answer Guidelines for Case Study on p. 176

Student Case Study
- Patient With Pressure Ulcers

Nursing Care Plans
- eNursing Care Plan 11-1: Patient With a Fever
- eNursing Care Plan 11-2: Patient With a Pressure Ulcer

Conceptual Care Map Creator
Audio Glossary
Content Updates

REFERENCES

1. Knowlton MC: Nurses know how to manage fever, but what about shivering? *Nursing* 43:49, 2013.
2. Atkins E: Fever: its history, cause, and function, *Yale J Biol Med* 55:283, 1982. (Classic)
3. LeBlanc K, Baranoski S: Skin tears: Best practices for care and prevention, *Nursing* 44:36, 2014.
4. Bergevin RC: Assessing wounds in palliative care, *Nursing* 44(8):67, 2014.

*5. Lisy K: Early vs. delayed removal of dressings covering surgical wounds, *AJN* 114:23, 2014.

*6. Ayello EA, Baranoski S: Wound care prevention, *Nursing* 44:32, 2014.

*7. Wilcox JR, Carter MJ, Covington S: Frequency of debridements and time to heal: a retrospective cohort study of 312,744 wounds, *JAMA Dermatol* 149(9):1050, 2013.

8. Negative pressure wound therapy: use with care. Retrieved from *www.fda.gov/MedicalDevices/Safety/AlertsandNotices/TipsandArticleson DeviceSafety/ucm225038.htm.*
9. Posthauer ME: Nutrition: fuel for pressure ulcer prevention and healing, *Nursing* 44:67, 2014.
10. Huddleston Cross H: Obtaining a wound swab culture specimen, *Nursing* 44:68, 2014.

*11. National Pressure Ulcer Advisory Panel. Retrieved from *www.npuap.org.*

12. Nightingale F: *Notes on nursing*, Philadelphia, 1859, Lippincott. (Classic)
13. Nelson M, Harris R: Pressure ulcer alert! *Nursing* 43:64, 2013.

*14. Roe E, Williams DL: Using evidence-based practice to prevent hospital-acquired pressure ulcers and promote wound healing, *AJN* 114:61, 2014.

*15. Paul R, McCutcheon SP, Tregarthen JP, et al: Sustaining pressure ulcer best practices in high-volume cardiac care unit, *AJN* 114:34, 2014.

*Evidence-based information for clinical practice.

12

Genetics and Genomics

Sharon L. Lewis

You inherit your environment just as much as your genes.

Johnny Rich

http://evolve.elsevier.com/Lewis/medsurg/

LEARNING OUTCOMES

1. Differentiate the common terms related to genetics and genetic disorders: autosomal, carrier, heterozygous, homozygous, mutation, recessive, and X-linked gene.
2. Differentiate between the two common causes of genetic mutations.
3. Compare and contrast the three most common inheritance patterns of genetic disorders.
4. Describe the most common classifications of genetic disorders.
5. Explore the complex ethical and social implications of genetic testing.
6. Analyze the role of pharmacogenomics and pharmacogenetics in developing personalized drug therapy.
7. Discuss your role in assisting the patient and family in dealing with genetic issues.

KEY TERMS

epigenetics, p. 183
genetics, p. 178
genomics, p. 178
hereditary, Table 12-1, p. 179
heterozygous, Table 12-1, p. 179
homozygous, Table 12-1, p. 179
mutation, Table 12-1, p. 179
pharmacogenetics, p. 186
pharmacogenomics, p. 186

GENETICS AND GENOMICS

In the 1860s an Austrian monk named Gregor Mendel, while experimenting with pea plants, discovered how traits are transmitted from parents to offspring. This discovery laid the foundation for modern **genetics**, the study of genes and their role in inheritance. Genetics determines the way that certain traits or conditions are passed down from one generation to another.

Genomics is the study of all of a person's genes (the *genome*), including interactions of these genes with each other and with the person's environment. (Common terms used in genetics and genomics are defined in Table 12-1.) Genomics includes the study of complex diseases such as heart disease, asthma, diabetes mellitus, and cancer, because these diseases are typically caused by a combination of genetic and environmental factors rather than by a single gene.

A person's genes can have a profound impact on health and disease. More than 4000 diseases are thought to be related to altered genes. Genomic factors play a role in 9 of the 10 leading causes of death in the United States, including heart disease, cancer, diabetes, stroke, and Alzheimer's disease.[1]

Genomics may help us understand why some people who eat healthy diets and exercise regularly still die at a young age of cancer, whereas some people eat unhealthy diets and never exercise and yet live to an old age.

The identification of a genetic basis for many human diseases has the potential to strongly influence the care of patients at risk for or diagnosed with a disease that has a genetic link. You need to know the basic principles of genetics, be familiar with the impact that genetics and genomics have on health and disease, and be prepared to assist the patient and family with genetic issues.

Basic Principles of Genetics

Genes. *Genes* are the basic units of heredity. There are more than 22,000 genes in each person's genetic makeup, or *genome.* Genes encode (carry the instructions) for proteins that direct the activities of cells and functions of the body. Genes control how a cell functions, including how quickly it grows, how often it divides, and how long it lives. To control these functions, genes produce proteins that perform specific tasks and act as messengers for the cell. Therefore it is essential that each gene have the correct instructions or "code" for making its protein so that the protein can perform the proper function for the cell.

Genes are arranged in a specific linear formation along a chromosome (Fig. 12-1). Each gene has a specific location on a chromosome, termed a *locus.* An *allele* is one of two or more alternative forms of a gene that occupy corresponding loci on *homologous chromosomes* (a pair of chromosomes having corresponding deoxyribonucleic acid [DNA] sequences, with one

Reviewed by Judy Carlyle, RN, MNSc, Faculty/Clinical Liaison, Arkansas Rural Nursing Education Consortium (ARNEC), Nashville, Arkansas; Laura A. Stokowski, RNC, MS, Inova Fairfax Hospital for Children, Falls Church, Virginia; and Kenneth Wysocki, PhD, FNP-BC, FAANP, Family Nurse Practitioner, Asthma and Genetics Researcher, Clinical Services, Matrix Medical Network, Scottsdale, Arizona.

TABLE 12-1 Glossary of Genetic and Genomic Terms

Term	Definition
Allele	An alternative form of a gene. Each person receives two alleles of a gene, one from each biologic parent. Different alleles produce variations in inherited traits such as eye color and blood type.
Autosome	Any chromosome that is not a sex chromosome. Humans have 22 pairs of autosomes.
Carrier	Individual who carries a copy of a mutated gene for a recessive disorder.
Chromosome	A compact structure containing DNA and proteins present in nearly all cells of the body. Normally each cell has 46 chromosomes in 23 pairs. Each biologic parent contributes one of each pair of chromosomes.
Codominance	Two dominant versions of a trait that are both expressed in the same individual (e.g., AB blood type).
Congenital disorder	Condition present at birth.
Dominant allele	Gene that is expressed in the phenotype of a heterozygous individual.
Familial disorder	Condition that affects more than one person in a family.
Gene	The basic unit of heredity information located on a specific part of a chromosome. Genes direct cells to make proteins and guide almost every aspect of operation and repair of cells.
Genetic risk factor	A change in a gene that increases a person's risk of developing a disease.
Genetics	Study of genes and their role in inheritance.
Genome	All the DNA contained in an individual.
Genome-wide association study (GWAS)	A study approach that involves scanning complete sets of DNA (genomes) of many individuals to find genetic variations associated with a particular disease.
Genomics	Study of how genes interact and influence people's biologic and physical characteristics.
Genotype	Genetic identity of an individual. This identity does not show as outward characteristics.
Hereditary	Transmission of a disease, condition, or trait from parent to children.
Heterozygous	Having two different alleles for one given gene, one inherited from each parent.
Homozygous	Having two identical alleles for one given gene, one inherited from each parent.
Locus	Position of a gene on a chromosome.
Mutation	A change in DNA or a gene. Sometimes these changes are passed from parent to children.
Oncogene	Gene that is able to initiate and contribute to the conversion of normal cells to cancer cells.
Pedigree	Family tree that contains the genetic characteristics and disorders of that particular family.
Pharmacogenetics	Study of variability of responses to drugs related to variations in single genes.
Pharmacogenomics	Study of variability of responses to drugs related to variations in and interactions of multiple genes.
Phenotype	Observable traits or characteristics of an individual (e.g., hair color).
Protooncogene	Normal cellular genes that are important regulators of normal cellular processes. Mutations can activate them to become oncogenes.
Recessive allele	Allele that has no noticeable effect on the phenotype in a heterozygous individual.
Trait	Physical characteristic that one inherits, such as hair or eye color.
X-linked gene	Gene located on the X chromosome. In general, sex-linked disorders are only seen in males.

coming from the mother and the other from the father). Each allele codes for a specific inherited characteristic.

When there are two different alleles, the allele that is fully expressed is the *dominant allele.* The other allele that lacks the ability to express itself in the presence of a dominant allele is the *recessive allele.* Physical traits expressed by an individual are termed the *phenotype,* and the actual genetic makeup of the individual is termed the *genotype.*

Chromosomes. *Chromosomes* are contained in the nucleus of a cell and occur in pairs. Humans have 23 pairs of chromosomes; 22 of the 23 pairs of chromosomes are *homologous* and are termed *autosomes.* Autosomes are the same in both males and females. The sex chromosomes make up the twenty-third pair of chromosomes. A female has two X chromosomes, and a male has one X and one Y chromosome. One chromosome of each pair is inherited from the mother and one from the father. One half of each child's chromosomes (and therefore the genetic makeup) comes from his or her father and one half from his or her mother.

DNA. Genes are made up of a nucleic acid called *deoxyribonucleic acid* (DNA). DNA stores genetic information and encodes the instructions for synthesizing specific proteins needed to maintain life. DNA also dictates the rate at which proteins are made. Every somatic cell in a person's body has the same DNA.

The information in DNA is stored as a code made up of four nitrogenous bases: adenine (A), guanine (G), cytosine (C), and thymine (T). Human DNA consists of about 3 billion bases, and more than 99% of those bases are the same in all people. The order (or sequence) of these bases determines the information for building and maintaining an organism. This is similar to the way letters of the alphabet are used to create words and sentences.

DNA bases pair up with each other, A with T and C with G, to form units called *base pairs.* Each base is also attached to a sugar molecule and a phosphate molecule (Fig. 12-2). Together, a base, sugar, and phosphate are called a *nucleotide.* Nucleotides are arranged in two long strands that form a spiral called a *double helix.* The structure of the double helix is somewhat like

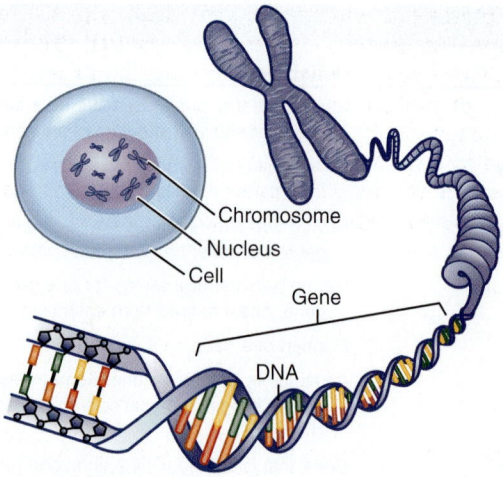

FIG. 12-1 The long, stringy DNA that makes up genes is spooled within chromosomes inside the nucleus of a cell. (Note that a gene would actually be a much longer stretch of DNA than what is shown here.) (Adapted from *The New Genetics,* National Institute of General Medical Science, National Institutes of Health, U.S. Department of Health and Human Services.)

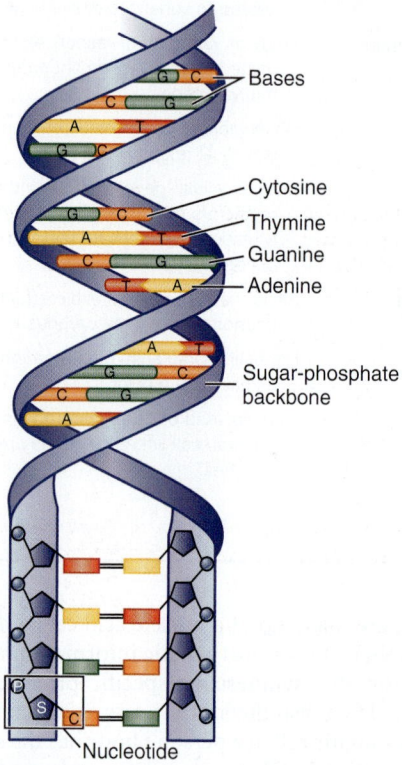

FIG. 12-2 DNA consists of two long, twisted chains made up of nucleotides. Each nucleotide contains one base, one phosphate molecule *(P),* and the sugar molecule deoxyribose *(S).* The bases in DNA nucleotides are adenine *(A),* thymine *(T),* cytosine *(C),* and guanine *(G).* (Adapted from *The New Genetics.* National Institute of General Medical Science, National Institutes of Health, U.S. Department of Health and Human Services.)

a ladder, with the base pairs forming the ladder's rungs and the sugar and phosphate molecules forming the ladder's vertical sidepieces.

DNA can *replicate* (make copies of itself). Each strand of DNA in the double helix can serve as a pattern for duplicating the sequence of bases. When cells divide, each new cell must have an exact copy of the DNA that was in the parent (original) cell.

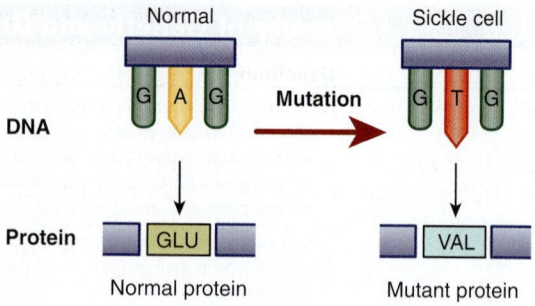

FIG. 12-3 In sickle cell disease a single gene mutation leads to mutant (incorrect) protein. The substitution of valine *(VAL)* for glutamic acid on the β-globin chain of hemoglobin produces abnormal hemoglobin, hemoglobin S *(Hb S).* In response to low O_2 levels, the erythrocytes with Hb S stiffen and elongate, taking on a sickle shape (see Fig. 30-3).

If the chromosomes in one of your cells were uncoiled and placed end to end, the DNA would be about 6 feet long. If all of the DNA in your body were connected, it would stretch about 67 billion miles.[2]

RNA. *Ribonucleic acid* (RNA) is similar to DNA but with some significant differences. Like DNA, RNA contains the nitrogenous bases adenine, guanine, and cytosine. However, RNA lacks the nitrogenous base thymine and instead contains uracil. RNA is single stranded and contains ribose instead of deoxyribose sugar. RNA transfers the genetic information obtained from DNA to the proper location for protein synthesis.

Protein Synthesis. Protein synthesis, or the making of proteins, occurs in two steps: *transcription* and *translation.* Transcription is the process by which messenger RNA (mRNA) is synthesized from single-stranded DNA. The mRNA becomes attached to a ribosome, where translation occurs. At this point another specialized type of RNA, transfer RNA (tRNA), arranges the amino acids in the correct sequence to assemble the protein. Once the protein is completed, it is released from the ribosome and is able to perform its specific function in the cell.

Mitosis. *Mitosis* is a type of cell division that results in the formation of genetically identical daughter cells. Before cell division, the chromosomes duplicate, and each new cell (called daughter cells) receives an exact replica of the chromosomes from the original cell (called the parent cell).

Meiosis. *Meiosis* occurs only in sexual reproductive cells. In meiosis the number of chromosomes is reduced, resulting in half of the usual number of chromosomes. Therefore oocytes and sperm contain only a single copy of each chromosome, whereas all other body cells contain duplicates of each chromosome.

Genetic Mutations

A *mutation* is any change in the usual DNA sequence. Subtle variations in DNA are called *polymorphisms* (meaning many forms). Many of these *gene* polymorphisms account for slight variations among people such as hair and eye color. However, some gene variations may result in disease or an increased risk for disease. These gene variations or changes are referred to as *mutations.*

A genetic mutation is like a spelling error in a gene's sequence. For example, in people with sickle cell disease, a substitution of a single base (adenine is replaced by thymine) in a single gene (β-globin gene) causes the disease (Fig. 12-3). Mutations range in size from a single DNA base (building block) to a large segment of a chromosome.

The change in gene structure may alter the type and/or amount of protein produced. The protein may not work at all, or it may work incorrectly. In some cases, genetic mutations do not have an obvious effect on the people who have them.

Types of Mutations. Genetic mutations occur in two ways. They can be inherited from a parent (germline mutation) or acquired (somatic mutation) during a person's lifetime.

Germline mutations are passed from parent to child. These mutations are present in the oocyte and sperm cells. This type of mutation is present throughout a person's life in virtually every cell in the body.

Acquired (somatic) mutations occur in the DNA of a cell at some time during a person's life. An acquired mutation is passed on to all cells that develop from that single cell. These mutations in somatic cells cannot be passed on to the next generation. Acquired mutations can occur if (1) a mistake is made as DNA replicates during cell division or (2) environmental factors alter the DNA.

Mutations can occur when a cell is dividing. Considering that 3 billion base pairs are replicated in each cell division, DNA replication is very accurate. However, during replication occasionally mistakes such as deletions, insertions, or duplication of DNA material can occur. Although DNA repair enzymes can correct replication errors, mistakes can go uncorrected.

In addition to cell division, DNA damage can also occur from environmental factors. For example, ultraviolet (UV) radiation can cause DNA damage, leading to skin cancer. Toxins in cigarettes can lead to lung cancer. Many chemotherapy drugs used to treat cancer target the DNA of cancer cells and healthy cells. In the process, these drugs increase a person's risk of developing secondary cancers (see Chapter 15).

Cells have built-in mechanisms that catch and repair most of the changes that occur during DNA replication or from environmental damage. However, as we age, our DNA repair does not work as effectively and we accumulate changes in our DNA.

Inheritance Patterns

Genetic disorders can be categorized into autosomal dominant, autosomal recessive, or X-linked (sex-linked) recessive disorders (Table 12-2). If the mutant gene is located on an autosome, the genetic disorder is called *autosomal.* If the mutant gene is on the X chromosome, the genetic disorder is called *X-linked.*

Family pedigrees for autosomal recessive and dominant disorders and X-linked recessive disorders are shown in Figs. 12-4 and 12-5.

Autosomal dominant disorders are caused by a mutation of a single gene pair (heterozygous) on a chromosome. A dominant allele prevails over a normal allele. Autosomal dominant disorders show variable expression. *Variable expression* means that the symptoms expressed by the individuals with the mutated gene vary from person to person even though they have the same mutated gene. Although autosomal dominant disorders have a high probability of occurring in families, sometimes these disorders cause a new mutation or skip a generation. This is termed *incomplete penetrance.*

Autosomal recessive disorders are caused by mutations of two gene pairs (homozygous) on a chromosome. A person who inherits one copy of the recessive allele does not develop the

TABLE 12-2 Comparison of Genetic Disorders

Characteristics	Examples
Autosomal Dominant	
• Males and females are affected* equally. • More common than recessive disorders and usually less severe. • Affected individuals show variable expression. • Affected individuals may have an affected parent. • Children of a heterozygous (affected) parent have a 50% chance of being affected. • Individuals are affected in successive generations.	• Breast and ovarian cancer related to *BRCA* genes • Familial hypercholesterolemia • Hereditary nonpolyposis colorectal cancer • Huntington's disease • Neurofibromatosis • Marfan's syndrome
Autosomal Recessive	
• Males and females are affected equally. • Heterozygotes are carriers and usually asymptomatic. • Affected individuals may have unaffected† parents who are heterozygous for trait. • Children of two heterozygous parents have 25% chance of being affected and 50% chance of being carriers (Fig. 12-9). • Frequently there is no family history of disease.	• Cystic fibrosis • Phenylketonuria • Sickle cell disease • Tay-Sachs disease • Thalassemia
X-Linked Recessive	
• Most affected individuals have unaffected parents. • Affected individuals are usually males. • Daughters of affected male are carriers. • Sons of affected male are unaffected (unless mother is a carrier).	• Duchenne muscular dystrophy • Hemophilia • Wiskott-Aldrich syndrome

*Have the disease.
†Do not have the disease.

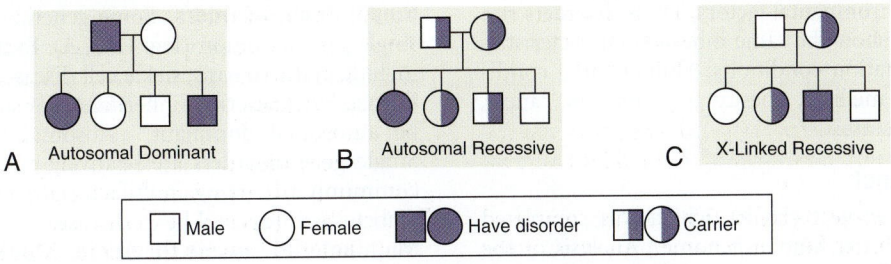

FIG. 12-4 Examples of family pedigrees showing inheritance of **(A)** autosomal dominant, **(B)** autosomal recessive, and **(C)** X-linked recessive disorders.

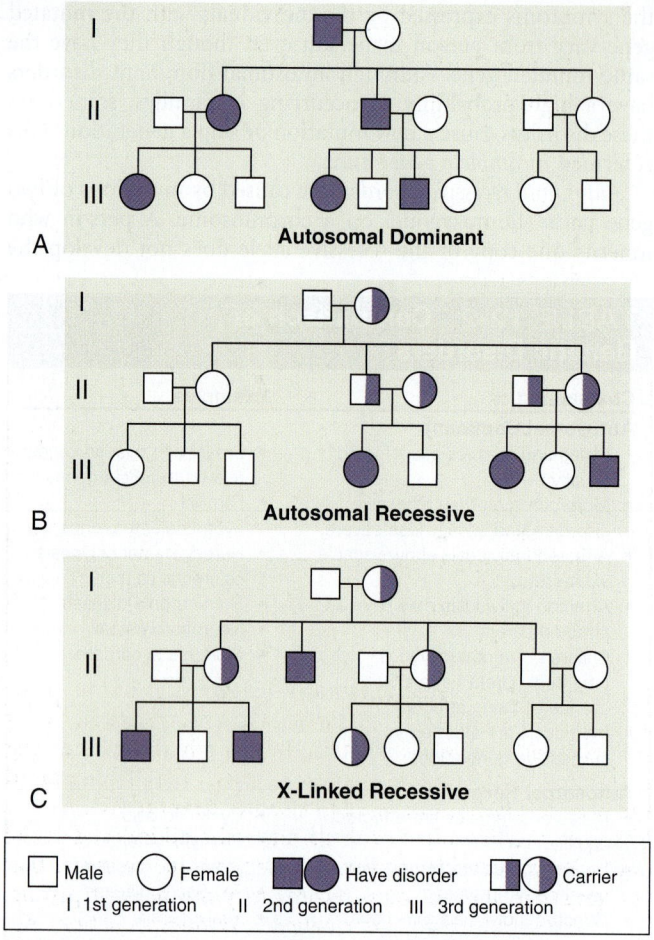

FIG. 12-5 Family pedigrees showing three generations. **A,** Family pedigree suggestive of an autosomal dominant disorder. **B,** Family pedigree suggestive of an autosomal recessive disorder. **C,** Family pedigree suggestive of an X-linked recessive disorder.

disease because the normal allele predominates.[3] However, this person is a *carrier.*

X-linked recessive disorders are caused by a mutation on the X chromosome. Usually only men are affected by this disorder because women who carry the mutated gene on one X chromosome have another X chromosome to compensate for the mutation. However, women who carry the mutated gene can transmit it to their offspring. It is possible for women to have X-linked recessive disorders, and this can occur when an affected male mates with an unaffected female carrier. This points to the importance of testing the carrier status of the female partner of affected males. *X-linked dominant disorders* do exist, but they are rare.

Multifactorial inherited conditions are caused by a combination of genetic and environmental factors. These disorders run in families but do not show the same inherited characteristics as the single gene mutation conditions. Multifactorial conditions include diabetes mellitus, obesity, hypertension, cancer, and coronary artery disease.

Human Genome Project

The Human Genome Project (HGP), which was completed in 2003, mapped the entire human genome.[4] Analysis of the data will continue for many years. The knowledge gained through the HGP will (1) help improve the diagnosis of

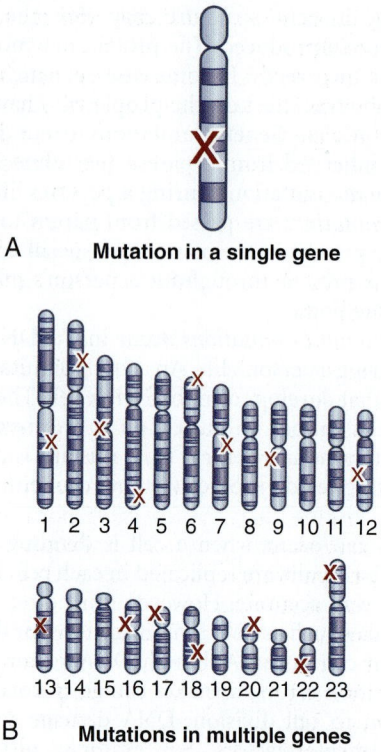

FIG. 12-6 **A,** Genetic disorders can be caused by a mutation in a single gene (e.g., sickle cell disease, cystic fibrosis, hemophilia). **B,** Most genetic disorders are multifactorial genetic disorders caused by a combination of mutations in multiple genes, often interacting with environmental factors. Examples include cancer, diabetes mellitus, obesity, and hypertension.

diseases, (2) allow for earlier detection of genetic predisposition to diseases, and (3) play a critical role in determining risk assessment for genetic-related diseases. In addition, the results of the HGP assist in matching organ donors with transplant recipients.

GENETIC DISORDERS

A *genetic disorder* is caused in whole or in part by an alteration in the DNA sequence. As discussed in the section on genetic mutations (pp. 180-181), genetic disorders can be inherited (person born with altered genetic code) or they can be acquired (e.g., replication errors, damage to DNA from toxins).[5] Genetic disorders can be caused by (1) a mutation in one gene (single gene disorder); (2) mutations in multiple genes (multifactorial inheritance disorder), which are often related to environmental factors; or (3) damage to chromosomes (changes in the number or structure of chromosomes).

Classification of Genetic Disorders

Single Gene Disorders. Some genetic disorders result from a single gene mutation (Fig. 12-6, *A*). Examples of these diseases include cystic fibrosis, sickle cell disease, and polycystic kidney disease. The pattern of inheritance for single gene disorders can be autosomal dominant, autosomal recessive, or X-linked. Single gene disorders are relatively rare compared with more commonly occurring multifactorial genetic disorders such as diabetes mellitus and heart disease.

Multifactorial Genetic Disorders. Multifactorial genetic disorders are complex diseases that result from small inherited variations in genes, often acting together with environmental factors

(Fig. 12-6, *B*). Heart disease, diabetes, and most cancers are examples of such disorders.

Although many common diseases are usually caused by inheritance of mutations in multiple genes, such diseases can also be caused by rare hereditary mutations in a single gene. In these cases, genetic mutations that cause or strongly predispose a person to these diseases run in a family. These mutations can significantly increase each family member's risk of developing the disease. One example is breast cancer, in which inheritance of a mutated *BRCA1* or *BRCA2* gene confers significant risk of developing the disease.

Epigenetics. Environmental factors can alter the way our genes are expressed (i.e., which genes are "switched" on or off). **Epigenetics** is the study of the chemical modification of specific genes or gene-associated proteins of an organism. Epigenetic modifications can define how the information in genes is expressed and used by cells. Genetic and environmental factors interact to influence a person's predisposition to different diseases. The expression of genes can be affected both positively and negatively by environmental factors, such as exercise, diet, chemicals, toxins, or smoking.

Identical twins, who have the same genetic makeup, do not always develop the same diseases or at the same rate. Twins share the same genes but their environments become more different as they age. This unique aspect of twins makes them an excellent model for understanding how genes and the environment contribute to certain traits, especially complex behaviors and diseases.[6]

Chromosome Disorders. *Chromosome disorders* are caused by structural changes within chromosomes or by an excess or deficiency of the genes that are located on chromosomes. For example, Down syndrome is caused by an extra copy of chromosome 21 (called trisomy 21), so there are three copies of this chromosome instead of two. In Down syndrome there is no individual abnormal gene on the chromosome.

Chronic myelocytic leukemia can be caused by a chromosomal translocation, in which portions of two chromosomes (chromosomes 9 and 22) are exchanged. This translocation is called the *Philadelphia chromosome*.

Throughout the book, genetic disorders are highlighted in Genetics in Clinical Practice boxes, Genetic Risk Alert boxes (in the assessment chapters), and Genetic Links content (in the management chapters).

GENETIC TESTING

Genetic testing includes any procedure done to analyze chromosomes, genes, or any gene product that can determine whether a mutation or predisposition to a condition exists. Genetic tests have been developed for more than 2000 diseases. A person's blood, skin, hair, or saliva can be used to obtain samples for genetic testing. Tissues and cells can also be obtained prenatally.

Genetic testing has been very useful in health care (Table 12-3). Most tests assess single genes and are used to diagnose genetic disorders such as cystic fibrosis or Duchenne muscular dystrophy.[7] Some genetic tests look at rare inherited mutations of otherwise protective genes, such as *BRCA1* and *BRCA2*, which are responsible for some types of hereditary breast and ovarian cancers.[8]

The results of these tests are used in diagnosing an illness or risk for a disorder and provide the basis for appropriate treatments. Other genetic tests identify people at high risk for conditions that may be preventable. For example, monitoring for and removing polyps or the entire colon in those inheriting a gene for familial adenomatous polyposis (FAP) have saved many lives.[8] (FAP is discussed in Chapter 42 on p. 953.)

Genetic testing of individuals may raise ethical and social issues. People considering genetic testing should be aware that test results in their medical records may not be kept private. However, the Genetic Information Nondiscrimination Act (GINA) protects people from discrimination by employers and health insurance companies.

If an individual has genetic testing, it may uncover information that may also affect a family member who was not tested. These individuals are frequently not a part of the decision-making process to undergo testing. Similarly, if a whole family is tested, the results may indicate that the biologic relationship is not what the family believed it to be. Some tests are used to help guide HCPs' recommendations for treatment in consultation with the patient (e.g., *BRCA* testing). Other tests allow families to make the decision about not having children with diseases (e.g., cystic fibrosis) or identify people at high risk for conditions that may be prevented by monitoring or having prophylactic surgery (e.g., familial adenomatous polyposis [FAP]).

Currently, many genetic tests are available from testing laboratories. In most cases, insurance companies will not cover the cost of genetic testing. For more information about genetic testing, see *www.cdc.gov/genomics/gtesting/index.htm*.

Interpreting Genetic Test Results

The results of genetic tests are not always straightforward, which often makes them challenging to interpret and explain. When interpreting test results, HCPs need to consider a person's medical history and family history and the type of genetic test that was done.

A *positive test* result means that the laboratory found a change in a particular gene, chromosome, or protein that was being tested. Depending on the purpose of the test, this result may confirm a diagnosis (e.g., Huntington's disease), indicate

GENETICS IN CLINICAL PRACTICE

Genetics in Clinical Practice Boxes Throughout Book

Genetic Disorder	Chapter	Page
α_1-Antitrypsin (AAT) Deficiency	28	559
Alzheimer's Disease (AD)	59	1402
Ankylosing Spondylitis	64	1536
Breast Cancer	51	1210
Cystic Fibrosis (CF)	28	576
Duchenne and Becker Muscular Dystrophy (MD)	63	1502
Familial Adenomatous Polyposis (FAP)	42	953
Familial Hypercholesterolemia	33	704
Genetic Information Nondiscrimination Act (GINA)	12	184
Hemochromatosis	30	620
Hemophilia A and B	30	627
Hereditary Nonpolyposis Colorectal Cancer (HNPCC) or Lynch Syndrome	42	954
Huntington's Disease (HD)	58	1396
Ovarian Cancer	53	1258
Polycystic Kidney Disease (PKD)	45	1051
Sickle Cell Disease	30	616
Types 1 and 2 Diabetes Mellitus and MODY	48	1122

TABLE 12-3 Use of Genetic Tests*

Type of Test	Description	Examples
Diagnostic testing	• Used to diagnose, rule out, or confirm a specific genetic or chromosomal condition • Used to confirm findings when patient's signs and symptoms suggest a genetic disorder • Can be performed at any time during a person's life but is not available for all genes or all genetic conditions	• Cystic fibrosis • Sickle cell disease • Polycystic kidney disease • Hemophilia • Familial hypercholesterolemia
Carrier screening	• Can be used to identify unaffected individuals who carry one copy of a gene • Offered to individuals who have a family history of a genetic disorder and to people in ethnic groups with an increased risk of specific genetic conditions • If both parents are tested, the test can provide information about a couple's risk of having a child with a genetic condition	• Cystic fibrosis • Sickle cell disease • Hemophilia
Preimplantation genetic diagnosis (PGD)	• Fertilized embryos tested before implantation and pregnancy • Allows embryos free of particular disorders to be placed into the uterus • Embryos that test positive for genetic disorders can be destroyed	• For individuals known to have or be a carrier for a genetic mutation (e.g., Huntington's disease)
Prenatal diagnostic testing	• Fluid obtained from amniocentesis or tissue from chorionic villus used to obtain fetal cells. Can also obtain fetal samples from mother's blood • Used to detect changes in genes or chromosomes of fetus before birth • Type of testing offered to couples with an increased risk of having a baby with a genetic or chromosomal disorder • Can decrease a couple's uncertainty or help them decide whether to terminate the pregnancy	• Down syndrome • Other genetic alterations in fetuses
Newborn screening	• Most widespread use of genetic testing • Early intervention to treat these disorders can eliminate or reduce symptoms that may otherwise cause a lifetime of disability	• Phenylketonuria • Congenital hypothyroidism • Cystic fibrosis
Presymptomatic testing	• Used to detect genetic mutations associated with disorders that appear later in life • Can be helpful to people who have a family member with a genetic disorder but who have no features of the disorder themselves at the time of testing • Results can provide information about a person's risk of developing a specific disorder and help with making decisions about treatment	• Huntington's disease • Adult polycystic kidney disease • Hemochromatosis • Familial adenomatous polyposis • Hereditary nonpolyposis colorectal cancer syndrome
Predictive testing	• Can identify mutations that increase a person's risk of developing disorders • If results are positive, person can have prophylactic measures (e.g., mastectomy, oophorectomy) to prevent development of cancer	• Breast cancer • Ovarian cancer
Forensic testing	• Done to identify an individual for legal purposes	• Identify crime or victims in catastrophic situations • Rule out or implicate a crime suspect
Parental testing	• Establish biologic relationships between people	• Paternity testing
Pharmacogenomic testing	• Identifies genetic variations that influence a person's response to drugs • Results provide information to help select drug therapy that is best for the person	• Warfarin (Coumadin) dose

*The laboratory performing the tests must, by law, keep your personal information and test results confidential.

GENETICS IN CLINICAL PRACTICE

Genetic Information Nondiscrimination Act (GINA)

What Is GINA?

The Genetic Information Nondiscrimination Act (GINA) prohibits discrimination in health care coverage and employment based on genetic information

Why Was GINA Needed?

- Decreases concerns about discrimination that might prevent people from getting genetic tests
- Enables people to take part in research studies without fear that their DNA information may be used against them in the workplace or prevent them from getting health insurance

What Is a Genetic Test?

- An analysis of human genes (DNA, RNA), chromosomes, proteins, or metabolites that detects genotypes, mutations, or chromosomal changes

What Is Genetic Information?

- Any information about a person's genetic tests, family members' genetic tests, and family history of a genetic disease or disorder
- Referral of a person or family for, or use of, genetic services and participation in clinical research that involves genetic services

What Does GINA Do?

- Prevents health insurers from denying health insurance coverage, adjusting premiums, and discriminating against a person based solely on his or her genetic or family history information
- Prevents health insurers from requesting that a person have a genetic test
- Prohibits most employers from using genetic information for hiring, firing, or promotion decisions, and for any decisions regarding terms of employment
- GINA's health coverage nondiscrimination protection does not extend to life insurance, disability insurance, and long-term care insurance

For more information see

- *www.genome.gov/Pages/PolicyEthics/GeneticDiscrimination/GINAInfoDoc.pdf*
- Frequently Asked Questions about GINA at *www.dnapolicy.org/gina/faqs.html*

that a person is a carrier of a particular genetic mutation (e.g., cystic fibrosis), identify an increased risk of developing a disease (e.g., breast cancer), or suggest a need for further testing. A positive result of a predictive or presymptomatic genetic test usually cannot establish the absolute risk of developing a disorder. In addition, a positive test cannot predict the course or severity of a condition.

In some situations, it is difficult to interpret a positive result because some people who have the genetic mutation being tested never develop the disease. For example, having the *apolipoprotein E-4 (Apo E-4)* allele increases the risk of developing Alzheimer's disease. However, many people who test positive for *Apo E-4* never develop Alzheimer's disease (see Chapter 59).

A *negative test* result means that the laboratory did not find an altered form of the gene, chromosome, or protein under consideration. This result can indicate that a person is not affected by a particular disorder, is not a carrier of a specific genetic mutation, or does not have an increased risk of developing a certain disease. However, it is possible that the test missed a disease-causing genetic alteration, since many tests cannot detect all the genetic changes that cause a particular disorder. Further testing may be required to confirm a negative result.

Direct-to-Consumer Genetic Tests

Direct-to-consumer genetic tests (at-home testing) are marketed directly to people (consumers) via television, print advertisements, or the Internet. The test kit is mailed to the person instead of being ordered through an HCP's office. The test typically involves collecting a DNA sample at home, often by swabbing the inside of the cheek, and mailing the sample back to the laboratory. In some cases, the person must visit a health clinic to have blood drawn.

Consumers are notified of their results by mail or over the telephone, or the results are posted online. In some cases a genetic counselor or other HCP is available to explain the results and answer questions. The cost of genetic testing can range from under $100 to more than $2,000, depending on the nature and complexity of the test. The cost increases if more than one test is necessary or if multiple family members must be tested to obtain a meaningful result.

Direct-to-consumer genetic tests have significant risks and limitations. People may want their genetic information, but they may not understand what it means. Consumers are vulnerable to being misled by the results of unproven or invalid tests. Without guidance from an HCP, they may make important decisions about disease treatment or prevention based on inaccurate, incomplete, or misunderstood information about their health. Consumers may also experience an invasion of genetic privacy if testing companies use their genetic information in an unauthorized way.

If your patients are considering using these kinds of genetic tests, let them know that they first need to discuss the issue with their HCP or a genetic counselor. Patient teaching related to genetic testing is presented in Table 12-4.

ETHICAL/LEGAL DILEMMAS

Genetic Testing

Situation

A 30-year-old woman informs you that she is 3 months pregnant. She has two children with her current husband. This pregnancy was unplanned, and her youngest child has cystic fibrosis (CF). She expresses concern regarding the possibility of having another child with CF. She mentions that she would like to have genetic testing on her fetus. Her husband asks you what the likelihood is of having another child with CF.

Ethical/Legal Points for Consideration

- With genetic testing, the patient and her family can find out whether their child will have CF. The woman and her husband can then make an informed decision.
- Genetic counseling is recommended before and after obtaining genetic testing because of the complexity of the information and the emotional issues involved with implications and options.
- Knowing that CF is an autosomal recessive condition, you can use Punnett squares (Fig. 12-9) or a family pedigree (Figs. 12-4 and 12-5) to show the woman and her husband the probability of having another child with CF.
- Be mindful of the privacy and confidentiality of genetic information and the potential conflict between one person's right to privacy and another person's right to information.

Discussion Questions

1. What information would you give the patient and her husband regarding genetic testing in order for them to make an informed decision?
2. What options are available for this couple?
3. How would you assist this couple as they are considering terminating the pregnancy if the results of the genetic testing reveal that the fetus will have CF?

TABLE 12-4 Patient & Family Teaching

Genetic Testing

Genetic Counselors

- Individuals who are considering genetic testing should meet with a genetic counselor who is specially trained in medical genetics and counseling.
- Counseling is advised to help you understand the purpose of genetic testing, considerations before testing, and the emotional and medical impact of the test results.
- Genetic counseling can help you understand the pros and cons of genetic testing before making a decision to undergo a genetic test.

General Information

The following includes some important general information about genetic testing.

- Genetic testing can be expensive and may not be included in your medical insurance policy.
- Genetic testing may determine whether you are predisposed to developing an inherited disease.
- A particular genetic test will only tell you whether there is a specific genetic variant or mutation. Positive tests do not mean you will develop that disease or disorder. Neither can the results tell you when you will develop the disease.
- If a genetic test demonstrates a genetic predisposition to an inherited disorder, the news can be depressing.
- Knowledge of a genetic predisposition to a disease may give you the motivation to take preventive measures (e.g., taking drugs for familial hypercholesterolemia) or make lifestyle changes to lower the risk of a disease (e.g., exercising to decrease the risk of type 2 diabetes).
- If a genetic test reveals a strongly negative result, you probably will not develop that disease.
- If a genetic test reveals you are at risk for a specific genetic disorder, there is the possibility that other family members may also be at risk.
- If a genetic test reveals you are at risk for developing an inherited disease, whether you decide to share that information with family members is a personal and an ethical decision that you will have to make.
- Genetic testing may provide important information that you can use when making decisions about having children.

Genetic Technology

DNA Fingerprinting. DNA (genetic) fingerprinting begins by extracting DNA from the cells in a sample of blood, saliva, semen, or other appropriate fluid or tissue. *Polymerase chain reaction (PCR)* is a quick, easy method to provide unlimited copies of a DNA or RNA sequence using only a small amount of sample. PCR involves the artificial replication of a DNA or RNA sequence. The DNA or RNA strands can be separated to form new templates that are used for replication.

PCR is a key element in *genetic fingerprinting.* It is an essential technique to finding mutations in genes. It is also used extensively in forensic medicine to identify DNA of criminal suspects by using samples from blood, hair, saliva, and semen. PCR has also been used in paternity testing and finding evidence to free wrongly incarcerated prisoners. PCR can also be used as a confirmatory test in HIV testing. This is especially important when an infant of a mother who is HIV-antibody positive also tests HIV positive. In this situation, it is not known whether the antibodies from the infant's blood are from the baby or the mother. PCR techniques can be used on the baby's lymphocytes to determine whether the baby is infected with HIV.

DNA Microarray (DNA Chip). Although all of a person's somatic cells contain identical genetic material, the same genes are not active in every cell. Studying which genes are active and which are inactive in different cell types helps to understand (1) how these cells function normally and (2) how they are affected when various genes do not perform properly.

Gene expression profiling uses a technology called *DNA microarrays* (DNA chips). This technology is used to measure the expression levels of large numbers of genes simultaneously or to genotype multiple regions of a genome. The chips are laid out by robots that can position DNA fragments so precisely that more than 20,000 of them can fit on one microscope slide.

Then fluorescent-tagged molecules are washed over the DNA fragments. Some molecules (with green fluorescent tags) bind to their complementary sequence. These molecules can be identified because they glow under fluorescent light when scanned using automated equipment. Complete patterns of gene activity can be captured with this technology.

Genome-Wide Association Study (GWAS)

Genome-wide association study (GWAS) is an approach that involves rapidly scanning complete sets of DNA, or genomes, of many individuals to find genetic variations associated with the development or progression of a particular disease.

Until recently, researchers looked at single genes and the proteins that they encode. With GWAS, researchers study large numbers of genes and proteins, including how they act and interact. This provides a more complete picture of what goes on in a person. After the genetic associations are identified, researchers may be able to learn how to stop or jump-start genes on demand, change the course of a disease, or prevent it from ever happening. GWAS is particularly useful in finding genetic variations that contribute to multifactorial inherited disorders such as asthma, cancer, diabetes, and heart disease.

To carry out a GWAS, researchers use two groups of participants: people with the disease being studied and similar people without the disease. Each person's complete set of DNA, or genome, is then purified from the blood or cells, placed on tiny chips, and scanned on automated laboratory machines. The machines quickly survey each participant's genome for strategically selected markers of genetic variation.

If certain genetic variations are found to be significantly more common in people with the disease compared to people without the disease, the variations are said to be "associated" with the disease. The associated genetic variations can serve as powerful pointers to the region of the human genome where the disease-causing problem resides.

The potential impact of GWAS is substantial, since it lays the groundwork for personalized medicine, in which the current one-size-fits-all approach to health care gives way to more customized strategies. Tools such as GWAS can provide patients with individualized information about their risks of developing certain diseases. The information will help health care professionals tailor prevention programs to each person's unique genetic makeup.

PHARMACOGENOMICS AND PHARMACOGENETICS

Patients vary widely in their response to drugs. Although the reasons for this are complex, genetic factors may account for a large percentage of patient variability in response to individual drugs. **Pharmacogenomics** is the study of genomic variation associated with drug responses.

Pharmacogenomics examines the entire genome and allows for the identification of variations in multiple genes affecting the drug response. **Pharmacogenetics** is the study of genetic variability of drug responses related to variations in single genes.

These two terms are frequently used interchangeably in describing the relationship between pharmacology and genetic variability in determining an individual's response to drugs. However, pharmacogenetics has a much narrower focus.[9]

Pharmacogenetic and pharmacogenomic studies can potentially lead to drugs that can be tailor-made or adapted to each person's particular genetic makeup. This makes it possible to have personalized medicine by choosing the right drug and the right dose for the right person.[9,10] Table 12-5 has examples of pharmacogenetics.

One important area of study has been focused on the cytochrome P450 (CYP450) family of major enzymes, which are important in drug metabolism. Alterations in the *CYP450* gene can affect how the liver breaks down certain drugs, such as warfarin (Coumadin). People with a less active form of the enzyme (who metabolize the drug slowly) may get too much of the drug, whereas people with a more active form of the enzyme (who metabolize the drug quickly) may get too little of the drug. Too much warfarin can lead to internal bleeding, whereas too little warfarin may still allow blood clots to form. Pharmacogenomic testing can assist HCPs in prescribing the right amount of a medicine based on a patient's particular genetic makeup (Fig. 12-7).

Currently a genetic test for identifying *CYP450* polymorphisms is available. In addition to maximizing the safety and effectiveness of drugs, this type of genetic testing can lead to individualized drug therapy.

HCPs are starting to use pharmacogenomic information to prescribe drugs, but at this time such tests are routine for only a few diseases or disorders (examples are presented in Table 12-5). However, given the field's rapid growth, pharmacogenomics may soon lead to personalized medicine and individualized drug therapy to manage heart disease, cancer, asthma, depression, and many other common diseases.

TABLE 12-5 Examples of Pharmacogenetics

Drug	Role of Pharmacogenetics
trastuzumab (Herceptin)	• In breast cancer, drug only works for women whose tumors have genes that lead to the overproduction of a protein called HER-2. • Drug is a monoclonal antibody to HER-2. After the antibody attaches to the antigen, it kills the cells. • Genetic testing provides information on which patients are good candidates for treatment with drug. • Drug does not work for patients whose tumor genes do not express HER-2.
crizotinib (Xalkori)	• Drug used to treat patients with late-stage (locally advanced or metastatic), non–small cell lung cancers (NSCLC) who express the abnormal anaplastic lymphoma kinase *(ALK)* gene. • *ALK* gene abnormality causes cancer development and growth. • Crizotinib works by blocking certain proteins called *kinases,* including the protein produced by the abnormal *ALK* gene. • Drug was approved for use with a companion genetic diagnostic test that determines whether a patient with NSCLC has the abnormal *ALK* gene.
vemurafenib (Zelboraf)	• Approved for patients with late-stage (metastatic) or unresectable melanoma. • Indicated for the treatment of patients with melanoma whose tumors express a gene mutation called *BRAF V600E.* • To be considered for treatment, patients must first have genetic testing to determine whether melanoma cells have the *BRAF V600E* mutation.
warfarin (Coumadin) (Fig. 12-7)	• Genetic variants in the genes *VKORC1* and cytochrome P450 2C9 *(CYP2C9)* have a significant impact on people's sensitivity to warfarin (Fig. 12-7) • Individuals with particular variations in these genes require a lower warfarin dose to maintain therapeutic levels of anticoagulation. • Individuals with other variations require higher doses. • Together these genetic variations explain about 50% of the required dose difference between individuals. • Testing for patient's *CYP2C9* and *VKORC1* genotype information can assist in selecting the starting dose.
abacavir (Ziagen)	• Some people are at greater risk for serious allergic reactions when first starting treatment with this drug. • Genetic testing for *HLA-B*5701* before taking the drug can identify people who carry a genetic marker that is associated with life-threatening hypersensitivity reactions.
clopidogrel (Plavix)	• For clopidogrel to work, cytochrome P450 enzymes in the liver (particularly CYP2C19) must convert the drug to its active form. • About 2% to 14% of the population are poor metabolizers of the drug, and these patients may not receive the full benefits of the drug. • Genetic tests are available to identify genetic differences in CYP2C19 function.

GENE THERAPY

Gene therapy is an experimental technique that uses genes to treat or prevent disease. Gene therapy is an approach to treating potentially lethal and disabling diseases that are caused by single gene deficiencies. With specialized techniques, gene expression can be manipulated to correct the problem in the particular patient, although the correction will not be passed along to offspring of that person. Approaches to gene therapy include the following:[11]

- Replacing a mutated gene that causes disease with a healthy copy of the gene
- Inactivating, or "knocking out," a mutated gene that is functioning improperly
- Introducing a new gene into the body to help fight a disease

A gene that is inserted directly into a cell usually does not function. A carrier molecule called a *vector* must be used to deliver the therapeutic gene to the patient's target cells. Currently, the most common vector is a virus that has been genetically altered to carry normal human DNA. The vector can be injected or given IV directly into specific tissue. The vector unloads its genetic material containing the therapeutic human gene into the target cell. If the treatment is successful, the new gene will make a functional protein and restore the target cell to a normal state. A diagram of gene therapy is depicted in Fig. 12-8.

Although gene therapy is a promising treatment option for a number of diseases (including inherited disorders, some types of cancer, and certain viral infections), the technique remains risky and is still under study to make sure that it will be safe and effective. Gene therapy is currently only being tested for the treatment of diseases that have no other cure.[11]

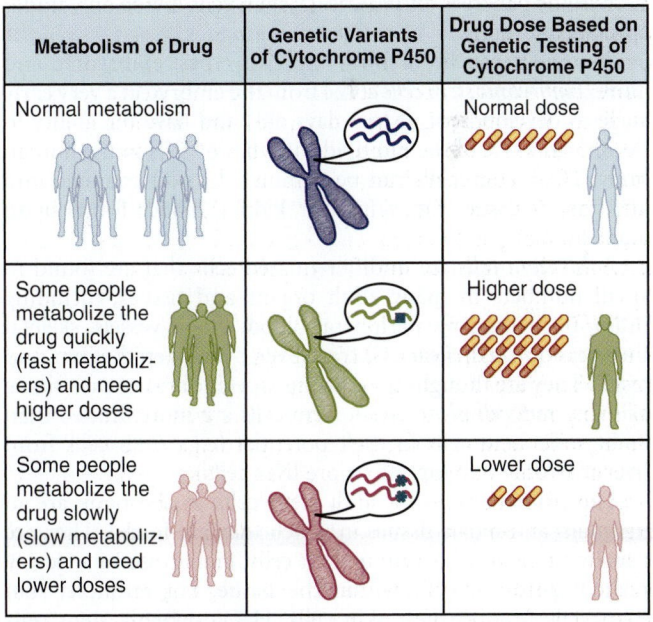

FIG. 12-7 Individuals respond differently to the drug warfarin (Coumadin). The diversity of responses is partially due to genetic variants in one of the cytochrome *P450* genes.

STEM CELL THERAPY

Stem cells are the subject of much discussion because they may offer treatment for many diseases. The use of stem cells may allow for the regeneration of lost tissue and restoration of function in various diseases.

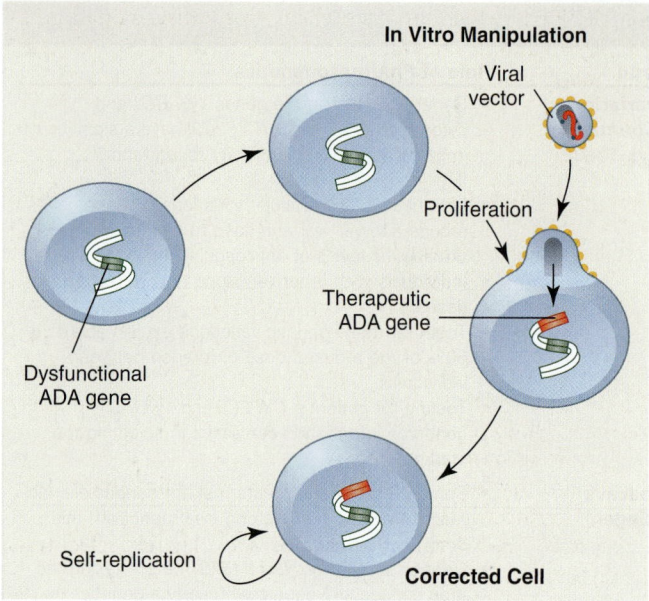

FIG. 12-8 Gene therapy for adenosine deaminase *(ADA)* deficiency attempts to correct this immunodeficiency state. The viral vector containing the therapeutic ADA gene is inserted into the patient's lymphocytes. These cells can then make the ADA enzyme.

Stem cells are unspecialized cells in the body that have the ability to (1) remain in their unspecialized state and divide or (2) differentiate and develop into specialized cells such as a brain cell or a muscle cell. In some body organs such as the gastrointestinal (GI) tract and bone marrow, stem cells divide to repair and replace damaged or old tissues. In other organs such as the pancreas and the heart, stem cells divide only under special conditions.

Stem cells can be divided into two types: embryonic and adult. *Embryonic stem cells* come from the embryo at a very early stage in development (4 to 5 days old) and have the ability to become any one of the hundreds of types of cells in the human body. These stem cells can be stimulated to differentiate into any type of tissue (e.g., skin, liver, kidney, blood) found in an adult human.

Adult stem cells are undifferentiated cells that are found in small numbers in many adult organs and tissues, including brain, bone marrow, peripheral blood, blood vessels, skeletal muscle, skin, teeth, heart, GI tract, liver, ovarian epithelium, and testes. They are thought to reside in a specific area of each tissue called a *stem cell niche.* Adult stem cells are more limited than embryonic stem cells in their potential (e.g., stem cells from liver may only develop into more liver cells).

The primary roles of adult stem cells in the body are to maintain and repair tissues in which they are found. They are usually thought of as multipotent cells, giving rise to a closely related family of cells within the tissue. For example, skin stem cells produce new skin cells. Hematopoietic stem cells found within the bone marrow are capable of forming all of the various blood cells. These cells are prolific by design and are already being used for bone marrow transplants (see Chapter 15).

Medical researchers are investigating the use of stem cells to repair or replace damaged body tissues, similar to whole organ transplants. Currently not enough donated organs are available to meet the demand for transplants. In organ transplants, when tissues from a donor are placed into a patient's body, the patient's immune system may react and reject the donated tissue as "foreign." However, using stem cells presents less risk of this immune rejection, and the therapy may be more successful.

In addition, stem cells could be directed to differentiate into specific cell types. They would then become a renewable source of replacement cells and tissues to treat conditions such as Alzheimer's disease, spinal cord injury, stroke, burns, heart disease, diabetes, osteoarthritis, and rheumatoid arthritis. It may become possible to generate healthy heart muscle cells in the laboratory and then transplant those cells into patients with chronic heart disease. Whether these cells can generate heart muscle cells or stimulate the growth of new blood vessels is under investigation.[12]

❖ NURSING MANAGEMENT: GENETICS AND GENOMICS

You must be knowledgeable about the fundamentals of genetics and genomics.[13,14] By understanding the profound influence that genetics has on health and illness, you can assist the patient and family in making critical decisions related to genetic issues, such as genetic testing. You also must collaborate with the health care team to involve a genetic nurse or a genetic counselor.

A genetic nurse is a licensed professional nurse with special education and training in genetics. Nurses with *GCN* after their names are baccalaureate-prepared licensed registered nurses who have received specialty credentialing as a Genetic Clinical Nurse (GCN). Nurses with *APNG* after their names are licensed registered nurses with a master's degree who have received specialty credentialing as an Advanced Practice Nurse in Genetics (APNG).

As a basic professional nurse, you should be an advocate for patients and families by facilitating access to genetics resources. In addition, you must provide or reinforce accurate information pertaining to genetics or a genetic disease or concern. This information should be tailored to the patient based on culture, religion, knowledge level, literacy, and preferred language.[15]

You can identify and assess inheritance patterns and explain them to the patient and family through the use of family pedigrees (see Figs. 12-4 and 12-5) and Punnett squares (Fig. 12-9). Maintain the patient's confidentiality and respect the patient's values and beliefs because genetic information may have major health and social implications.

Genetic testing may raise many psychologic and emotional issues. Knowledge of carrier status of a genetic disorder may influence a person's decisions for a career, marriage, and childbearing. It may also affect significant others in grappling with serious life and health care issues. For example, how should a wife deal with a husband who has tested positive for Huntington's disease and shows early signs of cognitive impairment but does not yet show any other neurologic manifestations of the disease? Should their children be tested for the disease? A 43-year-old woman who has a family history of breast cancer and is now diagnosed with breast cancer wants to know if she and her two teenage daughters should have *BRCA* testing. What do you tell her?

Furthermore, there are ethical concerns. Who should know the results of a genetic test? Who should protect the privacy of individuals' test results and prevent individuals from possible

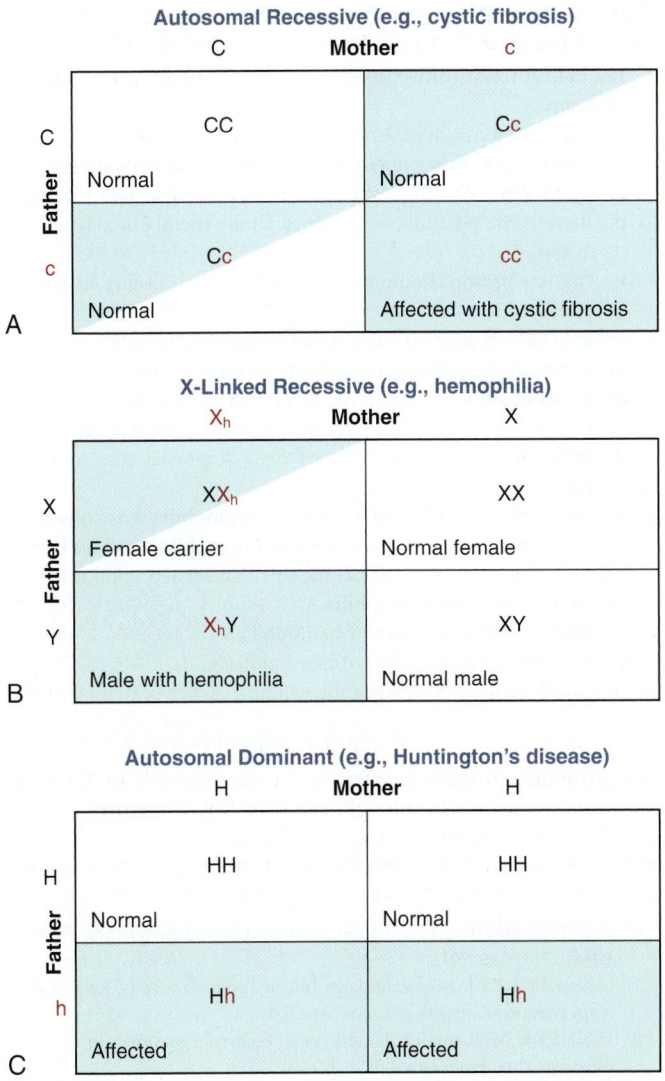

FIG. 12-9 Punnett squares illustrate inheritance possibilities. **A,** If the mother and father are both carriers for cystic fibrosis, there is a 25% chance that offspring will have cystic fibrosis. **B,** If the mother is a carrier for the hemophilia gene and the father has a normal genotype, there is a 50% chance that any male offspring will have hemophilia. There is a 50% chance that any female offspring will be a carrier. **C,** If the mother has a normal genotype and the father has Huntington's disease, there is a 50% chance that offspring will have the disease.

discrimination? Genetic information should not be misused to label individuals or particular ethnic groups. Close attention must be paid to better understand the psychosocial needs of individuals and societal responses and health care policy related to genetic testing.

People may be reluctant to share or disclose information about family history or genetic test results. They fear they are vulnerable to discrimination based on their DNA. Inform your patients about the Genetic Information Nondiscrimination Act (GINA), which protects them from discrimination by employers and health care insurance companies (see Genetics in Clinical Practice Box on p. 184).

◆ Nursing Assessment: Family History

Family history is one of the strongest influences on a person's risk of developing genetic-related disorders such as heart disease, stroke, diabetes, or cancer. The family history is a free genetic test. Even though a person cannot change his or her genetic makeup, knowing the family history can help in the prevention or early diagnosis and treatment of a disorder. For example, it is important to monitor cholesterol levels in a person with a family history of familial hypercholesterolemia.

The key features of a family history that may increase a person's risk for genetic-related diseases are

- Disease in more than one close relative
- Disease that does not usually affect a certain gender (e.g., breast cancer in a male)
- Diseases that occur at an earlier age than expected (e.g., myocardial infarction before age 35)
- Certain combinations of diseases within a family (e.g., breast and ovarian cancer, heart disease and diabetes)

If a family has one or more of these features, the family history may hold important clues about a person's risk for a genetic disease. People with a family history of disease may have the most to gain from lifestyle changes and screening tests. People cannot change their genes, but they can change unhealthy behaviors (e.g., smoking, poor eating habits). They can also get screening tests to detect diseases and disease risk factors (e.g., elevated cholesterol, hypertension) that can be treated.

Genetic Risk Alert boxes in the assessment chapters in this book highlight a patient's risks related to genetic diseases and disorders. Use the information in these boxes when obtaining a nursing history.

Family health history is a written or graphic record of the diseases and health conditions present in one's family (see Chapter 3). A useful family health history shows three generations of a person's biologic relatives, the age of diagnosis of a disease, and the age and cause of death of deceased family members. A family health history is a useful tool for understanding health risks and preventing disease in individuals and their close relatives.

Talk with your own family members about your family's health history. Record this information and update it periodically so that you and your family members will have organized and accurate information ready to share with your HCP. Family health history information may help HCPs determine which tests and screenings are recommended to help you and your family know your health risk.

To help individuals collect and organize their family history information, the Centers for Disease Control and Prevention (CDC) has collaborated with the U.S. Surgeon General and other federal agencies to develop a Web-based tool called *My Family Health Portrait (https://familyhistory.hhs.gov/fhh-web/home.action)*.

BRIDGE TO NCLEX EXAMINATION

The number of the question corresponds to the same-numbered outcome at the beginning of the chapter.

1. If a person is heterozygous for a given gene, it means that the person
   a. is a carrier for a genetic disorder.
   b. is affected by the genetic disorder.
   c. has two identical alleles for the gene.
   d. has two different alleles for the gene.
2. Common causes of genetic mutations include *(select all that apply)*
   a. DNA damage from toxins.
   b. DNA damage from UV radiation.
   c. inheritance of altered genes from father.
   d. inheritance of altered genes from mother.
   e. inheritance of somatic mutations from either parent.
3. A father who has an X-linked recessive disorder and a wife with a normal genotype will
   a. pass the carrier state to his male children.
   b. pass the carrier state to all of his children.
   c. pass the carrier state to his female children.
   d. not pass on the genetic mutation to any of his children.
4. What characterizes multifactorial genetic disorders?
   a. Genetic testing available for most disorders
   b. Commonly caused by single gene alterations
   c. Many family members report having the disorder
   d. Caused by complex interactions of genetic and environmental factors
5. If a person tests positive for a genetic mutation, it means *(select all that apply)*
   a. that the laboratory found an alteration in a gene.
   b. that the person is predisposed to develop a genetic disease.
   c. that the person will develop the disease at some point in time.
   d. there is the possibility that other family members may also be at risk.
   e. that the person should not have any children or any additional children.
6. What role does pharmacogenomics have in health care?
   a. It can assess individual variability to many drugs.
   b. It can be used to determine the effectiveness of a drug.
   c. It provides important assessment data for gene therapy.
   d. It can assess the variability of drug responses due to single genes.
7. A couple who recently had a son with hemophilia A is consulting with a nurse. They want to know if their next child will have hemophilia A. The nurse can tell the parents that if their child is a
   a. boy, he will have hemophilia A.
   b. boy, he will be a carrier of hemophilia A.
   c. girl, she will be a carrier of hemophilia A.
   d. girl, there is a 50% chance she will be a carrier of hemophilia A.

1. d, 2. a, b, c, d, 3. c, 4. d, 5. a, d, 6. d, 7. d

For rationales to these answers and even more NCLEX review questions, visit *http://evolve.elsevier.com/Lewis/medsurg.*

EVOLVE WEBSITE

http://evolve.elsevier.com/Lewis/medsurg

Review Questions (Online Only)
Key Points
Answer Key for Questions
- Rationales for Bridge to NCLEX Examination Questions

Conceptual Care Map Creator
Audio Glossary
Content Updates

REFERENCES

1. US Department of Health and Human Services: Genomics. Retrieved from *www.healthypeople.gov.*
2. The New Genetics, National Institute of General Medical Sciences, National Institutes of Health, US Department of Health and Human Services. Retrieved from *http://publications.nigms.nih.gov/thenewgenetics.*
3. Nakano S, Tluczek A: Genomic breakthroughs in the diagnosis and treatment of cystic fibrosis, *AJN* 114:36, 2014.
4. US Department of Energy: Human Genome Project information. Retrieved from *www.ornl.gov.*
5. Genes and diseases. Retrieved from *www.ncbi.nlm.nih.gov/books/NBK22183.*
6. Bell JT, Spector TD: A twin approach to unraveling epigenetics, *Trends Genet* 27(3):116, 2011.
7. National Center for Biotechnology Information: GeneTests. Retrieved from *www.ncbi.nlm.nih.gov/sites/GeneTests.*
8. Filipski KK, Mechanic LE, Long R, et al: Pharmacogenomics in oncology care, *Front Genet* 5:73, 2014.

*9. Knisely MR, Carpenter JS, Von Ah D: Pharmacogenonics in the nursing literature: an integrative review, *Nursing Outlook* 62(4):285, 2014.

10. Cheek DJ: What you need to know about pharmacogenomics, *Nursing* 43:44, 2013.
11. Gene therapy. Retrieved from *http://ghr.nlm.nih.gov/handbook/therapy/genetherapy.*
12. National Institutes of Health: Stem cell basics. Retrieved from *stemcells.nih.gov.*
13. Genetic Science Learning Center, University of Utah: Learning genetics. Retrieved from *http://learn.genetics.utah.edu.*
14. *Journal of Nursing Scholarship* Genomics Webinar Series (2013). Retrieved from *www.genome.gov/27552312#al-2.*

*15. International Society of Nurses in Genetics: *Position statements: genetic counseling for vulnerable populations: the role of nursing.* Retrieved from *www.isong.org.*

*Evidence-based information for clinical practice.

13

Altered Immune Responses and Transplantation

Sharon L. Lewis

Happiness is not something readymade. It comes from your own actions.

Dalai Lama

http://evolve.elsevier.com/Lewis/medsurg/

LEARNING OUTCOMES

1. Describe the functions and components of the immune system.
2. Compare and contrast humoral and cell-mediated immunity, including lymphocytes involved, types of reactions, and effects on antigens.
3. Characterize the five types of immunoglobulins.
4. Differentiate among the four types of hypersensitivity reactions in terms of immunologic mechanisms and resulting alterations.
5. Identify the clinical manifestations and emergency management of a systemic anaphylactic reaction.
6. Describe the assessment and interprofessional care of a patient with chronic allergies.
7. Explain the relationship between the human leukocyte antigen system and certain diseases.
8. Describe the etiologic factors, clinical manifestations, and treatment modalities of autoimmune diseases.
9. Describe the etiologic factors and categories of immunodeficiency disorders.
10. Differentiate among the types of rejections following transplantation.
11. Identify the types and side effects of immunosuppressive therapy.

KEY TERMS

anergy, p. 196
antigen, p. 191
autoimmunity, p. 204
cell-mediated immunity, p. 196
cytokines, p. 194
human leukocyte antigen (HLA), p. 206
humoral immunity, p. 195
hypersensitivity reactions, p. 197
immunocompetence, p. 196
immunodeficiency, p. 205
immunosuppressive therapy, p. 209

This chapter discusses the normal immune response and the altered immune responses of hypersensitivity (including allergies), autoimmunity, and immunodeficiency. Histocompatibility, organ transplantation, and immunosuppressive therapy are also presented.

NORMAL IMMUNE RESPONSE

Immunity is the body's ability to resist disease. Immune responses serve the following three functions:

1. *Defense:* The body protects against invasions by microorganisms and prevents the development of infection by attacking foreign antigens and pathogens.
2. *Homeostasis:* Damaged cellular substances are digested and removed. Through this mechanism, the body's different cell types remain uniform and unchanged.
3. *Surveillance:* Mutations continually arise in the body but are normally recognized as foreign cells and destroyed.

Antigens

An **antigen** is a substance that elicits an immune response. Most antigens are composed of protein. However, other substances such as large polysaccharides, lipoproteins, and nucleic acids can act as antigens. All of the body's cells have antigens on their surface that are unique to that person and enable the body to recognize itself. The immune system normally becomes "tolerant" to the body's own molecules. Therefore it is nonresponsive to "self" antigens.

Types of Immunity

Immunity is classified as innate or acquired.

Innate Immunity. *Innate immunity* is present at birth, and its primary role is first-line defense against pathogens. This type of immunity involves a nonspecific response, and neutrophils and monocytes are the primary white blood cells (WBCs) involved. Innate immunity is not antigen specific, so it can respond within minutes to an invading microorganism without prior exposure to that organism.

Reviewed by Kelly S. Grimshaw, RN, MSN, APRN, CCRN, CCTN, Acute Care Nurse Practitioner, Transplant Department, Yale New Haven Hospital, New Haven, Connecticut; and Allison J. Terry, RN, PhD, Associate Professor of Nursing, Assistant Dean of Clinical Practice, School of Nursing, Auburn University Montgomery, Montgomery, Alabama.

TABLE 13-1 Types of Acquired Specific Immunity

Type	Natural	Artificial
Active	Natural contact with antigen through actual infection (e.g., chickenpox, measles, mumps)	Immunization with antigen (e.g., vaccines for chickenpox, measles, mumps)
Passive	Transplacental and colostrum transfer from mother to child (e.g., maternal immunoglobulins passed to baby)	Injection of serum with antibodies from one person (e.g., injection of hepatitis B immune globulin) to another person who does not have antibodies

Acquired Immunity. *Acquired immunity* is the development of immunity, either actively or passively (Table 13-1).

Active Acquired Immunity. *Active acquired immunity* results from the invasion of the body by foreign substances such as microorganisms and subsequent development of antibodies and sensitized lymphocytes. With each reinvasion of the microorganisms, the body responds more rapidly and vigorously to fight off the invader. Active acquired immunity may result naturally from a disease or artificially through immunization. Because antibodies are synthesized, immunity takes time to develop but is long lasting.

Passive Acquired Immunity. *Passive acquired immunity* implies that the host receives antibodies to an antigen rather than synthesizing them. This may take place naturally through the transfer of immunoglobulins across the placental membrane from mother to fetus. Artificial passive acquired immunity occurs through injection with gamma globulin (serum antibodies). The benefit of this immunity is its immediate effect. Unfortunately, passive immunity is short lived because the person does not synthesize the antibodies and consequently does not retain memory cells for the antigen.

Lymphoid Organs

The lymphoid system is composed of central (or primary) and peripheral lymphoid organs. The *central lymphoid organs* are the thymus gland and bone marrow. The *peripheral lymphoid organs* are the lymph nodes; tonsils; spleen; and gut-, genital-, bronchial-, and skin-associated lymphoid tissues (Fig. 13-1).

Lymphocytes are produced in the bone marrow and eventually migrate to the peripheral organs. The thymus is involved in the differentiation and maturation of T lymphocytes and is therefore essential for a cell-mediated immune response. During childhood the thymus is large. It shrinks with age, and in the older person the thymus is a collection of lymphocytes and connective tissue.

When antigens are introduced into the body, they may be carried by the bloodstream or lymph channels to regional lymph nodes. The antigens interact with B and T lymphocytes and macrophages in the lymph nodes. The two important functions of lymph nodes are (1) filtration of foreign material brought to the site and (2) circulation of lymphocytes.

The tonsils are an example of lymphoid tissue. The spleen, a peripheral lymph organ, is important as the primary site for filtering foreign antigens from the blood. Lymphoid tissue is found in the submucosa of the gastrointestinal (GI) (gut-associated), genitourinary (genital-associated), and respiratory (bronchial-associated) tracts. This tissue protects the body from external microorganisms.

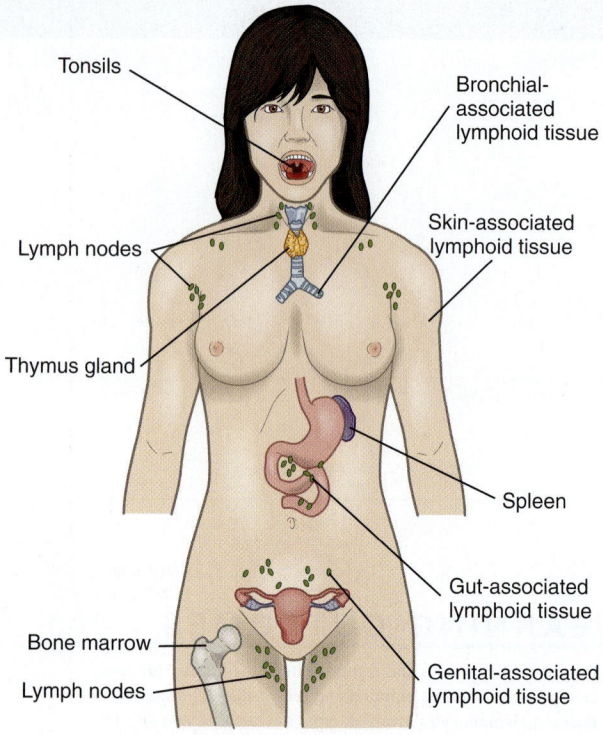

FIG. 13-1 Organs of the immune system.

The skin-associated lymph tissue consists primarily of lymphocytes and Langerhans' cells (type of dendritic cell) found in the epidermis of skin. When Langerhans' cells are depleted, the skin cannot initiate an immune response. Therefore a delayed hypersensitivity reaction (as determined by skin testing with injected antigens) does not occur.

Cells Involved in Immune Response

Mononuclear Phagocytes. The *mononuclear phagocyte system* includes monocytes in the blood and macrophages found throughout the body. Mononuclear phagocytes have a critical role in the immune system. They are responsible for capturing, processing, and presenting the antigen to the lymphocytes. This stimulates a humoral or cell-mediated immune response. Capturing is accomplished through phagocytosis. The macrophage-bound antigen, which is highly immunogenic, is presented to circulating T or B lymphocytes and thus triggers an immune response (Fig. 13-2).

Lymphocytes. Lymphocytes are produced in the bone marrow (Fig. 13-3). They then differentiate into B and T lymphocytes.

B Lymphocytes. In the early research on *B lymphocytes* (bursa-equivalent lymphocytes) in birds, it was discovered that they mature under the influence of the bursa of Fabricius, hence the name *B cells.* However, this lymphoid organ does not exist in humans. The bursa-equivalent tissue in humans is the bone marrow. B cells differentiate into *plasma cells* when activated. Plasma cells produce antibodies (immunoglobulins) (Table 13-2).

T Lymphocytes. Cells that migrate from the bone marrow to the thymus differentiate into *T lymphocytes* (thymus-dependent cells). The thymus secretes hormones, including thymosin, that stimulate the maturation and differentiation of T lymphocytes.

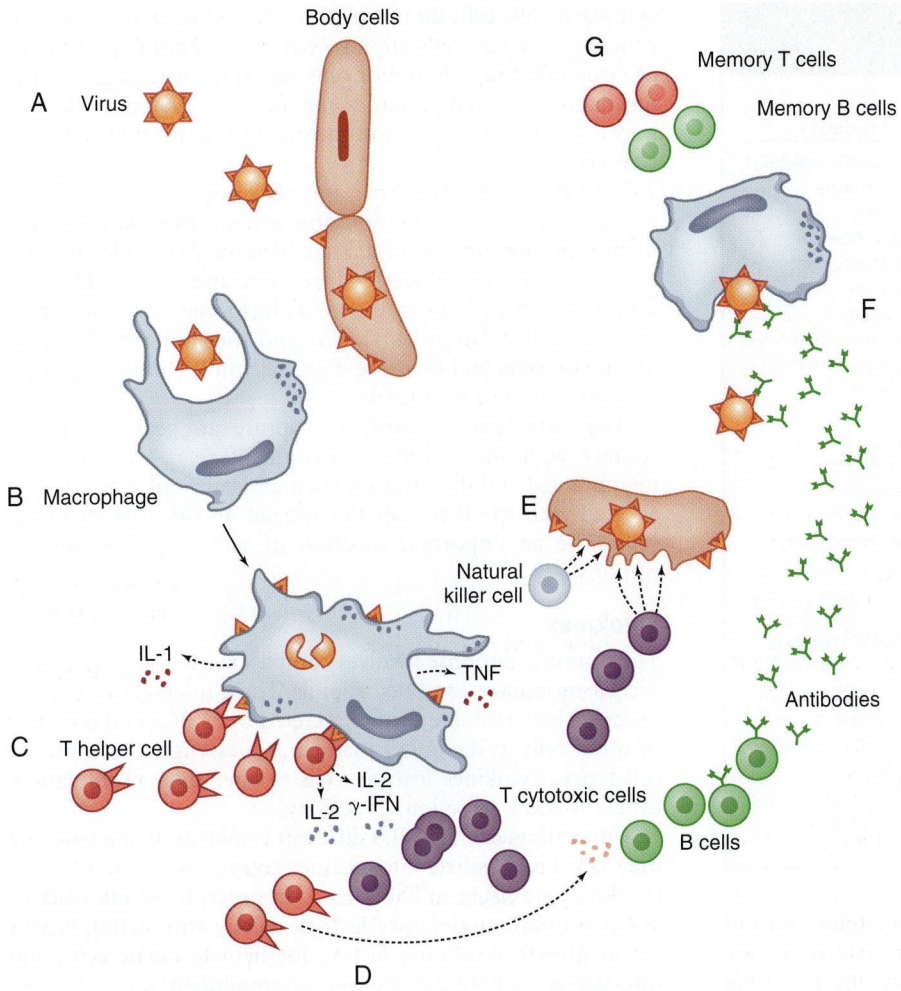

FIG. 13-2 The immune response to a virus. **A,** A virus invades the body through a break in the skin or another portal of entry. The virus must make its way inside a cell to replicate itself. **B,** A macrophage recognizes the antigens on the surface of the virus. The macrophage digests the virus and displays pieces of the virus (antigens) on its surface. **C,** T helper cell recognizes the antigen displayed and binds to the macrophage. This binding stimulates the production of cytokines (interleukin-1 *[IL-1]* and tumor necrosis factor *[TNF]*) by the macrophage and interleukin-2 *(IL-2)* and γ-interferon *(γ-IFN)* by the T cell. These cytokines are intracellular messengers that provide communication among the cells. **D,** IL-2 instructs other T helper cells and T cytotoxic cells to proliferate (multiply). T helper cells release cytokines, causing B cells to multiply and produce antibodies. **E,** T cytotoxic cells and natural killer cells destroy infected body cells. **F,** The antibodies bind to the virus and mark it for macrophage destruction. **G,** Memory B and T cells remain behind to respond quickly if the same virus attacks again.

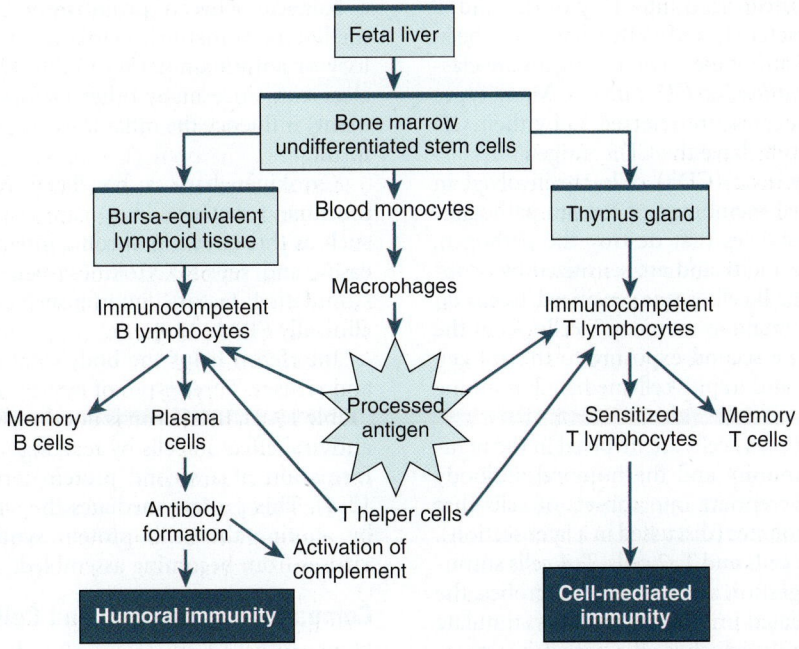

FIG. 13-3 Relationships and functions of macrophages, B lymphocytes, and T lymphocytes in an immune response.

TABLE 13-2 Characteristics of Immunoglobulins

Class	Serum Concentration	Location	Characteristics
IgG	76%	Plasma, interstitial fluid	Is only immunoglobulin that crosses placenta Is responsible for secondary immune response
IgA	15%	Body secretions, including tears, saliva, breast milk, colostrum	Lines mucous membranes and protects body surfaces
IgM	8%	Plasma	Is responsible for primary immune response Forms antibodies to ABO blood antigens
IgD	1%	Plasma	Is present on lymphocyte surface Assists in the differentiation of B lymphocytes
IgE	0.002%	Plasma, interstitial fluids	Causes symptoms of allergic reactions Fixes to mast cells and basophils Assists in defense against parasitic infections

T cells make up 70% to 80% of the circulating lymphocytes and are primarily responsible for immunity to intracellular viruses, tumor cells, and fungi. T cells live from a few months to the life span of an individual and account for long-term immunity.

T lymphocytes can be categorized into T cytotoxic and T helper cells. Antigenic characteristics of WBCs have now been classified using monoclonal antibodies. These antigens are classified as *clusters of differentiation,* or *CD antigens.* Many types of WBCs, especially lymphocytes, are referred to by their CD designations. All mature T cells have the CD3 antigen.

T cytotoxic cells. T cytotoxic (CD8) cells are involved in attacking antigens on the cell membrane of foreign pathogens and releasing cytolytic substances that destroy the pathogen. These cells have antigen specificity and are sensitized by exposure to the antigen. Much like B cells, some sensitized T cells do not attack the antigen but remain as memory T cells. As in the humoral immune response, a second exposure to the antigen results in a more intense and rapid cell-mediated immune response.

T helper cells. T helper (CD4) cells are involved in the regulation of cell-mediated immunity and the humoral antibody response. T helper cells differentiate into subsets of cells that produce distinct types of cytokines (discussed in a later section). These subsets are called T_H1 cells and T_H2 cells. T_H1 cells stimulate phagocyte-mediated ingestion and killing of microbes, the key component of cell-mediated immunity. T_H2 cells stimulate eosinophil-mediated immunity, which is effective against parasites and is involved in allergic responses.

Natural Killer Cells. Natural killer (NK) cells are also involved in cell-mediated immunity. These cells are not T or B cells but are large lymphocytes with numerous granules in the cytoplasm. NK cells do not require prior sensitization for their generation. These cells are involved in recognition and killing of virus-infected cells, tumor cells, and transplanted grafts. The mechanism of recognition is not fully understood. NK cells have a significant role in immune surveillance for malignant cell changes.

T Dendritic Cells. *Dendritic cells* make up a system of cells that are important to the immune system, especially the cell-mediated immune response. They have an atypical shape with extensive dendritic processes that form and retract. They are found in many places in the body, including the skin (where they are called *Langerhans' cells*) and the lining of the nose, lungs, stomach, and intestine. Especially in the immature state, they are found in the blood.[1]

They function primarily to capture antigens at sites of contact with the external environment (e.g., skin, mucous membranes) and then transport an antigen until it encounters a T cell with specificity for the antigen. In this role, dendritic cells have an important function in activating the immune response.

Cytokines

The immune response involves complex interactions of T cells, B cells, monocytes, and neutrophils. These interactions depend on **cytokines** (soluble factors secreted by WBCs and a variety of other cells in the body) that act as messengers between the cell types. Cytokines instruct cells to alter their proliferation, differentiation, secretion, or activity.

Currently more than 100 different cytokines are known, and they can be classified into distinct categories. Some of these cytokines are listed in Table 13-3. In general, the interleukins act as immunomodulatory factors, colony-stimulating factors act as growth-regulating factors for hematopoietic cells, and interferons are antiviral and immunomodulatory.

The net effect of an inflammatory response is determined by a balance between proinflammatory and antiinflammatory mediators. Sometimes cytokines are classified as proinflammatory or antiinflammatory (Table 13-3). However, it is not that clear-cut, since many other factors (e.g., target cells, environment) influence the inflammatory response to a given injury or insult.

Cytokines have a beneficial role in hematopoiesis and immune function. They can also have detrimental effects such as those seen in chronic inflammation, autoimmune diseases, and sepsis. Cytokines such as erythropoietin, colony-stimulating factors, interferons, and interleukin-2 are used clinically (Table 13-4).

Interferon helps the body's natural defenses attack tumors and viruses. Three types of interferon have now been identified (Table 13-3). Interferon is not directly antiviral but produces an antiviral effect in cells by reacting with them and inducing the formation of a second protein termed *antiviral protein* (Fig. 13-4). This protein mediates the antiviral action of interferon by altering the cell's protein synthesis and preventing new viruses from becoming assembled.

Comparison of Humoral and Cell-Mediated Immunity

Humans need both humoral and cell-mediated immunity to remain healthy. Each type of immunity has unique properties, different methods of action, and reactions against particular antigens. Table 13-5 compares humoral and cell-mediated immunity.

TABLE 13-3 Types and Functions of Cytokines

Type	Primary Functions
Interleukins (ILs)	
IL-1	Proinflammatory mediator. Promotes proliferation of B cells. Activates T cells, NK cells, and macrophages
IL-2	Activates T cells, NK cells, and macrophages. Stimulates release of other cytokines (α-IFN, TNF, IL-1, IL-6)
IL-3	Hematopoietic growth factor for hematopoietic precursor cells
IL-4	Antiinflammatory mediator. B cell growth and differentiation. Induces differentiation into T_H2 cells. Stimulates growth of mast cells
IL-5	B cell growth and differentiation. Promotes growth and differentiation of eosinophils
IL-6	Proinflammatory mediator. T- and B-cell growth factor, promotes differentiation of B cells into plasma cells and stimulates antibody secretion. Induces fever. Synergistic effects with IL-1 and TNF
Interferons (IFNs)	
α-IFN β-IFN	Inhibit viral replication, activate NK cells and macrophages, antiproliferative effects on tumor cells
γ-IFN	Proinflammatory mediator. Activates macrophages, neutrophils, and NK cells. Promotes B cell differentiation. Inhibits viral replication
Tumor Necrosis Factor (TNF)	Proinflammatory mediator. Activates macrophages and granulocytes. Promotes immune and inflammatory responses. Kills tumor cells. Responsible for weight loss associated with chronic inflammation and cancer
Colony-Stimulating Factors (CSFs)	
Granulocyte colony-stimulating factor (G-CSF)	Stimulates proliferation and differentiation of neutrophils, enhances functional activity of mature PMNs
Granulocyte-macrophage colony-stimulating factor (GM-CSF)	Stimulates proliferation and differentiation of PMNs and monocytes
Macrophage colony-stimulating factor (M-CSF)	Promotes proliferation, differentiation, and activation of monocytes and macrophages
Erythropoietin	Stimulates erythroid progenitor cells in bone marrow to produce red blood cells

NK, Natural killer; *PMNs,* polymorphonuclear neutrophils.

TABLE 13-4 Clinical Uses of Cytokines

Cytokine	Clinical Uses
α-Interferon (Roferon-A, Intron A)	Hairy cell leukemia, chronic myelogenous leukemia, malignant melanoma, renal cell carcinoma, ovarian cancer, multiple myeloma, Kaposi sarcoma, hepatitis B and C
β-Interferon (Betaseron, Avonex, Rebif)	Multiple sclerosis
Colony-Stimulating Factors	
G-CSF	
• filgrastim (Neupogen) • pegfilgrastim (Neulasta)	Chemotherapy-induced neutropenia
GM-CSF	
• sargramostim (Leukine)	Neutropenia, myeloid recovery after bone marrow transplantation
Soluble TNF Receptor	
etanercept (Enbrel)	Rheumatoid arthritis
Interleukin-2	
aldesleukin (Proleukin)	Metastatic renal cell carcinoma, metastatic melanoma
Interleukin 11 (platelet growth factor)	
oprelvekin (Neumega)	Thrombocytopenia related to chemotherapy
Erythropoietin	
epoetin alfa (Epogen, Procrit) darbepoetin alfa (Aranesp)	Anemia related to chronic kidney disease, cancer, and chemotherapy
IL-1 Receptor Antagonist	
anakinra (Kineret)	Rheumatoid arthritis

G-CSF, Granulocyte colony-stimulating factor; *GM-CSF,* granulocyte-macrophage colony-stimulating factor; *IL,* interleukin; *TNF,* tumor necrosis factor.

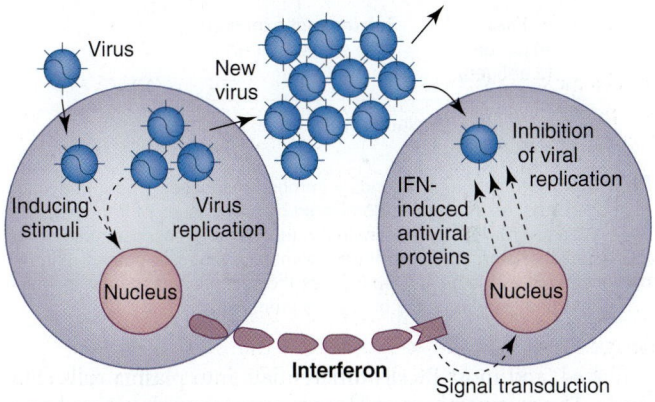

FIG. 13-4 Mechanism of action of interferon (IFN). When a virus attacks a cell, the cell begins to synthesize viral DNA and interferon. Interferon serves as an intercellular messenger and induces the production of antiviral proteins. Then the virus is not able to replicate in the cell.

Humoral Immunity. **Humoral immunity** consists of antibody-mediated immunity. The term *humoral* comes from the Greek word *humor,* which means body fluid. Since antibodies are produced by plasma cells (differentiated B cells) and found in plasma, the term *humoral immunity* is used. Production of antibodies is an essential component in a humoral immune response. Each of the five classes of immunoglobulins (Igs) (IgG, IgA, IgM, IgG, IgE) has specific characteristics (Table 13-2).

When a pathogen (especially bacteria) enters the body, it may encounter a B cell that is specific for antigens located on that bacterial cell wall. In addition, a monocyte or macrophage may phagocytize the bacteria and present its antigens to a B cell. The B cell recognizes the antigen because it has receptors on its cell surface specific for that antigen. When the antigen comes in contact with the cell surface receptor, the B cell becomes

TABLE 13-5 Comparison of Humoral and Cell-Mediated Immunity

Characteristics	Humoral Immunity	Cell-Mediated Immunity
Cells involved	B lymphocytes	T lymphocytes, macrophages
Products	Antibodies	Sensitized T cells, cytokines
Memory cells	Present	Present
Protection	Bacteria Viruses (extracellular) Respiratory and GI pathogens	Fungus Viruses (intracellular) Chronic infectious agents Tumor cells
Examples	Anaphylactic shock Atopic diseases Transfusion reaction Bacterial infections	Tuberculosis Fungal infections Contact dermatitis Graft rejection Destruction of cancer cells

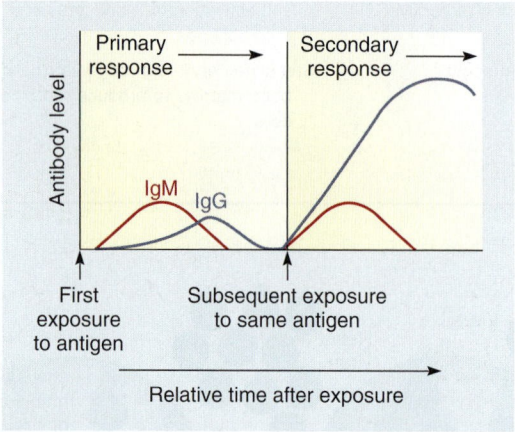

FIG. 13-5 Primary and secondary immune responses. The introduction of antigen induces a response dominated by two classes of immunoglobulins, IgM and IgG. IgM predominates in the primary response, with some IgG appearing later. After the host's immune system is primed, another challenge with the same antigen induces the secondary response, in which some IgM and large amounts of IgG are produced.

activated, and most B cells differentiate into plasma cells (Fig. 13-3). The mature plasma cell secretes immunoglobulins. Some stimulated B cells remain as memory cells.

The primary immune response becomes evident 4 to 8 days after the initial exposure to the antigen (Fig. 13-5). IgM is the first type of antibody formed. Because of the large size of the IgM molecule, this immunoglobulin is confined to the intravascular space. As the immune response progresses, IgG is produced, and it can move from intravascular to extravascular spaces.

When the individual is exposed to the antigen the second time, a secondary antibody response occurs. This response occurs faster (1 to 3 days), is stronger, and lasts for a longer time than a primary response. Memory cells account for the memory of the first exposure to the antigen and the more rapid production of antibodies. IgG is the primary antibody found in a secondary immune response.

IgG crosses the placental membrane and provides the newborn with passive acquired immunity for at least 3 months. Infants may also get some passive immunity from IgA in breast milk and colostrum.

TABLE 13-6 Gerontologic Assessment Differences

Effects of Aging on the Immune System

- Thymic involution
- ↓ Cell-mediated immunity
- ↓ Delayed hypersensitivity reaction
- ↓ IL-1 and IL-2 synthesis
- ↓ Expression of IL-2 receptors
- ↓ Proliferative response of T and B cells
- ↓ Primary and secondary antibody responses
- ↑ Autoantibodies

IL, Interleukin.

Cell-Mediated Immunity. Immune responses that are initiated through specific antigen recognition by T cells are termed **cell-mediated immunity**. Several cell types and factors are involved in cell-mediated immunity. The cell types involved include T cells, macrophages, and NK cells. Cell-mediated immunity is of primary importance in (1) immunity against pathogens that survive inside of cells, including viruses and some bacteria (e.g., mycobacteria); (2) fungal infections; (3) rejection of transplanted tissues; (4) contact hypersensitivity reactions; and (5) tumor immunity.

Gerontologic Considerations: Effects of Aging on the Immune System

With advancing age, there is a decline in the function of the immune response (Table 13-6). The primary clinical evidence of *immunosenescence* is the high incidence of malignancies in older adults. Older people are also more susceptible to infections (e.g., influenza, pneumonia) from pathogens that they were relatively immunocompetent against earlier in life. Bacterial pneumonia is the leading cause of death from infections in older adults. The antibody response to immunizations (e.g., flu vaccine) in older adults is considerably lower than in younger adults.[2]

The bone marrow remains relatively unaffected by increasing age. Immunoglobulin levels decrease with age and therefore lead to a suppressed humoral immune response in older adults. *Thymic involution* (shrinking) occurs with aging, along with decreased numbers of T cells. These changes in the thymus gland are a primary cause of immunosenescence. Both T and B cells show deficiencies in activation, transit time through the cell cycle, and subsequent differentiation. However, the most significant alterations involve T cells. As thymic output of T cells diminishes, the differentiation of T cells increases. Consequently, there is an accumulation of memory cells rather than new precursor cells responsive to previously unencountered antigens.

The delayed hypersensitivity reaction, as determined by skin testing with injected antigens, is frequently decreased or absent in older adults. This altered response reflects **anergy** (an immunodeficient condition characterized by lack of or diminished reaction to an antigen or a group of antigens).

ALTERED IMMUNE RESPONSE

Immunocompetence exists when the body's immune system can identify and inactivate or destroy foreign substances. When the immune system is incompetent or underresponsive, severe infections, immunodeficiency diseases, and malignancies may occur.

TABLE 13-7 Types of Hypersensitivity Reactions

Type I: IgE-Mediated	Type II: Cytotoxic	Type III: Immune-Complex	Type IV: Delayed Hypersensitivity
Antigen			
Pollen, food, drugs, dust	Cell surface of RBCs Cell basement membrane	Extracellular fungal, viral, bacterial	Intracellular or extracellular
Antibody Involved			
IgE	IgG, IgM	IgG, IgM	None
Complement Involved			
No	Yes	Yes	No
Mediators of Injury			
Histamine Mast cells Leukotrienes Prostaglandins	Complement lysis Macrophages in tissues	Neutrophils Complement lysis Monocytes, macrophages Lysosomal enzymes	Cytokines T cytotoxic cells
Examples			
Allergic rhinitis Asthma Atopic dermatitis Urticaria Angioedema	Transfusion reaction Goodpasture syndrome Immune thrombocytopenic purpura Graves' disease	Systemic lupus erythematosus Rheumatoid arthritis Acute glomerulonephritis	Contact dermatitis (e.g., to poison ivy)
Skin Test			
Wheal and flare	None	Erythema and edema in 3-8 hr	Erythema and edema in 24-48 hr (e.g., TB test)

When the immune system overreacts, hypersensitivity disorders such as allergies and autoimmune diseases may develop.

Hypersensitivity Reactions

Sometimes the immune response is overreactive against foreign antigens or reacts against its own tissue, resulting in tissue damage. These responses are termed **hypersensitivity reactions**. *Autoimmune diseases,* a type of hypersensitivity response, occur when the body fails to recognize self-proteins and reacts against self-antigens.

Hypersensitivity reactions can be classified according to the source of the antigen, time sequence (immediate or delayed), or immunologic mechanisms causing the injury. Four types of hypersensitivity reactions exist (Table 13-7). Types I, II, and III are immediate and are examples of humoral immunity. Type IV is a delayed hypersensitivity reaction and is related to cell-mediated immunity.

Type I: IgE-Mediated Reactions. *Anaphylactic reactions* are type I reactions that occur only in susceptible people who are highly sensitized to specific allergens. IgE antibodies, produced in response to the allergen, have a characteristic property of attaching to mast cells and basophils (Fig. 13-6; see Fig. 28-2). Within these cells are granules containing potent chemical mediators (histamine, serotonin, leukotrienes, eosinophil chemotactic factor of anaphylaxis [ECF-A], kinins, and bradykinin). (Chemical mediators of inflammation are discussed in Chapter 11 and Table 11-1.)

On the first exposure to the allergen, IgE antibodies are produced and bind to mast cells and basophils. On any subsequent exposures, the allergen links with the IgE bound to mast cells or basophils and triggers degranulation of the cells and the release of chemical mediators from the granules. In this process, the mediators that are released attack target tissues, causing clinical symptoms of an allergic response. These effects include smooth muscle contraction, increased vascular permeability, vasodilation, hypotension, increased secretion of mucus, and itching. Fortunately, the mediators are short acting and their effects are reversible. (The mediators are listed in Table 13-8.)

TABLE 13-8 Mediators of Allergic Response*

- Anaphylatoxins (C3a, C4a, C5a from complement activation)
- Histamine
- Kinins
- Leukotrienes†
- Platelet-activating factor
- Prostaglandins
- Serotonin

*Mediators of inflammation and their mechanism of action are presented in Table 11-1.
†See Chapter 11, Fig. 11-2.

A genetic predisposition to the development of allergic diseases exists. The capacity to become sensitized to an allergen, rather than the specific allergic disorder, appears to be the inherited trait. For example, a father with asthma may have a son who has allergic rhinitis.

The clinical manifestations of an anaphylactic reaction depend on whether the mediators remain local or become systemic, or whether they affect particular organs. When the mediators remain localized, a cutaneous response termed the *wheal-and-flare reaction* occurs. This reaction is characterized by a pale wheal containing edematous fluid surrounded by a red flare from the hyperemia. The reaction occurs in minutes or hours and is usually not dangerous. A classic example of a wheal-and-flare reaction is the mosquito bite. The wheal-and-flare reaction serves a diagnostic purpose as a means of demonstrating allergic reactions to specific allergens during skin tests.

Common allergic reactions include anaphylaxis and atopic reactions.

Anaphylaxis. *Anaphylaxis* can occur when mediators are released systemically (e.g., after injection of a drug, after an insect sting). The reaction occurs within minutes and can be life threatening because of bronchial constriction and subsequent airway obstruction and vascular collapse. The target organs affected are seen in Fig. 13-7. Initial symptoms include

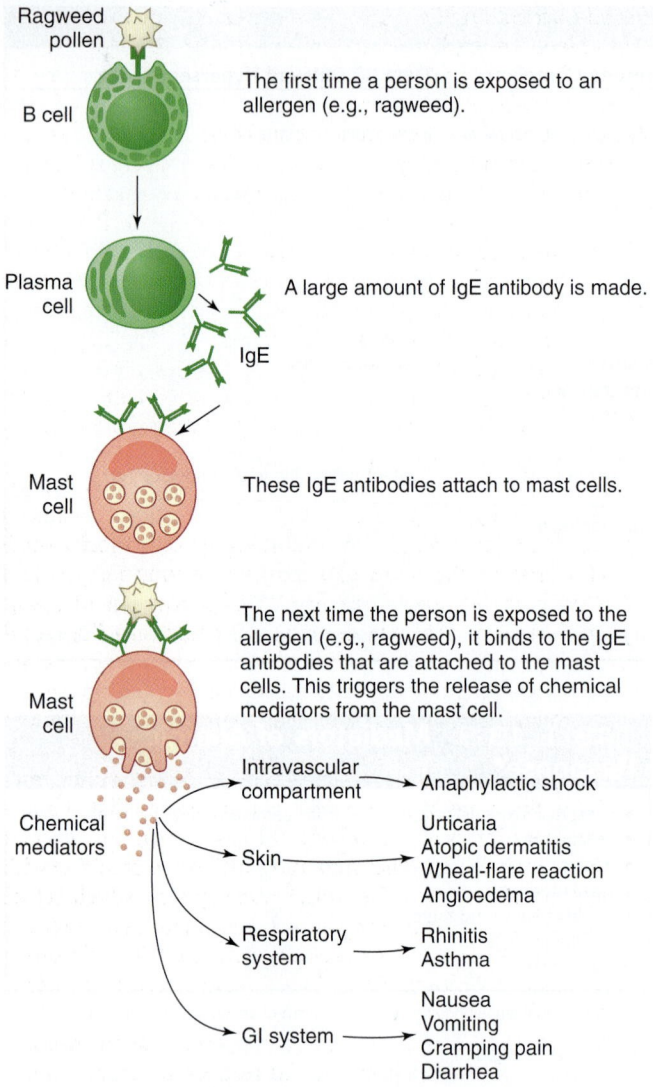

FIG. 13-6 Steps in a type I allergic reaction.

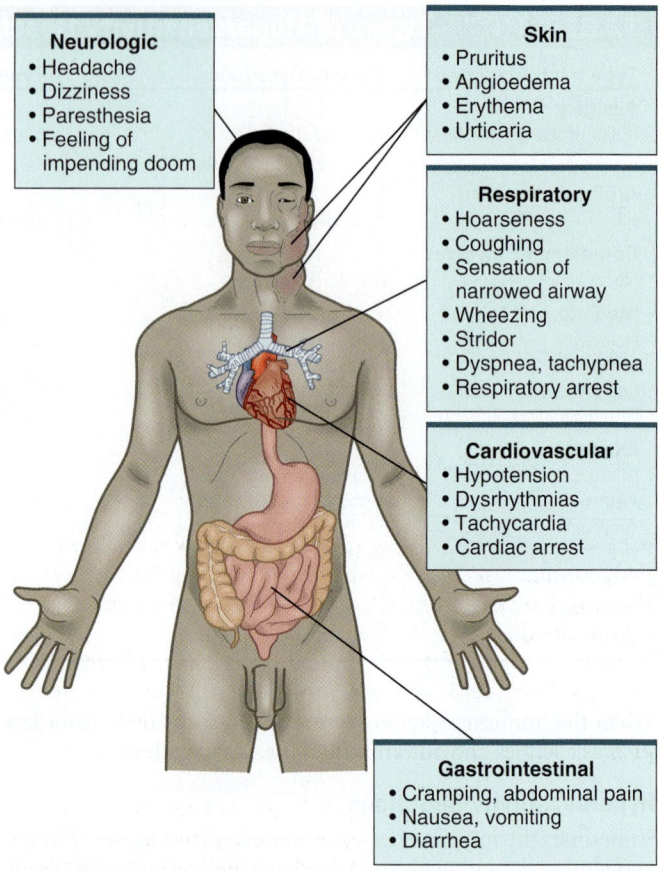

FIG. 13-7 Clinical manifestations of a systemic anaphylactic reaction.

TABLE 13-9 Allergens Causing Anaphylactic Shock

Drugs	Treatment Measures
• Aspirin • Cephalosporins • Chemotherapy drugs • Insulins • Local anesthetics • Nonsteroidal antiinflammatory drugs • Penicillins • Sulfonamides • Tetracycline	• Allergenic extracts used in immunotherapy • Blood products (whole blood and components) • Iodine-contrast media for CT scan or other radiologic procedures
Foods	**Insect Venoms**
• Eggs, milk, nuts, peanuts, shellfish, fish, chocolate, strawberries	• Wasps, hornets, yellow jackets, bumblebees, ants
	Animal Sera
	• Diphtheria antitoxin • Rabies antitoxin • Snake venom antitoxin • Tetanus antitoxin

edema and itching at the site of exposure to the allergen. Shock can occur rapidly and is manifested by rapid, weak pulse; hypotension; dilated pupils; dyspnea; and possibly cyanosis. This is compounded by bronchial edema and angioedema. Death will occur if emergency treatment is not initiated. Some of the important allergens that can cause anaphylactic shock in hypersensitive people are listed in Table 13-9. Drugs are the leading cause of anaphylaxis-related deaths.[3]

Atopic Reactions. An estimated 20% of the population is *atopic,* having an inherited tendency to become sensitive to environmental allergens. The atopic diseases that can result are allergic rhinitis, asthma, atopic dermatitis, urticaria, and angioedema.

Allergic rhinitis, or hay fever, is the most common type I hypersensitivity reaction. It may occur year-round (perennial allergic rhinitis), or it may be seasonal (seasonal allergic rhinitis). Airborne substances such as pollens, dust, and molds are the primary causes of allergic rhinitis. Perennial allergic rhinitis may be caused by dust, molds, and animal dander. Seasonal allergic rhinitis is commonly caused by pollens from trees, weeds, or grasses. The target areas affected are the conjunctiva of the eyes and the mucosa of the upper respiratory tract. Symptoms include nasal discharge; sneezing; lacrimation; mucosal swelling with airway obstruction; and pruritus around the eyes, nose, throat, and mouth. (Treatment of allergic rhinitis is discussed in Chapter 26 on p. 478.)

Many patients with *asthma* have an allergic component to their disease. These patients frequently have a history of atopic disorders (e.g., infantile eczema, allergic rhinitis, food intolerances). Inflammatory mediators produce bronchial smooth muscle constriction, excessive secretion of viscoid mucus, edema of the mucous membranes of the bronchi, and decreased

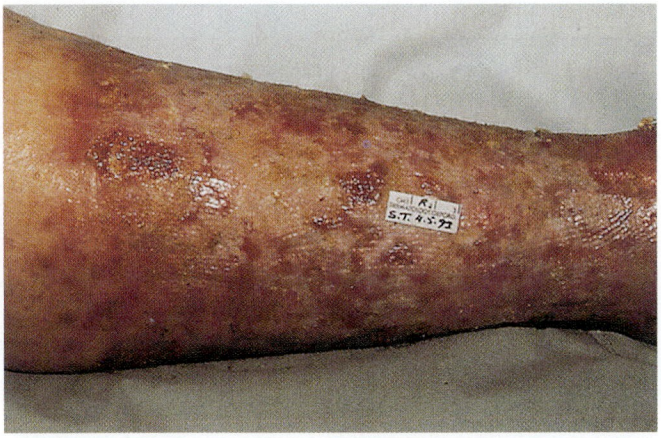

FIG. 13-8 Atopic dermatitis of the lower leg. (From Morison MJ: *Nursing management of chronic wounds,* Edinburgh, 2001, Mosby.)

lung compliance. Because of these physiologic alterations, patients manifest dyspnea, wheezing, coughing, tightness in the chest, and thick sputum. (Pathophysiology and management of asthma are discussed in Chapter 28.)

Atopic dermatitis is a chronic, inherited skin disorder characterized by exacerbations and remissions. It is caused by several environmental allergens that are difficult to identify. Although patients with atopic dermatitis have elevated IgE levels and positive skin tests, the histopathologic features do not represent the typical, localized wheal-and-flare type I reactions. The skin lesions are more generalized and involve vasodilation of blood vessels, resulting in interstitial edema with vesicle formation (Fig. 13-8). (Dermatitis is discussed in Chapter 23.)

Urticaria (hives) is a cutaneous reaction against systemic allergens occurring in atopic people. It is characterized by transient wheals (pink, raised, edematous, pruritic areas) that vary in size and shape and may occur all over the body. Urticaria develops rapidly after exposure to an allergen and may last minutes or hours. Histamine causes localized vasodilation (erythema), transudation of fluid (wheal), and flaring. Flaring is due to dilated blood vessels on the edge of the wheal. Histamine is responsible for the pruritus associated with the lesions. (Urticaria is discussed in Chapter 23.)

Angioedema is a localized cutaneous lesion similar to urticaria but involving deeper layers of the skin and submucosa. The principal areas of involvement include the eyelids, lips, tongue, larynx, hands, feet, GI tract, and genitalia. Swelling usually begins in the face and then progresses to the airways and other parts of the body. Dilation and engorgement of the capillaries secondary to the release of histamine cause the diffuse swelling. Welts are not apparent as in urticaria. The outer skin appears normal or has a reddish hue. The lesions may burn, sting, or itch and can cause acute abdominal pain if in the GI tract. The swelling may occur suddenly or over several hours and usually lasts for 24 hours.

Type II: Cytotoxic and Cytolytic Reactions. Cytotoxic and cytolytic reactions are type II hypersensitivity reactions involving the direct binding of IgG or IgM antibodies to an antigen on the cell surface. Antigen-antibody complexes activate the complement system, which mediates the reaction. Cellular tissue is destroyed in one of two ways: (1) activation of the complement system resulting in cytolysis or (2) enhanced phagocytosis.

Target cells frequently destroyed in type II reactions are erythrocytes, platelets, and leukocytes. The tissue damage usually occurs rapidly. Some of the antigens involved are the ABO blood group, Rh factor, and drugs. Pathophysiologic disorders characteristic of type II reactions include ABO incompatibility transfusion reaction, Rh incompatibility transfusion reaction, autoimmune and drug-related hemolytic anemias, leukopenias, thrombocytopenias, erythroblastosis fetalis (hemolytic disease of the newborn), and Goodpasture syndrome.

Hemolytic Transfusion Reactions. A classic type II reaction occurs when a recipient receives ABO-incompatible blood from a donor. Naturally acquired antibodies to antigens of the ABO blood group are in the recipient's serum but are not present on the erythrocyte membranes (see Table 29-8). For example, a person with type A blood has anti-B antibodies, a person with type B blood has anti-A antibodies, a person with type AB blood has no antibodies, and a person with type O blood has anti-A and anti-B antibodies.

If the recipient is transfused with incompatible blood, antibodies immediately coat the foreign erythrocytes, causing *agglutination* (clumping). The clumping of cells blocks small blood vessels in the body, uses existing clotting factors, and depletes them, leading to bleeding. Within hours, neutrophils and macrophages phagocytize the agglutinated cells. The complement system is activated and cell lysis occurs, which causes the release of hemoglobin into the urine and plasma. Acute kidney injury can result from the hemoglobinuria. (Blood transfusions are discussed in Chapter 30.)

Goodpasture Syndrome. *Goodpasture syndrome* is a disorder involving the lungs and kidneys. An antibody-mediated autoimmune reaction occurs involving the glomerular and alveolar basement membranes. The circulating antibodies combine with tissue antigen to activate the complement system, which causes deposits of IgG to form along the cell basement membranes of the lungs or kidneys. This reaction may result in pulmonary hemorrhage and glomerulonephritis. (Goodpasture syndrome is discussed in Chapter 45.)

Type III: Immune-Complex Reactions. Tissue damage in immune-complex reactions, which are type III reactions, occurs secondary to antigen-antibody complexes. Soluble antigens combine with immunoglobulins of the IgG and IgM classes to form complexes that are too small to be effectively removed by the mononuclear phagocyte system. Therefore the complexes deposit in tissue or small blood vessels. They cause activation of the complement system and release of chemotactic factors that lead to inflammation and destruction of the involved tissue.

Type III reactions may be local or systemic and immediate or delayed. The clinical manifestations depend on the number of complexes and the location in the body. Common sites for deposit are the kidneys, skin, joints, blood vessels, and lungs. Severe type III reactions are associated with autoimmune disorders such as systemic lupus erythematosus, acute glomerulonephritis, and rheumatoid arthritis. (Systemic lupus erythematosus and rheumatoid arthritis are discussed in Chapter 64, and acute glomerulonephritis is discussed in Chapter 45.)

Type IV: Delayed Hypersensitivity Reactions. A *delayed hypersensitivity reaction*—a type IV reaction—is a *cell-mediated immune response.* Although cell-mediated responses are usually protective mechanisms, tissue damage occurs in delayed hypersensitivity reactions.

The tissue damage in a type IV reaction does not occur in the presence of antibodies or complement. Rather, sensitized T cells attack antigens or release cytokines. Some of these cytokines attract macrophages into the area. The macrophages and

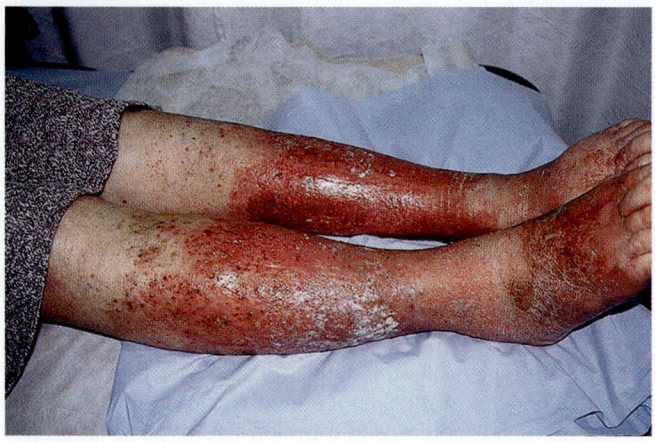

FIG. 13-9 Contact dermatitis to rubber. (From Morison MJ: *Nursing management of chronic wounds,* Edinburgh, 2001, Mosby.)

enzymes released by them are responsible for most of the tissue destruction. In the delayed hypersensitivity reaction, it takes 24 to 48 hours for a response to occur.

Clinical examples of a delayed hypersensitivity reaction include contact dermatitis (Fig. 13-9); hypersensitivity reactions to bacterial, fungal, and viral infections; and transplant rejections. Some drug sensitivity reactions also fit this category.

Contact Dermatitis. *Allergic contact dermatitis* is an example of a delayed hypersensitivity reaction involving the skin. The reaction occurs when the skin is exposed to substances that easily penetrate the skin to combine with epidermal proteins. The substance then becomes antigenic. Over a period of 7 to 14 days, memory cells form to the antigen. On subsequent exposure to the substance, a sensitized person develops eczematous skin lesions within 48 hours. The most common potentially antigenic substances are metal compounds (e.g., those containing nickel or mercury); rubber compounds; poison ivy, poison oak, and poison sumac; cosmetics; and some dyes.

In acute contact dermatitis, the skin lesions appear erythematous and edematous and are covered with papules, vesicles, and bullae. The involved area is pruritic but may also burn or sting. When contact dermatitis becomes chronic, the lesions resemble atopic dermatitis because they are thickened, scaly, and lichenified. The main difference between contact dermatitis and atopic dermatitis is that contact dermatitis is localized and restricted to the area exposed to the allergens, whereas atopic dermatitis is usually widespread.

Microbial Hypersensitivity Reactions. The classic example of a microbial cell-mediated immune reaction is the body's defense against the tubercle bacillus. Tuberculosis results from invasion of lung tissue by the highly resistant tubercle bacillus. The organism itself does not directly damage the lung tissue. However, antigenic material released from the tubercle bacilli reacts with T cells, initiating a cell-mediated immune response. The resulting response causes extensive caseous necrosis of the lung.

After the initial cell-mediated reaction, memory cells persist, so subsequent contact with the tubercle bacillus or an extract of purified protein from the organism causes a delayed hypersensitivity reaction. This is the basis for the purified protein derivative (PPD) tuberculosis skin test, which is read 48 to 72 hours after the PPD is injected intradermally. (Tuberculosis is discussed in Chapter 27.)

ALLERGIC DISORDERS

Assessment

For a thorough assessment of a patient with allergies, perform a comprehensive patient history, physical examination, diagnostic workup, and skin testing for allergens. Obtain information from the patient about family allergies, past and present allergies, and social and environmental factors.

Family history, including information about atopic reactions in relatives, is especially important in identifying at-risk patients. Note past and present allergies. In addition to identifying the allergen, also obtain information about the clinical manifestations and course of allergic reaction. The time of year when an allergic reaction occurs can be a clue to a seasonal allergen. Also obtain information about any over-the-counter or prescription medications used to treat the allergies.

Social and environmental factors, especially the physical environment, are important. Ask about pets, trees and plants on the property, pollutants in the air, floor coverings, houseplants, and cooling and heating systems in the home and workplace. In addition, a daily or weekly food diary with a description of any untoward reactions is important.[4] Of particular interest is a screening for any reaction to medication. Finally, ask about the patient's lifestyle and stress level in connection with the allergic symptoms.

Do a comprehensive head-to-toe physical examination, with particular attention focused on the site of the allergic manifestations. Obtain a comprehensive assessment that includes subjective and objective data (Table 13-10).

Diagnostic Studies

Many specialized immunologic techniques can be performed to detect abnormalities of lymphocytes, eosinophils, and immunoglobulins. A complete blood count (CBC) with WBC differential is done, with an absolute lymphocyte count and eosinophil count. Immunodeficiency is diagnosed if the lymphocyte count is below 1200/μL (1.2×10^9/L). T cell and B cell quantification is used to diagnose specific immunodeficiency syndromes. The eosinophil count is elevated in type I hypersensitivity reactions involving IgE. The serum IgE level is also generally elevated in type I hypersensitivity reactions and serves as a diagnostic indicator of atopic diseases.

Sputum and nasal and bronchial secretions may also be tested for the presence of eosinophils. If asthma is suspected, pulmonary function tests (especially for forced expiratory volume) are helpful.

Skin testing for allergens is the preferred method, but in some cases blood testing may be ordered. Allergy blood testing is recommended if a person (1) is using a drug that interferes with skin test results (e.g., antihistamines, corticosteroids) and cannot stop taking it for a few days, (2) cannot tolerate the many needle scratches required for skin testing, or (3) has a skin disorder (e.g., severe eczema, dermatitis, psoriasis).

Skin Tests. Skin testing is used to identify the specific allergens that are causing the allergy symptoms. With the use of empiric allergy medications as the treatment of choice for most allergic rhinitis, it has become common practice to omit skin testing for specific allergens in these patients. However, diagnosing an allergy to a specific antigen enables the patient to avoid an allergen and makes him or her a candidate for immunotherapy. Unfortunately, skin testing cannot be done on patients who cannot stop taking drugs that suppress the histamine response or patients with food allergies.

TABLE 13-10 Nursing Assessment

Allergies

Subjective Data

Important Health Information

Past health history: Recurrent respiratory problems, seasonal exacerbations. Unusual reactions to insect bites or stings; past and present allergies

Medications: Unusual reactions to any medications; use of over-the-counter drugs or medications for allergies

Functional Health Patterns

Health perception–health management: Family history of allergies; malaise

Nutritional-metabolic: Food intolerances, vomiting

Elimination: Abdominal cramps, diarrhea

Activity-exercise: Fatigue; hoarseness, cough, dyspnea

Cognitive-perceptual: Itching, burning, stinging of eyes, nose, throat, or skin; chest tightness

Role-relationship: Altered home and work environment, presence of pets

Objective Data

Integumentary

Rashes, including urticaria, wheal and flare, papules, vesicles, bullae; dryness, scaliness, scratches, irritation

Eyes, Ears, Nose, and Throat

Eyes: Conjunctivitis; lacrimation; rubbing or excessive blinking; dark circles under the eyes ("allergic shiner")

Ears: Diminished hearing; immobile or scarred tympanic membranes; recurrent ear infections

Nose: Nasal polyps, nasal voice, nose twitching, itchy nose, rhinitis; pale, boggy mucous membranes; sniffling, repeated sneezing; swollen nasal passages; recurrent, unexplained nosebleeds; crease across the bridge of nose ("allergic salute")

Throat: Continual throat clearing; swollen lips or tongue; red throat; palpable neck lymph nodes

Respiratory

Wheezing, stridor; thick sputum

Possible Diagnostic Findings

Eosinophilia of serum, sputum, or nasal and bronchial secretions; ↑ serum IgE levels; positive skin tests; abnormal chest and sinus x-rays

Procedure. Skin testing may be done by three different methods: (1) a scratch or prick test, (2) an intradermal test, or (3) a patch test. The areas of the body usually used in skin testing are the arms and back. Allergen extracts are applied to the skin in rows with a corresponding control site opposite the test site. Saline or another diluent is applied to the control site. In the *scratch test* a drop of allergen is placed on the skin, and then a pricking device is used so that the allergen can enter the skin. In the *intradermal test* the allergen extract is injected under the skin, similar to a PPD test for TB. In the *patch test* an allergen is applied to a patch that is placed on the skin (see Fig. 22-10).

Results. In the scratch and intradermal tests the reaction occurs in 5 to 10 minutes. In the patch test the patches must be worn for 48 to 72 hours. If the person is hypersensitive to the allergen, a positive reaction will occur within minutes after insertion in the skin and may last for 8 to 12 hours. A positive reaction is manifested by a local wheal-and-flare response.

The size of the positive reaction does not always correlate with the severity of allergy symptoms. False-positive and false-negative results may occur. Negative results from skin testing do not necessarily mean the person does not have an allergic disorder, and positive results do not necessarily mean that the allergen was causing the clinical manifestations. Positive results imply that the person is sensitized to that allergen. Therefore correlating skin test results with the patient's history is important.

Precautions. A highly sensitive person is always at risk for developing an anaphylactic reaction to skin tests. Therefore a patient should never be left alone during the testing period. Sometimes skin testing is completely contraindicated and blood allergy testing is used. If a severe reaction does occur with a skin test, the extract is immediately removed and antiinflammatory topical cream is applied to the site. For intradermal testing, the arm is used so that a tourniquet can be applied during a severe reaction. A subcutaneous injection of epinephrine may also be necessary.

Interprofessional Care

After an allergic disorder is diagnosed, treatment is aimed at reducing exposure to the offending allergen, treating the symptoms, and, if necessary, desensitizing the person through immunotherapy.

Anaphylaxis. Anaphylactic reactions occur suddenly in hypersensitive patients after exposure to the offending allergen. They may occur after parenteral injection of drugs (especially antibiotics) or blood products, and after insect stings. The cardinal principle in management is speed in (1) recognition of signs and symptoms of an anaphylactic reaction, (2) maintenance of a patent airway, (3) prevention of spread of the allergen by using a tourniquet, (4) administration of drugs, and (5) treatment for shock. Table 13-11 summarizes the emergency treatment of anaphylactic shock.

Severe cases of anaphylaxis may result in hypovolemic shock because of the loss of intravascular fluid into interstitial spaces that occurs secondary to increased capillary permeability.[5] Peripheral vasoconstriction and stimulation of the sympathetic nervous system occur to compensate for the fluid shift. However, unless shock is treated early, the body will no longer be able to compensate, and irreversible tissue damage will occur, leading to death. (Hypovolemic shock is discussed in Chapter 66.)

All health care workers must be prepared for the rare but life-threatening anaphylactic reaction, which requires immediate medical and nursing interventions. It is extremely important to list all of a patient's allergies on the chart, nursing care plan, and medication record.[6]

Chronic Allergies. Most allergic reactions are chronic and are characterized by remissions and exacerbations of symptoms. Treatment focuses on identification and control of allergens, relief of symptoms through drug therapy, and hyposensitization of a patient to an offending allergen.

Allergen Recognition and Control. You play an important role in helping the patient make lifestyle adjustments so that there is minimal exposure to offending allergens. Reinforce that, even with drug therapy and immunotherapy, the patient will never be totally desensitized or completely symptom free. Help the patient initiate various preventive measures to control the allergic symptoms.

Of primary importance is the need to identify the offending allergen. Sometimes this is done through skin testing. In the case of food allergies an elimination diet is sometimes valuable. If an allergic reaction occurs, all foods eaten shortly before the

TABLE 13-11 Emergency Management

Anaphylactic Shock

Etiology

- Injection of, inhalation of, ingestion of, or topical exposure to substance that produces profound allergic response (Table 13-9 for more complete listing).

Assessment Findings

Fig. 13-7.

Interventions

Initial

- Ensure patent airway. Intubation if evidence of impending obstruction.
- Remove insect stinger if present.
- Establish IV access.
- Epinephrine (1 mg/mL preparation): Give 0.3-0.5 mg IM preferably in the mid-outer thigh. Can repeat every 5-15 min.*
- Administer high-flow O_2 (8-10 L/min) via face mask. Can give up to 100% as needed.
- Nebulized albuterol (Proventil) for bronchospasm resistant to epinephrine.
- Diphenhydramine (Benadryl) IV for urticaria and itching.
- Corticosteroids: methylprednisolone (Solu-Medrol) IV.

Hypotension

- Place recumbent and elevate legs.
- IV normal saline rapid bolus of 1-2 L.
- Maintain BP with fluids, volume expanders, vasopressors (e.g., dopamine [Intropin]).

Ongoing Monitoring

- Monitor vital signs, respiratory effort, O_2 saturation, level of consciousness, cardiac rhythm, and urine output.
- Anticipate intubation with severe respiratory distress.
- Anticipate cricothyrotomy or tracheostomy with severe laryngeal edema.

*Patients receiving β-blockers may be resistant to treatment with epinephrine and can develop refractory hypotension and bradycardia. Glucagon should be administered in this setting because it has inotropic and chronotropic effects that are not mediated through β-receptors.

reaction should be eliminated and gradually reintroduced one at a time until the offending food is detected.

Many allergic reactions, especially asthma and urticaria, may be aggravated by fatigue and emotional stress. Assist the patient in planning a stress management program. Relaxation techniques can be practiced when the patient comes for frequent immunotherapy treatments.

Sometimes control of allergic symptoms requires environmental control, including changing an occupation, moving to a different climate, or giving up a favorite pet. In the case of airborne allergens, sleeping in an air-conditioned room, damp dusting daily, covering mattresses and pillows with hypoallergenic covers, and wearing a mask outdoors may be helpful.

If the allergen is a drug, instruct the patient to avoid the drug. The patient also has the responsibility to make his or her allergies well known to all health care providers. The patient should wear a Medic Alert bracelet listing the particular drug allergy and have the offending drug listed on all medical and dental records.

For a patient allergic to insect stings, commercial bee-sting kits containing preinjectable epinephrine and a tourniquet are available. Instruct the patient and family about the technique of applying the tourniquet and self-injecting the subcutaneous epinephrine. This patient also should wear a Medic Alert bracelet and carry a bee-sting kit whenever going outdoors.

Drug Therapy. The major categories of drugs used for symptomatic relief of chronic allergic disorders include antihistamines, sympathomimetic/decongestant drugs, corticosteroids, antipruritic drugs, and mast cell–stabilizing drugs. Many of these drugs can be obtained over the counter and are often misused by patients.

Antihistamines. Antihistamines are the best drugs for treatment of allergic rhinitis and urticaria (see Chapter 26, Table 26-2). They are less effective for severe allergic reactions. They act by competing with histamine for H_1-receptor sites and thus blocking the effect of histamine. Best results are achieved if they are taken as soon as allergy symptoms appear. Antihistamines can be used effectively to treat edema and pruritus but are relatively ineffective in preventing bronchoconstriction. With seasonal rhinitis, antihistamines should be taken during peak pollen seasons. (Antihistamines are discussed in Chapter 26.)

Sympathomimetic/Decongestant Drugs. The major sympathomimetic drug is epinephrine (Adrenalin), which is the drug of choice to treat an anaphylactic reaction. Epinephrine is produced by the adrenal medulla and stimulates α- and β-adrenergic receptors. Stimulation of the α-adrenergic receptors causes vasoconstriction of peripheral blood vessels. β-Receptor stimulation relaxes bronchial smooth muscles. Epinephrine also acts directly on mast cells to stabilize them against further degranulation. The action of epinephrine lasts only a few minutes. For the treatment of anaphylaxis, the drug must be given parenterally (IM, IV).

Several specific, minor sympathomimetic drugs differ from epinephrine because they can be taken orally or nasally and last for several hours. Included in this category are phenylephrine (Neo-Synephrine) and pseudoephedrine (Sudafed). The minor sympathomimetic drugs are used primarily to treat allergic rhinitis.

Corticosteroids. Nasal corticosteroid sprays are effective in relieving the symptoms of allergic rhinitis (see Chapter 26 and Table 26-2). Occasionally patients have such severe manifestations of allergies that they are truly incapacitated. In these situations, a brief course of oral corticosteroids can be used.

Antipruritic Drugs. Topically applied antipruritic drugs are most effective when the skin is not broken. These drugs protect the skin and provide relief from itching. Common over-the-counter drugs include calamine lotion, coal tar solutions, and camphor. Menthol and phenol may be added to other lotions to produce an antipruritic effect. Some more potent drugs that require a prescription include methdilazine (Tacaryl) and trimeprazine (Temaril).

Mast Cell–Stabilizing Drugs. Cromolyn (NasalCrom) is a mast cell–stabilizing agent that inhibits the release of histamines, leukotrienes, and other agents from the mast cell after antigen-IgE interaction. It is available as an inhalant nebulizer solution or a nasal spray. Cromolyn is used in the management of allergic rhinitis (see Chapter 27).

Leukotriene Receptor Antagonists. Leukotriene receptor antagonists (LTRAs) block leukotriene, one of the major mediators of the allergic inflammatory process (see Table 26-2). These medications can be taken orally. They may be used in the treatment of allergic rhinitis and asthma.

Immunotherapy. Immunotherapy is the recommended treatment for control of allergic symptoms when the allergen cannot be avoided and drug therapy is not effective. Relatively few patients with allergies have symptoms so intolerable that they require allergy immunotherapy. (In individuals with anaphylactic reactions to insect venom, immunotherapy is definitely indicated.)

Immunotherapy involves administration of small titers of an allergen extract in increasing strengths until hyposensitivity to the specific allergen is achieved. For best results, teach the patient to avoid the offending allergen whenever possible because complete desensitization is impossible. Unfortunately, not all allergy-related conditions respond to immunotherapy. Food allergies cannot be safely treated with this therapy, and eczema may worsen with immunotherapy.

Mechanism of Action. The IgE level is elevated in atopic individuals. When IgE combines with an allergen in a hypersensitive person, a reaction occurs, releasing histamine in various body tissues. Allergens more readily combine with IgG than with other immunoglobulins. Therefore immunotherapy involves injecting allergen extracts that will stimulate increased IgG levels. The goal of long-term immunotherapy is to keep "blocking" IgG levels high. By increasing the IgG levels, the IgE is blocked from binding to the allergen. Thus mast cell degranulation is prevented. In addition, allergen-specific T suppressor cells develop in individuals receiving immunotherapy.

Method of Administration. The allergens included in immunotherapy are chosen based on the results of skin testing with a panel of allergens.

Subcutaneous immunotherapy. *Subcutaneous immunotherapy (SCIT)* involves the subcutaneous injection of titrated amounts of allergen extracts biweekly or weekly. The dose is small at first and is increased slowly until a maintenance dosage is reached. Generally it takes 1 to 2 years of immunotherapy to reach the maximal therapeutic effect. Therapy may be continued for about 5 years. After that, discontinuing therapy is considered. In many patients a decrease in symptoms is sustained after the treatment is discontinued. For patients with severe allergies or sensitivity to insect stings, maintenance therapy is continued indefinitely. Best results are achieved when immunotherapy is administered throughout the year.

Sublingual immunotherapy. *Sublingual immunotherapy (SLIT)* involves allergen extracts taken under the tongue. SLIT has been used in Europe for decades. Recently the first sublingual products have become available in the United States. These include a five-grass pollen tablet (Oralair), a single grass pollen tablet (Grastek), and a ragweed pollen tablet (Ragwitek).[7]

SLIT is self-administered (usually daily) by patients at home, although the initial dose is usually given under medical supervision. Some patients experience local application site reactions (e.g., oral pruritus, throat irritation, tongue swelling), but systemic allergic reactions are markedly fewer than SCIT. Local reactions subside in many patients within a few days to a week.

SLIT has the advantage of being a convenient, self-administered oral therapy. Its primary disadvantage is that it requires the patient to be consistently compliant with therapy.[8]

❖ NURSING MANAGEMENT: IMMUNOTHERAPY

You will often be the person responsible for administering SCIT. Always anticipate adverse reactions, especially when using a new-strength dose, after a previous reaction, or after a missed dose. Early manifestations of a systemic reaction include pruritus, urticaria, sneezing, laryngeal edema, and hypotension. Emergency measures for anaphylactic shock should be initiated immediately. Describe a local reaction according to the degree of redness and swelling at the injection site. If the area is greater than the size of a quarter in an adult, report the reaction to the HCP so that the allergen dosage may be decreased.

Immunotherapy always carries the risk of a severe anaphylactic reaction. Therefore an HCP, emergency equipment, and essential drugs should be available whenever injections are given.

Record keeping must be accurate and can be invaluable in preventing an adverse reaction to the allergen extract. Before giving an injection, check the patient's name against the name on the vial. Next, determine the vial strength, amount of last dose, date of last dose, and any reaction information.

Always administer the allergen extract in an extremity away from a joint so that a tourniquet can be applied for a severe reaction. Rotate the site for each injection. Aspirate for blood before giving an injection to ensure that the allergen extract is not injected into a blood vessel. An injection directly into the bloodstream can potentiate an anaphylactic reaction. After giving the injection, carefully observe the patient for 20 to 30 minutes, since systemic reactions are most likely to occur immediately. However, warn the patient that a delayed reaction can occur as long as 24 hours later.

Latex Allergies

Allergies to latex products have become an increasing problem, affecting patients and health care professionals. The increase in allergic reactions has coincided with the sharp increase in glove use. The more frequent and prolonged the exposure to latex, the greater the likelihood of developing a latex allergy.[9]

In addition to gloves, many latex-containing products are used in health care, such as blood pressure cuffs, stethoscopes, tourniquets, IV tubing, syringes, electrode pads, O_2 masks, tracheal tubes, colostomy and ileostomy pouches, urinary catheters, anesthetic masks, and adhesive tape. Latex proteins can become aerosolized through powder on gloves and can result in serious reactions when inhaled by sensitized individuals. It is recommended that all health care facilities use powder-free gloves to avoid respiratory exposure to latex proteins.[10]

Types of Latex Allergies. Two types of latex allergies can occur: type IV allergic contact dermatitis and type I allergic reactions. *Type IV contact dermatitis* is caused by the chemicals used in the manufacturing process of latex gloves. It is a delayed reaction that occurs within 6 to 48 hours. Typically the person first has dryness, pruritus, fissuring, and cracking of the skin, followed by redness, swelling, and crusting at 24 to 48 hours. Chronic exposure can lead to lichenification, scaling, and hyperpigmentation. The dermatitis may extend beyond the area of physical contact with the allergen.

A *type I allergic reaction* is a response to the natural rubber latex proteins and occurs within minutes of contact with the proteins. The manifestations of these allergic reactions can vary from skin redness, urticaria, rhinitis, conjunctivitis, or asthma to full-blown anaphylactic shock. Systemic reactions to latex may result from exposure to latex protein via various routes, including the skin, mucous membranes, inhalation, and blood.

Latex-Food Syndrome. Because some proteins in rubber are similar to food proteins, some foods may cause an allergic reaction in people who are allergic to latex. This is called *latex-food syndrome.* The most common of these foods are banana, avocado, chestnut, kiwi, tomato, water chestnut, guava, hazelnut, potato, peach, grape, and apricot. Most people with latex allergy have a positive allergy test to at least one related food.

❖ NURSING AND INTERPROFESSIONAL MANAGEMENT: LATEX ALLERGIES

Identifying patients and health care workers sensitive to latex is crucial to prevent adverse reactions. Obtain a thorough health history and history of any allergies, especially for patients with any complaints of latex contact symptoms. Not all latex-sensitive individuals can be identified, even with a careful and thorough history. The greatest risk factor is long-term multiple exposures to latex products (e.g., health care personnel, individuals who have had multiple surgeries, rubber industry workers). Additional risk factors include a patient history of allergic rhinitis, asthma, and allergies to certain foods (listed earlier).

Use latex precaution protocols for those patients identified as having a positive latex allergy test or a history of signs and symptoms related to latex exposure. Many health care facilities have created latex-free product carts that can be used for patients with latex allergies. The National Institute for Occupational Safety and Health (NIOSH) has published recommendations for preventing allergic reactions to latex in the workplace (Table 13-12).

Because of the potential for severe symptoms of food allergy, teach patients to avoid those foods. Other recommendations for people with latex and food allergies include wearing a Medic Alert bracelet or necklace and carrying an injectable epinephrine pen.

Multiple Chemical Sensitivity

Multiple chemical sensitivity (MCS) is a subjective illness marked by recurrent, vague, nonspecific symptoms attributed to low levels of chemical, biologic, or physical agents.

Commonly accused substances include smoke, pesticides, plastics, synthetic fabrics, scented products, petroleum products, and paint fumes. Women between the ages of 30 and 50 are more likely to develop the symptoms. MCS is a controversial diagnosis and is not recognized as an illness by the American Medical Association or other authorities.[11]

The symptoms that people report are wide-ranging and not specific. They include headache, fatigue, dizziness, nausea, congestion, itching, sneezing, sore throat, chest pain, breathing problems, muscle pain or stiffness, skin rash, diarrhea, bloating, gas, confusion, difficulty concentrating, memory problems, and mood changes. These symptoms are usually subjective, and there is no evidence of a pathologic condition or physiologic dysfunction.

Diagnosis is usually made based on a patient's health history. There is no established test to diagnose MCS. The most effective treatment for MCS is to avoid the chemicals that may trigger the symptoms and create a chemical-free and odor-free home and workplace.

Psychotherapy is recommended as a primary option. In patients who are unwilling to undergo psychotherapy but willing to accept medications, antidepressants including selective serotonin reuptake inhibitors (SSRIs) (e.g., citalopram [Celexa]), have been used for treatment. Drugs for anxiety and sleep have also been used.

TABLE 13-12 Guidelines for Preventing Allergic Latex Reactions

- Use nonlatex gloves for activities that are not likely to involve contact with infectious materials (e.g., food preparation, housekeeping).
- Appropriate barrier protection is needed when handling infectious materials. If you choose latex gloves, use powder-free gloves with reduced protein content.
- When wearing latex gloves, do not use oil-based hand creams or lotions.
- Frequently clean work areas that are contaminated with latex-containing dust (e.g., carpets, ventilation ducts).
- Learn to recognize the symptoms of latex allergy: skin rash; hives; flushing; itching; nasal, eye, or sinus symptoms; asthma; and shock.
- If symptoms of latex allergy develop, avoid direct contact with latex gloves and products.
- Wear a Medic Alert bracelet and carry an epinephrine pen (e.g., EpiPen).

Source: National Institute for Occupational Safety and Health (NIOSH) (*www.cdc.gov/niosh*).

AUTOIMMUNITY

Autoimmunity is an immune response against self in which the immune system no longer differentiates self from nonself. For some unknown reason, immune cells that are normally unresponsive (tolerant to self-antigens) are activated. In autoimmunity, autoantibodies and autosensitized T cells cause pathophysiologic tissue damage.

The cause of autoimmune diseases is still unknown. Age is thought to play some role because the number of circulating autoantibodies increases in people over age 50. However, the principal factors in the development of autoimmunity are (1) the inheritance of susceptibility genes, which may contribute to the failure of self-tolerance; and (2) initiation of autoreactivity by triggers, such as infections, which may activate self-reactive lymphocytes.

Autoimmune diseases tend to cluster, so that a given person may have more than one autoimmune disease (e.g., rheumatoid arthritis, Addison's disease), or the same or related autoimmune diseases may be found in other members of the same family. This observation has led to the concept of genetic predisposition to autoimmune disease. Most of the genetic research in this area correlates certain human leukocyte antigen (HLA) types with an autoimmune condition. (HLAs and disease association are discussed later in this chapter on p. 207.)

Even in a genetically predisposed person, some trigger is required for the initiation of autoreactivity. This may include infectious agents such as a virus. Viral infections can cause an alteration of cells or tissues that are not normally antigenic. The virally induced changes can make the cells or tissues antigenic. Viruses may be involved in the development of diseases such as type 1 diabetes mellitus. Rheumatic fever and rheumatic heart disease are autoimmune responses triggered by streptococcal infection and mediated by antibodies against group A β-hemolytic streptococci that cross-react with heart muscles and valves and synovial membranes.

Drugs can also be precipitating factors in autoimmune disease. Hemolytic anemia can result from methyldopa (Aldomet) administration. Procainamide (Pronestyl) can induce the formation of antinuclear antibodies and cause a lupus-like syndrome.

Gender and hormones also have a role in autoimmune disease. More women than men have autoimmune disease. During pregnancy, many autoimmune diseases get better. After delivery, the woman with an autoimmune disease frequently has an exacerbation.

Autoimmune Diseases

Generally, autoimmune diseases are grouped according to organ-specific and systemic diseases (Table 13-13). Systemic lupus erythematosus (SLE) is a classic example of a systemic autoimmune disease characterized by damage to multiple organs. The cause is unknown, but there appears to be a loss of self-tolerance for the body's own DNA antigens.

In SLE, tissue injury appears to be the result of the formation of antinuclear antibodies. For some reason (possibly a viral infection), the cell membrane is damaged and deoxyribonucleic acid (DNA) is released into the systemic circulation, where it is viewed as nonself. This DNA is normally sequestered inside the nucleus of cells. On release into the circulation, the DNA antigen reacts with an antibody. Some antibodies are involved in immune complex formation, and others may cause damage directly. Once the complexes are deposited, the complement system is activated and further damages the tissue, especially the renal glomerulus. (SLE is discussed in Chapter 64.)

Apheresis

Apheresis has been effectively used to treat autoimmune diseases and other diseases and disorders. *Apheresis* is a procedure to separate components of the blood followed by the removal of one or more of these components. Compound words are often used to describe any particular apheresis procedure, depending on the blood components being collected. *Plateletpheresis* is the removal of platelets, usually for collection from normal individuals to infuse into patients with low platelet counts (e.g., patients taking chemotherapy who develop thrombocytopenia). *Leukocytapheresis* is a general term indicating the removal of WBCs and is used in chronic myelogenous leukemia to remove high numbers of leukemic cells.

Apheresis is also used in hematopoietic stem cell transplantation to collect stem cells from peripheral blood. These stem cells can then be used to repopulate a person's bone marrow after high-dose chemotherapy (see section on hematopoietic stem cell transplants in Chapter 15).

Plasmapheresis. *Plasmapheresis* is the removal of plasma containing components causing or thought to cause disease. It can also be used to obtain plasma from healthy donors to administer to patients as replacement therapy.

When plasma is removed, it is replaced by substitute fluids such as saline, fresh-frozen plasma, or albumin. Thus the term *plasma exchange* more accurately describes this procedure.

Plasmapheresis has been used to treat autoimmune diseases such as SLE, glomerulonephritis, Goodpasture syndrome, myasthenia gravis, thrombocytopenic purpura, rheumatoid arthritis, and Guillain-Barré syndrome. Many disorders for which plasmapheresis is used are characterized by circulating autoantibodies (usually of the IgG class) and antigen-antibody complexes. The rationale for performing therapeutic plasmapheresis in autoimmune disorders is to remove pathologic substances present in plasma. Immunosuppressive therapy has been used to prevent recovery of IgG production, and plasmapheresis has been used to prevent antibody rebound.

In addition to removing antibodies and antigen-antibody complexes, plasmapheresis may also remove inflammatory mediators (e.g., complement) that are responsible for tissue damage. In the treatment of SLE, plasmapheresis is usually reserved for the patient having an acute attack who is unresponsive to conventional therapy.

Plasmapheresis involves the removal of whole blood through an IV device, and then the blood circulates through the apheresis machine. Inside the machine the blood is divided into plasma and its cellular components by centrifugation or membrane filtration. The plasma is generally replaced with normal saline, lactated Ringer's solution, fresh-frozen plasma, plasma protein fractions, or albumin. When blood is manually removed, only 500 mL can be taken at one time. However, with the use of apheresis procedures, more than 4 L of plasma can be pheresed in 2 to 3 hours.

As with administration of other blood products, be aware of side effects associated with plasmapheresis. The most common complications are hypotension and citrate toxicity. Hypotension is usually the result of a vasovagal reaction or transient volume changes. Citrate is used as an anticoagulant and may cause hypocalcemia, which may manifest as headache, paresthesias, and dizziness.

TABLE 13-13 Examples of Autoimmune Diseases*

Systemic Diseases
- Rheumatoid arthritis
- Scleroderma (systemic sclerosis)
- Systemic lupus erythematosus

Organ-Specific Diseases

Blood
- Autoimmune hemolytic anemia
- Hemochromatosis
- Immune thrombocytopenic purpura (ITP)

Central Nervous System
- Guillain-Barré syndrome
- Multiple sclerosis

Muscle
- Myasthenia gravis

Heart
- Rheumatic fever

Endocrine System
- Addison's disease
- Graves' disease
- Hypothyroidism
- Thyroiditis
- Type 1 diabetes mellitus

Gastrointestinal System
- Celiac disease
- Inflammatory bowel disease
- Pernicious anemia

Kidney
- Glomerulonephritis
- Goodpasture syndrome

Liver
- Autoimmune hepatitis
- Primary biliary cirrhosis

Eye
- Uveitis

*These diseases are discussed in various chapters throughout the book.

IMMUNODEFICIENCY DISORDERS

When the immune system does not adequately protect the body, **immunodeficiency** exists. Immunodeficiency disorders involve an impairment of one or more immune mechanisms, which include (1) phagocytosis, (2) humoral response, (3) cell-mediated response, (4) complement, and (5) a combined humoral and cell-mediated deficiency. Immunodeficiency disorders are *primary* if the immune cells are improperly developed or absent and *secondary* if the deficiency is caused by illnesses or treatment. Primary immunodeficiency disorders are rare and often serious, whereas secondary disorders are more common and less severe.

Primary Immunodeficiency Disorders

The basic categories of primary immunodeficiency disorders are (1) phagocytic defects, (2) B cell deficiency, (3) T cell deficiency, and (4) a combined B cell and T cell deficiency (Table 13-14).

Secondary Immunodeficiency Disorders

Some of the important factors that may cause secondary immunodeficiency disorders are listed in Table 13-15. Drug-induced immunosuppression is the most common. Immunosuppressive therapy is prescribed for patients to treat autoimmune disorders and to prevent transplant rejection. In addition, immunosuppression is a serious side effect of drugs used in cancer chemotherapy. Generalized leukopenia often results, leading to a decreased humoral and cell-mediated response. Therefore secondary infections are common in immunosuppressed patients.

Malnutrition alters cell-mediated immune responses. When protein is deficient over a prolonged period, the thymus gland atrophies and lymphoid tissue decreases. In addition, an increased susceptibility to infections always exists.

Hodgkin's lymphoma greatly impairs the cell-mediated immune response, and patients may die from severe viral or fungal infections. (Hodgkin's lymphoma is discussed in Chapter 30.) Viruses, especially rubella, may cause immunodeficiency by direct cytotoxic damage to lymphoid cells. Systemic infections can place such a demand on the immune system that resistance to a secondary or subsequent infection is impaired.

Radiation can destroy lymphocytes either directly or through depletion of stem cells. As the radiation dose is increased, more bone marrow atrophies, leading to severe pancytopenia and suppression of immune function. Splenectomy in children is especially dangerous and may lead to septicemia simply from respiratory tract infections.

Stress may alter the immune response. This response involves interrelationships among the nervous, endocrine, and immune systems (see Chapter 6).

TABLE 13-14 Primary Immunodeficiency Disorders

Disorder	Affected Cells	Genetic Basis
Chronic granulomatous disease	PMNs, monocytes	X-linked
Job syndrome	PMNs, monocytes	—
Bruton's X-linked agammaglobulinemia	B	X-linked
Common variable hypogammaglobulinemia	B	—
Selective IgA, IgM, or IgG deficiency	B	Some X-linked
DiGeorge syndrome (thymic hypoplasia)	T	—
Severe combined immunodeficiency disease	Stem, B, T	X-linked or autosomal recessive
Ataxia-telangiectasia	B, T	Autosomal recessive
Wiskott-Aldrich syndrome	B, T	X-linked
Graft-versus-host disease	B, T	—

PMNs, Polymorphonuclear neutrophils.

TABLE 13-15 Causes of Secondary Immunodeficiency

Drug-Induced Immunodeficiency
- Chemotherapy drugs
- Corticosteroids

Age
- Infants
- Older adults

Malnutrition
- Dietary deficiency
- Cachexia

Therapies
- Radiation
- Surgery
- Anesthesia

Diseases or Disorders
- Acquired immunodeficiency syndrome (AIDS)
- Cirrhosis
- Chronic kidney disease
- Diabetes mellitus
- Hodgkin's lymphoma
- Malignancies
- Systemic lupus erythematosus
- Burns
- Trauma
- Severe infection

Stress
- Chronic stress
- Trauma (physical or emotional)

HUMAN LEUKOCYTE ANTIGEN SYSTEM

The antigens responsible for rejection of genetically unlike tissues are called the *major histocompatibility antigens.* These antigens are products of histocompatibility genes. In humans, they are called the **human leukocyte antigen (HLA)** system. The genes for the HLA antigens are linked and occur together on the sixth chromosome. HLAs are present on all nucleated cells and platelets. The HLA system is primarily used in matching organs and tissues for transplantation.

An important characteristic of HLA genes is that they are highly *polymorphic* (variable). Each HLA locus can have many different possible alleles, and thus many combinations exist. Each person has two alleles for each locus, one inherited from each parent. Both alleles of a locus are expressed independently (i.e., they are codominant). The proteins encoded by certain genes are known as *antigens.*

The entire set of A, B, C, D, and DR genes (the HLA genes) located on one chromosome is termed a *haplotype.* A complete set is inherited as a unit (haplotype). One haplotype is inherited from each parent (Fig. 13-10). This means that a person has HLA genes that are one-half identical to those of each parent. The HLA genes of one person have a 25% chance of being identical to the HLA genes of a sibling.

In organ transplantation A, B, and DR are primarily used for compatibility matching. The specific allele at each locus is identified by a number. For example, a person could have an HLA of A2, A6, B7, B27, DR4, and DR7. Currently more than 8000 HLA alleles have been identified for the various HLA genes.

Human Leukocyte Antigen and Disease Associations

The early interest in HLAs was stimulated by the role of HLAs in matching donors and recipients of organ transplants. Since that time, the interest in the association between HLAs and disease has grown.

A number of diseases show significant associations with specific HLA alleles. People who have these alleles are much more likely to develop the associated disease than those who do not have the allele. However, the possession of a particular HLA allele does not mean that the person will necessarily develop the associated disease—only that the relative risk is greater than in the general population.

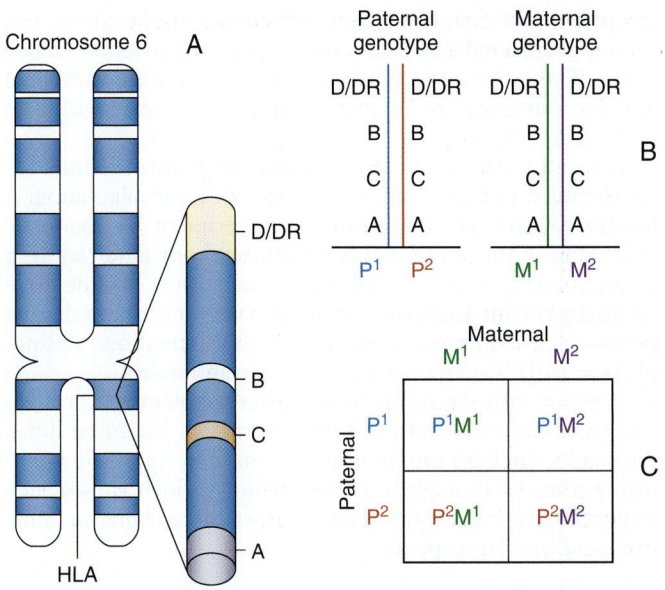

FIG. 13-10 Patterns of human leukocyte antigen (HLA) inheritance. **A,** HLA genes are located on chromosome 6. **B,** The two haplotypes of the father are labeled P^1 and P^2, and the haplotypes of the mother are labeled M^1 and M^2. Each child inherits two haplotypes, one from each parent. **C,** Therefore only four combinations—P^1M^1, P^1M^2, P^2M^1, and P^2M^2—are possible, and 25% of the offspring will have identical HLA haplotypes.

Most of the HLA-associated diseases are classified as autoimmune disorders. Examples of HLA types and disease associations include (1) HLA-B27 and ankylosing spondylitis, (2) HLA-DR2 and HLA-DR3 and SLE, (3) HLA-DR3 and HLA-DR4 and diabetes mellitus, and (4) HLA-DR2 and narcolepsy.

The discovery of HLA associations with certain diseases is a major breakthrough in understanding the genetic bases of these diseases. It is now known that at least part of the genetic bases of HLA-associated diseases lies in the HLA region, but the actual mechanisms involved in these associations are still unknown. However, most individuals who inherit a specific HLA type (e.g., HLA-DR3) that is associated with a disease will never develop that disease.

Currently the association between HLAs and certain diseases is of minimal practical clinical importance. Nevertheless, there is promise for the development of clinical applications in the future. For example, with certain autoimmune diseases, it may be possible to identify members of a family at greatest risk for developing the same or a related autoimmune disease. These people would need close medical supervision, implementation of preventive measures (if possible), and early diagnosis and treatment to prevent chronic complications.

ORGAN TRANSPLANTATION

Transplantation success has improved with advances in surgical technique, advances in histocompatibility testing, and more effective immunosuppressant drugs. Common tissue transplants include corneas, skin, bone marrow, heart valves, bone, and connective tissues (Fig. 13-11). Cornea transplants can prevent or correct blindness. Skin grafts are used in managing burn patients. Bone marrow is donated to help patients with leukemias and other malignancies.

Transplanted organs currently come from many different body systems. These organs include the heart, lung, liver, kidney,

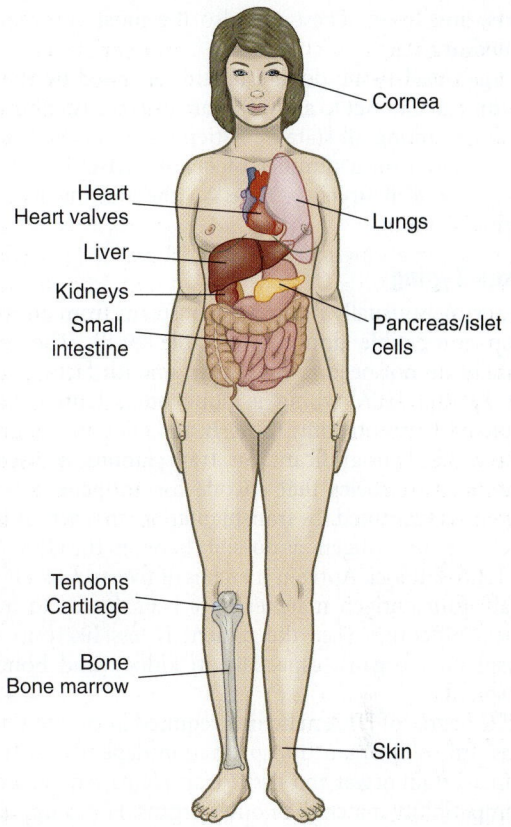

FIG. 13-11 Tissues and organs that can be transplanted.

pancreas, and intestine. Multiple organs can be transplanted together, such as kidney and pancreas, kidney and liver, kidney and heart, or the complete intestinal tract. For example, many patients with diabetes who receive a pancreas transplant also receive a kidney transplant because the diabetes has not only impaired the pancreas but also led to renal failure.

Some organs can be transplanted in parts or segments instead of transplanting an entire organ. Liver and lung lobes (rather than the whole organ) may be transplanted, or an intestine may be used in segments, thus allowing for one person's organ donation to benefit many recipients. This technique also enables living donors to donate part of an organ (or one of their organs in the case of kidneys).

Organ donations are taken from two sources: deceased (cadaver) and living donors. Most organs and tissues currently come from deceased donors. However, because of the shortage of organs from deceased donors, the use of related and living unrelated donor organs is increasing.

Individuals can make a decision to become a donor when they sign a donor card, the back of their driver's license, or a donor registry (depending on the state) and indicate their wish to donate organs. However, on their death or imminent death, the person's legal next of kin may need to consent to the donation regardless of whether the donor card is signed. Legal requirements and the facility's policy for a donor's legal next of kin to consent regardless of whether the donor card is signed vary from state to state and from facility to facility.

Currently more than 123,000 people are on the organ procurement and transplantation network's national waiting list, which is maintained by the United Network for Organ Sharing (UNOS). However, fewer than 30,000 people receive transplants annually. The organs in highest demand are kidneys, hearts, and livers. These are also the most commonly transplanted organs.[12]

Organ and tissue donations are regulated by the Uniform Anatomical Gift Act to allow for fair and consistent transplantation laws among all states.[13] Patients are matched to available donors based on a number of factors: ABO blood and HLA typing, medical urgency, time on the waiting list, and geographic location.

Tissue Typing

The recipient usually receives a transplant from an ABO blood group–compatible donor (see Table 29-8). The donor and recipient do not need to share the same Rh factor.

HLA Typing. HLA typing is done on potential donors and recipients. Currently only the A, B, and DR antigens are thought to be clinically significant for transplantation. Because each locus has two alleles that encode for antigens, a total of six antigens is identified. In transplantation an attempt is made to match as many antigens as possible between the HLA-A, HLA-B, and HLA-DR loci. Antigen matches of five and six antigens and certain four-antigen matches have been found to have better clinical outcomes (i.e., the patient is less likely to reject the transplanted organ), especially in kidney and bone marrow transplants.

The degree of HLA matching required or deemed suitable for successful solid organ transplantation depends on the type of organ. Certain organ and tissue transplants require a closer histocompatibility match than other organs. For example, a cornea transplant can be accepted by nearly any individual because corneas are avascular and therefore no antibodies reach the cornea to cause rejection. In kidney and bone marrow transplantation, HLA matching is very important, since these transplants are at high risk for graft rejection. On the other hand, for liver transplants, HLA mismatches have little impact on graft survival. Heart and lung transplants fall somewhere in between, but minimizing HLA mismatches significantly improves survival. In addition, for liver, lung, and heart transplants, few donors are available, and it is difficult to get good HLA matches.

Transporting and storing donated organs can take time. The "best" match may live many miles from the "ideal" recipient. The need to have the "best" matches has to be balanced against the time it takes to harvest and transport a donated organ and then transplant it.

Panel of Reactive Antibodies. A *panel of reactive antibodies (PRA)* indicates the recipient's sensitivity to various HLAs before receiving a transplant. To detect preformed antibodies to HLA, the recipient's serum is mixed with a randomly selected panel of donor lymphocytes to determine reactivity. The potential recipient may have been exposed to HLA antigens by means of previous blood transfusions, pregnancy, or a previous organ transplant.

PRA allows for the determination of whether a recipient is of high or low reactivity to potential donors. The results for the PRA are calculated in percentages. A high PRA indicates that the person has a large number of cytotoxic antibodies and is highly sensitized, which means there is a poor chance of finding a crossmatch-negative donor. In patients awaiting transplantation, a PRA panel is usually done on a regular basis. In highly sensitized patients (high PRA), plasmapheresis and IV immunoglobulin (IVIG) can be used to lower the number of antibodies.

Crossmatch. A crossmatch is done to determine the existence of antibodies against the potential donor. A crossmatch uses serum from the recipient mixed with donor lymphocytes to test for any preformed anti-HLA antibodies to the potential donor organ. The crossmatch can be used as a screening test when possible living donors are being considered or once a cadaver donor is selected.

A negative crossmatch indicates that no preformed antibodies are present and it is safe to proceed with transplantation. A positive crossmatch indicates that the recipient has cytotoxic antibodies to the donor and is an absolute contraindication in living donor transplants. Live donor transplants may be done for patients with a positive crossmatch if no other live donors (with a negative crossmatch) exist. In this situation, plasmapheresis or IVIG can be done to remove antibodies.

It is not always possible to complete a crossmatch prior to transplantation. If a retrospective crossmatch has to be done, the results will have implications for immunosuppression protocols after the transplant. Crossmatching, which is especially important for kidney transplants, may not be done for lung, liver, and heart transplants.

Transplant Rejection

Rejection is one of the major problems following organ transplantation. Rejection of organs occurs as a normal immune response to foreign tissue. The rejection can be prevented by using immunosuppression therapy, performing ABO and HLA matching, and ensuring that the crossmatch is negative. Unfortunately, many different HLAs exist, and a perfect match is nearly impossible unless the tissue is from oneself, an identical twin, or in some cases a sibling. Rejection can be hyperacute, acute, or chronic. Prevention, early diagnosis, and treatment of rejection are essential for long-term graft function.

Hyperacute Rejection. *Hyperacute rejection* occurs within 24 hours after transplantation because the blood vessels are rapidly destroyed. It occurs because the person had preexisting antibodies against the transplanted tissue or organ. There is no treatment for hyperacute rejection, and the transplanted organ is removed. Fortunately hyperacute rejection is a rare event because the final testing just before transplant usually determines whether the recipient is sensitized to any of the donor HLAs.

Acute Rejection. *Acute rejection* most commonly manifests in the first 6 months after transplantation. This type of rejection is usually a cell-mediated immune response by the recipient's lymphocytes, which have been activated against the donated (foreign) tissue or organ (Fig. 13-12). In addition to cell-mediated rejection, another type of acute rejection occurs when the recipient develops antibodies to the transplanted organ (humoral rejection).

It is not uncommon to have at least one rejection episode, especially with organs from deceased donors. These episodes are usually reversible with additional immunosuppressive therapy, which may include increased corticosteroid doses or polyclonal or monoclonal antibodies. Unfortunately, immunosuppressants increase the risk for infection. To combat acute rejection, all patients with transplants require long-term use of immunosuppressants, putting them at a high risk for infection, especially in the first few months after transplant when the immunosuppressive doses are highest.

Chronic Rejection. *Chronic rejection* is a process that occurs over months or years and is irreversible. Chronic rejection can occur for unknown reasons or from repeated episodes of acute rejection. The transplanted organ is infiltrated with large numbers of T and B cells characteristic of an ongoing,

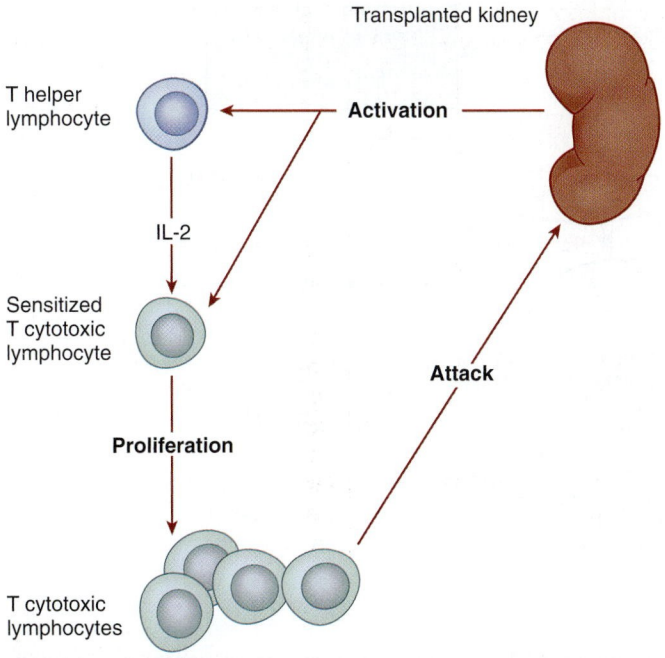

FIG. 13-12 Mechanism of action of T cytotoxic lymphocyte activation and attack of transplanted tissue. The transplanted organ (e.g., kidney) is recognized as foreign and activates the immune system. T helper cells are activated to produce interleukin-2 *(IL-2)*, and T cytotoxic lymphocytes are sensitized. After the T cytotoxic cells proliferate, they attack the transplanted organ.

low-grade, immune-mediated injury. Chronic rejection results in fibrosis and scarring. In heart transplants it manifests as accelerated coronary artery disease. In lung transplants it manifests as bronchiolitis obliterans. In liver transplants it is characterized by loss of bile ducts. In kidney transplants it manifests as fibrosis and glomerulopathy.

There is no definitive therapy for this type of rejection. Treatment is primarily supportive. This type of rejection is difficult to manage and is not associated with the optimistic prognosis of acute rejection.

Immunosuppressive Therapy

Immunosuppressive therapy requires a lifelong balance between rejection and infection. On one hand, the immune response must be suppressed to prevent rejection of the transplanted organ. On the other hand, an adequate immune response must be maintained to prevent overwhelming infection and the development of malignancies.[14]

Many of the drugs used to achieve immunosuppression have significant side effects. Because transplant recipients must take immunosuppressants for life, the risk of toxicity continues for the rest of their lives.

Immunosuppressant drugs are listed in Table 13-16. With the use of a combination of agents that work during different phases of the immune response (Fig. 13-13), lower doses of each drug can be given to produce effective immunosuppression while minimizing side effects.

The major immunosuppressive agents are (1) calcineurin inhibitors, including cyclosporine (Sandimmune, Neoral, Gengraf) and tacrolimus (Prograf); (2) corticosteroids (prednisone, methylprednisolone [Solu-Medrol] IV); (3) mycophenolate mofetil (CellCept, Myfortic); and (4) sirolimus (Rapamune). Azathioprine (Imuran) and cyclophosphamide (Cytoxan) can also be used. Muromonab-CD3 (Orthoclone OKT3) and either horse antithymocyte globulin (Atgam) or rabbit antithymocyte globulin (ATG) are IV medications used for short periods to prevent early rejection or reverse acute rejection.

Immunosuppression protocols are highly variable among transplant centers, with different combinations of medications being used. Most patients are initially on triple therapy. The standard triple therapy usually includes a calcineurin inhibitor, a corticosteroid, and mycophenolate mofetil.

The doses of immunosuppressant drugs are reduced over time after the transplant. Patients taking corticosteroids may be weaned off after a few years. The trend in many transplant centers is to use immunosuppression protocols that do not contain corticosteroids because of their many side effects.

Calcineurin Inhibitors. This group of drugs, including tacrolimus and cyclosporine, is the foundation of most immunosuppression regimens. As the most effective immunosuppressants, these drugs prevent a cell-mediated attack against the transplanted organ (Fig. 13-13). These drugs do not cause bone marrow suppression or alterations of the normal inflammatory response. They are generally used in combination with corticosteroids, mycophenolate mofetil, and sirolimus. Tacrolimus is the most widely used calcineurin inhibitor. Cyclosporine is being used less frequently.

Many of the side effects of calcineurin inhibitors are dose related. These drugs are potentially nephrotoxic. Drug levels are monitored closely to prevent toxicity.

DRUG ALERT Tacrolimus and Cyclosporine

- A substance in grapefruit and grapefruit juice prevents metabolism of these drugs.
- Consuming grapefruit or grapefruit juice while using these drugs could increase their toxicity.

Mycophenolate Mofetil. Mycophenolate mofetil inhibits purine synthesis with suppressive effects on T and B cells. The major limitation of this drug is its GI toxicities, including nausea, vomiting, and diarrhea. In many cases the side effects can be diminished by lowering the dose or giving smaller doses more frequently.

DRUG ALERT Mycophenolate Mofetil

- When given IV, it must be reconstituted in D_5W and no other solution.
- Do not give as IV bolus. Administer over 2 or more hours.

Sirolimus. Sirolimus is an immunosuppressive agent that suppresses T cell activation and proliferation. It is used in combination with corticosteroids, cyclosporine, and/or tacrolimus.

Monoclonal Antibodies. Monoclonal antibodies are used for preventing and treating acute rejection episodes. Muromonab-CD3 was the first of these monoclonal antibodies to be used in clinical transplantation. It is a mouse monoclonal antibody that binds with the CD3 antigen found on the surface of human thymocytes and mature T cells. It interferes with the function of T cells, the pivotal cells involved in rejection. It is administered via IV bolus. All T cells are affected, rather than just the subset active in graft rejection. Within minutes after the initial infusion of muromonab-CD3, the number of circulating T cells decreases significantly.

A flu-like syndrome occurs during the first few days of treatment because of cytokine release. Side effects include fever, rigors, headache, myalgias, and various GI disturbances. To reduce the expected side effects of muromonab-CD3, give patients acetaminophen (Tylenol), diphenhydramine

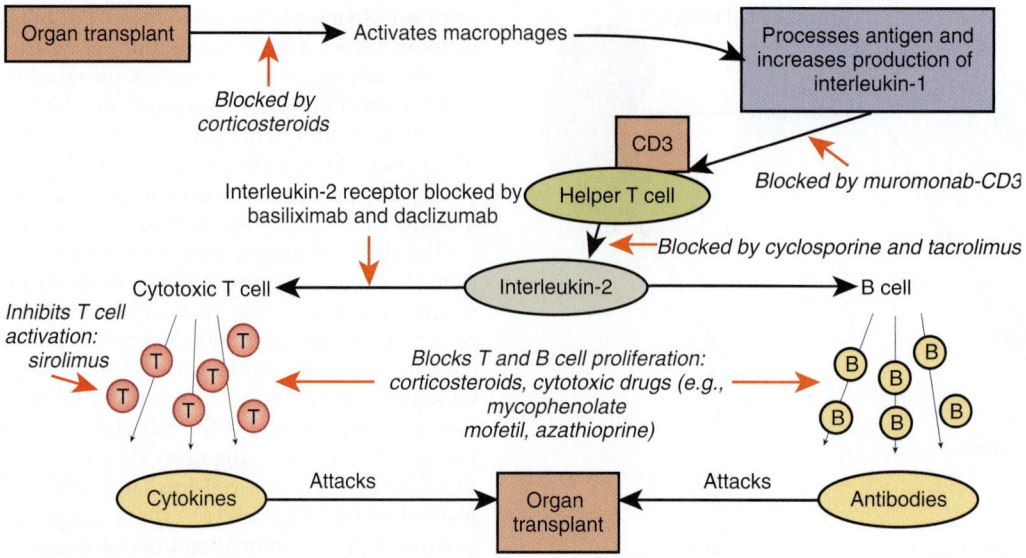

FIG. 13-13 Sites of action for immunosuppressive agents. (Adapted from McKenry L, Tessier E, Hogan M: *Mosby's pharmacology in nursing,* St Louis, 2006, Mosby.)

(Benadryl), and IV methylprednisolone before administering the dose.

Newer-generation monoclonal antibodies are a hybrid of mouse and human antibodies and have fewer side effects than muromonab-CD3 because they have been "humanized." These include daclizumab (Zenapax) and basiliximab (Simulect), which target the IL-2 receptor and impair lymphocyte proliferation. Another monoclonal antibody is alemtuzumab (Campath), which targets the CD52 antigen found on T and B cells, monocytes, and macrophages. It can cause prolonged T cell depletion.

Polyclonal Antibodies. Polyclonal antibodies to T cells include horse antithymocyte globulin (Atgam) and rabbit antithymocyte globulin (Thymoglobulin, ATG). These agents are derived by injecting animals (rabbit or horse) with human lymphoid cells, then harvesting and purifying the resultant antibody. They have been commonly used for induction immunosuppression and treatment of acute rejection.

Allergic reactions to the foreign proteins from the host animal, manifested by fever, arthralgias, and tachycardia, are common but usually not severe enough to preclude use. These side effects can be decreased by administering the preparation slowly, over 4 to 6 hours, and premedicating patients with acetaminophen, diphenhydramine, and methylprednisolone. The main toxicities of polyclonal antibodies are leukopenia and thrombocytopenia caused by antibody contaminants that are not completely removed during preparation of the antibodies.

GRAFT-VERSUS-HOST DISEASE

Graft-versus-host disease (GVHD) occurs when an immunoincompetent (immunodeficient) patient receives immunocompetent cells. A GVHD response is most commonly seen in hematopoietic stem cell transplants. In most transplantation situations, the biggest concern is the patient's (host's) rejection of the organ or transplant. However, in GVHD disease, the graft (donated tissue) rejects the host (recipient) tissue.[15]

The GVHD response may begin 7 to 30 days after transplantation. Once the reaction is started, little can be done to modify its course. The exact mechanism involved in this reaction is not completely understood. However, it involves donor T cells attacking and destroying vulnerable host (recipient) cells.

The target organs for the GVHD phenomenon are the skin, liver, and GI tract. The skin disease may be a maculopapular rash, which may be pruritic or painful. It initially involves the palms and soles of the feet but can progress to a generalized erythema with bullous formation and desquamation (shedding of the outer layer of skin). The liver disease may range from mild jaundice with elevated liver enzymes to hepatic coma. The GI manifestations may include mild to severe diarrhea, severe abdominal pain, GI bleeding, and malabsorption.

The biggest problem with GVHD is infection, with different types of infections seen in different periods. Bacterial and fungal infections predominate immediately after transplantation when granulocytopenia exists. The development of interstitial pneumonitis is the primary concern later in the course of the disease.

There is no adequate treatment of GVHD once it is established. Although corticosteroids are often used, they enhance the susceptibility to infection. The use of immunosuppressive agents (e.g., methotrexate, cyclosporine) has been most effective as a preventive rather than a treatment measure. Radiation of blood products before they are administered is another measure to prevent T cell replication.

TABLE 13-16 Drug Therapy

Immunosuppressive Therapy

Agent	Route	Mechanism of Action	Side Effects
Corticosteroids			
prednisone, methylprednisolone (Solu-Medrol)	PO, IV	Suppress inflammatory response. Inhibit cytokine production (IL-1, IL-6, TNF) and T cell activation and proliferation	Peptic ulcers, hypertension, osteoporosis, Na^+ and H_2O retention, muscle weakness, easy bruising, delayed healing, hyperglycemia, ↑ risk for infection
Calcineurin Inhibitors			
cyclosporine (Sandimmune, Neoral, Gengraf)	PO, IV	Acts on T helper cells to prevent production and release of IL-2. Inhibits proliferation of T and B cells	Nephrotoxicity, ↑ risk for infection, neurotoxicity (tremors, seizures), hepatotoxicity, lymphoma, hypertension, tremors, hirsutism, leukopenia, gingival hyperplasia
tacrolimus (Prograf)	PO, IV	Same as cyclosporine but more effective	Same as cyclosporine
Cytotoxic (Antiproliferative) Drugs			
mycophenolate mofetil (CellCept, Myfortic)	PO, IV	Inhibits purine synthesis. Suppresses proliferation of T and B cells	Diarrhea, nausea and vomiting, neutropenia, thrombocytopenia, ↑ risk for infection, ↑ incidence of malignancies
azathioprine (Imuran)	PO, IV	Inhibits purine synthesis. Suppresses proliferation of T and B cells	Bone marrow suppression (neutropenia, anemia, thrombocytopenia)
cyclophosphamide (Cytoxan, Neosar)	PO, IV	Cross-links DNA, leading to cell injury and death. Results in decrease in number and activity of T and B cells	Neutropenia, hemorrhagic cystitis
sirolimus (Rapamune)	PO	Binds to mechanistic target of rapamycin (mTOR), thereby suppressing T cell activation and proliferation	↑ Risk for infection, leukopenia, anemia, thrombocytopenia, hyperlipidemia, hypercholesterolemia, arthralgias, diarrhea. ↑ incidence of malignancies
everolimus (Zortress)	PO	Same as above	Peripheral edema, constipation, hypertension, nausea, anemia, urinary tract infection, hyperlipidemia
Monoclonal Antibodies			
muromonab-CD3 (Orthoclone OKT3)	IV push	Monoclonal antibody that binds to CD3 receptors on T cells, causing cell lysis. Inhibits function of T cells	Fever, chills, dyspnea, chest pain, nausea and vomiting Anaphylactic reactions include pulmonary edema, cardiac or respiratory arrest.
daclizumab (Zenapax)	IV	Monoclonal antibody that targets IL-2 receptor and inhibits T cell activation and proliferation	Can cause acute hypersensitivity reaction, including anaphylaxis
basiliximab (Simulect)	IV	Same as daclizumab	Same as daclizumab
alemtuzumab (Campath)	IV	Monoclonal antibody that targets the CD52 antigen on T and B cells, monocytes, and macrophages. Causes prolonged T cell depletion	Fever, chills, dyspnea, chest pain, nausea and vomiting. Neutropenia, anemia, thrombocytopenia Increased risk of opportunistic infections
Polyclonal Antibodies			
Horse antithymocyte globulin (Atgam) Rabbit antithymocyte globulin (Thymoglobulin, ATG)	IV	Prepared by immunizing horse or rabbit with human thymocyctes or T cells. Polyclonal antibodies directed against T cells, thus depleting them	Fever, chills, dyspnea, myalgia, chest pain, nausea and vomiting, anaphylaxis, leukopenia, thrombocytopenia, rash, ↑ risk for infection
Other			
belatacept (Nulojix)	IV	Prevents the activation of T cells	Anemia, diarrhea, constipation, urinary tract infection, peripheral edema

IL, Interleukin; *TNF*, tumor necrosis factor.

BRIDGE TO NCLEX EXAMINATION

The number of the question corresponds to the same-numbered outcome at the beginning of the chapter.

1. The function of monocytes in immunity is related to their ability to
   a. stimulate the production of T and B lymphocytes.
   b. produce antibodies on exposure to foreign substances.
   c. bind antigens and stimulate natural killer cell activation.
   d. capture antigens by phagocytosis and present them to lymphocytes.
2. One function of cell-mediated immunity is
   a. formation of antibodies.
   b. activation of the complement system.
   c. surveillance for malignant cell changes.
   d. opsonization of antigens to allow phagocytosis by neutrophils.
3. The reason newborns are protected for the first 6 months of life from bacterial infections is because of the maternal transmission of
   a. IgG.
   b. IgA.
   c. IgM.
   d. IgE.
4. In a type I hypersensitivity reaction the primary immunologic disorder appears to be
   a. binding of IgG to an antigen on a cell surface.
   b. deposit of antigen-antibody complexes in small vessels.
   c. release of cytokines used to interact with specific antigens.
   d. release of chemical mediators from IgE-bound mast cells and basophils.

5. The nurse is alerted to possible anaphylactic shock immediately after a patient has received IM penicillin by the development of
   a. edema and itching at the injection site.
   b. sneezing and itching of the nose and eyes.
   c. a wheal-and-flare reaction at the injection site.
   d. chest tightness and production of thick sputum.
6. The nurse advises a friend who asks him to administer his allergy shots that
   a. it is illegal for nurses to administer injections outside of a medical setting.
   b. he is qualified to do it if the friend has epinephrine in an injectable syringe provided with his extract.
   c. avoiding the allergens is a more effective way of controlling allergies, and allergy shots are not usually effective.
   d. immunotherapy should only be administered in a setting where emergency equipment and drugs are available.
7. Association between HLA antigens and diseases is *most* commonly found in what disease conditions?
   a. Malignancies
   b. Infectious diseases
   c. Neurologic diseases
   d. Autoimmune disorders
8. A patient is undergoing plasmapheresis for treatment of systemic lupus erythematosus. The nurse explains that plasmapheresis is used in her treatment to
   a. remove T lymphocytes in her blood that are producing antinuclear antibodies.
   b. remove normal particles in her blood that are being damaged by autoantibodies.
   c. exchange her plasma that contains antinuclear antibodies with a substitute fluid.
   d. replace viral-damaged cellular components of her blood with replacement whole blood.
9. The *most* common cause of secondary immunodeficiencies is
   a. drugs.
   b. stress.
   c. malnutrition.
   d. human immunodeficiency virus.
10. What accurately describes rejection following transplantation?
   a. Hyperacute rejection can be treated with OKT3.
   b. Acute rejection can be treated with sirolimus or tacrolimus.
   c. Chronic rejection can be treated with tacrolimus or cyclosporine.
   d. Hyperacute reaction can usually be avoided if crossmatching is done before the transplantation.
11. In a person having an acute rejection of a transplanted kidney, what would help the nurse understand the course of events *(select all that apply)*?
   a. A new transplant should be considered.
   b. Acute rejection can be treated with OKT3.
   c. Acute rejection usually leads to chronic rejection.
   d. Corticosteroids are the most successful drugs used to treat acute rejection.
   e. Acute rejection is common after a transplant and can be treated with drug therapy.

1. d, 2. c, 3. a, 4. d, 5. a, 6. d, 7. d, 8. c, 9. a, 10. d, 11. b, e

For rationales to these answers and even more NCLEX review questions, visit *http://evolve.elsevier.com/Lewis/medsurg.*

EVOLVE WEBSITE

http://evolve.elsevier.com/Lewis/medsurg

Review Questions (Online Only)
Key Points
Answer Key for Questions
- Rationales for Bridge to NCLEX Examination Questions

Conceptual Care Map Creator
Audio Glossary
Supporting Media
- Animations
  - Antibodies and Antigens
  - Vaccination

Content Updates

REFERENCES

1. Sparber F: Langerhans cells: an update, *J Dtsch Dermatol Ges* 12(12):1107, 2014.
2. Pritz T, Weinberger B, Grubeck-Loebenstein B: The aging bone marrow and its impact on immune responses in old age, *Immunol Lett* 162(1 Pt B): 310, 2014.
3. Moore LE, Kemp AM, Kemp SF: Recognition, treatment, and prevention of anaphylaxis, *Immunol Allergy Clin North Am* 35(2):363, 2015.
4. Simmons S: Taking the bite out of food allergies, *Nursing* 44(12):44, 2014.
5. Vacca VM, McMahon-Bowen E: Anaphylaxis, *Nursing* 43(11):16, 2013.
6. Yunker NS, Wagner BJ: A pharmacologic review of anaphylaxis, *Plast Surg Nurs* 34(4):183, 2014.
7. Lee S, Nolte H, Benninger MS: Clinical considerations in the use of sublingual immunotherapy for allergic rhinitis, *Am J Rhinol Allergy* 29(2):106, 2015.
8. Compalati E, Braido F, Walter Canonica G: Sublingual immunotherapy: recent advances, *Allergol Int* 62(4):415, 2013.
9. Latex allergies. Retrieved from *www.webmd.com/allergies/latex-allergies.*
10. Preventing allergic reactions to natural rubber latex in the workplace. Retrieved from *http://www.cdc.gov/niosh/docs/97-135/pdfs/97-135.pdf.*
11. Multiple chemical sensitivity. Retrieved from *www.webmd.com/allergies/multiple-chemical-sensitivity.*
12. United Network of Organ Sharing (UNOS). Retrieved from *www.unos.org.*
13. Uniform Anatomical Gift Act. Retrieved from *http://uniformlaws.org/Act.aspx?title=Anatomical%20Gift%20Act.*
14. Immunosuppression. Retrieved from *http://emedicine.medscape.com/article/432316-overview.*
15. Flowers ME, Martin PJ: How we treat chronic graft-versus-host disease, *Blood* 125(4):606, 2015.

14

Infection and Human Immunodeficiency Virus Infection

Jeffrey Kwong

Do not allow the pain of loss to stop the process of living.

Trent Thomas

http://evolve.elsevier.com/Lewis/medsurg/

LEARNING OUTCOMES

1. Evaluate the impact of emerging and reemerging infections on health care.
2. Identify appropriate interventions to reduce health care-associated infections (HAIs).
3. Explain the ways human immunodeficiency virus (HIV) is transmitted and factors that affect transmission.
4. Describe the pathophysiology of HIV infection.
5. Chart the spectrum of untreated HIV infection.
6. Identify the diagnostic criteria for acquired immunodeficiency syndrome (AIDS).
7. Describe methods used to test for HIV infection.
8. Discuss the interprofessional management of HIV infection.
9. Summarize the characteristics of opportunistic diseases associated with AIDS.
10. Describe the potential complications associated with long-term treatment of HIV infection.
11. Compare and contrast HIV prevention methods.
12. Describe the nursing management of HIV-infected patients and HIV-at-risk patients.

KEY TERMS

acquired immunodeficiency syndrome (AIDS), p. 221
antiretroviral therapy (ART), p. 219
emerging infection, p. 215
health care–associated infections (HAIs), p. 217
human immunodeficiency virus (HIV), p. 218
opportunistic diseases, p. 219
postexposure prophylaxis (PEP), p. 226
preexposure prophylaxis (PrEP) p. 223
reverse transcriptase, p. 219
standard precautions, p. 218
transmission-based precautions, p. 218
viral load, p. 220
window period, p. 222

This chapter presents a brief overview of emerging and health care–associated infections (HAIs). In addition, this chapter provides a comprehensive discussion of human immunodeficiency virus (HIV) infection, focusing on transmission, pathophysiology, interprofessional care, and nursing management.

INFECTIONS

Infections, such as lower respiratory tract infections, malaria, HIV, and tuberculosis (TB), are responsible for a significant number of deaths worldwide. Infection occurs when a *pathogen* (a microorganism that causes disease) invades the body, begins to multiply, and produces disease, usually causing harm to the host. The signs and symptoms of infection are a result of specific pathogen activity, which triggers inflammation and other immune responses.

Infections can be categorized as localized, disseminated, or systemic. A *localized* infection is limited to a small area. A *disseminated* infection has spread to areas of the body beyond the initial site of infection. *Systemic* infections have spread extensively throughout the body, often via the blood.

TYPES OF PATHOGENS

The many different kinds of pathogens can be classified into several groups, including bacteria, viruses, fungi, protozoa, and prions. *Bacteria* are one-celled organisms that are common throughout nature. Many bacteria are normal flora. They live harmoniously in or on the human body without causing disease under normal circumstances. Normal flora protect the human body by preventing the overgrowth of other microorganisms. For example, *Escherichia coli* is a bacteria that is part of the normal flora in the large intestine.

Bacteria cause disease in two ways: by entering the body and growing inside human cells (e.g., TB) or by secreting toxins that damage cells (e.g., *Staphylococcus aureus*). Bacteria are divided into categories based on the shape of their cells. *Cocci*, such as streptococci and staphylococci, are round. *Bacilli* are rod shaped

Reviewed by Suzanne Jed, MSN, FNP-BC, Senior Clinical Technical Advisor, International Training and Education Center for Health (I-TECH) South Africa, University of Washington, Pretoria, South Africa; Allison J. Terry, RN, PhD, Associate Professor of Nursing, Assistant Dean of Clinical Practice, School of Nursing, Auburn University Montgomery, Montgomery, Alabama; and Daniel Worrall, MSN, ANP-BC, Nurse Practitioner, Massachusetts General Hospital, Boston, Massachusetts.

TABLE 14-1 Disease-Causing Bacteria

Bacteria	Diseases Caused
Chlamydia trachomatis	Chlamydia, lymphogranuloma venereum
Clostridia	
• *Clostridium botulinum*	Food poisoning with progressive muscle paralysis
• *Clostridium tetani*	Tetanus (lockjaw)
Corynebacterium diphtheriae	Diphtheria
Escherichia coli	Urinary tract infections, peritonitis, hemolytic-uremic syndrome
Haemophilus	
• *Haemophilus influenzae*	Nasopharyngitis, meningitis, pneumonia
• *Haemophilus pertussis*	Pertussis (whooping cough)
Helicobacter pylori	Peptic ulcers, gastritis
Klebsiella-Enterobacter organisms	Urinary tract infections, peritonitis, pneumonia
Legionella pneumophila	Pneumonia (Legionnaires' disease)
Mycobacteria	
• *Mycobacterium leprae*	Hansen's disease (leprosy)
• *Mycobacterium tuberculosis*	Tuberculosis
Neisseriae	
• *Neisseria gonorrhoeae*	Gonorrhea, pelvic inflammatory disease, proctitis
• *Neisseria meningitidis*	Meningococcemia, meningitis
Proteus species	Urinary tract infections, peritonitis
Pseudomonas aeruginosa	Urinary tract infections, meningitis
Salmonella	
• *Salmonella typhi*	Typhoid fever
• Other *Salmonella* organisms	Food poisoning, gastroenteritis
Shigella	Shigellosis; diarrhea, abdominal pain, and fever (dysentery)
Staphylococcus aureus	Skin infections, pneumonia, urinary tract infections, acute osteomyelitis, toxic shock syndrome
Streptococci	
• *Streptococcus faecalis*	Genitourinary infection, infection of surgical wounds
• *Streptococcus pneumoniae*	Pneumococcal pneumonia
• *Streptococcus pyogenes* (group A β-hemolytic streptococci)	Pharyngitis, scarlet fever, rheumatic fever, acute glomerulonephritis, erysipelas, pneumonia
• *S. pyogenes* (group B β-hemolytic streptococci)	Urinary tract infections
• *Streptococcus viridans*	Bacterial endocarditis
Treponema pallidum	Syphilis

TABLE 14-2 Disease-Causing Viruses

Virus	Diseases Caused
Adenoviruses	Upper respiratory tract infection, pneumonia
Arbovirus	Syndrome of fever, malaise, headache, myalgia; aseptic meningitis; encephalitis
Coronavirus	Upper respiratory tract infection
Coxsackieviruses A and B	Upper respiratory tract infection, gastroenteritis, acute myocarditis, aseptic meningitis
Ebola	Hemorrhagic fever
Echoviruses	Upper respiratory tract infection, gastroenteritis, aseptic meningitis
Hepatitis A, B, C	Viral hepatitis
Herpesviruses	
• Cytomegalovirus (CMV)	Gastroenteritis; pneumonia and retinal damage in immunosuppressed individuals, infectious mononucleosis-like syndrome
• Epstein-Barr	Mononucleosis, Burkitt's lymphoma (possibly)
• Herpes simplex type 1	Herpes labialis ("fever blisters"), genital herpes infection
• Herpes simplex type 2	Genital herpes infection
• Varicella-zoster	Chickenpox, shingles
Human immunodeficiency virus (HIV)	HIV infection, AIDS
Influenza A and B	Upper respiratory tract infection, H1N1 (swine) flu, H5N1 avian (bird) flu
Mumps	Parotitis, orchitis in postpubertal males
Papillomavirus	Genital warts, cervical and anal cancer
Parainfluenza 1-4	Upper respiratory tract infection
Parvovirus	Gastroenteritis
Poliovirus	Poliomyelitis
Pox viruses	Smallpox, Molluscum contagiosum
Reoviruses 1, 2, 3	Upper respiratory tract infection
Respiratory syncytial virus	Gastroenteritis, respiratory tract infection
Rhabdovirus	Rabies
Rhinovirus	Upper respiratory tract infection, pneumonia
Rotaviruses	Gastroenteritis
Rubella	German measles
Rubeola	Measles
West Nile virus	Flu-like symptoms, meningitis, encephalitis

and include tetanus and TB. *Curved rods* include *Vibrio* bacteria, one of which causes cholera. *Spirochetes* are spiral shaped and include the organisms that cause leprosy and syphilis. Table 14-1 lists common bacteria that cause disease.

Viruses, unlike bacteria, do not have a cellular structure. They are simple infectious particles that consist of a small amount of genetic material (either ribonucleic acid [RNA] or deoxyribonucleic acid [DNA]) and a protein envelope. Viruses can reproduce only after releasing their genetic material into the cell of another living organism. Examples of diseases caused by viruses are presented in Table 14-2.

Fungi are organisms similar to plants, but they lack chlorophyll. *Mycosis* is any disease caused by a fungus. Pathogenic fungi cause infections that are usually localized but can become disseminated in an immunocompromised person. Tinea pedis (athlete's foot) and tinea corporis (ringworm) are two common mycotic infections. Some fungi are normal flora in the body, but when overgrowth occurs, disease can result. Overgrowth of *Candida albicans,* for example, can cause candidiasis in the mouth (thrush), esophagus, intestines, and vagina. Other fungi and their respective mycotic infections are listed in Table 14-3.

Protozoa are single-cell, animal-like microorganisms. Protozoa normally live in soil and bodies of water. When introduced into the human body, they can cause infection. Amoebic dysentery and giardiasis are caused by protozoal parasites. Malaria is caused by a sporozoa called *Plasmodium malariae.*

Prions are infectious particles that contain abnormally shaped proteins. Not all prions cause disease, but those that do

TABLE 14-3 Disease-Causing Fungi

Fungi	Diseases Caused	Organs Affected
Aspergillus fumigatus	Aspergillosis Otomycosis	Lungs* Ears
Blastomyces dermatitidis	Blastomycosis	Lungs, various organs
Candida albicans	Candidiasis	Intestines
	Vaginitis	Vagina
	Thrush	Skin,† mouth
Coccidioides immitis	Coccidioidomycosis	Lungs*
Pneumocystis jiroveci	Pneumocystis pneumonia (PCP)	Lungs*
Sporothrix schenckii	Sporotrichosis	Skin, lymph vessels
Trichophyton	Tinea pedis	Skin†
Microsporum	Tinea capitis	Skin†
Epidermophyton	Tinea corporis	Skin†

*See Table 27-14: Fungal Infections of the Lung.
†See Table 23-7: Common Fungal Infections of the Skin.

typically affect the nervous system. They can cause a group of illnesses called *transmissible spongiform encephalopathies (TSEs).* Examples of TSEs are Creutzfeldt-Jakob disease and bovine spongiform encephalopathy in cattle (also known as mad cow disease).

EMERGING INFECTIONS

An **emerging infection** is an infectious disease that has recently increased in incidence or that threatens to increase in the immediate future.[1] Examples of emerging infections are described in Table 14-4. Emerging infectious diseases can originate from unknown sources or from contact with animals, changes in known diseases, or biologic warfare. For example, severe acute respiratory syndrome (SARS) and the West Nile virus come from animal sources. Others emerged when a previously treatable organism (e.g., *S. aureus*) developed resistance to antibiotics.

The battle against infection is not new, but modern technologies have changed the rules of the game. Global travel, population density, encroachment into new environments, misuse of antibiotics, and bioterrorism have increased the risk for widespread distribution of emerging infections.

Additionally, some diseases thought to be under control, such as TB, measles, and pertussis, have reemerged.[2] Newer infections have also been identified, such as Middle Eastern Respiratory Syndrome (MERS), SARS, Ebola virus, Chikungunya (a self-limiting viral illness causing flu-like symptoms seen in Africa, Asia, and more recently the Caribbean), and influenza A (H1N1) virus.

Studies in *zoonosis* (science of transmission of diseases from animals to humans) have shown that many known infectious diseases come from animal and insect vectors. The SARS outbreak in China in 2003, for instance, was linked to the civet cat, a small carnivorous mammal found throughout much of Asia and Africa. (SARS is discussed in Chapter 67.)

West Nile virus is carried and transmitted by mosquitoes. Mosquitoes acquire the virus as they draw blood from infected animals and people. The virus does not cause illness in the mosquito but can be transferred to uninfected animals and humans as the mosquito continues to feed. Bird deaths are an early warning sign of a West Nile virus outbreak, which can spread quickly if action is not taken in a timely manner. (West Nile virus is discussed in Chapter 56.)

TABLE 14-4 Emerging Infections

Microorganism	Related Disease
Bacteria	
Borrelia burgdorferi	Lyme disease
Campylobacter jejuni	Diarrhea
Escherichia coli O157:H7	Hemorrhagic colitis, hemolytic-uremic syndrome
Helicobacter pylori	Peptic ulcer disease
Legionella pneumophila	Pneumonia (Legionnaires' disease)
Vibrio cholerae 0139	New strain associated with epidemic cholera
Virus	
Chikungunya	Fever, muscle aches, rash
Ebola virus	Ebola hemorrhagic fever
H1N1	H1N1 (swine) flu
Hantavirus	Hemorrhagic fever associated with severe pulmonary syndrome
Hepatitis C virus	Parenterally transmitted hepatitis
Hepatitis E virus	Enterically transmitted hepatitis
Human immunodeficiency virus (HIV)	HIV infection and AIDS
Human herpesvirus 6 (HHV-6)	Roseola subitum
Human herpesvirus 8 (HHV-8)	Associated with Kaposi sarcoma in immunosuppressed patients, including people with HIV infection
West Nile virus	West Nile fever
Zika virus	Fever, rash, muscle aches; possible microcephaly in children born to infected mothers
Parasite	
Cryptosporidium parvum	Acute and chronic diarrhea

Influenza viruses are examples of how disease can spread between animals and humans. Variants of influenza A viruses were responsible for influenza epidemics. These include the 2009 influenza A (H1N1) outbreak that was traced back to pigs, hence the name *swine flu.* In 1997 and 2003 outbreaks of the influenza A (H5N1) strain of avian flu resulted from transmission of influenza virus from chickens to humans.

Ebola virus has presented an ongoing challenge to public health since it was first seen in 1976. In 2014, rates of Ebola increased significantly in East Africa, and the first cases of Ebola were seen in the United States. These initial cases were primarily from travelers or medical aid workers who were working in Africa. Ebola virus can cause severe hemorrhagic fever and is usually lethal. Therapeutic and preventive measures are limited. The natural reservoir and path of transmission are unknown, which makes it impossible to effectively combat Ebola virus and the disease it causes.

Reemerging Infections

Advances in the development of medications and vaccines has led to the near eradication of some infections (e.g., smallpox, polio), but infective agents can reemerge under the right conditions. Table 14-5 presents some diseases that have shown resurgence in recent decades.[3] For example, there have been outbreaks and the resurgence of vaccine-preventable infections such as measles and pertussis in recent years. This is in part due to people not receiving recommended preventive vaccines.

International travel has created a new obstacle for the local eradication of diseases. For example, measles is no longer

TABLE 14-5 Reemerging Infections

Microorganism	Infection	Description
Bacteria		
Corynebacterium diphtheriae	Diphtheria	Localized infection of mucous membranes or skin
Bordetella pertussis	Pertussis	Acute, highly contagious respiratory disease characterized by loud whooping inspiration. Also known as whooping cough
Mycobacterium tuberculosis	Tuberculosis	Chronic infection transmitted by inhalation of infected droplets (see Chapter 27)
Virus		
Dengue viruses (flaviviruses)	Dengue fever	Acute infection transmitted by mosquitoes and occurring mainly in tropical and subtropical regions
Rubeola	Measles	Fever, malaise, cough, and maculopapular rash
Parasite		
Giardia	Giardiasis	Diarrheal illness that usually originates in water contaminated with fecal matter. Also known as traveler's diarrhea

TABLE 14-6 Common Antibiotic-Resistant Organisms and Treatment

Bacteria	Resistant to	Preferred Treatment
Staphylococcus aureus	methicillin*	vancomycin
Staphylococcus epidermidis	methicillin*	vancomycin
Enterococcus faecalis	vancomycin streptomycin gentamicin	penicillin G or ampicillin
Enterococcus faecium	vancomycin streptomycin gentamicin	penicillin G or ampicillin
Streptococcus pneumoniae	penicillin G	ceftriaxone (Rocephin) cefotaxime (Claforan)
Klebsiella pneumoniae	Third-generation cephalosporins (e.g., ceftazidime [Ceptaz, Fortaz])	imipenem and cilastatin (Primaxin) meropenem (Merrem IV)
Neisseria gonorrheae	Third-generation cephalosporins (e.g., cefixime and ceftriaxone)	gemifloxacin/ gentamicin plus azithromycin

*This drug is no longer available in the United States.

considered endemic in the United States but remains a leading cause of death in developing countries. Domestic outbreaks have typically occurred in areas with low vaccination rates. Some cases have been found in people who have recently traveled to measles-endemic areas outside the United States.[4]

Antimicrobial-Resistant Organisms

Resistance occurs when pathogenic organisms change in ways that decrease the ability of a drug (or a family of drugs) to treat disease.[5] Microorganisms can become resistant to classic treatments (e.g., penicillin) as well as to newer antibiotics and antiviral agents. Microorganisms are highly adaptable. They have evolved genetic and biochemical mechanisms to defend against antimicrobials. Genetic mechanisms include mutation and acquisition of new DNA or RNA. Biochemically, bacteria can resist antibiotics by producing enzymes that destroy or inactivate the drugs. Drug target sites are then altered so that the antibiotic cannot bind to or enter the bacteria. If the drug cannot enter the cell, it cannot kill the bacteria. Table 14-6 describes common antibiotic-resistant bacteria.

Methicillin-resistant *S. aureus* (MRSA), vancomycin-resistant enterococci (VRE), vancomycin-resistant *S. aureus* (VRSA), carbapenem-resistant enterobacteriaceae (CRE), and penicillin-resistant *Streptococcus pneumoniae* are examples of emerging strains of antibiotic-resistant organisms. These drug-resistant bacteria were initially seen primarily in health care settings but are becoming more prevalent in the community. For example, MRSA, a form of *S. aureus* that does not respond to methicillin- or penicillin-based therapies, was initially considered a health care–associated infection (HA-MRSA). However, a variant strain of MRSA that is primarily acquired in the community (community-acquired MRSA [CA-MRSA]) has emerged. This strain of MRSA is more *virulent* (able to cause disease or infection) compared with HA-MRSA.[6] CA-MRSA has been known to cause rapidly forming skin infections and systemic diseases, including pneumonia and sepsis. Rates of CA-MRSA infections appear to be on the rise. Conversely, there has been a reduction in HA-MRSA with the use of strict infection control measures in health care settings.

VRE is another antibiotic-resistant bacteria that has become a concern for patients and health care workers. VRE is more virulent than MRSA and can remain viable on environmental surfaces for weeks. Although antibiotic-resistant bacteria can infect anyone, patients who are hospitalized and those with a suppressed immune system are more likely to be exposed to these bacteria and to develop infection.

HCPs have contributed to the development of drug-resistant microorganisms by (1) administering antibiotics for viral infections, (2) succumbing to pressures from patients to prescribe unnecessary antibiotic therapy, (3) using inadequate drug regimens to treat infections, or (4) using broad-spectrum or combination agents for infections that should be treated with first-line medications.

Patients can also contribute to resistance development by (1) skipping doses, (2) not taking antibiotics for the full duration of prescribed therapy, or (3) saving unused antibiotics "in case I need them later." In addition, limited resources and access to medications make it difficult for some patients to get adequate treatment for infections. Teaching patients and their families the proper use of antibiotics (Table 14-7) is crucial to treatment success and prevention of drug-resistant pathogens. The Centers for Disease Control and Prevention (CDC), the Infectious Diseases Society of America (IDSA), and many health care organizations have been campaigning for greater vigilance in minimizing the misuse of antibiotics in reaction to this growing concern.

Although antibiotics are a class of drugs that are typically thought of when discussing drug-resistant organisms, any organism (virus, fungi, or parasite) can develop drug resistance to agents typically used to treat them. Hence, the term *antimicrobial resistance* is now used to describe the phenomena of resistance across different classes of organisms.

TABLE 14-7 Patient & Caregiver Teaching

Decrease Risk for Antibiotic-Resistant Infection

Include the following instructions when teaching patients or their caregivers how to decrease the risk for antibiotic-resistant infection.

1. Do Not Take Antibiotics to Prevent Illness (unless prescribed)

- Doing this increases your risk for developing resistant infection
- Exceptions include taking antibiotics as prescribed before certain surgeries and dental work or in the presence of immune dysfunction

2. Wash Your Hands Frequently

Hand washing is the single most important thing you can do to prevent infection.

3. Follow Directions When Taking Antibiotics

- Not taking your antibiotic as prescribed or skipping doses can allow antibiotic-resistant bacteria to develop.

4. Do Not Request an Antibiotic for Flu or Colds

- If your HCP says that you do not need an antibiotic, chances are you do not.
- Antibiotics are effective against bacterial infections but not viruses, which cause colds and flu.

5. Finish Your Antibiotic

- Do not stop taking your antibiotic when you feel better.
- If you stop taking your antibiotic early, the hardiest bacteria survive and multiply.
- Eventually you could develop an infection resistant to many antibiotics. You should never have leftover antibiotics.

6. Do Not Take Leftover Antibiotics

- Do not save unfinished antibiotics for later use or borrow leftover drugs from family or friends.
- This is dangerous because (1) the leftover antibiotic may not be appropriate for you, (2) your illness may not be a bacterial infection, (3) old antibiotics can lose their effectiveness and in some cases can even be fatal, and (4) there will not be enough doses in a leftover bottle to provide full treatment.

HEALTH CARE–ASSOCIATED INFECTIONS

Health care–associated infections (HAIs) are infections that are acquired as a result of exposure to microorganisms in a health care setting.[7] Approximately 722,000 HAIs occur annually, and nearly 1 out of every 25 hospitalized patients has at least one HAI. Improvements in infection control have resulted in fewer infections in recent years.[8,9] In recent years there were decreases in several of the major types of HAIs, including central line–associated bloodstream infections, surgical site infections, *Clostridium difficile* infections, and methicillin-resistant *S. aureus* bacteremia. Surgical and immunocompromised patients are at highest risk. Any organism can cause HAIs, but certain bacteria, including *E. coli, S. aureus, Enterobacter aerogenes,* and various types of streptococci, are the more common culprits. Some bacteria that do not normally cause disease can cause infections in high-risk patients as a result of illness or treatment of illness.

Approximately one third of HAIs are preventable. HCPs often transmit HAIs from patient to patient through direct contact. First lines of defense to prevent the spread of HAIs include hand washing (or using an alcohol-based hand sanitizer) before and after patient contact or procedures, appropriate use of protective equipment such as gloves, and decontamination of equipment used for patient care.[10] Isolated infections can also be caused when bacteria that normally stay in one area of the body are introduced into another area. Therefore care must be taken to change gloves and wash hands when moving from one task to another, even when working with the same patient. Guidelines on reducing and controlling the spread of disease in health care settings, especially of antimicrobial-resistant organisms, have been developed and are implemented in most institutions[11,12] (Table 14-8). Nurses and all HCPs have the responsibility of using appropriate measures, including transmission-based precautions, to help protect patients from HAIs.

TABLE 14-8 OSHA Requirements for Personal Protective Equipment

The following equipment is used to minimize exposure to blood-borne pathogens.

Equipment	Indications for Use
Gloves	• Must be used when the employee can reasonably anticipate having contact with blood or other potentially infectious materials, when performing vascular access procedures, and when handling or touching contaminated items or surfaces • Gloves must be replaced if torn, punctured, or contaminated or their ability to function as a barrier is compromised.
Clothing (gowns, aprons, caps, boots)	• Must be used when occupational exposure is anticipated • The type and characteristics depend on the task and degree of exposure anticipated.
Face protection (mask and glasses with solid side shields or a chin-length face shield)	• Must be used when splashes, sprays, spatters, or droplets of blood or other potentially infectious materials pose a hazard to the eyes, nose, or mouth

Source: Occupational Safety and Health Administration: Bloodborne pathogens and needlestick prevention. Retrieved from *www.osha.gov/SLTC/bloodbornepathogens.*
NOTE: Employers must provide, make accessible, and require the use of personal protective equipment (PPE) at no cost to the employee. PPE also must be provided in appropriate sizes. Hypoallergenic gloves or similar alternatives must be made available to employees who have an allergic sensitivity to gloves.
OSHA, Occupational Safety and Health Administration.

Gerontologic Considerations: Infections in Older Adults

For older adults, the rate of HAIs is two or three times higher than for younger patients. Individuals in long-term care facilities are at special risk for HAI. Age-related changes (e.g., impaired immune function, co-morbidities such as diabetes, physical disabilities) can contribute to higher infection rates in older adults.[13]

Infections common in older adults include pneumonia, urinary tract infections, skin infections, and TB. Urinary tract infections are more common in older adults who reside in long-term care facilities. Patients with indwelling catheters are at particular risk.

Infections in older adults often have atypical manifestations, such as cognitive and behavioral changes, before the emergence of fever, pain, or alterations in laboratory values. Do not rely on the presence of fever to indicate infection in older adults, because many have lower core body temperatures and decreased immune responses. Suspicion of disease should typically begin

CHECK YOUR PRACTICE

You are working in a long-term care facility and one of your residents, a 76-yr-old man who is recovering from a stroke, seems very confused today. You discuss your concerns with the unlicensed assistive personnel (UAP), explaining that he seemed so alert yesterday and you wonder if he may have an infection, such as pneumonia or a urinary tract infection. The UAP says, "I just took his temperature and it is normal so I don't think he has an infection."

- How should you follow up with this resident and UAP?

if a patient demonstrates changes in the ability to perform daily activities or in cognitive function. In addition, underlying diseases, increased frequency of drug reactions, and institutionalization can complicate the management of an older adult with infection.

INFECTION PREVENTION AND CONTROL

Occupational Safety and Health Administration (OSHA) Guidelines

OSHA is a federal agency that protects workers from injury and illness in places of employment and supports activities that minimize or eliminate exposure to infectious materials in the workplace. OSHA mandates that any employer whose employees could be exposed to potentially infectious materials implement standard policies and procedures for protection of those employees. Employees must be provided with appropriate personal protective equipment (PPE) and safety equipment.[11] These include gloves, gowns, facial protection, and disposal systems for sharps (Table 14-8). Appropriate PPE varies depending on the situation, and you need to use sound judgment when deciding when and how to use protective equipment.

Infection Precautions

If a patient is admitted with or develops an infection that is considered a risk to others, infection precautions may need to be implemented. The CDC has established guidelines with two levels of precautions: (1) **standard precautions**, designed for the care of all patients in hospitals and health care facilities and (2) **transmission-based precautions**, designed for specific diseases.[11] The purpose of these precautions is to prevent the transmission of organisms from patients to HCPs, from HCPs to patients, from patients to other patients, and from health care personnel and patients to people outside of the hospital (Table 14-9).

The *standard precautions* system applies to (1) blood; (2) all body fluids, secretions, and excretions; (3) non-intact skin; and (4) mucous membranes. Standard precautions are designed to reduce the risk of transmission of microorganisms in hospitals. Standard precautions should be applied to *all* patients regardless of diagnosis or presumed infection status. The CDC's standard precautions incorporate all of the OSHA blood-borne pathogens standard requirements.

Transmission-based precautions are used for patients known to be or suspected of being infected with highly transmissible or epidemiologically important pathogens that require additional precautions to interrupt transmission and prevent infection. Transmission-based precautions include airborne precautions, droplet precautions, and contact precautions. *Airborne precautions* are used if the organism can cause infection over long distances when suspended in the air (e.g., TB, rubeola).

TABLE 14-9 Types of Isolation Precautions Used in Health Care Settings

Type	Examples
Standard Precautions	
• Used for care of all patients, regardless of their diagnosis or presumed infection status	Includes the use of hand washing and appropriate personal protective equipment
Transmission-Based Precautions	
• Recommended to provide additional precautions beyond standard precautions to prevent transmission of pathogens • Can be used for patients known or suspected to be infected or colonized with pathogens that can be transmitted by airborne or droplet transmission, or by contact with dry skin or contaminated surfaces • These precautions should be used in addition to standard precautions.	**Airborne Precautions:** Used for infections spread in small particles in the air such as chickenpox (varicella), measles, and tuberculosis (TB) **Droplet Precautions:** Used for infections spread in large droplets by coughing, talking, or sneezing such as influenza and bacterial meningitis **Contact Precautions:** Used for infections spread by skin-to-skin contact or contact with other surfaces such as *C. difficile*, MRSA, and VRE

Droplet precautions are used to minimize contact with pathogens that are spread through the air at close contact and that affect the respiratory system or mucous membranes (e.g., influenza, pertussis). *Contact precautions* are used to minimize the spread of pathogens that are acquired from direct or indirect contact, especially multidrug-resistant organisms (e.g., MRSA, VRE, CRE). Transmission-based precautions may be combined for diseases that have multiple routes of transmission. Whether used alone or in combination, transmission-based precautions should always be used in conjunction with standard precautions.

HUMAN IMMUNODEFICIENCY VIRUS INFECTION

Human immunodeficiency virus (HIV) is a retrovirus that causes immunosuppression. People with HIV are more susceptible to infections that are normally controlled through immune responses. The term *HIV disease* is used interchangeably with HIV infection. With advances in treatment, HIV is managed as a chronic disease, since people with the disease are living longer.

More than 1 million people are currently living with HIV in the United States, with approximately 50,000 new infections occurring each year.[14] With the availability of effective HIV treatment, there has been a dramatic drop in the number of deaths attributable to HIV.

In North America HIV is most prevalent among men who have sex with men (MSM). However, increasing numbers of new HIV infections are occurring in women, people of color, people who live in poverty, and young adults.

Transmission of HIV

HIV can be transmitted through contact with infected blood, semen, vaginal secretions, or breast milk. HIV transmission occurs through sexual intercourse with an infected partner; exposure to HIV-infected blood or blood products; and perinatal transmission during pregnancy, at delivery, or through breastfeeding. HIV is not spread casually.[15] The virus cannot be transmitted through hugging, dry kissing, shaking hands, sharing eating utensils, using toilet seats, or casual encounters in any setting. It is not spread by tears, saliva, urine, emesis, sputum, feces, sweat, respiratory droplets, or enteric routes. Health care personnel have a low risk of acquiring HIV at work, even after a needle-stick injury.[16]

Sexual Transmission. The most common mode of HIV transmission is unprotected sexual contact with an HIV-infected partner. Sexual activity involves contact with semen, vaginal secretions, and/or blood, all of which have lymphocytes that may contain HIV. During any form of sexual intercourse (anal, vaginal, or oral), the risk of infection is greater for the partner who receives the semen, although infection can also be transmitted to the inserting partner. This occurs because the receiver has prolonged contact with infected fluids, and it helps explain why it is easier to infect women than men during heterosexual intercourse. Sexual activities that cause trauma to local tissues can increase the risk of transmission. In addition, genital lesions from other sexually transmitted infections (e.g., herpes, syphilis) significantly increase the likelihood of transmission.

Contact With Blood and Blood Products. HIV can be transmitted from exposure to blood when sharing drug-using paraphernalia. Needles, syringes, straws, and other equipment may be contaminated with HIV or other blood-borne organisms, and sharing this equipment can result in disease transmission.

Routine screening of blood donors to identify at-risk individuals and testing donated blood for the presence of HIV have improved the safety of the blood supply. In countries that routinely test donated blood, HIV infection as a result of blood transfusions or hemophilia clotting factors is unlikely.

Puncture wounds are the most common means of work-related HIV transmission. The risk of infection after a needle-stick exposure to HIV-infected blood is 0.3% to 0.4% (or 3 or 4 out of 1000).[16] The risk is higher if the exposure involves blood from a patient with a high level of circulating HIV, a deep puncture wound, a needle with a hollow bore and visible blood, or a device used for venous or arterial access. Splash exposures of blood on skin with an open lesion present some risk, but it is much lower than from a puncture wound.

Perinatal Transmission. Perinatal transmission from an HIV-infected mother to her infant can occur during pregnancy, delivery, or breastfeeding. On average, 25% of infants born to women with untreated HIV infection are born with HIV. Fortunately, the risk of transmission can be reduced to less than 2% in settings in which pregnant women are routinely tested for HIV infection and, if found to be infected, treated with **antiretroviral therapy (ART)**, a combination of medication used to control and suppress HIV replication.[17,18]

Pathophysiology

HIV is an RNA virus. RNA viruses are called *retroviruses* because they replicate in a "backward" manner (going from RNA to DNA). Like all viruses, HIV cannot replicate unless it is inside a living cell.[19] The *CD4⁺ T cell (CD4 cell)*, a type of lymphocyte, is the target cell for HIV. HIV enters the CD4⁺ T cell by binding to protein receptors on the outside of the cell (Fig. 14-1). This process is known as *fusion* (Fig. 14-2).

Once HIV is attached and fused with the CD4⁺ T cell, HIV RNA enters the CD4⁺ T cell. This triggers the release of **reverse transcriptase**, an enzyme that transforms HIV RNA into a single strand of DNA. This strand copies itself, becoming

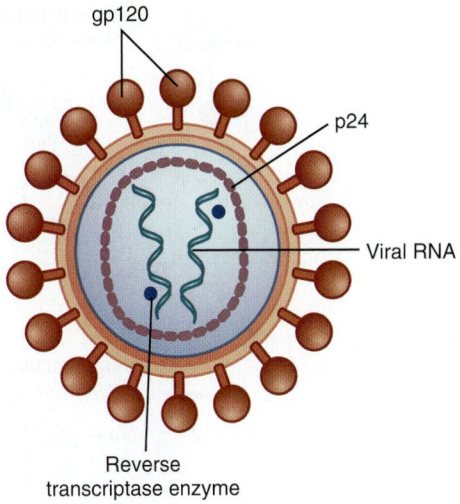

FIG. 14-1 HIV is surrounded by an envelope made up of proteins (including gp120) and contains a core of viral RNA and proteins.

double-stranded viral DNA. Another enzyme, called *integrase*, allows the newly formed double-stranded DNA to integrate itself into the host's genetic structure. This action has two consequences: (1) because all genetic material is replicated during cell division, all daughter cells are also infected and (2) viral DNA in the genome directs the cell to make new HIV.

Protease, another enzyme involved in the replication process, cleaves the newly formed strands of HIV genetic material into smaller pieces. New HIV virions are then formed and released. The CD4⁺ T cell is then destroyed after the HIV virions are released.[19]

HIV destroys about 1 billion CD4⁺ T cells every day. For many years the body can produce new CD4⁺ T cells to replace the destroyed cells. However, over time the ability of HIV to destroy CD4⁺ T cells exceeds the body's ability to replace the cells. The decline in the CD4⁺ T cell count impairs immune function. Generally, the immune system remains healthy with more than 500 CD4⁺ T cells/μL. Immune problems begin to occur when the count drops below 500 CD4⁺ T cells/μL. Severe problems develop with fewer than 200 CD4⁺ T cells/μL.

With HIV, a point is eventually reached where so many CD4⁺ T cells have been destroyed that not enough are left to regulate immune responses (Fig. 14-3). This allows **opportunistic diseases** (infections and cancers that occur in immunosuppressed patients) to develop. Opportunistic diseases are the main cause of disease, disability, and death in patients with HIV infection.

Clinical Manifestations and Complications

The typical course of untreated HIV infection follows the pattern shown in Fig. 14-4. It is important to remember that (1) disease progression is highly individualized, (2) treatment can significantly alter this pattern, and (3) an individual's prognosis is unpredictable.

Acute Infection. Approximately 2 to 4 weeks after someone becomes newly infected with HIV, individuals typically experience *acute HIV infection*, a period when people can have a mononucleosis-like syndrome of fever, swollen lymph nodes, sore throat, headache, malaise, nausea, muscle and joint pain, diarrhea, and/or a diffuse rash. Some people also develop neurologic complications, such as aseptic meningitis, peripheral neuropathy, facial palsy, or Guillain-Barré syndrome.[20] During

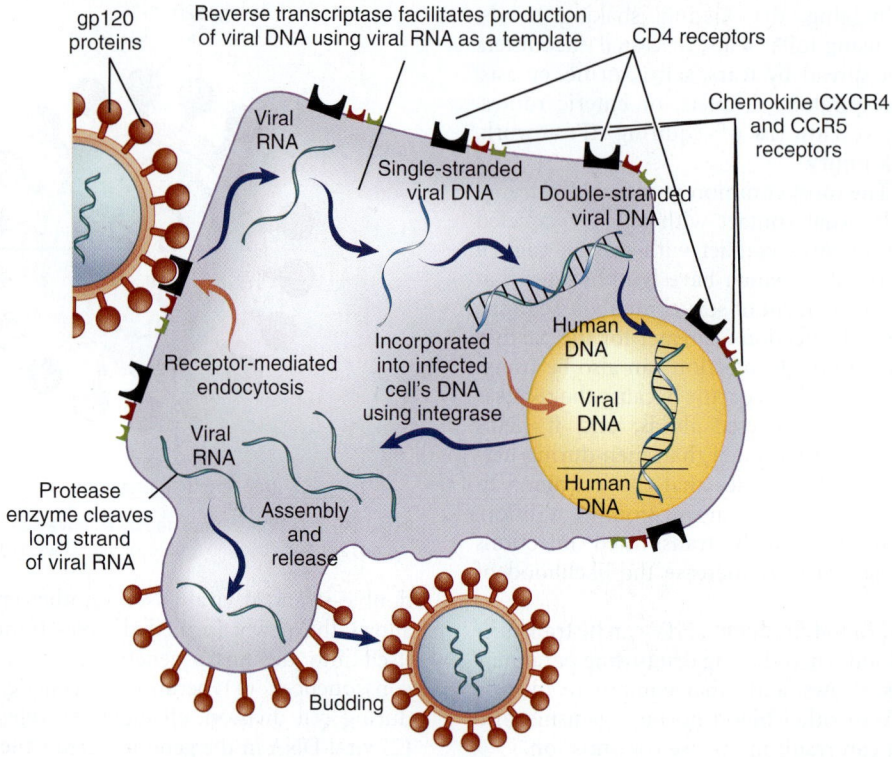

FIG. 14-2 HIV has gp120 glycoproteins that attach to CD4 and chemokine CXCR4 and CCR5 receptors on the surface of CD4+ T cells. Viral RNA then enters the cell, produces viral DNA in the presence of reverse transcriptase, and incorporates itself into the cellular genome in the presence of integrase, causing permanent cellular infection and the production of new virions. New viral RNA develops initially in long strands that are cut in the presence of protease and leave the cell through a budding process that ultimately contributes to cellular destruction.

this time a high **viral load** (the amount of HIV circulating in the blood) is noted, and CD4+ T cell counts fall temporarily but quickly return to baseline or near-baseline levels (Fig. 14-3). Many people, including HCPs, mistake acute HIV symptoms for a bad case of the flu. Individuals are most infectious during the acute infection stage because of the high amounts of circulating HIV.

Chronic HIV Infection

Asymptomatic Infection. The interval between initial HIV infection and a diagnosis of AIDS is about 10 years in untreated infection. During the first several years after initial infection, individuals are typically asymptomatic and have no symptoms or relatively limited signs of infection.

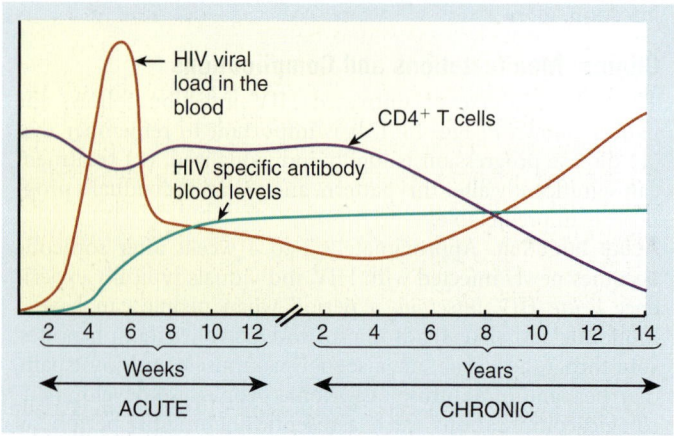

FIG. 14-3 Viral load in the blood in relationship to number of CD4+ T cells over the spectrum of untreated HIV infection.

Because most of the symptoms during early infection are vague and nonspecific for HIV, people may not be aware that they are infected. During this time, infected people continue their usual activities, which may include high-risk sexual and drug-using behaviors. This is a public health problem because infected individuals can transmit HIV to others even though they have no symptoms.[20] Personal health is also affected because people who do not know that they are infected have little reason to seek treatment and are less likely to make

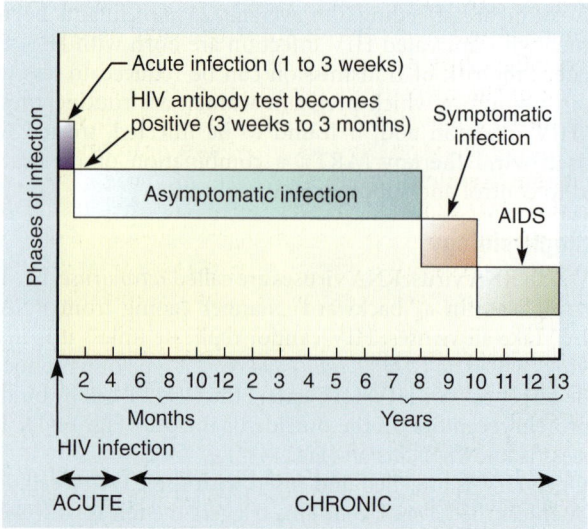

FIG. 14-4 Timeline for the spectrum of untreated HIV infection. The timeline represents the course of untreated illness from the time of infection to clinical manifestations of disease.

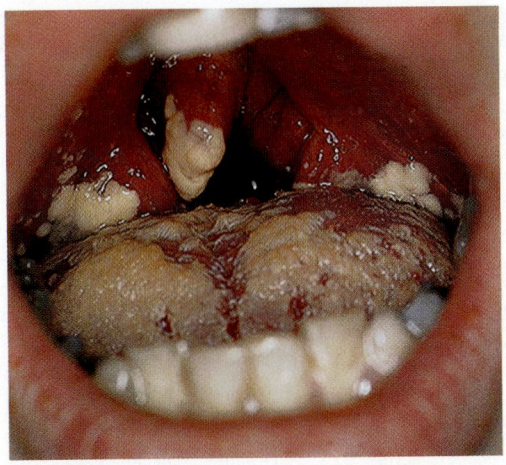

FIG. 14-5 Oral thrush involving hard and soft palate. (From Emond R, Welsby P, Rowland H: *Colour atlas of infectious diseases,* ed 4, Edinburgh, 2003, Mosby.)

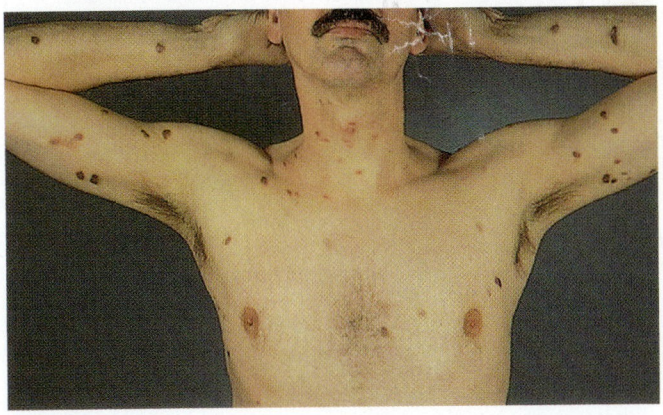

FIG. 14-6 Kaposi sarcoma (KS). The malignant vascular lesions of KS can appear anywhere on the skin surface or on internal organs. Lesions vary in size from pinpoint to large and may appear in a variety of shades. (From Friedman-Kien AE: *Color atlas of AIDS,* Philadelphia, 1989, Saunders.)

behavior changes that could improve the quality and length of their lives.

Symptomatic Infection. As the CD4$^+$ T cell count declines closer to 200 cells/μL and the viral load increases, HIV advances to a more active stage. Symptoms such as persistent fever, frequent night sweats, chronic diarrhea, recurrent headaches, and severe fatigue may develop.

One of the more common infections associated with this phase of HIV infection is oropharyngeal candidiasis (thrush) (Fig. 14-5). *Candida* organisms rarely cause problems in healthy adults but are more common in HIV-infected people. Other infections that can occur at this time include shingles (caused by the varicella-zoster virus); persistent vaginal candidal infections; outbreaks of oral or genital herpes; bacterial infections; and Kaposi sarcoma (KS), which is caused by human herpesvirus 8 (Fig. 14-6). *Oral hairy leukoplakia,* an Epstein-Barr virus infection that causes painless, white, raised lesions on the lateral aspect of the tongue (Fig. 14-7), is another indicator of disease progression.

AIDS. A diagnosis of **acquired immunodeficiency syndrome (AIDS)** is made when an HIV-infected patient meets criteria established by the CDC.[21] These criteria occur when the immune system becomes severely compromised (Table 14-10). Opportunistic diseases generally do not occur in the presence of a functioning immune system. Many infections, a variety of

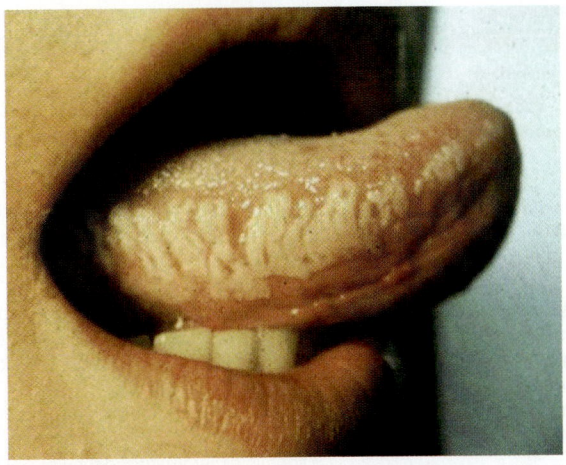

FIG. 14-7 Oral hairy leukoplakia on the lateral aspect of the tongue. (Set of slides published in 1992 by Jon Fuller, MD, and Howard Libman, MD, at Boston University School of Medicine, Boston.)

TABLE 14-10 Diagnostic Criteria for AIDS

AIDS is diagnosed when an individual with HIV develops at least one of the following conditions:

1. CD4$^+$ T cell count drops below 200 cells/μL.
2. One of the following opportunistic infections (OIs):
   - *Fungal:* candidiasis of bronchi, trachea, lungs, or esophagus; *Pneumocystis jiroveci* pneumonia (PCP); disseminated or extrapulmonary coccidioidomycosis; disseminated or extrapulmonary histoplasmosis
   - *Viral:* cytomegalovirus (CMV) disease other than liver, spleen, or nodes; CMV retinitis (with loss of vision); herpes simplex with chronic ulcer(s) or bronchitis, pneumonitis, or esophagitis; progressive multifocal leukoencephalopathy (PML); extrapulmonary cryptococcosis
   - *Protozoal:* toxoplasmosis of the brain, chronic intestinal isosporiasis, chronic intestinal cryptosporidiosis
   - *Bacterial: Mycobacterium tuberculosis* (any site); any disseminated or extrapulmonary mycobacteria, including *Mycobacterium avium* complex (MAC) or *Mycobacterium kansasii;* recurrent pneumonia; recurrent *Salmonella* septicemia
3. One of the following opportunistic cancers:
   - Invasive cervical cancer
   - Kaposi sarcoma (KS)
   - Burkitt's lymphoma
   - Immunoblastic lymphoma
   - Primary lymphoma of the brain
4. Wasting syndrome. *Wasting* is defined as a loss of 10% or more of ideal body mass.

Modified from Centers for Disease Control and Prevention: 1993 Revised classification system for HIV infection and expanded surveillance case definition for AIDS among adolescents and adults, 1993. Retrieved from *www.cdc.gov/mmwr/preview/mmwrhtml/rr5710a1.htm?s_cid=rr5710a1_e.*

malignancies, wasting, and HIV-related cognitive changes can occur in patients with immune impairment (Table 14-11). Organisms that do not cause severe disease in people with functioning immune systems can cause debilitating, disseminated, and life-threatening infections during this stage. Several opportunistic diseases may occur at the same time, compounding the difficulties of diagnosis and treatment. Advances in HIV treatment have decreased the occurrence of opportunistic diseases.

Diagnostic Studies

Diagnosis of HIV Infection. Diagnosis of HIV infection is made by testing for HIV antibodies and/or antigens in the blood.[22] HIV screening tests detect HIV-specific antibodies or antigens,

TABLE 14-11 Common Opportunistic Diseases Associated With HIV Infection

Organism or Disease	Clinical Manifestations
Candida albicans	Thrush (Fig. 14-5), esophagitis, vaginitis. Whitish yellow patches in mouth, esophagus, GI tract, vagina
Coccidioides immitis	Pneumonia and fever, weight loss, cough
CNS lymphoma	Cognitive dysfunction, motor impairment, aphasia, seizures, personality changes, headache
Cryptococcus neoformans	Meningitis, cognitive impairment, motor dysfunction, fever, seizures, headache
Cryptosporidium muris	Gastroenteritis, watery diarrhea, abdominal pain, weight loss
Cytomegalovirus (CMV)	*Retinitis:* retinal lesions, blurred vision, loss of vision *Esophagitis, stomatitis:* difficulty swallowing, colitis or gastritis: bloody diarrhea, pain, weight loss *Pneumonitis:* respiratory symptoms. *Neurologic disease:* CNS manifestations
Hepatitis B virus (HBV)	Jaundice, fatigue, abdominal pain, loss of appetite, nausea, vomiting, joint pain. Some have no signs or symptoms
Hepatitis C virus (HCV)	Jaundice, fatigue, abdominal pain, loss of appetite, nausea, vomiting, dark urine. Many have no signs or symptoms.
Herpes simplex	*HSV-1 (type 1):* orolabial and mucocutaneous vesicular and ulcerative lesions. Keratitis, visual disturbances, encephalitis, CNS manifestations *HSV-2 (type 2):* genital and perianal vesicular and ulcerative lesions
Histoplasma capsulatum	*Pneumonia:* fever, cough, weight loss *Meningitis:* CNS manifestations, disseminated disease
JC papovavirus	Progressive multifocal leukoencephalopathy (PML), CNS manifestations, mental and motor declines
Kaposi sarcoma (KS) caused by human herpesvirus 8 (HHV-8)	Vascular lesions on the skin (Fig. 14-6), mucous membranes, and viscera with wide range of presentation: firm, flat, raised, or nodular; pinpoint to several cm in size; hyperpigmented, multicentric. Can cause lymphedema and disfigurement, particularly when confluent. Usually not serious unless occurring in the respiratory or gastrointestinal system
***Mycobacterium avium* complex (MAC)**	Gastroenteritis, watery diarrhea, weight loss
***Mycobacterium tuberculosis* (MTB, TB)**	Respiratory and disseminated disease. Productive cough, fever, night sweats, weight loss
***Pneumocystis jiroveci* pneumonia (PCP)**	Pneumonia, nonproductive cough, hypoxemia, progressive shortness of breath, fever, night sweats, fatigue
Toxoplasma gondii	Encephalitis, cognitive dysfunction, motor impairment, fever, altered mental status, headache, seizures, sensory abnormalities
Varicella-zoster virus (VZV)	*Shingles:* erythematous maculopapular rash along dermatomal planes, pain, pruritus *Ocular:* progressive outer retinal necrosis (PORN)

but typically it takes several weeks after initial infection before evidence of HIV can be detected on a screening test (Fig. 14-3). This delay is known as the **window period**. HIV screening tests can be performed using blood or saliva. Combination antibody and antigen tests (also known as fourth-generation tests) are able to detect HIV earlier than previous versions of HIV screening tests. The fourth-generation test decreases the window period to within 3 weeks following infection (Table 14-12).

Laboratory Studies in HIV Infection. Two laboratory tests are used for monitoring HIV progression: $CD4^+$ T cell count and viral load. The $CD4^+$ T cell count provides a marker of immune function. As the disease progresses, the number of $CD4^+$ T cells usually decreases (Fig. 14-3). The normal range for $CD4^+$ T cells is 800 to 1200 cells/μL. Laboratory tests that measure viral levels provide an assessment of disease progression. The lower the viral load, the less active the disease. In HIV, viral loads are reported as real numbers (e.g., 1260 copies/μL). The goal of treatment is to suppress the viral load to the lowest level possible, which is below the level of detection on a commercial assay. This is often referred to as "undetectable." "Undetectable" does *not* mean that the virus has been eliminated from the body or that the individual can no longer transmit HIV to others. Rather, it refers to the fact that the amount of circulating HIV in the blood is below the level of detection of the test.

Abnormal blood test results are common in HIV infection and may be caused by HIV, opportunistic diseases, or complications of therapy. Decreased white blood cell (WBC) counts,

TABLE 14-12 HIV Testing

HIV-Antibody/Antigen Testing (Fourth-Generation Testing)

A highly sensitive test detects antibodies and antigens associated with HIV. Blood samples that are negative for HIV infection are reported as negative. The new fourth-generation testing algorithm includes confirmatory testing with HIV viral load testing for any indeterminate results.

- If the patient has a negative fourth-generation test, but reports recent risky behaviors, encourage retesting in 4 to 6 weeks. Individuals at ongoing risk should be assessed or counseled for risk reduction interventions including preexposure prophylaxis (PrEP).
- If the results are positive and consistent with HIV infection, assist the patient in getting appropriate counseling, support, and follow-up HIV primary care.

Rapid HIV-Antibody Testing

1. Rapid testing is strongly recommended by the Centers for Disease Control and Prevention. Results are highly accurate, and it can be done in a variety of settings (mobile health units, HCPs' offices, or even in the privacy of an individual's home). Results are typically available within 20 minutes.
2. In-home HIV test kits are available. Testing is done on saliva.
3. Rapid tests are screening tests for antibodies, not for antigen.
4. Negative rapid tests should be followed by a risk assessment to determine the need for repeat tests.
5. Positive rapid tests can be disclosed to the patient but must be confirmed with a standard HIV assay. This step necessitates a blood draw and a return appointment to get results.

especially below-normal numbers of lymphocytes (lymphopenia) and neutrophils (neutropenia), are often seen. Low platelet counts (thrombocytopenia) may be caused by HIV, antiplatelet antibodies, or drug therapy. Anemia is associated with the chronic disease process and with adverse effects of ART. Altered liver function, caused by HIV infection, drug therapy, or co-infection with a hepatitis virus, is common. Early identification of co-infection with hepatitis B virus (HBV) or hepatitis C virus (HCV) is extremely important because these infections have a more serious course in patients with HIV, may ultimately limit options for ART, and can cause liver-related morbidity and mortality.[23]

Resistance tests can determine if a patient's HIV is resistant to drugs used for ART. *Genotype* and *phenotype* assays are used to help HCPs know which medications can be used to control a patient's infection. These tests are similar to culture and sensitivity testing used for antibiotic selection.

Interprofessional Care

Interprofessional care of the HIV-infected patient focuses on (1) monitoring HIV disease progression and immune function, (2) initiating and monitoring ART, (3) preventing the development of opportunistic diseases, (4) detecting and treating opportunistic diseases, (5) managing symptoms, (6) preventing or decreasing complications of treatment, and (7) preventing further transmission of HIV. To accomplish these goals, ongoing assessment, clinician-patient interactions, and patient teaching and support are required.

The initial patient visit provides an opportunity to gather baseline data and to start establishing rapport. A complete history and physical examination, including an immunization history and psychosocial and dietary evaluations, should be conducted. Findings from the history, assessment, and laboratory tests help to determine patient needs. This is also a good time to complete the case reports required by the state health department. Patient teaching about the spectrum of HIV disease, treatment, prevention of transmission to others, improvements in health, and family planning can be initiated at this meeting. Use patient input to develop a plan of care and determine the need for referrals. Remember that a newly diagnosed patient may not be able to retain or understand information. Be prepared to repeat and clarify information over the course of several months.

Drug Therapy for HIV Infection. The goals of drug therapy in HIV infection are to (1) decrease the viral load, (2) maintain or increase $CD4^+$ T cell counts, (3) prevent HIV-related symptoms and opportunistic diseases, (4) delay disease progression, and (5) prevent HIV transmission. HIV cannot be cured, but ART can delay disease progression by decreasing viral replication.[24] When taken consistently and correctly, ART can reduce viral loads by 90% to 99%, which makes adherence to treatment regimens extremely important.

Drugs used to treat HIV work at various points in the HIV replication cycle (Table 14-13). The major advantage of using drugs from different classes is that combination therapy can inhibit viral replication in several different ways, making it more difficult for the virus to recover and decreasing the likelihood of drug resistance. A major problem with most drugs used in ART is that resistance develops rapidly when they are used alone *(monotherapy)* or taken in inadequate doses. For that reason, combinations of three or more drugs should be used.

SAFETY ALERT Interaction of ART With Other Drugs

- Many ARTs have interactions with other commonly used drugs and herbal therapies (e.g., St. John's wort).
- Significant interactions with ARTs also occur with over-the-counter drugs, including antacids, proton pump inhibitors, and certain supplements.
- Be sure to ask patients about prescribed and over-the-counter drugs as well as herbal products and supplements.

Drug Therapy for Opportunistic Diseases. Management of HIV is complicated by the many opportunistic diseases that can develop as the immune system deteriorates (Table 14-11). Prevention is the preferred approach to opportunistic diseases. A number of opportunistic diseases associated with HIV can be delayed or prevented with adequate ART, vaccines (including hepatitis B, influenza, and pneumococcal), and disease-specific prevention measures.[25] Although it is usually not possible to eradicate opportunistic diseases once they occur, prophylactic medications can significantly decrease morbidity and mortality rates. Advances in the prevention, diagnosis, and treatment of opportunistic diseases have contributed significantly to increased life expectancy.

Preventing Transmission of HIV. Preexposure prophylaxis (PrEP) is a comprehensive HIV prevention strategy to reduce the risk of sexually acquired HIV infection in adults at high risk.[26] PrEP should be used in conjunction with other proven prevention interventions such as condoms, risk reduction counseling, and regular HIV testing.

Tenofovir in combination with emtricitabine, also known as Truvada, is used to reduce the risk of HIV infection in uninfected individuals who are at significant risk of acquiring HIV. Tenofovir/emtricitabine is also currently used in combination with other antiretroviral agents for the treatment of HIV-infected people.

NURSING MANAGEMENT: HIV INFECTION

Nursing Assessment

Nursing assessment of individuals not known to be infected with HIV should focus on behaviors that put the person at risk for HIV and other sexually transmitted and blood-borne infections. Assess patients for risky behaviors on a regular basis. Do not assume that someone is without risk because he or she is too old, too young, heterosexual, or married.

Help individuals assess risk by asking some basic questions: (1) Have you ever had a blood transfusion or used clotting factors? If so, was it before 1985? (2) Have you ever shared drug-using equipment with another person? (3) Have you ever had a sexual experience in which your penis, vagina, rectum, or mouth came into contact with another person's penis, vagina, rectum, or mouth? (4) Have you ever had a sexually transmitted infection? (5) Have you ever had sexual contact with someone known to have HIV? These questions provide the minimum information needed to initiate a risk assessment. Follow up a positive response to any of these questions with an in-depth exploration of issues related to the identified risk.

Specific assessments are needed for an individual who has been diagnosed with HIV infection. Subjective and objective data that should be obtained are presented in Table 14-14. Repeated nursing assessments over time are essential because people's circumstances change. Early recognition and treatment can slow the progression of HIV infection and prevent new

TABLE 14-13 Drug Therapy

HIV Infection

Drug Classification	Mechanism of Action	Examples
Entry Inhibitors	Prevent binding of HIV to cells, thus preventing entry of HIV into cells where replication would occur	enfuvirtide (Fuzeon) maraviroc (Selzentry)
Reverse Transcriptase Inhibitors		
Nucleoside Reverse Transcriptase Inhibitors (NRTIs)	Insert a piece of DNA into the developing HIV DNA chain, blocking further development of the chain and leaving the production of the new strand of HIV DNA incomplete	zidovudine (AZT, ZDV, Retrovir) didanosine (ddI, Videx, Videx-EC [time-released]) stavudine (d4T, Zerit) lamivudine (3TC, Epivir) abacavir (Ziagen) emtricitabine (FTC, Emtriva)
Nonnucleoside Reverse Transcriptase Inhibitors (NNRTIs)	Inhibit the action of reverse transcriptase	nevirapine (Viramune XR) delavirdine (Rescriptor) efavirenz (Sustiva) etravirine (Intelence) rilpivirine (Edurant)
Nucleotide Reverse Transcriptase Inhibitor (NtRTI)	Combines with reverse transcriptase enzyme to block the process needed to convert HIV RNA into HIV DNA	tenofovir (Viread)
Integrase Inhibitors	Bind with integrase enzyme and prevent HIV from incorporating its genetic material into the host cell	raltegravir (Isentress) elvitegravir (Vitekta)† dolutegravir (Tivicay)
Protease Inhibitors (PIs)	Prevent the protease enzyme from cutting HIV proteins into the proper lengths needed to allow viable virions to assemble and bud out from the cell membrane	saquinavir (Fortovase, Invirase) indinavir (Crixivan) ritonavir (Norvir)‡ nelfinavir (Viracept) atazanavir (Reyataz) fosamprenavir (Lexiva) tipranavir (Aptivus) darunavir (Prezista) lopinavir + ritonavir (Kaletra)
Fixed-Dose Combination Products	More than one drug combined into a single tablet. Drugs may be from the same or different classes.	Atripla (tenofovir DF + emtricitabine + efavirenz) Combivir (lamivudine + zidovudine) Complera (tenofovir DF + emtricitabine + rilpivirine) Odefsky (tenofovir AF + emtricitabine + rilpivirine) Epzicom (abacavir + lamivudine) Triumeq (abacavir + lamivudine + dolutegravir) Trizivir (abacavir + lamivudine + zidovudine) Truvada (tenofovir DF + emtricitabine) Descovy (tenofovir AF + emtricitabine) Stribild (tenofovir DF + emtricitabine + elvitegravir + cobicistat§) Genvoya (tenofovir AF + emtricitabine + elvitegravir + cobicistat§) Evotaz (atazanavir + cobicistat§) Prezcobix (darunavir + cobicistat§)

AF, Alafenamide. *DF,* disoproxil fumarate.
†Vitekta must be administered with a boosted HIV protease inhibitor. Elvitegravir in other fixed dose combinations can be given with either a protease inhibitor or cobicistat.
‡Most often used in low doses with other PIs to boost effect.
§Cobicistat is a pharmacologic booster that enhances the potency of some HIV antiretrovirals. It has no direct effects against HIV.

infections. A complete history and thorough systems review can help identify and address problems in a timely manner.

◆ Planning

Nursing interventions can help the patient to (1) adhere to drug regimens; (2) adopt a healthy lifestyle that includes avoiding exposure to other sexually transmitted infections and blood-borne diseases; (3) protect others from HIV; (4) maintain or develop healthy and supportive relationships; (5) maintain activities and productivity; (6) explore spiritual issues; (7) come to terms with issues related to disease, disability, and death; and (8) cope with symptoms caused by HIV and its treatments.

◆ Nursing Implementation

The complexity of HIV disease is related to its chronic nature. As with most chronic and infectious diseases, primary prevention and health promotion are the most effective health care strategies. When prevention fails, disease results. Table 14-15 presents a summary of nursing goals, assessments, and interventions throughout the course of HIV infection.

◆ **Health Promotion.** Even with recent successes in HIV treatment, prevention remains a critical component to control the epidemic. In addition, health promotion encourages early detection of the disease so that, if primary prevention has failed, early intervention can be initiated.

◆ ***Prevention of HIV Infection.*** HIV infection is preventable. Avoiding or modifying risky behaviors is the most effective prevention tool. Nursing interventions to prevent disease transmission are based on an assessment of the individual's risk behaviors. Provide culturally sensitive, language-appropriate, and age-specific teaching and behavior change counseling. Nurses who are comfortable with and know how to talk about

TABLE 14-14 Nursing Assessment

HIV-Infected Patient

Subjective Data

Important Health Information

Past health history: Route of infection. Hepatitis, other sexually transmitted infections, tuberculosis. Frequent viral, fungal, and/or bacterial infections

Medications: Use of immunosuppressive drugs

Functional Health Patterns

Health perception–health management: Perception of illness. Alcohol and drug use. Malaise

Nutritional-metabolic: Weight loss, anorexia, nausea, vomiting. Lesions, bleeding, or ulcerations of lips, mouth, gums, tongue, or throat. Sensitivity to acidic, salty, or spicy foods. Difficulty swallowing, abdominal cramping. Skin rashes, lesions, or color changes

Elimination: Persistent diarrhea, change in character of stools. Painful urination, low back pain

Activity-exercise: Chronic fatigue, muscle weakness, difficulty walking. Cough, shortness of breath

Sleep-rest: Insomnia, night sweats, fatigue

Cognitive-perceptual: Headaches, stiff neck, chest pain, rectal pain, retrosternal pain. Blurred vision, photophobia, diplopia, loss of vision. Hearing impairment. Confusion, forgetfulness, attention deficit, changes in mental status, memory loss, personality changes Paresthesias, hypersensitivity in feet, pruritus

Role-relationship: Support system(s), career or job, financial resources

Sexuality-reproductive: Lesions on genitalia or anus (internal or external), pruritus or burning in vagina, penis, or anus. Painful sexual intercourse, rectal pain or bleeding, changes in menstruation, vaginal or penile discharge. Use of birth control measures, pregnancies, desire for future children

Coping–stress tolerance: Stress levels, previous losses, coping patterns, self-concept; social withdrawal

Objective Data

General

Lethargy, persistent fever, lymphadenopathy, peripheral wasting, fat deposits in truncal areas and upper back

Eyes

Presence of exudates, retinal lesions or hemorrhage, papilledema

Integumentary

Decreased skin turgor, dry skin, diaphoresis. Pallor, cyanosis. Lesions, eruptions, discolorations, bruises of skin or mucous membranes. Vaginal or perianal excoriation. Alopecia. Delayed wound healing

Respiratory

Tachypnea, dyspnea, intercostal retractions. Crackles, wheezing, productive or nonproductive cough

Cardiovascular

Pericardial friction rub, murmur, bradycardia, tachycardia.

Gastrointestinal

Mouth lesions, including blisters (HSV), white-gray patches (*Candida* infection), painless white lesions on lateral aspect of the tongue (hairy leukoplakia), discolorations (KS). Gingivitis, tooth decay or loosening. Redness or white patchy lesions of throat. Vomiting, diarrhea, incontinence, rectal lesions, hyperactive bowel sounds, abdominal masses, hepatosplenomegaly

Musculoskeletal

Muscle wasting, weakness

Neurologic

Ataxia, tremors, lack of coordination. Sensory loss, slurred speech, aphasia. Memory loss, peripheral neuropathy, apathy, agitation, depression, inappropriate behavior. Decreasing levels of consciousness, seizures, paralysis, coma

Reproductive

Genital lesions or discharge, abdominal tenderness secondary to pelvic inflammatory disease (PID)

Possible Diagnostic Findings

Positive HIV antibody/antigen assay. Detectable viral load. ↓ $CD4^+$ T cell count, ↓ WBC count, lymphopenia, anemia, thrombocytopenia. Electrolyte imbalances, abnormal liver function tests. ↑ cholesterol, triglycerides, and blood glucose

HSV, Herpes simplex virus; *KS,* Kaposi sarcoma; *WBC,* white blood cell.

sensitive topics such as sexuality and drug use are best prepared to provide prevention education.

A wide variety of activities can reduce the risk of HIV infection.[27] Individuals choose the methods that best fit their needs and circumstances. Prevention techniques can be divided into *safe sexual activities* (those that eliminate risk) and *risk-reducing sexual activities* (those that decrease, but do not eliminate, risk).

The goal is to develop safer, healthier, and less risky behaviors. The more consistently and correctly prevention methods are used, the more effective they are in preventing HIV infection. It is also a good idea to use a combination of prevention methods (e.g., using condoms and decreasing the number of sex partners) to increase the prevention effect.

◆ **Decreasing risks related to sexual intercourse.** *Safe sexual activities* eliminate the risk of exposure to HIV in semen and vaginal secretions. Abstaining from all sexual activity is an effective way to accomplish this goal, but there are safe options for those who cannot or do not wish to abstain. Limiting sexual behavior to activities in which the mouth, penis, vagina, or rectum does not come into contact with a partner's mouth, penis, vagina, or rectum eliminates contact with blood, semen, or vaginal secretions. Safe activities include masturbation, mutual masturbation ("hand job"), and other activities that meet the "no contact" requirements. *Insertive sex* between partners who are not infected with HIV and not at risk of becoming infected with HIV is also considered safe.

Risk-reducing sexual activities decrease the risk of contact with HIV through the use of barriers. Barriers should be used when engaging in insertive sexual activity (oral, vaginal, or anal) with a partner who has HIV or whose HIV status is not known. The most commonly used barrier is the male condom. Male condoms can be used for protection during anal, vaginal, and oral intercourse. Female condoms provide an alternative to male condoms. Squares of latex (known as dental dams) can be used as a barrier during oral sexual activity.

◆ **Decreasing risks related to drug use.** Drug use, including alcohol and tobacco, can cause immunosuppression, poor nutrition, and a host of psychosocial problems. However, drug use does not cause HIV infection. The major risk for HIV related to using drugs involves sharing equipment or having

ETHICAL/LEGAL DILEMMAS

Individual vs. Public Health Protection

Situation

A nurse in a community clinic is having a follow-up visit with V.T., a 38-year-old woman, who was found to have HIV during her annual examination 2 weeks ago. During the visit, V.T. discloses that she has been verbally and physically abused by her partner. V.T. also indicates that she had not yet told her partner about the HIV diagnosis because she is afraid that he will hurt her. She has not used any protection during sex with him since she learned of her test results because she suspects he infected her.

Ethical/Legal Points for Consideration

- You face a conflict between preventing further harm to V.T. (possible increase in intimate partner violence), providing care to her partner (his need for an HIV test, diagnosis, and treatment), and protecting the public health (potential spread of HIV infection to her partner or from her partner to others in the community). Patient teaching and support are essential because your primary obligation is to the patient.
- Because relevant law varies from state to state, your first step is to be familiar with your state law concerning mandated reporting for domestic partner abuse and infectious diseases.
- Laws regarding protection of privacy in HIV testing are federal and apply everywhere.
- In many states, reporting domestic abuse is mandatory only when the abuse is actually witnessed by the reporter or when the immediate effects of the abuse (e.g., wounds, contusions, broken bones) are witnessed.[1]
- You should be familiar with crisis counseling services for V.T. and offer her the following advice: collect and stash a set of car keys or taxi money in a safe place, keep a bag packed and hidden or even stored in a locker somewhere accessible, develop a code phrase to use with a friend or family member to call for help, keep a cell phone charged, and have money hidden in a safe place.

Discussion Questions

1. Within the parameters of your state's requirements for reportable conditions, how can you protect the patient's confidentiality to prevent further intimate partner violence?
2. What services are offered by your state to notify a partner without disclosing the source patient's name? How would V.T. access those services in your state?
3. How can you protect the partner from possible infection while also protecting V.T. from further violence?
4. How can you best address the issue of intimate partner violence? What resources would V.T. have in your community?
5. Discuss the benefits of universal, voluntary testing in light of V.T.'s case.

Reference

1. National Coalition Against Domestic Violence: *www.ncadv.com.*

unsafe sexual experiences while under the influence of drugs. Basic risk reduction rules are (1) do not use drugs; (2) if you use drugs, do not share equipment; and (3) do not have sexual intercourse when under the influence of any drug (including alcohol) that impairs decision making.[28]

The safest method is to abstain from drugs, but this may not be a viable option for users who are not prepared to quit or have no access to drug treatment services. The risk of HIV for these individuals can be eliminated if they do not share equipment. Injecting equipment ("works") includes needles, syringes, cookers (spoons or bottle caps used to mix the drug), cotton, and rinse water. Equipment used to snort (straws) or smoke (pipes) drugs can also be contaminated with blood and should not be shared.

HEALTHY PEOPLE

Prevention and Early Detection of HIV

- Increase safer sexual practices, including condom use.
- Decrease equipment sharing among IV drug users.
- Increase clinician skills to assess for risk factors for HIV infection, recommend HIV testing, and provide counseling for behavior change.
- Make voluntary HIV testing a routine part of health care.
- Increase access to new HIV testing technologies, especially rapid testing.
- Increase access to HIV testing facilities in traditional health care settings, as well as in alternative sites such as drug and alcohol treatment facilities and community-based organizations.
- Increase risk assessment and individualized behavior change messages to people with HIV to prevent new infections.
- Decrease perinatal HIV infection by offering voluntary HIV testing as a part of routine prenatal care.
- Provide counseling and appropriate HIV therapy to those who are infected.

Access to sterile equipment is an important risk elimination tactic. Some communities have needle and syringe exchange programs (NSEPs) that provide sterile equipment in exchange for used equipment. Opposition to these programs is related to the fear that access to injecting supplies will increase drug use. However, studies have shown that, in communities with NSEPs, drug use does not increase, rates of HIV and other blood-borne infections are controlled, and an overall cost benefit results.[29] Cleaning equipment before use can also reduce risk by decreasing the chance of blood contact.

In addition, providing support for patients with substance use and referring individuals to professionals who can assist patients manage the psychologic aspects of substance use is important. Other self-help programs (e.g., Narcotics Anonymous, Alcoholics Anonymous) may also be beneficial.

◆ **Decreasing risks of perinatal transmission.** The best way to prevent HIV infection in infants is to prevent HIV infection in women. Women who are already infected with HIV should be asked about their reproductive desires. Those who choose not to have children need to have family planning methods discussed in detail. Should they become pregnant, abortion may be desired and should be discussed in conjunction with other options, including the possibility of maintaining the pregnancy and using ART to decrease the risk of transmission.

If HIV-infected pregnant women are appropriately treated during pregnancy, the rate of perinatal transmission can be decreased from 25% to less than 2%. ART has significantly decreased the risk for infants born to HIV-infected women, and more of these women are now becoming mothers. The current standard of care is for all women who are pregnant or contemplating pregnancy to be counseled about HIV, routinely offered access to voluntary HIV-antibody testing, and, if infected, offered optimal ART.[24,30]

◆ **Decreasing risks at work.** The risk of infection from occupational exposure to HIV is small but real. OSHA requires employers to protect workers from exposure to blood and other potentially infectious materials (Table 14-8). Precautions and safety devices decrease the risk of direct contact with blood and body fluids. Should exposure to HIV-infected fluids occur, **postexposure prophylaxis (PEP)** with combination ART can significantly decrease the risk of infection.[16] The need for timely treatment and counseling makes it even more critical for nurses to report all blood exposures.

TABLE 14-15 Nursing Interventions in HIV Infection

Nursing Care and Goals	Assessment	Interventions
Health Promotion		
1. Prevent HIV infection.	*Risk factors:* What behaviors or social, physical, emotional, pathogenic, or immune factors place the patient at risk?	• Education, including knowledge, attitudes, and behaviors, with emphasis on risk reduction to the following: • *General population:* Cover general information • *Pregnant women:* General information and information specific to HIV infection and pregnancy • *Individual patient:* Specific to assessed need • Empower patients to take control of prevention measures.
2. Detect HIV infection early.	Does the patient need to be tested for HIV?	• Provide HIV antibody/antigen testing with appropriate counseling.
Acute Care		
1. Promote health and limit disability.	*Physical health:* Is the patient experiencing problems? *Mental health:* How is the patient coping? *Resources:* Does the patient have family or social support? Is the patient accessing community services? Is money or insurance a problem? Does the patient have access to spiritual support as desired?	• Provide case management or refer to interprofessional team, including social work. • Teach regarding HIV, the spectrum of infection, options for care, signs and symptoms to report, treatment options, immune enhancement, risk reduction, and ways to adhere to treatment regimens. • Establish long-term, trusting relationship with patient, family, and significant others. • Provide emotional and spiritual support. • Develop resources for legal needs: discrimination prevention, wills and advance directives, child care wishes. • Empower the patient to identify needs, direct care, and seek services.
2. Manage problems caused by HIV infection.	*Physical health:* Has the patient experienced acute exacerbation of problems related to immunodeficiency, opportunistic disease, or risk factors (e.g., substance use)? *Mental health status:* Has the patient's ability to cope with psychosocial issues deteriorated?	• Provide care during acute exacerbations: recognition of life-threatening developments, life support, rapid intervention with treatments and drugs, comfort, and hygiene needs. • Support patient and family during crisis. • Assist the patient with mental health issues and provide referral to mental health specialist as needed.
Ambulatory Care		
1. Maximize quality of life.	*Physical health:* Are new symptoms developing? Is the patient experiencing drug side effects or interactions?	• Continue case management. • Teach about changing treatment options and continued adherence. • Empower patient to continue to direct care and to make desires known to family members and significant others.
2. Resolve life and death issues.	*Mental health:* How is the patient coping? What adjustments have been made? *Finances:* Can the patient maintain health care and basic standards of living? *Family, social, and community support:* Are these available? Is the patient using support in an effective manner? Do family or significant others need teaching, encouragement, or stress relief? *Spirituality issues:* Does the patient desire support from a religious organization or spiritual counselor? What assistance does the patient desire?	• Continue physical care for chronic disease process: treatments, drugs, comfort, and hygiene needs. • Encourage health promotion measures (as above). • Refer the patient to resources to support finances. • Support patient and family or significant others in a trusting relationship. • Assist with end-of-life issues: resuscitation orders, comfort measures, funeral plans, estate planning, child care, etc. • Assess desires and refer to resources that will assist in meeting identified spiritual needs.

◆ ***HIV Testing.*** An estimated 14% of people living with HIV in the United States are not aware that they are infected. People who do not know they are infected are more likely to transmit the infection to others. Current guidelines recommend universal, voluntary testing as part of routine medical care.[31,32] The goal is to normalize the test, decrease the stigma related to HIV testing, find hidden cases, get infected individuals into care, and prevent new cases of infection.

◆ **Acute Care**

◆ ***Early Intervention.*** Early intervention after detection of HIV infection can promote health and limit disability. The nursing assessment in HIV disease should focus on early detection of symptoms, opportunistic diseases, and psychosocial problems (Table 14-15).

◆ **Initial response to diagnosis of HIV.** Reactions to an HIV diagnosis are similar to the reactions of people who are diagnosed with any life-threatening, debilitating, or chronic illness. These reactions include anxiety, panic, fear, depression, denial, hopelessness, anger, and guilt.[33] Unfortunately, all these emotions are overlaid with the stigma and discrimination that continue to pervade societal reactions to HIV. Many of these reactions are also seen in the patient's family members, friends, and caregivers. As time passes, patients and their loved ones will be confronted with complex treatment decisions; feelings of loss, anger, powerlessness, depression, and grief; social isolation; the possibility of death; and/or thoughts of suicide.

◆ **Antiretroviral therapy.** ART can significantly slow the progression of HIV. However, treatment regimens can be complex,

EVIDENCE-BASED PRACTICE

Applying the Evidence

Condom Use and HIV

As a nurse in an HIV clinic, you are counseling M.J., a 27-year-old gay man, and his partner. M.J. is on antiretroviral therapy. His viral load is very low and his CD4+ T cell count is normal. He tells you that since the medications are working, he and his partner (who is not infected with HIV) are considering not using condoms in the future.

Making Clinical Decisions

Best Available Evidence. One of the best ways to prevent HIV transmission from an infected person to an uninfected person is by using condoms.

Clinician Expertise. You know that risk-reducing sexual activities in this situation include the continued use of condoms. However, you also know that although a very low viral load decreases the risk of HIV transmission, a partner may become infected.

Patient Preferences and Values. M.J. tells you that he and his partner are in a committed relationship, have no other partners, and do not like using condoms.

Implications for Practice

1. What information would you discuss with M.J. related to HIV transmission, viral load, and the risks of unprotected sexual activity?
2. What measures besides condom use would you discuss with M.J. to reduce the risk of HIV transmission?

References for Evidence

Centers for Disease Control and Prevention: HIV prevention in the United States-proven HIV prevention methods. Retrieved from *www.cdc.gov/nchhstp/newsroom/HIVFactSheets/Prevention.*

Centers for Disease Control and Prevention: Condom fact sheet in brief. Retrieved from *www.cdc.gov/condomeffectiveness/brief.html.*

the drugs have side effects, ART does not work for everyone, and it is expensive. These factors can contribute to problems with adherence to treatment, a dangerous situation because of the high risk of developing drug resistance.

CHECK YOUR PRACTICE

You are working in an outpatient HIV clinic and one of the patients, a 34-yr-old single mother with HIV infection, tells you, "I've been feeling well lately, and I've been so busy taking care of my 2-year-old son, so I have not been taking my HIV meds."

- How would you respond to this patient?

As a nurse, you are often the person who works most closely with patients who are trying to cope with the issues of dealing with the diagnosis and treatment of HIV. Table 14-16 provides a guide to providing patient and caregiver teaching on HIV treatment and initial follow up.

Interventions include teaching about (1) advantages and disadvantages of new treatments, (2) dangers of poor adherence to therapeutic regimens, (3) how and when to take each drug, (4) drug interactions to avoid, and (5) side effects that must be reported to the HCP.

Clinical guidelines provide information on initial drug regimens.[24] However, one of the most important considerations for initiating therapy is patient readiness for treatment. *Adherence* to ART is a critical component of successful drug therapy for people with HIV infection. Nurses are uniquely prepared to provide assistance with adherence to the drug regimen (Table 14-17). Taking drugs as prescribed (right dose and time) is important for all drug therapy, but with HIV infection, missing even a few doses can lead to drug resistance. Patients can be helped to adhere to difficult treatment regimens with electronic reminders, beepers, timers on pillboxes, and calendars. Group support and individual counseling can also help, but the best approach is to learn about the patient's life and assist with problem solving related to taking medications within the confines of that life.

Delaying disease progression. HIV disease progression may be delayed by promoting a healthy immune system, whether the patient chooses to take ART or not. Useful interventions for HIV-infected patients include (1) getting nutritional support to maintain lean body mass and ensure appropriate levels of vitamins and micronutrients; (2) moderating or eliminating alcohol, tobacco, and drug use; (3) keeping up to date with recommended vaccines; (4) getting adequate rest and exercise; (5) reducing stress; (6) avoiding exposure to new infectious agents; (7)

TABLE 14-16 Patient & Caregiver Teaching

Antiretroviral Drugs

Resistance to antiretroviral drugs is a major problem in treating HIV infection. Include the following instructions when teaching the patient and/or caregiver to decrease the risk of developing resistance.

1. Discuss options with your HCP to find the best regimen for you. Your provider should order at least three different antiretroviral drugs from at least two different drug groups.
2. Know the drugs you are taking and how to take them (some have to be taken with food, some must be taken on an empty stomach, some cannot be taken together). If you do not understand, ask. Have your nurse write the instructions clearly for you.
3. Take the full dose prescribed, and take it on schedule. If you cannot take the drug because of side effects or other problems, report it to your HCP immediately.
4. Take all of your medications as prescribed. Do not quit taking one drug while continuing the others. If you cannot tolerate even one of your drugs, talk to your HCP, who will recommend a way to deal with the side effects or a new set of drugs.
5. Many antiretroviral drugs interact with other drugs, including a number of common drugs you can buy without a prescription. Be sure your HCP and pharmacist know all of the drugs that you are taking, and do not take any new drugs without checking for possible interactions.
6. The goals of antiretroviral therapy are to decrease the amount of virus in your blood (your viral load) and to keep your CD4+ T cell count high. The best results reduce your viral load below detectable levels and keep your CD4+ T cell count high. Most HCPs do routine laboratory work every 3 to 6 months whether you are taking antiretroviral agents or not.
7. Two to 4 weeks after you start on drug therapy (or change your therapy), your HCP will test your viral load to find out how the drugs are working.
   - Your viral load is reported in absolute numbers. All you need to know is that you want to see the viral load drop.
   - Your CD4+ T cell count is reported in absolute numbers or percentages. It is best for your CD4+ T cell count to be above 500 to 600 cells/μL. If reported in percentages, you would like your CD4+ T cell value to be above 14%.
8. An undetectable viral load means that the amount of virus is extremely low and HIV cannot be found in the blood using current testing technology. It does not mean that the virus is gone because the virus can be in lymph nodes and organs that blood tests cannot detect. It also does not mean that you are no longer able to transmit HIV to others. You will need to continue protecting all of your sexual and drug-using partners from HIV.

TABLE 14-17 Patient & Caregiver Teaching

Improving Adherence to Antiretroviral Therapy

The following are strategies that you can use to improve a patient's adherence to using antiretroviral therapy:

1. Determine whether the patient understands the importance of adherence and is ready to start therapy.
2. Provide teaching on medication dosing.
3. Review potential side effects of drugs.
4. Assure the patient that side effects can be treated. If not, medication regimens can be changed.
5. Use teaching and memory aids, including pictures, pillboxes, and calendars.
6. Engage family and friends in the teaching process. Solicit their support to help the patient take treatment.
7. Simplify regimens, dosing, and food requirements as much as possible.
8. Use a team of nurses, HCPs, pharmacists, case managers, and mental health and peer counselors to support the patient.
9. Help the patient integrate the medication regimen into his or her typical life activities and work schedules.

Modified from Centers for Disease Control and Prevention: Guidelines for the use of antiretroviral agents in HIV-1-infected adults and adolescents, 2015. Retrieved from *http://aidsinfo.nih.gov.*

INFORMATICS IN PRACTICE

Use of Internet and Mobile Devices to Manage HIV

- The Internet offers resources and support for patients that can assist them in coping with their illness and educate them about signs and symptoms of serious illness.
- By monitoring their health and quickly spotting warning signs of serious illnesses, patients are able to alert their HCPs and receive earlier treatment.
- These systems can help the patient manage antiretroviral therapy by sending medication reminders by text or e-mail.

accessing counseling; (8) getting involved in support groups and community activities; and (9) developing a consistent relationship with HCPs, including attendance at regular appointments.

Teach patients to recognize symptoms that may indicate disease progression and/or drug side effects so that prompt medical care can be initiated. Table 14-18 provides an overview of symptoms that patients should report.

◆ ***Acute Exacerbations.*** Chronic diseases are characterized by acute exacerbations of recurring problems. This is especially true in HIV disease in which infections, cancers, debility, and psychosocial or economic issues may interact to overwhelm the patient's ability to cope. Nursing care becomes more complex as the patient's immune system deteriorates and new problems arise to compound existing difficulties. When opportunistic diseases or difficult treatment side effects develop, symptom management, teaching, and emotional support are needed.

Nursing care can help prevent the many opportunistic diseases associated with HIV infection. The best way to prevent opportunistic disease is to ensure that the patient is adhering to an effective ART regimen and, if appropriate, taking prophylactic medications for opportunistic infections. Should an opportunistic disease occur, nursing care is an essential part of helping the patient adhere to medications and providing supportive care specific to the opportunistic disease. For example, if the patient has *Pneumocystis jiroveci* pneumonia (PCP)

TABLE 14-18 Patient & Caregiver Teaching

Signs and Symptoms HIV-Infected Patients Need to Report

Teach the patient with HIV infection and the caregiver to report the following signs and symptoms.

Report Immediately

- Any change in level of consciousness: lethargic, hard to arouse, unable to be aroused, unresponsive, unconscious
- Headache accompanied by nausea and vomiting, changes in vision, changes in ability to perform coordinated activities, or after any head trauma
- Vision changes: blurry or black areas in vision field, new floaters, double vision
- Persistent shortness of breath related to activity and not relieved by a short rest period
- Nausea and vomiting accompanied by abdominal pain
- Vomiting blood
- Dehydration: unable to eat or drink because of nausea, diarrhea, or mouth lesions; severe diarrhea or vomiting; dizziness when standing
- Yellow discoloration of the skin
- Any bleeding from the rectum that is not related to hemorrhoids or trauma (e.g., from anal sexual intercourse)
- Pain in the flank with fever and inability to urinate for more than 6 hr
- Blood in the urine
- New onset of weakness in any part of the body, new onset of numbness that is not obviously related to pressure, new onset of difficulty speaking
- Chest pain not obviously related to cough
- Seizures
- New rash accompanied by fever
- New oral lesions accompanied by fever
- Severe depression, anxiety, hallucinations, delusions, or thoughts of causing danger to self or others

Report the Following Signs and Symptoms Within 24 Hours

- New or different headache; constant headache not relieved by over-the-counter medication
- Headache accompanied by fever, nasal congestion, or cough
- Burning, itching, or discharge from the eyes
- New or productive cough
- Vomiting 2 or 3 times a day
- Vomiting accompanied by fever
- New, significant, or watery diarrhea (more than 6 times a day)
- Painful urination, bloody urine, urethral discharge
- Significant new rash (widespread; painful; or following a path down the leg or arm, around the chest, or on the face)
- Difficulty eating or drinking because of mouth lesions
- Vaginal discharge, pain, or itching

(Fig. 14-8), nursing interventions can ensure adequate oxygenation. If the patient has cryptococcal meningitis, an important nursing concern is maintaining a safe environment for a confused patient.

◆ **Ambulatory Care.** HIV infection has no cure, continues for life, causes physical disability, and contributes to impaired health. In many cases it can lead to death. HIV infection affects the entire range of a person's life from physical health to social, emotional, economic, and spiritual well-being.

◆ ***Stigma of HIV.*** HIV-infected patients share problems experienced by all individuals with chronic diseases, but these problems are exacerbated by negative social attitudes and beliefs surrounding HIV.[34] HIV-infected people may be thought to lack

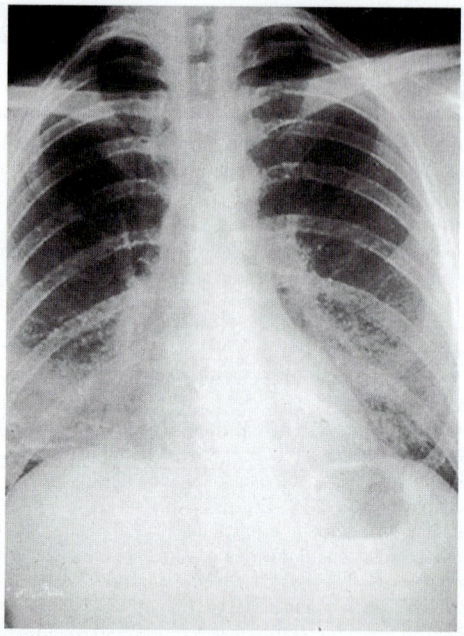

FIG. 14-8 Chest x-ray showing interstitial infiltrates as the result of *Pneumocystis jiroveci* pneumonia. (From the Centers for Disease Control and Prevention. Courtesy Jonathan W.M. Gold, MD, New York.)

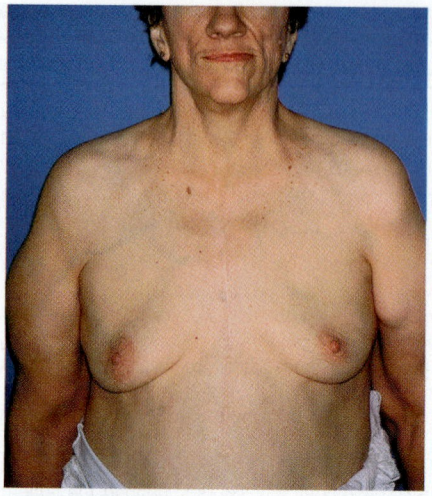

FIG. 14-9 Lipodystrophy manifestations. (From James WD, Berger T, Elston D: *Andrews' diseases of the skin: clinical dermatology,* ed 11, St Louis, 2011, Saunders.)

control over urges to have sex or use drugs. Some people conclude that people with HIV brought the disease upon themselves and deserve to be sick. Behaviors associated with HIV infection are viewed by some as immoral (e.g., homosexuality, promiscuity) and are sometimes illegal (e.g., using drugs, sex work). The fact that infected individuals can transmit HIV to others creates fear, which leads to stigma and discrimination in all facets of life.

In the United States, HIV-infected people have lost jobs, homes, and insurance, although these forms of discrimination are prohibited by the Americans with Disabilities Act (ADA). HIV-related stigma is a global problem that is often more severe for women. Discrimination can lead to social isolation, dependence, frustration, low self-image, loss of control, and economic pressures.

◆ ***Disease and Drug Side Effects.*** Physical problems related to HIV or its treatment can interfere with the patient's ability to maintain a desired lifestyle. HIV-infected patients frequently experience anxiety, fear, depression, diarrhea, peripheral neuropathy, pain, nausea, vomiting, and fatigue. Nursing interventions for these symptoms are similar to what they would be for the patient who does not have HIV infection. For example, nursing management of diarrhea includes helping patients collect specimens, recommending dietary changes, encouraging fluid and electrolyte replacement, instructing the patient about skin care, and managing skin breakdown around the perianal area. Nursing approaches for fatigue in HIV include teaching patients to assess fatigue patterns; determine contributing factors; set activity priorities; conserve energy; schedule rest periods; exercise regularly; and avoid substances such as caffeine, nicotine, alcohol, and other drugs that may disturb sleep.

Some HIV-infected patients, especially those who have been infected and on ART for a long time, may develop a set of metabolic disorders. These include (1) lipodystrophy (changes in body shape caused by a redistribution of fat in the abdomen, upper back, and breasts along with fat loss in the arms, legs, and face) (Fig. 14-9); (2) hyperlipidemia (elevated triglycerides, elevated low-density lipoproteins, and decreased high-density lipoproteins); (3) insulin resistance (4) hyperglycemia; (5) bone disease (osteoporosis, osteopenia, avascular necrosis); (6) lactic acidosis; (7) renal disease; and (8) cardiovascular disease.[35,36]

It is still not clear why these disorders develop, but it is probably a combination of factors such as long-term infection with HIV, side effects of ART, genetic predisposition, and chronic stress. Management of metabolic disorders focuses on detecting problems early, dealing with symptoms, and helping the patient cope with emerging problems and changes to treatment regimens. It is important to recognize and treat these problems early, especially because cardiovascular disease and lactic acidosis are potentially fatal complications.

A frequent first intervention is to change ART medications because some drugs are more often associated with these disorders. Lipid abnormalities are generally treated with lipid-lowering drugs (see Table 33-5), dietary changes, and exercise. Insulin resistance is treated with hypoglycemic drugs and weight loss. Bone disease may be improved with exercise, dietary changes, and calcium and vitamin D supplements.

◆ ***End-of-Life Care.*** Despite new developments in the treatment of HIV infection, many patients eventually experience disease progression, disability, and death. Sometimes these occur because treatments do not work for the patient. Sometimes the patient's HIV becomes resistant to all available drug therapies. In addition, ART is now allowing people living with HIV to live longer and to develop diseases of aging, such as cardiovascular and endocrine problems that lead to death.

Nursing care during the terminal phase of any disease should focus on keeping the patient comfortable, facilitating emotional and spiritual acceptance of the finite nature of life, helping the patient's significant others deal with grief and loss, and maintaining a safe environment.[37] As a nurse, you are the pivotal care provider during this phase of illness, whether at home, through hospice, or in a health care facility. (End-of-life care is discussed in Chapter 9.)

◆ Evaluation

The expected outcomes are that the patient at risk for HIV infection will

- Analyze personal risk factors
- Develop and implement a personal plan to decrease risks
- Get tested for HIV

The expected outcomes are that the patient with HIV infection will

- Describe basic aspects of the effects of HIV on the immune system
- Compare and contrast various treatment options for HIV disease
- Work with a team of HCPs to achieve optimal health
- Prevent transmission of HIV to others

Gerontologic Considerations: HIV Infection

The number of older adults who have HIV disease is increasing because (1) HIV treatment has been effective in reducing the number of deaths from HIV-related opportunistic infections and (2) people 60 and older are being infected at increasing rates. The number of people over the age of 60 living with HIV is expected to grow.

Remember that older people living with HIV are susceptible to the same diseases as non-HIV-infected older people. These include heart disease, cancer, diabetes, bone disease, arthritis, hypertension, kidney disease, and cognitive impairment. However, people with HIV infection may experience these diseases at an earlier age (compared with non-HIV-infected people) and may be at higher risk of co-morbidities related to the medications used to treat HIV.[38] For example, some of the HIV medications are associated with increased lipids and altered insulin metabolism. Focusing nursing care on early identification of these complications, and assisting patients in reducing their risk for heart disease, diabetes, or other chronic disease, are critical aspects of caring for the older HIV patient.

Another consideration with the aging HIV population is the impact of polypharmacy (taking multiple medications to treat a variety of conditions). In general, older adults are often prescribed multiple medications to manage various chronic diseases. Some of these medications may interact with or be potentiated by HIV medications. Therefore careful monitoring and assessment of possible drug interactions is important when providing care to this population.

Older adults may be ashamed and hesitate to tell anyone that they have an HIV infection. This may make it difficult for them to get the appropriate health care and support. As a nurse, you need to recognize that HIV is a chronic disease that will affect an increasing number of older adults and be prepared to help the older person who is living with HIV infection.

CHECK YOUR PRACTICE

You are receiving report on a newly admitted patient to the rehabilitation unit. He is a 68-yr-old male patient who had a hip replacement 3 days ago. The nurse giving the report casually mentions, "Oh, by the way, he has AIDS. Can you believe that an old man like that has HIV?"

- How would you respond?

CASE STUDY

HIV Infection

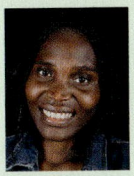

(©iStockphoto/Thinkstock)

Patient Profile

J.N., a 35-year-old African American woman, was admitted to the hospital in respiratory distress. AIDS and *Pneumocystis jiroveci* pneumonia (PCP) were both diagnosed 2 days ago.

Subjective Data

- Seen by an HCP 6 years ago for pain behind the sternum and difficulty swallowing, diagnosed as esophageal candidiasis; positive HIV-antibody test at that time
- Has consistently refused ART because, "We can't afford it"
- Married to Jim, a former IV drug user, for 15 years until his recent death from AIDS-related complications
- Has two children, ages 8 and 10; neither has been tested for HIV infection
- Experiences fatigue and frequent oral and vaginal candidiasis outbreaks
- Expresses concern about the welfare of her children, who are at home with her sister, and says, "Maybe I should take better care of myself for them"

Objective Data

Physical Examination

- 5 ft 6 in tall, 100 lb, temperature 100.4° F (38° C), O_2 saturation 92% on 3 L of O_2 via nasal cannula

Laboratory Studies

- $CD4^+$ T cell count 185 cells/μL
- Viral load 55,328 copies/μL
- Hematocrit 30%

Interprofessional Care

- Trimethoprim/sulfamethoxazole
- Combination antiretroviral therapy: tenofovir and emtricitabine (Truvada), with darunavir and cobicistat (Prezcobix)

Discussion Questions

1. Why did J.N.'s initial medical problem (esophageal candidiasis) lead to an HIV test?
2. Why was trimethoprim/sulfamethoxazole ordered, and what are its common side effects?
3. What diagnostic criteria for AIDS are present in J.N.?
4. Is there a potential advantage to J.N.'s refusal to take antiretroviral drugs in the past? If so, why or why not?
5. ***Priority Decision:*** What priority teaching needs should be covered before J.N. is discharged from the hospital to return home? What referrals must be made?
6. How can J.N. be helped to adhere to her medication schedule?
7. ***Priority Decision:*** What are the priority nursing interventions? What plans must be made for continued nursing care after discharge?
8. ***Evidence-Based Practice:*** J.N. asks you if her kids should be tested. She is afraid of what the results may be. How should you respond?
9. ***Teamwork and Collaboration:*** Women often put their children's welfare first. What barriers could this cause for J.N.'s treatment? How could an interprofessional team assist in addressing these issues?
10. ***Safety:*** The nurse needs to start an IV for fluid replacement on J.N. Before inserting the IV what type of personal protective equipment is recommended for this situation?

Answers available at *http://evolve.elsevier.com/Lewis/medsurg.*

BRIDGE TO NCLEX EXAMINATION

The number of the question corresponds to the same-numbered outcome at the beginning of the chapter.

1. Emerging and reemerging infections affect health care by *(select all that apply)*
   a. reevaluating vaccine practices.
   b. revealing antimicrobial resistance.
   c. limiting antibiotics to those with life-threatening infection.
   d. challenging researchers to discover new antimicrobial therapies.
2. Which types(s) of isolation precautions is (are) appropriate for a patient with tuberculosis (*select all that apply*)?
   a. contact precautions
   b. droplet precautions
   c. airborne precautions
   d. standard precautions
   e. neutropenic precautions
3. Transmission of HIV from an infected individual to another most commonly occurs as a result of
   a. unprotected anal or vaginal sexual intercourse.
   b. low levels of virus in the blood and high levels of $CD4^+$ T cells.
   c. transmission from mother to infant during labor and delivery and breastfeeding.
   d. sharing of drug-using equipment, including needles, syringes, pipes, and straws.
4. During HIV infection
   a. reverse transcriptase helps HIV fuse with the $CD4^+$ T cell.
   b. HIV RNA uses the $CD4^+$ T cell's mitochondria to replicate.
   c. the immune system is impaired predominantly by the eventual widespread destruction of $CD4^+$ T cells.
   d. a long period of dormancy develops during which HIV cannot be found in the blood and there is little viral replication.
5. Which statements accurately describe HIV infection (*select all that apply*)?
   a. Untreated HIV infection has a predictable pattern of progression.
   b. Late chronic HIV infection is called acquired immunodeficiency syndrome (AIDS).
   c. Untreated HIV infection can remain in the early chronic stage for a decade or more.
   d. Untreated HIV infection usually remains in the early chronic stage for 1 year or less.
   e. Opportunistic diseases occur more often when the $CD4^+$ T cell count is high and the viral load is low.
6. A diagnosis of AIDS is made when an HIV-infected patient has
   a. a $CD4^+$ T cell count below 200/μL.
   b. a high level of HIV in the blood and saliva.
   c. lipodystrophy with metabolic abnormalities.
   d. oral hairy leukoplakia, an infection caused by Epstein-Barr virus.
7. Screening for HIV infection generally involves
   a. detecting $CD8^+$ cytotoxic T cells in saliva.
   b. laboratory analysis of saliva to detect $CD4^+$ T cells.
   c. analysis of lymph tissues for the presence of HIV RNA.
   d. laboratory analysis of blood to detect HIV antigen or antibody.
8. HIV antiretroviral drugs are used to
   a. cure acute HIV infection.
   b. decrease viral RNA levels.
   c. treat opportunistic diseases.
   d. decrease pain and symptoms in terminal disease.
9. Opportunistic diseases in HIV infection
   a. are usually benign.
   b. are generally slow to develop and progress.
   c. occur in the presence of immunosuppression.
   d. are curable with appropriate drug interventions.
10. Which statement(s) about metabolic side effects of ART is (are) true (*select all that apply*)?
    a. These are annoying symptoms that are ultimately harmless.
    b. ART-related body changes include fat redistribution and peripheral wasting.
    c. Lipid abnormalities include increases in triglycerides and decreases in high-density cholesterol.
    d. Insulin resistance and hyperlipidemia can be treated with drugs to control glucose and cholesterol.
    e. Compared to uninfected people, insulin resistance and hyperlipidemia are more difficult to treat in HIV-infected patients.
11. Which strategy can the nurse teach the patient to eliminate the risk of HIV transmission?
    a. Using sterile equipment to inject drugs
    b. Cleaning equipment used to inject drugs
    c. Taking lamivudine (Epivir) during pregnancy
    d. Using latex or polyurethane barriers to cover genitalia during sexual contact
12. What is the *most* appropriate nursing intervention to help an HIV-infected patient adhere to a treatment regimen?
    a. "Set up" a drug pillbox for the patient every week.
    b. Give the patient a video and a brochure to view and read at home.
    c. Tell the patient that the side effects of the drugs are bad but that they go away after a while.
    d. Assess the patient's routines and find adherence cues that fit into the patient's life circumstances.

1. a, b, d, 2. c, d, 3. a, 4. c, 5. a, b, c, 6. a, 7. d, 8. b, 9. c, 10. b, c, d, 11. a, 12. d

For rationales to these answers and even more NCLEX review questions, visit *http://evolve.elsevier.com/Lewis/medsurg.*

EVOLVE WEBSITE

http://evolve.elsevier.com/Lewis/medsurg

Review Questions (Online Only)
Key Points
Answer Keys for Questions
- Rationales for Bridge to NCLEX Examination Questions
- Answer Guidelines for Case Study on p. 231

Student Case Study
- Patient With Human Immunodeficiency Virus (HIV) Infection and Acquired Immunodeficiency Syndrome (AIDS)

Conceptual Care Map Creator
Audio Glossary
Content Updates

REFERENCES

1. Centers for Disease Control and Prevention: Emerging infectious diseases. Retrieved from *http://wwwnc.cdc.gov/eid.*
2. Centers for Disease Control and Prevention: The reemergence of vaccine-preventable diseases—exploring the public health successes and challenges, 2015. Retrieved from *www.cdc.gov.*

3. Khabbaz RF, Moseley RR, Steiner RJ, et al: Challenges of infectious diseases in the USA, *Lancet* 384:53, 2014.
4. Clemons NS, Gastanaduy PA, Fiebelkorn AP, et al: Measles—United States, January 4–April 2, 2015, *MMWR* 64:373, 2015.
5. Infectious Disease Society of America: Antimicrobial resistance. Retrieved from *www.idsociety.org/topic_antimicrobial_resistance.*
6. Velez R, VanGraafeiland B, Sloand E: Using clinical guidelines and clinical acumen to manage community-acquired methicillin-resistant *Staphylococcus aureus* infection, *J Nurse Pract* 11:124, 2015.
7. Centers for Disease Control and Prevention: Healthcare-associated infections. Retrieved from *www.cdc.gov/HAI.*
8. Centers for Disease Control and Prevention: Healthcare-associated infections: Data and statistics. Retrieved from *www.cdc.gov/HAI/surveillance/index.html.*
9. US Department of Health and Human Services Agency for Healthcare Research & Quality: Healthcare-associated infections. Retrieved from *www.ahrq.gov.*
10. Centers for Disease Control and Prevention: Top CDC recommendations to prevent healthcare-associated infections. Retrieved from *www.cdc.gov/HAI.*
11. Centers for Disease Control and Prevention: Guidelines for isolation precautions: preventing transmission of infectious agents in healthcare settings, 2007. Retrieved from *www.cdc.gov/hicpac.*
12. Society of Healthcare Epidemiology of America: Compendium of strategies to prevent healthcare-associated infection in acute care hospitals—2014 update. Retrieved from *www.shea-online.org/View/ArticleId/289/Compendium-of-Strategies-to-Prevent-Healthcare-Associated-Infections-in-Acute-Care-Hospitals-2014-Up.aspx.*
13. High K: Evaluation of infection in the older adult. Retrieved from *www.uptodate.com.*
14. Centers for Disease Control and Prevention: HIV surveillance report: diagnosis of HIV infection in the United States and dependent areas, 2013. Retrieved from *www.cdc.gov/hiv/statistics/basics.*
15. US Department of Health and Human Services. HIV/AIDS basics. Retrieved from *www.aids.gov/hiv-aids-basics.*
*16. Kuhar DT, Henderson DK, Struble KA, et al: Updated US public health service guidelines for the management of occupational exposures to human immunodeficiency virus and recommendations for postexposure prophylaxis, *Infect Control Hosp Epidemiol* 34:875, 2013.
17. World Health Organization. Mother-to-child transmission of HIV. Retrieved from *www.who.int/hiv/topics/mtct/en.*
18. Centers for Disease Control and Prevention: US Public Health Service Task Force recommendations for use of antiretroviral drugs in pregnant HIV-1–infected women for maternal health and interventions to reduce perinatal HIV transmission in the United States—July 31, 2012. Retrieved from *www.aidsinfo.nih.gov.*
19. US Department of Health and Human Services. The HIV life cycle. Retrieved from *http://aidsinfo.nih.gov/education-materials/fact-sheets/19/73/the-hiv-life-cycle.*
20. Smith MK, Rutstein SE, Powers KA, et al: The detection and management of early HIV infection: a clinical and public health emergency, *J Acquir Immune Defic Syndr* 63:S187, 2013.
21. US Department of Health and Human Services. The stages of HIV infection. Retrieved from *http://aidsinfo.nih.gov/education-materials/fact-sheets/19/46/the-stages-of-hiv-infection.*
22. Branson BM, Owen SM, Weslowski LG, et al: Laboratory testing for the diagnosis of HIV infection: updated recommendations, 2014. Retrieved from *http://stacks.cdc.gov/view/cdc/23447.*
23. Kang W, Tong HI, Sun Y, et al: Hepatitis C virus infection in patients with HIV-1 infection: epidemiology, natural history and management, *Expert Rev Gastreoenterol Hepatol* 8:247, 2014.
*24. Panel on Antiretroviral Guidelines for Adults and Adolescents. Guidelines for the use of antiretroviral agents in HIV-1–infected adults and adolescents, 2015. Retrieved from *http://aidsinfo.nih.gov/guidelines/html/1/adult-and-adolescent-treatment-guidelines/0.*
25. Panel on Opportunistic Infections in HIV-infected Adults and Adolescents. Guidelines for the prevention and treatment of opportunistic infections in HIV-infected adults and adolescents, 2015. Retrieved from *www.aidsinfo.nih.gov.*
*26. Smith DK, Koenig LJ, Martin M, et al: Preexposure prophylaxis for the prevention of HIV infection – 2014: a clinical practice guideline. Retrieved from *http://stacks.cdc.gov/view/cdc/23109.*
27. Centers for Disease Control and Prevention, Health Resources and Services Administration, National Institutes of Health, American Academy of HIV Medicine, Association of Nurses in AIDS Care, the National Minority AIDS Council, and Urban Coalition for HIV/AIDS Prevention Services: Recommendations for HIV prevention with adults and adolescents with HIV in the United States, 2014. Retrieved from *http://stacks.cdc.gov/view/cdc/26062.*
28. US Department of Health and Human Services. Substance abuse/use. Retrieved from *www.aids.gov/hiv-aids-basics/prevention/reduce-your-risk/substance-abuse-use.*
29. Shoptaw S: HIV prevention for people who use substances: evidence-based strategies, *J Food Drug Anal* 21:S91, 2013.
*30. Panel on Treatment of HIV-infected Pregnant Women and Prevention of Perinatal Transmission. Recommendations for use of antiretroviral drugs in pregnant HIV-1-infected women for maternal health and interventions to reduce perinatal HIV transmission in the United States. Retrieved from *http://aidsinfo.nih.gov/guidelines/html/3/perinatal-guidelines/0#.*
31. Centers for Disease Control and Prevention: Revised guidelines for HIV testing of adults, adolescents, and pregnant women in health-care settings—September 22, 2006. (Classic) Retrieved from *www.aidsinfo.nih.gov.*
32. US Preventive Services Task Force. Human immunodeficiency virus (HIV) infection: screening, 2013. Retrieved from *www.uspreventiveservicestaskforce.org/Page/Topic/recommendation-summary/human-immunodeficiency-virus-hiv-infection-screening.*
33. US Department of Health and Human Services. Just diagnosed: next steps after testing positive for HIV. Retrieved from *http://aidsinfo.nih.gov/education-materials/fact-sheets/21/65/just-diagnosed–next-steps-after-testing-positive-for-hiv.*
34. French H, Greeff M, Watson MJ, et al: HIV stigma and disclosure experiences of people living with HIV in an urban and a rural setting, *AIDS Care* 8:1042, 2015.
35. Hemkens LG, Bucher HC: HIV infection and cardiovascular disease, *Eur Heart J* 35:1373, 2014.
36. Bociaga-Jasik M, Goralska J, Razny U, et al: Impact of antiretroviral therapy on selected metabolic disorders-pilot study, *Adv Clin Exp Med* 23:539, 2014.
37. Kirton C, Krakowski A, Witt Sherman D: Palliative care in HIV/AIDS. In Matzo M, editor: *Palliative care nursing: quality care to the end of life*, ed 4, New York, 2015, Springer.
*38. The HIV and Aging Consensus Project. Recommended treatment strategies for clinicians managing older patients with HIV. Retrieved from *http://hiv-age.org.*

*Evidence-based information for clinical practice.

15

Cancer

Carolee Polek

Every tomorrow has two handles. We can take hold of it by the handle of anxiety or by the handle of faith.

Author Unknown

http://evolve.elsevier.com/Lewis/medsurg/

LEARNING OUTCOMES

1. Describe the prevalence, incidence, survival, and mortality rates of cancer in the United States.
2. Describe the processes involved in the biology of cancer.
3. Differentiate among the three stages of cancer development.
4. Describe the role of the immune system related to cancer.
5. Discuss the role of the nurse in the prevention, detection, and diagnosis of cancer.
6. Explain the use of surgery, chemotherapy, radiation therapy, immunotherapy, targeted therapy, and hormone therapy in the treatment of cancer.
7. Identify the classifications of chemotherapy agents and methods of administration.
8. Differentiate between teletherapy (external beam radiation) and brachytherapy (internal radiation).
9. Describe the effects of radiation therapy and chemotherapy on normal tissues.
10. Identify the types and effects of immunotherapy and targeted therapy.
11. Describe the nursing management of patients receiving chemotherapy, radiation therapy, immunotherapy, and targeted therapy.
12. Describe nutritional therapy for patients with cancer.
13. Identify the complications associated with advanced cancer.
14. Describe support interventions for cancer patients, cancer survivors, and their caregivers.

KEY TERMS

bone marrow transplantation (BMT), p. 259
brachytherapy, p. 250
cancer, p. 234
carcinogens, p. 237
carcinoma in situ (CIS), p. 241
chemotherapy, p. 245
hematopoietic stem cell transplantation (HSCT), p. 259
histologic grading, p. 241
immunologic surveillance, p. 239
immunotherapy, p. 257
malignant neoplasms, p. 240
metastasis, p. 238
nadir, p. 253
oncogenes, p. 236
peripheral stem cell transplantation (PSCT), p. 259
protooncogenes, p. 236
radiation, p. 249
staging, p. 241
targeted therapy, p. 257
teletherapy, p. 250
tumor angiogenesis, p. 238
vesicants, p. 246

Cancer is a group of diseases characterized by uncontrolled and unregulated growth of cells. Although cancer is often considered a disease of aging, with the majority of cases diagnosed in those over age 55 years, it occurs in people of all ages. An estimated 1,658,370 people in the United States are diagnosed annually with invasive carcinoma (excluding basal and squamous cell skin cancers).[1]

Overall both the incidence and mortality rate of cancer have been declining.[2] The incidences of many cancers, such as colorectal, lung, breast, and oropharyngeal cancers, have declined largely as a result of preventive efforts. However, the incidence of other types of cancers, such as kidney, thyroid, pancreas, liver, uterus, skin melanoma, multiple myeloma, and non-Hodgkin's lymphoma, has been increasing.[3]

Overall cancer incidence is higher in men than women. Gender differences in incidence and in death rates for specific cancers are presented in Tables 15-1 and 15-2 and the Gender Differences box.

Although mortality rates from all cancers combined are on the decline, cancer is still the second most common cause of

Reviewed by Margaret Barton-Burke, RN, PhD, FAAN, Mary Ann Lee Professor of Oncology Nursing, College of Nursing, University of Missouri–St Louis, St. Louis, Missouri; Stephanie Jackson, RN, MSN, AOCNS, Oncology Clinical Nurse Specialist, Hematology/Stem Cell Transplant, UCLA Medical Center, Los Angeles, California; Laura A. Stokowski, RNC, MS, Inova Fairfax Hospital for Children, Falls Church, Virginia; Joseph Tariman, RN, PhD, ANP-BC, Assistant Professor, School of Nursing, De Paul University, Chicago, Illinois; Deborah Kirk Walker, DNP, FNP-BC, NP-C, AOCN, Assistant Professor/Nurse Practitioner, Coordinator of Dual Adult—Gerontology Primary Care and Oncology Nurse Practitioner Specialty Track, Acute, Chronic, and Continuing Care Department, University of Alabama at Birmingham School of Nursing, Birmingham, Alabama; and Linda H. Yoder, RN, PhD, AOCN, FAAN, Associate Professor and Director, Nursing Administration and Healthcare Systems Management, Robert Wood Johnson Executive Nurse Alumna, Luci Baines Johnson Fellow in Nursing, The University of Texas at Austin School of Nursing, Austin, Texas.

TABLE 15-1 Cancer Incidence by Site and Gender*

MALE		FEMALE	
Type	**%**	**Type**	**%**
Prostate	26	Breast	29
Lung	14	Lung	13
Colon/rectum	8	Colon/rectum	8
Urinary bladder	7	Uterus	7
Non-Hodgkin's lymphoma	5	Thyroid	6
Kidney and renal pelvis	5	Non-Hodgkin's lymphoma	4
Oral cavity and pharynx	4	Melanoma	4
Leukemia	4	Pancreas	3

Source: American Cancer Society: *Cancer facts & figures 2015*, Atlanta, 2015, American Cancer Society.
*Numbers are estimates excluding basal and squamous cell skin cancers and carcinoma in situ.

TABLE 15-2 Cancer Deaths by Site and Gender

MALE		FEMALE	
Type	**%**	**Type**	**%**
Lung and bronchus	28	Lung and bronchus	26
Prostate	9	Breast	15
Colon/rectum	8	Colon/rectum	9
Pancreas	7	Pancreas	7
Liver and intrahepatic bile ducts	5	Ovary	5
Leukemia	5	Leukemia	4
Esophagus	4	Uterus	4
Urinary bladder	4	Non-Hodgkin's lymphoma	3
Non-Hodgkin's lymphoma	4	Liver and intrahepatic bile ducts	3
Kidney and renal pelvis	3	Brain and other nervous system	2

Source: American Cancer Society: *Cancer facts & figures 2015*, Atlanta, 2015, American Cancer Society.

GENDER DIFFERENCES

Cancer

Men

- More men than women die from cancer-related deaths each year.
- Mortality rate from lung cancer is higher in men than in women.
- Cancer with the highest incidence among men is prostate cancer.
- Men are more likely to develop liver cancer than women.
- Head and neck cancer occurs more frequently in men than in women.

Women

- Cancer with the highest death rate among women is lung cancer.
- Cancer with the highest incidence among women is breast cancer.
- Thyroid cancer is more prevalent in women than in men.
- Women are less likely to have colon cancer screenings than men.

death in the United States (heart disease is the most common). However, in people 40 to 79 years of age, cancer is the leading cause of death. Annually about 589,400 Americans are expected to die as a result of cancer, which is more than 1600 people per day.[1,2]

Considerable progress has been made in controlling cancer for long periods. More than 14.5 million Americans are alive today who have a history of cancer. This statistic represents Americans living with cancer, including those who are disease free, in remission, or undergoing treatment.[2] (Cancer survivors are discussed in this chapter on pp. 266-267).

Statistics are helpful in describing the scope of cancer as a public health problem, but they cannot describe the combined physiologic, psychologic, and social impact of cancer on individual patients, their caregivers, and families. Considerable apprehension is associated with a cancer diagnosis, proportionately more than with other chronic diseases such as heart disease. Despite advances in treatment and care, a great deal of anxiety and fear continue to be associated with a diagnosis of cancer. Education of health care professionals and the public is essential to promote realistic attitudes about cancer and cancer treatment.

You are in a strategic position to lead efforts at changing attitudes about cancer. Furthermore, you can also (1) assist individuals in decreasing their risk of cancer development, (2) increase rates of cancer screening, (3) help patients comply with cancer management regimens, and (4) support patients and their families as they cope with the effects of cancer and related treatment. You need to be knowledgeable about specific types of cancer, treatment options, management of side effects of therapy, and supportive therapies for cancer.

BIOLOGY OF CANCER

Two major dysfunctions in the process of cancer development are defective cell proliferation (growth) and defective cell differentiation.

Defect in Cell Proliferation

Normally, most tissues contain a population of undifferentiated cells known as stem cells. These stem cells ultimately differentiate and become mature, functioning cells of that tissue and only that tissue.

Cell proliferation originates in the stem cell and begins when the stem cell enters the cell cycle (Fig. 15-1). The time from when a cell enters the cell cycle to when the cell divides into two identical cells is called the *generation time of the cell.* A mature cell continues to function until it degenerates and dies.

All of the body's cells are controlled by an intracellular mechanism that determines when cell proliferation is necessary. Under normal conditions, a state of dynamic equilibrium is constantly maintained (i.e., cell proliferation equals cell degeneration or death). Normally the process of cell division and proliferation is activated only in the presence of cell degeneration or death *(apoptosis).* Cell proliferation also occurs if the body has a physiologic need for more cells. For example, a normal increase in white blood cell (WBC) count occurs in the presence of infection.

Another mechanism for proliferation control in normal cells is *contact inhibition.* Normal cells respect the boundaries and territory of the cells surrounding them. They will not invade a territory that is not their own. The neighboring cells are thought to inhibit cell growth through the physical contact of the surrounding cell membranes. Cancer cells grown in tissue culture are characterized by loss of contact inhibition. These cells have no regard for cell boundaries and grow on top of one another and also on top of or between normal cells.

The rate of normal cell proliferation (from the time of cell birth to the time of cell death) differs in each body tissue. In some tissues, such as bone marrow, hair follicles, and epithelial lining of the gastrointestinal (GI) tract, the rate of cell proliferation is rapid. In other tissues, such as myocardium and cartilage, cell proliferation does not occur or is slow.

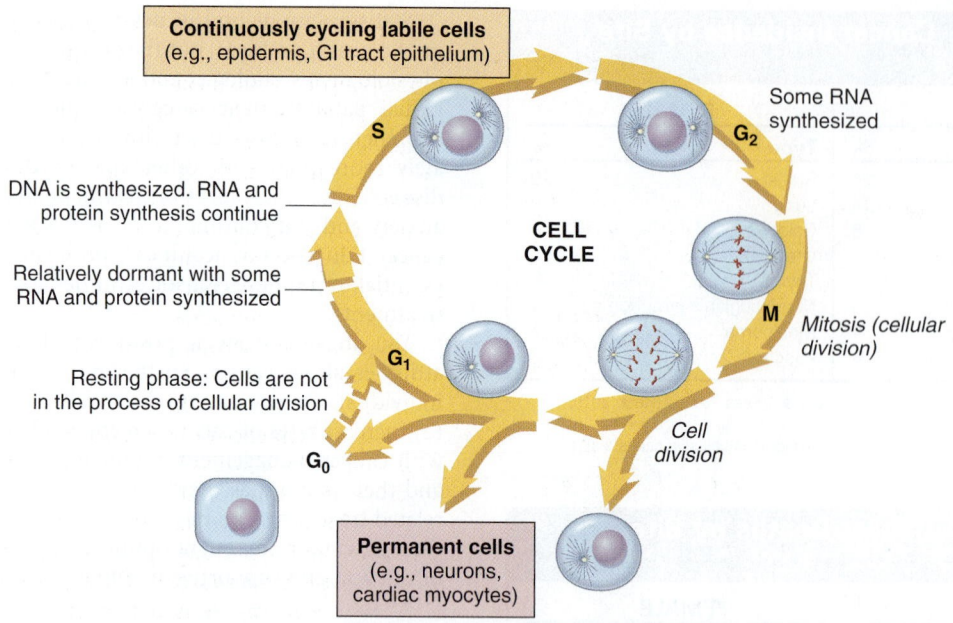

FIG. 15-1 Cell life cycle and metabolic activity. Generation time is the period from *M* phase to *M* phase. Cells not in the cycle but capable of division are in the resting phase *(G_0)*. (Adapted from Kumar V, Abbas AK, Fausto N, et al: *Robbins and Cotran pathologic basis of disease,* ed 8, Philadelphia, 2010, Saunders.)

Cancer cells proliferate at the same rate as the normal cells of the tissue from which they arise. However, cancer cells respond differently than normal cells to the intracellular signals that regulate the state of dynamic equilibrium. The difference is that proliferation of the cancer cells is indiscriminate and continuous. Sometimes they produce more than two cells at the time of mitosis. In this way, there is continuous growth of a tumor mass: $1 \times 2 \times 4 \times 8 \times 15$ and so on. This is termed the *pyramid effect.* The time required for a tumor mass to double in size is known as its *doubling time.*

Defect in Cell Differentiation

Cell differentiation is normally an orderly process that progresses from a state of immaturity to a state of maturity. Because all body cells are derived from the fertilized ova, all cells have the potential to perform all body functions. As cells differentiate, this potential is repressed, and the mature cell is capable of performing only specific functions. With cell differentiation, there is a stable and orderly phasing out of cell potential. Under normal conditions, the differentiated cell is stable and will not *dedifferentiate* (i.e., revert to a previous undifferentiated state).

Genetic Link

Cancer involves the malfunction of genes that control differentiation and proliferation. Two types of normal genes that can be affected by mutation are *protooncogenes* and *tumor suppressor genes.* **Protooncogenes** are normal cell genes that are important regulators of normal cell processes. Protooncogenes promote growth, whereas tumor suppressor genes suppress growth. Mutations that alter the expression of protooncogenes can activate them to function as **oncogenes** (tumor-inducing genes).

The protooncogene has been described as the genetic lock that keeps the cell in its mature functioning state. When this lock is "unlocked," as may occur through exposure to *carcinogens* (agents that cause cancer) or oncogenic viruses, genetic alterations and mutations occur. The abilities and properties that the cell had in fetal development are again expressed. Oncogenes can change a normal cell to a malignant one. This cell regains a fetal appearance and function. For example, some cancer cells produce new proteins, such as those characteristic of the embryonic and fetal periods of life. These proteins, located on the cell membrane, include carcinoembryonic antigen (CEA) and α-fetoprotein (AFP). They can be detected in human blood by laboratory studies (see Role of the Immune System later in this chapter). Other cancer cells, such as small cell carcinoma of the lung, produce hormones (see Complications of Cancer later in this chapter on pp. 261-267) that are ordinarily produced by cells arising from the same embryonic cells as the tumor cells.[4]

Tumor suppressor genes function to regulate cell growth. They prevent cells from going through the cell cycle. Mutations that alter tumor suppressor genes make them inactive, resulting in a loss of their tumor-suppressing action. Examples of tumor suppressor genes are *BRCA1* and *BRCA2.* Alterations in these genes increase a person's risk for breast and ovarian cancer. Another tumor suppressor gene is the *APC* gene. Alterations in this gene increase a person's risk for familial adenomatous polyposis, which is a precursor for colorectal cancer (see Chapter 42). Mutations in the *p53* tumor suppressor gene have been found in many cancers, including bladder, breast, colorectal, esophageal, liver, lung, and ovarian cancers.

Development of Cancer

The following is a theoretical model of the development of cancer. The cause and development of each type of cancer are likely to be multifactorial. A common misbelief is that the development of cancer is a rapid, haphazard event. However, cancer is usually an orderly process that occurs over time and has several stages: initiation, promotion, and progression (Fig. 15-2).

Initiation. Cancer cells arise from normal cells as a result of changes in genes. The first stage, *initiation,* involves a mutation in the cell's genetic structure. A *mutation* is any change in the usual DNA sequence.

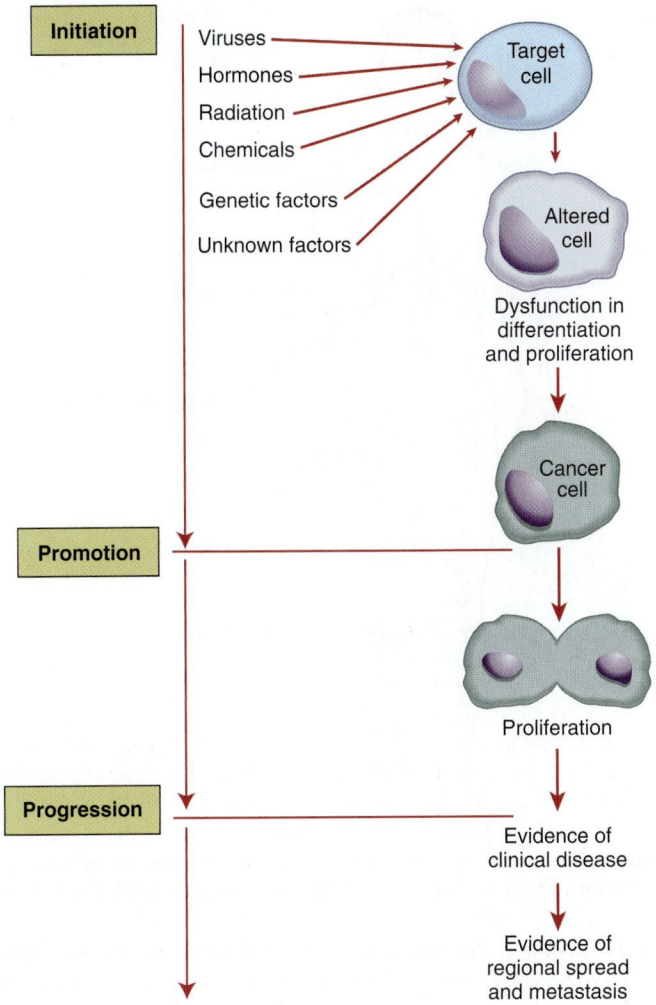

FIG. 15-2 Process of cancer development.

Genetic Link

Gene mutations can occur in two different ways: *inherited* from a parent (passed from one generation to the next) or *acquired* during a person's lifetime. (Mutations are discussed in Chapter 12.)

About 5% to 10% of all cancers or the predisposition to the cancer is inherited from one's parents.[5] These genetic alterations lead to a high risk of developing a specific type of cancer. However, most cancers do not result from inherited genes but are acquired from damage to genes occurring during one's lifetime. An acquired mutation is passed on to all cells that develop from that single cell. The damaged cell may die or repair itself. However, if cell death or repair does not occur before cell division, the cell will replicate into daughter cells, each with the same genetic alteration.

Carcinogens. Many **carcinogens** (cancer-causing agents capable of producing cell alterations) are detoxified by protective enzymes and are harmlessly excreted. If this protective mechanism fails, carcinogens can enter the cell's nucleus and alter deoxyribonucleic acid (DNA). Carcinogens may be chemical, radiation, or viral.

Chemical carcinogens. Chemicals were identified as cancer-causing agents in the latter part of the eighteenth century when Percival Pott noted that chimney sweeps had a higher incidence of cancer of the scrotum associated with exposure to soot residue in chimneys. As the years passed, many chemical agents have been identified as carcinogens (e.g., benzene, arsenic, formaldehyde). People exposed to certain chemicals over time have a greater incidence of certain cancers than others. The long latency period from the time of exposure to the development of cancer makes it difficult to identify cancer-causing chemicals.

Radiation. Radiation can cause cancer in almost any body tissue. When cells are exposed to a source of radiation, damage occurs to DNA. Certain malignancies have been correlated with radiation as a carcinogenic agent:

- Leukemia, lymphoma, thyroid cancer, and other cancers increased in incidence in the general population of Hiroshima and Nagasaki after the atomic bomb explosions.
- A higher incidence of bone cancer occurs in people exposed to radiation in certain occupations, such as radiologists, radiation chemists, and uranium miners.

Ultraviolet (UV) radiation has long been associated with melanoma and squamous and basal cell carcinoma of the skin. Sunlight is the main source of UV exposure giving off UVA and UVB rays. Skin cancer is the most common type of cancer among whites in the United States. Of great concern is the increase in the incidence of melanoma. Although the cause of melanoma is probably multifactorial, UV radiation secondary to sunlight exposure is linked to the development of melanoma. UV radiation from tanning beds can cause skin cancer (melanoma, basal cell and squamous cell carcinoma).[6]

Viral carcinogens. Certain DNA and ribonucleic acid (RNA) viruses, termed *oncogenic,* can transform the cells they infect and induce malignant transformation. Viruses have been identified as causative agents of cancer in animals and humans. Burkitt's lymphoma is associated with Epstein-Barr virus (EBV).[7] People with acquired immunodeficiency syndrome (AIDS), which is caused by human immunodeficiency virus (HIV), have a high incidence of Kaposi sarcoma (see Chapter 14). Other viruses that have been linked to the development of cancer include hepatitis B virus, which is associated with hepatocellular carcinoma; and human papillomavirus (HPV), which is believed to induce lesions that progress to squamous cell carcinomas, such as cervical, anal, and head and neck cancers.

Promotion. A single alteration of the genetic structure of the cell is not sufficient to result in cancer. However, the odds of cancer development are increased with the presence of promoting agents. *Promotion,* the second stage in the development of cancer, is characterized by the reversible proliferation of the altered cells. An increase in the altered cell population further increases the likelihood of additional mutations.

An important distinction between initiation and promotion is that the activity of promoters is reversible. This is a key concept in cancer prevention. Promoting factors include such agents as dietary fat, obesity, cigarette smoking, and alcohol consumption. Changing a person's lifestyle to modify these risk factors can reduce the chance of cancer development. Approximately one third of cancer-related deaths in the United States are related to tobacco use, unhealthy diet, physical inactivity, and obesity.[1]

Several promoting agents have activity against specific types of body tissues. Therefore these agents tend to promote specific kinds of cancer. For example, cigarette smoke is a promoting agent in bronchogenic carcinoma and, in conjunction with alcohol intake, promotes esophageal and bladder cancers.

Some carcinogens, termed *complete carcinogens,* are capable of both initiating and promoting the development of cancer. Cigarette smoke is an example of a complete carcinogen capable of initiating and promoting cancer.

A period of time, ranging from 1 to 40 years, elapses between the initial genetic alteration and the actual clinical evidence of cancer. This period, called the *latent* period, includes both the initiation and promotion stages in the natural history of cancer. The variation in the length of time that elapses before the cancer becomes clinically evident is associated with the mitotic rate of the tissue of origin and environmental factors. In most cancers, the process of developing cancer is years or even decades in length.

For the disease process to become clinically evident, the cells must reach a critical mass. A tumor that is 1.0 cm (0.4 inch) (the size usually detectable by palpation) contains 1 billion cancer cells. A 0.5-cm tumor is the smallest that can be detected by current diagnostic measures, such as MRI.

Progression. *Progression* is the final stage in the natural history of a cancer. This stage is characterized by increased growth rate of the tumor, increased invasiveness, and **metastasis** (spread of the cancer to a distant site). Certain cancers seem to have an affinity for a particular tissue or organ as a site of metastasis (e.g., colon cancer often spreads to the liver). Other cancers (e.g., melanoma) are unpredictable in their pattern of metastasis. The most frequent sites of metastasis are lungs, liver, bone, brain, and adrenal glands (Fig. 15-3).

Metastasis is a multistep process beginning with the rapid growth of the primary tumor (Fig. 15-4). As the tumor increases in size, development of its own blood supply is critical to its survival and growth. The process of the formation of blood vessels within the tumor itself is termed **tumor angiogenesis** and is facilitated by tumor angiogenesis factors produced by the cancer cells.

Tumor cells are able to detach from the primary tumor, invade the tissue surrounding the tumor, and penetrate the walls of lymph or vascular vessels for metastasis to a distant site. Once free from the primary tumor, metastatic tumor cells frequently travel to distant organ sites via hematogenous or lymphatic routes.

Hematogenous metastasis involves several steps beginning with primary tumor cells penetrating blood vessels. These tumor cells then enter the circulation, travel through the body, and adhere to and penetrate small blood vessels of distant organs. Most tumor cells do not survive this process and are destroyed by mechanical mechanisms (e.g., turbulence of blood flow) and cells of the immune system. However, the formation of a combination of tumor cells, platelets, and fibrin deposits may protect some tumor cells from destruction in blood vessels.

In the lymphatic system, tumor cells may be "trapped" in the first lymph node confronted and likely to spread from a tumor. This lymph node is referred to as the *sentinel lymph node.* A biopsy can be done of the sentinel node to help determine the extent of the cancer. The procedure is less extensive requiring the removal of fewer lymph nodes. The tumor cells may bypass regional lymph nodes and travel to more distant lymph nodes, a phenomenon termed *skip metastasis.* This phenomenon is exhibited in malignancies such as esophageal cancers. Tumor cells that do survive the process of metastasis must create an environment in the distant organ site that is conducive to their growth and development.

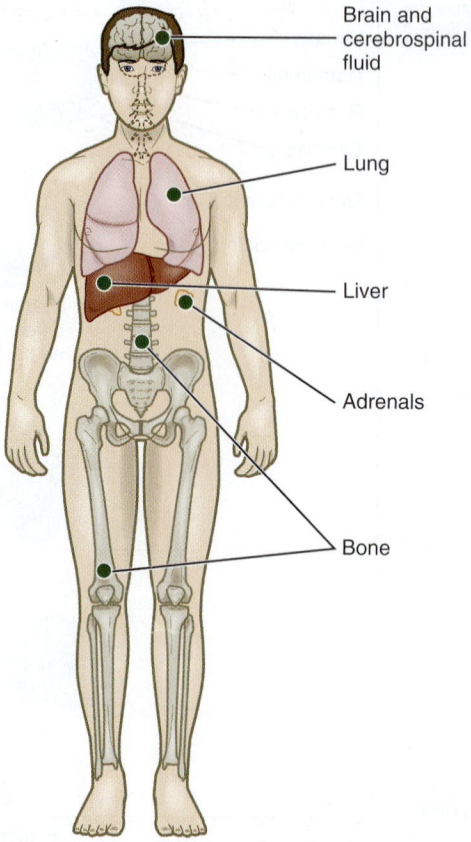

FIG. 15-3 Main sites of metastasis. (Adapted from Stevens A, Lowe J: *Pathology: an illustrated review in colour,* ed 2, London, 2000, Mosby.)

Growth and development are facilitated by the tumor cells' ability to evade cells of the immune system and to produce a vascular supply within the metastatic site similar to that developed in the primary tumor site. Vascularization is critical to the supply of nutrients to the metastatic tumor and to the removal of waste products. Vascularization of the metastatic site is also facilitated by tumor angiogenesis factors produced by the cancer cells.

Role of the Immune System

This section is limited to a discussion of the role of the immune system in the recognition and destruction of tumor cells. (For a detailed discussion of immune system function, see Chapter 13.)

The immune system has the potential to distinguish cells that are normal (self) from abnormal (nonself) cells. For example, cells of transplanted organs can be recognized by the immune system as *nonself* and thus elicit an immune response. This response can ultimately result in the rejection of the organ. Similarly, cancer cells can be perceived as nonself and elicit an immune response resulting in their rejection and destruction. However, unlike transplanted cells, cancer cells arise from normal human cells and, although they are mutated and thus different, the immune response that is mounted against cancer cells may be inadequate to effectively kill them.

Cancer cells may display altered cell-surface antigens as a result of malignant transformation. These antigens are termed *tumor-associated antigens (TAAs)* (Fig. 15-5). It is believed that one of the functions of the immune system is to respond to TAAs. The immune system's response to antigens of the

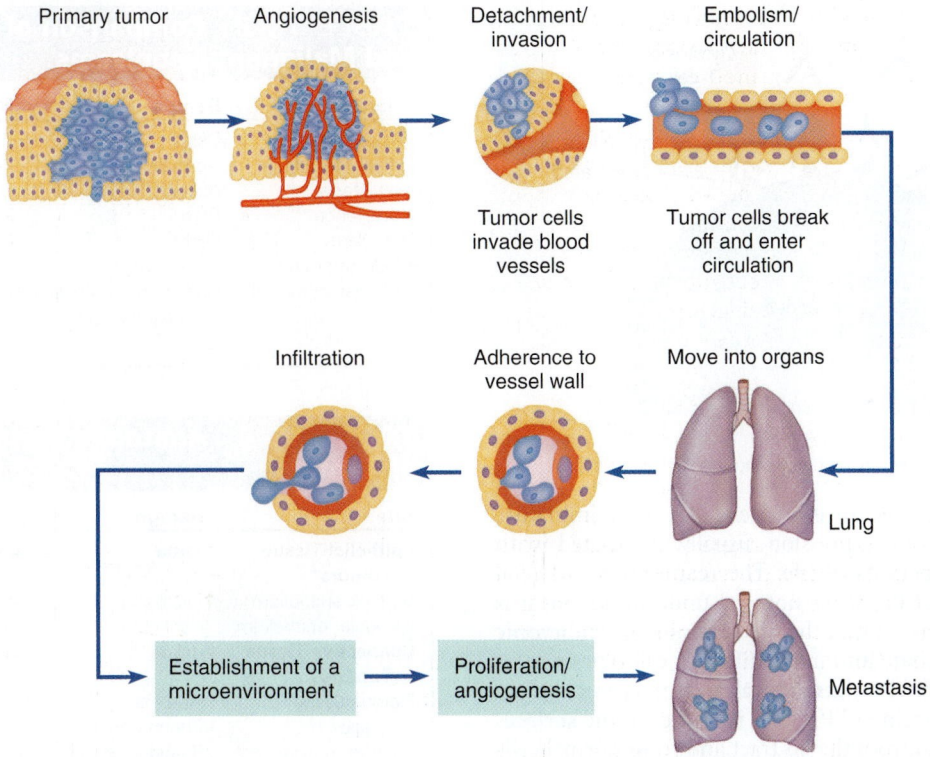

FIG. 15-4 The pathogenesis of cancer metastasis. To produce metastases, tumor cells must detach from the primary tumor and enter the circulation, survive in the circulation to rest in the capillary bed, adhere to capillary basement membrane, gain entrance into the organ parenchyma, respond to growth factors, proliferate and induce angiogenesis, and evade host defenses. (Adapted from Fidler IT: The pathogenesis of cancer metastasis: the "seed and soil" hypothesis revisited, *Nat Rev Cancer* 3(6):453, 2003.)

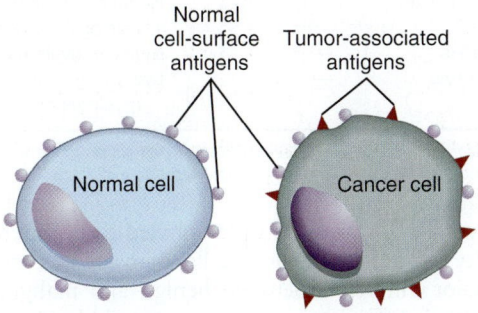

FIG. 15-5 Tumor-associated antigens appear on the cell surface of malignant cells.

malignant cells is termed **immunologic surveillance**. In this process, lymphocytes continuously check cell-surface antigens and detect and destroy cells with abnormal or altered antigenic determinants. Under most circumstances, immune surveillance prevents these transformed cells from developing into clinically detectable tumors.

Immune response to malignant cells involves cytotoxic T cells, natural killer (NK) cells, macrophages, and B cells. *Cytotoxic T cells* play a dominant role in resisting tumor growth. These cells are capable of killing tumor cells. T cells are also important in the production of cytokines (e.g., interleukin-2 [IL-2] and γ-interferon), which stimulate T cells, NK cells, B cells, and macrophages.

Natural killer (NK) cells are able to directly lyse tumor cells spontaneously without any prior sensitization. These cells are stimulated by γ-interferon and IL-2 (released from T cells), resulting in increased cytotoxic activity.

Monocytes and *macrophages* have several important roles in tumor immunity. Macrophages can be activated by γ-interferon (produced by T cells) to become nonspecifically lytic for tumor cells. Macrophages also secrete cytokines, including interleukin-1 (IL-1), tumor necrosis factor (TNF), and colony-stimulating factors (CSFs). The release of IL-1, coupled with the presentation of the processed antigen, stimulates T cell activation and production. α-Interferon augments the killing ability of NK cells. TNF causes hemorrhagic necrosis of tumors and exerts cytocidal or cytostatic actions against tumor cells. CSFs regulate the production of various blood cells in the bone marrow and stimulate the function of various WBCs.

B cells can produce specific antibodies that bind to tumor cells. These antibodies are often detectable in the patient's serum and saliva.

Escape Mechanisms From Immunologic Surveillance. The process by which cancer cells evade the immune system is termed *immunologic escape.* Possible mechanisms by which cancer cells can escape immunologic surveillance include (1) suppression of factors that stimulate T cells to react to cancer cells; (2) weak surface antigens allowing cancer cells to "sneak through" immunologic surveillance; (3) development of tolerance of the immune system to some tumor antigens; (4) suppression of the immune response by products secreted by cancer cells; (5) induction of suppressor T cells by the tumor; and (6) blocking antibodies that bind TAAs, thus preventing their recognition by T cells (Fig. 15-6).

Oncofetal Antigens and Tumor Markers. *Oncofetal antigens* are a type of tumor antigen. They are found on the surfaces and the inside of cancer cells and fetal cells. These antigens are an

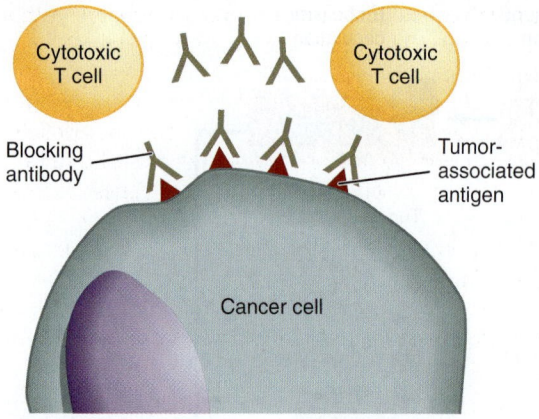

FIG. 15-6 Blocking antibodies prevent T cells from interacting with tumor-associated antigens and from destroying the malignant cell.

expression of the shift of cancerous cells to a more immature metabolic pathway, an expression usually associated with embryonic or fetal periods of life. The reappearance of fetal antigens in malignant disease is not well understood, but it is believed to occur as a result of the cell regaining its embryonic capability to differentiate into many different cell types.

Examples of oncofetal antigens are carcinoembryonic antigen (CEA) and α-fetoprotein (AFP). CEA is found on the surfaces of cancer cells derived from the GI tract and from normal cells from the fetal gut, liver, and pancreas. Normally, CEA disappears during the last 3 months of fetal life. CEA was originally isolated from colorectal cancer cells. However, elevated CEA levels have also been found in nonmalignant conditions (e.g., cirrhosis of the liver, ulcerative colitis, heavy smoking).

These oncofetal antigens can be used as *tumor markers* that may be clinically useful to monitor the effect of therapy and indicate tumor recurrence. However, oncofetal antigens are not 100% specific for tumor recurrence. Tumor markers are affected by various factors that must be accounted for when reviewing these results. For example, the persistence of elevated preoperative CEA titers after surgery indicates that the tumor is not completely removed. A rise in CEA levels after chemotherapy or radiation therapy may indicate recurrence or spread of the cancer and may be affected by chronic lung or liver disease and smoking.

AFP is produced by malignant liver cells and fetal liver cells. AFP levels have also been found to be elevated in some cases of testicular carcinoma, viral hepatitis, and nonmalignant liver disorders. AFP has diagnostic value in primary cancer of the liver (hepatocellular cancer), but it is also produced when metastatic liver growth occurs. The detection of AFP is of value in tumor detection and determination of tumor progression.

Other examples of oncofetal antigens are CA-125 (found in ovarian carcinoma), CA-19-9 (found in pancreatic and gallbladder cancer), prostate-specific antigen (PSA) (found in prostate cancer), and CA-15-3 and CA-27-29 (found in breast cancer). Molecular markers for specific tumors include kRAS (expression of oncogene in colon cancer), epidermal growth factor receptor (EGFR) often overexpressed in lung cancer, and human epidermal growth factor receptor-2 (HER-2) expression in breast cancer.

BENIGN VERSUS MALIGNANT NEOPLASMS

Tumors can be classified as benign or malignant. In general, *benign neoplasms* are well differentiated, and **malignant neoplasms** range from well differentiated to undifferentiated. The ability of malignant tumor cells to invade and metastasize is the major difference between benign and malignant neoplasms. Other differences are presented in Table 15-3.

TABLE 15-3 Comparison of Benign and Malignant Neoplasms

Characteristic	Benign	Malignant
Encapsulated	Usually	Rarely
Differentiated	Normally	Poorly
Metastasis	Absent	Capable
Recurrence	Rare	Possible
Vascularity	Slight	Moderate to marked
Mode of growth	Expansive	Infiltrative and expansive
Cell characteristics	Fairly normal, similar to parent cells	Cells abnormal, become more unlike parent cells

TABLE 15-4 Anatomic Classification of Tumors

Site	Benign	Malignant
Epithelial Tissue Tumors*	**-oma**	**-carcinoma**
Surface epithelium	Papilloma	Carcinoma
Glandular epithelium	Adenoma	Adenocarcinoma
Connective Tissue Tumors†	**-oma**	**-sarcoma**
Fibrous tissue	Fibroma	Fibrosarcoma
Cartilage	Chondroma	Chondrosarcoma
Striated muscle	Rhabdomyoma	Rhabdomyosarcoma
Bone	Osteoma	Osteosarcoma
Nervous Tissue Tumors	**-oma**	**-oma**
Meninges	Meningioma	Meningeal sarcoma
Nerve cells	Ganglioneuroma	Neuroblastoma
Hematopoietic Tissue Tumors		
Lymphoid tissue	—	Hodgkin's lymphoma, non-Hodgkin's lymphoma
Plasma cells	—	Multiple myeloma
Bone marrow	—	Lymphocytic and myelogenous leukemia

*Body surfaces, lining of body cavities, and glandular structures.
†Supporting tissue, fibrotic tissue, and blood vessels.

CLASSIFICATION OF CANCER

Tumors can be classified according to anatomic site, histology (grading), and extent of disease (staging). Tumor classification systems provide a standardized way to (1) communicate the status of the cancer to all members of the interprofessional care team, (2) assist in determining the most effective treatment plan, (3) evaluate the treatment plan, (4) predict prognosis, and (5) compare like groups for statistical purposes.

Anatomic Site Classification

In the *anatomic classification* of tumors, the tumor is identified by the tissue of origin, anatomic site, and behavior of the tumor (i.e., benign or malignant) (Table 15-4). *Carcinomas* originate from embryonal *ectoderm* (skin and glands) and *endoderm* (mucous membrane linings of the respiratory tract, GI tract, and genitourinary [GU] tract). *Sarcomas* originate from embryonal *mesoderm* (connective tissue, muscle, bone, and fat).

Lymphomas and leukemias originate from the hematopoietic system.

Histologic Classification

In **histologic grading** of tumors, the appearance of cells and degree of differentiation are evaluated pathologically. For many tumor types, four grades are used to evaluate abnormal cells based on the degree to which the cells resemble the tissue of origin. Tumors that are poorly differentiated (undifferentiated) have a poorer prognosis than those that are closer in appearance to the normal tissue of origin (well differentiated):

Grade I: Cells differ slightly from normal cells (mild dysplasia) and are well differentiated (low grade).

Grade II: Cells are more abnormal (moderate dysplasia) and moderately differentiated (intermediate grade).

Grade III: Cells are very abnormal (severe dysplasia) and poorly differentiated (high grade).

Grade IV: Cells are immature and primitive *(anaplasia)* and undifferentiated; cell of origin is difficult to determine (high grade).

Grade X: Grade cannot be assessed.

Extent of Disease Classification

Classifying the extent and spread of disease is termed **staging**. This classification system is based on the anatomic extent of disease rather than on cell appearance. Although there are similarities in the staging of various cancers, there are many differences for specific types of cancer.

Clinical Staging. The clinical staging classification system determines the anatomic extent of the malignant disease process by stages:

Stage 0: cancer in situ

Stage I: tumor limited to the tissue of origin; localized tumor growth

Stage II: limited local spread

Stage III: extensive local and regional spread

Stage IV: metastasis

Clinical staging has been used as a basis for staging a variety of tumor types, including cancer of the cervix (see Table 53-13) and Hodgkin's lymphoma (see Fig. 30-14). Other malignant diseases (e.g., leukemia) do not use this staging approach.

TNM Classification System. The *TNM classification system* (Table 15-5) is used to determine the anatomic extent of the disease involvement according to three parameters: tumor size and invasiveness (T), presence or absence of regional spread to the lymph nodes (N), and metastasis to distant organ sites (M). (Examples of the TNM classification system can be found in Tables 27-17 and 51-6.) TNM staging cannot be applied to all malignancies. For example, leukemias are not solid tumors and therefore cannot be staged using these guidelines.

Carcinoma in situ (CIS) refers to a neoplasm whose cells are localized and show no tendency to invade or metastasize to other tissues. CIS has its own designation in the system (T_{is}) because it has all the histologic characteristics of cancer except invasion—a primary feature of the TNM staging system.

Staging of the disease can be performed initially and at several evaluation points. Clinical staging is done at the completion of the diagnostic workup to guide effective treatment selection. Examples of diagnostic studies that may be performed to assess for extent of disease include radiologic studies, such as bone and liver scans; ultrasonography; and computed tomography (CT), MRI, and positron emission tomography (PET) scans.

Surgical staging refers to the extent of the disease as determined by surgical excision, exploration, and/or lymph node sampling. For example, a laparotomy and a splenectomy may be performed in staging of Hodgkin's lymphoma. During a staging laparotomy, lymph node biopsies may be done, and margins of any masses may be marked with metal clips for use during radiation therapy. However, exploratory surgical staging is being used less frequently as noninvasive diagnostic technology becomes increasingly sophisticated.

After the extent of the disease is determined, the stage classification is not changed. The original description of the extent of the tumor remains part of the record. If additional treatment is needed, or if treatment fails, retreatment staging is done to determine the extent of the disease process before retreatment. "Restaging" classification (rTNM) is differentiated from the stage at diagnosis, since the clinical significance may be different.

In addition to tumor classification systems, other rating scales can be used to describe and document the status of patients with cancer at the time of diagnosis, treatment, and retreatment and at each follow-up examination. For example, the Karnofsky Performance Scale[8] and Katz Index of Independence in Activities of Daily Living[9] describe patient's functional performance.

TABLE 15-5 TNM Classification System

Primary Tumor (T)	
T_0	No evidence of primary tumor
T_{is}	Carcinoma in situ
T_{1-4}	Ascending degrees of increase in tumor size and involvement
T_x	Tumor cannot be measured or found
Regional Lymph Nodes (N)	
N_0	No evidence of disease in lymph nodes
N_{1-4}	Ascending degrees of nodal involvement
N_x	Regional lymph nodes unable to be assessed clinically
Distant Metastases (M)	
M_0	No evidence of distant metastases
M_{1-4}	Ascending degrees of metastatic involvement, including distant nodes
M_x	Cannot be determined

NOTE: For examples of TNM classification system applied to diseases, see Fig. 30-14 and Table 27-17.

PREVENTION AND EARLY DETECTION OF CANCER

The war on cancer will not be won with drugs or radiation therapy. A stronger emphasis on prevention is needed.[10] As a nurse, you have an essential role in the prevention and early detection of cancer. Eliminating risk factors reduces the incidence of cancer. For example, rates of smoking-related cancers (e.g., lung and head and neck cancers) have declined following reduction in smoking rates.[1]

Early detection and prompt treatment are responsible for increased survival rates in patients with cancer. Colonoscopy is important in reducing colon cancer mortality both by early detection of colon cancers and by prevention (e.g., excision of adenomatous polyps).

Teach patients and the public about cancer prevention and early detection, including the following:

TABLE 15-6 Seven Warning Signs of Cancer

Change in bowel or bladder habits
A sore that does not heal
Unusual bleeding or discharge from any body orifice
Thickening or a lump in the breast or elsewhere
I ndigestion or difficulty in swallowing
Obvious change in a wart or mole
Nagging cough or hoarseness

- Reduce or avoid exposure to known or suspected carcinogens and cancer-promoting agents, including cigarette smoke, tanning beds, and sun exposure.
- Eat a balanced diet that includes vegetables and fresh fruits (see Fig. 39-1 and Table 39-1), whole grains, and adequate amounts of fiber. Reduce dietary fat and preservatives, including smoked and salt-cured meats containing high nitrite concentrations.
- Limit alcohol intake.
- Participate in regular exercise (i.e., 30 minutes or more of moderate physical activity five times weekly).
- Maintain a healthy weight.
- Obtain adequate, consistent periods of rest (at least 6 to 8 hours per night).
- Eliminate, reduce, or change the perception of stressors and enhance the ability to effectively cope with stressors (see Chapter 6).
- Have a regular physical examination that includes a health history. Be familiar with your own family history and your risk factors for cancer.
- Learn and follow the American Cancer Society's recommended cancer screening guidelines for breast, colon, cervical, and prostate cancer.[11]
- Learn and practice self-examination (e.g., breast or testicular self-examination).
- Know the seven warning signs of cancer, and inform the health care provider if they are present (Table 15-6). (These actually detect fairly advanced disease.)
- Seek immediate medical care if you notice a change in what is normal for you and if cancer is suspected.

The goals of public education are to (1) motivate people to recognize and modify behaviors that may negatively affect health and (2) encourage awareness of and participation in health-promoting behaviors. When you teach about cancer, try to minimize the fear that surrounds the diagnosis.

Diagnosis of Cancer

When a patient has a possible diagnosis of cancer, it is a stressful time for the patient and family. Patients may undergo several days to weeks of diagnostic studies. During this time, fear of the unknown may be more stressful than the actual diagnosis of cancer. Patients may also be overwhelmed or confused by the need for multiple diagnostic studies and consultations. Help to coordinate care between multiple specialists and explain the purpose of required tests and any special preparation needed for them.

Some facilities have comprehensive oncology teams and services that are all housed in the same building to help coordinate care among the cancer specialists. These centers consolidate appointments to make the experience convenient and comfortable for the patients and their families.

While patients are waiting for the results of diagnostic studies, be available to actively listen to their concerns. Their anxiety may arise from myths and misconceptions about cancer (e.g., cancer is a "death sentence," cancer treatment is worse than the illness). Correcting those misconceptions can help to minimize their anxiety.

Learn to recognize your own discomfort during difficult conversations. Avoid communication patterns that may hinder exploration of feelings and meaning, such as providing false reassurances (e.g., "It's probably nothing"), redirecting the discussion (e.g., "Let's discuss that later"), generalizing (e.g., "Everyone feels this way"), and using overly technical language as a means of distancing yourself from the patient. These self-protective strategies deny patients the opportunity to share the meaning of their experience. In addition, they can jeopardize your ability to build a trusting relationship with your patients.

During this time of high anxiety, the patient may need repeated explanations of the diagnostic workup. Include as much information as needed by the patient and family. Give clear, understandable explanations and reinforce them as needed. Written information is helpful for reinforcement of verbal information.

A diagnostic plan for the person suspected of having cancer includes the health history (including a history of present illness), identification of risk factors, the physical examination, and specific diagnostic studies. For many people, cancer is initially diagnosed after the findings of an abnormal screening test (e.g., mass on mammogram). For others, they are alerted to the presence of cancer by a presenting symptom or cluster of symptoms (e.g., cough and hemoptysis, anorexia and weight loss).

Concentrate on risk factors for cancer such as family or personal history of cancer, exposure to or use of known carcinogens (e.g., cigarette smoking, occupational pollutants or chemicals, radiation exposure), diseases characterized by chronic inflammation or immunosuppression (e.g., ulcerative colitis), and drug ingestion (e.g., hormone therapy, previous anticancer therapies). Also assess factors that may warrant additional supportive care during therapy, including alcohol or recreational drug use, living situation, social support, and coping strategies for perceived stressors.

Diagnostic studies depend on the suspected primary or metastatic site(s) of the cancer. (Specific procedures as they relate to each body system are discussed in the respective assessment chapters.) Examples of diagnostic studies include the following:

- Cytology studies (e.g., Papanicolaou [Pap] test, bronchial washings)
- Tissue biopsy
- Chest x-ray
- Complete blood count, chemistry profile

HEALTHY PEOPLE

Prevention and Early Detection of Cancer

- Limit alcohol use.
- Get regular physical activity.
- Maintain a normal body weight.
- Obtain regular colorectal screenings.
- Avoid cigarette smoking and other tobacco use.
- Get regular mammography screening and Pap tests.
- Use sunscreen with a sun protection factor of 15 or higher.
- Practice healthy dietary habits, such as reducing fat consumption, avoiding processed meats, and increasing fruit and vegetable consumption.

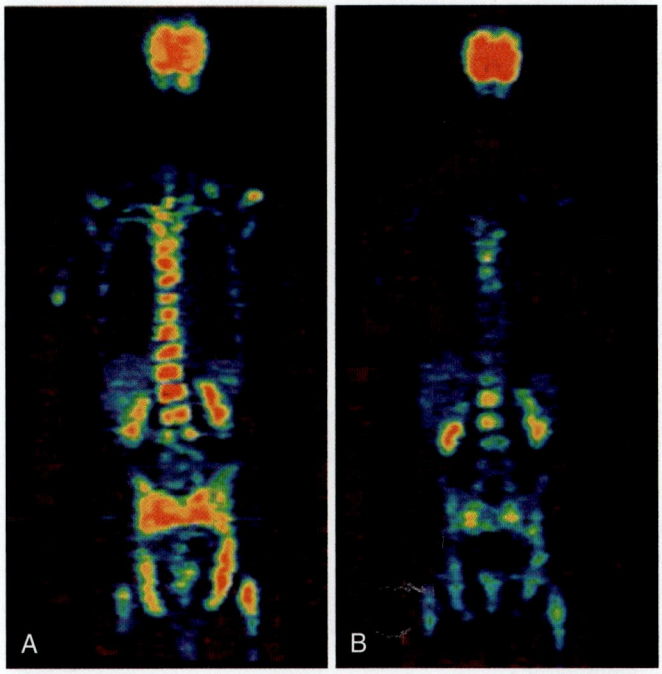

FIG. 15-7 Positron emission tomography (PET) scan before treatment **(A)** indicating metastasis throughout the body. PET scan after treatment **(B)** indicates the effects of therapy. More radioactive material accumulates in areas that have higher levels of activity. This often corresponds to areas of disease and shows up as brighter spots on the PET scan. (From Shimizu N, Masuda H, Yamanaka H, et al: Fluorodeoxyglucose positron emission tomography scan of prostate cancer bone metastases with flare reaction after endocrine therapy, *J Urol* 151[2]:609, 1999.)

- Liver function studies (e.g., aspartate aminotransferase [AST])
- Endoscopic examination: upper GI, sigmoidoscopy, or colonoscopy (including guaiac test for occult blood)
- Radiographic studies (e.g., mammography, ultrasound, CT scan, MRI)
- Radioisotope scans (e.g., bone, lung, liver, brain)
- PET scan (Fig. 15-7)
- Tumor markers (e.g., CEA, AFP, PSA, CA-125)
- Genetic markers (e.g., *BRCA1, BRCA2*)
- Molecular receptor status (e.g., estrogen and progesterone receptors)
- Bone marrow examination (if a hematolymphoid malignancy is suspected or to document metastatic disease)

Biopsy. A *biopsy* is the removal of a tissue sample for pathologic analysis. Various methods are used to obtain a biopsy depending on the location and size of the suspected tumor. *Percutaneous biopsy* is commonly performed for tissue that can be safely reached through the skin. *Endoscopic biopsy* may be used for lung or other intraluminal lesions (esophageal, colon, bladder). When a tumor is not easily accessible, a *surgical procedure* (laparotomy, thoracotomy, craniotomy) is often necessary to obtain a piece of the tumor tissue. Many radiographic techniques may be used in conjunction with the biopsy procedure (e.g., CT, MRI, ultrasound-guided biopsy, stereotactic biopsy, fluoroscopic-assisted biopsy) to improve tissue localization.

Various types and sizes of biopsy needles are available and are selected according to the type of tissue to be sampled. *Fine-needle aspiration* (FNA) may be accomplished with a small-gauge aspiration needle that provides cells from the mass for cytologic examination. *Large-core biopsy* cutting needles deliver an actual piece of tissue (core) that can be analyzed with the advantage of preserving the histologic architecture of the tissue specimen. *Excisional biopsy* involves the surgical removal of the entire lesion, lymph node, nodule, or mass. Therefore it is therapeutic as well as diagnostic. If an excisional biopsy is not feasible, an *incisional biopsy* (partial excision) may be performed with a scalpel or dermal punch.

Pathologic evaluation of a tissue sample is the only definitive means to diagnose cancer. The pathologist examines the tissue to determine (1) whether it is benign or malignant, (2) the anatomic tissue from which the tumor arises *(histology)*, and (3) the degree of cell differentiation *(histologic grade)*. Other information that can be obtained includes the extent of malignant involvement (size of tumor and depth), evidence of invasiveness (extracapsular, lymphatic), adequacy of surgical excision (positive or negative surgical margin status), nuclear grade (mitotic rate), and special staining techniques that may provide insight into responsiveness of the tumor to treatment or disease behavior (receptor status, tumor markers).

INTERPROFESSIONAL CARE

Treatment Goals

The goals of cancer treatment are cure, control, and palliation (Fig. 15-8). Primary factors that determine what therapy is used are the tumor histology and staging outcomes. Other important factors are the patient's physiologic status (e.g., presence of co-morbid illnesses), psychologic status, and personal desires (e.g., active treatment versus palliation of symptoms).

These factors influence (1) the modalities chosen for treatment (i.e., surgery, radiation therapy, chemotherapy, immunotherapy, targeted therapy, hormone therapy), (2) how therapies are sequenced, and (3) the length of time the treatment is prescribed. Each type of therapy can be used alone or in any combination during initial treatment or as maintenance therapy, as well as in retreatment if the disease does not respond or recurs after remission.

For many cancers, two or more of the treatment modalities (known as *multimodality therapy* or *combined modality therapy*) are used to achieve the goal of cure or control for a long time. Multimodality therapy has the benefit of being more effective (because it takes advantage of more than one mechanism of action), but often at the expense of greater toxicity.

Cure. When caring for the patient and family with cancer, know the treatment goals to appropriately communicate with, teach, and support the patient. When *cure* is the goal, treatment is expected to have the greatest chance of disease eradication. Curative cancer therapy differs according to the particular cancer being treated and may involve local therapies (i.e., surgery or radiation) alone or in combination, with or without periods of adjunctive systemic therapy (i.e., chemotherapy).

For example, basal cell carcinoma of the skin is usually cured by surgical removal of the lesion and/or several weeks of radiation therapy. In the treatment plan for acute promyelocytic leukemia (which has curative potential), several chemotherapy drugs are given on a scheduled basis over many months to several years. Testicular cancer can be cured with a combination of surgery, chemotherapy, and radiation.

Although there is no benchmark that ensures "cure" for most cancers, in general the risk for recurrent disease is highest after treatment completion and gradually decreases the longer the

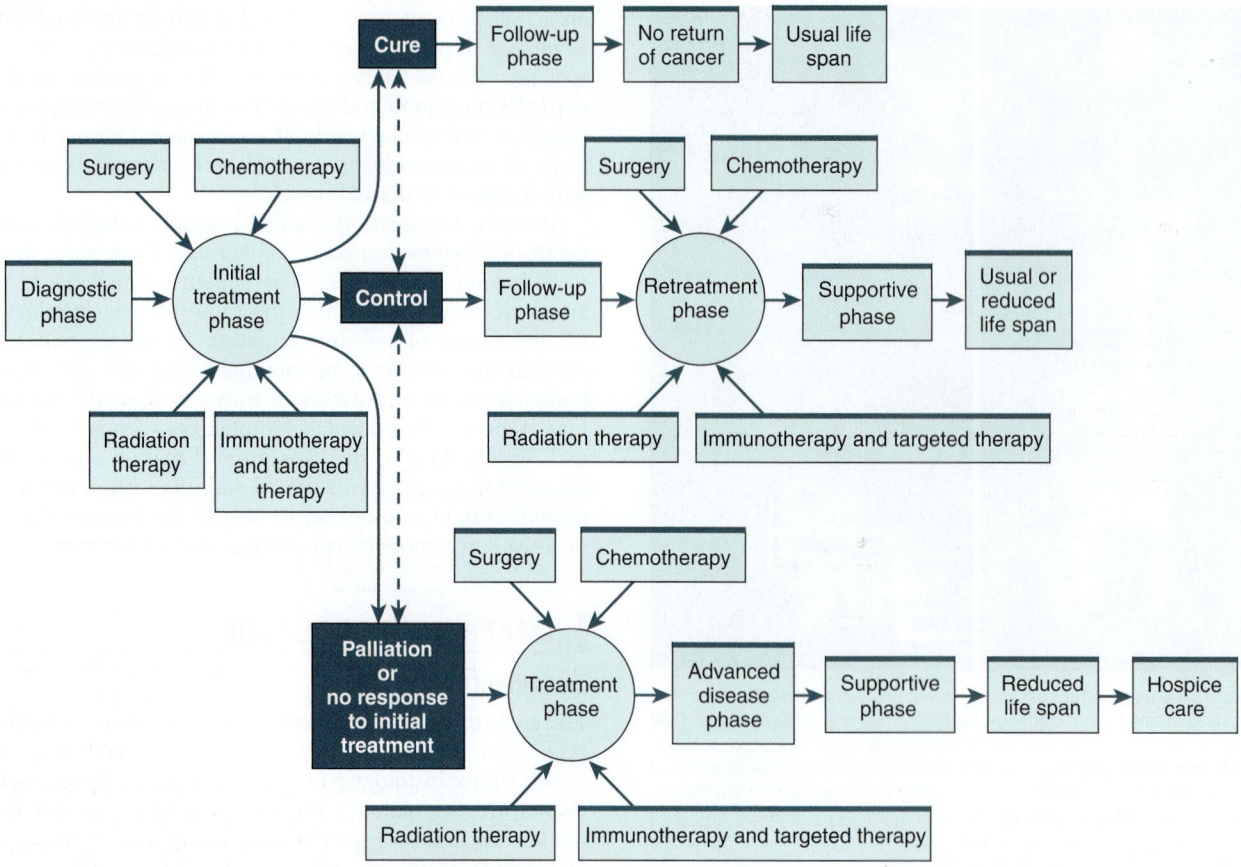

FIG. 15-8 Goals of cancer treatment.

patient remains disease free following treatment. Cancers with a higher mitotic rate (e.g., testicular cancer) are more likely to recur than cancers with slower mitotic rates (e.g., postmenopausal breast cancer). Therefore the timeframe to consider a person "cured" may differ according to the tumor and its characteristics.

Control. *Control* is the goal of the treatment plan for many cancers that cannot be completely eradicated but are responsive to anticancer therapies. As with other chronic illnesses (e.g., diabetes mellitus, heart failure), cancer can be controlled for long periods with therapy. Examples include multiple myeloma and chronic lymphocytic leukemia (see Chapter 30). Patients may undergo an initial course of treatment followed by maintenance therapy for as long as the disease is responding. Patients are monitored closely for early signs and symptoms of disease recurrence or progression and the cumulative effects of therapy. Evidence of tumor resistance (such as disease progression) may warrant changing to an alternative therapy.

Palliation. *Palliation* is the treatment goal when relief or control of symptoms and the maintenance of a satisfactory quality of life are the primary objectives. Palliative care and treatment are not mutually exclusive and can take place concurrently. An example of treatment in which palliation is the primary goal includes using radiation therapy or chemotherapy to reduce tumor size and relieve subsequent symptoms such as the pain of bone metastasis.

Personalized Cancer Medicine

An emerging trend in cancer care is *personalized medicine,* in which the patient's genetic information is used to guide (customize) decisions made about prevention, diagnosis, and treatment of cancer. Many of the diagnostic studies (tumor markers, genetic markers, molecular receptor status) are useful in determining treatment options for patients with cancer.

Before personalized medicine, most patients with a specific type and stage of cancer received the same treatment. However, some treatments worked well for some patients and not as well for others. With increasing research, it was found that genetic differences in people and their tumors explained many of these different responses to treatment. By performing more genetic tests and analysis, treatments can now be personalized.[12]

Targeted therapy (see Table 15-13 later in this chapter) targets a cancer's specific genes or proteins that contribute to cancer growth and survival. Treatment with a targeted therapy depends on assessing whether the tumor has the specific target. This is usually done by testing a sample of the tumor obtained through a biopsy.

Pharmacogenomics and *pharmacogenetics* is the study of genomic variation associated with drug responses.[13,14] Examples of how the results of genetic testing can be applied to the use of cancer drugs are presented in Table 12-5. For example, vemurafenib (Zelboraf) is used to treat patients with metastatic melanoma. However, it is indicated only for the treatment of patients with melanoma whose tumors express a gene mutation called *BRAF V600E.*

Despite the promises of personalized cancer treatments, not all types of cancer have personalized treatment options. Genetic testing of the patient and tumor sample may be costly and time consuming, and many insurance plans may not cover the costs

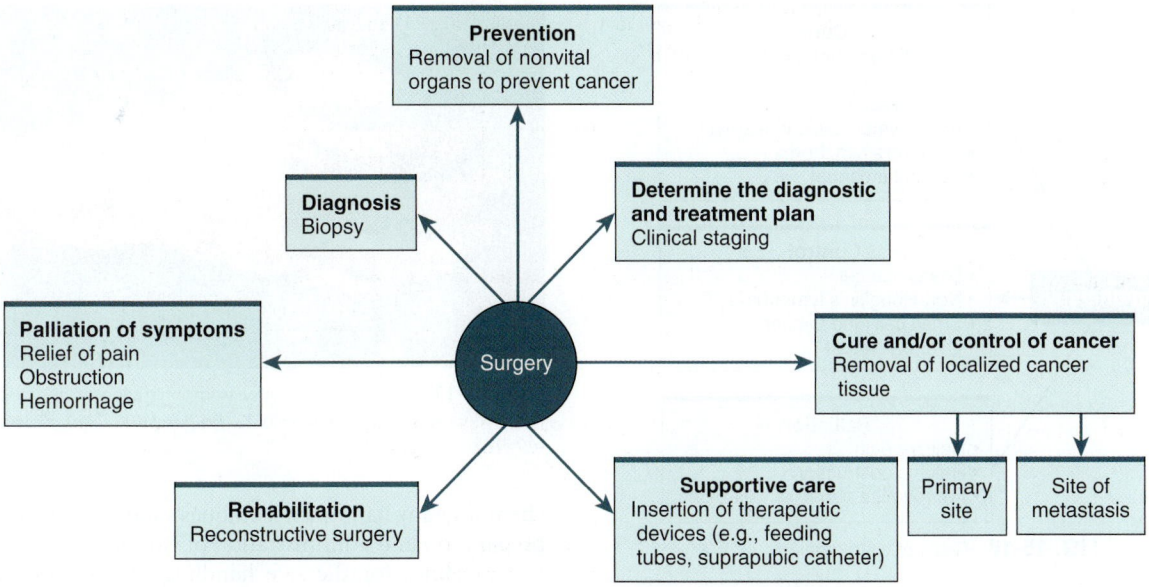

FIG. 15-9 Role of surgery in the treatment of cancer.

of these tests. Some personalized treatments, such as targeted treatments, can also be expensive.[12]

SURGICAL THERAPY

Surgery is the oldest form of cancer treatment. The treatment of choice for many years was to remove the cancer and as much of the surrounding normal tissue as possible. What this approach did not fully consider was the ability of cancer cells to travel from the original tumor site to other locations, making surgical cure possible only when the tumor was localized and relatively small. Today surgery is used to meet a variety of goals (Fig. 15-9), and the trend is toward less radical surgeries.

Prevention

Surgical intervention can be used to eliminate or reduce the risk of cancer development. Prophylactic removal of nonvital organs has been successful in reducing the incidence of some cancers. For example, patients who have adenomatous familial polyposis may benefit from a total colostomy to prevent colorectal cancer (see Chapter 42). Individuals who have genetic mutations of *BRCA1* or *BRCA2* and have a strong family history of early-onset breast cancer may consider having a prophylactic mastectomy (see Chapter 51).

Cure or Control

When the goal is cure or control, the objective is to remove all or as much resectable tumor as possible while sparing normal tissue. Examples of surgical procedures used for cure or control of cancer include radical neck dissection, mastectomy, orchiectomy, thyroidectomy, nephrectomy, hysterectomy, and/or oophorectomy.

A *debulking* or *cytoreductive procedure* may be used if the tumor cannot be completely removed (e.g., a tumor attached to a vital organ). When this occurs, as much tumor as possible is removed and the patient is given chemotherapy and/or radiation therapy. This type of surgical procedure can make chemotherapy or radiation therapy more effective, since the tumor mass is reduced before treatment is initiated. Other times, a patient may need to receive *neoadjuvant* (treatment before surgery) chemotherapy and/or radiation therapy to reduce tumor burden and improve the surgical outcome.

Supportive and Palliative Care

When cure or control of cancer is no longer possible, the focus shifts to supportive care and palliation of symptoms. Surgical procedures may be used to provide supportive care that maximizes bodily function or facilitates cancer treatment. Examples of supportive surgical procedures include the following:

- Insertion of feeding tube to maintain nutrition during head and neck cancer treatment
- Placement of central venous access devices to deliver chemotherapy agents
- Prophylactic surgical fixation of bones at risk for pathologic fracture

Effects of treatment or symptoms from metastatic cancer may necessitate surgical intervention for palliation. Examples include (1) debulking of tumor to relieve pain or pressure, (2) colostomy for the relief of a bowel obstruction (see Chapter 42), and (3) laminectomy for the relief of a spinal cord compression (see Chapter 60).

CHEMOTHERAPY

Chemotherapy (antineoplastic therapy) is the use of chemicals as a systemic therapy for cancer. In the 1940s nitrogen mustard, a chemical warfare agent used in World Wars I and II, was used in the treatment of lymphoma and acute leukemia. In the 1970s chemotherapy was established as an effective treatment modality for cancer. Chemotherapy is now a mainstay of cancer treatment for most solid tumors and hematologic malignancies (e.g., leukemias, lymphomas). Chemotherapy can offer cure for some cancers, control other cancers for long periods, and in some instances offer palliative relief of symptoms when cure or control is no longer possible (Fig. 15-10).

Effect on Cells

The goal of chemotherapy is to eliminate or reduce the number of cancer cells in the primary tumor and metastatic tumor site(s). All cells (cancer cells and normal cells) enter the cell

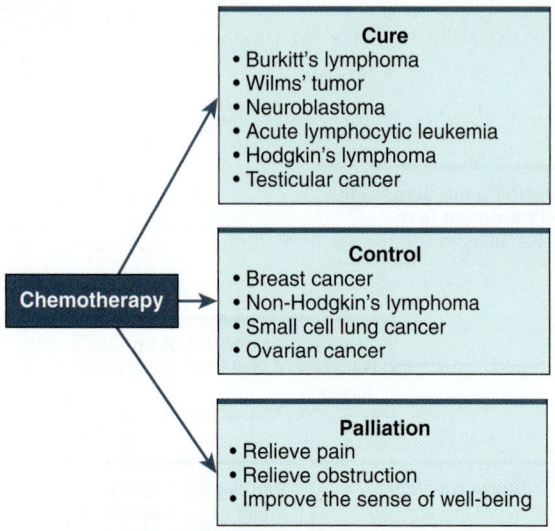

FIG. 15-10 Goals of chemotherapy.

cycle for replication and proliferation (Fig. 15-1). The effects of the chemotherapy drugs are described in relation to the cell cycle.

The two major categories of chemotherapy drugs are cell cycle phase–nonspecific and cell cycle phase–specific drugs. *Cell cycle phase–nonspecific chemotherapy drugs* have their effect on the cells during all phases of the cell cycle, including the process of cell replication and proliferation and the resting phase (G_0). *Cell cycle phase–specific chemotherapy drugs* exert their most significant effects during specific phases of the cell cycle (i.e., when cells are in the process of cell replication or proliferation during G_1, S, G_2, or M). Cell cycle phase–specific and cell cycle phase–nonspecific agents are often administered in combination to maximize effectiveness by using agents that function by differing mechanisms and throughout the cell cycle.

When cancer first begins to develop, most of the cells are actively dividing. As the tumor increases in size, more cells become inactive and convert to a resting state (G_0). Because most chemotherapy agents are most effective against dividing cells, cells can escape death by staying in the G_0 phase. A major challenge is to overcome the effect of resistant resting and non-cycling cells.

Classification of Chemotherapy Drugs

Chemotherapy drugs are classified in general groups according to their molecular structure and mechanisms of action (Table 15-7). Each drug in a particular classification has many similarities. However, there are major differences in how the drugs work and the unique side effects associated with drugs in each class.

Preparation of Chemotherapy

It is important to know the specific guidelines for administration of chemotherapy drugs. In addition, it is important to understand that drugs may pose an occupational hazard to health care professionals who do not follow safe handling guidelines. A person preparing, transporting, or administering chemotherapy may absorb the drug through inhalation of particles when reconstituting a powder and through skin contact from exposure to droplets or powder from oral agents. There may also be some risk in handling the body fluids and excretions of people receiving chemotherapy immediately after administration for 48 hours. Only those personnel specifically trained in chemotherapy handling techniques should be involved with the preparation and administration of cancer drugs.

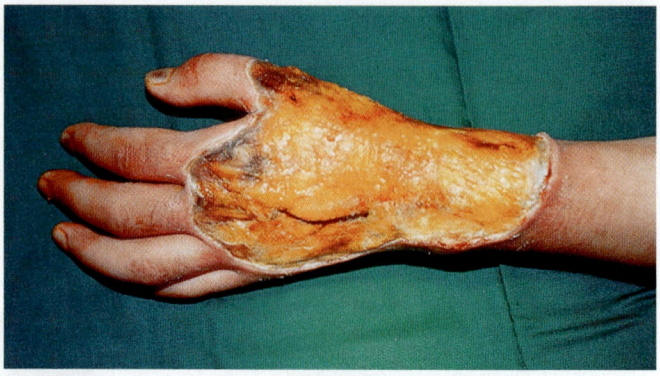

FIG. 15-11 Extravasation injury from infiltration of chemotherapy drug. (From Weinzweig N, Weinzweig J: *The mutilated hand,* Philadelphia, 2005, Mosby.)

Guidelines for the safe handling of chemotherapy agents have been developed by the National Institute for Occupational Safety and Health (OSHA)[15] and the Oncology Nursing Society (ONS).[16]

Methods of Administration

Chemotherapy can be administered by multiple routes (Table 15-8). With advances in drug formulation techniques, more oral chemotherapy agents are available. With oral agents, the patient will need to be taught about storage and side effects.

The IV route is the most common method of administering chemotherapy. Major concerns associated with the IV administration of antineoplastic drugs include venous access difficulties, device- or catheter-related infection, and *extravasation* (infiltration of drugs into tissues surrounding the infusion site) causing local tissue damage (Fig. 15-11).

Many chemotherapy drugs are either irritants or vesicants. *Irritants* will damage the intima of the vein, causing phlebitis and sclerosis and limiting future peripheral venous access but will not cause tissue damage if infiltrated. However, **vesicants**, if inadvertently infiltrated into the skin, may cause severe local tissue breakdown and necrosis. It is extremely important to monitor for and promptly recognize symptoms associated with extravasation of a vesicant and to take immediate action if it occurs. To minimize the associated physical discomforts, emotional distress, and risks of infection and infiltration, IV chemotherapy can be administered by a *central venous access device* (CVAD). CVADs are placed in large blood vessels and permit frequent, continuous, or intermittent administration of chemotherapy, immunotherapy, and targeted therapy, and other products, thus avoiding multiple venipunctures for vascular access. (CVADs are discussed in Chapter 16.)

Regional Chemotherapy Administration

Regional treatment with chemotherapy involves delivery of the drug directly to the tumor site. The advantage of this method is that higher concentrations of the drug can be delivered to the tumor with reduced systemic toxicity. Several regional delivery methods have been developed, including intraarterial, intraperitoneal, intrathecal or intraventricular, and intravesical bladder chemotherapy.

Intraarterial Chemotherapy. Intraarterial chemotherapy delivers the drug to the tumor via the arteries supplying the tumor. This method has been used for the treatment of osteogenic

TABLE 15-7 Drug Therapy

Chemotherapy

Mechanisms of Action	Examples
Alkylating Agents	
Cell Cycle Phase–Nonspecific Agents	
Damage DNA by causing breaks in the double-stranded helix. If repair does not occur, cells will die immediately (cytocidal) or when they attempt to divide (cytostatic).	bendamustine (Treanda), busulfan (Myleran), chlorambucil (Leukeran), cyclophosphamide, dacarbazine (DTIC-Dome), ifosfamide (Ifex), mechlorethamine (Mustargen), melphalan (Alkeran), temozolomide (Temodar), thiotepa
Nitrosoureas	
Cell Cycle Phase–Nonspecific Agents	
Like alkylating agents, break DNA helix, interfering with DNA replication. Cross blood-brain barrier.	carmustine (BiCNU, Gliadel), lomustine (Gleostine), streptozocin (Zanosar)
Platinum Drugs	
Cell Cycle Phase–Nonspecific Agents	
Bind to DNA and RNA, miscoding information and/or inhibiting DNA replication, and cells die.	carboplatin, cisplatin (Platinol-AQ), oxaliplatin (Eloxatin)
Antimetabolites	
Cell Cycle Phase–Specific Agents	
Mimic naturally occurring substances, thus interfering with enzyme function or DNA synthesis. Primarily act during S phase. Purine and pyrimidine are building blocks of nucleic acids needed for DNA and RNA synthesis	
• Interfere with purine metabolism	cladribine, clofarabine (Clolar), fludarabine, mercaptopurine (Purixan), nelarabine (Arranon), pentostatin (Nipent), thioguanine
• Interfere with pyrimidine metabolism	capecitabine (Xeloda); cytarabine (ara-C [Cytosar-U, DepoCyt]), floxuridine, 5-fluorouracil (5-FU), gemcitabine (Gemzar)
• Interfere with folic acid metabolism	methotrexate (Trexall), pemetrexed (Alimta)
• Interfere with DNA synthesis	hydroxyurea (Hydrea, Droxia)
Antitumor Antibiotics	
Cell Cycle Phase–Nonspecific Agents	
Bind directly to DNA, thus inhibiting the synthesis of DNA and interfering with transcription of RNA.	bleomycin, dactinomycin (Cosmegen), daunorubicin (Cerubidine, DaunoXome), doxorubicin (Doxil), epirubicin (Ellence), idarubicin, mitomycin, mitoxantrone, valrubicin (Valstar)
Mitotic Inhibitors	
Cell Cycle Phase–Specific Agents	
Taxanes	albumin-bound paclitaxel (Abraxane), docetaxel (Taxotere), paclitaxel (Taxol)
Antimicrotubule agents that interfere with mitosis. Act during the late G_2 phase and mitosis to stabilize microtubules, thus inhibiting cell division.	
Vinca Alkaloids	vinblastine, vincristine, vinorelbine (Navelbine)
Act in M phase to inhibit mitosis.	
Others	estramustine (Emcyt), ixabepilone (Ixempra), eribulin (Halaven)
Microtubular inhibitors.	
Topoisomerase Inhibitors	
Cell Cycle Phase–Specific Agents	
Inhibit topoisomerases (normal enzymes) that function to make reversible breaks and repairs in DNA that allow for flexibility of DNA in replication.	etoposide, irinotecan (Camptosar), teniposide (Vumon), topotecan (Hycamtin)
Miscellaneous	
Enzyme derived from the yeast Erwinia used to deplete the supply of asparagine (amino acid) for leukemic cells that are dependent on an exogenous source of this amino acid. Inhibits protein synthesis.	Erwinia asparaginase, L-asparaginase (Elspar)
Causes changes in DNA in leukemia cells and leads to cell death.	arsenic trioxide (Trisenox)
Suppresses mitosis. Appears to alter DNA, RNA, and protein.	procarbazine (Matulane)

NOTE: Many of these drugs are irritants or vesicants that require special attention during administration to avoid extravasation. It is important to know this information about a drug before administering it.

sarcoma; cancers of the head and neck, bladder, and cervix; melanoma; primary liver cancer; and metastatic liver disease. One method of intraarterial drug delivery involves the surgical placement of a catheter that is subsequently connected to an external infusion pump or an implanted infusion pump for infusion of the chemotherapy agent.

Intraperitoneal Chemotherapy. Intraperitoneal chemotherapy involves the delivery of chemotherapy to the peritoneal cavity for treatment of peritoneal metastases from primary colorectal and ovarian cancers and malignant ascites. Temporary Silastic catheters (Tenckhoff, Hickman, and Groshong) are percutaneously or surgically placed into the peritoneal cavity for short-term administration of chemotherapy. Alternatively, an implanted port can be used to administer chemotherapy intraperitoneally. Chemotherapy is generally infused into the peritoneum in 1 to 2 L of fluid and allowed to *dwell* in the peritoneum for 1 to 4 hours. After the *dwell time,* the fluid is drained from the peritoneum.

TABLE 15-8 Drug Therapy

Methods of Chemotherapy Administration

Method	Examples
Oral	cyclophosphamide, capecitabine (Xeloda), temozolomide (Temodar)
Intramuscular	bleomycin
Intravenous	doxorubicin, vincristine, cisplatin, 5-fluorouracil (5-FU), paclitaxel (Taxol)
Intracavitary (pleural, peritoneal)	Radioisotopes, alkylating agents, methotrexate
Intrathecal	methotrexate (preservative free), cytarabine
Intraarterial	dacarbazine, 5-FU, methotrexate
Perfusion	Alkylating agents
Subcutaneous	cytarabine, bortezomib
Topical	5-FU cream

TABLE 15-9 Cells With Rapid Rate of Proliferation

Cells	Generation Time	Effect of Cell Destruction
Bone marrow stem cell	6-24 hr	Myelosuppression (infection, bleeding, anemia)
Neutrophils	12 hr	Leukopenia, infection
Epithelial cells lining the gastrointestinal tract	12-24 hr	Anorexia, mucositis (including stomatitis, esophagitis), nausea and vomiting, diarrhea
Cells of the hair follicle	24 hr	Alopecia
Ova or testes	24-36 hr	Reproductive dysfunction

Intrathecal or Intraventricular Chemotherapy. Cancers that metastasize to the central nervous system (CNS) are difficult to treat because the blood-brain barrier often prevents distribution of chemotherapy to this area. One method used to treat metastasis to the CNS is intrathecal chemotherapy. This method involves a lumbar puncture and injection of chemotherapy into the subarachnoid space. To reduce the need for repeated lumbar punctures, patients may have an Ommaya reservoir inserted. An Ommaya reservoir is a Silastic, dome-shaped disk with an extension catheter that is surgically implanted through the cranium into a lateral ventricle.

Intravesical Bladder Chemotherapy. *Intravesical bladder chemotherapy* involves instillation of chemotherapy into the bladder. The chemotherapy agent is instilled into the bladder via a urinary catheter and retained for 1 to 3 hours.

Effects of Chemotherapy on Normal Tissues

Chemotherapy agents cannot selectively distinguish between normal cells and cancer cells. Chemotherapy-induced side effects are the result of the destruction of normal cells, especially those that are rapidly proliferating such as those in the bone marrow, lining of the GI system, and integumentary system (skin, hair, and nails) (Table 15-9). The general and drug-specific adverse effects of these drugs are classified as acute, delayed, or chronic.

Acute toxicity occurs during and immediately after drug administration and includes anaphylactic and hypersensitivity reactions, extravasation or a flare reaction, anticipatory nausea and vomiting, and cardiac dysrhythmias.

Delayed effects are numerous and include delayed nausea and vomiting, mucositis, alopecia, skin rashes, bone marrow suppression, altered bowel function (diarrhea or constipation), and a variety of cumulative neurotoxicities.

Chronic toxicities involve damage to organs such as the heart, liver, kidneys, and lungs. Chronic toxicities can be either long-term effects that develop during or immediately after treatment and persist or late effects that are absent during treatment and manifest later.

Some side effects fall into more than one category. For example, nausea and vomiting can be both acute and delayed.

Treatment Plan

Although single-drug chemotherapy is sometimes prescribed, the more common modality is combining agents in multidrug regimens. This approach to treatment targets more than one signaling pathway and has proven to be more effective in managing most cancers. The regimens with multiple agents involve drugs with different mechanisms of action and varying toxicity profiles. However, when chemotherapy agents are used in combination, patients can experience an increase in toxicities.

Drug regimens are selected based on evidence supporting their use in specific cancers. Sometimes they are customized to meet the needs of an individual patient. Chemotherapy is most effective when the tumor burden is low, therapy is not interrupted, and the patient receives the intended dose. The dose of each drug is based on the individual's body weight and height using the body surface area calculation.

Mutation of cancer cells within the tumor can result in cells that are resistant to chemotherapy. With the use of multiple drugs that work at different places in the cell cycle, cancer cells can be more effectively killed. Thus mutation and resistance of cancer cells can be prevented.

INFORMATICS IN PRACTICE

Managing Cancer Patients' Symptoms

- Patients arriving at some clinics are handed a tablet computer. While in the waiting room or chemotherapy infusion unit, with the touch of a finger they select the symptoms that they are experiencing.
- HCPs can review the information and provide care aimed at managing the patient's specific symptoms.
- After the visit, the notes are stored in the patient's electronic health record. This system can assist with quality of care by determining if standards of care were followed.

RADIATION THERAPY

Along with surgery, radiation therapy is one of the oldest methods of cancer treatment. It was first used by Emil Grubbe (a medical student) to treat an ulcerating breast cancer in 1896 (although the patient responded locally, she died later of metastatic disease). The observation that radiation exposure caused tissue damage led scientists to explore the use of radiation to treat tumors. The hypothesized association was that if radiation exposure resulted in the destruction of highly mitotic skin cells, it could be used in a controlled way to prevent the continued growth of cancer cells.

It was not until the 1960s that sophisticated equipment and treatment planning facilitated the delivery of adequate radiation doses to tumors and tolerable doses to normal tissues. Today many cancer patients receive radiation therapy at some point in their treatment.

Effects of Radiation

Radiation is energy that is emitted from a source and travels through space or some material. Delivery of high-energy beams, when absorbed into tissue, produces ionization of atomic particles. The energy in ionizing radiation acts to break the chemical bonds in DNA. The DNA is damaged, resulting in cell death.

Different types of ionizing radiation are used to treat cancer, including *electromagnetic radiation* (i.e., x-rays, gamma rays) and *particulate radiation* (alpha particles, electrons, neutrons, protons). High-energy x-rays (photons) are generated by an electric machine, such as a linear accelerator.

Technologic advances have expanded and refined the sources and methods of delivering radiation therapy, thus offering more accurate and less invasive radiation treatment options. Most radiation centers in the United States currently use megavoltage linear accelerator technology. Larger radiation facilities may offer a combination of machines that permit expanded options for patients at one treatment site.

Principles of Radiobiology

As the radiation beam passes through the treatment field, energy is deposited. *Low-energy beams* (such as electrons) expend energy quickly on impact with matter. Therefore they penetrate only a short distance. (They are clinically useful in treating superficial skin lesions.) *High-energy beams* (such as photons) have greater depth of penetration, not attaining full intensity until they reach a certain depth. Therefore they are suitable for delivering optimal doses to internal targets while sparing the skin.

Technically, all cancer cells could be killed with radiation given in high enough doses. However, to avoid serious toxicity and long-term complications of treatment, radiation to surrounding healthy tissue must be limited to the *maximal tolerated dose* for that specific tissue. Advances in planning and in delivery technology (such as *intensity-modulated radiation therapy [IMRT]* and *image-guided radiation therapy [IGRT]*) have greatly improved the ability to deliver maximal doses to the target volume while sparing critical structures (e.g., spinal cord, carotid arteries, optic chiasm) as much as possible.

Historically, the radiation dose was expressed in units called *rads* (radiation absorbed doses). Current nomenclature is *gray* (Gy) or centigray (cGy). A *centigray* is equivalent to 1 rad, and 100 centigray equals 1 gray. Once the total dose to be delivered is determined, that dose is divided into daily *fractions.* Doses between 180 and 200 cGy/day are considered *standard fractionation,* typically delivered once a day Monday through Friday for a period of 2 to 8 weeks (depending on the desired total dose).

Certain cancers are more susceptible to the effects of radiation than others (Table 15-10). In responsive tumors (such as lymphomas), even a large tumor burden is affected by radiation therapy. In less responsive tumors, a large tumor burden may result in a slower and perhaps incomplete response. Localized prostate cancer responds very slowly to radiation (several months after treatment is completed).

Simulation and Treatment Planning

Simulation is a process by which the radiation treatment fields are defined, filmed, and marked out on the skin. The radiation oncologist specifies the dose and volume of area to be treated. Treatment volumes include the (1) *gross target* volume (GTV), which is the gross extent of the tumor identified by examination or imaging; (2) the *clinical target* volume (CTV), which is the GTV plus additional margin to encompass any potential microscopic or subclinical disease; and (3) the *planning target volume* (PTV), which is the GTV/CTV plus additional margin to allow for organ motion or variance in daily set-up position.

TABLE 15-10 Tumor Radiosensitivity*

High Radiosensitivity
- Ovarian dysgerminoma
- Testicular seminoma
- Hodgkin's lymphoma
- Non-Hodgkin's lymphoma
- Wilms' tumor
- Neuroblastoma

Moderate Radiosensitivity
- Oropharyngeal carcinoma
- Esophageal carcinoma
- Breast adenocarcinoma
- Uterine and cervical carcinoma
- Prostate carcinoma
- Bladder carcinoma

Mild Radiosensitivity
- Soft tissue sarcomas (e.g., chondrosarcoma)
- Gastric adenocarcinoma
- Renal adenocarcinoma
- Colon adenocarcinoma

Poor Radiosensitivity
- Osteosarcoma
- Malignant melanoma
- Malignant glioma
- Testicular nonseminoma

*Radiosensitivity is the relative susceptibility of cells and tissues to the effects of radiation.

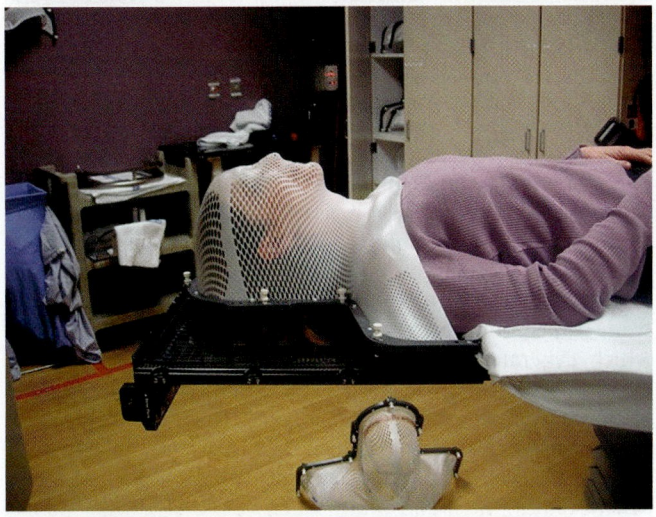

FIG. 15-12 Immobilization device. A head holder and an immobilization mask may be used to ensure accurate positioning for daily treatment of head and neck cancer. (Courtesy Jormain Cady, Virginia Mason Medical Center, Seattle, Wash.)

During the simulation, the patient is positioned on a simulator, which is a diagnostic x-ray machine that re-creates the actions of the linear accelerator and the radiation fields are marked on the patient's skin. Immobilization devices (e.g., casts, bite blocks, thermoplastic face masks) are typically used to help the patient maintain a stable position (Fig. 15-12).

The target is defined using a variety of possible imaging techniques (e.g., x-rays; CT, MRI, PET scans), physical examination, and surgical reports. Small tattoos may be placed to ensure the patient position is precisely reproduced on a daily basis.

Treatment

Radiation is used to treat a carefully defined area of the body. Since radiation only has an effect on tissues within the treatment field, it is not appropriate as the primary treatment for systemic disease. However, radiation may be used by itself, in combination with chemotherapy or surgery to treat primary tumors, or for palliation of metastatic lesions.

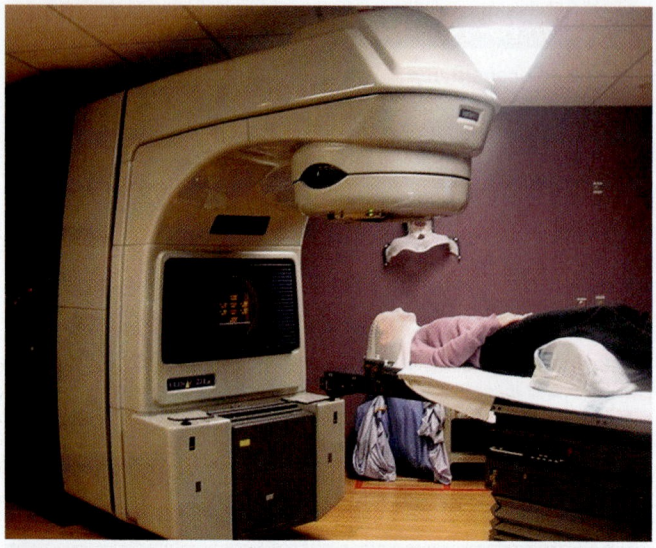

FIG. 15-13 Linear accelerator. Varian Clinac EX linear accelerator with multiple photon and electron energies available for use according to the treatment plan. Patient is positioned on radiation treatment table for treatment of head and neck cancer. (Courtesy Jormain Cady, Virginia Mason Medical Center, Seattle, Wash.)

External Radiation. Radiation can be delivered externally (known as *teletherapy* or *external beam radiation therapy*) or internally *(brachytherapy)*. **Teletherapy** *(external beam radiation)* is the most common form of radiation treatment delivery. With this technique, the patient is exposed to radiation from a megavoltage treatment machine. A linear accelerator, which generates ionizing radiation from electricity and can have multiple energies, is the most commonly used machine for delivering external beam radiation (Fig. 15-13). *Gamma knife technology* (used to deliver highly accurate stereotactic treatment to a localized treatment volume) uses a cobalt source.

Internal Radiation. Radiation can also be delivered as **brachytherapy**, which means "close" or internal radiation treatment. It consists of the implantation or insertion of radioactive materials directly into the tumor (interstitial) or in close proximity to the tumor (intracavitary or intraluminal). This allows for direct delivery of radiation to the target with minimal exposure to surrounding healthy tissues. (In external radiation, the beam has to pass through external tissues to reach the internal target.) Brachytherapy is commonly used in combination with external radiation as a supplemental "boost" treatment, but may also be used as primary or adjuvant therapy.

Sources of radiation for brachytherapy include temporary sealed sources such as iridium-192 and cesium-137 and permanent sealed sources such as iodine-125, gold-198, and palladium-103. These are supplied in the form of seeds or ribbons. With a temporary implant, the source may be placed into a special catheter or metal tube that has been inserted into the tumor area. It is left in place until the prescribed dose of radiation has been reached in the calculated number of hours.

Brachytherapy may be delivered as high-dose-rate (HDR) treatment (i.e., several doses administered at varying intervals over a few minutes each time) or low-dose-rate (LDR) treatment (i.e., continuous treatment over several hours or days). A remote "afterloading" technique (i.e., the source is inserted after the applicator is in place) is designed to enhance physician and patient safety and is used for HDR brachytherapy with iridium-192. These methods are commonly used for head and neck, lung, breast, and gynecologic cancers.

Permanent implants, such as for prostate brachytherapy, involve the insertion of radioactive seeds directly into the tumor tissue, where they remain permanently. As interstitial seeds used for treatment emit low energies with limited tissue penetration, patients are not considered radioactive. However, some initial radiation precautions may be recommended because of a small risk of seed dislodgement. Over time, the isotopes that are used decay and are no longer radioactive. The timeframe for side effects induced by treatment can be predicted based on the rate of decay for the specific isotope used.

Radiopharmaceutical therapy employs unsealed liquid radioactive sources that are administered orally as a drink, such as iodine-131 for thyroid cancer, or IV as with yttrium-90 given for refractory lymphomas or samarium-153 used to treat bone metastases.

Caring for the person undergoing brachytherapy or receiving radiopharmaceuticals requires that you be aware that the patient is emitting radioactivity. Patients with temporary implants are radioactive only while the source is in place. In patients with permanent implants, because the sources have short half-lives and are weak emitters, the radioactive exposure to the outside and to others is low. These patients may be discharged with minimal precautions.

The principles of *ALARA (as low as reasonably achievable)* and *time, distance,* and *shielding* are vital to health care professional safety when caring for the person with a source of internal radiation. Organize care to limit the time spent in direct contact with the patient. To minimize anxiety and confusion, tell the patient the reason for time and distance limitations before the procedure.

The radiation safety officer will indicate how much time at a specific distance can be spent with the patient. This is determined by the dose delivered by the implant. Because the source is nonpenetrating, small differences in distance are critical. Only care that must be delivered near the source, such as checking placement of the implant, is performed in close proximity. Use shielding, if available, and do not deliver care without wearing a film badge (dosimeter) indicating cumulative radiation exposure. Do not share the film badge, do not wear it anywhere but at work, and return it according to the agency's protocol.

❖ NURSING MANAGEMENT: CHEMOTHERAPY AND RADIATION THERAPY

You have an important role in helping patients deal with the side effects of chemotherapy and radiation therapy. Before initiating teaching, assess the patient's ability to process information. Customize teaching to meet the patient's and family's learning needs.[17,18]

Common side effects of chemotherapy and radiation are presented in Table 15-11. Bone marrow suppression, fatigue, GI disturbances, integumentary and mucosal reactions, and pulmonary and reproductive effects are discussed in this section.

◆ Nursing Implementation

◆ **Bone Marrow Suppression.** Myelosuppression is one of the most common effects of chemotherapy and, to a lesser extent,

TABLE 15-11 Nursing Management of Problems Caused by Chemotherapy and Radiation Therapy

Etiology	Nursing Management
Gastrointestinal System	
Stomatitis, Mucositis, Esophagitis	
Epithelial cells are destroyed by chemotherapy or radiation treatment when located in field (e.g., head and neck, stomach, esophagus). Inflammation and ulceration occur due to rapid cell destruction.	• Assess oral mucosa daily and teach patient to do this. • Encourage nutritional supplements (e.g., Ensure, Carnation Instant Breakfast) if intake decreasing. • Be aware that eating, swallowing, and talking may be difficult (may require analgesics). • Instruct in avoidance of irritating spicy or acidic foods or too hot or too cold food (extremes in temperature). • Instruct on how to select moist, bland, and softer foods. • Encourage patient to keep oral cavity clean and moist by performing frequent oral rinses with saline or salt and soda solution. • Encourage patient to use artificial saliva to manage dryness (radiation). • Discourage use of irritants such as tobacco and alcohol. • Apply topical anesthetics (e.g., viscous lidocaine, oxethazaine).
Nausea and Vomiting	
Release of intracellular breakdown products stimulates vomiting center in brain. Drugs also stimulate vomiting center in brain (see Fig. 41-1). GI lining destroyed with radiation and chemotherapy.	• Encourage patient to eat and drink when not nauseated. • Administer antiemetics prophylactically before chemotherapy and also on as-needed basis. • Instruct patient to take antiemetics on a scheduled basis for 2-3 days after highly emetogenic chemotherapy. • Use diversional activities (if appropriate).
Anorexia	
Release of TNF and IL-1 from macrophages has appetite-suppressant effect. Therapy-induced GI effects (mucositis, nausea and vomiting, bowel disturbances) and anxiety reduce appetite.	• Monitor weight. • Encourage patient to eat small, frequent meals of high-protein, high-calorie foods. • Gently encourage patient to eat, but avoid nagging. • Recommend keeping a food diary to track daily calories and fluids. • Serve food in pleasant environment.
Diarrhea	
From denuding of epithelial lining of intestines. Side effect of chemotherapy. Follows radiation to abdomen, pelvis, lumbosacral areas.	• Give antidiarrheal drugs as needed. • Encourage low-fiber, low-residue diet. • Encourage fluid intake of at least 3 L/day.
Constipation	
Decreased intestinal motility is related to autonomic nervous system dysfunction. Caused by neurotoxic effects of plant alkaloids (vincristine, vinblastine).	• Instruct patient to take stool softeners as needed, eat high-fiber foods, and increase fluid intake. • Instruct patient to increase activity (e.g., walking) if tolerated.
Hepatotoxicity	
Toxic effects from chemotherapy drugs (usually transient and resolve when drug is stopped).	• Monitor liver function tests.
Hematologic System	
Anemia	
Bone marrow depressed secondary to therapy. Malignant infiltration of bone marrow by cancer.	• Monitor hemoglobin and hematocrit levels. • Administer iron supplements and erythropoietin. • Encourage intake of foods that promote RBC production (see Table 30-5).
Leukopenia	
Depression of bone marrow secondary to chemotherapy or radiation therapy. Infection most frequent cause of morbidity and death in cancer patients. Respiratory and genitourinary system usual sites of infection.	• Monitor WBC count, especially neutrophils. • Tell patient to report temperature elevation and any other manifestations of infection. • Teach patient to avoid large crowds and people with infections. • Administer WBC growth factors (Table 15-15). • For patient teaching, see Table 30-23.
Thrombocytopenia	
Bone marrow depressed secondary to chemotherapy. Malignant infiltration of bone marrow crowds out normal marrow. Spontaneous bleeding can occur with platelet counts ≤20,000/μL.	• Observe for signs of bleeding (e.g., petechiae, ecchymosis). • Monitor platelet counts. • For patient teaching, see Table 30-15.
Integumentary System	
Alopecia	
Destruction of hair follicles by chemotherapy or radiation to scalp. Hair loss usually is temporary with chemotherapy, but usually permanent in response to radiation.	• Suggest ways to cope with hair loss (e.g., hair pieces, scarves, wigs). • Cut long hair before therapy. • Avoid excessive shampooing, brushing, and combing of hair. • Avoid use of electric hair dryers, curlers, and curling rods. • Discuss impact of hair loss on self-image.
Radiation Skin Changes (dry to moist desquamation)	
Radiation damages skin.	• See Table 15-12 for patient management details.

IL-1, Interleukin-1; *TNF*, tumor necrosis factor.

Continued

TABLE 15-11 Nursing Management of Problems Caused by Chemotherapy and Radiation Therapy—cont'd

Etiology	Nursing Management
Integumentary System—cont'd	
Chemotherapy-Induced Skin Changes	
Hyperpigmentation. Telangiectasia. Photosensitivity. Acneiform eruptions. Acral erythema.	• Alert patient to potential skin changes. • Encourage patient to avoid sun exposure. • Implement symptomatic management as needed depending on specific skin effect (e.g., application of lotions, benzoyl peroxide for acne, corticosteroid creams).
Genitourinary Tract	
Hemorrhagic Cystitis	
Cells lining bladder are destroyed by chemotherapy (e.g., cyclophosphamide, ifosfamide). Side effect of radiation when located in treatment field.	• Encourage increased fluid intake 24-72 hr after treatment as tolerated. • Monitor manifestations such as urgency, frequency, and hematuria. • Administer cytoprotectant agent (mesna [Mesnex]) and hydration. • Administer supportive care agents to manage symptoms (e.g., flavoxate [Urispas]).
Reproductive Dysfunction	
Cells of testes or ova are damaged by therapy.	• Discuss possibility with patients before treatment initiation. • Offer opportunity for sperm and ova banking before treatment for patients of childbearing age.
Nephrotoxicity	
Direct renal cell damage from exposure to nephrotoxic agents (cisplatin and high-dose methotrexate). Precipitation of metabolites of cell breakdown (tumor lysis syndrome [TLS]).	• Monitor BUN and serum creatinine levels. • Avoid potentiating drugs. • Alkalinize the urine by adding sodium bicarbonate to IV infusion and administer allopurinol (Zyloprim) or rasburicase for TLS prevention.
Nervous System	
Intracranial Pressure	
May result from radiation edema in central nervous system.	• Monitor neurologic status. • May be controlled with corticosteroids.
Peripheral Neuropathy	
Paresthesias, areflexia, skeletal muscle weakness, and smooth muscle dysfunction can occur as a side effect of plant alkaloids, taxanes, and cisplatin.	• Monitor for these manifestations in patients on these drugs. • Consider temporary chemotherapy dose interruption or reduction until symptoms improve. • Antiseizure drugs (e.g., gabapentin [Neurontin]) may be considered.
Cognitive Changes ("chemo brain")	

Occur during and after treatment (especially with chemotherapy).
Difficulties in concentration, memory lapses, trouble remembering details, taking longer to finish tasks.
May happen quickly and last a short time. Sometimes people have mild long-term effects.
	• Teach patients to do the following:
	  • Use detailed daily planner.
	  • Get enough sleep and rest.
	  • Exercise brain (learn something new, do word puzzles).
	  • Focus on one thing (no multitasking).

Respiratory System	
Pneumonitis	
Radiation pneumonitis develops 2-3 mo after start of treatment. After 6-12 mo, fibrosis occurs and is evident on x-ray. Side effect of some chemotherapy drugs.	• Monitor for dry, hacking cough; fever; and exertional dyspnea.
Cardiovascular System	
Pericarditis and Myocarditis	
Inflammation secondary to radiation injury. Complication when chest wall is irradiated. May occur up to 1 yr after treatment. Side effect of some chemotherapy drugs.	• Monitor for clinical manifestations of these disorders (e.g., dyspnea).
Cardiotoxicity	
Some chemotherapy drugs (e.g., anthracyclines, taxanes) can cause ECG changes and rapidly progressive heart failure.	• Monitor heart with ECG and cardiac ejection fractions. • Drug therapy may need to be modified for symptoms or deteriorating cardiac function studies.
Biochemical	
Hyperuricemia	
Increased uric acid levels due to chemotherapy-induced cell destruction. Can cause secondary gout and obstructive uropathy.	• Monitor uric acid levels. • Allopurinol may be given as a prophylactic measure. • Encourage increased fluid intake.
Psychoemotional	
Fatigue	
Anabolic processes result in accumulation of metabolites from cell breakdown.	• Assess for reversible causes of fatigue, and address them as indicated. • Reassure patient that fatigue is a common side effect of therapy. • Encourage patient to rest when fatigued, to maintain usual lifestyle patterns as much as possible, and to pace activities in accordance with energy level. • Encourage moderate exercise as tolerated.

BUN, Blood urea nitrogen; *ECG,* electrocardiogram.

it can also occur with radiation. Treatment-induced reductions in blood cell production can result in life-threatening and distressing effects, including infection, hemorrhage, and overwhelming fatigue. The major difference in manifestations between radiation therapy and chemotherapy is that with radiation (a local therapy), only bone marrow within the treatment field is affected, whereas chemotherapy (a systemic therapy) affects bone marrow function throughout the body. Therefore effects are more profound with chemotherapy and when the two therapies are combined.

In general, the onset of bone marrow suppression is related to the life span of the type of blood cell. WBCs (especially neutrophils) are affected most acutely (within 1 to 2 weeks), platelets in 2 to 3 weeks, and red blood cells (RBCs), with a longer life span of 120 days, at a later time. The severity of myelosuppression depends on the chemotherapy drugs used, dosages of drugs, and the specific radiation treatment field. Radiation to large marrow-containing regions of the body produces the most clinically significant myelosuppression. In the adult, most of the active marrow is in the pelvis or thoracic and lumbar vertebrae.

Monitor the complete blood count, particularly the neutrophil, platelet, and RBC counts, in patients receiving chemotherapy or radiation. Typically patients experience the lowest blood cell counts (called the **nadir**) between 7 and 10 days after initiation of therapy. However, the exact onset depends on the particular drug regimen.

Neutropenia is more common in patients receiving chemotherapy than radiation therapy. Neutropenia is a serious risk factor for life-threatening infection and sepsis. Significant neutropenia will prompt treatment delay or modification (i.e., lower dosages). Take every possible measure to prevent infections in these patients. Hand hygiene is the mainstay of patient protection. Patients and their contacts (including hospital staff) should follow hand-washing guidelines.

Monitor temperature routinely. Any sign of infection should be treated promptly, since fever in the setting of neutropenia is a medical emergency. WBC growth factors (i.e., filgrastim [Neupogen], pegfilgrastim [Neulasta]) are routinely used to reduce the duration of chemotherapy-induced neutropenia. They are also used as a prophylactic measure to prevent neutropenia when highly myelosuppressive chemotherapy drugs are used.[19] (Neutropenia is discussed in Chapter 30; see also the patient teaching guide in Table 30-23 and eNursing Care Plan 30-3 on the website for that chapter.)

Thrombocytopenia can result in spontaneous bleeding or major hemorrhage. Avoid invasive procedures and advise patients to avoid activities that place them at risk for injury or bleeding (including excessive straining). Risk of serious bleeding is generally not apparent until the platelet count falls below 50,000/μL. Platelet transfusions may be necessary and are usually administered when platelet counts fall below 20,000/μL. (Thrombocytopenia is discussed in Chapter 30; see also the patient teaching guide in Table 30-15 and eNursing Care Plan 30-2 on the website for that chapter.)

Anemia is common in patients undergoing either radiation therapy or chemotherapy. It generally has a later onset (about 3 to 4 months after treatment initiation). For patients with low hemoglobin levels, RBC growth factors (i.e., darbepoetin [Aranesp], epoetin [Procrit]) may be given according to clinical guidelines for use. In extreme circumstances (i.e., symptomatic anemia), RBC transfusions may also be indicated. However, in general, RBC transfusions should be avoided. (Hematopoietic growth factors are discussed later in this chapter and presented in Table 15-15.)

◆ **Fatigue.** *Fatigue* is the persistent subjective sense of tiredness associated with cancer and its treatment that interferes with usual day-to-day functioning. Fatigue is a nearly universal symptom affecting most patients with cancer. It is commonly reported by patients as the most distressful of treatment-related side effects. Furthermore, it may persist long after treatment has ended.

Anemia is one cause of fatigue. Other causes may be related to the (1) accumulation of toxic substances that are left in the body after cells are killed by cancer treatment, (2) need for extra energy to repair and heal body tissue damaged by treatment, and (3) lack of sleep caused by some chemotherapy drugs.

Assess for reversible causes of fatigue, such as anemia, hypothyroidism, depression, anxiety, insomnia, dehydration, or infection.

Help patients recognize that fatigue is a common side effect of therapy, and encourage energy conservation strategies. Help individuals identify days or times during the day when they typically feel better, and encourage them to remain more active during that time period.

Resting before activity and having others assist with work or home management may be necessary. Ignoring the fatigue or overstressing the body when fatigue is tolerable may lead to an increase in symptoms. However, maintaining exercise and activity within tolerable limits is often helpful in managing fatigue. Walking programs are a way for most patients to keep active without overtaxing themselves. Remaining active helps to improve mood and avoid the debilitating cycle of fatigue-depression-fatigue that can occur in patients with cancer. Guidelines for the evaluation and management of cancer-related fatigue are available.[20]

◆ **Gastrointestinal Effects.** The cells of the mucosal lining of the GI tract are highly proliferative, with epithelial cells being replaced every 2 to 6 days. The intestinal mucosa is one of the most sensitive tissues to radiation and chemotherapy. The etiology of GI reactions is related to a variety of mechanisms, including (1) the release of serotonin from the GI tract, which then stimulates the chemoreceptor trigger zone (CTZ) and the vomiting center in the brain and (2) cell death and resulting damage to GI mucosa. Additionally, radiation to treatment fields that contain GI structures (i.e., abdominopelvic, lumbosacral, and lower thoracic areas) and selected chemotherapy agents produce direct injury to GI epithelial cells. These injuries result in a variety of GI effects, including nausea and vomiting, diarrhea, mucositis, and anorexia. These problems can significantly affect the patient's hydration and nutritional status and sense of well-being.

◆ ***Nausea and Vomiting.*** Nausea and vomiting are common sequelae of chemotherapy and, in some instances, radiation therapy. Vomiting may occur within 1 hour of chemotherapy administration or a few hours after radiation therapy to the chest or abdomen and may persist for 24 hours or more. Several antiemetic drugs are available (see Table 41-1).

Metoclopramide (Reglan), prochlorperazine, serotonin ($5\text{-}HT_3$) receptor antagonists (ondansetron [Zofran], granisetron [Kytril], dolasetron [Anzemet], and palonosetron [Aloxi]), and dexamethasone have been used to decrease nausea and vomiting caused by chemotherapy. Aprepitant (Emend) and rolapitant (Varubi), substance P/neurokinin-1 receptor antagonists, are effective in preventing nausea and vomiting on the day of chemotherapy, as well as for delayed symptoms. Akynzeo is a fixed combination of two drugs: palonosetron and netupitant (a substance P/neurokinin-1 receptor antagonist).

Patients may also develop *anticipatory nausea and vomiting* if they experience poorly controlled nausea and vomiting after chemotherapy administration. In this phenomenon, encountering the cues even without receiving treatment may precipitate nausea and vomiting. Aggressive emesis control, including the prophylactic administration of antiemetic and antianxiety medication 1 hour before treatment, is recommended. The patient may find that eating a light meal of nonirritating food before treatment is also helpful.

Delayed nausea and vomiting can develop 24 hours to a week after treatment. Assess patients who are experiencing nausea and vomiting for signs and symptoms of dehydration and metabolic alkalosis. Nausea and vomiting can be successfully managed with antiemetic regimens, dietary modification, and other nondrug interventions (e.g., relaxation breathing).

◆ **Diarrhea.** Diarrhea is a reaction of the bowel mucosa to radiation and certain chemotherapy drugs. It is characterized by an increase in frequency and liquidity of stool. The small bowel is extremely sensitive and does not tolerate significant radiation doses. With pelvic radiation, patients may be treated with a full bladder to move the small bowel out of the treatment field. Both radiation- and chemotherapy-induced diarrhea are best managed with diet modification, antidiarrheals, antimotility agents, and antispasmodics (see Table 42-2).

Recommend a diet low in fiber and residue before treatment with chemotherapy known to cause diarrhea. This includes limiting foods that are high in roughage (e.g., fresh fruits, vegetables, seeds, nuts) (see Table 42-7). To prevent diarrhea, other foods to avoid include fried, fatty, or highly seasoned foods and other foods that are gas producing. Bowel mucosal injury from radiation may also result in temporary lactose intolerance. Therefore avoiding milk products is helpful for some patients during and immediately after treatment.

Depending on the severity of the diarrhea, hydration and electrolyte supplementation are also recommended. Lukewarm sitz baths may alleviate discomfort and cleanse the rectal area if significant rectal irritation has developed. The rectal area must be kept clean and dry to maintain skin integrity. You should visually inspect the perianal area for evidence of skin breakdown. Systemic analgesia may be used for the painful skin irritations that may develop. Note the number, volume, consistency, and character of stools per day. Teach patients to maintain a diary or log to record episodes and aggravating and alleviating factors.

◆ **Mucositis.** Mucositis (irritation, inflammation, and/or ulceration of the mucosa) is a common complication in almost all patients receiving radiation to the head and neck and in many patients receiving certain antineoplastic agents. Similar to the bowel mucosa, the mucosal linings of the oral cavity, oropharynx, and esophagus are extremely sensitive to the effects of radiation and chemotherapy.

Certain factors can compound the problem. For example, patients undergoing head and neck radiation may face the additional challenge of radiation-induced parotid gland dysfunction. This may result in decreased salivary flow, causing acute or chronic *xerostomia* (dry mouth). Dryness or thick saliva compromises the protective salivary functions of assisting with cleansing teeth, moistening food, and swallowing. Meticulous oral care during and for a long time after treatment reduces the risk of cavities related to the radiation, which may develop as a result of diminished saliva. Advise patients to continue regular dental follow-up every 6 months and to use fluoride supplements as recommended by their dentist. Saliva substitutes may be offered to patients with xerostomia, although many patients find that drinking small amounts of water frequently has a similar effect.

Dysgeusia (taste loss) may develop during therapy, and by the end of treatment, patients often report that all food has lost its flavor. Ultimately, nutritional status may be compromised. *Dysphagia* (difficulty swallowing), which characterizes pharyngeal and/or esophageal involvement, further impedes eating. Patients may report feeling that they have a "lump" as they swallow and that "foods get stuck." *Odynophagia* (painful swallowing) caused by oropharyngeal or esophageal irritation and ulceration may require the use of analgesics before meals.

Oral assessment and meticulous intervention to keep the oral cavity moist, clean, and free of debris are essential to prevent infection and to facilitate nutritional intake. Implementing standard oral care protocols that address prevention and management of mucositis facilitates routine assessment, patient and family teaching, and intervention.

Routinely assess the oral cavity, mucous membranes, characteristics of saliva, and ability to swallow. Having a dentist perform all necessary dental work before the initiation of treatment is also recommended. Teach the patient to self-examine the oral cavity as well as how to perform oral care (proper tooth brushing with a soft-bristle toothbrush, flossing, and use of fluoride trays to prevent caries). Oral care should be performed at least before and after each meal, at bedtime, and as needed through the day. A saline solution of 1 tsp of salt in 1 L of water is an effective cleansing agent. One tsp of sodium bicarbonate may be added to the oral care solution to decrease odor, alleviate pain, and dissolve mucin.

Mucositis or pain in the throat can be alleviated by systemic and/or topical analgesics and antibiotics if infection is present. Monitor and get prompt treatment for oral candidiasis (which often occurs with mucositis). Frequent cleansing with saline and water and topical application of anesthetic gels directly to the lesions are standard care.

◆ **Anorexia.** Anorexia (loss of appetite) is a common occurrence in patients with cancer. It is a side effect of the cancer itself as well as of cancer treatment. Anorexia may be related to an inflamed mouth or esophagus, which creates difficulty chewing or swallowing, or to emotions such as anxiety or depression. It is important to have a dietitian involved in patient care before cancer treatment begins.

Patients experiencing nausea and vomiting, bowel disturbances, mucositis, and taste alterations typically have little desire to eat. Although it is highly individual, anorexia seems to peak at about 4 weeks of treatment and to resolve more quickly than fatigue when treatment ends.

Monitor the patient with anorexia during and after treatment to ensure that weight loss does not become excessive. Also observe for dehydration. Small, frequent meals of high-protein, high-calorie foods are better tolerated than large meals. Nutritional supplements can be helpful as well. Enteral or parenteral nutrition may be indicated if the patient is severely malnourished, if symptoms are expected to interfere with nutrition for a time, or if the bowel is being rested. Monitor for and manage

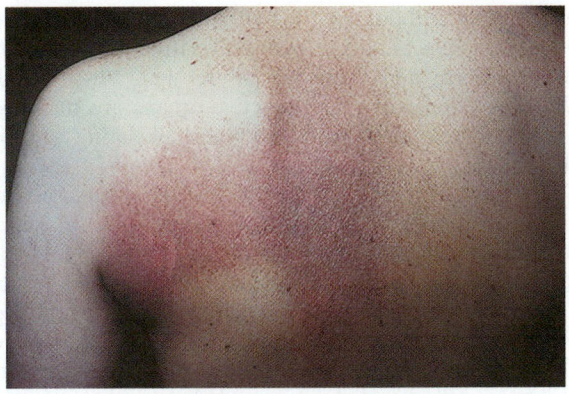

FIG. 15-14 Dry desquamation.

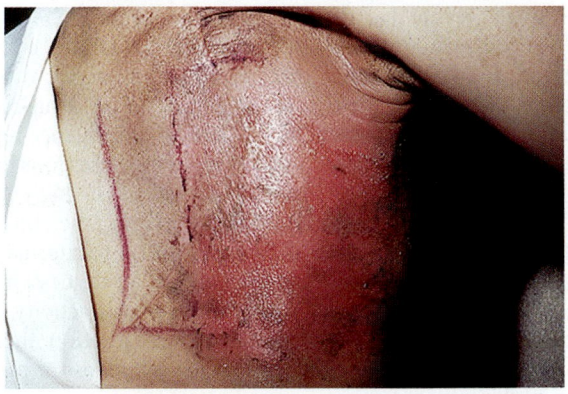

FIG. 15-15 Wet desquamation.

other symptoms that may interfere with appetite (e.g., nausea, vomiting, pain, depression).

Skin Reactions

Radiation Skin Changes. With radiation therapy, skin effects are local, occurring only in the treatment field. Radiation-induced skin changes can be acute or chronic depending on the area irradiated, dosage, and technique. The skin-sparing ability of modern radiation equipment limits the severity of these reactions.

Erythema may develop 1 to 24 hours after a single treatment but generally occurs progressively as the treatment dose accumulates. Erythema is an acute response followed by dry desquamation (Fig. 15-14). If the rate of cell sloughing is faster than the ability of the new epidermal cells to replace dead cells, a wet desquamation occurs with exposure of the dermis and weeping of serous fluid (Fig. 15-15). Skin reactions are particularly evident in areas of skinfolds or where skin is subjected to pressure, such as behind the ear; in gluteal folds; or on the perineum, breast, collar line, and bony prominences.

Although skin care protocols vary among institutions, basic skin care principles apply. The goal is to prevent infection and facilitate wound healing. Protect radiated skin from temperature extremes. Do not use heating pads, ice packs, and hot water bottles in the treatment field. Avoid constricting garments, rubbing, harsh chemicals, and deodorants, since they may traumatize the skin. Dry reactions are uncomfortable and result in pruritus. Lubricate dry skin with a nonirritating lotion emollient that contains no metal, alcohol, perfume, or additives, since these can be irritating. Calendula ointment and topical hyaluronic acid cream are effective for the management of radiation dermatitis. Aloe vera gel is also used, especially for prevention of skin problems.

TABLE 15-12 Patient & Caregiver Teaching

Radiation Skin Reactions

Include the following instructions when teaching the patient and caregiver to clean and protect the skin in a radiation treatment area.

1. Gently cleanse the skin in the treatment field using a mild soap (Ivory, Dove), tepid water, a soft cloth, and a gentle patting motion. Rinse thoroughly and pat dry.
2. Apply nonmedicated, nonperfumed, moisturizing lotion or cream, such as calendula ointment, aloe gel, Aquaphor, or Biafine cream, to alleviate dry skin. Some substances must be gently cleansed from the treatment field before each treatment and reapplied. Over-the-counter hydrocortisone cream 1% may reduce itching.
3. Rinse the area with saline solution. Expose the area to air as often as possible. If copious drainage is present, use astringent compresses (such as Domeboro solution) and nonadhesive absorbent dressings (they must be changed as soon as they become wet). Observe the area daily for signs of infection.
4. Avoid wearing tight-fitting clothing such as brassieres and belts over the treatment field.
5. Avoid wearing harsh fabrics, such as wool and corduroy. A lightweight cotton garment is best. If possible, expose the treatment field to air.
6. Use gentle detergents such as Dreft and Ivory Snow to wash clothing that will come in contact with the treatment field.
7. Avoid direct exposure to the sun. If the treatment field is in an area that is exposed to the sun, wear protective clothing such as a wide-brimmed hat when out in the sun and apply sunscreen lotion.
8. Avoid all sources of excessive heat (hot water bottles, heating pads, sunlamps) on the treatment field.
9. Avoid exposing the treatment field to cold temperatures (ice bags or cold weather).
10. Avoid swimming in saltwater or in chlorinated pools during the time of treatment.
11. Avoid the use of potential irritants (e.g., perfumes, powders, or cosmetics) on the skin in the treatment field; review use of other topical medications or lotions with your health care provider during treatment. Also avoid tape, dressings, and adhesive bandages unless permitted by the radiation therapist. Avoid shaving the hair in the treatment field.
12. Continue to protect sensitive skin after the treatment is completed. Do the following:
    - Avoid direct exposure to the sun. A sunscreen agent and protective clothing must be worn if the potential of exposure to the sun is present.
    - Use an electric razor if shaving is necessary in the treatment field.

Wet desquamation of tissues generally produces pain, drainage, and increased risk of infection. Skin care to manage most desquamation includes keeping tissues clean with normal saline compresses or modified Burow's solution soaks. Then protect the skin from further damage with moisture vapor–permeable dressings or Vaseline petrolatum gauze. Because protocols vary widely, the guidelines presented in Table 15-12 should be verified with your institution's radiation oncology department before using.

Chemotherapy Skin Changes. Chemotherapy produces a wide range of skin toxicities. These can range from mild erythema and hyperpigmentation to more distressing effects such as acral erythema and *erythrodysesthesia syndrome* (also called palmar-plantar erythrodysesthesia or hand-foot syndrome).

Erythrodysesthesia syndrome can cause mild symptoms of redness and tingling of the palms of the hands and soles of the feet. It may also cause severe symptoms of painful moist desquamation, ulceration, blistering, and pain.

Alopecia is an easily recognizable effect of cancer therapy. It is frequently associated with varying degrees of emotional distress. Hair loss associated with radiation is local, whereas chemotherapy affects hair throughout the body. The degree and duration of hair loss experienced by patients depend on the type and dose of the chemotherapy agent.

Alopecia caused by the administration of chemotherapy agents is usually reversible. Usually the hair does not grow back until 3 to 4 weeks after the drugs are discontinued. Often the new hair has a different color and texture than the hair that was lost.

Patients experience a range of emotions at the prospect of losing their hair and when hair loss actually occurs. These may include anger, grief, embarrassment, or fear. Hair loss is a visible reminder of their cancer and the challenges of treatment. For some people, the loss of hair is one of the most stressful events experienced during the course of treatment. The American Cancer Society's "Look Good, Feel Better" program is an excellent support and resource for people experiencing not just hair loss but body image changes in general.

- **Pulmonary Effects.** Both chemotherapy and radiation have the potential to produce pulmonary tissue damage that is irreversible and progressive. Distinguishing between the complications of treatment and those related to disease is challenging. The effects of radiation on the lung include both acute and late reactions. Immediate pulmonary effects of radiation can be alarming to patients because they may mimic symptoms (e.g., cough, dyspnea) that precipitated the cancer diagnosis.

  Pneumonitis is a delayed acute inflammatory reaction that may occur within 1 to 3 months after completion of thoracic radiation. This reaction is often asymptomatic, although an increase in cough, fever, and night sweats may occur. Some patients may develop pulmonary fibrosis (with or without prior pneumonitis), which is a late effect of therapy.

  The most common pulmonary toxicities associated with chemotherapy include pulmonary edema (noncardiogenic) related to capillary leak syndrome or fluid retention, hypersensitivity pneumonitis, interstitial fibrosis, and pneumonitis produced by an inflammatory reaction or destruction of alveolar-capillary endothelium.
- **Cardiovascular Effects.** Radiation to the thorax can damage the pericardium, myocardium, valves, and coronary blood vessels. The pericardium is most commonly involved, with pericardial effusion or pericarditis the key problems. Patients with preexisting coronary artery disease are especially vulnerable.

  Anthracyclines (e.g., doxorubicin [Adriamycin], daunorubicin) cause cardiotoxicity. Acute cardiotoxicities may cause electrocardiographic (ECG) abnormalities and late effects cause left ventricular dysfunction and heart failure. Baseline and periodic echocardiograms to monitor left ventricular function during treatment are usually done.
- **Cognitive Effects.** Cognitive effects can happen at any time during cancer, especially after treatment. This alteration in mental function, commonly described by patients as mental cloudiness or fog, is commonly called *chemo brain.*[21,22] Patients can experience thinking and memory problems. Although the brain will usually recover over time, the effects can last a short time or last for years. The effects can be so severe that patients may be unable to be involved in any activities that require mental effort such as school, work, or social activities.
- **Reproductive Effects.** Reproductive dysfunction secondary to radiation and chemotherapy varies according to the radiation treatment field and dosage, the particular chemotherapy agent and dose, and host factors (e.g., age). Treatment can cause temporary or permanent gonadal failure. Reproductive effects occur most often when reproductive organs are included in the radiation treatment field and when alkylating agents are used.

  The testes are highly sensitive to radiation and should be protected with a testicular shield whenever possible. Pretreatment status may be a significant factor because a low sperm count and loss of motility are seen in individuals with testicular cancer and Hodgkin's lymphoma before any therapy is begun. Combined modality treatment or prior chemotherapy with alkylating agents enhances and prolongs the effects of radiation on the testes. When radiation is used alone with conventional doses and appropriate shielding, testicular recovery often occurs. Compromise of reproductive function in men may also result from erectile dysfunction after pelvic radiation.

  The radiation dose that induces ovarian failure changes with age. Unlike the testes, there is no way to repair ovarian function. When radiation therapy is given, the ovaries are shielded whenever possible. Other factors that influence reproductive or sexual functioning in women include reactions in the cervix and endometrium. These tissues withstand a high radiation dose with minimal sequelae, accounting for the ability to treat endometrial and cervical cancer with high external and brachytherapy doses. Acute reactions such as tenderness, irritation, and loss of lubrication compromise sexual activity. Late effects of combined internal and external radiation therapy include vaginal shortening related to fibrosis and loss of elasticity and lubrication.

  The patient and her or his partner require information about the expected effects of treatment relative to reproductive and sexual issues. Fertility preservation should be addressed prior to the start of any cancer treatment. Pretreatment harvesting of sperm, ova, or ovarian tissue may be considered.[23]

  Potential infertility can be a significant consequence for the individual, and counseling may be indicated. However, in no case should the patient think that conception is not possible during treatment. Specific suggestions to manage side effects that have an impact on sexual functioning include using a water-soluble vaginal lubricant and routinely using a vaginal dilator after pelvic irradiation. Encourage discussion of issues related to reproduction and sexuality, offer specific suggestions, and make referrals for ongoing counseling when indicated.

LATE EFFECTS OF RADIATION AND CHEMOTHERAPY

Cancer survivors are achieving long-term remission and survival with advancements in treatment modalities. However, these forms of therapy (especially radiation therapy and chemotherapy) may produce long-term sequelae termed *late effects* that occur months to years after cessation of therapy.[24,25] Every body system can be affected to some extent by radiation therapy or chemotherapy.

Acute radiation effects generally manifest as transient inflammatory changes in highly proliferative cells (e.g., epithelial tissues). In contrast, late radiation effects occur most commonly in post-mitotic cells (e.g., liver, kidney, lung, heart, muscle, bone, and connective tissues). Once they occur, the late effects may be progressive and generally are permanent. Examples range from skin telangiectasias to strictures, fistulas, or radiation necrosis.

Alteration of the lymphatic channels (e.g., axillary lymph node dissection) may contribute to lymphedema.

Long-term effects of chemotherapy include cardiac toxicity, cataracts, arthralgias, endocrine alterations, renal insufficiency, hepatitis, osteoporosis, neurocognitive dysfunction, or other effects depending on the agents. The additive effects of multiagent chemotherapy before, during, or after a course of radiation therapy can significantly increase the resulting late effects.

The cancer survivor may also be at risk for secondary malignancies, including leukemia, angiosarcoma, and skin cancer. Patients treated with alkylating agents and those treated with high-dose radiation have an increased risk. The potential risk for developing a secondary malignancy does not contraindicate the use of cancer treatment.

IMMUNOTHERAPY AND TARGETED THERAPY

Immunotherapy uses the immune system, the body's main defense against infection and disease, to fight cancer. Some types of immunotherapy are called *biologic therapy*. Immunotherapy can (1) boost or manipulate the immune system and create an environment that is not conducive for cancer cells to grow or (2) attack cancer cells directly. Various types of immunotherapy include cytokines, vaccines, and monoclonal antibodies (Table 15-13). Monoclonal antibodies (drugs ending in -mab) are the most successful immunotherapy. Antibodies are proteins produced by the immune system that bind to a target antigen on the cell surface. Because each antibody is specific to an antigen, that mechanism is used to develop specific drugs to treat cancer. Many of the monoclonal antibodies are targeted therapies.

Targeted therapy interferes with cancer growth by targeting specific cell receptors and pathways that are important in tumor growth.[26,27] Targeted therapies work at sites that are on the cell surface, at the intracellular level, or in the extracellular domain (Fig. 15-16 and Table 15-13). Targeted therapies are more selective for specific molecular targets than chemotherapy drugs. Thus they act on specific targets that are associated with cancer. In comparison, chemotherapy acts on all rapidly dividing normal and cancer cells. A major advantage of targeted therapy (compared with chemotherapy) is that it does less damage to normal cells.

As more oncogene targets are identified, additional agents are being developed that target specific oncogenes. Targeted therapies provide for use of personalized therapy based on the biology of an individual's tumor. Examples of some targeted therapies are discussed in the next few paragraphs.

A major class of targeted therapy is tyrosine kinase inhibitors (Table 15-13). Tyrosine kinases are enzymes responsible for the activation of many proteins by signal transduction cascades. EGFR is a transmembrane molecule that works through activation of intracellular tyrosine kinase (TK). Overexpression of EGFR is associated with unregulated cell growth and a poor prognosis. Drugs that inhibit EGFR suppress cell proliferation and promote *apoptosis* (programmed cell death).

EGFRs belong to the same receptor family as human epidermal growth factor receptor-2 (HER-2), the target for trastuzumab (Herceptin), which is a drug primarily used to treat breast cancer. HER-2 is overexpressed in certain cancers (especially breast cancers) and is associated with more aggressive disease and decreased survival. Trastuzumab is a monoclonal antibody (MoAb) that binds to HER-2 and is given IV to inhibit the growth of breast cancer cells that overexpress the HER-2 protein. Lapatinib (Tykerb) is an oral agent used for breast cancer that overexpresses HER-2.

Chronic myeloid leukemia (CML) cells make an abnormal active enzyme called BCR-ABL tyrosine kinase. Drugs (e.g., imatinib [Gleevec]) that inhibit this enzyme suppress proliferation of CML cells and promote apoptosis.

Angiogenesis inhibitors work by preventing the mechanisms and pathways necessary for vascularization of tumors. Bevacizumab (Avastin), a recombinant human MoAb, binds with vascular endothelial growth factor (VEGF), a compound that stimulates blood vessel growth. When bevacizumab binds with VEGF, it prevents VEGF from binding with its receptors on vascular endothelial cells and promoting new vessel formation. As a result, further tumor growth is inhibited.

Proteasomes are intracellular multienzyme complexes that degrade proteins. In cancer cells, proteasome inhibitors (e.g., bortezomib [Velcade]) promote accumulation of proteins that leads to cell death.

Cancer cells can become resistant to targeted therapies. This can occur because the (1) target changes through mutation and the therapy no longer interacts with it and (2) tumor finds a new growth pathway and no longer depends on the target. Because of the possibility of resistance, targeted therapies work best in combination or in combination with a chemotherapy drug.

Side Effects of Immunotherapy and Targeted Therapy

The administration of one type of immunotherapy usually induces the endogenous release of other agents. The release and action of these agents result in systemic immune and inflammatory responses. The toxicities and side effects of these agents are related to dose and schedule.

Common side effects include constitutional flu-like symptoms, including headache, fever, chills, myalgias, fatigue, malaise, weakness, photosensitivity, anorexia, and nausea. With interferon therapy, these flu-like symptoms almost invariably appear, but their severity generally decreases over time. Acetaminophen administered every 4 hours, as prescribed, often reduces the severity of the flu-like syndrome. The patient is commonly premedicated with acetaminophen in an attempt to prevent or decrease the intensity of these symptoms. In addition, large amounts of fluids help decrease the symptoms.

Tachycardia and orthostatic hypotension are also commonly reported. IL-2 and MoAbs can cause *capillary leak syndrome,* which can result in pulmonary edema. Other toxic and side effects may involve the CNS, renal and hepatic systems, and cardiovascular system. These effects are found particularly with interferons and IL-2.

A wide range of neurologic deficits has been observed with interferon and IL-2 therapy. The nature and extent of these problems are not yet completely understood. However, these problems are understandably frightening to the patient and family, who must be taught to observe for neurologic problems (e.g., confusion, memory loss, difficulty making decisions, insomnia), report their occurrence, and institute appropriate safety and support measures.

MoAbs are administered by infusion. Patients may experience infusion-related symptoms, which can include fever, chills, urticaria, mucosal congestion, nausea, diarrhea, and myalgias.

Skin rashes are common in patients receiving EGFR inhibitors and manifest generally as erythema and acneiform-like

TABLE 15-13 Drug Therapy

Immunotherapy and Targeted Therapy*

Mechanism of Action	Examples
Cytokines (see Table 13-4)	
Inhibits DNA and protein synthesis. Suppresses cell proliferation. Increases cytotoxic effects of natural killer (NK) cells	α-interferon (Intron A)
Stimulates proliferation of T and B cells Activates NK cells	interleukin-2 (aldesleukin [Proleukin])
Vaccines	
Live attenuated strain of *Mycobacterium bovis* induces immune response. Used intravesically to treat bladder cancer (see Chapter 45)	BCG vaccine
Vaccine against prostate cancer that stimulates the immune system against the cancer (see Chapter 54)	sipuleucel-T (Provenge)
Kinase Inhibitors	
EGFR Tyrosine Kinase (TK) Inhibitors	
Inhibit epidermal growth factor receptor (EGFR) TK	cetuximab (Erbitux) erlotinib (Tarceva) gefitinib (Iressa) panitumumab (Vectibix)
Inhibit EGFR-TK and binds HER-2	lapatinib (Tykerb)
BCR-ABL Tyrosine Kinase Inhibitors	
Inhibit BCR-ABL TK. Primarily used in chronic myeloid leukemia	bosutinib (Bosulif) dasatinib (Sprycel) imatinib (Gleevec) nilotinib (Tasigna)
Multi-Tyrosine Kinase Inhibitors	
Inhibit multiple TKs	axitinib (Inlyta) cabozantinib (Cometriq) pazopanib (Votrient) regorafenib (Stivarga) sorafenib (Nexavar) sunitinib (Sutent) vandetanib (Caprelsa)
Anaplastic Lymphoma Kinase (ALK) Inhibitors	
Inhibit anaplastic lymphoma kinase (ALK)	ceritinib (Zykadia) crizotinib (Xalkori)
BRAF and MEK Kinase Inhibitors	
Inhibit BRAF and MEK enzymes	dabrafenib (Tafinlar) trametinib (Mekinist) vemurafenib (Zelboraf) cobimetinib (Cotellic)
mTOR Kinase Inhibitors	
Inhibits a specific protein known as the mechanistic target of rapamycin (mTOR)	everolimus (Afinitor) temsirolimus (Torisel)
Human Epidermal Growth Factor Receptor-2 (HER-2)	
Monoclonal antibody to HER-2 that attaches to the antigen. It is taken into the cells and eventually kills them	pertuzumab (Perjeta) trastuzumab (Herceptin)
Trastuzumab connected to a chemotherapy drug called DM1	ado-trastuzumab emtansine (Kadcyla)
CD20 Monoclonal Antibodies	
Binds CD20 antigen, causing cytotoxicity and radiation injury	ibritumomab tiuxetan/yttrium-90 (Zevalin)
Binds CD20 antigen, causing cytotoxicity	ofatumumab (Arzerra) rituximab (Rituxan)
CD52 Monoclonal Antibody	
Binds CD52 antigen (found on T and B cells, monocytes, NK cells, neutrophils)	alemtuzumab (Campath)
Angiogenesis Inhibitors	
Binds vascular endothelial growth factor (VEGF), thereby inhibiting angiogenesis	bevacizumab (Avastin) pazopanib (Votrient) ramucirumab (Cyramza)
Proteasome Inhibitors	
Inhibits proteasome activity, which functions to regulate cell growth	bortezomib (Velcade) carfilzomib (Kyprolis)
Immunomodulatory Drugs (IMiDs)	
Inhibit production of TNF, IL-6, and VEGF (which leads to its antiangiogenic effects). Stimulates T and NK cells and increases γ-interferon and IL-2 production	apremilast (Otezla) lenalidomide (Revlimid) pomalidomide (Pomalyst) thalidomide (Thalomid)
Programmed Death Receptor (PD)-1 Blockers	
Blocks PD-1, a protein on T cells that normally helps keep these cells from attacking other cells. Thus boosts immune response against cancer cells	nivolumab (Opdivo) pembrolizumab (Keytruda)

BRAF, B-Raf; *HER-2*, human epidermal growth factor receptor 2; *IL*, interleukin; *TNF*, tumor necrosis factor.
*This list is not all inclusive.

rash that can cover a large part of the upper body. Angiogenesis inhibitors can cause problems of arterial thrombi, hemorrhage, hypertension, impaired wound healing, and proteinuria. Other toxicities of MoAbs include hepatotoxicity, bone marrow depression, and CNS effects.

❖ NURSING MANAGEMENT: IMMUNOTHERAPY AND TARGETED THERAPY

Some problems experienced by the patient receiving immunotherapy and targeted therapy are different from those observed with more traditional forms of cancer therapy. These effects occur more acutely and are dose limited (i.e., effects resolve when the agent is discontinued). Patients may be hesitant to inform the HCP of intolerable side effects. Some patients may be afraid to discuss side effects because they may think that the drug will be stopped. Or they decide to discontinue the drug because of side effects. Assess and evaluate the patient's side effects and tolerance. Appropriate proactive nursing care can prevent these problems because you are in a position to intervene.

Capillary leak syndrome and pulmonary edema are problems that require critical care nursing. Bone marrow depression is generally more transient and less severe than that observed with chemotherapy. Fatigue associated with immunotherapy and targeted therapy can be so severe that it constitutes a dose-limiting toxicity. As these agents are increasingly combined with chemotherapy, the spectrum of therapy-related effects expands.

Nursing interventions for flu-like syndrome include the administration of acetaminophen before treatment and every 4

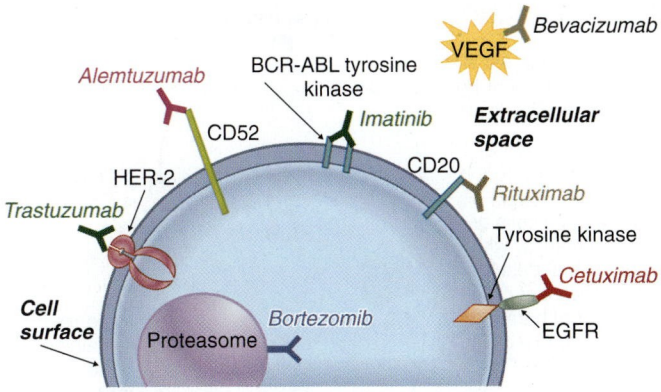

FIG. 15-16 Sites of action of targeted therapy. Examples of targeted therapy drugs that work at the specific site of action are indicated in colored, italicized font. *EGFR,* Epidermal growth factor receptor; *HER-2,* human epidermal growth factor receptor-2; *VEGF,* vascular endothelial growth factor.

hours after treatment. IV meperidine (Demerol) has been used to control the severe chills or rigors associated with some agents. Other nursing measures include monitoring vital signs and temperature, planning for periods of rest for the patient, assisting with activities of daily living (ADLs), and monitoring for adequate oral intake.

HORMONE THERAPY

Hormones are substances that are produced in endocrine glands and function as chemical messengers in the body. The hormones estrogen and progesterone can enhance the growth of some breast cancers, and androgen (testosterone) can enhance the growth of some prostrate cancers. When given as a cancer treatment, drugs (hormone therapy) can block the effects of the hormone and stop the growth of cancer cells (Table 15-14).

Corticosteroids are used in combination with many drug regimens for cancer. They are antiinflammatory agents that reduce swelling and inflammation, which may be contributing to cancer pain. They are used with other drugs, such as ondansetron and aprepitant, to control and prevent nausea and vomiting caused by chemotherapy.

In addition to drug manipulation of hormones, surgical interventions (oophorectomy, castration) can be used to remove the effects of the hormone on cancer growth.

HEMATOPOIETIC GROWTH FACTORS

Hematopoietic growth factors are used to support cancer patients through the treatment of the disease (Table 15-15). Colony-stimulating factors (CSFs) are a family of glycoproteins produced by various cells. CSFs stimulate production, maturation, regulation, and activation of cells of the hematologic system. The name of the CSF is based on the specific cell line it affects (Table 15-15).

Erythropoiesis-stimulating agents (ESAs) should be used only when treating anemia specifically caused by chemotherapy. ESA use is avoided in patients receiving chemotherapy with the intent to cure the disease. Use of these agents has raised safety concerns because they can cause potential harms (thromboembolic events, shorter survival) and increase the risk for death and for serious cardiovascular events when administered to achieve a target hemoglobin of greater than 12 g/dL. Therefore the lowest dose should be used that will gradually increase hemoglobin to the lowest level sufficient to avoid the need for blood transfusion. Monitor the hemoglobin level regularly.

TABLE 15-14 Drug Therapy

Hormone Therapy

Corticosteroids	
Disrupt the cell membrane and inhibit synthesis of protein. Decrease circulating lymphocytes, inhibit mitosis, depress immune system, increase sense of well-being.	cortisone, dexamethasone, hydrocortisone (Cortef), methylprednisolone (Medrol), prednisone
Estrogen Receptor Blockers	
Selectively attach to estrogen receptors, blocking estrogen from binding. Inhibits tumor growth.	fulvestrant (Faslodex), tamoxifen, toremifene (Fareston)
Estrogen Receptor Modulator	
Produces both estrogen-agonistic effects on bone and estrogen-antagonistic effects on breast tissue.	raloxifene (Evista)
Aromatase Inhibitors	
Inhibit aromatase, thus preventing the production of estrogen.	anastrozole (Arimidex), exemestane (Aromasin), letrozole (Femara)
Estrogens	
Interfere with effect of testosterone.	estradiol, estramustine (Emcyt), estrogen (Menest)
Androgen Receptor Blockers	
Selectively attach to androgen receptors, blocking androgen from binding, Inhibits tumor growth.	flutamide, bicalutamide (Casodex), enzalutamide (Xtandi)

HEMATOPOIETIC STEM CELL TRANSPLANTATION

Bone marrow transplantation (BMT) and **peripheral stem cell transplantation (PSCT)** are effective, lifesaving procedures for the treatment of a number of malignant and nonmalignant diseases (Table 15-16). BMT and PSCT allow for the safe use of very high doses of chemotherapy agents and/or radiation therapy in patients whose tumors have developed resistance (refractory) or failed to respond to standard doses of chemotherapy and radiation. Although these procedures are lifesaving, patients may have long-term or delayed complications that can affect their quality of life.

This therapeutic approach was typically referred to as BMT because the bone marrow was the original source of stem cells when the procedure was first developed. However, advances in harvesting and cryopreservation technologies have opened new pathways to the collection of stem cells from the peripheral blood.[28] Consequently, the terminology has changed, and the procedure is now referred to as **hematopoietic stem cell transplantation (HSCT)**. Overall cure rates are steadily increasing. Even when cure is not achieved, transplantation can result in a period of remission.

The approach in HSCT is to eradicate diseased tumor cells and/or clear the bone marrow of its components to make way for engraftment of the transplanted, healthy stem cells. This is accomplished by administering higher than usual dosages of chemotherapy with or without radiation therapy. Life-threatening consequences associated with pancytopenia and

TABLE 15-15 Drug Therapy

Hematopoietic Growth Factors Used in Cancer Treatment

Growth Factor	Drug Name	Indications	Side Effects
Granulocyte-macrophage colony-stimulating factor (GM-CSF)	sargramostim (Leukine)	Myeloid cell recovery after bone marrow transplantation	Nausea, vomiting, diarrhea, fever, chills, myalgia, headache, fatigue
Granulocyte colony-stimulating factor (G-CSF)	filgrastim (Neupogen) pegfilgrastim (Neulasta) tbo-filgrastim (Granix) filgrastim-sndz (Zarxio)	Chemotherapy-induced neutropenia	Bone pain, nausea, vomiting
Erythropoietin	epoetin α (Epogen, Procrit)	Anemia of chronic cancer	Hypertension, thrombosis, headache
	darbepoetin α (Aranesp)	Anemia related to chemotherapy	Hypertension, thrombosis, headache
Interleukin-11 (platelet growth factor)	oprelvekin (Neumega)	Thrombocytopenia related to chemotherapy	Fluid retention, peripheral edema, dyspnea, tachycardia, nausea, mouth sores

TABLE 15-16 Indications for Hematopoietic Stem Cell Transplantation

Malignant Diseases	Nonmalignant Diseases
• Acute and chronic myelogenous leukemia	• Aplastic anemia
• Acute and chronic lymphocytic leukemia	• Chronic granulomatous disease
• Hodgkin's lymphoma	• Fanconi's anemia
• Multiple myeloma	• Hematologic diseases
• Myelodysplastic syndrome	• Immunodeficiency diseases
• Non-Hodgkin's lymphoma	• Severe combined immunodeficiency disease (SCID)
	• Sickle cell disease (severe)
	• Thalassemia
	• Wiskott-Aldrich syndrome

other adverse effects can result from this procedure. After chemotherapy and radiation therapy are completed, healthy stem cells are infused. These healthy stem cells "rescue" the damaged bone marrow through subsequent proliferation and differentiation of the donated stem cells in the recipient.

HSCT is an intensive procedure with many risks. Some patients die from treatment-related complications or from recurrence of the original disease. Because it is a highly toxic therapy, the patient must weigh the significant risks of treatment-related death or treatment failure (relapse) against the hope of cure.

Types of Hematopoietic Stem Cell Transplants

HSCTs are categorized as allogeneic, syngeneic, or autologous. The sources of stem cells include the bone marrow, peripheral

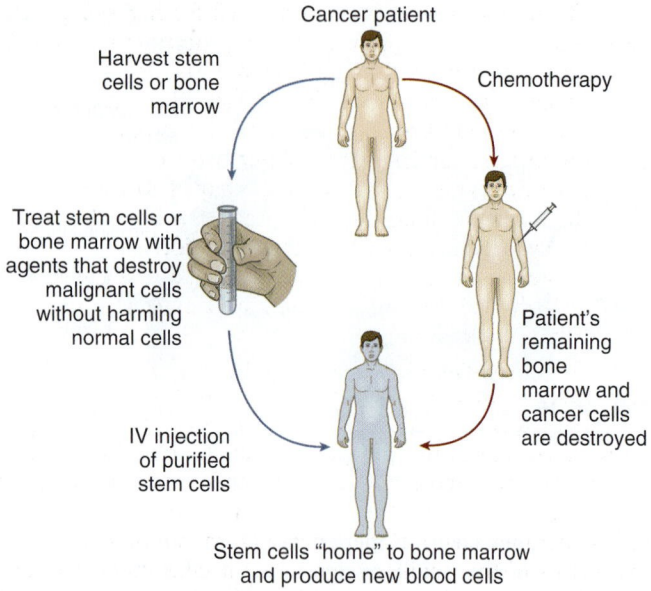

FIG. 15-17 Autologous stem cell transplant.

circulating blood, and umbilical cord blood. In *allogeneic transplantation,* stem cells are acquired from a donor (graft) who, through human leukocyte antigen (HLA) tissue typing, has been determined to be HLA matched to the recipient (host). HLA typing involves testing WBCs to identify genetically inherited antigens common to both donor and recipient that are important in compatibility of transplanted tissue. (HLA tissue typing is discussed in Chapter 13.) The donor is often a family member but may be an unrelated donor found through a national or international bone marrow registry (e.g., National Marrow Donor Program). These are known as MUD (matched unrelated donor) transplants. Increased risks and toxicities may be associated with an unrelated allogeneic transplant. Common indications for allogeneic transplant are certain leukemias, multiple myeloma, and lymphoma.

Syngeneic transplantation is a type of allogeneic transplant that involves obtaining stem cells from one identical twin and infusing them into the other. Identical twins have identical HLA types and are a perfect match

In *autologous transplantation,* patients receive their own stem cells back after *myeloablative* (destroying bone marrow) chemotherapy (Fig. 15-17). The aim of this approach is purely "rescue." It enables patients to receive intensive chemotherapy and/or radiation by supporting them with their previously harvested stem cells until their marrow generates blood cells again on its own. Restoration usually takes about 4 to 6 weeks. Autologous transplants are typically used to treat hematologic malignancies if there is no suitable donor or the patient cannot undergo allogeneic transplantation.

The newer, nonmyeloablative or reduced intensity transplant uses lower doses of radiation or chemotherapy that result in less toxicity and myelosuppression. HSCT continues to be investigated in the management of some solid tumors refractory to treatment.

Procedures

Harvest Procedures. Hematopoietic stem cells are *harvested* from a donor (for allogeneic transplantation) or from the recipient (for autologous transplantation) via two different methods. In one type of procedure, used for harvesting stem cells residing in bone marrow (as the process was originally developed), the procedure is performed in the operating room using general or spinal anesthesia. Multiple bone marrow aspirations (usually from the iliac crest, but sometimes from the sternum) are carried out to obtain stem cells. The entire bone marrow harvest procedure takes about 1 to 2 hours, and the patient can be discharged after recovery. Postharvest, the donor may experience pain at the collection site that lasts up to 7 days and can be treated with mild analgesics. The donor's body will replenish the removed bone marrow in a few weeks.

In the other type of procedure, peripheral stem cell transplants are obtained from the peripheral blood in an outpatient procedure. It is done using cell separator equipment that automatically separates the stem cells from the blood circulating through the machine and returns the remaining blood components to the donor. The process averages about 2 to 4 hours but can sometimes take longer depending on donor factors and the quality of the venous access. Often it takes more than one procedure to obtain enough stem cells. Because the blood has fewer stem cells than the bone marrow, "mobilization" of stem cells from the bone marrow into the peripheral blood can be accomplished using chemotherapy and/or hematopoietic growth factors.

To increase stem cell production for collection, common growth factors that are used are granulocyte-macrophage colony-stimulating factor (GM-CSF) and granulocyte colony-stimulating factor (G-CSF) (Table 15-15). When patients are given growth factors for mobilization, stem cells are harvested after 4 or 5 days of growth factor injections.

Harvested marrow is processed to strain out bone fragments (this is not necessary with peripheral collections). The marrow or peripherally collected stem cells are then bagged with preservative for cryopreservation and storage until they are needed, or they are used immediately. Since it is coming from the patient, autologous stem cells are sometimes treated (purged) to remove undetected cancer cells. Many different pharmacologic, immunologic, physical, and chemical agents have been used for this purpose.

Umbilical cord blood is also rich in hematopoietic stem cells, and successful allogeneic transplants have been performed using this source. Cord blood can be HLA-typed and cryopreserved. A disadvantage of cord blood is the possibility of insufficient numbers of stem cells to permit transplant to adults. Considerable research is currently ongoing to define the optimal application of this technology.

Preparative Regimens and Stem Cell Infusions. Patients receive myeloablative dosages of chemotherapy with or without adjunctive radiation to treat the underlying disease. Total-body irradiation (TBI) can be used for immunosuppression or to treat the disease. These preparative therapies are known as the *conditioning regimen.*

Stem cell infusions are administered IV, and can be injected via the slow bolus method or infused much like a blood transfusion (using tubing without a filter). The infused stem cells reconstitute the bone marrow elements, "rescuing" the recipient's hematopoietic system. Usually 2 to 4 weeks are required for the transplanted marrow to start producing hematopoietic blood cells. During this period, when the patient has pancytopenia, the patient must be protected from exposure to infectious agents and supported with electrolyte supplements, nutrition, and blood component transfusions (as needed) to maintain adequate levels of circulating RBCs and platelets.

Complications. Bacterial, viral, and fungal infections are common after HSCT, so prophylactic therapies are used to reduce their incidence. A potentially serious complication of allogeneic transplant is graft-versus-host disease. This occurs when the T cells from the donated marrow (graft) recognize the recipient (host) as foreign and begin to attack certain organs such as the skin, liver, and GI tract. (Graft-versus-host disease is discussed in Chapter 13.)

The occurrence and severity of posttransplant complications also depend on the drugs used (some are more toxic than others) and the stem cell source. Because stem cells in the peripheral blood are more mature than those harvested from the marrow, the hematologic recovery period in PSCT is shorter, and fewer, less severe complications are seen.

GENE THERAPY

Gene therapy is an experimental therapy that involves introducing genetic material into a person's cells to fight disease. At this time, the use of gene therapy is investigational. (Gene therapy is discussed in Chapter 12.)

COMPLICATIONS OF CANCER

The patient may develop complications related to the continual growth of the cancer into normal tissue or to the side effects of treatment.

NUTRITIONAL PROBLEMS

Malnutrition

The patient with cancer may experience protein and calorie malnutrition characterized by fat and muscle depletion. (Assessment of malnutrition is discussed in Chapter 39.)

Soft, nonirritating high-protein and high-calorie foods should be eaten throughout the day. Foods suggested for increasing the protein intake are presented in Table 15-17. High-calorie foods that provide energy and minimize weight loss are presented in Table 15-18. (A sample high-calorie, high-protein diet is presented in Table 39-10.)

Teach the patient to avoid extremes of temperature, tobacco, alcohol, spicy or rough foods, and other irritants. Encourage nutritional supplements (e.g., Ensure) as an adjunct to meals and fluid intake. Weigh the patient at least twice each week to monitor for weight loss.

Suggest a referral for individualized nutritional counseling to the patient or HCP as soon as a 5% weight loss is noted or if the patient has the potential for protein and calorie malnutrition. Monitor albumin and prealbumin levels. Once a 10-lb (4.5-kg) weight loss occurs, it may be difficult to maintain the patient's nutritional status.

Teach the patient to use nutritional supplements in place of milk when cooking or baking. Foods to which nutritional supplements can be easily added include scrambled eggs, pudding, custard, mashed potatoes, cereal, and cream sauces. Packages of instant breakfast can be used as indicated or sprinkled on cereals, desserts, and casseroles.

Families are an integral part of the health care team. As symptom severity increases, the family's role in helping the patient eat becomes increasingly critical.

TABLE 15-17 Nutritional Therapy

Protein Foods With High Biologic Value

Milk

- Whole milk: 1 cup = 9 g protein.
- Double-strength milk (1 quart of whole milk plus 1 cup of dried skim milk blended and chilled): 1 cup = 14 g protein.
- Milk shake (1 cup of ice cream plus 1 cup of milk): 15 g protein, 415 cal.
- Use evaporated milk, double-strength milk, or half-and-half to make casseroles, hot cereals, sauces, gravies, puddings, milk shakes, and soups.
- Yogurt (regular and frozen): check labels and purchase brand with highest protein content: 1 cup = 10 g protein

Eggs

- Egg: 6 g protein.
- Eggnog: 1 cup = 15.5 g protein.
- Add eggs to salads, casseroles, and sauces. Deviled eggs are especially well tolerated.
- Desserts that contain eggs include angel food cake, sponge cake, custard, and cheesecake.

Cheese

- Cottage: ½ cup = 15 g protein.
- American: 1 slice = 3 g protein.
- Cheddar: 1 slice = 6 g protein.
- Cream: 1 Tbsp = 1 g protein.
- Use cheese in a sandwich or as a snack.
- Add cheese to salads, casseroles, sauces, and baked potatoes.
- Cheese spread with crackers is a wholesome snack that can be made and stored in the refrigerator for easy accessibility.
- Advise patient that cheese can be constipating.

Meat, Poultry, Fish

- Pork: 3 oz = approx. 19 g protein.
- Chicken: ½ breast = approx. 26 g protein.
- Fish: 3 oz = approx. 30 g protein.
- Tuna fish: 6½ oz = approx. 44.5 g protein.
- Add meat, poultry, and fish to salads, casseroles, and sandwiches.
- Add strained and junior baby meats to soups and casseroles.
- Cocktail wieners and deviled ham on crackers are wholesome snacks. These snacks can be made and stored in the refrigerator for easy accessibility.

If the malnutrition cannot be treated with dietary intake, it may be necessary to use enteral or parenteral nutrition. (Enteral and parenteral nutrition are discussed in Chapter 39.)

Altered Taste Sensation (Dysgeusia)

Cancer cells may release substances that stimulate the bitter taste buds. The patient may also experience an alteration in the sweet, sour, and salty taste sensations. Meat may taste bitter or bland. The physiologic basis of these varied taste alterations is unknown.

Teach patients with altered taste problems to avoid foods that they dislike. Frequently the patient may feel compelled to eat certain foods that are believed to be beneficial. Tell the patient to experiment with spices and other seasoning agents in an attempt to mask the taste alterations. Lemon juice, onion, mint, basil, and fruit juice marinades may improve the taste of certain meats and fish. Ham may enhance the taste of vegetables. Increasing the amount of spice or seasoning agent is usually not an effective way to enhance the taste.

TABLE 15-18 Nutritional Therapy

High-Calorie Foods

Mayonnaise	1 Tbsp	=	101 cal
Butter or margarine	1 tsp	=	35 cal
Sour cream	1 Tbsp	=	72 cal
Peanut butter	1 Tbsp	=	94 cal
Whipped cream	1 Tbsp	=	53 cal
Corn oil	1 Tbsp	=	119 cal
Jelly	1 Tbsp	=	49 cal
Ice cream	1 cup	=	256 cal
Honey	1 Tbsp	=	64 cal

Cancer Cachexia

Cancer cachexia (wasting syndrome) is a complex, multifactorial syndrome characterized by anorexia and/or unintended loss of weight and appetite. It is accompanied by generalized tissue wasting, skeletal muscle atrophy, immune dysfunction, and metabolic abnormalities. The weight loss cannot be reversed nutritionally.

Cancer patients can suffer from cachexia, especially those with upper gastrointestinal and pancreatic cancers. As cancer progresses, cachexia can affect many cancer patients, and is associated with increased morbidity.[29]

The best management of cancer cachexia is to effectively treat the cancer. Unfortunately, this is not a realistic goal for patients with advanced cancer. A second option is to increase nutritional intake, but this does not completely reverse the wasting associated with cachexia. A third option is to use megestrol acetate (Megace), a synthetic form of the hormone progesterone, which stimulates appetite in patients with cachexia.

INFECTION

Infection is a primary cause of death in the patient with cancer. The usual sites of infection include the lungs, GU system, mouth, rectum, peritoneal cavity, and blood (septicemia). Infection occurs as a result of the ulceration and necrosis caused by the tumor, compression of vital organs by the tumor, and neutropenia caused by the disease process or the cancer treatment.

Instruct patients at risk for neutropenia to call their HCP if they have a temperature of 100.4° F (38° C) or greater. Assessment most often includes signs and symptoms of fever, determination of possible etiology (e.g., sinuses, mucous membranes, respiratory, GI, urinary, sites of any tubes or lines), and complete blood count.

Many patients are neutropenic when an infection develops. In these individuals, infection may cause significant morbidity and may be rapidly fatal if not treated promptly. The classic manifestations of infection are often subtle or absent in a patient with neutropenia and a depressed immune system. (Neutropenia was discussed earlier in this chapter on p. 253 and is also discussed in Chapter 30.)

ONCOLOGIC EMERGENCIES

Oncologic emergencies are life-threatening emergencies that can occur as a result of cancer or cancer treatment. These emergencies can be obstructive, metabolic, or infiltrative (Table 15-19).

TABLE 15-19 Oncologic Emergencies

Description	Manifestations	Management
Obstructive Emergencies		
Superior Vena Cava Syndrome (SVCS)		
• Results from obstruction of superior vena cava by tumor or thrombosis. • Common causes are lung cancer, non-Hodgkin's lymphoma, and metastatic breast cancer. • Presence of central venous catheter and previous mediastinal radiation increase risk of development.	• Facial edema, periorbital edema. • Distention of veins of head, neck, and chest (Fig. 15-18). • Headache, seizures. • Mediastinal mass on chest x-ray.	• Considered a serious medical problem. • Radiation therapy to site of obstruction. • Chemotherapy for tumors more sensitive to this therapy.
Spinal Cord Compression		
• Neurologic emergency caused by cancer in epidural space of spinal cord. • Common causes are breast, lung, prostate, GI, and renal cancers and melanomas. • Lymphomas can also invade epidural space.	• Intense, localized, and persistent back pain accompanied by vertebral tenderness. • Motor weakness, sensory paresthesia and loss. • Autonomic dysfunction (e.g., change in bowel or bladder function).	• Radiation therapy and corticosteroids. • Surgical decompressive laminectomy. • Activity limitations and pain management.
Third Space Syndrome		
• Shifting of fluid from vascular space to interstitial space. • Occurs secondary to extensive surgical procedures, immunotherapy, or septic shock.	• Signs of hypovolemia: hypotension, tachycardia, low central venous pressure, decreased urine output.	• Fluid, electrolyte, and plasma protein replacement. • During recovery hypervolemia can occur, resulting in hypertension, elevated central venous pressure, weight gain, and shortness of breath.
Metabolic Emergencies		
Syndrome of Inappropriate Antidiuretic Hormone (SIADH)		
• Tumor cells can produce abnormal or sustained production of antidiuretic hormone (ADH). • Many chemotherapy agents may also contribute to ectopic ADH production or potentiate ADH effects.	• Water retention and hyponatremia (hypotonic hyponatremia) (see Chapter 49). • Weight gain without edema, weakness, anorexia, nausea, vomiting, personality changes, seizures, oliguria, decrease in reflexes, and coma.	• Treat underlying malignancy. • Take measures to correct sodium-water imbalance, including fluid restriction, oral salt tablets or isotonic (0.9%) saline administration, and IV 3% sodium chloride solution (severe cases). • Furosemide (Lasix) used in initial phases. • Monitor sodium level because correcting SIADH rapidly may result in seizures or death.
Hypercalcemia		
• Occurs in metastatic disease of bone or multiple myeloma, or when a parathyroid hormone–like substance is secreted by cancer cells. • Immobility and dehydration can contribute to or exacerbate hypercalcemia.	• Serum calcium in excess of 12 mg/dL (3 mmol/L) often produces symptoms. • Apathy, depression, fatigue, muscle weakness, ECG changes, polyuria and nocturia, anorexia, nausea, and vomiting. • High calcium elevations can be life threatening. • Chronic hypercalcemia can result in nephrocalcinosis and irreversible renal failure.	• Treat primary disease. • Hydration (3 L/day) and bisphosphonate therapy. • Diuretics (particularly loop diuretics) used to prevent heart failure or edema. • Infusion of bisphosphonate zoledronate (Zometa) or pamidronate (Aredia).
Tumor Lysis Syndrome (TLS)		
• Metabolic complication characterized by rapid release of intracellular components in response to chemotherapy and radiation therapy (less commonly). • Massive cell destruction releases intracellular components (potassium, phosphate, DNA, RNA) that are metabolized to uric acid by liver.	• *Hallmark signs*: hyperuricemia, hyperphosphatemia, hyperkalemia, hypocalcemia. • Weakness, muscle cramps, diarrhea, nausea, and vomiting. • Occurs within first 24 to 48 hr after initiation of chemotherapy. • May persist for about 5 to 7 days. • Metabolic abnormalities and concentrated uric acid (which crystallizes in distal tubules of kidneys) can lead to acute kidney injury.	• Identify patients at risk. • Increase urine production using hydration therapy. • Decrease uric acid concentrations using allopurinol. • Use IV sodium bicarbonate to counter effects of acidic properties that are released.
Infiltrative Emergencies		
Cardiac Tamponade		
• Fluid accumulation in pericardium. • Caused by constriction of pericardium by tumor or pericarditis secondary to radiation therapy to the chest.	• Heavy feeling over chest, shortness of breath, tachycardia, cough, dysphagia, hiccups, hoarseness. • Nausea, vomiting, excessive perspiration. • Decreased level of consciousness, distant or muted heart sounds. • Extreme anxiety.	• Decrease fluid around heart using (1) surgery to create a pericardial window or an (2) indwelling pericardial catheter. • Administer O_2 therapy, IV hydration, and vasopressor therapy.
Carotid Artery Rupture		
• Invasion of arterial wall by tumor or erosion following surgery or radiation therapy. • Occurs most frequently in patients with head and neck cancer.	• Bleeding: ranges from minor oozing to spurting of blood in the case of a "blowout" of artery.	• Administer IV fluids and blood products. • Surgery: ligation of carotid artery above and below rupture site and reduction of local tumor.

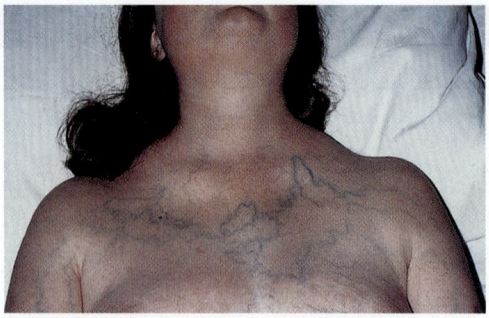

FIG. 15-18 Superior vena caval obstruction in bronchial carcinoma. Note the swelling of the face and neck and the development of collateral circulation in the veins. (From Forbes CD, Jackson WF: *Colour atlas and text of clinical medicine,* ed 3, London, 2003, Mosby.)

Obstructive Emergencies

Obstructive emergencies are primarily caused by tumor obstruction of an organ or blood vessel. Obstructive emergencies include superior vena cava syndrome (Fig. 15-18), spinal cord compression syndrome, third space syndrome, and intestinal obstruction.

Metabolic Emergencies

Metabolic emergencies are caused by the production of ectopic hormones directly from the tumor or are secondary to metabolic alterations caused by the tumor or by cancer treatment. Ectopic hormones arise from tissues that do not normally produce these hormones. Cancer cells return to a more embryonic form, thus allowing the cells' stored potential to become evident.

Metabolic emergencies include syndrome of inappropriate antidiuretic hormone secretion, hypercalcemia, tumor lysis syndrome, septic shock (discussed in Chapter 66), and disseminated intravascular coagulation (discussed in Chapter 30).

Infiltrative Emergencies

Infiltrative emergencies occur when malignant tumors infiltrate major organs or secondary to cancer therapy. The most common infiltrative emergencies are cardiac tamponade and carotid artery rupture.

CANCER PAIN

Moderate to severe pain occurs in approximately 50% of patients who are receiving active treatment for their cancer and in 80% to 90% of patients with advanced cancer.[30] What is concerning is that these statistics have not changed in the past 30 years. Undertreatment of cancer pain is common and causes needless suffering, decreases quality of life, and increases the burden on family caregivers.

Pain Assessment

Inadequate pain assessment is the single greatest barrier to effective pain management. Data such as vital signs and patient behaviors are not reliable indicators of pain, especially long-standing, chronic pain. It is important to distinguish between persistent and episodic, positional, or breakthrough pain. Therefore it is essential that a comprehensive pain assessment include a detailed history to elicit the following characteristics of pain: quality, location, intensity, duration, and precipitating and alleviating factors. Differentiating between types of pain (e.g., visceral, bone, neuropathic) is important in developing an effective pain management plan.

TABLE 15-20 Pain Assessment in Cancer Patients

Characteristic	Questions to Ask
Location	• Where is the pain? • Is the pain in more than one place? Is the pain in a new location? • Does location of pain correlate with known diagnosis?
Intensity	• How bad is the pain? • Rate the pain on a scale of 0 to 10. (See Chapter 8 for rating scales.)
Quality	• What does the pain feel like—sharp, dull, burning, shooting, aching, or other? (See Chapter 8 for descriptors.)
Pattern	• Has the pain changed? • Is the pain getting better, worse, or unchanged? • What makes the pain better or worse?
Relief measures	• What do you do to control your pain? • Do you use medications? • Do the relief measures help much? How much?

Assess pain on an ongoing basis to determine the effectiveness of the treatment plan. Obtain data and document at regular intervals the location and intensity of the pain, what it feels like, and how it is relieved. Assess change in pain (e.g., a significant change in the intensity, character, worsening, or location of pain) to determine the cause (e.g., progression of disease).

Always believe the patient report and accept it as the primary source of assessment data. Table 15-20 presents assessment questions that may facilitate data collection.

Pain Management

Pain management for the cancer patient must address both persistent and breakthrough components of pain if they are present. Adjuvant therapies need to be developed specific to the type or nature of the pain. In addition, teach patients how to keep a pain management diary.[30]

Drug therapy, including nonsteroidal antiinflammatory drugs, opioids, and adjuvant pain medications, should be used and selected based on the character and/or cause of the pain. Opioids normally are prescribed for the treatment of moderate to severe cancer pain. Analgesic medications (e.g., morphine, fentanyl) should be given on a regular schedule (around the clock) with additional doses available as needed for breakthrough pain. In general, oral administration of the medication is preferred, but other routes (e.g., transdermal, transmucosal) are also available.

It is critical for you to pay attention to common side effects of pain medications (e.g., constipation) to ensure the patient's well-being and adherence with the pain management program. Nonsteroidal antiinflammatories (e.g., ibuprofen) often serve as helpful adjuncts to opioid therapy, particularly for bone pain. Other adjuvant therapies, such as antidepressant and antiseizure drugs, may be beneficial in neuropathic pain, which is often resistant to opioids.

Radiopharmaceuticals (e.g., samarium-153) may benefit patients with diffuse bone pain (particularly if no further chemotherapy is planned). Patients may experience an initial pain *flare* after administration. Nerve blocks or epidural or intrathecal analgesia may also be used to treat patients with unrelieved pain or to minimize the requirements for opioids.

Remember that with opioid drugs (e.g., morphine) the appropriate dosage is whatever is necessary to control the pain with the fewest side effects. Fear of addiction is not warranted. However, it must be addressed as part of patient teaching, since it is a significant barrier for patients and nurses in appropriate pain management. In addition, you need to assess the patient for possible risk factors for opioid misuse/abuse.

Discuss the goals of analgesic therapy with patients, especially those requiring large or chronic doses of opioids. Treatment plans should be developed that balance analgesia and side effects to maintain optimal functional status.

Patient teaching should clarify myths and misconceptions and reassure patients and family caregivers that cancer pain can be effectively relieved. Furthermore, addiction and tolerance are not problems associated with effective cancer pain management. Nondrug interventions, including relaxation therapy and imagery, can be effectively used to manage pain (see Chapter 6). Additional strategies to relieve pain are discussed in Chapter 8.

COPING WITH CANCER AND TREATMENT

You have a key role in assisting patients in coping with the psychosocial issues associated with cancer and cancer treatment. The patient may experience a variety of concerns, including fears of dependency, loss of control, family and relationship stress, financial burden, and fear of death. Anxiety and fear may be experienced throughout the cancer continuum, including at diagnosis, during or after treatment, and in association with long-term follow-up.

Repetitive office visits or hospitalizations, continuing medications, and frequent laboratory testing force the individual to confront the cancer on a daily basis. Treatment-related uncertainties and fears are often most evident at the beginning of therapy. However, anxiety and fear may be present throughout treatment, and when therapy is completed (e.g., fear of recurrence, less available support).

Adaptation and coping with a cancer diagnosis may be influenced by a variety of patient factors, including demographics, prior coping skills and strategies, social support, and religious and spiritual beliefs (Table 15-21). You are in a key position to assess the patient's and family's responses and support positive coping strategies. To facilitate the development of effective coping and to support the patient and family during the various stages of cancer, you should do the following:

- Be available and continue to be available, especially during difficult times.
- Exhibit a caring attitude.
- Listen actively to fears and concerns.
- Help provide relief from distressing symptoms.
- Provide essential information regarding cancer and cancer care that is accurate and establishes realistic expectations about what the patient will experience.
- Maintain a relationship based on trust and confidence. Be open, honest, and caring in the approach.
- Use touch to exhibit caring. A squeeze of the hand or a hug may at times be more effective than words.
- Assist the patient in setting realistic, reachable short-term and long-term goals.
- Assist the patient in maintaining usual lifestyle patterns.

TABLE 15-21 Factors Affecting How Patients Cope With Cancer

Factor	Description
Ability to cope with stressful events in the past	How patients coped with previous stressful events (e.g., loss of job, major disappointment, significant traumatic event) affects how they cope with diagnosis of cancer.
Availability of significant others	Patients who have effective support systems cope more effectively than those who do not.
Ability to express feelings and concerns	Patients who express feelings and needs and ask for help cope more effectively than those who internalize feelings and needs.
Age at the time of diagnosis	Age determines coping strategies to a great degree. For example, a young mother with cancer may have concerns that differ from those of a 70-yr-old woman with cancer.
Extent of disease	Cure or control of the disease process is usually easier to cope with than the reality of terminal illness.
Disruption of body image	Disruption of the body image (e.g., radical neck dissection, alopecia, mastectomy) may intensify the psychologic impact of cancer.
Presence of symptoms	Symptoms such as fatigue, nausea, diarrhea, and pain may intensify the psychologic impact of cancer.
Past experience with cancer	Negative experiences with cancer (personal or in others) influence perceptions about the current situation.
Attitude associated with the cancer	Patients who feel in control and have a positive attitude about cancer and cancer treatment cope better with the diagnosis and treatment of cancer than those who feel hopeless, helpless, and out of control.

- Maintain hope, which is the key to effective cancer care. Hope varies, depending on the patient's status—hope that the symptoms are not serious, hope that the treatment is curative, hope for independence, hope for relief of pain, hope for a longer life, hope to achieve meaningful goals, or hope for a peaceful death. Hope provides control over what is occurring and is the basis of a positive attitude toward cancer and cancer care.

Tell patients that they will be followed and reassure them that support is ongoing. Provide information and support to help minimize the negative impact of cancer therapy on a person's quality of life. Patient teaching and symptom management help patients to self-manage their illness (e.g., adjusting treatment schedules to permit patients to work when possible, making referrals to support groups). Collaborate with the oncology nurse navigators who serve as the liaison between the patient and members of the interprofessional care team.

Arrange for patients to meet with individuals who have successfully completed therapy as this can increase their hopefulness and confidence. In addition, make regular supportive telephone contacts between office visits and assist with planning for transportation, nutrition, and emotional support.

Do not forget the caregiver and other family members. They need education and support throughout the trajectory of diagnosis, treatment, and follow-up.[31] Patients and caregivers may benefit from a variety of psychosocial interventions, such as supportive listening, stress management techniques, individual or group counseling, and cognitive-behavioral therapy. Assess

ETHICAL/LEGAL DILEMMAS

Medical Futility

Situation

D.M., a 65-year-old Asian woman, has breast cancer with metastasis to the liver and bone. The family asks you why their mother is not receiving chemotherapy. In addition, they want to make sure that she will be resuscitated should her heart stop. They are aware of her diagnosis and that she may have only a few months to live. In morning rounds you were told that D.M. does not want any treatment that would prolong her life.

Ethical/Legal Points for Consideration

- Although court decisions have varied, legally there is substantial consensus concerning the right to privacy (a constitutional right), right to informed consent and refusal of treatment, and rights pertaining to end-of-life decision making. The *Code of Ethics for Nurses* addresses the key components in the informed consent process that nurses must address.[1]
- A patient who is an adult and is competent (defined as capable of understanding and interpreting information, making choices, and communicating those choices) solely retains the right to make personal health care decisions.
- The Patient Self-Determination Act requires that the patient be asked on admission whether he or she has an advance directive. If available, it is placed in the medical record. If the patient does not have an advance directive, it must be documented.
- The National POLST Paradigm is an approach to end-of-life planning that emphasizes patients' wishes about the care they receive. The POLST Paradigm is an approach to end-of-life planning emphasizing the medical orders and includes coverage regardless of location (e.g., hospital, home, assisted living).[2]
- Often families have difficulty accepting the finality of a terminal diagnosis.
- Sometimes family members have conflicting interests (e.g., finances, property, inheritance rights) that influence their decision-making abilities.

Discussion Questions

1. How can you help D.M. communicate her wishes to her family?
2. How can you and the interprofessional care team assist the family in planning end-of-life care that incorporates the wishes of their mother?
3. What are the cultural issues in D.M.'s case?

References

1. Code of Ethics for Nurses. *www.nursingworld.org/MainMenu Categories/EthicsStandards/Ethics-Position-Statements.*
2. Physician Orders for Life Sustaining Treatment (POLST) Paradigm: *www.polst.org.*

the psychosocial concerns and emotional responses of patients, caregivers, and families so you can connect patients with appropriate supportive care resources. Use the available resources in the community such as the American Cancer Society, Cancer Lifeline, churches, and other community resources.

Gerontologic Considerations: Cancer

Cancer is usually a disease of aging with 78% of cancers occurring in people 55 years or older.[1] The cancer mortality rate is exceedingly high in older adults, with 70% of all deaths due to cancer occurring in those over age 65. This is especially important since the normal life span is increasing and the proportion of the population who are older than 65 years is increasing.

Clinical manifestations of cancer in older adults may be mistakenly attributed to age-related changes and ignored by the person.[32] Older adults are particularly vulnerable to the complications of both cancer and cancer therapy. This is due to their decline in physiologic functioning, social and emotional resources, and cognitive function.

The older adult's functional status should be taken into consideration when developing a treatment plan. Age alone is not a good predictor of tolerance or response to treatment. Advances in the treatment of cancer are making cancer therapies beneficial to an increasing number of older adults, including patients with suboptimal health.

Assess the patient at the time of diagnosis to identify important issues that may affect decisions about treatment options. Issues to assess include projected life expectancy, estimate of morbidity from cancer, co-morbidities that would affect treatment, and patient decision-making capacity and wishes.

Some important questions to consider when an older person is diagnosed with cancer include the following: Will the treatment provide more benefits than harm? Will he or she be able to tolerate the treatment safely? Is there need to optimize other co-morbidities or nutritional or functional status before starting treatment? What are the patient's preferences and wishes?

CANCER SURVIVORSHIP

Although the overall incidence and death rate from cancer has decreased, the number of cancer survivors continues to increase. It is estimated that there are currently more than 14.5 million cancer survivors in the United States. Some of these individuals are cancer free, whereas others still have evidence of cancer and may be undergoing treatment. The increase in survivorship is attributed to the aging and growth of the population as well as improvements in early detection and treatment. Survival statistics vary greatly by the type and stage of cancer.[1,33]

The rapid increase in cancer survivors has been accompanied by a greater awareness of the long-term health and quality-of-life issues that a cancer diagnosis imposes. Cancer survivors experience a variety of long-term and late sequelae following treatment (discussed earlier in this chapter on pp. 256-257). You need to be aware of the long-term late effects of the various treatments so that you can teach patients and their caregivers.

The impact of cancer and its treatment confers greater risk of non–cancer-related death and co-morbidities (e.g., heart disease, diabetes, metabolic syndrome, endocrine dysfunction, osteoporosis) among cancer survivors. Furthermore, cancer survivors may continue to experience symptoms or functional impairment related to treatment for years after treatment.

The impact of a cancer diagnosis can affect many aspects of a patient's life, with cancer survivors commonly reporting financial, vocational, marital, and spiritual concerns long after treatment is over. Psychosocial/emotional issues can play a profound role in a patient's life after cancer, with issues related to living in uncertainty being frequently encountered.

Some patients may wish to return to their normal lives as soon as possible, and they may fail to attend scheduled follow-up appointments. Other survivors may become cancer advocates or active members of a cancer support group. Still others may allow their lives to revolve around the cancer and may even resist giving up the illness role.

Tips to help cancer survivors are presented in Table 15-22. Connecting cancer survivors to online support and resources is a strategy to enhance positive health outcomes[34,35] (Table 15-23).

TABLE 15-22 Patient Teaching

Cancer Survivors

You can help cancer survivors by doing the following:

1. Provide all cancer patients with a treatment summary and care plan outlining treatment exposures, risk of late effects, preventive care recommendations, and follow-up surveillance plan after completion of treatment.
   - Care plans should clearly identify all members of the interprofessional team and their responsibilities for follow-up care.
   - Include referrals to appropriate supportive care and community resources that would benefit the patient in recovery or ongoing care.
2. Coordinate care among the oncology team, primary HCP, and other specialists.
3. Teach HCPs about the needs of cancer survivors, including long-term effects of cancer and cancer treatments.
4. Teach cancer survivors to look for and report any ongoing symptoms resulting from treatment, including late effects of radiation therapy and chemotherapy.
5. Promote healthy behaviors:
   - *Prevention:* good nutrition, exercise, smoking avoidance, maintenance of proper weight, cardiac risk reduction, bone health.
   - *Early detection:* routine health screenings (e.g., breast, colon), cholesterol, diabetes, osteoporosis screening as recommended.
6. Encourage cancer survivors to have regular follow-up examinations with their HCP.
7. Assess for psychoemotional, financial, health insurance, or vocational problems related to cancer. Assist patients in getting appropriate help if necessary.

TABLE 15-23 Resources for Cancer Survivors

Organization	Purpose
ACS Cancer Survivors Network	Provides survivorship information and resources and online forum for connecting with others affected by cancer. *(www.cancer.org/cancersurvivorsnetwork)*
CancerCare	Provides a variety of free support services delivered by professional oncology social workers for patients and anyone else affected by cancer. *(www.cancercare.org)*
Cancer.Net	American Society of Clinical Oncology (ASCO) patient support site that includes extensive information and resources for cancer survivors. *(www.cancer.net)*
National Cancer Institute Office of Cancer Survivorship	Supports research into the short- and long-term physical, social, emotional, and economic effects of cancer survivorship. Offers educational and support resources for cancer survivors, caregivers, and advocates. *(www.cancercontrol.cancer.gov/ocs/)*
National Coalition for Cancer Survivorship	Advocates for quality cancer care. Seeks to empower and educate patients and advocates on issues that affect the quality of life of cancer survivors. *(www.canceradvocacy.org)*

Culturally Competent Care: Cancer

Cancer incidence and death rates are disproportionately higher in African Americans than in whites and other minority groups (see Cultural & Ethnic Health Disparities box). Although overall racial disparities in cancer death rates have been declining, death rates continue to be higher among African Americans than whites. In addition, African Americans are more likely to have later stage disease at the time of diagnosis than whites.[1]

Differences in survival rates from cancer are attributed primarily to a combination of factors, including poverty, difficult access to and poorer quality of health care, more co-morbid conditions, and differences in tumor biology. Disparities in cancer care exist throughout the continuum from cancer prevention and screening to end-of-life care and survivorship. The disparity in prevention and screening results in cancer being in advanced stages at the time of diagnosis.[1,2]

CULTURAL & ETHNIC HEALTH DISPARITIES

Cancer

- Cancer incidence and death rates for men are highest among African Americans, followed by whites, Hispanics, and Asians/Pacific Islanders.
- Cancer incidence rates for women are highest among whites, followed by African Americans, Hispanics, and Asians/Pacific Islanders.
- However, cancer death rates for women are highest among African Americans, followed by whites, Hispanics, and Asians/Pacific Islanders.

Culturally competent care in oncology is needed to meet the needs of diverse groups. Culturally competent care involves awareness of personal background, how culture affects care delivery, and how to adapt to meet cultural needs. Nurses need to actively seek to understand cultural differences to meet the individualized needs. (Culture is discussed in Chapter 2 and culturally competent care related to specific cancers is presented in the chapters where the cancer is discussed.)

BRIDGE TO NCLEX EXAMINATION

The number of the question corresponds to the same-numbered outcome at the beginning of the chapter.

1. Trends in the incidence and death rates of cancer include the fact that
   a. lung cancer is the most common type of cancer in men.
   b. a higher percentage of women than men have lung cancer.
   c. breast cancer is the leading cause of cancer deaths in women.
   d. African Americans have a higher death rate from cancer than whites.
2. What features of cancer cells distinguish them from normal cells *(select all that apply)*?
   a. Cells lack contact inhibition.
   b. Oncogenes maintain normal cell expression.
   c. Cells return to a previous undifferentiated state.
   d. Proliferation occurs when there is a need for more cells.
   e. New proteins characteristic of embryonic stage emerge on cell membrane.

3. A characteristic of the stage of progression in the development of cancer is
   a. oncogenic viral transformation of target cells.
   b. a reversible steady growth facilitated by carcinogens.
   c. a period of latency before clinical detection of cancer.
   d. proliferation of cancer cells despite host control mechanisms.
4. The primary protective role of the immune system related to malignant cells is
   a. surveillance for cells with tumor-associated antigens.
   b. binding with free antigen released by malignant cells.
   c. production of blocking factors that immobilize cancer cells.
   d. reacting to a new set of antigenic determinants on cancer cells.
5. The nurse is caring for a 59-year-old woman who had surgery 1 day ago for removal of a malignant abdominal mass. The patient is awaiting the pathology report. She is tearful and says that she is scared to die. The *most* effective nursing intervention at this point is to use this opportunity to
   a. motivate change in an unhealthy lifestyle.
   b. teach her about the seven warning signs of cancer.
   c. instruct her about healthy stress relief and coping practices.
   d. let her communicate about the meaning of this experience.
6. The goals of cancer treatment are based on the principle that
   a. surgery is the single most effective treatment for cancer.
   b. initial treatment is always directed toward cure of the cancer.
   c. a combination of treatment modalities is effective for controlling many cancers.
   d. although cancer cure is rare, quality of life can be increased with treatment modalities.
7. The *most* effective method of administering a chemotherapy agent that is a vesicant is to
   a. give it orally.
   b. give it intraarterially.
   c. use an Ommaya reservoir.
   d. use a central venous access device.
8. The nurse explains to a patient undergoing brachytherapy of the cervix that she
   a. must undergo simulation to locate the treatment area.
   b. requires the use of radioactive precautions during nursing care.
   c. may experience desquamation of the skin on the abdomen and upper legs.
   d. requires shielding of the ovaries during treatment to prevent ovarian damage.
9. A patient on chemotherapy and radiation for head and neck cancer has a WBC count of $1.9 \times 10^3/\mu L$, hemoglobin of 10.8 g/dL, and a platelet count of $99 \times 10^3/\mu L$. Based on the CBC results, what is the *most* serious clinical finding?
   a. Cough, rhinitis, and sore throat
   b. Fatigue, nausea, and skin redness at site of radiation
   c. Temperature of 101.9° F, fatigue, and shortness of breath
   d. Skin redness at site of radiation, headache, and constipation
10. To prevent fever and shivering during an infusion of rituximab (Rituxan), the nurse should premedicate the patient with
    a. aspirin.
    b. acetaminophen.
    c. sodium bicarbonate.
    d. meperidine (Demerol).
11. The nurse counsels the patient receiving radiation therapy or chemotherapy that
    a. effective birth control methods should be used for the rest of the patient's life.
    b. if nausea and vomiting occur during treatment, the treatment plan will be modified.
    c. after successful treatment, a return to the person's previous functional level can be expected.
    d. the cycle of fatigue-depression-fatigue that may occur during treatment may be reduced by restricting activity.
12. A patient on chemotherapy for 10 weeks started at a weight of 121 lb. She now weighs 118 lb and has no sense of taste. Which nursing intervention would be a *priority*?
    a. Advise the patient to eat foods that are fatty, fried, or high in calories.
    b. Discuss with the physician the need for parenteral or enteral feedings.
    c. Advise the patient to drink a nutritional supplement beverage at least three times a day.
    d. Advise the patient to experiment with spices and seasonings to enhance the flavor of food.
13. A 70-year-old male patient has multiple myeloma. His wife calls to report that he sleeps most of the day, is confused when awake, and complains of nausea and constipation. Which complication of cancer is this *most* likely caused by?
    a. Hypercalcemia
    b. Tumor lysis syndrome
    c. Spinal cord compression
    d. Superior vena cava syndrome
14. A patient has recently been diagnosed with early stages of breast cancer. What is *most* appropriate for the nurse to focus on?
    a. Maintaining the patient's hope
    b. Preparing a will and advance directives
    c. Discussing replacement child care for the patient's children
    d. Discussing the patient's past experiences with her grandmother's cancer

1. d, 2. a, c, e, 3. d, 4. a, 5. d, 6. c, 7. d, 8. b, 9. c, 10. b, 11. c, 12. d, 13. a, 14. a

For rationales to these answers and even more NCLEX review questions, visit *http://evolve.elsevier.com/Lewis/medsurg.*

EVOLVE WEBSITE

http://evolve.elsevier.com/Lewis/medsurg

Review Questions (Online Only)
Key Points
Answer Keys for Questions
- Rationales for Bridge to NCLEX Examination Questions

Conceptual Care Map Creator
Supporting Media
- Animations
  - Chemotherapy
  - Radiation Therapy

Audio Glossary
Content Updates

REFERENCES

1. American Cancer Society: *Cancer facts & figures 2015*, Atlanta, 2015, American Cancer Society.
2. Siegel RL, Miller KD, Jemal A: Cancer statistics 2015, *CA Cancer J Clin* 65:5, 2015.
3. National Cancer Institute, NIH, DHHS: Cancer trends progress report, Bethesda, Md, March 2015. Retrieved from *http://progressreport.cancer.gov.*

4. Vockley JG, Niederhuber JE: Diagnosis and treatment of cancer using genomics, *BMJ* 350:h1832, 2015.
5. Ariga H: Common mechanisms of onset of cancer and neurodegenerative diseases, *Biol Pharm Bull* 38(6):795, 2015.
6. Cancer Prevention and Control, Centers for Disease Control and Prevention: Skin cancer. Retrieved from *www.cdc.gov/cancer/skin/index.htm.*
7. Casulo C, Friedberg J: Treating Burkitt lymphoma in adults, *Curr Hematol Malig Rep* 10(3):266, 2015.
8. Karnofsky Performance Scale. Retrieved from *www.pennmedicine.org/homecare/hcp/elig_worksheets/Karnofsky-Performance-Status.pdf.*
9. Katz Index of Independence in Activities of Daily Living. Retrieved from *http://consultgerirn.org/uploads/File/trythis/try_this_2.pdf.*
10. Stewart BW, Wild P: World cancer report. World Health Organization.
*11. American Cancer Society: Cancer screening guidelines. Retrieved from *www.cancer.org/healthy/findcancerearly/cancerscreeningguidelines/american-cancer-society-guidelines-for-the-early-detection-of-cancer.*
12. American Society of Clinical Oncology (ASCO): What is personalized cancer medicine? Retrieved from *www.cancer.net/navigating-cancer-care/how-cancer-treated/personalized-and-targeted-therapies/what-personalized-cancer-medicine.*
13. Low SK, Takahashi A, Mushiroda T, et al: Genome-wide association study: a useful tool to identify common genetic variants associated with drug toxicity and efficacy in cancer pharmacogenomics, *Clin Cancer Res* 20(10):2541, 2014.
14. McLeod HL: Cancer pharmacogenomics: early promise, but concerted effort needed, *Science* 339(6127):1563, 2013.
15. National Institute for Occupational Safety and Health: Safe handling of chemotherapy agents. Retrieved from *www.cdc.gov/niosh/topics/antineoplastic.*
16. Polovich M, Olsen M, LeFebvre K: *Chemotherapy and biotherapy guidelines and recommendations for practice*, ed 4, Pittsburgh, 2014, Oncology Nursing Society.
*17. Tariman JD, Doorenbos A, Schepp KG, et al: Information needs priorities in patients diagnosed with cancer: a systematic review, *J Adv Pract Oncol* 2014(5):115, 2014.
18. Matsuyama RK, Kuhn LA, Molisani A, et al: Cancer patients' information needs the first nine months after diagnosis, *Patient Educ Couns* 90(1):96, 2013.
*19. Mhaskar R, Clark OA, Lyman G, et al: Colony-stimulating factors for chemotherapy-induced febrile neutropenia, *Cochrane Database Syst Rev* 10:CD003039, 2014.
20. National Cancer Institute: Guidelines for the evaluation and management of cancer-related fatigue. Retrieved from *www.cancer.gov/cancertopics/pdq/supportivecare/fatigue/HealthProfessional/page4.*
21. Kaiser J, Bledowski C, Dietrich J: Neural correlates of chemotherapy-related cognitive impairment, *Cortex* 54C:33, 2014.
22. American Cancer Society: Chemo brain. Retrieved from *www.cancer.org/treatment/treatmentsandsideeffects/physicalsideeffects/chemotherapyeffects/chemo-brain.*
23. Wright CI, Coad J, Morgan S, et al: "Just in case": the fertility information needs of teenagers and young adults with cancer, *Eur J Cancer Care (Engl)* 23(2):189, 2014.
24. Armenian SH, Kremer LC, Sklar C: Approaches to reduce the long-term burden of treatment-related complications in survivors of childhood cancer, *Am Soc Clin Oncol Educ Book* 35:196, 2015.
*25. Salz T, Baxi SS, Raghunathan N, et al: Are we ready to predict late effects? A systematic review of clinically useful prediction models, *Eur J Cancer* 51(6):758, 2015.
26. American Cancer Society: How does targeted cancer therapy work? Retrieved from *www.cancer.org/treatment/treatmentsandsideeffects/treatmenttypes/targetedtherapy/targeted-therapy-how-work.*
27. National Cancer Institute: What are targeted cancer therapies? Retrieved from *www.cancer.gov/about-cancer/treatment/types/targeted-therapies/targeted-therapies-fact-sheet#q4.*
28. Ozkan MC, Sahin F, Saydam G: Peripheral blood stem cell mobilization from healthy donors, *Transfus Apher Sci* 53:13, 2015.
29. Aoyagi T, Terracina KP, Raza A, et al: Cancer cachexia, mechanism and treatment, *World J Gastrointest Oncol* 7(4):17, 2015.
30. National Council of Cancer Nurses' guidelines for management of adult cancer pain. Retrieved from *www.nccn.org/professionals/physician_gls/pdf/pain.pdf.*
31. Longacre ML: Cancer caregivers information needs and resource preferences, *J Cancer Educ* 28(2):297, 2013.
32. National Institute on Aging: Global health and aging. Retrieved from *www.nia.nih.gov/research/publication/global-health-and-aging/living-longer.*
33. DeSantis CE, Lin CC, Mariotto AB, et al:. Cancer treatment and survivorship statistics, 2014, *CA Cancer J Clin* 64(4):252, 2014.
34. Warren E, Footman K, Tinelli M, et al: Do cancer-specific websites meet patient's information needs? *Patient Educ Couns* 95(1):126, 2014.
35. Shea-Budgell MA, Kostaras X, Myhill KP, et al: Information needs and sources of information for patients during cancer follow-up, *Curr Oncol* 21(4):165, 2014.

*Evidence-based information for clinical practice.

16

Fluid, Electrolyte, and Acid-Base Imbalances

Mariann M. Harding

Water is the driving force in nature.

Leonardo da Vinci

http://evolve.elsevier.com/Lewis/medsurg/

LEARNING OUTCOMES

1. Describe the composition of the major body fluid compartments.
2. Define processes involved in the regulation of movement of water and electrolytes between the body fluid compartments.
3. Describe the etiology, laboratory diagnostic findings, clinical manifestations, and nursing and interprofessional management of the following disorders:
   a. Extracellular fluid volume imbalances: fluid volume deficit and fluid volume excess
   b. Sodium imbalances: hypernatremia and hyponatremia
   c. Potassium imbalances: hyperkalemia and hypokalemia
   d. Magnesium imbalances: hypermagnesemia and hypomagnesemia
   e. Calcium imbalances: hypercalcemia and hypocalcemia
   f. Phosphate imbalances: hyperphosphatemia and hypophosphatemia
4. Identify the processes involved in maintaining acid-base balance.
5. Discuss the etiology, laboratory diagnostic findings, clinical manifestations, and nursing and interprofessional management of the following acid-base imbalances: metabolic acidosis, metabolic alkalosis, respiratory acidosis, and respiratory alkalosis.
6. Describe the composition of and indications for common IV fluid solutions.
7. Discuss the types and nursing management of commonly used central venous access devices.

KEY TERMS

acidosis, p. 287
active transport, p. 272
alkalosis, p. 287
anions, p. 271
buffers, p. 287
cations, p. 271
central venous access devices (CVADs), p. 294
electrolytes, p. 271
fluid spacing, p. 274
hydrostatic pressure, p. 273
hypertonic, p. 273
hypotonic, p. 273
isotonic, p. 273
oncotic pressure, p. 273
osmolality, p. 272
osmosis, p. 272
osmotic pressure, p. 272

HOMEOSTASIS

Body fluids and electrolytes play an important role in maintaining *homeostasis,* the body's stable internal environment. Body fluids are in constant motion transporting nutrients, electrolytes, and oxygen to cells and carrying waste products away from cells. The body uses a number of adaptive responses to keep the composition and volume of fluids and electrolytes within narrow limits to maintain homeostasis and promote health.

Many diseases and their treatments affect fluid and electrolyte balance. For example, a patient with metastatic colon cancer may develop hypercalcemia because of bone destruction from tumor invasion. Chemotherapy used to treat the cancer may result in nausea and vomiting and, subsequently, dehydration and acid-base imbalances. When correcting dehydration with IV fluids, the patient requires close monitoring to prevent fluid overload.

It is important to anticipate the potential for fluid and electrolyte imbalances associated with certain disorders and medical therapies, recognize the signs and symptoms of imbalances, and intervene with the appropriate action. This chapter describes the (1) normal control of fluids, electrolytes, and acid-base balance; (2) conditions that disrupt homeostasis and resulting manifestations; and (3) actions that the health care provider and you can take to manage fluid, electrolyte, and acid-base imbalances and restore homeostasis.

WATER CONTENT OF THE BODY

The body is composed primarily of water. It accounts for about 50% to 60% of body weight in the adult. Water content varies with body mass, gender, and age (Fig. 16-1). Lean body mass has a higher percentage of water, while adipose tissue has a lesser percentage of water. So, the more fat present in the body, the less the total water content. Women generally have a lower percentage of body water because they tend to have less lean body mass than men. Older adults also tend to have less lean body mass, resulting in a lower percentage of body water when compared to younger adults. In older adults, body water content

Reviewed by Helene Harris, RN, MSN, Clinical Educator, Central Texas Veterans Healthcare System, Temple, Texas; Ellen Odell, DNP, ACNS-BC, CNE, APRN, Director of Nursing, Associate Professor, Department of Nursing, John Brown University, Siloam Springs, Arkansas; and Daryle Wane, PhD, ARNP, FNP-BC, RN to BSN Coordinator, Professor of Nursing, Department of Health Occupations, Pasco-Hernando State College, New Port Richey, Florida.

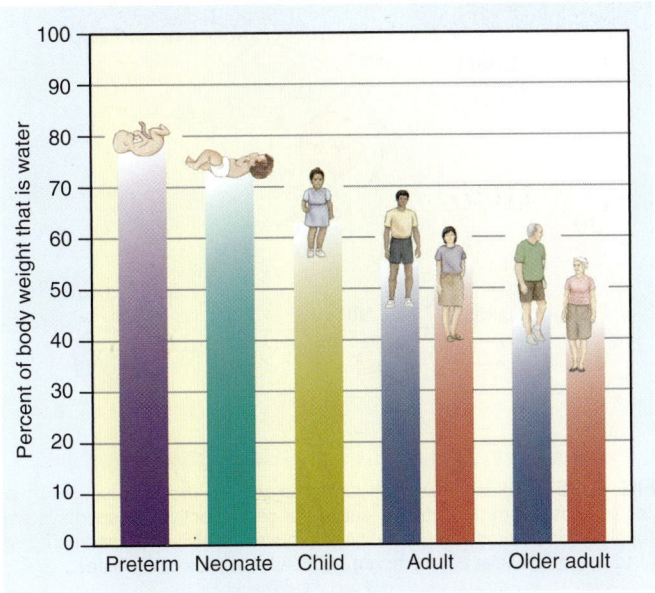

FIG. 16-1 Body water over the life span.

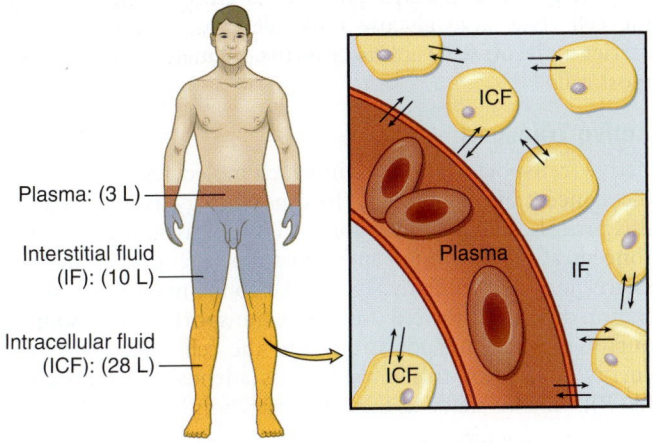

FIG. 16-2 Relative volumes of three body fluids. Values represent fluid distribution in a young male adult.

averages 45% to 50% of body weight. This places them at a higher risk for fluid-related problems than young adults.

Body Fluid Compartments

The two fluid compartments in the body are the *intracellular space* (inside the cells) and the *extracellular space* (outside the cells) (Fig. 16-2). About two thirds of the body water is located within cells and is termed *intracellular fluid* (ICF). ICF makes up about 40% of body weight of an adult. This means a 70-kg young man would have about 42 L of water, with about 28 L of that water located within his cells.

The fluid in the extracellular space is *extracellular fluid* (ECF). The two main compartments containing ECF are the *interstitial fluid*, or the fluid in the spaces between cells, and the intravascular fluid or *plasma*, the liquid part of blood. Other ECF compartments include lymph and *transcellular fluids*. Transcellular fluids include cerebrospinal fluid; fluid in the gastrointestinal (GI) tract and joint spaces; and pleural, peritoneal, intraocular, and pericardial fluid. ECF makes up about one third of the body water; this amounts to about 14 L in a 70-kg man. About one third of ECF is in the intravascular space as plasma (3 L in a 70-kg man), and two thirds is in the interstitial space (10 L in a 70-kg man). The fluid in the transcellular spaces totals about 1 L at any given time.

Calculation of Fluid Gain or Loss

One liter of water weighs 2.2 lb (1 kg). Body weight change, especially sudden change, is an excellent indicator of overall fluid volume loss or gain. For example, if a patient drinks 240 mL (8 oz) of fluid, weight gain will be 0.5 lb (0.23 kg). A patient receiving diuretic therapy who loses 4.4 lb (2 kg) in 24 hours has experienced a fluid loss of about 2 L. An adult patient who is fasting may lose 1 to 2 lb/day. A weight loss exceeding this is likely due to loss of body fluid.

ELECTROLYTES

Electrolytes are substances whose molecules dissociate, or split, into ions when placed in water. *Ions* are electrically charged particles. **Cations** are positively charged ions. Examples include sodium (Na^+), potassium (K^+), calcium (Ca^{2+}), and magnesium (Mg^{2+}) ions. **Anions** are negatively charged ions. Examples include bicarbonate (HCO_3^-), chloride (Cl^-), and phosphate (PO_4^{3-}) ions. Most proteins bear a negative charge and are thus anions.

Measurement of Electrolytes

The concentration of electrolytes in body fluids is expressed in milliequivalents (mEq) per liter. Since electrolytes are active chemicals, it is useful to express their concentration according to their chemical activity, or the number of electrolytes able to combine chemically. Ions combine milliequivalent for milliequivalent. For example, 1 mEq (1 mmol) of sodium combines with 1 mEq (1 mmol) of chloride.

Electrolyte Composition of Fluid Compartments

Electrolyte composition varies between ECF and ICF. The overall concentration of electrolytes is nearly the same in the two compartments. However, concentrations of specific ions differ greatly (Fig. 16-3). In ECF the main cation is sodium, with small amounts of potassium, calcium, and magnesium. The primary ECF anion is chloride, with small amounts of bicarbonate, sulfate, and phosphate anions.

In ICF the most prevalent cation is potassium, with small amounts of magnesium and sodium. The prevalent ICF anion is phosphate, with some protein and a small amount of bicarbonate. See Table 16-1 for normal serum electrolyte values.

MECHANISMS CONTROLLING FLUID AND ELECTROLYTE MOVEMENT

The movement of electrolytes and water between ICF and ECF to maintain homeostasis involves many different processes, including simple diffusion, facilitated diffusion, and active transport. Water moves as driven by two forces: hydrostatic pressure and osmotic pressure.

Diffusion

Diffusion is the movement of molecules from an area of high concentration to low concentration (Fig. 16-4). Net movement of molecules stops when the concentrations are equal in both areas. It occurs in liquids, gases, and solids. Simple diffusion requires no external energy.

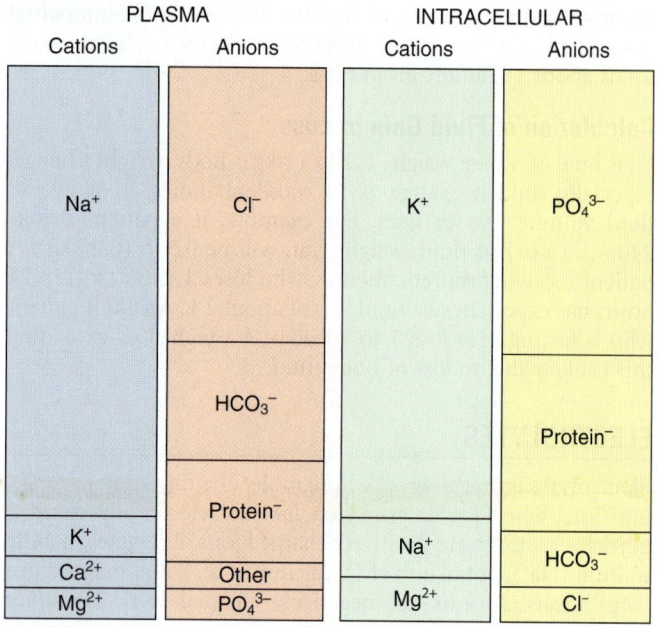

FIG. 16-3 The relative concentrations of the major cations and anions in the intracellular space and the plasma.

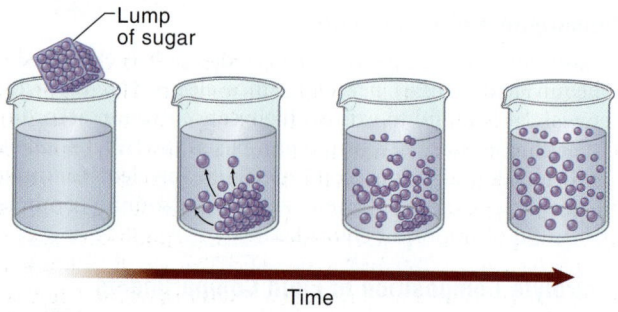

FIG. 16-4 Diffusion is the movement of molecules from an area of high concentration to an area of low concentration. Eventually the sugar molecules are evenly distributed.

TABLE 16-1 Normal Serum Electrolyte Values

Electrolyte	Reference Interval
Anions	
Bicarbonate (HCO_3^-)	22-26 mEq/L (22-26 mmol/L)
Chloride (Cl^-)	96-106 mEq/L (96-106 mmol/L)
Phosphate (PO_4^{3-})*	2.4-4.4 mg/dL (0.78-1.42 mmol/L)
Cations	
Potassium (K^+)	3.5-5.0 mEq/L (3.5-5.0 mmol/L)
Magnesium (Mg^{2+})	1.5-2.5 mEq/L (0.75-1.25 mmol/L)
Sodium (Na^+)	135-145 mEq/L (135-145 mmol/L)
Calcium (Ca^{2+}) (total)	8.6-10.2 mg/dL (2.15-2.55 mmol/L)
Calcium (ionized)	4.6-5.3 mg/dL (1.16-1.32 mmol/L)

*The majority of the phosphorus (P) in the body is found as phosphate (PO_4^{3-}). The terms are used interchangeably in this text.

Facilitated Diffusion

Facilitated diffusion involves the use of a protein carrier in the cell membrane. The protein carrier combines with a molecule, especially one too large to pass easily through the cell membrane, and assists in moving the molecule across the membrane from an area of high to low concentration. Like simple diffusion, facilitated diffusion is passive and requires no energy. An example of facilitated diffusion is glucose transport into the cell. The large glucose molecule must combine with a carrier molecule to be able to cross the cell membrane and enter most cells.

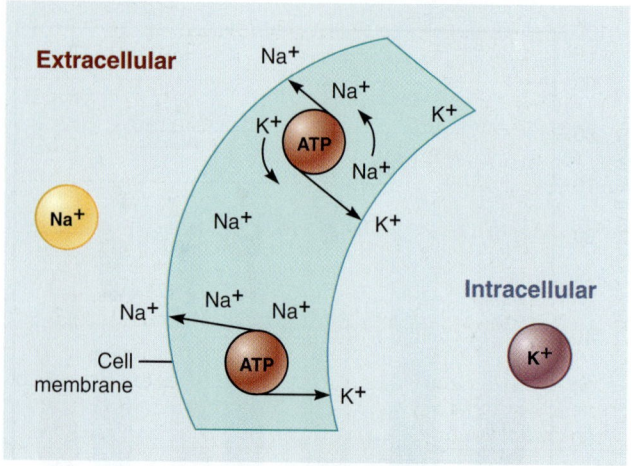

FIG. 16-5 Sodium-potassium pump. As sodium *(Na^+)* diffuses into the cell and potassium *(K^+)* diffuses out of the cell, an active transport system supplied with energy delivers Na^+ back to the extracellular compartment and K^+ to the intracellular compartment. *ATP,* Adenosine triphosphate.

Active Transport

Active transport is a process in which molecules move against the concentration gradient. External energy is required for this process. An example is the sodium-potassium pump. The concentrations of sodium and potassium differ greatly intracellularly and extracellularly (Fig. 16-3). To maintain this concentration difference, the cell uses active transport to move sodium out of the cell and potassium into the cell (Fig. 16-5). The energy source for this movement is adenosine triphosphate (ATP), which is made in the cell's mitochondria.

Osmosis

Osmosis is the movement of water "down" a concentration gradient, that is, from a region of low solute concentration to one of high solute concentration, across a semipermeable membrane. Osmosis requires no outside energy sources. It stops when the concentration differences disappear or when hydrostatic pressure builds and opposes any further movement of water. Imagine a chamber with two compartments separated by a semipermeable membrane, one that allows only the movement of water (Fig. 16-6). If you add albumin to one side, water will move from the less concentrated side (has more water) to the more concentrated side of the chamber water (has less water) until the concentrations are equal.

Whenever dissolved substances are contained in a space with a semipermeable membrane, they can pull water into the space by osmosis. The concentration of the solution determines the strength of the osmotic pull. The higher the concentration, the greater a solution's pull, or **osmotic pressure.** Osmotic pressure is measured in milliosmoles (mOsm). It may be expressed as either fluid osmolarity or fluid osmolality. Although you will often see the terms *osmolarity* and *osmolality* used interchangeably, they are different measurements. *Osmolarity* measures the total milliosmoles per liter of solution, or the concentration of molecules per volume of solution (mOsm/L). **Osmolality**

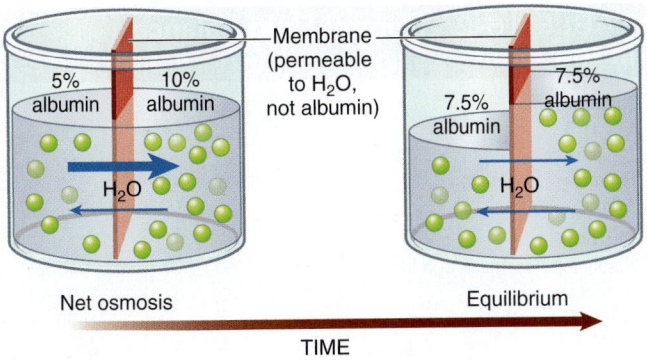

FIG. 16-6 Osmosis is the process of water movement through a semipermeable membrane from an area of low solute concentration to an area of high solute concentration.

measures the number of milliosmoles per kilogram of water, or the concentration of molecules per weight of water. Osmolality is the preferred measure to evaluate the concentration of plasma, urine, and body fluids.[1]

Measurement of Osmolality. Osmolality is nearly the same in the various body fluid spaces. Therefore measuring or estimating plasma osmolality is a useful way to assess the state of the body's water balance. Calculate the plasma osmolality using the following formula.[2]

$$\text{Plasma osmolality} = (2 \times \text{Na}) + \left(\frac{\text{BUN}}{2.8}\right) + \left(\frac{\text{Glucose}}{18}\right)$$

Normal plasma osmolality is between 280 and 295 mOsm/kg. A value greater than 295 mOsm/kg indicates that the concentration of solute is too great or the water content is too little. This condition is termed *water deficit.* A value less than 275 mOsm/kg indicates too little solute for the amount of water or too much water for the amount of solute. This condition is termed *water excess.* Both conditions are clinically significant.

Osmolality of urine can range from 100 to 1300 mOsm/kg. Urine osmolality depends on fluid intake, the amount of antidiuretic hormone (ADH) in circulation, and the renal response to ADH.

Osmotic Movement of Fluids. The osmolality of the fluid surrounding cells affects them. Fluids with the same osmolality as the cell interior are termed **isotonic.** Normally, ECF and ICF are isotonic to one another, so no net movement of water occurs.

Changes in the osmolality of ECF alter the volume of cells. Solutions in which the solutes are less concentrated than in the cells are termed **hypotonic** (hypoosmolar). If a cell is surrounded by hypotonic fluid, water moves into the cell, causing it to swell and possibly to burst. Fluids with solutes more concentrated than in cells, or an increased osmolality, are termed **hypertonic** (hyperosmolar). If hypertonic fluid surrounds a cell, water leaves the cell to dilute ECF; the cell shrinks and may eventually die (Fig. 16-7).

Hydrostatic Pressure

Hydrostatic pressure is the force of fluid in a compartment pushing against a cell membrane or vessel wall. In the blood vessels, hydrostatic pressure is the BP generated by the contraction of the heart. Hydrostatic pressure in the vascular system gradually decreases as the blood moves through the arteries until it is about 30 mm Hg in the capillary bed. At the capillary level, hydrostatic pressure is the major force that pushes water out of the vascular system and into the interstitial space.

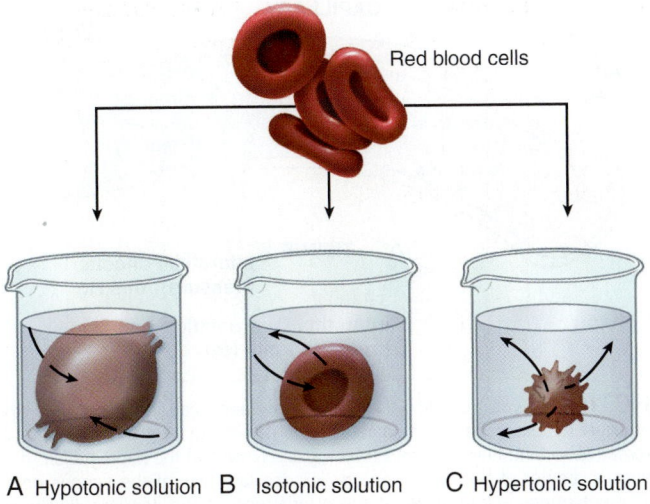

FIG. 16-7 Effects of water status on red blood cells. **A,** Hypotonic solution (H_2O excess) results in cellular swelling. **B,** Isotonic solution (normal H_2O balance) results in no change. **C,** Hypertonic solution (H_2O deficit) results in cellular shrinking.

Oncotic Pressure

Oncotic pressure (colloidal osmotic pressure) is the osmotic pressure caused by plasma colloids in solution. The major colloids in the vascular system contributing to osmotic pressure are proteins, such as albumin. Plasma has substantial amounts of protein, while the interstitial space has very little. The plasma protein molecules attract water, pulling fluid from the tissue space to the vascular space. Under normal conditions, plasma oncotic pressure is about 25 mm Hg. The small amount of protein found in the interstitial space exerts an oncotic pressure of about 1 mm Hg.

FLUID MOVEMENT IN CAPILLARIES

As plasma flows through the capillary bed, four factors determine if fluid moves out of the capillary and into the interstitial space or if fluid moves back into the capillary from the interstitial space. The amount and direction of movement are determined by the interaction of (1) capillary hydrostatic pressure, (2) plasma oncotic pressure, (3) interstitial hydrostatic pressure, and (4) interstitial oncotic pressure.

Capillary hydrostatic pressure and interstitial oncotic pressure move water out of the capillaries. Plasma oncotic pressure and interstitial hydrostatic pressure move fluid into the capillaries. At the arterial end of the capillary, capillary hydrostatic pressure exceeds plasma oncotic pressure, and fluid moves into the interstitial space. At the venous end of the capillary, the capillary hydrostatic pressure is lower than plasma oncotic pressure, drawing fluid back into the capillary by the oncotic pressure created by plasma proteins (Fig. 16-8).

Fluid Shifts

If capillary or interstitial pressures change, fluid may abnormally shift from one compartment to another, resulting in edema or dehydration.

Shifts of Plasma to Interstitial Fluid. *Edema,* an accumulation of fluid in the interstitial space, occurs if venous hydrostatic

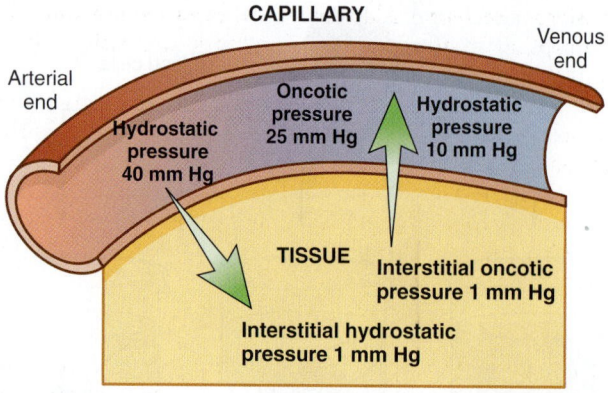

FIG. 16-8 Dynamics of fluid exchange between a capillary and tissue. An equilibrium exists between forces filtering fluid out of the capillary and forces absorbing fluid back into the capillary. Note that the hydrostatic pressure is greater at the arterial end of the capillary than at the venous end. The net effect of pressures at the arterial end of the capillary causes a movement of fluid into the tissue. At the venous end of the capillary, there is net movement of fluid back into the capillary.

pressure rises, plasma oncotic pressure decreases, or interstitial oncotic pressure rises. Edema may also develop if an obstruction of lymphatic outflow causes decreased removal of interstitial fluid.

Elevation of Venous Hydrostatic Pressure. Increasing the pressure at the venous end of the capillary inhibits fluid movement back into the capillary, which results in edema. Causes of increased venous pressure include fluid overload, heart failure, liver failure, obstruction of venous return to the heart (e.g., tourniquets, restrictive clothing, venous thrombosis), and venous insufficiency (e.g., varicose veins).

Decrease in Plasma Oncotic Pressure. Fluid remains in the interstitial space if the plasma oncotic pressure is too low to draw fluid back into the capillary. Low plasma protein content decreases oncotic pressure. This can result from excessive protein loss (renal disorders), deficient protein synthesis (liver disease), and deficient protein intake (malnutrition).

Elevation of Interstitial Oncotic Pressure. Trauma, burns, and inflammation can damage capillary walls and allow plasma proteins to accumulate in the interstitial space. This increases interstitial oncotic pressure, draws fluid into the interstitial space, and holds it there.

Shifts of Interstitial Fluid to Plasma. An increase in the plasma osmotic or oncotic pressure draws fluid into the plasma from the interstitial space. This could happen with administration of colloids, dextran, mannitol, or hypertonic solutions. Increasing the tissue hydrostatic pressure is another way of causing a shift of fluid into plasma. Wearing elastic compression gradient stockings or hose to decrease peripheral edema is a therapeutic application of this effect.

FLUID SPACING

Fluid spacing is a term used to describe the distribution of body water. *First spacing* describes the normal distribution of fluid in ICF and ECF compartments. *Second spacing* refers to an abnormal accumulation of interstitial fluid (i.e., edema). *Third spacing* occurs when excess fluid collects in the nonfunctional area between cells. This fluid is trapped where it is difficult or impossible for it to move back into the cells or blood vessels. Third spacing occurs with ascites; fluid leaking into the abdominal cavity with peritonitis or pancreatitis; and edema associated with burns, trauma, or sepsis.

TABLE 16-2 Normal Fluid Balance in the Adult

Intake	
Fluids	1200 mL
Solid food	1000 mL
Water from oxidation	300 mL
Total	2500 mL
Output	
Insensible loss (skin and lungs)	900 mL
In feces	100 mL
Urine	1500 mL
Total	2500 mL

REGULATION OF WATER BALANCE

A number of factors are involved in maintaining the finely tuned balance among water intake, use, and excretion. For proper fluid balance, an average healthy adult requires a daily water intake between 2000 and 3000 mL (Table 16-2). This amount replaces what is lost from the body in urinary output and insensible losses. Oral fluid intake accounts for most of the water intake. Water intake also includes water from food metabolism and water present in solid foods.

Insensible water loss, which is invisible vaporization from the lungs and skin, assists in regulating body temperature. Accelerated body metabolism, which occurs with increased body temperature and exercise, increases the amount of water lost and may result in the need for additional water replacement.

Do not confuse water loss through the skin with the vaporization of water excreted by sweat glands. Insensible perspiration causes only water loss. Excessive sweating *(sensible perspiration)* caused by exercise, fever, or high environmental temperatures may lead to large losses of water and electrolytes.

Hypothalamic-Pituitary Regulation

Water ingestion equals water loss in the individual who has free access to water, intact thirst and ADH mechanism, and normally functioning kidneys. A body fluid deficit or increase in plasma osmolality activates osmoreceptors in the hypothalamus, which stimulate thirst and the release of ADH from the posterior pituitary gland. ADH acts on the distal tubules and collecting ducts in the kidney by making them more permeable to water. The result is increased water reabsorption from the tubular filtrate into the blood and decreased excretion in the urine. Because ADH is only able to regulate how much water the body holds onto, an intact thirst mechanism is our main protection against developing dehydration or hyperosmolality. Thirst causes us to increase the amount of water we drink. Together these result in increased free water in the body, decreasing plasma osmolality and restoring fluid volume.

Many factors influence ADH secretion and thirst. Decreased BP, nausea, pain, hypoglycemia, and hypoxemia stimulate ADH release. In the postoperative patient, the stress response to surgery and receiving analgesics and anesthesia cause ADH release and decreased osmolality. The unconscious or cognitively impaired patient is at increased risk for fluid deficit and hyperosmolality because of an inability to express thirst and act on it. A dry mouth will cause a person to drink, even when there is no body water deficit.

Renal Regulation

The primary function of the kidneys is to regulate fluid and electrolyte balance by adjusting urine volume and the excretion of most electrolytes (see Chapter 44). The kidneys filter the total plasma volume many times each day. In the average adult, the kidneys reabsorb 99% of this filtrate, producing around 1.5 L of urine per day. Under the influence of ADH, aldosterone, and other hormones, selective reabsorption and secretion of water and electrolytes in the renal tubules results in urine that is greatly different in composition and concentration from plasma. This process helps maintain normal plasma osmolality, electrolyte balance, blood volume, and acid-base balance.

With severely impaired renal function, the kidneys cannot maintain fluid and electrolyte balance. This condition results in edema, potassium and phosphorus retention, acidosis, and other electrolyte imbalances (see Chapter 46).

Adrenal Cortical Regulation

Glucocorticoids and mineralocorticoids secreted by the adrenal cortex help regulate water and electrolyte balance. The glucocorticoids (e.g., cortisol) primarily have an antiinflammatory effect and increase serum glucose levels, while the mineralocorticoids (e.g., aldosterone) enhance sodium retention and potassium excretion (Fig. 16-9). When sodium is reabsorbed, water follows because of osmotic changes.

Aldosterone is a mineralocorticoid with strong sodium-retaining and potassium-excreting capabilities. Decreased renal perfusion or decreased sodium in the distal portion of the renal tubule activates the renin-angiotensin-aldosterone system (RAAS), resulting in aldosterone secretion. In addition to the RAAS, increased serum potassium, decreased serum sodium, and adrenocorticotropic hormone (ACTH) stimulate aldosterone secretion. Aldosterone increases sodium and water reabsorption in the renal distal tubules, decreasing plasma osmolality and restoring fluid volume.

Cortisol is the most abundant glucocorticoid. In large doses, cortisol has both glucocorticoid (glucose-elevating and antiinflammatory) and mineralocorticoid (sodium-retention) effects. Normally cortisol secretion is in a diurnal or circadian pattern. Increased cortisol secretion occurs in response to physical and psychologic stress. This affects many body functions, including fluid and electrolyte balance (Fig. 16-10).

Cardiac Regulation

Natriuretic peptides, including atrial natriuretic peptide (ANP) and b-type natriuretic peptide (BNP), are hormones produced by cardiomyocytes. They are produced in response to increased atrial pressure (increased volume, such as occurs in heart failure) and high serum sodium levels. They are natural antagonists to the RAAS and suppress secretion of aldosterone, renin, and ADH, and the action of angiotensin II. In the renal tubules, peptides promote excretion of sodium and water, decreasing blood volume and BP.

Gastrointestinal Regulation

In addition to oral intake, the GI tract normally secretes around 8000 mL of digestive fluids each day. The GI tract normally reabsorbs most of this fluid, with only a small amount eliminated in feces. This is why diarrhea and vomiting, which prevent GI reabsorption of secreted fluid, can lead to significant fluid and electrolyte loss.

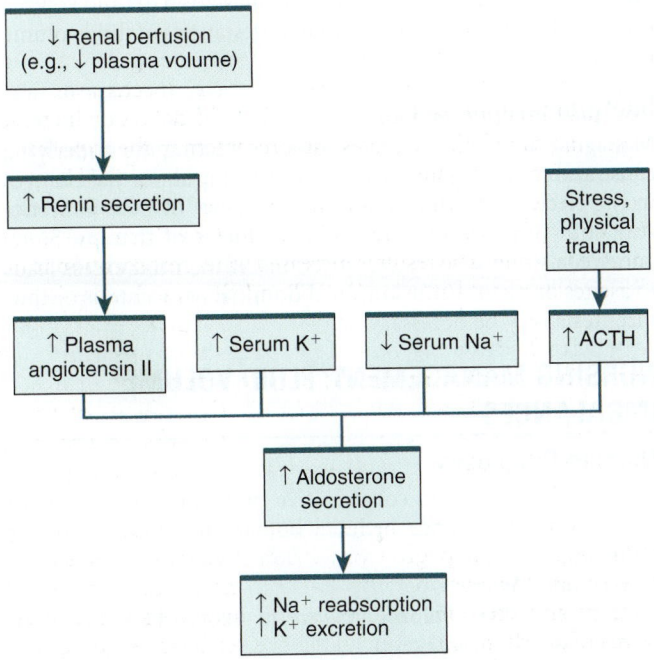

FIG. 16-9 Factors affecting aldosterone secretion. *ACTH,* Adrenocorticotropic hormone.

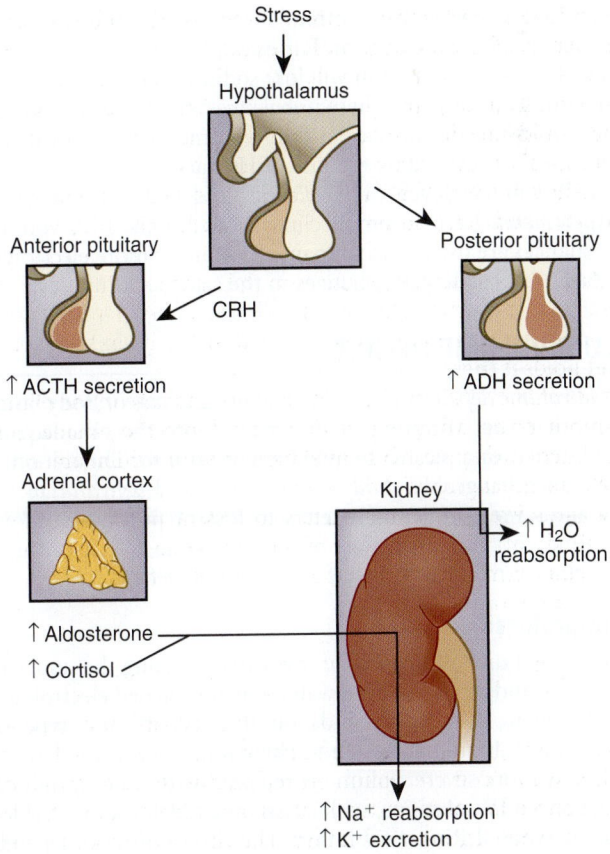

FIG. 16-10 Effects of stress on fluid and electrolyte balance. *ACTH,* Adrenocorticotropic hormone; *ADH,* antidiuretic hormone; *CRH,* corticotropin-releasing hormone.

Gerontologic Considerations: Fluid and Electrolytes

The older adult experiences normal physiologic changes that increase susceptibility to fluid and electrolyte imbalances. Structural changes to the kidneys and a decrease in the renal blood flow lead to decreased glomerular filtration rate and loss of the ability to concentrate urine and conserve water. Hormonal changes include a decrease in renin and aldosterone and an increase in ADH and ANP. The loss of subcutaneous tissue and thinning of the dermis lead to increased moisture lost through the skin and an inability to respond quickly to heat or cold.

Do not automatically attribute older patients' fluid and electrolyte problems to the natural processes of aging. Throughout this chapter are suggestions for adapting your assessment and nursing interventions when caring for the older adult.

FLUID VOLUME IMBALANCES

Fluid and electrolyte imbalances occur to some degree in most patients with a major illness or injury because illness disrupts normal homeostatic mechanisms. Illness or disease directly causes some fluid and electrolyte imbalances (e.g., burns, heart failure). Other times therapeutic measures (e.g., colonoscopy preparation, diuretics) cause or contribute to imbalances. Perioperative patients are at risk for developing fluid and electrolyte imbalances because of fluid restrictions, blood or fluid loss, and the stress of surgery.

Fluid and electrolyte imbalances are commonly classified as *deficits* or *excesses*. Although each imbalance is discussed separately in this chapter, it is common for more than one imbalance to occur in the same patient. For example, a patient with prolonged nasogastric suction will lose sodium, potassium, hydrogen, and chloride ions. These imbalances may result in sodium and potassium deficiencies, a fluid volume deficit, and metabolic alkalosis caused by the loss of HCl acid.

ECF volume deficit *(hypovolemia)* and ECF volume excess *(hypervolemia)* are common clinical conditions. ECF volume imbalances are usually accompanied by one or more electrolyte imbalances, particularly changes in the serum sodium level.

FLUID VOLUME DEFICIT

Fluid volume deficit can occur with abnormal loss of body fluids (e.g., diarrhea, vomiting, hemorrhage, polyuria), inadequate fluid intake, or a plasma to interstitial fluid shift. Though often used interchangeably, *fluid volume deficit* and *dehydration* are not the same. *Dehydration* refers to loss of pure water alone without a corresponding loss of sodium. Table 16-3 lists causes and clinical manifestations of fluid volume deficit.

Interprofessional Care

Managing fluid volume deficit involves correcting the underlying cause and replacing both water and any needed electrolytes. Replacement therapy depends on the severity and type of volume loss. In mild losses, oral rehydration may be used. If the deficit is more severe, volume is replaced with blood products or balanced IV solutions, such as isotonic (0.9%) sodium chloride or lactated Ringer's solution. The choice of fluid depends on the cause and patient's electrolyte status. For rapid volume replacement, 0.9% sodium chloride is preferred. Blood is administered when volume loss is due to blood loss.

TABLE 16-3 Extracellular Fluid Imbalances: Causes and Manifestations

ECF Volume Deficit	ECF Volume Excess
Causes	
• ↑ Insensible water loss or perspiration (high fever, heatstroke) • Diabetes insipidus • Osmotic diuresis • Hemorrhage • GI losses: vomiting, NG suction, diarrhea, fistula drainage • Overuse of diuretics • Inadequate fluid intake • Third-space fluid shifts: burns, pancreatitis	• Excessive isotonic or hypotonic IV fluids • Heart failure • Renal failure • Primary polydipsia • SIADH • Cushing syndrome • Long-term use of corticosteroids
Manifestations	
• Restlessness, drowsiness, lethargy, confusion • Thirst, dry mucous membranes • Cold clammy skin • Decreased skin turgor, ↓ capillary refill • Postural hypotension, ↑ pulse, ↓ CVP • ↓ Urine output, concentrated urine • ↑ Respiratory rate • Weakness, dizziness • Weight loss • Seizures, coma	• Headache, confusion, lethargy • Peripheral edema • Jugular venous distention • S3 heart sound • Bounding pulse, ↑ BP, ↑ CVP • Polyuria (with normal renal function) • Dyspnea, crackles, pulmonary edema • Muscle spasms • Weight gain • Seizures, coma

CVP, Central venous pressure; *ECF,* extracellular fluid; *SIADH,* syndrome of inappropriate antidiuretic hormone.

FLUID VOLUME EXCESS

Fluid volume excess may result from excess intake of fluids, abnormal retention of fluids (e.g., heart failure, renal failure), or a shift of fluid from interstitial fluid into plasma fluid. Weight gain is the most consistent manifestation of fluid volume excess. Table 16-3 lists causes and manifestations of fluid volume excess.

Interprofessional Care

Managing fluid volume excess involves treating the underlying cause and removing fluid without producing abnormal changes in the electrolyte composition or osmolality of ECF. Diuretics and fluid restriction are the primary forms of therapy. Some patients also need sodium restrictions. If the fluid excess leads to ascites or pleural effusion, an abdominal paracentesis or thoracentesis may be necessary.

❖ NURSING MANAGEMENT: FLUID VOLUME IMBALANCES

◆ Nursing Diagnoses

Nursing diagnoses and collaborative problems for the patient with a fluid imbalance include, but are not limited to, the following:

ECF volume deficit:

- Deficient fluid volume *related to* excess ECF losses or decreased fluid intake
- Decreased cardiac output *related to* excess ECF losses or decreased fluid intake

- Risk for impaired oral mucous membrane *related to* fluid volume deficit
- Potential complication: hypovolemic shock

ECF volume excess:

- Excess fluid volume *related to* increased water and/or sodium retention
- Impaired gas exchange *related to* water retention leading to pulmonary edema
- Risk for impaired skin integrity *related to* edema
- Activity intolerance *related to* increased water retention, fatigue, and weakness
- Disturbed body image *related to* altered body appearance secondary to edema
- Potential complications: pulmonary edema, ascites

Nursing Implementation

Daily Weights. Daily weights are the most accurate measure of volume status. An increase of 1 kg (2.2 lb) is equal to 1000 mL (1 L) of fluid retention, provided the person has maintained usual dietary intake or has not been on NPO status. Obtain the weight under standardized conditions. Weigh the patient at the same time every day, wearing the same garments and on the same carefully calibrated scale. Remove excess bedding and empty all drainage bags before the weighing. If items are present that are not there every day, such as bulky dressings or tubes, note this along with the weight.

Intake and Output. Intake and output records provide valuable information about fluid and electrolyte problems. An accurately recorded intake and output will identify sources of excessive intake or fluid losses. Intake should include oral, IV, and tube feedings and retained irrigants. Output includes urine, excess perspiration, wound or tube drainage, vomitus, and diarrhea. Estimate fluid loss from wounds and perspiration. Note the amount and color of the urine and measure the urine specific gravity. Readings greater than 1.025 indicate concentrated urine, while readings less than 1.010 indicate dilute urine.

Laboratory Findings. Monitor laboratory results when available and calculate the serum osmolality. The patient with a fluid volume deficit often has increased BUN, sodium, and hematocrit levels with increased plasma and urine osmolality. With fluid volume excess, the patient will have decreased BUN, sodium, and hematocrit levels with decreased plasma and urine osmolality.

Cardiovascular Care. Monitor vital signs and perform a thorough cardiovascular assessment as needed. Changes in BP, central venous pressure, pulse force, and jugular venous distention reflect ECF volume imbalances. In fluid volume excess, the pulse is full, bounding, and not easily obliterated. Increased volume causes distended neck veins (jugular venous distention), increased central venous pressure, and high BP. Auscultate heart sounds, being alert for the presence of an S3.

In mild to moderate fluid volume deficit, sympathetic nervous system compensation increases the heart rate and results in peripheral vasoconstriction in an effort to maintain BP within normal limits. Pulses may be weak and thready. Assess for orthostatic changes. A change in position from lying to sitting or standing may elicit a decrease in BP or a further increase in the heart rate (orthostatic hypotension). In more severe deficits, hypotension may be present.

Respiratory Care. Monitor pulse oximetry and auscultate lung sounds as needed. ECF excess can result in pulmonary congestion and pulmonary edema, as increased hydrostatic pressure in the pulmonary vessels forces fluid into the alveoli. The patient will experience shortness of breath and moist crackles on auscultation. The patient with ECF deficit will demonstrate an increased respiratory rate because of decreased tissue perfusion and resultant hypoxia. Administer oxygen as ordered.

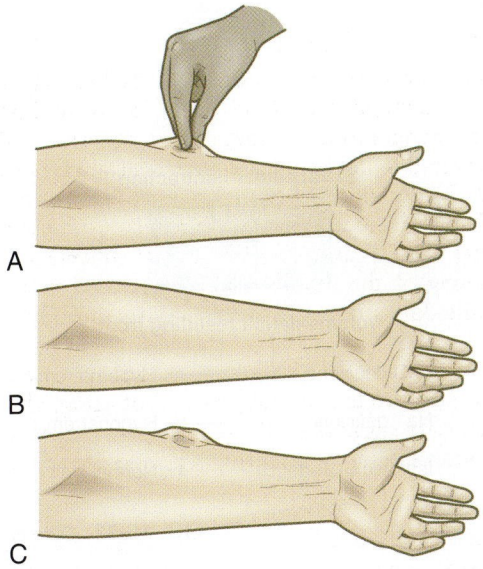

FIG. 16-11 Assessment of skin turgor. **A** and **B,** When normal skin is pinched, it resumes shape in seconds. **C,** If the skin remains wrinkled for 20 to 30 seconds, the patient has poor skin turgor.

Patient Safety. The patient with fluid volume deficit is at risk for falls because of orthostatic hypotension, muscle weakness, and changes in level of consciousness. Assess level of consciousness, gait, and muscle strength. Implement fall precautions. If orthostatic hypotension is present, teach the patient to change positions slowly when rising from a bed or chair. Place alarm monitors on patients who are confused and try to get out of bed without assistance.

Skin Care. Examine the skin for turgor and mobility. Normally a fold of skin, when pinched, will readily move and, on release, rapidly return to its former position. In ECF volume deficit, skin turgor is diminished, and there is a lag in the pinched skinfold's return to its original state (referred to as *tenting*). Skin areas over the sternum, abdomen, and anterior forearm are the usual sites for evaluation of tissue turgor (Fig. 16-11). In older people, decreased skin turgor is less predictive of fluid deficit because of the loss of tissue elasticity.[3]

In mild fluid deficits, the skin may appear warm, dry, and wrinkled. These signs may be difficult to evaluate in the older adult because the patient's skin may be normally dry, wrinkled, and nonelastic. In more severe deficits, the skin may be cool and moist if there is vasoconstriction to compensate for the decreased fluid volume. Oral mucous membranes will be dry, the tongue may be furrowed, and the individual often complains of thirst. Routine oral care is critical for the comfort of a patient who is dehydrated or on a fluid restriction.

Edematous skin may feel cool because of fluid accumulation and a decrease in blood flow secondary to the pressure of the fluid. The fluid can stretch the skin, causing it to feel taut and hard. Assess edema by pressing with a thumb or forefinger over the edematous area. A grading scale is used to standardize the description if an indentation (ranging from 1+ [slight edema; 2-mm indentation] to 4+ [pitting edema; 8-mm indentation]) remains when pressure is released. Evaluate for edema in areas

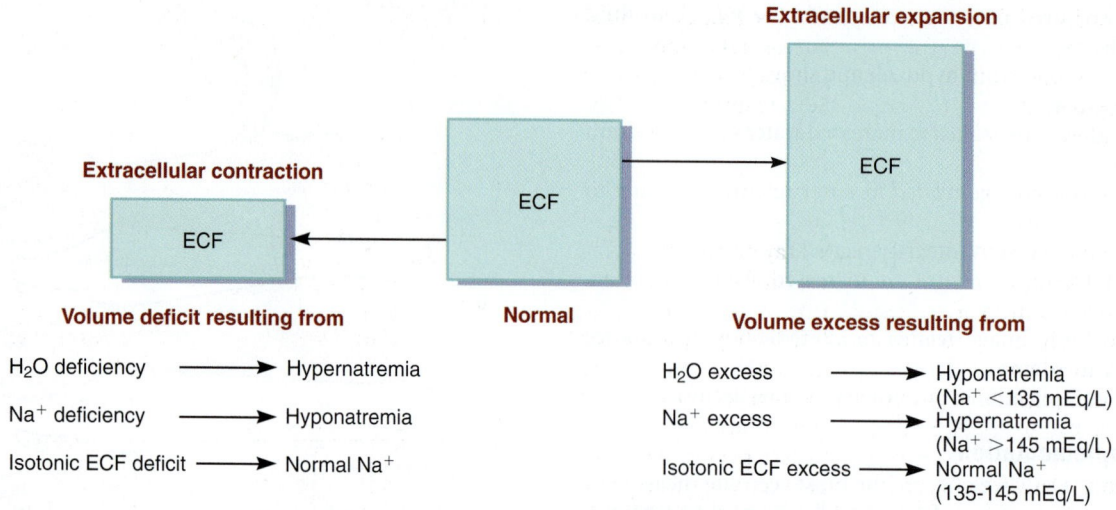

FIG. 16-12 Differential assessment of extracellular fluid (ECF) volume.

where soft tissues overlie a bone, particularly the tibia, fibula, and sacrum.

Good skin care is important. Protect tissues from extremes of heat and cold, prolonged pressure, and trauma. Frequent skin care and changes in position will prevent skin breakdown. Elevate edematous extremities to promote venous return and fluid reabsorption. Dehydrated skin needs frequent care without the use of soap. Applying moisturizing creams or oils increases moisture retention and stimulates circulation.

◆ **Fluid Therapy.** Administer IV fluids as ordered. Carefully monitor the rates of infusion of IV fluid solutions, especially when large volumes of fluid are being given. This is especially true in patients with cardiac, renal, or neurologic problems.

In the presence of fluid volume deficit, you can use several interventions to maintain adequate oral intake. Assess the patient's ability to obtain adequate fluids independently, express thirst, and swallow effectively. Fluids should be easily accessible. Provide a variety of fluids that the patient likes. Serve fluids at a temperature preferred by the patient. Offer fluids every 1 to 2 hours and at select times, such as when administering medications. Remind the patient to finish all drinks.

If the patient is choosing to limit intake to decrease nocturia or incontinence, make it easier for the patient to reach the toilet when needed.[3] Assist those with physical limitations, such as arthritis, to open and hold containers. Involve the dietitian, speech therapist, or occupation therapist for help with patients with dysphagia or physical limitations.

SODIUM IMBALANCES

Sodium, the main cation of ECF, plays a major role in maintaining the concentration and volume of ECF and influencing water distribution between ECF and ICF. Sodium has an important role in the generation and transmission of nerve impulses, muscle contractility, and regulation of acid-base balance.

The serum sodium level reflects the ratio of sodium to water, not necessarily the amount of sodium in the body. Changes in the serum sodium level can reflect a primary water imbalance, primary sodium imbalance, or combination of the two. Sodium imbalances are typically associated with imbalances in ECF volume (Figs. 16-12 and 16-13). Because sodium is the primary determinant of ECF osmolality, sodium imbalances are typically associated with parallel changes in osmolality.

The GI tract absorbs sodium from foods. Typically, daily intake of sodium far exceeds the body's daily requirements. Sodium leaves the body through urine, sweat, and feces. The

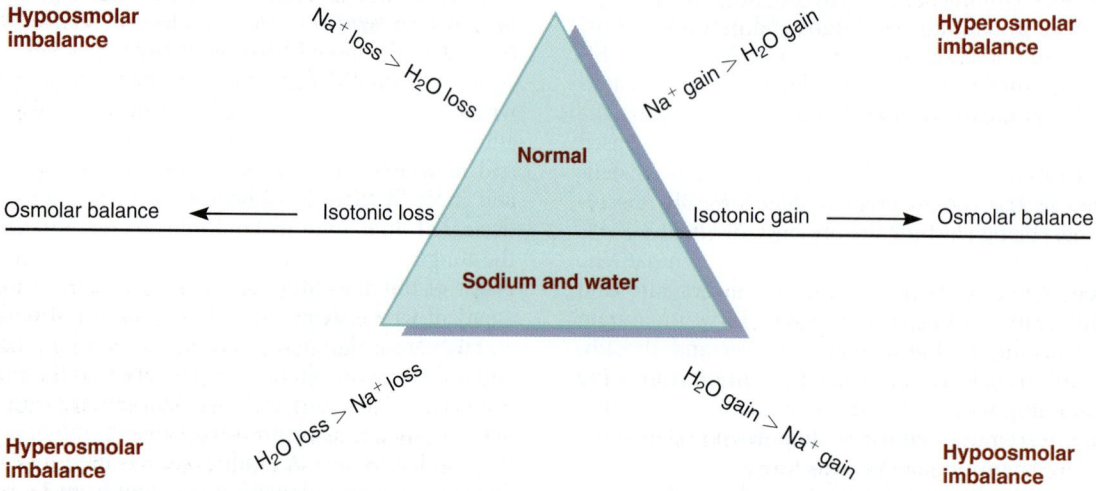

FIG. 16-13 Isotonic gains and losses affect mainly the extracellular fluid (ECF) compartment with little or no water movement into the cells. Hypertonic imbalances cause water to move from inside the cell into ECF to dilute the concentrated sodium, causing cell shrinkage. Hypotonic imbalances cause water to move into the cell, causing cell swelling.

kidneys primarily regulate sodium balance. The kidneys control ECF sodium concentration by excreting or retaining water under the influence of ADH. Aldosterone plays a smaller role in sodium regulation by promoting sodium reabsorption from the renal tubules.

HYPERNATREMIA

Hypernatremia (elevated serum sodium) may occur with inadequate water intake, excess water loss or, rarely, sodium gain. Because sodium is the major determinant of ECF osmolality, hypernatremia causes hyperosmolality. ECF hyperosmolality causes water to move out of the cells to restore equilibrium, leading to cellular dehydration. As discussed earlier, the primary protection against the development of hyperosmolality is thirst. Hypernatremia is not a problem in an alert person who has access to water, can sense thirst, and is able to swallow. Hypernatremia secondary to water deficiency is often the result of an impaired level of consciousness or an inability to obtain fluids.

Several clinical states can produce hypernatremia from water loss (Table 16-4). A deficiency in the synthesis or release of ADH from the posterior pituitary gland (central diabetes insipidus) or a decrease in kidney responsiveness to ADH (nephrogenic diabetes insipidus) can result in profound diuresis, producing a water deficit and hypernatremia. Hyperosmolality with osmotic diuresis can result from hyperglycemia associated with uncontrolled diabetes mellitus or administering concentrated hyperosmolar tube feedings.

Excess sodium intake with inadequate water intake can also lead to hypernatremia. Examples of sodium gain include IV administration of hypertonic saline or sodium bicarbonate, use of sodium-containing drugs, excessive oral intake of sodium (e.g., ingestion of seawater), and *primary aldosteronism* (hypersecretion of aldosterone) caused by a tumor of the adrenal glands.

Clinical Manifestations

The manifestations of hypernatremia are primarily the result of water shifting out of cells into ECF with resultant dehydration and shrinkage of cells (Table 16-4). Dehydration of brain cells results in alterations in mental status, ranging from agitation, restlessness, confusion, and lethargy to coma.[3] If there is any accompanying ECF volume deficit, manifestations such as postural hypotension, tachycardia, and weakness occur.

TABLE 16-4 Sodium Imbalances: Causes and Manifestations

Hypernatremia (Na^+ >145 mEq/L [mmol/L])	Hyponatremia (Na^+ <135 mEq/L [mmol/L])
Causes	
Excessive Sodium Intake	***Excessive Sodium Loss***
• IV fluids: hypertonic NaCl, excessive isotonic NaCl, IV sodium bicarbonate • Hypertonic tube feedings without water supplements • Near-drowning in salt water	• *GI losses:* diarrhea, vomiting, fistulas, NG suction • *Renal losses:* diuretics, adrenal insufficiency, Na^+ wasting renal disease • *Skin losses:* burns, wound drainage
Inadequate Water Intake	***Inadequate Sodium Intake***
• Unconscious or cognitively impaired individuals	• Fasting diets
Excessive Water Loss (↑ sodium concentration)	***Excessive Water Gain (↓ sodium concentration)***
• ↑ Insensible water loss (high fever, heatstroke, prolonged hyperventilation) • Osmotic diuretic therapy • Diarrhea	• Excessive hypotonic IV fluids • Primary polydipsia
Diseases	***Diseases***
• Diabetes insipidus • Primary hyperaldosteronism • Cushing syndrome • Uncontrolled diabetes mellitus	• SIADH • Heart failure • Primary hypoaldosteronism • Cirrhosis
Manifestations	
Hypernatremia With Decreased ECF Volume	***Hyponatremia With Decreased ECF Volume***
• Restlessness, agitation, lethargy, seizures, coma • Intense thirst, dry swollen tongue, sticky mucous membranes • Postural hypotension, ↓ CVP, weight loss, ↑ pulse • Weakness, muscle cramps	• Irritability, apprehension, confusion, dizziness, personality changes, tremors, seizures, coma • Dry mucous membranes • Postural hypotension, ↓ CVP, ↓ jugular venous filling, ↑ pulse, thready pulse • Cold and clammy skin
Hypernatremia With Normal or Increased ECF Volume	***Hyponatremia With Normal or Increased ECF Volume***
• Restlessness, agitation, twitching, seizures, coma • Intense thirst, flushed skin • Weight gain, peripheral and pulmonary edema, ↑ BP, ↑ CVP	• Headache, apathy, confusion, muscle spasms, seizures, coma • Nausea, vomiting, diarrhea, abdominal cramps • Weight gain, ↑ BP, ↑ CVP

CVP, Central venous pressure; *ECF,* extracellular fluid; *SIADH,* syndrome of inappropriate antidiuretic hormone.

❖ NURSING AND INTERPROFESSIONAL MANAGEMENT: HYPERNATREMIA

◆ Nursing Diagnoses

Nursing diagnoses and collaborative problems for the patient with hypernatremia include, but are not limited to, the following:

- Risk for electrolyte imbalance *related to* inadequate water intake, excess sodium intake and/or water loss injury *related to* altered sensorium and seizures
- Risk for fluid volume deficit *related to* inadequate water intake and/or water loss
- Risk for injury *related to* altered sensorium and seizures
- Potential complications: seizures and coma

◆ Nursing Implementation

Managing hypernatremia depends on the underlying cause and the patient's volume status. In primary water deficit, fluid replacement is provided either orally or IV with isotonic such as 0.9% sodium chloride.[2] If the problem is sodium excess, expect diluting the high sodium concentration with sodium-free IV fluids, such as 5% dextrose in water, and promoting sodium excretion with diuretics. Dietary sodium intake is often restricted. If the patient has an altered sensorium or is having seizures, initiate seizure precautions.

Monitor serum sodium levels, serum osmolality, and the patient's response to therapy. The serum sodium level should not decrease by more than 8 to 15 mEq/L in an 8-hour period.[2] Quickly reducing levels can cause a rapid shift of water back into the cells, resulting in cerebral edema and neurologic complications. This risk is greatest in the patient who developed hypernatremia over several days or longer.

HYPONATREMIA

Hyponatremia (low serum sodium) may result from a loss of sodium-containing fluids, water excess in relation to the amount of sodium (dilutional hyponatremia), or a combination of both (Table 16-4). Hyponatremia is usually associated with ECF hypoosmolality from the excess water. To restore balance, fluid shifts out of the ECF and into the cells, leading to cellular edema.

Common causes of hyponatremia from loss of sodium-rich body fluids include draining wounds, diarrhea, vomiting, and primary adrenal insufficiency. Inappropriate use of sodium-free or hypotonic IV fluids causes hyponatremia from water excess. This may occur in patients after surgery or major trauma or administering fluids to patients with renal failure. Patients with psychiatric disorders may have an excessive water intake. Syndrome of inappropriate antidiuretic hormone secretion (SIADH) results in dilutional hyponatremia caused by abnormal retention of water. See Chapter 49 for a discussion of the causes of SIADH.

Clinical Manifestations

The manifestations of hyponatremia are due to cellular swelling and first appear in the central nervous system (CNS). Mild hyponatremia has minor, nonspecific neurologic symptoms including headache, irritability, and difficulty concentrating. More severe hyponatremia can cause confusion, vomiting, seizures, and even coma. If hyponatremia is severe and develops rapidly, irreversible neurologic damage or death from brain herniation can occur.[4]

◆ NURSING AND INTERPROFESSIONAL MANAGEMENT: HYPONATREMIA

◆ Nursing Diagnoses

Nursing diagnoses and collaborative problems for the patient with hyponatremia include, but are not limited to, the following:

- Risk for electrolyte imbalance *related to* excess sodium loss and/or excess water intake or retention
- Risk for injury *related to* altered sensorium and decreased level of consciousness
- Risk for acute confusion *related to* electrolyte imbalance
- Potential complication: severe neurologic changes

◆ Nursing Implementation

Managing hyponatremia from fluid loss includes replacing fluid using isotonic sodium-containing solutions, encouraging oral intake, and withholding all diuretics.[2] In mild hyponatremia caused by water excess, fluid restriction is often the only treatment. The aim of the restriction is 500 mL less than the previous 24-hour urine output.[4] Loop diuretics and demeclocycline may be given. If hyponatremia is acute or more serious, small amounts of IV hypertonic saline solution (3% sodium chloride) can restore the serum sodium level while the body is returning to a normal water balance.

Vasopressor receptor antagonists (drugs that block the activity of ADH), are used to treat patients who cannot tolerate fluid restrictions or have more severe symptoms.[4] These drugs include conivaptan (Vaprisol) and tolvaptan (Samsca). Conivaptan is given IV to hospitalized patients with severe hyponatremia from water excess. Tolvaptan is an oral preparation used to treat hyponatremia from heart failure and SIADH.

Monitor serum sodium levels and the patient's response to therapy to avoid rapid or overcorrection. The level should not increase by more than 8 to 12 mEq/L in the first 24 hours.[4] Quickly increasing levels of sodium can cause osmotic demyelination syndrome with permanent damage to nerve cells in the brain. An accurate urine output record is essential. The patient may need a urinary catheter placed if unable to assist with monitoring output. If the patient has an altered sensorium or is having seizures, initiate seizure precautions.

POTASSIUM IMBALANCES

Potassium is the major ICF cation, with 98% of the body potassium being intracellular. For example, potassium concentration within muscle cells is around 140 mEq/L; potassium concentration in ECF is 3.5 to 5.0 mEq/L. The sodium-potassium pump in cell membranes maintains this concentration difference by pumping potassium into the cell and sodium out. Insulin helps by stimulating the sodium-potassium pump.

Because the ratio of ECF potassium to ICF potassium is the major factor in the resting membrane potential of nerve and muscle cells, neuromuscular and cardiac function are often affected by potassium imbalances. Potassium is involved with regulating intracellular osmolality and promoting cellular growth. It is required for glycogen to be deposited in muscle and liver cells. Potassium also plays a role in acid-base balance (discussed in the section on Acid-Base Regulation later in this chapter).

Diet is the source of potassium. The typical Western diet contains roughly 50 to 100 mEq of potassium daily, mainly from protein-rich foods and many fruits and vegetables. Many salt substitutes used in low-sodium diets contain substantial potassium. Patients may receive potassium from parenteral sources, including IV fluids; transfusions of stored, hemolyzed blood; and medications (e.g., potassium penicillin).

The kidneys are the primary route for potassium loss, eliminating about 90% of the daily potassium intake. Potassium excretion depends on the serum potassium level, urine output, and renal function. When serum potassium is high, urine potassium excretion increases and when serum levels are low, excretion decreases. Large urine output can cause excess potassium loss. Impaired kidney function can cause potassium retention. There is an inverse relationship between sodium and potassium reabsorption in the kidneys. Factors that cause sodium retention (e.g., low blood volume, hyponatremia, aldosterone secretion) cause potassium excretion.

HYPERKALEMIA

Hyperkalemia (high serum potassium) may result from impaired renal excretion, a shift of potassium from ICF to ECF, a massive intake of potassium, or a combination of these factors (Table 16-5). The most common cause of hyperkalemia is renal failure. Adrenal insufficiency with a subsequent aldosterone deficiency leads to potassium retention. Factors that cause potassium to move from ICF to ECF include acidosis, massive cell destruction (as in burn or crush injury, tumor lysis, severe infections), and intense exercise. In metabolic acidosis, potassium ions shift

TABLE 16-5 Potassium Imbalances: Causes and Manifestations

Hyperkalemia (K^+ >5.0 mEq/L [mmol/L])	Hypokalemia (K^+ <3.5 mEq/L [mmol/L])
Causes	
Excess Potassium Intake	***Potassium Loss***
• Excessive or rapid parenteral administration • Potassium-containing drugs (e.g., potassium penicillin) • Potassium-containing salt substitute	• *GI losses:* diarrhea, vomiting, fistulas, NG suction, ileostomy drainage • *Renal losses:* diuretics, hyperaldosteronism, magnesium depletion • *Skin losses:* diaphoresis • Dialysis
Shift of Potassium Out of Cells	***Shift of Potassium Into Cells***
• Acidosis • Tissue catabolism (e.g., fever, crush injury, sepsis, burns) • Intense exercise • Tumor lysis syndrome	• Increased insulin release (e.g., IV dextrose load) • Insulin therapy (e.g., with diabetic ketoacidosis) • Alkalosis • ↑ Epinephrine (e.g., stress)
Failure to Eliminate Potassium	***Lack of Potassium Intake***
• Renal disease • Adrenal insufficiency • *Medications:* Angiotensin II receptor blockers, ACE inhibitors, heparin, potassium-sparing diuretics, NSAIDs	• Starvation • Diet low in potassium • Failure to include potassium in parenteral fluids if NPO
Clinical Manifestations	
• Fatigue, irritability • Muscle weakness, cramps • Loss of muscle tone • Paresthesias, decreased reflexes • Abdominal cramping, diarrhea, vomiting • Confusion • Irregular pulse • Tetany	• Fatigue • Muscle weakness, leg cramps • Soft, flabby muscles • Paresthesias, decreased reflexes • Constipation, nausea, paralytic ileus • Shallow respirations • Weak, irregular pulse • Hyperglycemia
ECG Changes	***ECG Changes***
• Tall, peaked T wave • Prolonged PR interval • ST segment depression • Widening QRS • Loss of P wave • Ventricular fibrillation • Ventricular standstill	• Flattened T wave • Presence of U wave • ST segment depression • Prolonged QRS • Peaked P wave • Ventricular dysrhythmias • First- and second-degree heart block

ACE, Angiotensin-converting enzyme.

from ICF to ECF in exchange for hydrogen ions moving into the cell.

Digoxin-like drugs and β-adrenergic blockers (e.g., propranolol) can impair entry of potassium into cells, resulting in a higher ECF potassium concentration. Several drugs, such as heparin, potassium-sparing diuretics, angiotensin II receptor blockers (e.g., losartan), and angiotensin-converting enzyme (ACE) inhibitors (e.g., lisinopril), can contribute to hyperkalemia by reducing the kidney's ability to excrete potassium.[5]

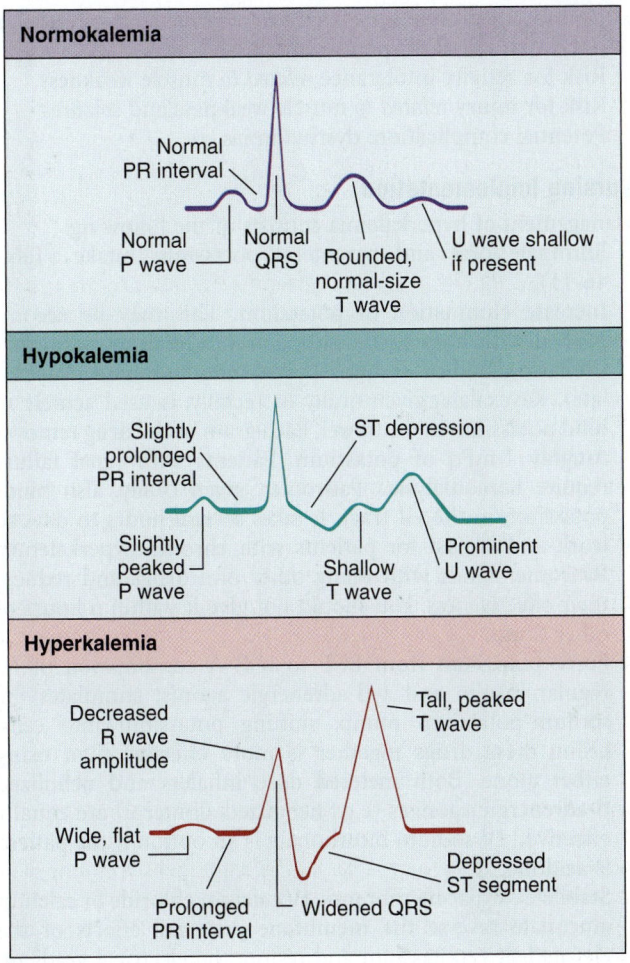

FIG. 16-14 ECG changes associated with alterations in potassium status.

Clinical Manifestations

The increased potassium concentration outside the cell changes the normal ECF and ICF ratio, resulting in increased cell excitability and changes in impulse transmission to the nerves and muscles. The most clinically significant problems are the disturbances in cardiac conduction. The initial finding is tall, peaked T waves. As potassium increases, cardiac depolarization decreases, leading to loss of P waves, a prolonged PR interval, ST segment depression, and widening QRS complex (Fig. 16-14). Heart block, ventricular fibrillation, or cardiac standstill may occur. Elevated potassium may cause failure to capture in a patient who has a pacemaker.[6]

The patient may experience fatigue, confusion, tetany, muscle cramps, paresthesias, and weakness. As potassium increases, loss of muscle tone and weakness or paralysis of other skeletal muscles, including the respiratory muscles can occur, leading to respiratory arrest. Abdominal cramping, vomiting, and diarrhea occur from hyperactivity of gastrointestinal smooth muscles.

❖ NURSING AND INTERPROFESSIONAL MANAGEMENT: HYPERKALEMIA

◆ Nursing Diagnoses

Nursing diagnoses and collaborative problems for the patient with hyperkalemia include, but are not limited to, the following.

- Risk for electrolyte imbalance *related to* excessive retention or cellular release of potassium
- Risk for activity intolerance *related to* muscle weakness
- Risk for injury *related to* muscle weakness and seizures
- Potential complication: dysrhythmias

Nursing Implementation

Management of hyperkalemia consists of the following:

1. Eliminate oral and parenteral potassium intake (Table 46-11).
2. Increase elimination of potassium. This may be accomplished with loop or thiazide diuretics, dialysis, patiromer (Veltassa), and/or sodium polystyrene sulfonate (Kayexalate). Kayexalate, given orally or rectally, is used acutely to bind potassium in the bowel. Each gram of the drug removes roughly 1 mEq of potassium. Patients with renal failure require hemodialysis.[6] Patiromer, given orally, also binds potassium in the GI tract. It takes several hours to days to work and is best for patients with chronic hyperkalemia. Patiromer binds with many other oral drugs and reduces their effectiveness. You should not give it within 6 hours of other drugs.
3. Force potassium from ECF to ICF. A combination of IV regular insulin and a β-adrenergic agonist stimulates the sodium-potassium pump, shifting potassium into cells. Using these drugs together is more effective than using either alone. Both metered dose inhalers and nebulized β-adrenergic agonists (e.g., nebulized albuterol) are equally effective.[5] IV sodium bicarbonate is an option if the patient is acidotic.
4. Stabilize cardiac membranes. IV calcium chloride or calcium gluconate reverse the membrane potential effects of the elevated ECF potassium and restore the electrical gradient. This protects the patient from life-threatening dysrhythmias.[6]

When the potassium elevation is mild and the kidneys are functioning, it may be sufficient to (1) withhold potassium from the diet and IV sources and (2) increase renal potassium elimination by administering fluids and loop or thiazide diuretics. Patients with severe hyperkalemia or symptomatic patients should receive one of the treatments to force potassium into cells.

Provide continuous ECG monitoring of all patients with clinically significant hyperkalemia to detect dysrhythmias and monitor the effects of therapy. The patient experiencing dangerous cardiac dysrhythmias should receive IV calcium immediately. Monitor BP because rapidly administering calcium can cause hypotension. When administering insulin, monitor for hypoglycemia and give glucose as needed.

HYPOKALEMIA

Hypokalemia (low serum potassium) can result from an increased loss of potassium, an increased shift of potassium from ECF to ICF, or rarely from deficient dietary potassium intake. The most common causes of hypokalemia are abnormal losses from either the kidneys or GI tract. GI tract losses are associated with diarrhea, laxative misuse, vomiting, and ileostomy drainage. Renal losses occur when a patient is diuresing or has a low magnesium level. Low plasma magnesium levels stimulate renin and aldosterone release, resulting in potassium excretion.

Among the factors causing potassium to move from ECF to ICF are insulin therapy, especially in conjunction with diabetic ketoacidosis, and β-adrenergic stimulation (catecholamine release in stress, coronary ischemia). Alkalosis can cause a shift of potassium into cells in exchange for hydrogen, lowering potassium in ECF and causing symptomatic hypokalemia.

Clinical Manifestations

Hypokalemia alters the resting membrane potential, resulting in hyperpolarization (an increased negative charge within the cell) and impaired muscle contraction. Therefore the manifestations of hypokalemia involve changes in cardiac and muscle function (Table 16-5).

The most serious clinical problems are cardiac changes, including impaired repolarization, resulting in a flattened T wave, depressed ST segment, and the presence of a U wave. The P waves peak and the QRS complex is prolonged (Fig. 16-14). There is an increased incidence of heart block and potentially lethal ventricular dysrhythmias.

As with hyperkalemia, skeletal muscle weakness and paresthesias may occur. Severe hypokalemia can cause paralysis. This usually involves the extremities but can involve the respiratory muscles, leading to shallow respirations and respiratory arrest. Alterations in smooth muscle function may lead to decreased GI motility (e.g., constipation, paralytic ileus). Finally, hypokalemia impairs insulin secretion, leading to glucose intolerance and hyperglycemia.

NURSING AND INTERPROFESSIONAL MANAGEMENT: HYPOKALEMIA

Nursing Diagnoses

Nursing diagnoses and collaborative problems for the patient with hypokalemia include, but are not limited to, the following:

- Risk for electrolyte imbalance *related to* excess potassium loss
- Risk for activity intolerance *related to* muscle weakness
- Risk for injury *related to* muscle weakness and hyporeflexia
- Potential complication: dysrhythmias

Nursing Implementation

Managing hypokalemia consists of oral or IV potassium chloride (KCl) supplements and increased dietary intake of potassium. Consuming potassium-rich foods can usually correct mild hypokalemia. Clinically significant hypokalemia requires administering oral or IV KCl.

SAFETY ALERT Administering IV KCl

- IV KCl must always be diluted and never given in concentrated amounts.
- Never give KCl via IV push or as a bolus.
- Invert IV bags containing KCl several times to ensure even distribution in the bag.
- Do not add KCl to a hanging IV bag to prevent giving a bolus dose.

IV KCl infusion rates should not exceed 10 mEq/hr unless the patient is in a critical care setting with continuous ECG monitoring and central line access for administration.[5] IV KCl must be given by infusion pump to ensure correct administration rate. Because KCl is irritating to the vein, assess IV sites at least hourly for phlebitis and infiltration. Infiltration can cause necrosis and sloughing of the surrounding tissue.

TABLE 16-6 Patient & Caregiver Teaching

Prevention of Hypokalemia

Include the following instructions when teaching at-risk patients how to prevent hypokalemia:

1. For all patients at risk:
   - Report the signs and symptoms of hypokalemia (Table 16-5) to the HCP.
   - Have serum potassium levels checked regularly.
   - Regularly include foods high in potassium in your diet (see Table 46-11).
   - Consume alcohol in moderation only.
   - Avoid consuming large amounts of licorice.
2. For patients taking oral potassium supplements:
   - Take the medication as prescribed to prevent overdosing.
   - Take the supplement with a full glass of water. Do not crush or chew tablets.

Patients who are critically ill and those at risk for hypokalemia should have continuous ECG monitoring to detect cardiac changes. Monitor serum potassium levels and urine output as appropriate.

CHECK YOUR PRACTICE

You are taking care of a 78-yr-old female patient with heart failure. She is taking furosemide (Lasix) and digitalis.

- What should you be alert for in a patient who takes both of these drugs?

KCl is usually given only if the urine output is at least 0.5 mL/kg of body weight per hour. Because patients on digoxin therapy have an increased risk of toxicity if their serum potassium level is low, monitor the patient for digitalis toxicity.

Teach patients ways to prevent hypokalemia (Table 16-6). Patients at risk for hypokalemia should have regular serum potassium levels monitored. Teach the patient taking digitalis to report signs and symptoms of digoxin toxicity immediately to the HCP.

CALCIUM IMBALANCES

Calcium is necessary for many metabolic processes. It is the major cation in bones and teeth. Calcium plays a role in blood clotting, transmission of nerve impulses, myocardial contractions, and muscle contractions. The source of calcium is dietary intake. Calcium absorption requires the active form of vitamin D. Vitamin D is obtained from foods or made in the skin by the action of sunlight on cholesterol.

The total body content of calcium is about 1200 g. The bones contain 99% of the body's calcium; the remainder is in plasma and body cells. Of the calcium in plasma, 50% is bound to plasma proteins, primarily albumin; 40% is in a free or ionized form, and the remainder is found bound with phosphate, citrate, or carbonate. The ionized or free calcium is biologically active. The serum pH influences how much calcium is ionized or bound to albumin. A decreased plasma pH (acidosis) decreases calcium binding to albumin, leading to more ionized calcium. An increased plasma pH (alkalosis) increases calcium binding, leading to decreased ionized calcium.

Serum calcium levels reflect the total level of all forms of plasma calcium. Serum albumin levels affect the interpretation of total calcium levels. Total calcium values increase or decrease directly with serum albumin levels. Ionized calcium levels are measured using special laboratory techniques or calculated using a formula. Albumin levels do not affect ionized calcium levels.

Parathyroid hormone (PTH) and calcitonin regulate calcium levels. Since the bones serve as a readily available store of calcium, the body is usually able to maintain normal serum calcium levels by regulating the movement of calcium into or out of the bone. Low serum calcium levels stimulate the parathyroid glands to produce and release PTH. PTH increases bone resorption (movement of calcium out of bones), increases GI absorption of calcium, and increases renal tubule reabsorption of calcium. High serum calcium levels stimulate the release of calcitonin from the thyroid gland. Calcitonin has the opposite effect of PTH. It lowers the serum calcium level by increasing calcium deposition into bone, increasing renal calcium excretion, and decreasing GI absorption.

HYPERCALCEMIA

Hypercalcemia (high serum calcium) is caused by hyperparathyroidism in about two thirds of persons. Malignancies, especially from hematologic, breast, and lung cancers, cause the remaining third. Malignancies lead to hypercalcemia through bone destruction from tumor invasion or tumor secretion of parathyroid-related proteins, which stimulate calcium release from bones.[7] More rare causes include thiazide diuretic use, prolonged immobilization, and increased calcium intake (e.g., use of calcium-containing antacids).

Excess calcium acts like a sedative, leading to reduced excitability of muscles and nerves. Neurologic manifestations begin with fatigue, lethargy, weakness, and confusion and progress to hallucinations, seizures, and coma. Disturbances in cardiac conduction can lead to dysrhythmias, including heart block and ventricular tachycardia. Table 16-7 lists the causes and manifestations of hypercalcemia.

❖ NURSING AND INTERPROFESSIONAL MANAGEMENT: HYPERCALCEMIA

◆ Nursing Diagnoses

Nursing diagnoses and collaborative problems for the patient with hypercalcemia include, but are not limited to, the following:

- Risk for electrolyte imbalance *related to* excessive bone destruction
- Risk for activity intolerance *related to* generalized muscle weakness
- Risk for injury *related to* neuromuscular and sensorium changes
- Potential complication: dysrhythmias

◆ Nursing Implementation

Management depends on the degree of hypercalcemia, patient's condition, and the underlying cause. Patients with mild hypercalcemia should stop any medications related to hypercalcemia, start a diet low in calcium, increase weight-bearing activity, and maintain adequate hydration. The patient must drink 3000 to 4000 mL of fluid daily to promote the renal excretion of calcium and decrease the chance of kidney stone formation. Fluids that promote urine acidity (cranberry or prune juice) will help to prevent formation of stones.

Managing severe hypercalcemia includes administering saline, a bisphosphonate, and calcitonin. Begin with hydrating

TABLE 16-7 Calcium Imbalances: Causes and Manifestations

Hypercalcemia (Ca^{2+} >10.2 mg/dL [2.55 mmol/L])	Hypocalcemia (Ca^{2+} <8.6 mg/dL [2.15 mmol/L])
Causes	
Increased Total Calcium	***Decreased Total Calcium***
• Hyperparathyroidism • Hematologic malignancy • Malignancies with bone metastasis • Prolonged immobilization • Vitamin A or D overdose • Paget's disease • Adrenal insufficiency • Thyrotoxicosis • Thiazide diuretics • Milk-alkali syndrome • Calcium-containing antacids • *Mycobacterium* infection	• Primary hypoparathyroidism • Renal insufficiency • Acute pancreatitis • Elevated phosphorus • Vitamin D deficiency, malnutrition • Magnesium deficiency • Bisphosphonates • Tumor lysis syndrome • Loop diuretics • Chronic alcoholism • Diarrhea • ↓ Serum albumin
Increased Ionized Calcium	***Decreased Ionized Calcium***
• Acidosis	• Alkalosis • Excess administration of citrated blood
Manifestations	
• Lethargy, weakness, fatigue • Decreased memory • Depressed reflexes • ↑ BP • Confusion, psychosis • Anorexia, nausea, vomiting • Bone pain, fractures • Polyuria, dehydration • Nephrolithiasis • Seizures, coma	• Weakness, fatigue • Depression, irritability, confusion • Hyperreflexia, muscle cramps • ↓ BP • Numbness and tingling in extremities and region around mouth • Chvostek's sign • Trousseau's sign • Laryngeal and bronchial spasms • Tetany, seizures
ECG Changes	***ECG Changes***
• Shortened ST segment • Shortened QT interval • Ventricular dysrhythmias • Increased digitalis effect	• Elongation of ST segment • Prolonged QT interval • Ventricular tachycardia

the patient with IV isotonic saline to maintain a urine output of 100 to 150 mL per hour.[8] IV saline therapy requires careful monitoring. Fluid overload can occur in patients who cannot excrete the excess sodium because of impaired renal function. Bisphosphonates (e.g., pamidronate, zoledronic acid) are the most effective agents in treating hypercalcemia, particularly when caused by a malignancy.[7] They interfere with the activity of osteoclasts, cells that break down bone. Because it takes 2 to 4 days for bisphosphonates to achieve maximum effect, patients receive IM or SC calcitonin for an immediate effect. Calcitonin rapidly increases renal calcium excretion. However, therapy is only effective for a few days and may cause tachycardia. Dialysis is an option in life-threatening situations.

HYPOCALCEMIA

Hypocalcemia (low serum calcium) can result from any condition associated with PTH deficiency. This may occur with surgical removal of a portion of or injury to the parathyroid glands during thyroid or neck surgery or with neck radiation. The patient who receives multiple blood transfusions can become

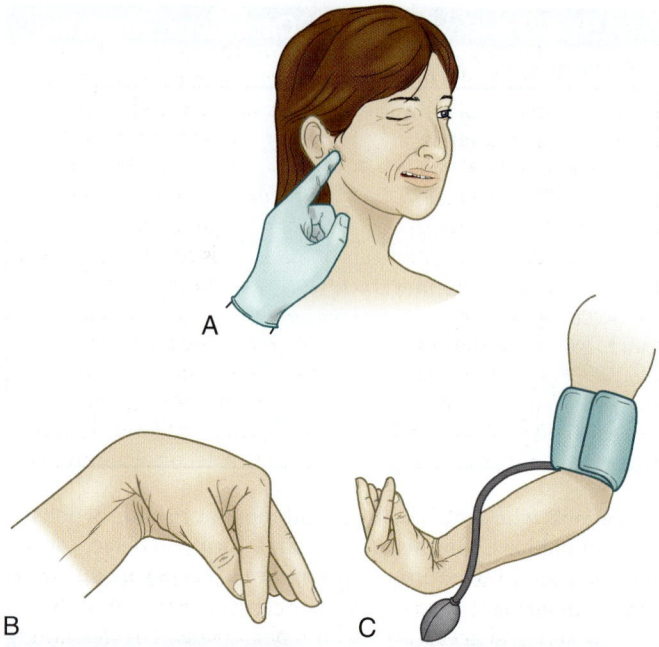

FIG. 16-15 Tests for hypocalcemia. **A,** Chvostek's sign is contraction of facial muscles in response to a light tap over the facial nerve in front of the ear. **B,** Trousseau's sign is a carpal spasm induced by **C,** inflating a BP cuff above the systolic pressure for a few minutes.

hypocalcemic because the citrate used to anticoagulate the blood binds with calcium, decreasing ionized calcium levels. Sudden alkalosis may result in symptomatic hypocalcemia despite a normal total serum calcium level. The high pH increases calcium binding to protein, decreasing the amount of ionized calcium. Table 16-7 lists causes and manifestations of hypocalcemia.

Low ionized calcium levels decrease the threshold for activating the sodium channels that cause cell membrane depolarization. This results in increased nerve excitability and sustained muscle contraction, or *tetany.* Clinical signs of tetany include Chvostek's sign and Trousseau's sign. *Chvostek's sign* is contraction of facial muscles in response to a tap over the facial nerve in front of the ear (Fig. 16-15, *A*). *Trousseau's sign* refers to carpal spasms induced by inflating a BP cuff on the arm (Fig. 16-15, *B* and *C*). When the cuff is inflated above the systolic pressure, carpal spasms occur within 3 minutes if hypocalcemia is present. Other manifestations of tetany are laryngeal stridor, dysphagia, paresthesia, and numbness and tingling around the mouth or in the extremities. Cardiac effects of hypocalcemia include decreased cardiac contractility and ECG changes. A prolonged QT interval may develop into ventricular tachycardia.

❖ NURSING AND INTERPROFESSIONAL MANAGEMENT: HYPOCALCEMIA

◆ Nursing Diagnoses

Nursing diagnoses and collaborative problems for the patient with hypocalcemia include, but are not limited to, the following:

- Risk for electrolyte imbalance *related to* decreased PTH level
- Ineffective breathing pattern *related to* laryngospasm
- Acute pain *related to* sustained muscle contractions
- Risk for injury *related to* tetany and seizures
- Potential complications: fracture, respiratory arrest

Nursing Implementation

Managing hypocalcemia depends on the underlying cause and the presence of symptoms. Treating mild or asymptomatic hypocalcemia involves a diet high in calcium-rich foods and calcium and vitamin D supplementation. Symptomatic hypocalcemia is treated with IV calcium gluconate.[9] Measures to promote CO_2 retention, such as breathing into a paper bag or sedating the patient, can control muscle spasm and other symptoms of tetany until the calcium level is corrected. Patients taking loop diuretics may need to change to thiazide diuretics to decrease urinary calcium excretion. Closely observe any patient who had thyroid or neck surgery in the immediate postoperative period for manifestations of hypocalcemia because of the proximity of the surgery to the parathyroid glands. Adequately treat pain and anxiety because hyperventilation-induced respiratory alkalosis can precipitate hypocalcemic symptoms.

PHOSPHATE IMBALANCES

Phosphorus is the primary anion in ICF and the second most abundant element in the body after calcium. Most phosphorus is in bones and teeth as calcium phosphate. The remaining phosphorus is metabolically active and essential to the function of muscle, red blood cells, and the nervous system. It is involved in the acid-base buffering system; the mitochondrial formation of ATP; cellular uptake and use of glucose; and carbohydrate, protein, and fat metabolism.

PTH maintains serum phosphorus levels and balance. Proper phosphate balance requires adequate renal functioning because the kidneys are the major route of phosphate excretion. When the phosphate level in the glomerular filtrate falls below normal or PTH levels are low, the kidneys reabsorb additional phosphorus. A reciprocal relationship exists between phosphorus and calcium. This means a low serum calcium level stimulates the release of PTH, decreasing reabsorption of phosphorus and lowering phosphorus levels.

HYPERPHOSPHATEMIA

Hyperphosphatemia (high serum phosphate) is common in patients with acute kidney injury or chronic kidney disease, which alters the kidney's ability to excrete phosphate. Other causes include excess phosphate intake from the use of phosphate-containing laxatives or enemas or a shift of phosphate from ICF to ECF. This may occur in patients with tumor lysis syndrome or rhabdomyolysis. Hypoparathyroidism and Vitamin D intoxication cause increased kidney phosphate reabsorption. Table 16-8 summarizes causes and clinical manifestations of hyperphosphatemia.

Hyperphosphatemia is often asymptomatic unless calcium binds with phosphate, leading to manifestations of hypocalcemia.[8] These manifestations include tetany, muscle cramps, paresthesias, and seizures. Long term, increased phosphate levels result in the development of calcified deposits outside of the bones. These calcium deposits can be found in soft tissues such as joints, arteries, skin, corneas, and kidneys and produce organ dysfunction, notably renal failure.

Managing hyperphosphatemia involves identifying and treating the underlying cause. Intake of foods and fluids high in phosphorus (e.g., dairy products) should be restricted. Oral phosphate-binding agents (e.g., calcium carbonate) limit intestinal phosphate absorption and increase phosphate secretion in the intestine. With severe hyperphosphatemia, hemodialysis may be used to rapidly decrease levels. Volume expansion and forced diuresis with a loop diuretic may increase phosphate excretion. If hypocalcemia is present, institute measures to correct calcium levels. See Chapter 46 for more information regarding treating hyperphosphatemia associated with kidney disease.

TABLE 16-8 Phosphate Imbalances: Causes and Manifestations

Hyperphosphatemia (PO_4^{3-} >4.4 mg/dL [1.42 mmol/L])	Hypophosphatemia (PO_4^{3-} <2.4 mg/dL [0.78 mmol/L])
Causes	
• Renal failure • Phosphate enemas (e.g., Fleet Enema) • Excessive ingestion (e.g., phosphate-containing laxatives) • Rhabdomyolysis • Tumor lysis syndrome • Thyrotoxicosis • Hypoparathyroidism • Sickle cell anemia, hemolytic anemia • Hyperthermia	• Malabsorption syndromes • Chronic diarrhea • Malnutrition, vitamin D deficiency • Parenteral nutrition • Chronic alcoholism • Phosphate-binding antacids • Diabetic ketoacidosis • Hyperparathyroidism • Refeeding syndrome • Respiratory alkalosis
Manifestations	
• Hypocalcemia • Numbness and tingling in extremities and region around mouth • Hyperreflexia, muscle cramps • Tetany, seizures • Calcium-phosphate precipitates in skin, soft tissue, cornea, viscera, blood vessels	• CNS depression (confusion, coma) • Muscle weakness, including respiratory muscle weakness • Polyneuropathy, seizures • Cardiac problems (dysrhythmias, heart failure) • Osteomalacia, rickets • Rhabdomyolysis

HYPOPHOSPHATEMIA

Hypophosphatemia (low serum phosphate) can result from decreased intestinal absorption, increased urinary excretion, or from ECF to ICF shifts. Malabsorption, diarrhea, and phosphate-binding antacids lead to decreased absorption. Phosphate shifts occur in respiratory alkalosis, treatment of diabetic ketoacidosis, and refeeding syndrome (reinstitution of nutrition to patients who are severely malnourished). Hypophosphatemia may occur in those who are malnourished or receive parenteral nutrition with inadequate phosphorus replacement. Table 16-8 lists causes and clinical manifestations of hypophosphatemia.

Most of the manifestations of hypophosphatemia result from impaired cellular energy and O_2 delivery due to low levels of cellular ATP and 2,3-diphosphoglycerate (2,3-DPG), an enzyme in RBCs that facilitates O_2 delivery to the tissues. Mild to moderate hypophosphatemia is often asymptomatic. Severe hypophosphatemia may be fatal because of decreased cellular function. Acute manifestations include CNS depression, muscle weakness and pain, respiratory failure, and heart failure. Chronic hypophosphatemia alters bone metabolism, resulting in rickets and osteomalacia.

Managing mild phosphorus deficiency involves increasing oral intake with dairy products or phosphate supplements. Dairy products are better tolerated because phosphate supplements are often associated with adverse GI effects.[10] Symptomatic hypophosphatemia can be fatal and usually requires IV administration of sodium phosphate or potassium phosphate.[8] Frequent monitoring is necessary during IV therapy as complications include hypocalcemia, hyperkalemia, hypotension, and dysrhythmias.

MAGNESIUM IMBALANCES

Magnesium, the second most abundant intracellular cation, plays an important role in essential cellular processes. It is a cofactor in many enzyme systems, including those responsible for carbohydrate metabolism, DNA and protein synthesis, blood glucose control, and BP regulation. Magnesium is required for the production and use of adenosine triphosphate (ATP), the energy source for the sodium-potassium pump. Muscle contraction and relaxation, normal neurologic function, and neurotransmitter release depend on magnesium.

About 50% to 60% of the body's magnesium is stored in muscle and bone; 30% is in cells. Only 1% is in ECF. The intestines and kidneys regulate magnesium levels. GI absorption increases when magnesium levels are low. The kidney regulates serum magnesium by controlling the amount of magnesium reabsorbed in the ascending loop of Henle and distal tubules.[8]

HYPERMAGNESEMIA

Hypermagnesemia (high serum magnesium level) usually occurs only with increased magnesium intake accompanied by renal insufficiency or failure. A patient with chronic kidney disease who ingests products containing magnesium (e.g., Maalox, milk of magnesia) will have a problem with excess magnesium. Magnesium excess could develop in a pregnant woman receiving magnesium sulfate for the treatment of eclampsia or in patients taking laxatives and antacids that contain magnesium. Table 16-9 lists the causes and manifestations of hypermagnesemia.

Excess magnesium inhibits acetylcholine release at the myoneural junction and calcium movement into cells, impairing nerve and muscle function. Initial manifestations include hypotension, facial flushing, lethargy, urinary retention, nausea, and vomiting. As the serum magnesium level increases, deep tendon reflexes are lost, followed by muscle paralysis and coma. Respiratory and cardiac arrest can occur.

Management begins with avoiding magnesium-containing drugs and limiting diet intake of magnesium-containing foods (e.g., green vegetables, nuts, bananas, oranges, peanut butter, chocolate). If renal function is adequate, increased fluids and diuretics promote urinary excretion. In the patient with impaired renal function, dialysis is required. If hypermagnesemia is symptomatic, giving IV calcium gluconate will oppose the effects of the excess magnesium on cardiac muscle.

TABLE 16-9 Magnesium Imbalances: Causes and Manifestations

Hypermagnesemia (Mg^+ >2.5 mEq/L [1.25 mmol/L])	Hypomagnesemia (Mg^+ <1.5 mEq/L [0.75 mmol/L])
Causes	
• Renal failure	• GI tract fluid losses (e.g., diarrhea, NG suction)
• IV administration of magnesium, especially for treatment of eclampsia	• Chronic alcoholism
• Tumor lysis syndrome	• Malabsorption syndromes
• Hypothyroidism	• Prolonged malnutrition
• Metastatic bone disease	• ↑ Urine output
• Adrenal insufficiency	• Hyperglycemia
• Antacids, laxatives	• Proton pump inhibitor therapy
Manifestations	
• Lethargy, drowsiness	• Confusion
• Muscle weakness	• Muscle cramps
• Urinary retention	• Tremors, seizures
• Nausea, vomiting	• Vertigo
• Diminished deep tendon reflexes	• Hyperactive deep tendon reflexes
• Flushed, warm skin, especially facial	• Chvostek's and Trousseau's signs
• ↓ Pulse, ↓ BP	• ↑ Pulse, ↑ BP, dysrhythmias

HYPOMAGNESEMIA

Hypomagnesemia (low serum magnesium level) occurs in patients with limited magnesium intake or increased gastrointestinal or renal losses. Causes of hypomagnesemia from insufficient food intake include prolonged fasting or starvation and chronic alcoholism. Another potential cause is prolonged parenteral nutrition without magnesium supplementation. Fluid loss from the GI tract, inflammatory bowel disease, and proton pump inhibitors interfere with magnesium absorption. Many diuretics and osmotic diuresis from high glucose levels may cause magnesium loss through increased urinary excretion.[11] Table 16-9 lists the causes and manifestations of hypomagnesemia.

Clinically, hypomagnesemia resembles hypocalcemia. Neuromuscular manifestations are common, such as muscle cramps, tremors, hyperactive deep tendon reflexes, Chvostek's sign, and Trousseau's sign. Neurologic manifestations include confusion, vertigo, and seizures.

Magnesium deficiency can lead to cardiac dysrhythmias, such as torsades de pointes and ventricular fibrillation. Hypomagnesemia is associated with digitalis toxicity.

Managing hypomagnesemia depends on the underlying cause and the patient's symptoms. Mild magnesium deficiencies involve oral supplements and increased dietary intake of foods high in magnesium. If hypomagnesemia is severe or if hypocalcemia is present, IV magnesium (e.g., magnesium sulfate) is given. Monitor vital signs and use an infusion pump, since rapid administration can lead to hypotension and cardiac or respiratory arrest.

ACID-BASE IMBALANCES

The body normally maintains a steady balance between the acids continually produced during normal metabolism and the bases that neutralize and promote the excretion of the acids. Because these acids alter the body's internal environment, their regulation is necessary to maintain homeostasis and acid-base balance. Many health problems may lead to acid-base imbalances. Patients with diabetes mellitus, chronic obstructive pulmonary disease, and kidney disease frequently develop acid-base imbalances.

Remember that an acid-base imbalance is not a disease but a symptom of an underlying health problem. Always consider the possibility of acid-base imbalance in patients with serious illnesses.

pH AND HYDROGEN ION CONCENTRATION

The acidity or alkalinity of a solution depends on its hydrogen ion (H^+) concentration. An increase in H^+ concentration leads

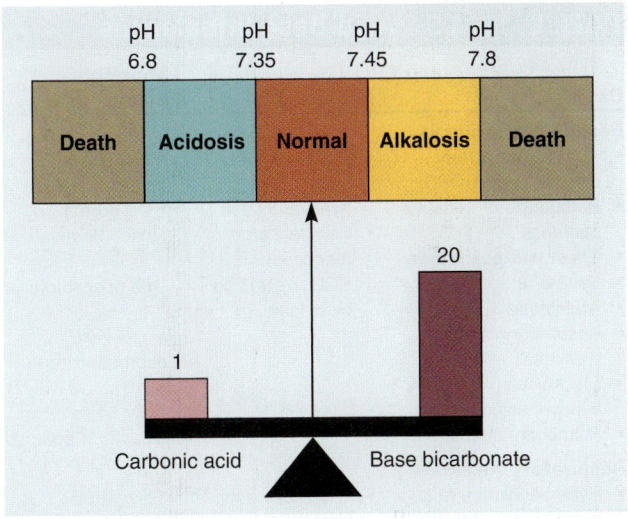

FIG. 16-16 The normal range of plasma pH is 7.35 to 7.45. A normal pH is maintained by a ratio of 1 part carbonic acid to 20 parts bicarbonate.

to acidity; a decrease leads to alkalinity. H^+ concentration is usually expressed as a negative logarithm (symbolized as *pH*). The use of the negative logarithm means that the lower the pH, the higher the H^+ concentration. In contrast to a pH of 7, a pH of 8 represents a 10-fold decrease in H^+ concentration.

The pH of a chemical solution may range from 1 to 14. A solution with a pH of 7 is considered neutral. An acid solution has a pH less than 7, and an alkaline solution has a pH greater than 7. Blood is slightly alkaline and has a normal arterial pH of 7.35 to 7.45. Medically, if the pH drops below 7.35, a person has **acidosis**. If the blood pH is greater than 7.45, the person has **alkalosis** (Fig. 16-16).

ACID-BASE REGULATION

The body uses three mechanisms to regulate acid-base balance and maintain the pH between 7.35 and 7.45. These are the buffer systems, respiratory system, and renal system. Each mechanism reacts at different speeds. Buffers are the fastest, reacting immediately. The respiratory system responds in minutes and reaches maximum effectiveness in hours. The renal response occurs hours to days after a change in pH, but the kidneys can maintain balance indefinitely in patients with chronic imbalances.

Buffer System

Buffering is the primary regulator of acid-base balance. **Buffers** act chemically to change strong acids into weaker ones or bind them to neutralize them. This minimizes the effect of acids on blood pH until their excretion from the body. Buffers can only maintain pH when the respiratory and renal systems function adequately.

All body fluids contain buffers. The major buffer system in ECF is carbonic acid–bicarbonate. Other buffers include phosphate, protein, and hemoglobin. The cell can act as a buffer by shifting H^+ in and out of the cell. When ECF levels of H^+ are increased, H^+ enters the cell in exchange for potassium. This may result in hyperkalemia. Conversely, with decreased H^+ levels, H^+ enters plasma in exchange for potassium. This is why alkalosis can cause hypokalemia.

A buffer consists of a weak acid, which releases H^+ when fluid is too alkaline, or a base and its salt, which takes up H^+ when fluid is too acidic. The carbonic acid–bicarbonate (H_2CO_3/HCO_3^-) buffer system neutralizes hydrochloric (HCl) acid in the following manner:

$$\underset{\text{Strong acid}}{HCl} + \underset{\text{Strong base}}{Na_2CO_3} \rightarrow \underset{\text{Salt}}{NaCl} + \underset{\text{Weak acid}}{H_2CO_3}$$

In this way, combining a strong acid with a strong base prevents the acid from making a large decrease in pH. The carbonic acid is broken down to H_2O and CO_2. The lungs excrete CO_2, either combined with insensible H_2O as carbonic acid, or alone as CO_2.

The phosphate, protein, and hemoglobin buffer systems act in the same way as the bicarbonate system. The main components of the phosphate system are monohydrogen phosphate (HPO_4^{2-}) and dihydrogen phosphate ($H_2PO_4^-$). A phosphate, combined with sodium, can neutralize a strong acid such as HCl, by forming sodium chloride (NaCl) and sodium biphosphate (NaH_2PO_4), a weak acid. If a strong base, such as sodium hydroxide (NaOH), is present, sodium biphosphate (NaH_2PO_4) neutralizes it to a weaker base (Na_2HPO_4) and H_2O.

Intracellular and extracellular proteins can act as acids or bases. Because the chemical structure of amino acids has an acid (the carboxyl group [COOH]) and a base (amine), they can accept H^+ if pH decreases or release H^+ if fluid is too alkaline. Some amino acids have basic radicals (NH_3OH [ammonium hydroxide]), which can dissociate into NH_3^+ (ammonia) and OH^- (hydroxide). The OH^- can combine with H^+ to form H_2O.

Hemoglobin is able to bind with both H^+, forming a weak acid, and CO_2, forming carbaminohemoglobin ($HbCO_2$). $HbCO_2$ dissociates in the lungs, releasing CO_2 for exhalation. Because H^+ can only combine with hemoglobin that has released its oxygen, hemoglobin less saturated with oxygen (venous blood) is a better buffer than saturated hemoglobin (arterial blood). Hemoglobin also assists in controlling pH by shifting chloride in and out of RBCs in exchange for bicarbonate.

The buffer system maintains a 20:1 ratio between HCO_3^- and carbonic acid in ECF. The body's ability to maintain this ratio is important in controlling pH. For example, excess carbonic acid increases the ratio and decreases pH, resulting in acidosis. In response, the body can increase HCO_3^- levels to keep the ratio 20:1 and maintain the pH near normal, a state called *compensation*. For example, a ratio of 40:2 would be present in compensated acid-base balance.

Respiratory System

The lungs help maintain a normal pH by excreting CO_2 and water, which are by-products of cellular metabolism. When released into the circulation, CO_2 enters RBCs and combines with H_2O to form H_2CO_3. This carbonic acid dissociates into H^+ and HCO_3^-. Hemoglobin buffers the free H^+, and the HCO_3^- diffuses into the plasma. This process is reversed in the pulmonary capillaries, forming CO_2 that is then excreted by the lungs. The overall reversible reaction is expressed in the following manner:

$$CO_2 + H_2O \rightarrow H_2CO_3 \rightarrow H_3 + HCO_3^-$$

The amount of CO_2 in the blood directly relates to carbonic acid concentration and subsequently to H^+ concentration. With increased respirations, more CO_2 is expelled and less remains in the blood. This leads to less carbonic acid and less H^+. With decreased respirations, more CO_2 remains in the blood. This leads to increased carbonic acid and more H^+.

The respiratory center in the medulla in the brainstem controls the rate of excretion of CO_2. If increased amounts of CO_2 or H^+ are present, the respiratory center stimulates an increased rate and depth of breathing to "blow off" CO_2 through hyperventilation. If the center senses low H^+ or CO_2 levels, respirations are inhibited and CO_2 retained. If a respiratory problem (e.g., respiratory failure) is the cause of an acid-base imbalance, the respiratory system loses ability to correct a pH alteration. The older adult has an impaired compensatory ability because of decreased respiratory function.

Renal System

Under normal conditions, the body depends on the kidneys to reabsorb and conserve all of the HCO_3^- they filter and excrete a portion of the acid produced by cellular metabolism. The three mechanisms of acid elimination are (1) secretion of small amounts of free hydrogen into the renal tubule, (2) combination of H^+ with ammonia (NH_3) to form ammonium (NH_4^+), and (3) excretion of weak acids.

The kidneys normally excrete acidic urine (average pH is 6). As a compensatory mechanism, the pH of the urine can decrease to 4 or increase to 8. To compensate for acidosis, the kidneys can reabsorb additional HCO_3^- and eliminate excess H^+. This increases the blood pH and decreases the urine pH. If the renal system is the cause of an acid-base imbalance (e.g., renal failure), it loses the ability to correct a pH alteration. In the older adult, the kidneys are less able to compensate for acid load.

ALTERATIONS IN ACID-BASE BALANCE

An acid-base imbalance results when there is an alteration in the ratio of 20:1 between base and acid content. This occurs when a disease or process alters one side of the ratio (e.g., CO_2 retention in pulmonary disease) and the compensatory processes that maintain the other side of the ratio (e.g., increased renal HCO_3^- reabsorption) either fail or are inadequate. The compensatory process may be inadequate because either the pathophysiologic process is overwhelming or there is insufficient time for the compensatory process to work.

Acid-base imbalances are classified as respiratory or metabolic. *Respiratory imbalances* result from the retention or an excess of CO_2 altering carbonic acid concentrations. *Metabolic imbalances* affect the base HCO_3^-. Acidosis occurs with an increase in carbonic acid (respiratory acidosis) or a decrease in HCO_3^- (metabolic acidosis). Alkalosis occurs with a decrease in carbonic acid (respiratory alkalosis) or an increase in HCO_3^- (metabolic alkalosis). Imbalances are further classified as acute or chronic. Chronic imbalances allow greater time for compensatory changes.

Respiratory Acidosis

Respiratory acidosis (carbonic acid excess) occurs whenever the person hypoventilates (Table 16-10). Hypoventilation leads to a buildup of CO_2, resulting in an accumulation of carbonic acid in the blood. Carbonic acid dissociates, releasing H^+ and decreasing pH. If CO_2 is not eliminated from the blood, acidosis results from the accumulation of carbonic acid (Fig. 16-17, *A*).

During acute respiratory acidosis, the renal compensatory mechanisms begin to operate within 24 hours. The kidneys conserve HCO_3^- and secrete increased concentrations of H^+ into the urine. Until the renal mechanisms have an effect, the serum HCO_3^- level will usually be normal, and then it will increase.

TABLE 16-10 Acid-Base Imbalances

Causes	Pathophysiology	Laboratory Findings
Respiratory Acidosis		
• Chronic respiratory disease (e.g., COPD) • Barbiturate or sedative overdose • Chest wall abnormality • Severe pneumonia • Atelectasis • Respiratory muscle weakness • Mechanical hypoventilation • Pulmonary edema	• ↑ CO_2 retention from hypoventilation • Compensatory response is ↑ HCO_3^- retention by kidney	↓ Plasma pH ↑ $PaCO_2$ HCO_3^- normal (uncompensated) ↑ HCO_3^- (compensated) *Sample ABG* Uncompensated: pH 7.31 $PaCO_2$ 54 mm Hg HCO_3^- 25 mEq/L
Respiratory Alkalosis		
• Hyperventilation (e.g., hypoxia, anxiety, fear, pain, exercise, fever) • Stimulated respiratory center (e.g., septicemia, stroke, meningitis, encephalitis, brain injury, salicylate poisoning) • Liver failure • Mechanical hyperventilation	• ↑ CO_2 excretion from hyperventilation • Compensatory response is ↑ HCO_3^- excretion by kidney	↑ Plasma pH ↓ $PaCO_2$ HCO_3^- normal (uncompensated) ↓ HCO_3^- (compensated) *Sample ABG* Uncompensated: pH 7.52 $PaCO_2$ 27 mm Hg HCO_3^- 24 mEq/L
Metabolic Acidosis		
• Diabetic ketoacidosis • Lactic acidosis • Starvation • Diarrhea • Renal tubular acidosis • Renal failure • Gastrointestinal fistulas • Shock	• Gain of fixed acid, inability to excrete acid or loss of base • Compensatory response is ↑ CO_2 excretion by lungs	↓ Plasma pH $PaCO_2$ normal (uncompensated) ↓ $PaCO_2$ (compensated) ↓ HCO_3^- *Sample ABG* Uncompensated: pH 7.29 $PaCO_2$ 38 mm Hg HCO_3^- 18 mEq/L
Metabolic Alkalosis		
• Vomiting • Nasogastric suctioning • Diuretic therapy • Hypokalemia • Excess $NaHCO_3$ intake • Mineralocorticoid use	• Loss of strong acid or gain of base • Compensatory response is ↑ CO_2 retention by lungs	↑ Plasma pH $PaCO_2$ normal (uncompensated) ↑ $PaCO_2$ (compensated) ↑ HCO_3^- *Sample ABG* Uncompensated: pH 7.50 $PaCO_2$ 40 mm Hg HCO_3^- 34 mEq/L

ABG, Arterial blood gas.

Respiratory Alkalosis

Respiratory alkalosis (carbonic acid deficit) occurs with hyperventilation, or an increase in respiratory rate or volume (Table 16-10). The primary cause of respiratory alkalosis is hypoxemia from acute pulmonary disorders (e.g., pneumonia, pulmonary embolus). Hyperventilation can occur as a physiologic response

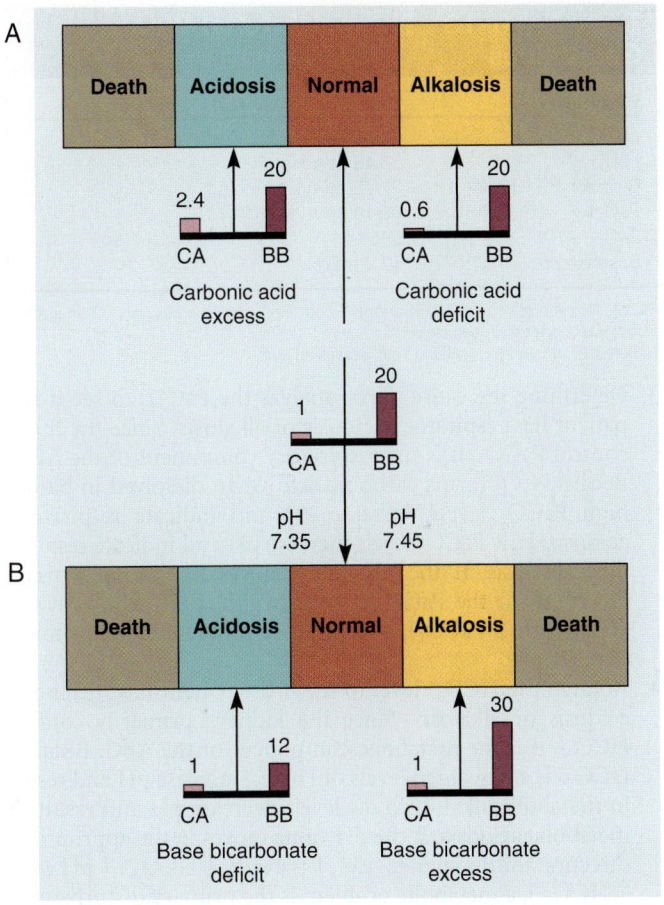

FIG. 16-17 Kinds of acid-base imbalances. **A,** Respiratory imbalances caused by carbonic acid (*CA*) excess and carbonic acid deficit. **B,** Metabolic imbalances caused by base bicarbonate (*BB*) deficit and base bicarbonate excess.

to metabolic acidosis and increased metabolic demands (e.g., fever). Pain, anxiety, and some CNS disorders can increase respirations without a physiologic need. The decrease in the arterial CO_2 level leads to decreased carbonic acid concentration in the blood and an increased pH (Fig. 16-17, *A*).

Compensated respiratory alkalosis is rare. In acute respiratory alkalosis, aggressive treatment of the cause of hypoxemia is essential and usually does not allow time for compensation to occur. Some buffering may occur with shifting of HCO_3^- into cells in exchange for chloride ions (Cl^-). In chronic respiratory alkalosis that occurs with pulmonary fibrosis or CNS disorders, compensation may include renal excretion of HCO_3^-.

Metabolic Acidosis

Metabolic acidosis (base bicarbonate deficit) occurs when an acid other than carbonic acid accumulates in the body or when bicarbonate is lost in body fluids (Table 16-10 and Fig. 16-17, *B*). Ketoacid accumulation in diabetic ketoacidosis and lactic acid accumulation with shock are examples of acid accumulation. Severe diarrhea results in loss of HCO_3^-. In renal disease, the kidneys lose their ability to reabsorb HCO_3^- and secrete H^+. To compensate for metabolic acidosis, the kidneys attempt to excrete additional acid and the lungs increase CO_2 excretion. The patient often develops *Kussmaul respirations* (deep, rapid breathing).

If metabolic acidosis is present, calculating the anion gap will help determine the source of the acidosis. The *anion gap* is the difference between the measured serum cations and anions in ECF. Calculate the anion gap using the following formula:

$$\text{Anion gap} = Na^+ - (HCO_3^- + Cl^-)$$

A normal anion gap is 8 to 12 mmol/L. The anion gap increases in metabolic acidosis associated with acid gain (e.g., lactic acidosis, diabetic ketoacidosis) but is normal in metabolic acidosis caused by bicarbonate loss (e.g., diarrhea).

Metabolic Alkalosis

Metabolic alkalosis (base bicarbonate excess) occurs when a loss of acid (e.g., from prolonged vomiting or gastric suction) or a gain in HCO_3^- (e.g., from ingestion of baking soda) occurs (Table 16-10 and Fig. 16-17, *B*). Renal excretion of HCO_3^- occurs in response to metabolic alkalosis. The lung's compensatory response is limited. The respiratory rate decreases in order to increase plasma CO_2. However, once hypoxemia occurs or plasma CO_2 reaches a certain level, stimulation of chemoreceptors increases respirations.

Mixed Acid-Base Disorders

A mixed acid-base disorder occurs when two or more disorders are present at the same time. The pH depends on the type, severity, and acuity of each disorder involved and any compensatory mechanisms at work. Respiratory acidosis combined with metabolic alkalosis (e.g., a patient with atelectasis and NG suction) may result in a near-normal pH, whereas respiratory acidosis combined with metabolic acidosis causes a greater decrease in pH than either disorder alone. An example of a mixed acidosis is a patient in severe shock with poor perfusion and hypoventilation. Mixed alkalosis can occur in a patient hyperventilating because of postoperative pain and losing acid secondary to NG suctioning.

CLINICAL MANIFESTATIONS OF ACID-BASE IMBALANCES

Clinical manifestations of acidosis and alkalosis are summarized in Tables 16-11 and 16-12. In both respiratory and metabolic acidosis, the CNS is depressed. Headache, lethargy, weakness, and confusion develop, leading eventually to coma and death. Compensatory mechanisms also produce specific clinical manifestations. For example, the deep, rapid respirations of a patient with metabolic acidosis occur with respiratory compensation.

In both types of alkalosis, symptoms usually result from an accompanying electrolyte abnormality rather than the alkalosis. Hypocalcemia occurs due to increased calcium binding with albumin, lowering the amount of ionized, active calcium. Therefore, muscle cramping, tingling and numbness of the fingers, and tetany occur. Once HCO_3^- levels are higher than 50 mEq/L, patients may develop seizures, hypoventilation, and coma.[12]

Blood Gas Values

Arterial blood gas (ABG) values provide objective information about a patient's acid-base status, the underlying cause of an imbalance, and the body's ability to regulate pH. Knowing the patient's clinical situation and the extent of renal and respiratory compensation allows you to identify acid-base disorders and the patient's ability to compensate. Blood gas analysis also

TABLE 16-11 Manifestations of Acidosis

Respiratory (↑ $PaCO_2$)	Metabolic (↓ HCO_3^-)
Neurologic	
Lethargy	Lethargy
Confusion	Confusion
Dizziness	Dizziness
Headache	Headache
Coma	Coma
Cardiovascular	
↓ BP	↓ BP
Ventricular fibrillation (related to hyperkalemia from compensation)	Dysrhythmias (related to hyperkalemia from compensation)
Warm, flushed skin	Cold, clammy skin
Gastrointestinal	
No significant findings	Nausea, vomiting, diarrhea, abdominal pain
Neuromuscular	
Seizures	Muscle weakness
Respiratory	
Hypoventilation with hypoxia	Deep, rapid respirations

TABLE 16-12 Manifestations of Alkalosis

Respiratory (↓ $PaCO_2$)	Metabolic (↑ HCO_3^-)
Neurologic	
Dizziness	Irritability
Light-headedness	Lethargy
Confusion	Confusion
Headache	Headache
Cardiovascular	
Tachycardia	Tachycardia
Dysrhythmias (related to hypokalemia from compensation)	Dysrhythmias (related to hypokalemia from compensation)
Gastrointestinal	
Nausea, vomiting, diarrhea	Nausea, vomiting
Epigastric pain	Anorexia
Neuromuscular	
Tetany	Tetany
Numbness	Tremors
Tingling of extremities	Tingling of fingers and toes
Hyperreflexia	Muscle cramps, hypertonic muscles
Seizures	Seizures
Respiratory	
Hyperventilation (lungs are unable to compensate if there is a respiratory problem)	Hypoventilation (compensatory action by lungs)

shows the partial pressure of arterial O_2 (PaO_2) and O_2 saturation. These values help you evaluate the patient's overall oxygenation status and identify hypoxemia.

To interpret the results of an ABG, perform the following six steps:

1. Look at each of the values. If the pH is between 7.35 and 7.45, and the CO_2, HCO_3^-, and PaO_2 are within normal limits, the ABGs are normal. If any value is out of normal, then continue.
2. Determine if the pH is acidotic or alkalotic. Values less than 7.35 are acidotic and values greater than 7.45 are alkalotic. A normal pH may indicate normal acid-base status, compensation is occurring, or a mixed disorder is present.

TABLE 16-13 Normal Arterial Blood Gas Values

Parameter	Reference Interval
pH	7.35-7.45
$PaCO_2$	35-45 mm Hg
Bicarbonate (HCO_3^-)	22-26 mEq/L (mmol/L)
PaO_2†	80-100 mm Hg
SaO_2	>95%
Base excess	±2.0 mEq/L

$PaCO_2$, Partial pressure of CO_2 in arterial blood; *PaO_2*, partial pressure of O_2 in arterial blood; *SaO_2*, arterial O_2 saturation.
†Decreases above sea level and with increasing age.

3. Determine the cause. First, analyze the $PaCO_2$ to see if the patient has respiratory acidosis or alkalosis. Since the lungs control $PaCO_2$, it is the respiratory component of the ABG. Because CO_2 forms carbonic acid when dissolved in blood, high $PaCO_2$ levels decrease pH and indicate respiratory acidosis. Low $PaCO_2$ levels increase pH and indicate respiratory alkalosis. If the pH value moves in the appropriate direction for the $PaCO_2$ change (e.g., ↓ pH with ↑ $PaCO_2$; ↑ pH with ↓ $PaCO_2$), a respiratory problem is the primary disturbance.
4. Analyze the HCO_3^- level to see if the patient has metabolic acidosis or alkalosis. Since the kidneys primarily control HCO_3^-, it is the metabolic component of the ABG. Because HCO_3^- is a base, high levels of HCO_3^- increase pH and result in metabolic alkalosis. Low levels decrease pH and result in metabolic acidosis. If the pH value moves in the appropriate direction for the change (e.g., ↓ pH with ↓ HCO_3^-; ↑ pH with ↑ HCO_3^-), a metabolic problem is the primary disturbance.
5. Determine if the patient is compensating or a mixed disorder is present. Look at the component (CO_2 or HCO_3^-) that is not the cause of the primary disturbance. If the component that does not match the pH is moving in the opposite direction, the body is attempting to compensate. For example, if the pH is slightly acidotic (7.33), the CO_2 is high (55 mm Hg), and the HCO_3^- is high (36 mEq/L), the CO_2 is the parameter that matches the acidotic pH. The patient's underlying acid-base imbalance is respiratory acidosis. The HCO_3^- level is alkalotic. Since this is in the opposite direction of respiratory acidosis, compensation is occurring. If both parameters match the pH, consider the possibility that a combined respiratory or metabolic acidosis or alkalosis is present. For example, if the pH is acidotic (7.28), the CO_2 is high (55 mm Hg), and the HCO_3^- is low (16 mEq/L), the patient's underlying acid-base imbalance is combined respiratory-metabolic acidosis.
6. Assess the PaO_2 and O_2 saturation. If these values are abnormal, hypoxemia is present.

Table 16-13 lists normal blood gas values. Table 16-14 explains how to analyze ABG results. The laboratory findings section of Table 16-10 provides ABG findings of the four major acid-base disturbances. Table 16-15 shows *ROME*, a quick memory device for understanding acid-base imbalances. See Chapter 25 for further discussion of ABGs.

ASSESSMENT OF FLUID, ELECTROLYTE, AND ACID-BASE IMBALANCES

Assessing patients for fluid, electrolyte, and acid-base imbalances is an important part of your nursing practice. In addition

TABLE 16-14 Arterial Blood Gas (ABG) Analysis

ABG Values	Analysis
pH 7.30 $PaCO_2$ 30 mm Hg HCO_3^- 16 mEq/L PaO_2 95 mm Hg on room air	1. The pH, $PaCO_2$, and HCO_3^- are abnormal. pH <7.35 indicates acidosis. 2. $PaCO_2$ is low, indicating respiratory alkalosis. 3. HCO_3^- is low, indicating metabolic acidosis. 4. HCO_3^- matches the pH, indicating metabolic acidosis is the primary problem. 5. The CO_2 is moving in the opposite direction, indicating the lungs are attempting to compensate for the metabolic acidosis. 6. PaO_2 is normal and does not indicate hypoxemia.

Interpretation
This ABG is interpreted as metabolic acidosis with partial compensation.

TABLE 16-15 ROME: Memory Device for Acid-Base Imbalances

For acid-base imbalances a quick memory device (mnemonic) can be used.

In ***Respiratory*** conditions, the pH and the $PaCO_2$ go in ***Opposite*** directions.
- In respiratory alkalosis, the pH is ↑ and the $PaCO_2$ is ↓.
- In respiratory acidosis, the pH is ↓ and the $PaCO_2$ is ↑.

In ***Metabolic*** conditions, the pH and the HCO_3^- go in the same direction (***Equal***). The $PaCO_2$ may also go in the same direction.
- In metabolic alkalosis, pH and HCO_3^- are ↑ and the $PaCO_2$ is ↑ or normal.
- In metabolic acidosis, pH and HCO_3^- are ↓ and the $PaCO_2$ is ↓ or normal.

		pH	$PaCO_2$
Respiratory			
Opposite	Acidosis	↓	↑
	Alkalosis	↑	↓
		pH	**HCO_3^-**
Metabolic			
Equivalent	Acidosis	↓	↓
	Alkalosis	↑	↑

to assessing for the clinical manifestations presented earlier in this chapter, obtain subjective and objective data from any patient with suspected fluid, electrolyte, or acid-base imbalances as discussed below.

Subjective Data

Important Health Information

Past Health History. Question the patient about any history of problems involving the kidneys, heart, GI system, or lungs that could affect the present fluid, electrolyte, and acid-base balance. Obtain information about specific diseases such as diabetes mellitus, diabetes insipidus, chronic obstructive pulmonary disease, renal failure, ulcerative colitis, and Crohn's disease. Ask the patient about any prior fluid, electrolyte, or acid-base disorders.

Medications. Assess the patient's current and past use of medications. The ingredients in many drugs, especially over-the-counter drugs, are often hidden sources of sodium, potassium, calcium, magnesium, and other electrolytes. Many prescription drugs, including diuretics, corticosteroids, and electrolyte supplements, can cause fluid and electrolyte imbalances.

Surgery or Other Treatments. Ask the patient about past or present renal dialysis, kidney surgery, or bowel surgery resulting in a temporary or permanent external collecting system such as an ileostomy.

Functional Health Patterns

Health Perception–Health Management Pattern. If the patient is currently experiencing a problem related to fluid, electrolyte, and acid-base balance, obtain a careful description of the illness, including onset, course, and treatment. Question the patient about any recent changes in body weight.

Nutritional-Metabolic Pattern. Ask the patient about diet and any special dietary practices. Weight reduction diets, fad diets, or any eating disorders, such as anorexia or bulimia, can lead to fluid and electrolyte problems. If the patient is on a special diet, such as low sodium or high potassium, assess the ability to adhere to the dietary prescription.

Elimination Pattern. Make note of the patient's usual bowel and bladder habits. Carefully document any deviations from the expected elimination pattern, such as diarrhea, oliguria, polyuria, or incontinence.

Activity-Exercise Pattern. Ask about the patient's exercise pattern and any complaints of excessive perspiration. Determine if the patient is exposed to extremely high temperatures during leisure or work activity. Ask the patient what he or she does to replace fluid and electrolytes lost through excessive perspiration. Assess the patient's activity level to determine any functional problems that could lead to lack of ability to obtain food or fluids.

Cognitive-Perceptual Pattern. Ask about any changes in sensations, such as numbness, tingling, or muscle weakness, which could indicate a fluid and electrolyte problem. Ask the patient and caregiver if there have been any changes in mentation or alertness, such as confusion, memory impairment, or lethargy.

Objective Data

Physical Examination. A complete physical examination is needed because fluid, electrolyte, and acid-base balance affects all body systems. As you assess each system, check for manifestations that you would expect with an imbalance. Common abnormal assessment findings of major body systems offer clues to possible imbalances (Table 16-16).

Laboratory Values. Assessing serum electrolyte values is a good starting point for evaluating fluid and electrolyte balance (Table 16-1). Serum electrolytes can also provide important information about a patient's acid-base balance. Changes in the serum HCO_3^- (often reported as total CO_2 or CO_2 content on an electrolyte panel) indicate metabolic acidosis (low HCO_3^- level) or alkalosis (high HCO_3^- level).

SAFETY ALERT Managing Critical Test Results
- Promptly report critical laboratory values to the HCP.
- Assess the patient and initiate appropriate actions (e.g., ECG monitoring).

Remember serum electrolyte values often provide limited information. They reflect the concentration of that electrolyte in ECF but not necessarily in ICF. For example, most potassium is found in the cells. Changes in serum potassium values may be the result of a true deficit or excess of potassium or reflect the movement of potassium into or out of the cell during acid-base imbalances. An abnormal serum sodium level may reflect a sodium problem or, more likely, a water problem.

Other useful laboratory tests include serum and urine osmolality, serum glucose, blood urea nitrogen, serum creatinine, venous blood gas sampling, urine specific gravity, and urine electrolytes.

TABLE 16-16 Assessment Abnormalities

Fluid and Electrolyte Imbalances

Finding	Possible Etiology
Skin	
Poor skin turgor	Fluid volume deficit
Cold, clammy skin	Fluid volume deficit, Na^+ deficit
Pitting edema	Fluid volume excess
Flushed, dry skin	Na^+ excess, Mg^{2+} excess
Pulse	
Bounding pulse	Fluid volume excess
Rapid, weak, thready pulse	Fluid volume deficit
Weak, irregular, rapid pulse	Severe K^+ deficit, Mg^{2+} deficit
Weak, irregular, slow pulse	Severe K^+ excess, Mg^{2+} excess
Blood Pressure	
Hypotension	Fluid volume deficit, Ca^{2+} deficit, Mg^{2+} excess
Hypertension	Fluid volume excess, Ca^{2+} excess, Mg^{2+} deficit
Respirations	
Rapid respirations	Fluid volume deficit
Shortness of breath	Fluid volume excess
Moist crackles	Fluid volume excess
Restricted airway	Ca^{2+} deficit, PO_4^{3-} excess
Skeletal Muscles	
Muscle cramping	K^+ excess , Ca^{2+} deficit, PO_4^{3-} excess, Mg^{2+} deficit
Muscle weakness	K^+ excess, K^+ deficit, Ca^{2+} excess, PO_4^{3-} deficit, Mg^{2+} excess
Trousseau's sign	Ca^{2+} deficit, Mg^{2+} deficit, PO_4^{3-} excess
Chvostek's sign	Ca^{2+} deficit, Mg^{2+} deficit, PO_4^{3-} excess
Neurologic	
Tremors, seizures	Na^+ excess, K^+ excess, Ca^{2+} deficit, PO_4^{3-} excess, Mg^{2+} deficit
Irritability	Na^+ deficit, K^+ excess, Ca^{2+} deficit, PO_4^{3-} excess
Fatigue	Fluid volume deficit, K^+ deficit, Ca^{2+} excess
Confusion	Fluid volume excess, Na^+ deficit, K^+ excess, K^+ deficit, Ca^{2+} excess, Mg^{2+} excess, Mg^{2+} deficit, PO_4^{3-} deficit
Decreased level of consciousness	Fluid volume deficit, fluid volume excess, Na^+ excess, Na^+ deficit, PO_4^{3-} deficit

ORAL FLUID AND ELECTROLYTE REPLACEMENT

In all cases of fluid, electrolyte, and acid-base imbalances, the primary treatment involves correcting the underlying cause. Oral rehydration solutions containing water, potassium, sodium, and glucose may be used to correct mild fluid and electrolyte deficits. Glucose not only provides calories, but also promotes sodium and water absorption in the small intestine. Commercial oral rehydration solutions are now available for home use. Cola drinks are avoided because they do not contain adequate electrolyte replacement and the sugar content may lead to osmotic diuresis.

IV FLUID AND ELECTROLYTE REPLACEMENT

IV fluid and electrolyte therapy is necessary to treat many different fluid and electrolyte imbalances. Many patients need maintenance IV fluid therapy when they cannot take oral fluids (e.g., during and after surgery). Other patients need corrective or replacement therapy for losses that are ongoing or have already occurred. The amount and type of solution is determined by the normal daily maintenance requirements and by imbalances identified by laboratory results. IV replacement solutions are classified by their concentration or tonicity (Table 16-17). Tonicity is an important factor in determining the appropriate solution to correct imbalances.

Solutions

Hypotonic. A hypotonic solution has more water than electrolytes, with an osmolality of less than 250 mOsm/kg.[13] Infusing a hypotonic solution dilutes ECF, lowering serum osmolality. Osmosis then produces a movement of water from ECF to interstitial spaces and cells, causing cells to swell. After achieving equilibrium, ICF and ECF have the same osmolality. Hypotonic solutions (e.g., 0.45% NaCl) are useful in treating patients with hypernatremia and are a good maintenance fluid because normal daily losses are hypotonic. They are not good for replacement because they can deplete ECF and lower BP. Because hypotonic solutions have the potential to cause cellular swelling, monitor patients for changes in mentation that may indicate cerebral edema.[13]

Although 5% dextrose in water is technically an isotonic solution, the dextrose quickly metabolizes. The net result is the administration of hypotonic free water with equal expansion of ECF and ICF. One liter of a 5% dextrose solution provides 50 g of dextrose, or 170 calories. While this amount of dextrose is not enough to meet caloric requirements, it helps prevent ketosis associated with starvation.

Isotonic. An isotonic solution has a similar concentration of water and electrolytes to plasma, with an osmolality of 250 to 375 mOsm/L.[13] Because of the similarity, administering an isotonic solution expands only ECF, and the fluid does not move into cells. This makes isotonic solutions the ideal fluid replacement for patients with ECF volume deficits. Examples of isotonic solutions include 0.9% NaCl and lactated Ringer's solution.

Isotonic saline (0.9% NaCl) or *normal saline* has a sodium concentration (154 mEq/L) somewhat higher than that of plasma (135 to 145 mEq/L) and a chloride concentration (154 mEq/L) significantly higher than the plasma chloride level (96 to 106 mEq/L). Therefore excessive administration of isotonic saline has the potential to increase sodium and chloride levels. Isotonic saline is used when a patient has experienced both fluid and sodium losses (e.g., diarrhea, vomiting). It is the fluid of choice for replacement.[13]

Lactated Ringer's solution contains sodium, potassium, chloride, calcium, and lactate (the precursor of bicarbonate) in about the same concentrations as ECF. This makes it the ideal fluid in certain situations, such as surgery, burns, or GI fluid losses. Patients with liver dysfunction, hyperkalemia, and severe hypovolemia should not receive lactated Ringer's because they have a decreased ability to convert lactate to bicarbonate.

Hypertonic. A hypertonic solution initially raises the osmolality of ECF and expands volume. The higher osmotic pressure draws water out of the cells into ECF. It is useful in the treatment of hyponatremia and trauma patients with head injury. Hypertonic solutions require frequent monitoring of BP, lung sounds, and serum sodium levels because of the risk for intravascular fluid volume excess.

Although concentrated dextrose and water solutions (10% dextrose or greater) are hypertonic solutions, once the dextrose

TABLE 16-17 Commonly Used Crystalloid Solutions

Solution	Tonicity	mOsm/kg	Contents	Indications and Considerations
Dextrose in Water				
5%	Isotonic, but physiologically hypotonic	278	50 g/L dextrose	• Contains free water only, no electrolytes • Provides 170 cal/L • Used to replace water losses and treat hypernatremia
10%	Hypertonic	556	100 g/L dextrose	• Contains free water only, no electrolytes • Provides 340 cal/L • Used with parenteral nutrition
Saline				
0.45%	Hypotonic	154	77 mEq/L Na^+ 77 mEq/L Cl^-	• Contains free water, Na^+ and Cl^-, no calories • Used to treat hypernatremia and uncontrolled hyperglycemia • Used as a maintenance solution
0.9%	Isotonic	308	154 mEq/L Na^+ 154 mEq/L Cl^-	• Contains Na^+ and Cl^- in excess of plasma levels • Does not contain free water or calories • Used to expand intravascular volume and replace extracellular fluid losses • Only solution that may be administered with blood products • May cause volume overload in patients with cardiac or renal disease
3.0%	Hypertonic	1026	513 mEq/L Na^+ 513 mEq/L Cl^-	• Contains Na^+ and Cl^- in excess of plasma levels • Used to treat symptomatic hyponatremia and trauma patients with head injury • Administer slowly because it may cause volume overload and pulmonary edema
Dextrose in Saline				
5% in 0.25%	Isotonic	355	50 g/L dextrose 34 mEq/L Na^+ 34 mEq/L Cl^-	• Provides Na^+, Cl^-, and free water • Used to replace hypotonic losses and treat hypernatremia • Provides 170 cal/L
5% in 0.45%	Hypertonic	432	50 g/L dextrose 77 mEq/L Na^+ 77 mEq/L Cl^-	• Provides Na^+, Cl^-, and free water • Used as a maintenance solution
5% in 0.9%	Hypertonic	586	50 g/L dextrose 154 mEq/L Na^+ 154 mEq/L Cl^-	• Contains Na^+ and Cl^- in excess of plasma levels • Used to treat metabolic alkalosis and volume deficits in patients with hyponatremia
Multiple Electrolyte Solutions				
Ringer's solution	Isotonic	309	147 mEq/L Na^+ 156 mEq/L Cl^- 4 mEq/L K^+ 4 mEq/L Ca^{2+}	• Similar in composition to plasma except that it has excess Cl^-, no Mg^{2+}, no HCO_3^- • Does not provide free water or calories • Used to expand the intravascular volume and replace extracellular fluid losses
Lactated Ringer's (Hartmann's) solution	Isotonic	273	130 mEq/L Na^+ 109 mEq/L Cl^- 4 mEq/L K^+ 3 mEq/L Ca^{2+} 28 mmol/L lactate	• Similar in composition to normal plasma except does not contain Mg^{2+} • Does not provide free water or calories • Used to treat hypovolemia, burns, and GI fluid losses • Cannot be used in patients with alkalosis or lactic acidosis

is metabolized, the net result is the administration of water. This free water ultimately expands ECF and ICF. The primary use of these solutions is providing calories as part of parenteral nutrition (see Chapter 39). You may administer solutions containing 10% dextrose or less through a peripheral line. You must use a central line to administer solutions with dextrose concentrations greater than 10%.

IV Additives. Additives in basic IV solutions replace specific losses. KCl, $CaCl_2$, $MgSO_4$, and HCO_3^- are common additives. The use of each was described earlier in the discussion of the specific electrolyte deficiencies. Many premixed IV solutions containing specific additives are available. Using these solutions reduces error as the solution contains the correct amount of the electrolyte in the proper volume and type of IV solution.

Colloids. Colloids solutions contain large molecules that increase oncotic pressure and pull fluid into the blood vessels. Because this action restores blood volume, colloids are also called volume expanders or plasma expanders. Colloids include human plasma products (albumin, fresh frozen plasma, blood) and semisynthetics (dextran, starches).

Albumin is available in 5% and 25% solutions. The 5% solution has an albumin concentration similar to plasma and results in plasma volume expansion equal to the volume infused. This makes the 5% concentration ideal for treating hypovolemic patients. In contrast, 25% albumin solution is hypertonic and draws fluid from the interstitial space. This makes it useful in treating patients with burns, hepatic failure, and ascites.

Dextrans are synthetic complex sugar solutions. There are two types: low-molecular-weight dextran (dextran 40) and high-molecular-weight dextran (dextran 70). Because dextran metabolizes slowly, it remains in the vascular system for a prolonged period. It pulls additional fluid into the intravascular space, expanding it by more volume than what is infused. Hydroxylethyl starches (e.g., Hespan) are synthetic colloids that work similarly to dextran to expand plasma volume.

Colloids can lead to circulatory overload because they pull fluid into ECF. Monitor vital signs and urine output frequently and assess for signs and symptoms of fluid volume excess. All colloids affect blood coagulation, with dextran and starches having the strongest anticoagulation effect. Monitor coagulation times and implement any necessary precautions. Fatal anaphylactic reactions have occurred with Hespan and dextran. Monitor the patient closely for a hypersensitivity reaction and discontinue an infusion immediately if a reaction occurs.

If the patient has lost blood, whole blood or packed RBCs are necessary. Packed RBCs have the advantage of giving the patient primarily RBCs rather than RBCs and fluid volume. Although packed RBCs have a decreased plasma volume, they increase the oncotic pressure and pull fluid into the intravascular space. The use of whole blood, with its additional fluid volume, may cause circulatory overload, particularly in patients who are susceptible to complications from excess circulating volume (e.g., heart failure). To prevent fluid volume excess, loop diuretics may be administered with blood and colloids. See Chapter 30 for more information on the administration of blood and blood products.

TEAMWORK & COLLABORATION

IV Therapy

Although many states permit licensed practical nurses (LPNs) to administer IV fluids and drugs, the registered nurse (RN) should administer IV fluids or medications to unstable or critically ill patients.

Role of Nursing Personnel

Registered Nurse (RN)

- Assess patient for clinical manifestations of fluid and electrolyte disturbances.
- Determine if ordered IV therapies are appropriate.
- Choose and insert appropriate IV catheters and infusion devices.
- Administer IV fluids and medications to unstable and critically ill patients.
- Evaluate patient for clinical manifestations of fluid overload or hypovolemia and initiate appropriate changes in IV fluids.
- Evaluate if IV therapies are addressing patient's fluid and electrolyte needs.

Licensed Practical/Vocational Nurse (LPN/LVN)

- Administer IV fluids and medications to stable patients (consider state nurse practice act and agency policy).
- Adjust IV flow rate for stable patients according to HCP orders (consider state nurse practice act and agency policy).
- Insert IV catheters (consider state nurse practice act and agency policy).
- Monitor for clinical manifestations of adverse reactions to IV fluids or medications.

Unlicensed Assistive Personnel (UAP)

- Measure and record oral intake and output.
- Report swelling or redness at IV site or patient complaints of discomfort at IV site to RN.

Role of Other Team Members

Pharmacist

- Determine appropriateness of IV therapies and need for dose adjustments.
- Prepare IV infusions and medications.
- Screen for potential problems, such as compatibility issues.
- Monitor response to therapy.

CENTRAL VENOUS ACCESS DEVICES

Central venous access devices (CVADs) are catheters placed in large blood vessels (e.g., subclavian vein, jugular vein) of people who require frequent or special access to the vascular system. There are three main types of CVADs: centrally inserted catheters, peripherally inserted central catheters (PICCs), and implanted ports.

Advantages of CVADs include immediate access to the central venous system, a reduced need for multiple venipunctures, and decreased risk of extravasation injury. CVADs permit frequent, continuous, rapid, or intermittent administration of fluids and medications. They allow for the administration of drugs that are potential *vesicants* (agents that can cause tissue damage), blood and blood products, and parenteral nutrition. CVADs can provide a means to perform hemodynamic monitoring and obtain venous blood samples. They are useful with patients who have limited peripheral vascular access or who have a projected need for long-term vascular access. CVADs can also be used for injections of radiopaque contrast media. Table 16-18 provides examples of conditions where CVADs are used.

The major disadvantages of CVADs are an increased risk of systemic infection and the invasiveness of the procedure. Extravasation (leakage of fluid) can still occur if there is displacement of or damage to the device.

Centrally Inserted Catheters

The tip of centrally inserted catheters (also called central venous catheters [CVCs]) rests in the distal end of the superior vena cava near its junction with the right atrium (Fig. 16-18). The other end of the catheter exits through a separate incision on the chest or abdominal wall. *Nontunneled catheters* are usually placed in the subclavian or internal jugular vein, more rarely in the femoral vein. They are best for patients with short-term needs in an acute care setting. *Surgically placed tunneled catheters* (e.g., Hickman) are suitable for long-term needs. Tunneling of the catheter through subcutaneous tissue and the synthetic cuff used to anchor the catheter provide stability and decrease infection risk. After the site heals, the catheter does not require a dressing, making it easier for the patient to maintain the site at home.

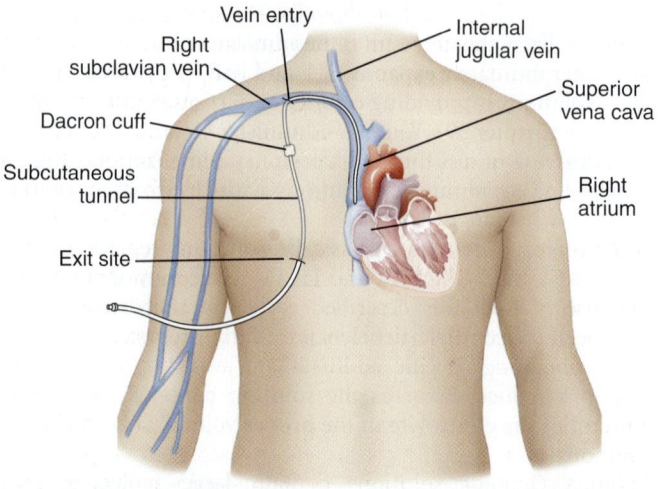

FIG. 16-18 Tunneled central venous catheter. Note tip of the catheter in the superior vena cava.

TABLE 16-18 Indications for Central Venous Access Devices (CVADs)*

Condition	Indications for Use
Medication administration	
• Cancer	• Chemotherapy, infusion of irritating or vesicant medications
• Infection	• Long-term administration of antibiotics
• Pain	• Long-term administration of pain medication
• Drugs at risk for causing phlebitis	• Epoprostenol (Flolan) • Calcium chloride • Potassium chloride • Amiodarone (Cordarone)
Nutritional replacement	• Infusion of parenteral nutrition • Infusion of high percentage dextrose solutions
Blood samples	• Multiple blood draws for diagnostic tests over time
Blood transfusions	• Infusion of blood or blood products
Renal failure	• Perform hemodialysis (especially on an acute basis) or continuous renal replacement therapy
Shock, burns	• Infusion of high volumes of fluid and electrolyte replacement
Hemodynamic monitoring	• Used to measure central venous pressure to assess fluid balance
Heart failure	• Perform ultrafiltration
Autoimmune disorders	• Perform plasmapheresis

*This list is not all-inclusive, and these are examples only.

CVCs are available with single-, double-, triple-, or quad-lumens. Multi-lumen catheters are useful in the critically ill patient because each lumen can be simultaneously used to provide a different therapy. For example, incompatible drugs infuse in separate lumens without mixing while a third lumen provides access for blood sampling.

Peripherally Inserted Central Catheters

Peripherally inserted central catheters (PICCs) are central venous catheters inserted into a vein in the arm. The basilic vein is preferred because of its large diameter (Fig. 16-19). The cephalic, median cubital, or brachial veins are other options. Single-, double-, or triple-lumens are available; double lumens are preferred, because they allow for simultaneous uses. PICCs are used with patients who need vascular access for 1 week to 6 months, but they can be in place for longer periods.

Advantages of a PICC over a CVC are lower infection rate, fewer insertion-related complications, decreased cost, and ability to insert at the bedside or in an outpatient area. PICCs, however, are associated with an increased risk of deep vein thrombosis and phlebitis (Table 16-19). If phlebitis occurs, it usually happens within 7 to 10 days after insertion. Do not use the arm with the PICC to obtain a BP reading or draw blood. When the BP cuff is inflated, the PICC can touch the vein wall, increasing the risk of vein damage and thrombosis.

Implanted Infusion Ports

An implanted infusion port consists of a surgically implanted central venous catheter connected to a reservoir or port (Fig. 16-20, *A*). The catheter tip lies in the desired vein. The port lies in a surgically created subcutaneous pocket on the upper chest or arm. It consists of a titanium or plastic reservoir covered with a self-sealing silicone septum. You access the port by using a special noncoring needle with a deflected tip. This prevents damage to the septum that could make the port useless (Fig. 16-20, *B*).

Drugs are placed in the reservoir either by a direct injection or through injection into an established IV line. The reservoir then slowly releases the medicine into the bloodstream. Implanted ports are good for long-term therapy and have a low risk of infection. The hidden port offers the patient cosmetic advantages and overall has less maintenance than other types of CVADs. Monitor accessed ports for infiltration that can occur if the needle is not in place or dislodges.

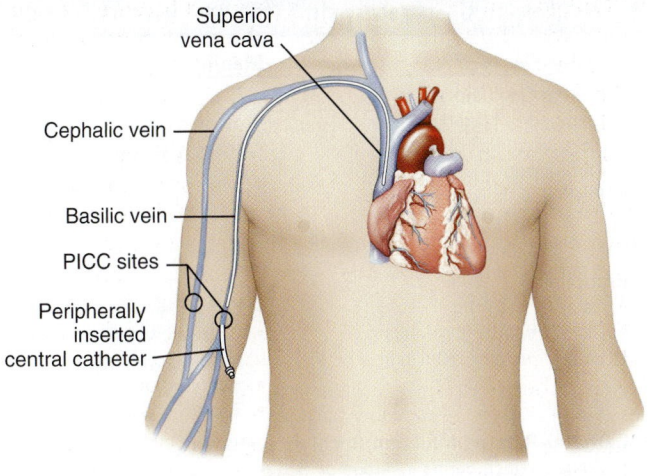

FIG. 16-19 Peripherally inserted central catheter (PICC) can be inserted using the basilic or cephalic vein.

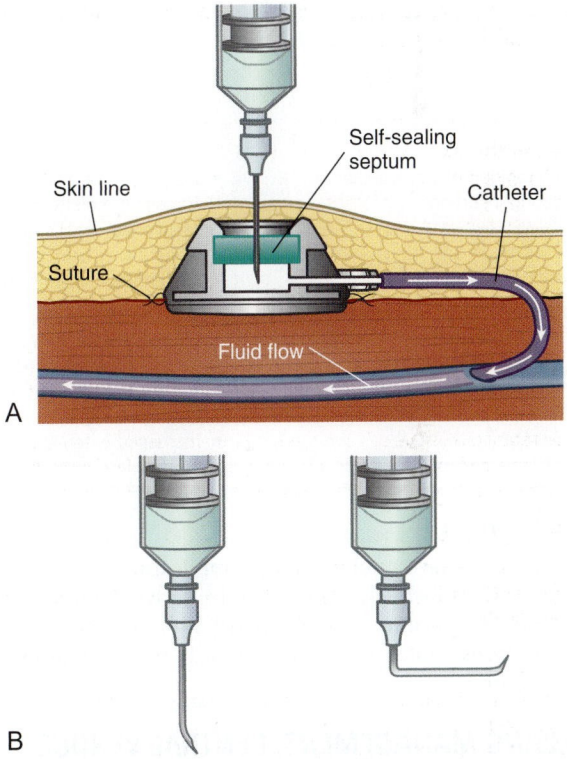

FIG. 16-20 **A,** Cross section of implantable port displaying access of the port with the Huber-point needle. Note the deflected point of the Huber-point needle, which prevents coring of the port's septum. **B,** Two Huber-point needles used to enter the implanted port. The 90-degree needle is used for top-entry ports for continuous infusion.

TABLE 16-19 Complications of Central Venous Access Devices (CVADs)

Possible Cause	Manifestations	Management
Catheter Occlusion		
• Clamped or kinked catheter • Tip against wall of vessel • Thrombosis • Precipitate buildup in lumen	• Sluggish infusion or aspiration • Inability to infuse and/or aspirate	• Instruct patient to change position, raise arm, and cough. • Assess for and alleviate clamping or kinking. • Flush with normal saline using a 10-mL syringe. Do not force flush. • Perform fluoroscopy to determine cause and site. • Instill anticoagulant or thrombolytic agent.
Embolism		
• Catheter breaking • Dislodgment of thrombus • Entry of air into circulation	• Chest pain • Respiratory distress (dyspnea, tachypnea, hypoxia, cyanosis) • Hypotension • Tachycardia	• Administer O_2. • Clamp catheter. • Place patient on left side with head down (air emboli). • Notify physician.
Catheter-Related Infection (local or systemic)		
• Contamination during insertion or use • Migration of organisms along catheter • Immunosuppressed patient	• *Local:* redness, tenderness, purulent drainage, warmth, edema • *Systemic:* fever, chills, malaise	***Local*** • Culture drainage from site. • Apply warm, moist compresses. • Remove catheter if indicated. ***Systemic*** • Take blood cultures. • Give antibiotic therapy. • Give antipyretic therapy. • Remove catheter if indicated.
Pneumothorax		
• Perforation of visceral pleura during insertion	• Decreased or absent breath sounds • Respiratory distress (cyanosis, dyspnea, tachypnea) • Chest pain • Distended unilateral chest	• Administer O_2. • Position in semi-Fowler's position. • Prepare for chest tube insertion.
Catheter Migration		
• Improper suturing • Insertion site trauma • Changes in intrathoracic pressure • Forceful catheter flushing • Spontaneous	• Sluggish infusion or aspiration • Edema of chest or neck during infusion • Patient complaint of gurgling sound in ear • Dysrhythmias • Increased external catheter length	• Perform fluoroscopy to verify position. • Assist with removal and new CVAD placement.

Complications

CVADs always have a potential for complications. Careful monitoring and assessment may assist in early identification of potential complications. Table 16-19 lists common possible complications, potential causes, clinical manifestations, and interventions.

❖ NURSING MANAGEMENT: CENTRAL VENOUS ACCESS DEVICES

Nursing management of CVADs includes assessment, dressing changes and cleansing, injection cap changes, and maintenance of catheter patency. The exact frequency and procedures for these requirements vary by type of CVAD and institution, so it is important to follow your specific institution's policies and procedures. The following section discusses some general guidelines.

Catheter and insertion site assessment includes inspecting the site for redness, edema, warmth, drainage, and tenderness or pain. Observing the catheter for misplacement or slippage is important. Perform a comprehensive pain assessment, particularly noting any complaints of chest or neck discomfort, arm pain, or pain at the insertion site. Do not use a newly placed CVAD until the tip position is verified with a chest x-ray.

Before manipulating a catheter for any reason, perform hand hygiene. Perform dressing changes and cleanse the catheter insertion site using strict sterile technique. Typical dressings include transparent semipermeable dressings or gauze and tape. If the site is bleeding, a gauze dressing may be preferable. Otherwise, transparent dressings are preferred. They allow observation of the site without having to remove the dressing. Transparent dressings may be left in place for up to 1 week. Change any dressing immediately if it becomes damp, loose, or soiled.

Cleanse the skin around the catheter insertion site according to institution policy. A chlorhexidine-based preparation is the cleansing agent of choice. Its effects last longer than either povidone-iodine or isopropyl alcohol, offering improved killing of bacteria.[14] When using chlorhexidine, cleansing the skin with friction is critical to preventing infection. When applying a new dressing, allow the area to air dry completely. Secure the lumen ports to the skin above the dressing site. Document the date and time of the dressing change and initial the dressing.

Disinfect catheter hubs, needleless connectors, and injection ports before accessing the catheter. Use an alcoholic chlorhexidine preparation, 70% alcohol, or povidone-iodine. Change injection caps at regular intervals according to institution policy or if they have damage from excessive punctures. Use strict sterile technique. Teach the patient to turn the head to the opposite side of the CVAD insertion site during cap change. If you cannot clamp the catheter, instruct the patient to lie flat in bed and perform the Valsalva maneuver whenever the catheter is open to air to prevent an air embolism.

Flushing is one of the most effective ways to maintain catheter patency. It also keeps incompatible drugs or fluids from mixing. Use a normal saline solution in a syringe that has a barrel capacity of 10 mL or more to avoid excess pressure on the catheter. If you feel resistance, do not apply force. This could result in a ruptured catheter or create an embolism if a thrombus is present. Because of the risk of contamination and infection, prefilled syringes or single-dose vials are preferred over multiple-dose vials. If you are not using a positive-pressure valve cap, clamp any unused lines after flushing.

Use the push-pause technique when flushing all catheters. Push-pause creates turbulence within the catheter lumen, promoting the removal of debris that adheres to the catheter lumen and decreasing the chance of occlusion. This technique involves injecting saline with a rapid alternating push-pause motion, instilling 1 to 2 mL with each push on the syringe plunger. If you are using a negative-pressure cap or neutral pressure cap, clamp the catheter while maintaining positive pressure while instilling the last 1 mL of saline. This prevents reflux of blood back into the catheter. If a positive-pressure valve cap is present, it works to prevent the reflux of blood and resultant catheter lumen occlusion. Remove the syringe before clamping the catheter to allow the positive pressure valve to work correctly.

Removal of CVADs

Removing a CVAD is done according to institution policy and the nurse's scope of practice. In many agencies, nurses with demonstrated competency can remove PICCs and nontunneled central venous catheters. The procedure involves removing any sutures and then gently withdrawing the catheter. Instruct the patient to perform the Valsalva maneuver as the last 5 to 10 cm of the catheter is withdrawn. Immediately apply pressure to the site with sterile gauze to prevent air from entering and to control bleeding. Inspect the catheter tip to determine that it is intact. After bleeding has stopped, apply an antiseptic ointment and sterile dressing to the site.

CASE STUDY

Fluid and Electrolyte Imbalance

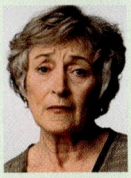

(©Kevin Peterson/ Photodisc/ Thinkstock)

Patient Profile

S.S., a 63-year-old white woman with acute lymphocytic leukemia, has been receiving chemotherapy on an outpatient basis. She completed her third treatment 5 days ago and has been experiencing nausea and vomiting for 2 days despite using ondansetron (Zofran). S.S.'s daughter brings her to the hospital, where she is admitted to the medical unit. As the admitting nurse, you perform a thorough assessment.

Subjective Data

- Complains of lethargy, weakness, dizziness, and dry mouth
- States she has been too nauseated to eat or drink anything for 2 days

Objective Data

- Heart rate 110 beats/min, pulse thready
- BP 100/65
- Weight loss of 5 lb since she received her chemotherapy treatment 5 days ago
- Dry oral mucous membranes

Discussion Questions

1. Based on her clinical manifestations, what fluid imbalance does S.S. have?
2. What additional assessment data should you obtain?
3. What are her risk factors for fluid and electrolyte imbalances?
4. You draw blood for a serum chemistry evaluation. What electrolyte imbalances are likely and why?
5. S.S. is at risk for which acid-base imbalance? Describe the changes that would occur in S.S.'s ABGs with this acid-base imbalance. How would the body compensate?
6. ***Teamwork and Collaboration:*** What is the interprofessional team's priority at this time for S.S.?
7. The physician orders dextrose 5% in 0.45% saline to infuse at 100 mL/hr. What type of solution is this, and how will it help S.S.'s fluid imbalance?
8. ***Priority Decision:*** What are the priority nursing interventions for S.S.?
9. ***Evidence-Based Practice:*** S.S. has a double-lumen PICC in her left arm. One lumen is connected to the IV infusion; the other is unused. What is the recommended practice for maintaining the patency of the unused lumen?
10. ***Quality Improvement:*** What outcomes will indicate that interprofessional care was effective?

Answers available at *http://evolve.elsevier.com/Lewis/medsurg.*

BRIDGE TO NCLEX EXAMINATION

The number of the question corresponds to the same-numbered outcome at the beginning of the chapter.

1. During the postoperative care of a 76-year-old patient, the nurse monitors the patient's intake and output carefully, knowing that the patient is at risk for fluid and electrolyte imbalances primarily because

a. older adults have an impaired thirst mechanism and need reminding to drink fluids.
b. water accounts for a greater percentage of body weight in the older adult than in younger adults.
c. older adults are more likely than younger adults to lose extracellular fluid during surgical procedures.
d. small losses of fluid are significant because body fluids account for 45% to 50% of body weight in older adults.

2. During administration of a hypertonic IV solution, the mechanism involved in equalizing the fluid concentration between ECF and the cells is

a. osmosis.
b. diffusion.
c. active transport.
d. facilitated diffusion.

3a. An older woman was admitted to the medical unit with GI bleeding and fluid volume deficit. Clinical manifestations of this problem are (*select all that apply*)

a. weight loss.
b. dry oral mucosa.
c. full bounding pulse.
d. engorged neck veins.
e. decreased central venous pressure.

3b. The nursing care for a patient with hyponatremia and fluid volume excess includes
- **a.** fluid restriction.
- **b.** administration of hypotonic IV fluids.
- **c.** administration of a cation-exchange resin.
- **d.** placement of an indwelling urinary catheter.

3c. The nurse should be alert for which manifestations in a patient receiving a loop diuretic?
- **a.** Restlessness and agitation
- **b.** Paresthesias and irritability
- **c.** Weak, irregular pulse and poor muscle tone
- **d.** Increased blood pressure and muscle spasms

3d. Which patient is at *greatest* risk for developing hypermagnesemia?
- **a.** 83-year-old man with lung cancer and hypertension
- **b.** 65-year-old woman with hypertension taking β-adrenergic blockers
- **c.** 42-year-old woman with systemic lupus erythematosus and renal failure
- **d.** 50-year-old man with benign prostatic hyperplasia and a urinary tract infection

3e. It is important for the nurse to assess for which clinical manifestation(s) in a patient who has just undergone a total thyroidectomy (*select all that apply*)?
- **a.** Confusion
- **b.** Weight gain
- **c.** Depressed reflexes
- **d.** Circumoral numbness
- **e.** Positive Chvostek's sign

3f. The nurse expects the long-term treatment of a patient with hyperphosphatemia secondary to renal failure will include
- **a.** fluid restriction.
- **b.** calcium supplements.
- **c.** magnesium supplements.
- **d.** increased intake of dairy products.

4. The lungs act as an acid-base buffer by
- **a.** increasing respiratory rate and depth when CO_2 levels in the blood are high, reducing acid load.
- **b.** increasing respiratory rate and depth when CO_2 levels in the blood are low, reducing base load.
- **c.** decreasing respiratory rate and depth when CO_2 levels in the blood are high, reducing acid load.
- **d.** decreasing respiratory rate and depth when CO_2 levels in the blood are low, increasing acid load.

5. A patient has the following arterial blood gas results: pH 7.52, $PaCO_2$ 30 mm Hg, HCO_3^- 24 mEq/L. The nurse determines that these results indicate
- **a.** metabolic acidosis.
- **b.** metabolic alkalosis.
- **c.** respiratory acidosis.
- **d.** respiratory alkalosis.

6. The typical fluid replacement for the patient with a fluid volume deficit is
- **a.** dextran.
- **b.** 0.45% saline.
- **c.** lactated Ringer's.
- **d.** 5% dextrose in 0.45% saline.

7. The nurse is unable to flush a central venous access device and suspects occlusion. The *best* nursing intervention would be to
- **a.** apply warm moist compresses to the insertion site.
- **b.** attempt to force 10 mL of normal saline into the device.
- **c.** place the patient on the left side with head-down position.
- **d.** instruct the patient to change positions, raise arm, and cough.

1. d, 2. a, 3a. a, b, e, 3b. a, 3c. c, 3d. c, 3e. a, d, e, 3f. b, 4. a, 5. d, 6. c, 7. d

For rationales to these answers and even more NCLEX review questions, visit *http://evolve.elsevier.com/Lewis/medsurg.*

EVOLVE WEBSITE

http://evolve.elsevier.com/Lewis/medsurg

Review Questions (Online Only)

Key Points

Answer Keys for Questions
- Answer Guidelines for Case Study on p. 297
- Rationales for Bridge to NCLEX Examination Questions
- Answer Guidelines for Managing Care of Multiple Patients Case Study (Section 2) on p. 299

Student Case Study
- Patient With Hyponatremia/Fluid Volume Imbalance

Conceptual Care Map Creator

Audio Glossary

Fluids and Electrolytes Tutorial

Content Updates

REFERENCES

1. McCance K, Huether SE: *Pathophysiology: the biologic basis for disease in adults and children*, ed 7, St Louis, 2014, Mosby.
2. Harring TR, Deal NS, Kuo DC: Disorders of sodium and water balance, *Emerg Med Clin N Am* 32:379, 2014.
3. Hooper L, Bunn D, Jimoh FO, Fairweather-Tait SJ: Water-loss dehydration and ageing, *Mech Ageing Dev* 136:50, 2014.

*4. Verbalis JG, Goldsmith SR, Greenberg A, et al: Diagnosis, evaluation, and treatment of hyponatremia: expert panel recommendations, *Am J Med* 126:S1, 2013.

5. Medford-Davis L, Rafique Z: Derangements of potassium, *Emerg Med Clin North Am* 32:329, 2014.
6. Crawford AH: Hyperkalemia: recognition and management of a critical electrolyte disturbance, *J Infus Nurs* 37:167, 2014.
7. Reagan P, Pani A, Rosner MH: Approach to the diagnosis and treatment of hypercalcemia in a patient with malignancy, *Am J Kidney Dis* 63:141, 2014.
8. Chang WT, Radin B, McCurdy MT: Calcium, magnesium, and phosphate abnormalities in the emergency department, *Emerg Med Clin North Am* 31:349, 2014.
9. Kelly A, Levine MA: Hypocalcemia in the critically ill patient, *J Int Care Med* 28:166, 2013.
10. Patel R, Taylor A, Pile T: Management of hypophosphataemia, *Br J Hosp Med* 74:C66, 2013.
11. Demssie Y, Patel L, Kumar M, Syed A: Hypomagnesemia: clinical relevance and management, *Br J Hosp Med* 75:39, 2014.
12. Soifer JT, Hyung TK: Approach to metabolic alkalosis, *Emerg Med Clin North Am* 32:453, 2014.

*13. Davison D, Rajit KB, Goldstein SL, Chawla LS: Fluid management in adults: core curriculum 2014, *Am J Kidney Dis* 63:700, 2014.

*14. Marschall J, Mermel LA, Fakih M, et al: Strategies to prevent central line–associated bloodstream infections in acute care hospitals: 2014 update, *Strategies* 35:753, 2014.

*Evidence-based information for clinical practice.

CASE STUDY

Managing Care of Multiple Patients

You and another RN are assigned to care for the following three patients in the intensive care unit (ICU). There is also a UAP (unlicensed assistive personnel) on duty.

Patients

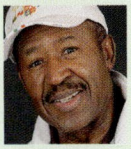

(©Stockphoto/ Thinkstock)

G.N., a 65-yr-old African American man, was admitted to the ICU after falling out of a tree onto a lit gas grill. He has partial-thickness burns on his face, neck, and upper trunk. He has undergone surgical repair of right tibia and left hip fractures as well as debridement of a severely lacerated right leg. His voice is slightly hoarse and he is coughing up sooty sputum. He is receiving O_2 at 4 L/min via nasal cannula, and his O_2 saturation is 93%. His WBC count is 26,400/μL (26.4 × 10^9/L) with 80% neutrophils (10% bands).

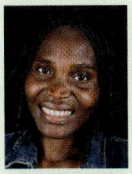

(©Stockphoto/ Thinkstock)

J.N., a 35-yr-old African American woman, was transferred to the ICU from the clinical unit last evening with acute respiratory failure. She was diagnosed 2 days ago with AIDS and *Pneumocystis jiroveci* pneumonia (PCP). Prior to this hospital admission she had consistently refused antiretroviral therapy (ART) because she could not afford it. She was started on oral trimethoprim/sulfamethoxazole (Bactrim) and combination antiretroviral therapy. However, her respiratory distress worsened and she was transferred to the ICU for intubation and mechanical ventilation. She is now receiving IV Bactrim.

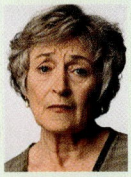

(© Kevin Peterson/ Photodisc/ Thinkstock)

S.S., a 63-yr-old white woman with acute lymphocytic leukemia, has been receiving chemotherapy on an outpatient basis. She completed her third treatment 5 days ago and has been experiencing nausea and vomiting for 2 days despite using ondansetron (Zofran). She was initially admitted to the clinical unit but was transferred to the ICU for close monitoring after becoming severely hypotensive overnight. Her most recent blood pressure was 98/50, HR 82 and regular, O_2 saturation 95% on 2L via nasal cannula, RR 22 and regular.

Discussion Questions

1. ***Priority Decision:*** After receiving report, which patient should you see first? Provide rationale.
2. ***Teamwork and Collaboration:*** Which morning tasks should you delegate to the UAP *(select all that apply)*?
   a. Take blood pressure readings on S.S.
   b. Perform respiratory assessment on G.N.
   c. Document strict intake and output on S.S.
   d. Provide oral care around the endotracheal tube for J.N.
   e. Titrate S.S.'s IV infusion rate based on her blood pressure reading.
3. ***Priority and Teamwork and Collaboration:*** When you enter J.N.'s room, the ventilator alarms are going off. The UAP had just finished providing oral care and she tells you that J.N. has become increasingly agitated within the last 5 minutes. Which *initial* action would be *most* appropriate?
   a. Suction J.N.'s endotracheal tube.
   b. Have the UAP stay with J.N. while you obtain IV sedation for her.
   c. Ask the UAP to describe exactly what she did when she was performing oral care.
   d. Assess the ventilator to identify what alarm is going off and to make sure all connections are secure.

Case Study Progression

J.N.'s ventilator tubing became disconnected. You quickly reconnect her tubing, and as she settles down her oxygenation improves. You ask the UAP to obtain vital signs on all your patients while you begin a more thorough assessment of J.N.

4. During your assessment of J.N., you note gray-white patches on the inside of her mouth. You recognize these as *most* likely caused by
   a. *Candida albicans.*
   b. poor oral hygiene.
   c. *Coccidioides immitis.*
   d. irritation from recent mouth care.
5. G.N.'s family asks you why surgery was performed on his leg wound. Your response is based on the knowledge that debridement *(select all that apply)*
   a. is used to remove infected tissue.
   b. is used to remove nonviable tissue.
   c. prepares the wound bed for healing.
   d. can only be accomplished in surgery.
   e. is necessary in any burn wound involving the skin.
6. S.S.'s morning laboratory results reveal a serum potassium level of 2.8 mEq/L. You notify the health care provider and obtain an order for IV potassium. During infusion of the potassium replacement, you prioritize assessment of S.S.'s
   a. bowel function.
   b. cardiac rhythm.
   c. muscle strength.
   d. level of consciousness.
7. ***Management Decision:*** While sitting at the computer charting your patients' morning assessments, you overhear the UAP telling a nursing student that J.N. deserves what she got because HIV is God's way of punishing those who sin. Your *most* appropriate response would be to
   a. report the UAP's actions to your supervisor.
   b. ask the UAP to keep her opinions to herself.
   c. ignore the conversation because it does not affect patient care.
   d. talk to the UAP and student about keeping personal feelings separate from patient care.

Answers available at *http://evolve.elsevier.com/Lewis/medsurg.*

SECTION 3

Perioperative Care

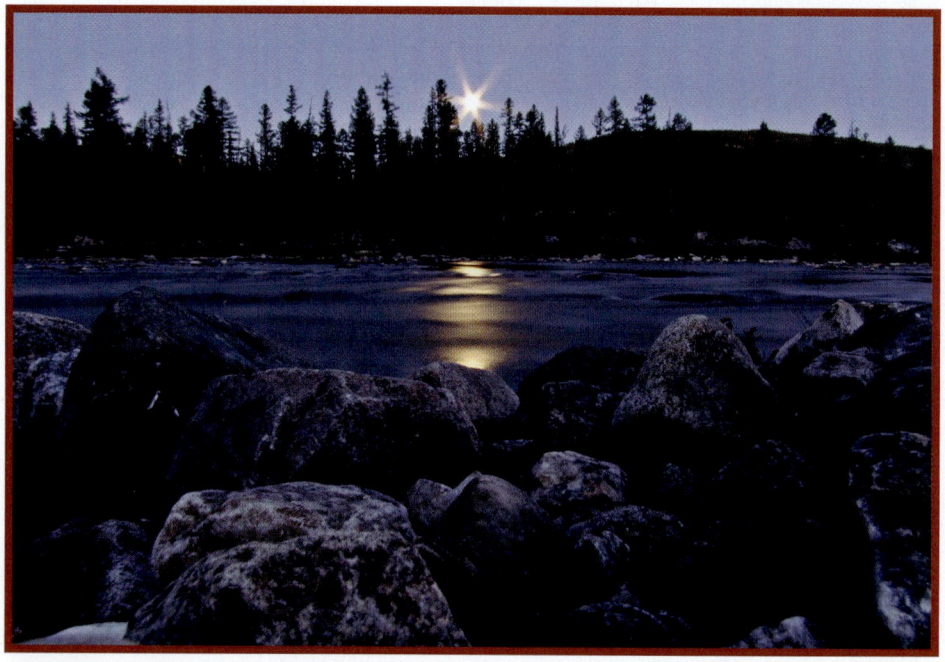

Thinkstock

I choose to listen to the river for a while, thinking river thoughts,
before joining the night and the stars.

Edward Abbey

Chapter 17 Preoperative Care, 301

Chapter 18 Intraoperative Care, 315

Chapter 19 Postoperative Care, 330

17

Preoperative Care

Janice A. Neil

The oldest and strongest emotion of mankind is fear, and the oldest and strongest kind of fear is fear of the unknown.

H.P. Lovecraft

http://evolve.elsevier.com/Lewis/medsurg/

LEARNING OUTCOMES

1. Differentiate the common purposes and settings of surgery.
2. Apply knowledge of the purpose and components of a preoperative nursing assessment.
3. Interpret the significance of data related to the preoperative patient's health status and operative risk.
4. Analyze the components and purpose of the patient's informed consent for surgery.
5. Examine the nursing role in the physical, psychologic, and educational preparation of the surgical patient.
6. Prioritize the nursing responsibilities related to day-of-surgery preparation for the surgical patient.
7. Differentiate the purposes and types of common preoperative medications.
8. Apply knowledge of the special considerations of preoperative preparation for the older adult surgical patient.

KEY TERMS

ambulatory surgery, p. 302
elective surgery, p. 301
emergency surgery, p. 301
informed consent, p. 309
same-day admission, p. 301
surgery, p. 301

Preparation of patients for surgery is an important nursing role. This chapter discusses preoperative care that is applicable to all surgical patients regardless of where the surgery is performed. Preparation measures for specific surgical procedures (e.g., abdominal, thoracic, or orthopedic surgery) are discussed in appropriate chapters of this text.

Surgery is the art and science of treating diseases, injuries, and deformities by operation and instrumentation. The surgical experience involves an interprofessional team, including the patient, surgeon, anesthesia care provider (ACP), nurse, and other health care team members. Surgery may be performed for any of the following purposes:

- *Diagnosis:* Determination of the presence and extent of a pathologic condition (e.g., lymph node biopsy, bronchoscopy)
- *Cure:* Elimination or repair of a pathologic condition (e.g., removal of ruptured appendix or benign ovarian cyst)
- *Palliation:* Alleviation of symptoms without cure (e.g., cutting a nerve root [rhizotomy] to remove symptoms of pain, creating a colostomy to bypass an inoperable bowel obstruction)
- *Prevention* (e.g., removal of a mole before it becomes malignant, removal of the colon in a patient with familial polyposis to prevent cancer)
- *Cosmetic improvement* (e.g., repairing a burn scar, breast reconstruction after a mastectomy)
- *Exploration:* Surgical examination to determine the nature or extent of a disease (e.g., laparotomy). With the advent of advanced diagnostic tests, exploration is less common because many problems can be identified noninvasively.

Specific suffixes are commonly used in combination with a body part or organ in naming surgical procedures (Table 17-1).

SURGICAL SETTINGS

Surgery may be a carefully planned event (**elective surgery**) or may arise with unexpected urgency (**emergency surgery**). Both elective and emergency surgeries are performed in a variety of settings. The setting where a surgical procedure may be safely performed is influenced by the type of surgery, potential complications, and the patient's health status. (Specific surgeries are described in chapters throughout the text in discussions of interventions for specific problems.)

For inpatient surgery, patients who are going to be admitted to the hospital are usually admitted on the day of surgery (**same-day admission**). Patients who are in the hospital before surgery are usually there because of acute or chronic medical conditions.

Reviewed by Janie Corbitt, RN, MLS, Retired Instructor of Nursing, Milledgeville, Georgia; Shari Gould, RN, MSN, Associate Professor of Nursing, Victoria College, Victoria, Texas; and Lisa Spruce, DNP, ACNS, ACNP, ANP, CNOR, CNS-CP, Director of Evidence-Based Perioperative Practice, Association of periOperative Registered Nurses, Denver, Colorado.

TABLE 17-1 Suffixes Describing Surgical Procedures

Suffix	Meaning	Example
-ectomy	Excision or removal of	Appendectomy
-lysis	Destruction of	Electrolysis
-orrhaphy	Repair or suture of	Herniorrhaphy
-oscopy	Looking into	Endoscopy
-ostomy	Creation of opening into	Colostomy
-otomy	Cutting into or incision of	Tracheotomy
-plasty	Repair or reconstruction of	Mammoplasty

The majority of surgical procedures are performed as **ambulatory surgery** (also called *same-day* or *outpatient surgery*). Many of these surgeries use minimally invasive techniques (e.g., laparoscopic techniques). Ambulatory surgery may be conducted in endoscopy clinics, physicians' offices, freestanding surgical clinics, and outpatient surgery units in hospitals. These procedures can be performed using general, regional, or local anesthetic and require less than a 24-hour stay postoperatively. Many patients go home with a caregiver within hours of surgery.

Ambulatory surgery is often preferred by patients and health care providers (HCPs). Generally, it requires fewer laboratory tests and preoperative and postoperative drugs and reduces the patient's risk for health care–associated infections. Patients like the convenience of recovering at home, HCPs prefer the flexibility in scheduling, and the cost is usually less for the patient and the insurer.

You play an essential role in preparing the patient for surgery, caring for the patient during surgery, and aiding the patient's recovery after surgery. To perform these functions effectively, first know the nature of the disorder requiring surgery and any co-morbidities. Second, identify the individual patient's response to the stress of surgery. Third, know the results of appropriate preoperative diagnostic tests. Last, identify potential risks and complications associated with the surgical procedure and any co-morbidities that should be included in the plan of care. The nurse caring for the patient preoperatively is likely to be different from the nurse in the operating room (OR), postanesthesia care unit (PACU), surgical intensive care unit (SICU), or surgical unit. Thus communication and documentation of important preoperative assessment findings are essential for quality care.

PATIENT INTERVIEW

One of the most important nursing actions is the preoperative interview. The nurse who works in the physician's office, ambulatory surgery center, or hospital may do the interview.

The preoperative interview can occur in advance or on the day of surgery. The primary purposes of the patient interview are to (1) obtain the patient's health information, including drug and food allergies; (2) provide and clarify information about the planned surgery, including anesthesia; and (3) assess the patient's emotional state and readiness for surgery, including his or her expectations about the surgical outcomes. The interview also provides the patient and caregiver an opportunity to ask questions about surgery, anesthesia, and postoperative care. Often patients ask about taking their routine drugs, such as insulin, anticoagulants, or heart medications, and if they will experience pain. By being aware of the patient's and caregiver's needs, you can provide the information and support needed during the perioperative period.

NURSING ASSESSMENT OF PREOPERATIVE PATIENT

The overall goal of the preoperative assessment is to identify risk factors and plan care to ensure patient safety throughout the surgical experience. To achieve this, you will need to do the following:

- Establish baseline data for comparison in the intraoperative and postoperative period.
- Determine the patient's psychologic status to reinforce the use of coping strategies during the surgical experience.
- Determine physiologic factors directly or indirectly related to the surgical procedure that may contribute to operative risk factors.
- Participate in the identification and documentation of the surgical site according to agency protocol.
- Identify prescription drugs, over-the-counter drugs, and herbs taken by the patient that may result in drug interactions affecting the surgical outcome.
- Review the results of all preoperative diagnostic studies in the patient's record, and share this information with the appropriate HCPs.
- Identify cultural and ethnic factors that may affect the surgical experience.
- Determine if the patient received adequate information from the surgeon to make an informed decision to have surgery and that the consent form is signed and witnessed.

Subjective Data

Psychosocial Assessment. Surgery is a stressful event, even when the procedure is minor. The psychologic and physiologic reactions to surgery may elicit the stress response (e.g., elevated BP and heart rate). The stress response enables the body to meet the demands in the perioperative period. If stressors or the responses to the stressors are excessive, the stress response can be magnified and may affect recovery. Many factors influence the patient's reaction to stress, including age, past experiences with illness and pain, current health, and socioeconomic status.

The use of common language and avoidance of medical jargon are essential. Use words and language that are familiar to the patient to help the patient understand the surgery. Familiar language also helps reduce preoperative anxiety.

Your role in psychologically preparing the patient for surgery is to assess the patient for potential or actual stressors that could negatively affect surgery (Table 17-2). Communicate all concerns to the appropriate surgical team member, especially if the concern requires intervention later in the surgical experience. Because many patients are admitted directly into the preoperative area from their homes, you must be skilled in assessing important psychologic factors in a short time. The most common psychologic factors are anxiety, fear, and hope.

Anxiety. Most people are anxious when facing surgery because of the unknown. This is normal and is an inborn survival mechanism. However, if the anxiety level is high, cognition, decision making, and coping abilities can be reduced.

Anxiety can arise from lack of knowledge. This can range from not knowing what to expect to uncertainty about the outcome and may result from past experiences or stories heard through friends or the media. You can decrease some anxiety

TABLE 17-2 Psychosocial Assessment of Preoperative Patient

Situational Changes

- Define current degree of personal control, decision making, and independence.
- Determine the presence of hope and anticipation of positive results.
- Consider the impact of surgery and hospitalization and possible effects on lifestyle.
- Identify support systems, including family, other caregivers, group and institutional structures, and religious and spiritual groups.

Concerns With the Unknown

- Identify specific areas and degree of anxiety and fears related to the surgery (e.g., pain).
- Identify expectations of surgery, changes in current health status, effects on daily living, and sexual activity (if appropriate).

Concerns With Body Image

- Identify current roles or relationships and view of self.
- Determine perceived or potential changes in roles or relationships and their impact on body image.

Past Experiences

- Review previous surgical experiences, hospitalizations, and treatments.
- Determine responses to those experiences (positive and/or negative).
- Identify current perceptions of surgical procedure in relation to the above and information from others (e.g., a friend's view of a personal surgical experience).

Knowledge Deficit

- Identify the amount and type of preoperative information the patient wants.
- Assess understanding of surgical procedure, including preparation, care, interventions, preoperative activities, restrictions, and expected outcomes.
- Identify the accuracy of information the patient has received from others, including health care team, family, friends, and media.

for the patient by providing information about what to expect. This is often done through classes or Web-based or audiovisual teaching materials before surgery. Inform the surgeon if the patient requires any additional information or if anxiety is excessive.

Patients may experience anxiety when surgery is in conflict with their religious or cultural beliefs. In particular, identify, record, and communicate patient decisions regarding the possibility of blood transfusions. For example, Jehovah's Witnesses may choose to refuse blood or blood products.[1]

Common Fears. Patients fear surgery for a number of reasons. The most common fear is the risk of death or permanent disability resulting from surgery. Sometimes the fear comes after hearing or reading about the risks during the informed consent process. Other fears are related to pain, change in body image, or results of diagnostic procedures.

Fear of death can be extremely harmful. Notify the HCP if the patient has a strong fear of death. A patient's strong fear of impending death may prompt the HCP to delay the surgery because the emotional state influences the stress response and thus the surgical outcome.

Fear of pain and discomfort during and after surgery is common. If the fear is extreme, notify the ACP or the surgeon. Reassure the patient that drugs are available for anesthesia and analgesia during surgery. For pain after surgery, tell patients to ask for pain medication before pain becomes severe. Teach the patient how to use a pain intensity scale (e.g., 0 to 10, FACES). (Pain scales are explained in Chapter 8.)

Drugs may also be given that provide an amnesic effect so that the patient will not remember what occurs during surgery. Tell the patient that this effect assists in decreasing anxiety after surgery.

Fear of mutilation or *alteration in body image* can occur whether the surgery is radical, such as amputation, or minor, such as a breast biopsy. Even a small scar on the body can upset some, and others fear keloid development (overgrowth of a scar). Listen to and assess the patient's concern about this fear with an accepting attitude.

Fear of anesthesia may arise from the unknown, personal experience, or tales of others' bad experiences. These concerns can also result from information about the risks of anesthesia (e.g., brain damage, paralysis). Many patients fear losing control while under anesthesia. If these fears are identified, inform the ACP immediately so that he or she can talk further with the patient.

Fear of disruption of life functioning may be present in varying degrees. It can range from fear of permanent disability to concern about not being able to engage in activities of daily living for a few weeks. Concerns about loss of role function, separation from family, and how the family will manage may be revealed. Financial concerns may be related to an anticipated loss of income or the costs of surgery.

If you identify any of these fears, a consult with the patient's caregiver, a social worker, a spiritual advisor, or a psychologist

EVIDENCE-BASED PRACTICE

Applying the Evidence

Music and Preoperative Anxiety

You are taking care of D.G., a 74-year-old woman scheduled for aortic valve replacement surgery. She was admitted early this morning to the preoperative unit. Unfortunately, an emergency surgery has resulted in at least a 4-hour delay of her surgery. You note that she is currently experiencing a high level of anxiety.

Making Clinical Decisions

Best Available Evidence. Music intervention in the preoperative period, including listening to pre-recorded music or individually tailored music administered by a trained therapist, may be effective in reducing anxiety.

Clinician Expertise. Anxiety can increase BP and pulse rate and may lengthen postoperative recovery. Excessive anxiety in a patient can even result in surgery being cancelled. Nonpharmacologic methods of reducing preoperative anxiety, such as listening to music, may help patients reduce their anxiety.

Patient Preference and Values. D.G. tells you that she is not able to relax and would like "a strong pill" to reduce her anxiety. D.G.'s family mentioned to you earlier that she enjoys listening to classical music at home.

Implications for Practice

1. What information would you share with D.G. related to the use of drugs to reduce her anxiety?
2. How would you respond to D.G. when she asks how music could possibly help in reducing her anxiety?

Reference for Evidence

Bradt J, Dileo C, Shim M: Music interventions for preoperative anxiety, *Cochrane Database Syst Rev* 6:CD006908, 2013.

CHECK YOUR PRACTICE

Your 19-year-old male patient is in the holding area. He is scheduled for an orchiectomy for testicular cancer. He is visibly sweating and agitated. When you ask him how he is doing, he responds, "I am scared. Wouldn't you be?"

- What can you do to reduce his fear?

may be appropriate. Financial advisors at the hospital may be able to provide information about financial support.

Hope. Although many psychologic factors related to surgery seem to be negative, hope is a positive attribute.[2] Hope may be the patient's strongest method of coping. To deny or minimize hope may negate the positive mental attitude necessary for a quick and full recovery. Some surgeries are hopefully anticipated. These can be the surgeries that repair (e.g., plastic surgery for burn scars), rebuild (e.g., total joint replacement to reduce pain and improve function), or save and extend life (e.g., repair of aneurysm, organ transplant). Assess and support the presence of hope and the patient's anticipation of positive results.

Past Health History. Ask the patient about any previous health problems and surgeries. Determine if the patient understands the need for surgery. For example, the patient scheduled for a total knee replacement may indicate that increasing pain and immobility are the reasons for the surgery.

Document the reason for any past hospitalizations, including previous surgeries and the dates. Also identify any problems with previous surgeries. For example, the patient may have experienced a wound infection or a reaction to a drug.

Ask women about their menstrual and obstetric history. This includes the date of their last menstrual period, the number of pregnancies, and any history of cesarean section.

When obtaining a family health history, ask the patient and caregiver about any inherited traits, since they may contribute to the surgical outcome. Record any family history of heart and endocrine diseases. For example, if a patient reports a parent with hypertension, sudden cardiac death, or myocardial infarction, this should alert you to the possibility that the patient may have a similar predisposition or condition. Also obtain information about the patient's family history of adverse reactions to or problems with anesthesia. For example, malignant hyperthermia has a genetic predisposition. Measures to decrease complications associated with this condition can be taken. (For further information on malignant hyperthermia, see Chapter 18.)

Medications. Document all current medication use, including over-the-counter drugs and herbs. In many ambulatory surgery centers, patients are asked to bring their medications with them when reporting for surgery. This helps to accurately assess and document the name and dosage of medications.

The interaction of the patient's current drugs and anesthetics can increase or decrease the desired physiologic effect of anesthetics. Consider the effects of opioids and prescribed drugs for chronic health conditions (e.g., heart disease, hypertension, depression, seizure disorder, diabetes). For example, certain antidepressants can potentiate the effect of opioids, agents that can be used for anesthesia. Antihypertensive drugs may predispose the patient to shock from the combined effect of the drug and the vasodilator effect of some anesthetic agents. Insulin or oral hypoglycemic drugs may require adjustments during the perioperative period because of increased body metabolism, decreased oral intake, stress, and anesthesia. Antiplatelet drugs (e.g., aspirin, clopidogrel [Plavix]) and nonsteroidal antiinflammatory drugs (NSAIDs) inhibit platelet aggregation and may contribute to postoperative bleeding.

Surgeons may instruct patients to withhold these drugs before surgery. Specific timeframes for withholding drugs depend on the drug and the patient. Patients on long-term anticoagulation therapy (e.g., warfarin [Coumadin], rivaroxaban [Xarelto], dabigatran [Pradaxa], apixaban [Eliquis]) present a unique challenge. The options for these patients include (1) continuing therapy, (2) withholding therapy for a time before and after surgery, or (3) withholding the therapy and starting subcutaneous or IV heparin therapy during the perioperative period. The management strategy selected is determined by patient history and the nature of the surgery.[3]

Ask about the use of herbs and dietary supplements because their use is so common. Many patients do not think to include supplements in their list of medications. They believe that herbal and dietary supplements are "natural" and do not pose a surgical risk.[4] (See the Complementary & Alternative Therapies box in Chapter 3 on p. 38 on how to assess for the use of herbal supplements.) Excessive use of vitamins and herbs can cause harmful effects in patients undergoing surgery. In patients taking anticoagulants or antiplatelets, herbal supplements can produce excessive postoperative bleeding that may require a return to the OR.[5] The effects of specific herbs that are of concern during the perioperative period are listed in the Complementary & Alternative Therapies box.

COMPLEMENTARY & ALTERNATIVE THERAPIES

Herbal Products and Surgery

The following can be used as a guide for patient teaching:

- Notify your HCP of all vitamins, herbs, and dietary supplements that you are taking.
- Avoid astragalus and ginseng, since they can increase BP before and during surgery.
- Avoid garlic, vitamin E, ginkgo, and fish oils because they can increase bleeding.
- Avoid kava and valerian because they can cause excess sedation.
- In general, discontinue all herbs 2 to 3 weeks before any surgical procedure. Consult your HCP for specific instructions.

Helpful Herbs and Vitamins

- Arnica is a homeopathic remedy useful in soft tissue healing.
- Multivitamins can be taken until the day before surgery. Taking them on the day of surgery on an empty stomach may contribute to nausea and vomiting after surgery.

Also ask the patient about any recreational drug use. The substances most likely to be used include tobacco, alcohol, opioids, marijuana, cocaine, and amphetamines. Ask questions about the use of these substances in a frank manner. Stress that recreational drug use may affect the type and amount of anesthesia that will be needed. When patients become aware of the potential interactions of these substances with anesthetics, most patients respond honestly about using them.

Chronic alcohol use can place the patient at risk because of lung, gastrointestinal, or liver damage. When liver function is decreased, metabolism of anesthetic agents is prolonged, nutritional status is altered, and the potential for postoperative complications is increased. Alcohol withdrawal can also occur during lengthy surgery or in the postoperative period. Although this can be a life-threatening event, it can be avoided with appropriate planning and management (see Chapter 10).

Record and share all findings of the drug history with the perioperative health care team. The ACP will determine the appropriate schedule and dose of the patient's routine drugs before and after surgery. Ensure that all of the patient's drugs are identified, implement any changes in the medication plan, and monitor the patient for potential interactions and complications.

Allergies. Ask the patient about drug intolerances and drug allergies. Drug intolerance usually results in side effects that are unpleasant for the patient but are not life threatening. These effects can include nausea, constipation, diarrhea, or *idiosyncratic* (opposite than expected) reactions. A true drug allergy produces hives and/or an anaphylactic reaction, causing cardiopulmonary compromise (e.g., hypotension, tachycardia, bronchospasm). Being aware of drug intolerances and drug allergies aids the health care team to maintain patient comfort and safety.

Record all drug intolerances and allergies and, if appropriate, place an allergy identification band on the patient on the day of surgery.

! SAFETY ALERT Allergies

- Some local anesthetic agents contain bisulfite preservatives.
- Notify the ACP if the patient reports an allergy to sulfur-containing drugs.

Also inquire about nondrug allergies, specifically food and environmental (e.g., latex, pollen, animals) allergies. The patient with a history of any allergic reactions has a greater potential for hypersensitivity reactions to drugs given during anesthesia. Patients need to be screened specifically for latex allergies by gathering data in the following areas:

- Risk factors
- Contact dermatitis
- Contact urticaria (e.g., hives)
- Aerosol reactions
- History of reactions that suggest an allergy to latex

Risk factors for latex allergy include long-term, multiple exposures to latex products, such as those experienced by health care and rubber industry workers. Additional risk factors include a history of hay fever, asthma, and allergies to certain foods (e.g., eggs, avocados, bananas, chestnuts, potatoes, peaches).[6] (Latex allergies are discussed in Chapter 13.)

Review of Systems. The last component of the patient history is the body systems review. Ask specific questions to confirm the presence or absence of any diseases. Current health problems can alert you to areas that should be more closely examined in the preoperative physical examination. The combined review of systems and patient history provide essential data to determine the specific preoperative tests that need to be ordered.

Cardiovascular System. Evaluate cardiovascular (CV) function to determine preexisting disease or problems (e.g., coronary artery disease, prosthetic heart valve). In reviewing the CV system, you may find a history of hypertension, angina, dysrhythmias, heart failure, or myocardial infarction. Inquire about the patient's current treatment for any CV condition (e.g., drugs) and the level of functioning. A cardiology consult is often required before surgery if the patient has a significant CV history (e.g., recent myocardial infarction [MI], valvular heart disease, implantable cardioverter-defibrillator).

If indicated, a 12-lead electrocardiogram (ECG) and coagulation studies should be ordered, and the results should be on the chart before surgery. The CV assessment provides data on what other measures have to be done. For example, the patient who is on diuretic therapy needs to have a serum potassium level drawn preoperatively. If the patient has a history of hypertension, the ACP may give vasoactive drugs to maintain adequate BP during surgery. If the patient has a prosthetic heart valve, antibiotic prophylaxis may be needed before surgery to decrease the risk of infective endocarditis (see Chapter 36).

Postoperative venous thromboembolism (VTE), a condition that includes deep vein thrombosis and pulmonary embolism, is a concern for any surgical patient. Patients at high risk for VTE include those with a history of previous thrombosis, blood-clotting disorders, cancer, varicosities, obesity, tobacco use, heart failure, or chronic obstructive pulmonary disease (COPD).[7] People are also at risk for developing a VTE because of immobility and positioning during the operative procedure. Antiembolism stockings or sequential compression devices (SCDs) may be applied in the preoperative holding area.

Respiratory System. Ask the patient about any recent or chronic respiratory disease or infections. Elective surgery may be postponed if the person has an upper respiratory tract infection. Upper airway infections increase the risk of bronchospasm, laryngospasm, decreased O_2 saturation, and problems with respiratory secretions. Also report a patient's history of dyspnea at rest or with exertion, coughing (dry or productive), or hemoptysis (coughing blood) to the ACP and surgeon.

If a patient has a history of asthma, ask about the use of inhaled or oral corticosteroids and bronchodilators, as well as the frequency and triggers of asthma attacks. The patient with a history of COPD is at high risk for postoperative pulmonary complications, including hypoxemia and atelectasis.

Gather information about the patient's tobacco use. The patient should be encouraged to stop smoking at least 6 weeks preoperatively by the HCP, as smoking increases the risk for pulmonary complications during and after surgery. Report conditions likely to affect respiratory function such as sleep apnea, obesity, and spinal, chest, and airway deformities. For example, patients may be asked to bring their sleep apnea devices with them to the hospital or surgical center. Depending on the patient's history and physical examination, baseline pulmonary function tests and arterial blood gases may be ordered preoperatively.

Neurologic System. Preoperative evaluation of neurologic functioning includes assessing the patient's ability to respond to questions, follow commands, and maintain orderly thought patterns. Alterations in the patient's hearing and vision may affect responses and the ability to follow directions throughout the perioperative assessment and evaluation. Record the patient's ability to pay attention, concentrate, and respond appropriately to establish a preoperative baseline for postoperative comparison.

If you note deficits in cognitive function, determine the extent of the problems and whether they can be corrected before surgery. If the problems cannot be corrected, it is important to involve a legal guardian or person with durable power of attorney for health care to assist the patient and provide informed consent for surgery.

Preoperative assessment of the older person's baseline cognitive function is especially crucial for intraoperative and postoperative evaluation. The older adult may have intact mental abilities preoperatively but is more prone to adverse outcomes during and after surgery than the younger adult. This is due to the additional stressors of the surgical procedure, dehydration, hypothermia, and anesthesia and adjunctive drugs. These factors may contribute to the development of *emergence delirium,* a condition that may be falsely labeled as senility or dementia. Thus preoperative findings are critical for postoperative comparison.

In the review of the neurologic system, inquire about any history of strokes, transient ischemic attacks, or spinal cord injury. Also ask about neurologic diseases, such as myasthenia gravis, Parkinson's disease, and multiple sclerosis, and any treatments used.

Genitourinary System. Assess for a history of renal or urinary tract diseases, such as chronic kidney disease or repeated urinary tract infections. Record the present disease state and current treatment of the disease. Renal dysfunction is associated with a number of alterations, including fluid and electrolyte imbalances, coagulopathies, increased risk for infection, and impaired wound healing. Because many drugs are metabolized and excreted by the kidneys, a decrease in renal function can lead to an altered response to drugs and unpredictable drug elimination. Renal function tests (e.g., serum creatinine, blood urea nitrogen [BUN]) are commonly ordered preoperatively.

Record and share with the perioperative team if the patient has problems voiding (e.g., incontinence, hesitancy). Older male patients may have an enlarged prostate that can interfere with the insertion of a bladder catheter or impair voiding in the postoperative period.

For a woman of childbearing age, determine if she is pregnant or thinks she could be pregnant. Most agencies require a pregnancy test for all women of childbearing age before surgery.[8] Immediately inform the surgeon if the patient states that she may be pregnant, since maternal and fetal exposure to anesthetics during the first trimester should be avoided.

Hepatic System. The liver is involved in glucose homeostasis, fat metabolism, protein synthesis, drug and hormone metabolism, and bilirubin formation and excretion. The liver detoxifies many anesthetics and adjunctive drugs. The patient with hepatic dysfunction may have an increased perioperative risk for clotting abnormalities and adverse responses to drugs. Consider the presence of liver disease if there is a history of jaundice, hepatitis, alcohol abuse, or obesity.

Integumentary System. Ask about a history of skin problems. Assess the current condition of the skin, especially at the incision site, for rashes, breakdown, or other dermatologic conditions. A patient with a history of pressure ulcers may require extra padding during surgery. Skin problems can affect postoperative healing.

Body art such as tattoos and piercings are increasingly common. When possible, select pigment-free areas for injections, IV sites, and laboratory draws.

Musculoskeletal System. Note any musculoskeletal and mobility problems, especially in the older adult. If the patient has arthritis, identify all affected joints. Mobility restrictions may influence intraoperative and postoperative positioning and ambulation. Spinal anesthesia may be difficult if the patient cannot flex the lumbar spine adequately to allow easy needle insertion. If the neck is affected, intubation and airway management may be difficult. Any mobility aids (e.g., cane, walker) should be brought with the patient on the day of surgery.

Endocrine System. The patient with diabetes mellitus is especially at risk for adverse effects of anesthesia and surgery. Hypoglycemia, hyperglycemia, delayed wound healing, and infection are common complications of diabetes during the perioperative period. Clarify with the patient's surgeon or ACP whether the patient should take the usual dose of insulin or oral hypoglycemic agents on the day of surgery. ACPs may vary the usual insulin dose based on the patient's current status and history of glucose control. Regardless of the preoperative insulin or oral hypoglycemic orders, measure serum or capillary glucose levels the morning of surgery to establish baseline levels. Assess the patient's glucose levels regularly and, if necessary, manage according to agency protocol.

Determine if the patient has a history of thyroid dysfunction. Hyperthyroidism or hypothyroidism can place the patient at surgical risk because of alterations in metabolic rate. If the patient takes a thyroid replacement drug, check with the ACP about administration of the drug on the day of surgery. If the patient has a history of thyroid dysfunction, laboratory tests may be ordered to determine current levels of thyroid function.

The patient with Addison's disease also requires special consideration during surgery. Addisonian crisis or shock can occur if a patient abruptly stops taking replacement corticosteroids, and the stress of surgery may require additional IV corticosteroid therapy[9] (see Chapter 49).

Immune System. If the patient has a history of a compromised immune system or takes immunosuppressive drugs, record it. Corticosteroids used in immunosuppressive doses may be tapered before surgery. Impairment of the immune system can lead to delayed wound healing and increased risk for postoperative infections.[10] If the patient has an acute infection (e.g., upper respiratory tract infection, sinusitis, influenza), elective surgery is often cancelled. Patients with active chronic infections such as hepatitis B or C, acquired immunodeficiency syndrome, or tuberculosis may have surgery if indicated. However, when preparing the patient for surgery, remember to take infection control precautions for the protection of the patient and staff.[11] (Infection control guidelines are discussed in Chapter 14.)

Fluid and Electrolyte Status. Ask the patient about any recent conditions that increase the risk for fluid and electrolyte imbalances, such as vomiting, diarrhea, or preoperative bowel preps. For example, surgery may be planned for a patient with cholecystitis who has been vomiting for several days. Also identify drugs that alter fluid and electrolyte status, such as diuretics. Serum electrolyte levels are often assessed before surgery. Many patients may have restricted fluids for some time before surgery. If the surgery is delayed, they could develop dehydration. A patient with or at risk for dehydration may need additional fluids and electrolytes before or during surgery.

Although a preoperative fluid balance history should be completed for all patients, it is especially critical for older adults. Their reduced adaptive capacity leaves a narrow margin of safety between overhydration and underhydration.

Nutritional Status. Nutritional deficits include overnutrition and undernutrition, both of which require considerable time to correct. However, knowing that a patient has a nutritional deficit can help the health care team provide more individualized care. For example, if the patient is thin, provide more padding than usual (pressure points on all patients are protected routinely) on the OR table. Notify the team if a patient is severely obese (body mass index [BMI] greater than 40 kg/m^2) to allow time to obtain special equipment needed for the patient's care (e.g., longer instruments for abdominal surgery).

Obesity stresses the cardiac and pulmonary systems and makes access to the surgical site and anesthesia administration more difficult.[12] It predisposes the patient to wound dehiscence, wound infection, and incisional herniation postoperatively. Adipose tissue is less vascular than other types of tissue. In addition, the patient may be slower to recover from anesthesia because inhalation agents are absorbed and stored by adipose tissue, thus leaving the body more slowly. (See Chapter 40 for special needs of obese patients undergoing surgery.)

Nutritional deficiencies impair the ability to recover from surgery. Remember that the obese patient and the very thin patient can also be protein and vitamin deficient. If the nutritional problem is severe, surgery may be postponed. Protein and vitamins A, C, and B complex deficiencies are particularly significant because these substances are essential for wound healing.[13]

TABLE 17-3 American Society of Anesthesiologists' Physical Classification System

Rating	Definition
P1	Normal healthy person
P2	Patient with mild systemic disease
P3	Patient with severe systemic disease
P4	Patient with severe systemic disease that is a constant threat to life
P5	Moribund patient who is not expected to survive without surgery
P6	Declared brain-dead patient whose organs are being removed for donor purposes

Source: American Society of Anesthesiologists: ASA physical status classification system, 2014. Retrieved from *www.asahq.org/clinical/physicalstatus.htm.*
NOTE: Patients selected for surgery in ambulatory or outpatient settings generally have ratings of P1, P2, or P3.

Supplemental nutrition may be given during the perioperative period to patients who are malnourished. The older adult is often at risk for malnutrition and fluid volume deficits.[8]

Identify patients who consume large quantities of coffee or caffeinated soft drinks. In many cases, withholding caffeinated beverages preoperatively or for some time postoperatively can lead to severe withdrawal headaches.[14] Caffeine withdrawal headaches can be confused with spinal headaches if the preoperative data are not recorded. Giving caffeinated beverages postoperatively, when possible, may prevent these headaches.

Objective Data

Physical Examination. The Joint Commission requires that all patients admitted to the OR have a documented history and physical examination (H&P) in their chart.[15] This may be done in advance of surgery or on the day of surgery. It may be performed by any qualified person, including advanced practice nurses, physicians, physician assistants, or ACPs. Findings from the patient's H&P will enable the ACP to assign the patient a physical status rating for anesthesia administration (Table 17-3). This rating is an indicator of the patient's perioperative risk and may influence perioperative decisions.

In addition to the health assessment, also complete a physical examination of the patient before surgery (Table 17-4). Review

TABLE 17-4 Health Assessment and Physical Examination of Preoperative Patient*

Cardiovascular System
- Identify acute or chronic problems. Note presence of angina, hypertension, heart failure, recent myocardial infarction, renal disease, diabetes.
- Identify any drugs (e.g., aspirin) or herbs (e.g., ginkgo) that may affect coagulation.
- Identify patients with prosthetic heart valves, pacemakers, or implantable cardioverter-defibrillators.
- Assess for edema (including dependent areas), noting location and severity.
- Inspect neck veins for distention.
- Obtain bilateral baseline BPs.
- Assess capillary refill and pulses (bilaterally when appropriate) for rate, rhythm, and quality: apical, radial, and pedal.

Respiratory System
- Identify acute or chronic problems. Note presence of infection, chronic obstructive pulmonary disease, or asthma. Note use of CPAP machine.
- Assess tobacco history, including date/time of last cigarette and number of pack-years.
- Determine baseline O_2 saturation and respiratory rate and rhythm.
- Observe for cough, dyspnea, and use of accessory muscles of respiration.
- Auscultate lungs for normal and adventitious breath sounds.

Neurologic System
- Determine orientation to person, place, and time.
- Assess baseline mental status. Note presence of confusion, disorderly thinking, or inability to follow commands.
- Identify past history of strokes, transient ischemic attacks, or neurologic diseases (e.g., Parkinson's disease, multiple sclerosis).

Genitourinary System
- Identify any infection or preexisting disease.
- Determine ability to void.
- Note color, amount, and characteristics of urine (if appropriate).
- Determine pregnancy status (if appropriate).

Hepatic System
- Review past history of substance abuse, especially alcohol and IV drug use.
- Inspect skin color and sclera of eyes for any signs of jaundice.

Integumentary System
- Determine skin status. Note any current or previous skin disorders (e.g., pressure ulcers, eczema, bruising).
- Inspect skin for rashes, boils, or infection, especially around the planned surgical site.
- Inspect mucous membranes and skin turgor for signs of dehydration.
- Assess skin moisture and temperature.

Musculoskeletal System
- Examine skin around bone pressure points.
- Assess for limitations in joint range of motion and muscle strength.
- Assess for joint or muscle pain.
- Assess mobility, gait, and balance.

Gastrointestinal System
- Determine patterns of food and fluid intake and any recent changes in weight.
- Determine usual pattern of bowel movements, including date of last bowel movement.
- Assess for presence of dentures and bridges (loose dentures or teeth may be dislodged during intubation).
- Weigh patient.
- Auscultate abdomen for presence of bowel sounds.

Immune System
- Identify any immunodeficiency or autoimmune disorders.
- Assess for use of corticosteroids or other immunosuppressant drugs.

Laboratory and Diagnostic Studies
- Review results of all laboratory and diagnostic studies completed preoperatively (see Table 17-5).

CPAP, Continuous positive airway pressure.
*See specific body system chapters for more detailed assessments and related laboratory studies.

TABLE 17-5 Common Preoperative Diagnostic Studies

Test	Assessment
ABGs, pulse oximetry	Respiratory and metabolic function, oxygenation status
Blood glucose	Metabolic status, diabetes
Blood urea nitrogen, creatinine	Renal function
Chest x-ray	Pulmonary disorders, cardiac enlargement, heart failure
CBC: RBCs, Hgb, Hct, WBCs	Anemia, immune status, infection
Electrocardiogram	Cardiac disease, dysrhythmias
Electrolytes	Metabolic status, renal function, diuretic side effects
hCG	Pregnancy status
Liver function tests	Liver status
PT, PTT, INR, platelet count	Coagulation status
Pulmonary function studies	Pulmonary status
Serum albumin	Nutritional status
Type and crossmatch	Blood available for replacement (elective surgery patients may have own blood available)
Urinalysis	Renal status, hydration, urinary tract infection

CBC, Complete blood count; *hCG,* human chorionic gonadotropin; *Hct,* hematocrit; *Hgb,* hemoglobin; *INR,* international normalized ratio; *PT,* prothrombin time; *PTT,* partial thromboplastin time.

the documentation already present in the patient's chart, including the H&P, to better proceed with your examination. Record all findings and share any relevant findings immediately with the surgeon or ACP.

Diagnostic Studies. Obtain and assess the results of diagnostic studies ordered preoperatively (Table 17-5). For example, if the patient is taking an antiplatelet drug (e.g., aspirin), a coagulation profile is ordered; if the patient is on diuretic therapy, a potassium level is assessed; if the patient is of childbearing age, a pregnancy test is done; or if the patient is taking drugs for dysrhythmias, a preoperative ECG is obtained. Blood glucose is monitored for patients with diabetes. In many settings, tests for methicillin-resistant *Staphylococcus aureus* are done preoperatively. Patients with positive results are prescribed antibiotics for several days before surgery.[16]

Ideally, preoperative tests are ordered based on the patient's H&P. However, many agencies and insurers have protocols for preoperative tests, which may not include all those in Table 17-5. In addition, the preoperative tests may be done days before surgery. Ensure that all laboratory and diagnostic reports are in the patient's chart. Missing reports may result in a delay or cancellation of the surgery.

❖ NURSING MANAGEMENT: PREOPERATIVE PATIENT

Preoperative nursing interventions are derived from the nursing assessment and must reflect each patient's specific needs. Physical preparations are determined by the pending surgery and routines of the surgery setting. Preoperative teaching may be minimal or extensive. The Association of periOperative Registered Nurses (AORN) provides standards and recommended practices to guide nursing interventions in all perioperative settings.[7]

◆ Preoperative Teaching

The patient has a right to know what to expect and how to participate effectively during the surgical experience. Preoperative teaching increases patient satisfaction and can reduce postoperative fear, anxiety, and stress.[17] Teaching may also decrease the development of complications, length of hospitalization, and recovery time after discharge.

In most surgical settings, patients often arrive only a short time before surgery is scheduled. Preoperative teaching for these patients is generally done in the surgeon's office or a preadmission surgical clinic and reinforced on the day of surgery. After ambulatory surgery the patient usually goes home several hours after recovery, depending on the patient's progress and procedure-specific needs. Teaching must include information that focuses on the patient's safety. Provide written materials for patients and caregivers to use for review and reinforcement at home. Discharge teaching is required for all patients[18] and is discussed in Chapter 19.

When doing preoperative teaching, find a balance between explaining so much that the patient is overwhelmed and telling so little that the patient is unprepared. If you observe and listen carefully to the patient, you can usually determine how much information is enough. Remember that anxiety and fear may limit learning ability. Also assess what the patient wants to know and give priority to those concerns.

Generally, preoperative teaching includes three types of information: sensory, process, and procedural. Different patients, with varying cultures, backgrounds, and experience, may want different types of information. See Table 4-7 for factors affecting patient teaching.

With *sensory information,* patients find out what they will see, hear, smell, and feel during the surgery. For example, you may tell them that the OR will be cold, but they can ask for a warm blanket; the lights in the OR are bright; or many unfamiliar sounds and specific smells will be present.

Patients wanting *process information* may not want specific details but just the general flow of what is going to happen. This information would include the patient's transfer to the holding area, visits by the nurse and the ACP before transfer to the OR, and waking up in the PACU.

With *procedural information,* patients desire details that are more specific. For example, this information would include that an IV line will be started while the patient is in the holding area and the surgeon will mark the operative area with an indelible marker to verify the surgical site.[7]

Share the preoperative teaching given to the patient with the nurses providing postoperative care to evaluate learning and avoid duplication of teaching. Because the time for teaching is limited, the team approach is often used. For example, teaching may be started in the outpatient setting. Your responsibility is to assess the patient's understanding of this teaching and fill in the gaps at this point in the surgical process.

Record all teaching in the patient's chart. A guide for preoperative patient and caregiver teaching is presented in Table 17-6. See Chapter 4 for additional information on patient and caregiver teaching.

◆ **General Surgery Information.** Unless contraindicated (e.g., after craniotomy, tonsillectomy), all patients should receive instruction about deep breathing, coughing, and early ambulation postoperatively. This is essential because patients may not want to do these activities postoperatively unless they know the reason for them and practice them preoperatively. Tell patients

TABLE 17-6 Patient & Caregiver Teaching

Preoperative Preparation

Include the following information in the preoperative teaching plan for the patient and caregiver.

Sensory Information

- Preoperative holding area may be noisy.
- Drugs and cleaning solutions may be odorous.
- Operating room (OR) can be cold. Forced air warming devices may be used. Warm blankets are also available and can be requested.
- Talking may be heard in OR but may be distorted because of masks. Ask questions if something is not understood.
- OR bed will be narrow. A safety strap will be applied over the thighs.
- Lights in the OR may be bright.
- Monitoring machines may be heard (e.g., beeping noises) when awake.

Procedural Information

- What to bring and what type of clothing to wear to the surgery center
- Any changes in time of surgery.
- Fluid and food restrictions.
- Physical preparation required (e.g., shower, bowel, or skin preparation).
- Purpose of frequent vital signs assessment.
- Pain control and other comfort measures.
- Why turning, deep breathing, and coughing postoperatively are important. Practice sessions must be done preoperatively.
- Insertion of IV lines.
- Procedure for anesthesia administration.
- Expect surgical site to be marked with indelible ink or marker.

Process Information

Information About General Flow of Surgery

- Admission area.
- Preoperative holding area, OR, and postanesthesia care unit (PACU).
- Caregivers can usually stay in preoperative holding area until surgery.
- Caregivers will be able to see patient after discharge from the PACU or possibly in PACU once the patient is awake.
- Identification of any technology that may be present on awakening, such as monitors, central lines, sequential compression devices.

Where Caregivers Can Wait During Surgery

- Encourage caregivers to ask questions and express any concerns.
- OR staff will update caregivers during surgery and when surgery is completed.
- Surgeon will usually talk with caregivers after surgery.

and caregivers if tubes, drains, monitoring devices, or special equipment will be used after surgery. Explain that these devices help you to safely care for the patient. Examples of individualized teaching may include how to use incentive spirometers or postoperative patient-controlled analgesia pumps. Patients should have a clear understanding of how to rate their pain and how their pain will be managed.[19] (See Chapter 8 for additional information on pain.)

The patient should also receive accurate surgery-specific information. For example, a patient having a total joint replacement may have an immobilizer after surgery, or a patient having heart surgery should be told about waking up in the intensive care unit.

◆ **Ambulatory Surgery Information.** The ambulatory surgery patient or the patient admitted to the hospital the day of surgery needs to receive information before admission. Some ambulatory surgical centers telephone the patients several days before the procedure to obtain health information, give instructions, and answer questions. Each center has policies and procedures that direct this communication in a timely manner.

TABLE 17-7 Preoperative Fasting Recommendations*

Liquid and Food Intake	Minimum Fasting Period (Hr)
Clear liquids (e.g., water, clear tea, black coffee, carbonated beverages, fruit juice without pulp)	2
Breast milk	4
Nonhuman milk, including infant formula	6
Light meal (e.g., toast and clear liquids)	6
Regular meal (may include fried or fatty food, meat)	8 or more

Source: Practice guidelines for preoperative fasting and the use of pharmacologic agents to reduce the risk of pulmonary aspiration: application to healthy patients undergoing elective procedures: an updated report by the American Society of Anesthesiologists Task Force on Preoperative Fasting. Retrieved from *http://anesthesiology.pubs.asahq.org/Article.aspx?articleid=1933410.*
*For healthy patients of all ages undergoing elective surgery (excluding women in labor).

In addition to specifics on the procedure, patients need information on day-of-surgery events such as arrival time, registration, parking, what to wear, what to bring, and the need to have a responsible adult present for transportation home after surgery.

Traditionally, patients having elective surgery are told to have nothing by mouth (NPO) starting at midnight on the night before surgery. Evidence-based guidelines published by the American Society of Anesthesiologists are less strict[20] (Table 17-7). Restriction of fluids and food is designed to reduce the risk of pulmonary aspiration and postoperative nausea and vomiting. Protocols may vary for patients having local anesthesia or surgery scheduled late in the day. Follow the NPO protocol of each surgical setting. The patient who has not followed the NPO instructions may have surgery delayed or cancelled. It is critical that the patient understands the reason for and follows all restrictions.

◆ Legal Preparation for Surgery

Legal preparation for surgery consists of checking that all required forms have been correctly signed and are present in the patient's chart, and that the patient and caregiver clearly understand what is going to happen. Standard consent forms include those for the surgical procedure and blood transfusions. Other forms may include advance directives and durable power of attorney for health care (see Chapter 9).

◆ **Consent for Surgery.** Before nonemergency surgery can be legally performed, the patient must voluntarily sign an informed consent form in the presence of a witness. **Informed consent** is an active, shared decision-making process between the HCP and recipient of care. Three conditions must be met for consent to be valid. First, there must be *adequate disclosure* of the (1) diagnosis; (2) nature and purpose of the proposed treatment; (3) risks and consequences of the proposed treatment; (4) probability of a successful outcome; (5) availability, benefits, and risks of alternative treatments; and (6) prognosis if treatment is not instituted. Second, the patient must demonstrate clear *understanding* of the information being provided before receiving sedating preoperative drugs. If a patient is sedated prior to signing the consent, surgery may be cancelled or delayed. Third, the recipient of care must *give consent voluntarily.* The patient must not be persuaded or coerced in any way by anyone to undergo the procedure.[21]

The surgeon is ultimately responsible for obtaining the patient's consent for surgical treatment. You may be asked to witness the patient's signature on the consent form. At this time, you must be a patient advocate, verifying that the patient understands the information in the consent and the implications of consent, and that consent for surgery is truly voluntary. If the patient is unclear about the surgical plans, contact the surgeon about the patient's need for additional information. The patient should also be aware that consent, even when signed, can be withdrawn at any time.

If the patient is a minor, unconscious, or mentally incompetent to sign the permit, a legally appointed representative or responsible family member may give written permission. An *emancipated minor* is one who is younger than the legal age of consent but is recognized as having the legal capacity to provide consent.[19] Procedures for obtaining consent vary among states and agencies. Follow specifics required by your state's nurse practice act and agency policies that apply to an individual situation.

ETHICAL/LEGAL DILEMMAS

Informed Consent

Situation

J.S., a 72-year-old woman, is waiting in the preoperative holding area. You are discussing her impending surgery when you realize that this competent adult does not fully understand her surgery and was not informed of the alternatives to this surgery. Although she has previously signed a consent form, your assessment is that she was not fully informed about her treatment options or does not recall them.

Ethical/Legal Points for Consideration

- Informed consent requires that patients have complete information about the proposed treatment, as well as alternative treatments, risks and benefits of each treatment option, and possible consequences of the surgical procedure. The person (usually the surgeon) performing the procedure usually has this responsibility.
- An opportunity to have questions answered about the various treatment options and their possible outcomes is also an important element of informed consent.
- A patient can revoke the consent at any time, even at the very last minute. It is essential that you report any circumstance that suggests that the patient does not understand the information or is revoking the informed consent to the person who obtained the consent.
- In most states, the registered nurse's legal role is to witness the signing of the document. This means that as a nurse, you attest to the fact that the patient's signature was valid.

Discussion Questions

1. What do you think you should do next?
2. What is your role as a patient advocate in the informed consent process?
3. What should you do if the patient states that she does not want to know about the surgical procedure or alternatives to surgery?

A true medical emergency may override the need to obtain consent.[19] When immediate medical treatment is needed to preserve life or prevent serious impairment to life or limb and the patient is incapable of giving consent, the next of kin may give consent. If reaching the next of kin is not possible, the HCP may begin treatment without written consent. A note is written in the chart documenting the medical necessity of the procedure. In the case of an emergency in which consent cannot be obtained, you will usually need to complete an event report because it is an occurrence that is inconsistent with routine agency practices.

◆ Day-of-Surgery Preparation

◆ **Nursing Role.** Day-of-surgery preparation varies a great deal depending on whether the patient is an inpatient or an ambulatory surgical patient. Your responsibilities immediately before surgery include final preoperative teaching, assessment, and communication of pertinent findings. In addition, ensure that all preoperative orders are done and that the chart is complete and accompanies the patient to the OR. It is especially important to verify the presence of a signed informed consent, results of laboratory and diagnostic studies, an H&P, a record of any consultations, baseline vital signs, proper skin preparation, and completed nursing notes. In addition, the surgical site is identified and marked with an indelible marker by the surgeon and documented to indicate that the patient agrees.[7]

Hospitals often require that a patient wear a hospital gown with no underclothes. Surgical centers may allow the patient to wear underwear, depending on the procedure to be performed. The patient should remove any cosmetics, since observation of skin color is important. Nail polish and artificial nails should be removed so that capillary refill and pulse oximetry can be assessed. Place an identification band on the patient and, if applicable, an allergy band (Fig. 17-1). Return all patient valuables to a caregiver or secure according to agency policy. All prostheses, including dentures, contact lenses, and glasses, are generally removed to prevent loss or damage. If electrocautery devices will be used during surgery, jewelry in piercings must be removed as a safety measure. Hearing aids should be left in place to allow the patient to better follow instructions. Return glasses to the patient as soon as possible after surgery.

Encourage the patient to void before preoperative drugs are given and before transfer to the OR. An empty bladder prevents involuntary elimination under anesthesia and reduces the risk of urinary retention during the early postoperative recovery.

Many preoperative drugs interfere with balance and increase the risk for a fall during ambulation. Carefully assess each patient for responses to preoperative drugs and adjust the plan of care accordingly.

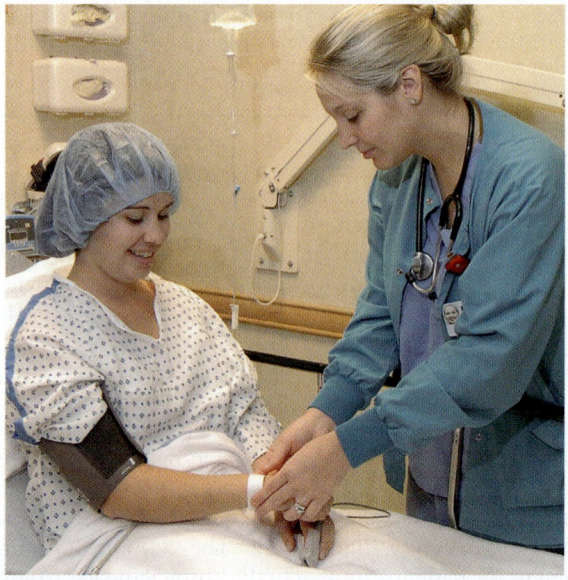

FIG. 17-1 The nurse performs a safety check by verifying that the patient has an identification band (wristband) as part of the preoperative preparations before she goes to surgery. (Courtesy Susan R. Volk, RN, MSN, CCRN, CPAN, Staff Development Specialist, Christiana Care Health System, Newark, Del.)

CHECK YOUR PRACTICE

You are caring for an older female patient who received a dose of alprazolam (Xanax) for preoperative anxiety. One hour later, she requests to use the bathroom. You ask her if she can walk and she replies "yes." When assisting her to stand, she becomes dizzy and almost falls. You return her to bed.

- Instead of trying to help this patient ambulate to the bathroom, what should have you done?

Preoperative Medications. Preoperative medications are used for a variety of reasons (Table 17-8). A patient may receive a single drug or a combination of drugs. Benzodiazepines are used for their sedative and amnesic properties. Anticholinergics are sometimes given to reduce secretions. Opioids may be given to decrease pain and intraoperative anesthetic requirements. Antiemetics may be given to decrease nausea and vomiting.

Other drugs that may be given preoperatively include antibiotics, eyedrops, and routine prescription drugs. Antibiotics may be given throughout the perioperative period for patients with a history of prosthetic heart valve to prevent infective endocarditis and for patients with previous joint replacement. Antibiotics may also be ordered for the patient undergoing surgery where wound contamination is a potential risk (e.g., gastrointestinal surgery). Antibiotics are most often given IV and are usually started preoperatively (e.g., 30 to 60 minutes before the surgical incision).

INFORMATICS IN PRACTICE

Computer-Based Timing for Antibiotic Administration

- A patient who receives the appropriate preoperative antibiotic has a decreased risk of a health care–associated infection.
- Using a computer to time the administration of preoperative antibiotics can decrease the incidence of wound infections.
- Computer-based timing systems assist with quality of care by tracking patient outcomes.
- You can look at the time patients received antibiotics and compare the rate of wound infections for those who did and did not receive timely treatment.

β-Adrenergic blockers (β-blockers) are sometimes used in people with known hypertension or coronary artery disease to control BP or reduce the chances of MI and cardiac arrest.[22] People with diabetes are also carefully monitored and may receive insulin in the preoperative period.[19] Eyedrops are often ordered and given preoperatively for the patient undergoing cataract and other eye surgery. Many times the patient will require multiple sets of eyedrops given at 5-minute intervals. It is important to give these drugs as ordered and on time to adequately prepare the eye for surgery.

Drugs that patients routinely take may or may not be used on the day of surgery. To aid patient teaching and remove confusion about which drugs should be taken, carefully check written preoperative orders and clarify the orders with the surgeon and/or ACP if there is any question.

Preoperative drugs may be ordered by mouth (PO), IV, or subcutaneously. Provide PO drugs with a small sip of water 60 to 90 minutes before the patient goes to the OR unless otherwise ordered. Subcutaneous injections (e.g., insulin) and IV drugs are usually given to the patient after arrival in the preoperative holding area or OR. Inform the patient about the expected effects of the drugs (e.g., drowsiness).

TABLE 17-8 Drug Therapy

Commonly Used Preoperative Medications

Class	Drug	Purpose
Antibiotics	cefazolin (Ancef)	Prevent postoperative infection
Anticholinergics	atropine glycopyrrolate (Robinul) scopolamine (Transderm-Scop)	↓ Oral and respiratory secretions Prevent nausea and vomiting Provide sedation
Antidiabetics	insulin (Humulin R)	Stabilize blood glucose
Antiemetics	metoclopramide (Reglan) ondansetron (Zofran)	↑ Gastric emptying Prevent nausea and vomiting
Benzodiazepines	midazolam diazepam (Valium) lorazepam (Ativan)	↓ Anxiety, induce sedation, amnesic effects
β-Blockers	labetalol	Manage hypertension
Histamine (H_2)-receptor antagonists	famotidine (Pepcid) ranitidine (Zantac)	↓ HCl acid secretion, ↑ pH, ↓ gastric volume
Opioids	morphine (Duramorph) fentanyl (Sublimaze)	Relieve pain during preoperative procedures

SAFETY ALERT Preoperative Checklist

- Use a preoperative checklist (Table 17-9) to ensure that all preoperative preparations have been completed.
- This is especially important to do before the patient is given any sedating drugs.

Transportation to Operating Room

For inpatients, transport staff move the patient by stretcher to the OR. Assist the patient in moving from the bed to the stretcher, raise the side rails, and ensure that the completed chart and any ordered preoperative equipment (e.g., SCDs) goes with the patient. In many agencies the caregiver may go with the patient to the holding area.

In an ambulatory surgical center the patient may be transported to the OR by stretcher or wheelchair. If no sedatives have been given, the patient may even walk accompanied to the OR. In all cases it is important to ensure patient safety during transport. Record the method of transportation and the person who transports the patient to the OR. Provide the hand-off communication to the nurse receiving the patient. This allows each of you to ensure that all pertinent information regarding the patient has been shared.[23] To avoid adverse events related to miscommunication, AORN recommends the use of the Situation-Background-Assessment-Recommendation (SBAR) model for the hand-off process in this setting[19] (see Table 1-6).

Show the caregiver where to wait for the patient during surgery. Many hospitals have a surgical waiting room where OR staff communicate the patient's status to the caregiver(s) and notify them when the surgery is complete. The surgeon also can locate the caregiver in this room after surgery to discuss the outcome. Some hospitals provide pagers to caregivers so that they may eat or do errands during the surgery.

Culturally Competent Care: Preoperative Patient

Include cultural considerations when assessing and implementing care for the patient's preoperative needs. For example, culture often determines one's expression of pain, family expectations, and ability to verbally express needs. One's culture may

TABLE 17-9 Preoperative Checklist

Preoperative Data	Initials
Height ____ Weight ____	
Isolation Y or N Type ____	
Allergies noted on chart Y or N	
Vital signs (baseline) T ____ P ____ R ____ BP ____ Pulse Ox ____	
Chart Review	
H&P on chart	
H&P within 30 days? Y or N	
Signed and witnessed informed consent form on chart Y or N	
Signed consent for blood administration Y or NA	
Blood type and crossmatch Y or NA	
Diagnostic Results	
Hgb/Hct ____ /____ NA	
PT/INR/PTT ____ /____ /____ NA	
CXR ____ NA	
ECG ____ NA hCG ____ Negative ____ Positive ____NA	
Other labs:	
Final Chart Review	
Additional forms attached:	

Day of Surgery	Initials
Surgical site marked Y or NA	
ID band on patient Y or N	
Allergy band on patient Y or NA	
Vital signs Time _____ T ____ P ____ R ____ BP ____ Pulse Ox ____	
Procedures	
NPO since ____	
Capillary blood glucose Time _____ Result: ____ NA	
Voided/catheter Time ____	
Preoperative drugs given Time ____ NA	
Preoperative antibiotics given Time ____ NA	
Preoperative skin prep Y or NA Shower____ Scrub____ Clip____	
Makeup, nail polish, false fingernails, and false eyelashes removed Y or NA	
Hospital gown applied Y or NA	
Valuables	
Dentures Y or N	
Wig or hairpiece Y or N	
Eyeglasses Y or N	
Contact lenses Y or N	
Hearing aid Y or N	
Prosthesis Y or N	
Jewelry Y or N Piercings with jewelry Y or N	
Clothing Y or N	
Disposition of valuables: Hearing aid in place Y or NA	

Time to OR _____ Date _____
Transported to OR by _____
Final check by _____ RN _____

require that the family be included in any decision making. For example, many older Hispanic women may defer to their family for the decision whether or not to have surgery. Respect these decisions. If the patient or caregiver does not speak English, it is mandated that a qualified interpreter or translator communication system be used.[24] (Culturally competent care is discussed in Chapter 2.)

Gerontologic Considerations: Preoperative Patient

Many surgical procedures are done on patients older than 65 years of age. Surgery on older adults requires careful evaluation.[25] Frequently performed procedures in older adults include cataract extraction, coronary and vascular procedures, prostate surgery, herniorrhaphy, cholecystectomy, and joint repair or replacement.

Be particularly alert when assessing and caring for the older adult surgical patient. An event that has little effect on a younger adult may be overwhelming to the older patient. Emotional reactions to impending surgery and hospitalization often intensify in the older adult. Hospitalization may represent a physical decline and loss of health, mobility, and independence. The older adult may view the hospital as a place to die or as a stepping-stone to a nursing home. Help to decrease anxieties and fears while maintaining the self-esteem of the older adult during the surgical experience.

The risks associated with anesthesia and surgery increase in the older patient. In general, the older the patient, the greater the risk of complications after surgery. In planning care, consider the patient's physiologic status, not only the chronologic age. The surgical risk in the older adult relates to normal physiologic aging and changes that compromise organ function, reduce reserve capacity, and limit the body's ability to adapt to stress. This decreased ability to cope with stress, often compounded by the burden of one or more chronic illnesses, and the surgery itself increase the risk of complications.[25]

When preparing the older adult for surgery, obtain a detailed H&P. Preoperative laboratory tests, an ECG, and a chest x-ray are important in planning the choice and type of anesthesia. The patient's primary HCP is usually not the surgeon, and frequently several HCPs are involved in the patient's care.

Older adults may have some sensory deficits. Vision and hearing may be reduced, and bright lights may bother those with eye problems. Thought processes and cognitive abilities may be slowed or impaired. Assess and record baseline sensory and cognitive function. Physical reactions are often slowed as a result of mobility and balance problems. All these changes may require more time for the older adult to complete preoperative testing and understand preoperative instructions. These changes also require attention to promote patient safety and prevent injury. (See Chapter 5 for more discussion about older adults.)

When older adults live in a long-term care or assisted living facility, you may need to coordinate transportation from these facilities so that timely arrival allows for surgery preparation. A legal representative of the patient must be present to provide consent for surgery if the patient cannot sign for himself or herself.

Finally, determine the presence of or need for caregiver support for the older adult undergoing surgery. With the increase in outpatient surgical procedures and shorter postoperative length of stays, caregiver support is critical in the continuity of care for this population.

CASE STUDY

Preoperative Patient

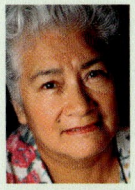

(©Ryan McVay/ Photodisc/ Thinkstock)

Patient Profile

F.D., a 72-year-old Hispanic retired librarian, is admitted to the hospital with compromised circulation of the right lower leg and a necrotic right foot. She has diabetes and takes insulin to maintain appropriate blood glucose levels. She has been NPO since midnight. It is now 10 AM on the morning of the surgery.

Subjective Data

- History of type 2 diabetes for 30 years; states, "My blood sugar is hard to control" and "I just started taking insulin"
- History of hypertension
- History of stage 2 chronic kidney disease
- History of peripheral vascular disease
- History of macular degeneration in right eye; reports poor vision
- Surgical history: cesarean section at age 30, cholecystectomy at age 65; reports poor wound healing after last surgery
- States her Social Security checks barely cover her living expenses
- States she often runs out of her drugs and cannot always afford to refill them right away
- Reports chronic burning pain in both legs and has trouble sleeping at night
- Lives alone but has family who want her to move in with them after surgery
- Uses herbs to control blood glucose levels and frequently skips her insulin

Objective Data

Physical Examination

- Alert, cognitively intact, anxious, older woman with complaints of numbness and lack of feeling in right leg
- Weight 190 lb, height 5 ft 3 in
- BP 180/94, pulse 84 and slightly irregular
- Wears glasses for close work and reading

Diagnostic Studies

- Admission serum blood glucose level 272 mg/dL (15.2 mmol/L), glycosylated hemoglobin (Hb A1C) 14%
- Morning capillary blood glucose level 198 mg/dL (11 mmol/L)
- Doppler pulses for right lower leg weak, absent in right foot
- Doppler pulses in left lower leg present, weak in left foot
- Serum creatinine 2.0 mg/dL (176 mmol/L)

Interprofessional Care

- Scheduled for a below-the-knee amputation of the right leg at 1 PM today

Discussion Questions

1. What factors may influence F.D.'s response to hospitalization and surgery?
2. ***Priority Decision:*** Given F.D.'s history, what priority preoperative nursing assessments would you want to complete and why?
3. What potential perioperative complications may you expect for F.D.?
4. ***Priority Decision:*** What priority topics would you include in F.D.'s preoperative teaching plan?
5. ***Priority Decision:*** Based on the assessment data presented, identify the priority nursing diagnoses and related interventions. Are there any collaborative problems?
6. ***Teamwork and Collaboration:*** Identify appropriate preoperative interventions that must be completed and could be delegated to unlicensed assistive personnel (UAP).
7. ***Safety:*** To ensure F.D.'s safety, what preoperative nursing interventions are essential?
8. ***Evidence-Based Practice:*** F.D. asks you why she received insulin this morning when she has not eaten anything since midnight. How would you respond to her?

Answers available at *http://evolve.elsevier.com/Lewis/medsurg.*

BRIDGE TO NCLEX EXAMINATION

The number of the question corresponds to the same-numbered outcome at the beginning of the chapter.

1. An overweight patient (BMI 28.1 kg/m^2) is scheduled for a laparoscopic cholecystectomy at an outpatient surgery setting. The nurse knows that
   a. surgery will involve multiple small incisions.
   b. this setting is not appropriate for this procedure.
   c. surgery will involve removing a portion of the liver.
   d. the patient will need special preparation because of obesity
2. The patient tells the nurse in the preoperative setting that she has noticed she has a reaction when wearing rubber gloves. What is the *most* appropriate intervention?
   a. Notify the surgeon so that the case can be cancelled.
   b. Ask additional questions to assess for a possible latex allergy.
   c. Notify the OR staff immediately so that latex-free supplies can be used.
   d. No intervention is needed because the patient's rubber sensitivity has no bearing on surgery.
3. A 59-year-old man scheduled for a herniorrhaphy in 2 days reports that he takes ginkgo daily. What is the *priority* intervention?
   a. Inform the surgeon, since the procedure may have to be rescheduled.
   b. Notify the anesthesia care provider, since this herb interferes with anesthetics.
   c. Ask the patient if he has noticed any side effects from taking this herbal supplement.
   d. Tell the patient to continue to take the herbal supplement up to the day before surgery.
4. A 17-year-old patient with a leg fracture who is scheduled for surgery is an emancipated minor. She has a statement from the court for verification. Which intervention is *most* appropriate?
   a. Witness the permit after consent is obtained by the surgeon.
   b. Call a parent or legal guardian to sign the permit, since the patient is under 18.
   c. Obtain verbal consent, since written consent is not necessary for emancipated minors.
   d. Investigate your state's nurse practice act related to emancipated minors and informed consent.

5. A *priority* nursing intervention to assist a preoperative patient in coping with fear of postoperative pain would be to
   a. inform the patient that pain medication will be available.
   b. teach the patient to use guided imagery to help manage pain.
   c. describe the type of pain expected with the patient's particular surgery.
   d. explain the pain management plan, including the use of a pain rating scale.
6. A patient is scheduled for surgery requiring general anesthesia at an ambulatory surgical center. The nurse asks him when he ate last. He replies that he had a light breakfast a couple of hours before coming to the surgery center. What should the nurse do *first*?
   a. Tell the patient to come back tomorrow, since he ate a meal.
   b. Proceed with the preoperative checklist, including site identification.
   c. Notify the anesthesia care provider of when and what the patient last ate.
   d. Have the patient void before administering any preoperative medications.
7. A patient who normally takes 40 units of glargine insulin (long acting) at bedtime asks the nurse what to do about her dose the night before surgery. The *best* response would be to have her
   a. skip her insulin altogether the night before surgery.
   b. get instructions from her surgeon or HCP on any insulin adjustments.
   c. take her usual dose at bedtime and eat a light breakfast in the morning.
   d. eat a moderate meal before bedtime and then take half her usual insulin dose.
8. Preoperative considerations for older adults include (*select all that apply*)
   a. using only large-print educational materials.
   b. speaking louder for patients with hearing aids.
   c. recognizing that sensory deficits may be present.
   d. providing warm blankets to prevent hypothermia.
   e. teaching important information early in the morning.

1. a, 2. b, 3. a, 4. a, 5. d, 6. c, 7. b, 8. c, d

For rationales to these answers and even more NCLEX review questions, visit *http://evolve.elsevier.com/Lewis/medsurg.*

EVOLVE WEBSITE

http://evolve.elsevier.com/Lewis/medsurg

Review Questions (Online Only)
Key Points
Answer Keys for Review Questions
- Rationales for Bridge to NCLEX Examination Questions
- Answer Guidelines for Case Study on p. 313

Conceptual Care Map Creator
Audio Glossary
Content Updates

REFERENCES

1. Jehovah's Witness Official Website: Why don't Jehovah's Witnesses accept blood transfusions? Retrieved from *www.jw.org/en/jehovahs-witnesses/faq/jehovahs-witnesses-why-no-blood-transfusions/#?insight[search_id]=b9ef370f-ef34-4500-a973-7cbe6fe12c54&insight[search_result_index]=2.*
2. Seyedfatemi N, Rafii F, Rezaer M, et al: Comfort and hope in the preanesthesia stage in patients undergoing surgery, *J Perianesth Nurs* 29:213, 2014.
3. Tran H, Joseph J, Young L, et al: New oral anticoagulants: a practical guide on prescription, laboratory testing and peri-procedural/bleeding management, *Intern Med J* 44:525, 2014.
4. Society of Gastroenterology Nurses and Associates: Patient safety issues with use of herbal supplements. Retrieved from *www.sgna.org/issues/sedationfactsorg/patientcare_safety/herbalsupplements.aspx.*
5. Erian M, McLaren G: Be wary of "natural" therapy in gynecological surgery, *Int J Womens Health* 5:345, 2013.
6. American College of Allergy, Asthma, and Immunology: Latex allergy. Retrieved from *www.acaai.org/ALLERGIST/ALLERGIES/TYPES/LATEX-ALLERGY/Pages/default.aspx.*

*7. Association of periOperative Registered Nurses: *Guidelines for perioperative practice*, Denver, 2015, The Association.

8. Hepner DL: The role of testing in the preoperative evaluation, *Cleve Clin J Med* 76:s22, 2009.
9. Yalamarthi S: Perioperative steroids in surgical patients. Retrieved from *www.hmjanaesthesia.4t.com/periopsteroid.htm.*
10. Neil JA: Perioperative care of the immunocompromised patient, *AORN J* 85:544, 2007.
11. Neil JA: Perioperative care of the patient with tuberculosis, *AORN J* 88:942, 2008.
12. Neil JA: Perioperative care of the bariatric revision surgery patient, *AORN J* 97:210, 2013.
13. Evans DC, Martindale RG, Kiraly LN, et al: Nutrition optimization prior to surgery, *Nutr Clin Prac* 29:10, 2014.
14. Lack L, Johannson K: Caffeine withdrawal: cost or benefit? *Sleep Med* 14:e53, 2013.
15. Department of Health and Human Services: CMS manual. Retrieved from *www.cms.gov/Regulations-and-Guidance/Guidance/Transmittals/downloads/R71SOMA.pdf.*
16. Marimuthu K, Harbarth S: Screening for methicillin-resistant *Staphylococcus aureus* … all doors closed? *Curr Opin Infect Dis* 27:356, 2014.

*17. Ping G: Preoperative education interventions to reduce anxiety and improve recovery among cardiac surgery patients: a review of randomised controlled trials, *J Clin Nurs* 24:34, 2014.

18. American Hospital Association: The patient care partnership: understanding expectations, rights and responsibilities. Retrieved from *www.aha.org/content/00-10/pcp_english_030730.pdf.*
19. Rothrock JC, editor: *Alexander's care of the patient in surgery*, ed 15, St Louis, 2015, Mosby.

*20. American Society of Anesthesiologists Committee: Practice guidelines for preoperative fasting and the use of pharmacologic agents to reduce the risk of pulmonary aspiration: application to healthy patients undergoing elective procedures: an updated report by the American Society of Anesthesiologists Committee on Standards and Practice Parameters, *Anesthesiology* 114:3, 2011.

21. American College of Surgeons: Informed consent. Retrieved from *www2.facs.org/public_info/operation/consent.html.*
22. Sear JW: Perioperative renin-angiotensin blockade: to continue or discontinue, that is the question! *Anesth Analg* 118:909, 2014.
23. Association of periOperative Registered Nurses: Patient hand off tool kit. Retrieved from *www.aorn.org/PracticeResources/ToolKits/PatientHandOffToolKit.*
24. Wilson-Stronks A, Lee KK, Cordero CL, et al: One size does not fit all: meeting the health care needs of diverse populations, Washington, DC, 2008, The Joint Commission. Retrieved from *www.jointcommission.org/assets/1/6/HLCOneSizeFinal.pdf.*

*25. Chow WB, Ko CY, Rosenthal RA, et al: American College of Surgeons NSQIP®/AGS best practice guidelines: optimal preoperative assessment of the geriatric surgical patient. Retrieved from *http://site.acsnsqip.org/wp-content/uploads/2011/12/ACS-NSQIP-AGS-Geriatric-2012-Guidelines.pdf.*

*Evidence-based information for clinical practice.

18

Intraoperative Care

*Anita Jo Shoup, David M. Horner**

Do not go where the path may lead, go instead where there is no path and leave a trail.

Ralph Waldo Emerson

http://evolve.elsevier.com/Lewis/medsurg/

LEARNING OUTCOMES

1. Differentiate the purposes of the various areas of the surgery department and the proper attire for each area.
2. Differentiate the roles and responsibilities of the interprofessional surgical team members.
3. Prioritize needs of patients undergoing surgery.
4. Analyze the role of the perioperative nurse in the management of patients undergoing surgery.
5. Apply basic principles of aseptic technique used in the operating room.
6. Evaluate the importance of safety in the operating room related to patients, equipment, and anesthesia.
7. Differentiate among the various anesthesia techniques and commonly used anesthesia drugs.

KEY TERMS

anesthesia care provider (ACP), p. 318
anesthesiology, p. 318
epidural block, p. 326
general anesthesia, p. 322
local anesthesia, p. 324
malignant hyperthermia (MH), p. 327
nurse anesthetist, p. 318
regional anesthesia, p. 324
spinal anesthesia, p. 325

Historically, surgery took place in the traditional environment of the hospital operating room (OR). Now, the majority of surgical procedures are done as ambulatory surgery (outpatient surgery). In addition, the use of *minimally invasive surgery* (MIS) is rapidly increasing. More procedures use endoscopes and other advanced technology (e.g., robotics). Incisions are smaller, blood loss is reduced, postoperative pain is decreased, recovery time is shorter, and patients are discharged sooner. This chapter discusses the intraoperative care that is applicable to all surgical patients regardless of where or how the surgery is performed.

PHYSICAL ENVIRONMENT OF THE OPERATING ROOM

Department Layout

The *surgical suite* is a controlled environment designed to minimize the spread of pathogens and allow a smooth flow of patients, staff, and equipment needed to provide safe patient care. The suite is divided into three distinct areas: unrestricted, semirestricted, and restricted areas. The *unrestricted area* is where people in street clothes can interact with those in surgical attire. These areas typically include the points of entry for patients (e.g., holding area), staff (e.g., locker rooms), and information (e.g., nursing station or control desk). The *semirestricted area* includes the surrounding support areas and corridors. Only authorized staff are allowed access to the semirestricted areas. All staff in the semirestricted area must wear surgical attire and cover all head and facial hair. In the *restricted area* masks are required to supplement surgical attire.[1] The restricted area can include the OR, scrub sink area, and sterile core.

In addition, the physical layout is designed to reduce cross-contamination. The flow of clean and sterile supplies and equipment is separated from contaminated supplies, equipment, and waste by space, time, and traffic patterns. Staff members move supplies from clean areas, such as the sterile core, through the OR for surgery, and on to the surrounding areas, such as the instrument decontamination area.

Holding Area

The *holding area,* frequently called the *preoperative holding area,* is a special waiting area inside of or next to the surgical suite. The size can range from a centralized area to handle numerous patients to a small designated area immediately outside the actual room scheduled for the surgical procedure. In the holding area you will identify and assess the patient before transferring him or her to the OR.

The *Surgical Care Improvement Project* (SCIP) is a national quality partnership of organizations focused on improving

*Contributed section on anesthesia content.

Reviewed by Judith M. Lewis, DNP, APRN, CRNA, Co-Chief Nurse Anesthetist, Akron's Children's Hospital, Akron, Ohio; Angela M. Martinelli, RN, PhD, CNOR, Clinical Professor, College of Nursing, Sacred Heart University, Fairfield, Connecticut; Crystal R. Sherman, DNP, CNP, FNP-BC, APHN-BC, Assistant Professor of Nursing, Shawnee State University, Portsmouth, Ohio; and Olga Van Dyke, RN, MSN, CAGS, Assistant Professor, School of Nursing, Massachusetts College of Pharmacy and Health Sciences, Boston, Massachusetts.

surgical care by significantly reducing the number of complications from surgery.[2] Several SCIP measures may be completed in the holding area, such as drug administration, patient warming, and application of sequential compression devices (SCDs). Many minor procedures (e.g., inserting IV catheters) can also be performed here.

The National Patient Safety Goals (NPSGs) require a preprocedure verification process, including the verification of relevant documentation (e.g., history and physical examination, signed consent forms, nursing and preanesthesia assessment).[3] In addition, any required blood products, implants, devices, and special equipment must be available. Further, the results of any diagnostic studies (e.g., x-rays, biopsy reports) must be included. In addition, the NPSGs require that the surgeon mark the procedure site. If possible, the marking should be done with the patient's involvement.[3]

In some settings, another area for holding is identified as the *admission, observation, and discharge* (AOD) area. This area is designed to allow early morning admission for outpatient surgery, same-day admission, and inpatient holding before surgery. In this area you can assess preoperative information, observe the patient before and after surgery, and allow sufficient recovery time before the patient is discharged to either the home or an inpatient room. The AOD area is important in the patient's stay throughout outpatient surgery and prevents unnecessary overnight stays in the inpatient setting.

Separation from caregivers just before surgery can produce anxiety for the patient. This anxiety can be reduced when the caregiver is permitted to wait with the patient in the holding area until the patient is transferred to the OR.

Operating Room

The traditional surgical environment, or OR, is a unique setting separate from other clinical units. It is controlled geographically, environmentally, and aseptically, and it is restricted in terms of the flow of staff (Fig. 18-1). It is preferred to have the OR next to the postanesthesia care unit (PACU) and the surgical intensive care unit. This allows for quick transport of the postoperative patient and close proximity to anesthesia staff if complications arise.

Several methods are used to prevent the transmission of infection. Filters and controlled airflow in the ventilating systems provide dust control. Positive air pressure in the rooms prevents air from entering the OR from the halls and corridors. Ultraviolet (UV) lighting may be used because UV radiation reduces the number of microorganisms in the air. Dust-collecting surfaces such as open shelves and tables are omitted. Materials that are resistant to the corroding effects of strong disinfectants are used.

Overall safety and comfort are aided by the use of OR furniture that is adjustable, easy to clean, and easy to move. All equipment is checked frequently to ensure proper functioning and electrical safety. The lighting is designed to provide a low- to high-intensity range for a precise view of the surgical site (Fig. 18-2). A communication system provides a means for the delivery of routine and emergency messages.[4]

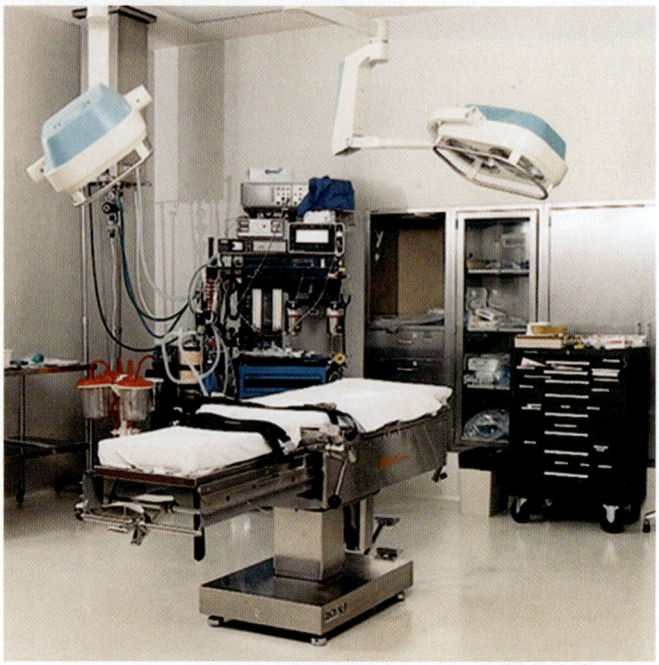

FIG. 18-1 Typical operating room. (Courtesy Greg McVicar.)

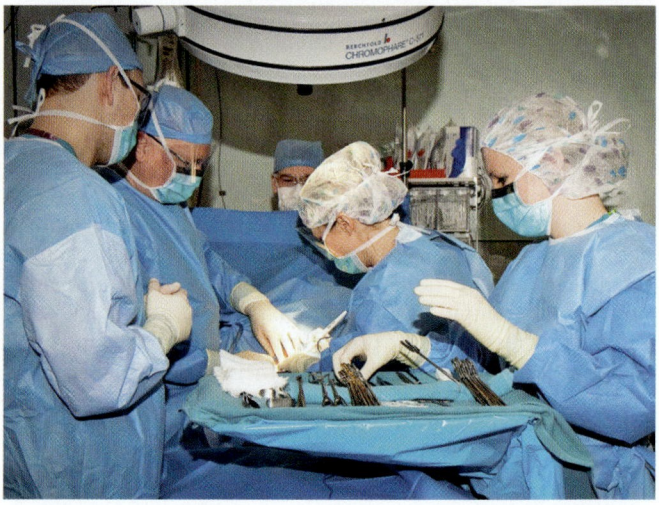

FIG. 18-2 The complexity of surgery requires maintaining asepsis. (Courtesy Swedish Edmonds Hospital, Edmonds, Wash. Photograph by Amy Wesley.)

SURGICAL TEAM

Registered Nurse

The *perioperative nurse* is a registered nurse (RN) who implements the patient's plan of care during the perioperative period. Through close collaboration with the other members of the surgical team, you prepare the OR for patients before they arrive. You are usually the first member of the surgical team who meets the patient. You are the patient's advocate throughout the intraoperative experience. This includes (1) maintaining the patient's safety, privacy, dignity, and confidentiality; (2) communicating with the patient; and (3) providing physical care.

Assess the patient to determine any additional needs or tasks to complete before surgery. Provide physical and emotional comfort for the patient and teaching regarding the upcoming surgery for the patient and caregivers. In addition, work with the patient's caregivers, keeping them informed and answering questions. This is particularly important in day-surgery settings, where caregivers must assume greater responsibility for preoperative and postoperative care.

In the perioperative role, you assume functions that involve either sterile or unsterile activities (Table 18-1). When you

TABLE 18-1 Intraoperative Nursing Activities

Circulating, Nonsterile Activities

- Reviews anatomy, physiology, and surgical procedure
- Assists in preparing room, ensuring that supplies and equipment are available, in working order, and sterile (if required)
- Maintains aseptic technique in all required activities
- Monitors practices of aseptic technique in self and others
- Checks mechanical and electrical equipment and environmental factors
- Conducts a preprocedure verification process
- Assesses patient's physical and emotional status
- Confirms and implements ordered SCIP measures
- Plans and coordinates intraoperative nursing care
- Checks chart and relates pertinent data to team members
- Helps with the application of monitoring devices and insertion of invasive lines and other devices
- Assists with and ensures patient safety in transferring and positioning patient
- Assists with induction of anesthesia
- Monitors draping procedure
- Participates in surgical time-out
- Records intraoperative care
- Prepares, records, labels, and sends blood, pathology, and any anatomic specimens to proper locations
- Measures blood, urine output, and other fluid loss
- Confirms, dispenses, and records drugs used, including local anesthetics
- Coordinates all intraoperative activities with team members and other staff and departments
- Maintains accurate count of sponges, needles, instruments, and medical devices that could be retained in the patient
- Goes with patient to PACU
- Gives hand-off report to PACU nurse with information relevant to care of patient

Scrubbed, Sterile Activities

- Reviews anatomy, physiology, and surgical procedure
- Assists in preparing the operating room
- Completes surgical hand antisepsis and gowns and gloves self and other members of surgical team
- Prepares instrument table and arranges sterile equipment for functional use
- Assists with draping procedure
- Participates in surgical time-out procedure
- Passes instruments to surgeon and assistants by anticipating their needs
- Maintains accurate count of sponges, needles, instruments, and medical devices that could be retained in the patient
- Monitors practices of aseptic technique in self and others
- Keeps track of irrigation solutions used for calculation of blood loss
- Accepts, verifies, and reports drugs used by surgeon and/or ACP, including local anesthetics

ACP, Anesthesia care provider; *PACU*, postanesthesia care unit; *SCIP*, Surgical Care Improvement Project.

serve in the role of *scrub nurse*, you follow the designated surgical hand antisepsis procedure, are gowned and gloved in sterile attire, and remain in the sterile field (Fig. 18-2). When you serve in the role of *circulating nurse*, you remain in the unsterile field and so you are not gowned and gloved in sterile attire.

Ongoing assessment of the patient is essential because the patient's condition may change quickly. You respond to these changes and revise the plan of care as needed. Examples of nursing activities that characterize each phase surrounding the surgical experience are presented in Table 18-2.

As patients move through the surgical experience, they are cared for by many team members. Chances for error arise whenever clinical information is shared among these members.[5] The Joint Commission requires that all health care providers use a standardized approach to hand-off communication. The perioperative RN ensures that a complete and accurate hand-off using a consistent format, such as SBAR (see Table 1-6), occurs every time patient care is transferred to another professional. Examples of such transfers include change of shift, surgeon to nurse, and OR nurse to postanesthesia nurse.

You have the opportunity to become a certified perioperative nurse (CNOR). Nursing certification is an objective measure (written test) that validates that a nurse has the essential knowledge needed to provide perioperative nursing care.[6]

Licensed Practical/Vocational Nurse and Surgical Technologist

Depending on your state nurse practice act, the role of the circulating or scrub nurse may be filled by a licensed practical/vocational nurse or a surgical technologist. Surgical technologists may attend an associate degree program, a vocational training program, or a hospital or military training program. The Association of Surgical Technologists sets the standards for education, provides continuing education opportunities, and offers certification for surgical technologists.[7]

If the circulating nurse is not an RN, the licensed practical/vocational nurse or surgical technologist must have access to an RN at all times. You are responsible for supervising the licensed practical/vocational nurse or surgical technologist in the performance of all delegated nursing tasks.[8]

Surgeon and Assistant

The *surgeon* is the physician who performs the surgical procedure. The surgeon is primarily responsible for the following:

- Preoperative medical history and physical assessment, including need for surgical intervention, choice of surgical procedure, management of preoperative testing, and discussion of the risks of and alternatives to surgical intervention
- Patient safety and management in the OR
- Postoperative management of the patient

The *surgeon's assistant* can be a physician who functions in an assisting role during the surgical procedure. The assistant usually holds retractors to expose surgical areas and assists with hemostasis and suturing. In some instances, especially in educational settings, the assistant may perform some portions of the surgery under the surgeon's direct supervision. In many institutions the surgeon's assistant is a registered nurse first assistant or a physician's assistant (PA) who functions under the physician's direct supervision.

Registered Nurse First Assistant

The *registered nurse first assistant* (RNFA) works in collaboration with the surgeon to produce an optimal surgical outcome for the patient. The Association of periOperative Registered Nurses (AORN) position statement on RNFAs states that the perioperative nurse must have formal education for this role and works collaboratively with the surgeon, patient, and surgical team by preparing and using instruments, providing exposure to the surgical site, handling tissue, assisting with hemostasis, and suturing.[9] RNFA education programs provide RNs with the education necessary to assume this expanded role. The RNFA can also obtain certification.

TABLE 18-2 Perioperative Nursing Activities*

BEFORE SURGERY	DURING SURGERY	AFTER SURGERY
Assessment and Planning	**Implementation**	**Evaluation**
Home, Clinic, Holding Area • Initiates preoperative assessment • Plans teaching appropriate to patient's needs • Involves caregiver **Surgical Unit** • Completes preoperative assessment • Coordinates patient teaching with staff • Develops a plan of care that reflects patient's level of function and ability • Safely gives ordered drugs **Surgical Suite** • Conducts preprocedure verification • Assesses patient's level of consciousness, skin integrity, mobility, emotional status, and functional limitations • Reviews chart • Ensures all supplies and equipment needed are available, functioning, and sterile, if appropriate	**Safety Maintenance** • Ensures integrity of sterile field • Ensures that sponge, needle, instrument, and medical device counts are correct • Positions patient to ensure correct alignment, exposure of surgical site, and prevention of injury • Prevents chemical injury from prepping solutions, drugs, etc. • Ensures safe use of electrical equipment • Safely gives ordered drugs **Monitoring Physical Status** • Monitors and reports changes in patient's vital signs • Monitors blood loss and urine output **Monitoring Psychologic Status** • Provides emotional support to patient • Ensures patient's right to privacy is maintained • Communicates patient's emotional status to health care team	**Postanesthesia, Discharge Area** • Determines patient's response to surgical intervention • Monitors ABCs, vital signs, level of consciousness • Safely gives ordered drugs **Clinical Unit** • Evaluates effectiveness of nursing care in OR using patient outcome criteria • Determines patient's level of satisfaction with care given during perioperative period • Assesses patient's psychologic status • Assists with discharge planning **Home, Clinic** • Seeks patient's perception of surgery in terms of effects of anesthetic agents, impact on body image, immobilization • Determines caregiver's perceptions of surgery

ABCs, Airway, breathing, circulation.
*List of activities is not all-inclusive.

Anesthesia Care Provider

The **anesthesia care provider (ACP)** is a person who administers anesthesia and can be an anesthesiologist, nurse anesthetist, or anesthesiologist assistant (AA). ACPs are responsible for giving anesthetic agents to provide a temporary state of depressed or loss of consciousness, relieve pain, and manage vital life functions (e.g., breathing, BP during surgery). After surgery, they provide care during recovery.[10]

Anesthesiology is a specialty within the practice of medicine that focuses on the following:

- Medically managing patients who are rendered unconscious or insensible to pain and emotional stress during surgical and other medical procedures
- Protecting functions and vital organs under the stress of anesthetic, surgical, or other medical procedures
- Managing pain
- Managing cardiopulmonary resuscitation
- Managing problems in pulmonary care
- Managing critically ill patients in special care units

A **nurse anesthetist** is a master's-prepared RN who has graduated from an accredited nurse anesthesia program and completed a national certification examination to become a certified registered nurse anesthetist (CRNA).

The CRNA scope of practice includes the following[11]:

- Performing and documenting a preanesthetic assessment and evaluation
- Developing and implementing a plan for delivering anesthesia
- Selecting and starting the planned anesthetic technique
- Selecting, obtaining, and administering the anesthesia, adjuvant drugs, and fluids
- Selecting, applying, and inserting appropriate noninvasive and invasive monitoring devices
- Managing a patient's airway and pulmonary status
- Managing emergence and recovery from anesthesia
- Releasing or discharging patients from a PACU
- Ordering, starting, or modifying pain relief therapy
- Responding to emergency situations by providing airway management, and giving emergency fluids and drugs
- Assuming additional responsibilities within the expertise of the individual

An AA is a master's-prepared health professional who serves under the direction of an anesthesiologist. The AA has graduated from an accredited program and completed a national certification examination. AAs participate in all types of anesthesia, including giving drugs, obtaining vascular access, applying and interpreting monitors, establishing and maintaining airways, and assisting with preoperative assessments.

❖ NURSING MANAGEMENT: PATIENT BEFORE SURGERY

The preoperative assessment of the surgical patient provides baseline data for intraoperative and postoperative care and is used to plan the intraoperative care. Preoperative care of the patient is discussed in Chapter 17.

◆ Psychosocial Assessment

Knowing about the activities that occur when a patient is moved into the surgical suite allows you to provide explanations and reassurances, especially to the anxious patient. You can usually answer general questions regarding surgery or anesthesia, such as, "When will I go to sleep?" "Who will be in the room?" "When will my surgeon arrive?" "How much of my body will be exposed?" "Will I be cold?" "When will I wake up?" Specific questions relating to details of the surgical procedure and anesthesia may be referred to the surgeon or ACP. For patients who do not speak English, a qualified interpreter must be used (see Table 2-10).

◆ Physical Assessment

Perform a thorough physical assessment during the preoperative preparation of the patient (see Chapter 17).

Chart Review

Required chart data vary with agencies, patient conditions, and surgical procedures. Because ambulatory surgery centers tend to have a healthier patient population, fewer tests may be needed. Examples of data that are obtained during the preoperative assessment are found in Tables 17-2 and 17-4. This information provides an understanding of past and present history, current health status, and potential for infection and other complications.

Admitting the Patient

Agency policy guides the protocol to be followed when admitting the patient to the holding area and OR. A general routine includes initial greeting, proper identification, and offer of human contact and warmth. A preprocedure verification process is conducted before the start of surgery. In some agencies this takes place in the holding area; in others it takes place in the OR itself.

The admitting procedure is continued with reassessment of the patient and with time allowed for last-minute questions. Complete the chart review for the previously mentioned data and note any abnormalities or changes. Question the patient concerning valuables, prostheses, and last intake of food and fluid. Confirm that the correct preoperative drugs were given (if ordered). Provide a pillow or adjust the patient's position if requested. Most hospitals require the patient's hair to be covered just before transfer to the OR suite to reduce potential shedding. Specific SCIP measures may include (1) a prophylactic antibiotic started within 30 to 60 minutes before the surgical incision and (2) application of a warming blanket and SCDs.

Complementary and alternative therapies such as therapeutic touch, aromatherapy, music therapy, guided imagery, and even movies may be used for surgical patients (see the Complementary & Alternative Therapies box). These therapies may decrease anxiety, promote relaxation, reduce pain, and facilitate the healing process.[12] In some agencies these therapies are started before the patient is admitted to the OR. In others, such as ambulatory settings, they may be started after the patient arrives in the holding area.

CHECK YOUR PRACTICE

Your patient has arrived in the holding area. As you review the chart, you realize that the consent for blood has not been signed. You also know that the patient has Alzheimer's disease and is not mentally competent to give consent.

- How would you proceed?

COMPLEMENTARY & ALTERNATIVE THERAPIES

Music Therapy

Music is an ancient healing tool recognized in the writings of Plato.

Scientific Evidence

Strong scientific evidence for use in reducing stress and anxiety and enhancing mood.*

Nursing Implications

- To be effective, the music selected must be appropriate for the situation. Music can have many different physiologic effects.
- Listening to calming music can result in slower, deeper breathing and a decrease in heart rate and BP. Both of these indicate relaxation.
- Music with a faster pace can energize a person and promote mental alertness.
- Music therapy is safe in combination with other treatment approaches.

*Based on a systematic review of scientific literature. Retrieved from *www.naturalstandard.com.*

NURSING MANAGEMENT: PATIENT DURING SURGERY

Whether surgery is only minutes long or lasts several hours, the circulating nurse is responsible for implementing the intraoperative plan of care. Patient care in the perioperative setting is dynamic and depends on the knowledge, skills, and judgment of the perioperative RN.[4] One of the critical duties of the circulating nurse is to serve as the patient's advocate. While each member of the perioperative team is focused on their specific activities, the circulating nurse focuses on the patient as a whole. This involves ongoing assessment, reassessment, and adjustment of the care plan so that the patient achieves a level of wellness equal to or improved from the preoperative level.

Room Preparation

Before transferring the patient into the OR, prepare the room to ensure privacy, prevention of infection, and safety. Individualization of this preparation is essential to achieve the expected patient outcomes.

CHECK YOUR PRACTICE

You are assigned to observe in the OR. A severely obese patient is admitted to the holding area. The circulating nurse tells you that the unique needs of each patient must be addressed for a safe surgical experience.

- What special considerations are needed for this patient?

When a patient is severely obese, special equipment is needed to safely transfer the patient to and from the OR table. Extra staff may also be needed for the positioning of the patient for the procedure. During surgery, special equipment (e.g., extra-long instrumentation) may be used.

Surgical attire (pants and shirts, masks, protective eyewear, and caps or hoods) is worn by all people entering the OR (Fig. 18-3). All electrical and mechanical equipment is checked for proper functioning. Aseptic technique is practiced as each surgical item is opened and placed on the instrument table. Sponges, needles, instruments, and small medical devices (e.g., surgical clip cartridges, universal adapters) are counted according to strict processes to ensure accurate retrieval at the end of the procedure. Any retained surgical supplies, devices, or instruments are sentinel events (never events) or serious reportable events that can result in negative outcomes for the patient.[1,4] (Sentinel events and serious reportable events are discussed in Chapter 1.)

During room preparation and the surgical procedure, the scrub person performs surgical hand antisepsis, dons sterile gown and gloves, and touches only those items in the sterile field. The circulating nurse remains in the unsterile field and performs those activities that permit touching all unsterile items and the patient. This coordinated effort allows for smooth functioning throughout the procedure.

Transferring Patient

Once the patient's identity has been confirmed and the OR has been prepared, the patient is moved into the room for the surgery. Each time a patient is transferred from one bed to another, the wheels of the stretcher must be locked. A sufficient number of staff members using ergonomic tools for safe patient handling and movement should be available to lift, guide, and

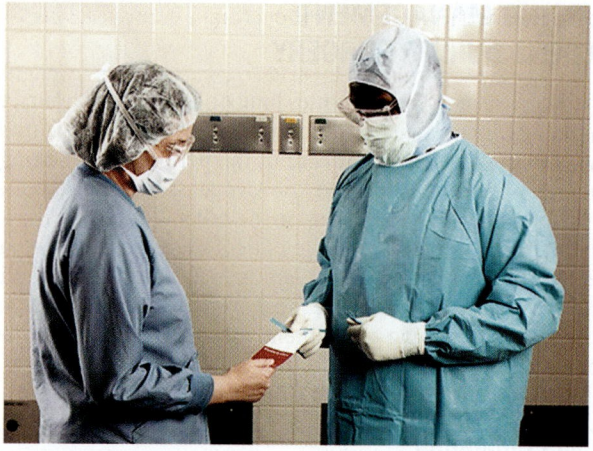

FIG. 18-3 Surgical attire is worn by all people entering the operating room.

prevent accidental falling or injury to self, other staff, or the patient. Once the patient is on the OR bed, place safety straps snugly across the patient's thighs. At this time the monitor leads (e.g., ECG leads), BP cuff, and pulse oximeter are usually applied and an IV catheter is inserted if it was not done in the holding area.

Scrubbing, Gowning, and Gloving

Surgical hand antisepsis is required of all sterile members of the surgical team (scrub nurse, surgeon, and assistant). When the procedure of scrubbing is the chosen method for surgical hand antisepsis (often for the first case of the day), your fingers and hands should be scrubbed first with progression to the forearms and elbows. The hands should be held away from surgical attire and higher than the elbows at all times to prevent contamination from clothing or detergent suds and water from draining from the unclean area above the elbows to the clean and previously scrubbed areas of the hands and fingers.

Waterless, alcohol-based agents are replacing soap and water in many agencies. When using an alcohol-based surgical handscrub product, prewash hands and forearms with soap and dry completely before applying the alcohol-based product. After application of the alcohol-based product, rub hands and forearms thoroughly until dry before donning sterile gloves.[1,4]

Once surgical hand antisepsis is completed, the team members enter the OR to put on surgical gowns and two pairs of gloves to protect patients and themselves from the transmission of microorganisms.[1,4] Because the gowns and gloves are sterile, those who have scrubbed can manipulate and organize all sterile items for use during the procedure.

Basic Aseptic Technique

Aseptic technique is practiced in the OR to prevent infection. This is implemented through the creation and maintenance of a sterile field (Fig. 18-4). The center of the sterile field is the site of the surgical incision. Items used in the sterile field, including surgical instruments and equipment, have been sterilized by appropriate sterilization methods.

Team members must understand specific principles to practice aseptic technique (Table 18-3). Unless these principles are followed, the patient's safety is compromised and the potential for postoperative infection is increased.[1,4]

In addition to following the principles of aseptic technique, the surgical team is responsible for following the guidelines

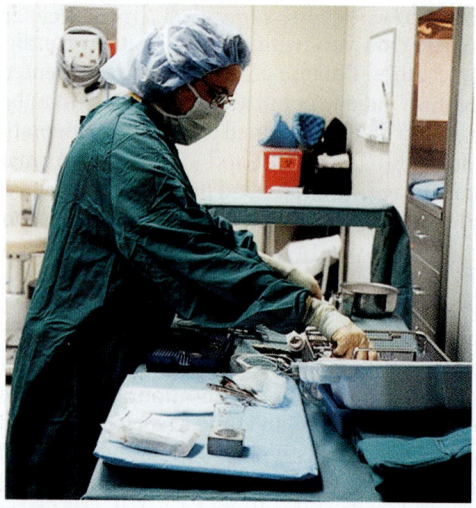

FIG. 18-4 A sterile field is created before surgery. (Courtesy The Methodist Hospital, Houston, Tex. Photograph by Donna Dahms, RN, CNOR.)

TABLE 18-3 Principles of Aseptic Technique in Operating Room

- All materials that enter the sterile field must be sterile.
- If a sterile item comes in contact with an unsterile item, it is contaminated.
- Contaminated items are removed immediately from the sterile field. If the unsterile item is small (e.g., unopened suture), once it is removed, the area is marked off (i.e., covered with a sterile drape). If the entire field is contaminated, it should be set up again with all new materials.
- The surgical team working in the operative field must wear sterile gowns and gloves. Once dressed for procedure, they must recognize that the only parts of the gown considered sterile are the front from chest to table level and sleeves to 2 inches above elbow.
- A wide margin of safety must be maintained between sterile and unsterile fields.
- Tables are considered sterile only at tabletop level. Items extending beneath this level are considered contaminated.
- The edges of a sterile package are considered contaminated once the package has been opened. If a sterile package (e.g., package of sutures) is placed on the sterile field, that entire package remains sterile even when opened.
- Microorganisms travel on airborne particles and will enter the sterile field with excessive air movements and currents.
- Microorganisms travel by capillary action through moist fabrics, resulting in contamination.
- Microorganisms harbor on the patient's and team members' hair, skin, and respiratory tracts and must be confined by appropriate attire.

established by the U.S. Occupational Safety and Health Administration (OSHA) and the AORN to protect the patient and the team from exposure to blood-borne pathogens.[13] These guidelines emphasize (1) standard and transmission-based precautions; (2) engineering and work practice controls; and (3) the use of personal protective equipment such as gloves, gowns, caps, face shields, masks, and protective eyewear. This is especially important in the OR because of the high potential for exposure to blood-borne pathogens.

Assisting Anesthesia Care Provider

While you check the OR to complete the final preparations, the ACP prepares the patient for the administration of the anesthetic. You need to understand the effects of the anesthetic agents and know the location of all emergency drugs and equipment.

If you are the circulating nurse, you may be involved in placing monitoring devices to be used during the surgical procedure (e.g., ECG leads). If the patient is to have general anesthesia, remain at the patient's side to ensure safety and assist the ACP. These responsibilities may include measuring BP and assisting in the maintenance of the patient's airway. During the surgical procedure, you also provide a vital communication link for the ACP to other departments, such as the laboratory or blood bank.

Safety Considerations

All surgical procedures, regardless of where they take place, can put the patient at risk for injury. These injuries can be infections, physical trauma from positioning or equipment used, or physiologic effects of surgery itself. Be alert to all safety issues, since the patient in the OR is often compromised from the effects of anesthesia.

Fire in the OR can have devastating consequences for the patient. Fortunately, surgical fires can be prevented with awareness of the hazards and emphasis on safe practices.[14] Care must be taken to correctly place the grounding pad and all electrosurgical equipment to prevent injury from burns or fire (Fig. 18-5). The electrosurgery plume of smoke contains toxic gas and vapors, bio-aerosols, and viruses as well as additional hazardous chemical compounds. These airborne contaminants can cause problems with visibility of the surgical site and tissue irritation and have mutagenic and carcinogenic potential.[1] Smoke evacuators may be used to minimize this exposure.

The *Universal Protocol,* one of the NPSGs, is followed to prevent wrong site, wrong procedure, and wrong surgery.[15] A patient safety checklist for ORs is the cornerstone of a major focus to make surgery safer. The use of the World Health Organization (WHO) Surgical Safety Checklist has improved compliance with standards and decreased complications from surgery.[16]

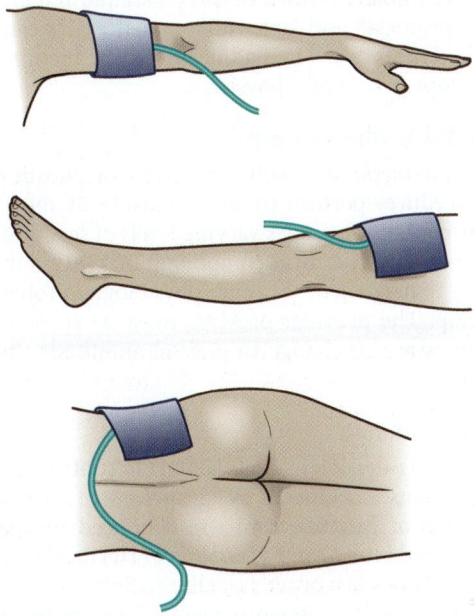

FIG. 18-5 When an electrosurgical unit is used, the patient must be properly grounded to prevent unintended injury. A well-vascularized muscle mass is an optimal site. Safety can be compromised by excessive hair, adipose tissue, bony prominences, fluid (edema), adhesive failure, and scar tissue. (Courtesy Covidien, Mansfield, Mass.)

Similarly, the AORN has developed a position statement regarding correct site surgery and guidelines for implementing the Universal Protocol.[17] All members of the surgical team stop what they are doing during a *surgical time-out* just before the procedure starts to verify patient identification, surgical procedure, and surgical site. In addition, OR staff complete a fire risk assessment (per agency protocol) to identify and reduce the potential for an OR fire.

! SAFETY ALERT Surgical Time-Out

- Before the induction of anesthesia, ask the patient to confirm name, birthdate, surgical procedure and site, and consent.
- Wrong surgical procedure and surgery performed on the wrong body part or wrong patient are *sentinel events (never events)* or *serious reportable events* (described in Chapter 1).

Positioning Patient

Positioning the patient is a critical part of every procedure and usually follows administration of the anesthetic. The ACP indicates when to begin the positioning. The patient's position should allow for accessibility to the operative site, administration and monitoring of anesthetic agents, and maintenance of the patient's airway. When positioning for the surgical procedure, take care to (1) provide correct musculoskeletal alignment; (2) prevent undue pressure on nerves, skin over bony prominences, earlobes, and eyes; (3) provide for adequate thoracic excursion; (4) prevent occlusion of arteries and veins; (5) provide modesty in exposure; and (6) recognize and respect individual needs such as previously assessed aches, pains, or deformities. It is your responsibility to secure the extremities, provide adequate padding and support, and obtain sufficient physical or mechanical help to avoid unnecessary straining of self or patient.

The patient may be placed in various positions, including supine, prone, lateral, lithotomy, or sitting. The supine is the most common position used. It is suited for surgery involving the abdomen, heart, and breast. The prone position allows easy access for back surgery (e.g., laminectomy). The lithotomy position is used for some types of pelvic organ surgery (e.g., vaginal hysterectomy).

Whatever position is needed for the procedure, take great care to prevent injury to the patient. Because anesthesia blocks the sensory nerve impulses, the patient will not feel pain, discomfort, or stress being placed on nerves, muscles, bones, and skin. Improper positioning could potentially result in muscle strain, joint damage, pressure ulcers, nerve damage, and other untoward effects.

Pressure ulcers are costly and debilitating complications of surgery. They are also considered preventable events.[18] Hypoperfusion of tissue under pressure in an immobile patient plays a major role in the development of pressure ulcers in the OR. A primary safety consideration for positioning is the redistribution of pressure, especially at the patient's bony prominences.

General anesthesia causes peripheral vessels to dilate. Position changes affect where the pooling of blood occurs. If the head of the OR bed is raised, the lower torso will have increased blood volume and the upper torso may become compromised. Hypovolemia and cardiovascular disease can further compromise the patient's status. Consequently, the entire surgical team carefully plans and implements the patient's positioning and then closely monitors the patient throughout the surgical procedure.

◆ Preventing Hypothermia

Research has shown a relationship between unintended hypothermia and impaired wound healing, adverse cardiac events, altered drug metabolism, and coagulopathies.[19] To prevent hypothermia, the surgical team needs to closely monitor the patient's temperature. A thermal warming blanket and warm IV fluids may be used to maintain the patient's normal body temperature.

◆ Preparing Surgical Site

The purpose of skin preparation, or "prepping," is to reduce the number of microorganisms available to migrate to the surgical wound. The task of prepping is completed intraoperatively by the circulating nurse, surgeon, or surgical assistant.

The skin is prepared by mechanically scrubbing or cleansing around the surgical site with an antimicrobial agent identified as one that reduces microorganisms on intact skin, contains a nonirritating antimicrobial agent, has broad-spectrum activity, is fast acting and persistent, and is nonallergenic to the patient. A liberal area is scrubbed in a circular motion. The principle of scrubbing from the clean area (site of the incision) to the dirty area (distal to the incision) is observed at all times.

Antiseptic agents used for skin preparation may contain alcohol and be flammable. Skin injury can occur if these agents are allowed to pool under the patient. Care must be taken to ensure that these agents are properly confined and allowed to fully dry. After the skin is prepped and the fumes are allowed to dispel to reduce the risk of fire, the sterile members of the surgical team drape the area. Only the site to be incised is left exposed.

❖ NURSING MANAGEMENT: PATIENT AFTER SURGERY

Through constant observation of the surgical process, the ACP anticipates the end of the surgical procedure. Appropriate types and doses of anesthetic agents are used so that their effects will be minimal at the end of the surgical procedure. This also allows greater physiologic control of the patient during the transfer to the PACU.

The patient's response to your care is evaluated based on outcome criteria established during the development of the patient's plan of care. These outcome criteria are published as the *Perioperative Nursing Data Set (PNDS)* by AORN. The PNDS reflects standards and recommended practices related to the delivery of nursing care in any perioperative setting.[20]

The ACP and you or another member of the surgical team go with the patient to the PACU. A hand-off of the patient that includes his or her status and the procedure performed is communicated to the nurse receiving the patient in the PACU to promote safe, ongoing care.

ANESTHESIA

The American Society of Anesthesiologists (ASA) defines anesthesia according to the effect that it has on the patient's sensorium and pain perception. These definitions include minimal sedation (e.g., anxiolysis), moderate sedation/analgesia, deep sedation/analgesia, and general anesthesia. The art and science of providing anesthesia continues to evolve. For example, noninvasive electroencephalogram-based technology allows ACPs to track the level of patient awareness (i.e., *awareness monitoring*) during surgery and adjust anesthesia as needed.

The anesthetic technique and agents are selected by the ACP in collaboration with the surgeon and patient. The ACP has ultimate responsibility for the choice of anesthesia. Factors contributing to the decision include the patient's current physical and mental status, age, allergy and pain history, expertise of the ACP, and factors relating to the operative procedure (e.g., length, site, discharge plans). An absolute contraindication to any anesthetic technique or agent is patient refusal.

The ACP obtains anesthesia consent, writes orders for preoperative and postoperative drugs, and assigns the patient an anesthesia classification. The ASA physical status classification system is based on the patient's physiologic status with no regard to the surgical procedure to be performed. A scale of P1 to P6 is used, with a rating of P6 reserved for a brain-dead patient undergoing organ harvest (see Table 17-3). An intraoperative complication is more likely to develop with a higher classification number.

Other designations can be added to the ASA status (e.g., "E" to designate an "emergent" procedure). ASA physical status is dynamic and represents the patient's status immediately before surgery. For example, a healthy 26-year-old adult who is severely injured in an automobile collision may be classified as ASA P5E because life-threatening injuries require emergent surgery.

ANESTHESIA TECHNIQUES

Types of anesthesia techniques include moderate to deep sedation, monitored anesthesia care (MAC), general anesthesia, and local and regional anesthesia[21] (Table 18-4).

Moderate to Deep Sedation

Moderate to deep sedation is used for procedures performed outside of the OR (e.g., reduction of dislocated joints in the emergency department) and does not require the presence of an ACP. RNs who are trained in this technique and are allowed by agency protocols and state nurse practice acts can provide this type of anesthesia.[22] It is administered by the nurse under the direct supervision of a physician.

Monitored Anesthesia Care

Monitored anesthesia care (MAC) is used for diagnostic or therapeutic procedures performed in or outside of the OR (e.g., endoscopy clinic). It includes varying levels of sedation, analgesia, and anxiolysis. A critical component of MAC is the assessment and management of any physiologic problems that may develop. The provider of MAC must be an ACP, since it may be necessary to change to general anesthesia during the procedure.

General Anesthesia

The goals of anesthesiology include the (1) control of excessive biologic responses induced by a variety of stressors and (2) protection of patients from stress-induced complications. To this end, *total intravenous anesthesia (TIVA)* and newer inhalation agents have a fast onset, fast elimination, and fewer undesirable side effects than previous agents. These factors facilitate early discharge from the PACU and ambulatory surgery centers.

General anesthesia is the technique of choice for patients who are having surgical procedures that are of significant duration, require skeletal muscle relaxation, require uncomfortable

TABLE 18-4 Anesthesia Techniques and Effects

Technique	Patient Effects
Moderate to deep sedation (formerly called *conscious sedation*)	• Sedative, anxiolytic, and/or analgesic drugs used • Does not include use of inhalation agents • Patients responsive and breathe without assistance • Not expected to induce levels of sedation that would impair patients' ability to protect their airway • Most often used for minor therapeutic procedures (e.g., realignment of a fracture in the emergency department)
Monitored anesthesia care (MAC)	• Sedative, anxiolytic, and/or analgesic drugs used • Does not usually involve inhalation agents • Patients less responsive and may require airway management • Provides maximum flexibility to match sedation level to patient needs and procedural requirements • Often used in conjunction with regional or local anesthesia • Often used for minor therapeutic and diagnostic procedures (e.g., eye surgery, colonoscopy)
General anesthesia	• Loss of sensation with loss of consciousness • Combination of hypnosis, analgesia, and amnesia • Usually involves use of inhalation agents • Skeletal muscle relaxation • Elimination of coughing, gagging, vomiting, and sympathetic nervous system responsiveness • Requires advanced airway management
Local anesthesia	• Loss of sensation without loss of consciousness • Induced topically or via infiltration, intracutaneously, or subcutaneously • Topical applications may be aerosolized or nebulized
Regional anesthesia	• Loss of sensation to a region of body without loss of consciousness • Involves blocking a specific nerve or group of nerves with administration of a local anesthetic • Includes spinal, caudal, and epidural anesthesia and IV and peripheral nerve blocks (e.g., interscalene, axillary, infraclavicular or supraclavicular, popliteal, femoral, sciatic)

Source: American Society of Anesthesiologists: *Distinguishing monitored anesthesia care ("MAC") from moderate sedation/analgesia (conscious sedation)*, Schaumburg, Ill, 2013, The Society.

operative positions because of the location of the incision site, or require control of ventilation. Additional reasons for general anesthesia include patient refusal of local or regional techniques, contraindications to other techniques, and uncooperative patients. Patients may be uncooperative due to intoxication, emotional lability, head injury, impaired cognition, or inability to remain immobile for any length of time. Phases of general anesthesia are presented in Table 18-5.

General anesthesia may be induced by IV or inhalation, and maintained by either one or a combination of the two (Table 18-6). A *balanced technique*, using adjunctive drugs to complement the induction, is the most common approach used for general anesthesia.

IV Agents. All routine general anesthetics begin with an IV induction agent, whether it is a hypnotic, an anxiolytic, or a dissociative agent. When used during the initial period of anesthesia, these agents induce a pleasant sleep with a rapid onset of action that patients find desirable. A single dose lasts only a few minutes, which is long enough for a laryngeal mask airway (LMA) or an endotracheal (ET) tube to be placed. Once this is done, the ACP uses the selected inhalation and IV agent(s).

Recent advances in IV hypnotics (e.g., dexmedetomidine [Precedex]) and opioids (e.g., remifentanil [Ultiva]) have led to the more frequent use of TIVA. However, the patient may still require advanced airway management (e.g., LMA, ET tube) and will receive oxygen/air mixtures via this route.

Inhalation Agents. Inhalation agents are the cornerstone of general anesthesia. They may be volatile liquids or gases. Volatile liquids are given through a specially designed vaporizer after being mixed with oxygen as a carrier gas. This gas mixture is then delivered to the patient via the anesthesia circuit. Waste gases are removed using negative evacuation pressure venting to the outside of the agency.

Inhalation agents enter the body through the alveoli in the lungs. Ease of administration and rapid excretion by ventilation make them desirable agents. One undesirable trait is the irritating effect some inhalation agents (e.g., desflurane [Suprane]) have on the respiratory tract. Possible complications include coughing, laryngospasm, and increased secretions.[23]

Once the patient has been induced with an IV agent, the choice for delivering inhalation agents is usually through an ET tube or LMA. The ET tube permits control of ventilation and protects the airway from aspiration. LMAs are currently an important option for patients with difficult airways, but they do not provide access to the trachea or airway protection with the same certainty as ETs. Complications of ET tube or LMA include those associated primarily with insertion and removal. These include failure to intubate, damage to teeth and lips, laryngospasm, laryngeal edema, postoperative sore throat, and hoarseness caused by injury or irritation of the vocal cords or surrounding tissues.

Adjuncts to General Anesthesia. The administration of general anesthesia is rarely limited to one agent. Drugs added to an inhalation anesthetic (other than an IV induction drug) are termed *adjuncts*. These drugs are added to the anesthetic regimen specifically to achieve unconsciousness, analgesia, amnesia, muscle relaxation, or autonomic nervous system control. Adjuncts include opioids, benzodiazepines, neuromuscular blocking agents (muscle relaxants), and antiemetics (Table 18-7). It is important to know that these drugs are often given in combination and may have synergistic or antagonistic effects. You may observe deeper levels of sedation or more drug-related side effects beyond those seen with inhalation anesthetics alone. If needed, drugs are available to reverse the effects of some of these adjuncts.

Dissociative Anesthesia. *Dissociative anesthesia* interrupts associative brain pathways while blocking sensory pathways. The patient may appear catatonic, is amnesic, and experiences profound analgesia that lasts into the postoperative period. Ketamine (Ketalar) (given IV or IM) is a common dissociative anesthetic. It is a potent analgesic and amnesic. Ketamine is used in asthmatic patients undergoing surgery because it promotes bronchodilation and in trauma patients requiring surgery because it increases heart rate and helps maintain cardiac output. Because ketamine is a phenylcyclohexyl piperidine (PCP) derivative, the drug may cause hallucinations and nightmares, greatly limiting its usefulness. Concurrent use of midazolam (Versed) can reduce or eliminate hallucinations associated with ketamine.

TABLE 18-5 Phases of General Anesthesia

Preinduction	Induction	Maintenance	Emergence
Description			
• Period starting with initiation of IV or arterial access, application of monitors (e.g., ECG), administration of preoperative drugs	• Initiation of drugs that make patient unconscious • Airway secured with airway assist devices	• Period during which surgical procedure is performed • Patient remains in an unconscious state with measures to ensure airway safety	• Period when surgical procedure is completed • Patient is prepared for return to consciousness and removal of airway assist devices
Role of Anesthesia Care Provider			
• Determine final anesthetic care plan • Insert and monitor IV or arterial access • Confirm antibiotic prophylaxis • Give drugs for anxiety, aspiration prophylaxis	• Give appropriate drugs • Secure airway • Position patient appropriately for surgical procedure	• Monitor patient's physiologic status • Give drugs and titrate fluids as appropriate	• Reverse residual neuromuscular blocking agents • Assess for return of all protective reflexes • Remove airway assist devices • Assess pain
Role of Perioperative Nurse			
• Complete preoperative assessment • Check and confirm signed informed consent • Complete surgical time-out.	• Assist with application of monitors (noninvasive and invasive) • Assist with airway management	• Adjust patient position as necessary • Monitor patient safety	• Assist in placement of dressing • Protect patient during return of reflexes • Prepare patient to move to postanesthesia care unit
Classes of Drugs Used (Tables 17-8, 18-6, and 18-7)			

• Benzodiazepines
• Opioids
• Antibiotics
• Aspiration prophylaxis:
  • H_2 receptor blockers (e.g., ranitidine [Zantac])
  • Gastric motility agents (e.g., metoclopramide [Reglan])
  • Anticholinergics (e.g., scopolamine [Transderm-Scōp])
	• Benzodiazepines
	• Opioids
	• Barbiturates
	• Hypnotics
	• Volatile gases
		• Benzodiazepines
		• Opioids
		• Barbiturates
		• Hypnotics
		• Volatile gases
		• Neuromuscular blocking agents
			• Reversal agents (PRN):
			  • Anticholinesterases (e.g., neostigmine)
			  • Opioid antagonists (e.g., naloxone)
			  • Benzodiazepine antagonists (e.g., flumazenil)
			  • Neuromuscular block reversal of rocuronium [Zemuron] and vecuronium [Norcuron] (e.g., sugammadex [Bridon])
			• Supplemental opioids (PRN)
			• Antiemetics (PRN)

Provide a quiet, unhurried environment in the PACU for all patients receiving dissociative anesthesia.[24]

Local and Regional Anesthesia

Local anesthesia interrupts the generation of nerve impulses by altering the flow of sodium into nerve cells. The result is autonomic nervous system blockade, anesthesia, and skeletal muscle flaccidity or paralysis. Local anesthetics are topical, ophthalmic, nebulized, or injectable. A local anesthetic, such as lidocaine (Xylocaine), is applied to a specific area of the body by the surgeon or ACP and does not require sedation or loss of consciousness.

Regional anesthesia (or block) using a local anesthetic is always injected. It involves a central nerve (e.g., spinal) or group of nerves (e.g., plexus) that innervate a site remote to the point of injection. Administration of a local or regional anesthetic may involve concurrent use of MAC or moderate to deep sedation (Table 18-4), either preinjection or intraoperatively. Regional blocks are used as preoperative analgesia, intraoperatively to manage surgical pain, and postoperatively to control pain. Indwelling catheters that deliver local anesthetic via a pump to the surgical site may be implanted before the patient emerges from anesthesia to provide continuous pain relief up to 72 hours postoperatively.

Advantages of local and regional anesthesia include rapid recovery and discharge with continued postoperative analgesia without any accompanying cognitive dysfunction. Local and regional anesthesia can be safely used in patients who have co-morbidities that would preclude the use of general anesthesia.

Disadvantages of local and regional anesthesia include the potential for technical difficulties; discomfort at the injection site; and the risk of inadvertent vascular injection leading to refractory hypotension, dysrhythmias, and possible seizures. Another disadvantage is the inability to precisely match the agent's duration of action to the duration of the surgical procedure.

In ambulatory or outpatient procedures, you may assist the ACP in the administration of a peripheral or regional block. Consequently, you must be familiar with the drugs, including the methods of administration and adverse and toxic effects. Initial assessment of the patient should include detailed questioning of the patient's history with the use of local anesthetics and any adverse events associated with their use by the patient or blood relatives.

Many patients report "allergies" to local anesthetics. Although true allergies to local anesthetics occur, they are rare. Allergies are likely to be a result of additives or preservatives in the preparation. Moreover, some local anesthetics are combined with epinephrine to provide localized vasoconstriction. This decreases absorption and extends the action of the agent. However, if the local anesthetic is absorbed in the tissues or inadvertently injected IV and enters the general circulation, the patient may experience tachycardia, hypertension, and a general perception of panic.

Methods of Administration. Local anesthetics are injected at the surgical site, nebulized, or applied topically. Topical applications of creams, ointments, aerosols, and liquids are standard methods of administration. The drug is applied directly to the skin, mucous membranes, or open surface. Eutectic mixture of

TABLE 18-6 Drug Therapy

General Anesthesia

Drugs	Advantages	Disadvantages	Nursing Interventions
IV Agents			
Barbiturates			
methohexital (Brevital)	Rapid induction, duration of action <5 min.	Adverse cardiac effects (e.g., myocardial depression), hypotension, respiratory depression, excitation, involuntary movement.	Usually have minimal postoperative effects because of short duration of action. Increased incidence of postoperative nausea in patients with barbiturate sensitivity, histamine-triggered nausea, vomiting.
Nonbarbiturate Hypnotics			
etomidate (Amidate)	Produces little change in cardiovascular dynamics. Useful for hemodynamically unstable patients. Only minor respiratory depression. No histamine release.	Associated with adverse effects of myoclonia, nausea and vomiting, hiccups, and adrenocortical inhibition.	Observe for transient skeletal muscle movements (myoclonia), nausea and vomiting, hiccups, hypotension, hypoglycemia.
propofol (Diprivan)	Ideal for short outpatient procedures because of rapid onset of action, metabolic clearance. May be used for induction and maintenance of anesthesia.	May cause bradycardia and other dysrhythmias, hypotension, apnea, transient phlebitis, nausea and vomiting, hiccups. May cause hypertriglyceridemia.	Monitor for postoperative hypotension, bradycardia. Monitor serum triglycerides q24hr when sedated >24 hr.
Inhalation Agents			
Volatile Liquids			
isoflurane (Forane) desflurane (Suprane) sevoflurane (Ultane)	All cause skeletal muscle relaxation. *isoflurane:* No increase in ventricular irritability. Does not cause liver or renal toxicity. Resistant to metabolic breakdown. *desflurane:* Fastest onset and emergence, widely used in ambulatory settings. Least postoperative cognitive dysfunction. Potential airway irritant. *sevoflurane:* Predictable effects on cardiovascular and respiratory systems, rapid acting. Preferred for inhalation induction as nonirritating to respiratory tract.	All cause respiratory depression, hypotension, myocardial depression. *isoflurane and desflurane:* May be unsuitable for patients with coronary artery disease. *sevoflurane:* May be associated with emergence delirium (see Chapter 19). Atypical seizure-like activity has been reported.	Assess and treat pain during early anesthesia recovery. Assess for adverse reactions such as cardiopulmonary depression with hypotension and prolonged respiratory depression. Monitor for nausea and vomiting.
Gaseous Agents			
nitrous oxide	Potentiates volatile agents, thus speeding induction and reducing total dosage and side effects. Good analgesic potency. Produces little or no toxicity at therapeutic concentrations.	Weak anesthetic, rarely used alone. Must be given with O_2 to prevent hypoxemia. Avoid in patients with strong history of nausea and vomiting.	Avoid in patients with bone marrow depression.
Dissociative Anesthetic			
ketamine (Ketalar)	Can be given IV or IM. Potent analgesic and amnesic.	May cause hallucinations and nightmares, increased intracranial and intraocular pressure, ↑ heart rate, ↑ BP.	Anticipate administration of a benzodiazepine if agitation and hallucinations occur. Calm, quiet environment is essential in postoperative care.

local anesthetics (EMLA cream, a combination of prilocaine and lidocaine) is an example of a cream applied to the site 30 to 60 minutes before the procedure for analgesia. The success of injected local anesthetics may be limited by prolonged duration of procedure or infection at the injection site, thus interfering with drug absorption.

When a patient is prepared for regional anesthesia, airway equipment, emergency drugs, and a cardiac monitor/defibrillator should be immediately available to provide advanced airway and cardiopulmonary support if necessary. Inadvertent IV injection of the agent or excessive absorption of bupivacaine (Sensorcaine), in particular, may lead to cardiac depression, severe dysrhythmias, or cardiac arrest.[25]

Examples of common regional nerve blocks include brachial plexus block; IV regional anesthesia (IVRA) or Bier block anesthesia; and femoral, axillary, cervical, sciatic, ankle, and retrobulbar blocks. For IVRA or Bier block, the patient has a double-cuff tourniquet applied as a safety measure. You can aid the success of regional anesthesia by assisting in patient positioning, monitoring vital signs during block delivery, administering oxygen therapy, and using supporting devices (at the direction of the ACP) that contribute to the anesthesia (e.g., ultrasound imaging, nerve stimulator, tourniquets).

Spinal and Epidural Anesthesia. Spinal anesthesia and epidural anesthesia are also types of regional anesthesia. **Spinal anesthesia** involves the injection of a local anesthetic into the cerebrospinal fluid in the subarachnoid space, usually below the level of L2 (Fig. 18-6, *A*). The local anesthetic mixes with cerebrospinal fluid. Depending on the extent of its spread, various levels of anesthesia are achieved. Because the local anesthetic is given directly into the cerebrospinal fluid, a spinal anesthetic produces an autonomic, sensory, and motor blockade. Patients experience vasodilation and may become hypotensive as a result of the autonomic block. They feel no pain as a result of the

TABLE 18-7 Drug Therapy

Adjuncts to General Anesthesia

Agents	Uses During Anesthesia	Adverse Effects	Nursing Interventions
Opioids			
fentanyl (Sublimaze) sufentanil (Sufenta) morphine sulfate hydromorphone (Dilaudid) alfentanil (Alfenta) remifentanil (Ultiva) methadone (Dolophine)	Induce and maintain anesthesia, reduce stimuli from sensory nerve endings, provide analgesia during surgery and recovery in PACU.	Respiratory depression, stimulation of vomiting center, possible bradycardia and peripheral vasodilation (when combined with anesthetics). High incidence of pruritus in both regional and IV administration.	• Assess respiratory rate and rhythm, monitor pulse oximetry, protect airway in anticipation of vomiting. • Use standing orders for antipruritics and antiemetics. • Reverse opioid-induced respiratory depression with naloxone (Narcan). If used, reversal of analgesic effects also occurs.
Benzodiazepines			
midazolam (Versed) diazepam (Valium) lorazepam (Ativan)	Reduce anxiety preoperatively and postoperatively, induce and maintain anesthesia, induce amnesia, treat emergence delirium. Supplement sedation in local and regional anesthesia and MAC.	Synergistic effect with opioids, increasing potential for respiratory depression. Hypotension and tachycardia. Prolonged sedation or confusion.	• Monitor level of consciousness. Assess for respiratory depression, hypotension, and tachycardia. • Reverse severe benzodiazepine-induced respiratory depression with flumazenil (Romazicon).
Neuromuscular Blocking Agents			
Depolarizing agent: succinylcholine (Anectine)	Facilitate endotracheal intubation, promote skeletal muscle relaxation (paralysis) to enhance access to surgical sites.	Apnea related to paralysis of respiratory muscles. Duration of action of nondepolarizing agents may be longer than surgery. Reversal agents may not completely eliminate effects. Confusion and nausea. Recurrence of muscle weakness with correction of hypothermia.	• If intubated, monitor return of muscle strength, level of consciousness, and ventilation. • Maintain patent airway. Monitor respiratory rate and rhythm until patient able to cough and return to previous levels of muscle strength. Ensure availability of nondepolarizing reversal agents (e.g., neostigmine [Prostigmin]) and emergency respiratory support equipment. • Monitor temperature and levels of muscle strength with temperature changes.
Nondepolarizing agents: pancuronium rocuronium atracurium cisatracurium (Nimbex)	Effects of nondepolarizing agents are usually reversed toward end of surgery by administration of anticholinesterase agents (e.g., neostigmine, pyridostigmine).		
Antiemetics			
ondansetron (Zofran) dolasetron (Anzemet) granisetron (Kytril) metoclopramide (Reglan) prochlorperazine promethazine scopolamine (Transderm-Scōp)	Counteract emetic effects of inhalation agents and opioids. Prophylactic prevention of nausea and vomiting related to histamine release, vagal stimulation, vestibular disturbance, surgical procedure (e.g., abdominal and laparoscopic procedures).	Headache, dizziness, IV irritation, dysrhythmias, dysphoria, dystonia, dry mouth, central nervous system sedation.	• Monitor heart rhythm, cardiopulmonary status, level of central nervous system excitation or sedation, ability to move limbs, presence of nausea or vomiting.
Miscellaneous			
dexmedetomidine (Precedex)	Induces and maintains sedation in nonintubated patients prior to and/or during surgical procedures.	Hypotension, bradycardia, sinus arrest, transient hypertension during administration of loading dose.	• Monitor heart rate and rhythm, and BP for possible side effects.
dexamethasone	Counteracts emetic effects of inhalation agents and opioids (off-label use).*	Insomnia, nervousness, abdominal distention.	• Monitor for possible side effects.

MAC, Monitored anesthesia care; *PACU,* postanesthesia care unit.
*For an explanation of off-label drug use, see *www.cancer.org/docroot/ETO/content/ETO_1_2x_Off-Label_Drug_Use.asp.*

sensory block. They cannot move as a result of the motor block. The duration of action of the spinal anesthetic depends on the drug selected and the dose given. A spinal anesthetic may be used for procedures involving the extremities (e.g., joint replacements) and lower gastrointestinal, prostate, and gynecologic surgeries.[23]

An **epidural block** involves injection of a local anesthetic into the epidural space via a thoracic or lumbar approach (Fig. 18-6, *B*). The anesthetic agent does not enter the cerebrospinal fluid but binds to nerve roots as they enter and exit the spinal cord. With the use of a low concentration of local anesthetic, sensory pathways are blocked but motor fibers remain intact. In higher doses, sensory and motor fibers are blocked. Epidural anesthesia may be used as the sole anesthetic for a surgical procedure. In addition, a catheter may be placed to allow for intraoperative use and continued analgesia in the postoperative period (Fig. 18-6, *C*). For postoperative analgesia, lower doses of epidurally administered local anesthetic, usually in combination with an opioid, are used. Epidural anesthesia is commonly used for analgesia, or in combination with MAC or general anesthesia, in obstetrics, vascular procedures involving the lower extremities, lung resections, and renal and midabdominal surgeries. The desirable effects of vasodilation and analgesia contribute to better surgical outcomes.

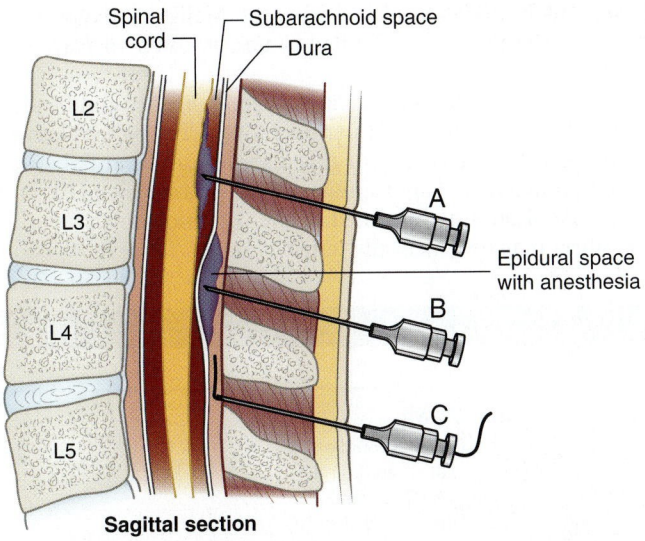

FIG. 18-6 Location of needle point and injected anesthetic relative to dura and spinal cord. **A,** Spinal anesthesia. **B,** Single-injection epidural. **C,** Epidural catheter. (Interspaces most commonly used are L2-3, L4-5, L3-4.)

When spinal or epidural anesthesia is used, the patient can remain fully conscious, receive MAC, or choose general anesthesia. The onset of spinal anesthesia is more rapid than that of epidural anesthesia. Spinal and epidural anesthesia may be extended in duration using indwelling catheters, thus allowing for additional doses of anesthetic.

When spinal or epidural anesthesia is used, closely observe the patient for manifestations of autonomic nervous system blockade. These include hypotension, bradycardia, nausea, and vomiting. There is less autonomic nervous system blockade with epidural anesthesia than with spinal anesthesia. Should "too high" a block be achieved, the patient may experience tingling in the arms and hands or inadequate breathing and apnea.[23] Other complications of spinal or epidural anesthesia include postdural puncture headache, back pain, isolated nerve injury, and meningitis.

Gerontologic Considerations: Patient During Surgery

Although anesthetic agents have become safer and more predictable, the aging process affects the pharmacokinetics of drugs, specifically the absorption, distribution, and metabolism of medications. This results in alterations in the onset, peak, and duration of drugs independent of the route of administration. Because of this, anesthetic drugs should be carefully titrated when given to older adults. Physiologic changes in aging may alter the patient's response not only to the anesthetic but also to blood and fluid loss and replacement, hypothermia, pain, and tolerance of the surgical procedure and positioning. Carefully monitor the older adult's response to all anesthetic agents. Assess the postoperative recovery from these agents before the patient is transferred out of the PACU.

Some older adults may have difficulty communicating and following directions as a result of alterations in hearing or vision. These factors increase the need for clear and concise communication in the OR, especially when preoperative sedation is combined with already existing sensory deficits. Because of decreased ability to perceive discomfort or pressure on vulnerable areas and a loss of skin elasticity, the older adult's skin is at risk for injury from tape, electrodes, warming and cooling blankets, and certain types of dressings. In addition, pooling of solutions used to prepare the skin in dependent areas can quickly create skin burns or abrasions.

The care and vigilance of the entire surgical team are needed in preparing and positioning the older patient. The older adult often has osteoporosis and/or osteoarthritis. Misalignment, pressure, or other insults to arthritic joints that may be desensitized from administration of an anesthetic may create long-term injury and disability. Older adults are also at a greater risk of perioperative hypothermia. Consider the use of a variety of warming devices and carefully monitor them if used.

CATASTROPHIC EVENTS IN THE OPERATING ROOM

Unanticipated intraoperative events occasionally occur. Although some may be anticipated (e.g., cardiac arrest in an unstable patient, massive blood loss during trauma surgery), others may occur without warning, demanding immediate intervention by all members of the OR team. Two such events are anaphylactic reactions and malignant hyperthermia.

Anaphylactic Reactions

Anaphylaxis is the most severe form of an allergic reaction, manifesting with life-threatening pulmonary and circulatory complications. The initial clinical manifestations of anaphylaxis may be masked by anesthesia. ACPs give a variety of drugs to patients, such as anesthetics, antibiotics, blood products, and plasma expanders. Because any parenterally administered material can stimulate an allergic response, vigilance and rapid intervention are essential. An anaphylactic reaction causes hypotension, tachycardia, bronchospasm, and possibly pulmonary edema. Anesthetic agents, antibiotics, and latex are responsible for many perioperative allergic reactions. (Anaphylaxis is discussed in Chapter 13.)

Latex allergy has become a particular concern in the perioperative setting, given the use of gloves, catheters, and many other devices containing natural rubber latex. Reactions to natural rubber latex range from urticaria to anaphylaxis with symptoms appearing immediately or at some time during the surgical procedure. Latex allergy protocols should be set up in each agency to provide a latex-safe environment for susceptible individuals.[26] (Latex allergies are discussed in Chapter 13.)

Malignant Hyperthermia

Malignant hyperthermia (MH) is a rare disorder characterized by hyperthermia with rigidity of skeletal muscles that can result in death. It occurs in susceptible people when they are exposed to certain anesthetic agents. Succinylcholine (Anectine), especially when given with volatile inhalation agents, appears to be the primary trigger of the disorder. Other factors, such as stress, trauma, and heat, also have been implicated. When MH does occur, it is usually during general anesthesia, but it may manifest in the recovery period as well.[27]

MH is an autosomal dominant trait but is variable in its genetic manifestation, so predictions based on family history are important but not reliable. (Autosomal dominant disorders are discussed in Chapter 12.) The fundamental defect is hypermetabolism of skeletal muscle resulting from altered control of intracellular calcium. This leads to muscle contracture, hyperthermia, hypoxemia, lactic acidosis, and hemodynamic and cardiac alterations.

Tachycardia, tachypnea, hypercarbia, and ventricular dysrhythmias are generally seen but are nonspecific to MH. MH is generally diagnosed after all other causes of the hypermetabolism are ruled out. The rise in body temperature is not an early sign of MH. Unless promptly detected and treated, MH can result in cardiac arrest and death. The definitive treatment of MH is prompt administration of dantrolene (Dantrium). Dantrolene slows metabolism, reduces muscle contraction, and mediates the catabolic processes associated with MH.[25] A treatment protocol, available from the Malignant Hyperthermia Association of the United States, is often displayed in the OR.[28]

To prevent MH, obtain a careful family history and be alert to the development of MH perioperatively. The patient known or suspected to be at risk for this disorder can be anesthetized with minimal risks if appropriate precautions are taken. Patients with MH should be informed of the condition so that family members may be genetically tested.

CASE STUDY

Intraoperative Patient

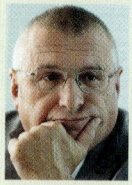

(©shironosov/ iStock/ Thinkstock)

Patient Profile

G.S., a 63-year-old retired accountant, was admitted to the hospital for severe pain from acute cholecystitis. G.S.'s medical history includes hypertension and type 2 diabetes. His pain has been managed with hydromorphone (Dilaudid) using patient-controlled analgesia. His intractable nausea and vomiting required the placement of a nasogastric (NG) tube. He is scheduled for a laparoscopic cholecystectomy. The surgery will be performed under general anesthesia.

Subjective Data

- G.S. is awake and able to identify himself, his birth date, surgical procedure, and surgical site
- States pain is controlled and rates it a 4 on a 0 to 10 scale on arrival to the holding area

Objective Data

- Admitted to the holding area with an NG tube in place and one peripheral IV catheter
- Capillary blood glucose 1 hour ago was 125 mg/dL
- Oxygen saturation 96% on room air

Interprofessional Care

- Vital signs per holding area routine
- 0.9 normal saline solution at 100 mL/hr
- Titrate O_2 therapy to keep O_2 saturation >90%
- Provide low, intermittent suction to NG tube

Discussion Questions

1. What are the potential intraoperative problems that you may expect with G.S.?
2. ***Priority Decision:*** What priority nursing interventions would be appropriate to prevent these complications from occurring?
3. ***Teamwork and Collaboration:*** What are the interprofessional team's priorities for G.S.?
4. ***Evidence-Based Practice:*** G.S. tells you that he is cold in spite of a blanket in place. Why is it important that G.S. remains warm?
5. ***Safety:*** Identify two areas of risk for injury to G.S. What actions can be taken to ensure patient safety?

Answers available at *http://evolve.elsevier.com/Lewis/medsurg.*

BRIDGE TO NCLEX EXAMINATION

The number of the question corresponds to the same-numbered outcome at the beginning of the chapter.

1. Proper attire for the semirestricted area of the surgery department is
   a. street clothing.
   b. surgical attire and head cover.
   c. surgical attire, head cover, and mask.
   d. street clothing with the addition of shoe covers.
2. Activities that the nurse might perform in the role of a scrub nurse during surgery include (*select all that apply*)
   a. checking electrical equipment.
   b. preparing the instrument table.
   c. passing instruments to the surgeon and assistants.
   d. coordinating activities occurring in the operating room.
   e. maintaining accurate counts of sponges, needles, and instruments.
3. The nurse is caring for a patient undergoing surgery for a knee replacement. What is critical to the patient's safety during the procedure (*select all that apply*)?
   a. Universal protocol is followed.
   b. The ACP is an anesthesiologist.
   c. The patient has adequate health insurance.
   d. The patient's family is in the surgery waiting area.
   e. The patient's allergies are conveyed to the surgical team.
4. The nurse's *primary* responsibility for the care of the patient undergoing surgery is
   a. developing an individualized plan of nursing care for the patient.
   b. carrying out specific tasks related to surgical policies and procedures.
   c. ensuring that the patient has been assessed for safe administration of anesthesia.
   d. performing a preoperative history and physical assessment to identify patient needs.
5. When scrubbing at the scrub sink, the nurse should
   a. scrub from elbows to hands.
   b. scrub without mechanical friction.
   c. scrub for a minimum of 10 minutes.
   d. hold the hands higher than the elbows.
6. When positioning a patient in preparation for surgery, the nurse understands that injury to the patient is *most* likely to occur as a result of
   a. incorrect musculoskeletal alignment.
   b. loss of perception of pain or pressure.
   c. pooling of blood in peripheral vessels.
   d. disregarding the patient's need for modesty.

7. IV induction for general anesthesia is the method of choice for *most* patients because
   a. the patient is not intubated.
   b. the agents are nonexplosive.
   c. induction is rapid and pleasant.
   d. emergence is longer but with fewer complications.

1. b, 2. b, c, e, 3. a, e, 4. a, 5. d, 6. a, 7. c

For rationales to these answers and even more NCLEX review questions, visit *http://evolve.elsevier.com/Lewis/medsurg.*

EVOLVE WEBSITE

http://evolve.elsevier.com/Lewis/medsurg

Review Questions (Online Only)

Key Points

Answer Keys for Questions

- Rationales for Bridge to NCLEX Examination Questions
- Answer Guidelines for Case Study on p. 328

Conceptual Care Map Creator

Audio Glossary

Content Updates

REFERENCES

*1. Association of periOperative Registered Nurses: *Perioperative standards and recommended practices*, Denver, 2012, The Association.
2. The Joint Commission: Surgical care improvement project, 2014. Retrieved from *www.jointcommission.org/surgical_care_improvement_project.*
3. The Joint Commission: Hospital national patient safety goals. Retrieved from *www.jointcommission.org/assets/1/6/2015_NPSG_HAP.pdf.*
4. Rothrock JC: *Alexander's care of the patient in surgery*, ed 15, St Louis, 2015, Mosby.
5. Agency for Healthcare Research and Quality: Patient safety network. Retrieved from *http://psnet.ahrq.gov/primer.aspx?primerID=9.*
6. Competency and Credentialing Institute: CNOR certification, 2014. Retrieved from *www.cc-institute.org/cnor/aboutabout.*
7. Association of Surgical Technologists: About the profession, 2014. Retrieved from *www.ast.org/AboutUs/About_AST.*
8. Association of periOperative Registered Nurses: AORN position statement on allied health care providers and support personnel in the perioperative practice setting, 2011. Retrieved from *www.aorn.org/TwoColumnInsert.aspx?id=21939&terms=POSITION%20STATEMENTS.*
9. Association of periOperative Registered Nurses: AORN position statement on RN first assistants, 2013. Retrieved from *www.aorn.org/TwoColumnInsert.aspx?id=21939&terms=POSITION%20STATEMENTS.*
10. American Society of Anesthesiologists: Anesthesia fast facts, 2014. Retrieved from *www.asahq.org/For-the-Public-and-Media/Press-Room/Anesthesia-Fast-Facts.aspxaspx.*
11. American Association of Nurse Anesthetists: Qualifications and capabilities of the certified Registered Nurse anesthetist, 2014. Retrieved from *www.aana.com/ceandeducation/becomeacrna/Pages/Qualifications-and-Capabilities-of-the-Certified-Registered-Nurse-Anesthetist-.aspx.*
*12. Jiménez-Jiménez M, García-Escalona A, Martín-López A, et al: Intraoperative stress and anxiety reduction with music therapy: a controlled randomized clinical trial of efficacy and safety, *J Vasc Nurs* 31:101, 2013.
13. Occupational Safety and Health Administration: Occupational safety and health standards, toxic and hazardous substances: bloodborne pathogens, 29 CFR §1910.1030 2012. Retrieved from *www.osha.gov/pls/oshaweb/owadisp.show_document?p_table=STANDARDS&p_id=10051.*
14. ECRI Institute: Surgical fire prevention. Retrieved from *www.ecri.org/Accident_Investigation/Pages/Surgical-Fire-Prevention.aspx.*
15. The Joint Commission: Universal protocol, 2014. Retrieved from *www.jointcommission.orghttp://www.jointcommission.org/standards_information/up.aspx..*
*16. Collins SJ, Newhouse R, Porter J, Talsma A: Effectiveness of the surgical safety checklist in correcting errors: a literature review applying Reason's Swiss cheese model, *AORN J* 100:65, 2014.
17. Association of periOperative Registered Nurses: Preventing wrong-patient, wrong-site, wrong-procedure events. Retrieved from *www.aorn.org/Clinical_Practicehttps://www.aorn.org/TwoColumnInsert.aspx.*
*18. Lumbley J, Ali S, Tchokouani L: Retrospective review of predisposing factors for intraoperative pressure ulcer development, *J Clin Anesth* 26:368, 2014.
*19. Leeds I, Wick E, Melton GB: Does close temperature regulation affect surgical site infection rates? *Adv Surg* 48:65, 2014.
20. Association of periOperative Registered Nurses: *Perioperative nursing data set: the perioperative nursing vocabulary*, ed 3, Denver, 2011, The Association.
21. American Society of Anesthesiologists: *Distinguishing monitored anesthesia care ("MAC") from moderate sedation/analgesia (conscious sedation)*, Schaumburg, Ill, 2013, The Society.
22. American Association of Nurse Anesthetists: Registered nurses engaged in the administration of sedation and analgesia, 2013. Retrieved from *www.aana.com/resources2/professionalpractice/Documents/PPM%20Consid%204.2%20RNs%20Engaged%20in%20Sedation%20Analgesia.pdf*
23. Naglehout JJ, Plaus KL, editors: *Nurse anesthesia*, ed 5, St Louis, 2014, Saunders.
24. Skidmore-Roth L: *Mosby's 2015 nursing drug reference*, ed 28, St Louis, 2015, Mosby.
25. Morrell RC: Intralipid might save lives as a rescue from bupivacaine toxicity, 2007. Retrieved from *www.apsf.org/newsletters/html/2007/summer/03_intralipid.htm.*
26. Shoup AJ: Latex allergy. In Watson DS, editor: *Perioperative safety*, St Louis, 2011, Mosby.
27. Seifert P, Wahr J, Pace M, et al: Crisis management of malignant hyperthermia in the OR, *AORN J* 100:189, 2014.
28. Malignant Hyperthermia Association of the United States: Emergency treatment for an acute MH event. Retrieved from *www.mhaus.org/healthcare-professionals/managing-a-crisis.*

*Evidence-based information for clinical practice.

19

Postoperative Care

Christine R. Hoch

You may have to fight a battle more than once to win it.

Margaret Thatcher

http://evolve.elsevier.com/Lewis/medsurg/

LEARNING OUTCOMES

1. Prioritize nursing responsibilities related to managing patients in the postanesthesia care unit (PACU).
2. Prioritize nursing responsibilities related to maintaining patient safety and preventing postoperative complications in the PACU and clinical unit.
3. Apply data from the initial nursing assessment to the management of the patient after transfer from the PACU to the clinical unit.
4. Select appropriate nursing interventions to manage potential problems during the postoperative period.
5. Differentiate discharge criteria from Phase I and Phase II postanesthesia care.

KEY TERMS

airway obstruction, p. 332
atelectasis, p. 334
delayed emergence, p. 338
emergence delirium, p. 338
fast-tracking, p. 331
patient-controlled analgesia (PCA), p. 340
postoperative ileus (POI), p. 341
rapid postanesthesia care unit progression (RPP), p. 331

The postoperative period begins immediately after surgery and continues until the patient is discharged from medical care. This chapter focuses on the common features of postoperative nursing. Specific surgical procedures and the related postoperative care are discussed in the appropriate chapters of this text.

POSTOPERATIVE CARE OF SURGICAL PATIENT

The patient's immediate recovery period is managed in a *postanesthesia care unit* (*PACU*), which is located adjacent to the operating room (OR). This location limits transportation of the patient immediately after surgery and provides ready access to anesthesia and OR staff. During the three phases of postanesthesia care, different levels of care are provided depending on the patient's needs[1] (Table 19-1).

Postanesthesia Care Unit Admission

The patient's initial admission to the PACU is a joint effort among the anesthesia care provider (ACP), OR nurse, and PACU nurse. This collaborative effort fosters a smooth transfer of care to the PACU and helps determine the phase to which the patient is assigned.

PACU Progression. How patients move through the phases of care in the PACU is determined by their condition. If a patient assigned to Phase I care on admission to the PACU is stable and recovering well, the patient may rapidly progress through Phase

TABLE 19-1 Phases of Postanesthesia Care

Phase I
- Care during the immediate postanesthesia period
- ECG and more intense monitoring (e.g., arterial BP monitoring, mechanical ventilation)

Goal: Prepare patient for transfer to Phase II level of care, an inpatient unit, or intensive care setting

Phase II
- Ambulatory surgery patients
- Fast-tracking (i.e., patients who have bypassed Phase I level of care)

Goal: Prepare patient for transfer to extended observation, home, or extended care facility

Extended Observation
- Extended care or observation after transfer/discharge from Phase I or Phase II levels of care

Goal: Prepare patient for self-care

Blended Levels of Care
- Various levels of care offered in the same environment

Source: American Society of PeriAnesthesia Nurses: 2015-2017 *Perianesthesia nursing standards, practice recommendations and interpretive statements,* Cherry Hill, NJ, 2015, The Society.

Reviewed by Diane Marie Rudolphi, RN, MS, Continuing Non-Tenure Track Nursing Faculty, University of Delaware, Newark, Delaware; and Lisa Spruce, DNP, ACNS, ACNP, ANP, CNOR, CNS-CP, Director of Evidence-Based Perioperative Practice, Association of periOperative Registered Nurses, Denver, Colorado.

TABLE 19-2 PACU Hand-Off Report

General Information
- Patient name and age
- Surgeon and ACP
- Surgical procedure
- Presence of tubes, drains, catheters, and IV lines
- Type of anesthesia (e.g., general, regional, monitored anesthesia care)
- Use of any reversal agents
- Airway status (artificial airway and/or interventions to maintain adequate oxygenation)
- Pain management interventions
- NPO status and postoperative orders to be started

Patient History
- Indication for surgery
- Medical history, medications, allergies
- Preoperative or baseline vital signs, laboratory and diagnostic findings
- Level of consciousness, orientation
- Specific patient characteristics (e.g., hearing loss, vision impairment, mobility limitations)
- Patient preferences (e.g., cultural, personal beliefs/restrictions)
- Patient emotional status on arrival to OR

Intraoperative Management
- Anesthetic agents
- Other drugs received preoperatively or intraoperatively
- Last dose of opioid administration/pain management plan
- Total fluid replacements, including blood transfusions
- Total fluid losses (e.g., blood, nasogastric drainage)
- Urine output

Intraoperative Course
- Unexpected anesthetic events or reactions
- Unexpected surgical events
- Most recent vital signs and monitoring trends
- Results of intraoperative laboratory tests and x-rays

ACP, Anesthesia care provider; *PACU,* postanesthesia care unit.

TABLE 19-3 Initial PACU Assessment

Airway
- Patency
- Oral or nasal airway
- Laryngeal mask airway
- Endotracheal tube with ventilator settings

Breathing
- Respiratory rate and quality
- Auscultated breath sounds
- Pulse oximetry
- Capnography or other technology supported monitoring if indicated
- Supplemental O_2

Circulation
- ECG monitoring: rate and rhythm
- BP: noninvasive or arterial line
- Hemodynamic pressure readings (if applicable)
- Temperature
- Capillary refill
- Color, temperature, moisture of skin
- Apical and peripheral pulses

Genitourinary
- Urine output

Neurologic
- Level of consciousness
- Orientation
- Sensory and motor status
- Pupil size and reaction

Gastrointestinal
- Nausea, vomiting
- Intake (fluids, irrigations)
- Output (vomitus)
- Bowel sounds

Surgical Site
- Dressings and visible incisions
- Drains: type, patency, and drainage
- IV assessment: location and condition of sites, solutions infusing

Pain
- Incision
- Other

Patient Safety Needs
- Patient position
- Fall risk assessment

TABLE 19-4 Signs of Inadequate Oxygenation

Central Nervous System
- Restlessness
- Agitation
- Confusion
- Muscle twitching
- Seizures
- Coma

Respiratory System
- Increased to absent respiratory effort
- Use of accessory muscles
- Abnormal breath sounds
- Abnormal arterial blood gases

Cardiovascular System
- Hypertension
- Hypotension
- Tachycardia
- Bradycardia
- Dysrhythmias
- Delayed capillary refill
- Weak peripheral pulses
- Decreased O_2 saturation

Integumentary System
- Flushed, cool, or moist skin
- Cyanosis

Renal System
- Urine output <0.5 mL/kg/hr

I to either Phase II care or an inpatient unit. This accelerated progress is called **rapid postanesthesia care unit progression (RPP)**. Another accelerated system of care is **fast-tracking**, which involves admitting ambulatory surgery patients directly to Phase II care.[1] Although both RPP and fast-tracking can potentially result in time and cost savings, the patient's safety is the primary determining factor of where and at what level postoperative care is provided.

Phase I Initial Assessment. On admission of the patient to the PACU, the ACP gives you a postanesthesia hand-off report (Table 19-2). Hand-off reports should be standardized and interactive allowing for questions and clarification of information.[2] The ACP should remain in the PACU until you accept responsibility for the nursing care of the patient. The goals of PACU care are to maintain patient safety during recovery from anesthesia, identify actual and potential patient problems that may occur as a result of anesthesia and surgery, and to intervene appropriately. Potential problems in the postoperative period are identified in Fig. 19-1. Table 19-3 identifies key components of a PACU assessment.

Begin your initial assessment with an evaluation of the patient's airway, breathing, and circulation (ABC) status. Oxygenation and ventilation can be affected by residual neuromuscular blockade, use of opioids, and patient characteristics such as sleep-disordered breathing (e.g., central or obstructive sleep apnea [OSA], abnormal airway anatomy). Identify signs of inadequate oxygenation and ventilation (Table 19-4). Any evidence of respiratory distress requires prompt intervention.

Pulse oximetry monitoring provides a noninvasive means of assessing oxygenation and can provide an early warning of hypoxemia. *Transcutaneous carbon dioxide ($PtcCO_2$)* and *end-tidal CO_2 ($PetCO_2$) (capnography) monitoring* are used to detect respiratory depression in high-risk patients.[3] Volumetric capnography and acoustic respiratory rate monitoring have also demonstrated benefit in early identification of postoperative respiratory distress.[4] (Pulse oximetry, capnography, $PtcCO_2$, and $PetCO_2$ are discussed in Chapter 25.)

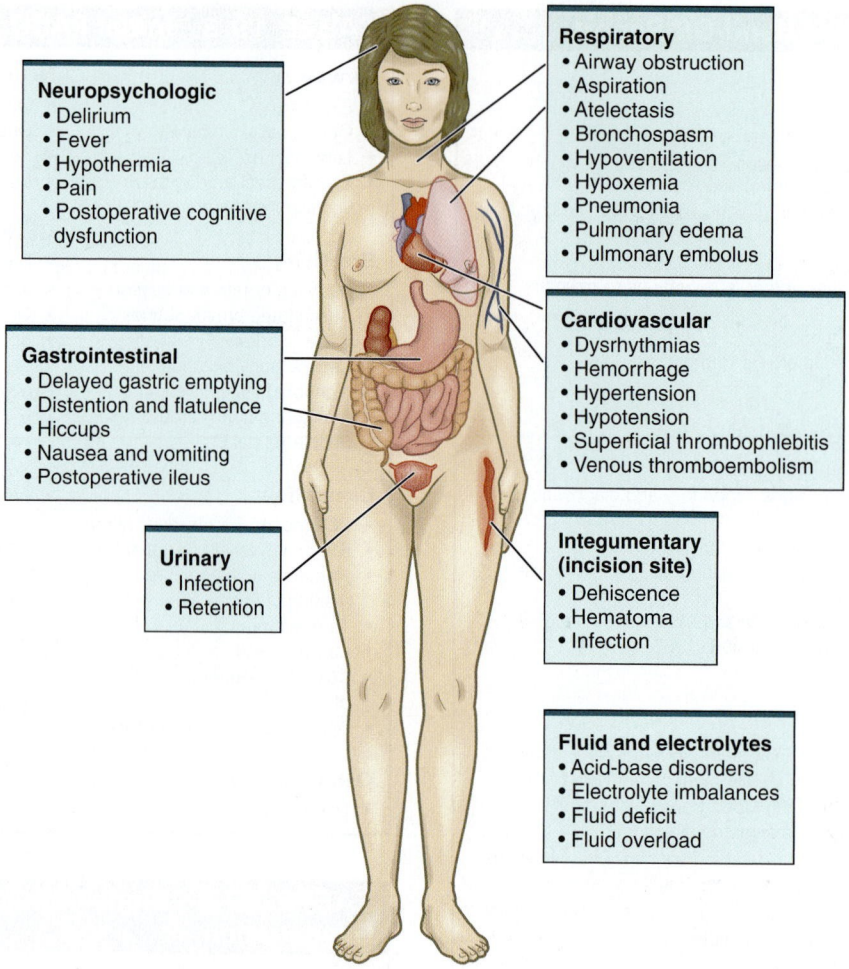

FIG. 19-1 Potential problems in the postoperative period.

Note and assess changes in ECG findings from the preoperative baseline. Measure the BP and compare it with baseline readings. Invasive monitoring (e.g., arterial BP) is started if needed. Also assess body temperature, peripheral pulses, capillary refill, and skin condition (e.g., color, moisture). Any signs of inadequate tissue perfusion require prompt intervention.

Focus the initial neurologic assessment on level of consciousness; orientation; sensory and motor status; and size, equality, and reactivity of the pupils. The patient may be awake, drowsy but arousable, or asleep. Because hearing is the first sense to return in the unconscious patient, explain all activities to the patient from the moment of admission to the PACU. If the patient received a regional anesthetic (e.g., spinal, epidural), sensory and motor blockade may still be present, and you should check a dermatome level (see Fig. 55-7). (Dermatomes are also discussed in Chapter 8.) During recovery from regional anesthesia, sensory and motor function returns from the extremities to the site where the anesthetic was given. Therefore the areas near the site of injections are the last to recover.

Assess the urinary system by measuring intake and output and determining fluid balance. Intraoperative fluid totals are part of the anesthesia report. Note the presence of all IV lines; all irrigation solutions and infusions; and all output devices, including catheters and wound drains. Assess the surgical site, noting the condition of any dressings and the type and amount of any drainage. Implement postoperative orders related to incision care.

Nursing management of select problems is discussed in the following pages and can be applied to patients in both the PACU and clinical unit.

RESPIRATORY PROBLEMS

Etiology

PACU. In the immediate postanesthesia period the most common causes of airway compromise include obstruction, hypoxemia, and hypoventilation (Table 19-5). Patients at high risk include those who (1) have had general anesthesia; (2) are older than 55 years of age; (3) have a history of tobacco use; (4) have preexisting lung disease and/or sleep-disordered breathing; (5) are obese; (6) have co-morbidities (e.g., renal disease, diabetes, hypertension); or (7) have undergone airway, thoracic, or abdominal surgery. However, respiratory problems may occur with any patient who has been anesthetized. The greatest risk for respiratory distress occurs in the first 24 hours following surgery.[5]

Airway obstruction is commonly caused by blockage of the airway by the patient's tongue (Fig. 19-2). The base of the tongue falls backward against the soft palate and occludes the pharynx. It is most pronounced in the supine position and in the patient who is extremely sleepy after surgery.

Hypoxemia, a partial pressure of arterial oxygen (PaO_2) less than 60 mm Hg, is characterized by a variety of nonspecific clinical signs and symptoms, ranging from agitation to

TABLE 19-5 Postoperative Respiratory Complications

Complications	Mechanisms	Manifestations	Interventions
Airway Obstruction			
Tongue falling back	Muscular flaccidity associated with ↓ consciousness and muscle relaxants	Use of accessory muscles Snoring respirations ↓ Air movement	• Patient stimulation • Head tilt, jaw thrust (Fig. 19-2) • Artificial airway
Retained thick secretions	Secretion stimulation by anesthetic agents Dehydration of secretions	Noisy respirations Coarse crackles	• Suctioning • Deep breathing and coughing • IV hydration • Chest PT
Laryngospasm	Irritation from endotracheal tube, anesthetic gases, or gastric aspiration Most likely to occur after removal of endotracheal tube	Inspiratory stridor (crowing respirations) Sternal retraction Acute respiratory distress	• O_2 therapy • Positive pressure ventilation • IV muscle relaxant • Lidocaine • Corticosteroids
Laryngeal edema	Allergic drug reaction Mechanical irritation from intubation Fluid overload	Similar to laryngospasm	• O_2 therapy • Antihistamines • Corticosteroids • Sedatives • Possible intubation
Hypoxemia			
Atelectasis	Bronchial obstruction caused by retained secretions or ↓ lung volumes	↓ Breath sounds ↓ O_2 saturation	• Humidified O_2 therapy • Deep breathing • Incentive spirometry • Early mobilization
Pulmonary edema	Fluid overload ↑ Hydrostatic pressure ↓ Interstitial pressure ↑ Capillary permeability	↓ O_2 saturation Crackles Infiltrates on chest x-ray	• O_2 therapy • Diuretics • Fluid restriction
Pulmonary embolism	Thrombus dislodged from peripheral venous system and lodged in pulmonary arterial system	Acute tachypnea Dyspnea Tachycardia Hypotension ↓ O_2 saturation Bronchospasm	• O_2 therapy • Cardiopulmonary support • Anticoagulant therapy
Aspiration	Inhalation of gastric contents into lungs	Unexplained tachypnea Bronchospasm ↓ O_2 saturation Atelectasis Interstitial edema Alveolar hemorrhage Respiratory failure	• O_2 therapy • Cardiopulmonary support • Antibiotics
Bronchospasm	↑ Smooth muscle tone with closure of small airways	Wheezing Dyspnea Tachypnea ↓ O_2 saturation	• O_2 therapy • Bronchodilators
Hypoventilation			
Depression of central respiratory drive	Medullary depression from anesthetics, opioids, sedatives	Shallow respirations ↓ Respiratory rate, apnea ↓ PaO_2 ↑ $PaCO_2$	• Initiate capnography or other technology supported respiratory monitoring • Stimulation • Reversal of opioids or benzodiazepines • Mechanical ventilation
Poor respiratory muscle tone	Neuromuscular blockade Neuromuscular disease	As above	• Reversal of paralysis • Mechanical ventilation
Mechanical restriction	Tight casts, dressings, abdominal binders Positioning and obesity preventing lung expansion	As above	• Elevate head of bed • Repositioning • Loosen dressings
Pain	Shallow breathing to prevent incisional pain	↑ Respiratory rate Hypotension Hypertension ↓ $PaCO_2$ ↓ PaO_2 Complaints of pain Guarding behavior	• Opioid analgesic drug therapy • Nonsteroidal antiinflammatory drug therapy • Complementary and alternative therapies (e.g., music, imagery)

$PaCO_2$, Partial pressure of arterial carbon dioxide; *PaO_2*, partial pressure of arterial oxygen.

TEAMWORK & COLLABORATION

Caring for the Postoperative Patient

In the PACU, patients require frequent assessment and intervention by RNs. On the clinical units, the RN is responsible for assessment, development of an individualized plan of care, implementation and evaluation of the plan of care, and discharge teaching. Much of the care can be delegated to LPNs/LVNs and UAP. Respiratory and physical therapy may also have a role in the patient's care, depending on the type of surgery and the patient's past medical history.

PACU	Clinical Unit
Role of Nursing Personnel	
Registered Nurse (RN)	
• Assess patient's initial airway, breathing, and circulation status. • Evaluate for the return to consciousness, ability to maintain airway and breathing. • Provide ongoing assessments for postoperative problems (e.g., airway obstruction, hypoventilation, hypotension or hypertension, dysrhythmias, emergence delirium). • Evaluate patient's readiness to be transferred to clinical unit or be discharged from ambulatory surgery. • Provide hand-off report about patient status when transferring patient to RN on clinical unit. • Provide discharge teaching for patient and caregiver after ambulatory surgery.	• Assess patient on initial admission to clinical unit. • Assess for postoperative complications (e.g., atelectasis, hemodynamic instability, cognitive dysfunction, pain, fluid and electrolyte imbalance, fever or hypothermia, nausea and vomiting, urinary retention, wound infection). • Develop and implement an individualized plan of care based on identification of patient risk factors and potential complications. • Develop and implement individualized patient and caregiver education, including discharge teaching.
Licensed Practical/Vocational Nurse (LPN/LVN)	
• Administer and titrate O_2 based on agency protocols. • Give analgesics and IV fluids (consider state nurse practice act and agency policy).	• Titrate O_2 administration according to prescribed parameters. • Monitor pain level and give prescribed analgesics. • Give medications (consider state nurse practice act and agency policy for medications). • Provide wound care, including dressing changes. • Use bladder ultrasound to check for urinary retention. • Insert catheter as prescribed for urinary retention.
Unlicensed Assistive Personnel (UAP)	
• Assist with positioning of patients in the lateral recovery position. • Obtain vital signs, pulse oximetry and capillary blood glucose levels (per agency policy). Report abnormal levels to RN. • Assist patient with elimination needs. • Assist in transfer of patient to clinical unit.	• Record oral intake and output. • Assist patient with deep breathing and coughing exercises. • Report complaints of pain to RN or LPN/LVN. • Reposition and ambulate patients as instructed. • Provide hygiene, including oral care. • Assist with nutrition and elimination needs.
Role of Other Team Members	
Respiratory Therapist	
• Provide respiratory care modalities that support patient recovery from anesthesia (e.g., O_2 therapy, nebulizer treatments, pulmonary drainage procedures, mechanical ventilation, and airway support). • Institute extubation protocols. • Monitor pulse oximetry, capnography, or other technology-assisted means of assessing hypoxemia or hypoventilation. • Assist with O_2 and/or ventilation management during patient transport. • Perform arterial blood gas sampling in the absence of an arterial line.	• Institute rapid intubation protocols if necessary in the absence of ACP. • Provide respiratory care modalities (e.g., O_2 therapy, nebulizer treatments, pulmonary drainage procedures). • Assist with O_2 and/or ventilation support during patient transport. • Monitor pulse oximetry and capnography and titrate O_2 as needed. • Perform arterial blood gas sampling as needed.
Physical Therapist	
• Perform initial assessment to ascertain normal functioning level if surgery was emergent. • Support patient motion and joint mobility.	• Support patient motion and joint mobility. • Support patient return to baseline functional mobility following surgery. • Support nursing staff on best measures for joint positioning, transferring from bed to chair, and/or ambulation.

somnolence, hypertension to hypotension, and tachycardia to bradycardia. Pulse oximetry will indicate low O_2 saturation (less than 90%).

The most common cause of postoperative hypoxemia is atelectasis. **Atelectasis** (alveolar collapse) may be the result of bronchial obstruction caused by retained secretions, decreased respiratory excursion, or general anesthesia. Atelectasis occurs when mucus blocks bronchioles or when the amount of alveolar surfactant (substance that holds the alveoli open) is reduced (Fig. 19-3). As air becomes trapped beyond the plug and is eventually absorbed, the alveoli collapse. Atelectasis may affect a portion of or an entire lobe of the lungs.

Other causes of hypoxemia include pulmonary edema, pulmonary embolism (PE), aspiration, and bronchospasm. *Pulmonary edema* is caused by an accumulation of fluid in the alveoli. It may be the result of fluid overload, heart failure, prolonged airway obstruction, sepsis, or aspiration.

Aspiration of gastric contents into the lungs is a potentially serious emergency. Gastric aspiration may also cause laryngospasm, infection, and pulmonary edema. Because of the serious consequences of aspiration of gastric fluids, prevention is the goal.

Bronchospasm is the result of an increase in bronchial smooth muscle tone with resultant closure of small airways. Airway edema develops, causing secretions to build up in the airway. The patient will have wheezing, dyspnea, use of accessory muscles, hypoxemia, and tachypnea. Bronchospasm may be due to aspiration, endotracheal intubation, pharyngeal suctioning, or an allergic response. (Allergic responses are discussed in Chapter 13.) Bronchospasm

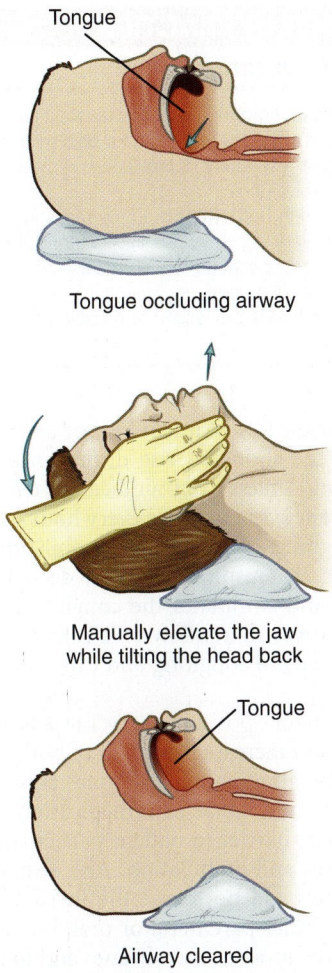

FIG. 19-2 Etiology and relief of airway obstruction.

may occur in any patient but is seen more frequently in patients with asthma and chronic obstructive pulmonary disease (COPD).

Hypoventilation, a common complication in the PACU, is characterized by a decreased respiratory rate or effort, hypoxemia, and an increasing partial pressure of arterial carbon dioxide ($PaCO_2$) (*hypercapnia*). Hypoventilation may result from depression of the central respiratory drive (secondary to anesthesia or use of opioids), poor respiratory muscle tone (secondary to neuromuscular blockade or disease), or a combination of both.

SAFETY ALERT Hypoventilation

- Always monitor for respiratory depression when giving opioids.
- Use a sedation assessment scale (e.g., Richmond Agitation and Sedation Scale) to assess for levels of sedation and promote patient safety when giving opioids in the PACU.

Richmond Agitation Scale available at *www.icudelirium.org/docs/RASS.pdf.*

Clinical Unit. Common causes of respiratory problems for postoperative patients in the clinical unit are atelectasis and pneumonia, especially in patients with co-morbidities (e.g., OSA, COPD, heart failure)[6,7] and following abdominal and thoracic surgery. The postoperative development of mucous plugs and decreased surfactant production is directly related to hypoventilation, immobility and bed rest, ineffective coughing, and history of tobacco use. Increased bronchial secretions occur when the respiratory passages have been irritated by heavy smoking; acute or chronic pulmonary infection or disease; and

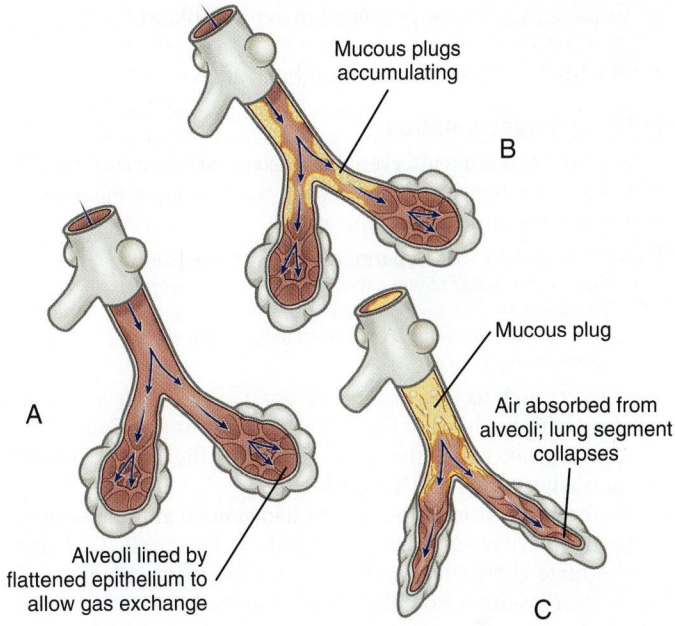

FIG. 19-3 Postoperative atelectasis. **A,** Normal bronchiole and alveoli. **B,** Mucous plug in bronchiole. **C,** Collapse of alveoli resulting from atelectasis after absorption of air.

the drying of mucous membranes that occurs with intubation, inhalation anesthesia, and dehydration. Without intervention, atelectasis can progress to pneumonia.

❖ NURSING MANAGEMENT: RESPIRATORY PROBLEMS

◆ Nursing Assessment

For an adequate respiratory assessment, evaluate airway patency; chest symmetry; and depth, rate, and character of respirations. Observe the chest wall for symmetry of movement. Impaired ventilation may first be seen as slowed breathing or reduced chest and abdominal movement during breathing. Also assess for the use of abdominal or accessory muscles, which may indicate respiratory distress. Auscultate breath sounds, since decreased or absent breath sounds are found when airflow is diminished or obstructed. Patients with poor respiratory effort, noisy respirations, or other signs of respiratory distress should be aroused immediately and instructed to take deep breaths.

Regular monitoring of vital signs, including pulse oximetry, capnography or other technology-supported monitoring (e.g., acoustic monitoring), and a thorough respiratory assessment permit you to recognize early signs of respiratory problems. Manifestations of hypoxemia include tachypnea, gasping, anxiety, restlessness, confusion, and a rapid or thready pulse.

Note and record the characteristics of sputum or mucus. Mucus from the trachea and throat is normally colorless and thin in consistency. Sputum from the lungs and bronchi is normally thick with a pale yellow tinge. Changes in sputum (e.g., color) may indicate a respiratory infection.

◆ Nursing Diagnoses

Nursing diagnoses and collaborative problems related to respiratory problems include, but are not limited to, the following:

- Ineffective airway clearance *related to* ineffective cough, obstruction, pain
- Ineffective breathing pattern *related to* anesthetic agents, pain, use of opioids

- Impaired gas exchange *related to* hypoventilation
- Risk for aspiration
- Potential complications: pneumonia, atelectasis

Nursing Implementation

In the PACU, nursing interventions are aimed at preventing and treating respiratory problems. Proper positioning of the patient aids breathing and protects the airway.

SAFETY ALERT Postoperative Patient Positioning

- Position the unconscious patient in a lateral "recovery" position (Fig. 19-4).
- This position keeps the airway open and reduces the risk of aspiration if vomiting occurs.

Once conscious, the patient is usually placed in a supine position with the head of the bed elevated. This position maximizes expansion of the thorax by decreasing the pressure of the abdominal contents on the diaphragm.

O_2 therapy is used if the patient had general anesthesia or if ordered. Give oxygen via nasal cannula or face mask. O_2 helps to eliminate anesthetic gases and meet the increased demand for oxygen resulting from decreased blood volume or increased metabolism.

Deep breathing is encouraged to aid gas exchange and promote the return to consciousness. Once the patient is more awake, deep breathing, coughing, and use of an incentive spirometer help prevent alveolar collapse and move respiratory secretions to larger airway passages for expectoration. One technique, known as *sustained maximal inspiration,* requires the patient to inhale as deeply as possible and, at the peak of inspiration, hold the breath for a few seconds, and then exhale. This should be followed by a second deep breath and cough.

The use of an incentive spirometer helps by giving visual feedback of respiratory effort (Fig. 19-5). Diaphragmatic or abdominal breathing involves inhaling slowly and deeply through the nose, holding the breath for a few seconds, and then exhaling slowly and completely through the mouth. Place the patient's hands lightly over the lower ribs and upper abdomen so that the patient can feel the abdomen rise during inspiration and fall during expiration. Unless contraindicated, tell the patient to perform these maneuvers 10 times every hour while awake.

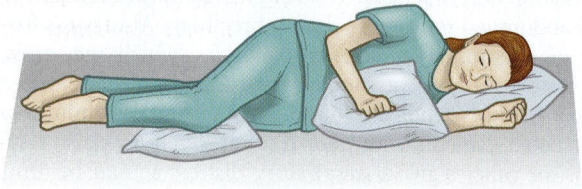

FIG. 19-4 Position of patient during recovery from general anesthesia.

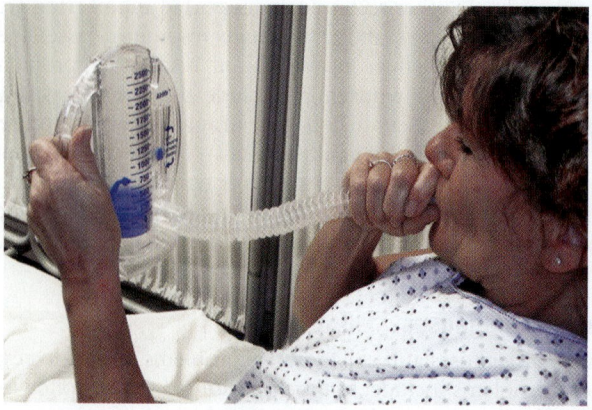

FIG. 19-5 Proper use of an incentive spirometer. (Courtesy Christine R. Hoch, MSN, RN, ACNS-BC, Nursing Instructor, University of Delaware, Newark, Del.)

INFORMATICS IN PRACTICE

Respiratory Monitoring

- Continuous monitoring of respiratory rate is especially important for postoperative patients receiving PCA for pain management, as opioids can cause respiratory depression and place patients at risk of serious injury or death.
- Acoustic Respiration Rate (RRa) is a new measurement that allows for the noninvasive and continuous assessment of patients' breathing. RRa uses a sensor with an acoustic transducer that is applied to the patient's neck.
- The respiratory signal is processed to display a continuous respiration rate.

Source: *www.masimo.com/rra*

Effective coughing is essential in mobilizing secretions. If secretions are in the respiratory tract, deep breathing often moves them up and stimulates the cough reflex. Splinting an abdominal incision with a pillow or a rolled blanket supports the incision and aids in coughing and expectorating secretions (Fig. 19-6).

Change the patient's position every 1 to 2 hours to allow full chest expansion and increase perfusion of both lungs. Sitting in a chair and ambulating should be done as soon as ordered. Provide adequate and regular pain medication. Incisional pain often is the greatest barrier to patient participation in effective breathing exercises and ambulation. Also reassure the patient that these activities will not cause the incision to open. Adequate hydration, either parenteral or oral, is essential to maintain the integrity of mucous membranes and to keep secretions thin and loose for easy expectoration.

Other nursing interventions appropriate for specific respiratory problems are detailed in Table 19-5. A nursing care plan for the postoperative patient (eNursing Care Plan 19-1) is available on the website for this chapter.

CARDIOVASCULAR PROBLEMS

Etiology

PACU. In the immediate postanesthesia period the most common cardiovascular problems include hypotension, hypertension, and

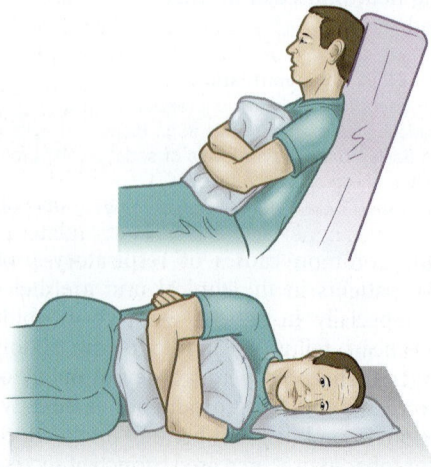

FIG. 19-6 Techniques for splinting incision when coughing.

dysrhythmias. Patients at greatest risk for alterations in cardiovascular function include those with alterations in respiratory function, those with a history of cardiovascular disease, older adults, the debilitated, and the critically ill.

Hypotension is evidenced by signs of hypoperfusion to the vital organs, especially the brain, heart, and kidneys. Clinical signs of disorientation, loss of consciousness, chest pain, and oliguria reflect hypoperfusion, hypoxemia, and the loss of physiologic compensation. Intervention must be timely to prevent the devastating complications of cardiac ischemia or infarction, cerebral ischemia, renal ischemia, and bowel infarction.

The most common cause of hypotension in the PACU is fluid and blood loss, which may lead to hypovolemic shock. Hemorrhage is always a risk of surgery. Marked blood loss is possible when cauterization or sutures fail. Hemorrhage most often occurs internally, requiring assessment for changes in level of consciousness and vital signs. If changes are detected, treatment is directed toward restoring circulating volume. If there is no response to fluid administration, heart dysfunction should be considered the cause of hypotension.

Primary heart dysfunction, as may occur in myocardial infarction, cardiac tamponade, or pulmonary embolism, results in an acute drop in cardiac output. Secondary heart dysfunction occurs as a result of the negative *chronotropic* (rate of heart contraction) and negative *inotropic* (force of heart contraction) effects of drugs, such as β-adrenergic blockers, digoxin, or opioids. Other causes of hypotension include decreased systemic vascular resistance, dysrhythmias, and measurement errors (e.g., taking BP with an incorrectly sized cuff).

Hypertension, a common finding in the PACU, is most frequently the result of sympathetic nervous system stimulation that may be the result of pain, anxiety, bladder distention, or respiratory distress. Hypertension may also be the result of hypothermia and preexisting hypertension.

In the PACU, *dysrhythmias* are caused by hypoxemia, hypercapnia, electrolyte and acid-base imbalances, circulatory instability, and preexisting heart disease. Hypothermia, pain, surgical stress, and many anesthetic agents can also cause dysrhythmias.

Clinical Unit. In the clinical unit, postoperative fluid and electrolyte imbalances are contributing factors to heart problems. Such imbalances may result from a combination of the body's normal response to the stress of surgery, excessive fluid losses, and improper IV fluid replacement. The body's fluid status directly affects cardiac output.

Fluid retention during postoperative days 1 to 3 can result from the stress response, which maintains both blood volume and BP. Fluid retention is caused by the secretion and release of two hormones by the pituitary—antidiuretic hormone (ADH) and adrenocorticotropic hormone (ACTH)—and activation of the renin-angiotensin-aldosterone system (RAAS). ADH release leads to increased water reabsorption and decreased urine output, increasing blood volume. ACTH stimulates the adrenal cortex to secrete cortisol and, to a lesser degree, aldosterone (see Figs. 16-9 and 16-10). Fluid losses resulting from surgery decrease kidney perfusion, stimulating the RAAS and causing marked release of aldosterone (see Chapter 16). Both mechanisms that increase aldosterone lead to significant sodium and fluid retention, thus increasing blood volume.

Fluid overload may occur during this period of fluid retention when IV fluids are infused too rapidly, when chronic (e.g., heart, kidney) disease exists, or when the patient is an older adult. Fluid deficits from untreated preoperative dehydration, intraoperative blood losses, or slow or inadequate fluid replacement can lead to decreases in cardiac output and tissue perfusion. Postoperative losses from vomiting, bleeding, wound drainage, or suctioning can also contribute to fluid deficits.

Hypokalemia can be a consequence of urinary and gastrointestinal (GI) tract losses. Low serum potassium levels directly affect the contractility of the heart and may contribute to decreases in cardiac output and tissue perfusion. Potassium replacement, usually 40 mEq/day, should not be given until renal function is assessed. A urine output of at least 0.5 mL/kg/hr is generally considered indicative of adequate renal function.

Cardiovascular status is also affected by the state of tissue perfusion or blood flow. The stress response contributes to an increase in clotting tendencies by increasing platelet production. In addition, general anesthesia causes peripheral vasodilation, which may contribute to damage of the vascular lining.

A *venous thromboembolism* (VTE) may form in leg veins as a result of inactivity, body position, and pressure, all of which lead to venous stasis and decreased perfusion. VTE is especially common in older adults, obese individuals, immobilized patients, and patients with a history of PE. It is a potentially life-threatening complication, because it may lead to PE and infarction. Suspect PE in any patient with tachypnea, dyspnea, and tachycardia, particularly when the patient is already receiving O_2 therapy. Other manifestations may include agitation, chest pain, hypotension, hemoptysis, dysrhythmias, and heart failure. Superficial thrombophlebitis is an uncomfortable but less serious complication that may develop in a leg vein as a result of venous stasis or in the arm veins as a result of irritation from IV catheters or solutions. (PE and VTE are discussed in Chapters 27 and 37, respectively.)

Syncope (fainting) may indicate decreased cardiac output, fluid deficits, or defects in cerebral perfusion. Syncope frequently occurs as a result of postural hypotension when the patient ambulates. It is more common in the older adult or in the patient who has been immobile for long periods. Normally when the patient stands up quickly, the arterial baroreceptors respond to the accompanying fall in BP with sympathetic nervous system stimulation. This produces vasoconstriction and thereby maintains BP. These sympathetic and vasomotor functions may be diminished in the older adult and the immobile or postanesthesia patient.

❖ NURSING MANAGEMENT: CARDIOVASCULAR PROBLEMS

◆ Nursing Assessment

The most important aspect of the cardiovascular assessment is frequent monitoring of vital signs. They are usually monitored every 15 minutes in Phase I, or more often until stabilized, and then less frequently in Phase II. Compare postoperative vital signs with pre- and intraoperative findings to determine when the signs are returning to baseline. Notify the ACP or surgeon if any of the following occurs:

- Systolic BP <90 mm Hg or >160 mm Hg
- Pulse rate <60 beats/minute or >120 beats/minute
- Pulse pressure (difference between systolic and diastolic BP) narrows
- BP trends gradually decrease or increase over several consecutive readings
- Change in heart rhythm

Hypotension accompanied by a normal pulse and warm, dry, pink skin usually represents the residual vasodilating effects of anesthesia and suggests only a need for continued observation. Hypotension accompanied by a rapid or weak pulse and cold, clammy, pale skin may indicate impending hypovolemic shock and requires immediate treatment.

ECG monitoring is recommended for patients who have a history of heart disease and for all older patients who have undergone major surgery, regardless of whether they have heart problems. Assess the apical-radial pulse carefully, and report any deficits or irregularities. Assess peripheral pulses and skin color, temperature, and moisture to gain valuable information about tissue perfusion.

◆ Nursing Diagnoses

Nursing diagnoses and collaborative problems related to cardiovascular problems include, but are not limited to, the following:

- Decreased cardiac output *related to* hypovolemia, dysrhythmias
- Ineffective peripheral tissue perfusion *related to* prolonged immobility, venous stasis
- Risk for imbalanced fluid volume
- Risk for impaired cardiovascular function
- Potential complications: hypovolemic shock, venous thromboembolism

◆ Nursing Implementation

◆ **PACU.** Begin treatment of hypotension with O_2 therapy to promote oxygenation of hypoperfused organs. Inspect the surgical incision to determine if excessive bleeding is the cause of volume loss. Because the most common cause of hypotension is fluid loss, give IV fluid boluses to normalize BP. Primary heart dysfunction may require drug intervention. Peripheral vasodilation and hypotension may require vasoconstrictive agents to increase systemic vascular resistance.

Treatment of hypertension centers on removing the cause of sympathetic nervous system stimulation. Treatment may include the use of analgesics, assistance in voiding, and correction of respiratory problems. Rewarming corrects hypothermia-induced hypertension. If the patient has preexisting hypertension or has undergone heart or vascular surgery, drug therapy to reduce BP is usually needed.

Because the majority of dysrhythmias seen in the PACU have identifiable causes, treatment is directed toward removing the cause. Correction of these physiologic alterations usually corrects the dysrhythmias. In the event of life-threatening dysrhythmias (e.g., ventricular tachycardia), follow the agency's protocol for advanced cardiac life support.

◆ **Clinical Unit.** Maintain an accurate intake and output record, monitor laboratory findings (e.g., electrolytes, hematocrit), and manage IV therapy during the postoperative period. Ongoing assessment of the potential complications associated with IV therapy (e.g., extravasation; redness, pain at the site) is essential.

Early ambulation is the most significant general nursing measure to prevent postoperative complications. The exercise associated with walking (1) increases muscle tone; (2) stimulates circulation, which prevents venous stasis and VTE, and speeds wound healing; and (3) increases vital capacity and maintains normal respiratory function. Progression to ambulation can be achieved by first raising the head of the patient's bed for 1 to 2 minutes and then assisting the patient to sit, with legs dangling, while monitoring the pulse rate. If no changes or complaints are noted, start ambulation with ongoing monitoring of the pulse. If changes in the pulse are noted or dizziness occurs, sit the patient in a nearby chair. The patient should remain in this location until the BP and pulse are stable. Then help the patient back to the bed. If dizziness occurs, it is often frightening for the patient and you. Injury can result from a fall, so take measures to ensure patient and staff safety.

CHECK YOUR PRACTICE

You are caring for an older, obese male patient who is 1 day post colon resection with activity orders for moving out of the bed to a chair. While he is in bed, you help him to a sitting position with his legs dangling. He tells you that he feels dizzy. You take his BP and it is 108/64 and his pulse is 124.

- What should you do?

NEUROLOGIC AND PSYCHOLOGIC PROBLEMS

Etiology

PACU. Postoperatively, **emergence delirium** is a short-term neurologic alteration manifested by behaviors such as restlessness, agitation, disorientation, thrashing, and shouting. This condition may be caused by hypoxia, anesthetic agents, bladder distention, postoperative pain, long duration of preoperative fasting, residual neuromuscular blockade, or the presence of an endotracheal tube.[8] If delirium occurs, first suspect hypoxia.

Delayed emergence may also be a problem postoperatively. The most common cause of delayed emergence is prolonged drug action, particularly of opioids, sedatives, residual neuromuscular blockade, and inhalation anesthetics. It is not usually due to neurologic injury. Delayed emergence is associated with longer PACU and hospital length of stay.[8]

Clinical Unit. Two types of postoperative cognitive impairments seen in surgical patients are *postoperative cognitive dysfunction* (POCD) and *delirium.* POCD is a decline in the patient's cognitive function (e.g., memory, ability to concentrate) for weeks or months after surgery. POCD is seen primarily in the older surgical patient. Preexisting cognitive impairment, age, duration of anesthesia, intraoperative complications, and postoperative infections are related to the development of POCD. Any changes in mental status should be quickly and thoroughly investigated, as the causes may be life threatening.

Postoperative delirium is more common in the older patient, but it can occur in patients of any age. Delirium may be the result of severe postoperative pain, fluid and electrolyte imbalances, hypoxemia, drug effects, sleep deprivation, and sensory deprivation or overload. It is characterized by cognitive dysfunction, varying levels of consciousness, altered psychomotor activity, and a disturbed sleep/wake cycle. (Delirium is discussed in Chapter 59.)

Anxiety and depression may also occur in postoperative patients. Patients may experience depressive symptoms and delirium at the same time. This increases the likelihood of postoperative complications.[9] Any patient may have these responses as part of grieving for lost body parts or functions or for loss of independence during recovery and rehabilitation.

Alcohol withdrawal delirium results from alcohol withdrawal in a postoperative patient. It is characterized by restlessness, insomnia and nightmares, irritability, and auditory or visual hallucinations. Chapter 10 discusses the identification and management of alcohol withdrawal delirium.

NURSING MANAGEMENT: NEUROLOGIC AND PSYCHOLOGIC PROBLEMS

Nursing Assessment

Assess the patient's level of consciousness, orientation, memory, and ability to follow commands. Determine the size, reactivity, and equality of the pupils. Also assess the patient's sleep/wake cycle and sensory and motor status. If the neurologic status is altered, try to determine possible causes. If the patient was mentally alert before surgery and becomes cognitively impaired postoperatively, you should suspect delirium or POCD.

Nursing Diagnoses

Nursing diagnoses related to neurologic or psychologic problems include, but are not limited to, the following:

- Acute confusion *related to* hypoxia, postoperative cognitive dysfunction, delirium
- Anxiety *related to* change in health status, hospital environment
- Disturbed body image *related to* loss of body part(s), function
- Disturbed sleep pattern *related to* pain, hospital environment

Nursing Implementation

PACU. The most common cause of postoperative agitation in the PACU is hypoxemia. As a result, focus your attention on evaluating respiratory function. Once you have ruled out hypoxemia or other known causes of postoperative delirium, sedation may be beneficial in controlling the agitation. Because the most common cause of delayed emergence is prolonged drug action, delays in awakening usually spontaneously resolve with time. If necessary, benzodiazepines and opioids may be reversed with drug antagonists.

Until the patient is awake and able to communicate effectively, be a patient advocate and maintain patient safety at all times. This includes monitoring physiologic status, having the side rails up and the call bell available, securing equipment (e.g., IV lines, artificial airways), using two unique patient identifiers before giving drugs or completing treatments, and verifying allergies.

Clinical Unit. To prevent or manage postoperative delirium or POCD, address factors that are known to contribute to the condition. Maintain normal physiologic function by achieving fluid and electrolyte balance, adequate nutrition and sleep, pain management, proper bowel and bladder function, and early mobilization. To help orient the patient, use specific aids, such as clocks, calendars, and photos.

To prevent or limit psychologic problems, provide adequate support for the patient. This includes listening to and talking with the patient, offering explanations and reassurance, and encouraging the presence and assistance of the patient's caregiver(s). Evaluate the patient's behavior to distinguish a normal reaction to a stressful situation from one that is becoming abnormal or excessive. The recognition of alcohol withdrawal delirium presents a particular challenge. Record and report any unusual or disturbed behavior so that a diagnosis can be made and treatment started.

PAIN AND DISCOMFORT

Etiology

Despite the availability of pain-relieving drugs and techniques, pain remains a common problem and a significant fear for patients. Postoperative pain is caused by the interaction of a number of physiologic and psychologic factors. The skin and underlying tissues have been traumatized by the incision and retraction during surgery. In addition, there may be reflex muscle spasms around the incision. Anxiety and fear, sometimes related to the anticipation of pain, create tension and further increase muscle tone and spasm. Positioning during surgery or the use of internal devices such as an endotracheal tube or catheters may also cause discomfort. The effort and movement associated with deep breathing, coughing, and ambulating may aggravate pain by creating tension on the incision area. Other sources of discomfort include nausea and vomiting, environmental noises, noxious odors, and shivering.

When the internal viscera are cut, no pain is felt. However, pressure in the internal viscera causes pain. Therefore deep visceral pain may signal a complication such as intestinal distention, bleeding, or abscess formation. Pain also increases the risk of atelectasis and impaired respiratory function.

NURSING MANAGEMENT: PAIN

Nursing Assessment

The patient's self-report is the single most reliable indicator of pain. Pain scales such as a numeric or FACES pain scale can assist with assessing the severity or intensity of pain. (Pain scales are discussed in Chapter 8.) Assess pain levels at rest and during activities. Since verbalization of pain is not always possible in the PACU, observe the patient for other indications of pain (e.g., restlessness, grimacing, changes in vital signs). You should expect that patients will experience incisional pain, especially with movement, and with certain procedures (e.g., removal of drains).

Assessment of patients from different cultures or who do not speak English may be challenging. Take extra time to explore the pain experience with these patients. (Chapter 2 discusses the use of an interpreter.) Adapt care as needed to meet the patient's unique needs and expectations for pain control.

Assess the patient on arrival to the PACU and at frequent intervals. Identifying the location of the pain is important. Incisional pain is to be expected, but other causes of pain, such as a full bladder, may also be present. Always involve patients in the assessment and management of their pain.

Nursing Diagnoses

Nursing diagnoses for the patient experiencing pain include, but are not limited to, the following:

- Acute pain *related to* inflammation or injury in surgical area
- Chronic pain *related to* preexisting conditions (e.g., arthritis)

Nursing Implementation

A plan for pain control that includes behavioral modalities and control of anxiety is developed preoperatively. Adjustments to or continuation of drugs used to treat any chronic pain is also evaluated in the preoperative phase of care. During this time, patients are taught to report pain and how it will be managed postoperatively. Pain management plans should be shared during the hand-off report.

Postoperative pain control techniques include the use of single modalities (e.g., opioid drugs, patient-controlled analgesia [PCA], regional analgesic [local anesthetic infiltration]) and multimodal analgesia. *Multimodal analgesia,* or the use of two or more analgesics with different mechanisms of action (e.g., opioid and a nonsteroidal antiinflammatory drug [NSAID]), is recommended when possible to achieve better pain relief with fewer or less severe side effects.[10] These drugs may be given via the same or different routes. The choice of modalities should be procedure and patient specific.

Orders for pain medication and other comfort measures are often written on an as-needed (PRN) basis. Time the administration of analgesics to ensure that they are in effect during activities that may be painful, such as walking. Although opioid analgesics are often essential for the postoperative patient's comfort, there are undesirable side effects. The most common include constipation, nausea and vomiting, respiratory and cough depression, and hypotension.

Before giving any analgesic, first assess the patient's pain, including location, quality, and intensity; vital signs; and level of consciousness. Treat incisional pain as ordered. If the patient reports chest or leg pain, analgesics may mask a complication (e.g., VTE). If it is gas pain, opioids can aggravate it. If the analgesic either fails to relieve the pain or makes the patient lethargic or somnolent, notify the health care provider (HCP) and request a change in the order.

Patient-controlled analgesia (PCA) is a method of pain management that allows the self-administration of predetermined doses of analgesia by the patient. The goals of PCA are to provide immediate analgesia and maintain an acceptable level of pain control. A continuous infusion in addition to patient-administered bolus doses may also be ordered especially in opioid tolerant patients.[10] Continuous infusions allow for a steady blood level of analgesia with the additional patient doses used prior to anticipated painful events (e.g., walking, deep breathing, and coughing) or for breakthough pain. The route of delivery may be IV, oral, epidural, or transdermal. The transdermal route is designed for short-term pain management and may offer advantages over the IV route (e.g., needleless, low infection risk, decreased drug errors associated with pump malfunction or inaccurate programming). Some advantages of PCA are early ambulation, better pain management than with PRN analgesia, and greater patient satisfaction. (PCA is discussed in Chapter 8.)

CHECK YOUR PRACTICE

Although PCA is infusing as ordered, your postoperative patient reports ongoing pain that is rated 8 on a 0 to 10 scale.

- What steps would you take next to manage this patient's pain more effectively?

Epidural analgesia is the infusion of opioid analgesics through a catheter placed into the epidural space surrounding the spinal cord. The goal of epidural analgesia is delivery of the drug directly to opiate receptors in the spinal cord. Administration methods include intermittent bolus dosing, continuous infusion, and patient-controlled epidural analgesia. This technique results in a constant circulating level and a reduced total dose of medication. The use of epidural analgesia for postoperative pain is increasing.

Perineural local anesthesia, the infiltration of a nonopioid drug into the surgical site, is another method of managing postoperative pain. A disposable or mechanical infusion pump delivers the local anesthetic via a catheter directly to the surgical incision site. A single dose of bupivacaine liposome injectable suspension (Exparel) provides pain relief with reduced opioid needs for up to 72 hours.

The acute pain of surgery almost always requires the use of analgesics. However, nondrug approaches such as repositioning, massage, and distraction can enhance pain management. Complementary and alternative therapies such as music therapy, guided imagery, relaxation exercises, and aromatherapy are effective adjuncts in pain management.

Organizational approaches have also demonstrated a reduction in postoperative pain intensity with decreases in side effects associated with the use of analgesia. These approaches include the use of procedure-specific, multimodal pain management guidelines with titration of analgesia based on specific patient needs.[10,11]

SAFETY ALERT Patient-Controlled Analgesia (PCA)

- Carefully check the HCP's order for PCA and properly program the pump to deliver the ordered dose of analgesic (e.g., continuous rate, bolus dose, maximum dose).
- A patient's death or serious injury associated with a drug error (e.g., wrong drug, wrong dose, wrong patient, wrong rate) is a serious reportable event (never event) or sentinel event. (See Chapter 1 for discussion of these events.)

ALTERATIONS IN TEMPERATURE

Etiology

The patient's temperature in the postoperative period provides valuable information (Table 19-6).

Hypothermia. Perioperative *hypothermia* is a core body temperature less than 96.8°F (36°C). Hypothermia occurs when heat loss exceeds heat production. Heat loss may occur due to skin exposure by the surgical procedure, use of cold irrigants and skin preparations, as well as unwarmed inhaled gases. Although all patients are at risk for hypothermia, patients with low preoperative core body temperatures, systolic BP less than 140 mm Hg, older patients, female patients, and patients who receive epidural or spinal anesthesia are at a higher risk of developing hypothermia postoperatively.[12] Long surgical procedures and prolonged anesthetic administration lead to redistribution of body heat from the core to the periphery. This places the patient at an increased risk for hypothermia.

Hypothermia can affect the patient's perception of the perioperative experience. The complications associated with hypothermia can include vasoconstriction with resultant hypertension, compromised immune function, bleeding, untoward cardiac events, surgical site infection (SSI), altered drug metabolism, and postoperative pain and shivering. Shivering can increase resting energy expenditure and O_2 consumption up to 500%, which can lead to hypoxemia and myocardial ischemia (angina). Shivering can also increase carbon dioxide production, contribute to increased heart rate, BP, and intracranial pressure, as well as significantly affect the patient's comfort level.

Fever. Fever may occur at any time during the postoperative period (Table 19-6). Wound infection, particularly from aerobic

TABLE 19-6 Postoperative Temperature Changes

Time After Surgery	Temperature	Possible Causes
Up to 12 hr	Hypothermia: ≤96.8°F (36°C)	Effects of anesthesia, body heat loss during surgical procedure
First 48 hr (postop days 1 and 2)	Mild elevation: ≤100.4°F (38°C)	Inflammatory response to surgical stress
	Moderate elevation: >100.4°F (38°C)	Lung congestion, dehydration
After first 48 hr (postop day 3 and later)	Elevation >100°F (37.8°C)	Infection (e.g., wound, urinary, respiratory)

organisms, is often accompanied by a fever that spikes in the afternoon or evening and returns to near-normal levels in the morning. The respiratory tract may be infected secondary to stasis of secretions in areas of atelectasis. The urinary tract may be infected secondary to catheterization. Superficial thrombophlebitis may occur at the IV site. VTE in the leg veins may produce a temperature elevation.

Surgical patients who take antibiotics for a period of time are at risk for *Clostridium difficile* infections. Manifestations of *C. difficile* may include fever, diarrhea, and abdominal pain.

Intermittent high fever accompanied by shaking chills and diaphoresis suggests septicemia. This may occur at any time during the postoperative period because microorganisms may have been introduced into the bloodstream during surgery, especially in GI or genitourinary (GU) procedures. Septicemia may also occur later from a wound or urinary tract infection.

Malignant hyperthermia (MH) causes a rapid rise in core body temperature to 105° F (40.5° C) or higher and severe muscle contractions after receiving general anesthesia. Additional signs of MH include tachycardia, hypercarbia, metabolic and respiratory acidosis, myoglobinuria, and elevated creatine kinase levels. MH is a life-threatening complication. While most cases of MH occur during general anesthesia, the 1-hour period immediately following surgery (e.g., in the PACU) is also a critical time.[13]

❖ NURSING MANAGEMENT: ALTERED TEMPERATURE

◆ Nursing Assessment

Record the patient's temperature on arrival to the PACU and every hour if the patient remains normothermic. Temperature may be taken orally, temporally, or via the tympanic membrane. Use the same route of measuring temperature during the patient's stay in the PACU. If the patient is hypothermic, measure the temperature every 15 minutes until normothermia is reached. Unintended hypothermia is an independent risk factor for surgical site infections (SSIs). Perioperative temperature management remains a quality measure by the Surgical Care Improvement Project (SCIP), a national partnership of organizations whose goal is to reduce SSIs.[14]

Risk factors for hypothermia or MH should be communicated to all members of the perioperative team. Supplies recommended by the Malignant Hyperthermia Association of the United States should be readily available to manage MH. Assess the color and temperature of the skin. Observe the patient for early signs of inflammation and infection that may precede a fever so that any complications can be treated in a timely manner.

◆ Nursing Diagnoses

Nursing diagnoses related to an altered temperature include, but are not limited to, the following:

- Hypothermia *related to* long surgical procedures, prolonged use of anesthetics
- Hyperthermia *related to* hypermetabolic state, infection
- Risk for imbalanced body temperature
- Risk for perioperative hypothermia

◆ Nursing Implementation

Passive warming measures include the use of warmed cotton blankets, socks, and reflective blankets and limiting skin exposure. *Active warming measures* involve the application of external warming devices, including forced air warmers; heated water mattresses; radiant warmers; heated, humidified O_2; and warmed IV fluids. When using any external warming device, record body temperature and the patient's comfort level at 15-minute intervals. In addition, take care to prevent skin injuries.

O_2 therapy via nasal prongs or mask is used to treat the increased demand for O_2 caused by shivering. Shivering can be treated with opioids (e.g., meperidine [Demerol]). Treatment for MH includes the administration of dantrolene (Dantrium) with the onset of symptoms in addition to measures to cool the patient (e.g., ice packs, cold IV solutions). Acid-base imbalances should also be corrected to reverse signs of MH.

Meticulous asepsis is required with wound and IV site care. Airway clearance is encouraged with deep breathing, coughing, and the use of the incentive spirometer. If fever develops, chest x-rays may be taken and antipyretic drugs given. Depending on the suspected cause of the fever, obtain cultures of the wound, sputum, urine, or blood. If a bacterial infection is the source of the fever, antibiotics are started as soon as cultures have been obtained. If the fever rises above 103° F (39.4° C), body-cooling measures may be used.

GASTROINTESTINAL PROBLEMS

Etiology

Postoperative nausea and vomiting (PONV) are the most common complications affecting as many as 80% of high-risk patients. Risk factors include younger age (less than 50 years of age), gender (female), history of motion sickness or previous PONV, nonsmoking status, action of anesthetics or opioids, and duration and type of surgery.[15] Delayed gastric emptying and slowed peristalsis that result from handling of the bowel during abdominal surgery also contribute to PONV, as does starting oral intake too soon after surgery.

Constipation may also occur postoperatively and can be due to anesthetics used during surgery that may paralyze the intestine; immobility; alterations in diet and fluid intake pre- and postoperatively; and the use of opioids for pain relief. Opioids contribute to constipation by decreasing peristalsis and slowing fecal transport through the intestinal tract. Opioids may also decrease a patient's urge to defecate. (Constipation is discussed in Chapter 42).

Postoperative ileus (POI), or the temporary impairment of gastric and bowel motility after surgery, results from the handling or reconstruction of the intestine during surgery and limited dietary intake before and after surgery. After abdominal surgery, motility in the large intestine may be reduced for 3 to 5 days, although motility in the small intestine resumes within several hours following surgery. Although POI is expected following abdominal surgery, it may occur following non-abdominal surgery.

Risk factors for POI include the use of opioids, immobility, older age, previous abdominal surgery, and early postoperative feeding. Use of opioid analgesia may prolong the duration of POI. Abdominal cramps, increasing abdominal distention, complaints of constipation or vomiting, and dehydration often accompany POI.

Hiccups (singultus) are intermittent spasms of the diaphragm caused by irritation of the phrenic nerve, which innervates the diaphragm. The phrenic nerve may be irritated postoperatively by gastric distention, intestinal obstruction, intraabdominal bleeding, and a subphrenic abscess. Indirect irritation of the phrenic nerve may be produced by acid-base and electrolyte imbalances. Reflex irritation may come from drinking hot or cold liquids or from the presence of a nasogastric (NG) tube. Hiccups usually last a short time and stop spontaneously.

❖ NURSING MANAGEMENT: GASTROINTESTINAL PROBLEMS

◆ Nursing Assessment

Ask the patient about feelings of nausea. If nausea is present, assess the severity using a verbal descriptor or numerical scale. If vomiting occurs, determine the quantity, characteristics, and color of the vomitus. Assess the abdomen for distention and presence of bowel sounds. Because bowel sounds are frequently absent or diminished in the immediate postoperative period, auscultate all four quadrants to determine the presence, frequency, and characteristics of the sounds. The return of normal bowel motility is usually accompanied by the passage of gas or stool and the patient's ability to tolerate oral intake without complaints of nausea or vomiting.

◆ Nursing Diagnoses

Nursing diagnoses and collaborative problems related to GI problems include, but are not limited to, the following:

- Nausea *related to* anesthetic agents, manipulation of abdominal contents
- Imbalanced nutrition: less than body requirements *related to* vomiting, decreased appetite, decreased peristalsis
- Constipation *related to* anesthetics, opioid analgesics, immobility, and dietary changes
- Risk for imbalanced fluid volume
- Risk for electrolyte imbalance
- Potential complications: POI, hiccups

◆ Nursing Implementation

In the PACU when the patient is NPO, IV fluids are given to maintain fluid and electrolyte balance. Begin oral fluids as ordered and tolerated. Depending on the type of the surgery, the patient may begin oral intake as soon as the gag reflex returns. When oral intake is allowed, offer clear liquids first and continue the IV fluids, usually at a reduced rate. If oral intake is well tolerated, the IV fluids are stopped.

Be alert to prevent aspiration if the patient vomits while still sleepy from anesthesia. Position the patient in the lateral recovery position and have suction equipment available. Interventions for PONV include verifying hydration status and BP and giving appropriate antiemetic or prokinetic drugs (see Chapter 41, Table 41-1). Consider complementary and alternative therapy interventions for PONV (e.g., imagery, music, aromatherapy, acupressure).

Constipation may be prevented using bowel protocols that include the use of a stool softener and laxative. Assess the patient regularly to detect the return of peristalsis. Encourage the patient to expel gas. Gas pains, which tend to become pronounced on the second or third postoperative day, may be relieved by ambulation and frequent repositioning. Positioning the patient on the right side permits gas to rise along the transverse colon and aids its release. Bisacodyl (Dulcolax) suppositories may be ordered to stimulate colonic peristalsis and expulsion of gas and stool. Resuming a normal diet after bowel sounds have returned also aids the return of normal peristalsis.

The goal of treatment for POI is the relief of associated symptoms and return of normal gastrointestinal function. Management includes bowel rest or the withholding of solid foods with a gradual reintroduction of food starting with clear liquids. Diet is advanced to solid food with an ongoing assessment of tolerance to oral intake.

An NG tube may be needed to decompress the stomach to prevent nausea, vomiting, and abdominal distention. Oral care is critical for comfort and stimulation of salivary glands when the patient is NPO or has an NG tube. Chewing gum has been studied as a treatment strategy for POI in select populations. Chewing gum mimics the act of eating, which is thought to stimulate gastric and bowel motility. This adjunctive intervention has been found to decrease the time for passage of flatus and stool for patients who undergo abdominal surgery.[16]

URINARY PROBLEMS

Etiology

Low urine output (800 to 1500 mL) in the first 24 hours after surgery may be expected, regardless of fluid intake. This low output is caused by increased aldosterone and ADH secretion resulting from the stress of surgery; fluid restriction before surgery; and fluid loss through surgery, drainage, and diaphoresis. By the second or third day, after fluid has been mobilized and the immediate stress reaction subsides, the patient will begin to have increasing urine output.

Acute urinary retention can occur in the postoperative period for a variety of reasons. Anesthesia depresses the nervous system, including the micturition reflex arc and the higher centers that influence it. This allows the bladder to fill more completely than normal before the urge to void is felt. Anesthesia also impedes voluntary micturition. Anticholinergic and opioid drugs may also interfere with the ability to initiate voiding or to empty the bladder completely.

Urinary retention is more likely to occur after lower abdominal or pelvic surgery because spasms or guarding of the abdominal and pelvic muscles interferes with their normal function in micturition. Pain may alter perception and interfere with the patient's awareness of bladder filling. Voiding ability is probably impaired to the greatest extent by immobility and bed rest. The supine position reduces the ability to relax the perineal muscles and external sphincter.

Oliguria (diminished output of urine) can be a sign of renal failure and is a less common, although more serious, problem after surgery. It may result from renal ischemia caused by inadequate renal perfusion.

❖ NURSING MANAGEMENT: URINARY PROBLEMS

◆ Nursing Assessment

Examine the urine for both quantity and quality. Note the color, amount, and odor of the urine. Assess indwelling catheters for patency. Urine output should be at least 0.5 mL/kg/hr. To decrease the risk of catheter-associated urinary tract infection (CAUTI), remove the catheter as soon as possible or within 24 hours, unless there is a reason to continue its use. Most patients void within 6 to 8 hours after surgery. If no voiding occurs, scan or percuss the suprapubic area for signs of bladder fullness or distention.

◆ Nursing Diagnoses

Nursing diagnoses and collaborative problems related to urinary problems include, but are not limited to, the following:

- Urinary retention *related to* anesthetic agents, pain
- Potential complication: acute kidney injury, CAUTI

Nursing Implementation

You can aid voiding by normal positioning of the patient—sitting for women and standing for men. Reassure the patient regarding the ability to void. Helpful techniques include providing privacy, running water, offering water for the patient to drink, or pouring warm water over the perineum. Walking, preferably to the bathroom, and the use of a bedside commode are additional helpful measures to assist in voiding.

The surgeon often leaves an order to catheterize the patient in 6 to 8 hours if voiding has not occurred. Because of the possibility of CAUTI, first try to confirm that the bladder is actually full. Consider fluid intake during and after surgery and determine bladder fullness (e.g., discomfort when the bladder is palpated). Scan the bladder with a portable ultrasound to assess volume of urine in the bladder and avoid unnecessary catheterization. If catheterization is required, a straight catheterization (as compared to an indwelling catheter) is preferred to limit the risk of CAUTI.

INTEGUMENTARY PROBLEMS

Etiology

Surgery generally involves an incision through the skin and underlying tissues, disrupting the protective skin barrier. One of the greatest risks during the perioperative period is *surgical site infection (SSI).* SSIs continue to be the most common health care–acquired infection and have been associated with prolonged hospitalizations, increased cost of care, and poor patient outcomes.[17] Wound healing is therefore a major concern during the postoperative period. The majority of SSIs are preventable with evidence-based strategies to prevent them (e.g., selection, timing, and duration of prophylactic antibiotics, surgical site skin preparation including hair removal, perioperative blood glucose management). Adherence to these strategies is known to reduce the incidence of SSIs and is a major goal of the SCIP initiative.

Wound infection may result from contamination of the wound from three major sources: (1) exogenous flora present in the environment and on the skin, (2) oral flora, and (3) intestinal flora. The incidence of wound sepsis is higher in patients who are malnourished, immunosuppressed, or older, or who have had a long hospital stay or a lengthy surgical procedure (more than 3 hours). Patients needing bowel surgery, particularly after a traumatic injury, are at high risk. Infection may involve the entire incision and may extend downward through deeper tissues. An abscess may form locally, or it may spread throughout entire body cavities, as in peritonitis.

Evidence of wound infection usually does not become apparent before the third to fifth postoperative day. Local manifestations include redness, swelling, and increasing pain and tenderness at the site. Systemic manifestations are fever and leukocytosis.

An accumulation of fluid in a wound may create pressure, impair circulation and wound healing, and predispose the patient to infection. To allow for drainage, the surgeon may place a drain in the incision or make a stab wound adjacent to the incision. These drains may be made of soft rubber and drain into a dressing, or they may be firm catheters attached to a Hemovac or other source of gentle suction.

An adequate nutritional state is essential for wound healing. The patient who is well nourished preoperatively can tolerate the postoperative delay in nutritional intake for several days. However, the patient with preexisting nutritional deficits that occur with chronic diseases (e.g., diabetes, ulcerative colitis, alcoholism) is more prone to problems of wound healing. The patient who cannot meet postoperative nutritional needs may be given enteral or parenteral nutrition to promote healing.

NURSING MANAGEMENT: SURGICAL WOUNDS

Nursing Assessment

Nursing assessment of the wound and dressing requires knowledge of the type of wound, the drains inserted, and expected drainage related to the specific type of surgery. Immediately postoperatively, check the wound every 15 to 30 minutes or as ordered. A small amount of serous drainage is common from any type of wound. If a drain is in place, a moderate to large amount of drainage may be expected. For example, an abdominal incision with an accompanying drain is expected to have a moderate amount of serosanguineous drainage in the first 24 hours. In contrast, an inguinal herniorrhaphy should have only minimal serous drainage during the postoperative period.

In general, drainage is expected to change from sanguineous (red) to serosanguineous (pink) to serous (clear yellow). The drainage should decrease over hours or days, depending on the type of surgery. Wound infection may be accompanied by purulent drainage. *Wound dehiscence* (separation and disruption of previously joined wound edges) may be preceded by a sudden discharge of brown, pink, or clear drainage. (Wound dehiscence is discussed in Chapter 11.)

Nursing Diagnoses

Nursing diagnoses related to surgical wounds include, but are not limited to, the following:

- Impaired skin integrity *related to* surgical incision
- Risk for infection: SSI

Nursing Implementation

When drainage appears on the dressing, record the type, amount, color, and odor of drainage. Expected drainage from tubes is outlined in Table 19-7. Also assess the effect of position changes on drainage. Notify the surgeon of any excessive or abnormal drainage or significant changes in vital signs.

The incision may be covered with a dressing immediately after surgery. Many surgeons prefer to change the first postoperative dressing. If the initial operative dressing is saturated, follow agency policy to determine whether you may change the dressing or simply reinforce it. Skin graft dressings may stay in place for 3 to 5 days to avoid disturbing the graft site and promote graft acceptance. These dressings may be changed by specially trained nurses. (Skin grafts are discussed in Chapter 23.)

When a dressing is changed, note the number and type of drains present and avoid dislodging the drains. Inspect the incision site carefully. The area around the sutures may be slightly reddened and swollen, which is an expected inflammatory response. However, the skin around the incision should be of normal color and temperature. If the wound is healing by primary intention, has little or no drainage, or has no drains in place, a single-layer dressing or no dressing is sufficient. A multilayer dressing is used when drains are in place, when moderate to heavy drainage is occurring, or when healing occurs other than by primary intention. (Wound healing and care are discussed in Chapter 11.)

TABLE 19-7 Output From Tubes, Drains, and Catheters

Substance	Daily Amount	Color	Odor	Consistency
Indwelling Catheter				
Urine	800-1500 mL for first 24 hr Minimum expected output: 0.5 mL/kg/hr	Clear, yellow	Ammonia	Watery
Nasogastric Tube or Gastrostomy Tube				
Gastric contents	<1500 mL/day	Pale, yellow-green Bloody after GI surgery	Sour	Watery
Open Drains (e.g., Penrose)				
Wound drainage	Varies with procedure May decrease over hours or days	Varies with procedure Initially may be sanguineous or serosanguineous, changing to serous	Same as wound dressing Foul odor may indicate infection	Thin, watery
Closed Suction Drains (e.g., Hemovac, Jackson-Pratt)				
Wound drainage	Varies with procedure May decrease over hours or days	Varies with procedure Initially may be sanguineous or serosanguineous, changing to serous	Little to no odor Foul odor may indicate infection	Thin, watery
T-Tube				
Bile	500 mL	Bright yellow to dark green	Acid	Thick
Mediastinal Chest Tube				
Wound drainage post cardiothoracic surgery	Varies with procedure Should decrease over several hours postoperatively	Sanguineous or serosanguineous	N/A	Thin
Pleural Chest Tube				
Fluid that has collected in the pleural space	Varies with procedure Decreases over hours or days >100 mL/hr is considered excessive	Varies with indication for insertion and fluid collected in the pleural spaces	N/A	Varies with indication for insertion

TABLE 19-8 Surgery Discharge Criteria

PACU Discharge Criteria (Phase I)

- Patient awake, easily arousable (or baseline)
- Vital signs at baseline or stable
- No excess bleeding or drainage
- No respiratory depression
- O_2 saturation >90%
- Pain controlled or acceptable
- Nausea and vomiting controlled
- Report given

Ambulatory Surgery Discharge Criteria (Phase II or Extended Observation)

- All PACU discharge criteria (Phase I) met
- No IV opioid drugs for last 30 min
- Voided if appropriate to surgical procedure or orders
- Able to ambulate if not contraindicated
- Responsible adult present to accompany and drive patient home
- Written discharge instructions given and patient and caregiver understanding confirmed

DISCHARGE FROM THE PACU

The choice of discharge site is based on patient acuity, access to follow-up care, and the potential for postoperative complications. The decision to discharge the patient from the PACU is based on written discharge criteria approved by the agency's anesthesiology and medical staff[1] (Table 19-8). Standardized scoring systems (e.g., *Modified Aldrete Scoring System*) are often used to determine the patient's general condition and readiness for discharge from the PACU.

Discharge to Clinical Unit

Before discharging the patient from the PACU to the clinical unit, provide a hand-off report about the patient to the receiving nurse. The report summarizes the operative and postanesthesia period. It should also include information as to where the patient's caregivers are waiting. Nurse-to-nurse communication must be accurate and allow for questions. The use of a standardized communication tool, such as SBAR (*Situation-Background-Assessment-Recommendation*), provides a complete report and enhances a safe transfer of the patient from PACU to the clinical unit (Table 19-9). (Hand-off communication is discussed in Chapter 1, and SBAR is presented in Table 1-6.)

As the nurse who receives the patient on the clinical unit, assist the PACU transport staff to safely move the patient from the stretcher to the bed. Take care to protect IV lines, drains, and traction devices. Obtain vital signs and compare the patient status with the report provided by the PACU nurse. After this, perform a more focused assessment and initiate postoperative orders and nursing care as appropriate (Table 19-10).

AMBULATORY SURGERY

Phase II and Extended Observation

Advances in minimally invasive and noninvasive procedures, anesthesia, and analgesia have resulted in an increase in ambulatory surgical procedures. Ambulatory surgery patients include those patients receiving Phase II and extended observation postoperative care (Table 19-1). PONV and pain are significant problems after ambulatory surgery. These can lead to delirium, prolonged PACU stay, delayed discharge, readmission, delayed resumption of usual activities, and decreased patient satisfaction.

Ambulatory Surgery Discharge

The patient leaving an ambulatory surgery setting must be mobile and alert to provide a degree of self-care when discharged to home (Table 19-8). PONV and pain must be controlled. Overall, the patient must be stable and near the level of preoperative functioning for discharge from the unit. At discharge, provide teaching for the patient and caregiver

TABLE 19-9 Postoperative SBAR Hand-Off Communication

Situation

Patient transferring to Room # _____ Date _____
Surgeon _____ Anesthesia _____
Procedure _____
Surgical site(s) _____

Background

Allergies _____
Medications received in PACU _____
IV site/fluids _____
Dressings and/or drains _____
Operative comments _____

Assessment

PACU vital signs T ____ P ____ RR ____ BP ____ O_2 Sat _____
O_2 source _____ FIO_2 _____
Pain rating at discharge _____
Method of pain management _____
Last dose of pain medication _____
Nausea/vomiting at discharge _____
Intake _____ Output _____
Recovery comments _____

Recommendations

Equipment needed _____
Physician orders to be completed _____
Other notes _____
Transferring RN _____ Phone # for questions _____
Receiving RN _____

Modified from Sandlin D: Improving patient safety by implementing a standardized and consistent approach to hand-off communication, *J Perianesth Nurs* 22:290, 2007.

TABLE 19-10 Nursing Assessment

Care of Patient on Admission to Clinical Unit

1. Record time of patient's return to unit and assess airway, breathing, and circulation.
2. Obtain baseline vital signs, including O_2 saturation.
3. Assess neurologic status, including level of consciousness and movement of extremities.
4. Assess level of pain:
   - Last dose and type of pain control
   - Current pain rating
5. Assess wound, dressing, and drainage tubes:
   - Type and amount of drainage
   - Tubing connected to gravity or suction drainage (per orders)
6. Assess color, temperature, and appearance of skin.
7. Assess urinary status:
   - Time of voiding
   - Presence of catheter, patency, and total output
   - Bladder distention or urge to void
8. Position for airway maintenance, comfort, and safety (bed in low position, side rails up).
9. Check IV infusion:
   - Type of solution
   - Amount of fluid remaining
   - Patency and flow rate
   - Condition of insertion site and size of catheter
10. Position call bell within reach, and orient patient to use of call bell.
11. Assess for any nausea or vomiting.
    - Availability of emesis basin and tissues
12. Determine emotional state and provide support as needed.
13. Check for presence of caregiver.
    - Patient and caregiver oriented to immediate environment
14. Check and carry out postoperative orders.

specific to the type of anesthesia and surgery, and reinforce with written instructions. The patient may not drive and must be accompanied by an adult at the time of discharge. A follow-up evaluation of the patient's status is made by telephone, and any specific questions and concerns are addressed.

Carefully assess the patient's readiness for discharge and home care needs. Determine availability of caregivers (e.g., family, friends) and access to (1) a pharmacy for prescriptions, (2) a phone in the case of an emergency, and (3) follow-up care.

Discuss the patient's expectations regarding activity and assistance needed after discharge. The patient and caregiver must be included in discharge planning and provided with the information and support to make informed decisions about ongoing care.

INFORMATICS IN PRACTICE

Discharge Teaching

- When discharging a patient who requires a complex dressing change and the written instructions are not adequate, consider using a video. This may be available on the hospital's television system or the Internet (e.g., YouTube). You could also take a series of pictures that show how to perform the procedure.
- If using a video from the Internet, check it to ensure that the procedure is properly performed.
- The patient and caregiver can view the video or pictures at home as a reference when performing the procedure.

Planning for Discharge and Follow-up Care

Preparation for the patient's discharge is an ongoing process that begins during the preoperative phase. The informed patient is prepared as events unfold and gradually assumes more responsibility for self-care during the postoperative period. As discharge approaches, be sure that the patient and caregiver(s) have the following information:

- Symptoms to be reported (e.g., fever, increased incisional drainage, unrelieved incisional pain, discomfort in other parts of the body)
- When and how to take prescribed drugs and possible side effects
- Care of incision and any dressings, including bathing recommendations
- Activities allowed and prohibited. When various activities can be resumed safely (e.g., driving, return to work, sexual intercourse, leisure activities)
- Dietary restrictions or modifications
- Where and when to return for follow-up appointment
- Answers to any individual questions or concerns

Common reasons patients seek help after discharge include unrelieved pain, need for advice about drugs, and wound issues (e.g., drainage). Attention to complete discharge instructions may prevent needless distress for the patient and caregiver. Standardized, preprinted discharge instructions that are surgery specific and easy to read ensure that information is complete.

Record the discharge teaching in the chart. For the patient, the postoperative phase of care continues and extends into the recuperative period. Assessment and evaluation of the patient after discharge may be done with a follow-up call or by a visit from a home health nurse.

Increasingly, patients are being discharged from the hospital with many care needs. They may be transferred to transitional care facilities, to long-term care facilities, or directly to their homes. When discharged directly to home, the patient is expected to continue self-care, with assistance from caregivers or home health care personnel (e.g., nurses, physical therapists). The care may include dressing changes, wound care, catheter or drain care, home antibiotics, or continued physical therapy. Working together with the discharge planner or case manager, ensure the patient's safe transition from hospital-based care to community- or home-based care.

Gerontologic Considerations: Postoperative Patient

The older postoperative patient deserves special consideration. The older adult has decreased respiratory function, including decreased ability to cough and decreased thoracic compliance. These alterations lead to an increase in the work of breathing and a decreased ability to eliminate drugs. Carefully monitor reactions to anesthetic drugs. Pneumonia is a common postoperative complication in older adults.

Vascular function in the older adult is altered due to atherosclerosis and decreased elasticity in the blood vessels. Cardiac function is often compromised, and compensatory responses to changes in BP and volume are limited. Circulating blood volume is decreased, and hypertension is common. Cardiovascular status must be closely monitored throughout surgery and the postoperative period.

Drug toxicity is a potential problem in the older adult. Renal perfusion in the older adult normally decreases, along with a reduced ability to remove drugs that are excreted by the kidneys. Decreased liver function also leads to reduced drug metabolism and increased drug activity. Carefully assess renal and liver function in the postoperative phase to prevent drug overdose and toxicity.

Observing for changes in mental status is an important part of postoperative care in older adults. Factors such as age, history of alcohol abuse, poor baseline cognition, hypoxia, metabolic imbalances, hypotension, and polypharmacy can contribute to postoperative delirium. Anesthetics, especially anticholinergic drugs and benzodiazepines, also increase the risk for delirium. Despite knowledge of risk factors, postoperative delirium in older adults is poorly understood.

Pain control in the older patient is challenging because of possible preexisting cognitive deficits, impaired communication, and physiologic changes that affect how drugs are metabolized. Older patients may hesitate to ask for pain medication because they believe that pain should be tolerated because it is an inevitable result of surgery. Some older patients may be nervous about using PCA machines.

Thoroughly assess pain in a surgical patient who does not report any pain. Encourage the use of analgesics, and explain to the patient and caregiver that untreated pain has a negative effect on recovery.

CASE STUDY

Postoperative Patient

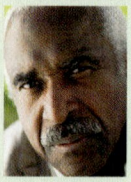

(©BananaStock/ BananaStock/ Thinkstock)

Patient Profile

E.G., a 74-year-old, African American, retired college professor, has just undergone surgery for a fractured hip. He fell off a ladder while painting his house. E.G.'s medical history includes type 2 diabetes and COPD. The surgery, performed while the patient was under general anesthesia, lasted 3 hours.

Subjective Data

- Active walker in his home community
- Smokes 1 pack of cigarettes per day × 58 years
- Always had problems sleeping
- Difficulty hearing, wears hearing aid
- Upset with injury and its impact on life
- Is a widower and has no relatives nearby or friends to assist with care
- Reports pain is 8 on a 0 to 10 scale on arrival to PACU

Objective Data

- Admitted to PACU with abduction pillow between his legs, one peripheral IV catheter, a self-suction drain from the hip dressing, an indwelling urinary catheter
- O_2 saturation 91% on 40% O_2 face mask

Interprofessional Care

Postoperative Orders

- Vital signs per PACU routine
- Capillary blood glucose level on arrival and every 4 hours. Call for blood glucose level <70 mg/dL or >250 mg/dL. Follow agency guidelines for management of hypoglycemia.
- 0.45 normal saline at 100 mL/hr
- Morphine via patient-controlled analgesia 1 mg q10min (20 mg max in 4 hr) for pain
- Advance diet as tolerated
- Incentive spirometry q1hr × 10 while awake
- O_2 therapy to keep O_2 saturation >90%
- Respiratory: Albuterol 2.5 mg via nebulizer every 4 hours PRN for wheezing
- Neurovascular checks q1hr × 4 hr
- Empty and measure self-suction drain every shift
- Strict intake and output

Discussion Questions

1. What are the potential postanesthesia problems that you may expect with E.G.?
2. ***Priority Decision:*** What priority nursing interventions would be appropriate to prevent these problems from occurring?
3. ***Teamwork and Collaboration:*** Which of these interventions could you delegate to unlicensed assistive personnel (UAP)?
4. What factors may predispose E.G. to the following problems: atelectasis, infection, pulmonary embolism, nausea and vomiting?
5. How can you determine when E.G. is sufficiently recovered from general anesthesia to be discharged to the clinical unit?
6. What potential postoperative problems on the clinical unit might you expect?
7. What are risk factors for this patient developing postoperative delirium? What are the signs and symptoms of delirium?
8. Why is drug toxicity a potential problem for E.G.?
9. ***Priority Decision:*** Based on the assessment data presented, identify two priority nursing diagnoses. Are there any collaborative problems?
10. ***Evidence-Based Practice:*** E.G. tells you he doesn't want the "catheter" to be removed because he doesn't want anyone to help him to the bathroom. How would you respond to this request?
11. ***Patient-Centered Care:*** What teaching will you provide so that E.G. can successfully self-manage his care?
12. ***Teamwork and Collaboration:*** What referrals may be indicated based on E.G.'s medical history?
13. ***Safety:*** Identify two areas of risk for injury to E.G. What actions can be taken to ensure patient safety?
14. ***Quality Improvement:*** What outcomes would indicate that interprofessional care with respiratory therapy was effective?

Answers available at *http://evolve.elsevier.com/Lewis/medsurg.*

BRIDGE TO NCLEX EXAMINATION

The number of the question corresponds to the same-numbered outcome at the beginning of the chapter.

1. When a patient is admitted to the PACU, what are the *priority* interventions the nurse performs?
   a. Assess the surgical site, noting presence and character of drainage.
   b. Assess the amount of urine output and the presence of bladder distention.
   c. Assess for airway patency and quality of respirations and obtain vital signs.
   d. Review results of intraoperative laboratory values and medications received.
2. A patient is admitted to the PACU after major abdominal surgery. During the initial assessment the patient tells the nurse he thinks he is going to "throw up." A *priority* nursing intervention is to
   a. increase the rate of the IV fluids.
   b. obtain vital signs, including O_2 saturation.
   c. position patient in lateral recovery position.
   d. administer antiemetic medication as ordered.
3. After admission of the postoperative patient to the clinical unit, which assessment data require the *most* immediate attention?
   a. O_2 saturation of 85%
   b. Respiratory rate of 13/min
   c. Temperature of 100.4°F (38°C)
   d. Blood pressure of 90/60 mm Hg
4. A 70-kg postoperative patient has an average urine output of 25 mL/hr during the first 8 hours. The *priority* nursing intervention(s) given this assessment would be to
   a. perform a straight catheterization to measure the amount of urine in the bladder.
   b. notify the physician and anticipate obtaining blood work to evaluate renal function.
   c. continue to monitor the patient because this is a normal finding during this time period.
   d. evaluate the patient's fluid volume status since surgery and obtain a bladder ultrasound.
5. Discharge criteria for the Phase II patient include (*select all that apply*)
   a. no nausea or vomiting.
   b. ability to drive self home.
   c. no respiratory depression.
   d. written discharge instructions understood.
   e. opioid pain medication given 45 minutes ago.

1. c, 2. c, 3. a, 4. d, 5. c, d, e

For rationales to these answers and even more NCLEX review questions, visit *http://evolve.elsevier.com/Lewis/medsurg.*

EVOLVE WEBSITE

http://evolve.elsevier.com/Lewis/medsurg

Review Questions (Online Only)
Key Points
Answer Keys for Questions
- Rationales for Bridge to NCLEX Examination Questions
- Answer Guidelines for Case Study on p. 346
- Answer Guidelines for Managing Care of Multiple Patients Case Study (Section 3) on p. 348

Student Case Study
- Patient Undergoing Surgery

Nursing Care Plan
- eNursing Care Plan 19-1: Postoperative Patient

Conceptual Care Map Creator
Audio Glossary
Content Updates

REFERENCES

*1. American Society of PeriAnesthesia Nurses: *2015-2017 Perianesthesia nursing standards, practice recommendations and interpretive statements*, Cherry Hill, NJ, 2015, The Society.
2. Joint Commission Center for Transforming Healthcare: Hand-off communications, 2014. Retrieved from *www.centerfortransforming healthcare.org/projects/detail.aspx?Project=1*.
3. Tusman G, Groisman I, Fiolo FE, et al: Noninvasive monitoring of lung recruitment maneuvers in morbidly obese patients: the role of pulse oximetry and volumetric capnography, *Anesth Analg* 118:137, 2014.
*4. Atkins JH, Mandel JE: Performance of Masimo rainbow acoustic monitoring for tracking changing respiratory rates under laryngeal mask airway general anesthesia for surgical procedures in the operating room: a prospective observational study, *Anesth Analg* 119:1307, 2014.
*5. ASPAN US PR Strategic Work Team: The APSAN prevention of unwanted sedation in the adult patient. Evidence-based practice recommendation, *J Perianesth Nurs* 29:344, 2014.
*6. American Society of Anesthesiologists: Practice guidelines for the perioperative management of patients with obstructive sleep apnea: an updated report by the American Society of Anesthesiologists Task Force on perioperative management of patients with obstructive sleep apnea, *Anesthesiology* 120:268, 2014.
*7. Maile MD, Engoren MC, Trempor KK, et al: Worsening preoperative heart failure is associated with mortality and noncardiac complications, but not myocardial infarction after noncardiac surgery: a retrospective cohort study, *Anesth Analg* 119:522, 2014.
8. Xara D, Acacio S, Mendoca J, et al: Inadequate emergence after anesthesia: emergence delirium and hypoactive emergence in the postanesthesia care unit, *J Clin Anesth* 25:439, 2013.
*9. Radinovic KS, Markovic-Denic L, Dubljanin-Raspopovic E, et al: Effect of the overlap syndrome of depressive symptoms and delirium on outcomes in elderly adults with hip fracture: a prospective cohort study, *J Am Geriatr Soc* 62:1640, 2014.
10. Chou R, Gordon DB, de Leon-Casasola OA, et al: Management of postoperative pain: A clinical practice guideline from the American Pain Society, the American Society of Regional Anesthesia and Pain Medicine, and the American Society of Anesthesiologists' Committee on Regional Anesthesia, Executive Committee, and Administrative Council, *J Pain* 17:131, 2016.
*11. Usichenko TI, Rottenbacher I, Kohlmann T, et al: Implementation of the quality management system improves postoperative pain treatment: a prospective pre-/post-interventional questionnaire study, *Br J Anaesth* 110:87, 2013.
*12. Hooper VD, Chard R, Clifford T, et al: ASPAN's evidence-based clinical practice guideline for the promotion of perioperative normothermia, ed 2, *J Perianesth Nurs* 25:346, 2010.
13. Larach MG, Brandom BW, Allen GC, et al: Malignant hyperthermia deaths related to inadequate temperature monitoring, 2007-2012: a report from the North American malignant hyperthermia registry of

the malignant hyperthermia association of the United States, *Anesth Analg* 119:1359, 2014.
14. The Joint Commission: Specifications manual for national hospital inpatient quality measures. Retrieved from *http://www.jointcommission.org/specifications_manual_for_national_hospital_inpatient_quality_measures.aspx.*
*15. Gan TJ, Diemunsch P, Habib AS, et al: Consensus guidelines for the management of postoperative nausea and vomiting, *Anesth Analgesia* 118:85, 2014.
16. Wronski S: Chew on this: reducing postoperative ileus with chewing gum, *Nursing* 44:19, 2014.
17. Magill SS, Hellinger W, Cohen J, et al: Prevalence of healthcare-associated infections in acute care hospitals in Jacksonville, Florida, *Infect Control Hosp Epidemiol* 33:283, 2012.

*Evidence-based information for clinical practice.

CASE STUDY

Managing Care of Multiple Patients

You have been called into work at 10:00 AM to cover patients for a nurse who had a family emergency. You take over care for the following three patients on a surgical unit. You have one UAP available who is assigned to help you and two other RNs.

Patients

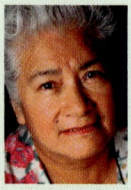

(©Ryan McVay/ Photodisc/ Thinkstock)

F.D., a 72-yr-old woman, was admitted to the hospital with compromised circulation of the right lower leg and a necrotic right foot as a complication of her diabetes. She is scheduled for a below-the-knee amputation of the right leg at 1:00 PM today. She has been NPO since midnight. Her morning capillary blood glucose level was 198 mg/dL. She received 4 units of regular insulin at 8 AM. She has an IV of normal saline infusing at 125 mL/hr.

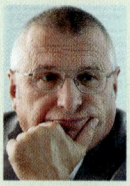

(©shironosov/ iStock/ Thinkstock)

G.S., a 63-yr-old male, was admitted to the hospital for severe pain and intractable vomiting from acute cholecystitis. G.S.'s medical history includes hypertension and type 2 diabetes. He had a laparoscopic cholecystectomy yesterday. His capillary blood glucose 1 hour ago was 135 mg/dL.

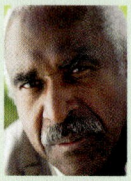

(©BananaStock/ BananaStock/ Thinkstock)

E.G., a 74-yr-old man, underwent surgery for a fractured hip yesterday. He is currently receiving dextrose 5% in 0.45 normal saline at 100 mL/hr, morphine via patient-controlled analgesia at 1 mg q10min (20 mg max in 4 hr) for pain, heparin 5000 units subcutaneously every 12 hours, and O_2 to keep O_2 saturation >93%. He has a self-suction drain in place at the surgical site. He has good respiratory effort when using his incentive spirometer.

Discussion Questions

1. ***Priority Decision:*** After receiving report, which patient should you see first? Provide a rationale for your decision.
2. ***Teamwork and Collaboration:*** Which tasks should you delegate to the UAP? *(select all that apply)*
   a. Explain discharge instructions to G.S.
   b. Obtain noon vital signs on E.G. and F.D.
   c. Obtain capillary blood glucose levels on F.D. and G.S.
   d. Confirm E.G.'s understanding of how to use the PCA pump.
   e. Remind E.G. and G.S. to use their incentive spirometers every hour.
3. ***Priority Decision and Teamwork and Collaboration:*** When you enter F.D.'s room, you find her somewhat withdrawn and lethargic. Her face is cool and slightly clammy. What initial action would be most appropriate?
   a. Give 1 ampule of D_{50} IV stat.
   b. Increase F.D.'s IV rate to 150 mL/hour.
   c. Obtain a stat capillary blood glucose level.
   d. Ask the UAP to give F.D. a glass of orange juice.

Case Study Progression

F.D.'s capillary blood glucose reading was 64 mg/dL. You notify her HCP and administer 1 ampule of D_{50} IV dextrose as ordered. You also change her IV infusion to D_5 ½NS. You check her capillary blood glucose within 15 minutes and then monitor her blood glucose levels on an hourly basis.

4. A preoperative checklist for F.D. is used to ensure completion of *(select all that apply)*
   a. removal of nail polish and jewelry.
   b. signed and witnessed informed consent.
   c. patient understanding of sensory information.
   d. identification of surgical site with surgical skin marker.
   e. notification of family of where to wait for the surgeon postoperatively.
5. F.D. tells you that she is afraid they may amputate the wrong leg. She tells you she has read stories of that happening at other hospitals. Your *best* response to F.D. would be to
   a. ask her if she would like a sedative to calm her fears.
   b. reassure her that it has never happened in this hospital.
   c. explain the "time-out" procedure for preventing such errors.
   d. offer to go to the operating room with her to ensure the correct leg is amputated.
6. ***Priority Decision:*** The charge nurse on the unit reports that E.G.'s aPTT (activated partial thromboplastin time) is 84 seconds. Upon assessing him, the nurse notes that the dressing on his hip is saturated with serosanguinous drainage. The next dose of heparin is due at 2100 this evening; the last dose was at 0900 this morning. The patient's blood pressure is 92/54 with a heart rate of 110 bpm. Respiratory rate is 30 breaths/minute and O_2 saturation is 98% on 2 L of O_2. The nursing *priority* for this patient would be to
   a. notify physical therapy that the patient's session today will have to be postponed until tomorrow.
   b. notify the previous RN that a medication error may have occurred with the patient's heparin dose at 0900.
   c. send an order to the laboratory for stat CBC and type and screen for 4 units of packed red blood cells.
   d. notify the health care provider of the laboratory result and anticipate orders for reversal agent such as protamine.
7. ***Management Decision:*** When providing discharge instructions to G.S., he tells you that the UAP told him that he could do whatever activity he was comfortable doing—to let pain guide his progress. Your *initial* reaction to this statement should be to
   a. ask the UAP to clarify what was said to G.S.
   b. report the UAP's actions to the nurse manager.
   c. teach G.S. about the reason for activity restrictions.
   d. clarify the discharge instructions with the health care provider.

Answers available at *http://evolve.elsevier.com/Lewis/medsurg.*

SECTION 4

Problems Related to Altered Sensory Input

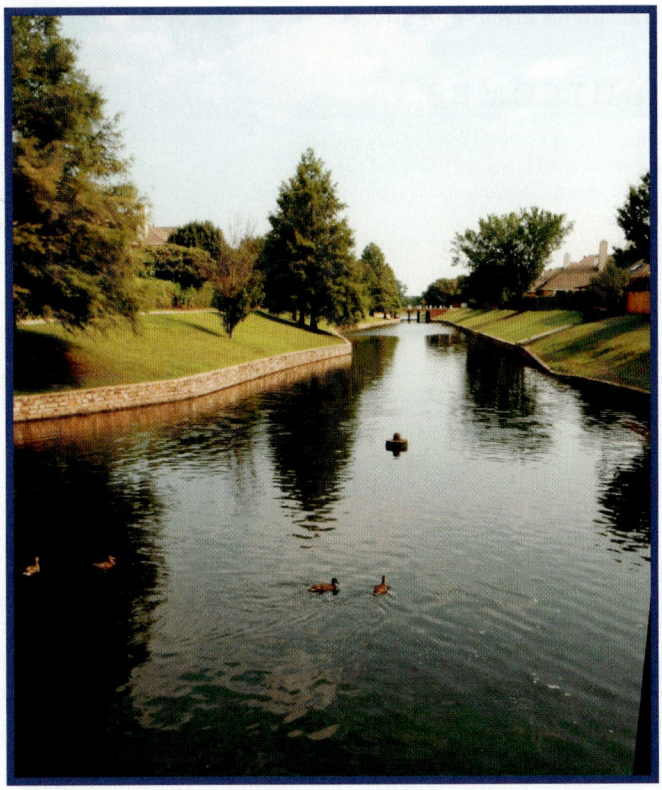

Peter Bonner

Rivers know this.
There is no hurry.
We will get there someday.

Winnie the Pooh

Chapter 20 Assessment of Visual and Auditory Systems, 350

Chapter 21 Visual and Auditory Problems, 367

Chapter 22 Assessment of Integumentary System, 394

Chapter 23 Integumentary Problems, 407

Chapter 24 Burns, 429

20

Assessment of Visual and Auditory Systems

Sharon L. Lewis

The most pathetic person in the world is someone who has sight, but has no vision.

Helen Keller

http://evolve.elsevier.com/Lewis/medsurg/

LEARNING OUTCOMES

1. Describe the structures and functions of the visual and auditory systems.
2. Explain the physiologic processes involved in normal vision and hearing.
3. Obtain significant subjective and objective assessment data related to the visual and auditory systems from a patient.
4. Perform a physical assessment of the visual and auditory systems using the appropriate techniques.
5. Differentiate normal from common abnormal findings of a physical assessment of the visual and auditory systems.
6. Link the age-related changes in the visual and auditory systems to differences in assessment findings.
7. Describe the purpose, significance of results, and nursing responsibilities related to diagnostic studies of the visual and auditory systems.

KEY TERMS

astigmatism, p. 351
conjunctiva, p. 352
hyperopia, p. 351
lens, p. 352
myopia, p. 351
nystagmus, p. 361
presbycusis, p. 361
presbyopia, p. 351
refraction, p. 351
retina, p. 352
sclera, p. 352
tinnitus, p. 361
vertigo, p. 361

VISUAL SYSTEM

STRUCTURES AND FUNCTIONS OF VISUAL SYSTEM

The visual system consists of the external tissues and structures surrounding the eye, external and internal structures of the eye, refractive media, and visual pathway in the brain. The external structures are the eyebrows, eyelids, eyelashes, lacrimal system, conjunctiva, cornea, sclera, and extraocular muscles. The internal structures are the iris, lens, ciliary body, choroid, and retina. The entire visual system is important for visual function. Light reflected from an object in the field of vision passes through the transparent structures of the eye and, in doing so, is *refracted* (bent) so that a clear image can fall on the retina. From the retina, the visual stimuli travel through the visual pathway to the occipital cortex, where they are perceived as an image.

Structures and Functions of Vision

Eyeball. The eyeball, or globe, is composed of three layers (Fig. 20-1). The tough outer layer is composed of the sclera and transparent cornea. The middle layer consists of the uveal tract (iris, choroid, and ciliary body), and the innermost layer is the retina. The *anterior cavity* is divided into the anterior and posterior chambers. The anterior chamber lies between the iris and posterior surface of the cornea, and the posterior chamber lies between the anterior surface of the lens and posterior surface of the iris. The *posterior cavity* lies in the large space behind the lens and in front of the retina.

Refractive Media. For light to reach the retina, it must pass through a number of structures: the cornea, aqueous humor, lens, and vitreous. All these structures must remain clear for light to reach the retina and stimulate the photoreceptor cells. The transparent cornea is the first structure through which light passes. It is responsible for the majority of light refraction necessary for clear vision.

Acknowledgment: We would like to acknowledge the contributions of Sarah Smith, RN, MA, CRNO, COT, Nurse Manager, Department of Ophthalmology, University of Iowa Health Care, Iowa City, Iowa, to this chapter over the past six editions of the book.
Reviewed by Hope Bussenius, DNP, APRN, FNP-BC, Clinical Assistant Professor, Nell Hodgson Woodruff School of Nursing, Emory University, Atlanta, Georgia; Deborah Ehlers, RN, MSN, Director of Nursing and Administrator of The Eye Center, Yakima, Washington; Deena Hollingsworth, MSN, FNP-BC, CORLN, Family Nurse Practitioner, ENT Specialists of Northern Virginia, Arlington, Virginia; Michelle Smeltzer, RN, MSN, DNPc, CEN, Clinical Education Specialist, Emergency Department, Einstein Medical Center Montgomery, East Norriton, Pennsylvania; Allison J. Terry, RN, PhD, Associate Professor of Nursing, Assistant Dean of Clinical Practice, School of Nursing, Auburn University Montgomery, Montgomery, Alabama; and Robert M. Welch, RN, MSN, FNP, CRNO, Family Nurse Practitioner, Nevada Retina Associates, Reno, Nevada.

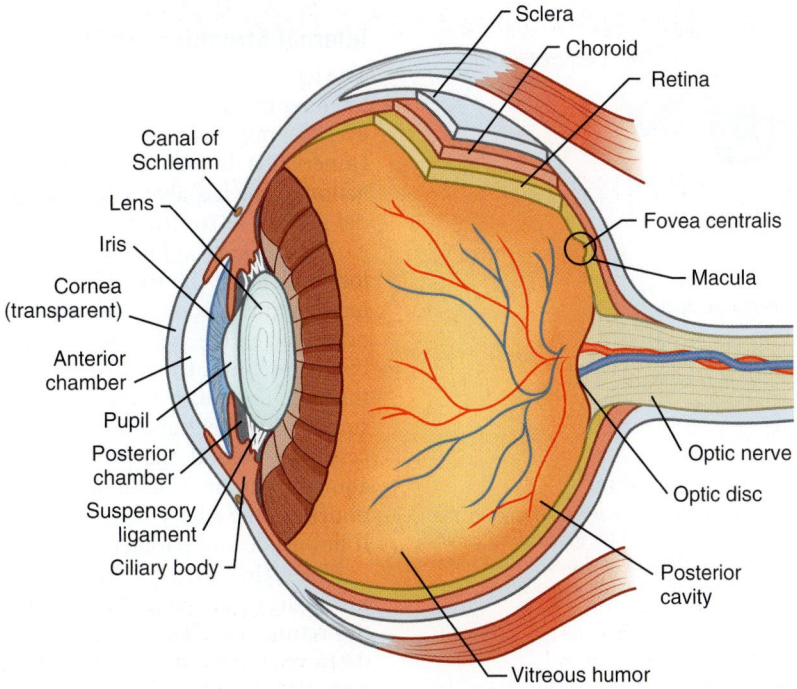

FIG. 20-1 The human eye. (Modified from Patton KT, Thibodeau GA: *Anatomy and physiology,* ed 8, St Louis, 2013, Mosby.)

Aqueous humor, a clear watery fluid, fills the anterior and posterior chambers of the anterior cavity of the eye. Aqueous humor is produced from capillary blood in the ciliary body. It is drained away by the scleral veins *(canal of Schlemm),* which enter the circulation of the body. The aqueous humor bathes and nourishes the lens and endothelium of the cornea. Excess production or decreased outflow can elevate intraocular pressure above the normal 10 to 21 mm Hg, a condition termed *glaucoma.*

The lens is a biconvex structure located behind the iris and supported in place by small fibers collectively called the *suspensory ligament* (also called *zonule*). The ligament is a "scaffolding," a series of microscopic wire-like threads that connect the lens to the ciliary body. The primary function of the lens is to bend light rays, allowing the rays to fall onto the retina. The lens shape is modified by action of the ciliary body as part of *accommodation,* a process that allows a person to focus. An example of accommodation is the ability to focus on near objects, such as when reading. Anything altering the clarity of the lens affects light transmission.

Vitreous humor is a transparent gel-like substance that fills the posterior cavity (Fig. 20-1). Light passing through the vitreous may be blocked by any nontransparent substance within the vitreous. The effect on vision varies, depending on the amount, type, and location of the substance blocking the light.

Refractive Errors. **Refraction** is the eye's ability to bend light rays so that they fall on the retina. In the normal eye, parallel light rays are focused through the lens into a sharp image on the retina. When the light does not focus properly, it is called a *refractive error.*

The individual with **myopia** (nearsightedness) can see near objects clearly, but objects in the distance are blurred. The individual with **hyperopia** (farsightedness) can see distant objects clearly, but close objects are blurred. **Astigmatism** is an uneven curvature of the cornea, which results in visual distortion.

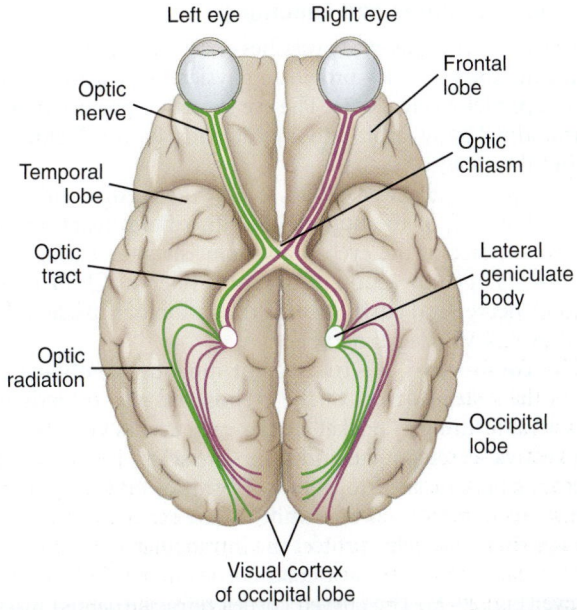

FIG. 20-2 The visual pathway. Fibers from the nasal portion of each retina cross over to the opposite side of the optic chiasma, terminating in the lateral geniculate body of the opposite side. Location of a lesion in the visual pathway determines the resulting visual defect.

Presbyopia is a loss of accommodation, causing an inability to focus on near objects. Manifestations of presbyopia appear around age 40.

Visual Pathways. Once the image travels through the refractive media, it is focused on the retina (Fig. 20-2). From the retina, the impulses travel through the optic nerve to the optic chiasm, where the nasal fibers of each eye cross over to the other side. Fibers from the left field of both eyes form the left optic tract and travel to the left occipital cortex. The fibers from the right field of both eyes form the right optic tract and travel to the

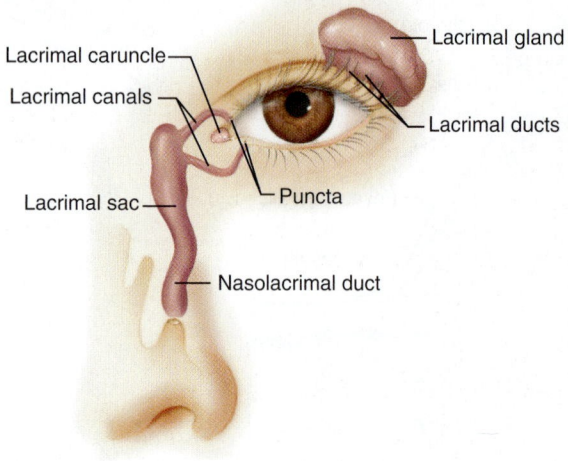

FIG. 20-3 External eye and lacrimal apparatus. Tears produced in the lacrimal gland pass over the surface of the eye and enter the lacrimal canal. From there the tears are carried through the nasolacrimal duct to the nasal cavity. (Modified from Patton KT, Thibodeau GA: *Anatomy and physiology*, ed 8, St Louis, 2013, Mosby.)

right occipital cortex. This arrangement of the nerve fibers in the visual pathways allows determination of the anatomic location of abnormalities.

External Structures and Functions

The eyebrows, eyelids, and eyelashes serve an important role in protecting the eye. They provide a physical barrier to dust and foreign particles (Fig. 20-3). The eye is further protected by the surrounding bony orbit and by fat pads located below and behind the *globe*, or eyeball.

The upper and lower eyelids join at the medial and lateral canthi. Blinking of the upper eyelid distributes tears over the anterior surface of the eyeball and nourishes the surface cells. The eyelids open by action of the cranial nerve (CN) III (oculomotor nerve) and close through the action of muscles innervated by CN VII (facial nerve).

The **conjunctiva** is a transparent mucous membrane that covers the inner surfaces of the eyelids and also extends over the sclera, forming a "pocket" under each eyelid. Glands in the conjunctiva secrete mucus and tears. The **sclera** is composed of collagen fibers meshed together to form an opaque structure commonly referred to as the "white" of the eye. The sclera forms a tough shell that helps protect the intraocular structures.

The transparent and avascular cornea allows light to enter the eye (Fig. 20-1). The curved cornea refracts (bends) incoming light rays to help focus them on the retina. The cornea consists of six layers: epithelium, Bowman's layer, stroma, Descemet's membrane, Dua's layer, and endothelium.[1] The lacrimal system consists of the lacrimal gland and ducts, lacrimal canals and puncta, lacrimal sac, and nasolacrimal duct (Fig. 20-3). In addition to the lacrimal gland, other glands provide secretions to make up the mucous, aqueous, and lipid layers of the tear film. The tear film moistens the eye and provides oxygen to the cornea.

Each eye is moved by three pairs of extraocular muscles: (1) superior and inferior rectus muscles, (2) medial and lateral rectus muscles, and (3) superior and inferior oblique muscles. Neuromuscular coordination produces simultaneous movement of the eyes in the same direction.

Internal Structures and Functions

The iris provides the color of the eye. The iris has a small round opening in its center, the *pupil*, which allows light to enter the eye. The pupil constricts via action of the iris sphincter muscle (innervated by CN III [oculomotor nerve]) and dilates via action of the iris dilator muscle (innervated by CN V [trigeminal nerve]) to control the amount of light that enters the eye.

The **lens** is a biconvex, avascular, transparent structure located behind the iris. The primary function of the lens is to bend light rays so that they focus on the retina. *Accommodation* occurs when the eye focuses on a near object and is facilitated by contraction of the ciliary body, which changes the shape of the lens. The ciliary body consists of the ciliary muscles, which surround the lens and lie parallel to the sclera. The ciliary processes lie behind the peripheral part of the iris and secrete aqueous humor. The *choroid* is a highly vascular structure that nourishes the ciliary body, iris, and outer portion of the retina. It lies inside and parallel to the sclera (Fig. 20-1).

The **retina** is the innermost layer of the eye that extends and forms the optic nerve. Neurons make up the major portion of the retina. Therefore retinal cells are unable to regenerate if destroyed. The retina lines the inside of the eyeball, extending from the area of the optic nerve to the ciliary body (Fig. 20-1). It is responsible for converting images into a form that the brain can understand and process as vision.

The retina is composed of two types of photoreceptor cells: rods and cones. Rods provide vision in dim or darkened environments, and cones are receptive to colors in bright environments. The central region of the retina is called the *macula*, a 6-mm diameter area that is responsible for the central visual field. The *fovea centralis*, located at the center of the macula, is composed only of densely packed cones. This area of the retina provides the sharpest visual acuity, which is necessary for activities in which visual detail is of primary importance, such as reading and driving.[2]

Gerontologic Considerations: Effects of Aging on Visual System

Every structure of the visual system is subject to changes as the individual ages. Whereas many of these changes are relatively benign, others may result in severely compromised visual acuity in the older adult. The psychosocial impact of poor vision or blindness can be highly significant. Age-related changes in the visual system and differences in assessment findings are presented in Table 20-1.

ASSESSMENT OF VISUAL SYSTEM

Assessment of the visual system may be as simple as determining a patient's visual acuity or as complex as collecting complete subjective and objective data pertinent to the visual system. To perform an appropriate visual evaluation, determine which parts of the data collection are important for each patient.

Subjective Data

Important Health Information

Past Health History. Obtain information about the patient's past health history, including the ocular and nonocular history. Question the patient specifically about systemic diseases, such as diabetes, hypertension, cancer, rheumatoid arthritis, syphilis and other sexually transmitted infections (STIs), acquired

TABLE 20-1 Gerontologic Assessment Differences

Visual System

Changes	Differences in Assessment Findings
Eyebrows and Eyelashes	
Loss of pigment in hair	Graying of eyebrows, eyelashes
Eyelids	
Loss of orbital fat, decreased muscle tone	Entropion, ectropion, mild ptosis
Tissue atrophy, prolapse of fat into eyelid tissue	Blepharodermachalasis (excessive upper lid skin)
Conjunctiva	
Tissue damage related to chronic exposure to ultraviolet light or to other chronic environmental exposure	Pinguecula (small yellowish spot usually on medial aspect of conjunctiva)
Sclera	
Lipid deposition	Scleral color yellowish as opposed to bluish
Cornea	
Cholesterol deposits in peripheral cornea	Arcus senilis (milky white-gray ring encircling periphery of cornea) (Fig. 20-4)
Tissue damage related to chronic exposure	Pterygium (thickened, triangular bit of pale tissue that extends from inner canthus of eye to nasal border of cornea)
Decrease in water content, atrophy of nerve fibers	Decreased corneal sensitivity and corneal reflex
Epithelial changes	Loss of corneal luster
Accumulation of lipid deposits	Blurring of vision
Lacrimal Apparatus	
Decreased tear secretion	Dryness
Malposition of eyelid resulting in tears overflowing lid margins instead of draining through puncta	Tearing, irritated eyes
Iris	
Increased rigidity of iris	Decreased pupil size
Dilator muscle atrophy or weakness	Slower recovery of pupil size after light stimulation
Loss of pigment	Change of iris color
Ciliary muscle becoming smaller, stiffer	Decrease in near vision and accommodation
Lens	
Biochemical changes in lens proteins, oxidative damage, chronic exposure to ultraviolet light	Cataracts
Increased rigidity of lens	Presbyopia
Opacities in lens (may also be related to opacities in cornea and vitreous)	Complaints of glare, night vision impaired
Accumulation of yellow substances	Yellow color of lens
Retina	
Retinal vascular changes related to atherosclerosis and hypertension	Narrowed, pale, straighter arterioles. Acute branching
Decrease in number of cones	Changes in color perception, especially blue and violet
Loss of photoreceptor cells, retinal pigment, epithelial cells, and melanin	Decreased visual acuity
Age-related macular degeneration as a result of vascular changes	Loss of central vision, presence of drusen, atrophy of macular retinal pigment
Vitreous	
Liquefaction and detachment of vitreous	Increased complaints of "floaters"

CASE STUDY

Patient Introduction

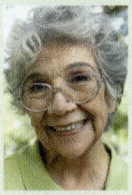

(©Jack Hollingsworth/ Photodisc/ Thinkstock)

F.M. is an 81-year-old Hispanic woman who comes to the emergency department with complaints of visual disturbances. F.M. states that her vision "looks like everything is covered with a spider web." She also reports seeing periodic light flashes and small white spots "floating" in the air.

Discussion Questions

1. What are the possible causes of F.M.'s visual disturbances?
2. Is her condition stable or an emergency?

You will learn more about F.M. and her condition as you read through this assessment chapter.

(See p. 356 for more information on F.M.)

Answers available at *http://evolve.elsevier.com/Lewis/medsurg.*

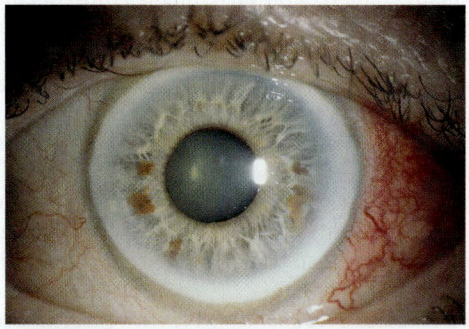

FIG. 20-4 Arcus senilis, or age-related degeneration of the cornea. (From Kanski JJ: *Clinical ophthalmology: a synopsis,* ed 2, New York, 2009, Butterworth-Heinemann.)

immunodeficiency syndrome (AIDS), muscular dystrophy, myasthenia gravis, multiple sclerosis, inflammatory bowel disease, and hypothyroidism or hyperthyroidism. Many of these diseases have ocular manifestations. It is particularly important to determine whether the patient has any history of cardiac or pulmonary disease because β-adrenergic blockers (β blockers) are often used to treat glaucoma. These medications can slow heart rate, decrease BP, and exacerbate asthma or chronic obstructive pulmonary disease (COPD).

Obtain a history of tests for visual acuity, including the date of the last examination and change in glasses or contact lenses. Ask the patient about a history of strabismus, amblyopia, cataracts, retinal detachment, refractive surgery, or glaucoma. Note any trauma to the eye, its treatment, and sequelae.

The patient's nonocular history can be significant in assessing or treating the ophthalmic condition. Ask the patient about previous surgeries, treatments, or trauma related to the head.

TABLE 20-2 Health History

Visual System

Health Perception–Health Management
- Describe the change in your vision. Describe how this affects your daily life.
- Do you wear protective eyewear (sunglasses, safety goggles, hats)?*
- Do you wear contact lenses? If so, how do you take care of them?
- If you use eyedrops, how do you instill them?
- Do you have any allergies that cause eye symptoms?*
- Do you have a family history of cataracts, glaucoma, or macular degeneration?*

Nutritional-Metabolic
- Do you take any nutritional supplements?*
- Does your visual problem affect your ability to obtain and prepare food?*

Elimination
- Do you have to strain to void or defecate?*

Activity-Exercise
- Are your activities limited in any way by your eye problem?*
- Do you participate in any leisure activities that have the potential for eye injury?*

Sleep-Rest
- Is your vision affected by the amount of sleep you get?*
- Does your eye problem affect your sleeping patterns?*

Cognitive-Perceptual
- Does your eye problem affect your ability to read?*
- Do you have any eye pain?* Do you have any eye itching, burning, or foreign body sensation?*

Self-Perception–Self-Concept
- How does your eye problem make you feel about yourself?

Role-Relationship
- Do you have any problems at work or home because of your eyes?*
- Have you made any changes in your social activities because of your eyes?*

Sexuality-Reproductive
- Has your eye problem caused a change in your sex life?*
- For women: Are you pregnant? Do you use birth control pills?*
- For men: Do you use any erectile dysfunction drugs? Any vision problems with their use?*

Coping–Stress Tolerance
- Do you feel able to cope with your eye problem?*
- How do you feel that your eye problem has affected your life, and how do you cope with these changes?*

Value-Belief
- Do you have any conflicts about the treatment of your eye problem?*

*If yes, describe.

Medications. If a patient takes medication, obtain a complete list, including dosage and frequency of over-the-counter (OTC) medicines, eye drops, and herbal therapies or dietary supplements. Many patients do not think of these as "real" drugs and may not mention their use unless specifically questioned. However, many of these drugs have ocular effects. For example, many cold preparations contain a form of epinephrine (e.g., pseudoephedrine) that can dilate the pupil. Note the use of any antihistamine or decongestant, since these drugs can cause ocular dryness. In addition, specifically ask whether the patient uses any prescription drugs such as corticosteroids, thyroid medications, or agents such as oral hypoglycemics and insulin to lower blood glucose levels. Long-term use of corticosteroid preparations can contribute to the development of glaucoma or cataracts.[3] Also note whether the patient is taking any β blockers, since these can be potentiated by the β blockers used to treat glaucoma.

Surgery or Other Treatments. Note any surgical procedures related to the eye or brain. Brain surgery and the subsequent swelling can cause pressure on the optic nerve or tract, resulting in visual alterations. Also document any laser procedures on the eye. The effect of any eye surgery or laser treatment on visual acuity is important information to obtain.

Functional Health Patterns. Ocular problems do not always affect the patient's visual acuity. For example, patients with blepharitis or diabetic retinopathy may not have noticeable visual deficits. The focus of the functional health pattern assessment depends on the presence or absence of vision loss and whether the loss is permanent or temporary. Table 20-2 lists suggested health history questions related to the functional health patterns.

Health Perception–Health Management Pattern. Patient characteristics such as gender, ethnicity, and age are important in assessing ophthalmic conditions. Men are more likely than women to have color blindness. The leading cause of blindness among African Americans is glaucoma.[4] Older individuals are also at greater risk for glaucoma.

The ophthalmic patient in a clinic or office setting is often seeking routine eye care or a change in the prescription of eyewear. However, the patient may have some underlying concerns that he or she does not mention or even recognize. Ask the patient, "Why are you here today?"

The patient's visual health can affect activities at home or at work. It is important to know how the patient perceives the current health problem. As outlined in Table 20-2, guide the patient in describing the current problem. Assess the patient's ability to accomplish necessary self-care, especially any eye care related to the patient's ophthalmic problem.

The patient may not recognize the importance of eye-safety practices, such as wearing protective eyewear during potentially hazardous activities or avoiding noxious fumes and other eye irritants. Obtain information about the use of sunglasses in bright light. Prolonged exposure to ultraviolet (UV) light can affect the retina. Ask about night driving habits and any problems encountered. Today, millions of people wear contact lenses, but many do not care for them properly. The type of contact lenses used and the patient's wearing and care habits may provide information for teaching.

Obtain information about allergies. Allergies often cause eye symptoms such as itching, burning, watering, drainage, and blurred vision.

Hereditary systemic diseases (e.g., sickle cell anemia) can significantly affect ocular health. In addition, many refractive errors and other eye problems are hereditary. Specifically, ask whether the patient has a family history of diseases such as arteriosclerosis, diabetes, thyroid disease, hypertension, arthritis, or cancer. In addition, determine whether the patient has a family history of ocular problems such as cataracts, tumors, glaucoma, refractive errors (especially myopia and hyperopia), or retinal degenerative conditions (e.g., macular degeneration, retinal detachment).

GENETIC RISK ALERT

Glaucoma

- Certain types of glaucoma have a strong genetic link. Many different glaucoma genes have been discovered.
- People with a family history of glaucoma have a much greater risk of developing it.

Age-Related Macular Degeneration (AMD)

- Some cases of AMD have a genetic link. Multiple genes may be associated with AMD.

Nutritional-Metabolic Pattern. High doses of vitamins containing antioxidants (vitamins C and E and beta-carotene) may be important to ocular health. Some patients with AMD may benefit from supplements of these vitamins.

Elimination Pattern. Straining to defecate (Valsalva maneuver) can raise the intraocular pressure. After patients have eye surgery, many surgeons do not want them to strain. Assess the patient's usual pattern of elimination and determine whether there is the potential for constipation in the patient who has had ophthalmic surgical procedures.

Activity-Exercise Pattern. The patient's usual level of activity or exercise may be affected by reduced vision, symptoms accompanying an ocular problem, or activity restrictions after a surgical procedure. Inquire about leisure activities during which the patient may incur an ocular injury. For example, gardening, woodworking, and other craft activities can result in corneal or conjunctival foreign bodies or even penetrating injuries of the globe. Sports activities such as racquetball, baseball, and tennis carry risks for blunt trauma to the eyes. Protection goggles should be worn for these sports.

Sleep-Rest Pattern. In the otherwise healthy person, lack of sleep may cause ocular irritation, especially if the patient wears contact lenses. Normal sleep patterns may be disrupted in the patient with painful eye problems such as corneal abrasions.

Cognitive-Perceptual Pattern. The entire assessment of the ophthalmic patient focuses on the sense of sight but does not overlook other cognitive or perceptual problems. For example, the functional ability of a patient with a visual deficit will be further compromised if the patient also has hearing problems. The patient who cannot see to read has increased difficulty following postoperative instructions if he or she also has trouble hearing or remembering verbal instructions. Eye pain is always an important symptom to assess. If eye pain is present, question the patient about treatment and response.

Self-Perception–Self-Concept Pattern. The loss of independence that can follow a partial or complete loss of vision, even if the condition is temporary, can have devastating effects on the patient's self-concept. Carefully evaluate the potential effect of vision loss on the patient's self-image. For instance, disabling glare from a cataract may prevent nighttime driving. In today's highly mobile society, the loss of the ability to drive can represent a significant loss of independence and self-esteem.

Role-Relationship Pattern. Ocular problems can negatively affect the patient's ability to maintain the necessary or desired roles and responsibilities in the home, work, and social environments. For example, AMD may decrease visual acuity so that the patient can no longer adequately function at work. Many occupations place workers in conditions in which eye injury may occur. For example, factory workers may be at risk from flying metal debris. Eye-safety practices, such as the use of goggles or safety glasses, are now a legal requirement in the workplace. The patient with diabetes may not be able to see well enough to self-administer insulin. This patient may resent dependence on a family member who takes over this function. Sensitively inquire if the ocular problem has affected the patient's preferred roles and responsibilities.

Sexuality-Reproductive Pattern. The patient with severe vision loss may develop such a poor self-image that the ability to be sexually intimate is lost. Assure the patient that low vision or blindness does not affect a person's ability to be sexually expressive. Often touch is more important than vision.

Coping–Stress Tolerance Pattern. The patient with temporary or permanent visual problems may experience emotional stress. Assess the patient's coping strategies and availability of support systems.

Value-Belief Pattern. Be sensitive to each patient's individual values and spiritual beliefs, since these may guide the patient's decisions regarding ophthalmic care. It can be difficult to understand why a patient refuses treatment that has potential benefit or wants treatment that may have limited potential benefit.

Objective Data

Physical Examination. Physical examination of the visual system includes inspecting the ocular structures and determining the status of their respective functions. Physiologic functional assessment includes (1) determining the patient's visual acuity, ability to judge closeness and distance, and extraocular muscle (EOM) function; (2) evaluating visual fields; (3) observing pupil function; and (4) measuring the intraocular pressure. Assessment of ocular structures should include examining the ocular adnexa, external eye, and internal structures. Some structures, such as the retina, blood vessels, and optic disc, must be assessed with an ophthalmoscope.

Assessment of the visual system may include all of the components discussed in the following sections, or it may be as brief as measuring the patient's visual acuity. Assess what is appropriate and necessary for the specific patient. Many of the following assessments are within your scope of practice, but some require special training.

Normal physical assessment of the visual system is outlined in Table 20-3. Age-related visual changes and differences in assessment findings are listed in Table 20-1. Assessment techniques related to vision are summarized in Table 20-4, and assessment abnormalities are listed in Table 20-5 on p. 357.

A *focused assessment* is used to evaluate the status of previously identified visual problems and to monitor for signs of new problems (see Table 3-7). A focused assessment of the visual system is presented in the box on p. 356.

Initial Observation. Your initial observation of the patient can provide information that will help focus the assessment. When first encountering the patient, you may observe that the patient is dressed in clothing with unusual color combinations. This may indicate a color-vision deficit. Also note an unusual head position. The patient with diplopia may hold the head in a skewed position in an attempt to see a single image. The patient with a corneal abrasion or photophobia will cover the eyes with the hands to try to block out room light. Make a crude estimate of depth perception by extending a hand for the patient to shake.

CASE STUDY

Subjective Data

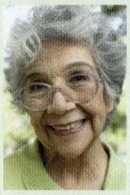

(©Jack Hollingsworth/ Photodisc/ Thinkstock)

A focused subjective assessment of F.M. revealed the following information:

- ***PMH:*** Extraocular extraction of cataract on R eye with implantation of intraocular lens 2 mo ago. Type 2 diabetes mellitus, hypothyroidism, and hypertension.
- ***Medications:*** Glyburide (DiaBeta) 5 mg/day, levothyroxine (Synthroid) 100 mcg/day, metoprolol (Lopressor) 50 mg PO daily.
- ***Health Perception–Health Management:*** States she was compliant with postoperative antibiotic and corticosteroid eyedrops and with office follow-up with eye surgeon. Recovery from surgery was uneventful, and eyedrops were discontinued 2 wk ago. Does not have allergies. Had excellent eyesight until today.
- ***Elimination:*** Has had difficulty moving bowels with increased straining. Trying prune juice to help.
- ***Activity-Exercise:*** Walks in the mall at least ½ mile three times a week. No resistance or isotonic exercises.
- ***Cognitive-Perceptual:*** Denies eye pain, itching, or tearing. Having difficulty reading.
- ***Coping–Stress Tolerance:*** Afraid she is having a stroke.

Discussion Questions

1. What type of assessment would be most appropriate for F.M.: comprehensive, focused, or emergency?
2. What assessment questions will you ask her?
3. How will you individualize the assessment based on her age, ethnic/cultural background, and condition?
4. Which subjective assessment findings are of most concern to you?
5. Based on the subjective assessment findings, what type of physical assessment should be performed?

You will learn more about the physical assessment of the visual system in the next section.

(See p. 359 for more information on F.M.)

Answers available at *http://evolve.elsevier.com/Lewis/medsurg.*

FOCUSED ASSESSMENT

Visual System

Use this checklist to make sure the key assessment steps have been done.

Subjective

Ask the patient about any of the following and note responses.

Changes in vision (e.g., acuity, blurred)	Y	N
Eye redness, itching, discomfort	Y	N
Drainage from eyes	Y	N

Objective: Physical Examination

Inspect

Eyes for any discoloration or drainage	✓
Conjunctiva and sclera for color and vascularity	✓
Lens for clarity	✓
Eyelid for ptosis	✓

Assess

Vision based on patient looking at nurse or Snellen chart	✓
Extraocular movements	✓
Peripheral vision	✓
PERRLA	✓

PERRLA, Pupils equal, round, reactive to light and accommodation.

TABLE 20-3 Normal Physical Assessment of Visual System

- Visual acuity 20/20 OU. No diplopia.
- External eye structures symmetric and without lesions or deformities.
- Lacrimal apparatus nontender and without drainage.
- Conjunctiva clear. Sclera white.
- PERRLA.
- Lens clear.
- EOMI.
- Optic disc margins sharp.
- Retinal vessels without AV nicking, with no hemorrhages or spots.

EOMI, Extraocular movements intact; *OU,* both eyes; *PERRLA,* pupils equal, round, reactive to light and accommodation.

TABLE 20-4 Nursing Assessment

Assessment Techniques: Visual System

Description	Purpose
Visual Acuity Testing	
Patient reads from Snellen chart at 20 ft (distance vision test) or Jaeger chart at 14 in (near vision test). Examiner notes smallest print patient can read on each chart.	Determines distance and near visual acuity
Confrontation Visual Field Test	
Patient faces examiner, covers one eye, fixates on examiner's face, and counts number of fingers that examiner brings into patient's field of vision.	Determines if patient has a full field of vision, without obvious scotomas
Pupil Function Testing	
Examiner shines light into patient's pupil and observes pupillary response. Each pupil is examined independently. Examiner also checks for consensual and accommodative response.	Determines if patient has normal pupillary response
Intraocular Pressure Testing: Tonometry	
Covered end of probe is gently touched several times to anesthetized corneal surface. Examiner records several readings to obtain a mean intraocular pressure.	Measures intraocular pressure (normal pressure is 10-21 mm Hg)
Ophthalmoscopy	
Examiner holds ophthalmoscope close to patient's eye, shining light into back of eye and looking through aperture on ophthalmoscope. Examiner adjusts dial to select one of lenses in ophthalmoscope that produces desired amount of magnification to inspect retina.	Provides magnified view of retina and optic nerve head (Fig. 20-5)
Color Vision Testing	
In the Ishihara test, a patient identifies numbers or paths formed by pattern of dots in series of color plates.	Determines ability to distinguish colors
Keratometry	
Examiner aligns projection and notes readings of corneal curvature.	Measures corneal curvature. Often done before fitting contact lenses, before refractive surgery, or after corneal transplantation

TABLE 20-5 Assessment Abnormalities

Visual System

Finding	Description	Possible Etiology and Significance
Subjective Data		
Pain	Foreign body sensation	Superficial corneal erosion or abrasion. Can result from contact lens wear or trauma. Conjunctival or corneal foreign body
	Severe, deep, throbbing	Anterior uveitis, acute glaucoma, infection. Acute glaucoma also associated with nausea, vomiting
Photophobia	Persistent abnormal intolerance to light	Inflammation or infection of cornea or anterior uveal tract (iris and ciliary body)
Blurred vision	Gradual or sudden inability to see clearly	Refractive errors, corneal opacities, cataracts, migraine aura, retinal changes (detachment, macular degeneration)
Spots, floaters	Patient describes seeing spots, "spider webs," "curtain," or floaters within the field of vision	Most common cause is vitreous liquefaction (benign phenomenon). Other possible causes include hemorrhage into the vitreous humor, retinal holes or tears.
Dryness	Discomfort, sandy, gritty, irritation, or burning	Decreased tear formation or changes in tear composition because of aging or various systemic diseases
Diplopia	Double vision	Abnormalities of extraocular muscle action related to muscle or cranial nerve pathologic condition
Objective Data		
Eyelids		
Allergic reactions	Redness, excessive tearing, and itching of lid margins	Many possible allergens. Associated eye trauma can occur from rubbing itchy eyelids.
Hordeolum (sty)	Small, superficial white nodule along lid margin	Infection of sebaceous gland of eyelid. Causative organism is usually bacterial (most commonly *Staphylococcus aureus*).
Blepharitis	Redness, swelling, and crusting along lid margins	Bacterial invasion of lid margins. Often chronic
Ptosis	Drooping of upper lid margin, unilateral or bilateral	Mechanical causes as a result of eyelid tumors or excess skin. Myasthenia gravis
Entropion	Inward turning of upper or lower lid margin, unilateral or bilateral	Congenital causes resulting in development abnormalities
Ectropion	Outward turning of lower lid margin	Mechanical causes as a result of eyelid tumors, herniated orbital fat, or extravasation of fluid
Conjunctiva		
Conjunctivitis	Redness, swelling of conjunctiva. May be itchy	Bacterial or viral infection. May be allergic response or inflammatory response to chemical exposure
Subconjunctival hemorrhage	Appearance of blood spot on sclera. May be small or can affect entire sclera	Conjunctival blood vessels rupture, leaking blood into the subconjunctival space.
Cornea		
Corneal abrasion	Localized painful disruption of the epithelial layer of cornea. Can be visualized with fluorescein dye	Trauma. Overwear or improper fit of contact lenses
Globe		
Exophthalmos	Protrusion of globe beyond its normal position within bony orbit. Sclera often visible above iris when eyelids are open	Intraocular or periorbital tumors. Hyperthyroidism
Pupil		
Anisocoria	Pupils unequal (constricted)	Central nervous system disorders. Slight difference in pupil size is normal in some people.
Abnormal response to light or accommodation	Pupils respond asymmetrically or abnormally to light stimulus or accommodation.	Central nervous system disorders, general anesthesia
Extraocular Muscles		
Strabismus	Deviation of eye position in one or more directions	Overaction or underaction of one or more extraocular muscles
Lens		
Cataract	Opacification of lens. Pupil can appear cloudy or white when opacity is visible behind pupil opening.	Aging, trauma, diabetes, long-term systemic corticosteroid therapy
Visual Field Defect		
Peripheral	Partial or complete loss of peripheral vision	Glaucoma. Interruption of visual pathway (e.g., tumor). Migraine headache
Central	Loss of central vision	Macular disease

During the initial observation, observe the patient's overall facial and ophthalmic appearance. The eyes should be symmetric and normally placed on the face. The globes should not have a bulging or sunken appearance.

Assessing Functional Status

Visual acuity. Always record the patient's visual acuity for medical and legal reasons. When doing a physical examination of the eyes, assess the right eye first and then the left eye. Document the patient's visual acuity before the patient receives any ophthalmic care.

To assess visual acuity, position the person on a mark exactly 20 ft (6 m) from the Snellen eye chart. If the person wears glasses or contacts, leave them on. Cover one eye at a time during the test. Ask the person to read down the lines of the chart to the smallest line of letters possible. Record the result using the numeric fraction at the end of the last successful line read. Indicate whether any letters were missed and if corrective lenses were worn (e.g., "Right eye, 20/30-2, with contacts"). Next ask the patient to cover the other eye, and repeat the process. Normal visual acuity is 20/20. The first number indicates the distance the person is standing or sitting from the chart; the second number gives the distance at which a normal eye can read the particular line. *Legal blindness* is defined as the best-corrected vision in the better eye of 20/200 or less.

If the patient reports near vision difficulty or is 40 years of age or older, you would also use a hand-held vision screener with varying print sizes (e.g., a Jaeger chart). Hold the card at 14 in (35 cm) from the eye in good light to assess near vision. Examine each eye separately with glasses on. A normal result is "14/14" in each eye, read without hesitancy and without the patient moving the card.

Hand motion or light perception may be used for distance vision assessment if a specific vision chart for distance assessment is not available. If you must assess near visual acuity without access to a Jaeger eye chart, an accurate assessment is still possible using newsprint or the label on a container. Record the acuity as "reads newspaper headline at X inches."

Extraocular muscle functions. Observe the corneal light reflex to evaluate for weakness or imbalance of the extraocular muscles (EOM). In a darkened room, ask the patient to look straight ahead while shining a penlight directly on the cornea. The light reflection should be located in the center of both corneas as the patient faces the light source.

To assess eye movement, hold a finger or an object within 10 to 12 inches of the patient's nose. Ask the patient to follow with eyes only the movement of the object or finger in the six cardinal positions of gaze. This test can indicate weakness or paralysis in the EOM and cranial nerves (oculomotor nerve [CN III], trochlear nerve [CN IV], and abducens nerve [CN VI]).[5]

Pupil function and intraocular pressure. Pupil function is determined by inspecting the pupils and their reactions to light. The normal finding is commonly abbreviated as PERRL (pupils are equal [in size], round, and reactive to light). To test for accommodation, ask the person to focus on a distant object. This process dilates the eyes. Then have the person shift the focus to a near object (e.g., your finger held about 3 inches from the person's nose). A normal response is constriction of the eyes and convergence (inward movement of both eyes toward each other). When accommodation is assessed in addition to the pupillary light reflex, a normal response is *PERRLA* (pupils are equal, round, and reactive to light and accommodation).

In a small percentage of the population, the pupils are unequal in size (*anisocoria*). The pupils should react to light directly (pupil constricts when a light shines into the eye) and consensually (pupil constricts when a light shines into the opposite eye).

Intraocular pressure (Table 20-4) can be measured by a variety of methods, including tonometry. Normal intraocular pressure ranges from 10 to 21 mm Hg.

Assessing Structures. The visual system structures are assessed primarily by inspection. The visual system is unique because not only the external structures but also many of the internal structures can be directly inspected. The iris, lens, vitreous, retina, and optic nerve can be visualized directly through the clear cornea and pupil opening.

This direct inspection requires special observation equipment, such as the slit lamp microscope and ophthalmoscope. This equipment permits examination of the conjunctiva, sclera, cornea, anterior chamber, iris, lens, vitreous, and retina under magnification. The *ophthalmoscope* is a hand-held instrument with a light source and magnifying lenses that is held close to the patient's eye to visualize the posterior part of the eye. Little pain or discomfort is associated with these examinations.

Eyebrows, eyelashes, and eyelids. All structures should be present and symmetric, without deformities, redness, or swelling. Eyelashes extend outward from the lid margins. In normal closing, the upper and lower eyelid margins just touch. The lacrimal puncta should be open and positioned properly against the globe.

Conjunctiva and sclera. The conjunctiva and sclera can easily be examined at the same time. Evaluate the color, smoothness, and presence of lesions or foreign bodies. The conjunctiva covering the sclera is normally clear, with fine blood vessels visible. These blood vessels are more common in the periphery.

The sclera is normally white, but it may take on a yellowish hue in the older adult because of lipid deposition. A pale blue cast caused by scleral thinning can also be normal in older adults. A slight yellow cast may also be found in some dark-skinned people, such as African Americans and Native Americans.

Cornea. The cornea should be clear, transparent, and shiny. The iris should appear flat and not bulge toward the cornea. The area between the cornea and iris should be clear, with no blood or purulent material visible in the anterior chamber.

Iris. Both irides should be of similar color and shape. However, a color difference between the irides occurs normally in a small portion of the population.

Retina and optic nerve. An ophthalmoscope is used to magnify the retina and optic nerves and bring them into crisp focus (Fig. 20-5). Examine the optic nerve or disc for size, color, and abnormalities. The optic disc is creamy yellow with distinct margins. A central depression in the disc, called the *physiologic cup*, may be seen. This area is the exit site for the optic nerve. The cup should be less than one half the diameter of the disc. Normally, no hemorrhages or exudates are present in the fundus (retinal background). Careful inspection of the fundus can reveal retinal holes, tears, detachments, or lesions. Small hemorrhages can be associated with diabetes or hypertension and can appear in various shapes, such as dots or flames. Finally, examine the macula for shape and appearance. This area of high reflectivity is devoid of any blood vessels.

Important information about the vascular system and central nervous system (CNS) can be obtained through direct

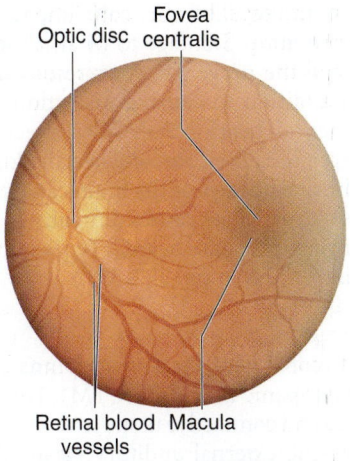

FIG. 20-5 Magnified view of retina through the ophthalmoscope. (From Newell FW: *Ophthalmology: principles and concepts*, ed 7, St Louis, 1992, Mosby.)

visualization with an ophthalmoscope. Skilled use of this instrument requires practice.

Special Assessment Techniques

Color Vision. Testing the patient's ability to distinguish colors can be an important part of the overall assessment because some occupations may require accurate color discrimination. The Ishihara color test determines the patient's ability to distinguish a pattern of color in a series of color plates.[6]

Stereopsis. Stereoscopic vision allows a patient to see objects in three dimensions. Any event that causes a patient to have monocular vision (e.g., enucleation, patching) results in the loss of stereoscopic vision. Without stereopsis, the individual's ability to judge distances or the height of a step is impaired. This disability can have serious consequences if the patient trips over a step when walking or follows too closely behind another vehicle when driving.

CASE STUDY

Objective Data: Physical Examination

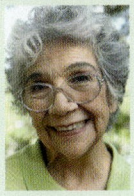

(©Jack Hollingsworth/ Photodisc/ Thinkstock)

Physical examination findings of F.M. were as follows:

- PERRL. No abnormalities noted on visual examination of external eye structures. EOM intact and symmetric.

Discussion Questions

1. What should be included in the physical assessment? For what would you be looking?
2. What diagnostic studies might you expect to be ordered?

As you continue to read this chapter, consider diagnostic studies that you would anticipate being performed for F.M.

Answers available at *http://evolve.elsevier.com/Lewis/medsurg.*

DIAGNOSTIC STUDIES OF VISUAL SYSTEM

Diagnostic studies of the visual system provide important information in monitoring the patient's condition and planning appropriate interventions. These studies are considered objective data. Table 20-6 presents common diagnostic studies of the visual system.

TABLE 20-6 Diagnostic Studies

Visual System

Study	Description, Purpose, and Nursing Responsibility*
Refractometry	Measure of refractive error. Patient sits looking through apertures at Snellen acuity chart and lenses are changed. Patient chooses lenses that make acuity sharpest. Dilation of eyes may help visualize retina and optic nerves. Procedure is painless. Pupil dilation, which may last 3-4 hr, makes it difficult to focus on near objects.
Ultrasonography	*A-scan* determines the right power of a lens implant before cataract surgery. *B-scan* used to diagnose ocular pathologic conditions such as intraocular foreign bodies or tumors, vitreous opacities, retinal detachments
Fluorescein Angiography	Fluorescein injected IV into peripheral vein followed by serial photographs (over 10-min period) of retina through dilated pupils Provides diagnostic information about flow of blood through retinal vessels If extravasation occurs, fluorescein is toxic to tissue. Tell patient that dye can sometimes cause transient nausea or vomiting. Yellow-orange discoloration of urine and skin may occur.
Amsler Grid Test	Self-administered test using a hand-held card printed with a grid of lines (similar to graph paper) (Fig. 20-6). Using one eye at a time, patient fixates on center dot and records any abnormalities of grid lines, such as wavy, missing, or distorted areas. Used to monitor macular problems
Perimetry (Visual Field) Testing	Can detect alterations in central and peripheral vision, which may be caused by various conditions such as glaucoma, stroke, brain tumors, or other neurologic deficits. Person sits and looks inside a bowl-shaped instrument called a *perimeter*. While staring at the center of bowl, a light flashes and the person presses a button each time flash is seen. A computer records the results, and a printout shows if there are areas where flashes of light are not seen.

*Patient teaching regarding the purpose and method of testing is a nursing responsibility for all diagnostic procedures.

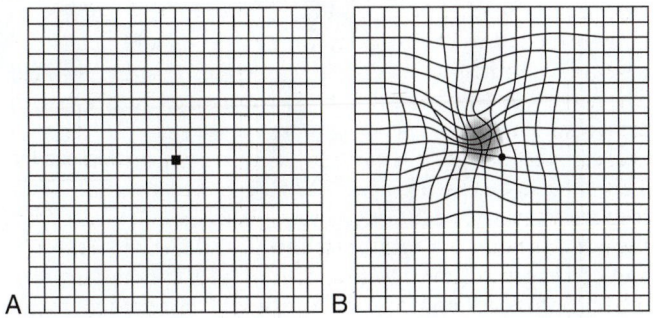

FIG. 20-6 Amsler grid. **A,** Normal grid. **B,** Abnormal grid as seen by person with macular degeneration.

CASE STUDY

Objective Data: Diagnostic Studies

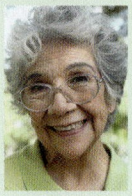

(©Jack Hollingsworth/ Photodisc/ Thinkstock)

The health care provider performs an ophthalmoscopic examination on F.M. and identifies a partial retinal detachment. This diagnosis is confirmed via ultrasonography.

Discussion Questions

1. Are these the diagnostic studies that you expected to be ordered?
2. Which diagnostic study results are of most concern to you?

Answers available at *http://evolve.elsevier.com/Lewis/medsurg.*

AUDITORY SYSTEM

STRUCTURES AND FUNCTIONS OF AUDITORY SYSTEM

The auditory system is composed of the peripheral auditory system and central auditory system. The peripheral auditory system includes the structures of the ear itself: external, middle, and inner ear (Fig. 20-7). This system is concerned with the reception and perception of sound. The inner ear functions in hearing and balance.

The central auditory system integrates and assigns meaning to what is heard. This system includes the vestibulocochlear nerve (CN VIII) and auditory cortex of the brain. The brain and its pathways transmit and process sound and sensations that maintain a person's equilibrium.

The role of the external and middle portion of the ear is to conduct and amplify sound waves from the environment. This portion of sound conduction is termed *air conduction.* Problems in these two parts of the ear may cause *conductive hearing loss,* resulting in a decrease in sound intensity and/or a distortion in sound.[7]

Disturbances in equilibrium can impair coordination, balance, and orientation. Damage to or an abnormality of the inner ear or along the nerve pathways results in *sensorineural hearing loss.* In addition to causing distortion or faintness of sound, sensorineural hearing loss may affect the ability to understand speech or cause complete hearing loss. Impairment within the auditory pathways of the brain causes *central hearing loss.* This type of hearing loss causes difficulty in understanding the meaning of words that are heard. (Types of hearing loss are discussed in Chapter 21 on pp. 387-388.)

External Ear

The external ear consists of the *auricle* (pinna), external auditory canal, and tympanic membrane (TM). The auricle is composed of cartilage and connective tissue covered with epithelium, which also lines the external auditory canal (Fig. 20-7). The external auditory canal is a slightly S-shaped tube about 1 inch (2.5 cm) in length in the adult. The lining of the proximal one third of the canal contains fine hairs (cilia), sebaceous (oil) glands, and ceruminous (wax) glands. The oil and wax lubricate the ear canal, keep it free from debris, and kill bacteria. The distal two thirds of the canal is lined with thin epithelium over the bone and is very sensitive.

The function of the external ear and canal is to collect and transmit sound waves to the *tympanic membrane* (eardrum). This shiny, translucent, pearl-gray membrane is composed of epithelial cells, connective tissue, and mucous membrane. It serves as a partition and an instrument of sound transmission between the external auditory canal and middle ear.

Middle Ear

The middle ear cavity is an air space located in the temporal bone. Mucous membrane lines the middle ear and is continuous from the nasal pharynx via the eustachian (auditory) tube. The eustachian tube equalizes atmospheric air pressure between the middle ear and throat and allows the tympanic membrane to move freely. It is normally closed and opened with the movement of the jaw, usually during yawning and swallowing.

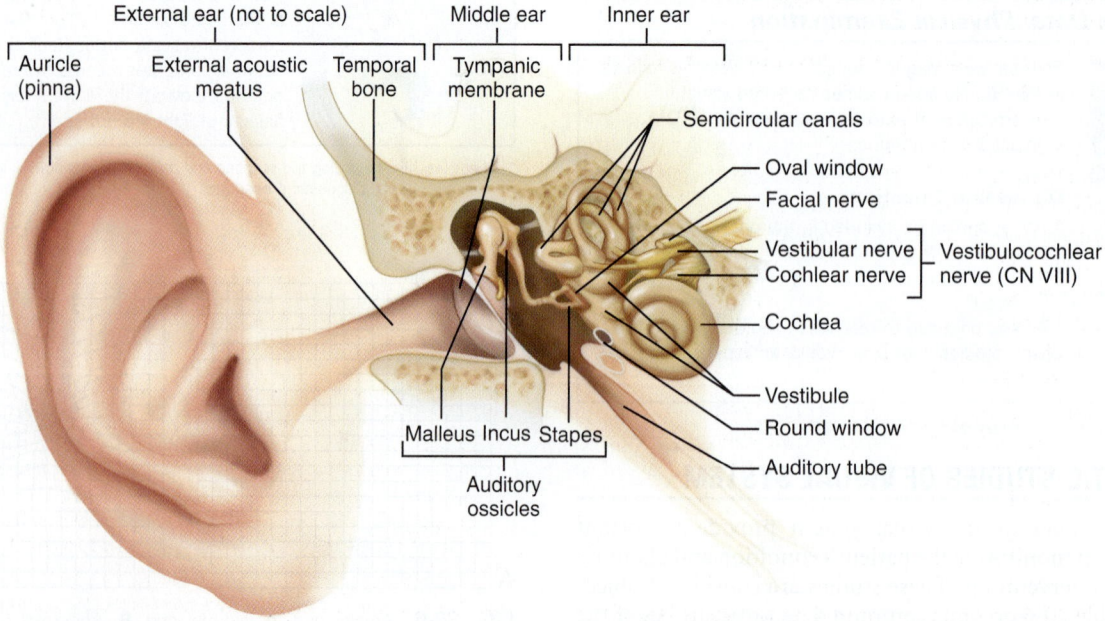

FIG. 20-7 External, middle, and inner ear. (Modified from Patton KT, Thibodeau GA: *Anatomy and physiology,* ed 8, St Louis, 2013, Mosby.)

Blockage of this tube can occur with allergies, nasopharyngeal infections, or enlarged adenoids. When the eustachian tube remains open, it is referred to as *patulous*. When this occurs, a person can hear one's own voice (autophony).

The middle ear contains the three smallest bones in the body: *malleus, incus,* and *stapes* (ossicles). Vibrations of the TM cause the ossicles to move and transmit sound waves to the oval window. The superior part of the middle ear is called the *epitympanum,* or the attic. It also communicates with air cells within the mastoid bone. The mastoid is the posterior part of the temporal bone. The facial nerve (CN VII) traverses above the oval window of the middle ear. The thin, bony covering of the facial nerve can become damaged by chronic ear infection, skull fracture, or trauma during ear surgery. Problems may occur related to voluntary facial movements, eyelid closure, and taste discrimination. Permanent damage to the facial nerve can also result.

Inner Ear

The inner ear is composed of a bony labyrinth (maze) surrounding a membrane. Perilymphatic fluid lies between the bone and membrane. The fluid inside the membrane is called *endolymph.* The inner ear contains the functional organs for hearing and balance. The receptor organ for hearing is the *cochlea,* which is a coiled structure. It contains the *organ of Corti,* whose tiny hair cells respond to stimulation of selected portions of the basilar membrane according to pitch. This stimulus is converted into an electrochemical impulse and then transmitted by the acoustic portion of the vestibulocochlear nerve (CN VIII) to the temporal lobe of the brain to process and interpret the sound.

Three semicircular canals and the vestibule make up the organ of balance, the membranous labyrinth, which is housed within the bony labyrinth. The membranous labyrinth is filled with endolymphatic fluid, and the bony labyrinth is filled with perilymphatic fluid. Nervous stimuli are communicated by the vestibular portion of CN VIII. Debris such as loose crystals of calcium or excessive pressure within the lymphatic fluid can produce disorders such as benign paroxysmal positional vertigo (BPPV). (BPPV is discussed in Chapter 21.)

Transmission of Sound. Sound waves travel by air (air conduction) and are picked up by the auricles and auditory canal. Sound waves strike the TM, causing it to vibrate. The central area of the TM is connected to the malleus, which also starts to vibrate. The malleus transmits the vibration to the incus and then the stapes. As the stapes moves back and forth, it pushes the membrane of the oval window in and out. Movement of the oval window produces waves in the perilymph.

Once sound waves are transmitted to the liquid medium of the inner ear, the vibration is picked up by the tiny sensory hair cells of the cochlea, which initiate nerve impulses. These impulses are carried by nerve fibers to the main branch of the acoustic portion of CN VIII and then to the brain.

The bones of the skull can also transmit sound directly to the inner ear (bone conduction). (Tuning fork tests are discussed in Table 20-11.)

Gerontologic Considerations: Effects of Aging on Auditory System

Approximately 20% of American adults report some degree of hearing loss, with aging being the primary cause.[8] **Presbycusis**, or hearing loss due to aging, can result from a variety of sources. Noise exposure, systemic diseases, poor nutrition, ototoxic drugs, and pollution exposure over the life span can damage the delicate hair cells of the organ of Corti or atrophy lymph-producing cells. Sound transmission is also diminished by calcification of the ossicles. The loss associated with presbycusis is usually greater for high-pitched sounds. Accumulation of dry cerumen (earwax) in the external canal can also interfere with the transmission of sound. **Tinnitus**, or ringing in the ears, may accompany the hearing loss that results from the aging process. As the average life span increases, the number of people with hearing loss will also increase. Prevention and early identification of problems ensure a more active and healthy aging population.

Age-related changes in the auditory system and differences in assessment findings are presented in Table 20-7.

ASSESSMENT OF AUDITORY SYSTEM

Assessment of the auditory system should include assessment of hearing and equilibrium because the auditory and *vestibular* (balance) systems are closely related. It is often difficult to separate symptoms related to these two systems. Help the patient describe symptoms and problems to differentiate the source of the problems. Health history questions to ask a patient with an auditory problem are listed in Table 20-8.

Problems with balance may manifest as vertigo or nystagmus. **Vertigo** is a sense that the person or objects around the person are moving or spinning and is usually stimulated by movement of the head. *Dizziness* is a sensation of being off-balance that occurs when standing or walking. **Nystagmus** is an abnormal eye movement that may be observed as a twitching of the eyeball or described by the patient as a blurring of vision with head or eye movement.

Initially try to categorize symptoms related to balance and separate them from symptoms related to hearing loss or

TABLE 20-7 Gerontologic Assessment Differences

Auditory System

Changes	Differences in Assessment Findings
External Ear	
Increased production of and drier cerumen	Impacted cerumen, potential hearing loss
Increased hair growth	Visible hair, especially in men
Loss of elasticity in cartilage	Collapsed ear canal
Middle Ear	
Atrophic changes of tympanic membrane	Conductive hearing loss
Inner Ear	
Hair cell degeneration, neuron degeneration in auditory nerve and central pathways, reduced blood supply to cochlea, calcification of ossicles	Presbycusis, diminished sensitivity to high-pitched sounds, impaired speech reception, tinnitus
Less effective vestibular apparatus in semicircular canals	Alterations in balance and body orientation
Brain	
Decline in ability to filter out unwanted and unnecessary sound	Difficulty hearing in a noisy environment, heightened sensitivity to loud sounds

tinnitus. The symptoms can be combined later in the assessment to help make the diagnosis and plan for the patient.

Subjective Data

Important Health Information

Past Health History. Many problems related to the ear may result from childhood illnesses or problems of adjacent organs. Consequently, a careful assessment of past health problems is important.

Ask the patient about previous problems regarding the ears, especially during childhood. Record the (1) frequency of acute middle ear infections (otitis media); (2) surgical procedures (e.g., myringotomy); (3) perforations of the eardrum; (4) drainage; and (5) history of mumps, measles, or scarlet fever. Congenital hearing loss can result from infectious diseases (e.g., rubella, influenza, syphilis), teratogenic medications, or hypoxia in the first trimester of pregnancy. Document head injury because it may result in hearing loss. Information about food and environmental allergies is important because they can cause the eustachian tube to become edematous and prevent aeration of the middle ear.

Record symptoms such as vertigo, tinnitus, and hearing loss in the patient's words. Guide the description by asking for specific details of the sensations and situations that may cause them or make them worse. Information regarding family members with hearing loss and type of hearing loss is important. Some congenital hearing loss is hereditary. The age of onset of presbycusis also follows a familial pattern.

Medications. Obtain information about present or past medications that are ototoxic (cause damage to CN VIII) and can produce hearing loss, tinnitus, and vertigo. The amount and frequency of aspirin use are important because tinnitus can result from high aspirin intake. Aminoglycosides and many other antibiotics, salicylates, antimalarial agents, chemotherapy drugs, diuretics, and nonsteroidal antiinflammatory drugs (NSAIDs) are groups of drugs that are potentially ototoxic. Monitor for hearing and balance problems in patients receiving these drugs. Many drugs produce hearing loss that may be reversible if treatment is stopped.

Surgery or Other Treatments. Document previous hospitalizations for ear surgery, including myringotomy (ventilation holes placed in the TM with or without tubes), tympanoplasty (surgical repair of TM), tonsillectomy, and adenoidectomy (removal of tonsils and adenoids). Record the use of and satisfaction with a hearing aid. Also note any problems with impacted cerumen.

Functional Health Patterns. Hearing and balance problems can affect all aspects of a person's life. To assess the impact of hearing loss, ask health history questions based on a functional health patterns approach (Table 20-8).

TABLE 20-8 Health History

Auditory System

Health Perception–Health Management

Hearing

- Have you had a change in your hearing?* If yes, how does this change affect your daily life?
- Do you use any devices to improve your hearing (e.g., hearing aid, special volume control, headphones for television or stereo)?*
- How do you protect your hearing?
- Do you have any allergies that result in ear problems?*

Equilibrium

- When did the dizziness or spinning sensation first occur?
- Does this sensation occur when you first stand up, when you are lying down, or both?
- Have you ever fallen because of the dizziness?*
- Can you drive or walk alone? If no, elaborate.
- Are there any times of the day when your symptoms are worse?*

Tinnitus

- How long have you experienced ringing in your ears? Has it changed?* Describe the ringing (e.g., buzzing, ringing, roaring). Do you also have a feeling of fullness or pressure?*
- When does it bother you the most?
- What things have you tried that help or have not helped?
- What medications are you taking?

Nutritional-Metabolic

- Do you notice any differences in symptoms with changes in diet?*
- Does your ear problem cause nausea that interferes with your food intake?*
- Does chewing or swallowing cause you any ear discomfort?*

Elimination

- Does straining during a bowel movement cause ear pain?*

Activity-Exercise

- Do you need help with certain activities (e.g., lifting, bending, climbing stairs, driving, speaking) because of symptoms?*

Sleep-Rest

- Is your sleep disturbed by noises or ringing in the ears or by a sensation of spinning?*

Cognitive-Perceptual

- Do you experience ear pain?* What relieves the pain? What makes it worse? Does the pain affect your hearing or balance?
- Have you noticed any problem with communicating or understanding what people are saying?*

Self-Perception–Self-Concept

- Have changes in your hearing affected how you feel about yourself or your feeling of independence?*

Role-Relationship

- What effect has your ear problem had on your work, family, or social life?
- Are you able to recognize the effects of your ear problems on your life?*

Sexuality-Reproductive

- Has your ear problem caused a change in your sex life?*

Coping–Stress Tolerance

- Do you consider your ear problem a source of stress?*
- How do you cope when you are experiencing symptoms?

Value-Belief

- Do you have a conflict between what your health care provider would like you to do and what you believe you should do?

*If yes, describe.

Health Perception–Health Management Pattern. Note the onset of hearing loss, whether sudden or gradual, and who noted the onset (e.g., patient, family, significant others). Gradual hearing losses are most often noted by those who communicate with the patient. Sudden losses and those exacerbated by some other condition are most often reported by the patient.

Assess the patient for personal measures used to preserve hearing. The use of protective ear covers or earplugs is good practice for people in high-noise environments. Document if the patient is a swimmer and the frequency and duration of swimming and use of ear protection. Note the type of water (pool, lake, or ocean) in which the swimming takes place to help identify contact with contaminated water. Assess for the placement of any item in the ear, including hearing aids, which can cause trauma to the canal and TM.

Nutritional-Metabolic Pattern. Alcohol, sodium, and dietary supplements affect the amount of endolymph in the inner ear system. Patients with Ménière's disease may notice some improvement in their symptoms with alcohol restriction and a low-sodium diet. Note changes in symptoms with food intake. Question the patient about any ear pain (otalgia) or discomfort associated with chewing or swallowing that may decrease nutritional intake. This situation is often associated with a problem in the middle ear.

Assessment of clenching or grinding of the teeth helps differentiate problems of the ear from referred pain of the temporomandibular joint (TMJ). Ask about dental problems and dentures.

Elimination Pattern. Elimination patterns are mainly of interest in the patient with perilymph fistula and after surgical procedures. Frequent constipation or straining with bowel or bladder elimination may interfere with healing or repair of a perilymph fistula. After middle ear surgery (stapedectomy) the patient needs to prevent increased intracranial (and consequent inner ear) pressure associated with straining during bowel movements. Stool softeners may be ordered postoperatively for the patient who reports chronic problems with constipation.

Activity-Exercise Pattern. A review of the patient's activity-exercise pattern is essential when assessing for equilibrium problems. Question the patient specifically about the onset, duration, and frequency of symptoms. Identify activities that relieve or worsen symptoms and how they relate to the time of the day. For example, patients with Ménière's disease are less able to compensate for environmental input as the day progresses.

Sleep-Rest Pattern. Ask the patient with chronic tinnitus about sleep problems. Find out if the patient has tried any techniques to modify the tinnitus (e.g., having fan on, using white noise devices). Also assess for snoring because it can be caused by swelling or hypertrophy of tissue in the nasopharynx. This excessive tissue can impair the functioning of the eustachian tube and cause the sensation of ear fullness or pain.

Cognitive-Perceptual Pattern. Pain is associated with some ear problems, particularly those involving the middle ear and auditory canal. If pain is present, ask the patient to describe the pain, presence of drainage *(otorrhea)*, history of teeth grinding, and the treatments used for relief. Note the effect on the pain level when the auricle is moved or the tragus is palpated.

Note the patient's ability to pay attention and follow directions. Problems with these tasks may be an early indicator of hearing loss. The patient may not recognize a gradual hearing loss. Ask significant others if they have noted any change in the patient's hearing.

Self-Perception–Self-Concept Pattern. Ask the patient to describe how the ear problem has affected his or her personal life and feelings about himself or herself. Hearing loss and chronic vertigo are particularly distressing for the patient. Hearing loss can result in embarrassing social situations that affect the patient's self-concept. Sensitively question the patient about such situations.

At times the patient with chronic vertigo may be accused of acting intoxicated. Clarify the symptom history with the patient and consider an evaluation with a hearing specialist.

Role-Relationship Pattern. Question the patient about the effect that the ear problem has had on family life, work responsibilities, and social relationships. Hearing loss can result in strained family relations and misunderstandings.

Also ask about employment or contact with environments that have excessive noise levels, such as work with jet engines and machinery and electronically amplified music. Document the use of preventive devices worn in noisy environments. Many jobs rely on the ability to hear accurately and respond appropriately. If a hearing loss is present, gather detailed information on the effect this has on the patient's job.

The unpredictability of vertigo attacks can have devastating effects on all aspects of a patient's life. Ordinary activities such as driving or cooking and work that requires balance all have an element of danger. Assess the effect of the vertigo on the patient's many roles and responsibilities.

Sexuality-Reproductive Pattern. Determine whether hearing loss or vertigo has interfered with the establishment of a satisfactory sex life. Although intimacy does not depend on the ability to hear, a hearing loss could interfere with establishing or maintaining a relationship.

Coping–Stress Tolerance Pattern. Ask the patient about his or her usual coping style, stress management strategies, and available support. If the patient seems unable to manage the situation, outside intervention may be required. Denial is a common response to a hearing problem and should be assessed.

Value-Belief Pattern. Question the patient about any conflicts produced by the problem or treatment related to values or beliefs. Every effort should be made to resolve the problem so that the patient does not experience additional stress. Ask about the use of home remedies such as hot oil in the ear.

Objective Data

Physical Examination. During the interview to obtain a health history, obtain objective data regarding the patient's ability to hear. Note clues such as posturing of the head and appropriateness of responses. Does the patient ask to have certain words repeated? Does the patient intently watch the examiner but miss comments when *not* looking at the examiner? Is the patient lip reading? Record these significant observations. This is also important because the patient is often unaware of hearing loss or does not admit to changes in hearing until moderate losses have occurred.

A normal assessment of the auditory system is listed in Table 20-9. Age-related changes of the auditory system and differences in assessment findings are listed in Table 20-7.

A *focused assessment* is used to evaluate the status of previously identified auditory problems and to monitor for signs of new problems (see Table 3-7). A focused assessment of the auditory system is presented in the box on p. 364.

TABLE 20-9 Normal Physical Assessment of Auditory System

- Ears symmetric in location and shape
- Auricles and tragus nontender, without lesions
- Canal clear, tympanic membrane intact, landmarks and light reflex intact
- Able to hear low whisper at 30 cm. Weber test results, no lateralization. Rinne test results AC > BC

AC, Air conduction; *BC,* bone conduction.

FOCUSED ASSESSMENT

Auditory System

Use this checklist to make sure the key assessment steps have been done.

Subjective

Ask the patient about any of the following and note responses.

Changes in hearing	Y	N
Ear pain	Y	N
Ear drainage	Y	N

Objective: Physical Examination

Inspect

Alignment and position of ears on head	✓
Size, shape, symmetry, color, and skin intactness	✓
External auditory meatus for discharge or lesions	✓

Assess

Hearing based on ability to respond to conversation, respond to a whisper, or hear a ticking watch	✓

External Ear. Inspect and palpate the external ear before examining the external canal and tympanum. Observe the auricle, preauricular area, and mastoid area for symmetry, color of skin, swelling, redness, and lesions. Then palpate the auricle and mastoid areas for tenderness and nodules. Grasping the auricle or pressing on the tragus may elicit pain, especially if the external ear or canal is inflamed.

External Auditory Canal and Tympanum. Before inserting an otoscope, inspect the canal opening for patency, palpate the tragus, and gently move the auricle to check for discomfort. Select a speculum slightly smaller than the size of the ear canal. Tip the patient's head to the opposite shoulder. Grasp the top of the auricle and gently pull up and backward to straighten the canal. Hold the otoscope while stabilizing it with your fingers on the patient's cheek, and then insert it slowly. A pneumatic otoscope creates negative pressure to pull at the TM and is helpful in confirming TM retraction or fluid behind the membrane. A tight seal of the speculum is essential during this step of the examination. Observe the canal for size and shape and the color, amount, and type of cerumen. Be careful when clearing the canal of cerumen. Damage can occur to the middle ear if the TM is perforated.

Inspect the TM for color, fluid behind the membrane, landmarks, contour, and intactness (Fig. 20-8). The TM is normally pearl gray, white, or pink; shiny; and translucent. The handle (manubrium) of the malleus and its short process (umbo) should be visible through the membrane. The position and dome (concave) shape of the TM cause the light from the otoscope to reflect back in a cone shape with crisp edges. If the TM is bulging or retracted, the edges of the light reflex will be fuzzy (diffuse) and may spread over the TM. The middle and inner ear cannot be examined with the otoscope because of the TM.

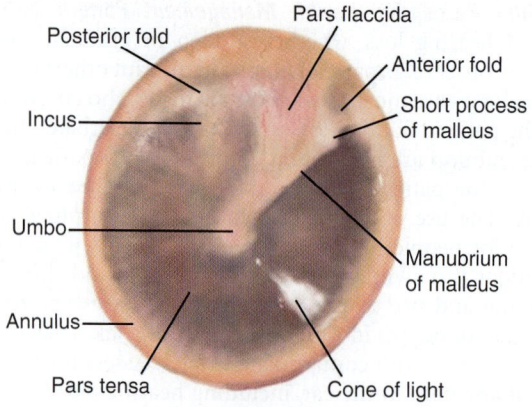

TYMPANIC MEMBRANE

FIG. 20-8 Normal tympanic membrane. (Jarvis C: *Physical examination and health assessment,* ed 7, St Louis, 2015, Elsevier.)

Table 20-10 summarizes assessment abnormalities of the auditory system.

DIAGNOSTIC STUDIES OF AUDITORY SYSTEM

Table 20-11 describes diagnostic studies commonly used to assess the auditory system.

Audiometry

Audiometry is beneficial as a screening test for hearing acuity and as a diagnostic test to determine the degree and type of hearing loss. The most common test performed by the audiologist is pure-tone audiometry.[9] The audiometer produces pure tones at varying intensities to which the patient can respond. Sound is characterized by the number of vibrations or cycles that occur each second. Hertz (Hz) is the unit of measurement used to classify the frequency of a tone. The higher the frequency is, the higher the pitch.

Hearing loss can affect certain sound frequencies. The specific pattern produced on the audiogram by these losses can assist in the diagnosis of the type of hearing loss. The intensity or strength of a sound wave is expressed in terms of decibels (dB), ranging from 0 to 110 dB. The intensity of a sound required to make any frequency barely audible to the average normal ear is 0 dB. Threshold refers to the signal level at which pure tones are detected (pure-tone thresholds) or the signal level at which the patient correctly hears 50% of the signals (speech detection thresholds).

Normal speech is approximately 40 to 65 dB; a soft whisper is 20 dB. Normally, a child and a young adult can hear frequencies from about 16 to 20,000 Hz, but hearing is most sensitive between 500 and 4000 Hz. This is similar to the frequencies of normal speech. A 40- to 45-dB loss in these frequencies causes moderate difficulty in hearing normal speech. A hearing aid may be helpful because it makes sound information louder but not clearer. A hearing aid may not be helpful to the patient who has problems with discrimination of sounds or sound information because the consonants are still not heard enough to make speech understandable.

Specialized Tests

More sophisticated tests are available to determine the cause of certain hearing losses (Table 20-11). CT scan and MRI are used to diagnose the site of a lesion, such as a tumor of the auditory nerve.

TABLE 20-10 Assessment Abnormalities

Auditory System

Finding	Description	Possible Etiology and Significance
External Ear and Canal		
Sebaceous cyst behind ear	Usually within skin, possible presence of black dot (opening to sebaceous gland)	Removal or incision and drainage if painful
Tophi	Hard nodules in the helix or antihelix consisting of uric acid crystals	Associated with gout, metabolic disorder. Further diagnosis needed
Impacted cerumen	Wax that has not normally been excreted from the ear. No visualization of eardrum	Decreased hearing possible, pain, sensation of fullness in auditory canal, removal necessary before otoscopic examination
Discharge in canal	Infection of external ear, usually painful	Swimmer's ear, infection of external ear. Possibly caused by ruptured eardrum and otitis media
Swelling of pinna, pain	Infection of glands of skin, hematoma caused by trauma	Aspiration (for hematoma)
Scaling or lesions	Change in usual appearance of skin	Seborrheic dermatitis, actinic keratosis, basal or squamous cell carcinoma
Exostosis	Bony growth extending into canal causing narrowing of canal	Possible interference with visualization of tympanum. Usually asymptomatic
Tympanum		
Retracted eardrum	Appearance of shorter, more horizontal malleus. Absent or bent cone of light	Vacuum in middle ear, blockage of eustachian tube, negative pressure in middle ear
Hairline fluid level, yellow-amber bubbles above fluid level	Caused by transudate of blood and serum, meniscus of fluid producing hairline appearance	Serous otitis media
Bulging red or blue eardrum, lack of landmarks	Fluid-filled middle ear, pus, blood	Acute otitis media, perforation possible
Perforation of eardrum (Fig. 20-8)	Previous perforations of the eardrum that have failed to heal. Thin, transparent layer of epithelium surrounding eardrum	Chronic otitis media, mastoiditis, drainage
Recruitment	Perception that sounds are getting too loud too fast	Sensorineural hearing loss. Hearing aid difficult to use

TABLE 20-11 Diagnostic Studies

Auditory System

Study	Description, Purpose, and Nursing Responsibility*
Auditory	
Audiometry	*Pure-tone audiometry* quantifies hearing loss. Sounds are presented through earphones in soundproof room. Patient responds when sound is heard. Response is recorded on an audiogram. Purpose is to determine patient's hearing range in terms of decibels (dB) and Hertz (Hz) for diagnosing hearing loss. Tinnitus can cause inconsistent results. *Speech audiometry* includes speech reception threshold (measure of intensity at which speech is recognized) and word recognition score (ability to discriminate among various speech sounds).
Auditory evoked potential (AEP)	Procedure is similar to electroencephalogram (see Chapter 55 and Table 55-7). Electrodes are attached to patient in a darkened room. Electrodes are placed typically at vertex, mastoid process, or earlobes and forehead. A computer is used to isolate auditory from other electrical activity of brain.
Electrocochleography	Test records electrical activity in cochlea and auditory nerve. Electrode placed on or through the eardrum. Used to assess and monitor patients with dizziness.
Auditory brainstem response (ABR)	Study measures electrical peaks along auditory pathway of inner ear to brain and provides diagnostic information related to acoustic neuromas, brainstem problems, and stroke.
Tympanometry	Used to check middle ear and mobility of eardrum. A probe is placed snugly into external ear canal, and positive and negative pressures are then applied. Measurements are made of movement of eardrum.
Tuning Fork Tests	
Weber test	Stem of vibrating tuning fork is placed on midline of skull or forehead. Patient asked to indicate where the sound is heard best. In normal auditory function, the patient perceives a midline tone and the sound is heard equally in both ears. If a patient has conductive hearing loss in one ear, the sound will be heard louder (lateralizes) in that ear. If sensorineural loss is present, the sound is louder (lateralizes) in the normal (unaffected) ear.
Rinne test	Hearing by bone conduction (BC) and air conduction (AC) is compared. Stem of vibrating tuning fork held against mastoid bone (for BC of sound) and time noted. When the sound is no longer perceived behind the ear (BC of sound), time is noted once again and the still-vibrating fork is moved close to the pinna (AC of sound). Have the patient report when the sound next to the ear canal (AC) is no longer heard and note time. Normally, the sound is heard twice as long in front of the ear as it is on the bone. With conductive hearing loss, the relationship is reversed; BC is longer than AC. With sensorineural hearing loss, both AC and BC are reduced, but AC remains longer.

Continued

TABLE 20-11 Diagnostic Studies

Auditory System—cont'd

Study	Description, Purpose, and Nursing Responsibility*
Vestibular Tests	
Electronystagmography (ENG)	Used to diagnose diseases of vestibular system such as dizziness and balance disorders. Electrodes are placed near patient's eyes, and movement of eyes (nystagmus) is recorded on graph during specific eye movements and when ear is irrigated. Caloric test may be part of testing to measure responses to warm and cold water circulated into the ear canal. Instruct patient to eat light meal before test to avoid nausea. Observe patient for vomiting. Ensure patient safety.
Posturography	Balance test that can isolate one semicircular canal from others to determine site of lesion. Test is done in a boxlike device in which floor moves in response to a correction in balance by patient. Inform patient that test may be uncomfortable. Test can be discontinued at any time at patient's request.
Rotary chair testing	Evaluates peripheral vestibular system. Patient is seated in a chair driven by a motor under computer control. Test is usually done in the dark. Instruct patient to eat light meal before test to avoid nausea. Observe patient for vomiting. Ensure patient safety.

*Patient teaching regarding the purpose and method of testing is a nursing responsibility for all diagnostic procedures.

BRIDGE TO NCLEX EXAMINATION

The number of the question corresponds to the same-numbered outcome at the beginning of the chapter.

1. In a patient who has a hemorrhage in the posterior cavity of the eye, the nurse knows that blood is accumulating
   a. in the aqueous humor.
   b. between the lens and retina.
   c. between the cornea and lens.
   d. in the space between the iris and lens.
2. Increased intraocular pressure may occur as a result of
   a. edema of the corneal stroma.
   b. dilation of the retinal arterioles.
   c. blockage of the lacrimal canals and ducts.
   d. increased production of aqueous humor by the ciliary process.
3. Question patients using eye drops to treat their glaucoma about
   a. use of corrective lenses.
   b. their usual sleep pattern.
   c. a history of heart or lung disease.
   d. sensitivity to opioids or depressants.
4. Always assess the patient with an ophthalmic problem for
   a. visual acuity.
   b. pupillary reactions.
   c. intraocular pressure.
   d. confrontation visual fields.
5. During an assessment of hearing, the nurse would expect that a normal finding would be
   a. absent cone of light.
   b. bluish purple tympanic membrane.
   c. midline tone heard equally in both ears.
   d. fluid level at hairline in the tympanum.
6. Age-related changes in the auditory system commonly include *(select all that apply)*
   a. drier cerumen.
   b. tinnitus in both ears.
   c. auditory nerve degeneration.
   d. atrophy of the tympanic membrane.
   e. greater ability to hear high-pitched sounds.
7. Before injecting fluorescein for angiography, it is important for the nurse to *(select all that apply)*
   a. obtain an emesis basin.
   b. ask if the patient is fatigued.
   c. administer a topical anesthetic.
   d. inform patient that skin may turn yellow.
   e. assess for allergies to iodine-based contrast media.

1. b, 2. d, 3. c, 4. a, 5. c, 6. a, c, d, 7. a, d

For rationales to these answers and even more NCLEX review questions, visit *http://evolve.elsevier.com/Lewis/medsurg.*

EVOLVE WEBSITE

http://evolve.elsevier.com/Lewis/medsurg

Review Questions (Online Only)

Key Points

Answer Keys for Questions

- Rationales for Bridge to NCLEX Examination Questions
- Answer Guidelines for Case Study on pp. 353, 356, 359, and 360

Conceptual Care Map Creator

Audio Glossary

Supporting Media

- Animation
  - Weber Test

Content Updates

REFERENCES

1. Dua HS, Fara LA, Said DG, et al: Human corneal anatomy redefined: a novel pre-Descmet's layer (Dua's layer), *Ophthalmology* 120(9):1778, 2013.
2. Thibodeau G, Patton K: *Structure and function of the body*, ed 14, St Louis, 2012, Mosby.
3. *Saunders nursing drug handbook 2015*, St Louis, 2015, Saunders.
4. American Foundation for the Blind: AFB senior site. Retrieved from *www.afb.org.*
5. Goldman L, Schafer A, editors: *Goldman's Cecil medicine*, ed 25, St Louis, 2016, Saunders.
6. Rakel R, Rakel D, editors: *Textbook of family medicine*, ed 9, St Louis, 2015, Saunders.
7. National Institute on Deafness and Other Communication Disorders: Quick statistics. Retrieved from *www.nidcd.nih.gov/health/statistics/Pages/quick.aspx.*
8. Hearing Loss Association of America. Retrieved from *http://hearingloss.org.*
9. Bope E, Kellerman R, editors: *Conn's current therapy 2015*, St Louis, 2015, Saunders.

21

Visual and Auditory Problems

Sharon L. Lewis

It is only with the heart that one can see rightly; what is essential is invisible to the eye.

Antoine de Saint-Exupery

http://evolve.elsevier.com/Lewis/medsurg/

LEARNING OUTCOMES

1. Compare and contrast the types of refractive errors and appropriate corrections.
2. Describe the etiology and nursing and interprofessional management of extraocular disorders.
3. Explain the pathophysiology, clinical manifestations, interprofessional care, and nursing management of the patient with intraocular disorders.
4. Discuss the nursing measures that promote the health of the eyes and ears.
5. Discuss the general preoperative and postoperative care of patients undergoing surgery of the eye or ear.
6. Summarize the action and uses of drug therapy for treating problems of the eyes and ears.
7. Explain the pathophysiology, clinical manifestations, and nursing and interprofessional management of common ear problems.
8. Compare the causes, management, and rehabilitative potential of conductive and sensorineural hearing loss.
9. Explain the use, care, and patient teaching related to assistive devices for eye and ear problems.
10. Describe the common causes and assistive measures for severe visual impairment and deafness.
11. Describe the measures used to assist the patient in adapting psychologically to decreased vision and hearing.

KEY TERMS

acoustic neuroma, p. 387
age-related macular degeneration (AMD), p. 378
astigmatism, p. 368
benign paroxysmal positional vertigo (BPPV), p. 386
cataract, p. 373
conjunctivitis, p. 371
enucleation, p. 382
external otitis, p. 383
glaucoma, p. 379
hordeolum, p. 370
hyperopia, p. 368
keratitis, p. 372
Ménière's disease, p. 386
myopia, p. 367
otosclerosis, p. 385
presbycusis, p. 391
presbyopia, p. 368
refractive error, p. 367
retinal detachment, p. 376
retinopathy, p. 376
strabismus, p. 373

The chapter describes visual and auditory problems, with an emphasis on their pathophysiology, clinical manifestations, interprofessional care, and nursing management. Assistive devices for visual and hearing impairment are also discussed.

VISUAL PROBLEMS

REFRACTIVE ERRORS

The most common visual problem is **refractive error**. This defect prevents light rays from converging into a single focus on the retina. Defects are a result of irregularities of the corneal curvature, focusing power of the lens, or length of the eye. The major symptom is blurred vision. In some cases, the patient may also complain of ocular discomfort, eyestrain, or headaches. Most refractive errors can be corrected by the use of lenses in the form of eyeglasses or contact lenses, refractive eye laser surgery, or surgical implantation of an artificial lens.

Myopia (nearsightedness) is an inability to accommodate for objects at a distance. It causes light rays to be focused in front of the retina. Myopia may occur because of excessive light refraction by the cornea or lens or because of an abnormally long eye. Myopia is the most common refractive error, with approximately 25% of Americans having this disorder.

Acknowledgment: We would like to acknowledge the contributions of Sarah Smith, RN, MA, CRNO, COT, Nurse Manager, Department of Ophthalmology, University of Iowa Health Care, Iowa City, Iowa, to this chapter over the past six editions of the book.
Reviewed by Marylee Bressie, RN, DNP, CCRN, CCNS, CEN, Core Faculty/Nurse Planner, Department of Nursing, School of Public Service Leadership, Capella University, Minneapolis, Minnesota; Hope Bussenius, DNP, APRN, FNP-BC, Clinical Assistant Professor, Nell Hodgson Woodruff School of Nursing, Emory University, Atlanta, Georgia; Deborah Ehlers, RN, MSN, Director of Nursing and Administrator of The Eye Center, Yakima, Washington; Deena Hollingsworth, MSN, FNP-BC, CORLN, Family Nurse Practitioner, ENT Specialists of Northern Virginia, Arlington, Virginia; Michelle Smeltzer, RN, MSN, DNPc, CEN, Clinical Education Specialist, Emergency Department, Einstein Medical Center Montgomery, East Norriton, Pennsylvania; and Robert M. Welch, RN, MSN, FNP, CRNO, Family Nurse Practitioner, Nevada Retina Associates, Reno, Nevada.

Hyperopia (farsightedness) is an inability to accommodate for near objects. It causes the light rays to focus behind the retina and requires the patient to use accommodation to focus the light rays on the retina for near objects. This type of refractive error occurs when the cornea or lens does not have adequate focusing power or when the eyeball is too short.

Presbyopia is the loss of accommodation associated with age. This condition generally appears at about age 40. As the eye ages, the lens becomes larger, firmer, and less elastic. These changes, which progress with aging, result in an inability to focus on near objects.

Astigmatism is caused by an irregular corneal curvature. This irregularity causes the incoming light rays to be bent unequally. Consequently, the light rays do not come to a single point of focus on the retina. Astigmatism can occur in conjunction with any of the other refractive errors.

Aphakia is the absence of the lens. Rarely, the lens may be absent congenitally, or it may be removed during cataract surgery. A lens that is traumatically injured is removed and replaced with an intraocular lens (IOL) implant. The absence of the lens generally results in a significant refractive error. Without the focusing ability of the lens, images are projected behind the retina.

Nonsurgical Corrections

Corrective Glasses. Myopia, hyperopia, presbyopia, and astigmatism can be modified by using the appropriate corrective lenses. Glasses for presbyopia are often called "reading glasses" because they are usually only worn for close work. The presbyopic correction may also be combined with a correction for another refractive error, such as myopia or astigmatism. In these combined glasses, the presbyopic correction is in the lower portion of the spectacle lens. A traditional bifocal or trifocal has visible lines. However, most lenses today that correct vision at various distances do not have visible lines. The prescription varies throughout the lens, allowing distance focusing in the top two thirds and near focus in the bottom one third of the lens.

Contact Lenses. Contact lenses are another way to correct refractive errors. Contact lenses are made from various plastic and silicone substances that are highly permeable to oxygen and have a high water content. These features allow for increased wearing time with greater comfort. If the oxygen supply to the cornea is decreased, it becomes swollen, visual acuity decreases, and the patient experiences severe discomfort.

In general, you need to know whether the patient wears contact lenses, the pattern of wear (daily versus extended), and care practices. Shining a light obliquely on the eyeball can help visualize a contact lens. Contact lenses are associated with microbial keratitis, a severe sight-threatening complication. Risk factors for keratitis include poor hand cleaning, poor lens case hygiene, and inadequate lens cleaning. Teach the patient the importance of following recommended cleaning practices and reporting redness, sensitivity, vision problems, and pain to the eye care professional. Instruct the patient to remove contact lenses immediately if any of these problems occur.

Surgical Therapy

Surgical procedures are designed to eliminate or reduce the need for eyeglasses or contact lenses and correct refractive errors by changing the focus of the eye. Surgical management for refractive errors includes laser surgery and IOL implantation.

Laser. *Laser-assisted in situ keratomileusis* (LASIK) may be considered for patients with low to moderately high amounts of myopia or hyperopia, with or without astigmatism.[1] The procedure first involves using a laser or surgical blade to create a flap in the cornea. The flap is folded back, exposing the middle section (stroma) of the cornea. Pulses from a computer-controlled laser vaporize a part of the stroma. The flap is then repositioned, adhering on its own without sutures in a few minutes.[2]

Photorefractive keratectomy (PRK) is indicated for low to moderate amounts of myopia or hyperopia, with or without astigmatism and is a good option for a patient with insufficient corneal thickness for a LASIK flap. In PRK only the epithelium is removed, and the laser sculpts the cornea to correct the refractive error. *Laser-assisted subepithelial keratomileusis* (LASEK) is similar to PRK, except that the epithelium is replaced after surgery.

Implant. *Refractive intraocular lens* (refractive IOL) implantation is an option for patients with a high degree of myopia or hyperopia. Like cataract surgery, it involves removal of the patient's natural lens and implantation of an IOL, which is a small plastic lens to correct a patient's refractive error. Accommodating IOLs correct both myopia and presbyopia.

Phakic intraocular lenses (phakic IOLs) are sometimes referred to as *implantable contact lenses.* They are implanted into the eye without removing the eye's natural lens. They are used for patients with high degrees of myopia or hyperopia. Unlike refractive IOLs, the phakic IOL is placed in front of the eye's natural lens. Leaving the natural lens in the eye preserves the eye's ability to focus for reading vision.

CULTURAL & ETHNIC HEALTH DISPARITIES

Visual and Auditory Problems

- Whites have a higher incidence of hearing impairment than African Americans or Asian Americans.
- Glaucoma has an increased incidence and severity among African Americans compared with whites.
- Hispanic Americans have an increased incidence of diabetic retinopathy.
- Native Americans have an increased incidence of otitis media when compared with whites.
- Whites have a higher incidence of macular degeneration than Hispanics, African Americans, and Asian Americans.

VISUAL IMPAIRMENT

Visual impairment describes vision that cannot be fully corrected by corrective lenses, medical treatment, or surgery. The term *visual impairment* includes conditions ranging from low vision to the absence of any sight at all (total blindness).[3] Many terms are used when people refer to visual impairment, including:

- *Low vision* is a term used to describe impaired vision that cannot be improved by conventional eyeglasses, contact lenses, medications, or surgery in which some good usable vision remains.
- *Severe visual impairment* describes visual impairment in people who are unable to read ordinary newsprint even with correction. People with a severe visual impairment may or may not be legally blind.
- *Legal blindness* refers to central visual acuity of 20/200 or less in the better eye with correction, or a peripheral visual field of 20 degrees or less.

Almost all blindness in the United States is the result of common eye diseases, including cataracts, glaucoma, age-related macular degeneration, and diabetic retinopathy.

NURSING MANAGEMENT: VISUAL IMPAIRMENT

Nursing Assessment

It is important to assess how long the patient has had a visual impairment, since recent loss of vision has different implications for nursing care. Determine how the patient's visual impairment affects normal functioning. Question the patient about the level of difficulty involved in doing certain tasks. For example, ask how much difficulty the patient has when reading a newspaper, writing a check, moving from one room to the next, or viewing television. Other questions can help determine the personal meaning that the patient attaches to the visual impairment. Ask how the vision loss has affected specific aspects of the patient's life, whether the patient has lost a job, or what activities the patient does not engage in because of the visual impairment.

Determine the patient's emotional reactions, coping strategies, and support systems. The patient may attach many negative meanings to the impairment because of societal views of blindness. For example, the patient may view the impairment as punishment or view himself or herself as useless and burdensome.

Planning

The overall goals are that the patient with impaired vision will (1) make a successful adjustment to the impairment, (2) verbalize feelings related to the loss, (3) identify personal strengths and support systems, and (4) use appropriate coping strategies. If the patient has been functioning at an appropriate or acceptable level, the goal is to maintain the current level of function.

Nursing Implementation

- **Health Promotion.** Encourage the patient with preventable causes of further visual impairment to seek appropriate health care. For example, the patient with vision loss from glaucoma may prevent further visual impairment by complying with prescribed therapies and ophthalmic evaluations.
- **Acute Care.** Provide emotional support and direct care to the patient with recent visual impairment. Allow the patient to express fear, anger, and grief. Help the patient identify appropriate coping strategies. The family is intimately involved in the experiences that occur with vision loss. With the patient's knowledge and permission, include family members in discussions and encourage them to express their concerns.

  Many people are uncomfortable around an individual with visual impairment because they are not sure what behaviors are appropriate. Being sensitive to the patient's feelings without being overly worried or smothering the patient's independence is vital in creating a therapeutic nursing presence. Always communicate in a normal conversational tone and manner with the patient, and address the patient, not the caregiver. Common courtesy dictates introducing oneself and any other people who approach patients with visual impairment. It is also important to say good-bye when leaving the presence of the visually impaired person. Making eye contact with the patient accomplishes several objectives. It ensures that you are speaking while facing the patient so that the patient has no difficulty hearing. Your head position validates that you are attentive to the patient. In addition, establishing eye contact ensures that you can observe the patient's facial expressions and reactions.

  Assist the patient using a *sighted-guide technique.* Stand slightly in front and to one side of the patient, and offer an elbow for the patient to hold. Serve as the sighted guide, walking slightly ahead of the patient with the patient holding the back of your arm. As you walk, describe the environment to help orient the patient. For example, "We're going through an open doorway and approaching two steps down." Help the patient sit by placing one of his or her hands on the seat of the chair.
- **Ambulatory Care.** In working with the patient who is visually impaired, remember that a person classified as legally blind may have some useful vision. Rehabilitation after partial or total loss of vision can foster independence, self-esteem, and productivity. Know what services and devices are available for the patients with visual impairments, and make appropriate referrals. For the legally blind patient the primary resource for services is the state agency for rehabilitation of the blind. Legally blind individuals are often eligible for federal and state assistance and income tax benefits. A list of agencies that serve the partially sighted or blind patient is available from the American Foundation for the Blind *(www.afb.org).*

  Braille or audio books for reading and a cane or guide dog for ambulation are examples of vision substitution techniques. These are usually most appropriate for the patient with no functional vision. For most patients who have some remaining vision, vision enhancement techniques can provide help in learning to ambulate, read printed material, and accomplish activities of daily living (ADLs).
- ***Optical Devices for Vision Enhancement.*** A wide range of newer technologies are available to assist people with low vision. These devices include desktop video magnification/closed circuit units, electronic hand-held magnifiers, text-to-speech scanners (material read aloud to you), E-readers, and computer tablets (material read aloud, magnification, image zooming, brighter screen, voice recognition). Many of these devices require some training by an assistive technology professional. Encourage patients to practice with the technologic device to ensure they can use it successfully.
- ***Nonoptical Methods for Vision Enhancement.*** *Approach magnification* is a simple way to enhance the patient's residual vision. Recommend that the patient sit closer to the television or hold books closer to the eyes. Contrast enhancement techniques include watching television in black and white, using a black felt-tip marker, and using contrasting colors (e.g., a red stripe at the edge of steps or curbs). Increased lighting can be provided by halogen lamps, direct sunlight, or gooseneck lamps that can be aimed directly at the reading material or other near objects. Large type is often helpful, especially in conjunction with other optical or nonoptical vision enhancements.
- ***Non–24-Hour Sleep-Wake Disorder.*** A common problem that can occur in blind people (especially those who are totally blind) is *non–24-hour sleep-wake disorder (Non-24).* It is a circadian rhythm sleep disorder in which an individual's biologic clock fails to synchronize to a 24-hour day.[4] (Sleep and sleep disorders are discussed in Chapter 7.) It is caused by lack of light input to the circadian clock.

  People with this disorder have difficulty falling asleep or staying asleep at night. During the day they may have an uncontrollable urge to sleep. This disorder can result in severe sleep issues including insomnia, excessive sleepiness, changing patterns of when a person sleeps, and social and work consequences.

Melatonin is used to shift the circadian clock earlier (an advance) or later (a delay). Tasimelteon (Hetlioz), a melatonin receptor agonist, can also be used for treatment. It works by targeting receptors in the brain that control the timing of the sleep-wake cycle.

Evaluation

The overall expected outcomes are that the patient with visual impairment will

- Follow treatment plan to prevent further loss of vision
- Be able to use adaptive coping strategies
- Not experience low self-esteem or a decrease in social interactions
- Function safely within her or his own environment

HEALTHY PEOPLE

Health Impact of Responsible Eye Care

- Regular hand washing prevents the spread of disease from one eye to the other.
- Seeking appropriate health care can lead to early detection of disease and prevent further loss of vision in patients with certain types of partial vision loss.
- Wearing sunglasses and practicing proper nutrition may help prevent cataract development and age-related macular degeneration.
- Wearing eye protection during potentially hazardous work, hobby, and sport activities reduces the risk of eye injuries.

Gerontologic Considerations: Visual Impairment

The older adult is at an increased risk for vision loss caused by eye disease.[5] This older person may have other deficits, such as cognitive impairment or limited mobility, that further affect the ability to function in usual ways. Societal devaluation of the older adults may compound the self-esteem or isolation issues associated with the older patient's visual impairment. Financial resources may be inadequate to meet the increased demands of vision services or assistive devices.

The older patient may become increasingly confused or disoriented when visually compromised. The combination of decreased vision and confusion increases the risk of falls, which have potentially serious consequences for the older adult. Decreased vision may compromise the older patient's ability to function, resulting in concerns about maintaining independence and a diminished self-image. Decreased manual dexterity may make the instillation of prescribed eye drops difficult for some older adults. Those with low vision are more likely to make medication errors that are potentially dangerous, such as taking too much insulin or mistaking one drug for another.

EYE TRAUMA

Although the eyes are well protected by the bony orbit and fat pads, everyday activities can result in ocular trauma. The most common ocular injuries in the United States occur in the home due to gardening, power tool use, and home repair work. Sport- and work-related injuries are additional causes of eye trauma.[6]

Table 21-1 outlines emergency management of the patient with an eye injury. A *Morgan lens* may be used to provide continuous irrigation of an injured eye. It consists of a sterile plastic device resembling a contact lens that floats over the eye (never physically touches it) and allows copious irrigation of the eye. The device is connected to tubing that delivers irrigating solution. The Morgan lens provides relief for chemical or thermal burns and removes nonembedded foreign materials in the eye.

CHECK YOUR PRACTICE

You are working in your garden when your neighbor comes running into your yard. She is screaming and waving her arms. Her husband was using a chain saw to cut down a tree when a piece of wood chip flew into his eye. When you go to your neighbor's yard, the husband is on the ground crying in pain and you assess that the wood chip is embedded in his eye.

- What should you do next?

Trauma is often a preventable cause of visual impairment. Many eye injuries could be prevented by wearing protective eyewear. Your role in individual and community education is extremely important in reducing the incidence of ocular trauma.

EXTRAOCULAR DISORDERS

INFLAMMATION AND INFECTION

One of the most common eye conditions is inflammation or infection of the external eye. Many external irritants or microorganisms can affect the eye, conjunctiva, and avascular cornea.

An external **hordeolum** (commonly called a *sty*) is an infection of the sebaceous glands in the lid margin (Fig. 21-1). The most common bacterial infective agent is *Staphylococcus aureus.* A red, swollen, circumscribed, and acutely tender area develops rapidly. Instruct the patient to apply warm, moist compresses at least four times a day until it improves. This may be the only treatment necessary. If it tends to recur, teach the patient to perform lid scrubs daily. In addition, appropriate antibiotic ointments or drops may be indicated.

A *chalazion* is a chronic inflammatory granuloma of the meibomian (sebaceous) glands in the lid. It may evolve from a hordeolum or occur in response to the material released into the lid when a blocked gland ruptures. The chalazion usually appears on the upper lid as a swollen, tender, reddened area that may be painful. Initial treatment is similar to that for a hordeolum. If warm, moist compresses are ineffective in promoting spontaneous drainage, the ophthalmologist may drain the lesion (this is normally an office procedure) or inject the lesion with corticosteroids.

Blepharitis is a common chronic bilateral inflammation of the lid margins. The lids are red rimmed with many scales or

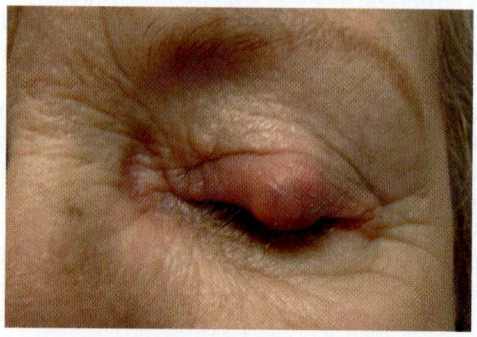

FIG. 21-1 Hordeolum (sty) on the upper eyelid caused by staphylococcal infection. (Courtesy Cory J. Bosanko, OD, FAAO, Eye Centers of Tennessee, Crossville, Tenn.)

TABLE 21-1 Emergency Management

Eye Injury

Etiology	Assessment Findings	Interventions
Trauma • Blunt (e.g., fist) • Penetrating (e.g., glass, metal, or wood fragments. Knife, stick, or other object) **Chemical Burn** • Alkaline • Acid **Thermal Burn** • Direct burn from hot surface • Indirect burn from UV light (e.g., welding torch, looking directly at sun) **Foreign Bodies** • Glass • Metal • Wood • Plastic • Ceramics	• Pain • Photophobia • Redness—diffuse or localized • Swelling • Ecchymosis • Tearing • Blood in the anterior chamber • Absent eye movements • Fluid drainage from eye (e.g., blood, CSF, aqueous humor) • Abnormal or decreased vision • Visible foreign body • Prolapsed globe • Abnormal intraocular pressure • Visual field defect	**Initial** • Determine mechanism of injury. • Ensure airway, breathing, and circulation. • Assess for other injuries. • Assess for chemical exposure. • Begin ocular irrigation *immediately* in case of chemical exposure. Do not stop until emergency personnel arrive to continue irrigation. Use sterile saline or water if saline is unavailable. • Assess visual acuity. • Do not put pressure on the eye. • Instruct patient not to blow nose. • Do not attempt to treat the injury (except as noted above for chemical exposure). • Stabilize foreign objects. • Cover the eye(s) with dry, sterile patches and a protective shield. • Do not give the patient food or fluids. • Elevate head of bed 45 degrees. • Do not put medication or solutions in the eye unless ordered by physician. • Administer analgesia as appropriate. **Ongoing Monitoring** • Reassure the patient. • Monitor pain. • Anticipate surgical repair for penetrating injury, globe rupture, or globe avulsion.

CSF, Cerebrospinal fluid; *UV,* ultraviolet.

crusts on the lid margins and lashes. The patient may primarily complain of itching but may also experience burning, irritation, and photophobia. Conjunctivitis may occur simultaneously.

If blepharitis is caused by a staphylococcal infection, an appropriate ophthalmic antibiotic ointment must be used. Often blepharitis is caused by both staphylococcal and seborrheal microorganisms, and the treatment must be more vigorous to avoid hordeolum, *keratitis* (inflammation of the cornea), and other eye infections. Emphasize thorough cleaning practices of the skin and scalp. Gentle cleansing of the lid margins with baby shampoo can effectively soften and remove crusting.

Conjunctivitis

Conjunctivitis is an infection or inflammation of the conjunctiva. These infections may be caused by bacteria or viruses.[7] Conjunctival inflammation may result from exposure to allergens or chemical irritants. The tarsal conjunctiva (lining the interior surface of the lids) may become inflamed as a result of a chronic foreign body in the eye, such as a contact lens. Careful hand washing and use of individual or disposable towels help prevent spreading the condition.

Bacterial Infections. Acute bacterial conjunctivitis *(pinkeye)* is a common infection. Although it occurs in every age group, epidemics are common among children. *S. aureus* is the most common cause. The patient with bacterial conjunctivitis may complain of discomfort, pruritus, redness, and a mucopurulent drainage. Although it typically occurs initially in one eye, it generally spreads to the unaffected eye. It is usually self-limiting, but treatment with antibiotic drops (e.g., besifloxacin [Besivance]) shortens the course of the disorder. Teach patients the importance of hand washing and avoiding contact with an infected person.

Viral Infections. Conjunctival infections may be caused by many different viruses. The patient with viral conjunctivitis may complain of tearing, foreign body sensation, redness, and mild photophobia. This condition is usually mild and self-limiting. However, it can be severe, with increased discomfort and subconjunctival hemorrhaging. Adenovirus conjunctivitis may be contracted in contaminated swimming pools and through direct contact with an infected patient. Treatment is usually palliative. If the patient is severely symptomatic, topical corticosteroids can provide temporary relief.

Chlamydial Infections. *Trachoma* is a chronic conjunctivitis caused by *Chlamydia trachomatis* (serotypes A through C). It is a major cause of blindness worldwide. This preventable eye disease is transmitted mainly by the hands and by flies. Adult inclusion conjunctivitis (AIC) is caused by *C. trachomatis* (serotypes D through K). AIC is becoming more prevalent in the United States because of the increase in sexually transmitted chlamydial infection.[8]

Manifestations of both trachoma and AIC are mucopurulent ocular discharge, irritation, redness, and lid swelling. For unknown reasons, AIC does not carry the long-term consequences of trachoma. AIC also differs from trachoma in that it is common in economically developed countries, whereas trachoma is most commonly seen in underdeveloped countries. Antibiotic therapy is usually effective for trachoma and AIC.

Although antibiotic treatment may be successful, patients with AIC have a high risk of concurrent chlamydial genital infection, as well as other sexually transmitted infections.

Allergic Conjunctivitis. Conjunctivitis caused by exposure to an allergen can be mild and transitory, or it can be severe enough to cause significant swelling, sometimes ballooning the conjunctiva beyond the eyelids. The defining symptom of allergic conjunctivitis is itching. The patient may also complain of burning, redness, and tearing. In addition to pollens, the patient may develop allergic conjunctivitis in response to animal dander, ocular solutions, and medications. Instruct the patient to avoid the allergen if it is known. Artificial tears can be effective in diluting the allergen and washing it from the eye. Effective topical medications include antihistamines and corticosteroids.

Keratitis

Keratitis is an inflammation or infection of the cornea that is caused by a variety of microorganisms or by other factors. The condition may involve the conjunctiva and/or the cornea. When it involves both, the disorder is termed *keratoconjunctivitis.*

Bacterial Infections. The cornea can become infected by a variety of bacteria. Topical antibiotics are generally effective, but eradicating the infection may require subconjunctival antibiotic injection or, in severe cases, IV antibiotics. Risk factors include mechanical or chemical corneal epithelial damage, contact lens wear, nutritional deficiencies, immunosuppressed states, and contaminated products (e.g., lens care solutions and cases, topical medications, cosmetics).

Viral Infections. Herpes simplex virus (HSV) keratitis is the most frequently occurring infectious cause of corneal blindness in the Western hemisphere. It is a growing problem, especially with immunosuppressed patients. The corneal ulcer has a characteristic dendritic (tree-branching) appearance. Pain and photophobia are common.

Antiviral treatments include trifluridine drops (Viroptic), oral acyclovir (Zovirax), and topical vidarabine (Vira-A) ointment. Therapy may also involve corneal debridement. Topical corticosteroids are usually contraindicated because they contribute to a longer course and possible deeper ulceration of the cornea.

The varicella-zoster virus (VZV) causes both chickenpox and herpes zoster ophthalmicus (HZO). HZO may occur by reactivation of an endogenous infection that has persisted in a latent form after an earlier attack of varicella or by contact with a patient with chickenpox or herpes zoster. It occurs most frequently in the older adult and in the immunosuppressed patient. Care of the patient with acute HZO may include analgesics for pain, topical corticosteroids to reduce inflammation, antiviral agents such as acyclovir to reduce viral replication, mydriatic agents to dilate the pupil and relieve pain, and topical antibiotics to combat secondary infection. The patient may apply warm compresses and povidone-iodine gel to the affected skin (gel should not be applied near the eye).

Epidemic keratoconjunctivitis (EKC) is the most serious ocular adenoviral disease. EKC is spread by direct contact, including sexual activity. In the medical setting, contaminated hands and instruments can be the source of spread. The patient may complain of tearing, redness, photophobia, and foreign body sensation. In most patients the disease involves only one eye. Treatment is primarily palliative and includes ice packs and dark glasses. In severe cases therapy can include mild topical corticosteroids to temporarily relieve symptoms and topical antibiotic ointment. Teach the patient the importance of good hygiene practices to avoid spreading the disease.

Other Causes of Keratitis. Keratitis may also be caused by fungi (most commonly *Aspergillus, Candida,* and *Fusarium* species), especially in the case of ocular trauma in an outdoor setting where fungi are prevalent in the soil and moist organic matter.

Acanthamoeba keratitis is caused by a parasite that is associated with contact lens wear, probably as a result of contaminated lens care solutions or cases. Homemade saline solution is particularly susceptible to *Acanthamoeba* contamination. Instruct the patient who wears contact lenses about good lens care practices. Medical treatment of *Acanthamoeba* keratitis is difficult, since the organism is resistant to most drugs. Antifungal agents (e.g., ketoconazole [Nizoral] and polyhexamethylene biguanide [PHMB]) may be used. If antimicrobial therapy fails, the patient may require a corneal transplant.

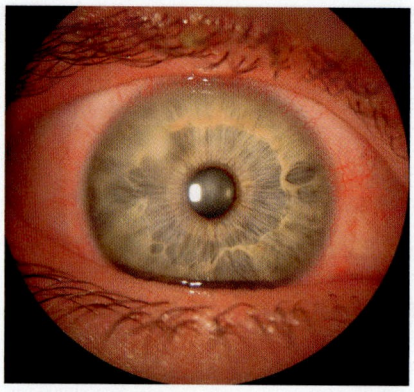

FIG. 21-2 Corneal ulcer. Infection associated with poor contact lens care. (Courtesy Cory J. Bosanko, OD, FAAO, Eye Centers of Tennessee, Crossville, Tenn.)

Exposure keratitis occurs when the patient cannot adequately close the eyelids. The patient with *exophthalmos* (protruding eyeball) from thyroid eye disease or masses posterior to the globe is susceptible to exposure keratitis.

Corneal Ulcer. Tissue loss caused by infection of the cornea produces a *corneal ulcer* (infectious keratitis) (Fig. 21-2). The infection can be due to bacteria, viruses, or fungi. Corneal ulcers are often painful, and patients may feel as if there is a foreign body in their eye. Other symptoms can include tearing, purulent or watery discharge, redness, and photophobia. Treatment is generally aggressive to avoid permanent loss of vision. Antibiotic, antiviral, or antifungal eye drops may be prescribed as frequently as every hour night and day for the first 24 hours. An untreated corneal ulcer can result in corneal scarring and perforation (hole in the cornea). A corneal transplant may be indicated.

❖ NURSING MANAGEMENT: INFLAMMATION AND INFECTION

Assess ocular changes, such as edema, redness, decreased visual acuity, feelings that a foreign body is present, or discomfort. Document the findings in the patient's record. Also consider the psychosocial aspects of the patient's condition, especially when vision is impaired.

Careful asepsis and frequent, thorough hand washing are essential to prevent spreading organisms from one eye to the other, to other patients, to family members, and to health care professionals. Teach the patient and family about avoiding sources of ocular irritation or infection and responding appropriately if an ocular problem occurs. Inform the patient about appropriate use and care of lenses and lens care products. The patient with infective disorders that may have a sexual mode of transmission needs specific information about those disorders.

Apply warm or cool compresses if indicated for the patient's condition. Darkening the room and providing an appropriate analgesic are other comfort measures. If the patient's visual acuity is decreased, modify the patient's environment or activities for safety.

The patient may require eye drops as frequently as every hour. If the patient receives two or more different drops, stagger the eye drops to promote maximum absorption. For example, if two different eye drops are ordered hourly, administer one drop on the hour and one drop on the half hour (unless otherwise prescribed). The patient who needs frequent eye drop administration may experience sleep deprivation.

The patient's primary need is for information about required care and how to accomplish that care. Also instruct the patient and caregiver about the proper techniques for medication administration. If the patient's vision is compromised, suggest alternative ways to accomplish necessary daily activities and self-care. Inform the patient who wears contact lenses and develops infections to discard all opened or used lens care products and cosmetics to decrease the risk of reinfection from contaminated products (a common problem and a probable source of infection for many patients).

DRY EYE DISORDERS

Keratoconjunctivitis sicca (dry eyes) is a common complaint, particularly of older adults and individuals with certain systemic diseases such as scleroderma and systemic lupus erythematosus. Patients with dry eyes complain of irritation or "sand in my eye" and that the sensation typically worsens through the day. This condition is caused by a decrease in the quality or quantity of the tear film, and treatment is directed at the underlying cause.

With decreased tear secretion, the patient may use artificial tears or ointments. Restasis (cyclosporine ophthalmic emulsion) helps to increase the eyes' natural ability to produce tears. In severe cases, closure of the lacrimal puncta may be necessary. Patients with dry eyes associated with dry mouth may have Sjögren's syndrome (see Chapter 64).

STRABISMUS

Strabismus is a condition in which the patient cannot consistently focus two eyes simultaneously on the same object. One eye may deviate in *(esotropia)*, out *(exotropia)*, up *(hypertropia)*, or down *(hypotropia)*. Strabismus in the adult may be caused by thyroid disease, neuromuscular problems of the eye muscles, retinal detachment repair, or cerebral lesions. In the adult the primary complaint with strabismus is double vision.

CORNEAL DISORDERS

Corneal Scars

The cornea is an optically transparent tissue that allows light rays to enter the eye and focus on the retina, thus producing a visual image. Any wound (trauma, infection) to the cornea can cause it to become scarred and opacified, thus decreasing the normal transparency. The treatment for corneal scars is a corneal transplant.

Keratoconus

Keratoconus is a noninflammatory, usually bilateral disease that has a familial tendency. Keratoconus usually appears during adolescence and slowly progresses between ages 20 and 60 years. The anterior cornea thins and protrudes forward, taking on a cone shape. The only symptom is blurred vision. The astigmatism may be corrected with glasses or rigid contact lenses.

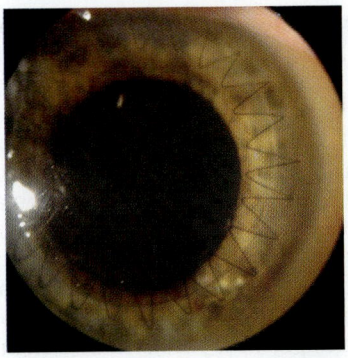

FIG. 21-3 Sutures on a donated cornea after penetrating keratoplasty (corneal transplant). (Courtesy Cory J. Bosanko, OD, FAAO, Eye Centers of Tennessee, Crossville, Tenn.)

Intacs inserts are two clear plastic lenses surgically inserted on the cornea perimeter to reduce astigmatism and myopia. Intacs are generally used to delay the need for a corneal transplant when contact lenses or glasses no longer help a patient achieve adequate vision.

In keratoconus the cornea can perforate as central corneal thinning progresses. In advanced cases, a corneal transplant is indicated before the cornea perforates.

Corneal Transplant. Indications for corneal transplants (keratoplasty) are corneal scarring and keratoconus. Types of corneal transplants include penetrating (full thickness) corneal transplant and lamellar corneal transplant.

Penetrating (full thickness) cornea transplant involves transplanting all the layers of the cornea using a donor cornea. In this procedure, the ophthalmic surgeon removes the full thickness of the patient's cornea and replaces it with a donor cornea that is sutured into place (Fig. 21-3). Vision may not be restored for up to 12 months.

During a *lamellar cornea transplant*, only some layers of the cornea are replaced with the transplant. This can include the deepest layer, called the *endothelium* (posterior lamellar cornea transplant). Commonly performed versions of this procedure include Descemet's stripping endothelial keratoplasty (DSEK) or Descemet's membrane endothelial keratoplasty (DMEK). Lamellar transplants may be more appropriate than full penetrating transplants when the disease process is limited to only a portion of the cornea.

Approximately 40,000 corneal transplants are performed in the United States each year. The surgery is one of the fastest and safest of all tissue or organ transplant surgeries.[9] The time between the donor's death and the removal of the tissue should be as short as possible. The eye banks test donors for human immunodeficiency virus (HIV) and hepatitis B and C. The tissue is preserved in a special nutritive solution. Improved methods of tissue procurement and preservation, postoperative topical corticosteroids, and careful follow-up have decreased graft rejection. Matching the blood type of the donor and recipient may also improve the success rate.

INTRAOCULAR DISORDERS

CATARACT

A **cataract** is an opacity within the lens. The patient may have a cataract in one or both eyes. If cataracts are present in both eyes, one may affect the patient's vision more than the other.

Cataract removal is the most common surgical procedure in the United States.[10]

Etiology and Pathophysiology

Although most cataracts are age related *(senile cataracts)*, they can be associated with other factors. These include blunt or penetrating trauma, congenital factors such as maternal rubella, radiation or ultraviolet (UV) light exposure, certain drugs such as systemic corticosteroids or long-term topical corticosteroids, and ocular inflammation. The patient with diabetes mellitus tends to develop cataracts at a younger age.

Cataract development is mediated by a number of factors. In senile cataract formation altered metabolic processes within the lens cause an accumulation of water and alterations in the lens fiber structure. These changes affect lens transparency, causing vision changes.

Clinical Manifestations and Diagnostic Studies

The patient with cataracts may complain of a decrease in vision, abnormal color perception, and glare. Glare is due to light scatter caused by the lens opacities, and it may be significantly worse at night when the pupil dilates. The visual decline is gradual, but the rate of cataract development varies from patient to patient.

Diagnosis is based on decreased visual acuity or other complaints of visual dysfunction. The opacity is directly observable by ophthalmoscopic or slit lamp microscopic examination. A totally opaque lens creates the appearance of a white pupil. Table 21-2 lists other diagnostic studies that may be helpful in evaluation of a cataract.

Interprofessional Care

The presence of a cataract does not necessarily indicate a need for surgery. For many patients the diagnosis is made long before they actually decide to have surgery. Nonsurgical therapy may postpone the need for surgery. Interprofessional care for cataracts is presented in Table 21-2.

TABLE 21-2 Interprofessional Care

Cataract

Diagnostic Assessment

- History and physical examination
- Visual acuity measurement
- Ophthalmoscopy (direct and indirect)
- Slit lamp microscopy
- Glare testing, potential acuity testing in selected patients
- Keratometry and A-scan ultrasound (if surgery is planned)
- Other tests (e.g., visual field perimetry) to determine cause of visual loss

Management

Nonsurgical

- Change in glasses prescription
- Strong reading glasses or magnifiers
- Increased lighting
- Lifestyle adjustment

Acute Care: Surgical Therapy

Preoperative

- Mydriatic, cycloplegic agents
- Nonsteroidal antiinflammatory drugs
- Topical antibiotics
- Antianxiety medications

Surgery

- Removal of lens
- Phacoemulsification
- Extracapsular extraction
- Correction of surgical aphakia
- Intraocular lens implantation (most frequent type of correction)
- Contact lenses

Postoperative

- Topical antibiotic
- Topical corticosteroid or other antiinflammatory agent
- Mild analgesia if necessary
- Eye patch or shield and activity as prescribed by patient's surgeon

Nonsurgical Therapy. Currently, no treatment is available to "cure" cataracts other than surgical removal. Often changing the patient's eyewear prescription can improve visual acuity, at least temporarily. Other visual aids, such as strong reading glasses or magnifiers of some type, may help the patient with near vision. Increasing the amount of light to read or accomplish other near-vision tasks is another useful measure. The patient may be willing to adjust his or her lifestyle to adjust to visual decline. For example, if glare makes it difficult to drive at night, a patient may elect to drive only during daylight hours or to have a family member drive at night. Sometimes informing and reassuring the patient about the disease process makes the patient comfortable about choosing nonsurgical measures, at least temporarily.

Surgical Therapy. When palliative measures no longer provide an acceptable level of visual function, the patient is an appropriate candidate for surgery. The patient's occupational needs and lifestyle changes are also factors affecting the decision to have surgery. In some instances, factors other than the patient's visual needs may influence the need for surgery. Lens-induced problems such as increased intraocular pressure (IOP) may require lens removal. Opacities may prevent the ophthalmologist from obtaining a clear view of the retina in the patient with diabetic retinopathy or other sight-threatening pathologic conditions. In those cases, the cataract may be removed to allow visualization of the retina and adequate management of the problem.

Preoperative Phase. The patient's preoperative preparation should include an appropriate history and physical examination. Because almost all patients have local anesthesia, many physicians and surgical facilities do not require an extensive preoperative physical assessment. However, most patients with cataracts are older adults who may have several medical problems that should be evaluated and controlled before surgery. Almost all patients with cataracts are admitted to a surgical facility on an outpatient basis. The patient is normally admitted several hours before surgery to allow time for preoperative procedures.

The patient receives dilating drops and a nonsteroidal antiinflammatory eye drop to reduce inflammation (depends on ophthalmologist's preference). One type of drug used for dilation is a *mydriatic*, an α-adrenergic agonist that produces pupillary dilation by contraction of the iris dilator muscle. Another type of drug is a *cycloplegic*, an anticholinergic agent that produces paralysis of accommodation (cycloplegia) by blocking the effect of acetylcholine on the ciliary body muscles. Cycloplegics (tropicamide [Mydriacyl, Tropicacyl]) produce pupillary dilation (mydriasis) by blocking the effect of acetylcholine on the iris sphincter muscle. The patient may receive preoperative antianxiety medication.

DRUG ALERT Cycloplegics and Mydriatics

- Instruct patient to wear dark glasses to minimize photophobia.
- Monitor for signs of systemic toxicity (e.g., tachycardia, central nervous system [CNS] effects).

Intraoperative Phase. Cataract extraction is an intraocular procedure using an operating microscope. The most common form of cataract surgery is *phacoemulsification*. In this procedure, a very small incision is made in the surface of the eye in or near the cornea. A thin ultrasound probe is inserted into the

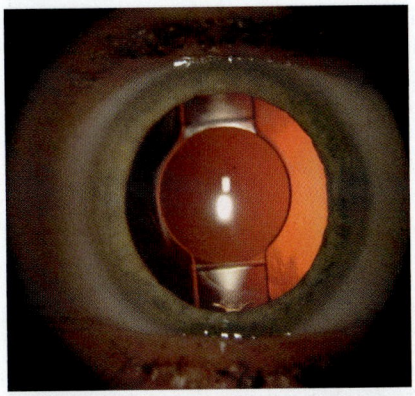

FIG. 21-4 Intraocular lens implant after cataract surgery. (Courtesy Cory J. Bosanko, OD, FAAO, Eye Centers of Tennessee, Crossville, Tenn.)

eye and ultrasonic vibrations are used to dissolve (phacoemulsify) the clouded lens into fragments. These pieces are then suctioned out through the same ultrasound probe. The small incisions are self-sealing and usually do not require sutures.

An *extracapsular cataract extraction procedure* is used mainly for very advanced cataracts where the lens is too dense to dissolve into fragments. This technique requires a larger incision so that the cataract can be removed in one piece without being fragmented inside the eye. This surgical technique requires sutures to close the larger wound, and visual recovery is often slower.

Almost all patients have an IOL implanted at the time of cataract extraction surgery (Fig. 21-4). The lens of choice is a posterior chamber lens that is implanted in the capsular bag behind the iris. At the end of the procedure, additional medications such as antibiotics and corticosteroids may be administered.

Postoperative Phase. Unless complications occur, the patient is usually ready to go home as soon as the effects of sedative agents have worn off. Postoperative medications usually include antibiotic drops to prevent infection and corticosteroid drops to decrease the postoperative inflammatory response. Recommendations for postoperative activity restrictions and nighttime eye shielding vary based on the ophthalmologist's preference. Many still prefer that the patient avoid activities that increase the IOP, such as bending or stooping, coughing, or lifting.

During each postoperative examination the ophthalmologist measures the patient's visual acuity, checks anterior chamber depth, assesses corneal clarity, and measures intraocular pressure (IOP). Even on the operative day the patient's uncorrected visual acuity in the operative eye may be good. However, it is not unusual or indicative of any problem if the patient's visual acuity is reduced immediately after surgery.

The postoperative eye drops are gradually reduced in frequency and finally discontinued when the eye has healed. Multifocal IOL can correct for both near and far vision. Regardless of the type of IOL used, patients may still need glasses or contact lenses to achieve their best visual acuity.

❖ NURSING MANAGEMENT: CATARACTS

◆ Nursing Assessment

Assess the patient's distance and near visual acuity. If the patient is going to have surgery, especially note the visual acuity in the patient's unoperated eye. Use this information to determine how visually compromised the patient may be while the operative eye is healing. In addition, assess the psychosocial impact of the patient's visual disability and the level of knowledge regarding the disease process and therapeutic options. Postoperatively, assess the patient's level of comfort and ability to follow the postoperative regimen.

◆ Nursing Diagnoses

Nursing diagnoses for the patient with a cataract include, but are not limited to, the following:

- Self-care deficits *related to* visual deficit
- Anxiety *related to* lack of knowledge about the surgical and postoperative experience

◆ Planning

Preoperatively, the overall goals are that the patient with a cataract will (1) make informed decisions regarding therapeutic options and (2) experience minimal anxiety. Postoperatively, the overall goals are that the patient with a cataract will (1) understand and comply with postoperative therapy, (2) maintain an acceptable level of physical and emotional comfort, and (3) remain free of infection and other complications.

◆ Nursing Implementation

◆ **Health Promotion.** There are no proven measures to prevent cataract development. However, it is probably wise (and certainly does no harm) to suggest that the patient wear sunglasses, avoid extraneous or unnecessary radiation, and maintain appropriate intake of antioxidant vitamins (e.g., vitamins C and E) and good nutrition. Also provide information about vision enhancement techniques for the patient who chooses not to have surgery.

◆ **Acute Care.** Preoperatively, the patient with cataracts needs accurate information about the disease process and treatment options, especially because cataract surgery is considered an elective procedure. Be available to give the patient and family information to help them make an informed decision about appropriate treatment. For the patient who elects to have surgery, provide information, support, and reassurance about the surgical and postoperative experience to reduce or alleviate anxiety.

Photophobia is common when administering pupil dilation medications. Therefore decreasing the room lighting is helpful. These medications produce transient stinging and burning. Table 21-3 outlines patient and caregiver teaching after eye surgery.

If a patch is used, inform patients that they will not have depth perception until the patch is removed. This necessitates special considerations to avoid falls or other injuries. The patient with significant visual impairment in the unoperated eye requires more assistance while the operative eye is patched. Some patients may require 1 or 2 weeks for the visual acuity in the operated eye to reach an adequate level for most visual needs. These patients also need some special assistance until the vision improves.

After cataract surgery the patient usually experiences little or no pain but may have some scratchiness or blurriness in the operative eye. Mild analgesics are usually sufficient to relieve any pain. If the pain is intense, the patient should notify the surgeon because this may indicate hemorrhage, infection, or increased IOP. Also instruct the patient to notify the surgeon if there is increased or purulent drainage, increased redness, or any decrease in visual acuity. A nursing care plan for the patient

TABLE 21-3 Patient & Caregiver Teaching

After Eye Surgery

Include the following information in the teaching plan for the patient and caregiver after eye surgery.

- Proper hygiene and eye care techniques to ensure that medications, dressings, and/or surgical wound is not contaminated during eye care
- Signs and symptoms of infection and when and how to report these to allow for early recognition and treatment of possible infection
- Importance of complying with postoperative restrictions on head positioning, bending, coughing, and Valsalva maneuver to optimize visual outcomes and prevent increased intraocular pressure
- How to instill eye medications using aseptic techniques and adherence with prescribed eye medication routine to prevent infection
- How to monitor pain, take pain medication, and report pain not relieved by medication
- Importance of continued follow-up as recommended to maximize potential visual outcomes

after eye surgery (eNursing Care Plan 21-1) is available on the website for this chapter.

◆ **Ambulatory Care.** Patients with cataracts who have surgery remain in the surgical facility for only a few hours. The patient and caregiver are responsible for almost all postoperative care. Give them written and verbal instructions before discharge, including information about postoperative eye care, activity restrictions, medications, follow-up visit schedule, and signs and symptoms of possible complications. Include the patient's caregiver in the instructions because some patients may have difficulty with self-care activities, especially if the vision in the unoperated eye is poor. Provide an opportunity for the patient and caregiver to perform return demonstrations of any self-care activities.

Most patients experience little visual impairment after surgery. IOL implants provide immediate visual rehabilitation, and many patients achieve a usable level of visual acuity within a few days after surgery.

A few patients may have significant visual impairment postoperatively. These include patients who do not have an IOL implanted at the time of surgery, those who require several weeks to achieve a usable level of visual acuity following surgery, or those with poor vision in their unoperated eye. For those patients the time between surgery and receiving glasses or contacts can be a period of significant visual disability. Suggest ways the patient and caregiver can modify activities and the environment to maintain an adequate level of safe functioning. Suggestions may include getting assistance with steps, removing area rugs and other potential obstacles, preparing meals for freezing before surgery, or obtaining audio books for diversion until visual acuity improves.

◆ Evaluation

The overall expected outcomes are that the patient following cataract surgery will

- Have improved vision
- Be better able to take care of self
- Have minimal to no pain
- Be optimistic about expected outcomes

Gerontologic Considerations: Cataracts

Most patients with cataracts are older. When the older patient is visually impaired, even temporarily, the patient may experience a loss of independence, lack of control over her or his life, and a significant change in self-perception. Societal devaluation of the older individual complicates these experiences. The older patient often needs emotional support and encouragement, as well as specific suggestions to allow a maximum level of independent function. Assure the older patient that cataract surgery can be accomplished safely and comfortably with minimal sedation.

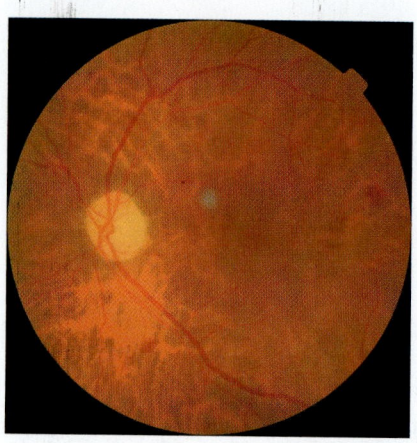

FIG. 21-5 Diabetic retinopathy. Intraretinal dot or blot hemorrhages. (Courtesy Cory J. Bosanko, OD, FAAO, Eye Centers of Tennessee, Crossville, Tenn.)

RETINOPATHY

Retinopathy is a process of microvascular damage to the retina. It can develop slowly or rapidly and lead to blurred vision and progressive vision loss. Retinopathy occurs most often in adults with diabetes mellitus or hypertension.

Diabetic retinopathy is a common complication of diabetes mellitus, especially in patients with long-standing uncontrolled diabetes.[11] *Nonproliferative retinopathy* is the most common form of diabetic retinopathy and is characterized by capillary microaneurysms, retinal swelling, and hard exudates. Macular edema represents a worsening of the retinopathy as plasma leaks from macular blood vessels. As capillary walls weaken, they can rupture, leading to intraretinal "dot or blot" hemorrhaging (Fig. 21-5). A severe loss in central vision can result. As the disease advances, *proliferative retinopathy* may occur. New blood vessels grow, but they are abnormal, fragile, and predisposed to leak, thus causing severe vision loss. (Diagnosis and treatment of diabetic retinopathy are discussed in Chapter 48.)

Hypertensive retinopathy is caused by high BP creating blockages in retinal blood vessels. (Hypertension is discussed in Chapter 32.) These changes may not initially affect a person's vision. On a routine eye examination, retinal hemorrhages, anoxic cotton-wool spots, and macular swelling can be noted. Sustained, severe hypertension can cause sudden visual loss from swelling of the optic disc and nerve *(papilledema)*. Treatment, which may be an emergency, focuses on lowering the BP. Normal vision is restored in most patients with treatment of the underlying cause of the hypertension.

RETINAL DETACHMENT

A **retinal detachment** is a separation of the sensory retina and the underlying pigment epithelium, with fluid accumulation between the two layers. In the patient with no other risk factors who has had a retinal detachment in one eye, the risk of detachment in the second eye is as high as 25%.[12] Almost all patients with an untreated, symptomatic retinal detachment become blind in the involved eye.

Etiology and Pathophysiology

Retinal detachment has many causes, the most common of which is a retinal break. *Retinal breaks* are an interruption in the full thickness of the retinal tissue, and they can be classified as tears or holes. *Retinal holes* are atrophic retinal breaks that occur spontaneously. *Retinal tears* can occur as the vitreous humor shrinks during aging and pulls on the retina. The retina tears when the traction force exceeds the strength of the retina. Once the retina has a break, liquid vitreous can enter the subretinal space between the sensory layer and the retinal pigment epithelium layer, causing a *rhegmatogenous* retinal detachment. Risk factors for retinal detachment are listed in Table 21-4.

Clinical Manifestations and Diagnostic Studies

Patients with a detaching retina describe symptoms that include *photopsia* (light flashes); floaters; and a "cobweb," "hairnet," or ring in the field of vision. Once the retina has detached, the patient describes a painless loss of peripheral or central vision, "like a curtain" coming across the field of vision.

The area of visual loss corresponds inversely to the area of detachment. For example, if the retinal detachment involves the superior retina, the defect is seen in the inferior visual field. If the detachment is small or develops slowly, the patient may not be aware of a visual problem.

Visual acuity measurements should be the first diagnostic procedure with any complaint of vision loss (Table 21-5). The retinal detachment can be directly visualized using direct and indirect ophthalmoscopy or slit lamp microscopy in conjunction with a special lens to view the far periphery of the retina.

TABLE 21-4 Risk Factors for Retinal Detachment

- Increasing age
- Severe myopia
- Eye trauma
- Cataract surgery
- Family or personal history of retinal detachment

Source: National Eye Institute, National Institutes of Health: Retinal detachment. Retrieved from *www.nei.nih.gov/health/retinaldetach.*

TABLE 21-5 Interprofessional Care

Retinal Detachment

Diagnostic Assessment

- History and physical examination
- Visual acuity measurement
- Ophthalmoscopy (direct and indirect)
- Slit lamp microscopy
- Ultrasound if cornea, lens, or vitreous is hazy or opaque

Management

Preoperative

- Mydriatic, cycloplegic agents
- Photocoagulation of retinal break that has not progressed to detachment

Surgery

- Laser photocoagulation
- Cryopexy
- Scleral buckling procedure
- Vitrectomy
- Intravitreal bubble

Postoperative

- Topical antibiotic
- Topical corticosteroid
- Analgesia
- Mydriatics
- Positioning and activity as prescribed by patient's surgeon

Ultrasound may be useful in identifying a retinal detachment if the retina cannot be directly visualized (e.g., when the cornea, lens, or vitreous is hazy or opaque).

Interprofessional Care

Some retinal breaks are not likely to progress to detachment. In these situations the ophthalmologist simply monitors the patient, giving precise information about the warning signs and symptoms of impending detachment and instructing the patient to seek immediate evaluation if any of those signs or symptoms is recognized. The ophthalmologist usually refers the patient with a detachment to a retinal specialist. Treatment objectives are to seal any retinal breaks and relieve inward traction on the retina. Several techniques are used to accomplish these objectives.

Surgical Therapy

Laser Photocoagulation and Cryopexy. These techniques seal retinal breaks by creating an inflammatory reaction that causes a chorioretinal adhesion or scar. *Laser photocoagulation* involves using an intense, precisely focused light beam to create an inflammatory reaction. The light is directed at the area of the retinal break. *Cryopexy* involves freezing (cryotherapy) the retinal break by placing a probe on the ocular surface at the location of the break. The probe is activated with compressed nitrous oxide gas that temporarily freezes the break. The freeze thaw reaction creates scarring in the area that will seal the break.

For retinal breaks accompanied by significant detachment, the retinal specialist may use photocoagulation or cryopexy intraoperatively in conjunction with scleral buckling. Tears or holes without accompanying retinal detachment may be treated prophylactically with laser photocoagulation or cryopexy if there is a high risk of progression to a retinal detachment. When used alone, laser photocoagulation or cryopexy therapy is an outpatient procedure that usually requires only topical anesthesia. The patient may experience minimal adverse symptoms during or after the procedure.

Scleral Buckling. *Scleral buckling* is an extraocular surgical procedure that involves indenting the globe so that the pigment epithelium, choroid, and sclera move toward the detached retina. The retinal surgeon sutures a silicone implant against the sclera, causing the sclera to buckle inward. The surgeon may place an encircling band over the implant if there are multiple retinal breaks, if suspected breaks cannot be located, or if there is widespread inward traction on the retina (Fig. 21-6). If present, subretinal fluid may be drained by inserting a small-gauge needle to facilitate contact between the retina and buckled sclera. Scleral buckling is usually done as an outpatient procedure.

Intraocular Procedures. In addition to the extraocular procedures described, retinal surgeons may also use one or more intraocular procedures in treating some retinal detachments. *Pneumatic retinopexy* is the intravitreal injection of a gas to form a temporary bubble in the vitreous that closes retinal breaks and provides apposition of the separated retinal layers. Because the intravitreal bubble is temporary, this technique is combined with laser photocoagulation or cryopexy. The patient with an intravitreal bubble must position the head so that the bubble is in contact with the retinal break. The patient may need to maintain this position as much as possible for up to several weeks.

Vitrectomy (surgical removal of the vitreous) may be used to relieve traction on the retina, especially when the traction results from proliferative diabetic retinopathy. Vitrectomy may

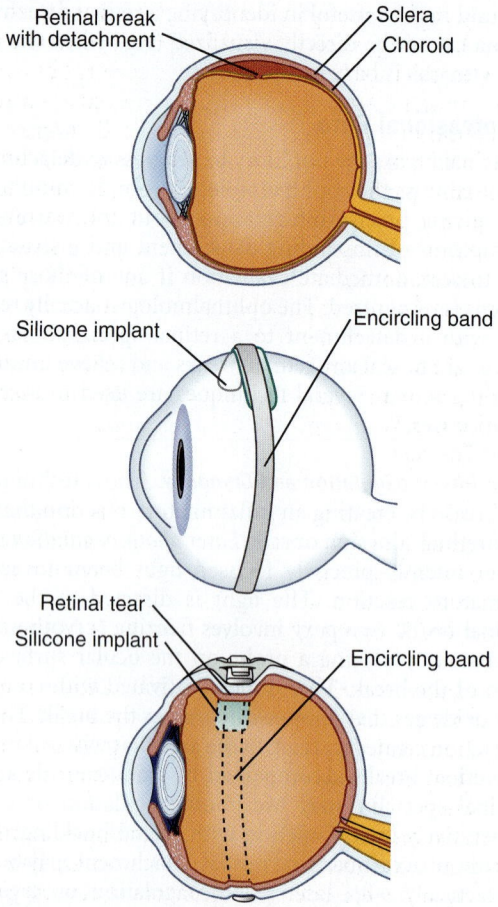

FIG. 21-6 Retinal break with detachment and surgical repair by scleral buckling technique.

be combined with scleral buckling to provide a dual effect in relieving traction.

Postoperative Considerations. Visual prognosis varies, depending on the extent, length, and area of detachment. Postoperatively the patient may be on bed rest and may require special positioning to maintain proper position of an intravitreal bubble. The patient may need multiple topical medications, including antibiotics, antiinflammatory agents, or dilating agents. The level of activity restriction after retinal detachment surgery varies greatly. Verify the prescribed level of activity with each patient's surgeon, and help the patient plan for any necessary assistance related to activity restrictions.

In most cases, retinal detachment is an urgent situation, and the patient is suddenly confronted with the need for surgery. The patient needs emotional support, especially during the immediate preoperative period when preparations for surgery can lead to additional anxiety. When the patient experiences postoperative pain, administer prescribed pain medications and teach the patient to take the medication as necessary after discharge. The patient may go home within a few hours of surgery or may remain in the hospital for several days, depending on the surgeon and type of repair.

Discharge planning and teaching are important and should begin as early as possible because the patient does not remain hospitalized long. Patient and caregiver teaching after eye surgery is discussed in Table 21-5. Because the patient is at increased risk for retinal detachment in the other eye, teach the patient the signs and symptoms of retinal detachment. Also promote the use of proper protective eyewear to help avoid ocular damage related to trauma.

AGE-RELATED MACULAR DEGENERATION

Age-related macular degeneration (AMD) is the most common cause of irreversible central vision loss in people over age 60 in the United States. AMD is divided into two forms: dry (nonexudative) and wet (exudative). People with *dry AMD,* which is the more common form (90% of all cases), often notice that close vision tasks are becoming more difficult. In this form of AMD the macular cells start to atrophy, leading to a slowly progressive and painless vision loss.

Wet AMD is the more severe form. Wet AMD accounts for the majority of the cases of AMD-related blindness. Wet AMD has a more rapid onset of vision loss and is characterized by the development of abnormal blood vessels in or near the macula. Patients with wet AMD had dry AMD first.

Etiology and Pathophysiology

AMD is related to retinal aging. Genetic factors also play a major role, and family history is a major risk factor for AMD.[13] Increased risk factors for AMD include white ethnicity, family history of AMD, chronic inflammation conditions, smoking, and hypertension.

Nutritional factors may play a role in the progression of AMD. A dietary supplement of vitamin C, vitamin E, lutein, zeaxanthin, and zinc decreases the progression of advanced AMD but has no effect on people with minimal AMD or those with no evidence of AMD. Eating lots of dark green, leafy vegetables containing lutein (e.g., kale and spinach) may help reduce the risk of AMD *(www.nei.nih.gov/health/maculardegen/armd_facts.asp)*.

The dry form of AMD starts with the abnormal accumulation of yellowish extracellular deposits called *drusen* in the retinal pigment epithelium. Over time atrophy and degeneration of macular cells occur. Wet AMD is characterized by the growth of new blood vessels in an abnormal location in the retinal epithelium. As the new blood vessels grow, they leak fluid and can bleed, causing scar tissue to gradually form. Acute vision loss may occur from either the dry or wet forms of AMD.

Clinical Manifestations and Diagnostic Studies

The patient may complain of blurred and darkened vision, *scotomas* (blind spots in the visual field), and *metamorphopsia* (distortion of vision). If patients have only one eye affected, they may not notice early changes in their vision. In addition to visual acuity measurement, the primary diagnostic procedure is ophthalmoscopy. The examiner looks for drusen and other fundus changes associated with AMD. The Amsler grid test may help define the involved area, and it provides a baseline for future comparison (see Fig. 20-6). Fundus photography and IV angiography with fluorescein and/or indocyanine green dyes may help to further determine the extent and type of AMD. Retinal anatomy can also be analyzed using optical coherence tomography (OCT) or scanning laser ophthalmoscopy.

Interprofessional Care

Visual prognosis varies greatly for people with AMD. Limited treatment options for patients with wet AMD include several medications that are injected directly into the vitreous cavity. Ranibizumab (Lucentis), bevacizumab (Avastin), aflibercept

(Eylea), and pegaptanib (Macugen) are selective inhibitors of endothelial growth factor, thus helping to slow vision loss in wet AMD. Side effects can include blurred vision, eye irritation, eye pain, and photosensitivity. Injections are given at 4- to 6-week intervals, depending on treatment response. Disease stability is determined by OCT, which allows the physician to identify pathology in the macula. The findings determine the need for continued intravitreal injections.

Photodynamic therapy (PDT) uses verteporfin (Visudyne) IV and a "cold" laser to excite the dye. The PDT procedure is used in wet AMD and damages the abnormal blood vessels in wet AMD. Verteporfin is a photosensitizing drug that becomes active when exposed to the low-level laser light wave. Until the drug is completely excreted by the body, it can be activated by exposure to sunlight or other high-intensity light such as halogen. Therefore caution patients to avoid direct exposure to sunlight and other intense forms of light for 5 days after treatment. After receiving therapy, patients must be completely covered because any exposure of the skin to sunlight could activate the drug in that area, resulting in a chemical burn.

People at risk for developing advanced AMD should consider supplements of vitamins and minerals (in consultation with their HCP). The cessation of smoking may also help in halting the progression of dry AMD to a more advanced stage.

Many patients with low-vision assistive devices can continue reading and retain a license to drive during the daytime and at lowered speeds. The permanent loss of central vision has significant psychosocial implications for nursing care. Management of the patient with visual impairment is discussed on p. 369 and is appropriate for the patient with AMD. Avoid giving the impression that "nothing can be done" about the problem when caring for the patient with AMD. Although therapy may not recover lost vision, much can be done to augment the remaining vision.

GLAUCOMA

Glaucoma is a group of disorders characterized by increased IOP and the consequences of elevated pressure, optic nerve atrophy, and peripheral visual field loss. Glaucoma is the second leading cause of permanent blindness in the United States and the leading cause of blindness among African Americans.[14] Many people with glaucoma are unaware of their condition. The incidence of glaucoma increases with age. Blindness from glaucoma is largely preventable with early detection and appropriate treatment. Genetic factors have been identified in some types of glaucoma.[13]

Etiology and Pathophysiology

A proper balance between the rate of aqueous production (referred to as *inflow*) and the rate of aqueous reabsorption (referred to as *outflow*) is essential to maintain the IOP within normal limits. The place where the outflow occurs is called the *angle* because it is the angle where the iris meets the cornea. When the rate of inflow is greater than the rate of outflow, IOP can increase above the normal limits. If IOP remains elevated, permanent vision loss may occur.

Primary open-angle glaucoma (POAG) is the most common type of glaucoma. In POAG the outflow of aqueous humor is decreased in the trabecular meshwork. The drainage channels become clogged, like a clogged kitchen sink. Damage to the optic nerve can then result.

Primary angle-closure glaucoma (PACG) is due to a reduction in the outflow of aqueous humor that results from angle closure. Usually this is caused by the lens bulging forward as a result of the aging process. Angle closure may also occur as a result of pupil dilation in the patient with anatomically narrow angles. An acute attack may be precipitated by situations in which the pupil remains partially dilated long enough to cause an acute and significant rise in the IOP. This may occur because of drug-induced mydriasis, emotional excitement, or darkness. Drug-induced mydriasis may occur not only from topical ophthalmic preparations but also from many systemic medications (both prescription and over-the-counter [OTC] drugs). Check drug records and documentation before administering medications to the patient with angle-closure glaucoma, and instruct the patient not to take any mydriatic medications.

Clinical Manifestations

POAG develops slowly and without symptoms of pain or pressure. The patient usually does not notice the gradual visual field loss until peripheral vision has been severely compromised. Eventually the patient with untreated glaucoma has "tunnel vision," in which only a small center field can be seen and all peripheral vision is absent.

Acute angle-closure glaucoma causes definite symptoms, including sudden, excruciating pain in or around the eye. This is often accompanied by nausea and vomiting. Visual symptoms include seeing colored halos around lights, blurred vision, and ocular redness.

Manifestations of subacute or chronic angle-closure glaucoma appear more gradually. The patient who has had a previous, unrecognized episode of subacute angle-closure glaucoma may report a history of blurred vision, seeing colored halos around lights, ocular redness, or eye or brow pain.

Diagnostic Studies

IOP is usually elevated in glaucoma (normal is 10 to 21 mm Hg). In the patient with elevated pressures, the ophthalmologist usually repeats the measurements over time to verify the elevation. In open-angle glaucoma, IOP is usually between 22 and 32 mm Hg. In acute angle-closure glaucoma, IOP may be more than 50 mm Hg.

In open-angle glaucoma, slit lamp microscopy reveals a normal angle. In angle-closure glaucoma the examiner may note a markedly narrow or flat anterior chamber angle, an edematous cornea, a fixed and moderately dilated pupil, and ciliary injection (hyperemia of the ciliary blood vessels produces a red color).

Measures of peripheral and central vision provide additional diagnostic information. Whereas central acuity may remain 20/20 even in the presence of severe peripheral visual field loss, visual field perimetry may reveal subtle changes in the peripheral vision early in the disease process, long before actual scotomas develop. In acute angle-closure glaucoma, central visual acuity is reduced if the patient has corneal edema, and the visual fields may be markedly decreased. As glaucoma progresses, *optic disc cupping* may be one of the first signs of chronic open-angle glaucoma. The optic disc becomes wider, deeper, and paler (light gray or white), which is visible with direct or indirect ophthalmoscopy (Fig. 21-7).

Interprofessional Care

The primary focus of glaucoma therapy is to keep the IOP low enough to prevent the patient from developing optic nerve

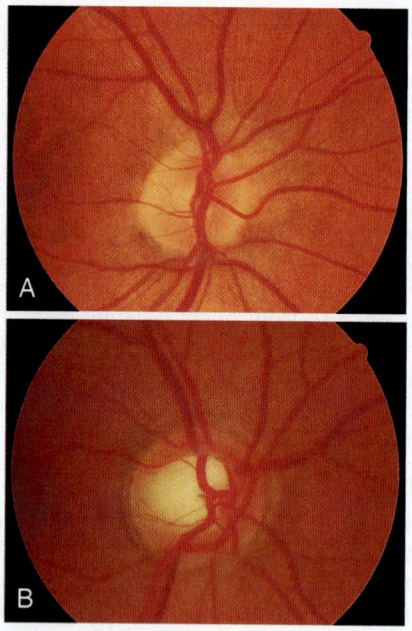

FIG. 21-7 **A,** In the normal eye the optic cup is pink with little cupping. **B,** In glaucoma the optic cup is bleached and optic cupping is present. (Note the appearance of the retinal vessels, which travel over the edge of the optic cup and appear to dip into it.)

TABLE 21-6 Interprofessional Care

Glaucoma

Diagnostic Assessment
- History and physical examination
- Visual acuity measurement
- Tonometry
- Ophthalmoscopy (direct and indirect)
- Slit lamp microscopy
- Gonioscopy
- Visual field perimetry

Management

Chronic Open-Angle Glaucoma

Drug Therapy (Table 21-7)
- β-Adrenergic blockers
- α-Adrenergic agonists
- Cholinergic agents (miotics)
- Carbonic anhydrase inhibitors

Surgical Therapy
- Argon laser trabeculoplasty (ALT)
- Trabeculectomy with or without filtering implant

Acute Angle-Closure Glaucoma
- Topical cholinergic agent
- Hyperosmotic agent
- Laser peripheral iridotomy
- Surgical iridectomy

damage. Therapy varies with the type of glaucoma. The diagnostic and interprofessional care of glaucoma is summarized in Table 21-6.

Chronic Open-Angle Glaucoma. Initial treatment in chronic open-angle glaucoma is with drugs (Table 21-7). The patient must understand that continued treatment and supervision are necessary because the drugs control, but do not cure, glaucoma.

Argon laser trabeculoplasty (ALT) is a noninvasive option to lower IOP when medications are not successful or when the patient either cannot or will not use the drug therapy as recommended. ALT is an outpatient procedure that requires only topical anesthetic. The laser stimulates scarring and contraction of the trabecular meshwork, which opens the outflow channels. ALT reduces IOP most of the time. The patient uses topical corticosteroids for 3 to 5 days after the procedure. The most common postoperative complication is an acute rise in IOP. The ophthalmologist examines the patient 1 week and again at 4 to 6 weeks after surgery.

Filtration surgery, also called a *trabeculectomy,* may be indicated if medical management and laser therapy are not successful.

Acute Angle-Closure Glaucoma. Acute angle-closure glaucoma is an ocular emergency that requires immediate intervention. Miotics (Table 21-7) and oral or IV hyperosmotic agents, including glycerin liquid (Ophthalgan), isosorbide solution (Ismotic), and mannitol solution (Osmitrol), are usually successful in immediately lowering the IOP. A laser peripheral iridotomy or surgical iridectomy is necessary for long-term treatment and prevention of subsequent episodes. These procedures allow the aqueous humor to flow through a newly created opening in the iris and into normal outflow channels. One of these procedures may also be performed on the other eye as a precaution because many patients often experience an acute attack in the other eye.

DRUG ALERT Miotics
- Warn patients about decreased visual acuity, especially in dim light.

NURSING MANAGEMENT: GLAUCOMA

Nursing Assessment

Because glaucoma is a chronic condition requiring long-term management, assess the patient's ability to understand and adhere to the rationale and regimen of the prescribed therapy. In addition, assess the patient's psychologic reaction to the diagnosis of a potentially sight-threatening chronic disorder. Include the patient's caregiver in the assessment process because the chronic nature of this disorder affects the family in many ways. Some families may become the primary care providers, such as eye drop administration, if the patient is unwilling or unable to accomplish these self-care activities.

Nursing Diagnoses

Nursing diagnoses for the patient with glaucoma include, but are not limited to, the following:
- Risk for injury *related to* visual acuity deficits
- Self-care deficits *related to* visual acuity deficits
- Acute pain *related to* pathophysiologic process and surgical correction
- Noncompliance *related to* the inconvenience and side effects of glaucoma medications

Planning

The overall goals are that the patient with glaucoma will (1) have no progression of visual impairment, (2) understand the disease process and rationale for therapy, (3) comply with all aspects of therapy (including medication administration and follow-up care), and (4) have no postoperative complications.

Nursing Implementation

Health Promotion. Loss of vision as a result of glaucoma is a preventable problem. Teach the patient and caregiver about the risk of glaucoma and that it increases with age. Stress the importance of early detection and treatment in preventing visual impairment. A comprehensive ophthalmic examination is important in identifying people with glaucoma or those at risk of developing glaucoma. The current recommendation is for an ophthalmologic examination every 2 to 4 years for people between ages 40 and

TABLE 21-7 Drug Therapy

Acute and Chronic Glaucoma

Drug	Action	Side Effects	Nursing Considerations
β-Adrenergic Blockers			
betaxolol (Betoptic)	β_1 cardioselective blocker. ↓ IOP, ↓ aqueous humor production	Transient discomfort. Systemic reactions rarely reported but include bradycardia, heart block, pulmonary distress, headache, depression	Topical drugs. Minimal effect on pulmonary and cardiovascular parameters. Contraindicated in patient with bradycardia, cardiogenic shock, or overt cardiac failure. Systemic absorption can have additive effect with systemic β_1-blocking agents.
levobunolol (Betagan) timolol maleate (Timoptic, Istalol)	β_1 and β_2 noncardioselective blockers. ↓ IOP, ↓ aqueous humor production	Transient ocular discomfort, blurred vision, photophobia, bradycardia, decreased BP, bronchospasm, headache, depression	Topical drops. Same as betaxolol. These noncardioselective β_2-blockers are also contraindicated in patients with asthma or COPD.
α-Adrenergic Agonists			
dipivefrin (Propine)	α- and β-adrenergic agonist. Converted to epinephrine inside the eye. ↓ aqueous humor production, enhances outflow facility	Ocular discomfort and redness, tachycardia, hypertension	Topical drops. Contraindicated in patient with narrow-angle glaucoma. Teach punctal occlusion if patient at risk of systemic reactions.
epinephrine	Same as dipivefrin	Same as dipivefrin, but can be more pronounced	Topical drops. Same as dipivefrin
apraclonidine (Iopidine) brimonidine	α-Adrenergic agonists. ↓ aqueous humor production	Ocular redness. Irregular heart rate	Topical drops. Used to control or prevent acute postlaser IOP rise (used before and immediately after ALT and iridotomy, Nd:YAG laser capsulotomy). Teach patient at risk of systemic reactions to occlude puncta.
latanoprost (Xalatan) travoprost bimatoprost (Lumigan)	Prostaglandin F analogs	Increased brown iris pigmentation, ocular discomfort and redness, dryness, itching, and foreign body sensation	Topical drops. Teach patient to not exceed 1 drop per evening. Have patient remove contact lens 15 min before instilling.
Cholinergic Agents (Miotics)			
carbachol (Miostat, Isopto Carbachol)	Parasympathomimetic. Stimulates iris sphincter contraction, causing miosis and opening of trabecular meshwork, facilitating aqueous outflow. Also partially inhibits cholinesterase	Transient ocular discomfort, headache, blurred vision, decreased adaptation to the dark, syncope, salivation, dysrhythmias, vomiting, diarrhea, hypotension	Topical drops. Caution patient about ↓ visual acuity caused by miosis, particularly in dim light.
pilocarpine (Isopto Carpine, Pilocar)	Parasympathomimetic. Stimulates iris sphincter contraction, causing miosis and opening of trabecular meshwork, facilitating aqueous humor outflow	Same as carbachol	Topical drops. Same as carbachol
Carbonic Anhydrase Inhibitors			
Systemic			
acetazolamide (Diamox) dichlorphenamide (Daranide) methazolamide	↓ Aqueous humor production	Paresthesias, especially "tingling" in extremities. Hearing dysfunction or tinnitus. Loss of appetite, taste alteration, GI disturbances. Drowsiness, confusion	Oral nonbacteriostatic sulfonamides. Anaphylaxis and other sulfa-type allergic reactions may occur in patient allergic to sulfa. Diuretic effect can ↓ electrolyte levels. Should not be given to patient on high-dose aspirin therapy
Topical			
brinzolamide (Azopt) dorzolamide (Trusopt)	—	Transient stinging, blurred vision, redness	Same as above

ALT, Argon laser trabeculoplasty; *IOP,* intraocular pressure.

64 years, and every 1 to 2 years for people age 65 years or older. African Americans in every age category should have examinations more often because of the increased incidence and more aggressive course of glaucoma in these individuals.[13]

- **Acute Care.** Acute nursing interventions are directed primarily toward the patient with acute angle-closure glaucoma and the surgical patient. The patient with acute angle-closure glaucoma requires immediate medication to lower the IOP. It must be administered in a timely and appropriate manner according to the ophthalmologist's prescription. Most surgical procedures for glaucoma are outpatient procedures. The patient needs postoperative instructions and may require nursing measures to relieve discomfort related to the procedure. Patient and caregiver teaching after eye surgery is discussed in Table 21-3.
- **Ambulatory Care.** Because of the chronic nature of glaucoma, remind the patient to follow the therapeutic regimen and follow-up recommendations prescribed by the ophthalmologist. Provide accurate information about the disease process and treatment options, including the rationale underlying each option. In addition, the patient needs information about the purpose, frequency, and technique for administration of antiglaucoma drugs. Encourage adherence by helping the patient identify the most convenient and appropriate times for medication administration or advocating a change in therapy if the patient reports unacceptable side effects.

Evaluation

The overall expected outcomes are that the patient with glaucoma will

- Have no further loss of vision
- Adhere to the recommended therapy
- Safely function within own environment
- Obtain relief from pain associated with the disease and surgery

Gerontologic Considerations: Glaucoma

Many older patients with glaucoma have systemic illnesses or take systemic medications that may affect their therapy. In particular, the patient using a β-adrenergic blocking glaucoma agent may experience an additive effect if a systemic β-adrenergic blocking drug is also being taken. All β-adrenergic blocking glaucoma agents are contraindicated in the patient with bradycardia, heart block greater than first-degree heart block, cardiogenic shock, and overt cardiac failure. The noncardioselective β-adrenergic blocking glaucoma agents are also contraindicated in the patient with chronic obstructive pulmonary disease (COPD) or asthma. The hyperosmolar agents may precipitate heart failure or pulmonary edema in the susceptible patient. The older patient on high-dose aspirin therapy for rheumatoid arthritis should not take carbonic anhydrase inhibitors. The α-adrenergic agonists can cause tachycardia or hypertension, which may have serious consequences in the older patient. Teach the older patient to occlude the puncta to limit the systemic absorption of glaucoma medications.

INTRAOCULAR INFLAMMATION AND INFECTION

The term *uveitis* is used to describe inflammation of the uveal tract, retina, vitreous body, or optic nerve. This inflammation may be caused by bacteria, viruses, fungi, or parasites. *Cytomegalovirus retinitis* (CMV retinitis) is an opportunistic infection that occurs in patients with acquired immunodeficiency syndrome (AIDS) and in other immunosuppressed patients. The etiology of sterile intraocular inflammation includes autoimmune disorders, AIDS, malignancies, or those disorders associated with systemic diseases such as inflammatory bowel disease. Pain and photophobia are common symptoms.

Endophthalmitis is an extensive intraocular inflammation of the vitreous cavity. Bacteria, viruses, fungi, or parasites can induce this serious inflammatory response. The mechanism of infection may be endogenous, in which the infecting agent arrives at the eye through the bloodstream, or exogenous, in which the infecting agent is introduced through a surgical wound or a penetrating injury. Although rare, endophthalmitis is a devastating complication of intraocular surgery or penetrating ocular injury. It can lead to irreversible blindness within hours or days. Manifestations include ocular pain, photophobia, decreased visual acuity, headaches, reddened and swollen conjunctiva, and corneal edema.

Treatment of intraocular inflammation depends on the underlying cause. Intraocular infections require antimicrobial agents, which may be delivered topically, subconjunctivally, intravitreally, systemically, or in some combination. Sterile inflammatory responses require antiinflammatory medications such as corticosteroids. The patient with intraocular inflammation is usually uncomfortable and may be noticeably anxious and frightened. Provide accurate information and emotional support to the patient and family. In severe cases, enucleation may be necessary. When the patient has lost visual function or even the entire eye, the patient will grieve the loss. Your role includes helping the patient through the grieving process.

OCULAR TUMORS

Benign and malignant tumors can occur in many areas of the eye, including the conjunctiva, retina, and orbit.[15] Malignancies of the eyelid include basal cell and squamous cell carcinomas (see Chapter 23).

Uveal melanoma is a cancerous neoplasm of the iris, choroid, or ciliary body. It is more frequently found in light-skinned people over age 60 with chronic UV exposure. Genetic factors may also increase a person's risk.[16] Uveal melanoma can arise from preexisting nevi in the eye. Tumors may be asymptomatic or associated with vision loss depending on their size and location and presence of hemorrhage and retinal detachment. As with other cancers, cancer stage and cell type are important variables in the patient's prognosis. Diagnostic testing may include ultrasound, MRI, and fine-needle aspiration biopsy. Uveal melanoma commonly appears as a dome-shaped, well-circumscribed, solid brown to golden pigment in the iris, choroid, or ciliary body (Fig. 21-8). Many patients do not lose their eye, and some may experience good vision after treatment in the affected eye.

Depending on the status of the involved eye, treatment options can include enucleation, radiation therapy (brachytherapy), external beam radiation, transpupillary photocoagulation, eye wall resection, and exenteration.

ENUCLEATION

Enucleation is the removal of the eye. The primary indication for enucleation is a blind, painful eye. This may result from glaucoma, infection, or trauma. Enucleation may also be indicated in ocular malignancies. The surgical procedure includes severing the extraocular muscles close to their insertion on the globe, inserting an implant to maintain the intraorbital anatomy, and suturing the ends of the extraocular muscles over the

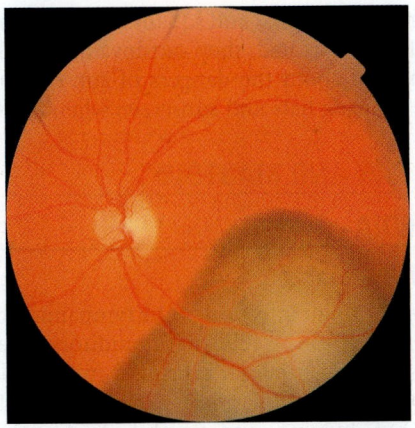

FIG. 21-8 Uveal melanoma. A large tumor in the choroid, the most common location in the eye for melanoma. (Courtesy Cory J. Bosanko, OD, FAAO, Eye Centers of Tennessee, Crossville, Tenn.)

implant. The conjunctiva covers the joined muscles, and a clear conformer is placed over the conjunctiva until the permanent prosthesis is fitted. A pressure dressing helps prevent postoperative bleeding.

Postoperatively, observe the patient for signs of complications, including excessive bleeding or swelling, increased pain, displacement of the implant, or temperature elevation. Patient teaching should include the instillation of topical ointments or drops and wound cleansing. Instruct the patient in the method of inserting the conformer into the socket in case it falls out. The patient is often devastated by the loss of an eye, even when enucleation occurs after a lengthy period of painful blindness. Recognize and validate the patient's emotional response and provide support to the patient and family.

Approximately 6 weeks after surgery the wound is sufficiently healed for the permanent prosthesis. The prosthesis is fitted by an ocularist and designed to match the remaining eye. Teach the patient how to remove, cleanse, and insert the prosthesis. Special polishing is required periodically to remove dried protein secretions.

OCULAR MANIFESTATIONS OF SYSTEMIC DISEASES

Many systemic diseases have significant ocular manifestations. Ocular signs and symptoms may be the first finding or complaint in the patient with a systemic disease. One example is the patient with undiagnosed diabetes who seeks ophthalmic care for blurred vision. A careful history and examination of the patient can reveal that the underlying cause of the blurred vision is lens swelling caused by hyperglycemia. Another example is the patient who seeks care for a conjunctival lesion. The ophthalmologist may be the first health care professional to make the diagnosis of AIDS based on the presence of a conjunctival Kaposi sarcoma (KS).

AUDITORY PROBLEMS: EXTERNAL EAR AND CANAL

TRAUMA

Trauma to the external ear can cause injury to the subcutaneous tissue that may result in a hematoma. If the hematoma is not aspirated, inflammation of the membranes of the ear cartilage (perichondritis) can result. Blows to the ear can also cause conductive hearing loss if the ossicles in the middle ear are damaged or the tympanic membrane (TM) is perforated. Head trauma that injures the temporal lobe of the cerebral cortex can impair the ability to understand the meaning of sounds.

EXTERNAL OTITIS

The skin of the external ear and canal is subject to the same problems as skin anywhere on the body. **External otitis** involves inflammation or infection of the epithelium of the auricle and ear canal. Swimming may alter the flora of the external canal because of chemicals and contaminated water. This can result in an infection often referred to as "swimmer's ear." Trauma from picking the ear or using sharp objects (e.g., hairpins) frequently causes the initial break in the skin. Piercing of cartilage in the upper part of the auricle also places the patient at higher risk for infection.

Infections and skin conditions may cause external otitis. Bacteria or fungi may be the cause. *Pseudomonas aeruginosa* is the most common bacterial cause. Fungi, especially *Candida albicans* and *Aspergillus,* thrive in warm, moist climates. The warm, dark environment of the ear canal provides a good growth medium for microorganisms.

Malignant external otitis is a serious infection caused by *P. aeruginosa.* It occurs mainly in older patients with diabetes. The infection, which can spread from the external ear to the parotid gland and temporal bone (osteomyelitis), is usually treated with antibiotics.

Ear pain *(otalgia)* is one of the first signs of external otitis. Even in mild cases, the patient may experience significant discomfort with chewing, moving the auricle, or pressing on the tragus. Swelling of the ear canal can muffle hearing. There may be serosanguineous (blood-tinged fluid) or purulent (white to green thick fluid) drainage. Fever occurs when the infection spreads to surrounding tissue.

❖ NURSING AND INTERPROFESSIONAL MANAGEMENT: EXTERNAL OTITIS

Diagnosis of external otitis is made by otoscopic examination of the ear canal. Care must be taken to avoid pain when pulling on the pinna to straighten out the canal or when inserting the otoscope speculum. The eardrum may be difficult to see due to swelling in the canal. Culture and sensitivity studies of the drainage may be done. Moist heat, mild analgesics, and topical anesthetic drops usually control the pain. Topical treatments may include antibiotics for infection and corticosteroids for inflammation. If the surrounding tissue is involved, systemic antibiotics are prescribed. Improvement should occur in 48 hours, but the patient needs to adhere to the prescribed therapy for 7 to 14 days for complete resolution.

Hands should be washed before and after administration of otic drops (eardrops). The drops should be administered at room temperature. Cold drops can cause vertigo due to stimulation of the semicircular canals, and heated drops can burn the tympanum. The tip of the dropper should not touch the ear during administration to prevent contamination of the entire bottle of drops. The ear is positioned so that the drops can run into the canal. The patient should maintain this position for 2 minutes to allow the drops to spread. Sometimes the drops are placed onto a wick of cotton that is placed in the canal. Instruct the patient not to push the cotton farther into the ear. Careful

TABLE 21-8 Patient & Caregiver Teaching

Prevention of External Otitis

Include the following instructions when teaching the patient and caregiver.

1. Do not put anything in your ear canal unless requested by your health care provider.
2. Report itching if it becomes a problem.
3. Earwax is normal.
   - It lubricates and protects the canal.
   - Report chronic excessive cerumen if it impairs your hearing.
4. Keep your ears as dry as possible.
   - Use earplugs if you are prone to swimmer's ear.
   - Turn your head to each side for 30 seconds at a time to help water run out of the ears.
   - Do not dry with cotton-tipped applicators.
   - A hair dryer set to low and held at least 6 in from the ear can speed water evaporation.

handling and disposal of material saturated with drainage are important. Instruct the patient on methods to reduce the risk of external otitis (Table 21-8).

CERUMEN AND FOREIGN BODIES IN EXTERNAL EAR CANAL

Impacted cerumen (earwax) can cause discomfort and decreased hearing. In the older person the cerumen becomes dense and drier. The hair in the ear becomes thicker and coarser, entrapping the hard, dry cerumen in the canal. Symptoms of cerumen impaction include hearing loss, otalgia, tinnitus, and vertigo.

Management of impacted cerumen involves irrigation of the canal with body-temperature solutions to soften the cerumen. Special syringes can be used and vary from a simple bulb syringe to special irrigating equipment. Place the patient in a sitting position with an emesis basin under the ear. Pull the auricle up and back, and direct the flow of solution above or below the impaction. It is important that the ear canal not be completely occluded with the syringe tip. If irrigation does not remove the wax, mild lubricant drops may be used to soften the earwax. Severe impactions may need to be removed by the HCP.

Attempts to remove a foreign object from the ear may result in pushing it farther into the canal. Vegetable matter in the ear tends to swell and may create a secondary inflammation, making removal more difficult. Mineral oil or lidocaine drops can be used to kill an insect before removal with microscope guidance. Removal of impacted objects should be performed by an HCP.

Ears should be cleaned with a washcloth and finger. Cotton-tipped applicators should be avoided. Penetration of the middle ear by a cotton-tipped applicator can cause serious injury to the TM and ossicles. The use of cotton-tipped applicators can also cause cerumen to become impacted against the TM and impair hearing.

MALIGNANCY OF EXTERNAL EAR

Skin cancers are the only common malignancies of the ear. Rough sandpaper-like changes to the upper border of the auricle are premalignant lesions (actinic keratoses) associated with chronic sun exposure. They are often treated with liquid nitrogen. Malignancies in the external ear canal include basal cell carcinoma in the pinna and squamous cell carcinoma in the ear canal. If left untreated, they can invade underlying tissue. Teach the patient about the dangers of sun exposure and the importance of using hats and sunscreen when outdoors.

MIDDLE EAR AND MASTOID

OTITIS MEDIA

Acute Otitis Media

Acute otitis media is an infection of the tympanum, ossicles, and space of the middle ear. Swelling of the auditory tube from colds or allergies can trap bacteria, causing a middle ear infection. Pressure from the inflammation pushes on the TM, causing it to become red, bulging, and painful. Acute otitis media is usually a childhood disease because in children the auditory tube that normally drains fluid and mucus from the middle ear is shorter and narrower and its position is flatter than in adults. Infection can be due to viruses or bacteria. Pain, fever, malaise, and reduced hearing are signs and symptoms of infection. Referred pain from the temporomandibular joint, teeth, gums, sinuses, or throat may also cause ear pain.

Antibiotics are used if an infection is present. Surgical intervention is generally reserved for the patient who does not respond to medical treatment. A *myringotomy* involves an incision in the tympanum to release the increased pressure and exudate from the middle ear. A tympanostomy tube may be placed for short- or long-term use. Prompt treatment of an episode of acute otitis media generally prevents spontaneous perforation of the TM. If allergies are a causative factor, antihistamines may also be prescribed.

Otitis Media With Effusion

Otitis media with effusion is an inflammation of the middle ear with a collection of fluid in the middle ear space. The fluid may be thin, mucoid, or purulent. If the auditory tube does not open and allow equalization of atmospheric pressure, negative pressure within the middle ear pulls fluid from surrounding tissues. This problem commonly follows upper respiratory tract or chronic sinus infections, barotrauma (caused by pressure change), or otitis media.

Complaints include a feeling of fullness of the ear, a "plugged" feeling or popping, and decreased hearing. The patient does not experience pain, fever, or discharge from the ear. It is common to have otitis media with effusion for weeks to months after an episode of acute otitis media. It usually resolves without treatment but may recur.

Chronic Otitis Media and Mastoiditis

Repeated attacks of otitis media may lead to chronic otitis media, especially in adults who have a history of recurrent otitis media in childhood. Because the mucous membrane of the middle ear is continuous with the air cells of the mastoid bone, both can be involved in the chronic infectious process.

Chronic otitis media is characterized by a purulent exudate and inflammation that can involve the ossicles, auditory tube, and mastoid bone. It is often painless. Hearing loss, nausea, and episodes of dizziness can occur. Hearing loss is a complication from inflammatory destruction of the ossicles, a TM perforation, or accumulation of fluid in the middle ear space. A mass of epithelial cells and cholesterol in the middle ear *(cholesteatoma)* may also develop. The cholesteatoma enlarges and can

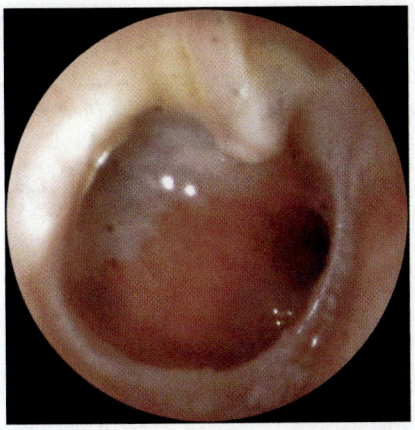

FIG. 21-9 Perforation of the tympanic membrane (TM). (From Flint P, Haughey B, Lund V, Niparko JK, editors: *Cummings otolaryngology: head and neck surgery,* ed 5, St Louis, 2010, Mosby.)

TABLE 21-9 Interprofessional Care

Chronic Otitis Media

Diagnostic Assessment	Management

• History and physical examination
• Otoscopic examination
• Culture and sensitivity of middle ear drainage
• Mastoid x-ray
	• Ear irrigations
	• Otic, oral, or parenteral antibiotics
	• Analgesics
	• Antiemetics
	• Surgery
	  • Tympanoplasty
	  • Mastoidectomy

destroy the adjacent bones. Unless removed surgically, it can cause extensive damage to the ossicles and impair hearing.

Otoscopic examination of the TM may reveal changes in color and mobility or a perforation (Fig. 21-9). Culture and sensitivity tests of the drainage are necessary to identify the organisms involved so that appropriate antibiotic therapy can be prescribed. The audiogram may demonstrate a hearing loss as great as 50 to 60 dB if the ossicles have been damaged or separated. Sinus x-rays, MRI, or a CT scan of the temporal bone is done to assess for bone destruction and the presence of a mass.

❖ NURSING AND INTERPROFESSIONAL MANAGEMENT: CHRONIC OTITIS MEDIA

The goals of treatment are to clear the middle ear of infection, repair any perforations, and preserve hearing (Table 21-9). Otic and systemic (oral and IV) antibiotic therapy is started based on the culture and sensitivity results. In many cases of chronic otitis media, antibiotic resistance is present. The patient may need to undergo frequent evacuation of drainage and debris in an outpatient setting.

Often chronic TM perforations do not heal with conservative treatment, and surgery is necessary. *Tympanoplasty (myringoplasty)* involves reconstruction of the TM and/or the ossicles. A *mastoidectomy* is often performed with a tympanoplasty to remove infected portions of the mastoid bone. Removal of tissue stops at the middle ear structures that appear capable of conducting sound. Sudden pressure changes in the ear and postoperative infections can disrupt the surgical repair during the healing phase or cause facial nerve paralysis.

TABLE 21-10 Interprofessional Care

Otosclerosis

Diagnostic Assessment	Management

• History and physical examination
• Otoscopic examination
• Rinne test
• Weber test
• Audiometry
• Tympanometry
	• Hearing aid
	• Surgery (stapedectomy or stapes prosthesis)
	• Drug therapy
	  • Sodium fluoride with vitamin D
	  • Calcium carbonate

Impaired hearing is expected during the postoperative period if there is packing in the ear. A cotton ball dressing is used for the incision made through the external auditory canal (endaural). Instruct the patient to change the cotton packing as needed. If a postauricular (behind the ear) incision is used and a drain is in place, place a dressing over the mastoid area. A small gauze pad is cut to fit behind the ear, and soft dressing material is applied over the ear to prevent the outer circular head dressing from placing pressure on the auricle. Monitor the tightness of the dressing to prevent tissue necrosis and assess the amount and type of drainage. Keep the suture line dry.

OTOSCLEROSIS

Otosclerosis is a hereditary autosomal dominant disease. It is the most common cause of hearing loss in young adults. Spongy bone develops from the bony labyrinth, preventing movement of the footplate of the stapes in the oval window. This reduces the transmission of vibrations to the inner ear fluids and results in conductive hearing loss. Although otosclerosis is typically bilateral, one ear may show faster progression of hearing loss. The patient is often unaware of the problem until the loss becomes so severe that communication is difficult.

Otoscopic examination may reveal a reddish blush of the tympanum (Schwartz's sign) caused by the vascular and bony changes within the middle ear. Tuning fork tests (e.g., Rinne) and an audiogram demonstrate good hearing by bone conduction but poor hearing by air conduction (air-bone gap). (These diagnostic tests are discussed in Table 20-11). Usually a difference of at least 20 to 25 dB between air and bone conduction levels of hearing is seen in otosclerosis.

The hearing loss associated with otosclerosis may be stabilized by the oral administration of sodium fluoride with vitamin D and calcium carbonate. These medications retard bone resorption and encourage the calcification of bony lesions. Amplification of sound by a hearing aid can be effective because the inner ear function is normal.

Interprofessional care of otosclerosis is presented in Table 21-10. Microdrill or laser surgical treatment involves opening the footplate (stapedotomy) or replacing the stapes with a metal or Teflon substitute (prosthesis). These procedures are usually performed with the patient under conscious sedation. The ear with poorer hearing is repaired first, and the other ear may be operated on within a year. Immediately after surgery the patient often reports a significant improvement in hearing in the operative ear. Because of the accumulation of blood and fluid in the middle ear during the postoperative period, the hearing level decreases initially, but it improves gradually with healing.

Nursing management of the patient undergoing surgery to correct otosclerosis is similar to that for the patient having a tympanoplasty. Use Gelfoam on the incision flap to limit bleeding. Place a cotton ball in the ear canal, and cover the ear with a small dressing. The patient may experience dizziness, nausea, and vomiting as a result of stimulation of the labyrinth during surgery. Some patients demonstrate nystagmus because of disturbance of the perilymph fluid. The patient should take care to avoid sudden movements that may bring on or exacerbate vertigo. Actions that increase inner ear pressure, such as coughing, sneezing, lifting, bending, and straining during bowel movements, should be avoided.

INNER EAR PROBLEMS

Three manifestations that indicate disease of the inner ear are vertigo, sensorineural hearing loss, and tinnitus. Symptoms of vertigo arise from the vestibular labyrinth, whereas hearing loss and tinnitus arise from the auditory labyrinth. There is an overlap between manifestations of inner ear problems and CNS disorders.

MÉNIÈRE'S DISEASE

Ménière's disease (endolymphatic hydrops) is characterized by symptoms caused by inner ear disease, including episodic vertigo, tinnitus, fluctuating sensorineural hearing loss, and aural fullness. The patient experiences significant disability because of sudden, severe attacks of vertigo with nausea, vomiting, sweating, and pallor. Symptoms usually begin between 30 and 60 years of age.[17]

The cause of the disease is unknown, but it results in an excessive accumulation of endolymph in the membranous labyrinth. The volume of endolymph increases until the membranous labyrinth ruptures. Attacks may be preceded by a sense of fullness in the ear, increasing tinnitus, and muffled hearing. The patient may experience the feeling of being pulled to the ground ("drop attacks"). Some patients report that they feel like they are whirling in space. Attacks may last hours or days and may occur several times a year. The clinical course of the disease is highly variable.

❖ NURSING AND INTERPROFESSIONAL MANAGEMENT: MÉNIÈRE'S DISEASE

Interprofessional care of Ménière's disease (Table 21-11) includes diagnostic tests to rule out other causes of the symptoms, including CNS disease. Results that suggest Ménière's disease include a mild, low-frequency sensorineural hearing loss on audiogram and abnormalities with vestibular tests. A glycerol test may aid in diagnosis. An oral dose of glycerol is given, followed by serial audiograms over 3 hours. Improvement in hearing or speech discrimination supports a diagnosis of Ménière's disease. The improvement is attributed to the osmotic effect of glycerol that pulls fluid from the inner ear.

During the acute attack, antihistamines (e.g., diphenhydramine), anticholinergics (e.g., atropine), and benzodiazepines (e.g., lorazepam [Ativan]) can be used to decrease the abnormal sensation and lessen nausea and vomiting. Acute vertigo is treated symptomatically with bed rest, sedation, and antiemetics (e.g., prochlorperazine) or antivertigo drugs (e.g., meclizine [Antivert]) for motion sickness. The patient requires reassurance and counseling that the condition is not life threatening. Management between attacks may include diuretics, antihistamines, calcium channel blockers, and a low-sodium diet. Diazepam (Valium), meclizine, and fentanyl with droperidol may be used to reduce the vertigo. Over time, most patients respond to the prescribed medications but must learn to live with the unpredictability of the attacks and the loss of hearing.

Frequent and incapacitating attacks are indications for surgical intervention. Decompression of the endolymphatic sac and shunting are performed to reduce the pressure on the cochlear hair cells and to prevent further damage and hearing loss. If relief is not achieved, vestibular nerve section (cutting the nerve) may be performed. When involvement is unilateral, surgical ablation of the labyrinth, resulting in loss of the vestibular and hearing cochlear function, is performed. Some patients with severe attacks of vertigo have shown improvement with the injection of gentamicin through the TM. This results in inner ear damage and a reduction in endolymph production.

Plan nursing interventions to minimize vertigo and provide for patient safety. During an acute attack keep the patient in a quiet, darkened room in a comfortable position. Teach the patient to avoid sudden head movements or position changes. Fluorescent or flickering lights or a television may exacerbate symptoms and should be avoided. Make an emesis basin available because vomiting is common. To minimize the risk of falling, keep the side rails up and the bed in a low position when the patient is in bed. Instruct the patient to call for assistance when getting out of bed. Medications and fluids are administered parenterally, and intake and output are monitored. When the attack subsides, assist the patient with ambulation because unsteadiness may remain.

TABLE 21-11 Interprofessional Care

Ménière's Disease

Diagnostic Assessment
- History and physical examination
- Audiometric studies (including speech discrimination, tone decay)
- Vestibular tests (including caloric test, positional test)
- Electronystagmography
- Neurologic examination
- Glycerol test

Management

Acute Care

Drug Therapy
- Sedatives
- Benzodiazepines
- Anticholinergics
- Antihistamines
- Antiemetics

Surgical Therapy
- Endolymphatic sac decompression
- Endolymphatic shunt
- Vestibular nerve section
- Labyrinthectomy

Ambulatory Care
- Diuretics
- Antihistamines
- Calcium channel blockers
- Sedatives
- Hydrops diet: restriction of sodium, caffeine, nicotine, alcohol, and foods with monosodium glutamate (MSG)

BENIGN PAROXYSMAL POSITIONAL VERTIGO

Benign paroxysmal positional vertigo (BPPV) is a common cause of vertigo. Approximately 50% of the cases of vertigo may be due to BPPV. In BBPV, free-floating debris in the semicircular canal causes vertigo with specific head movements, such as getting out of bed, rolling over in bed, and sitting up from lying down. The debris ("ear rocks") is composed of small crystals of calcium carbonate that derive from the utricle in the inner ear. The utricle may be injured by head trauma, infection, or degeneration from the aging process. However, for many patients, a cause cannot be found.

Symptoms of BPPV include nystagmus, vertigo, lightheadedness, loss of balance, and nausea. There is no hearing loss, and symptoms tend to be intermittent. The symptoms of BPPV may be confused with those of Ménière's disease. Diagnosis is based on the results of auditory and vestibular tests.

Although BPPV is bothersome, it is rarely serious unless a person falls. The Epley maneuver, or canalith repositioning procedure, is effective in providing symptom relief for many patients. In this maneuver, the ear debris is moved from areas in the inner ear that cause symptoms and repositioned into less sensitive areas where they do not cause these problems. The Epley maneuver does not address the actual presence of debris but rather changes their location. A trained HCP can instruct the patient how to perform the maneuver.

ACOUSTIC NEUROMA

An **acoustic neuroma** is a unilateral benign tumor that occurs where the vestibulocochlear nerve (cranial nerve [CN] VIII) enters the internal auditory canal. Early diagnosis is important because the tumor can compress the trigeminal and facial nerves and arteries within the internal auditory canal. Symptoms usually begin between 40 and 60 years of age.

Early symptoms are associated with CN VIII compression and destruction. They include unilateral, progressive, sensorineural hearing loss; reduced touch sensation in the posterior ear canal; unilateral tinnitus; and mild, intermittent vertigo. Diagnostic tests include neurologic, audiometric, and vestibular tests; CT scans; and MRI.

Surgery to remove small tumors generally preserves hearing and vestibular function. Large tumors (larger than 3 cm) and the surgery required to remove them can leave the patient with permanent hearing loss and facial paralysis. Stereotactic radiosurgery may slow tumor growth and preserve the facial nerve. Instruct the patient to report any clear, colorless discharge from the nose. This may be cerebrospinal fluid (CSF), which increases the risk of infection. Teach the importance of follow-up care after surgery to monitor hearing and for recurrence of the tumor.

HEARING LOSS AND DEAFNESS

Hearing disorders are a common cause of disability in the United States. Nearly half of the people who need assistance with hearing disorders are 65 years of age or older. With the aging of the population, the incidence of hearing loss is increasing.[18] Causes of hearing loss are shown in Fig. 21-10.

Types of Hearing Loss

Conductive Hearing Loss. *Conductive hearing loss* occurs when conditions in the outer or middle ear impair the transmission of sound through air to the inner ear. A common cause is otitis media with effusion. Other causes are impacted cerumen, perforation of the TM, otosclerosis, and narrowing of the external auditory canal.

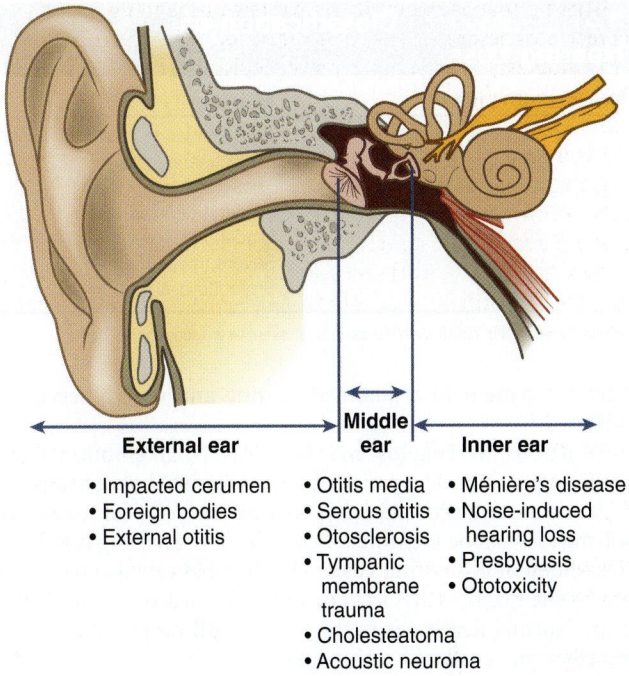

FIG. 21-10 Causes of hearing loss.

The audiogram demonstrates better hearing through bone than through air (air-bone gap). The patient often speaks softly because hearing his or her own voice (which is conducted by bone) seems loud. This patient hears better in a noisy environment. The first step is to identify and treat the cause if possible. If correction of the cause is not possible, a hearing aid may help if the loss is greater than 40 to 50 dB.

Sensorineural Hearing Loss. *Sensorineural hearing loss* is caused by impairment of function of the inner ear or the vestibulocochlear nerve (CN VIII). Congenital and hereditary factors, noise trauma over time, aging (presbycusis), Ménière's disease, and ototoxicity can cause sensorineural hearing loss. Ototoxic drugs include aspirin, nonsteroidal antiinflammatory drugs, antibiotics (aminoglycosides, erythromycin, vancomycin), loop diuretics, and chemotherapy drugs (e.g., vincristine [Oncovin], cisplatin [Platinol]).

Systemic infections, such as Paget's disease of the bone, immune diseases, diabetes mellitus, bacterial meningitis, and trauma, are associated with this type of hearing loss. The main problems are the ability to hear sound but not to understand speech, and the lack of understanding of the problem by others. The ability to hear high-pitched sounds (including consonants) diminishes. Sounds become muffled and difficult to understand. An audiogram demonstrates a loss in decibel levels of the 4000-Hz range and eventually the 2000-Hz range. A hearing aid may help some patients, but it only makes sounds and speech louder, not clearer.

Mixed Hearing Loss. Mixed hearing loss occurs due to a combination of conductive and sensorineural causes. Careful evaluation is needed if corrective surgery for conductive loss is planned because the sensorineural component of the hearing loss will still remain.

Central and Functional Hearing Loss. Central hearing loss involves an inability to interpret sound, including speech, because of a problem in the brain (CNS). A careful history is helpful because there are usually cases of deafness in the family.

TABLE 21-12 Classification of Hearing Loss

Decibel (dB) Loss	Meaning
0-15	Normal hearing
16-25	Slight hearing loss
26-40	Mild impairment
41-55	Moderate impairment
56-70	Moderately severe impairment
71-90	Severe impairment
>90	Profound deafness*

*Most people in this category have been deaf since birth (congenitally deaf).

Refer the patient to a qualified hearing and speech service if indicated.

Functional hearing loss may be caused by an emotional or a psychologic factor. The patient does not seem to hear or respond to pure-tone subjective hearing tests, but no physical reason for hearing loss can be identified. Psychologic counseling may help.

Classification of Hearing Loss. Hearing loss can also be classified by the decibel (dB) level or loss as recorded on the audiogram. Normal hearing is in the 0- to 15-dB range. Table 21-12 describes the levels of hearing loss.

Clinical Manifestations

Common early signs of hearing loss are answering questions inappropriately, not responding when not looking at the speaker, asking others to speak up, and showing irritability with others who do not speak up. Other behaviors that suggest hearing loss include straining to hear, cupping the hand around the ear, reading lips, and an increased sensitivity to slight increases in noise level. Often the patient is unaware of minimal hearing loss. Family and friends who get tired of repeating or talking loudly are often the first to notice the hearing loss. Pressure exerted by significant others is a significant factor in whether the patient seeks help for hearing impairment.

Sudden hearing loss, commonly known as sudden deafness, occurs as an unexplained, rapid loss of hearing (usually in one ear) either at once or over several days. It is a medical emergency, and the patient should see an HCP immediately.[19]

Deafness is often called the "unseen handicap" because the difficulty in communication with a deaf person is not realized until you initiate a conversation with that person. You need to thoroughly validate the deaf person's understanding of health teaching. Descriptive visual aids can be helpful. If the significantly hearing-impaired individual uses sign language to communicate, the Americans with Disabilities Act requires providing an interpreter when significant information is presented such as for patient consent or discharge teaching.[20]

Interference in communication and interaction with others can be the source of many problems for the patient and caregiver. Often the patient refuses to admit or may be unaware of impaired hearing. Irritability is common because the patient must concentrate so hard to understand speech. The loss of clarity of speech in the patient with sensorineural hearing loss is most frustrating. The patient may hear what is said but not understand it. Withdrawal, suspicion, loss of self-esteem, and insecurity are commonly associated with advancing hearing loss.[21]

Tinnitus and Hearing Loss. *Tinnitus* is the perception of *sound* in the ears where no external source is present. It is "ringing in the ears" or "head noise" (see *www.ata.org*). Tinnitus is sometimes the first symptom of hearing loss, especially in older people. It may be soft or loud, high pitched or low pitched.

Tinnitus and hearing loss are directly related. Both are caused by inner ear nerve damage. The main difference between tinnitus and hearing loss is the extent of the damage (since tinnitus can still be heard).

Although the most common cause of tinnitus is noise, it can also be a side effect of medications (see discussion on drugs causing sensorineural hearing loss on p. 387). More than 200 drugs are known to cause tinnitus.

❖ NURSING AND INTERPROFESSIONAL MANAGEMENT: HEARING LOSS AND DEAFNESS

Health Promotion

Environmental Noise Control. Noise is the most preventable cause of hearing loss. (Fig. 21-11 lists the levels of environmental noise generated by common indoor and outdoor sounds.) Sudden severe loud noise (acoustic trauma) and chronic exposure to loud noise (noise-induced hearing loss) can damage hearing. Acoustic trauma causes hearing loss by destroying the hair cells of the organ of Corti. Sensorineural hearing loss as a result of increased and prolonged environmental noise, such as amplified sound, is occurring in young adults at an increasing rate. Amplified music (e.g., on iPods or MP3 players) should not exceed 50% of maximum volume. Ear protection should be worn when firing a gun and during other recreational pursuits with high noise levels. Health teaching regarding avoidance of continued exposure to noise levels greater than 70 dB is essential.

In work environments known to have high noise levels (more than 85 dB), ear protection should be worn. Occupational Safety and Health Administration (OSHA) standards require ear protection for workers in environments where the noise levels consistently exceed 85 dB. Periodic audiometric screening should be part of the health maintenance policies of industry. This provides baseline data on hearing to measure subsequent hearing loss.

Employees should participate in hearing conservation programs in work environments. Such programs should include noise exposure analysis, provision for control of noise exposure (hearing protectors), measurements of hearing, and employee-employer notification and education. Young adults should be encouraged to keep amplified music at a reasonable level and limit their exposure time. Hearing loss caused by noise is not reversible.

CHECK YOUR PRACTICE

Your newly assigned 68-yr-old female patient is being discharged today following a hip replacement. Before going to her room, you prepared the materials and information for her discharge. You sit down by her bed and start talking with her. She shakes her head and says, "No, no." You are perplexed until she flashes a bracelet that says *I am deaf.*

- How will you proceed?

HEALTHY PEOPLE

Health Impact of Wearing Ear Protection

- Ear protection should be worn during all recreational and work activities involving high noise levels.
- Ear protection can greatly reduce the damage to the ear from loud noise.
- Periodic audiometric screening is important to detect hearing loss before it progresses.

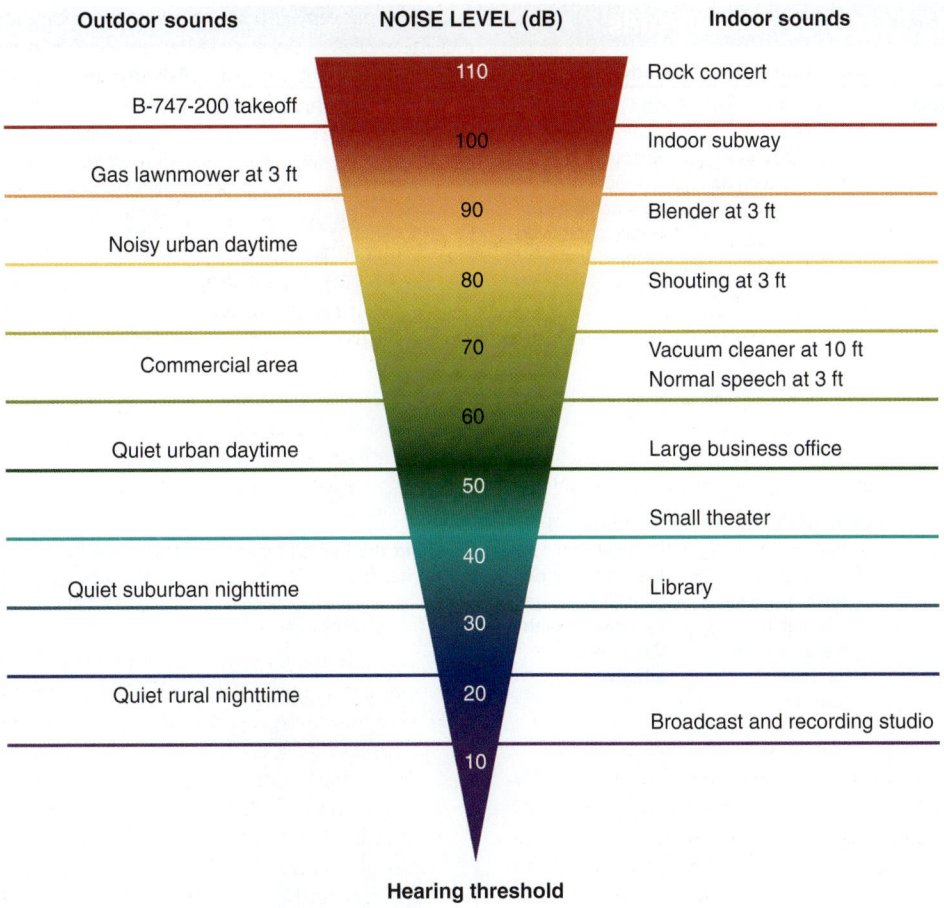

FIG. 21-11 Range of common environmental sounds.

Immunizations. Various viruses can cause deafness as a result of fetal damage and malformations affecting the ear. Promote childhood and adult immunizations, including the measles, mumps, and rubella (MMR) vaccine. Rubella infection during the first 8 weeks of pregnancy is associated with a high incidence of congenital rubella syndrome, which causes sensorineural deafness. Women of childbearing age should be tested for antibodies to these viral diseases. Women should avoid pregnancy for at least 3 months after being immunized. Immunization must be delayed if the woman is pregnant. Women who are susceptible to rubella can be vaccinated safely during the postpartum period.

Ototoxic Substances. Drugs commonly associated with ototoxicity include salicylates, loop diuretics, chemotherapy drugs, and antibiotics. Chemicals used in industry (e.g., toluene, carbon disulfide, mercury) may damage the inner ear. The patient who is receiving ototoxic drugs or is exposed to ototoxic chemicals should be monitored for signs and symptoms associated with ototoxicity, including tinnitus, diminished hearing, and changes in equilibrium. If these symptoms develop, immediate withdrawal of the drug may prevent further damage and may cause the symptoms to disappear.

Assistive Devices and Techniques

Hearing Aids. The patient with a suspected hearing loss should have a hearing assessment by a qualified audiologist. If a hearing aid is indicated, it should be fitted by an audiologist or a speech and hearing specialist. Many types of hearing aids are available, each with advantages and disadvantages (Table 21-13). The conventional hearing aid serves as a simple amplifier. For the patient with bilateral hearing impairment, binaural hearing aids provide the best sound lateralization and speech discrimination.

The goal of hearing aid therapy is improved hearing with consistent use. Patients who are motivated and optimistic about using a hearing aid are more successful users. Determine the patient's readiness for hearing aid therapy, including acknowledgment of a hearing problem, the patient's feelings about wearing a hearing aid, the degree to which the hearing loss affects life, and any difficulties the patient has manipulating small objects such as putting a battery in a hearing aid.

Initially, use of the hearing aid should be restricted to quiet situations in the home. The patient must first adjust to voices (including the patient's own voice) and household sounds. The patient should also experiment by increasing and decreasing the volume as situations require. As the patient adjusts to the increase in sounds and background noise, he or she can progress to situations where several people will be talking simultaneously. Next, the environment can be expanded to the outdoors and then a shopping mall or grocery store. Adjustment to different environments occurs gradually, depending on the individual patient.

When the hearing aid is not being worn, it should be placed in a dry, cool area where it will not be inadvertently damaged or lost. The battery should be disconnected or removed when not in use. A standard hearing aid battery lasts anywhere from 3 to 22 days, depending on the hearing aid type, battery type and capacity, and the amount of hearing aid use. Battery life

TABLE 21-13 Types of Hearing Aids

Type	Advantages	Disadvantages
Completely in the canal (mild to moderate hearing loss)	Smallest and least visible aid. Protected from sounds such as wind noise.	Costly. No space for add-ons such as directional microphones or volume controls. Small, short-lived batteries.
In the canal (mild to severe hearing loss)	More powerful than aids completely in the canal. Has adjustable features such as noise reduction.	Small size of aid with its additional features may be difficult to operate for patients with visual loss or arthritis.
In the ear (mild to severe hearing loss)	Powerful amplification. Inserts and adjusts easily. Longer-lasting batteries.	Visible. May pick up wind noise readily.
Behind the ear (all types of hearing loss)	Most powerful aid. Adjusts easily. Longest battery life.	Largest, most visible aid. Newer models may be smaller and less obvious.

averages 1 week (depends on hearing aid, battery, and amount of use), and patients should be advised to purchase only a month's supply at a time. Ear molds should be cleaned weekly or as needed. Toothpicks or pipe cleaners may be used to clear a clogged ear tip.

An *implantable hearing device* or aid is available to patients who cannot or will not use traditional hearing aids or cochlear implants. Implanted hearing devices amplify sound and transmit the sound vibrations through the ear. The device does not have external components that are visible. There are two types of implantable hearing devices: fully implantable and partially implantable. The fully implantable devices are surgically placed and nothing is visible externally. Partially implanted devices have an internal device that is implanted surgically but have an external device that is worn behind or in the ear.

Speech Reading. *Speech reading,* commonly called *lip reading,* can be helpful in increasing communication. It allows for approximately 40% understanding of the spoken word. The patient is able to use visual cues associated with speech, such as gestures and facial expression, to help clarify the spoken message. In speech reading, many words look alike to the patient (e.g., rabbit, woman). Help the patient by using and teaching verbal and nonverbal communication techniques as described in Table 21-14.

TABLE 21-14 Communication With Patients With Hearing Impairment

Nonverbal Aids	Verbal Aids
• Draw attention with hand movements. • Have speaker's face in good light. • Avoid covering mouth or face with hands. • Avoid chewing, eating, smoking while talking. • Maintain eye contact. • Avoid distracting environments. • Avoid careless expression that the patient may misinterpret. • Use touch. • Move close to better ear. • Avoid light behind speaker.	• Speak normally and slowly. • Do not overexaggerate facial expressions. • Do not overenunciate. • Use simple sentences. • Rephrase sentence. Use different words. • Write name or difficult words. • Do not shout. • Speak in normal voice directly into better ear.

Sign Language. *Sign language* is used as a form of communication for people with profound hearing impairment. It involves gestures and facial features such as eyebrow motion and lip-mouth movements. Sign language is not universal. American Sign Language (ASL) is used in the United States and the English-speaking parts of Canada.

Cochlear Implant. The *cochlear implant* is used as a hearing device for people with severe to profound sensorineural hearing

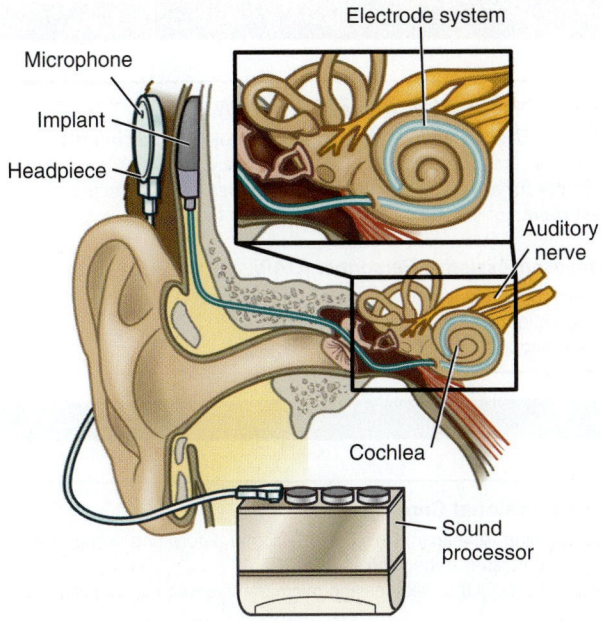

FIG. 21-12 Cochlear implant.

loss in one or both ears.[22] The ideal candidate is one who has become deaf after acquiring speech and language. The system consists of an external microphone placed behind the ear, a speech processor and a transmitter implanted under the skin that change sounds into electrical impulses, and a group of electrodes placed within the cochlea that stimulate the auditory nerves in the ear (Fig. 21-12). Cochlear implants send information that covers the entire range of sound frequencies. The cochlear implant electrodes are inserted as far as possible into the cochlea to send both high- and low-frequency information. For patients with conductive and mixed hearing loss, the cochlear Baha system may be surgically implanted. The system works through direct bone conduction and integrates with the skull bone over time.

Extensive training and rehabilitation are essential to receive maximum benefit from these implants. The positive aspects of a cochlear implant include providing sound to the person who heard none, improving lip-reading ability, monitoring the loudness of the person's own speech, improving the sense of security, and decreasing feelings of isolation.

Assistive Listening Devices. Numerous devices are now available to assist the hearing-impaired person. Direct amplification devices, amplified telephone receivers, alerting systems that flash when activated by sound, an infrared system for amplifying the sound of the television, and a combination FM receiver and hearing aid are all devices that you can explore based on patient needs. People with profound deafness may be assisted by text-telephone alerting systems that flash when activated by sound, closed captioning on television, and a specially trained dog. The dogs are trained to alert their owners to specific sounds within the environment, thus increasing the person's safety and independence.

TABLE 21-15 Classification of Presbycusis

Type	Hearing Change and Prognosis
Sensory	
Atrophy of auditory nerve. Loss of sensory hair cells	Loss of high-pitched sounds. Little effect on speech understanding. Good response to sound amplification
Neural	
Degenerative changes in cochlea and spinal ganglion	Loss of speech discrimination. Amplification alone not sufficient
Metabolic	
Atrophy of blood vessels in wall of cochlea with interruption of essential nutrient supply	Uniform loss for all frequencies accompanied by recruitment.* Good response to hearing aid
Cochlear	
Stiffening of basilar membrane, which interferes with sound transmission in the cochlea	Hearing loss increases from low to high frequencies. Speech discrimination affected with higher-frequency losses. Helped by appropriate forms of amplification

*Abnormally rapid increase in loudness as sound intensity increases.

Gerontologic Considerations: Hearing Loss

Presbycusis, hearing loss associated with aging, includes the loss of peripheral auditory sensitivity, a decline in word recognition ability, and associated psychologic and communication issues. Because consonants (high-frequency sounds) are the letters by which spoken words are recognized, the older person with presbycusis has a diminished ability to understand the spoken word. Vowels are heard, but some consonants fall into the high-frequency range and cannot be differentiated. This may lead to confusion and embarrassment because of the difference in what was said and what was heard.[23]

The cause of presbycusis is related to degenerative changes in the inner ear. Noise exposure is thought to be a common factor. Table 21-15 describes the classification of specific causes and associated hearing changes of presbycusis. Often a person may have more than one type of presbycusis. The prognosis for hearing depends on the cause of the loss. Sound amplification with the appropriate device is often helpful in improving the understanding of speech. In other situations, an audiologic rehabilitation program can be valuable.

The older adult is often reluctant to use a hearing aid for sound amplification. Reasons cited most often include cost, appearance, insufficient knowledge about hearing aids, amplification of competing noise, and unrealistic expectations. Most hearing aids and batteries are small, and neuromuscular changes such as stiff fingers, enlarged joints, and decreased sensory perception often make the care and handling of a hearing aid difficult and frustrating for an older person. Some older adults may also tend to accept their losses as part of getting older and believe there is no need for improvement.

TEAMWORK & COLLABORATION

Corrective Lenses and Hearing Aids

Role of Nursing Personnel

Registered Nurse (RN)

- Assess patient vision and hearing with and without corrective devices.
- Teach patient about the use of and care for corrective lenses and hearing aids.
- Evaluate whether corrective lenses or hearing aids are effective in maintaining or improving vision or hearing.
- Evaluate for problems that may occur with contact lenses (e.g., conjunctivitis) or with hearing aids (e.g., external ear irritation).

Licensed Practical/Vocational Nurse (LPN/LVN)

- Perform Snellen and/or Jaeger testing as delegated by the RN (consider state nurse practice act and agency policy).
- Monitor for adverse effects of contact lenses (e.g., redness, complaints of irritation) and report these to the RN.

Unlicensed Assistive Personnel (UAP)

- Clean corrective lenses with ordered solutions.
- Help patients with hearing aid placement.
- Clean and replace batteries in hearing aids.

CASE STUDY

Glaucoma and Diabetic Retinopathy

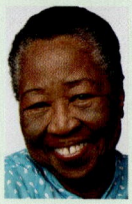

(©Kevin Peterson/ Stockbyte/ Thinkstock)

Patient Profile

J.K. is a 68-year-old African American woman who has been diagnosed with osteoarthritis and type 2 diabetes mellitus for the past 15 years. She now has diabetic retinopathy. She returns to the eye clinic with her daughter for continued care of primary open-angle glaucoma (POAG) and reexamination for changes in diabetic retinopathy. Her current medical regimen for POAG includes topical timolol maleate 0.5% extended (Timoptic-XE) once daily OU and latanoprost (Xalatan) 0.005% OU at bedtime. At her last examination it was noted that she had microaneurysms and hard exudates of the retina.

Subjective Data

- She can no longer read the newspaper and reports that medication labels are difficult to read.
- States she is not always successful in getting the eye drops instilled because her hands are gnarled and painful from osteoarthritis.

Objective Data

- Distant and near visual acuity are stable at 20/60 (OD) and 20/50 (OS). This is a reduction from 20/40 (OU) at her last visit.
- Intraocular pressures are stable at 20 mm Hg (OU). There is a new scotoma on visual field testing in the OS.
- Fluorescein angiography reveals diabetic macular edema OU.

Interprofessional Care

- Brimonidine (Alphagan) 0.15% (OS) 15 min before and immediately after argon laser trabeculoplasty (ALT)
- Argon laser (OU) to seal leaking microaneurysms from macular edema
- Check intraocular pressure (IOP) 1 hr after ALT
- Continue previous glaucoma drop regimen
- Follow-up examination for glaucoma in 2 wk for possible ALT (OD)
- Follow-up examination for diabetic macular edema in 8 wk

Discussion Questions

1. Explain the etiology of the new scotoma.
2. Why may ALT be an appropriate therapy for J.K.?
3. What is the purpose of the eye drops before and immediately after ALT?
4. ***Patient-Centered Care:*** What are the priority topics that should be discussed in discharge teaching with J.K.?
5. What is the etiology of the vision loss from diabetic retinopathy?
6. ***Priority Decision:*** What are the priority nursing interventions for J.K.?
7. ***Priority Decision:*** Based on the assessment data, what are the priority nursing diagnoses? Are there any collaborative problems?
8. ***Evidence-Based Practice:*** J.K. wants to know if her glaucoma is related to her diabetes. How would you respond to her question?

Answers available at *http://evolve.elsevier.com/Lewis/medsurg.*

BRIDGE TO NCLEX EXAMINATION

The number of the question corresponds to the same-numbered outcome at the beginning of the chapter.

1. Presbyopia occurs in older individuals because
   a. the eyeball elongates.
   b. the lens becomes inflexible.
   c. the corneal curvature becomes irregular.
   d. light rays are focusing in front of the retina.
2. The *most* important intervention for the patient with epidemic keratoconjunctivitis is
   a. cleansing the affected area with baby shampoo.
   b. monitoring spread of infection to the opposing eye.
   c. regular instillation of artificial tears to the affected eye.
   d. teaching the patient and family members good hygiene techniques.
3. Inflammation and infection of the eye
   a. are caused by irritants and microorganisms.
   b. have a higher incidence in sexually active patients.
   c. are chronic problems that result in a loss of vision.
   d. are frequently treated with cold compresses and antibiotics.
4. Which patient behaviors would the nurse promote for healthy eyes and ears *(select all that apply)*?
   a. Wearing protective sunglasses when bicycling
   b. Supplemental intake of B vitamins and magnesium
   c. Playing amplified music at 75% of maximum volume
   d. Patient notifying the health care provider of tinnitus while on antibiotics
   e. A woman avoiding pregnancy for 4 weeks after receiving MMR immunization
5. What should be included in the postoperative teaching of the patient who has undergone cataract surgery *(select all that apply)*?
   a. Eye discomfort is often relieved with mild analgesics.
   b. A decline in visual acuity is common for the first week.
   c. Stay on bed rest and limit activity for the first few days.
   d. Notify surgeon if an increase in redness or drainage occurs.
   e. Nighttime eye shielding and activity restrictions are essential to prevent eyestrain.

6. What should be included in the nursing plan for a patient who needs to administer antibiotic eardrops?
   a. Cool the drops so that they decrease swelling in the canal.
   b. Avoid placing a cotton wick to assist in administering the drops.
   c. Be careful to avoid touching the tip of the dropper bottle to the ear.
   d. Keep the head tilted 5 to 7 minutes after administration of the drops.
7. What is *important* for the nurse to include in the postoperative care of the patient following tympanoplasty?
   a. Check the gag reflex.
   b. Encourage independence.
   c. Avoid changing the cotton padding.
   d. Instruct patient to refrain from forceful nose blowing.
8. The patient who has a conductive hearing loss
   a. hears better in a noisy environment.
   b. hears sound but does not understand speech.
   c. often speaks loudly because his or her own voice seems low.
   d. experiences clearer sound with a hearing aid if the loss is less than 30 dB.
9. Instruct the patient who is newly fitted with bilateral hearing aids to *(select all that apply)*
   a. replace the batteries monthly.
   b. clean the ear molds weekly or as needed.
   c. clean ears with cotton-tipped applicators daily.
   d. disconnect or remove the batteries when not in use.
   e. initially restrict usage to quiet listening in the home.
10. Which strategies would *best* assist the nurse in communicating with a patient who has a hearing loss *(select all that apply)*?
    a. Overenunciate speech.
    b. Speak normally and slowly.
    c. Exaggerate facial expressions.
    d. Raise the voice to a higher pitch.
    e. Write out names or difficult words.
11. Patients with permanent visual impairment
    a. feel most comfortable with other visually impaired people.
    b. may feel threatened when others make eye contact during a conversation.
    c. usually need others to speak louder so that they can communicate appropriately.
    d. may experience the same grieving process that is associated with other losses.

1. b, 2. d, 3. a, 4. a, d, 5. a, d, 6. c, 7. d, 8. a, 9. b, d, e, 10. b, e, 11. d

For rationales to these answers and even more NCLEX review questions, visit *http://evolve.elsevier.com/Lewis/medsurg.*

EVOLVE WEBSITE

http://evolve.elsevier.com/Lewis/medsurg

Review Questions (Online Only)

Key Points

Answer Keys for Review Questions

- Rationales for Bridge to NCLEX Examination Questions
- Answer Guidelines for Case Study on p. 392

Student Case Study

- Patient Undergoing Cataract Surgery

eNursing Care Plan

- eNursing Care Plan 21-1: Patient After Eye Surgery

Conceptual Care Map Creator

Audio Glossary

Supporting Media

- Animations
  - Cataract Removal
  - LASIK
  - Myringotomy
  - Scleral Buckling

Content Updates

REFERENCES

1. Sutton G, Lawless M, Hodge C: Laser in situ keratomileusis in 2012: a review, *Clin Exp Optom* 97(1):18, 2014.
2. FDA: Lasik. Retrieved from *www.fda.gov/MedicalDevices/ProductsandMedicalProcedures/SurgeryandLifeSupport/LASIK/default.htm.*
3. American Foundation for the Blind: Aging and vision fact sheet. Retrieved from *www.afb.org/info/programs-and-services/public-policy-center/directconnect-newsletter/new-learning-opportunity-from-afb-finding-the-numbers-we-need/1235.*
4. National Sleep Foundation: Non-24. Retrieved from *https://sleepfoundation.org/non-24/content/non-24.*
5. Akpek EK, Smith RA: Overview of age-related ocular conditions, *Am J Manag Care* 19(5 Suppl):S67, 2013.
6. Lin A, Confait C, Ahmad M, et al: Severe ocular trauma in the emergency room, *J Miss State Med Assoc* 55(6):176, 2014.
7. Durning MV: Conjunctivitis, *Nursing* 43:39, 2013.
*8. Lockwood C, Stern C: Interventions for the treatment of trachoma: an overview of Cochrane systematic reviews, *Int J Nurs Pract* 20(6):709, 2014.
*9. Güell JL, El Husseiny MA, Manero F, et al: Historical review and update of surgical treatment for corneal endothelial diseases, *Ophthalmol Ther* 3(1-2):1, 2014.
10. National Eye Institute: Facts about cataracts. Retrieved from *www.nei.nih.gov/health/cataract/cataract_facts.*
11. Nentwich MM, Ulbig MW: Diabetic retinopathy—ocular complications of diabetes mellitus, *World J Diabetes* 6(3):489, 2015.
12. Steel D: Retinal detachment, *BMJ Clin Evid* 3;2014. pii: 0710.
13. Mackey DA, Hewitt AW: Genome-wide association study success in ophthalmology, *Curr Opin Ophthalmol* 25(5):386, 2014.
14. Glaucoma Research Foundation: African Americans and glaucoma. Retrieved from *www.glaucoma.org/glaucoma/african-americans-and-glaucoma.php.*
15. American Cancer Society: Eye cancer. Retrieved from *www.cancer.org/cancer/eyecancer.*
16. Nielsen M, Dogrusöz M, Bleeker JC, et al: The genetic basis of uveal melanoma, *J Fr Ophthalmol* 38(6):516, 2015.
*17. Tassinari M, Mandrioli D, Gaggioli N, et al: Ménière's disease treatment: a patient-centered systematic review, *Audiol Neurootol* 20(3):153, 2015.
18. Hearing Loss Association of America: *http://hearingloss.org.*
19. Sudden deafness. Retrieved from *www.nidcd.nih.gov/health/hearing/pages/sudden.aspx.*ssw
20. American Disabilities Act. Retrieved from *www.ada.gov/pubs/ada.htm.*
21. Shuler GK, Mistler LA, Torrey K, et al: Bridging communication gaps with the deaf, *Nursing* 43:24, 2013.
22. National Institute on Deafness and Other Communication Disorders: Cochlear implants. Retrieved from *www.nidcd.nih.gov.*
23. Öberg M: Hearing care for older adults: beyond the audiology clinic, *Am J Audiol* 2015 Apr 7. doi:10.1044/2015_AJA-14-0077. [Epub ahead of print]

*Evidence-based information for clinical practice.

22

Assessment of Integumentary System

Diana L. Gallagher

Nobody grows old merely by living a number of years. We grow old by deserting our ideals. Years may wrinkle the skin, but to give up enthusiasm wrinkles the soul.

Samuel Ullman

http://evolve.elsevier.com/Lewis/medsurg/

LEARNING OUTCOMES

1. Describe the structures and functions of the integumentary system.
2. Link the age-related changes in the integumentary system to differences in assessment findings.
3. Obtain significant subjective and objective data related to the integumentary system from a patient.
4. Describe specific assessments to be made during the physical examination of the skin and appendages.
5. Compare and contrast the critical components for describing primary and secondary lesions.
6. Perform a physical assessment of the integumentary system using appropriate techniques.
7. Specify the structural and assessment differences in light- and dark-skinned persons.
8. Differentiate normal from common abnormal findings of a physical assessment of the integumentary system.
9. Describe the purpose, significance of results, and nursing responsibilities related to diagnostic studies of the integumentary system.

KEY TERMS

alopecia, Table 22-8, p. 403
dermis, p. 395
epidermis, p. 394
erythema, Table 22-8, p. 403
hirsutism, Table 22-8, p. 403
intertriginous, p. 399
keloid, p. 403
keratinocytes, p. 394
melanocytes, p. 395
mole (nevus), Table 22-8, p. 403
pruritus, p. 399
sebaceous glands, p. 396

The integumentary system is the largest organ of the body. It is composed of the skin, hair, nails, and certain glands. The skin has two major layers: epidermis (outer layer) and dermis (inner layer). The subcutaneous tissue (layer) lies under the dermis (Fig. 22-1). The skin is as complex as any organ, but unlike the others, it is readily visible. Being able to see and touch the skin helps you assess your patients. You can see abnormalities, understand their significance, and intervene early.

STRUCTURES AND FUNCTIONS OF SKIN AND APPENDAGES

Structures

Epidermis. The **epidermis**, the outer layer of the skin, is relatively thin, ranging from 0.05 mm on the eyelids to 0.1 mm on the soles.[1] There are no lymphatic or vascular structures in the epidermis. It is supported by passive circulation from the dermis.

The epidermis can be divided into five distinct but interrelated layers. Two of the layers are the stratum corneum (the surface layer) and the stratum germinativum (deepest, basal layer) (Fig. 22-1).

The major cells in the epidermis are the keratinocytes (90%) and melanocytes (5%). The remaining cells are Langerhans' cells and Merkel cells.

Keratinocytes are synthesized from epidermal cells in the basal layer. Initially they are undifferentiated and shaped like columns. As they mature (keratinize), they move to the surface, where they flatten and die to form the outer skin layer (stratum corneum). Keratinocytes produce a fibrous protein, keratin, which is vital to the skin's protective barrier function. The upward movement of keratinocytes from the basal layer to the outermost levels of the stratum corneum takes about 14 days. The keratinocytes remain there for another 14 days, allowing the epidermis to regenerate every 28 days. (Each month you have a new layer of skin.)

Many skin problems result from changes in this cell cycle. If dead cells slough off too rapidly, the skin appears thin and eroded. If new cells form faster than old cells are shed, the skin becomes scaly and thickened. Failure of the epidermis to

Reviewed by Patricia Gable Burke, RN, BSN, CWOCN, Patient Educator Wound, Ostomy, Continence Care, Bethesda North Hospital, Cincinnati, Ohio; Kim Clevenger, RN, EdD, BC, Associate Professor of Nursing, BSN Program Coordinator, Morehead State University, Morehead, Kentucky; and Allison J. Terry, RN, PhD, Associate Professor of Nursing, Assistant Dean of Clinical Practice, School of Nursing, Auburn University Montgomery, Montgomery, Alabama.

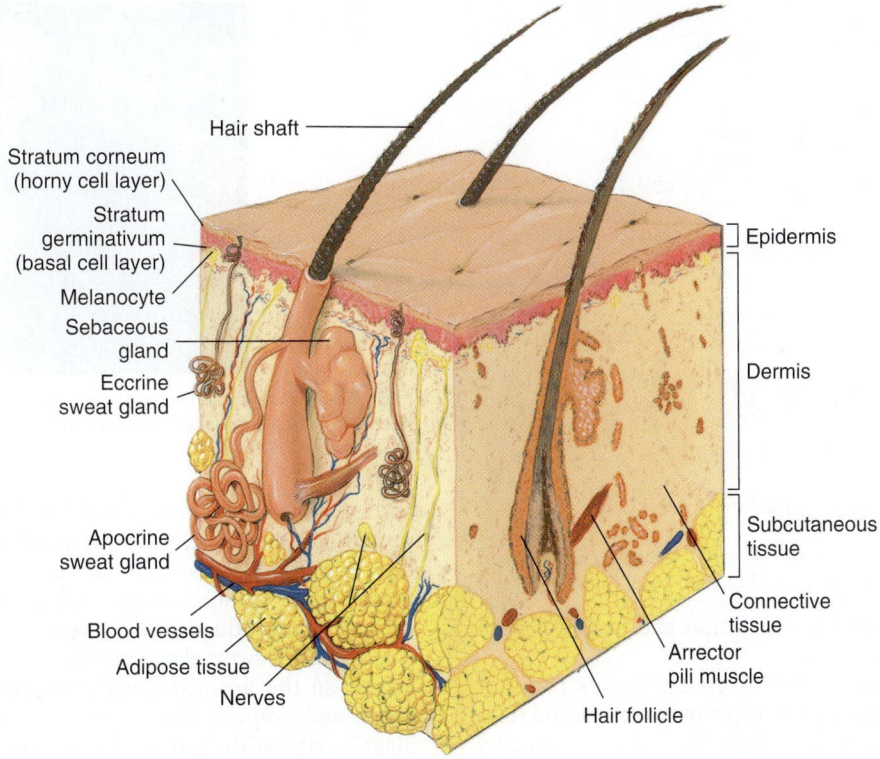

FIG. 22-1 Microscopic view of the skin in longitudinal section. (From Jarvis C: *Physical examination and health assessment,* ed 6, St Louis, 2012, Saunders.)

function normally occurs with skin cancer and psoriasis (discussed in Chapter 23).

Melanocytes are also found in the deep, basal layer. They contain melanin, a pigment that gives color to the skin and hair and protects the body from damaging ultraviolet (UV) sunlight. Sunlight and hormones stimulate the melanosome (within the melanocyte) to increase the production of melanin. People of all races have similar numbers of melanocytes. In darker skin, the melanosomes are larger and more numerous, thus producing more melanin.[1] This increased melanin forms a natural sun shield for dark skin and results in a decreased incidence of skin cancer in these persons. The distribution of melanocytes varies from one area of the body to another. For example, the face has more melanocytes than the abdomen.

Langerhans' cells are a type of dendritic cell (discussed in Chapter 13 on p. 194). They are immunocompetent cells that are essential to recognize antigens. When they are depleted, the skin cannot initiate an immune response. The Langerhans' cells in bioengineered skin grafts have been removed to prevent graft rejection. In skin diseases such as psoriasis and sarcoidosis, there are decreased numbers of Langerhans' cells.

Merkel cells are touch receptors found in the epidermis and involved in the sensation of light touch. They are used when feeling the texture of an object and determining what it is. High concentrations of Merkel cells are found in the fingertips and also in the lips, but they are also present in areas of hairy skin.[2]

The basement membrane zone is between the epidermis and dermis. This structure provides for the (1) exchange of fluids between the epidermis and dermis and (2) structural support for the epidermis. The basement membrane also helps to secure the two layers together. Inflammation and separation of the epidermal and dermal layers result in the blisters seen with problems such as burns, full-thickness wounds, and mechanical trauma.

Dermis. The **dermis** is the connective tissue below the epidermis. Dermal thickness ranges from 0.3 mm on the eyelid to 3.0 mm on the back.[3] The dermis is very vascular, containing many blood vessels. It also contains nerves, lymphatic vessels, hair follicles, sebaceous glands, and specialized cells such as mast cells and macrophages that protect the body from external stimuli.

The dermis is made of three types of connective tissue: collagen, elastic fibers, and reticular fibers. Collagen forms the greatest part of the dermis. It is responsible for the skin's mechanical strength. The primary cell type in the dermis is the *fibroblast,* which produces collagen and elastin. Collagen is critical in wound healing.

The dermis has two layers: upper thin papillary layer and a deeper, thicker reticular layer. The papillary layer is arranged haphazardly in ridges, or papillae, which extend into the outer epidermal layer. These elevated surface ridges form fingerprints and footprints. The reticular layer forms the bulk of the dermis. It is made up of thick collagen bundles arranged perpendicular to the skin's surface.

Subcutaneous Tissue. The subcutaneous tissue lies below the dermis. It is made of loose connective tissue and fat cells that provide insulation, cushioning, temperature regulation, and energy storage. The subcutaneous tissue attaches the skin to underlying tissues, such as muscle and bone. The distribution pattern of subcutaneous tissue varies with gender, heredity, age, and nutritional status.

Skin Appendages. *Skin appendages* include the hair, nails, and glands (sebaceous, apocrine, and eccrine). These appendages are epidermal extensions that have their roots in the dermis. These structures receive nutrients, electrolytes, and fluids from the dermis. Hair and nails form from specialized keratin.

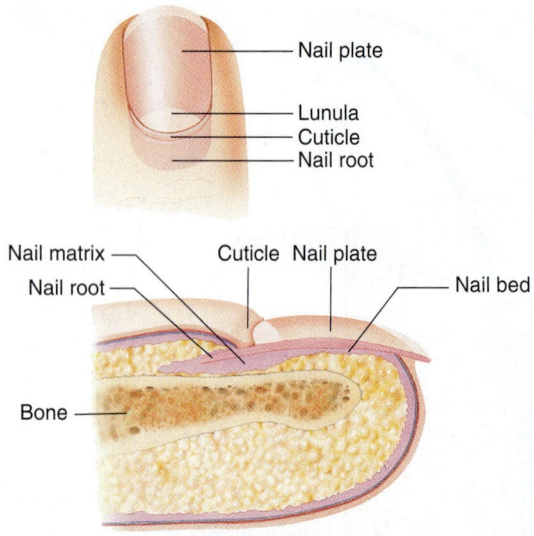

FIG. 22-2 Structure of a nail. (From Patton KT, Thibodeau GA, Douglas M: *Essentials of anatomy and physiology,* St Louis, 2012, Mosby.)

Systemic diseases can affect the condition and health of both hair and nails.

Hair grows on most of the body except for the lips, palms of the hands, interdigital spaces, portions of the genitalia, and soles of the feet. Hair color is a result of heredity and determined by the type and amount of melanin in the hair shaft. Hair grows approximately 1 cm per month. People lose an average of 25 to 100 hairs each day.[1] When lost hair is not replaced, baldness, or *alopecia,* results.

Fingernails and toenails are made of heavily keratinized cells. The part of the nail that you can see is the nail body. The rest is the nail root. A fold of skin hides most of the nail root. The cuticle borders this skin fold. Nail growth begins in the nail root. The portion of the nail root you can see is the *lunula.* This white, crescent-shaped area is the site of mitosis and nail growth (Fig. 22-2). Under the nail is an area of epidermis called the *nail bed.* The nail bed contains many blood vessels. Fingernails grow at a rate of 0.7 to 0.84 mm per week, with toenail growth 30% to 50% slower.[4] A lost fingernail usually regenerates in 3 to 6 months, while a lost toenail may require 12 months or longer to regenerate. Nail growth varies based on a person's age and health. Nails grow faster in men and in warm weather. Nail color ranges from pink to yellow or brown depending on skin color. Color and texture variations in the nails may represent normal or abnormal conditions. Pigmented longitudinal bands *(melanonychia striata)* occur in the nail bed in approximately 90% or more of people with dark skin[2] (Fig. 22-3).

Two major types of glands are associated with the skin: sebaceous and sweat (apocrine and eccrine) glands. **Sebaceous glands** secrete *sebum,* which is emptied into the hair follicles. Sebum waterproofs and lubricates the skin and promotes the absorption of fat-soluble substances. Sebum is somewhat bacteriostatic and fungistatic. These glands depend on sex hormones, particularly testosterone, to regulate sebum secretion and production. Actual production varies depending on age, sex, and testosterone and estrogen levels. Sebaceous glands are present on all areas of the skin except the palms and soles and dorsum of the feet. These glands are most abundant on the face, scalp, upper chest, and back.

The *apocrine sweat glands* are located in the axillae, breast areolae, umbilical and anogenital areas, external auditory canals, and eyelids. They secrete a thick milky substance containing protein, carbohydrate, and other substances.[5] The secretions are odorless. Odor occurs when skin surface bacteria alter the secretions. These glands enlarge and become active at puberty because of reproductive hormones.

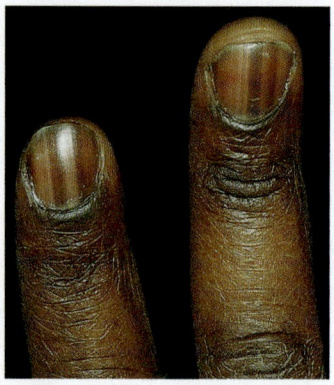

FIG. 22-3 Pigmented nail bed normally seen with dark skin color. (From Habif TP: *Clinical dermatology: a color guide to diagnosis and therapy,* ed 5, St Louis, 2011, Mosby.)

The *eccrine sweat glands* are widely distributed over the body, except on the lips, ear canals, nail beds, labia minora, glans penis, and prepuce. One square inch of skin contains about 3000 eccrine sweat glands. Their main function is to cool the body by evaporation, excrete waste products, and moisturize surface cells. Sweat is a transparent watery solution composed of salts, ammonia, urea, and other wastes. In extreme situations, the body can produce 2 to 4 L of sweat per hour or up to 12 liters in 24 hours. Heat, certain mental stimuli, and ingestion of hot, spicy foods stimulate sweat secretion.

Functions of Integumentary System

The skin's primary function is to protect the underlying body tissues by serving as a barrier to the external environment. The skin acts as a barrier against invasion by bacteria and viruses and prevents excessive water loss. The fat in the subcutaneous layer insulates the body and provides protection from trauma. Melanin screens and absorbs ultraviolet radiation.

The skin with its nerve endings and special receptors provides sensory perception for environmental stimuli. These highly specialized nerve endings supply information to the brain related to pain, heat and cold, touch, pressure, and vibration.

The skin controls heat regulation by responding to changes in internal and external temperature with vasoconstriction or vasodilation. The skin's excretory function and heat regulation are related. Between 600 and 900 mL of water is lost daily through insensible water loss (invisible vaporization from the lungs and skin), which assists in regulating body temperature. Sebum and sweat lubricate the skin surface. Endogenous synthesis of vitamin D, which is critical to calcium and phosphorus balance, occurs in the epidermis. Vitamin D is synthesized by the action of UV light on vitamin D precursors in epidermal cells.

The skin is a delivery system for drugs. An increasing number of systemic drugs are effectively delivered via patches or creams applied directly to the skin.

Gerontologic Considerations: Effects of Aging on Integumentary System

Many skin changes are associated with aging. Depending on a person's view of themselves, the normal, visible effects of aging

TABLE 22-1 Gerontologic Assessment Differences

Integumentary System

Changes	Differences in Assessment Findings
Skin	
Decreased subcutaneous fat, muscle laxity, degeneration of elastic fibers, collagen stiffening	Increased wrinkling, sagging breasts and abdomen, redundant flesh around eyes, slowness of skin to flatten when pinched (tenting)
Decreased extracellular water, surface lipids, and sebaceous gland activity	Dry, flaking skin with possible signs of excoriation caused by scratching
Decreased activity of apocrine and sebaceous glands	Dry skin with minimal to no perspiration, skin color uneven
Increased capillary fragility and permeability	Bruising
Increased focal melanocytes in basal layer with pigment accumulation	Solar lentigines on face and back of hands
Diminished blood supply	Decrease in rosy appearance of skin and mucous membranes. Skin cool to touch. Diminished awareness of pain, touch, temperature, peripheral vibration
Decreased proliferative capacity	Diminished rate of wound healing
Decreased immunocompetence	Increase in neoplasms
Hair	
Decreased melanin and melanocytes	Gray or white hair
Decreased oil	Dry, coarse hair. Scaly scalp
Decreased density of hair	Thinning and loss of hair
Cumulative androgen effect; decreasing estrogen levels	Facial hirsutism, baldness
Nails	
Decreased peripheral blood supply	Thick, brittle nails with diminished growth
Increased keratin	Longitudinal ridging
Decreased circulation	Prolonged return of blood to nails on blanching

on the skin and hair may have a profound psychologic effect. Having a youthful look may affect a person's self-image. The appearance of the signs of aging can be a threat to self-concept. Other changes in skin structure related to normal changes with aging can pose serious risk. Age-related changes of the integumentary system and differences in assessment findings are listed in Table 22-1.

Chronic UV exposure is the major contributor to the photoaging and wrinkling of skin.[6] Sun damage to the skin is cumulative (Fig. 22-4). The wrinkling of sun-exposed areas such as the face and hands is more marked than that of a sun-shielded area, such as the buttocks. Poor nutrition, with decreased intake of protein, calories, and vitamins, contributes to skin aging. Collagen fibers stiffen, elastic fibers degenerate, and the amount of subcutaneous tissue decreases. These changes, with the added effects of gravity, lead to wrinkling.

The junction between the dermis and epidermis flattens. This causes the two layers to lose their tight bond. Skin tears and other trauma become common as the epidermis slides separately from the dermis. Fewer free fatty acids in the epidermis results in dry, scaly, itchy skin. Dryness, combined with trauma caused by scratching, increases the risk of fissures (cracks) in the skin and secondary infections. Decreased subcutaneous fat

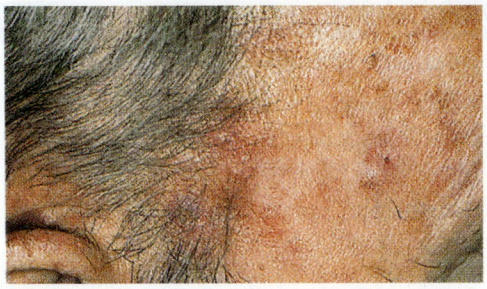

FIG. 22-4 Photoaging. Irregular pigmentation and keratoses occur on sun-damaged skin on forehead. (From Gawkrodger D, Ardern-Jones MR: *Dermatology*, ed 5, Edinburgh, 2012, Churchill Livingstone.)

TABLE 22-2 Normal Physical Assessment of Integumentary System

Skin	• Evenly pigmented. No petechiae, purpura, lesions, or excoriations • Warm, good turgor
Nails	• Pink, oval, adhere to nail bed with 160-degree angle
Hair	• Shiny and full; amount and distribution appropriate for age and gender • No flaking of scalp, forehead, or pinna

increases the risk of traumatic injury, hypothermia, and skin shearing, which may lead to pressure ulcers.

Fewer melanocytes are present, and with decreased levels of melanin, hair color fades. Hormonal and vitamin deficiencies can cause dry, thin hair and alopecia. The growth rate of the hair and nails decreases because of atrophy. The nail plate thins, and nails become brittle and more prone to splitting and yellowing. Nails, especially the toenails, may thicken with age. With aging, the apocrine and eccrine sweat glands atrophy, causing dry skin and decreased body odor.

Benign neoplasms related to the aging process can occur. These growths include seborrheic keratoses, vascular lesions such as cherry angiomas, and skin tags. *Actinic keratoses* appear on areas of chronic sun exposure, especially in the person who has a fair complexion and light eyes (blue, green, or hazel). These premalignant cutaneous lesions place a person at increased risk for squamous cell and basal cell carcinomas. A photoaged person is more susceptible to skin cancers because UV exposure decreases the capacity to repair cellular damage. Chronic UV exposure from tanning beds causes the same damage as UV from the sun.

ASSESSMENT OF INTEGUMENTARY SYSTEM

The general skin assessment begins with your initial contact with the patient and continues throughout the examination. As you are meeting your patient for the first time, take a moment to note the overall condition of their skin and hair. Specific areas of the skin are assessed during the examination of other body systems, unless the chief complaint is a dermatologic problem. Record a general statement about the skin's physical condition (Table 22-2). In addition, ask the health history questions presented in Table 22-3 when a skin problem is noted.

Subjective Data

People with skin problems may have complaints that you are not able to readily observe. A thorough health history yields information about possible causes and the effect of the problem on the person's life.

TABLE 22-3 Health History

Integumentary System

Health Perception–Health Management
- Describe your daily hygiene practices.
- What skin products are you currently using?
- Describe any current skin condition, including onset, course, and treatment (if any).

Nutritional-Metabolic
- Describe any changes in the condition of your skin, hair, nails, and mucous membranes.
- Have you noticed any recent changes in the way sores or wounds heal?*
- Have you had any weight loss or dietary changes, including supplemental vitamins and minerals?*

Elimination
- Have you noticed recent changes in your skin related to excessive sweating, dryness, or swelling?*

Activity-Exercise
- Do your leisure or work activities involve the use of any chemicals that are irritating to your skin?*
- Do you do anything to protect yourself from the sun?*

Sleep-Rest
- Does your skin condition keep you awake or awaken you after you have fallen asleep?*

Cognitive-Perceptual
- Do you have any unusual sensations of heat, cold, or touch?*
- Do you have any pain associated with your skin condition?*
- Do you have any joint pain?*

Self-Perception–Self-Concept
- How does your skin condition make you feel about yourself?

Role-Relationship
- Has your skin condition changed your relationships with others?*
- Have you changed your lifestyle because of your skin condition?*

Sexuality-Reproductive
- Has your skin condition changed your intimate relationships with others?*
- Has your birth control method (if used) caused a skin problem?*

Coping–Stress Tolerance
- Are you aware of any situation or stressor that changes your skin condition?*
- Do you think that stress plays a role in your skin condition?*
- How do you handle stress?

Value-Belief
- Are there any cultural beliefs that influence your thinking or feelings about your skin condition?*
- Are there any treatment options that you would be opposed to using?

*If yes, describe.

CASE STUDY

Patient Introduction

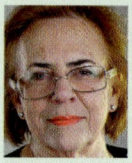

(©iStockphoto/Thinkstock)

D.A. is a 74-year-old woman who comes to the medical clinic with concerns related to various "spots" on her face. She says they have been there for a while and she thought they were just "age spots" but got concerned after her friend was diagnosed with a malignant melanoma.

Discussion Questions

1. What type of assessment should you perform: comprehensive, focused, or emergency?
2. What are the possible causes of D.A.'s facial lesions?
3. What questions would you ask D.A. to determine the possible causes?

You will learn more about D.A. and her condition as you read through this assessment chapter.

(See p. 400 for more information on D.A.)

Answers available at *http://evolve.elsevier.com/Lewis/medsurg.*

Important Health Information

Past Health History. Past health history reveals previous trauma, surgery, or disease that involves the skin. Many diseases have dermatologic manifestations (Table 22-4). Determine if the patient has noticed any problems such as jaundice (liver disease), delayed wound healing (diabetes mellitus), cyanosis (respiratory disorder), or pallor (anemia). Obtain specific information related to food sensitivities, pet or drug allergies, and skin reactions to insect bites and stings. Note any history of chronic or unprotected exposure to UV light, including tanning bed use and radiation treatments.

Medications. A thorough medication history is important. Ask the patient about skin-related problems that occurred because of taking prescription or over-the-counter (OTC) medications. Many vitamins, hormones, antibiotics, corticosteroids, and antimetabolites have side effects that are manifested in the skin. Document the use of medications specifically used to treat a primary skin problem, such as acne, or a secondary skin problem, such as itching. Record the drug's name, length of use, method of application, and effectiveness.

Surgery or Other Treatments. Determine if any surgical procedures, including cosmetic surgery, were done on the skin. Record any previous biopsy results. Note any treatments specific for a skin problem (e.g., phototherapy) or for a health problem (e.g., radiation therapy). Document any treatments undergone primarily for cosmetic purposes, such as tanning booth use, laser resurfacing, or cosmetic "peels."

Functional Health Patterns

Health Perception–Health Management Pattern. Question the patient about health practices, such as self-care habits related to daily hygiene. Document the frequency of use and sun protection factor (SPF) of sunscreen products. Assess the use of personal care products (e.g., shampoos, moisturizing agents, cosmetics), including brand name, quantity, and frequency. Record a description of any current skin problem, including onset, symptoms, course, and treatment. Note any medications used for treating hair loss.

Obtain information about the family history of any skin diseases, including congenital and familial diseases (e.g., alopecia, psoriasis) and systemic diseases with dermatologic manifestations (e.g., diabetes, thyroid disease, cardiovascular diseases, immune disorders). Note any family and personal history of skin cancer, particularly melanoma.

TABLE 22-4 Diseases With Dermatologic Manifestations

Systemic Problem	Dermatologic Manifestations
Endocrine	
Hyperthyroidism	Increased sweating, warm skin with persistent flush, thin nails, alopecia. Fine, soft hair
Hypothyroidism	Cold, dry, pale to yellow skin. Generalized nonpitting edema. Dry, coarse, brittle hair. Brittle, slow-growing nails
Glucocorticoid excess (Cushing syndrome)	Atrophy, striae, epidermal thinning, telangiectasia, acne. Decreased subcutaneous fat over extremities. Thin, loose dermis. Impaired wound healing. Increased vascular fragility. Mild hirsutism. Excessive collection of fat over clavicles, back of neck, abdomen, and face
Addison's disease	Loss of body hair (especially axillary), generalized hyperpigmentation (accentuated in folds)
Androgen excess	Enlarged facial pores, male sex characteristics, acne, acceleration of coarse hair growth
Androgen deficiency	Development of sparse hair. Marked reduction in sebum production
Hypoparathyroidism	Opaque, brittle nails with transverse ridges. Coarse, sparse hair with patchy alopecia
Hyperpituitarism (acromegaly)	Coarsened skin, deepened lines. Increased oiliness and sweating, acne. Increased number of nevi, hyperpigmentation; hypertrichosis (excess hair growth)
Diabetes mellitus	Erythematous plaques of shins, delayed wound healing, neuropathy, acanthosis nigricans (velvety, dark skin on the neck and in skin folds)
Reproductive Organs	
Primary syphilis	Chancre
Secondary syphilis	Generalized skin lesions, alopecia
Tertiary syphilis	Gummas
Paget's disease	Eczematous patch of nipple and areola
Gastrointestinal	
Inflammatory bowel disease	Mouth ulcers, erythema nodosum
Liver disease and biliary tract obstruction	Jaundice, itching, pigmentary abnormalities, alterations in nails and hair, spider angiomas, telangiectasia
Deficiency of essential fatty acids	Scaly skin
Malabsorption syndrome	Acquired ichthyosis (dry, scaly skin)
Cystic fibrosis	Abnormal sweat gland function
Musculoskeletal and Connective Tissue	
Systemic lupus erythematosus	Discoid lesions, maculopapular semiconfluent rash (butterfly rash), alopecia, mouth ulcers
Scleroderma	Leathery hardening and stiffness of skin
Dermatomyositis	Edema; purplish-red upper eyelids; scaly, macular erythema over knuckles
Metabolic	
Vitamin B_1 (thiamine) deficiency	Edema, redness of soles of feet
Vitamin B_2 (riboflavin) deficiency	Red fissures at corner of mouth, glossitis
Nicotinic acid (niacin) deficiency	Redness of exposed areas of skin of hand or foot, face, or neck; infected dermatitis
Vitamin C deficiency	Petechiae, purpura, bleeding gums
Immune	
Hodgkin's lymphoma	Pruritus, sensitive skin
Non-Hodgkin's lymphoma	Papules, nodules, plaques, pruritus
HIV infection	Kaposi sarcoma, eosinophilic folliculitis
Cardiovascular	
Rheumatic heart disease	Petechiae, urticaria, nodules, erythema
Thromboangiitis obliterans (Buerger's disease)	Pallor or cyanosis, gangrene, ulceration
Peripheral vascular disease	Loss of hair on hands and feet. Delayed capillary filling. Dependent rubor (redness), pain
Venous ulcers	Leathery, brownish skin on lower leg; pruritus, concave lesion with edema. Scar tissue with healing
Respiratory	
Inadequate oxygenation due to respiratory disease	Cyanosis
Hematologic	
Anemia	Pallor, hyperpigmentation, pale mucous membranes, hair loss, nail dystrophy
Clotting disorders	Purpura, petechiae, ecchymosis
Renal	
Chronic kidney disease	Dry skin, pruritus, uremic frost, pallor, bruises
Neurologic	
Chronic sensory polyneuropathies	Trophic changes in skin resulting from sensory denervation, pressure ulcers, anesthesia, paresthesias
Spinal cord trauma	

GENETIC RISK ALERT

- The primary risk factor leading to skin cancer and melanoma is environmental exposure to UV radiation. UV radiation damages DNA, causing an error in the genetic code and resulting in abnormal skin cells.[6]
- Inherited genetic factors can increase the risk for skin cancer. A person has an increased risk for developing melanoma if he or she has a first-degree relative (e.g., parent, full sibling) who had a melanoma.
- The risk for skin cancer is increased in people who have a fair complexion (light-colored skin that easily freckles, red or blond hair, and blue or light-colored eyes).

Nutritional-Metabolic Pattern. Question the patient about any changes in the condition of skin, hair, nails, and mucous membranes and whether they are related to dietary changes. A diet history reveals the adequacy of nutrients essential to healthy skin such as vitamins A, D, E, and C; dietary fat; and protein. Note any food allergies that cause a skin reaction. Ask obese patients if they have areas of chafing or a rash in **intertriginous** areas, where skin surfaces overlap and rub on each other (e.g., below the breasts, axillae, and groin). Note any excessive or absent sweating. Question the patient about poor or delayed wound healing.

Elimination Pattern. Ask the patient about conditions of the skin such as dehydration, edema, and **pruritus** (itching), which can indicate alterations in fluid balance. If urinary or fecal incontinence is a problem, determine the condition of the skin in the anal and perineal areas.

Activity-Exercise Pattern. Obtain information about environmental hazards in relation to hobbies and recreational activities, including exposure to known carcinogens, chemical irritants, and allergens. Ask the patient if any changes occur in the skin during exercise or other activities.

Sleep-Rest Pattern. Question the patient about disturbances in sleep patterns caused by a skin condition. For example, pruritus can be distressing and cause major alterations in normal sleep patterns. Poor sleep and resulting tiredness are often reflected in a patient's face by dark circles under the eyes and a decreased firmness in the facial skin.

Cognitive-Perceptual Pattern. Determine the patient's perception of the sensations of heat, cold, pain, and touch. Note any discomfort associated with a skin condition, especially when observed in intact skin, or any complaints of unusual skin sensations. Patients with neuropathy may describe numbness, tingling, or crawling sensations in their arms or legs. Assess and record any joint pain. Assess the mobility of the joints, since the patient's skin condition may cause alterations in mobility.

Self-Perception–Self-Concept Pattern. Assess any feelings related to the patient's skin condition such as sadness, anxiety, despair, or altered body image. These feelings can occur with classic signs of aging or visible skin problems such as acne, rosacea, and psoriasis, which alter physical appearance.

Role-Relationship Pattern. Determine how the patient's skin condition affects relationships with family members, peers, and work associates. In addition, question the patient regarding the effect of environmental factors on the skin such as occupational exposure to irritants, sun, and unusually cold or unhygienic conditions. Contact dermatitis caused by allergens and irritants is a common problem associated with occupation.

Sexuality-Reproductive Pattern. Tactfully question and assess the effect of the patient's skin condition on sexual activity. In particular, note the reproductive status of the female patient relative to possible therapeutic interventions. For example, isotretinoin (Accutane), used to treat acne, and topical fluorouracil (Efudex, Fluoroplex), used to treat actinic keratoses, are teratogenic drugs that may cause abnormal fetal development. Pregnant women or women who could become pregnant should not use them.

Coping–Stress Tolerance Pattern. Assess and question the patient about the role that stress may play in creating or exacerbating the skin condition. Ask the patient what coping strategies are used to manage the skin condition.

Value-Belief Pattern. Ask about cultural or religious beliefs that could influence the patient's self-image as related to the skin condition. Assess values and beliefs that may influence or limit the choice of treatment options.

Objective Data

Physical Examination. A physical examination of the skin begins with a systematic, general inspection and then a more specific assessment of problem areas. A normal range of differences exists in the skin, hair, and nails. Your assessment should note normal skin changes related to age, genetic factors, and environmental exposures from other changes. Look for changes in the color of the skin, turgor, temperature, dryness, thickness, and vascularity. General principles when assessing the skin are as follows:

- Have a private examination room of moderate temperature with good lighting; a room with exposure to daylight is preferred.
- Ensure that the patient is comfortable and in a dressing gown that allows easy access to all skin areas.
- Be systematic and proceed from head to toe.

CASE STUDY

Subjective Data

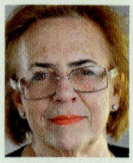

(©iStockphoto/Thinkstock)

A focused subjective assessment of D.A. reveals the following:

- ***PMH:*** Negative except for an appendectomy at age 16.
- ***Medications:*** None at present. NKA.
- ***Health Perception–Health Management:*** Currently washes her face with a skin cleanser in the morning and nighttime. After cleansing, she applies a moisturizer with SPF 15. She has used these facial products for the past 3 years since she first started noticing small age spots appearing. Before that, she just used soap and water.
- ***Nutritional:*** D.A. reports that her skin seems to be drier as she ages but otherwise no changes besides the "age spots" or "whatever they are." Denies any changes in the way cuts or sores heal. No weight loss. Does not take any supplemental vitamins or minerals.
- ***Elimination:*** Although skin is a little dry, D.A. does not perceive it to be excessively dry. Denies excessive sweating or any swelling.
- ***Activity-Exercise:*** Loves to garden and go for walks outdoors. Reports a history of frequent, sometimes severe, sunburns as a child. No use of sunscreen growing up but does remember her mother making her wear T-shirts over her bathing suits to help prevent sunburn. Has used sunscreen for the past 20 years when outdoors. Reapplies as needed.
- ***Cognitive-Perceptual:*** Denies any pain or discomfort associated with skin lesions.
- ***Coping–Stress Tolerance:*** Fearful that she might have skin cancer.

Discussion Questions

1. Which subjective assessment findings are of most concern to you?
2. What should be included in the physical assessment? What specific characteristics of the skin lesions would you be looking for?

You will learn more about the physical examination of the skin in the next section.

(See p. 404 for more information on D.A.)

Answers available at *http://evolve.elsevier.com/Lewis/medsurg.*

- Compare symmetric parts.
- Perform a general inspection and then a lesion-specific examination.
- Use the metric system when taking measurements.
- Use appropriate terminology and nomenclature when reporting or documenting.

Photographs are useful when accurate findings are needed. Follow clinical agency protocol regarding obtaining a patient's consent to photograph skin lesions for inclusion in the medical record.

Inspection. Inspect the skin for general color and pigmentation, vascularity, bruising, and lesions or discolorations. The critical factor in assessment of skin color is change. A skin color that is normal for a particular patient can be a sign of a pathologic condition in another patient. The skin color depends on the amount of melanin (brown), carotene (yellow), oxyhemoglobin (red), and reduced hemoglobin (bluish red) present at a particular time. The most reliable areas to assess erythema, cyanosis, pallor, and jaundice are the areas of least pigmentation, such as the sclera, conjunctivae, nail beds, lips, and buccal mucosa. The true skin color is best observed in photo-protected areas such as the buttocks. Activity, sun (UV) exposure, emotions, cigarette smoking, and edema, as well as respiratory, renal, cardiovascular, and hepatic disorders, can all directly affect skin color.

In your general inspection, note the presence of body art such as piercings and tattoos. The nose, ears, eyebrows, lips, navel, and nipples are common sites of piercing. Examine tattoos and needle-track marks and note the location and characteristics of the surrounding skin area. Tattoo pigments deposited in the skin may cause itching, pain, and sensitivity for several weeks after the tattoo is placed.

Examine the skin for possible problems related to vascularity, including bruising and vascular and purpuric lesions such as *angioma* (benign tumor of blood or lymph vessels), *petechiae* (tiny, flat, purplish red pinpoint lesions on skin), *ecchymosis* (bruise larger than petechiae), or *purpura* (purple colored spots and patches characterized by ecchymosis or other small hemorrhages). Note the reaction to direct pressure on the lesion. If a lesion blanches on direct pressure and then refills, the redness is due to dilated blood vessels. If the discoloration remains, it is the result of subcutaneous or intradermal bleeding or a nonvascular lesion. Note any pattern of bruising such as discoloration in the shape of the hand or fingers or bruises at different stages of resolution. These may indicate other health problems or abuse and require further investigation.

Record the color, size, height, distribution, location, and shape of any lesions. Lesions may be primary or secondary lesions. *Primary skin lesions* develop on previously unaltered skin. The common characteristics of primary skin lesions are shown in Table 22-5. *Secondary skin lesions* are lesions that change with time or occur because of factors such as scratching or infection. Secondary skin lesions are shown in Table 22-6.

Skin lesions are usually described in terms related to the lesions' configuration (solitary or pattern in relation to other lesions) and distribution (arrangement of lesions over an area of skin) (Table 22-7). Note any unusual odors. Skin sites with lesions, such as rashes, may be colonized with yeast or bacteria, which can be associated with distinctive odors in intertriginous areas (Fig. 22-5).

Inspect all body hair. Note the distribution, texture, and quantity of hair. Changes in the normal distribution of body hair and growth may indicate an endocrine or vascular disorder. Carefully inspect the nails, including nail shape, thickness, curvature, and surface. Note any grooves, pitting, ridges, or detachment from nail bed. Changes in nail smoothness or thickness can occur with anemia, psoriasis, thyroid problems, decreased vascular circulation, and some infections.

Palpation. Palpate the skin to obtain information about temperature, turgor, moisture, and texture. Use the back of your hand to gauge skin temperature. The skin should be warm, not hot. Skin temperature increases when blood flow to the dermis is increased. A localized temperature increase occurs with burns and local inflammation. A generalized increase occurs when a person has a fever. A decreased body temperature may occur when shock or other circulatory problems, chilling, or infection are present.

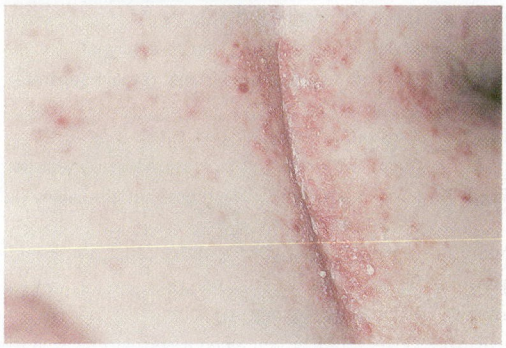

FIG. 22-5 Intertrigo. Rash in body folds with *Candida* infection. (From Graham-Brown R, Bourke J, Cunliffe T: *Dermatology: fundamentals of practice,* Edinburgh, 2008, Mosby Ltd.)

Turgor refers to the elasticity of the skin. Assess turgor by gently pinching an area of skin under the clavicle or on the back of the hand. Skin with good turgor should move easily when lifted and immediately return to its original position when released. In patients with dehydration and aging, a loss of turgor occurs and can cause tenting of the skin.

Skin moisture (dampness or dryness of the skin) increases in intertriginous areas and with high humidity. Skin moisture

TABLE 22-5 Primary Skin Lesions

Lesion	Description
Macule 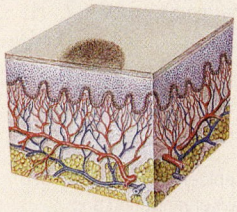	Circumscribed, flat area with a change in skin color. <0.5 cm in diameter. If lesion >0.5 cm, it is a *patch.* *Examples:* freckles, petechiae, measles, flat mole (nevus), café-au-lait spots, vitiligo (complete depigmentation)
Papule 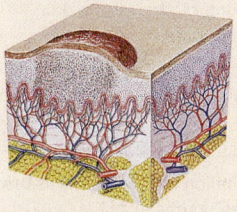	Elevated, solid lesion. <0.5 cm in diameter. If lesion is >0.5 cm in diameter, it is a *nodule.* *Examples:* wart (verruca), elevated moles, lipoma, basal cell carcinoma
Vesicle 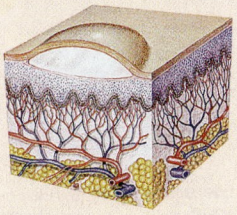	Circumscribed, superficial collection of serous fluid. <0.5 cm in diameter *Examples:* varicella (chickenpox), herpes zoster (shingles), second-degree burn
Plaque 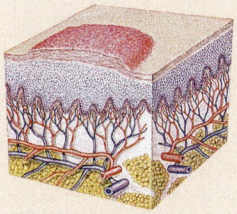	Circumscribed, elevated, superficial, solid lesion. >0.5 cm in diameter *Examples:* psoriasis, seborrheic and actinic keratoses
Wheal 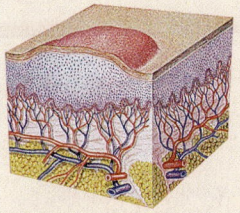	Firm, edematous, irregularly shaped area. Diameter variable *Examples:* insect bite, urticaria
Pustule 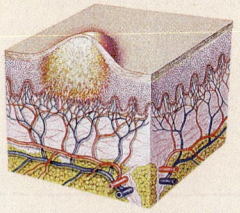	Elevated, superficial lesion filled with purulent fluid *Examples:* acne, impetigo

varies with environmental temperature, muscular activity, body weight, and body temperature. The skin should be intact with no flaking, scaling, or cracking. Skin generally becomes drier with increasing age.

Texture refers to the fineness or coarseness of the skin. The skin should feel smooth and firm with the surface evenly thin in most areas. Thickened callus areas are normal on the soles and palms and relate to weight bearing. Increased skin thickness is often work related and the result of excessive pressure. Excessive calluses on the soles of patients with neuropathy or diabetes predispose them to developing lesions.

Use a *focused assessment* to evaluate the status of previously identified skin problems and to monitor for signs of new problems. A focused assessment of the skin is presented in the box below. Assessment abnormalities of the skin are described in Table 22-8.

TABLE 22-6 Secondary Skin Lesions

Lesion	Description
Fissure 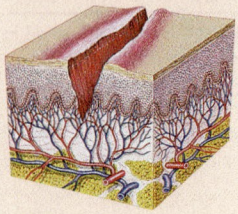	Linear crack or break from the epidermis to the dermis. Dry or moist *Examples:* athlete's foot, cracks at corner of the mouth
Scale 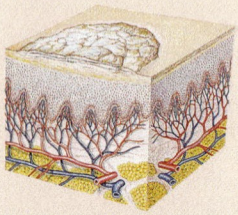	Excess, dead epidermal cells produced by abnormal keratinization and shedding *Examples:* flaking of skin after a drug reaction or sunburn
Scar 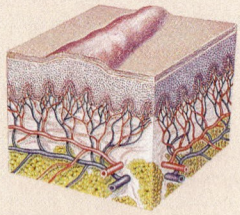	Abnormal formation of connective tissue that replaces normal skin *Examples:* surgical incision, healed wound
Ulcer 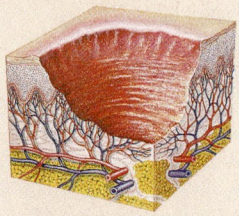	Loss of the epidermis, extending into the dermis. Crater-like, irregular shape *Examples:* pressure ulcer, chancre
Atrophy 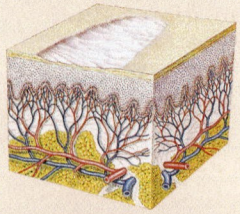	Depression in skin resulting from thinning of the epidermis or dermis *Examples:* aged skin, striae
Excoriation 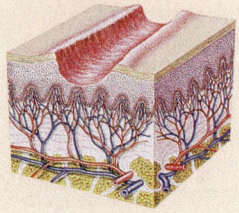	Area in which epidermis is missing, exposing the dermis *Examples:* abrasion, scratch

Assessment of Dark Skin

The structures of dark skin are no different from those of lighter skin, but they are often more difficult to assess (Table 22-9). Color is easiest to assess in areas where the epidermis is thin and pigmentation is not influenced by sun exposure, such as

FOCUSED ASSESSMENT

Integumentary System

Use this checklist to make sure the key assessment steps have been done.

Subjective

Ask the patient about any of the following and note responses.

Hair loss (unusual or rapid)	Y	N
Changes in skin (e.g., lesions, bruising)	Y	N
Nail discoloration	Y	N

Objective: Diagnostic

Check the following for results and critical values.

Biopsy results	✓
Albumin	✓

Objective: Physical Examination

Inspect

Skin for color, integrity, scars, lesions, signs of breakdown	✓
Facial and body hair for distribution, color, quantity, hygiene	✓
Nails for shape, contour, color, thickness, cleanliness	✓
Dressings if present	✓

Palpate

Skin for temperature, texture, moisture, thickness, turgor, mobility	✓

TABLE 22-7 Lesion Distribution Terminology

Term	Description
Annular	Circular, begins in center and spreads to periphery (e.g., tinea corporis [ringworm])
Asymmetric	Unilateral distribution
Confluent	Merging together (e.g., urticaria [hives])
Discrete	Distinct individual lesions that remain separate (e.g., acne)
Gyrate	Twisted, coiled spiral, snakelike
Grouped	Clusters of lesions (e.g., vesicles of contact dermatitis)
Localized	Limited areas of involvement that are clearly defined (confined to one area)
Polycyclic	Annular lesions grow together (e.g., psoriasis)
Solitary	Single lesion
Symmetric	Bilateral distribution
Zosteriform	Linear arrangement along a dermatome area (e.g., herpes zoster)

TABLE 22-8 Assessment Abnormalities

Integumentary System

Finding	Description	Possible Etiology and Significance
Alopecia	Loss of hair (localized or general)	Heredity, friction, rubbing, traction, trauma, stress, infection, inflammation, chemotherapy, pregnancy, emotional shock, tinea capitis, immunologic factors
Angioma	Tumor consisting of blood or lymph vessels	Normal increase in incidence with aging, liver disease, pregnancy, varicose veins
Carotenemia (carotenosis)	Yellow discoloration of skin, no yellowing of sclerae, most noticeable on palms and soles	Vegetables containing carotene (e.g., carrots, squash), hypothyroidism
Comedo (acne lesion)	Enlarged hair follicle plugged with sebum, bacteria, and skin cells; can be open (blackhead) or closed (whitehead)	Heredity, certain drugs, hormonal changes with puberty and pregnancy
Cyanosis	Slightly bluish gray or dark purple discoloration of the skin and mucous membranes caused by excessive amounts of reduced hemoglobin in capillaries	Cardiorespiratory problems, vasoconstriction, asphyxiation, anemia, leukemia, and malignancies
Cyst	Sac containing fluid or semisolid material	Obstruction of a duct or gland, parasitic infection
Ecchymosis	Large, bruise-like lesion caused by collection of extravascular blood in dermis and subcutaneous tissue	Trauma, bleeding disorders
Erythema	Redness occurring in patches of variable size and shape	Heat, certain drugs, alcohol, ultraviolet rays, any problem that causes dilation of blood vessels in the skin
Hematoma	Extravasation of blood of sufficient size to cause visible swelling	Trauma, bleeding disorders
Hirsutism	Male distribution of hair in women	Abnormality of ovaries or adrenal glands, decrease in estrogen level, familial trait
Hypopigmentation	Loss of pigmentation resulting in lighter patches than the normal skin	Chemical agents, nutritional factors, burns, inflammation, infection
Intertrigo	Dermatitis of overlying surfaces of the skin	Moisture, irritation, obesity; may be complicated by *Candida* infection (Fig. 22-5)
Jaundice	Yellow (in white patients) or yellowish brown (in African Americans) discoloration of the skin, best observed in the sclera, secondary to increased bilirubin in the blood	Liver disease, red blood cell hemolysis, pancreatic cancer, common bile duct obstruction
Keloid	Hypertrophied scar beyond wound margins (Fig. 22-6)	Predisposition more common in African Americans
Lichenification	Thickening of the skin with accentuated normal skin markings	Repeated scratching, rubbing, and irritation usually as a result of pruritus or neurosis
Mole (nevus)	Benign overgrowth of melanocytes	Defects of development; excessive numbers and large, irregular moles; often familial
Petechiae	Pinpoint, discrete deposits of blood <1-2 mm in the extravascular tissues and visible through the skin or mucous membrane	Inflammation, marked vasodilation, blood vessel trauma, blood dyscrasia that results in bleeding tendencies (e.g., thrombocytopenia)
Telangiectasia	Visibly dilated, superficial, cutaneous small blood vessels, commonly found on face and thighs	Aging, acne, sun exposure, alcohol, liver failure, corticosteroids, radiation, certain systemic diseases, skin tumors
Tenting	Failure of skin to return immediately to normal position after gentle pinching	Aging, dehydration, cachexia
Varicosity	Increased prominence of superficial veins	Interruption of venous return (e.g., from tumor, incompetent valves, inflammation), commonly found on lower legs with aging
Vitiligo	Complete absence of melanin (pigment) resulting in chalky white patch (Fig. 22-7)	Autoimmune, familial, thyroid disease

the lips, mucous membranes, nail beds, and protected areas (e.g., buttocks). Palmar and plantar surfaces are lighter than other skin areas in darker-skinned persons. Rashes are often more difficult to observe and may have to be palpated. Wrinkling is less apparent in those with dark skin.

Persons with dark skin are predisposed to certain skin and hair conditions. **Keloid** is an overgrowth of collagenous tissue at the site of a skin injury (e.g., ear piercing) (Fig. 22-6). *Vitiligo* is total loss of pigment in the affected area (Fig. 22-7). In *dermatosis papulosa nigra,* the person has small, pigmented wart-like papules, commonly on the face. *Nevus of Ota* is a slate-gray or blue-gray birthmark located on the forehead and face around the eye area. It may also involve the sclera (Fig. 22-8). *Traction alopecia* may be the result of trauma from hair rollers or from tight braiding of the hair (Fig. 22-9). The hair loss may be temporary or permanent. *Pseudofolliculitis* is an inflammatory response to ingrown hairs that occurs after shaving too closely

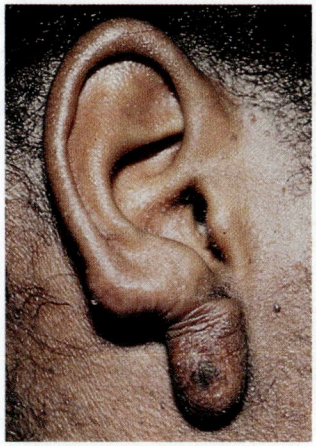

FIG. 22-6 Keloid. Hypertrophic scarring after skin injury, which is more common in dark-skinned persons. (From Habif TP: *Clinical dermatology: a color guide to diagnosis and therapy,* ed 5, St Louis, 2011, Mosby.)

TABLE 22-9 Nursing Assessment

Assessment Variations in Light- and Dark-Skinned Persons

Light Skin	Dark Skin
Cyanosis	
Grayish blue tone, especially in nail beds, earlobes, lips, mucous membranes, palms, and soles	Ashen or gray color most easily seen in the conjunctiva of the eye, mucous membranes, and nail beds
Ecchymosis	
Dark red, purple, yellow, or green color, depending on age of bruise	Purple to brownish black. Difficult to see unless occurring in an area of light pigmentation
Erythema	
Reddish tone, possibly accompanied by increased skin temperature secondary to localized inflammation	Deeper brown or purple skin tone with evidence of increased skin temperature secondary to inflammation
Jaundice	
Yellowish color of skin, sclera, fingernails, palms, and oral mucosa	Yellowish green color most obviously seen in sclera of eye (do not confuse with yellow eye pigmentation, which may be evident in dark-skinned patients), palms, and soles
Pallor	
Pale skin color that may appear white or ashen; also evident on lips, nail beds, and mucous membranes	Lack of underlying red tone in brown or black skin. In light-skinned African Americans, yellowish brown skin. In dark-skinned African Americans, ashen or gray skin
Petechiae	
Lesions appearing as small, reddish purple pinpoints, best observed on abdomen and buttocks	Difficult to see. May be evident in the buccal mucosa of the mouth or conjunctiva of the eye
Rash	
May be visualized and felt with light palpation	Not easily visualized, but may be felt with light palpation
Scar	
Generally heals, showing narrow scar line	Higher incidence of keloid development, resulting in a thickened, raised scar (Table 22-6)

CASE STUDY

Objective Data: Physical Examination

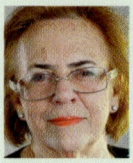

(©iStockphoto/Thinkstock)

- Physical examination findings of D.A.'s skin are as follows:
  - Complexion fair. Wrinkles around eyes, above upper lip, and on sides of cheeks bilaterally. Normal skin temperature and turgor.
  - Lesions: on upper right forehead measuring 2 × 3 mm; on left forehead near hairline measuring 1 × 2 mm; and on left lower cheek measuring 2 × 2.5 mm.

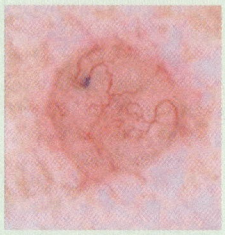

Cheek lesion. (From Bolognia JL, Schaffer JV, Duncan KO, et al: *Dermatology essentials,* Philadelphia, 2014, Saunders.)

- The lesions are slightly erythematous but do not blanch when direct pressure is applied. Borders distinct. The lesions on the forehead have minimal elevation noted on palpation. The lesion on the cheek is slightly elevated.
- No other skin lesions noted on rest of body.

Discussion Questions

1. Which physical assessment findings are of most concern to you?
2. Based upon the subjective and objective assessment data presented so far, what would be three priority nursing diagnoses?
3. What diagnostic studies do you think may be ordered for D.A.?

You will learn more about diagnostic studies related to the skin in the next section.

(See p. 406 for more information on D.A.)

Answers available at *http://evolve.elsevier.com/Lewis/medsurg.*

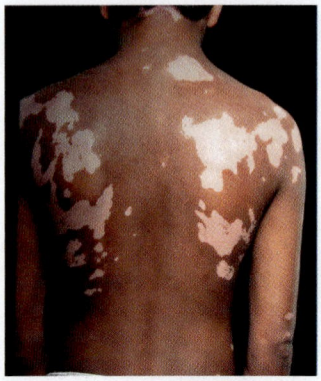

FIG. 22-7 Vitiligo. Total loss of pigment in the affected area. (From Graham-Brown R, Bourke J, Cunliffe T: *Dermatology: fundamentals of practice,* Edinburgh, 2008, Mosby Ltd.)

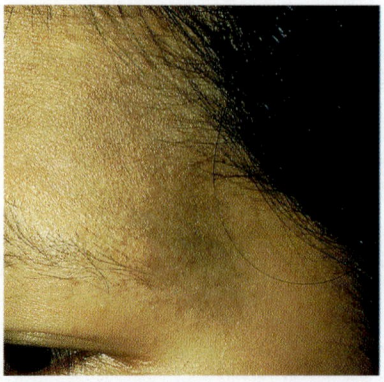

FIG. 22-8 Nevus of Ota. Flat gray to blue pigmentation in the upper trigeminal area, which is more common in dark-skinned persons. (From Gawkrodger D, Ardern-Jones MR: *Dermatology,* ed 5, Edinburgh, 2012, Churchill Livingstone.)

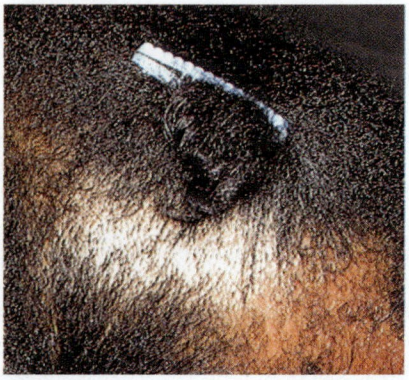

FIG. 22-9 Traction alopecia. Hair loss in scalp because of prolonged tension from hair rollers, braiding, or straightening combs. (From Hurwitz S: *Clinical pediatric dermatology: a textbook of skin disorders of childhood and adolescence,* ed 2, Philadelphia, 1993, Saunders.)

in the beard area. The ingrown hairs result in pustules and papules.

Because of the darkness of the skin in some people, color may not be a reliable indicator of systemic conditions (e.g., flushed skin with fever). Cyanosis may be difficult to determine because a normal bluish hue occurs in dark-skinned people. Dark skin rarely shows a blanch response, making it more difficult to identify pressure ulcers.

DIAGNOSTIC STUDIES OF INTEGUMENTARY SYSTEM

Table 22-10 presents diagnostic studies commonly used for the integumentary system. The main diagnostic techniques related to skin problems are inspection of an individual lesion and a careful history related to the problem. If a definitive diagnosis cannot be made by these techniques, additional tests may be indicated, such as *dermatoscopy* (examination of the skin through a lighted instrument with optical magnification).[7]

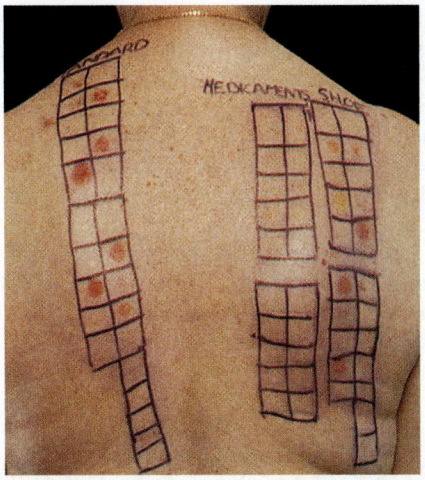

FIG. 22-10 Patch test. Results from an application of possible allergens to the skin shows positive reactions in the sites labeled "standard" and "shoe." (From Graham-Brown R, Bourke J, Cunliffe T: *Dermatology: fundamentals of practice,* Edinburgh, 2008, Mosby Ltd.)

TABLE 22-10 Diagnostic Studies

Integumentary System

Study	Description and Purpose	Nursing Responsibility
Biopsy		
Punch	Special punch biopsy instrument of appropriate size used. Instrument rotated to appropriate level to include dermis and some fat. Suturing may or may not be done. Provides full-thickness skin for diagnostic purposes	*Before:* Verify that consent form is signed (if needed). *During:* Assist with site preparation, anesthesia, procedure, and hemostasis. Properly identify specimen. *After:* Apply dressing, give postprocedure instructions to patient.
Excisional	Used when good cosmetic results and/or entire lesion removal desired. Skin closed with subcutaneous and skin sutures	Same as above
Incisional	Wedge-shaped incision made in lesion too large for excisional biopsy. Useful when larger specimen than shave or punch biopsy is needed	Same as above
Shave	Single-edged razor blade used to shave off superficial lesions or small sample of a large lesion. Provides thin specimen for diagnostic purposes	Same as above
Microscopic Tests		
Potassium hydroxide (KOH)	Hair, scales, or nails examined for superficial fungal infection. Specimen put on glass slide and 10%-20% concentration of KOH added	*Before:* Instruct patient regarding purpose of test. *During:* Prepare slide.
Tzanck test (Wright's and Giemsa's stain)	Fluid and cells from vesicles examined. Used to diagnose herpes infections. Specimen put on slide, stained, and examined microscopically	*Before:* Inform patient of purpose of test. *During:* Use sterile technique for collection of fluid.
Culture	Test identifies fungal, bacterial, and viral organisms. For *fungi,* scraping or swab of skin performed. For *bacteria,* material obtained from intact pustules, bullae, or abscesses. For *viruses,* vesicle or bulla and exudate taken from base of lesion	*Before:* Instruct patient regarding purpose and procedure. *During:* Properly identify specimen. Follow instructions for storing specimen if not immediately sent to laboratory.
Mineral oil slides	To check for infestations, scrapings are placed on slide with mineral oil and viewed microscopically.	*Before:* Instruct patient about purpose of test. *During:* Prepare slide.
Immunofluorescent studies	Some skin diseases have specific, abnormal antibody proteins that can be identified by fluorescent studies. Both skin tissue and serum can be examined.	*Before:* Inform patient about purpose of test. *During:* Assist in obtaining specimen. For punch biopsy, place specimen in special fixative (e.g., Michel's) and not formalin.
Miscellaneous		
Wood's lamp (black light)	Examination of skin with long-wave ultraviolet light causes specific substances to fluoresce (e.g., *Pseudomonas* fungal, infections, vitiligo).	*Before:* Explain purpose of examination. Inform patient it is not painful. *During:* Darken room.
Patch test (Fig. 22-10)	Used to assess for allergic dermatitis and photoallergic reactions. Application of allergens to the patient's skin (usually on the back) for 48 hr. Test sites examined 48 hr later for a reaction, characterized by the presence of erythema, papules, vesicles, or all of these. Additional readings beyond 48 hr may be done.	*Before:* Explain purpose and procedure to patient. *After:* Instruct patient that patches are left in place for 48 hr, during which time it is important not to wash the area or play vigorous sport because if the adhesive tapes peel off the process will have to be repeated. The patches should not be exposed to sunlight or other sources of ultraviolet (UV) light.

Biopsy is one of the most common diagnostic tests used to evaluate a skin lesion. A biopsy is indicated when a malignancy is suspected or a specific diagnosis is questionable. Techniques include punch, incisional, excisional, and shave biopsies. The method used depends on factors such as the site of the biopsy, cosmetic result desired, and type of tissue needed.

Other diagnostic procedures include stains and cultures for fungal, bacterial, and viral infections. Direct immunofluorescence is a special diagnostic technique used on biopsy specimens and may be indicated in certain conditions such as bullous diseases and systemic lupus erythematosus. Indirect immunofluorescence is performed on a sample of blood.

CASE STUDY

Objective Data: Diagnostic Studies

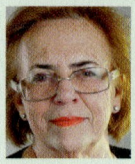

(©iStockphoto/Thinkstock)

The HCP examines the lesion via dermatoscopy and uses a Wood's lamp to rule out a fungal infection. The HCP suspects basal cell carcinoma.

Discussion Questions

1. Are these the diagnostic tests you expected the HCP to perform?
2. What, if any, additional diagnostic studies would you anticipate being ordered for D.A.?
3. What are the interprofessional team's priorities for D.A. at this time?

Answers available at *http://evolve.elsevier.com/Lewis/medsurg.*

BRIDGE TO NCLEX EXAMINATION

The number of the question corresponds to the same-numbered outcome at the beginning of the chapter.

1. The primary function of the skin is
   a. insulation.
   b. protection.
   c. sensation.
   d. absorption.
2. Age-related changes in the hair and nails include *(select all that apply)*
   a. oily scalp.
   b. scaly scalp.
   c. thinner nails.
   d. thicker, brittle nails.
   e. longitudinal nail ridging.
3. When assessing the nutritional-metabolic pattern in relation to the skin, the nurse questions the patient regarding
   a. joint pain.
   b. the use of moisturizing shampoo.
   c. recent changes in wound healing.
   d. self-care habits related to daily hygiene.
4. During the physical examination of a patient's skin, the nurse would
   a. use a flashlight in a poorly lit room.
   b. note cool, moist skin as a normal finding.
   c. pinch up a fold of skin to assess for turgor.
   d. perform a lesion-specific examination first and then a general inspection.
5. The nurse assessed the patient's skin lesions as firm, edematous, irregularly shaped with a variable diameter. They would be called
   a. wheals.
   b. papules.
   c. pustules.
   d. plaques.
6. To assess the skin for temperature and moisture, the *most* appropriate technique for the nurse to use is
   a. palpation.
   b. inspection.
   c. percussion.
   d. auscultation.
7. Persons with dark skin are more likely to develop
   a. keloids.
   b. wrinkles.
   c. skin rashes.
   d. skin cancer.
8. On inspection of a patient's dark skin, the nurse notes a blue-gray birthmark on the forehead and eye area. This assessment finding is called
   a. vitiligo.
   b. intertrigo.
   c. Nevus of Ota.
   d. telangiectasia.
9. Diagnostic testing is recommended for skin lesions when
   a. a health history cannot be obtained.
   b. a more definitive diagnosis is needed.
   c. percussion reveals an abnormal finding.
   d. treatment with prescribed medication has failed.

1. b, 2. b, d, e, 3. c, 4. c, 5. a, 6. a, 7. a, 8. c, 9. b

For rationales to these answers and even more NCLEX review questions, visit *http://evolve.elsevier.com/Lewis/medsurg.*

EVOLVE WEBSITE

http://evolve.elsevier.com/Lewis/medsurg

Review Questions (Online Only)
Key Points
Answer Keys for Questions
- Rationales for Bridge to NCLEX Examination Questions
- Answer Guidelines for Case Study on pp. 398, 400, 404, and 406

Conceptual Care Map Creator
Audio Glossary
Content Updates

REFERENCES

1. Marks JG, Miller JJ: *Principles of dermatology*, ed 5, St Louis, 2013, Mosby.
2. Bryant R, Nix D: *Acute and chronic wounds: current management concepts*, ed 4, St Louis, 2012, Elsevier. (Classic)
3. Habif TP: *Clinical dermatology*, ed 5, St Louis, 2011, Mosby. (Classic)
4. Patton KT, Thibodeau GA: *Anatomy and physiology*, ed 8, St Louis, 2013, Mosby.
5. Ball JW, Dains JE, Flynn JA, et al: *Seidel's guide to physical examination*, ed 8, St Louis, 2014, Mosby.
6. Han A, Chien AL, Kang S: Photoaging, *Dermatol Clin* 32:291, 2014.
7. Marchetti MA, Marghoob AA: Dermoscopy, *CMAJ* 186:1167, 2014.

23

Integumentary Problems

Diana L. Gallagher

I am tired of all this nonsense about beauty being skin deep. That is deep enough. What do you want, an adorable pancreas?

Jean Kerr

http://evolve.elsevier.com/Lewis/medsurg/

LEARNING OUTCOMES

1. Specify health promotion practices related to the integumentary system.
2. Explain the etiology, clinical manifestations, and nursing and interprofessional management of malignant dermatologic disorders.
3. Explain the etiology, clinical manifestations, and nursing and interprofessional management of bacterial, viral, and fungal infections of the integument.
4. Describe the etiology, clinical manifestations, and nursing and interprofessional management of infestations and insect bites.
5. Explain the etiology, clinical manifestations, and nursing and interprofessional management of allergic dermatologic disorders.
6. Explain the etiology, clinical manifestations, and nursing and interprofessional management related to benign dermatologic disorders.
7. Select appropriate nursing interventions to manage the patient with a dermatologic disorder.
8. Summarize the psychologic effects of chronic dermatologic conditions.
9. Explain the indications and nursing management related to common cosmetic procedures and skin grafts.

KEY TERMS

acne vulgaris, Table 23-10, p. 419
actinic keratosis, p. 411
basal cell carcinoma (BCC), p. 411
cellulitis, Table 23-5, p. 414
cryosurgery, p. 422
curettage, p. 422
dysplastic nevi (DN), p. 413
herpes zoster, Table 23-6, p. 415
impetigo, Table 23-5, p. 414
lichenification, p. 424
malignant melanoma, p. 411
psoriasis, p. 417
squamous cell carcinoma (SCC), p. 411
sun protection factor (SPF), p. 408

This chapter discusses health promotion of the skin, common dermatologic conditions, and malignant skin neoplasms. An emphasis is placed on the nursing management of patients with dermatologic conditions.

HEALTH PROMOTION

Health promotion practices related to the skin often parallel practices for general good health. The skin reflects both physical and psychologic well-being. Specific health promotion activities appropriate to good skin health include avoiding environmental hazards, attention to hygiene, good nutrition, adequate hydration, skin self-exam, and periodic professional exams for areas that are difficult to see.

Environmental Hazards

Sun Exposure. Exposure to the sun comes with serious risk. Sun exposure results in permanent sun damage. The damage caused by ultraviolet (UV) rays is cumulative. It results in degenerative changes in the dermis, premature aging (e.g., loss of elasticity, thinning, wrinkling, abnormal dryness), and an impaired immune response. Prolonged and repeated sun exposure is a major factor in precancerous and cancerous lesions. Other problems directly associated with sun exposure include actinic keratosis, basal cell carcinoma, squamous cell carcinoma, and malignant melanoma.

Specific wavelengths (Table 23-1) have different effects on the skin. Sunlight is composed of visible light and UV light. There are two types of UV light: UVA and UVB. UVA light is responsible for tanning, UVB for sunburn. Both types can damage the skin, increase the risk of skin cancer, and accelerate the aging of skin. Tanning is the skin's response to injury. It is caused by the increased production of melanin. When sun exposure is excessive, the skin's turnover time becomes shortened, which can result in peeling. Fair-skinned persons and those with light-colored eyes should be especially cautious about excess sun exposure. They have less melanin and thus less natural protection.

Reviewed by Patricia Gable Burke, RN, BSN, CWOCN, Patient Educator Wound, Ostomy, Continence Care, Bethesda North Hospital, Cincinnati, Ohio; Kim Clevenger, RN, EdD, BC, Associate Professor of Nursing, BSN Program Coordinator, Morehead State University, Morehead, Kentucky; and Allison J. Terry RN, PhD, Associate Professor of Nursing, Assistant Dean of Clinical Practice, School of Nursing, Auburn University Montgomery, Montgomery, Alabama.

TABLE 23-1 Wavelengths of Sun and Effects on Skin

Wavelength	Effect
Long (ultraviolet A [UVA])	Can produce elastic tissue damage and actinic skin damage. Contributes to formation of skin cancer.
Middle (ultraviolet B [UVB])	Causes sunburn and cumulative effect of sun damage. Major factor in development of skin cancer.
Short (ultraviolet C [UVC])	Does not reach earth, since it is blocked by atmosphere.

Other factors that increase the possibility of sunburn include being at a high altitude, being in snow (reflects 80% of the sun's rays), or being in or near water. Warn people of the dangers of tanning booths and sun lamps, which emit UVA. Tanning booths increase the risk of sunburn, cataracts, and skin cancer.[1]

Your patient teaching should include information on sun protection. People often do not understand the serious risks of sun exposure. Education is important. Teach patients sun safety guidelines, including sun avoidance, wearing protective clothing, and using appropriate sunscreen. Avoiding exposure to the midday sun and using protective clothing and sunscreens beginning early in life can prevent the formation of skin cancer later in life.

Teach the patient ways to avoid the damaging effects of the sun. This includes wearing sunglasses, a large-brimmed hat, and a darker-colored, long-sleeved shirt of a tightly woven fabric or carrying an umbrella. The greatest risk is between the hours of 10:00 AM and 2:00 PM, regardless of the latitude. This is when 80% of UV rays occur. Even on overcast days, serious sunburn can occur because up to 80% of the sun's UV rays can penetrate the clouds.

EVIDENCE-BASED PRACTICE

Applying the Evidence

Tanning Booths and Skin Cancer

You are a nurse working in a dermatology clinic. D.F., a 30-year-old female with fair skin (blonde hair and blue eyes), is completing her health history before a skin screening examination. She says she regularly visits an indoor tanning salon every other week. She tells you that being tan makes her feel "more healthy and attractive."

Making Clinical Decisions

Best Available Evidence. There is a strong link between exposure to UV from indoor tanning booth use and increased risk of skin cancer and melanoma.

Clinician Expertise. You note that D.F. has the following skin cancer risk factors: fair skin, blue eyes, frequent use of tanning booths.

Patient Preferences and Values. After listening, D.F. tells you that she will consider reducing the frequency of her visits, going only when she has an important event to attend.

Implications for Nursing Practice

1. How would you respond to D.F., given the information that she has provided to you?
2. What resources can help address her view that a "tan looks healthy"?
3. What sun safe precautions should she take when outdoors to prevent skin cancer?

Reference for Evidence

Wehner M, Chren M, Nameth D, et al: International prevalence of indoor tanning: a systematic review and meta-analysis, *JAMA Dermatol* 150:390, 2014.

TABLE 23-2 Drug Therapy

Drugs That May Cause Photosensitivity

Categories	Examples
Antidepressants	amitriptyline, doxepin, venlafaxine
Antidysrhythmics	quinidine, amiodarone (Cordarone)
Antihistamines	diphenhydramine, chlorpheniramine, clemastine, cetirizine (Zyrtec)
Antimicrobials	tetracycline, sulfamethoxazole, azithromycin (Zithromax), ciprofloxacin (Cipro)
Antifungals	griseofulvin, ketoconazole
Antipsychotics	chlorpromazine, haloperidol
Chemotherapy	methotrexate, dacarbazine (DTIC), 5-fluorouracil (5-FU)
Diuretics	furosemide (Lasix), hydrochlorothiazide
Hypoglycemics	tolbutamide, glipizide (Glucotrol), glyburide
Nonsteroidal antiinflammatory drugs	diclofenac (Voltaren), piroxicam (Feldene), sulindac

Sunscreens can filter both UVA and UVB wavelengths. The two types of topical sunscreens are chemical and physical. Chemical sunscreens are light creams or lotions designed to absorb or filter UV light, resulting in decreased UV light penetration. Physical sunscreens are thick, opaque, heavy creams that reflect UV radiation. Regular sunscreen use decreases the risk of developing melanoma.

The U.S. Food and Drug Administration (FDA) rates sunscreen products on their **sun protection factor (SPF)**. The SPF measures the effectiveness of a sunscreen in filtering and absorbing UV radiation. All sunscreen labels in the United States must state which rays they protect against. Products labeled with "broad spectrum" block both UVA and UVB.[2] Sunscreens with broad spectrum labeling must have an SPF of at least 15. Sunscreens with an SPF of 15 or more filter 92% of the UVB rays and make sunburn unlikely when applied appropriately.

People need to select the sunscreen most appropriate for their needs. Para-aminobenzoic acid (PABA) and PABA esters, cinnamates, salicylates, and methyl anthranilate block UVB rays. Many sunscreen products no longer contain PABA because it stains clothing and can cause allergic reactions, including contact dermatitis. Avobenzone (Parsol) blocks UVA rays and has been added to some sunscreens. Benzophenones block both UVA and UVB rays.

The general recommendation is that everyone should use daily sunscreen with a minimum SPF of 15. Teach patients to look for the term *broad spectrum* on sunscreen packaging. Patients who have a history of skin cancer or problems with sun sensitivity should use a product with an SPF of at least 30. Sunscreens should be applied 20 to 30 minutes before going outdoors, even in cloudy weather. The SPF value of all sunscreens decreases with time. Sunscreen must be reapplied every 2 hours in a sufficient amount. One ounce per total body application is recommended. The ears, toes, and lips also need sunscreen. Sunscreens are not "waterproof" and must be reapplied immediately after swimming.

Certain medications potentiate the sun's effects, even with brief exposure. Drug categories that contain common photosensitizing medications are listed in Table 23-2. Be aware

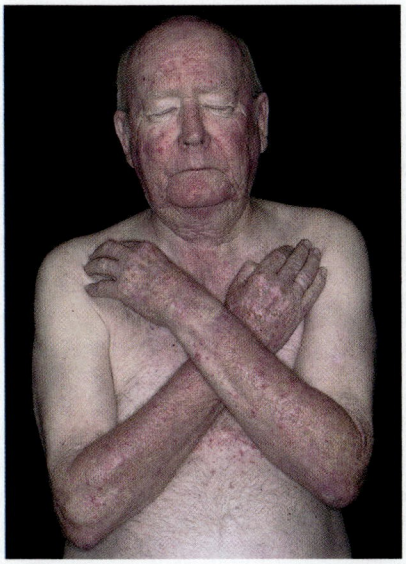

FIG. 23-1 Intense eruption in areas exposed to sunlight after patient started on hydrochlorothiazide. (From Habif TP: *Clinical dermatology: a color guide to diagnosis and therapy,* ed 5, St Louis, 2011, Mosby.)

that many drugs are included in these categories. Assess the photosensitivity of each individual drug. The chemicals in these medications absorb light when exposed to natural sunlight and release energy that harms cells and tissues. The clinical manifestations of drug-induced photosensitivity (Fig. 23-1) are similar to those of exaggerated sunburn. These include swelling, erythema, vesicles, and papular, plaquelike lesions. Teach patients who are taking these drugs about their photosensitizing effect and the need to protect the skin from photosensitivity reactions by using sunscreen products.

Irritants and Allergens. Patients can seek treatment for irritant or allergic dermatitis, which are two types of contact dermatitis. *Irritant contact dermatitis* results from direct chemical injury to the skin. *Allergic contact dermatitis* is an antigen-specific, type IV delayed hypersensitivity response. This response requires sensitization and occurs only in those who are predisposed to react to a particular antigen (see Chapter 13).

Teach patients to avoid known irritants (e.g., ammonia, harsh detergents). Skin patch testing (application of allergens) can sometimes help determine the most likely sensitizing agent. Sometimes the HCP is the first to detect a contact allergy to various metals or medical products, such as gloves (latex) and adhesives in wound or ostomy products. Medications used to treat a variety of conditions may contain fragrances and preservatives that can cause dermatologic reactions.

Radiation. Although most radiology departments are extremely cautious in protecting both themselves and their patients from the effects of excessive radiation, it is important for you to help the patient make decisions about radiologic procedures. X-rays are valuable in both diagnosis and therapy. They can cause serious side effects to the skin, including erythema, dry and moist desquamation, edema, and changes in pigmentation.

Rest and Sleep

Sleep is restorative to the skin. Pruritic skin diseases often interfere with sleep. Therefore helping patients obtain high-quality sleep is an important health-promotion consideration. Adequate rest increases the patient's ability to tolerate itching, thereby decreasing skin damage from the resultant scratching.

Exercise

Exercise increases circulation and dilates the blood vessels. In addition to the healthy glow produced by exercise, the psychologic effects can improve one's appearance and mental outlook. However, caution must be used to prevent overexposure to heat, cold, and sun during outdoor exercise.

Hygiene

The patient's skin type, lifestyle, culture, age, and gender influence hygienic practices. The normal acidity of the skin and perspiration protect against bacterial overgrowth. Most soaps are alkaline and neutralize the skin surface, leading to a loss of protection. Using mild, moisturizing soaps and lipid-free cleansers, and avoiding hot water and vigorous scrubbing can noticeably decrease local skin irritation and inflammation. Skin piercings in which jewelry has been inserted can be cared for with antibacterial soaps that do not contain sulfites.

In general, skin and hair must be washed often enough to remove excess oil and excretions and to prevent odor. Older persons should avoid harsh soaps and shampoos and frequent bathing because of the dryness of their skin and scalp. Moisturizers used immediately after a bath or shower (while the skin is still damp) seal in the moisture.

Nutrition

A well-balanced diet adequate in all food groups can produce healthy skin, hair, and nails. Important elements of skin nutrition include the following:

- *Vitamin A:* Essential for maintenance of normal cell structure, specifically epithelial cells. It is necessary for normal wound healing. The absence of vitamin A causes dryness of the conjunctiva and poor wound healing.
- *Vitamin B complex:* Essential for complex metabolic functions. Deficiencies of niacin and pyridoxine (B_6) manifest as dermatologic symptoms such as erythema, bullae, and seborrhea-like lesions.
- *Vitamin C (ascorbic acid):* Essential for connective tissue formation and normal wound healing. Absence of vitamin C causes symptoms of scurvy, including petechiae, bleeding gums, and purpura.
- *Vitamin D_3 (cholecalciferol):* Essential for bone health. It is produced naturally by cutaneous photosynthesis after UVB exposure. A deficiency manifests as bone and muscle weakness and pain.
- *Vitamin K:* Essential for synthesizing blood clotting factors. A deficiency can lead to bruising.
- *Protein:* Necessary in amounts adequate for cell growth and maintenance and normal wound healing. A deficiency can lead to decreased wound healing.

Obesity has adverse effects on the skin. The increase in subcutaneous fat can lead to stretching and overheating (see Chapter 40). Overheating secondary to the greater insulation provided by fat causes increased sweating, which inflames and dries the skin. Obesity is a risk factor for poor wound healing and is associated with developing type 2 diabetes mellitus. Increased skin folds contribute to skin problems. Skin in these intertriginous (skin on skin) areas is predisposed to skin tags *(acrochordons),* and candidiasis (yeast), intertrigo (bacteria, fungi, yeast), and erythrasma (bacteria) infections.

Self-Treatment

Determine if the patient is aware of the dangers of ignoring a skin problem, self-diagnosis, and treatment. The increasing variety of OTC skin preparations can be confusing.

In your general instructions to the patient, stress the duration of the treatment and the need to follow package directions. Skin problems may be slow to produce symptoms and slow to resolve. Tell the patient to follow package directions when using OTC drugs. If the package insert says its use should not exceed 7 days, patients should heed this warning. Teach the patient to stop self-care and seek the help of a HCP if any systemic signs of inflammation or extensions of the skin problem (e.g., an increasing number of lesions, increased erythema, increased swelling) develop.

SKIN CANCER

Skin cancer is the most commonly diagnosed cancer.[3] Skin cancers are either nonmelanoma or melanoma. The fact that skin lesions are so visible increases the likelihood of early detection and diagnosis. Early detection and treatment can often lead to a highly favorable prognosis.

Teach patients to self-examine their skin at least on a monthly basis. The cornerstone of skin self-examination is the ABCDE rule.[4] Examine skin lesions for ***A**symmetry, **B**order* irregularity, ***C**olor* change and variation, ***D**iameter* of 6 mm or more, and ***E**volving* in appearance (Fig. 23-2). Emphasize that a persistent skin lesion that does not heal and lesions once flat and now raised, once small and recently growing, or changing in appearance are warning signs. These lesions must be examined by an HCP.

Risk Factors

Risk factors for skin cancer include having fair skin, blond or red hair, light eye color, history of chronic sun exposure, family or personal history of skin cancer, and indoor tanning.[5] The Fitzpatrick Classification of Skin Type can assist you in determining a skin complexion and how likely a person is to get skin cancer (Table 23-3).

Because of genetic markers, people of Celtic ancestry (fair skin, blue eyes, red or fair hair, an inability to tan) are at a higher risk for squamous cell carcinoma. Environmental factors that increase the risk of skin cancer include living near the equator, outdoor occupations, and frequent outdoor recreational activities. Using indoor tanning booths and outdoor sunbathing are controllable risk factors for skin cancer. Patients treated with oral methoxsalen (psoralen) and psoralen plus ultraviolet A radiation (PUVA) may be at greater risk for melanoma.

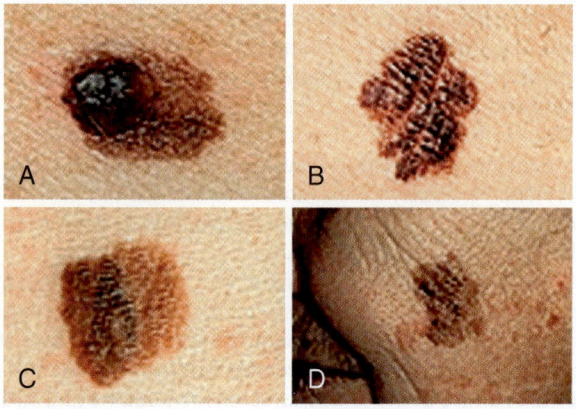

FIG. 23-2 The ABCDEs of melanoma. **A,** Asymmetry: one half unlike the other half. **B,** Border irregularity: edges are ragged, notched, or blurred. **C,** Color: varied pigmentation; shades of tan, brown, and black. **D,** Diameter: greater than 6 mm (diameter of a pencil eraser). **E,** (not pictured) Evolving; changing appearance (change in shape, size, color, or other characteristic is noted over time). (From The Skin Cancer Foundation, New York, N.Y.)

CULTURAL & ETHNIC HEALTH DISPARITIES

Integumentary Problems

- African Americans and Hispanics have a lower incidence of skin cancer than whites.
- In the United States, rates of BCC and SCC are increasing among Hispanic and Asian women.
- Melanoma can occur in dark-skinned persons but often goes unrecognized until the advanced stages.
- When darker skin heals after injury or inflammation, it tends to be hypopigmented or hyperpigmented.
- African Americans and Asians are more likely to develop a keloid at the site of an injury.

Dark-skinned persons are less susceptible to skin cancer because of their increased melanin, which acts like a sunscreen. However, there is still a risk and a need to wear sunscreen. They often have melanomas on areas with less melanin, such as the palms, soles, mucous membranes, and under the nails. Since it is common for people with dark skin to have pigmented, longitudinal bands on their nails, assess and follow any nail discoloration.

NONMELANOMA SKIN CANCER

Nonmelanoma skin cancers (basal cell and squamous cell carcinomas) are the most common forms of skin cancer. More than 3.5 million new cases are diagnosed each year.[3] Nonmelanoma skin cancers do not develop from melanocytes. They develop in the basement membrane of the skin. Although there are few deaths from nonmelanoma skin cancer, they have the potential for severe local destruction, permanent disfigurement, and disability.

Nonmelanoma skin cancers usually develop in sun-exposed areas, such as the face, head, neck, back of the hands, and arms. The most common causative factor is sun exposure. There are some differences between basal and squamous cell cancers. Squamous cell cancers usually occur on the head and neck where there is the highest degree of UV radiation. Basal cell

TABLE 23-3 Fitzpatrick Classification of Skin Type

Skin Type	Skin Color	Characteristics
I	White, freckles, very fair. Red or blond hair. Blue eyes	Always burns, never tans
II	White, fair. Red or blond hair. Blue, hazel, or green eyes	Usually burns, tans with difficulty
III	Cream white, fair. Any eye or hair color	Sometimes mild burn, gradually tan
IV	Brown, typical Mediterranean skin	Rarely burns, tans with ease
V	Dark brown, Middle Eastern skin types	Very rarely burns, tans very easily
VI	Black	Never burns, tans very easily

cancers do not follow that pattern and may occur in sun-protected areas.

Actinic Keratosis

Actinic keratosis, also known as *solar keratosis,* consists of hyperkeratotic papules and plaques on sun-exposed areas. Actinic keratoses are premalignant skin lesions that affect nearly all of the older white population. These are the most common of all precancerous skin lesions. The clinical appearance of actinic keratoses can be highly varied. The typical lesion is an irregularly shaped, flat, slightly erythematous papule with indistinct borders and an overlying hard keratotic scale or horn (Table 23-4). Actinic keratoses may spontaneously resolve when exposure to sunlight is reduced. Sun exposure is a key factor. They are often first noticed in the summer.

Because actinic keratosis is impossible to differentiate from squamous cell carcinoma, treatment should be aggressive. Nonsurgical procedures are the first-line treatment (Table 23-4). Any lesion that persists should be evaluated for a possible biopsy.

Basal Cell Carcinoma

Basal cell carcinoma (BCC) is a locally invasive malignancy arising from epidermal basal cells. It is the most common type of skin cancer but the least deadly. BCC usually occurs in middle-aged to older adults. It commonly develops at the site of earlier trauma, such as scarring, thermal burns, and injuries.[6]

Clinical manifestations are described in Table 23-4. Some BCC are pigmented, with curled borders and an opaque appearance. They may be hard to distinguish from melanoma. A tissue biopsy is needed to confirm the diagnosis. BCC rarely metastasize (Fig. 23-3). However, if BCC is left untreated, massive tissue destruction may result.

Treatment depends on the tumor location and histologic type, history of recurrence, and patient characteristics (Table 23-4). Location and size are important factors in determining the best treatment.

Squamous Cell Carcinoma

Squamous cell carcinoma (SCC) is a malignant neoplasm of keratinizing epidermal cells. It frequently occurs on sun-exposed skin at the base of an actinic keratosis or another lesion. SCC is less common than BCC. It can be highly aggressive, has the potential to metastasize, and may lead to death if not treated early and correctly. Pipe, cigar, and cigarette smoking contribute to the formation of SCC on the mouth and lips. Immunosuppression leads to a dramatic increase in the incidence of SCC. Renal transplant recipients have a 253-fold increase in the risk of SCC.[6] The clinical manifestations of SCC are described in Table 23-4. A biopsy should always be performed when a lesion is suspected to be SCC.

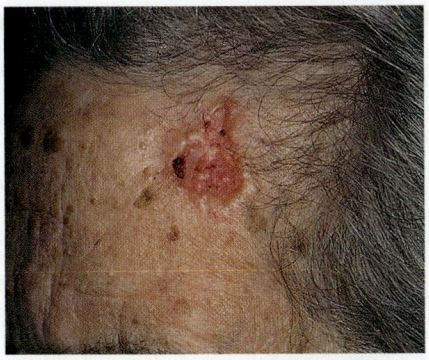

FIG. 23-3 Basal cell carcinoma. Rolled, well-defined border and central erosion. (From Swartz MH: *Textbook of physical diagnosis: history and examination,* ed 6, Philadelphia, 2010, Saunders.)

MALIGNANT MELANOMA

Malignant melanoma is a tumor arising in melanocytes, the cells producing melanin. Melanoma causes the majority of skin cancer deaths. More than 132,000 new cases are diagnosed every year worldwide.[3] The incidence of melanoma in whites has tripled in the last 40 years. Non-whites have a decreased incidence of melanoma, but they often have more advanced disease at initial diagnosis and a higher mortality rate than whites.[7] Melanoma can occur in the eyes, ears, gastrointestinal tract, leptomeninges, and oral and genital mucous membranes. When it begins in the skin, it is called *cutaneous melanoma.* Melanoma has the ability to metastasize to any organ, including the brain and heart.

Although the exact cause of melanoma is unknown, a combination of environmental and genetic factors is involved. UV radiation from the sun is the main cause of melanomas, but artificial sources of UV radiation, such as sunlamps and tanning booths, play a role. UV radiation damages the deoxyribonucleic acid (DNA) in skin cells, causing "misspellings" (mutations) in their genetic code. This alters the cells. Although anyone can develop melanoma, the risk is greatest for people who have red or blond hair, blue or light-colored eyes, and light-colored skin that freckles easily. These people have less melanin and thus less protection from UV radiation. The use of immunosuppressive drugs and a history of dysplastic nevi also increase a person's risk.

A person may have a genetic predisposition toward getting melanoma. Between 5% and 10% of people with melanoma have a first-degree relative (e.g., parent, full sibling) who had melanoma. This risk increases significantly if multiple relatives have a history of melanoma. Mutated genes have been identified in some families who have a high familial incidence of melanoma.

Clinical Manifestations

About one fourth of melanomas occur in existing nevi or moles; about 20% occur in dysplastic nevi (Table 23-4). Melanoma frequently occurs on the lower legs and backs in women and on the trunk, head, and neck in men. Because most melanoma cells continue to produce melanin, melanoma tumors are often dark brown or black. Patients should consult their HCP immediately if their moles or lesions show any of the clinical signs (ABCDEs) of melanoma (Fig. 23-2). Any sudden or progressive change or increase in the ABCDE rule must be evaluated.

Interprofessional Care

One of the initial steps in correctly diagnosing a suspicious lesion is dermoscopic examination. Dermoscopes use magnification to see patterns and structures not visible with the naked eye. Handheld screening devices (e.g., MelaFind) can assist the HCP in determining if a lesion without the obvious ABCDE signs should be biopsied. Biopsy is a critical tool for identifying a lesion. All suspicious lesions should be biopsied using an excisional biopsy technique. They should not be shave-biopsied, shave-excised, or electrocauterized. These techniques fail to provide an accurate measurement of depth.

The most important prognostic factor is tumor thickness at the time of diagnosis. Two methods to determine thickness are currently in use. The *Breslow measurement* indicates the depth of the tumor in millimeters (Fig. 23-4). The *Clark level* indicates the depth of invasion of the tumor; the higher the number, the deeper the melanoma.

Treatment depends on the site of the original tumor, stage of the cancer, and patient's age and general health. The staging

TABLE 23-4 Premalignant and Malignant Conditions of the Skin

Etiology and Pathophysiology	Clinical Manifestations	Treatment and Prognosis
Actinic Keratosis • Actinic (sun) damage • Premalignant skin lesions • Common in older whites	• Flat or elevated, dry, hyperkeratotic scaly papule. Often multiple • Possibly flat, rough, or verrucous (wartlike) • Rough adherent scale on red base, which returns when removed • Often on erythematous sun-exposed area • Increase in number with age	• Cryosurgery. Topical application of 5-FU, imiquimod (Aldara) or diclofenac (Solaraze), chemical peels, laser resurfacing, photodynamic therapy (PDT, with 5-aminolevulinic acid [5-ALA] or methyl aminolevulinate [MAL] followed by light irradiation) • Recurrence possible even with adequate treatment
Atypical or Dysplastic Nevi • Morphologically between common acquired nevi and melanoma • May be precursor of malignant melanoma	• Often >5 mm. Irregular border, possibly notched. Frequently multiple • Variegated color of tan, brown, black, red, or pink within single mole • Presence of at least one flat portion, often at edge of mole • Most common site on back, but possible in uncommon mole sites such as scalp or buttocks (Fig. 23-5)	• Increased risk for melanoma • Careful monitoring of persons suspected of familial tendency to melanoma or dysplastic nevi • Excisional biopsy for suspicious lesions
Basal Cell Carcinoma • Change in basal cells. No maturation or normal keratinization • Continuing division of basal cells and formation of enlarging mass • Related to excessive sun exposure, genetic skin type, x-ray radiation, scars, and some types of nevi	*Nodular and ulcerative:* • Small, slowly enlarging papule • Borders semitranslucent or "pearly" with overlying telangiectasia • Erosion, ulceration, and depression of center • Normal skin markings lost (Fig. 23-3) *Superficial:* • Erythematous, pearly, sharply defined, barely elevated plaques	• Surgical excision, electrodessication and curettage, cryosurgery, radiation therapy, topical or systemic chemotherapy, and photodynamic therapy • 90% cure rate with primary lesions • Slow-growing tumor that invades local tissue. Metastasis rare • 5-FU and imiquimod for superficial lesions, photodynamic therapy for small lesions, vismodegib (Erivedge) or sonidegib (Odomzo) for metastatic or recurrent locally invasive lesions
Squamous Cell Carcinoma • Frequent occurrence on previously damaged skin (e.g., from sun, radiation, scar) • Malignant tumor of squamous cell of epidermis. Invasion of dermis, surrounding skin	• Most common on sun-exposed areas such as face and hands • *Superficial:* Thin, scaly erythematous plaque without invasion into the dermis • *Early:* Firm nodules with indistinct borders, scaling, and ulceration • *Late:* Covering of lesion with scale or horn from keratinization, ulceration	• Surgical excision, cryosurgery, radiation therapy, chemotherapy, electrosurgery • Untreated lesion may metastasize to regional lymph nodes and distant organs. • 13-*cis*-retinoic acid and interferon alfa-2A for metastatic lesions • High cure rate with early detection and treatment
Malignant Melanoma • Neoplastic growth of melanocytes anywhere on skin, eyes, or mucous membranes • Classification according to major histologic mode of spread • Potential invasion and widespread metastases	• Irregular color, surface, and border Variegated color, including red, white, blue, black, gray, brown • Flat or elevated. Eroded or ulcerated • Often <1 cm in size • Most common sites in males are back, then chest. In females are legs, then back (Fig. 23-2)	• Surgical excision and possible sentinel lymph node evaluation • Possible use of adjuvant therapy after surgery if lesion >1.5 mm in depth • Correlation between survival rate and depth of invasion • Poor prognosis unless diagnosed and treated early • Spreading by local extension, regional lymphatic vessels, and bloodstream
Cutaneous T-Cell Lymphoma • Origins in skin. Localized chronic, slowly progressing disease • Possibly related to environmental toxins and chemical exposure • Mycosis fungoides (MF) is most common form. • Sézary syndrome is an advanced form of MF. • Prevalence twice as high in men as in women	• Classic presentation involves 3 stages: patch (early), plaque, and tumor (advanced). • History of persistent macular eruption followed by gradual appearance of indurated erythematous plaques on trunk that appears similar to psoriasis • Pruritus, lymphadenopathy	• Treatment usually controls symptoms but is not curative. UVB, PUVA, corticosteroids, topical nitrogen mustard, radiation therapy in patch and plaque stage of disease • Interferon, systemic chemotherapy, extracorporeal photopheresis, romidepsin (Istodax) for progressive disease • Bexarotene (Targretin), denileukin diftitox (Ontak), and vorinostat (Zolinza) for advanced disease • Disease course is unpredictable. 10% will have progressive disease.

5-FU, Fluorouracil; *PUVA,* psoralen ultraviolet A; *UVB,* ultraviolet B.

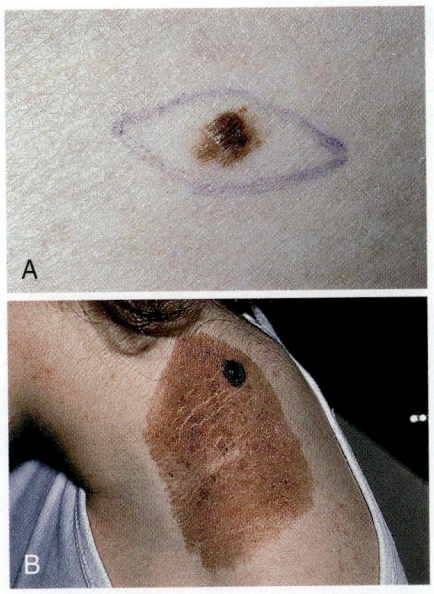

FIG. 23-4 Breslow measurement of tumor thickness. **A,** Thin (0.08-mm) superficial spreading melanoma, good prognosis. **B,** Thick nodular melanoma with lymph node involvement, poor prognosis. (From Gawkrodger D, Ardern-Jones MR: *Dermatology,* ed 5, Edinburgh, 2012, Churchill Livingstone.)

of melanoma (stages 0 to IV) is based on tumor size (thickness), nodal involvement, and metastasis. In stage 0 the melanoma is confined to one place (in situ) in the epidermis. Melanoma is nearly 100% curable by excision if diagnosed at stage 0. The 5-year survival rate depends on sentinel node biopsy results, which indicate if metastasis has occurred. The presence of metastasis in the sentinel lymph node is the most important prognostic factor for recurrence.[6]

The initial treatment of malignant melanoma is wide surgical excision. Melanoma that has spread to the lymph nodes or nearby sites usually requires additional (adjuvant) therapy such as chemotherapy, immunotherapy, targeted therapy, and/or radiation therapy. Chemotherapy includes dacarbazine (DTIC) and temozolomide (Temodar). Adding combinations of cisplatin, carmustine, carboplatin (Paraplatin), or vincristine improves response rate.

Immunotherapy can include cytokines (α-interferon, interleukin-2), PD-1 inhibitors, and CTLA-4 inhibitors. PD-1 inhibitors include nivolumab (Opdivo) and pembrolizumab (Keytruda). These drugs block PD-1, a protein on T cells that normally keeps these cells from attacking other cells in the body. By blocking PD-1, these drugs boost the immune response against melanoma cells. Ipilimumab (Yervoy), a CTLA-4 inhibitor, also boosts the immune system, but it has a different target. It blocks CTLA-4, a protein that normally helps keep T cells in check. By blocking the action of CTLA-4, ipilimumab boosts the immune response against melanoma cells.[8]

Targeted therapy for melanoma includes BRAF and MEK inhibitors. About half of all melanomas have mutations in the *BRAF* gene, which makes an altered BRAF protein that signals melanoma cells to proliferate. Vemurafenib (Zelboraf), dabrafenib (Tafinlar), and cobimetinib (Cotellic) are BRAF inhibitor drugs that attack the BRAF protein directly.

The *MEK* gene is involved in the activation of the BRAF pathway. Therefore a MEK inhibitor drug, trametinib (Mekinist), can be used to treat melanomas with *BRAF* gene changes.

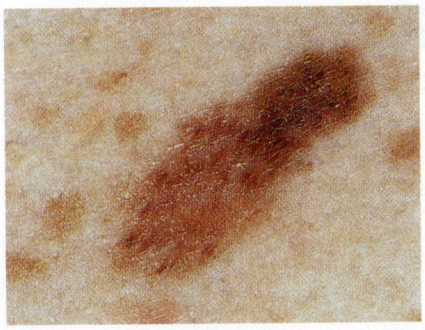

FIG. 23-5 Dysplastic nevus. Irregular border and color. (From Graham-Brown R, Bourke J, Cunliffe T: *Dermatology: fundamentals of practice,* Edinburgh, 2008, Mosby Ltd.)

Atypical or Dysplastic Nevus

An abnormal nevus pattern called *dysplastic nevus syndrome* identifies a person at increased risk of melanoma. Approximately 2% to 8% of the white population have moles classified as atypical or dysplastic nevi. **Dysplastic nevi (DN)**, or atypical moles, are nevi that are larger than usual (greater than 5 mm across) with irregular borders and various shades of color (Fig. 23-5). These nevi may have the same ABCDE characteristics as melanoma, but they are less pronounced. A difference between DN and common nevi is that DN do not appear until a person is nearing puberty and continue to develop beyond the fourth decade. The average number of normal nevi in adults is about 40. Those with DN may have more than 100 normal-appearing nevi.

Obtain a detailed family history related to melanoma and DN. The risk of developing melanoma doubles with the presence of one DN, and having multiple DN increases the risk up to 12-fold.

CHECK YOUR PRACTICE

You are working in a dermatology clinic, and your assigned patient is a 78-yr-old white man. He is worried about his many "brown" spots on his face and arms. He tells you that they probably developed because he worked outside in construction most of his life.

- How do you distinguish among an age spot (lentigo), normal mole, and malignant melanoma?
- What risk factors would you assess for in a patient with a suspected cancerous lesion?

SKIN INFECTIONS AND INFESTATIONS

Bacterial Infections

The skin provides an ideal environment for bacterial growth with an abundant supply of nutrients, water, and warm temperature. Bacterial infection occurs when the balance between the host and microorganisms is altered. This can occur as a primary infection after a break in the skin. It can occur as a secondary infection in already damaged skin or as a sign of a systemic disease (Table 23-5). *Staphylococcus aureus* and group A β-hemolytic streptococci are the major types of bacteria responsible for primary and secondary skin infections. Streptococci cause impetigo, erysipelas, cellulitis, and lymphangitis. *S. aureus* causes impetigo, folliculitis, cellulitis, and furuncles (Fig. 23-6).

Healthy persons can develop bacterial skin infections. Predisposing factors such as moisture, obesity, atopic dermatitis,

TABLE 23-5 Common Bacterial Infections of the Skin

Etiology and Pathophysiology	Clinical Manifestations	Treatment and Prognosis
Impetigo • Group A β-hemolytic streptococci, staphylococci, or combination of both • Associated with poor hygiene • Primary or secondary infection. Contagious	• Vesiculopustular lesions that develop thick, honey-colored crust surrounded by erythema • Pruritic • Most common on face as primary infection	*Topical:* • Wound care with warm saline or aluminum acetate soaks followed by soap-and-water removal of crusts and application of topical antibiotic cream or ointment (mupirocin [Bactroban], retapamulin [Altabax]) • Meticulous hygiene essential *Systemic:* • Systemic antibiotics (e.g., cephalosporins, amoxicillin, clindamycin) for widespread infections or systemic manifestations
Folliculitis • Usually staphylococci • Present in areas subjected to friction, moisture, rubbing, or oil • Increased incidence in patients with diabetes mellitus	• Small pustule at hair follicle opening with minimal erythema • Development of crusting • Most common on scalp, beard, extremities in men • Tender to touch	• Antistaphylococcal soap (e.g., Hibiclens, Lever 2000, Dial) and water cleansing • Topical antibiotics (e.g., mupirocin) • Warm compresses of water or aluminum acetate solution • Usually heals without scarring • If lesions extensive and deep, possible scarring, loss of involved hair follicles, and treatment with systemic antibiotics
Furuncle • Deep infection with staphylococci around hair follicle • Often associated with severe acne or seborrheic dermatitis	• Tender erythematous area around hair follicle that is painful • Draining pus and core of necrotic debris on rupture • Most common on face, back of neck, axillae, breasts, buttocks, perineum, thighs	• Incision and drainage (possibly with packing), antibiotics, meticulous care of involved skin, frequent application of warm, moist compresses
Furunculosis • Increased incidence in patients who are obese, diabetic, chronically ill, or regularly exposed to moisture, pressure	• Lesions as above • Malaise, regional adenopathy, elevated body temperature	*Topical:* • Incision and drainage of painful nodules • Warm, moist compresses to erythematous plaques • Measures to reduce surface staphylococci include antimicrobial cream to nares, armpits, and groin and antiseptic to entire skin. • Meticulous personal hygiene *Systemic:* • Systemic antibiotic effective against MRSA pending culture and sensitivity results • Often recurrent with scarring
Carbuncle • Multiple, interconnecting furuncles	• Many pustules appearing in erythematous area • Most common at nape of neck	• Treatment same as for furuncles • Often recurrent despite production of antibodies • Heal slowly with scar formation
Cellulitis • Inflammation of subcutaneous tissues • Possibly secondary complication or primary infection • Often following break in skin • *Staphylococcus aureus* and streptococci usual causative agents • Deep inflammation of subcutaneous tissue from enzymes produced by bacteria	• Hot, tender, erythematous, and edematous area with diffuse borders • Chills, malaise, and fever (Fig. 23-6)	*Topical:* • Moist heat, immobilization, and elevation *Systemic:* • Systemic antibiotic therapy • Hospitalization if severe for IV antibiotic therapy (dalbavancin [Dalvance], vancomycin, linezolid [Zyvox], ceftaroline fosamil [Teflaro], daptomycin [Cubicin]) • Progression to gangrene possible if untreated
Erysipelas • Superficial cellulitis primarily involving the dermis • Group A β-hemolytic streptococci	• Red, hot, sharply demarcated plaque that is indurated and painful • Bacteremia possible • Most common on face and extremities • Toxic signs: fever, ↑ WBC count, headache, malaise	• Systemic antibiotics, usually penicillin • Hospitalization often required

MRSA, Methicillin-resistant *S. aureus.*

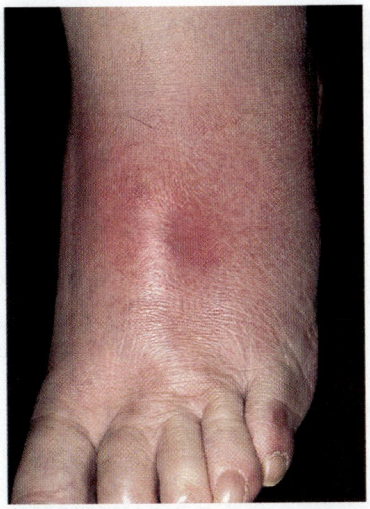

FIG. 23-6 Cellulitis with characteristic erythema, tenderness, and edema. (From Habif TP: *Clinical dermatology: a color guide to diagnosis and therapy*, ed 5, St Louis, 2011, Mosby.)

systemic corticosteroids and antibiotics, and chronic disease such as diabetes mellitus increase the likelihood of infection. Good hygiene practices and general good health inhibit bacterial infections. If an infection is present, the resulting drainage is infectious. Good skin hygiene and infection control practices are necessary to prevent the spread of the infection.

Viral Infections

Similar to viral infections anywhere in the body, viral infections of the skin are difficult to treat. When a virus infects a cell, a skin lesion may develop. Lesions can also result from an inflammatory response to viral infections. Herpes simplex, herpes zoster (Fig. 23-7), and warts (Fig. 23-8) are the most common viral infections affecting the skin (Table 23-6).

Infestations and Insect Bites

The possibilities for exposure to *infestations* (harboring insects or worms) and insect bites are numerous (Table 23-7). In many instances, an allergy to the venom plays a major role in the reaction. In other cases, the clinical manifestations are a

TABLE 23-6 Common Viral Infections of the Skin

Etiology and Pathophysiology	Clinical Manifestations	Treatment and Prognosis
Herpes Simplex Virus (HSV) Types 1 and 2 • Oral or genital HSV infections serotyped as either HSV-1 or HSV-2 • Both are recurrent lifelong viral infections. • Exacerbated by sunlight, trauma, menses, stress, and systemic infection • Contagious to those not previously infected • Transmitted by respiratory droplets or virus-containing fluid (e.g., saliva, cervical secretions) • Infection in one area readily transmitted to another site by contact	*First episode:* • Symptoms occurring 2 days to 2 weeks after contact • Painful local reaction • Single or grouped vesicles on erythematous base • Systemic symptoms (e.g., fever, malaise) possible or no symptoms possible *Recurrent:* • Recurrence in similar spot • Characteristic grouped vesicles on erythematous base	• Symptomatic • Soothing, moist compresses. White petroleum to lesions • Scarring not usual result • Antiviral agents such as acyclovir (Zovirax), famciclovir (Famvir), and valacyclovir (Valtrex) • Vaccine not currently available for HSV-1 or HSV-2
Herpes Zoster (Shingles) • Activation of the varicella-zoster virus • Incidence increases with age. • Potentially contagious to anyone who has not had varicella or who is immunosuppressed	• Linear distribution along a dermatome of grouped vesicles and pustules on erythematous base resembling chickenpox (Fig. 23-7) • Usually unilateral on trunk, face, and lumbosacral areas • Burning, pain, and neuralgia preceding outbreak • Mild to severe pain during outbreak	• Symptomatic *Topical:* • Wet compresses, silver sulfadiazine (Silvadene) to ruptured vesicles *Systemic:* • Antiviral agents (e.g., acyclovir, famciclovir, valacyclovir) within 72 hr to prevent postherpetic neuralgia • Analgesia. Mild sedation at bedtime • Gabapentin (Neurontin) to treat postherpetic neuralgia • Usually heals without complications, but scarring and postherpetic neuralgia possible • Vaccine (Zostavax) to prevent shingles for adults ≥50 yr
Verruca Vulgaris • Caused by human papillomavirus (HPV) • Spontaneous disappearance in 1-2 yr possible • Mildly contagious by autoinoculation • Specific response dependent on body part affected • Prevalence greater in youth and immunosuppressed	• Circumscribed, hypertrophic, flesh-colored papule limited to epidermis • Painful on lateral compression	• Multiple treatments, including surgery using blunt dissection with scissors or curette • Liquid nitrogen therapy • Blistering agent (cantharidin) • Keratolytic agent (salicylic acid) • CO_2 laser destruction
Plantar Warts • Caused by HPV	• Wart on bottom surface of foot, growing inward because of pressure of walking or standing (Fig. 23-8) • Painful when pressure applied • Interrupted skin markings • Cone shaped with black dots (thrombosed vessels) when wart removed	• Topical immunotherapy (imiquimod), cryosurgery, salicylic acid, duct tape

TABLE 23-7 Common Infestations and Insect Bites

Etiology and Pathophysiology	Clinical Manifestations	Treatment and Prognosis
Bees and Wasps *Hymenoptera* species	• Intense, burning, local pain • Swelling and itching • Severe hypersensitivity possibly leading to anaphylaxis	• Cool compresses • Local application of antipruritic lotion • Antihistamines if indicated • Usually uneventful recovery
Bedbugs • *Cimicidae* species • Feeding periodic, usually at night • Present in furniture, walls during day	• Wheal surrounded by vivid flare • Firm urticaria transforming into persistent lesion • Severe pruritus • Often grouped in threes appearing on uncovered parts of body	• Bedbug controlled by chlorocyclohexane • Lesions usually require no treatment • Severe itching possibly requires use of antihistamines or topical corticosteroids
Pediculosis (Head Lice, Body Lice, Pubic Lice) • *Pediculus humanus* var. capitis, *Pediculus humanus* var. corporis, *Phthirus pubis* • Obligate parasites that suck blood, leave excrement and eggs on skin and hair, live in seams of clothing (if body lice) and in hair as nits. Transmission of pubic lice often by sexual contact	• Minute, red, noninflammatory • Points flush with skin. Progression to papular wheal-like lesions • Pruritus • Secondary excoriation, especially parallel linear excoriations in intrascapular region • Nits and eggs are firmly attached to hair shaft in head and body.	• γ-Benzene hexachloride or pyrethrins to treat various parts of body • Spinosad (Natroba) topical suspension 0.9% to treat scalp and hair • Close contacts (e.g., bed partners and playmates) should be screened and treated. • Do not share head gear.
Scabies • *Sarcoptes scabiei* • Mite penetrates stratum corneum, deposits eggs. • Allergic reaction to eggs, feces, mite parts • Transmission by direct physical contact, only occasionally by shared personal items • Rarely seen in dark-skinned people	• Severe itching, especially at night, usually not on face • Presence of burrows, especially in interdigital webs, flexor surface of wrists, genitalia, and anterior axillary folds • Erythematous papules (may be crusted), possible vesiculation, interdigital web crusting	• 5% permethrin topical lotion, one overnight application with second application 1 wk later, may yield 95% eradication. • Treat all family members, treat environment with plastic covering for 5 days, launder all clothes and linen with bleach. • Treat sexual partner. • Antibiotics if secondary infections present • Possible residual pruritus up to 4 wk after treatment • Recurrence possible if inadequately treated
Ticks • *Borrelia burgdorferi* (spirochete transmitted by ticks in certain areas) causes Lyme disease. • Endemic areas include Northeast, Mid-Atlantic states, parts of Midwest and West (see Chapter 64).	• Spreading, ringlike rash 3-4 wk after bite (see Fig. 64-7) • Rash commonly in groin, buttocks, axillae, trunk, and upper arms and legs • Warm, itchy, or painful rash • Flu-like symptoms • Cardiac, arthritic, and neurologic manifestations possible • Unreliable laboratory test	• Oral antibiotics, such as doxycycline, tetracycline • IV antibiotics for arthritic, neurologic, and cardiac symptoms • Rest and healthy diet • Most patients recover.

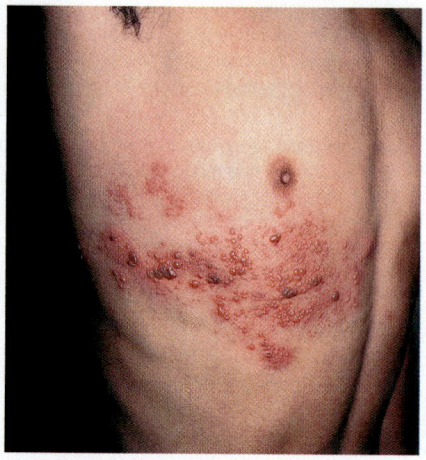

FIG. 23-7 Herpes zoster (shingles) on the anterior chest, classic dermatomal distribution. (From James WD, Berger T, Elston DMD: *Andrews' diseases of the skin,* ed 11, Philadelphia, 2011, Saunders.)

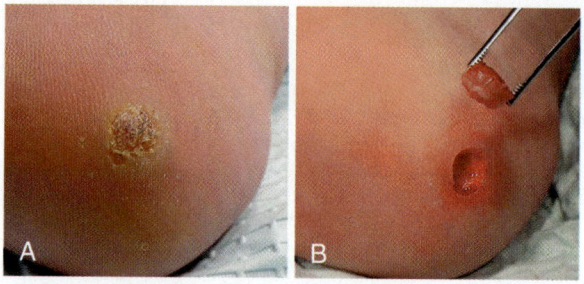

FIG. 23-8 Plantar wart. **A,** Keratotic lesion. **B,** After excision. (From Swartz MH: *Textbook of physical diagnosis: history and examination,* ed 6, Philadelphia, 2010, Saunders.)

reaction to the eggs, feces, or body parts of the invading organism. Some people react with a severe hypersensitivity (anaphylaxis), which can be life threatening. (Anaphylaxis is discussed in Chapter 13.)

Preventing insect bites by avoidance or using repellents is somewhat effective. Meticulous hygiene related to personal articles, clothing, bedding, and examination and care of pets, as well as careful selection of sexual partners, can reduce the incidence of infestations. Prompt, routine skin inspection is necessary in geographic areas where there is a risk of tick bite. (Lyme disease, which is caused by a tick, is discussed in Chapter 64.)

Fungal Infections

Because of the large number of fungi that are present everywhere, exposure to some pathologic varieties may occur. Skin, hair, and nails can become infected with fungi, including candidiasis and tinea unguium (Fig. 23-9). Common fungal infections of the skin are presented in Table 23-8. Most infections are relatively harmless in healthy adults, but they can be embarrassing and distressing to the patient.

The microscopic examination of the scraping of suspicious scaly skin lesions in 10% to 20% potassium hydroxide (KOH) is an inexpensive diagnostic measure to determine the presence of a fungus. The appearance of microscopic hyphae (threadlike structures) is indicative of a fungal infection.

ALLERGIC DERMATOLOGIC PROBLEMS

Dermatologic problems associated with allergies and hypersensitivity reactions may present a challenge to the clinician (Table 23-9). (The pathophysiology related to allergic and contact dermatitis is discussed in Chapter 13.) A careful family history and discussion of exposure to possible offending agents can provide valuable data. Patch testing is used to help to determine possible causative agents (see Fig. 22-10). The best treatment of allergic dermatitis is avoidance of the causative agent. The extreme pruritus and its potential for chronicity make it a frustrating problem for you and the patient, especially if the offending agent cannot be identified.

BENIGN DERMATOLOGIC PROBLEMS

Although the list of benign dermatoses is extensive, some of the most commonly seen and distressing problems include acne vulgaris (Fig. 23-10), psoriasis, and seborrheic keratoses. Benign problems are summarized in Table 23-10.

Psoriasis is an autoimmune disease. Men and women develop psoriasis at equal rates. It occurs in all racial groups, but at varying rates. About 1.3% of African Americans have psoriasis, compared to 2.5% of whites.[9] It usually develops in persons between 15 and 35 years old. One third of people with psoriasis have at least one relative with the disease.

Diagnosis is often based on the skin's appearance (Fig. 23-11). Lesions are distinctive and appear as red, scaling papules that merge to form plaques. The affected area is normally rounded, with adherent silver scales that bleed easily when removed.

While most people have mild disease, many with severe disease often have a weakened immune system, diabetes mellitus, depression, and cardiovascular disease. Psoriatic arthritis affects 10% to 30% of all persons with psoriasis. (Psoriatic arthritis is discussed in Chapter 64.) The chronicity of psoriasis can be severe and disabling. People withdraw from social contacts because of visible lesions, and quality of life can diminish.

DRUG ALERT Isotretinoin (Accutane)

- Used to treat acne (Table 23-10)
- Can cause serious damage to fetus
- Contraindicated in women who are pregnant or want to become pregnant while on the drug
- Blood donation prohibited for those taking the drug and for 1 month after treatment ends
- Linked to liver function test abnormalities

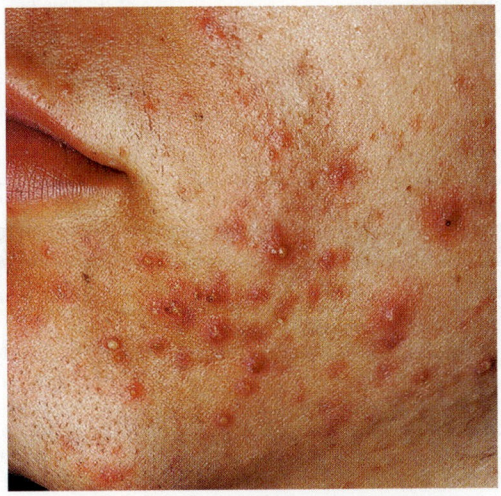

FIG. 23-10 Acne vulgaris. Papules and pustules. (From James WD, Berger T, Elston DMD: *Andrews' diseases of the skin,* ed 11, Philadelphia, 2011, Saunders.)

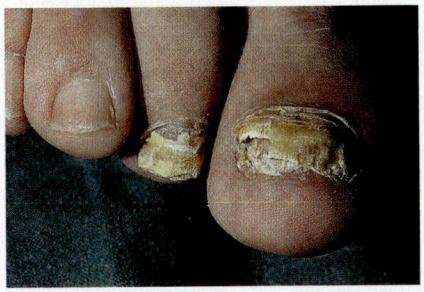

FIG. 23-9 Tinea unguium (onychomycosis). Fungal infection of toenails. Crumbly, discolored, and thickened nails. (From Gawkrodger D, Ardern-Jones MR: *Dermatology,* ed 5, Edinburgh, 2012, Churchill Livingstone.)

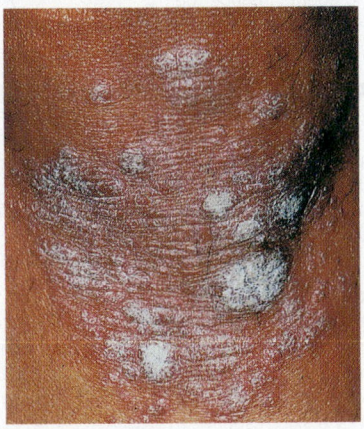

FIG. 23-11 Psoriasis. Characteristic inflammation and scaling. (From Habif TP: *Clinical dermatology: a color guide to diagnosis and therapy,* ed 5, St Louis, 2011, Mosby.)

TABLE 23-8 Common Fungal Infections of the Skin

Etiology and Pathophysiology	Clinical Manifestations	Treatment and Prognosis
Candidiasis • Caused by *Candida albicans* • Also known as *moniliasis* • 50% of adults symptom-free carriers • Appears in warm, moist areas such as groin area, oral mucosa, and submammary folds • Immunosuppression (e.g., from HIV infection, chemotherapy, radiation, and organ transplantation) allows yeast to become pathogenic.	*Mouth:* White, cheesy plaque, resembles milk curds *Vagina:* Vaginitis with red, edematous, painful vaginal wall, white patches. Vaginal discharge. Pruritus. Pain on urination and intercourse *Skin:* Diffuse papular erythematous rash with pinpoint satellite lesions around edges of affected area	• Azole antifungals (e.g., fluconazole, ketoconazole) or other specific medication such as vaginal suppository or oral lozenge • Sexual abstinence or use of condom • Skin hygiene to keep area clean and dry • Powder is effective on nonmucosal surfaces of skin to prevent recurrence.
Tinea Corporis • Various dermatophytes, commonly referred to as *ringworm*	• Typical annular (ringlike) scaly appearance, well-defined margins • Erythematous	• Cool compresses • Topical antifungals for isolated patches. Creams or solutions of miconazole, ketoconazole, clotrimazole, butenafine
Tinea Cruris • Various dermatophytes • Commonly referred to as *jock itch*	• Well-defined scaly plaque in groin area • Does not affect mucous membranes	• Topical antifungal cream or solution
Tinea Pedis • Various dermatophytes • Commonly referred to as *athlete's foot*	• Interdigital scaling and maceration • Scaly plantar surfaces sometimes with erythema and blistering • May be pruritic. Possibly painful	• Topical antifungal cream, gel, solution, spray, or powder
Tinea Unguium (Onychomycosis) • Various dermatophytes • Incidence increases with age.	• Only few nails on one hand may be affected. Toenails more commonly affected • Scaliness under distal nail plate • Brittle, thickened, broken, or crumbling nails with yellowish discoloration (Fig. 23-9)	• Oral antifungal (terbinafine [Lamisil], itraconazole [Sporanox]) • Topical antifungal cream or solution (minimal effectiveness) if unable to tolerate systemic treatment • Thinning of toenails if needed • Nail avulsion (removal) is an option.

TABLE 23-9 Common Allergic Conditions of the Skin

Etiology and Pathophysiology	Clinical Manifestations	Treatment and Prognosis
Allergic Contact Dermatitis • Type IV delayed hypersensitivity response (see Chapter 13) • Absorbed agent acts as antigen. • Sensitization occurs after one or more exposures. • Appearance of lesions 2-7 days after contact with allergen	• Red papules and plaques • Sharply circumscribed with occasional vesicles (see Fig. 13-9) • Usually pruritic • Area of dermatitis frequently takes shape of causative agent (e.g., metal allergy and bandlike dermatitis on ring finger).	• Topical or oral corticosteroids, antihistamines • Skin lubrication • Elimination of contact allergen • Avoidance of irritating affected area • Systemic corticosteroids if sensitivity severe
Urticaria • Usually allergic phenomenon • Erythema and edema in upper dermis resulting from a local increase in permeability of capillaries (usually from histamine release)	• Spontaneously occurring, raised or irregularly shaped wheals, varying size, usually multiple • A single lesion usually resolves in 24 hr. • Can occur anywhere on the body	• Removal of triggering agent, if known • Oral antihistamine therapy • Possibly systemic corticosteroids
Drug Reaction • May be caused by any drug that acts as antigen and causes hypersensitivity reaction • Certain drugs (e.g., penicillin) more likely to cause reactions • Not all reactions are allergic, some are intolerance (e.g., gastric upset).	• Rash of any morphology • Often red, macular and papular, semiconfluent, generalized rash with abrupt onset • Appearance as late as 14 days after cessation of drug. Possibly pruritic • Some reactions may be life threatening requiring immediate and intensive care.	• Withdrawal of drug if possible • Antihistamines, topical or systemic corticosteroids may be necessary depending on severity of symptoms.
Atopic Dermatitis • Type 1 hypersensitivity response (see Chapter 13) • Genetically influenced, chronic, relapsing disease • Exaggerated by a skin response to environmental allergens • Associated with allergic rhinitis and asthma	• Multiple presentations, including acute, subacute, and chronic stages. All are pruritic. • *Acute stage:* Bright erythema, oozing vesicles, with extreme pruritus (see Fig. 13-8) • *Subacute stage:* Scaly, light red to red-brown plaques • *Chronic stage:* Thickened skin with accentuation of skin markings (lichenification), possible hypopigmentation, or hyperpigmentation. Dry skin. Common in antecubital and popliteal space	• Lubrication of dry skin • Topical immunomodulators (pimecrolimus [Elidel], tacrolimus [Protopic]) • Reduction of stress reduces flares • Corticosteroids, phototherapy for severe inflammation and pruritus • Antibiotics for secondary infection as needed

TABLE 23-10 Common Benign Conditions of the Skin

Etiology and Pathophysiology	Clinical Manifestations	Treatment and Prognosis
Acne Vulgaris • Inflammatory disorder of sebaceous glands • More common in teenagers but possible development and persistence in adulthood • Flare can occur with use of corticosteroids and androgen-dominant birth control pills and before menses.	• Noninflammatory lesions, including open comedones (blackheads) and closed comedones (whiteheads) • Inflammatory lesions, including papules and pustules • Most common on face, neck, and upper back (Fig. 23-10)	*Topical:* • Mechanical removal of multiple lesions with comedo extractor • Topical benzoyl peroxide, retinoids, or antimicrobials (clindamycin, erythromycin) *Systemic:* • Systemic antibiotics • Use of isotretinoin (Accutane) for severe nodulocystic acne to possibly provide lasting remission. Pregnancy tests, monitor liver function, cholesterol, triglycerides, and for depression • Aim of treatment to suppress new lesions and minimize scarring • Spontaneous remission possible • Often improvement with exposure to sun • May last many years
Nevi (Moles) Grouping of normal cells derived from melanocyte-like precursor cells	• Hyperpigmented areas that vary in form and color • Flat, slightly elevated, verrucoid, polypoid, dome-shaped, sessile, or papillomatous • Preservation of normal skin markings • Hair growth possible	• No treatment necessary except for cosmetic reasons • Skin biopsy for suspicious nevi
Psoriasis • Autoimmune chronic dermatitis that involves excessively rapid turnover of epidermal cells • Family predisposition • Usually develops before age 40	• Sharply demarcated silvery scaling plaques on reddish colored skin commonly on the scalp, elbows, knees, palms, soles, and fingernails (Fig. 23-11) • Itching, burning, pain • Localized or general, intermittent or continuous • Symptoms vary in intensity from mild to severe.	Goal to reduce inflammation and suppress rapid turnover of epidermal cells. No cure, but control is possible *Topical treatments:* • Corticosteroids, tar, salicylic acid, calcipotriene, anthralin • Intralesional injection of corticosteroids for chronic plaques *Systemic treatments:* • Natural or artificial UVB. PUVA (UVA with topical or systemic photosensitizer (psoralen) • Antimetabolite (methotrexate), PDE-4 inhibitor (apremilast [Otezla]), retinoid (acitretin), immunosuppressant (cyclosporine), biologic therapy (adalimumab [Humira], etanercept [Enbrel], infliximab [Remicade], ustekinumab [Stelara], certolizumab pegol [Cimzia], secukinumab [Cosentyx], golimumab [Simponi]), and ixekizumab (Taltz) for moderate to severe plaque disease
Seborrheic Keratoses • Benign, familial, exact etiology unknown • Usually occur after age 40, increase in number with age	• Irregularly round or oval, often verrucous papules or plaques • Well-defined shape, appearance of being stuck on • Increase in pigmentation with time • Usually multiple and possibly itchy	• Removal by curettage or cryosurgery for cosmetic reasons or to eliminate source of irritation • Biopsy if unable to distinguish from melanoma
Acrochordons (Skin Tags) • Common after midlife • Appearance on neck, axillae, and upper trunk secondary to mechanical friction or redundant skin (associated with obesity)	• Small, skin-colored, soft, pedunculated papules • May become irritated	• No treatment medically necessary • Surgical removal when needed • Usually just snipping without anesthesia
Lipoma • Benign tumor of adipose tissue, often encapsulated • Most common in 40- to 60-yr-old age group	• Rubbery, compressible, round mass of adipose tissue • Single or multiple • Variable in size, possibly extremely large • Most common on trunk, back of neck, and forearms	• Usually no treatment • Biopsy to differentiate from liposarcoma • Excision usual treatment (when indicated)
Lentigo • Increased number of normal melanocytes in basal layer of epidermis related to sun exposure and aging • Also called "liver spots" or "age spots"	• Hyperpigmented, brown to black macule or patch (flat lesion) on sun-exposed areas	• Evaluate carefully for progression. • Treatment only for cosmetic purposes: liquid nitrogen, laser resurfacing • May recur • Biopsy when suspicious of melanoma.

PUVA, Psoralen ultraviolet A; *UVA,* ultraviolet A; *UVB,* ultraviolet B.

INTERPROFESSIONAL CARE: DERMATOLOGIC PROBLEMS

Diagnostic Studies

A careful history is of prime importance in diagnosing skin problems. The HCP must be skilled at detecting any evidence that could lead to the cause of many different skin diseases and conditions. After a careful history and physical examination, inspect individual lesions. The history, physical examination, and appropriate diagnostic test results guide therapy.

Interprofessional Therapy

Many different treatment methods are used in dermatology. Advances in this field have brought relief to many previously chronic, untreatable conditions. Many of the specific therapeutic treatments require specialized equipment and are usually reserved for use by a dermatologist.

Phototherapy. Ultraviolet light (UVL) of different wavelengths may be used to treat many dermatologic conditions, including psoriasis, cutaneous T-cell lymphoma, atopic dermatitis, vitiligo, and pruritus. Light sources available include broadband UVB, narrowband UVB, and long-wave UV (UVA1). One form of phototherapy involves the use of psoralen plus UVA light (PUVA). Psoralen is a photosensitizing drug given to patients for a prescribed amount of time before exposure to UVA.

Treatments are generally given two to four times a week. Side effects of oral psoralen include nausea and vomiting, sunburn, and persistent pruritus. Perform frequent skin assessments on all patients receiving phototherapy, since erythema is a side effect of treatment. Topical corticosteroids may reduce painful erythema. Use psoralen with extreme caution in patients with liver or renal disease because slower metabolism and excretion can lead to prolonged photosensitivity.

Since there is risk with any UV exposure, discuss the risks and benefits with the patient prior to initiating phototherapy. Caution patients about the potential hazards of using photosensitizing chemicals and further exposure to UV rays from sunlight or artificial UVL during therapy. Because the lens of the eye absorbs psoralen, patients receiving PUVA need prescription protective eyewear that blocks 100% of UVL. Using the eyewear prevents cataract formation. Instruct patients to use the eyewear for 24 hours after taking the medication when outdoors or near a bright window because UVA penetrates glass. Ongoing monitoring is essential because of the immunosuppressive effects of PUVA, including an increased risk of SCC, BCC, and melanoma.

CHECK YOUR PRACTICE

You are working in a dermatology clinic preparing a 64-yr-old woman for phototherapy to treat multiple actinic keratoses on her nose and both cheeks. She says the first lesion appeared a few years ago. She then got worried about all of the time she spent in her garden without sunscreen. She thought the lesions were just "age spots" and was unconcerned until a few started to grow and periodically bleed.

- Prior to therapy, what teaching will you do to get her ready for the procedure and to take care of herself after the procedure?

Photodynamic therapy is a special type of phototherapy used to treat actinic keratosis and some malignant skin tumors. This therapy uses a photosensitizing agent in a different way than other phototherapy treatments. The patient receives the photosensitizing agent IV or topically, depending on the area treated. Time is allowed for the drug to be absorbed by the target cells. Light is then applied to the area, causing the drug to react with oxygen. This starts a reaction that kills the cells.[10]

TABLE 23-11 Skin Conditions Treated by Laser

• Acne scars	• Psoriasis
• Hair removal	• Resurfacing of skin
• Hemangiomas	• Rosacea
• Leg veins	• Skin lesions
• Pigment discoloration in epidermis	• Tattoo removal
• Pigmented nevi	• Vascular lesions
• Port wine stain	• Wrinkles

Radiation Therapy. The use of radiation therapy to treat BCC, SCC, and malignant melanoma varies greatly according to local practice and availability. Radiation may be given to reduce tumor size or as palliative treatment. One advantage of radiation therapy is minimal damage to surrounding tissue. This is of prime consideration in locations such as the nose, eyelids, and canthal areas. Radiation therapy is particularly effective for the older adult or debilitated patient who cannot tolerate even a minor surgical procedure.

Radiation therapy usually requires multiple visits to a radiology department. It can produce permanent hair loss *(alopecia)* of the irradiated areas. Other adverse effects, depending on anatomic location and dose of radiation delivered, include telangiectasia, atrophy, hyperpigmentation, depigmentation, ulceration, hearing loss, ocular damage, atrophy, and mucositis. Careful shielding is necessary to prevent ocular lens damage if the irradiated area is around the eyes. (Radiation therapy is discussed in Chapter 15.)

Total-body skin irradiation (body is bombarded with high-energy electrons) is one treatment for cutaneous T-cell lymphoma. Treatment follows a lengthy course and causes premature aging of the skin. Patients experience varying degrees of permanent alopecia and radiation dermatitis with a transient loss of sweat gland function.

Laser Technology. Laser treatment is expanding rapidly as an efficient surgical tool for many types of dermatologic problems (Table 23-11). Depending on the type of laser and the wavelength, lasers serve a wide variety of functions. Lasers are able to produce measurable, repeatable, consistent zones of tissue damage. They can cut, coagulate, and vaporize tissue to some degree. Laser light does not accumulate in body cells and cannot cause cumulative cellular changes or damage. With less damage to surrounding tissue, there is a decreased risk of scarring.

The surgical use of laser energy requires a focusing device to produce a small, high-density spot of energy. Several types of lasers are available. The CO_2 laser, the most common, has numerous applications as a vaporizing and cutting tool for most tissues. The argon laser emits light that is primarily absorbed by hemoglobin. It helps in the treatment of vascular and other pigmented lesions. Other, less common lasers include copper and gold vapors and neodymium: yttrium-aluminum-garnet (Nd:YAG). Written policies and procedures should cover laser safety and be reviewed by all personnel working with laser equipment.

Drug Therapy

Antibiotics. A number of topical and systemic antibiotics are used to treat dermatologic problems. Sometimes topical and systemic antibiotics are used concurrently. Common OTC topical antibiotics include bacitracin-neomycin-polymyxin (Neosporin), bacitracin, and polymyxin B. Many HCPs do not recommend Neosporin because of the risk of allergic contact dermatitis. Prescription topical antibiotics include mupirocin (for superficial *Staphylococcus* infections such as impetigo), gentamicin (used for *Staphylococcus* and most gram-negative organisms), and erythromycin (used for gram-positive cocci [staphylococci and streptococci] and gram-negative cocci and bacilli). Topical erythromycin and clindamycin (Cleocin solutions or gels) are used in the treatment of acne vulgaris. Topical metronidazole is used to treat rosacea and bacterial vaginosis. Many popular systemic antibiotics are not used topically because of the danger of allergic contact dermatitis.

If there are manifestations of systemic infection, a systemic antibiotic is used. Frequently used drugs include penicillin, minocycline, erythromycin, tetracycline, and for severe infections, vancomycin. These drugs are particularly useful for acne vulgaris and bacterial infections, such as erysipelas, cellulitis, carbuncles, and severe infected eczema. Teach patients drug-specific instructions on the proper technique of taking or applying antibiotics.

Corticosteroids. Corticosteroids are effective in treating a wide variety of dermatologic conditions. They can be used topically, intralesionally, or systemically. Topical corticosteroids have local antiinflammatory and antipruritic effects. Since corticosteroids may alter the clinical manifestations, attempt to diagnose a skin problem before applying a corticosteroid preparation. Accurate and adequate topical therapy is often the key to a successful outcome. Once a sufficient amount of medication is dispensed, limits should be set on the duration and frequency of application.

The potency of a particular preparation depends on the concentration of active drug. With prolonged use, more potent corticosteroid formulations can cause adrenal suppression, especially if a large surface area is covered and occlusive dressings are used. Over time, high-potency corticosteroids may produce side effects, including skin atrophy resulting from impaired cell mitosis, capillary fragility, and susceptibility to bruising. In general, dermal and epidermal atrophy does not occur until a corticosteroid has been used for 2 to 3 weeks. If drug use is discontinued at the first sign of atrophy, recovery usually occurs in several weeks. Rosacea eruptions and severe exacerbations of acne vulgaris may also occur. Rebound dermatitis is common when therapy is stopped. Tapering the use of high-potency topical corticosteroids when improvement is noted reduces the risk.

Low-potency corticosteroids such as hydrocortisone act more slowly but can be used for a longer time without producing serious side effects. Low-potency corticosteroids are safe to use on the face and intertriginous areas, such as the axillae and groin.

The most potent delivery system for a topical corticosteroid is an ointment form. Apply creams and ointments in thin layers and slowly massage into the site 1 to 3 times a day.

Intralesional corticosteroids are injected directly into or just beneath the lesion. This method provides a reservoir of medication with an effect lasting several weeks to months. Intralesional injection is common in the treatment of psoriasis, alopecia areata (patchy hair loss), cystic acne, hypertrophic scars, and keloids. Triamcinolone acetonide (Kenalog) is the most common drug used for intralesional injection.

Systemic corticosteroids can have remarkable results in the treatment of skin conditions. However, they often have undesirable systemic effects (see Chapter 49). Corticosteroids can be given as short-term therapy for acute conditions such as contact dermatitis caused by poison ivy. Long-term corticosteroid therapy for dermatologic conditions is reserved for severe disease such as bullous (blistering) disorders.

Antihistamines. Oral antihistamines are helpful in treating urticaria, angioedema, and pruritus that can occur in problems such as atopic dermatitis, allergic dermatitis, and other allergic cutaneous reactions. Several different antihistamines may be tried before the satisfactory therapeutic effect is achieved. Antihistamines may have sedative effects. Sedating antihistamines, such as hydroxyzine and diphenhydramine, are often preferred for pruritic conditions because the tranquilizing and sedative effects offer symptomatic relief. Warn the patient about sedative effects, a problem when driving or operating heavy machinery. Antihistamines, such as loratadine (Claritin), fexofenadine (Allegra), and cetirizine (Zyrtec), bind to peripheral histamine receptors, providing antihistamine action without sedation. They are not effective for controlling pruritus. All antihistamines should be used with caution in older adults because of their long half-life and anticholinergic effects.

Topical Fluorouracil. Fluorouracil (5-FU) is a topical cytotoxic agent with selective toxicity for sun-damaged cells. It is used to treat premalignant (especially actinic keratosis) and some malignant skin diseases. Because systemic absorption of the drug is minimal, systemic side effects are not a problem. Patient compliance is a consideration in the use of 5-FU. The medication produces erythema and pruritus within 3 to 5 days. Painful, eroded areas over the damaged skin occur within 1 to 3 weeks, depending on skin thickness at the site. Low-potency topical corticosteroids are often applied 20 minutes after 5-FU to reduce erythema and pruritus and increase patient adherence with therapy. 5-FU is available in four strengths (0.5%, 1%, 2%, and 5%). Treatment must continue with applications 1 (only in the 0.5% strength) or 2 times a day for 2 to 4 weeks. Healing may take up to 4 weeks after medication is stopped.[11]

Because 5-FU is a photosensitizing drug, instruct the patient to avoid sunlight during treatment. Teach patients about the effect of the medication. Tell them they will look worse before they look better. Adherence depends on thoroughness of your instruction, which should include a written handout. After treatment, skin should be smooth and free of actinic keratosis. Actinic keratosis may recur in treated areas, and multiple courses of therapy may be necessary over the years for those with severely sun-damaged skin.

Immunomodulators. Topical immunomodulators, such as pimecrolimus (Elidel) and tacrolimus (Protopic), are used to treat atopic dermatitis. They work by suppressing an overreactive immune system. The side effects are minimal and may include a transient burning or feeling of heat at the application site. An increased risk of skin cancer and precancerous lesions may be associated with these drugs.

Another topical immunomodulator, imiquimod (Aldara), acts to stimulate the production of α-interferon and other cytokines to enhance cell-mediated immunity. It boosts the immune response only where applied and is safe for transplant patients. Imiquimod is used for external genital warts, actinic keratoses, and superficial BCC. Most patients using this cream experience skin reactions, including redness, swelling, blistering, excoriations, peeling, itching, and burning. Dosing varies depending on the type of lesion treated and the strength of medication prescribed.[11]

Diagnostic and Surgical Therapy

Skin Scraping. Scraping with a scalpel blade is done to obtain a sample of surface cells (stratum corneum) for microscopic inspection and diagnosis. The most common tests of skin scrapings are mineral oil examination for scabies and 10% to 20% potassium hydroxide (KOH) for fungus.

Electrodessication and Electrocoagulation. Electrical energy can be converted to heat with the tip of an electrode. The heat burns and destroys tissue. The major uses of this type of therapy are coagulation of bleeding vessels to obtain hemostasis and destruction of small *telangiectasias* (dilation of groups of superficial capillaries and venules). *Electrodessication* usually involves more superficial destruction, and a monopolar electrode is used. *Electrocoagulation* uses a dipolar electrode. It has a deeper effect, with better hemostasis but an increased possibility of scarring. While minor electrosurgery on patients with a pacemaker poses minimal risk, both pacemakers and internal defibrillators can be affected by the electrical energy being used.

Curettage. Curettage is the removal and scooping away of tissue using an instrument called a *curette.* A curette looks like a small spoon with very sharp edges. Although a curette is not usually strong enough to cut normal skin, it can remove many types of small, soft skin tumors and superficial lesions, such as warts, actinic keratoses, seborrheic keratosis, and small BCC and SCC. The area to be curetted is anesthetized before the procedure. The lesion is removed, and then the skin is cauterized. The removed tissue is usually biopsied. A dressing may be applied, and you will need to teach the patient wound care. A small scar and hypopigmentation can result.

Punch Biopsy. Punch biopsy is a common procedure used to obtain a tissue sample for histologic study or to remove small lesions (Fig. 23-12). The procedure is simple. The biopsy area is marked and then anesthetized so that the anesthetizing agent will not obscure the landmarks. The HCP rotates the punch into the skin and removes a small cylinder of skin. Hemostasis is achieved with pressure or absorbable gelatin (Gelfoam) packing. Sites of 4 mm or larger are usually closed with sutures. Punch biopsies are not done below the knee if other sites are available. Circulatory changes can make evaluation of the tissue sample more difficult.

Cryosurgery. Cryosurgery is the use of subfreezing temperatures to destroy epidermal lesions. Cryosurgery is a useful treatment for common benign, precancerous conditions, including common and genital warts, cutaneous tags, thin seborrheic keratoses, lentigines, actinic keratoses, BCC, and SCC. Topical liquid nitrogen (−196° F) is the agent most commonly used for cryosurgery.[12] The mechanism of injury involves direct cellular freezing and vascular stasis (stoppage or slowdown in the flow of blood), which develops after thawing. Intracellular ice formation causes the cell to rupture during thaw, leading to cell death and necrosis of the treated tissue.

Liquid nitrogen is applied topically (directly onto the lesion) with a direct spray or a cotton-tipped applicator. Tell patients that they will feel a stinging cold sensation. The lesion first becomes swollen and red, and it may blister. A scab forms and falls off in 1 to 3 weeks. The skin lesion sloughs along with the scab. Growth of new skin follows.

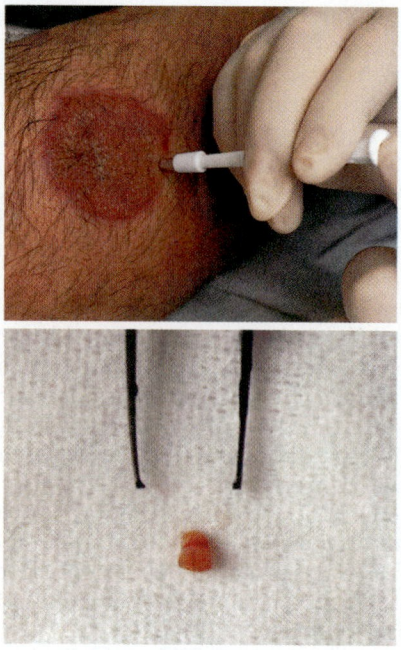

FIG. 23-12 Punch biopsy. **A,** Removal of skin for diagnostic purposes. **B,** Specimen obtained. (From Graham-Brown R, Bourke J, Cunliffe T: *Dermatology: fundamentals of practice,* Edinburgh, 2008, Mosby Ltd.)

The low temperature of liquid nitrogen can easily destroy melanocytes, leaving an area of hypopigmentation resembling a scar. The size of an affected area to be treated may limit the use of cryotherapy. The disadvantages of this treatment are the lack of a tissue specimen for histologic confirmation of cell type before destruction and the potential for destruction of adjacent healthy tissue.

Excision. Excision is an option if the lesion involves the dermis. Complete closure of the excised area usually results in a good cosmetic result.

A specific type of excision is *Mohs surgery,* which is a microscopically controlled removal of a skin malignancy. In this procedure, the HCP removes tissue sections in thin horizontal layers. All of the specimen's margins are examined to determine whether any malignant cells remain (Fig. 23-13). Any residual tumor not removed by the first surgical excision is removed in serial excisions performed the same day. Benefits of Mohs surgery are preserving normal tissue, producing the smallest possible wound, and completely removing the cancer before surgical closure. Although this can become a lengthy procedure, it is done in an outpatient setting using local anesthesia.

❖ NURSING MANAGEMENT: DERMATOLOGIC PROBLEMS

◆ Ambulatory Care

Dermatologic conditions are not usually the primary reason for hospitalization. Nevertheless, many hospitalized patients have skin problems that need nursing intervention and patient education. Nursing interventions related to skin conditions fall into broad categories. They are applicable to many problems in both inpatient and outpatient settings. A nursing care plan for the patient with chronic skin lesions (eNursing Care Plan 23-1) is available on the website for this chapter.

◆ **Wet Compresses.** For superficial skin problems that involve inflammation, itching, and infection, wet compresses are

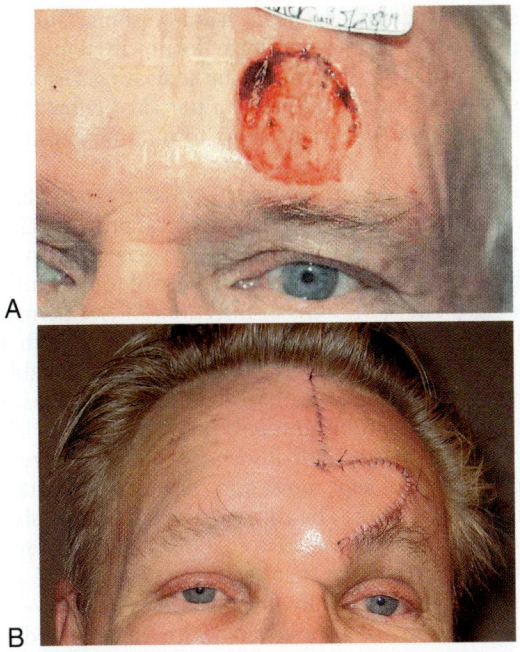

FIG. 23-13 **A,** Removal of melanoma by Mohs surgery. **B,** After plastic surgery using a skin flap to repair defect. (Courtesy Peter Bonner, Placitas, N. Mex.)

commonly used. They are appropriate for damaged, oozing skin. Wet compresses are an excellent way to remove crusts and scabs that are adhering to the wound surface. Wet compresses provide comfort and treatment of conditions such as poison ivy, insect bites, and skin infections.

It is important to understand how to do a wet compress (dressing) correctly. Unless there is a concern about water quality, tap water at room temperature is the best choice. If drinkable water is not available, filtered, bottled, or sterile water may be used. Depending on the problem, additives may be used. Antibacterial solutions may contain aluminum acetate (Domeboro powder), silver nitrate, or acetic acid. Concentrations are critical when additives are used. For example, the desired concentration for acetic acid (vinegar) for a compress is 1% to 2.5%. Kitchen vinegar is 5% and must be diluted. Either white or brown vinegar using ½ cup diluted in 1 pint of water will yield a 1% concentration. Wet compresses should be tepid. However, when an antiinflammatory effect is desired, the wet dressing should be cool.

The material you select for wet compresses should be four to eight layers thick and slightly larger than the area that you are treating. Use gauze or any clean material (e.g., thin cotton sheeting, thermal underwear, tube socks). Ingenuity is sometimes required when covering odd-shaped body parts. Do not use gauze sponges with fillers (abdominal pads), because they will retain too much solution, and fibers can be left in the wound if the skin is open. Place the prescribed compress material into fresh solution and squeeze out excess water. Your goal is a wet compress—not simply damp and not dripping.

Wet compresses are applied continuously or intermittently. When used continuously, use new solution as needed. Do not add additional solution. This can alter the concentration and damage the skin. Depending on the desired effect, intermittent compresses are placed for 10 to 30 minutes, 2 to 4 times a day. Careful monitoring of the skin is important. If the skin appears *macerated* (softens and turns white), discontinue the dressings for 2 to 3 days. Change and wash daily any material used repeatedly throughout the day. Protect the patient from discomfort and chilling. A water-resistant pad will help protect the mattress, linens, and furniture.

TABLE 23-12 Drug Therapy

Common Bases for Topical Medications

Agent	Therapeutic Considerations
Powder	Promotion of dryness. Lubricates skinfold areas to prevent irritation. Base for antifungal preparations. Protect patient from inhaling.
Lotion	Emulsions of water, alcohol, and/or oil. Cooling and drying. Some leave residual powder film after evaporation of water. Useful in subacute pruritic eruptions
Cream	Emulsions of oil and water. Most common base for topical medications. Lubrication and protection
Ointment	Oil with differing amounts of water added in suspension. Lubrication and prevention of dehydration. Petrolatum most common
Paste	Mixture of powder and ointment, used when drying effect necessary because moisture is absorbed
Gel	Nongreasy combination of propylene glycol and water. May contain alcohol

◆ **Baths.** Baths are an appropriate intervention when large areas of the body need treatment. Baths may be relaxing and will help decrease itching. Agents such as colloidal oatmeal (Aveeno) and sodium bicarbonate can be added directly to bath water. Fill the tub with tepid water to cover the affected areas. Depending on the severity of the problem and the patient's discomfort, have the patient soak for 15 to 20 minutes 3 or 4 times a day. Stress to the patient not to rub the skin dry with a towel but gently pat to prevent increased irritation and inflammation. Avoid adding oils as their use increases the risk of falls. To sustain the hydrating effect, apply cream, ointment emollients (moisturizers), or other prescribed topical agents after the bath. This helps seal the moisture in the hydrated cells and increases the absorption of any topical medications.

◆ **Topical Medications.** Topical medications are commonly used to treat cutaneous problems. The effectiveness of topical therapy depends on which base the medication is prepared in. Table 23-12 summarizes the common agents used as bases for topical preparations and their therapeutic considerations. The base selected depends on the properties needed.

Creams are very versatile and most commonly prescribed. They are a mix of organic oils, water, and usually a preservative. Ointments are primarily organic oils with little or no water. Many are preservative free. They are more lubricating than creams and offer enhanced potency of the active ingredient. They may be too occlusive for conditions with high levels of exudate or in body creases. Gels work well on the scalp, where other compounds may mat the hair and for acute exudative conditions such as poison ivy. Lotions can be a mix of water, alcohols, and/or oils. They are also appropriate for the scalp but may cause stinging and drying when used in skin folds. Pastes are a compound of 50% or more powder in an ointment base. They are good for protecting the skin but are messy. A limited number of foams are available.

Apply topical medications as directed. Proper administration will yield best results, maintain consistency, and avoid waste. Some are very costly. As a general rule, topical medication should be applied in a thin film to clean skin and spread evenly in a downward motion in the direction of hair growth. Thick creams will spread easier if the skin is still damp. If a secondary dressing is going to be used, you can apply the medication directly onto a dressing. Teach the patient and caregiver proper dosing, application technique, anticipated results, and common reactions.

Occlusion with a plastic wrap is an effective way of increasing the absorption of topical corticosteroids or simple emollients. The plastic wrap traps perspiration against the outer layer of the epidermis. Applying preparations to moist skin increases absorption 10-fold. Use tape or stretch wraps to keep the plastic wrap in place. For conditions on the feet or lower legs, socks can be worn over the plastic wrap. Wraps applied multiple times daily are kept in place for 2 to 8 hours. Some patients choose to use the occlusion technique at bedtime. Recommend occlusion with discretion. It is not appropriate in areas prone to infection, such as skin creases.

◆ **Control of Pruritus.** *Pruritus* (itching) can be caused by dry skin, almost any physical or chemical stimulus to the skin (such as drugs or insects), and any scaling skin disorder. The itch sensation is carried by the same nonmyelinated nerve fibers as pain and temperature. The patient will have pain rather than an itch if the epidermis is damaged or absent.

The itch/scratch cycle must be broken to prevent excoriation and lichenification. Control of pruritus is important because it is difficult to diagnose an excoriated and inflamed lesion. Certain circumstances make itching worse. Have the patient avoid anything that causes vasodilation, such as heat or rubbing. Dryness of the skin lowers the itch threshold and increases the itch sensation.

Teach the patient ways to help break the itch/scratch cycle. A cool environment may cause vasoconstriction and decrease itching. Hydration, wet compresses, and moisturizers (including antipruritic lotions) are normally helpful. Apply wet compresses for 30 to 60 minutes, pat the skin dry, and apply a lubricant or medication. Topical and injectable corticosteroids are occasionally ordered. Topically applied menthol, camphor, or phenol numb the itch receptors. Systemic antihistamines may provide relief. The principal side effect of most antihistamines is sedation. This may be desirable because pruritus is often worse at night and can interfere with sleep.

Lichenification is a thickening of epidermis with exaggerated markings resembling a washboard. It is caused by chronic scratching or rubbing of the skin. Lichenification is often associated with atopic dermatoses and other pruritic conditions. Although any area of the body may be affected, the hands, forearms, shins, and nape of the neck are common sites. Itching may become habitual. The persistent scratching can cause excoriations. Treating the cause of the itching is the key to preventing lichenification.

◆ **Prevention of Spread.** Although most skin problems are not contagious, infection control precautions indicate wearing gloves when working with any open wounds or lesions with drainage. Not all infected drainage is purulent. Careful hand washing and properly disposing of soiled dressings are the best means of preventing the spread of infections or infestations. The most common contagious lesions include impetigo, streptococcal infections, staphylococcal infections (e.g., methicillin-resistant *S. aureus* [MRSA]), fungal infections, primary chancre, scabies, and pediculosis.

◆ **Prevention of Secondary Infections.** Open skin lesions are susceptible to invasion by other viral, bacterial, or fungal organisms. Meticulous hygiene, hand washing, and dressing changes are important to minimize the potential for secondary infections. Warn the patient about scratching lesions, which can cause excoriations and create a portal of entry for pathogens. Trim the patient's nails short to minimize trauma from scratching.

◆ **Specific Skin Care.** You are often in a position to teach patients skin care after simple dermatologic surgical procedures, such as skin biopsy, excision, and cryosurgery. In general, your instructions should include dressing changes, use of topical antibiotics, and the signs and symptoms of infection. After a dermatologic procedure, any oozing wound should be cleansed with a saline solution twice daily or as ordered by the HCP. Potable (safe, drinking water) is a safe alternative in some situations. Antibiotic or plain petrolatum ointment may be applied with a secondary dressing that is both absorbent and nonadherent.

Wounds that are kept moist and covered heal more rapidly and with less scarring. The initial crust that forms should be left undisturbed as a protective coating for the damaged skin beneath it. Healing crusts that have been moisturized and protected will separate naturally from healed epidermis.

A sutured wound may be covered with a variety of dressings. Sutures are generally removed in 4 to 14 days, depending on the placement site. Sometimes alternating sutures are removed after the third day. Incision lines may require daily cleansing, usually with plain water. If necessary, a topical antibiotic is applied and the wound either is covered with a dry dressing or left open to air. The patient may experience some swelling and discomfort in the first 24 hours. Intermittent application of cold (ice packs) over the surgical dressing may reduce edema. Mild analgesics such as acetaminophen or a nonsteroidal antiinflammatory medication should control discomfort. Teach the patient how to differentiate normal inflammation from an infection. A slight red border during the first few days after a procedure is normal inflammation. Redness that persists longer than a week or extends beyond a 1 cm border, a fever above 101° F, increased pain, pronounced swelling, and purulent drainage are all signs and symptoms of a possible infection. If these occur, they should be promptly reported to the HCP.

◆ **Psychologic Effects of Chronic Dermatologic Problems.** Emotional stress can occur for persons who suffer from chronic skin problems such as psoriasis, atopic dermatitis, or acne. The sequelae of chronic skin problems could result in social and employment problems with subsequent financial implications, a poor self-image, problems with sexuality, and increasing and progressive frustration. The usual lack of systemic illness coupled with the visibility of the skin lesions often presents a real problem to the patient.

Help the patient comply with the prescribed regimen. Allow the patient to verbalize the "Why me?" question, even though there is no ready answer. Refer the patient to dermatology support groups. Many are listed on the American Academy of Dermatology website *(www.aad.org)*. These groups are extremely helpful for patient support and accurate education materials.

The location of lesions and scars is the determining factor with respect to its cosmetic implications. Facial scars are the most damaging psychologically because they are so visible. Creative use of cosmetics can do much to mask lesions and scarring. Consider individual sensitivity to product ingredients when selecting cosmetics. Oil-free, hypoallergenic cosmetics are available and may be beneficial for the allergic patient.

TEAMWORK & COLLABORATION

Skin Care

Role of Nursing Personnel

Registered Nurse (RN)

- Assess patient's skin for acute and chronic integumentary problems.
- Assess patient's risk factors for integumentary problems.
- Document skin condition and risk factor assessment, and develop a plan of care.
- Determine whether patient is taking drugs that increase photosensitivity.
- Teach about risks associated with sun exposure and methods for decreasing exposure to the sun.
- Teach about therapies used for integumentary disorders, including dressings, baths, and oral or topical medications used on an outpatient basis.
- Evaluate treatment for effectiveness and any adverse effects.

Licensed Practical/Vocational Nurse (LPN/LVN)

- Administer prescribed therapies such as dressings and oral or topical medications.
- Monitor the skin for changes in appearance or texture that may indicate worsening of integumentary problem or adverse reactions to treatment.
- Reinforce teaching done by the RN.

Unlicensed Assistive Personnel (UAP)

- Assist patient with bathing.
- Apply wet dressings to skin or add medications (such as oilated oatmeal) to patient baths (consider state nurse practice act and agency policy).
- Report changes in skin appearance or patient complaints of discomfort to the RN.

Rehabilitative cosmetics are available to help camouflage and deemphasize such lesions as *vitiligo* (loss of pigmentation), *melasma* (tan to brown patches on the face), or healed postoperative wound sites. These commercially available products are opaque, smudge resistant, and water resistant.

COSMETIC PROCEDURES

A vast array of cosmetic procedures is available, including chemical peels, toxin injections, fillers, laser surgery, breast enlargement and reduction (see Chapter 51), face-lift, eyelid-lift, and liposuction. Common cosmetic topical procedures are presented in Table 23-13. Other types of cosmetic procedures include the injection of botulinum toxin (Botox), deoxycholic acid (Kybella), calcium hydroxylapatite (Radiesse), collagen (Zyplast), and hyaluronic acid fillers (e.g., Restylane, Perlane, Juvéderm). Transitory side effects may occur, such as mild redness, pain, swelling, and bruising. Uncommon side effects from cosmetic procedures include allergic reaction, infection, or lumps at the injection sites; undercorrection or overcorrection of wrinkles; and reactivation of human papillomavirus (HPV). Tell the patient that he or she will need to repeat the procedure at prescribed intervals to maintain the desired appearance.

The reasons for undergoing these procedures are as varied as the techniques. The most common reason that people suffer the discomfort and financial expense (most are not covered by health insurance) of a cosmetic procedure is to improve their body image. If they feel better about themselves after having cosmetic procedures, they often act more confident and self-assured. Often social position and economic considerations are part of the decision. Increased longevity provides a larger population to whom cosmetic procedures are especially appealing.

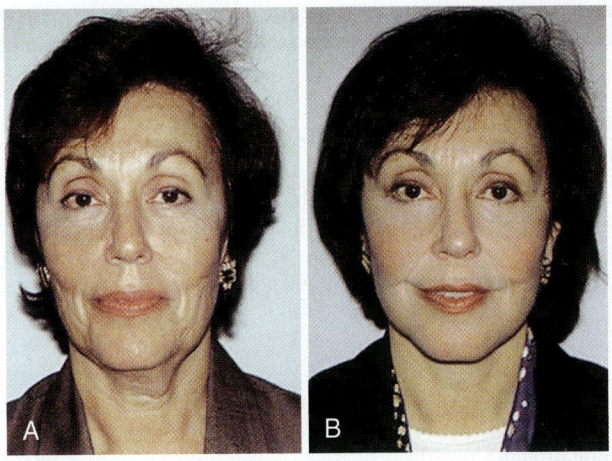

FIG. 23-14 Face-lift. **A,** Preoperative. **B,** Postoperative. (From Pastorek N, Bustillo A: Deep plane face-lift, *Facial Plast Surg Clin North Am* 13:433-449, 2005.)

Regardless of the patient's reasons for seeking cosmetic procedures, maintain a supportive, nonjudgmental attitude about these procedures. If the patient wishes to change or enhance a body feature perceived as unattractive and has realistic expectations about the outcome, you should support this decision.

Elective Surgery

Laser Surgery. Laser surgery is used to treat congenital and acquired vascular lesions (cherry angiomas, spider leg veins, hemangiomas, port wine stains, and tattoo removal) and for skin resurfacing and hair removal. Lasers can reduce scarring and fine wrinkles around the lips or eyes and remove facial lesions (Table 23-11). Swelling, redness, and bruising are common after treatment. The treated areas usually are kept moist with ointment or occlusive dressings for the first few days. The patient must protect treated skin from the sun.

Face-Lift. A face-lift *(rhytidectomy)* is the lifting and repositioning of the lower two thirds of the face and neck to improve appearance (Fig. 23-14). Indications for this procedure include the following:

- Redundant soft tissue or scarring resulting from disease (e.g., acne scarring)
- Asymmetric redundancy of soft tissues (e.g., facial palsy)
- Redundant soft tissue resulting from trauma
- Preauricular lesions
- Redundant soft tissues resulting from *solar elastosis* (sagging of the skin from sun damage), changes in body weight, and the effects of gravity
- Restoration of body image

The surgical approach and lines of incisions vary according to the desired correction and the position of the hairline. Eyelid-lifts *(blepharoplasty)* can remove redundant tissue and possibly improve the field of vision. Preventing hematoma formation is the most important postoperative consideration. Ice packs are usually applied for the first 24 to 48 hours to reduce swelling and decrease the possibility of hematoma formation. Usually the pain is minimal. Antibiotics are used at the surgeon's discretion. Complications can occur if the person smokes or is involved in vigorous exercise.

TABLE 23-13 Common Cosmetic Topical Procedures

Tretinoin (Retin-A, Renova)	Chemical Peels (e.g., Beta Hydroxy Acid, Jessner's Peel, TCA)	Microdermabrasion	α-Hydroxy Acids (e.g., Glycolic Acid, Lactic Acid)
Indications			
Improves appearance of photodamaged skin, especially fine wrinkling. Reduces actinic keratoses	Improves appearance of photodamaged skin, acne scarring, actinic and seborrheic keratoses	Smoothes appearance of photodamaged and wrinkled skin, acne scarring	Smoothes appearance of photodamaged and wrinkled skin, acne scarring
Description			
Initially applied every 2 to 3 days. Treatment stopped if severe inflammation occurs. Maximum response in 8-12 mo	Solution applied in varying amounts to the skin, causing a controlled burn with a loss of melanin.	Epidermis and top dermal layer removed by applying aluminum oxide or baking soda crystals. Re-epithelialization of abraded surface then occurs.	Low concentrations (<10%) in many skin care products consumers can apply to the skin. Higher concentrations (50%-70%) applied only by an HCP
Side Effects			
Erythema, swelling, flaking, pigmentation changes. Teratogenic. Increases phototoxicity if taking other photosensitive drugs	Moderate swelling and crusting for 1 wk. Redness for 6-8 wk. Pink tone possible for several mo. Photosensitivity	Light pink tone that resolves within 24 hr. Photosensitivity	Photosensitivity, slight irritation at lower concentrations, severe redness, oozing, and flaking skin possible with higher concentrations
Patient Teaching			
Apply at night since preparation is inactivated by light. Apply emollients, use sunscreen, use sun avoidance measures, avoid using abrasive or drying facial cleansers for severe sensitivity (e.g., excess irritation).	Use sunscreen. Avoid sun for 6 mo to prevent hyperpigmentation.	Generous application of emollients and sunscreen	Use sunscreen and sun avoidance measures.

Liposuction. Liposuction is a technique for removing subcutaneous fat to improve facial and body contours. Although not a substitute for diet and exercise, it can be successful in removing areas of fat from virtually any body area that is resistant to other techniques.

Liposuction is relatively free of complications. Possible contraindications include the use of anticoagulants, uncontrolled hypertension, diabetes mellitus, and poor cardiovascular status. Persons under 40 years of age with good skin elasticity are the best candidates. However, patients over 40 can be treated successfully.

The procedure is usually done on an outpatient basis under local anesthesia. One or more sessions may be necessary, depending on the size of the area to be treated. The HCP inserts a blunt-tipped cannula through a small incision and pushes into the fat to break it loose from the fibrous stroma. Multiple repeated thrusts disrupt the fat and create tunnels. The loosened fat is removed with a powerful suction. Afterwards, firm pressure is applied to the wounds and compression garments are worn for 3 to 4 weeks.[13] Bandaging also helps to contour the skin. It may take several months for the results to be evident.

❖ NURSING MANAGEMENT: COSMETIC SURGERY

Many cosmetic surgical procedures are done in well-equipped day-surgery units or in dermatologist or plastic surgeon in-office surgery suites.

◆ Preoperative Management

A major preoperative consideration relates to informed consent and realistic expectations of what cosmetic surgery can accomplish. Although the HCP should provide this information, reinforce it and answer questions and concerns. For instance, a face-lift has little or no effect on deep wrinkling of the forehead and temples, deep nasolabial grooves, or vertical lip wrinkles. Before-and-after treatment photographs of similar cases are often useful in helping the patient to set realistic expectations.

Your teaching plan should include the timeframe for healing. Explain the oozing, crusting stage of an abrasive procedure so the patient can plan time off from work if necessary. Since wound healing may not be complete for 1 year, the patient should not anticipate complete results immediately. The final result is affected by the patient's age, general state of health, and skin type and the extent (severity) of the condition being treated. Efforts should be made to correct or control any existing health problem before the procedure.

◆ Postoperative Management

Most cosmetic procedures are not extremely painful. Usually mild analgesics are sufficient to keep the patient comfortable. Although infection is not a common problem after cosmetic surgery, assess the sites for signs of infection. Teach the patient signs and symptoms of infection with instructions to report them immediately so that appropriate antibiotic intervention can be started.

If the surgery involved an alteration in the skin's circulation, as in a face-lift, carefully monitor for adequate circulation. Warm, pink skin that blanches on pressure indicates that adequate circulation is present in the surgical area. Supportive, compressive dressings and ice packs may be necessary early in the postoperative period.

SKIN GRAFTS

Uses

Skin grafts may be necessary to protect underlying structures or to reconstruct areas for cosmetic or functional purposes.

They may be used to facilitate rapid closure and minimize complications. Ideally, wounds heal by primary intention. However, large wounds, surgically created wounds, trauma, and chronic wounds can result in extensive tissue destruction, making healing by primary intention impossible. In these cases, skin grafting may be necessary to close the defect. Improved surgical techniques make it possible to graft skin, bone, cartilage, fat, fascia, muscles, and nerves. For cosmetically pleasing results, the color, thickness, texture, and hair-growing nature of skin used for grafting should match the recipient site. (See Chapter 24 for a discussion of skin grafting for patients with burn injuries.)

Types

The two types of traditional skin grafts are free grafts and skin flaps. Free grafts are further classified according to the method of providing a blood supply to the grafted skin. One method is to transfer the graft (epidermis and part or all of the dermis) to the recipient site from the donor site. The *autograft* (from the patient's own body) or *isograft* (from an identical twin) revascularizes and becomes fixed to the new site. The other method of free skin grafting is by *reconstructive microsurgery.* With the use of an operating microscope, circulation is established immediately in the graft by anastomosis of the blood vessels from the skin flap to the vessels in the recipient site.

Skin flaps involve moving a section of skin and subcutaneous tissue from one part of the body to another without terminating the vascular attachment *(pedicle).* Skin flaps are used to cover wounds with a poor vascular bed, provide padding when needed, and cover wounds over cartilage and bone. The patient may need intermediate flap placement if the recipient site is far removed from the donor site. For instance, a skin flap from the thigh to the head would require an intermediate graft. The flap is advanced to the recipient site when circulation is well established at the intermediate site. The patient's needs and the type of defect determine the type of flap and the route of transfer.

Soft tissue expansion is a technique for providing skin (1) for resurfacing of a defect, such as a burn scar; (2) for removal of a disfiguring mark (e.g., a tattoo); or (3) as a preliminary step in breast reconstruction. A subcutaneous tissue expander of an appropriate size and shape is placed under the skin, usually as an outpatient procedure. Weekly expansion with saline solution can be done in a health care setting or by the patient at home. This expansion procedure is repeated until the skin reaches the size needed for the repair. This may take from several weeks to 3 to 4 months. Once sufficient skin is available, the old incision is opened, the expander is removed, and the soft tissue is ready to be used as an advancement flap. The tissue expander next to a defect retains the primary tissue characteristics such as color and texture.

Newer engineered skin substitutes (e.g., Apligraf, Dermagraft, Integra, Alloderm) are gaining popularity. There are a number available and each offers its own benefits. Some are two-layered membranes with both dermal and epidermal components. Others are only one layer. The skin is engineered from neonatal foreskins and cadavers. Because the tissue is engineered, Langerhans' cells are removed, reducing the risk of rejection.[14] Engineered skin grafts have an extended shelf life. Some are cryopreserved, others shipped overnight as they are needed. Advantages include ready availability, the avoidance of a donor site, application in outpatient settings, minimal scarring, and less pain.

CASE STUDY

Malignant Melanoma and Dysplastic Nevi

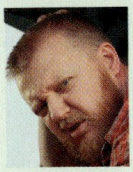

(©Dimedrol68/ iStock/ Thinkstock)

Patient Profile

G.L. is a 44-year-old white, fair-skinned man who is a long-distance truck driver. In his leisure time, he enjoys swimming. He comes to the clinic for evaluation of a changing lesion on his left arm.

Subjective Data

- History of a basal cell carcinoma (BCC) on his left ear in the last 4 years
- Father treated for metastatic malignant melanoma in the last 2 years
- First noted the lesion 5 months ago when it started changing size
- Anxious the lesion might have spread and require extensive, disfiguring surgery

Objective Data

Physical Examination

- Has a 4-mm lesion, dark brown, scalloped with vaguely defined borders
- Four dysplastic nevi found on back

Diagnostic Studies

- Excisional biopsy confirmed malignant melanoma.
- Sentinel node biopsy results were negative.
- Diagnostic tests indicate melanoma stage I.

Discussion Questions

1. What risk factors for malignant melanoma does he have?
2. What are the usual clinical manifestations associated with malignant melanoma?
3. What is the prognosis for a patient with this stage of malignant melanoma?
4. What treatment options are available for him?
5. ***Priority Decision:*** Based on the assessment data presented, what are the priority nursing diagnoses? Are there any collaborative problems?
6. ***Patient-Centered Care:*** How would you help G.L. deal with his anxiety over the treatment outcomes?
7. ***Priority Decision:*** What is the priority of care for G.L.?
8. ***Safety:*** What would you include in his patient teaching plan to address future sun exposure?
9. ***Teamwork and Collaboration:*** Which of the following nursing personnel should be responsible for teaching G.L.: RN, LPN/LVN, or UAP?
10. ***Evidence-Based Practice:*** G.L. wants to know whether regularly applying sunscreen will reduce his risk for developing a second melanoma. How would you reply?

Answers available at *http://evolve.elsevier.com/Lewis/medsurg.*

BRIDGE TO NCLEX EXAMINATION

The number of the question corresponds to the same-numbered outcome at the beginning of the chapter.

1. Which safe sun practices would the nurse include in the teaching plan for a patient who has photosensitivity *(select all that apply)*?
   a. Wear protective clothing.
   b. Apply sunscreen liberally and often.
   c. Emphasize the short-term use of a tanning booth.
   d. Avoid exposure to the sun, especially during midday.
   e. Wear any sunscreen as long as it is purchased at a drugstore.
2. When teaching a patient with malignant melanoma about this disorder, the nurse recognizes that the patient's prognosis is *most* dependent on
   a. the thickness of the lesion.
   b. the degree of asymmetry in the lesion.
   c. the amount of ulceration in the lesion.
   d. how much the lesion has spread superficially.
3. The nurse determines that a patient with a diagnosis of which disorder is *most* at risk for spreading the disease?
   a. Tinea pedis
   b. Impetigo on the face
   c. Candidiasis of the nails
   d. Psoriasis on the palms and soles
4. A mother and her two children have been diagnosed with pediculosis corporis at a health care center. An appropriate measure in treating this condition is
   a. applying pyrethrins to the body.
   b. topical application of griseofulvin.
   c. moist compresses applied frequently.
   d. administration of systemic antibiotics.
5. A common site for the lesions associated with atopic dermatitis is the
   a. buttocks.
   b. temporal area.
   c. antecubital space.
   d. plantar surface of the feet.
6. During the assessment of a patient, you note an area of red, sharply defined plaques covered with silvery scales that are mildly itchy on the patient's knees and elbows. You recognize this finding as
   a. lentigo.
   b. psoriasis.
   c. actinic keratosis.
   d. seborrheic keratosis.
7. In teaching a patient who is using topical corticosteroids to treat acute dermatitis, the nurse should tell the patient that *(select all that apply)*
   a. the cream form is the most efficient system of delivery.
   b. short-term use of topical corticosteroids usually does not cause systemic side effects.
   c. apply creams and ointments with a glove in small amounts to prevent further infection.
   d. abruptly discontinuing the use of topical corticosteroids may cause a reappearance of the dermatitis.
   e. systemic side effects may be experienced from topical corticosteroids if the person is malnourished.
8. A patient with acne vulgaris tells the nurse that she has quit her job as a receptionist because she believes her facial appearance is unattractive to customers. The nursing diagnosis that *best* describes this patient response is
   a. ineffective coping related to lack of social support.
   b. impaired skin integrity related to presence of lesions.
   c. anxiety related to lack of knowledge of the disease process.
   d. social isolation related to decreased activities secondary to fear of rejection.
9. Important patient teaching after a chemical peel includes
   a. avoidance of sun exposure.
   b. application of firm bandages.
   c. limitation of vigorous exercise.
   d. use of moist heat to relieve discomfort.

1. a, b, d, 2. a, 3. b, 4. a, 5. c, 6. b, 7. b, d, 8. d, 9. a

For rationales to these answers and even more NCLEX review questions, visit *http://evolve.elsevier.com/Lewis/medsurg.*

EVOLVE WEBSITE

http://evolve.elsevier.com/Lewis/medsurg

Review Questions (Online Only)
Key Points
Answer Keys for Questions
- Rationales for Bridge to NCLEX Examination Questions
- Answer Guidelines for Case Study on p. 427

Nursing Care Plan
- eNursing Care Plan 23-1: Patient With Chronic Skin Lesions

Conceptual Care Map Creator
Audio Glossary
Supporting Media
- Animation
  - Mohs Surgery

Content Updates

REFERENCES

1. Centers for Disease Control: Indoor tanning is not safe. Retrieved from *www.cdc.gov/cancer/skin/basic_info/indoor_tanning.htm.*
2. US Food and Drug Administration: Sunscreen drug products for over-the-counter human use. Retrieved from *www.fda.gov/drugs/guidancecomplianceregulatoryinformation/guidances/ucm330694.htm.*
3. American Cancer Society: Skin cancer facts. Retrieved from *www.cancer.org/cancer/cancercauses/sunanduvexposure/skin-cancer-facts.*
4. Tsao H, Olazagasti J, Cordoro KM, et al: Early detection of melanoma: reviewing the ABCDEs, *J Am Acad Dermatol* 72:717, 2015.
5. CDC: What are the risk factors for skin cancer? Retrieved from *www.cdc.gov/cancer/skin/basic_info/risk_factors.htm.*
6. Habif TP: *Clinical dermatology*, ed 5, St Louis, 2011, Elsevier. (Classic)
7. Stubblefield J, Kelly B: Melanoma in Non-Caucasian populations, *Surg Clin N Am* 94:1115, 2014.
*8. Kim DW, Trinh VA, Hwu WJ: Ipilimumab in the treatment of advanced melanoma, *Expert Opin Biol Ther* 14:1709, 2014.
9. National Psoriasis Foundation: About psoriasis. Retrieved from *www.psoriasis/org/about.*
10. Rkein AM, Ozog DM: Photodynamic therapy, *Dermatol Clin* 32:415, 2014.
*11. Micali G, Lacarrubba F, Nasca MR, et al: Topical pharmacotherapy for skin cancer, *J Am Acad Derm* 70:979, 2014.
12. Marks JG, Miller JJ: *Principles of dermatology*, ed 5, St Louis, 2013, Elsevier.
13. Afrooz PN, Pozner JN, DiBernado BE: Noninvasive and minimally invasive techniques in body contouring, *Clin Plastic Surg* 41:789, 2014.
14. Nathoo R, Howe N, Cohen G: Skin substitutes: An overview of the key players in wound management, *J Clin Aesthet Derm* 7:44, 2014.

*Evidence-based information for clinical practice.

24

Burns

Judy Knighton

With the new day comes new strength and new thoughts.

Eleanor Roosevelt

http://evolve.elsevier.com/Lewis/medsurg/

LEARNING OUTCOMES

1. Relate the causes of burns to the prevention strategies for burn injuries.
2. Differentiate between partial-thickness and full-thickness burns.
3. Apply tools used to determine the severity of burns.
4. Compare the pathophysiology, clinical manifestations, complications, and interprofessional care throughout the three burn phases.
5. Compare the fluid and electrolyte shifts during the emergent and acute burn phases.
6. Differentiate the nutritional needs of the burn patient throughout the three burn phases.
7. Compare the various burn wound care techniques and surgical options for partial-thickness and full-thickness burn wounds.
8. Prioritize nursing interventions in the management of the burn patient's physiologic and psychosocial needs.
9. Examine the various physiologic and psychosocial aspects of burn rehabilitation.
10. Design a plan of care to prepare the burn patient and caregiver for discharge.

KEY TERMS

burn, p. 429
carboxyhemoglobin, p. 430
chemical burns, p. 429
contracture, p. 446
cultured epithelial autograft (CEA), p. 445
debridement, p. 439
electrical burns, p. 431
escharotomy, p. 437
excision and grafting, p. 444
full-thickness burns, p. 432
partial-thickness burns, p. 432
smoke and inhalation injuries, p. 430
thermal burns, p. 429

The focus of this chapter is the care of patients who have experienced a burn. A **burn** is an injury to the tissues of the body caused by heat, chemicals, electric current, or radiation. The resulting effects are influenced by the temperature of the burning agent, duration of contact time, and type of tissue that is injured.

An estimated 450,000 Americans seek medical care each year for burns.[1] Approximately 40,000 people are hospitalized, one half of whom requires care in specialized burn centers. About 3400 Americans die annually as a direct result of their injuries. The highest fatality rates occur in children ages 4 years and younger and adults over age 65. Around the world, nearly 11 million people need medical attention annually for burn injuries, and about 265,000 die.[2]

Although burn incidence has decreased over the past 20 years, burn injuries still occur too frequently and mainly to those at a lower socioeconomic level and with histories of substance abuse and mental health illness. Most burn incidents are preventable. The focus of burn prevention has shifted from blaming individuals and changing behaviors to making legislative changes and collecting global burn data to address the unique prevention needs of low- and middle-income countries.[3]

Coordinated national programs in developed countries have focused on child-resistant lighters, nonflammable children's clothing, tap water anti-scald devices, stricter building codes, hardwired smoke detectors and alarms, and fire sprinklers. As a nurse, you can advocate for and teach about burn risk–reduction strategies in the home and at work (Tables 24-1 and 24-2).

TYPES OF BURN INJURY

Thermal Burns

Thermal burns, caused by flame, flash, scald, or contact with hot objects, are the most common type of burn injury (Fig. 24-1). The severity of the injury depends on the temperature of the burning agent and duration of contact time. Scald injuries can occur in the bathroom or while cooking. Flash, flame, or contact burns can occur while cooking, smoking, burning leaves in the backyard, or using gasoline or hot oil.

Chemical Burns

Chemical burns are the result of contact with acids, alkalis, and organic compounds. In addition to tissue damage, eyes can be

Reviewed by Cecilia M. Bidigare, RN, MSN, CNS-BC, CNE, Associate Professor of Nursing, Sinclair Community College, Dayton, Ohio; Patricia S. Regojo, RN, MSN, Nurse Manager, Burn Intensive Care Unit and Thoracic Surgery Unit, Temple University Hospital, Philadelphia, Pennsylvania; and Olga Van Dyke, RN, MSN, CAGS, Assistant Professor, School of Nursing, Massachusetts College of Pharmacy and Health Sciences, Boston, Massachusetts.

injured if they are splashed with the chemical. Acids are found in the home and at work and include hydrochloric, oxalic, and hydrofluoric acid. Alkali burns can be more difficult to manage than acid burns, since alkalis adhere to tissue, causing protein hydrolysis and liquefaction. Alkalis are found in cement, oven and drain cleaners, and heavy industrial cleansers.[4] Organic compounds, including phenols (chemical disinfectants) and petroleum products (creosote and gasoline), produce contact burns and systemic toxicity.

TABLE 24-1 Sources of Burn Injury*

Home Hazards

Kitchen and Bathroom

- Microwaved food
- Steam, hot grease or liquids from cooking
- Hot water heaters set at 140°F (60°C) or higher

General Household

- Heat lamps
- Fireplaces (e.g., gas, wood)
- Open space heaters
- Radiators (e.g., home, automobile)
- Outdoor grills (e.g., propane, charcoal)
- Frayed or defective wiring
- Multiple extension cords per outlet
- Flammables (e.g., starter fluid, gasoline, kerosene)
- Carelessness with cigarettes, matches, candles

Occupational Hazards

- Tar
- Cement
- Chemicals
- Hot metals
- Steam pipes
- Combustible fuels
- Fertilizers, pesticides
- Electricity from power lines
- Sparks from live electric sources

*List is not all-inclusive.

TABLE 24-2 Strategies to Reduce Burn Injury

Flame or Contact

- Never smoke in bed.
- Use "child-resistant" lighters.
- Hold regular home fire exit drills.
- Never leave hot oil unattended while cooking.
- Never use gasoline or other flammable liquids to start a fire.
- Never leave candles unattended or near open windows or curtains.
- Consider a flame-retardant smoking apron for older or "at-risk" people.
- Exercise caution when microwaving food and beverages as they can get very hot.

Scald

- Use "anti-scald" devices with showerhead or faucet fixtures.
- Lower hot water temperature to the "lowest point" or 120°F (49°C).
- After running bath water, check temperature with back of hand or bath thermometer.
- Supervise bathing with small children, older adults, or anyone with impaired physical movement, physical sensation, or judgment.

Inhalation

- Install smoke and carbon monoxide detectors and change batteries annually (if appropriate).

Chemical

- Store chemicals safely in approved containers and label clearly.
- Ensure safety of workers handling chemicals (education, protective eyewear, gloves, masks, clothing).

Electrical

- Avoid or repair frayed wiring.
- Avoid outdoor activities during electrical (i.e., lightning) storms.
- Ensure electrical power source is shut off before beginning repairs.
- Wear protective eyewear and gloves when making electrical repairs.

Smoke and Inhalation Injury

Smoke and inhalation injuries from breathing noxious chemicals or hot air can cause damage to the respiratory tract. Three types of smoke and inhalation injuries can occur: metabolic asphyxiation, upper airway injury, and lower airway injury. Smoke inhalation injuries are a major predictor of mortality in burn patients. Rapid initial and ongoing assessment is critical. Airway compromise and pulmonary edema can develop over the first 12 to 48 hours.[5]

Metabolic Asphyxiation. The majority of deaths at a fire scene are the result of inhaling certain smoke elements, primarily carbon monoxide (CO) or hydrogen cyanide. Oxygen delivery to or consumption by tissues is impaired. The result is hypoxia and, ultimately, death when **carboxyhemoglobin** (i.e., hemoglobin combined with CO) blood levels are greater than 20%. CO and hydrogen cyanide poisoning may occur in the absence of burn injury to the skin.

Upper Airway Injury. Upper airway injury results from an inhalation injury to the mouth, oropharynx, and/or larynx. The injury may be caused by thermal burns or the inhalation of hot

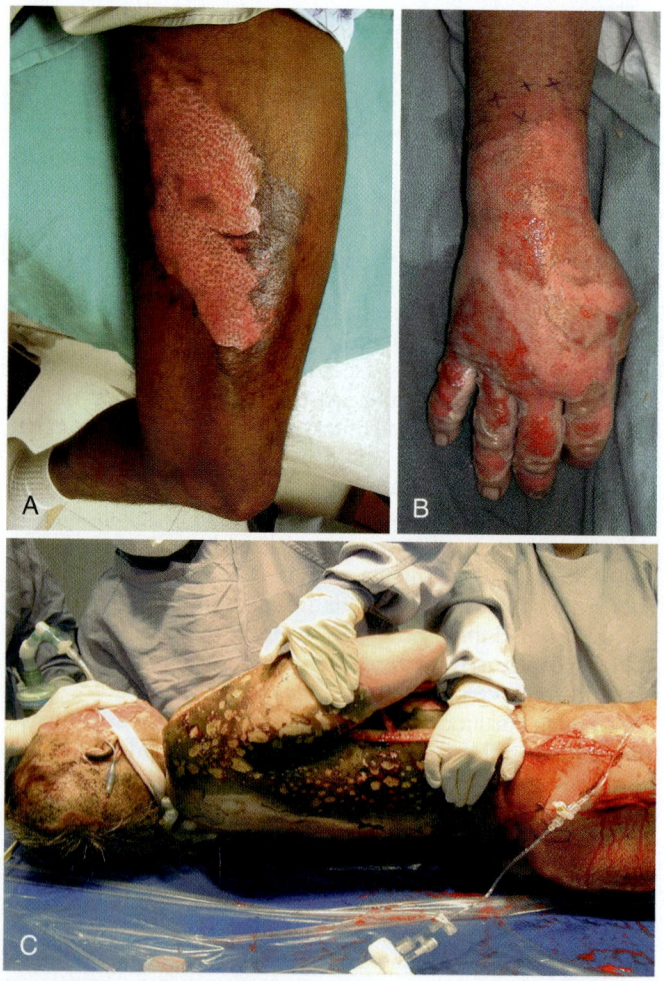

FIG. 24-1 Types of burn injury. **A,** Superficial, partial-thickness scald burn to thigh. **B,** Deep, partial-thickness flame burn to hand. **C,** Full-thickness flame burn to posterior chest and arm. (Courtesy Judy Knighton, Toronto, Canada.)

TABLE 24-3 Manifestations of Lung Injury Associated With Burns

Upper Airway	Lower Airway
• Blisters, edema • Hoarseness • Difficulty swallowing • Copious secretions • Stridor • Substernal and intercostal retractions • Total airway obstruction	• High degree of suspicion if patient was trapped in a fire in an enclosed space or clothing caught fire • Presence of facial burns or singed nasal or facial hair • Dyspnea • Carbonaceous sputum • Wheezing • Hoarseness • Altered mental status

air, steam, or smoke. Mucosal burns of the oropharynx and larynx are manifested by redness, blistering, and edema (Table 24-3). The swelling can be massive and the onset rapid. Flame burns to the neck and chest may make breathing more difficult because of the burn eschar, which becomes tight and constricting from the underlying edema. Swelling from scald burns to the face and neck can also be lethal, as can external pressure from edema pressing on the airway. Mechanical obstruction can occur quickly, presenting a true airway emergency.

Lower Airway Injury. An inhalation injury to the trachea, bronchioles, and alveoli is usually caused by breathing in toxic chemicals or smoke. Tissue damage is related to the duration of exposure to toxic fumes or smoke. Clinical manifestations of lower airway lung injury are presented in Table 24-3. Carefully assess the patient for facial burns, singed nasal hair, hoarseness, painful swallowing, darkened oral and nasal membranes, carbonaceous sputum, history of being burned in an enclosed space, and clothing burns around the neck and chest. Pulmonary edema may not appear until 12 to 48 hours after the burn, and then it may manifest as acute respiratory distress syndrome (ARDS) (see Chapter 67).

Electrical Burns

Electrical burns result from intense heat generated from an electric current. Direct damage to nerves and vessels, causing tissue anoxia and death, can also occur. The severity of the electrical injury depends on the amount of voltage, tissue resistance, current pathways, surface area in contact with the current, and length of time that the current flow was sustained (Fig. 24-2). Tissue densities offer various amounts of resistance to electric current. For example, fat and bone offer the most resistance, whereas nerves and blood vessels offer the least resistance. Current that passes through vital organs (e.g., brain, heart, kidneys) produces more life-threatening sequelae than that which passes through other tissues. In addition, electric sparks may ignite the patient's clothing, causing a flash injury.

As with inhalation injury, perform a rapid assessment of the patient with an electrical injury. Transfer to a burn center is indicated. The severity of an electrical injury can be difficult to determine, since most of the damage is below the skin (known as the *iceberg effect*). Determination of electric current contact points and history of the injury may help reveal the likely path of the current and potential areas of injury. Contact with electric current can cause muscle contractions strong enough to fracture the long bones and vertebrae. Another reason to suspect long bone or spinal fractures is a fall resulting from the electrical injury. For this reason, consider all patients with electrical burns at risk for a cervical spine injury. Use cervical spine immobilization during transport and subsequent diagnostic testing until injury is ruled out.

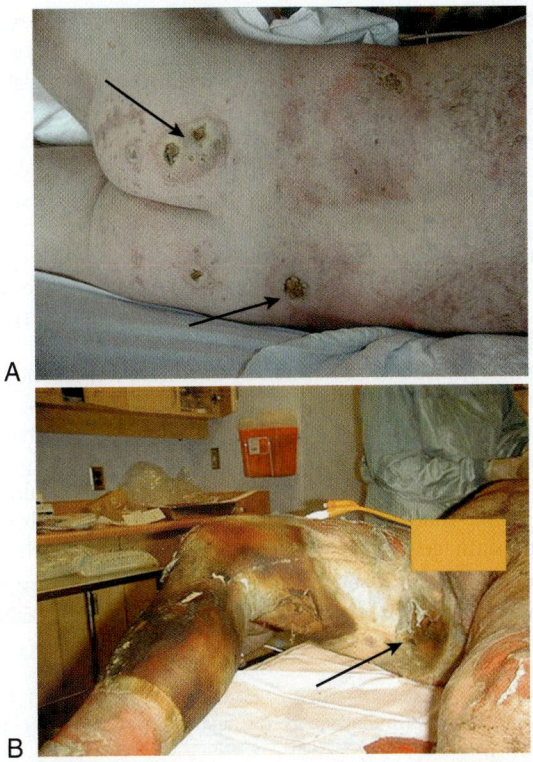

FIG. 24-2 Electrical injury produces heat coagulation of blood supply and contact area as electric current passes through the skin. **A,** Back and buttock *(arrows)*. **B,** Leg *(arrow)*. (Courtesy Judy Knighton, Toronto, Canada.)

Electrical injury puts the patient at risk for dysrhythmias or cardiac arrest, severe metabolic acidosis, and myoglobinuria.[6] The electric shock can cause immediate heart standstill or ventricular fibrillation. Delayed dysrhythmias or arrest can also occur without warning during the first 24 hours after injury. Myoglobin from injured muscle and hemoglobin from damaged red blood cells (RBCs) are released into the circulation whenever massive muscle and blood vessel damage occurs. The released myoglobin travels to the kidneys and can block the renal tubules. This can result in acute tubular necrosis (ATN) and acute kidney injury (see Chapter 46).

Cold Thermal Injury

Cold thermal injury, or frostbite, is discussed in Chapter 68.

CLASSIFICATION OF BURN INJURY

The treatment of burns is related to the severity of the injury.[7] Severity is determined by (1) depth of burn, (2) extent of burn calculated in percent of total body surface area (TBSA), (3) location of burn, and (4) patient risk factors (e.g., age, past medical history). The American Burn Association (ABA) uses referral criteria to determine which burn injuries should be treated in burn centers (Table 24-4). The majority of patients with minor burn injuries can be managed in community hospitals.[8]

Depth of Burn

Burn injury involves the destruction of the integumentary system. The skin is divided into three layers: epidermis, dermis, and subcutaneous tissue (Fig. 24-3). The *epidermis,* or nonvascular protective outer layer of the skin, is approximately as thick as a sheet of paper. (The structure and function of the skin are discussed in Chapter 22.)

The *dermis,* which lies below the epidermis, is approximately 30 to 45 times thicker than the epidermis. The dermis contains connective tissues with blood vessels, hair follicles, nerve endings, sweat glands, and sebaceous glands.

Under the dermis lies the *subcutaneous tissue,* which contains major vascular networks, fat, nerves, and lymphatics. The subcutaneous tissue acts as a heat insulator for underlying structures, including muscles, tendons, bones, and internal organs.

Burns continue to be defined by degrees: first, second, third, and fourth degree. The ABA recommends a more precise definition and classifies burns according to depth of skin destruction: **partial-thickness burns** and **full-thickness burns** (Fig. 24-3). Skin-reproducing (re-epithelializing) cells are located along the shafts of the hair follicles, sweat glands, and oil glands. If significant damage occurs to the dermis (i.e., a full-thickness burn), not enough skin cells remain to regenerate new skin. A permanent, alternative source of skin must be found. Table 24-5 compares the various burn classifications according to the depth of injury.

TABLE 24-4 Burn Center Referral Criteria

Burn injuries that should be referred to a burn center include the following:

1. Partial-thickness burns >10% of total body surface area (TBSA)
2. Burns that involve the face, hands, feet, genitalia, perineum, or major joints
3. Third-degree burns in any age group
4. Electrical burns, including lightning injury
5. Chemical burns
6. Inhalation injury
7. Burn injury in patients with preexisting medical disorders that could complicate management, prolong recovery, or affect mortality risk (e.g., heart or kidney disease, diabetes)
8. Any patients with burns and concomitant trauma (e.g., fractures) in which the burn injury poses the greatest risk of morbidity or mortality. In such cases, if the trauma poses the greater immediate risk, the patient may be initially stabilized in a trauma center before being transferred to a burn center. The HCP will need to use his or her judgment, in consultation with the regional medical control plan and triage protocols.
9. Burn injury in children in hospitals without qualified personnel or equipment needed to care for them
10. Burn injury in patients who will require special social, emotional, or long-term rehabilitative intervention

Source: American Burn Association: Guidelines for the operation of burn centers. Retrieved from *http://www.ameriburn.org/Chapter14.pdf.*

Extent of Burn

Two commonly used tools for determining the TBSA affected or the extent of a burn wound are the *Lund-Browder chart* (Fig. 24-4, *A*) and the *Rule of Nines* (Fig. 24-4, *B*). (First-degree burns, equivalent to a sunburn, are not included when calculating TBSA.) The Lund-Browder chart is considered more accurate because it considers the patient's age in proportion to relative body-area size. The Rule of Nines is often used for initial assessment of a burn patient because it is easy to remember. For irregular- or odd-shaped burns, the patient's hand (including the fingers) is approximately 1% TBSA. The *Sage Burn Diagram* is a free, web-based tool for estimating TBSA burned (*www.sagediagram.com*). There are also mobile applications (e.g., uBurn, Mersey Burns) available to estimate the percentage of burn and fluid resuscitation needs.[9]

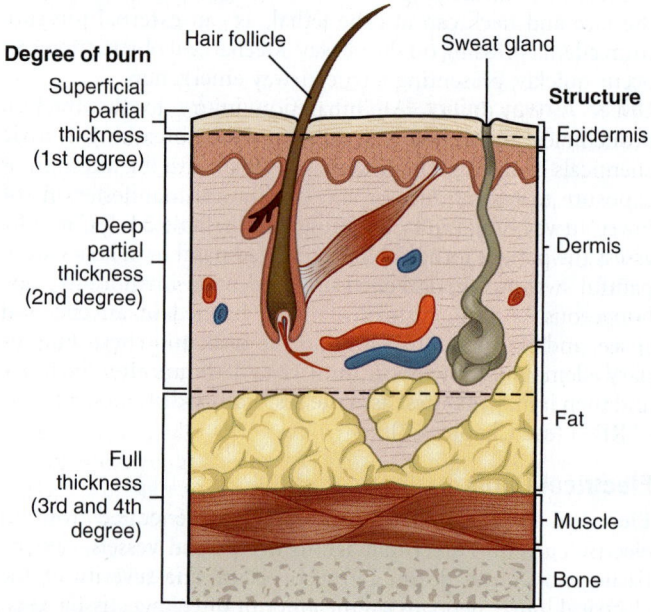

FIG. 24-3 Cross section of skin indicating the depth of burn and structures involved.

TABLE 24-5 Classification of Burn Injury Depth

Classification	Appearance	Possible Cause	Structures Involved
Partial-Thickness Skin Destruction			
Superficial (first-degree) burn	Erythema, blanching on pressure, pain and mild swelling, no vesicles or blisters (although after 24 hr skin may blister and peel)	Superficial sunburn Quick heat flash	Superficial epidermal damage with hyperemia. Tactile and pain sensation intact
Deep (second-degree) burn	Fluid-filled vesicles that are red, shiny, wet (if vesicles have ruptured). Severe pain caused by nerve injury. Mild to moderate edema	Flame Flash Scald Contact burns Chemicals Tar, cement Electric current	Epidermis and dermis involved to varying depths. Skin elements, from which epithelial regeneration occurs, remain viable.
Full-Thickness Skin Destruction			
Third- and fourth-degree burns	Dry, waxy white, leathery, or hard skin. Visible thrombosed vessels. Insensitivity to pain because of nerve destruction. Possible involvement of muscles, tendons, and bones	Flame Scald Chemical Tar, cement Electric current	All skin elements and local nerve endings destroyed. Coagulation necrosis present. Surgical intervention required for healing

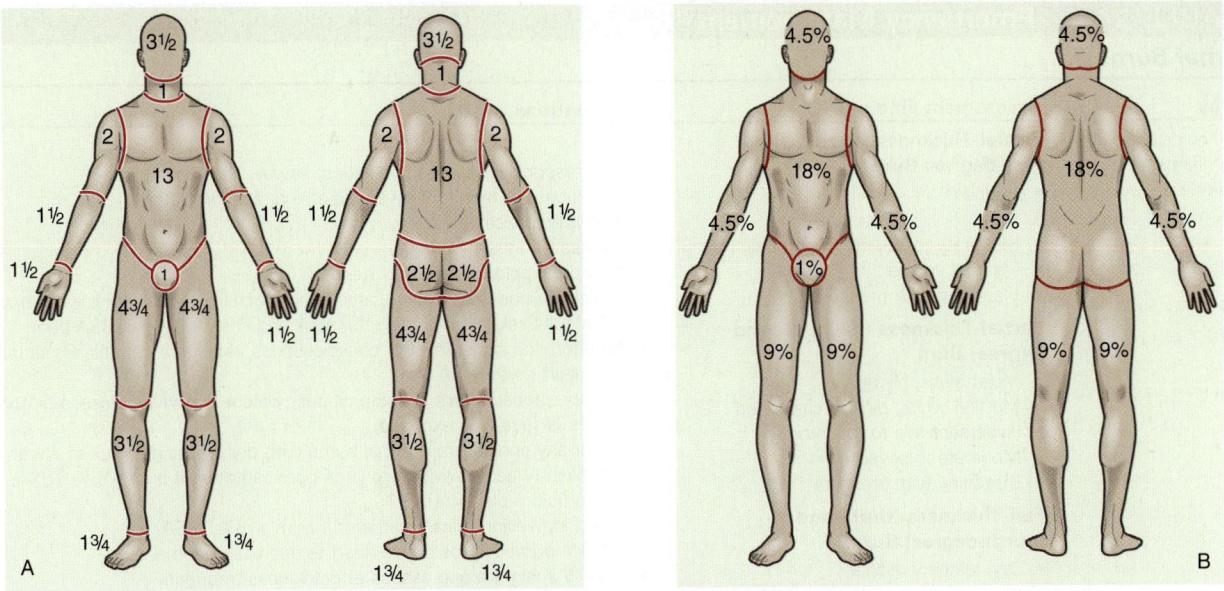

FIG. 24-4 **A,** Lund-Browder chart. By convention, areas of partial-thickness injury are colored in blue and areas of full-thickness injury in red. Superficial partial-thickness burns are not calculated. **B,** Rule of Nines chart.

Location of Burn

The severity of the burn injury is also determined by the location of the burn. Burns to the face and neck and circumferential burns to the chest or back may interfere with breathing as a result of mechanical obstruction from edema or leathery, devitalized burn tissue *(eschar)*. These burns may also indicate possible smoke or inhalation injury.

Burns to the hands, feet, joints, and eyes are of concern because they make self-care difficult and may jeopardize future function. Burns to the hands and feet are challenging to manage because of superficial vascular and nerve supply systems that must be protected while the burn wounds are healing.

Burns of the ears and nose are at risk for infection as the skin is very thin and the underlying skeleton is frequently exposed. Burns to the buttocks or perineum are at high risk for infection from urine or feces contamination. Circumferential burns to the extremities can cause circulation problems distal to the burn, with possible nerve damage to the affected extremity. Patients may also develop compartment syndrome (see Chapter 62) from direct heat damage to the muscles, swelling, and/or preburn vascular problems.

Patient Risk Factors

Any patient with preexisting heart, lung, or kidney disease has a poorer prognosis for recovery because of the increased demands placed on the body by a burn injury. The patient with diabetes or peripheral vascular disease is at high risk for poor healing, especially with foot and leg burns.[10] General physical weakness from any chronic disease, including alcoholism, drug abuse, or malnutrition, makes it challenging for the patient to fully recover from a burn injury. In addition, the burn patient who has also sustained fractures, head injuries, or other trauma has a more difficult recovery.

PREHOSPITAL AND EMERGENCY CARE

At the scene of the injury, priority is given to removing the person from the source of the burn and stopping the burning process. Rescuers must also protect themselves from being injured. In the case of electrical and chemical injuries, initial care involves removal of the patient from contact with the electrical or chemical source.

Small thermal burns (10% or less of TBSA) should be covered with a clean, cool, tap water–dampened towel for the patient's comfort and protection until medical care is available. Cooling of the injured area (if small) within 1 minute helps minimize the depth of the injury. If the burn is large (greater than 10% TBSA) or an electrical or inhalation burn is suspected and the patient is unresponsive, first focus your attention on CAB:

- *Circulation:* Check for presence of pulses and elevate the burned limb(s) above the heart to decrease pain and swelling.
- *Airway:* Check for patency, soot around nares and on the tongue, singed nasal hair, darkened oral or nasal membranes.
- *Breathing:* Check for adequacy of ventilation.

If the patient is responsive, your priorities would follow the order of the ABCs: airway, breathing, and circulation.

To prevent hypothermia, cool large burns for no more than 10 minutes. Do not immerse the burned body part in cool water because it may cause extensive heat loss. Never cover a burn with ice, since this can cause hypothermia and vasoconstriction of blood vessels, thus further reducing blood flow to the injury. Gently remove as much burned clothing as possible to prevent further tissue damage. Leave adherent clothing in place until the patient is transferred to a hospital. Wrap the patient in a dry, clean sheet or blanket to prevent further contamination of the wound and to provide warmth.

Chemical burns are best treated by quickly removing any chemical particles or powder from the skin. Remove all clothing containing the chemical because the burning process continues while the chemical is in contact with the skin. Flush the affected area with copious amounts of water to irrigate the skin anywhere from 20 minutes to 2 hours postexposure. Tap water is acceptable for flushing eyes exposed to chemicals. Tissue destruction may continue for up to 72 hours after contact with some chemicals.

Watch patients with inhalation injuries closely for signs of respiratory distress. These patients need to be treated quickly and efficiently if they are to survive. If CO poisoning is suspected, treat the patient with 100% humidified O_2. Patients who have both body burns and an inhalation injury must be transferred to the nearest burn center.

TABLE 24-6 Emergency Management

Thermal Burns

Etiology	Assessment Findings	Interventions
• Hot liquids or solids • Flash flame • Open flame • Steam • Hot surface • Ultraviolet rays	**Partial-Thickness (superficial; first-degree) Burn** • Redness • Pain • Moderate to severe tenderness • Minimal edema • Blanching with pressure **Partial-Thickness (deep; second-degree) Burn** • Moist blebs, blisters • Mottled white, pink to cherry-red • Hypersensitive to touch or air • Moderate to severe pain • Blanching with pressure **Full-Thickness (third- and fourth-degree) Burns** • Dry, leathery eschar • Waxy white, dark brown, or charred appearance • Strong burn odor • Impaired sensation when touched • Absence of pain with severe pain in surrounding tissues • Lack of blanching with pressure	**Initial** • If unresponsive, assess circulation, airway, and breathing. • If responsive, monitor airway, breathing, and circulation. • Stabilize cervical spine. • Assess for inhalation injury. • Provide supplemental O_2 as needed. • Anticipate endotracheal intubation and mechanical ventilation with circumferential full-thickness burns to the neck and chest or large TBSA burn. • Monitor vital signs, level of consciousness, respiratory status, O_2 saturation, and heart rhythm. • Remove nonadherent clothing, shoes, watches, jewelry, glasses or contact lenses (if face was exposed). • Cover any concurrent thermal burns with dry dressings or clean sheet. • Establish IV access with two large-bore catheters if burn >15% TBSA. • Begin fluid replacement. • Insert indwelling urinary catheter if burn >15% TBSA. • Elevate burned limbs above heart to decrease edema. • Give IV analgesia and assess effectiveness frequently. • Identify and treat other associated injuries (e.g., fractures, head injury). **Ongoing Monitoring** • Monitor airway, breathing, and circulation. • Monitor vital signs, O_2 saturation, heart rhythm, and level of consciousness. • Monitor pain level. • Monitor urine output.

TBSA, Total body surface area.

Always remember that the burn patient may also have sustained other injuries that could take priority over the burn itself. Persons involved in the prehospital phase of burn care must fully share the circumstances of the injury to emergency department (ED) staff. This is especially important if the patient was trapped in a closed space, exposed to hazardous chemicals or electricity, or suffered a possible traumatic injury (e.g., fall).

Prehospital and emergency care are presented in tables that describe thermal burns (Table 24-6), inhalation injury (Table 24-7), electrical burns (Table 24-8), and chemical burns (Table 24-9).

PHASES OF BURN MANAGEMENT

Burn management can be organized chronologically into three phases: emergent (resuscitative), acute (wound healing), and rehabilitative (restorative). Overlap in care does exist. For example, the emergent phase begins at the time of the burn injury, and care often begins prehospital or in the ED. Wound care is the primary focus of the acute phase, but wound care also takes place in both the emergent and rehabilitation phases. Planning for rehabilitation begins on the day of the burn injury or admission to the burn center. Formal rehabilitation begins as soon as functional assessments can be performed.

EMERGENT PHASE

The *emergent (resuscitative) phase* is the time required to resolve the immediate, life-threatening problems resulting from the burn injury.[11] This phase usually lasts up to 72 hours from the time the burn occurred. The primary concerns are the onset of hypovolemic shock and edema formation. The emergent phase ends when fluid mobilization and diuresis begin.

Pathophysiology

Fluid and Electrolyte Shifts. The greatest initial threat to a patient with a major burn is hypovolemic shock (Fig. 24-5). It is caused by a massive shift of fluids out of the blood vessels as a result of increased capillary permeability and can begin as early as 20 minutes postburn. As the capillary walls become more permeable, water, sodium, and plasma proteins (especially albumin) move into the interstitial spaces and other surrounding tissue. The colloidal osmotic pressure decreases with progressive loss of protein from the vascular space. This results in more fluid shifting out of the vascular space into the interstitial spaces (Fig. 24-6).

Fluid also moves to areas that normally have minimal to no fluid, a phenomenon termed *third spacing.* Examples of third spacing in burn injury are exudate and blister formation, as well as edema in unburned areas.

Other sources of fluid loss are insensible losses by evaporation from large, denuded body surfaces and the lungs. The normal insensible loss of 30 to 50 mL/hr is increased in the severely burned patient. The net result of the fluid shifts and losses is termed *intravascular volume depletion.* Clinical signs of hypovolemic shock are decreased BP and increased heart rate. If hypovolemic shock is not corrected, refractory shock and death may result. (Shock is discussed in Chapter 66.)

The circulatory system is also affected by the hemolysis of RBCs from circulating factors (e.g., oxygen free radicals) released at the time of the burn, as well as by the direct insult of the burn injury. Thrombosis in the capillaries of burned tissue causes an additional loss of circulating RBCs. An elevated hematocrit is commonly caused by hemoconcentration due to fluid loss. After fluid balance is restored, the hematocrit levels drop.

Major electrolyte shifts of sodium and potassium also occur during this phase. A potassium shift develops first because

TABLE 24-7 Emergency Management

Inhalation Injury

Etiology	Assessment Findings	Interventions
• Exposure of respiratory tract to intense heat or flames • Inhalation of noxious chemicals, smoke, or CO	• History of being trapped in an enclosed space, being in an explosion, or having clothing catch fire • Rapid, shallow respirations • Increasing hoarseness • Coughing • Singed nasal or facial hair • Darkened oral or nasal membranes • Smoky breath • Carbonaceous sputum • Productive cough with black, gray, or bloody sputum • Irritation of upper airways or burning pain in throat or chest • Difficulty swallowing • Cherry-red skin color (CO levels >20%) • Restlessness, anxiety • Altered mental status, including confusion, coma • Decreased O_2 saturation • Dysrhythmias	**Initial** • If unresponsive, assess circulation, airway, and breathing. • If responsive, monitor airway, breathing, and circulation. • Stabilize cervical spine. • Assess for concurrent thermal burn. • Provide 100% humidified O_2. • Anticipate endotracheal intubation and mechanical ventilation with significant inhalation injury. • Monitor vital signs, level of consciousness, O_2 saturation, and heart rhythm. • Remove nonadherent clothing, jewelry, glasses, or contact lenses (if face was exposed). • Establish IV access with two large-bore catheters if burn >15% TBSA. • Begin fluid replacement. • Insert indwelling urinary catheter if burn >15% TBSA. • Elevate burned limb(s) above heart to decrease edema. • Obtain arterial blood gas, carboxyhemoglobin levels, and chest x-ray. • Give IV analgesia and assess effectiveness frequently. • Identify and treat other associated injuries (e.g., fractures, pneumothorax, head injury). • Cover concurrent burned areas with dry dressings or clean sheet. • Anticipate need for fiberoptic bronchoscopy or intubation. **Ongoing Monitoring** • Monitor airway, breathing, and circulation. • Monitor vital signs, O_2 saturation, heart rhythm, and level of consciousness. • Monitor pain level. • Monitor urine output.

CO, Carbon monoxide; *TBSA,* total body surface area.

TABLE 24-8 Emergency Management

Electrical Burns

Etiology	Assessment Findings	Interventions
• Electric wires • Utility wires • Lightning • Defibrillator	• Leathery, white, or charred skin • Burn odor • Loss of consciousness • Impaired touch sensation • Minimal or absent pain • Dysrhythmias • Cardiac arrest • Location of contact points • Diminished peripheral circulation in injured extremity • Thermal burns if clothing ignites • Fractures or dislocations from force of current • Head or neck injury if fall occurred • Depth and extent of wound difficult to visualize. Assume injury greater than what is seen.	**Initial** • Remove patient from electrical source while protecting rescuer. • If unresponsive, assess circulation, airway, and breathing. • If responsive, monitor airway, breathing, and circulation. • Stabilize cervical spine. • Provide supplemental O_2 as needed. • Monitor vital signs, heart rhythm, level of consciousness, respiratory status, and O_2 saturation. • Check pulses distal to burns. • Remove nonadherent clothing, shoes, watches, jewelry, glasses or contact lenses (if face was exposed). • Cover burned areas with dry dressings or clean sheet. • Establish IV access with two large-bore catheters if burn >15% TBSA. • Begin fluid replacement. • Obtain arterial blood gas to assess acid-base balance. • Insert indwelling urinary catheter if burn >15% TBSA. • Elevate burned limb(s) above heart to decrease edema. • Give IV analgesia and assess effectiveness frequently. • Identify and treat other associated injuries (e.g., fractures, head injury, thermal burns). **Ongoing Monitoring** • Monitor airway, breathing, and circulation. • Monitor vital signs, O_2 saturation, heart rhythm, level of consciousness, and neurovascular status of injured limbs. • Monitor pain level. • Monitor urine output. • Monitor urine for development of myoglobinuria secondary to muscle breakdown and hemoglobinuria secondary to RBC breakdown. • Anticipate possible administration of $NaHCO_3$ to alkalinize the urine and maintain serum pH >6.0.

$NaHCO_3$, Sodium bicarbonate; *TBSA,* total body surface area.

TABLE 24-9 Emergency Management

Chemical Burns

Etiology	Assessment Findings	Interventions
• Acids • Alkalis • Organic compounds	• Burning • Redness, swelling of injured tissue • Degeneration of exposed tissue • Discoloration of injured skin • Localized pain • Edema of surrounding tissue • Tissue destruction continuing for up to 72 hr • Respiratory distress if chemical inhaled • Decreased muscle coordination (if organophosphate) • Paralysis	**Initial** • If unresponsive, assess circulation, airway, and breathing before decontamination procedures. • If responsive, monitor airway, breathing, and circulation. • Stabilize cervical spine. • Provide supplemental O_2 as needed. • Brush dry chemical from skin before irrigation. • Remove nonadherent clothing, shoes, watches, jewelry, glasses or contact lenses (if face was exposed). • Flush chemical from wound and surrounding area with copious amounts of saline solution or water. • For chemical burn of the eye(s), flush from inner to outer corner of eye with water or lactated Ringer's (if available). • Cover burned areas with dry dressings or clean sheet. • Establish IV access with two large-bore catheters if burn >15% TBSA. • Begin fluid replacement. • Insert indwelling urinary catheter if burn >15% TBSA. • Elevate burned limb(s) above heart to decrease edema. • Give IV analgesia and assess effectiveness frequently. • Contact poison control center for assistance. **Ongoing Monitoring** • Monitor airway if exposed to chemicals. • Monitor pain level. • Monitor urine output. • Consider possibility of systemic impact of identified chemical, and monitor and treat accordingly. • Monitor pH of eye if exposed to chemicals.

TBSA, Total body surface area.

PATHOPHYSIOLOGY MAP

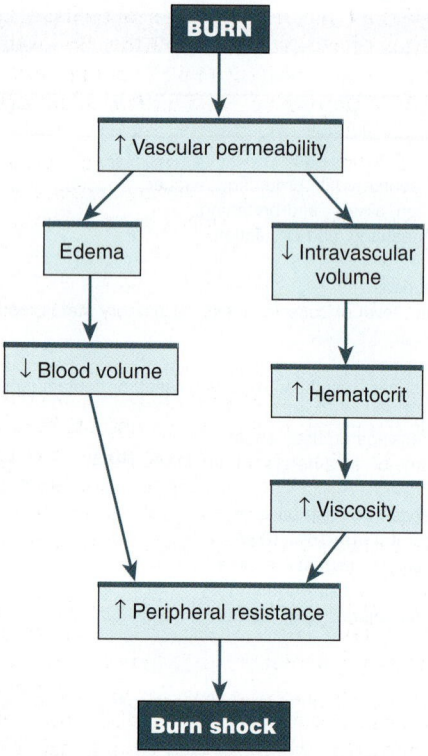

FIG. 24-5 At the time of major burn injury, there is increased capillary permeability. All fluid components of the blood begin to leak into the interstitium, causing edema and a decreased blood volume. Hematocrit increases, and the blood becomes more viscous. The combination of decreased blood volume and increased viscosity produces increased peripheral resistance. Burn shock, a type of hypovolemic shock, rapidly ensues and, if not corrected, can result in death.

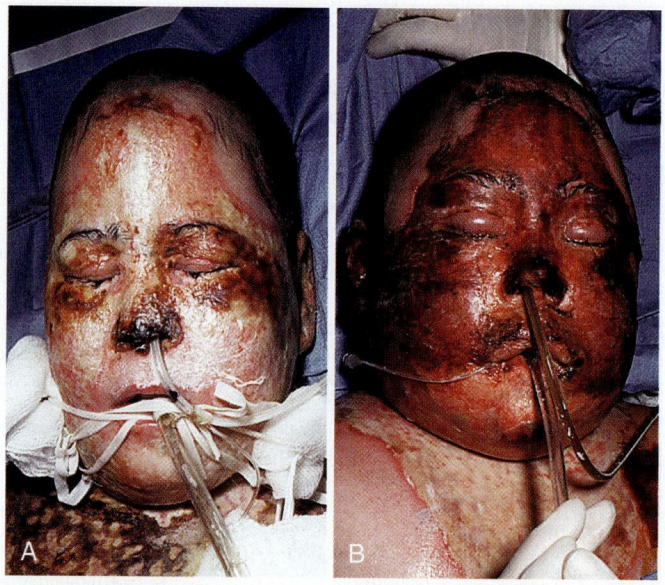

FIG. 24-6 **A,** Facial edema before fluid resuscitation. **B,** Facial edema after 24 hours. (Courtesy Judy Knighton, Toronto, Canada.)

injured cells and hemolyzed RBCs release potassium into the circulation. Sodium rapidly moves to the interstitial spaces and remains there until edema formation ends (Fig. 24-7).

Toward the end of the emergent phase, capillary membrane permeability is restored if fluid replacement is adequate. Fluid loss and edema formation end. Interstitial fluid gradually returns to the vascular space (Fig. 24-7). Diuresis occurs, and the urine has a low specific gravity.

Inflammation and Healing. Burn injury to tissues and vessels causes coagulation necrosis. Neutrophils and monocytes accumulate at the site of injury. Fibroblasts and newly formed collagen fibrils appear and begin wound repair within the first 6

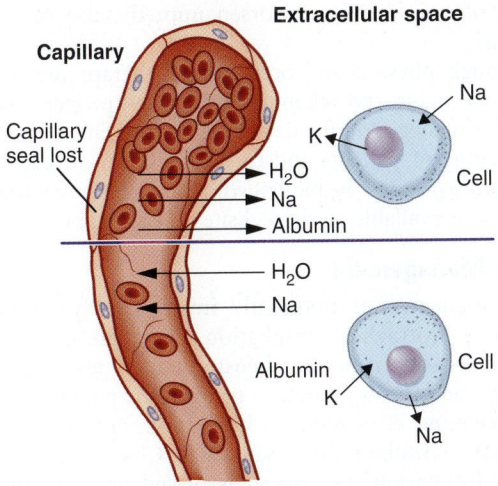

FIG. 24-7 The effects of burn shock are shown above the blue line. As the capillary seal is lost, interstitial edema develops. The cellular integrity is also altered, with sodium *(Na)* moving into the cell in abnormal amounts and potassium *(K)* leaving the cell. The shifts after the resolution of burn shock are shown below the blue line. The water and sodium move back into the circulating volume through the capillary. The albumin remains in the interstitium. Potassium is transported into the cell and sodium is transported out as the cellular integrity returns.

to 12 hours after injury. (The inflammatory response is discussed in Chapter 11.)

Immunologic Changes. The body's immune system is challenged when a burn injury occurs. The skin barrier to invading organisms is destroyed, bone marrow depression occurs, and circulating levels of immunoglobulins are decreased. Defects occur in the function of white blood cells (WBCs). The inflammatory cytokine cascade, triggered by tissue damage, impairs the function of lymphocytes, monocytes, and neutrophils. Thus the patient is at a greater risk for infection.

Clinical Manifestations

The patient with severe burns is likely to be in shock from hypovolemia. Often the areas of full-thickness and deep partial-thickness burns are at first painless because the nerve endings have been destroyed. Superficial to moderate partial-thickness burns are very painful. Blisters, filled with fluid and protein, are common in partial-thickness burns. The patient with a larger burn area may develop a paralytic ileus, with absent or decreased bowel sounds. Shivering may occur as a result of chilling that is caused by heat loss, anxiety, or pain.

The patient may be alert and able to answer questions shortly after admission or until he or she is intubated (if there is respiratory compromise). Patients are often frightened and need your calm reassurances. Give simple explanations of what to expect as you provide care. Unconsciousness or altered mental status in a burn patient usually results from hypoxia associated with smoke inhalation. Other possibilities include head trauma, substance abuse, or excessive amounts of sedation or pain medication.

Complications

The three major organ systems most susceptible to complications during the emergent phase of burn injury are the cardiovascular, respiratory, and urinary systems.

Cardiovascular System. Cardiovascular system complications include dysrhythmias and hypovolemic shock, which, if untreated, may progress to refractory shock. Circulation to the extremities

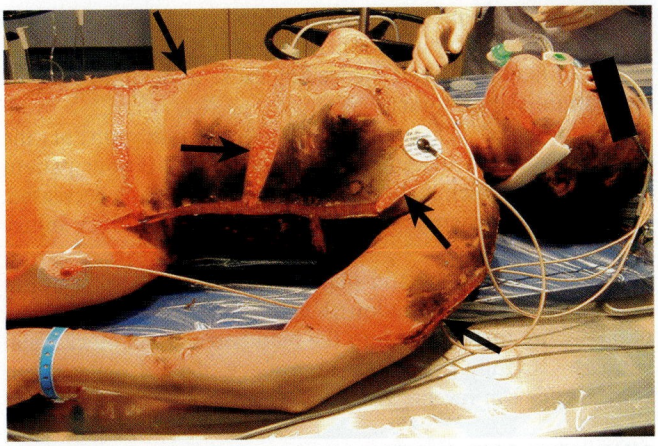

FIG. 24-8 Escharotomies of the anterior and lateral chest and arm (indicated by *arrows*). (Courtesy Judy Knighton, Toronto, Canada.)

can be severely impaired by deep circumferential burns and subsequent edema formation, which act like a tourniquet. If untreated, ischemia, paresthesias, and necrosis can occur. An escharotomy (an incision through the full-thickness eschar) is frequently done after transfer to a burn center to restore circulation to compromised extremities (Fig. 24-8).

Initially, blood viscosity increases because of the fluid loss. Microcirculation is impaired because of the damage to skin structures that contain small capillary systems. These two events result in a phenomenon termed *sludging*. Sludging is corrected by adequate fluid replacement.

Burn patients are at an increased risk for venous thromboembolism (VTE) if one or more of the following conditions are present: advanced age, obesity, extensive or lower-extremity burns, concomitant lower-extremity trauma, and prolonged immobility. VTE prophylaxis with anticoagulant drugs should be started, unless contraindicated.[12]

Respiratory System. The respiratory system is vulnerable to two types of injury: (1) upper airway burns and (2) lower airway injury (Table 24-3). Upper airway distress may occur with or without smoke inhalation, and airway injury at either level may occur in the absence of burn injury to the skin. (Smoke and inhalation injuries are discussed earlier in this chapter on pp. 430-431.)

The patient may need a fiberoptic bronchoscopy and carboxyhemoglobin blood levels to confirm a suspected inhalation injury. Look in the prehospital and ED notes to see if the patient was exposed to smoke or fumes. Examine any sputum for carbon. Watch for signs of respiratory distress, such as increased agitation, anxiety, restlessness, or a change in the rate or character of the patient's breathing, since symptoms may not be present immediately.

In general, there is no correlation between the percentage TBSA burn (% TBSA) and the severity of inhalation injury. In a patient with inhalation injury, a chest x-ray may appear normal on admission, but changes usually occur over the next 24 to 48 hours. Arterial blood gas (ABG) values may also be within the normal range on admission and change over time.

Other Cardiopulmonary Problems. Patients with preexisting heart disease (e.g., myocardial infarction) or lung disease (e.g., chronic obstructive pulmonary disease [COPD]) are at an increased risk for complications. If fluid replacement is too vigorous, watch for early signs of heart failure or pulmonary edema. Invasive measures (e.g., hemodynamic monitoring) may be necessary to monitor fluid resuscitation.

Patients with preexisting lung disease are more likely to develop a respiratory infection. Pneumonia, a common complication of major burns, is the leading cause of death in patients with an inhalation injury.

Urinary System. The most common complication of the urinary system in the emergent phase is ATN. If your patient becomes hypovolemic, blood flow to the kidneys is decreased, causing renal ischemia. If this continues, acute kidney injury may develop.

With full-thickness and major electrical burns, myoglobin (from muscle cell breakdown) and hemoglobin (from RBC breakdown) are released into the bloodstream and block renal tubules. Carefully monitor the adequacy of fluid replacement because this can reverse the obstruction of the tubules.

❖ NURSING AND INTERPROFESSIONAL MANAGEMENT: EMERGENT PHASE

In the emergent phase the patient's survival depends on rapid and thorough assessment and appropriate interventions.[13] Usually the health care provider (HCP) and you make an initial assessment of the depth and extent of the burn and coordinate the actions of others on the health care team. In a community hospital, determine whether the patient requires inpatient or outpatient care. In the case of inpatient care, decide whether the patient remains in the hospital or should be transferred to a burn center (Table 24-4). Care predominantly focuses on airway management, fluid therapy, and wound care (Table 24-10). Patients often improve and worsen, unpredictably, on an almost daily basis.

Although physical and occupational therapy are important in both the acute and rehabilitation phases, proper positioning and splinting begin on the day of admission. Emotional support and teaching of patients and caregivers begin on admission. A nursing care plan for the patient with burn injury (eNursing Care Plan 24-1) is available on the website for this chapter.

◆ Airway Management

Airway management frequently involves early endotracheal (preferably orotracheal) intubation. Early intubation removes the need for emergency tracheostomy after respiratory problems have become apparent. In general, the patient with burns to the face and neck requires intubation within 1 to 2 hours after injury. (Intubation is discussed in Chapter 65.)

After intubation the patient is placed on ventilatory support, with the oxygen concentration based on ABG values.

INFORMATICS IN PRACTICE

Staff Training Using Gaming

1. Preparing burn center staff for a mass casualty incident involving burn victims is essential.
2. Interactive, video game–based training modules simulate real-life emergency events surrounding a mass casualty burn incident.
3. Critical skills for triage and initial resuscitation (emergent phase) for multiple victims can be practiced.

TABLE 24-10 Interprofessional Care

Burn Injury

Emergent Phase	Acute Phase	Rehabilitation Phase
Fluid Therapy (Table 24-11) • Assess fluid needs. • Begin IV fluid replacement. • Insert indwelling urinary catheter. • Monitor urine output. **Wound Care** • Start daily shower and wound care. • Debride as necessary. • Assess extent and depth of burns. • Administer tetanus toxoid or tetanus antitoxin. **Pain and Anxiety** • Assess and manage pain and anxiety. **Physical and Occupational Therapy** • Place patient in position that prevents contracture formation and reduces edema. • Assess need for splints. **Nutritional Therapy** • Assess nutritional needs and begin feeding patient by most appropriate route as soon as possible. **Respiratory Therapy** • Assess oxygenation needs. • Provide supplemental O_2 as needed. • Intubate if necessary. • Monitor respiratory status. **Psychosocial Care** • Provide support to patient and caregiver during initial crisis phase.	**Fluid Therapy** • Continue to replace fluids, depending on patient's clinical response. **Wound Care** • Continue daily shower and wound care. • Continue debridement (if necessary). • Assess wound daily and adjust dressing protocols as necessary. • Observe for complications (e.g., infection). **Early Excision and Grafting** • Provide temporary allografts. • Provide permanent autografts. • Care for donor sites. **Pain and Anxiety** • Continue to assess for and treat pain and anxiety. **Physical and Occupational Therapy** • Begin daily therapy program for maintenance of range of motion. • Assess need for splints and anticontracture positioning. • Encourage and assist patient with self-care as possible. **Nutritional Therapy** • Continue to assess diet to support wound healing. **Respiratory Therapy** • Continue to assess oxygenation needs. • Continue to monitor respiratory status. • Monitor for signs of complications (e.g., pneumonia). **Psychosocial Care** • Provide ongoing support, counseling, and teaching to patient and caregiver about physical and emotional aspects of care and recovery. • Begin to anticipate discharge needs. **Drug Therapy** (Table 24-13) • Assess need for drugs (e.g., antibiotics). • Continue to monitor effectiveness and adjust dosage as needed.	• Continue to counsel and teach patient and caregiver about wound care. • Continue to encourage and assist patient in resuming self-care. • Continue to prevent or minimize contractures and assess likelihood for scarring (surgery, physical and occupational therapy, splinting, pressure garments). • Discuss possible reconstructive surgery. • Prepare for discharge home or transfer to rehabilitation hospital. • Discuss possible need for home care nursing.

Extubation may be indicated when the edema resolves, usually 3 to 6 days after burn injury, unless severe inhalation injury exists. Escharotomies of the chest may be needed to relieve respiratory distress secondary to circumferential, full-thickness burns of the neck and chest (Fig. 24-8).

Within 6 to 12 hours after injury in which smoke inhalation is suspected, a fiberoptic bronchoscopy should be done to assess the lower airway. When intubation is not done, treatment of inhalation injury includes giving 100% humidified O_2. Place the patient in a high Fowler's position, unless contraindicated (e.g., spinal injury), and encourage deep breathing and coughing every hour. Reposition the patient every 1 to 2 hours. Provide suctioning and chest physiotherapy (as ordered).

If severe respiratory distress (e.g., hoarseness, shortness of breath) develops, intubation and mechanical ventilation are started. Positive end-expiratory pressure (PEEP) may be used to prevent collapse of the alveoli and progressive respiratory failure (see Chapters 65 and 67). Bronchodilators may be given to treat severe bronchospasm. CO poisoning is treated by administering 100% O_2 until carboxyhemoglobin levels return to normal.

! SAFETY ALERT Pulse CO Oximetry Monitoring

- Standard pulse oximetry (SpO_2) does not distinguish oxyhemoglobin from carboxyhemoglobin. A patient with CO poisoning will have normal SpO_2 readings in spite of elevated carboxyhemoglobin levels.
- For patients with suspected or confirmed CO poisoning, use a pulse CO oximetry (SpCO) device.[14]

Fluid Therapy

Obtaining IV access is critical for fluid resuscitation and drug administration. At least two large-bore IVs must be in place for patients with burns that are 15% TBSA or more. It is critical to obtain IV access that can handle large volumes of fluid. For patients with burns greater than 30% TBSA, consider a central line for fluid and drug administration and blood sampling (central lines are discussed in Chapter 16). An arterial line is often placed if frequent ABGs or invasive BP monitoring is needed.

Assess the extent of the burn wound using a standardized tool (Fig. 24-4). Then use a standardized formula to estimate the patient's fluid resuscitation needs. Fluid replacement is achieved with crystalloid solutions (usually lactated Ringer's), colloids (albumin), or a combination of the two. IV saline is usually started during the prehospital phase.

The Parkland (Baxter) formula for fluid replacement is the most common formula used (Table 24-11 or *www.mdcalc.com/parkland-formula-for-burns*). Remember that all formulas are estimates. Fluids are titrated based on the patient's response (e.g., hourly urine output, vital signs). Patients with an electrical injury have greater than normal fluid needs. They generally require an osmotic diuretic (mannitol [Osmitrol]) to increase their urine output and overcome high levels of hemoglobin and myoglobin in the urine. Too much fluid and overestimation of TBSA contribute to over-resuscitation of fluids or "fluid creep."[15] For the first 24 hours, the recommendation is 2 to 4 mL lactated Ringer's/kg/%TBSA burned.

Colloidal solutions (e.g., 5% albumin) may also be given. However, administration is recommended after the first 12 to 24 hours postburn when capillary permeability returns to normal or near normal. After this time, the plasma remains in the vascular space and expands the circulating volume. The replacement volume is calculated based on the patient's body weight and TBSA burned (e.g., 0.3 to 0.5 mL/kg/%TBSA burned).

TABLE 24-11 Fluid Resuscitation

Parkland (Baxter) Formula*

4 mL lactated Ringer's solution per kilogram (kg) of body weight per percent of total body surface area (% TBSA) burned = Total fluid requirements for first 24 hr after burn

Application

½ of total in first 8 hr
¼ of total in second 8 hr
¼ of total in third 8 hr

Example

For a 70-kg patient with a 50% TBSA burn:

4 mL × 70 kg × 50 (%TBSA) burned = 14,000 mL in 24 hr

½ of total in first 8 hr = 7000 mL (875 mL/hr)
¼ of total in second 8 hr = 3500 mL (437 mL/hr)
¼ of total in third 8 hr = 3500 mL (437 mL/hr)

*Formulas are guidelines. Fluid is given at a rate to produce 0.5-1.0 mL/kg/hr of urine output. The American Burn Association Consensus Fluid Resuscitation Formula has suggested 2-4 mL lactated Ringer's solution per kg of body weight per %TBSA burned = total fluid requirements for first 24 hr after burn. This strategy avoids over-resuscitation of fluids or "fluid creep."

Assess for the adequacy of fluid resuscitation hourly using clinical parameters. Urine output, the most commonly used parameter, and cardiac parameters are defined as follows.

- *Urine output:* 0.5 to 1 mL/kg/hr; 75 to 100 mL/hr for electrical burn patient with evidence of hemoglobinuria or myoglobinuria.
- *Cardiac parameters:* Mean arterial pressure (MAP) greater than 65 mm Hg, systolic BP greater than 90 mm Hg, heart rate less than 120 beats/minute. MAP and BP are best measured by an arterial line. Manual BP measurement is often invalid because of edema and vasoconstriction.

CHECK YOUR PRACTICE

You are assigned to a new male burn patient who weighs 72 kg and has 45% TBSA burn.

- What rate (mL/hr) should fluids be infused over the second 8 hours of fluid resuscitation for him?

Wound Care

Once a patent airway, effective circulation, and adequate fluid replacement have been achieved, priority is given to care of the burn wound. Partial-thickness burn wounds appear pink to cherry-red and are wet and shiny with serous exudate. These wounds may or may not have intact blisters; are painful when touched; and have only minor, localized sensation because nerve endings may have been destroyed in the burned dermis.

You and unlicensed assistive personnel (UAP) can perform cleansing and gentle debridement (using scissors and forceps) on a shower cart (Fig. 24-9), in a regular shower, or on a patient's bed or stretcher. Extensive, surgical debridement is done in the operating room (OR) (Fig. 24-10). During **debridement**, necrotic skin is removed. Releasing escharotomies and fasciotomies are done in the emergent phase, usually in burn centers by burn physicians.

Patients find the first wound care to be both physically and mentally demanding. Provide emotional support and begin to build trust during this activity. A once-daily shower and dressing change in the morning, with an evening dressing change in

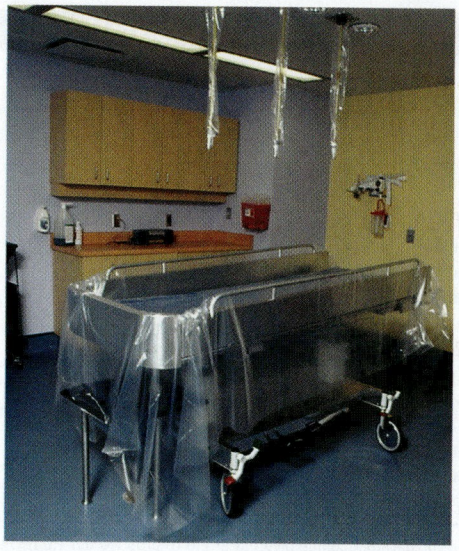

FIG. 24-9 Shower cart. Showering presents an opportunity for wound care and physical therapy. (Courtesy Judy Knighton, Toronto, Canada.)

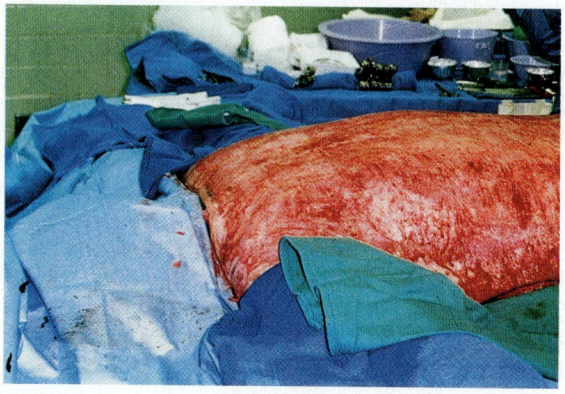

FIG. 24-10 Surgical debridement of full-thickness burns is necessary to prepare the wound for grafting. (Courtesy Judy Knighton, Toronto, Canada.)

the patient's room, are part of the routine in many burn centers. Others opt to shower the patient on admission and then perform all other dressing changes in the patient's room. Some of the newer antimicrobial dressings can be left in place from 3 to 14 days, thereby reducing the frequency of dressing changes.

Infection can cause further tissue injury and possible sepsis.[16] The source of infection in burn wounds is likely the patient's own flora, mostly from the skin and respiratory and gastrointestinal (GI) systems. Preventing cross-contamination from one patient to another is a priority.

Two approaches to burn wound treatment are (1) the open method and (2) the use of multiple dressing changes (closed method). In the *open method* the patient's burn is covered with a topical antimicrobial and has no dressing over the wound. This approach is usually limited to the care of facial burns. In the *multiple dressing change,* or *closed method,* sterile gauze dressings are impregnated with or laid over a topical antimicrobial (Fig. 24-11). These dressings are changed anywhere from every 12 to 24 hours to once every 14 days (depending on the product). Most burn centers support the concept of moist wound healing and use dressings to cover the burned areas, with the exception of facial burns.

When the patient's open burn wounds are exposed, always wear personal protective equipment (PPE) (e.g., disposable hats, masks, gowns, gloves). When removing contaminated dressings

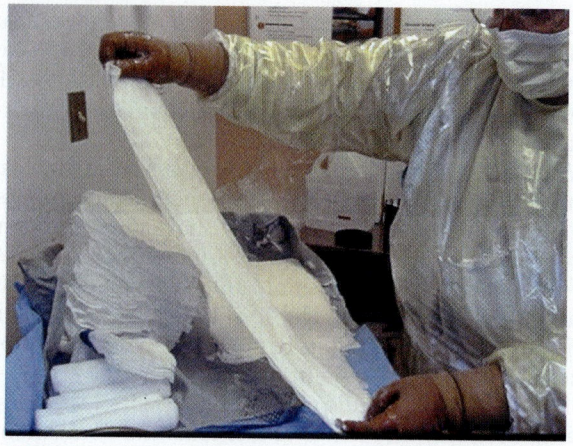

FIG. 24-11 Application of silver sulfadiazine cream to saline-moistened gauze. (Courtesy Judy Knighton, Toronto, Canada.)

TABLE 24-12 Skin Grafts Used for Burn Injury

Graft Type	Source and Description	Coverage
Xenograft (or heterograft) (different species)	Porcine skin	Temporary (3 days to 2 wk)
Allograft (or homograft) (same species)	Cadaveric skin	Temporary (3 days to 2 wk)
Autograft	Patient's own skin	Permanent
Cultured epithelial autograft (CEA)–Epicel	Patient's own skin cell cultures	Permanent
Biobrane	Semipermeable silicone membrane bonded to nylon fabric	Temporary (10-21 days)
Integra	Biodegradable dermal layer made of bovine collagen and glycosaminoglycan bonded to silicone membrane	Permanent
AlloDerm	Acellular dermal matrix derived from donated human skin	Permanent
OrCel	Donated neonatal foreskin fibroblasts and keratinocytes in bovine collagen sponge	Permanent
Apligraf	Donated neonatal foreskin fibroblasts and keratinocytes in bovine collagen gel	Permanent
Matriderm	Bovine collagen and elastin matrix	Permanent

and washing the wound, use nonsterile, disposable gloves. Use sterile gloves when applying ointments and sterile dressings. In addition, prevent shivering by keeping the room warm (approximately 85°F [29.4°C]). Before leaving one patient, remove your PPE. Don new PPE before you treat another patient. Thoroughly wash your hands both before and after patient contact to prevent cross-contamination.

Permanent skin coverage is the primary goal for burn wound care. There is rarely enough unburned skin in the major (greater than 50% TBSA) burn patient for immediate skin grafting. In this situation, temporary wound closure methods are needed. *Allograft (homograft) skin* (from skin donor cadavers) is used, along with newer biosynthetic options. Treatment approaches vary among burn centers (Table 24-12).

Other Care Measures

Certain parts of the body (e.g., face, eyes, hands, arms, ears, perineum) need vigilant nursing care. The face is highly vascular and can become very swollen. It is often covered with ointments and gauze but not wrapped to limit pressure on delicate facial structures. An ophthalmology exam should occur soon after admission for all patients with facial burns. Periorbital edema can prevent eye opening and is often frightening for the patient. Always check that the patient's eyelashes are not turned inward towards the eyeball. Provide assurance that the swelling is not permanent. Instill methylcellulose drops or artificial tears into the eyes for moisture and additional comfort. Apply antibiotic eye ointment for corneal burns or edema as ordered.

Ears should be kept free from pressure because of their poor vascularization and tendency to become infected. Do not use pillows for the patient with ear burns. The pressure on the cartilage may cause chondritis. Further, the ear may stick to the pillowcase, causing pain and bleeding. Raise your patient's head using a rolled towel placed under the shoulders, being careful to avoid pressure necrosis. Follow the same strategy for the patient with neck burns to hyperextend the neck and prevent neck contracture.

Extend your patient's burned hands and arms and raise them on pillows or plastic-covered foam wedges to reduce edema. Ask the physical therapist and the HCP if splints should be applied to burned hands and feet to keep them in positions of function. Remove the splints often and inspect the skin and bony prominences to avoid areas of pressure from inappropriate or prolonged application.

Keep your patient's perineum as clean and dry as possible after each voiding or bowel movement. In addition to monitoring hourly urine outputs, an indwelling catheter prevents urine contamination of the perineal area. Regular once- or twice-daily perineal care, in the presence or absence of a perineal burn wound, is essential. Assess the need for an indwelling urinary catheter on a daily basis. Remove when no longer needed to limit the risk of a urinary tract infection. If your patient has frequent, loose stools, consider using a fecal diversion device.

Perform necessary laboratory tests to monitor fluid and electrolyte balance. Draw ABGs, as necessary, to assess adequacy of ventilation and oxygenation in patients with suspected or confirmed inhalation or electrical injury.

Work with the physical therapist to perform range-of-motion (ROM) exercises during dressing changes and throughout the day. Movement aids the shift of the leaked fluid back into the vascular bed. Active and passive exercise of body parts also maintains function, prevents skin and joint contractures, and reassures the patient that movement is still possible.

Drug Therapy

Analgesics and Sedatives. Promote the use of analgesics for the patient's comfort. Early in the postburn period, IV pain medications should be given because (1) onset of action is fastest with this route; (2) oral drugs have a slower onset of action and are not as effective when GI function is slowed or impaired because of shock or paralytic ileus; and (3) IM injections are not absorbed well in burned or edematous areas, causing pooling of drugs in the tissues. Consequently, when fluid mobilization starts, the patient could be inadvertently overdosed from the interstitial accumulation of previous IM drugs.

Common drugs used for pain control are listed in Table 24-13. Initially, opioids are the drug of choice for pain control.

TABLE 24-13 Drug Therapy

Burns

Drugs	Purpose
Analgesics	
morphine (Avinza)	Relieve pain
sustained-release morphine (MS Contin)	
hydromorphone (Dilaudid)	
sustained-release hydromorphone (Dilaudid CR)	
fentanyl (Sublimaze)	
oxycodone and acetaminophen (Percocet)	
methadone (Dolophine)	
Nonsteroidal antiinflammatory (e.g., ketorolac)	
Adjuvant analgesics (e.g., gabapentin [Neurontin])	
Sedatives/Hypnotics	
lorazepam (Ativan)	Reduce anxiety
midazolam	Provide short-acting amnesic effects
zolpidem (Ambien)	Promote sleep
Antidepressants	
sertraline (Zoloft)	Reduce depression, improve mood
citalopram (Celexa)	
Anticoagulants	
enoxaparin (Lovenox)	Prevent venous thromboembolism
heparin	
Nutritional Support	
Vitamins A, C, E, and multivitamins	Promote wound healing
Minerals: zinc, iron (ferrous sulfate)	Promote cell integrity and hemoglobin formation
Gastrointestinal Support	
ranitidine (Zantac)	Decrease stomach acid and risk of Curling's ulcer
esomeprazole (Nexium)	
calcium carbonate and magnesium carbonate (Mylanta)	Neutralize stomach acid
aluminum hydroxide and magnesium hydroxide (Maalox)	
nystatin	Prevent overgrowth of *Candida albicans* in oral mucosa

When given appropriately, these drugs should provide adequate pain relief. Evaluate the pain management plan often, since the patient's needs may change and tolerance to drugs may develop over time. Remember that the patient's pain level may not directly correlate with the extent and depth of burn. Analgesic needs vary from one patient to another. Consider a multimodal approach to pain control. Sedatives/hypnotics and antidepressants can also be given with analgesics to control the anxiety, insomnia, or depression that patients may experience (Table 24-13).

Tetanus Immunization. Tetanus toxoid is given routinely to all burn patients because of the likelihood of anaerobic burn wound contamination. If the patient has not received an active immunization within 10 years before the burn injury, tetanus immunoglobulin should be considered. (Tetanus immunization is discussed in Table 68-6.)

Antimicrobial Agents. After the wound is cleansed, topical antimicrobial agents may be applied (Fig. 24-11) and covered with a light dressing. Systemic antibiotics are not routinely used to control burn wound flora because the burn eschar has little or no blood supply, and consequently little antibiotic is delivered to the wound. In addition, the routine use of systemic antibiotics increases the chance of developing multidrug-resistant organisms.

Some topical burn agents penetrate the eschar and inhibit bacterial invasion of the wound. Silver-impregnated dressings can be left in place from 3 to 14 days, depending on the patient's clinical situation and the particular product. Silver sulfadiazine (Silvadene) and mafenide acetate (Sulfamylon) creams are also used.[17]

SAFETY ALERT Drug Allergy Check

- Check the patient for any allergies to sulfa, since many burn antimicrobial creams contain sulfa.

Sepsis remains a primary cause of death in the patient with major burns and may lead to multiple organ dysfunction syndrome (see Chapter 66). Systemic antibiotic therapy is started when the diagnosis of sepsis is made or when some other source of infection is identified (e.g., pneumonia).

Fungal infections may develop in the patient's mucous membranes (mouth and genitalia) as a result of systemic antibiotic therapy and low resistance. The offending organism is usually *Candida albicans.* Oral infection is treated with nystatin (Mycostatin) mouthwash. When a normal diet is resumed, yogurt or *Lactobacillus* (Lactinex) may be given to reintroduce the normal intestinal flora that was destroyed by antibiotic therapy.

◆ **Venous Thromboembolism Prophylaxis.** Burn patients are at risk for VTE. If there are no contraindications, it is recommended that low-molecular-weight heparin (enoxaparin) or low-dose unfractionated heparin be started as soon as it is considered safe. For burn patients who have a high bleeding risk, VTE prophylaxis with sequential compression devices and/or graduated compression stockings are used until the bleeding risk decreases and heparin can be started (Table 24-13). (VTE prophylaxis is discussed in Chapter 37.)

◆ Nutritional Therapy

Once fluid replacement needs have been addressed, nutrition takes priority in the initial emergent phase. Early and aggressive nutritional support within several hours of the burn injury can decrease complications and mortality, optimize burn wound healing, and minimize the negative effects of hypermetabolism and catabolism.[18] Nonintubated patients with a burn of less than 20% TBSA will usually be able to eat enough to meet their nutritional needs.

Intubated patients and those with larger burns require additional support. Enteral feedings have almost entirely replaced parenteral feeding. Early enteral feeding, usually with smaller-bore tubes, preserves GI function, increases intestinal blood flow, and promotes optimal conditions for wound healing. In general, begin the feedings slowly at a rate of 20 to 40 mL/hr and increase to the goal rate within 24 to 48 hours. If a large nasogastric tube is used, gastric residuals should be checked to rule out delayed gastric emptying. Assess bowel sounds every 8 hours.

A *hypermetabolic state* proportional to the size of the wound occurs after a major burn injury. Resting metabolic expenditure may be increased by 50% to 100% above normal in patients with major burns. Core temperature is elevated. Catecholamines, which stimulate catabolism and heat production, are increased. Massive catabolism can occur and is characterized by protein breakdown and increased gluconeogenesis.

Failure to supply adequate calories and protein leads to malnutrition and delayed healing. Calorie-containing nutritional supplements are often given to meet the caloric needs. Protein powder can also be added to food and liquids. Supplemental vitamins may be started in the emergent phase, with iron supplements often given in the acute phase[19] (Table 24-13).

ACUTE PHASE

The *acute phase* of burn care begins with the mobilization of extracellular fluid and subsequent diuresis. It concludes when partial-thickness wounds are healed or full-thickness burns are covered by skin grafts. This may take weeks or months.

Pathophysiology

A healing burn injury causes many pathophysiologic changes in the body. Diuresis from fluid mobilization occurs, and the patient is less edematous. Bowel sounds return. The depth of the burn wounds may be more apparent as they "declare" themselves as partial or full thickness. The patient may now become more aware of the enormity of his or her situation and will benefit from emotional support and information.

Some healing begins as WBCs surround the burn wound and phagocytosis occurs. Necrotic tissue begins to slough. Fibroblasts lay down matrices of the collagen precursors that eventually form granulation tissue. A partial-thickness burn will heal, from both the wound edges and the dermal bed below, if kept free from infection and *desiccation* (dryness). However, full-thickness burn wounds, unless extremely small, must have the burn eschar surgically removed (excised) and skin grafts applied in order to heal. In some cases, healing time and length of hospitalization are decreased by early excision and grafting.

Clinical Manifestations

Partial-thickness wounds form eschar, which begins separating fairly soon after injury. Once the eschar is removed, re-epithelialization begins at the wound margins and appears as red or pink scar tissue. Epithelial buds, from the hair follicles and glands in the dermal bed, eventually close the wound. Healing is spontaneous and usually occurs within 10 to 21 days.

Margins of full-thickness eschar take longer to separate. As a result, full-thickness burn wounds require surgical debridement and skin grafting to heal.

Laboratory Values

Because the body is attempting to reestablish fluid and electrolyte balance in the initial acute phase, it is important to follow serum electrolyte levels closely.

Sodium. *Hyponatremia* can develop from excessive GI suction and diarrhea. Manifestations of hyponatremia include weakness, dizziness, muscle cramps, fatigue, headache, tachycardia, and confusion. The patient may also develop a *dilutional hyponatremia* called *water intoxication* from excess water intake. To avoid this condition, offer the patient fluids other than water, such as juice or nutritional supplements, to drink.

Hypernatremia may be seen after successful fluid resuscitation if large amounts of hypertonic solutions were used. Hypernatremia may also be caused by tube feedings or inappropriate fluid administration. Manifestations of hypernatremia include thirst; dried, furry tongue; lethargy; confusion; and possibly seizures. Sodium restrictions may be applied to IV fluids and enteral or oral feedings until levels return to safe limits.

Potassium. *Hyperkalemia* may occur if the patient has renal failure, adrenocortical insufficiency, or massive deep muscle injury (e.g., electrical burn) with large amounts of potassium released from damaged cells. Heart dysrhythmias and arrest can occur with elevated potassium levels. Check for muscle weakness, cramping, and paralysis.

Hypokalemia occurs with vomiting, diarrhea, prolonged GI suction, and IV therapy without potassium supplementation. Potassium is also lost through the patient's burn wounds. Signs and symptoms of hypokalemia include fatigue, muscle weakness, leg cramps, heart dysrhythmias, paresthesias, and decreased reflexes (see Chapter 16).

Complications

Infection. A burn injury destroys the body's first line of defense, the skin. The burn wound is now colonized with the person's own organisms that were on the skin before the burn. If the levels of bacteria between the eschar and viable wound bed rise to greater than 10^5 per gram of tissue, the patient has a burn wound infection. Localized inflammation, induration, and sometimes suppuration can be seen at the burn wound margins. Partial-thickness burns can change to full-thickness wounds when these bacteria invade viable, unburned tissue. Wound infections may be treated with systemic antibiotics based on wound culture and sensitivity results.

Watch for signs and symptoms, including hypothermia or hyperthermia, increased heart and respiratory rate, decreased BP, and decreased urine output. The patient may have mild confusion, chills, malaise, and loss of appetite. The WBC count usually is between 10,000/μL (10×10^9/L) and 20,000/μL (20×10^9/L). The WBCs have functional defects and the patient is immunosuppressed for many months after the burn injury.

The causative organisms of sepsis are usually gram-negative bacteria (e.g., *Pseudomonas, Proteus*), putting the patient at further risk for septic shock. When sepsis is suspected, immediately obtain cultures from all possible sources, including the burn wound, blood, urine, sputum, oropharynx and perineal regions, and IV site. Treatment immediately begins with antibiotics. When the culture and sensitivity results are known, the antibiotic in use may be continued or changed based on the results. At this stage the patient's condition is considered critical, and close monitoring of vital signs and mental status is needed.

Cardiovascular and Respiratory Systems. The same cardiovascular and respiratory system complications present in the emergent phase may continue into the acute phase of care. In addition, new problems might arise, requiring timely intervention.

Neurologic System. Neurologically, the patient probably has no physical symptoms, unless severe hypoxia from respiratory injuries or complications from electrical injuries occur. Probable causes of neurologic complications include electrolyte imbalance, stress, cerebral edema, sepsis, sleep disturbances, and the use of analgesics and antianxiety drugs. However, some patients may demonstrate certain behaviors that are not completely understood.

The patient may become extremely disoriented, may withdraw or become combative, and may have hallucinations and frequent nightmare-like episodes. Delirium is more acute at night and occurs more often in the older patient. Start appropriate nursing interventions to prevent delirium and use a screening tool to diagnose delirium (see Table 59-18). Orient and reassure your patient if he or she is confused or agitated. This state is usually transient, lasting from a day or two to several weeks, but complications and sequelae can last for years and be serious.

Musculoskeletal System. The musculoskeletal system is particularly prone to complications during the acute phase, and the involvement of both the physical and occupational therapist is vitally important. As the burns begin to heal and scar tissue forms, the skin is less supple and pliant. ROM may be limited, and skin and joint contractures can occur. Because of pain, the patient prefers a flexed position for comfort. Have the patient stretch and move the burned body parts as much as possible. Consult with the physical or occupational therapist about proper positioning and splinting to prevent or reduce contracture formation.

Gastrointestinal System. The GI system may also experience complications during this phase. Paralytic ileus can be caused by sepsis. Diarrhea may result from the use of enteral feedings or antibiotics. Constipation can occur as a side effect of opioids, decreased mobility, and a low-fiber diet. *Curling's ulcer* is a type of gastroduodenal ulcer characterized by diffuse superficial lesions (including mucosal erosion). It is caused by a generalized stress response to decreased blood flow to the GI tract. The patient has increased gastric acid secretion.

Aim to prevent Curling's ulcer by feeding the patient as soon as possible after the burn injury. Antacids, H_2-histamine blockers (e.g., ranitidine [Zantac]), and proton pump inhibitors (e.g., esomeprazole [Nexium]) are used prophylactically to neutralize stomach acids and inhibit histamine and the secretion of hydrochloric acid (Table 24-13). Patients with major burns may also have occult blood in their stools during the acute phase and require close monitoring for bleeding.

Endocrine System. Watch for transient increases in the patient's blood glucose levels as a result of stress-mediated cortisol and catecholamine release. There is an increased mobilization of glycogen stores and gluconeogenesis. Subsequently, glucose is produced, along with an increase in insulin production. However, insulin's effectiveness is decreased because of relative insulin insensitivity. This results in an elevated blood glucose level. Hyperglycemia may also be caused by the increased caloric intake necessary to meet some patients' metabolic requirements. When this occurs, treat with IV or subcutaneous insulin, not decreased feeding. Check blood glucose levels and give insulin as ordered. Point-of-care testing of glucose can be done, but serum glucose testing is more accurate. As the patient's metabolic demands are met and less stress is placed on the entire system, this stress-induced condition is reversed.

◆ NURSING AND INTERPROFESSIONAL MANAGEMENT: ACUTE PHASE

The major therapeutic interventions in the acute phase are (1) wound care, (2) excision and grafting, (3) pain management, (4) physical and occupational therapy, and (5) nutritional therapy.

◆ Wound Care

The goals of wound care are to (1) prevent infection by cleansing and debriding the area of necrotic tissue that would promote bacterial growth and (2) promote wound re-epithelialization and/or successful skin grafting.

Wound care consists of ongoing observation, assessment, cleansing, debridement, and dressing reapplication. Nonsurgical debridement, dressing changes, topical antimicrobial therapy, graft care, and donor site care are performed as often as necessary, depending on the topical cream or dressing ordered. Enzymatic debriding agents made of natural ingredients, such as collagen, may be used for *enzymatic debridement* of burn wounds, which speeds up the removal of dead tissue from the healthy wound bed.

Cleanse wounds with soap and water or normal saline-moistened gauze to gently remove the old antimicrobial agent and any loose necrotic tissue, scabs, or dried blood. During the debridement phase, cover the wound with topical antimicrobial creams (e.g., silver sulfadiazine) or silver-impregnated dressings. When the partial-thickness burn wounds have been fully debrided, a protective, coarse or fine-meshed, greasy-based (paraffin or petroleum) gauze dressing is applied to protect the re-epithelializing keratinocytes as they resurface and close the open wound bed.

If grafting is necessary, protect the skin graft (discussed later) with the same greasy gauze dressings next to the graft, followed by saline-moistened middle dressing, and dry gauze outer dressings. With facial grafts the unmeshed sheet graft is left open, so it is possible for *blebs* (serosanguineous exudate) to form between the graft and recipient bed. Blebs prevent the graft from permanently attaching to the wound bed. The evacuation of blebs is best performed by aspiration with a tuberculin syringe and only by those trained in this specialized skill. (Dressings are discussed in Table 11-9.)

◆ Excision and Grafting

Management of full-thickness burn wounds involves early removal (surgical excision) of the necrotic tissue followed by application of split-thickness autograft skin.[20] This approach has improved the management and survival rate of burn patients. In the past, patients with major burns had low rates of survival because healing and wound coverage took so long that the patient usually died of sepsis or malnutrition.

Many patients, especially those with major burns, are taken to the OR for wound excision on day 1 or 2 (emergent phase). The wounds are covered with a biologic dressing or allograft for temporary coverage until permanent grafting can occur (Table 24-12).

During the procedure of **excision and grafting**, devitalized tissue (eschar) is excised down to the subcutaneous tissue or fascia, depending on the degree of injury. Surgical excision can result in massive blood loss. To decrease surgical blood loss, topical application of epinephrine or thrombin, injection of saline and epinephrine, application of extremity tourniquets, or application of a new fibrin sealant (Artiss) is used.

Once hemostasis has been achieved, a graft is then placed on clean, viable tissue to achieve good adherence. Whenever possible, the freshly excised wound is covered with *autograft* (the person's own) skin (Table 24-12). Recently, fibrin sealant has been used to attach skin grafts to the wound bed. Grafts can also be stapled or sutured into place (Fig. 24-12, *A*). Negative pressure wound therapy dressings are often placed on top of skin grafts to optimize adherence of the graft to the excised wound bed.[21] A temporary allograft can be used to test the suitability of the recipient site to accept a graft. The allograft is then removed several days later in the OR and an autograft applied.

With early excision, function is restored and scar tissue formation is minimized. Clots between the graft and wound keep the graft from adhering to the wound. Outer occlusive dressings apply just enough pressure to promote adherence of the graft to the wound bed and help control bleeding. Protect the grafted area from shearing, friction, and pressure. Facial, neck, and hand burns require skilled nursing care to identify and manage clots quickly for the best functional and esthetic outcomes.

Donor skin is taken from the patient for grafting by means of a *dermatome,* which removes a thin (14/1000 to 16/1000 inch) split-thickness layer of skin from an unburned site (Fig. 24-12, *B*). The donor skin can be meshed (usually ratio of 1.5 : 1) to allow for greater wound coverage, or it may be applied as an unmeshed sheet for a better cosmetic result when grafting the face, neck, and hands. The donor site now becomes a new open wound.

The goals of donor site care are to promote rapid, moist wound healing; decrease pain at the site; and prevent infection.

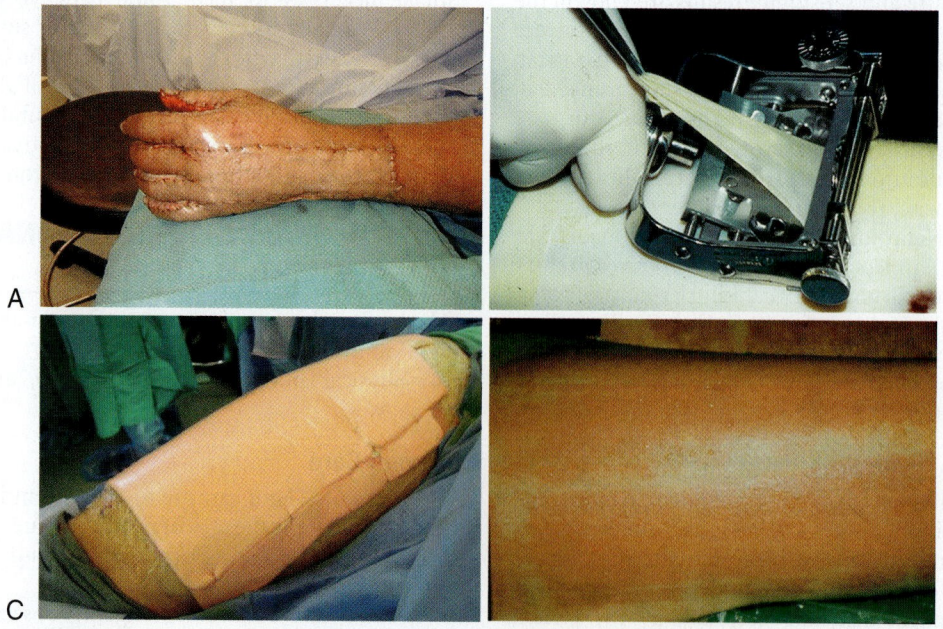

FIG. 24-12 **A,** Freshly applied split-thickness sheet skin graft to the hand. **B,** Split-thickness skin graft is harvested from a patient's thigh using a dermatome. **C,** Donor site is covered with a hydrophilic foam dressing after harvesting. **D,** Healed donor site. (Courtesy Judy Knighton, Toronto, Canada.)

The choices of dressings for donor sites include transparent dressings (e.g., OpSite), xenograft, silver sulfadiazine, silver-impregnated dressings, calcium alginate, and hydrophilic foam dressings (Fig. 24-12, *C*). Nursing care of the donor site is specific to the dressing selected. Several of the newer dressings decrease healing time, which allows earlier reharvesting of skin at the same site. The average healing time for a donor site is 10 to 14 days (Fig. 24-12, *D*).

◆ **Cultured Epithelial Autografts.** In the patient with large body burns, only a limited amount of unburned skin may be available as donor sites for grafting, and some of that skin may not be suitable for harvesting. **Cultured epithelial autograft (CEA)** is a method of getting permanent skin from a person with limited skin available for harvesting. CEA is grown from biopsies obtained from the patient's unburned skin. This procedure is performed in suitable patients in some burn centers as soon as possible. The specimens are sent to a commercial laboratory, where the biopsied keratinocytes are grown in a culture medium containing epidermal growth factor. After approximately 18 to 25 days, the keratinocytes have expanded up to 10,000 times and form sheets that can be used as skin grafts. The cultured skin is returned to the burn center, where it is placed on the patient's excised burn wounds (Fig. 24-13, *A*). CEA grafts generally form a seamless, smooth replacement skin tissue (Fig. 24-13, *B*). Problems related to CEA include a poor graft take because of thin epidermal skin, graft loss during healing, infection, and contracture development.

◆ **Artificial Skin.** Artificial skin can replace all functions of the skin and consists of both dermal and epidermal elements.[22] The Integra artificial skin dermal regeneration template is an example of a skin replacement system. As with CEA, it is indicated for use in the treatment of life-threatening, full-thickness or deep partial-thickness burn wounds when a conventional autograft is not available or advisable, as in older or high anesthetic-risk patients. It has also been successfully used in reconstructive burn surgery procedures. It must be applied within a few days postburn for greatest success.

Integra artificial skin has a bilayer membrane composed of acellular dermis and silicone. The wound is excised, the bilayer membrane is placed dermal layer down, and the wound is wrapped with dressings in the OR. The dermal layer functions as a biodegradable template that induces organized regeneration of new dermis by the body. The silicone layer remains intact for 3 weeks as the dermal layer degrades and epidermal autografts become available. At this point, the silicone is removed during a second surgical procedure and replaced by the patient's own epidermal autografts. Some burn centers use CEA as the source of the epidermis.

Another dermal replacement is AlloDerm, a cryopreserved allogenic dermis. Human allograft dermis, harvested from cadavers, is decellularized to make it immunogenic and then freeze-dried. Once thawed, AlloDerm is rehydrated with ultrathin epidermal autografts immediately before placement on a freshly excised wound.

◆ Pain Management

Many aspects of burn care cause pain. However, patients will experience acceptable levels of relative comfort if they receive adequate analgesia. To provide effective pain management, you must understand both the physiologic and psychologic aspects of pain. (Pain management is discussed in Chapter 8.)

Burn patients experience two kinds of pain: (1) *continuous, background pain* that might be present throughout the day and night; and (2) *treatment-induced pain* associated with dressing changes, ambulation, and rehabilitation activities. The first line of pain treatment is drugs (Table 24-13). With background pain, a continuous IV infusion of an opioid (e.g., hydromorphone [Dilaudid]) provides a steady, therapeutic level of the drug. If an IV infusion is not ordered, slow-release, twice-a-day opioids (e.g., morphine [MS Contin]) are used.

Breakthrough doses of analgesia must be available regardless of the regimen selected. Anxiolytics, which can enhance analgesics, are also indicated and include lorazepam (Ativan) and midazolam. Adjuvant analgesics, such as gabapentin (Neurontin) and pregabalin (Lyrica), also enhance opioids. The use of these drugs can help reduce the opioid dosage and undesirable side effects.

For treatment-induced pain, premedicate with an analgesic and possibly an anxiolytic via the IV or oral route. For patients with an IV, a short-acting analgesic is often used.

Elimination of all pain is difficult, and most patients will accept a "tolerable" level of discomfort. Some pain can be managed using

CHECK YOUR PRACTICE

Your patient with a burn injury is ordered fentanyl (Sublimaze) before a dressing change. The patient has multiple IV lines and you are not sure which line to use to insert the drug. You know that mixing up IV lines can lead to serious drug errors.

- How would you determine which IV line to use to give the drug?

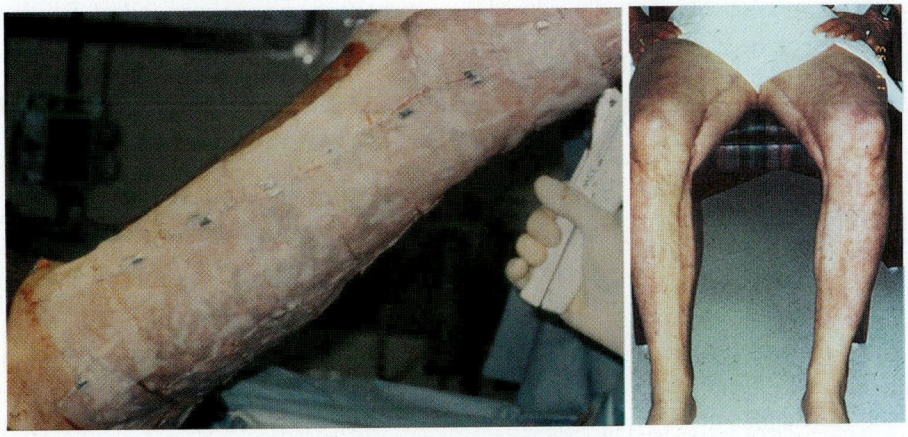

FIG. 24-13 Patient with cultured epithelial autograft (CEA). **A,** Intraoperative application of CEA. **B,** Appearance of healed CEA.

nondrug strategies. Relaxation breathing, guided imagery, hypnosis, biofeedback, computerized gaming, and music therapy can also help patients cope with pain[23] (see Chapters 6 and 8).

Remember, the more control the patient has in managing pain, the more successful the chosen strategies will be. Active participation in asking for time-outs and scheduling treatments and rest periods can help the patient manage feelings of anticipatory pain. Patient-controlled analgesia (PCA) is used in some burn centers, with varying degrees of success. (PCA is discussed in Chapter 8.)

◆ Physical and Occupational Therapy

Continuous physical therapy throughout burn recovery is imperative if the patient is to regain and maintain muscle strength and optimal joint function. A good time for exercise is during and after wound cleansing, when the skin is softer and bulky dressings are removed. Passive and active ROM should be performed on all joints. Ensure that the patient with neck burns continues to sleep without pillows or with the head hanging slightly over the top of the mattress to encourage hyperextension.

Maintain the occupational therapy schedule for wearing custom-fitted splints, which are designed to keep joints in functional position. Check the splints often to ensure an optimal fit, with no undue pressure that may lead to skin breakdown or nerve damage.

◆ Nutritional Therapy

The goal of nutritional therapy during the acute burn phase is to provide adequate calories and protein to promote healing. When the wounds are still open, the burn patient is in a hypermetabolic and highly catabolic state.

The patient may benefit from an antioxidant protocol, which includes selenium, vitamin E, acetylcysteine, ascorbic acid, zinc, and a multivitamin. Meeting daily caloric requirements is crucial and should start within the first 1 to 2 days postburn. The daily estimated caloric needs must be regularly calculated by a dietitian and readjusted as the patient's condition changes (e.g., wound healing improves, sepsis develops). Monitor laboratory values (e.g., albumin, prealbumin, total protein, transferrin) on a regular basis.

If the patient is mechanically ventilated or unable to eat enough calories by mouth, a small-bore feeding tube is placed and enteral feedings are started. When the patient is extubated, contact the speech pathologist for a swallowing assessment before an oral diet is started. Encourage the patient to eat high-protein, high-carbohydrate foods to meet caloric goals. Ask caregivers to bring in favorite foods from home. Appetite is usually reduced, and you will need to reinforce whatever steps are taken to achieve adequate intake. Ideally, weight loss should not be more than 10% of preburn weight. Record the patient's daily caloric intake using calorie count sheets, which are reviewed by the dietitian. Weigh your patient weekly to evaluate progress.

REHABILITATION PHASE

The formal *rehabilitation phase* begins when the patient's wounds have healed and he or she is engaging in some level of self-care. This may happen as early as 2 weeks or as long as 7 to 8 months after a major burn injury. Goals for the patient now are to (1) work toward resuming a functional role in society and (2) rehabilitate from any functional and cosmetic postburn reconstructive surgery that may be necessary.[24]

Pathophysiologic Changes and Clinical Manifestations

Burn wounds heal either by spontaneous re-epithelialization or by skin grafting. Layers of keratinocytes begin rebuilding the tissue structure destroyed by the burn injury. Collagen fibers, present in the new scar tissue, assist with healing and add strength to weakened areas. The new skin appears flat and pink. In about 4 to 6 weeks, the area becomes raised and hyperemic. If adequate ROM is not started, the new tissue will shorten, causing a **contracture**. Mature healing is reached in about 12 months when suppleness has returned, and the pink or red color has faded to a slightly lighter hue than the surrounding unburned tissue.

Tell patients who have more heavily pigmented skin that it will take longer for it to regain its color because many of the melanocytes have been destroyed. Frequently, the skin does not regain its original color. Provide teaching and emotional support to assist the patient with grieving about these changes to his or her body. Cosmetic camouflage, the implantation of pigment within the skin, can help even out unequal skin tones and improve the patient's overall appearance and self-image.

Scarring has two characteristics: discoloration and contour. The discoloration of scars fades somewhat with time. However, scar tissue tends to develop altered contours; that is, it is no longer flat or slightly raised but becomes elevated and enlarged above the original burned area. Some burn care providers believe that pressure can eventually help keep a scar flat. Gentle pressure is maintained on the healed burn with custom-fitted pressure garments and clear, thermoplastic face masks. Pressure garments and masks should never be worn over unhealed wounds. Once a wearing schedule has been set, they are removed only for short periods while bathing. Pressure garments are worn up to 24 hours a day for as long as 12 to 18 months.

The patient typically reports discomfort from itching where healing is occurring. Teach your patient about the application of water-based moisturizers and selective, short-term use of oral antihistamines (e.g., hydroxyzine [Atarax]) to help reduce the itching. Massage oil, silicone gel sheeting (e.g., Biodermis), gabapentin, and injectable corticosteroids also may help.[25]

As "old" epithelium is replaced by new cells, flaking occurs. The newly formed skin is extremely sensitive to trauma. Blisters and skin tears are likely to develop from slight pressure or friction. Additionally, these newly healed areas can be hypersensitive or hyposensitive to cold, heat, and touch. Grafted areas are more likely to be hyposensitive until peripheral nerve regeneration occurs. Teach your patients to protect healed burn areas from direct sunlight for about 3 months to prevent hyperpigmentation and sunburn injury. Tell them to always wear sunscreen when outside.

Complications

The most common complications during the rehabilitation phase are skin and joint contractures and hypertrophic scarring.[26] A *joint contracture* (an abnormal condition of a joint characterized by flexion and fixation) develops as a result of the shortening of scar tissue in the flexor tissues of a joint. Areas that are most susceptible to skin and joint contractures include the anterior and lateral neck areas, axillae, antecubital fossae, fingers, groin areas, popliteal fossae, knees, and ankles (Fig. 24-14). Some areas encompass major joints. Not only does the skin over these areas develop contractures, but the underlying tissues, such as the ligaments and tendons, also have a tendency to shorten during the healing process.

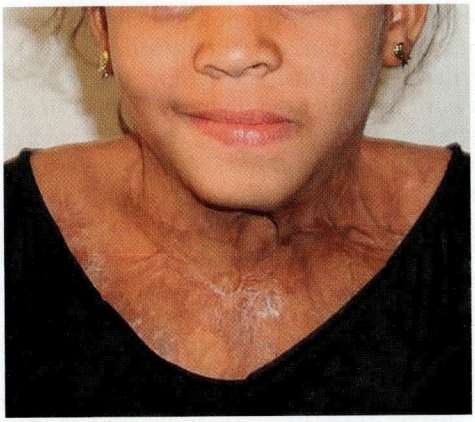

FIG. 24-14 Neck contracture. (Courtesy Linda Bucher, RN, PhD, CEN, CNE, Staff Nurse, Virtua Memorial Hospital, Mt. Holly, N.J.)

Carefully watch the patient for these potential problems. Encourage proper positioning, splinting, and exercise to minimize this complication. Tell the patient to continue with these strategies until the skin matures at around 1 year posthealing. Rehabilitative therapy is aimed at the extension of body parts because the flexors are stronger than the extensors. Burned legs may first be wrapped with elastic (e.g., tensor, Ace) bandages to assist with circulation to leg-graft and donor sites before ambulation. Burned arms can be wrapped with a layer of tubular elastic gauze (e.g., Tubigrip). This interim pressure prevents blister formation, promotes venous return, and decreases pain and itchiness. Once the skin is completely healed and less fragile, custom-fitted pressure garments replace the elastic bandages and tubular gauze.

❖ NURSING AND INTERPROFESSIONAL MANAGEMENT: REHABILITATION PHASE

During the rehabilitation phase, encourage both the patient and caregiver to participate in care. Since the patient may go home with unhealed wounds, teach your patient and caregiver the skills for wound care. Before discharge, have the patient or caregiver return demonstrate (show-back) the proper dressing change. In addition, make sure the patient or caregiver knows when to contact the burn team (e.g., signs of infection, increased pain) and the need to keep outpatient visits to ensure good wound healing.

If needed, arrange home care nursing to assist with care. The newly discharged patient will need to know how to gently remove the dressings in the shower, once daily, if a nonadherent, greasy gauze dressing is used or twice daily, if a topical, antimicrobial cream is ordered. Teach that showering, not bathing, with mild soap and warm water keeps the wounds clean.

Give advice on scar management, moisturizing, and sun protection. Suggest using water-based creams that penetrate into the dermis (e.g., Vaseline Intensive Rescue) on healed areas to keep the skin supple and moisturized. This will decrease itching and flaking. Occasionally antihistamines are used at bedtime if itching persists.

Base ongoing pain management and nutritional needs on individual patient status. Continue to encourage the patient to perform the physical and occupational therapy routines. Suggest computerized gaming devices for breaks from the exercise routines.[27] Encourage and reassure the patient to maintain morale, particularly once the patient realizes that recovery can be slow. Rehabilitation may have to be a primary focus for at least the next 6 to 12 months.

Postburn reconstructive surgery is frequently required after a major burn. The need for further surgery is reviewed at the outpatient burn clinic appointments after discharge.

Gerontologic Considerations: Burns

The older patient presents many challenges for the burn team. The normal aging process puts the patient at risk for injury because of unsteady gait, limited eyesight, and diminished hearing. As people age, skin becomes drier and more wrinkled. Older adults have thinning of the dermal layer, a loss of elastic fibers, a reduction in subcutaneous adipose tissue, and a decrease in vascularity. As a result, the thinner dermis, with reduced blood flow, sustains deeper burns with poorer rates of healing.

Once injured, the older adult has more complications in the emergent and acute phases of burn resuscitation because of preexisting co-morbidities. For example, older patients with diabetes, heart failure, or COPD have morbidity and mortality rates exceeding those of healthy, younger patients. In older patients, pneumonia is a frequent complication, burn wounds and donor sites take longer to heal, and surgical procedures are not well tolerated. Weaning from a ventilator can be a challenge. Although usually self-limiting, delirium, if it develops, may be distressing. It usually takes longer for these patients to rehabilitate to the point where they can safely return home. For some, a return home to independent living may not be possible. As the population ages, developing strategies to prevent burn injuries in older adults is a priority.

EMOTIONAL/PSYCHOLOGIC NEEDS OF PATIENTS AND CAREGIVERS

Patients and caregivers have many emotional/psychologic needs during the often lengthy, unpredictable, and complex course of care.[28] You have an important supportive and counseling role as patients struggle to get their lives back on track.

To manage the enormous range of emotional responses that the burn patient may exhibit, assess the circumstances of the burn (e.g., cause, people involved), family relationships, and previous coping experiences with stressful stimuli. At any time the patient may experience a variety of emotions such as fear, anxiety, anger, guilt, and depression (Table 24-14).

Burn survivors frequently experience thoughts and feelings that are frightening and disturbing, such as guilt about the burn incident, reliving the burn experience, fear of dying, concern about future therapy and surgery, frustrations with ongoing discomfort and treatment, and hopelessness about the future. During recovery, as more independence is expected from the patient, new fears may occur: "Can I really do this?" "Am I a desirable person?" "How can I go outside looking like this?" These challenges confront patients throughout their recovery and often for years to come.

A person's self-esteem may be adversely affected by a burn injury. Some individuals may fear the loss of relationships because of perceived or actual physical disfigurement. In a society that values physical beauty, alterations in body image can result in psychologic distress.

Open and frequent communication among the patient, caregivers, close friends, and burn team members is essential. Because of the tremendous psychologic impact of a burn injury, be particularly sensitive to the patient's emotions and concerns. Encourage the patient to discuss fears regarding loss of life as

TABLE 24-14 Emotional Responses of Burn Patients*

Emotion	Possible Verbal Expression
Fear	• Will I die? • What will happen next? • Will I be disfigured? • Will my family and friends still love me?
Anxiety	• I feel out of control. • What's going to happen to me? • When will I look normal again?
Anger	• Why did this happen to me? • The nurses enjoy hurting me. • I hope the person who did this to me dies.
Guilt	• If only I'd been more careful • I'm being punished because I did something wrong.
Hopefulness	• What do I need to do to survive this injury emotionally and return to my life/family/friends? • What am I meant to learn from this injury?
Depression	• It's no use going on like this. • I don't care what happens to me. • I wish people would leave me alone.

*List is not all-inclusive.

he or she once knew it, loss of function, temporary or permanent deformity and disfigurement, return to work and home life, and financial burdens resulting from a long and costly hospitalization and rehabilitation.[29]

Encourage appropriate independence and an eventual return to preburn activities, such as school or work. Peer counseling and informal interactions with other burn survivors may bring comfort and help to restore confidence.[30] Reassure patients that their feelings, during this period of adjustment, are a normal reaction to an extraordinary life event. Their frustration and impatience are to be expected as they work to establish a new life. Assist patients in adapting to a realistic, yet positive appraisal of their particular situation, emphasizing what they *can* do instead of what they *cannot* do.

Caregivers may share some or all of these challenges and feelings. At times, they may feel helpless or too exhausted to assist their loved one. Continued support from trusted and familiar burn team members is essential. Helping caregivers assist with aspects of the patient's care helps them to reconnect with their loved one and eases the transition home. Many burn survivors and their caregivers remark on the powerful learning experience of the burn and a renewed appreciation of life, despite the ongoing challenges of a prolonged recovery. You must acknowledge that their feelings are real and common. Most burn survivors speak of a real satisfaction with their post-burn life and are more empowered as time goes on.

It is important to address individual spiritual and cultural needs because both have a role in treatment decisions and recovery. Pastoral care may be a helpful resource for the patient and caregiver. The need for support, information, and family involvement may vary among cultures. Identify what is important to your patient and caregiver, and communicate that information in the patient's plan of care. Encourage the burn care team to remain culturally aware of and sensitive to the individual patient's and caregiver's cultural needs.

The difficult issue of sexuality must be met with honesty.[31] Physical appearance is altered in the patient who has sustained a major burn. Acceptance of any changes is difficult at first for the patient and significant other. The nature of skin injury in itself can cause modifications in processing sexual stimuli. Touch is an important part of sexuality, and immature scar tissue may make the sensation of touch unpleasant or may dull it. This may only be transient, but the patient and partner need to know that it is normal and receive anticipatory guidance from the burn team to avoid undue emotional strain.

A significant number of burn survivors have preexisting mental health or substance abuse issues, any of which may have contributed to the burn incident. The stress of the burn injury can precipitate a psychologic crisis. Assessment by a psychiatrist who can prescribe appropriate drugs, if needed, and begin counseling is often helpful. Early psychiatric intervention is essential if the patient has been previously treated for a psychiatric illness or if the injury was a suicide attempt. The diagnosis of posttraumatic stress disorder is made in a number of burn patients. However, it has been noted that distress and trauma symptoms can act as a catalyst for positive posttraumatic growth. Coping styles and social support appear to assist in these positive changes postburn.[32]

Psychologic care typically begins in the hospital, but links to community resources must be made before discharge to ensure continuity of treatment. A referral to a psychiatrist, psychologist, psychiatric advanced practice nurse (APN), mental health counselor, or social worker should be discussed if concerns are raised at burn clinic follow-up.

Caregiver and patient support groups may be beneficial in meeting the patient's and caregiver's emotional needs at any phase of the recovery process. Speaking with others who have experienced burn trauma can be beneficial, both in terms of confirming that the patient's feelings are normal and in sharing helpful advice. The Phoenix Society *(www.phoenix-society.org)* is an international, highly respected burn survivors' support group. For many years the society has offered valuable support and resources (e.g., annual World Burn Congress conference) to burn survivors, caregivers, and burn team staff.

SPECIAL NEEDS OF NURSES

Warm, trusting, and mutually satisfying relationships frequently develop between burn patients and nursing staff, not only during hospitalization but also during the long-term rehabilitation period. Sometimes the bond can be so strong that the patient has difficulty separating from the hospital and staff. The frequency and intensity of family contact can be rewarding as well as draining to you. You may find it difficult to cope with the deformities caused by the burn injury, odors, unpleasant sight of the wound, and reality of the pain that accompanies the burn and its treatment. Do not hesitate to seek help from co-workers, a manager, or the employee assistance program should you feel the need.

In time, you will come to know that the specialized burn care you provide makes a critical difference in helping patients not only survive but also cope with and triumph over an intense and complex injury.

Ongoing support services or critical incident stress debriefings led by a psychiatrist, psychologist, psychiatric APN, or social worker may also be helpful. Peer support groups (e.g., ABA, International Society for Burn Injuries) can serve a similar purpose by helping you cope with difficult feelings experienced when caring for burn patients. Because burn nursing is physically, psychologically, and intellectually demanding, it has many challenges and inherent rewards.[33] Attention to your own self-care is important to maintain a positive attitude and healthy work-life balance. Time with family and friends and rest and relaxation at home are essential parts of self-care and a balanced life with purpose and meaning.

CASE STUDY

Burn Injury

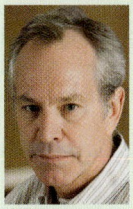

(©Comstock/ Thinkstock)

Patient Profile

G.M., a 52-year-old married white man, arrives at the emergency department with burns to his face, neck, chest, right arm and hand, and right foot. He was burning brush on his farm when the fire went out of control. He has an 18-gauge IV with NSS running at 100 mL/hr, and he is receiving 100% humidified O_2 by mask.

Subjective Data

- Complains of blurry vision and trouble swallowing
- States his burns are painful and that he is scared
- States he is a "diabetic" and has "high blood pressure"

Objective Data

Physical Examination

- Is awake, alert, and oriented, but in some distress
- Eyes are red, irritated
- Voice is hoarse; nasal hair is singed
- Face is reddened with blisters noted on the nose and forehead
- Right arm, right hand, anterior chest, neck, and right foot have shiny, bright red, wet wounds
- Is shivering

Discussion Questions

1. ***Priority Decision:*** What are the priorities of care in the prehospital setting and emergency department? How should his airway, breathing, and circulation be managed?
2. ***Priority Decision:*** What factors place G.M. at high risk for an inhalation injury? What priority interventions can be anticipated?
3. ***Patient-Centered Care:*** What pain medications might be considered to relieve his pain?
4. Which of the criteria for burn center referral does G.M. meet for admission to the hospital burn unit?
5. What metabolic disturbances would be expected soon after G.M.'s admission? Explain the physiologic basis for these changes.
6. How might G.M.'s co-morbidities affect his burn care and rehabilitation?
7. ***Patient-Centered Care:*** What measures should be taken to support G.M.'s caregivers?
8. ***Priority Decision:*** Based on the assessment data presented, what are the priority nursing diagnoses? Identify any collaborative problems.
9. ***Evidence-Based Practice:*** What are the most effective wound care strategies to manage G.M.'s burn wounds?
10. ***Patient-Centered Care:*** Prior to discharge what teaching should be provided to G.M. and his family so they can successfully manage his care at home?
11. ***Safety:*** To ensure G.M.'s safety at home, what interventions are necessary prior to discharge?
12. ***Quality Improvement:*** What outcomes will indicate that interprofessional care was effective?

Answers available at *http://evolve.elsevier.com/Lewis/medsurg.*

BRIDGE TO NCLEX EXAMINATION

The number of the question corresponds to the same-numbered outcome at the beginning of the chapter.

1. Knowing the most common causes of household fires, which prevention strategy would the nurse focus on when teaching about fire safety?
   a. Set hot water temperature at 140° F.
   b. Use only hardwired smoke detectors.
   c. Encourage regular home fire exit drills.
   d. Never permit older adults to cook unattended.
2. The injury that is *least* likely to result in a full-thickness burn is
   a. sunburn.
   b. scald injury.
   c. chemical burn.
   d. electrical injury.
3. When assessing a patient with a partial-thickness burn, the nurse would expect to find *(select all that apply)*
   a. blisters.
   b. exposed fascia.
   c. exposed muscles.
   d. intact nerve endings.
   e. red, shiny, wet appearance.
4. A patient is admitted to the burn center with burns to his head, neck, and anterior and posterior chest after an explosion in his garage. On assessment, the nurse auscultates wheezes throughout the lung fields. On reassessment, the wheezes are gone and the breath sounds are greatly diminished. Which action is the *most* appropriate for the nurse to take *next*?
   a. Encourage the patient to cough and auscultate the lungs again.
   b. Obtain vital signs, oxygen saturation, and a STAT arterial blood gas.
   c. Document the findings and continue to monitor the patient's breathing.
   d. Anticipate the need for endotracheal intubation and notify the physician.
5. Fluid and electrolyte shifts that occur during the early emergent phase of a burn injury include
   a. adherence of albumin to vascular walls.
   b. movement of potassium into the vascular space.
   c. sequestering of sodium and water in interstitial fluid.
   d. hemolysis of red blood cells from large volumes of rapidly administered fluid.
6. To maintain a positive nitrogen balance in a major burn, the patient must
   a. eat a high-protein, high-carbohydrate diet.
   b. increase normal caloric intake by about three times.
   c. eat at least 1500 calories/day in small, frequent meals.
   d. eat a gluten-free diet for the chemical effect on nitrogen balance.
7. A patient has 25% TBSA burn from a car fire. His wounds have been debrided and covered with a silver-impregnated dressing. The nurse's *priority* intervention for wound care would be to
   a. reapply a new dressing without disturbing the wound bed.
   b. observe the wound for signs of infection during dressing changes.
   c. apply cool compresses for pain relief in between dressing changes.
   d. wash the wound aggressively with soap and water three times a day.

8. Pain management for the burn patient is *most* effective when *(select all that apply)*
   a. a pain rating tool is used to monitor the patient's level of pain.
   b. painful dressing changes are delayed until the patient's pain is completely relieved.
   c. the patient is informed about and has some control over the management of the pain.
   d. a multimodal approach is used (e.g., sustained-release and short-acting opioids, NSAIDs, adjuvant analgesics).
   e. nonpharmacologic therapies (e.g., music therapy, distraction) replace opioids in the rehabilitation phase of a burn injury.
9. A therapeutic measure used to prevent hypertrophic scarring during the rehabilitation phase of burn recovery is
   a. applying pressure garments.
   b. repositioning the patient every 2 hours.
   c. performing active ROM at least every 4 hours.
   d. massaging the new tissue with water-based moisturizers.
10. A patient is recovering from second- and third-degree burns over 30% of his body and the burn care team is planning for discharge. The *first* action the nurse should take when meeting with the patient would be to
   a. arrange a return-to-clinic appointment and prescription for pain medications.
   b. teach the patient and the caregiver proper wound care to be performed at home.
   c. review the patient's current health care status and readiness for discharge to home.
   d. give the patient written information and websites for information for burn survivors.

1. c, 2. a, 3. a, d, e, 4. d, 5. c, 6. a, 7. b, 8. a, c, d, 9. a, 10. c

For rationales to these answers and even more NCLEX review questions, visit *http://evolve.elsevier.com/Lewis/medsurg.*

EVOLVE WEBSITE

http://evolve.elsevier.com/Lewis/medsurg

Review Questions (Online Only)

Key Points

Answer Keys for Questions

- Rationales for Bridge to NCLEX Examination Questions
- Answer Guidelines for Case Study on p. 449
- Answer Guidelines for Managing Care of Multiple Patients Case Study (Section 4) on p. 451

Student Case Study

- Patient With Burns

Nursing Care Plan

- eNursing Care Plan 24-1: Patient With a Thermal Burn Injury

Conceptual Care Map Creator

Audio Glossary

Content Updates

REFERENCES

1. American Burn Association: Burn incidence and treatment in the US: 2013 fact sheet. Retrieved from *www.ameriburn.org/resources?factsheet.php.*
2. WHO International: Burns fact sheet number 365, updated April 2014. Retrieved from *www.Who.int/mediacentrefactsheets/fs365/en.*
3. Peck M: Epidemiology and prevention of burns throughout the world. In Jeschke MG, Kamolz L-P, Sjoberg F, et al, editors: *Handbook of burns: acute burn care,* vol 1, Wein, Austria, 2012, Springer-Verlag.
4. Summers A: Treating cement burns in the emergency department, *Emerg Nurse* 20:30, 2013.
5. Jeschke MG: Critical care of burn victims including inhalation injury. In Jeschke MG, Kamolz L-P, Shahrokhi S, editors: *Burn care and treatment: a practical guide,* Wein, Austria, 2013, Springer-Verlag.

*6. Saracogli A, Kuzucuoglu T, Yakupoglu S, et al: Prognostic factors in electrical burns: a review of 101 patients, *Burns* 40:702, 2014.

7. Burn injury. Retrieved from *www.burninjury.org.*
8. Payne S, Cole E: Treatment of acute burn blisters in unscheduled care settings, *Emerg Nurse* 20:32, 2012.

*9. Morris R, Javed M, Bodger O, et al: A comparison of two smartphone applications and the validation of smartphone applications as tools for fluid calculation for burns resuscitation, *Burns* 40:826, 2014.

10. Somerset A, Coffee R, Jones L, et al: The impact of prediabetes on glycemic control and clinical outcomes post-burn injury, *J Burn Care Res* 35:5, 2014.
11. Rice PL, Orgill DP: Emergency care of moderate and severe thermal burns in adults, 2014. Retrieved from *www.uptodate.com.*
12. Faraklas I, Ghanem M, Brown A, et al: Evaluation of an enoxaparin dosing calculator using burn size and weight, *J Burn Care Res* 34:621, 2013.
13. Culleiton AL, Simko LM: Caring for patients with burn injuries, *Nursing* 43:27, 2013.

*14. Hampson NB, Piantadosi CA, Thom SR, et al: Practice recommendations in the diagnosis, management, and prevention of carbon monoxide poisoning, *Am J Resp Crit Care Med* 186:1095, 2012.

15. Fahlstrom K, Boyle C, Makic MBF: Implementation of a nurse-driven burn resuscitation protocol: a quality improvement project, *Crit Care Nurse* 33:25, 2013.
16. Shahrokhi S: Infections in burns. In Jeschke MG, Kamolz L-P, Shahrokhi S, editors: *Burn care and treatment: a practical guide,* Germany, 2014, Springer Wien.

*17. Scheckter CC, VanVliet MM, Krishnan NM, et al: Cost effectiveness comparison between topical silver sulfadiazine and enclosed silver dressings for partial-thickness burn treatment, *J Burn Care Res* 35:284, 2014.

18. Jeschke MG: Nutrition of the burn patient and treatment of the hypermetabolic response. In Jeschke MG, Kamolz L-P, Shahrokhi S, editors: *Burn care and treatment: a practical guide,* Germany, 2014, Springer Wien.

*19. Nordlund MJ, Pham TN, Gibran NS: Micronutrients after burn injury: a review, *J Burn Care Res* 35:121, 2014.

20. Kamolz L-P: Acute burn surgery. In Jeschke MG, Kamolz L-P, Shahrokhi S, editors: *Burn care and treatment: a practical guide,* Germany, 2014, Springer Wien.

*21. Waltzman JT, Bell DE: Vacuum-assisted closure device as a split-thickness skin graft bolster in the burn population, *J Burn Care Res* 35:e338, 2014.

22. Jeschke MG, Finerty CC, Shahrokhi S, et al: Wound coverage technologies in burn care: novel technologies, *J Burn Care Res* 34:612, 2013.

*23. Jeffs D, Dorman D, Brown S, et al: Effect of virtual reality on adolescent pain during burn wound care, *J Burn Care Res* 35:39, 2014.

*24. Stergiou-Kita M, Grigorovich A, Gomez M: Development of an interprofessional clinical practice guideline for vocational evaluation following severe burn, *Burns* 40:1149, 2014.

*25. Carrougher GJ, Martinez EM, McMullen KS, et al: Pruritus in adult burn survivors: post-burn prevalence and risk factors associated with increased intensity, *J Burn Care Res* 34:94, 2013.

*26. Godleski M, Oeffling A, Bruflat AK, et al: Treating burn-associated joint contracture: results of an inpatient rehabilitation stretching protocol, *J Burn Care Res* 34:420, 2013.

27. Perry IS, Carbullido C, Kowada J, et al: Keeping up with video game technology: objective analysis of XBox Kinect™ and PlayStation 3 Move™ for use in burn rehabilitation, *Burns* 40:852, 2014.
28. Kornhaber R, Wilson A, Abu-Kumar MZ, et al: Coming to terms with it all: adult burn survivors' "lived experience" of acknowledgement and acceptance, *Burns* 40:589, 2014.

*29. Stavrou D, Weissman O, Tessone A, et al: Health-related quality of life in burn patients: a review of the literature, *Burns* 40:788, 2014.

*30. Tolley JS, Foroushani PS: What do we know about one-to-one peer support for adults with a burn injury? A scoping review, *J Burn Care Res* 35:233, 2014.
*31. Goncalves N, Melo A, Caltran MP, et al: Sexuality in burn victims: an integrative literature review, *Burns* 40:552, 2014.
32. Baillie SE, Sellwood W, Wisely JA: Post-traumatic growth in adults following a burn, *Burns* 40:1089, 2014.
*33. Leggatt JM, Wassa K, Sinacore JM, et al: A pilot study examining moral distress in nurses working in one United States burn center, *J Burn Care Res* 34:521, 2013.

*Evidence-based information for clinical practice.

CASE STUDY

Managing Care of Multiple Patients

Introduction

You are working the day shift on a medical-surgical unit and have been assigned to care for the following five patients. You have one UAP who is assigned to work with you. There are 15 other patients on the unit being cared for by an additional 3 RNs and 3 UAP.

Patients

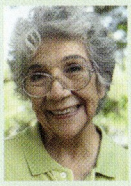

(©Jack Hollingsworth/ Photodisc/ Thinkstock)

F.M., an 81-yr-old Hispanic woman, had pneumatic retinopexy surgery yesterday to repair a partial detached retina. She has a history of type 2 diabetes, hypothyroidism, and hypertension. She is scheduled to be discharged today, but the night nurse is concerned because her BP is elevated at 150/94 mm Hg.

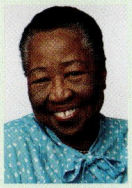

(©Kevin Peterson/ Stockbyte/ Thinkstock)

J.K., a 68-yr-old African American woman with osteoarthritis and type 2 diabetes mellitus for the past 15 years, now has diabetic retinopathy. She had argon laser therapy to her right eye yesterday to seal leaking microaneurysms from macular edema. She was admitted with uncontrolled postoperative hyperglycemia.

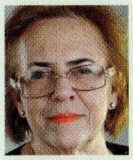

(©Stockphoto/ Thinkstock)

D.A., a 74-yr-old woman, is admitted to the hospital with complaints of chest tightness and shortness of breath. Her past medical history is negative except for a recent diagnosis of basal cell carcinoma (BCC) on her face. She was scheduled to have the BCC surgically removed tomorrow. The health care provider suspects D.A.'s symptoms are caused by anxiety but first needs to rule out any coronary artery disease before surgery.

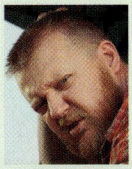

(©Dimedrol68/ iStock/ Thinkstock)

G.L., a 51-yr-old white man, just arrived for admission. He is scheduled for surgical removal of malignant melanoma lesions on his face at 1200. He is worried that the surgery will be disfiguring.

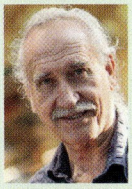

(©Stockphoto/ Thinkstock)

D.B., a 74-yr-old white man, was admitted 3 hours ago from the ED with partial thickness burns on his chest and arms (estimated to be 6% TBSA). He was burning leaves and branches using gasoline. The pile exploded and his clothes caught fire.

Discussion Questions

1. ***Priority Decision:*** After receiving report, which patient should you see first? Provide rationale.
2. ***Teamwork and Collaboration:*** Which tasks could you delegate to the UAP *(select all that apply)*?
   a. Obtain vital signs on F.M.
   b. Take a blood pressure reading on D.B.
   c. Perform an admission assessment on G.L.
   d. Explain planned diagnostic testing to D.A.
   e. Obtain a capillary blood glucose reading on J.K.
3. ***Priority Decision and Teamwork and Collaboration:*** When you enter D.B.'s room, he tells you he is not feeling well. He says he has a headache and his legs are "cramping up." He is also somewhat confused as he is unaware that he is in the hospital. What initial action would be *most* appropriate?
   a. Administer acetaminophen for headache relief.
   b. Have the UAP obtain a stat capillary blood glucose reading.
   c. Notify D.B.'s health care provider of his altered level of consciousness.
   d. Ask the UAP to obtain vital signs on D.B. while you look at his most recent lab work.

Case Study Progression

D.B.'s vital signs are BP 154/88 mm Hg, heart rate is 112 bpm, respirations are 18 breaths/min, and temperature is 98°F (36.8°C). His most recent lab work reveals a serum sodium level of 128 mEq/L (128 mmol/L). You notify his health care provider, who orders a normal saline IV to infuse at 100 mL/hr.

4. D.B. complains of thirst and asks for something to drink. Which fluid would be appropriate to give him *(select all that apply)*?
   a. Gatorade
   b. Tap water
   c. Cola soda
   d. Apple juice
   e. Orange juice
5. In addition to teaching F.M. how to administer postoperative eye drops, you will also explain
   a. position and activity restrictions.
   b. how to change the dressing on her eye.
   c. the necessity for restricting fluid intake.
   d. that protective eyewear will no longer be required.
6. When giving report to your UAP regarding your assigned patients, you are asked by the UAP if there is a significant difference between D.A. and G.L.'s skin cancers. You reply based on knowledge that
   a. basal cell carcinoma is the most deadly form of skin cancer.
   b. malignant melanoma typically appears as red, rough patches on the skin.
   c. basal cell carcinoma typically presents during the second and third decades of life.
   d. melanoma has the ability to metastasize to any organ, including the brain and heart.
7. ***Management Decision:*** Another RN offers to help you by providing care for F.M. Which observed action by the RN would require your immediate intervention?
   a. The RN assists F.M. to lie flat on her back.
   b. The RN gives F.M. oral medication for pain.
   c. The RN assures F.M. that retinal reattachment is usually successful.
   d. The RN explains to F.M. that she is at risk for detachment in the other eye.

Answers available at *http://evolve.elsevier.com/Lewis/medsurg.*
TBSA, Total body surface area.

Problems of Oxygenation: Ventilation

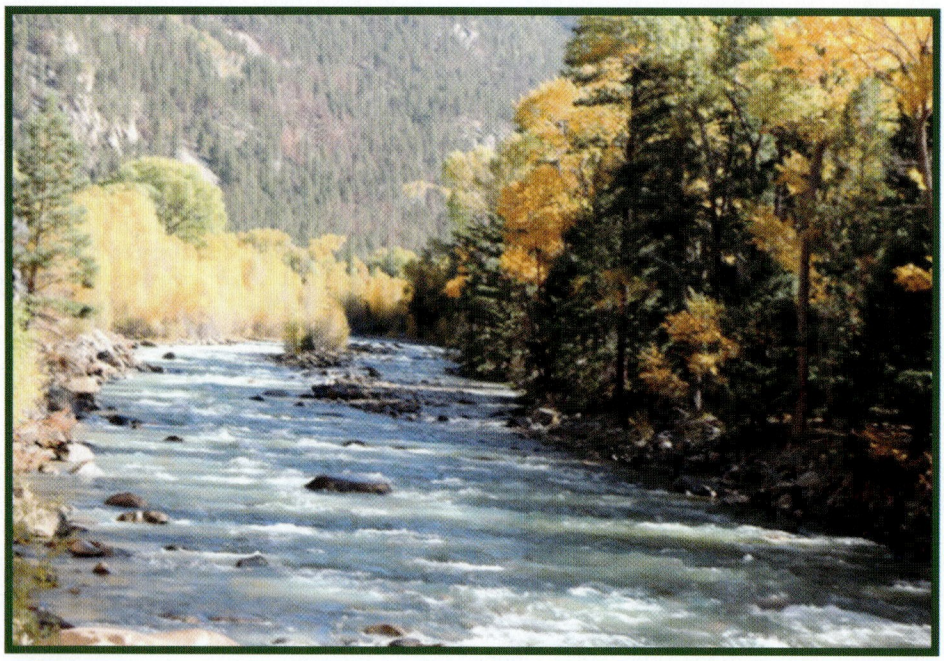

Peter Bonner

The mark of a successful man is one that has spent an entire day on the bank of a river without feeling guilty about it.

Chinese Philosopher

Chapter 25 Assessment of Respiratory System, 453

Chapter 26 Upper Respiratory Problems, 475

Chapter 27 Lower Respiratory Problems, 499

Chapter 28 Obstructive Pulmonary Diseases, 538

25

Assessment of Respiratory System

Eugene E. Mondor

For breath is life, and if you breathe well you will live long on earth.

Sanskrit Proverb

http://evolve.elsevier.com/Lewis/medsurg/

LEARNING OUTCOMES

1. Differentiate among the structures and functions of the upper respiratory tract, lower respiratory tract, and chest wall.
2. Describe the process that initiates and controls inspiration and expiration.
3. Describe the process of oxygenation and ventilation within the lungs.
4. Identify the respiratory defense mechanisms.
5. Describe the significance of arterial blood gas values in relation to respiratory function.
6. Relate the signs and symptoms of inadequate oxygenation to physical assessment findings.
7. Link the age-related changes of the respiratory system to the differences in assessment findings.
8. Obtain significant subjective and objective assessment data related to the respiratory system from a patient.
9. Perform a physical assessment of the respiratory system using the appropriate techniques.
10. Differentiate normal from common abnormal findings in a physical assessment of the respiratory system.
11. Describe the purpose, significance of results, and nursing responsibilities related to diagnostic studies of the respiratory system.

KEY TERMS

adventitious breath sounds, p. 466
chemoreceptor, p. 458
compliance, p. 456
crackles, Table 25-8, p. 468
dyspnea, p. 456
elastic recoil, p. 456
fremitus, p. 464
mechanical receptors, p. 458
oxygenation, p. 456
pleural friction rub, Table 25-8, p. 468
resistance, p. 456
surfactant, p. 455
tidal volume (V_T), p. 454
ventilation, p. 456
wheezes, Table 25-8, p. 468

STRUCTURES AND FUNCTIONS OF RESPIRATORY SYSTEM

The primary purpose of the respiratory system is gas exchange. This involves the transfer of O_2 and CO_2 between the atmosphere and blood. The respiratory system is divided into two parts: upper respiratory tract and lower respiratory tract (Fig. 25-1).

Upper Respiratory Tract

The *upper respiratory tract* includes the nose, mouth, pharynx, epiglottis, larynx, and trachea. Air enters into the respiratory tract through the nose. The nose is made of bone and cartilage and is divided into two nares by the nasal septum. The inside of the nose is shaped into three passages by projections called *turbinates.* The turbinates increase the surface area of the nasal mucosa, which warms and moistens the air as it enters the nose. The internal nose opens directly into the sinuses. The nasal cavity connects with the pharynx, a tubular passageway that is subdivided into three parts: the *nasopharynx, oropharynx,* and *laryngopharynx.*

The nose functions to protect the lower airway by warming and humidifying air and filtering small particles before air enters the lungs. Olfactory nerve endings, located in the roof of the nose, are responsible for the sense of smell.

Air moves through the oropharynx to the laryngopharynx. It then travels through the epiglottis to the larynx before moving into the trachea. The *epiglottis* is a small flap located behind the tongue that closes over the larynx during swallowing. This prevents solids and liquids from entering the lungs. The vocal cords are located in the larynx. Air passes through the glottis (the opening between the vocal cords) and into the trachea. The trachea is a cylindrical tube about 5 in (10 to 12 cm) long and 1 in (1.5 to 2.5 cm) in diameter. U-shaped cartilages keep the trachea open but allow the adjacent esophagus to expand for swallowing. The trachea bifurcates into the right and left mainstem bronchi at a point called the *carina.* The carina is located at the level of the manubriosternal junction, also called the

Reviewed by Donna C. Bond, RN, DNP, CCNS, AE-C, CTTS, Pulmonary Clinical Nurse Specialist, Carilion Clinic, Roanoke, Virginia; Deborah Cline, RN, MS, Nursing Faculty, Carrington College, Reno, Nevada; and Cynthia M. Steinwedel, RN, PhD, CNE, Assistant Professor, Department of Nursing, Bradley University, Peoria, Illinois.

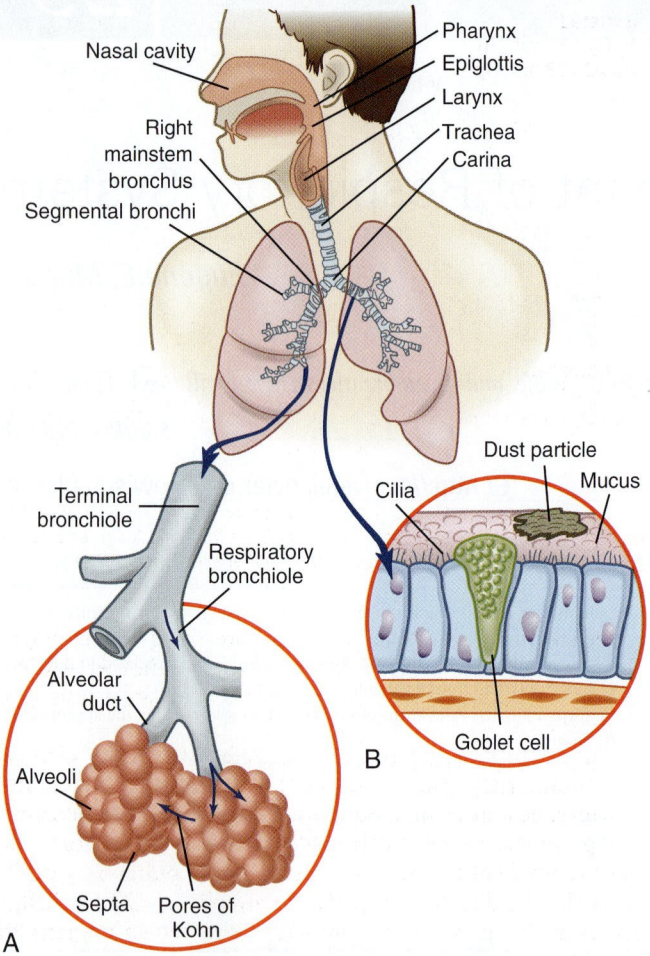

FIG. 25-1 Structures of the respiratory tract. **A,** Pulmonary functional unit. **B,** Ciliated mucous membrane. (Redrawn from Price SA, Wilson LM: *Pathophysiology: clinical concepts of disease processes,* ed 6, St Louis, 2003, Mosby.)

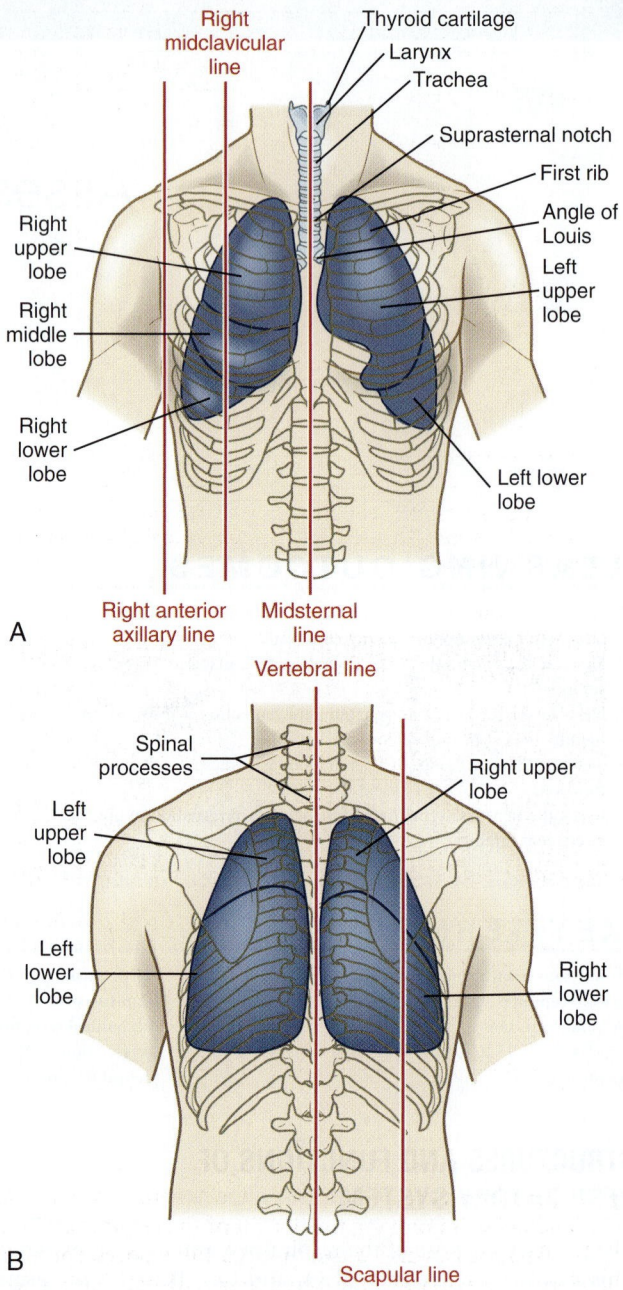

FIG. 25-2 Landmarks and structures of the chest wall. **A,** Anterior view. **B,** Posterior view. (Redrawn from Thompson JM, McFarland GK, Hirsch JE, Tucker SM: *Mosby's clinical nursing,* ed 5, St Louis, 2002, Mosby.)

angle of Louis. The carina is highly sensitive, and stimulation of this area during suctioning causes vigorous coughing.[1]

Lower Respiratory Tract

Once air passes the carina, it is in the lower respiratory tract. The *lower respiratory tract* consists of the bronchi, bronchioles, alveolar ducts, and alveoli. With the exception of the right and left mainstem bronchi, all lower airway structures are located inside the lungs. The right lung is divided into three lobes (upper, middle, and lower) and the left lung into two lobes (upper and lower) (Fig. 25-2). The structures of the chest wall (ribs, pleura, muscles of respiration) are also important for respiration.

The mainstem bronchi, pulmonary vessels, and nerves enter the lungs through a slit called the *hilus.* The right mainstem bronchus is shorter, wider, and straighter than the left mainstem bronchus. For this reason, aspiration is more likely to occur in the right lung than in the left lung.

The mainstem bronchi subdivide several times to form the lobar, segmental, and subsegmental bronchi. Further divisions form the bronchioles. The most distant bronchioles are called the respiratory bronchioles. Beyond these lie the alveolar ducts and alveoli (Fig. 25-3). The bronchioles are encircled by smooth muscles that constrict and dilate in response to various stimuli. The terms *bronchoconstriction* and *bronchodilation* refer to a decrease or increase in the diameter of the airways caused by contraction or relaxation of these muscles.

The trachea and bronchi act as a pathway to conduct gases to and from the alveoli. The trachea plus the bronchi are called *anatomic dead space* (V_D). The air filling this space does not participate in gas exchange. In adults a normal tidal volume (V_T), or volume of air exchanged with each breath, is about 500 mL (in a 150-lb man). Of each 500 mL inhaled, about 150 mL is V_D.

After moving through the V_D, air reaches the respiratory bronchioles and alveoli (Fig. 25-4). *Alveoli* are small sacs in the lungs that are the primary site of gas exchange for O_2 and CO_2. The adult lung has over 300 million alveoli, each 0.3 mm in diameter. The alveoli are interconnected by pores of Kohn,[1,2]

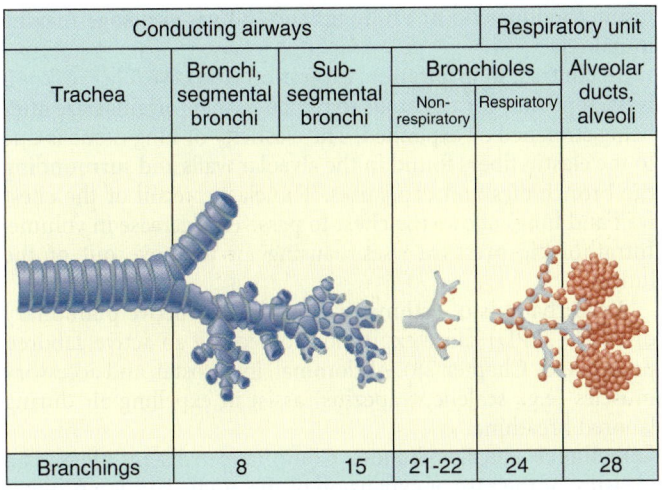

FIG. 25-3 Structures of lower airways. (Redrawn from Thompson JM, McFarland GK, Hirsch JE, Tucker SM: *Mosby's clinical nursing,* ed 5, St Louis, 2002, Mosby.)

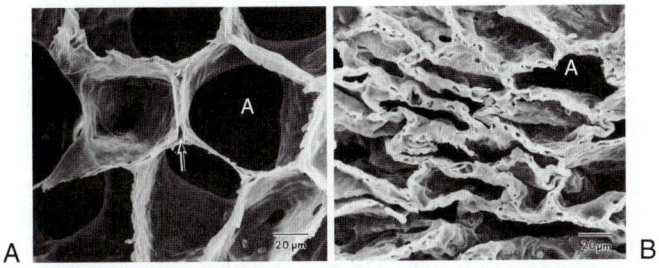

FIG. 25-4 Scanning electron micrograph of lung parenchyma. **A,** Alveoli *(A)* and alveolar-capillary membrane *(arrow).* **B,** Effects of atelectasis. Alveoli *(A)* are partially or totally collapsed. (*A,* From Dantzker DR, Bone RC, George RB, editors: *Pulmonary and critical care medicine,* vol 1, St Louis, 1993, Mosby. *B,* From Albertine KH, Williams MC, Hyde DM: Anatomy of the lungs. In RJ Mason, VC Broaddus, JF Murray, et al, editors: *Murray and Nadel's textbook of respiratory medicine,* ed 4, Philadelphia, 2005, Saunders.)

which allow movement of air from alveolus to alveolus (Fig. 25-1). Deep breathing promotes air movement through these pores and assists in moving mucus out of the respiratory bronchioles. Bacteria can also move through these pores, spreading infection to previously uninfected areas. Alveoli have a total volume of about 2500 mL and a surface area for gas exchange that is about the size of a tennis court.

Gases are exchanged at the alveolar-capillary membrane, where the alveoli come in contact with pulmonary capillaries (Fig. 25-5). In conditions such as pulmonary edema, excess fluid fills the interstitial space and alveoli, markedly reducing gas exchange.

Surfactant. Because alveoli are unstable, they have a natural tendency to collapse. Alveolar cells secrete surfactant. **Surfactant** is a lipoprotein that lowers the surface tension in the alveoli.[3] It reduces the amount of pressure needed to inflate the alveoli and makes them less likely to collapse. Normally, each person takes a slightly larger breath, termed a *sigh,* after every five or six breaths. This sigh stretches the alveoli and promotes surfactant secretion.

When not enough surfactant is present, the alveoli collapse. The term *atelectasis* refers to collapsed, airless alveoli (Fig. 25-4, *B*). The postoperative patient is at risk for atelectasis because of

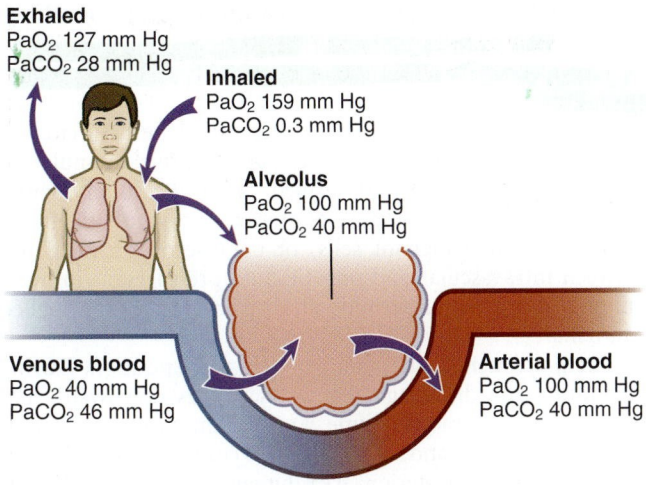

FIG. 25-5 Partial pressure of respiratory gases in normal respiration. The pressures are shown in inhaled and exhaled air from the lungs and at the level of the alveoli and pulmonary venous and arterial blood vessels.

the effects of anesthesia and restricted breathing with pain (see Chapter 19). In acute respiratory distress syndrome (ARDS), lack of surfactant contributes to widespread atelectasis (see Chapter 67).

Blood Supply. The lungs have two different types of circulation: pulmonary and bronchial. The pulmonary circulation provides the lungs with blood that participates in gas exchange. The pulmonary artery receives deoxygenated blood from the right ventricle of the heart and delivers it to pulmonary capillaries that lie directly alongside the alveoli. O_2–CO_2 exchange occurs at this point. The pulmonary veins return oxygenated blood to the left atrium, which then delivers it to the left ventricle. This oxygenated blood is pumped by the left ventricle into the aorta, which supplies the arteries of the systemic circulation. Venous blood is collected from capillary networks of the body and returned to the right atrium by way of the superior and inferior vena cava.

The *bronchial circulation* starts with the bronchial arteries, which arise from the thoracic aorta. The bronchial circulation provides O_2 to the bronchi and other pulmonary tissues. Deoxygenated blood returns from the bronchial circulation through the azygos vein into the superior vena cava.

Chest Wall

The chest wall is shaped, supported, and protected by 24 ribs (12 on each side). The ribs and sternum protect the lungs and the heart from injury and are called the *thoracic cage.* The *mediastinum* is the space in the middle of the thoracic cavity. It contains many major organs of the chest, including the heart, aorta, and esophagus. The mediastinum physically separates the right and left lungs into two separate compartments.

The chest cavity is lined with a membrane called the *parietal pleura,* and the lungs are lined with a membrane called the *visceral pleura.* The parietal and visceral pleurae join to form a closed, double-walled sac. The visceral pleura does not have any sensory pain fibers or nerve endings, whereas the parietal pleura does have sensory pain fibers. Therefore irritation and inflammation of the parietal pleura causes pain with each breath.

The space between the pleural layers is called the *intrapleural space.* Normally this space contains 20 to 25 mL of fluid. This fluid serves two purposes: (1) it provides lubrication, allowing the pleural layers to slide over each other during breathing; and (2) it increases cohesion between the pleural layers, thereby facilitating expansion of the pleurae and lungs during inspiration.

Fluid drains from the pleural space by the lymphatic circulation. Several pathologic conditions may cause the accumulation of greater amounts of fluid, termed a *pleural effusion.* Pleural fluid may accumulate because of blockage of lymphatic drainage (e.g., from malignant cells) or because of an imbalance between intravascular and oncotic fluid pressures, as in heart failure. Purulent pleural fluid with bacterial infection is called *empyema.*

The *diaphragm* is the major muscle of respiration. During inspiration the diaphragm contracts, moves downward, and increases intrathoracic volume. At the same time the external intercostal muscles and scalene muscles contract, increasing the lateral and anteroposterior (AP) dimension of the chest. This causes the size of the thoracic cavity to increase and intrathoracic pressure to decrease, so air is pulled into the lungs.

The diaphragm is made up of two hemidiaphragms, each innervated by the right and left phrenic nerves. The phrenic nerves arise from the spinal cord between C3 and C5, the third and fifth cervical vertebrae. Injury to the phrenic nerve results in hemidiaphragm paralysis on the side of the injury. Complete spinal cord injuries above the level of C3 result in total diaphragm paralysis and dependence on a mechanical ventilator.

Physiology of Respiration

Oxygenation. Oxygenation refers to the process of obtaining O_2 from the atmospheric air and making it available to the organs and tissues of the body. The lungs' ability to oxygenate arterial blood adequately is assessed by clinical assessment of the patient (Table 25-2), partial pressure of O_2 in arterial blood (PaO_2), and arterial O_2 saturation (SaO_2).

O_2 is carried in the blood in two forms: dissolved O_2 and hemoglobin-bound O_2. The PaO_2 represents the amount of O_2 dissolved in the plasma and is expressed in millimeters of mercury (mm Hg). The SaO_2 is the amount of O_2 bound to hemoglobin in comparison with the amount of O_2 the hemoglobin can carry. The SaO_2 is expressed as a percentage. For example, if the SaO_2 is 90%, this means that 90% of the hemoglobin attachments for O_2 have O_2 bound to them.

O_2 and CO_2 move back and forth across the alveolar-capillary membrane by diffusion. The overall direction of movement is from the area of higher concentration to the area of lower concentration. Thus O_2 moves from alveolar gas (atmospheric air) into the arterial blood and CO_2 from the arterial blood into the alveolar gas. Diffusion continues until equilibrium is reached.

Ventilation. Ventilation involves *inspiration,* or inhalation (movement of air into the lungs), and *expiration,* or exhalation (movement of air out of the lungs). Air moves in and out of the lungs because intrathoracic pressure changes in relation to pressure at the airway opening. Contraction of the diaphragm and intercostal and scalene muscles increases chest dimensions, thereby decreasing intrathoracic pressure. Gas flows from an area of higher pressure (atmospheric) to one of lower pressure (intrathoracic). When dyspnea (shortness of breath) occurs, neck and shoulder muscles can assist the effort. Some conditions (e.g., phrenic nerve paralysis, rib fractures, neuromuscular disease) may limit diaphragm or chest wall movement and cause the patient to breathe with smaller tidal volumes. As a result, the lungs do not fully inflate, and gas exchange may be impaired.

In contrast to inspiration, expiration is passive. Elastic recoil is the tendency for the lungs to return to their original size after being stretched or expanded. The elasticity of lung tissue is due to the elastin fibers found in the alveolar walls and surrounding the bronchioles and capillaries. The elastic recoil of the chest wall and lungs allows the chest to passively decrease in volume. Intrathoracic pressure rises, causing air to move out of the lungs.

Exacerbations of asthma or chronic obstructive pulmonary disease (COPD) cause expiration to become an active, labored process (see Chapter 28). Abdominal, intercostal, and accessory muscles (e.g., scalene, trapezius) assist in expelling air during labored breathing.

Compliance and Resistance. Compliance (distensibility) is a measure of the ease of expansion of the lungs. This is a product of the elasticity of the lungs and elastic recoil of the chest wall.[4] When compliance is decreased, the lungs are more difficult to inflate. Examples include conditions that increase fluid in the lungs (e.g., pulmonary edema, ARDS, pneumonia), conditions that make lung tissue less elastic or distensible (e.g., pulmonary fibrosis, sarcoidosis), and conditions that restrict lung movement (e.g., pleural effusion). Compliance is increased when there is destruction of alveolar walls and loss of tissue elasticity, as in COPD.

On the other hand, resistance refers to any impediment to airflow during inspiration and expiration. Airway resistance is primarily affected by changes in the diameter (size) of the airways. For example, a patient with an acute asthma attack has narrowed airways, resulting in increased resistance. Smaller-size airways make it more difficult for patients to get air into their lungs. The presence of secretions in the bronchi also increases resistance. The administration of bronchodilators decreases resistance by increasing the diameter of the bronchi, facilitating air entry into the lungs.

Changes in either compliance and/or resistance have the ability to seriously affect both oxygenation and ventilation of the patient.

Arterial Blood Gases. Two methods are used to assess the efficiency of gas transfer in the lung and tissue oxygenation: (1) analysis of *arterial blood gases* (ABGs) and (2) pulse oximetry. ABGs are measured to determine oxygenation status and acid-base balance. ABG analysis includes measurement of the PaO_2, $PaCO_2$ (the partial pressure of CO_2 in arterial blood), acidity (pH), bicarbonate (HCO_3^-), and SaO_2. Normal values for ABGs are given in Table 25-1.

Blood for ABG analysis can be obtained by arterial puncture or from an arterial catheter, which is usually in the radial or femoral artery. Both techniques allow only intermittent analysis. Continuous intraarterial blood gas monitoring is also possible via a fiberoptic sensor or an O_2 electrode inserted into an arterial catheter. An arterial catheter permits ABG sampling without repeated arterial punctures.

The normal PaO_2 decreases with advancing age. It also varies in relation to the distance above sea level. At higher altitudes the barometric pressure is lower, resulting in a lower inspired O_2 pressure and a lower PaO_2 (Table 25-1).

Mixed Venous Blood Gases. For the patient with a normal or near-normal cardiac status, assessment of PaO_2 or SaO_2 is usually sufficient to determine the level of oxygenation. The patient with impaired cardiac output or hemodynamic

TABLE 25-1 Normal Arterial and Venous Blood Gas Values*

	ARTERIAL BLOOD GASES		VENOUS BLOOD GASES	
Laboratory Value	**Sea Level BP 760 mm Hg**	**1 Mile Above Sea Level BP 629 mm Hg**	**Mixed Venous Blood Gases**	
pH	7.35-7.45	7.35-7.45	pH	7.32-7.43
PaO_2†	80-100 mm Hg	65-75 mm Hg	PvO_2	38-42 mm Hg
SaO_2†	>95%‡	>95%‡	SvO_2	60%-80%‡
$PaCO_2$	35-45 mm Hg	35-45 mm Hg	$PvCO_2$	38-55 mm Hg
HCO_3^-	22-26 mEq/L (mmol/L)	22-26 mEq/L (mmol/L)	HCO_3^-	22-26 mEq/L (mmol/L)

BP, Barometric pressure; *HCO_3^-*, bicarbonate; *PaO_2*, partial pressure of O_2 in arterial blood; *$PaCO_2$*, partial pressure of arterial CO_2; *$PvCO_2$*, partial pressure of CO_2 in venous blood; *PvO_2*, partial pressure of O_2 in venous blood; *SaO_2*, arterial O_2 saturation; *SvO_2*, venous O_2 saturation.
HCO_3^-, BE (base excess), and SaO_2 are all calculated values unless identified as "measured."
*Assumes patient is ≤60 yr of age and breathing room air.
†Values decrease with age.
‡The same normal values apply when SpO_2 and SvO_2 are obtained by oximetry.

instability (e.g., altered level of consciousness, alterations in heart rate and rhythm, low BP) may have inadequate tissue O_2 delivery or abnormal O_2 consumption.

The amount of O_2 delivered to the tissues or consumed can be calculated. A catheter positioned in the pulmonary artery, termed a *pulmonary artery (PA) catheter*, is used for mixed venous sampling (see Chapter 65). Blood drawn from a PA catheter is termed a *mixed venous blood gas* (SvO_2) sample because it consists of venous blood that has returned to the right side of the heart from all parts of the body and "mixes" in the right ventricle. Normal SvO_2 is 60% to 80%. Other normal mixed venous values are given in Table 25-1.

SvO_2 can be monitored intermittently by obtaining a blood sample from the PA catheter. A decrease in SvO_2 suggests that less O_2 is being delivered to the tissues or that more O_2 is being consumed. Changes in SvO_2 provide an early warning of a change in cardiac output or tissue O_2 delivery.

Oximetry. Arterial O_2 saturation can be monitored noninvasively and continuously using a *pulse oximetry* probe on the finger, toe, ear, or bridge of the nose. The abbreviation SpO_2 is used to indicate the O_2 saturation of hemoglobin as measured by pulse oximetry.[5] SpO_2 and heart rate are displayed on the monitor as digital readings. Normal SpO_2 values are 94% to 99%.

SpO_2 is assessed with each routine vital sign check in many inpatient areas. Oximetry is also used during exercise testing and when adjusting flow rates during long-term O_2 therapy. Pulse oximetry is particularly valuable in intensive care and perioperative situations, in which sedation or decreased consciousness may mask hypoxia (Table 25-2). Changes in SpO_2 can be detected quickly and treated immediately (Table 25-3).

Values obtained by pulse oximetry are less accurate if the SpO_2 is less than 70%. At this level the oximeter may display a value that is ±4% of the actual value. For example, if the SpO_2 reading is 70%, the actual value can range from 66% to 74%. Pulse oximetry is also inaccurate if hemoglobin variants (e.g., carboxyhemoglobin, methemoglobin) are present. Other factors that can alter the accuracy of pulse oximetry include motion, low perfusion, anemia, cold extremities, bright fluorescent lights, intravascular dyes, thick acrylic nails, and dark skin color. If there is doubt about the accuracy of the SpO_2 reading, obtain an ABG analysis to verify the results.

CO_2 Monitoring. CO_2 can be monitored using transcutaneous CO_2 ($PtcCO_2$) and end-tidal CO_2 ($PetCO_2$) capnography. Transcutaneous measurement of CO_2 is a noninvasive method of estimating arterial pressure of CO_2 ($PaCO_2$) using an electrode placed on the skin.

TABLE 25-2 Manifestations of Inadequate Oxygenation

	ONSET	
Manifestations	**Early**	**Late**
Central Nervous System		
Unexplained apprehension	X	
Unexplained restlessness or irritability	X	
Unexplained confusion or lethargy	X	X
Combativeness		X
Coma		X
Respiratory		
Tachypnea	X	
Dyspnea on exertion	X	
Dyspnea at rest		X
Use of accessory muscles		X
Retraction of interspaces on inspiration		X
Pause for breath between sentences, words		X
Cardiovascular		
Tachycardia	X	
Mild hypertension	X	
Dysrhythmias	X	X
Hypotension		X
Cyanosis		X
Cool, clammy skin		X
Other		
Diaphoresis	X	X
Decreased urine output	X	X
Unexplained fatigue	X	X

$PetCO_2$ is the noninvasive measurement of alveolar CO_2 during exhalation when CO_2 concentration is at its peak. It is used to monitor and assess trends in the patient's ventilatory status. Expired gases are sampled from the patient's airway and are analyzed by a CO_2 sensor that uses infrared light to measure exhaled CO_2.[6] The sensor may be attached to an adaptor on the endotracheal tube or the tracheostomy tube. A nasal cannula with a sidestream capnometer can be used in patients without an artificial airway. Capnography is usually presented as a graph of expiratory CO_2 plotted against time.

In the past, capnography was used mainly intraoperatively, postoperatively, and in critical care units. Today's monitors are portable and practical for use in emergency departments and on inpatient units.

Measurement of O_2 saturation (oximetry) is primarily used to assess for hypoxia. CO_2 monitoring assesses for hypercapnia. The use of both measures together is important in determining the patient's oxygenation and ventilatory status.

TABLE 25-3 Normal and Critical Values for PaO_2 and SpO_2

PaO_2 (mm Hg)	SpO_2 (%)	Significance	Manifestations	Management
80-100	≥94	Normal value	Asymptomatic	• Routine assessment of patient
60-79	90	Mild hypoxemia	Restlessness, tachycardia, dysrhythmias, dyspnea, hypertension	• Assess patient condition as necessary • Supplemental O_2 may be required
40-59	88	Moderate hypoxemia	Confusion, lethargy, dysrhythmias, hypotension, respiratory distress, accessory muscle use	• O_2 required • Escalate level of care. Obtain critical care consult • Monitor frequently for sudden deterioration in condition
<40	75	Severe hypoxemia	Cyanosis, coma, respiratory and/or cardiac arrest possible	• High FIO_2, intubation, mechanical ventilation • Continuous patient assessment and evaluation

Control of Respiration

The respiratory center in the medulla (located in the brainstem) responds to chemical and mechanical signals. Impulses are sent from the medulla to the respiratory muscles through the spinal cord and phrenic nerves.

Chemoreceptors. A **chemoreceptor** is a receptor that responds to a change in the chemical composition ($PaCO_2$ and pH) of the fluid around it. Central chemoreceptors are located in the medulla and respond to changes in the hydrogen ion (H^+) concentration. An increase in the H^+ concentration *(acidosis)* causes the medulla to increase the respiratory rate and tidal volume (V_T). A decrease in H^+ concentration *(alkalosis)* has the opposite effect. Changes in $PaCO_2$ regulate ventilation primarily by their effect on the pH of the cerebrospinal fluid. When the $PaCO_2$ level is increased, more CO_2 is available to combine with H_2O and form carbonic acid (H_2CO_3). This lowers the cerebrospinal fluid pH and stimulates an increase in respiratory rate. The opposite process occurs with a decrease in $PaCO_2$ level.

Peripheral chemoreceptors are located in the carotid bodies at the bifurcation of the common carotid arteries and in the aortic bodies above and below the aortic arch. The peripheral chemoreceptors respond to decreases in PaO_2 and pH and to increases in $PaCO_2$. These changes also stimulate the respiratory center.

In a healthy person an increase in $PaCO_2$ or a decrease in pH causes an immediate increase in the respiratory rate. The $PaCO_2$ does not vary more than about 3 mm Hg if lung function is normal. Conditions such as COPD alter lung function and may result in chronically elevated $PaCO_2$ levels. In these instances, the patient is relatively insensitive to further increases in $PaCO_2$ as a stimulus to breathe and may be maintaining ventilation largely because of a hypoxic drive from the peripheral chemoreceptors (see Chapter 28).

Mechanical Receptors. **Mechanical receptors** (juxtacapillary and irritant) are located in the lungs, upper airways, chest wall, and diaphragm. They are stimulated by a variety of physiologic factors, such as irritants, muscle stretching, and alveolar wall distortion. Signals from the stretch receptors aid in the control of respiration. As the lungs inflate, pulmonary stretch receptors activate the inspiratory center to inhibit further lung expansion. This is termed the *Hering-Breuer reflex,* and it prevents overdistention of the lungs. Impulses from the mechanical sensors are sent through the vagus nerve to the brain. The stimulation of juxtacapillary receptors causes the rapid respiration (tachypnea) seen in pulmonary edema. These receptors are stimulated by fluid entering the pulmonary interstitial space.

Respiratory Defense Mechanisms

Respiratory defense mechanisms are efficient in protecting the lungs from inhaled particles, microorganisms, and toxic gases. The defense mechanisms include the filtration of air, mucociliary clearance system, cough reflex, reflex bronchoconstriction, and alveolar macrophages.

Filtration of Air. Nasal hairs filter inspired air. In addition, the abrupt changes in direction of airflow that occur as air moves through the nasopharynx and larynx increase air turbulence. This causes particles and bacteria to contact the mucosa lining these structures. Most large particles (greater than 5 μm) are less dangerous because they are removed in the nasopharynx or bronchi and do not reach the alveoli.

The velocity of airflow slows greatly after it passes the larynx, facilitating the deposition of smaller particles (1 to 5 μm). They settle out the way that sand does in a river, a process termed *sedimentation.* Particles less than 1 μm in size are too small to settle in this manner and are deposited in the alveoli. An example of small particles that can build up is coal dust, which can lead to pneumoconiosis (see Chapter 27).

Mucociliary Clearance System. Below the larynx, the movement of mucus is accomplished by the mucociliary clearance system, commonly referred to as the *mucociliary escalator.* This term is used to indicate the relationship between the secretion of mucus and the ciliary activity. Mucus is continuously secreted at a rate of about 100 mL/day by goblet cells and submucosal glands. It forms a mucous blanket that contains the impacted particles and debris from distal lung areas (Fig. 25-1). The small amount of mucus normally secreted is swallowed without being noticed. Secretory immunoglobulin A (IgA) in the mucus helps protect against bacteria and viruses.

Cilia cover the airways from the level of the trachea to the respiratory bronchioles (Fig. 25-1). Each ciliated cell contains approximately 200 cilia, which beat rhythmically about 1000 times per minute in the large airways, moving mucus toward the mouth. The ciliary beat is slower further down the tracheobronchial tree. As a consequence, particles that penetrate more deeply into the airways are removed less rapidly. Ciliary action is impaired by dehydration, smoking, inhalation of high O_2 concentrations, infection, and ingestion of drugs such as atropine, anesthetics, alcohol, or cocaine. Patients with COPD and cystic fibrosis have repeated lower respiratory tract infections. In these conditions cilia are often destroyed, resulting in impaired secretion clearance, a chronic productive cough, and chronic colonization by bacteria, which leads to frequent respiratory tract infections.

Cough Reflex. The cough is a protective reflex action that clears the airway by a high-pressure, high-velocity flow of air. It is a backup for mucociliary clearance, especially when this clearance mechanism is overwhelmed or ineffective. Coughing is only effective in removing secretions above the subsegmental level (large or main airways). Secretions below this level must be moved upward by the mucociliary mechanism before they can be removed by coughing.

Reflex Bronchoconstriction. *Reflex bronchoconstriction* is another defense mechanism. In response to the inhalation of large amounts of irritating substances (e.g., dusts, aerosols), the bronchi constrict in an effort to prevent entry of the irritants. A person with hyperreactive airways, such as a person with asthma, may experience bronchoconstriction after inhalation of triggers such as cold air, perfume, or other strong odors.

Alveolar Macrophages. Because ciliated cells are not found below the level of the respiratory bronchioles, the primary defense mechanism at the alveolar level is alveolar macrophages. *Alveolar macrophages* rapidly phagocytize inhaled foreign particles such as bacteria. The debris is moved to the level of the bronchioles for removal by the cilia or removed from the lungs by the lymphatic system. Particles (e.g., coal dust, silica) that cannot be adequately phagocytized tend to remain in the lungs for indefinite periods and can stimulate inflammatory responses (see Chapter 27). Because alveolar macrophage activity is impaired by cigarette smoke, the smoker who is employed in an occupation with heavy dust exposure (e.g., mining, foundries) is at an especially high risk for lung disease.

Gerontologic Considerations: Effects of Aging on Respiratory System

Age-related changes in the respiratory system can be divided into alterations in structure, defense mechanisms, and respiratory control (Table 25-4). Structural changes include calcification of the costal cartilages, which can interfere with chest expansion. The outward curvature of the spine is marked, especially with osteoporosis, and the lumbar curve flattens. Therefore the chest may appear barrel shaped, and the older person may need to use accessory muscles to breathe. Respiratory muscle strength progressively declines after age 50. Overall, the lungs in the older adult are harder to inflate.

Within the lung, the number of functional alveoli decreases, and they become less elastic. Small airways in the lung bases close earlier in expiration. As a consequence, more inspired air is distributed to the lung apices and ventilation is less well matched to perfusion, lowering the PaO_2. Therefore older adults have less tolerance for exertion, and dyspnea can occur if their activity exceeds their normal exercise.

In older adults *respiratory defense mechanisms* are less effective because of a decline in both cell-mediated and humoral immunity (ability to produce antibodies). The alveolar macrophages are less effective at phagocytosis. An older patient has a less forceful cough and fewer and less functional cilia. Mucous membranes tend to be drier. Retained mucus predisposes the older adult to respiratory tract infections. Formation of secretory IgA, an important defense mechanism, is diminished. Swallowing is slower because of transit time in the pharyngeal area, and there is reduced sensation in the pharynx. If the older adult patient has a superimposed neurologic condition (e.g., stroke), aspiration is more likely.

Respiratory control is also altered as a result of the aging process, resulting in a more gradual response to changes in blood O_2 or CO_2 level. The PaO_2 may drop to a slightly lower than normal level, and the $PaCO_2$ may rise to a slightly higher than normal level before the respiratory rate changes.

The extent of these changes in people of the same age varies greatly. The older adult who has a significant smoking history, is obese, and has a chronic illness is at greatest risk of adverse outcomes.

TABLE 25-4 Gerontologic Assessment Differences

Respiratory System

Changes	Differences in Assessment Findings
Structures	
Chest wall stiffening Costal cartilage calcification ↑ Anteroposterior diameter ↓ Elastic recoil ↓ Chest wall compliance ↓ Functioning alveoli ↓ Respiratory muscle strength	Barrel chest appearance, kyphotic posture, ↓ chest wall movement, ↓ deep breathing Mucus thickened ↓ Vital capacity, ↑ residual volume, ↑ functional residual capacity Diminished breath sounds, particularly at lung bases ↓ PaO_2 and SaO_2, normal pH and $PaCO_2$
Defense Mechanisms	
↓ Cell-mediated immunity ↓ Specific antibodies ↓ Cilia function ↓ Cough force ↓ Alveolar macrophage function ↓ Sensation in pharynx	↓ Cough effectiveness, ↓ secretion clearance ↑ Risk of upper respiratory aspiration, infection, influenza, pneumonia Respiratory infections may be more severe and last longer
Respiratory Control	
↓ Response to hypoxemia ↓ Response to hypercapnia	Slight ↓ in PaO_2 and ↑ in $PaCO_2$ before respiratory rate changes ↓ Ability to maintain acid-base balance Significant hypoxemia or hypercapnia may develop from relatively small incidents Retained secretions, excessive sedation, or positioning that impairs chest expansion may substantially alter PaO_2 or SpO_2 values

ASSESSMENT OF RESPIRATORY SYSTEM

Determining a patient's needs related to the respiratory system requires an accurate health history and a thorough physical examination.[7] A respiratory assessment can be done as part of a comprehensive physical examination or as a focused respiratory examination. Use judgment in determining whether all or part of the history and physical examination will be completed based on the patient's problems and degree of respiratory distress. If respiratory distress is severe, only obtain pertinent information and defer a thorough assessment until the patient's condition stabilizes.

Subjective Data

Important Health Information

Past Health History. It is important to determine the frequency of upper respiratory problems (e.g., colds, sore throats, sinus problems, allergies) and whether seasonal changes have an effect on these problems. Question the patient with allergies about possible precipitating factors or triggers such as medications, pollen, smoke, mold, or pet exposure. Document the characteristics and severity of the allergic reaction such as runny nose, wheezing, scratchy throat, or chest tightness. Inquire about a past history of lower respiratory problems, such as asthma, COPD, pneumonia, and tuberculosis (TB). Also determine the frequency of asthma exacerbations and triggers, if

CASE STUDY

Patient Introduction

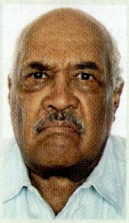

(©Fuse/ Thinkstock)

F.T. is a 70-year-old African American man who comes to the emergency department (ED) complaining of increased shortness of breath. He states that he started using his albuterol inhaler every 4 hours a few days ago, but it does not seem to be helping. He has been having trouble sleeping or doing any activity because of his shortness of breath.

Discussion Questions

1. What are the possible causes of F.T.'s shortness of breath?
2. Does F.T. require urgent admission to the hospital or is his condition stable and he can be seen by an HCP in a few hours?

You will learn more about F.T. and his condition as you read through this assessment chapter.

(See p. 463 for more information on F.T.)

Answers available at *http://evolve.elsevier.com/Lewis/medsurg.*

known. Because respiratory symptoms are often manifestations of problems that involve other body systems, it is important to ask about a history of additional health problems. For example, the patient with cardiac dysfunction may experience dyspnea (shortness of breath) as a consequence of heart failure. The patient with human immunodeficiency virus (HIV) infection may experience frequent respiratory tract infections because immune function is compromised.

Medications. Take a thorough medication history, including both prescription and over-the-counter medications. Ask about the reason for taking the medication, its name, the dose and frequency, length of time taken, its effect, and any side effects. Assess for overuse of short-term bronchodilators as a key indicator of symptom control, since this information will help guide management. Inquire about the use of an angiotensin-converting enzyme (ACE) inhibitor, since cough is a relatively common side effect of this class of drugs. Encourage the patient to bring her or his medication bottles and any inhalers to each visit with an HCP.

If the patient is using O_2 for a breathing problem, document the fraction of inspired O_2 concentration (FIO_2), flow rate (liters per minute), method of administration, number of hours used per day, and effectiveness of the therapy. Assess safety practices, including the patient's cognitive and physical ability related to using O_2 and any metered-dose inhalers.

Surgery or Other Treatments. Determine if the patient has been hospitalized for a respiratory problem. Note the dates, therapy (including surgery), and current status of the problem. Determine if the patient has ever been intubated because of a respiratory problem. Ask about the use of and response to respiratory treatments such as a nebulizer, humidifier, airway clearance modalities (see Chapter 28), high-frequency chest wall oscillation, postural drainage, and percussion.

Functional Health Patterns. Health history questions to ask a patient with a respiratory problem are presented in Table 25-5.

Health Perception–Health Management Pattern. Ask the patient if there has been a perceived change in health status within the last several days, months, or years. In COPD, lung function declines slowly over many years. The patient may not notice this decline because activity is altered to accommodate reduced exercise tolerance. If an upper respiratory tract infection is superimposed on a chronic problem, dyspnea and decreased exercise tolerance may occur very quickly. In asthma, symptoms may occur or worsen during exercise, in the presence of mold, or following changes in temperature or air pollution.

Explore and document common manifestations of respiratory problems (e.g., cough, dyspnea). Also describe the course of the patient's illness, including when it began, type of symptoms, and factors that alleviate or aggravate these symptoms. Because of the chronic nature of respiratory problems, the patient may relate a change in symptoms rather than the onset of new symptoms when describing the present illness. Carefully document any changes because they often suggest the cause of illness. For example, increased shortness of breath or increased purulence of sputum may suggest an acute exacerbation of COPD.

If a cough is present, evaluate its quality. For example, a loose-sounding cough indicates secretions; a dry, hacking cough indicates airway irritation or obstruction; a harsh, barky cough suggests upper airway obstruction from inhibited vocal cord movement related to subglottic edema. Assess whether the cough is strong enough to clear secretions, and note whether it is productive or nonproductive of secretions. Determine if a cough is acute or chronic (longer than 3 weeks in duration) or if it first began with an upper respiratory tract infection. The pattern and etiology of the cough are determined by asking questions such as the following: What has been the pattern of coughing? Has it been regular or paroxysmal (i.e., sudden, periodic onset), or related to a time of day, the weather, certain activities, talking, or deep breathing? Any change over time? Do you clear your throat a lot? What have you tried to alleviate the coughing? Did you try any prescription or over-the-counter drugs?

If the patient has a productive cough, evaluate the following characteristics of sputum: amount, color, consistency, and odor. Quantify the amount of sputum in teaspoons, tablespoons, or cups per day. Note any recent increases or decreases in the amount. The normal color is clear or slightly whitish. If a patient is a cigarette smoker, the sputum is usually clear to gray with occasional specks of brown. The patient with COPD may exhibit clear, whitish, or slightly yellow sputum, especially in the morning on rising. If the patient reports any change from baseline color, suspect pulmonary complications. Note any changes in consistency of sputum to thick, thin, or frothy and pink tinged. These changes may indicate dehydration, postnasal drip or sinus drainage, or possible pulmonary edema. Normally sputum should be odorless. A foul odor or exceptionally bad breath or taste in the mouth suggests an infectious process. Ask the patient if sputum production has increased or decreased with a change in position (e.g., increased with lying down) or activity.

When assessing mucus, determine if the patient has a history of spitting or coughing up blood *(hemoptysis)*. Hemoptysis can range from a slight streaking of blood in the mucus to massive coughing up of blood, in which the patient loses more than 600 mL of blood in a 24-hour period. Massive hemoptysis is an immediate medical emergency.

Frequently the patient cannot differentiate between hemoptysis and *hematemesis* (vomiting blood). Hemoptysis can be found with a variety of conditions such as pneumonia, TB, lung cancer, and severe bronchiectasis.

Assess for a history of any difficulty breathing. For example, *wheezes* are musical sounds that can be audible. Wheezing indicates some degree of airway obstruction, such as asthma, foreign body aspiration, and emphysema. Assess for any history of family exposure to *Mycobacterium tuberculosis.*

TABLE 25-5 Health History

Respiratory System

Health Perception–Health Management

- Describe your daily activities. Have breathing problems prevented you from doing activities that you used to be able to do?* Are your breathing problems better, worse, or about the same compared with 6 months ago?
- How do your breathing problems affect your self-care abilities?
- Have you ever smoked? Do you smoke now? If so, what have you smoked? Cigarettes? Cigars? Pipes? Electronic cigarettes?
- If yes, how many cigarettes each day and for how long? Are you interested in stopping smoking? Are there aids we can tell you about that would assist your quitting? Would you be willing to come back for a visit so that we can explore your quitting? If you stopped smoking, did you do so because of your health?* How did you stop?
- Have you ever used chewing tobacco?
- Have you ever smoked street drugs?*
- Do you get the flu shot yearly? When was your last flu shot? Have you had a Pneumovax vaccination?
- What equipment helps you manage your respiratory problems? How often do you use it? Does it help? Cause problems?
- Do you feel that your respiratory problem is getting better or worse?

Nutritional-Metabolic

- Have you recently lost weight because of difficulty eating related to your respiratory problem? How much weight have you lost? Have you lost this weight voluntarily?
- Do any particular foods affect your breathing?* Sputum production?*

Elimination

- Does your breathing problem make it difficult for you to get to the toilet?*
- Are you inactive because of shortness of breath to the point that it causes incontinence?* Constipation?*

Activity-Exercise

- Are you ever short of breath during exercise?* At rest?*
- Do you get too short of breath to do the things you want to do?*
- Is your home one story? Two stories? How many steps from the street to your door?
- Can you walk up a flight of steps without stopping?
- Are you able to maintain your typical activities of daily living? If not, what are you able to do independently? What do you need help with? What have you had to give up?
- What do you do when you get short of breath? Does this help? How long does it take you to recover after you have been short of breath?

Sleep-Rest

- Do breathing problems cause you to wake up during the night?*
- Can you lie flat at night? If not, how many pillows do you use?
- Do you need to sleep upright in a chair?*
- Are you or your partner aware of any snoring?
- Do you awaken in the morning feeling rested?
- Do you ever wake up in the morning with a headache?*
- Do you fall asleep easily during the day?*

Cognitive-Perceptual

- Do you have any pain associated with breathing?* On a scale from 0 to 10, with 0 being "no pain" and 10 being "the worst pain you can imagine," where would you rate your pain? Does it hurt more on inspiration?* Expiration?* Or both?*
- If you are experiencing pain with breathing, describe the pain.
- Has the pain gotten better, worse, or stayed about the same over the past 6 months?
- Do you ever feel restless, irritable, or confused without a reason?*
- Do you have difficulty remembering things?*

Self-Perception–Self-Concept

- Describe how your respiratory problems have changed your life.
- If you use O_2, do you ever go out without bringing it with you? How often does this occur? Why?

Role-Relationship

- Has your respiratory problem caused any difficulties in your work, family, or social relationships?*

Sexuality-Reproductive

- Has your respiratory problem caused a change in your sexual activity?*
- Have you and your partner talked about ways to minimize your breathing problems during sexual activity?

Coping–Stress Tolerance

- On a daily/weekly basis, how often do you leave your home?
- Do you feel under any stress right now?
- Does stress have an effect on your breathing?*
- Do you notice if your emotions have any effect on your respiratory problems?
- Are you aware of any respiratory support groups in your area?

Value-Belief

- What do you think causes/has caused your respiratory problem(s)?
- How are you feeling right now?
- Do you think the things you have been told to do for your respiratory problems really help? If not, why?
- What are you looking for/expecting from the HCP today, in terms of your breathing problem(s)?

*If answer "yes" to any of the above questions, ask patient to describe.

GENETIC RISK ALERT

- Respiratory problems that have a strong genetic link include cystic fibrosis, COPD resulting from α_1-antitrypsin deficiency, and asthma.
- If people have a family history of these respiratory problems, they have a much greater risk of developing them.
- Although cigarette smoking is a major risk factor for COPD, only a minority of cigarette smokers develop symptomatic disease. The risk for COPD related to cigarette smoking is genetically related.
- Determine if there is a family history of any of these respiratory problems that may have genetic or familial tendencies.

Smoking is the most important risk factor for COPD and lung cancer. Ask about cigarette use, and find out about the use of any tobacco products, including cigars, pipes, chewing tobacco, electronic cigarettes (e-cigarettes), and hookah (instrument for vaporizing and smoking flavored tobacco). Also find out about exposure to secondhand smoke. Determine if the patient has tried to quit using tobacco products, including using prescription, over-the-counter, and herbal remedies.

Discuss current and past smoking habits. Quantify smoking habits in *pack-years.* This is done by multiplying the number of packs smoked per day by the number of years smoked. For example, a person who smoked 1 pack per day for 15 years has a 15 pack-year history.

Assess if the patient received immunizations for influenza (flu) and pneumococcal pneumonia. Influenza vaccine should be administered yearly in the fall. Recommendations for pneumococcal vaccines are presented in Table 27-5.

Ask where the patient has lived and traveled. Risk factors for TB include prior residence in China, India, Africa, the former Soviet Republics, Latin America, or any developing country. Other TB risk factors include exposure to people with high rates of TB transmission such as the homeless, injection drug users, and people with HIV infection. Risk factors for fungal infections of the lung include individuals who may be exposed to bird and rodent feces and/or live or travel in the Southwest (coccidioidomycosis) and the Mississippi River Valley (histoplasmosis).

Ask the patient about the use of equipment to manage respiratory symptoms (e.g., home O_2 therapy equipment, inhalers, devices for sleep apnea). Question the patient about the type of equipment used, cleaning of the device, frequency of use, its effect, and any side effects. Have patients demonstrate the use of their inhalers. Many patients do not know how to use these devices correctly (see Chapter 28).

Nutritional-Metabolic Pattern. Weight loss is a symptom of many respiratory diseases. Determine if weight loss was intentional and, if not, if food intake is altered by anorexia (from medications), fatigue (from hypoxemia, increased work of breathing), or feeling full quickly (from lung hyperinflation). Anorexia, weight loss, and chronic malnutrition are common in patients with COPD, lung cancer, TB, and chronic severe infection (bronchiectasis). Also note fluid intake. Dehydration can cause mucus to thicken and obstruct the airway. Rapid weight gain from fluid retention may decrease pulmonary gas exchange.

Elimination Pattern. Healthy elimination habits depend on the ability to reach a toilet when necessary. Activity intolerance secondary to dyspnea could result in incontinence. Dyspnea can also be the cause of limited mobility, which can cause constipation. Question the patient with dyspnea about incontinence and constipation. People with a chronic cough, especially women, may be troubled with urinary incontinence during paroxysms of coughing.

Activity-Exercise Pattern. Determine if the patient's activity is limited by dyspnea at rest or during exercise. Also note whether the patient's residence (e.g., number of steps, levels) poses a problem that increases social isolation. Record and objectively measure the degree of the patient's dyspnea. For example, can the patient walk up one flight of stairs without stopping because of dyspnea? Is dyspnea that is associated with an activity better, worse, or about the same in the last few months? Determine if the patient has difficulty breathing in a certain position, or if relief of dyspnea can be obtained by assuming a different position (e.g., tripod position in COPD).

Discuss whether the patient is able to carry out activities of daily living without dyspnea or other respiratory symptoms. If unable, document the amount and type of care needed. Immobility and sedentary habits can be risk factors for hypoventilation leading to atelectasis or pneumonia.

Sleep-Rest Pattern. Determine if the patient wakes up because of pulmonary problems. The patient with asthma or COPD may awaken at night with chest tightness, wheezing, or coughing. This suggests a need for adjunct therapy or other medication changes. The patient with cardiovascular disease (e.g., heart failure) may sleep with the head elevated on several pillows to avoid respiratory problems brought on by lying flat *(orthopnea)*. Excessive weight interferes with normal ventilation and may cause sleep apnea (see Chapter 7). Extremely obese individuals may hypoventilate while awake or asleep, and weight loss can improve respiratory function. Manifestations of sleep apnea include snoring, insomnia, abrupt awakenings, daytime drowsiness, and early morning headaches. Night sweats may be a manifestation of TB.

Cognitive-Perceptual Pattern. Because hypoxia can cause neurologic symptoms, ask the patient about apprehension, restlessness, irritability, and memory changes, which can indicate inadequate cerebral oxygenation (Table 25-2). Hypoxemia interferes with the ability to learn and retain information. For this reason, teaching may be more effective if the caregiver is present during teaching sessions to provide reinforcement at a later date.

Assess the patient's cognitive ability to cooperate with treatment. Failure or inability to participate in needed therapy may result in exacerbation of respiratory problems.

Inquire about any discomfort or pain with breathing. Explore a complaint of chest pain carefully to rule out cardiac involvement. Problems such as pleurisy, fractured ribs, and costochondritis cause chest pain. Careful assessment of the patient experiencing pain with breathing, such as onset, exact location of the pain, and factors that make the pain with breathing better or worse can help establish an accurate diagnosis.

Self-Perception–Self-Concept Pattern. Dyspnea limits activity, impairs ability to fulfill normal roles, and often alters self-esteem. A patient may be reluctant to appear in public with a highly visible nasal cannula and O_2 equipment. Discuss with the patient his or her personal body image. A barrel chest, clubbed fingers, pursed-lip breathing, and frequent expectoration of sputum or throat clearing can be embarrassing and can lead to social isolation. Referral to a support group or pulmonary rehabilitation program may be beneficial in developing a support system and coping strategies.

Role-Relationship Pattern. Acute and chronic respiratory problems can seriously affect performance in work or other activities. Discuss the impact of medications, O_2 therapy, and special routines (e.g., pulmonary hygiene for cystic fibrosis) on the patient's family, job, and social life.

Document the nature of the patient's work and frequency and intensity of exposure to fumes, toxins, asbestos, coal, fibers, or silica. Inquire whether symptoms are worse in specific situations (e.g., home versus work environments). Investigate any patient-specific allergens, such as dust or fumes, that could be present in the work environment. Hobbies such as woodworking (sawdust) or pottery (silica) and exposure to animals (allergies) may also cause respiratory problems. Because of hyperreactive airways, exposure to fumes, smoke, and other chemicals may trigger an attack in the patient with asthma.

Sexuality-Reproductive Pattern. Most patients can continue to have satisfactory sexual relationships despite marked physical limitations. In a tactful manner, determine whether breathing difficulties have caused alterations in sexual activity. If so, provide teaching about positions that decrease dyspnea during sexual activity and alternative strategies for sexual fulfillment. Many patients need to perform good pulmonary hygiene (bronchodilators, coughing, and deep breathing) before intimacy. This is similar to what they would do before strenuous physical activity. They may need to use O_2 therapy equipment during intercourse.

Coping–Stress Tolerance Pattern. Dyspnea causes anxiety, and anxiety exacerbates dyspnea. The result is a vicious cycle—the patient avoids activities that cause dyspnea, becoming more

CASE STUDY

Subjective Data

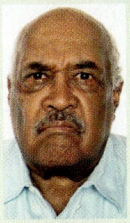

(©Fuse/ Thinkstock)

A focused subjective assessment of F.T. revealed the following information:

PMH: COPD, hypertension, and benign prostatic hyperplasia. No history of allergies.

Medications: metoprolol (Lopressor) 50 mg/day PO, furosemide (Lasix) 20 mg PO daily, finasteride (Proscar) 5 mg/day PO, Advair inhaler (fluticasone and salmeterol) 2 puffs bid, and albuterol inhaler 2 puffs q4hr PRN. Does not use O_2 at home.

Health Perception–Health Management: F.T. states he usually manages his COPD well with the Advair inhaler and occasional use of albuterol inhaler PRN. He thinks he caught a cold from his granddaughter last week. Increasing difficulty breathing, even with albuterol. Has a history of 30 pack-years of smoking, quitting 5 years ago.

Nutritional-Metabolic Pattern: Not eating, drinking very little over past 2 to 3 days.

Activity-Exercise: At present, cannot walk 100 feet without feeling short of breath, nor walk up one flight of stairs without stopping to catch his breath.

Sleep-Rest: Difficulty sleeping at present. Last night he slept upright in his recliner.

Cognitive-Perceptual: Denies any pain associated with shortness of breath. Feels slightly irritable because of lack of sleep.

Coping–Stress Tolerance: Denies any stress or emotional disturbance.

Discussion Questions

1. What type of assessment would be most appropriate for F.T.: comprehensive, focused, or emergency?
2. From the information provided by F.T., what other information would you ask him about his condition (time permitting)?
3. How will you individualize the assessment based on his current physiologic condition?
4. What considerations will you make based on his age? Ethnic/cultural background?
5. Of the information provided, which subjective assessment findings are of most concern to you?
6. F.T. cannot use his inhaler appropriately while he is talking with you. Is this an appropriate time to teach him about the proper use of his inhaler?
7. What should be included in the physical assessment? What do you think will be the priorities in your physical assessment?

You will learn about the physical assessment of the respiratory system in the next section.

(See p. 464 for more information on F.T.)

Answers available at *http://evolve.elsevier.com/Lewis/medsurg.*

deconditioned and more dyspneic. The outcome is often physical and social isolation. Assess how often the patient leaves home and interacts with others. Referral to a support group or pulmonary rehabilitation program may be beneficial.

The chronic nature of many respiratory problems such as COPD and asthma can cause prolonged stress. Inquire about the patient's coping strategies to manage this stress.

Value-Belief Pattern. Determine the patient's adherence to the management regimen. Explore reasons for lack of adherence, including conflict with cultural beliefs, financial constraints (e.g., costs of prescriptions), or failure to understand benefit. Including the patient and caregiver in the planning of care can improve adherence.

Objective Data

Physical Examination. Vital signs, including temperature, pulse, respirations, BP, and SpO_2 are important data to collect before examination of the respiratory system.

Nose. Inspect the nose for patency, inflammation, deformities, symmetry, and discharge. Check each naris for air patency with respiration while the other naris is briefly occluded. Tilt the patient's head backward and push the tip of the nose upward gently. With a nasal speculum and a good light, inspect the interior of the nose. The mucous membrane should be pink and moist, with no evidence of edema (bogginess), exudate, or bleeding. Inspect the nasal septum for deviation, perforations, and bleeding. Some septal deviation is normal in an adult. Inspect the turbinates for polyps, which are abnormal, finger-like projections of swollen nasal mucosa. Polyps may result from long-term irritation of the mucosa (e.g., from allergies). Assess any discharge for color and consistency. Purulent and malodorous discharge could indicate the presence of a foreign body. Watery discharge could be secondary to allergies or from cerebrospinal fluid. Bloody discharge could be from trauma or dryness. Thick mucosal discharge could indicate infection.

Mouth and Pharynx. Using a good light source, inspect the interior of the mouth for color, lesions, masses, gum retraction, bleeding, and poor dentition. Inspect the tongue for symmetry and lesions. Observe the pharynx by pressing a tongue blade against the middle of the back of the tongue. If the oropharynx is tight, have the patient yawn, since this usually allows more structures to be visible. The pharynx should be smooth and moist, with no evidence of exudate, ulcerations, swelling, or postnasal drip. Note the color, symmetry, and any enlargement of the tonsils. Stimulate the gag reflex by placing a tongue blade along the side of the pharynx behind the tonsil. A normal response (gagging) indicates that cranial nerves IX (glossopharyngeal) and X (vagus) are intact and that the airway is protected.[8]

Neck. Inspect the neck for symmetry and tender or swollen areas. Palpate the lymph nodes while the patient is sitting erect with the neck slightly flexed. Progression of palpation is from the nodes around the ears, to the nodes at the base of the skull, and then to those located under the angles of the mandible to the midline. The patient may have small, mobile, nontender nodes *(shotty nodes),* which are not a sign of a pathologic condition. Tender, hard, or fixed nodes indicate disease. Describe the location and characteristics of any palpable nodes.

Thorax and Lungs. Picture imaginary lines on the chest to help identify abnormalities (Fig. 25-2). Describe abnormalities in terms of their location relative to these lines (e.g., 2 cm from the right midclavicular line).

Chest examination is best performed in a well-lit, warm room with measures taken to ensure the patient's privacy. The patient's chest is exposed. Perform all physical assessment maneuvers (inspection, palpation, percussion, auscultation) on either the anterior or the posterior chest first rather than moving from anterior to posterior or vice versa with each maneuver. It is best to begin on the posterior chest, particularly with female patients, since more information can be obtained without interference from the breast tissue. In addition, if the patient tires or you are interrupted, baseline data with the most information will have been obtained from examining the posterior of the chest.

Inspection. When inspecting the *anterior chest,* have the patient sit upright, or, position the patient supine with the head of the bed elevated to thirty degrees (semi-Fowler's position). The patient may need to lean forward for support on the bedside table to facilitate breathing.

First, observe the patient's appearance and note any evidence of respiratory distress, such as tachypnea or use of accessory muscles. Next, determine the shape and symmetry of the chest. Chest movement should be equal on both sides, and the anterior-posterior (AP) diameter should be less than the side-to-side or transverse diameter. Normal AP ratio is 1:2. An increase in AP diameter (e.g., barrel chest) may be due to normal aging or result from lung hyperinflation. Observe for abnormalities in the sternum (e.g., *pectus carinatum* [a prominent protrusion of the sternum] and *pectus excavatum* [an indentation of the lower sternum above the xiphoid process]).

Next observe the respiratory rate, depth, and rhythm. The normal adult respiratory rate is 12 to 20 breaths/minute. Inspiration (I) should take half as long as expiration (E) (I:E ratio = 1:2). Observe for abnormal breathing patterns, such as *Kussmaul* (rapid, deep breathing), *Cheyne-Stokes* (abnormal respirations characterized by alternating periods of apnea and deep, rapid breathing), or *Biot's* (irregular breathing with apnea every four to five cycles) respirations.

Skin color provides clues to respiratory status. Cyanosis, a late sign of hypoxemia, is best observed in light-skinned patients as a bluish tinge to the mucous membranes, lips, and palms of the hands. In dark-skinned individuals, cyanosis may be reflected as a gray or white discoloration in the conjunctivae or around the mouth. Causes of cyanosis include hypoxemia or decreased cardiac output. Inspect the fingers for evidence of long-standing hypoxemia known as *clubbing* (an increase in the angle between the base of the nail and the fingernail to 180 degrees or more, usually accompanied by an increase in the depth, bulk, and sponginess of the end of the finger).

When inspecting the *posterior chest,* ask the patient to lean forward with arms folded. This position moves the scapulae away from the spine, exposing more of the area to be examined. The same sequence of observations that was done on the anterior part of the chest is performed on the posterior part. In addition, any spinal curvature is noted. Spinal curvatures that affect breathing include kyphosis, scoliosis, and kyphoscoliosis.

Palpation. Determine tracheal position by gently placing the index fingers on either side of the trachea just above the suprasternal notch and gently pressing backward. Normal tracheal position is midline; deviation to the left or right is abnormal. Tracheal deviation occurs away from the side of a tension pneumothorax or a neck mass, but toward the side of a pneumonectomy or lobar atelectasis.

Symmetry of chest expansion and extent of movement are determined at the level of the diaphragm. Place your hands over the lower anterior chest wall along the costal margin and move them inward until the thumbs meet at midline. Ask the patient to breathe deeply. Observe the movement of the thumbs away from each other. Normal expansion is 1 in (2.5 cm). Hand placement on the posterior side of the chest is at the level of the tenth rib. Move the thumbs until they meet over the spine (Fig. 25-6). Check expansion anteriorly or posteriorly, but it is not necessary to check both.

Normal chest movement is equal. Unequal expansion occurs when air entry is limited by conditions involving the lung (e.g., atelectasis, pneumothorax) or the chest wall (e.g., incisional pain). Equal but diminished expansion occurs in conditions that produce a hyperinflated or barrel chest or in neuromuscular diseases (e.g., amyotrophic lateral sclerosis, spinal cord lesions). Movement may be absent or unequal over a pleural effusion, an atelectasis, or a pneumothorax.

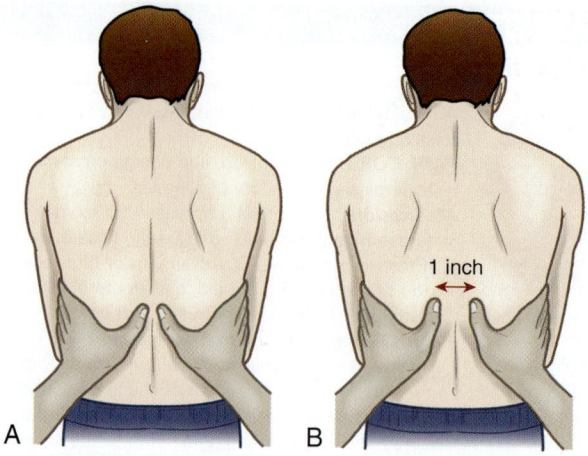

FIG. 25-6 Estimation of thoracic expansion. **A,** Exhalation. **B,** Maximal inhalation.

CASE STUDY

Objective Data: Physical Examination

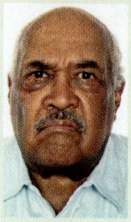

(©Fuse/ Thinkstock)

Physical examination findings of F.T. are as follows: Temperature: 38°C (100.4°F), apical pulse 110, respiratory rate 30 (regular, shallow, slightly labored), BP 170/90. O_2 saturation (SpO_2) 87% on room air. Patient sitting on edge of bed with arms resting on bedside table. Skin color normal for race with no signs of cyanosis. Slight use of accessory muscles in neck and shoulders noted. Trachea midline. Chest expansion equal. Prolonged expiration. No clubbing noted. Lungs: adequate air entry at apices bilaterally with fine crackles; decreased air entry to both bases with coarse crackles. Slight expiratory wheeze heard throughout all lung fields. F.T. has a moist, productive cough with yellow-tinged sputum.

Discussion Questions

1. What physical assessment findings are of most concern to you?
2. Based upon the subjective and objective assessment data presented so far, what would be three priority nursing diagnoses?
3. Identify three interventions that may be considered immediately post-assessment?
4. Can any of your priority interventions be delegated to unlicensed assistive personnel (UAP)?
5. With this additional physical assessment information, what diagnostic studies would you now anticipate being ordered for F.T.?

You will learn more about diagnostic studies of the respiratory system in the next section.

(See p. 473 for more information on F.T.)

Answers available at *http://evolve.elsevier.com/Lewis/medsurg.*

Fremitus is the vibration of the chest wall produced by vocalization. Tactile fremitus can be felt by placing the palmar surface of the hands against the patient's chest with the fingers hyperextended. Ask the patient to repeat a phrase such as "boy-oh-boy" in a deeper, louder-than-normal voice. Move your hands from side to side at the same time from top to bottom on the patient's chest (Fig. 25-7). Palpate all areas of the chest and compare vibrations from similar areas. Tactile fremitus is most intense adjacent to the sternum and between the scapulae because these areas are closest to the major bronchi. Fremitus is less intense farther away from these areas.

Note any increase, decrease, or absence of fremitus. Increased fremitus occurs when the lung becomes filled with fluid or is

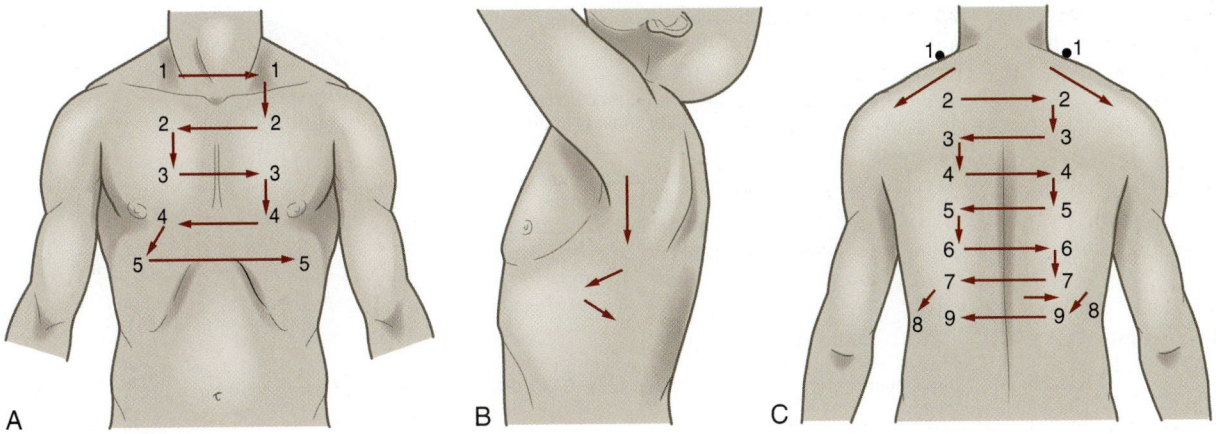

FIG. 25-7 Sequence for examination of the chest. **A,** Anterior sequence. **B,** Lateral sequence. **C,** Posterior sequence. For palpation, place the palms of the hands in the position designated as *"1"* on the right and left sides of the chest. Compare the intensity of vibrations. Continue for all positions in each sequence. For percussion, tap the chest at each designated position, moving downward from side to side. Compare percussion sounds at all positions. For auscultation, place the stethoscope at each position and listen to at least one complete inspiratory and expiratory cycle. Keep in mind that, with a female patient, the breast tissue will modify the completeness of the anterior examination.

TABLE 25-6 Percussion Sounds

Sound	Description
Resonance	Low-pitched sound heard over normal lungs
Hyperresonance	Loud, lower-pitched sound than normal resonance heard over hyperinflated lungs, such as in chronic obstructive pulmonary disease and acute asthma
Tympany	Drum-like, loud, empty quality sound heard over pneumothorax
Dull	Sound with medium-intensity, pitch and duration heard over areas of "mixed" solid and lung tissue, such as top area of liver, partially consolidated lung tissue (pneumonia), or fluid-filled pleural space
Flat	Soft, high-pitched sound of short duration heard over very dense tissue where air is not present, such as posterior chest below level of diaphragm

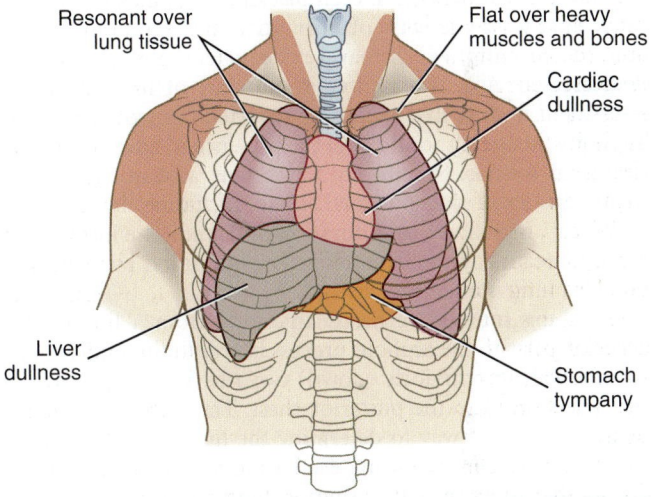

FIG. 25-8 Diagram of percussion areas and sounds on the anterior side of the chest. (Redrawn from Thompson JM, McFarland GK, Hirsch JE, Tucker SM: *Mosby's clinical nursing,* ed 5, St Louis, 2002, Mosby.)

denser. As the patient's voice moves through a dense tissue or fluid, you can feel that the vibration is increased. This is found in pneumonia, in lung tumors, with thick bronchial secretions, and above a pleural effusion (the lung is compressed upward). Fremitus is decreased if the hand is farther from the lung (e.g., pleural effusion) or the lung is hyperinflated (e.g., barrel chest). Absent fremitus may be noted with pneumothorax or atelectasis. The anterior of the chest is more difficult to palpate for fremitus because of the large muscles and breast tissue.

Percussion. Percussion is performed to assess the density or aeration of the lungs. Percussion sounds are described in Table 25-6. (The technique for percussion is described in Chapter 3 and Fig. 3-3.)

The anterior chest is usually percussed with the patient in a semi-sitting or supine position. Starting above the clavicles, percuss downward, interspace by interspace (Fig. 25-7). The area over lung tissue should be resonant, with the exception of the area of cardiac dullness (Fig. 25-8). For percussion of the posterior chest, have the patient sit leaning forward with arms folded. The posterior chest should be resonant over lung tissue to the level of the diaphragm (Fig. 25-9).

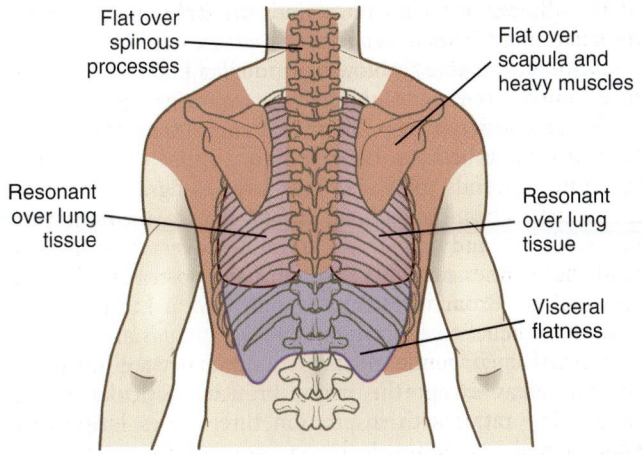

FIG. 25-9 Diagram of percussion areas and sounds on the posterior side of the chest. Percussion proceeds from the lung apices to the lung bases while comparing sounds in opposite areas of the chest. (Redrawn from Thompson JM, McFarland GK, Hirsch JE, Tucker SM: *Mosby's clinical nursing,* ed 5, St Louis, 2002, Mosby.)

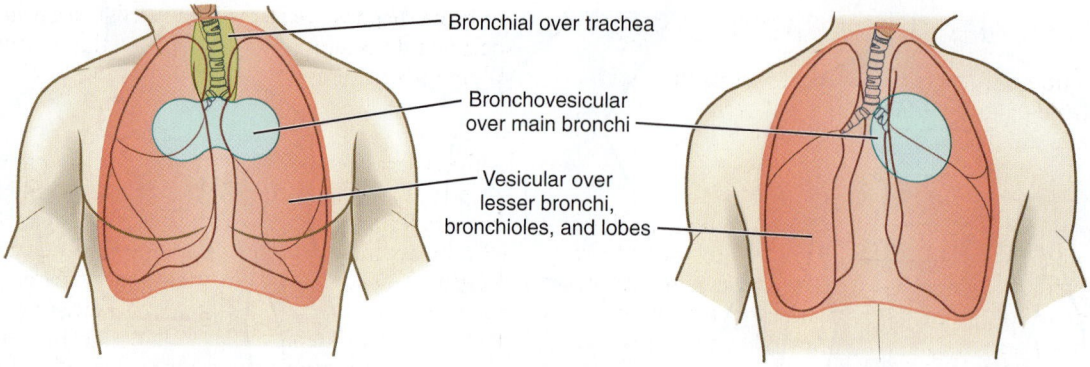

FIG. 25-10 Normal auscultatory sounds. (Redrawn from Beare PG, Myers JL: *Adult health nursing,* ed 3, St Louis, 1998, Mosby.)

Auscultation. During chest auscultation, instruct the patient to breathe slowly and a little more deeply than normal through the mouth. Auscultation should proceed from the lung apices to the bases, comparing opposite areas of the chest, unless the patient is in respiratory distress or will tire easily; if so, start at the bases (Fig. 25-7). Place the stethoscope over lung tissue, not over bony prominences. At each placement of the stethoscope, listen to at least one cycle of inspiration and expiration. First, note the air entry, which may be adequate, slightly decreased, or decreased. Absent air entry in any part of the lung is an assessment finding that should be reported immediately. Next, listen for the breath sound, and the presence of adventitious or abnormal sounds. Specifically focus your assessment on the characteristics of the abnormal sound, including the location, pitch (e.g., high, low), and duration of sound. The location of normal breath sounds is more easily understood by visualization of a lung model (Fig. 25-10).

The lung sounds are heard anteriorly from a line drawn perpendicular to the xiphoid process lateral to the midclavicular line. Palpate inferiorly (down) two ribs in the midaxillary line and around to the posterior chest. This gives you a fairly accurate and easy way to determine the lung fields to be auscultated. When documenting the location of the lung sounds, divide the anterior and posterior lung into thirds (upper, middle, and lower) and note, for example, "crackles posterior right lower lung field." You are not expected to define which lobe of the lung has particular lung sounds.

The three normal breath sounds are bronchial, bronchovesicular, and vesicular.[9] *Bronchial sounds* are loud, high-pitched sounds that resemble air blowing through a hollow pipe. Bronchial sounds have an inspiratory to expiratory ratio of 2:3, with a gap between inspiration and expiration. This reflects the short pause between the respiratory cycles. To hear bronchial breath sounds, place the stethoscope alongside the trachea in the neck. *Bronchovesicular sounds* have a medium pitch and intensity and are heard anteriorly over the mainstem bronchi on either side of the sternum and posteriorly between the scapulae. Bronchovesicular sounds have a 1:1 ratio, with inspiration equal to expiration. *Vesicular sounds* are relatively soft, low-pitched, gentle, rustling sounds. They are heard over all lung areas except the major bronchi. Vesicular sounds have a 3:1 ratio, with inspiration three times longer than expiration.

A variety of terms have been used inconsistently over time to describe breath sounds.[10] Rales are now referred to as *crackles,* and rhonchi are referred to as *wheezes.* Breath sounds are categorized into two main categories: normal and abnormal (adventitious).[11] **Adventitious breath sounds** include fine crackles, coarse crackles, wheezes, stridor, and pleural friction rub (Table 25-8).

A record of the normal physical assessment of the respiratory system is shown in Table 25-7. Assessment abnormalities of the thorax and lungs are presented in Table 25-8. Chest examination findings in common pulmonary problems are presented in Table 25-9. Age-related changes in the respiratory system and assessment findings are presented in Table 25-4.

A *focused assessment* is used to evaluate the status of previously identified respiratory problems and to monitor for signs of new problems (see Chapter 3, Table 3-7). A focused assessment of the respiratory system is presented in the box on this page.

FOCUSED ASSESSMENT

Respiratory System

Use this checklist to make sure the key assessment steps have been done.

Subjective

Ask the patient about any of the following and note responses.

Shortness of breath	Y	N
Wheezing	Y	N
Sputum production (color, quantity)	Y	N
Pain with breathing	Y	N
Cough	Y	N

Objective: Diagnostic

Check the following diagnostic tests for critical values.

Arterial blood gases	✓
Chest x-ray	✓
Hct, Hgb	✓

Objective: Physical Examination

Observe

Respirations: Rate, quality, and pattern	✓

Inspect

Skin and nails for integrity and color	✓
Neck for position of trachea	✓
Shape, symmetry, and movement of chest wall	✓

Palpate

Chest and back for masses	✓

Auscultate

Lung (breath) sounds	✓

Hct, Hematocrit; *Hgb,* hemoglobin.

DIAGNOSTIC STUDIES OF RESPIRATORY SYSTEM

Numerous diagnostic studies are available to assess the respiratory system. Table 25-10 identifies the most common studies, and select studies are described in more detail below.

Sputum Studies

Sputum samples can be obtained by expectoration, tracheal suction, or bronchoscopy (discussed later). When the patient is unable to expectorate spontaneously, sputum may also be collected by inhalation of an irritating aerosol, usually hypertonic saline. This is called *sputum induction*. The specimens may be examined for culture and sensitivity to identify an infecting organism (e.g., *Mycobacterium, Pneumocystis jiroveci*) or to confirm a diagnosis (e.g., malignant cells). Regardless of whether specimen tests are ordered, observe the sputum for color, volume, viscosity, and presence or absence of blood.

TABLE 25-7 Normal Physical Assessment of the Respiratory System

Nose	• Symmetric with no deformities • Nasal mucosa pink, moist with no edema, exudate, blood, or polyps • Nasal septum straight (slight nasal deviation possible). Nares patent bilaterally
Oral mucosa	• Light pink, moist, no exudate or ulcerations
Pharynx	• Smooth, moist, and pink
Neck	• Trachea midline
Chest	• AP (anteroposterior to lateral) diameter 1:2 • Respirations nonlabored at 12-20 breaths/min • Breath sounds vesicular without crackles or wheezes • Excursion equal bilaterally with no increase in tactile fremitus

Skin Tests

Skin tests may be performed to test for allergic reactions (see Chapter 13) or exposure to TB bacilli or fungi. Skin tests involve the intradermal injection of an antigen. A positive result on a TB skin test indicates that the patient has been exposed to the antigen. It does not indicate that TB is currently present. A negative result indicates either no exposure or a depression of cell-mediated immunity such as occurs in HIV infection (Table 25-11 for interpreting responses to tuberculin skin testing).

Nursing responsibilities are similar for all skin tests. First, to prevent a false-negative reaction, be certain that the injection is intradermal and not subcutaneous. After the injection, circle the site(s) and instruct the patient not to remove the marks. When charting administration of the antigen, draw a diagram of the forearm and hand and label the injection site. The diagram is especially helpful when more than one test is administered.

When reading test results, use a good light. If an induration is present, use a marking pen to indicate the periphery on all four sides of the induration. As the pen touches the raised area, make a mark. Then determine the diameter of the induration in millimeters. Reddened, flat areas are not measured.

Endoscopy

Bronchoscopy. *Bronchoscopy* is a procedure in which the bronchi are visualized through a fiberoptic tube (Fig. 25-11). Bronchoscopy may be used for diagnostic purposes to obtain biopsy specimens and assess results of treatment. Bronchoscopy is also

TABLE 25-8 Assessment Abnormalities

Respiratory System

Finding	Description	Possible Etiology and Significance*
Inspection		
Pursed-lip breathing	Exhalation through mouth with lips pursed together to slow exhalation.	COPD, asthma. Suggests ↑ breathlessness Strategy taught to slow expiration, ↓ dyspnea
Tripod position. Inability to lie flat	Leaning forward with arms and elbows supported on overbed table.	COPD, asthma exacerbation, pulmonary edema Indicates moderate to severe respiratory distress
Accessory muscle use. Intercostal retractions	Neck and shoulder muscles used to assist breathing; muscles between ribs pull in during inspiration.	COPD, asthma exacerbation, secretion retention Indicates severe respiratory distress/failure, hypoxemia
Splinting	Voluntary ↓ in tidal volume to ↓ pain on chest expansion	Thoracic or abdominal incision, chest trauma, pleurisy
↑ AP diameter	AP chest diameter equal to lateral. Slope of ribs more horizontal (90 degrees) to spine	COPD, asthma, cystic fibrosis, lung hyperinflation, advanced age
Tachypnea	Rate >20 breaths/min	Fever, anxiety, hypoxemia, restrictive lung disease Magnitude of ↑ above normal rate reflects increased work of breathing.
Kussmaul respirations	Regular, rapid, and deep respirations	Metabolic acidosis. Increases CO_2 excretion
Cyanosis	Bluish color of skin best seen in lips and on the palpebral conjunctiva (inside the lower eyelid)	Reflects 5-6 g of hemoglobin not bound with O_2. ↓ O_2 transfer in lungs, ↓ cardiac output. Nonspecific, unreliable indicator
Finger clubbing	↑ Depth, bulk, sponginess of distal portion of finger	Chronic hypoxemia, cystic fibrosis, lung cancer, bronchiectasis
Abdominal paradox	Inward (rather than normal outward) movement of abdomen during inspiration	Inefficient and ineffective breathing pattern. Nonspecific indicator of severe respiratory distress
Palpation		
Tracheal deviation	Leftward or rightward movement of trachea from normal midline position	Nonspecific indicator of change in position of mediastinal structures. Medical emergency if caused by tension pneumothorax (trachea deviates to side opposite collapsed lung)

Continued

TABLE 25-8 Assessment Abnormalities

Respiratory System—cont'd

Finding	Description	Possible Etiology and Significance*
Palpation—cont'd		
Altered tactile fremitus	Increase or decrease in vibrations	↑ In pneumonia, pulmonary edema. ↓ in pleural effusion, lung hyperinflation. Absent in pneumothorax, atelectasis
Altered chest movement	Unequal or equal but diminished movement of two sides of chest with inspiration	Unequal movement caused by atelectasis, pneumothorax, pleural effusion, splinting. Equal but diminished movement caused by barrel chest, restrictive disease, neuromuscular disease
Percussion		
Hyperresonance	Loud, lower-pitched sound over areas that normally produce a resonant sound	Lung hyperinflation (COPD), lung collapse (pneumothorax), air trapping (asthma)
Dullness	Medium-pitched sound over areas that normally produce a resonant sound	↑ Density (pneumonia, large atelectasis), ↑ fluid in pleural space (pleural effusion)
Auscultation		
Fine crackles	Series of short-duration, discontinuous, high-pitched sounds heard just before the end of inspiration. Result of rapid equalization of gas pressure when collapsed alveoli or terminal bronchioles suddenly snap open. Similar sound to that made by rolling hair between fingers	Interstitial edema (early pulmonary edema), alveolar filling (pneumonia), loss of lung volume (atelectasis), early phase of heart failure, idiopathic pulmonary fibrosis
Coarse crackles	Series of long-duration, discontinuous, low-pitched sounds caused by air passing through airway intermittently occluded by mucus, unstable bronchial wall. Evident on inspiration and, at times, expiration. Similar sound to blowing through straw under water. Increase in bubbling quality with more fluid	Excessive fluid within the lungs, heart failure, pulmonary edema, pneumonia with severe congestion, COPD
Wheezes	Continuous high-pitched squeaking or musical sound caused by rapid vibration of bronchial walls. First evident on expiration but possibly evident on inspiration as obstruction of airway increases. Possibly audible without stethoscope	Bronchospasm (caused by asthma), airway obstruction (caused by foreign body, tumor), COPD
Stridor	Continuous musical or crowing sound of constant pitch. Result of partial obstruction of larynx or trachea	Croup, epiglottitis, vocal cord edema after extubation, foreign body
Absent breath sounds	No sound evident over entire lung or area of lung	Pneumothorax, pleural effusion, mainstem bronchi obstruction, large atelectasis, pneumonectomy, lobectomy
Pleural friction rub	Creaking or grating sound from roughened, inflamed pleural surfaces rubbing together. Evident during inspiration, expiration, or both and no change with coughing. Often uncomfortable, especially on deep inspiration	Pleurisy, pneumonia, pulmonary infarct
Bronchophony, whispered pectoriloquy	Spoken or whispered syllable more distinct than normal on auscultation	Pneumonia.
Egophony	Spoken "E" similar to "A" on auscultation because of altered transmission of voice sounds	Pneumonia, pleural effusion

*Limited to common etiologic factors. (Further discussion of conditions listed may be found in Chapters 26 through 28.)

TABLE 25-9 Chest Examination Findings in Respiratory Problems

Problem	Inspection	Palpation	Percussion	Auscultation
Chronic obstructive pulmonary disease	Barrel chest, cyanosis, tripod position, use of accessory muscles	↓ Movement	Hyperresonant or dull if consolidation	Crackles, wheezes, distant breath sounds
Asthma				
Exacerbation	Prolonged expiration, tripod position, pursed lips	↓ Movement	Hyperresonance	Wheezes, ↓ breath sounds ominous sign (severely diminished air movement)
No exacerbation	Normal	Normal	Normal	Normal
Pneumonia	Tachypnea, use of accessory muscles, duskiness or cyanosis	↑ Fremitus over affected area	Dull over affected areas	*Early:* Bronchial sounds *Later:* Fine and/or coarse crackles, egophony, whispered pectoriloquy
Atelectasis	No change unless involves entire segment, lobe	If small, no change If large, ↓ movement, ↓ fremitus	Dull over affected area	Fine crackles (may disappear with deep breaths) Absent sounds if large
Pulmonary edema	Tachypnea, labored respirations, cyanosis, blood-tinged sputum	↓ Movement or normal movement	Dull or normal depending on amount of fluid	Fine or coarse crackles
Pleural effusion	Tachypnea, use of accessory muscles	↑ Movement ↑ Fremitus above effusion Absent fremitus over effusion	Dull	Diminished or absent over effusion, egophony above effusion
Pulmonary fibrosis	Tachypnea	↓ Movement	Normal	Crackles or sounds like Velcro being pulled apart

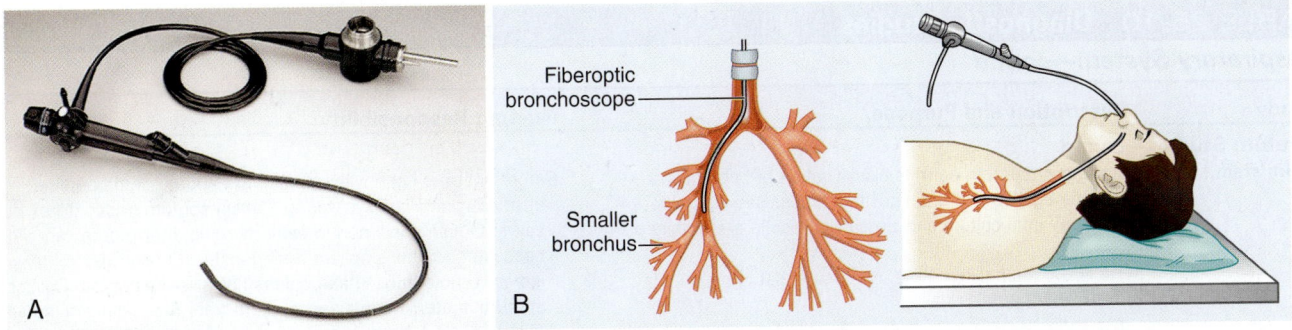

FIG. 25-11 Fiberoptic bronchoscope. **A,** The transbronchoscopic balloon-tipped catheter and the flexible fiberoptic bronchoscope. **B,** The catheter is introduced into a small airway and the balloon inflated with 1.5 to 2 mL of air to occlude the airway. Bronchoalveolar lavage is performed by injecting and withdrawing 30-mL aliquots of sterile saline solution, gently aspirating after each instillation. Specimens are sent to the laboratory for analysis. *(A,* Courtesy Olympus America Inc, Melville, N.Y.)

TABLE 25-10 Diagnostic Studies

Respiratory System

Study	Description and Purpose	Nursing Responsibility
Blood Studies		
Hemoglobin	Test reflects amount of hemoglobin available for combination with O_2. Venous blood sample obtained. *Male:* 13.2-17.3 g/dL (132-173 g/L) *Female:* 11.7-16.0 g/dL (117-160 g/L)	*Before:* Explain procedure and its purpose.
Hematocrit	Test reflects ratio of RBCs to plasma. Increased hematocrit (polycythemia) found in chronic hypoxemia. Venous blood sample obtained. *Male:* 39%-50% (0.39-0.50) *Female:* 35%-47% (0.35-0.47)	*Before:* Explain procedure and its purpose.
Arterial blood gases (ABGs)	Arterial blood is obtained through puncture of radial or femoral artery or through arterial catheter. Performed to assess acid-base balance, oxygenation/ventilation status, need for and/or change in O_2 therapy, or change in ventilator settings.*	*Before:* Indicate whether patient is using O_2 (flow rate in L/min). Avoid change in O_2 therapy or interventions (e.g., suctioning, position change) for 15 min before obtaining sample. *During:* Assist with positioning (e.g., palm up, wrist slightly hyperextended if radial artery is used). Collect blood in heparinized syringe. To ensure accurate results, expel all air bubbles. *After:* Apply pressure to radial artery for at least 5 min after specimen is obtained to prevent hematoma at the arterial puncture site. Send sample to lab promptly for analysis.
O_2 Monitoring		
Oximetry	Monitors arterial or venous O_2 saturation. Probe attaches to finger, toe, earlobe, bridge of the nose for SpO_2 monitoring or is contained in a pulmonary artery catheter for SvO_2 monitoring. Oximetry is used for intermittent or continuous monitoring and exercise testing. *Normal SpO_2:* 94%-99%; *normal SvO_2:* 60%-80%.	*During:* Apply probe. When interpreting SpO_2 and SvO_2 values, first assess patient status and presence of factors that can alter accuracy of pulse oximeter reading. For SpO_2 these include motion, low perfusion, cold extremities, bright lights, acrylic nails, dark skin color, carbon monoxide, and anemia. For SvO_2, these include change in O_2 delivery or O_2 consumption.
CO_2 Monitoring		
End-tidal CO_2 ($PetCO_2$) (capnography)	Assesses the level of CO_2 in exhaled air. Graphically displays partial pressure of CO_2 Expired gases are sampled from patient's airway and analyzed by a CO_2 sensor that uses infrared light to measure exhaled CO_2. Sensor may be attached to an adaptor on endotracheal or tracheostomy tube. A nasal cannula with a sidestream capnometer can be used in patients without an artificial airway. Can be used as a diagnostic measure to detect lung disease and for monitoring patients. Normal difference between $PaCO_2$ and $PetCO_2$ is 2-5 mm Hg ($PaCO_2$: 35-45 mm Hg; $PetCO_2$: 37-50 mm Hg).	*Before:* Teach patient and caregiver about purpose of capnography monitoring, emphasizing the benefit of continuous monitoring. *During:* Make sure that sensor is properly attached. Record and document data per institution policy.
Sputum Studies		
Culture and sensitivity	Purpose is to diagnose bacterial infection, select antibiotic, and evaluate treatment. Sputum specimen is collected in a sterile container. Takes 48-72 hr for results.	*Before:* Instruct patient on how to produce a good specimen (see Gram stain in this table). If patient cannot produce specimen, bronchoscopy may be used (Fig. 25-11). *After:* Send specimen to laboratory promptly for analysis.

Continued

*For reference intervals, see Table 25-1.

TABLE 25-10 Diagnostic Studies

Respiratory System—cont'd

Study	Description and Purpose	Nursing Responsibility
Sputum Studies—cont'd		
Gram stain	Staining of sputum permits classification of bacteria into gram-negative and gram-positive types. Results guide therapy until culture and sensitivity results are obtained.	*Before:* Instruct patient to expectorate sputum into container after coughing deeply. *During:* Obtain sputum (mucoidlike), not saliva. Obtain specimen in early morning after mouth care because secretions collect during night. If unsuccessful, try increasing oral fluid intake unless fluids are restricted. Collect sputum in sterile container (sputum trap) during suctioning via endotracheal tube or by aspirating secretions from the trachea. *After:* Send specimen to laboratory promptly for analysis.
Acid-fast bacteria (AFB) smear and culture	Two different tests used to assess sputum for acid-fast bacilli (e.g., *Mycobacterium tuberculosis*). In AFB smear (a rapid test), sputum sample spread thinly on glass slide, treated with a fluorochrome stain, and examined under a microscope for AFB. Culture for AFB may take up to 6 wk.	*Before:* Instruct patient how to produce a good specimen (see Gram stain in this table). *After:* Send specimen to laboratory promptly for analysis.
Cytology	Determines presence of abnormal cells that may indicate malignant condition. Single sputum specimen is collected in special container with fixative solution.	*Before:* Instruct patient on how to produce a good specimen (see Gram stain in this table). If patient cannot produce specimen, bronchoscopy may be used (Fig. 25-11). *After:* Send specimen to laboratory promptly for analysis.
Radiology		
Chest x-ray	Used to screen, diagnose, and evaluate changes in respiratory system. Most common views are anteroposterior (AP) and lateral.	*Before:* Instruct patient to undress to waist, put on gown, and remove any metal between neck and waist.
Computed tomography (CT) scan	Performed for diagnosis of suspicious lesions difficult to assess (e.g., mediastinum, hilum, pleura) by conventional x-ray. Common types are helical or spiral CT (contrast medium is usually used) and high-resolution CT scan (contrast medium is not used). Spiral CT used to diagnose a pulmonary embolism.	Same as for chest x-ray. Contrast medium may be given IV. *Before:* Before contrast medium used evaluate BUN and serum creatinine to assess renal function. Assess if patient is allergic to shellfish (iodine), since the contrast is iodine based. Be sure the patient is well hydrated before and after procedure (to excrete contrast). *During:* Warn patient that contrast injection may cause a feeling of being warm and flushed. Instruct patient to lie still on a hard table and that scanner will revolve around body with clicking noises.
Magnetic resonance imaging (MRI)	Used for in-depth diagnosis of lesions difficult to assess by CT scan (e.g., lung apex) and for differentiating vascular from nonvascular structures.	Same as for chest x-ray and CT scan, except contrast medium is not iodine based. *Before:* Explain MRI unit will be close to patient's body. If patient has claustrophobia, provide relaxation suggestions to help cope. Patient must remove all metal (e.g., jewelry, watch) before test. Patients with pacemakers and implantable cardioverter-defibrillators may not be able to have MRI.
Ventilation-perfusion (V/Q) scan	Used to assess ventilation and perfusion of lungs. IV radioisotope given to assess perfusion. For the ventilation portion, patient inhales a radioactive gas (xenon or krypton) that outlines alveoli. Normal scans show homogeneous radioactivity. Diminished or absent radioactivity suggests lack of perfusion or airflow. Ventilation without perfusion suggests a pulmonary embolus.	Same as for chest x-ray. No precautions needed afterward because the gas and isotope transmit radioactivity for only a brief interval. Not useful for patients in critical care who are intubated and mechanically ventilated.
Pulmonary angiogram	Used to visualize pulmonary vasculature and locate obstruction or pathologic conditions (e.g., pulmonary embolus). Contrast medium is injected through a catheter threaded into pulmonary artery or right side of heart. Series of x-rays are taken after contrast medium is injected into pulmonary artery. Chest CT is replacing angiography, since it is less invasive.	Same as for chest x-ray. (See CT scan in this table for contrast media precautions.) *After:* Check pressure dressing site after procedure. Monitor BP, pulse, and circulation distal to injection site. Report and record significant changes.
Positron emission tomography (PET) scan	Used to distinguish benign from malignant pulmonary nodules. Because malignant lung cells have an increased uptake of glucose, the PET scan, which uses an IV radioactive glucose preparation, can demonstrate increased uptake of glucose in malignant lung cells.	*Before:* Patient is NPO at least 4-6 hr preprocedure. Check the blood glucose levels as high levels may interfere with test. *After:* Encourage fluids to excrete radioactive substance.
Endoscopy		
Bronchoscopy (Fig. 25-11)	Flexible fiberoptic scope is used for diagnosis, biopsy, specimen collection, or assessment of changes. It may also be done to suction mucous plugs, lavage lungs, or remove foreign objects.	*Before:* Obtain signed consent. Instruct patient to be NPO for 6-12 hr before the test. Give sedative (as ordered). *After:* Keep patient NPO until gag reflex returns. Monitor for recovery from sedation. Blood-tinged mucus is not abnormal. If biopsy was done, monitor for hemorrhage and pneumothorax.

TABLE 25-10 Diagnostic Studies
Respiratory System—cont'd

Study	Description and Purpose	Nursing Responsibility
Mediastinoscopy	Scope is inserted through a small incision in suprasternal notch and advanced into mediastinum to inspect and biopsy lymph nodes. Used to diagnose lung cancer, non-Hodgkin's lymphoma, granulomatous infections, and sarcoidosis.	*Before:* Obtain signed consent. Prepare patient for surgical intervention. Performed in OR using a general anesthetic *After:* Monitor as for bronchoscopy.
Lung Biopsy	Specimens may be obtained by transbronchial or percutaneous biopsy or via transthoracic needle aspiration (TTNA), video-assisted thoracoscopic surgery (VATS), or open lung biopsy. Transbronchial biopsy and VATS can be performed in the bronchoscopy suite. TTNA is done under CT guidance in radiology department. Open lung is performed in the OR. VATS can also be done in the OR. These tests are used to obtain specimens for laboratory analysis.	*Before:* Obtain signed consent. Same as bronchoscopy if procedure done with bronchoscope, and same as thoracotomy if open lung biopsy done *After TTNA:* Check breath sounds q4hr for 24 hr and report any respiratory distress. Check incision site for bleeding. A chest x-ray should be done after TTNA or transbronchial biopsy to check for pneumothorax. *After VATS:* A chest tube may be placed postprocedure until lung has reexpanded. Monitor breath sounds to follow chest reexpansion. Encourage deep breathing for lung reinflation.
Thoracentesis (Fig. 25-13)	Used to obtain specimen of pleural fluid for diagnosis, remove pleural fluid, or instill medication. Chest x-ray is always obtained after procedure to check for pneumothorax.	*Before:* Explain procedure to patient and obtain signed consent before procedure. *During:* Usually performed in patient's room. Position patient upright with elbows on an overbed table and feet supported. Instruct patient not to talk or cough during procedure. *After:* Observe for signs of hypoxia and pneumothorax, and verify breath sounds in all fields. Encourage deep breaths to expand lungs. Send labeled specimens to laboratory promptly for analysis.
Pulmonary Function Tests	Used to evaluate lung function. Involves use of spirometer to assess air movement as patient performs prescribed respiratory maneuvers.†	*Before:* Avoid scheduling immediately after mealtime. Avoid administration of inhaled bronchodilator 6 hr before procedure. Explain procedure to patient. Assess for respiratory distress. *During:* Assess for respiratory distress. *After:* Assess for respiratory distress. Provide rest after procedure.
Exercise Testing	Used in diagnosis and determining exercise capacity. A *complete test* involves walking on a treadmill while expired O_2 and CO_2, respiratory rate, heart rate, and heart rhythm are monitored. In a *modified test* (desaturation test) only SpO_2 is monitored.	*Before:* Instruct patient to wear comfortable shoes. *During:* Encourage patient to hold handlebars on treadmill and walk as quickly as possible.
6-Min walk test	Used to measure functional capacity and response to treatment in patients with heart or lung disease. Pulse oximetry is usually monitored during walk. Distance walked is measured and used to monitor progression of disease or improvement after rehabilitation.	*During:* Patient is instructed by a trained practitioner to walk as far as possible during 6 min, stopping when short of breath and continuing when able. Continually assess and observe patient tolerance to test.

†For reference intervals, see Tables 25-12 and 25-13.

used for treatment (e.g., to remove mucous plugs or foreign bodies). Laser therapy, electrocautery, cryotherapy, and stents may be placed through a bronchoscope to achieve patency of an airway that has been completely or partially obstructed by tumors.

Bronchoscopy can be performed in an outpatient procedure room, in a surgical suite, or at the bedside in the intensive care unit or on a medical-surgical unit, with the patient lying down or seated. The bronchoscope may be inserted through either the nose or the mouth. Depending upon the approach, after the nasopharynx or oropharynx are anesthetized with local anesthetic spray, the bronchoscope is coated with water-soluble lubricant and inserted down into the airways. Small amounts (30 mL) of sterile saline may be injected through the scope and withdrawn and examined for cells, a technique termed *bronchoalveolar lavage* (BAL). On mechanically ventilated patients in ICU, bronchoscopy can be done through the endotracheal tube.

Lung Biopsy

Lung biopsy may be done (1) transbronchially, (2) percutaneously or via transthoracic needle aspiration (TTNA), (3) by video-assisted thoracic surgery (VATS), or (4) as an open lung biopsy. The purpose of a lung biopsy is to obtain tissue, cells, or secretions for evaluation. Transbronchial lung biopsy involves passing a forceps or needle through the bronchoscope for a specimen (Fig. 25-12). Specimens can be cultured or examined for malignant cells. A combination of transbronchial lung biopsy and BAL is used to differentiate infection and rejection in lung transplant recipients.

The procedure for percutaneous or TTNA involves inserting a needle through the chest wall, usually under CT guidance. Because of the risk of a pneumothorax, a chest x-ray is ordered after TTNA.

In VATS a rigid scope with a lens is passed through a trocar placed into the pleura via one or two small incisions in the intercostal muscles. The physician views the lesions on a monitor directly via the scope, and biopsy specimens can be taken. A chest tube is kept in place until the lung expands. Lesions in the pleura or peripheral lung are biopsied via VATS. VATS is much less invasive than open lung biopsy and is the procedure of choice when appropriate.

TABLE 25-11 Interpreting Responses to Tuberculin Skin Testing

Types of Responses	Consider Positive in the Following Groups
Positive Reactions	
≥5-mm induration	• HIV-infected people • People who had recent contact with a person with TB disease • People with fibrotic lesions on chest x-ray consistent with prior TB • Patients with organ transplants • People who are immunosuppressed (e.g., taking the equivalent of ≥15 mg/day of prednisone for ≥1 mo)
≥10-mm induration	• Recent immigrants (<5 yr) from high-prevalence countries • Injecting drug users • Residents and employees of high-risk congregate settings • Mycobacteriology laboratory personnel • People with clinical conditions (e.g., diabetes mellitus, end-stage kidney disease) that place them at high risk
≥15-mm induration	• Any person (including those with no known risk factors for TB)
False Reactions	**Possible Causes**
False-negative reactions (do not react even though infected)	• Anergy, immunosuppression • Recent TB infection (within 8-10 wk of exposure) • Overwhelming TB infection • Very old TB infection (many years) • Recent live virus vaccination (e.g., measles, chickenpox)
False-positive reactions (react even though not infected)	• Nontuberculous mycobacteria (e.g., *Mycobacterium avium-intracellulare* [MAI] or *Mycobacterium avium* complex [MAC]) • Previous BCG vaccine

Source: Centers for Disease Control and Prevention: Tuberculosis (TB) fact sheet: tuberculin skin testing. Retrieved from *www.cdc.gov/tb/publications/factsheets/testing/skintesting.htm.*

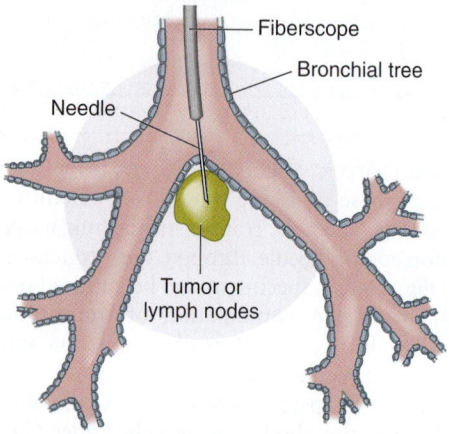

FIG. 25-12 Transbronchial biopsy needle penetrating the bronchial wall and entering a mass of subcarinal lymph nodes or tumor. (Redrawn from Du Bois RM, Clarke SW: *Fiberoptic bronchoscopy in diagnosis and management,* Orlando, 1987, Grune & Stratton.)

Open lung biopsy is used when pulmonary disease cannot be diagnosed by other procedures. The patient is anesthetized, the chest is opened with a thoracotomy incision, and a biopsy specimen is obtained. Nursing care for the procedure is the same as after thoracotomy (see Chapter 27).

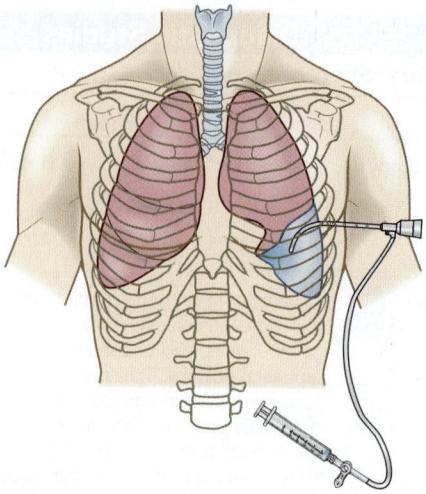

FIG. 25-13 Thoracentesis. A catheter is positioned in the pleural space to remove accumulated fluid.

Thoracentesis

Thoracentesis is the insertion of a large-bore needle through the chest wall into the pleural space to obtain specimens for diagnostic evaluation, remove pleural fluid, or instill medication (Fig. 25-13). The patient is positioned sitting upright with elbows on an overbed table and feet supported. The skin is cleansed and a local anesthetic (lidocaine) is injected subcutaneously. A chest tube may be inserted to permit further drainage of fluid.

Pulmonary Function Tests

Pulmonary function tests (PFTs) measure lung volumes and airflow. The results of PFTs are used to diagnose pulmonary disease, monitor disease progression, evaluate disability, and assess response to bronchodilators. Airflow measurement is administered by trained personnel using a spirometer. The patient inserts a mouthpiece, takes as deep a breath as possible, and exhales as hard, fast, and for as long as possible. Verbal coaching is given to ensure that the patient continues blowing out until exhalation is complete.

The computer calculates the patient's percentage of predicted values, that is, how well the performance compares with an average based on age, gender, race, and height.[12] Normal values are approximately 80% to 120% of the predicted value. Normal values for PFTs are shown in Tables 25-12 and 25-13.

Spirometry may be ordered before and after the administration of a bronchodilator to determine the patient's response. This may help document reversibility of airway obstruction (e.g., asthma). A positive response to the bronchodilator is greater than 200 mL increase or greater than 12% increase between preadministration and postadministration values.

Home spirometry may be used to monitor lung function in people with asthma, cystic fibrosis, or COPD, as well as before and after lung transplantation or other thoracic surgeries. A peak flow meter is the instrument used at home. It is a hand-held device through which one blows forcefully and quickly after taking a deep breath. Spirometry changes at home can warn of early lung transplant rejection or infection. Data from a peak flow meter provide important feedback to patients with asthma so that they can learn to modify activities and medications in response to changes in peak expiratory flow rates (see Chapter 28).

More specific pulmonary function parameters can be directly assessed at the bedside in the high-acuity or critical care unit to determine the need for or liberation (weaning and extubation) from mechanical ventilation (see Table 65-13).

TABLE 25-12 Lung Volumes and Capacities

Parameter	Definitions	Normal Value*
Volumes		
Tidal volume (VT)	Volume of air inhaled and exhaled with each breath. Only a small proportion of total capacity of lungs	0.5 L
Expiratory reserve volume (ERV)	Additional air that can be forcefully exhaled after normal exhalation is complete	1.0 L
Residual volume (RV)	Amount of air remaining in lungs after forced expiration. Air available in lungs for gas exchange between breaths	1.5 L
Inspiratory reserve volume (IRV)	Maximum volume of air that can be inhaled forcefully after normal inhalation	3.0 L
Capacities		
Total lung capacity (TLC)	Maximum volume of air that lungs can contain (TLC = IRV + VT + ERV + RV)	6.0 L
Functional residual capacity (FRC)	Volume of air remaining in lungs at end of normal exhalation (FRC = ERV + RV). Increase or decrease possible with lung disease	2.5 L
Vital capacity (VC)	Maximum volume of air that can be exhaled after maximum inspiration (VC = IRV + VT + ERV). Higher VC for men (generally)	4.5 L
Inspiratory capacity (IC)	Maximum volume of air that can be inhaled after normal expiration (IC = VT + IRV)	3.5 L

*Normal values vary with patient's height, weight, age, race, and gender.

TABLE 25-13 Pulmonary Function Airflow

Measure	Description	Normal Value*
Forced vital capacity (FVC)	Amount of air that can be quickly and forcefully exhaled after maximum inspiration	>80% of predicted
Forced expiratory volume in first second of expiration (FEV_1)	Amount of air exhaled in first second of FVC. Grades severity of airway obstruction	>80% of predicted
FEV_1/FVC ratio	Dividing value for FEV_1 by value for FVC. Useful in differentiating obstructive and restrictive pulmonary dysfunction	*Age <50:* ≥75% of predicted *Age ≥50:* ≥70% of predicted
Forced midexpiratory flow rate ($FEF_{25\%-75\%}$)	Measurement of airflow rate in middle half of forced expiration. Early indicator of disease of small airways	*Age <50:* ≥75% of predicted *Age ≥50:* ≥70% of predicted
Maximal voluntary ventilation (MVV)	Deep breathing as rapidly as possible for specified period. Fairly nonspecific test that gives information about exercise capacity. Used in conjunction with exercise stress test	About 170 L/min
Peak expiratory flow rate (PEFR)	Maximum airflow rate during forced expiration. Aids in monitoring bronchoconstriction in asthma. Can be measured with peak flow meter	Up to 600 L/min

*Normal values vary with patient's height, weight, age, race, and gender.

CASE STUDY

Objective Data: Diagnostic Studies

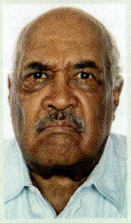

(©Fuse/ Thinkstock)

The HCP orders the following diagnostic studies for F.T.:

- CBC, basic metabolic panel (electrolytes, BUN, creatinine)
- ABGs
- Chest x-ray
- Sputum for culture and sensitivity

The ABGs indicate a compensated respiratory alkalosis with hypoxemia. The WBC is 17,350/μL, potassium 2.9 mEq/L, and chest x-ray shows bilateral consolidation to both lower lobes. F.T. is admitted to the cardiopulmonary medical-surgical nursing unit.

Discussion Questions

1. Are these the diagnostic studies that you expected to be ordered?
2. Of the diagnostic test results, is anything abnormal?
3. Of the diagnostic test results, which ones are of most concern to you?
4. What do you think is the pathophysiologic cause of F.T.'s problems?
5. F.T. asks you what he could have done differently to prevent this problem from happening. What will you tell him?
6. F.T. will be admitted to the hospital. What patient teaching can you do with F.T. as he is waiting to be admitted?
7. What is the interprofessional team's top priority for F.T. at this time?
8. What patient outcomes would indicate that the interprofessional team was effective?

You will learn more about the upper and lower respiratory problems and chronic obstructive pulmonary disease (COPD) in the next three chapters.

Answers available at *http://evolve.elsevier.com/Lewis/medsurg.*

BRIDGE TO NCLEX EXAMINATION

The number of the question corresponds to the same-numbered learning outcome identified at the beginning of this chapter.

1. To promote the release of surfactant, the nurse encourages the patient to
   a. take deep breaths.
   b. cough five times per hour to prevent alveolar collapse.
   c. decrease fluid intake to reduce fluid accumulation in the alveoli.
   d. sit with head of bed elevated to promote air movement through the pores of Kohn.
2. A patient with a respiratory condition asks, "How does air get into my lungs?" The nurse bases her answer on knowledge that air moves into the lungs because of
   a. increased CO_2 and decreased O_2 in the blood.
   b. contraction of the accessory abdominal muscles.
   c. stimulation of the respiratory muscles by the chemoreceptors.
   d. decrease in intrathoracic pressure relative to pressure at the airway.

3. The nurse can *best* determine adequate arterial oxygenation of the blood by assessing
   a. heart rate.
   b. hemoglobin level.
   c. arterial oxygen partial pressure.
   d. arterial carbon dioxide partial pressure.
4. When teaching a patient about the *most* important respiratory defense mechanism distal to the respiratory bronchioles, which topic would the nurse discuss?
   a. Alveolar macrophages
   b. Impaction of particles
   c. Reflex bronchoconstriction
   d. Mucociliary clearance mechanism
5. A student nurse asks the RN what can be measured by arterial blood gas (ABG). The RN tells the student that the ABG can measure *(select all that apply)*
   a. acid-base balance.
   b. oxygenation status.
   c. acidity of the blood.
   d. bicarbonate (HCO_3^-) in arterial blood.
   e. overall balance of electrolytes in arterial blood.
6. To detect early signs or symptoms of inadequate oxygenation, the nurse would examine the patient for
   a. dyspnea and hypotension.
   b. apprehension and restlessness.
   c. cyanosis and cool, clammy skin.
   d. increased urine output and diaphoresis.
7. During the respiratory assessment of an older adult, the nurse would expect to find *(select all that apply)*
   a. a vigorous reflex cough.
   b. increased chest expansion.
   c. increased residual volume.
   d. diminished lung sounds at base of lungs.
   e. increased anteroposterior (AP) chest diameter.
8. When assessing activity-exercise patterns related to respiratory health, the nurse inquires about
   a. dyspnea during rest or exercise.
   b. recent weight loss or weight gain.
   c. ability to sleep through the entire night.
   d. willingness to wear O_2 equipment in public.
9. When auscultating the chest of an older patient in respiratory distress, it is *best* to
   a. begin listening at the apices.
   b. begin listening at the lung bases.
   c. begin listening on the anterior chest.
   d. Ask the patient to breathe through the nose with the mouth closed.
10. Which assessment finding of the respiratory system does the nurse interpret as abnormal?
    a. Inspiratory chest expansion of 1 inch
    b. Symmetric chest expansion and contraction
    c. Resonance (to percussion) over the lung bases
    d. Bronchial breath sounds in the lower lung fields
11. The nurse is preparing the patient for a diagnostic procedure to remove pleural fluid for analysis. The nurse would prepare the patient for which test?
    a. Thoracentesis
    b. Bronchoscopy
    c. Pulmonary angiography
    d. Sputum culture and sensitivity

1. a, 2. d, 3. c, 4. a, 5. a, b, c, d, 6. b, 7. c, d, e, 8. a, 9. b, 10. d, 11. a

For rationales to these answers and even more NCLEX review questions, visit *http://evolve.elsevier.com/Lewis/medsurg.*

EVOLVE WEBSITE

http://evolve.elsevier.com/Lewis/medsurg

Review Questions (Online Only)

Key Points

Answer Keys for Questions

- Rationales for Bridge to NCLEX Examination Questions
- Answer Guidelines for Case Study on pp. 460, 463, 464, and 473

Conceptual Care Map Creator

Audio Glossary

Supporting Media

- Animations
  - Inhalation
  - Oxygenation
  - Pulse Oximetry
  - Respiration Cycle
  - Respiratory System Overview
- Audio
  - Bronchial Breath Sounds
  - Bronchovesicular Breath Sounds
  - High-Pitched Crackles
  - High-Pitched Wheeze
  - Low-Pitched Crackles
  - Low-Pitched Wheeze
  - Pleural Friction Rub
  - Stridor
  - Vesicular Breath Sounds

Content Updates

REFERENCES

1. McCance KL, Huether SE: *Pathophysiology: the biological basis for disease in adults and children*, ed 7, St Louis, 2014, Mosby.
2. Urden LD, Stacy KM, Lough ME: *Critical care nursing: diagnosis and management*, ed 7, St Louis, 2013, Mosby.
3. Patton KT, Thibodeau GA. *The human body in health and disease*, ed 6, St Louis, 2014, Mosby.
4. Heuer AJ, Scanlan CL: *Wilkins' clinical assessment in respiratory care*, ed 7, St Louis, 2014, Mosby.
5. Mechem CC: Pulse oximetry. Retrieved from *www.uptodate.com/contents/pulse-oximetry*.
6. Press CD: End tidal capnography. Retrieved from *http://emedicine.medscape.com/article/2116444*.
7. Jarvis C: *Physical examination and health assessment*, ed 7, St Louis, 2015, Elsevier.
8. Ball JW, Dains JE, Flynn JA, et al: *Seidel's guide to physical examination*, ed 8, St Louis, 2015, Saunders.
9. Bohadana A, Izbicki G, Kraman SS: Fundamentals of lung auscultation, *NEJM* 370:744, 2014.
10. Mikami R, Murao M, Cugell DW, et al: International symposium on lung sounds: Synopsis of proceedings, *Chest* 2:342, 1987. (Classic)
11. Stahlheber CL: Breath sound assessment. Retrieved from *http://emedicine.medscape.com/article/1894146*.
12. Dancer R, Thickett D: Pulmonary function tests, *Medicine* 40:186, 2012.

26

Upper Respiratory Problems

Eugene E. Mondor

When you own your breath, nobody can steal your peace.

Author unknown

http://evolve.elsevier.com/Lewis/medsurg/

LEARNING OUTCOMES

1. Describe the clinical manifestations and nursing and interprofessional management of problems of the nose.
2. Discuss the clinical manifestations and nursing and interprofessional management of problems of the paranasal sinuses.
3. Describe the clinical manifestations and nursing and interprofessional management of problems of the pharynx and larynx.
4. Discuss the nursing and interprofessional management of the patient who requires a tracheostomy.
5. Identify the steps involved in performing tracheostomy care and suctioning an airway.
6. Describe the risk factors for and clinical manifestations of head and neck cancer.
7. Discuss the nursing and interprofessional management of patients requiring surgery for head and neck cancer.
8. Explain essential components of discharge teaching for the patient going home with a permanent tracheostomy after total laryngectomy for cancer.

KEY TERMS

allergic rhinitis, p. 477
decannulation, p. 490
deviated septum, p. 475
epistaxis, p. 476
nasal polyps, p. 483
rhinoplasty, p. 476
sinusitis, p. 482
tracheostomy, p. 485

Disorders of the upper respiratory system, including nose, sinuses, pharynx, and larynx, are presented in this chapter. Nursing management of patients with a tracheostomy or requiring surgery for head and neck cancer is also discussed.

PROBLEMS OF NOSE AND PARANASAL SINUSES

DEVIATED SEPTUM

Deviated septum is a deflection of the normally straight nasal septum. Although up to 80% of adults may have septa that are slightly off center, the diagnosis of deviated septum is generally reserved for those whose septa are severely shifted.[1] Trauma to the nose, either at birth or later in life, is the most common cause of deviated septum.[2] Deviation of the septum from midline can interfere with both airflow and sinus drainage through the narrowed passageway.

Symptoms vary depending on the degree of deviation. Minor septal deviations may be asymptomatic. Manifestations of severe septal deviation include obstruction to nasal breathing, nasal congestion, frequent sinus infections, nosebleeds *(epistaxis)*, and facial pain.

The diagnosis of deviated septum is made by an HCP during physical examination with a nasal speculum. Medical management of minor septal deviation is focused on symptom control of nasal inflammation and congestion using saline rinses and decongestants to clear nasal passages. For severe septal deviation, a nasal septoplasty, performed under local or general anesthetic, reconstructs and properly aligns the deviated septum.

NASAL FRACTURE

Nasal fracture is the most common facial fracture and the third most common fracture of any bone.[3] Fracture of the nose most often occurs as a result of blunt trauma, including fights, automobile accidents, falls, and sports injuries. Complications associated with nasal fractures include airway obstruction, epistaxis, meningeal tears causing cerebrospinal fluid (CSF) leakage, septal hematoma, and cosmetic deformity. Many cases of facial trauma can be prevented by using protective sports equipment and protecting against falls.

There is no standardized classification system for nasal fractures. Most nasal fractures, however, can be classified as simple or complex. *Simple fractures* may be unilateral or bilateral and

Reviewed by Donna C. Bond, RN, DNP, CCNS, AE-C, CTTS, Pulmonary Clinical Nurse Specialist, Carilion Clinic, Roanoke, Virginia; Marylee Bressie, RN, DNP, CCRN, CCNS, CEN, Core Faculty/Nurse Planner, Department of Nursing, School of Public Service Leadership, Capella University, Minneapolis, Minnesota; Deborah Cline, RN, MS, Nursing Faculty, Carrington College, Reno, Nevada; and Cynthia M. Steinwedel, RN, PhD, CNE, Assistant Professor, Department of Nursing, Bradley University, Peoria, Illinois.

typically produce little or no displacement. Powerful frontal blows can cause *complex fractures,* which may also involve subsequent damage to adjacent facial structures such as the teeth or eyes. Patients with complex nasal fractures should be evaluated for possible injury to the cervical spine and orbital or mandibular fractures.[4]

Diagnosis of a nasal fracture is based on the health history and physical examination. Clinical manifestations suggestive of a nasal fracture include localized pain, crepitus on palpation, swelling, difficulty breathing out of the nostrils, epistaxis, ecchymosis, and cosmetic deformity. Although facial deformity with a nasal fracture is common, often epistaxis may be the only initial manifestation of a nasal fracture.

On inspection, assess the patient's ability to breathe through each side of the nose and note the presence of edema, bleeding, or hematoma. Ecchymosis may be under one or both eyes. Ecchymosis involving both eyes is often termed *raccoon eyes* and may suggest a basilar skull fracture (see Chapter 56). Inspect the nose internally for evidence of septal deviation, hemorrhage, or clear drainage.

Clear, pink-tinged, or persistent drainage after control of epistaxis suggests a possible CSF leak. Checking this fluid for glucose at the bedside to help confirm the presence of CSF is highly unreliable and influenced by many factors. If possible, send a specimen to the laboratory to determine the fluid type. Goals of nursing management are to maintain the airway, reduce edema and pain, prevent complications, and provide emotional support.

The best way to maintain the airway is to keep the patient sitting upright. Apply ice to the face and nose in 10- to 20-minute intervals to help reduce edema and bleeding. Administer analgesia as ordered to control pain. Acetaminophen is preferred over nonsteroidal antiinflammatory drugs (NSAIDs) or acetylsalicylic acid (ASA; aspirin) for the first 48 hours to avoid prolonging clotting time and increasing the risk for bleeding. Nasal stuffiness may be relieved with nasal decongestants, saline nasal sprays, and a humidifier. The patient should avoid hot showers and alcohol for the first 48 hours to prevent an increase in swelling. Encourage the patient to quit or decrease smoking to facilitate tissue healing.

When a fracture is confirmed, the goals are to realign the fracture using closed or open reduction.[5] Simple fractures are often reduced with manual manipulation. With complex nasal fractures, considerable swelling of soft tissues occurs, and it may be necessary to wait to repair the fracture until after the edema subsides, which may be 5 to 10 days.

Septoplasty and rhinoplasty are surgical options. These procedures provide an adequate airway and function of the nose, and help to reestablish a person's cosmetic appearance. The presence of septal hematoma increases the patient's risk for infection, which may necessitate drainage and antibiotic therapy.

RHINOPLASTY

Rhinoplasty, surgical reconstruction of the nose, is performed to improve airway function (when trauma or developmental deformities result in nasal obstruction) or for cosmetic reasons. When caring for rhinoplasty patients before surgery, assess the patient's expectations of the surgery. Actual or perceived alterations in body image (e.g., deformed or enlarged nose) can affect self-esteem and interactions with others. Computerized photographs can be used to show the patient's appearance after the surgery. These images can help patients decide whether to undergo rhinoplasty.

Rhinoplasty is often performed as an outpatient procedure using regional or general anesthesia. Nasal tissue is added or removed, and the nose may be lengthened or shortened. Plastic implants are sometimes used to reshape the nose. Incisions are typically inside the nose and hidden. Sonic rhinoplasty incorporates the use of an ultrasonic device to gently aspirate bone, enabling a refined cosmetic result.[6]

After surgery, nasal packing may be inserted in some patients to apply pressure and prevent bleeding or septal hematoma formation. An external plastic splint protects and supports the new shape of the nose during the healing process. If present, nasal packing is usually removed 1 or 2 days after surgery. The splint may be left in place for approximately 1 to 2 weeks.

❖ NURSING MANAGEMENT: NASAL SURGERY

Before surgery, instruct patients to notify the HCP about any medications that they take at home. Aspirin-containing drugs and NSAIDs may have to be discontinued for 5 days to 2 weeks preoperatively to reduce the risk of bleeding. Encourage smoking cessation to promote postoperative wound healing. During the immediate postoperative period, nursing interventions include maintenance of the airway; assessment of respiratory status; pain management; and observation of the surgical site for bleeding, infection, and edema.

Teaching is important because the patient must be able to detect complications at home. The patient typically experiences temporary edema and ecchymosis. Cold compresses and elevation of the head can help minimize swelling and discomfort. Teach about activity restrictions aimed at preventing bleeding and injury (no nose blowing, swimming, heavy lifting, strenuous exercise). Subtle swelling may be slow to resolve, delaying the achievement of a full cosmetic result for up to 1 year.

EPISTAXIS

Epistaxis (nosebleed) most often occurs in adults over age 50. Epistaxis can be caused by trauma, hypertension, low humidity, upper respiratory tract infections, allergies, sinusitis, foreign bodies, chemical irritants (such as street drugs), overuse of decongestant nasal sprays, facial or nasal surgery, anatomic malformation, and tumors.[7] Conditions that prolong bleeding time or alter platelet counts will predispose the patient to epistaxis. Bleeding time may be prolonged if the patient takes aspirin, NSAIDs, warfarin, or other anticoagulant drugs.

Approximately 90% of nosebleeds occur in the anterior portion of the nasal cavity and are easily visualized. Anterior bleeding can be self-treated and usually stops spontaneously. Posterior bleeding may require medical treatment.

Posterior bleeding occurs more commonly with older adults secondary to other health problems (e.g., hypertension). Since posterior nosebleeds occur closer to the throat, it is often difficult to determine how much blood loss has occurred.

❖ NURSING AND INTERPROFESSIONAL MANAGEMENT: EPISTAXIS

Use simple first aid measures to control epistaxis including (1) calm the patient; (2) place the patient in a sitting position, leaning slightly forward with head tilted forward; and (3) apply direct pressure by squeezing the entire soft lower portion of the nose (nostrils) together for 5 to 15 minutes. If bleeding does not stop within 15 minutes, seek medical assistance.

Medical management involves attempting to identify the location of the bleed. For anterior bleeds, a pledget (nasal tampon) impregnated with anesthetic solution (lidocaine) and/or vasoconstrictive agents such as epinephrine may be placed into the nasal cavity. Alternatively, absorbable materials such as oxidized cellulose (surgical), gelatin foam (Gelfoam), or a gelatin-thrombin combination (Floseal) may be used. Packing for anterior bleeds can remain in place for 48 to 72 hours. Silver nitrate may also be used to chemically cauterize an identified bleeding point. Thermal cauterization is reserved for more severe bleeding and may require the use of local or general anesthesia.[8]

It may be much more difficult to identify the location of a posterior bleed. Posterior bleeds often require packing. Packing with compressed nasal sponges (e.g., Merocel) or epistaxis balloons (e.g., Rapid Rhino) is preferred over the use of traditional Vaseline ribbon gauze because of the ease of placement. Packing is inserted into the nares and advanced along the floor of the nasal cavity. The sponge expands with moisture to fill the nasal cavity and tamponade bleeding. The epistaxis balloon is inflated with air to achieve the same pressure effect (Fig. 26-1). In the absence of a specific nasal device, a size 10F, 12F, or 14F Foley catheter with a 30 mL balloon may be used. A nasal sling (folded 2 × 2-inch gauze pad) may be gently taped under the nares to absorb drainage. If packing fails to stop the bleeding, arterial embolization may be required.

Nasal sponges, packing, and balloons may impair respiratory status. Closely monitor the level of consciousness, heart rate and rhythm, respiratory rate, O_2 saturation using pulse oximetry (SpO_2), and observe for any signs of difficulty breathing or swallowing. Because of the risk of complications, all patients with posterior packing should be admitted to a monitored unit for close observation.

Nasal packing is painful because sufficient pressure must be applied to stop the bleeding. Nasal packing predisposes patients to infection from bacteria (e.g., *Staphylococcus aureus*) present in the nasal cavity. The patient should receive a mild opioid analgesic for pain (e.g., acetaminophen with codeine). Antibiotics effective against staphylococci may be prescribed.

Nasal packing may be left in place for 2 to 3 days. Before removal, medicate the patient for pain because this procedure is uncomfortable. After removal, cleanse the nares gently and lubricate them with water-soluble jelly.

Before discharge teach the patient and caregiver about home care. Teach the patient to use saline nasal spray and/or a humidifier, sneeze with the mouth open, and avoid the use of aspirin-containing products or NSAIDs. Instruct the patient to avoid vigorous nose blowing, engaging in strenuous activity, lifting, and straining for 4 to 6 weeks.

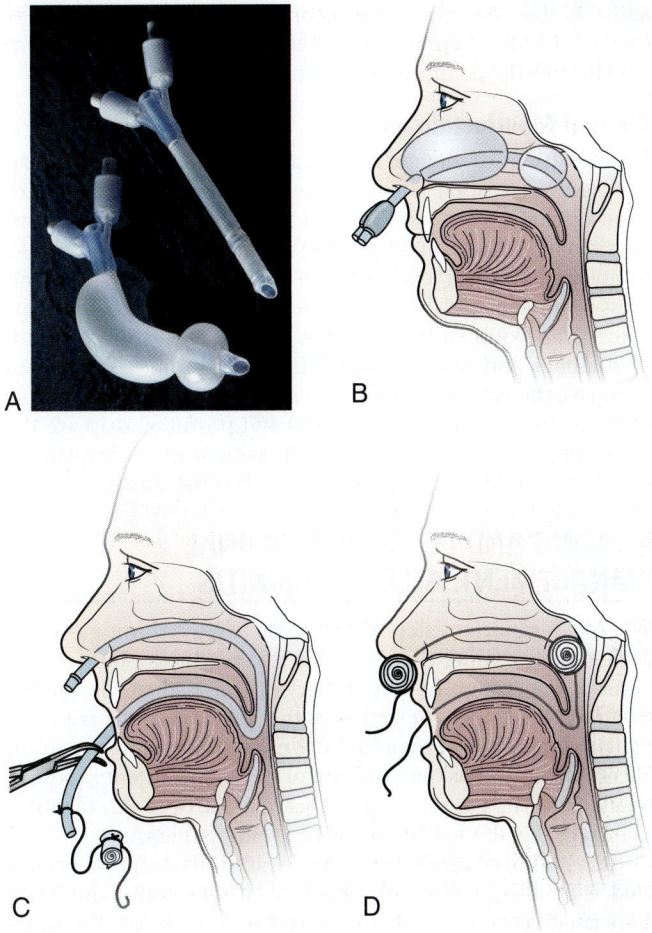

FIG. 26-1 **A,** Epistaxis balloon. The balloon is inflated after insertion. (Courtesy Boston Medical, Westborough, Mass.) **B,** Epistaxis balloon in proper position in nares. (From Roberts JR, Hedges JR: *Clinical procedures in emergency medicine,* ed 5, Philadelphia, 2009, Saunders.) **C,** Method for placing posterior nasal pack. Catheter is passed through the bleeding side of the nose and pulled out through the mouth with a hemostat. Strings are tied to the catheter, and the pack is pulled up behind the soft palate and into the nasopharynx. **D,** Nasal pack in position in the posterior nasopharynx. Dental roll at the nose helps maintain correct position.

ALLERGIC RHINITIS

Allergic rhinitis is inflammation of the nasal mucosa in response to a specific allergen. Allergic rhinitis can be classified according to the causative allergen (seasonal or perennial) or the frequency of symptoms (episodic, intermittent, or persistent). *Episodic* refers to symptoms related to sporadic exposure to allergens not typically encountered in the patient's normal environment, such as exposure to animal dander when visiting another person's home. *Intermittent* means that the symptoms are present less than 4 days a week or less than 4 weeks per year. *Persistent* means that symptoms are present more than 4 days a week and for more than 4 weeks per year.

Seasonal rhinitis usually occurs in the spring and fall, and is caused by allergy to pollens from trees, flowers, grasses, or weeds. The typical attack lasts for several weeks during times when pollen counts are high; then it disappears and recurs at the same time the following year. *Perennial rhinitis* occurs year round from exposure to environmental allergens, such as animal dander, dust mites, cockroaches, fungi, and molds. Both seasonal and perennial rhinitis can be classified as episodic, intermittent, or persistent, depending on the duration and frequency of symptoms.

Sensitization to an allergen occurs with initial allergen exposure, which results in the production of antigen-specific immunoglobulin E (IgE) (see Fig. 13-6). After exposure, mast cells and basophils release histamine, cytokines, prostaglandins, and leukotrienes, which cause the early symptoms of sneezing, itching, rhinorrhea, and congestion.[9] Four to 8 hours after exposure, inflammatory cells infiltrate the nasal tissues, causing and maintaining the inflammatory response. Because symptoms of rhinitis resemble those of the common cold, the patient may believe the condition is a continuous or repeated cold.

Clinical Manifestations

Manifestations of allergic rhinitis are initially sneezing; watery, itchy eyes and nose; altered sense of smell; and thin, watery nasal discharge that can lead to a more sustained mucus production and nasal congestion. The nasal turbinates appear pale, boggy, and swollen. The turbinates may fill the air space and press against the nasal septum. The posterior ends of the turbinates can become so enlarged that they obstruct sinus aeration or drainage and result in sinusitis. With chronic exposure to allergens, the patient may develop a headache, stuffy nose, congestion, and pressure. Nasal polyps and postnasal drip are the most common causes of cough. The patient may complain of hoarseness and the recurrent need to clear the throat.

❖ NURSING AND INTERPROFESSIONAL MANAGEMENT: ALLERGIC RHINITIS

The most important step in managing allergic rhinitis is identifying and avoiding triggers of allergic reactions (Table 26-1). Instruct the patient to keep a diary of times when the allergic reaction occurs and the activities that precipitate the reaction. Patients are often more aware of intermittent exposure to an allergen such as pets than they are of a more persistent exposure to allergens such as dust mites, cockroaches, or mold. Identifying triggers is the first step toward avoiding them.

The goal of drug therapy is to reduce inflammation associated with allergic rhinitis, reduce nasal symptoms, minimize associated complications, and maximize quality of life. Nasal corticosteroid sprays are the first line and most effective treatment for allergic rhinitis.[10] Appropriate oral medication options include H_1-antihistamines, decongestants, and leukotriene receptor antagonists (LTRAs). Intranasal medications include antihistamines, anticholinergics, corticosteroids, cromolyn, and decongestants[11] (Table 26-2).

Second-generation antihistamines are preferred over first-generation antihistamines because of their nonsedating effects. Remind patients who are taking antihistamines to have adequate fluid intake to reduce adverse symptoms. Nasal corticosteroid sprays are used to decrease inflammation locally with little absorption in the systemic circulation. Therefore systemic side effects are rare. If symptoms are not relieved with monotherapy, a two-drug combination (such as an oral H_1-antihistamine and an intranasal corticosteroid) may be helpful.

DRUG ALERT Antihistamines

- First-generation antihistamines (e.g., chlorpheniramine [Chlor-Trimeton]) can cause drowsiness and sedation.
- Warn patients that operating machinery and driving may be dangerous because of the sedative effect.

DRUG ALERT Pseudoephedrine (Sudafed)

- Large doses may produce tachycardia and palpitations, especially in patients with cardiac disease.
- Overdose in those over 60 years of age may result in central nervous system depression, seizures, and hallucinations.

Immunotherapy (allergy shots) may be used when a specific, unavoidable allergen is identified and drugs are not tolerated or are ineffective in controlling symptoms. Immunotherapy involves controlled exposure to small amounts of the known allergen through frequent (at least weekly) injections with the goal of decreasing sensitivity. Sublingual or intranasal administration of allergen immunotherapy may be appropriate for selected patients. (Immunotherapy is discussed in Chapter 13.)

TABLE 26-1 Patient & Caregiver Teaching

Avoiding Allergens in Allergic Rhinitis

Include the following instructions when teaching a patient or caregiver about allergic rhinitis.

What to Avoid	Specific Approaches
House dust	• Focus on the bedroom. Remove carpeting. Limit furniture. • Put the pillows, mattress, and springs in airtight vinyl bags or containers. • Limit clothing in the bedroom to items used frequently. Place clothing in airtight, zipper-sealed vinyl clothes bags. • Install an air filter. Close the air conditioning vent into room. Use blinds rather than draperies.
House dust mites	• Wash bedding in hot water (130° F [54° C]). • Wear a mask when vacuuming. Install a filter on the outlet port of vacuum cleaner. • Avoid sleeping or lying on upholstered furniture. • Keep house temperature and conditions cool and dry.
Pet allergens	• Remove pets from interior of home. • Clean living area thoroughly. • Do not expect instant relief. Symptoms usually do not improve significantly for 2 months after pet removal.
Mold spores	• The three *D*s that promote growth of mold spores are darkness, dampness, and drafts. • Ventilate closed rooms and open doors. Consider adding windows to dark rooms. Consider keeping a small light on in closets. • Basement light with a timer that provides light several hours a day may decrease mold growth. • Avoid places where humidity is high (e.g., basements, clothes hampers, greenhouses, barns). Dehumidifiers are rarely helpful.
Pollens	• Stay inside with closed doors and windows during high-pollen season. • Install an air conditioner with a good air filter. Wash filters weekly during high-pollen season. • Put the car air conditioner on "recirculate" when driving. • Avoid having plants, especially in the bedroom.
Smoke	• Presence of a smoker will sabotage the best of all possible symptom reduction programs.

ACUTE VIRAL RHINITIS

Acute viral rhinitis (common cold or acute coryza) is an infection of the upper respiratory tract that can be caused by more than 200 different viruses. The majority of colds, caused by rhinoviruses, are mild and self-limiting. Other viruses, such as coxsackieviruses and adenoviruses, can cause a more severe illness. Acute viral rhinitis is the most prevalent infectious disease, with the average adult contracting one to three colds per year.

The virus is spread by airborne droplets emitted by the infected person while breathing, talking, sneezing, or coughing. Because the virus can survive on inanimate objects for up to 3 days, transmission can also occur by direct hand contact. Frequency of the infection increases in the winter months when

TABLE 26-2 Drug Therapy

Rhinitis and Sinusitis

Drug	Mechanism of Action	Side Effects	Nursing Actions
Corticosteroids			
Nasal Spray beclomethasone budesonide (Rhinocort) ciclesonide (Omnaris) flunisolide fluticasone (Flonase) fluticasone furoate (Veramyst) mometasone (Nasonex) triamcinolone	Inhibits inflammatory response of allergic rhinitis. At recommended dose, systemic side effects are unlikely because of low systemic absorption. Systemic effects may occur with higher than recommended doses.	Mild transient nasal burning and stinging, mucosal drying. In rare instances, localized fungal infection with *Candida albicans.*	• Instruct patient to use on regular basis and not PRN. • Instruct patient to clear nasal passages before use. • Reinforce that spray acts to decrease inflammation and it may take several days or weeks to achieve maximum effects. • Discontinue use if nasal infection develops.
Mast Cell Stabilizer			
Nasal Spray cromolyn spray	Suppresses release of histamine and other inflammatory mediators from mast cells.	Minimal side effects. Occasional burning or nasal irritation.	• Reinforce that spray prevents symptoms. • Begin 2 wk before pollen season starts and use throughout pollen season. • If isolated allergy, such as cat, use prophylactically before exposure to allergen.
Leukotriene Receptor Antagonists (LTRAs) and Inhibitors			
Antagonists zafirlukast (Accolate) montelukast (Singulair) ***Inhibitors*** zileuton (Zyflo)	Suppress leukotriene activity, thereby inhibiting airway edema, bronchoconstriction, mucus production, and inflammation (see Fig. 11-2).	Generally well tolerated May cause headaches, dizziness, rash, altered liver function tests, GI disturbances *Zafirlukast and zileuton:* Monitor PT levels and theophylline levels if patient is taking warfarin or theophylline.	• Monitor liver function tests periodically while on therapy. Discontinue if elevated. • Administer on empty stomach. • Do not discontinue therapy without consulting HCP. • Not to be used for acute attacks.
Anticholinergic			
Nasal Spray ipratropium bromide (Atrovent)	Blocks nasal cholinergic receptors, reducing nasal secretions in the common cold and nonallergic rhinitis.	Nasal dryness and irritation may occur. Does not cause systemic side effects.	• Need to prime pump with seven actuations before initial use • May reduce the need for other rhinitis medications.
Antihistamines			
First-Generation Agents (Oral) brompheniramine chlorpheniramine (Chlor-Trimeton) clemastine dexchlorpheniramine diphenhydramine levocetirizine (Xyzal)	Bind with H_1 receptors on target cells, blocking histamine binding. Relieve acute symptoms of allergic response (itching, sneezing, rhinorrhea).	Cross blood-brain barrier, frequently causing sedation and somnolence. Can also cause paradoxic stimulation (restlessness, nervousness, insomnia). Anticholinergic side effects (e.g., palpitations, dry mouth, constipation, urinary hesitancy).	• Warn patient that operating machinery and driving may be dangerous because of sedative effect. • Teach patient to report palpitations, change in heart rate, change in bowel or bladder habits. • Instruct patient not to use alcohol with antihistamines because of additive depressant effect. • Rapid onset of action, no drug tolerance with prolonged use.
Second-Generation Agents (Oral) loratadine (Claritin) cetirizine (Zyrtec) fexofenadine (Allegra) desloratadine (Clarinex) levocetirizine (Xyzal)	Same as above.	Limited affinity for brain H_1 receptors. Cause minimal sedation, few effects on psychomotor activities or bladder function.	• Teach patient to expect few, if any, side effects. • More expensive than traditional antihistamines • Rapid onset of action, no drug tolerance with prolonged use.
Second-Generation Agents (Intranasal) azelastine (Astelin) olopatadine (Patanase)	Same as above.	Headache, bitter taste, somnolence, nasal irritation.	• Longer use increases risk of rebound vasodilation, which can increase congestion.
Decongestants			
Oral pseudoephedrine (Sudafed)	Stimulates adrenergic receptors on blood vessels, promotes vasoconstriction, reduces nasal congestion.	CNS stimulation, causing insomnia, excitation, headache, irritability, increased blood and ocular pressure, dysuria, palpitations, tachycardia.	• Advise patient of adverse reactions. • Advise that some preparations are contraindicated for patients with cardiovascular disease, hypertension, diabetes, glaucoma, benign prostatic hyperplasia, hepatic and renal disease.
Topical (Nasal Spray) oxymetazoline phenylephrine	Same as above.	Same as above, plus rebound nasal congestion.	• Teach patient that these drugs should not be used for >3 days or >3-4 times/day.

PT, Prothrombin time.

Continued

TABLE 26-2 Drug Therapy

Rhinitis and Sinusitis—cont'd

Drug	Mechanism of Action	Side Effects	Nursing Actions
Combination Cold Medications			
Zutripro oral solution (hydrocodone, chlorpheniramine, and pseudoephedrine) Rezira oral solution (hydrocodone and pseudoephedrine)	Hydrocodone suppresses cough. Mechanism of action of chlorpheniramine and pseudoephedrine discussed above.	See individual drugs above.	• Avoid in patients with head injury or increased intracranial pressure. • Use with caution in patients with acute abdominal conditions.

people stay indoors and overcrowding is more common. Other factors that increase susceptibility include fatigue, physical and emotional stress, allergies that affect the nose and throat, and compromised immune status. Exercise may reduce the number of upper respiratory tract infections.

Symptoms of acute viral rhinitis typically begin 2 or 3 days after infection and may include runny nose, watery eyes, nasal congestion, sneezing, cough, sore throat, fever, headache, and fatigue. Symptoms may last 2 to 14 days, with typical recovery in 7 to 10 days.

COMPLEMENTARY & ALTERNATIVE THERAPIES

Echinacea

Scientific Evidence

- Echinacea may have some benefit in reducing the incidence and duration of the common cold.
- However, there is conflicting evidence on its use in prevention and treatment of upper respiratory tract infections.

Nursing Implications

- Echinacea is considered safe when used on a short-term basis in recommended doses.
- Patients with asthma or allergies to plants in the daisy family (including ragweed, mums, marigolds, and daisies) are more likely to have allergic reactions.
- It may interfere with drugs that suppress the immune system and those that are metabolized by the liver.
- Caution is advised for patients with autoimmune disorders using this herb.

Source: *www.nlm.nih.gov/medlineplus/druginfo/natural/981.html.*

NURSING AND INTERPROFESSIONAL MANAGEMENT: ACUTE VIRAL RHINITIS

Interventions are directed at relieving symptoms. Rest, oral fluids, antipyretics, and analgesics are recommended. Warm salt water gargles, ice chips, lozenges, or sprays may help alleviate a sore throat. Petroleum jelly soothes a raw nose. Saline nasal spray reduces nasal congestion. Antihistamine and decongestant therapy reduces postnasal drip and significantly decreases the severity of cough, nasal obstruction, and nasal discharge. Caution patients to use intranasal decongestant sprays for no more than 3 days to prevent rebound congestion from occurring. Cough suppressants, such as dextromethorphan, and expectorants, such as guaifenesin, may be used.

Complications of acute viral rhinitis include pharyngitis, sinusitis, otitis media, tonsillitis, and lung infections. Unless complications are present, antibiotic therapy is not indicated. Antibiotics have no effect on viruses. If symptoms remain for 10 to 14 days with no improvement, an HCP should be consulted.

Teach the patient to recognize the manifestations of secondary bacterial infection, such as a temperature higher than 103° F (39.4° C); tender, swollen glands; severe sinus or ear pain; or significantly worsening symptoms. Green, purulent nasal drainage during the later stages of a cold is not uncommon and is not always indicative of bacterial infection. In the patient with pulmonary disease, signs of infection often include a change in consistency, color, or volume of the sputum. Because infection can progress rapidly, teach the patient with chronic respiratory disease to immediately report sputum changes, increased shortness of breath, and chest tightness.

During the cold season, advise patients with a chronic illness or a compromised immune system to avoid crowded situations and other individuals who have obvious cold symptoms. Frequent hand washing and avoiding hand-to-face contact can help prevent direct spread.

INFLUENZA

Influenza (flu) is a highly contagious respiratory illness that causes significant morbidity and mortality. Millions of Americans (about 5% to 20% of U.S. population) contract influenza each year. The flu season begins in September and continues through April of each year, peaking anywhere from November to March. More than 225,000 people are hospitalized each year for flu-related complications.[12] On average, influenza is responsible for 20,000 deaths annually. Vaccination of high-risk groups can prevent many of these deaths.

Etiology and Pathophysiology

Influenza viruses are classified into three serotypes (A, B, and C), but only A and B cause significant illness in humans. Influenza A is subtyped based on the presence of two surface proteins: hemagglutinin (H) and neuraminidase (N). The H antigens enable the virus to enter the cell, and the N antigens facilitate cell-to-cell transmission. As a result, influenza A viruses are named according to their H and N type (e.g., H3N2).

Influenza A is the most common and most virulent flu virus and can infect a variety of animals as well as humans. More than 100 types of influenza A are found in birds (avian flu), pigs (swine flu), horses, seals, and dogs. The virus mutates (changes) to allow it to infect different species. When a new viral strain reaches humans, people do not have immunity, and the virus can spread quickly around the globe, causing a *pandemic.* For example, type A H1N1 influenza (swine flu) emerged in 2009 and had never been seen in humans before. A worldwide pandemic resulted. Pandemics can also be triggered by the reemergence of a viral strain that has not circulated for many years. *Epidemics* are more localized outbreaks, usually occurring yearly, caused by variants of already circulating strains.

Influenza B and C viruses are not divided into subtypes and only infect humans. Outbreaks of influenza B can also cause regional epidemics, but the disease it produces is generally milder than that caused by influenza A. Influenza C causes mild illness and does not cause epidemics or pandemics.

Every flu season is different. Several different strains of influenza viruses exist, and the viruses are able to mutate over time; this explains the need for annual vaccination. Fewer cases of influenza result when a minor change in the virus occurs because most persons have partial immunity.

Influenza is transmitted from animals to humans by direct or indirect contact with infected animals (e.g., animal feces). Influenza is communicable between humans primarily through infected droplets and inhalation of aerosolized particles and to a lesser extent through direct contact with contaminated surfaces. The virus has an incubation period of 1 to 4 days, with peak transmission risk starting approximately 1 day before onset of symptoms and continuing for 5 to 7 days after a person first becomes sick.[13]

Clinical Manifestations

For some patients, it may be difficult to distinguish between the common cold and flu (Table 26-3). The onset of flu is typically abrupt, with systemic symptoms of chills, fever, and generalized myalgia, often accompanied by a headache, cough, sore throat, and fatigue. Physical examination findings are usually minimal, with normal assessment on chest auscultation. In uncomplicated cases, symptoms often subside within 7 days. Dyspnea and diffuse crackles are signs of pulmonary complications. Some patients, particularly older adults, experience weakness or lethargy that may persist for weeks.

Common complications of influenza include pneumonia (which can be either primary influenza [viral] pneumonia or secondary bacterial pneumonia) and ear or sinus infections. The patient who develops secondary bacterial pneumonia usually experiences gradual improvement of influenza symptoms, then worsening cough and purulent sputum. Treatment with antibiotics is usually effective if started early. Older adults are particularly prone to dehydration.

Diagnostic Studies

Influenza is commonly diagnosed based on the patient's health history, clinical findings, and the knowledge of other cases of influenza in the community.

Viral cultures are considered the "gold standard" for diagnosing influenza. However, they can take up to 3 to 10 days for results. Viral cultures may be obtained from a throat swab, nasopharyngeal swab, expectorated sputum, ET tube sample, or bronchoscopy (bronchial wash).[14] A viral culture has the advantage of identifying which virus (A, B, or another respiratory virus) and which strains of virus are present. These data are used in the formulation of the following season's flu vaccine.

Rapid flu tests can help in the diagnosis by detecting the virus in nasal secretions. Depending on the method, the test may be completed in the HCP's office in less than 30 minutes or be sent to a laboratory, with results available the same day. The test can help differentiate influenza from other viral and bacterial infections with similar manifestations that may be serious and must be treated differently. Rapid flu tests are best used within the first 48 hours of the onset of symptoms to help diagnose influenza and determine whether antiviral drugs are a treatment option.[15] The main disadvantages of the rapid flu test are that it will miss some cases or occasionally be positive when a person does not actually have the flu.

TABLE 26-3 Comparison of Common Cold and Influenza

Manifestations and Treatment	Common Cold (Viral Rhinitis)	Influenza
Symptom onset	Appear gradually	Abrupt onset. Within 3 to 6 hr
Fever	Rare	Characteristically high 102-104° F (38.9-40° C]). Lasts 3-4 days
Headache	Uncommon	Common (can be severe)
General aches and pains	Slight	Usual. Often severe
Fatigue and weakness	Sometimes. Usually mild	Usual. Starts early and can last up to 2-3 wk
Exhaustion	Uncommon	Usual at beginning of illness
Stuffy nose	Common	Sometimes
Sneezing	Common	Sometimes
Sore throat	Common	Sometimes
Chest discomfort, cough	Common. Mild to moderate hacking cough	Common
Complications	Sinus congestion. Earache	Bronchitis, pneumonia, acute respiratory failure. Can be life-threatening
Prevention	Hand washing. Avoid close contact with anyone who has a cold	Hand washing. Annual vaccination. Antiviral drugs. Avoid close contact with anyone who has the flu
Treatment	Temporary relief of symptoms: rest, hydration, decongestants, acetaminophen or ibuprofen for headache, aches, and pains	Antiviral drugs if given within 24-48 hr of onset. Rest, hydration, acetaminophen or ibuprofen for headache, aches, and pains

Adapted from Johnson K: Is it a cold or the flu? Retrieved from *www.webmd.com/cold-and-flu/is-it-a-cold-or-flu.*

❖ NURSING AND INTERPROFESSIONAL MANAGEMENT: INFLUENZA

The most effective strategy for managing influenza is prevention. Two types of flu vaccines are available: inactivated and live attenuated (Table 26-4). Administration of the flu vaccine results in the production of antibodies against the viruses contained in the vaccine.

The influenza vaccine is changed on a yearly basis, depending on the virus strains identified by the Centers for Disease Control and Prevention (CDC) as being most likely to cause illness in the upcoming flu season. The best time to receive the vaccine is in September (before flu exposure) because it takes 2 weeks for full protection to occur. However, the vaccine can be administered at any time during the flu season.

TABLE 26-4 Types of Influenza Immunization

Trivalent Inactivated Influenza Vaccine (TIV)	Live Attenuated Influenza Vaccine (LSIV)
Given by injection Approved for use in people ≥6 mo of age	Given by nasal spray Approved for healthy people ages 2-49 yr
Can be used in people at increased risk: • People of any age with chronic medical conditions • Residents of nursing homes and long-term care facilities • People who are immunocompromised • Pregnant women	Should NOT be used in: • Children <2 yr or adults >50 yr • Pregnant women • People with known immunodeficiency • Children or adolescents receiving aspirin or other salicylates • People who have medical conditions that place them at increased risk for complications from influenza (chronic cardiovascular, pulmonary, or neurologic diseases; diabetes mellitus; renal or hepatic dysfunction; hemoglobinopathies) • HCPs of high-risk patients because of risk of viral transmission from vaccine (should not care for high-risk patients for 7 days after vaccination)
Most common side effects are injection site reactions, such as pain, redness, and swelling	Most common side effects are runny nose and nasal congestion in all ages, fever in children ages 2-6 yr old and sore throat in adults

SAFETY ALERT Influenza Vaccination

- Advocate for vaccination of all people older than 6 months of age, but especially for those at high risk (e.g., health care workers, residents of long-term care facilities).
- Give high priority to groups, such as health care workers, who can transmit influenza to high-risk persons.

Vaccination of healthy people decreases the incidence and risk of transmitting influenza to those who have less ability to cope with the effects of this illness. Despite obvious benefits, many persons are reluctant to be vaccinated. Current vaccines are highly purified, and reactions are extremely rare. Soreness at the injection site is usually the most frequently reported adverse effect. Contraindications are a history of severe allergic reactions to previous flu vaccine. Patients with anaphylactic hypersensitivity to eggs should discuss the vaccine with their HCP, as alternatives for vaccinating patients with egg allergies are now available.

The primary nursing goals in influenza are relief of symptoms and prevention of secondary infection. Unless the patient with influenza is at high risk or complications develop, only supportive therapy is necessary. Rest, hydration, analgesics, and antipyretics can provide symptom relief. Older adults and those with a chronic illness may require hospitalization.

To treat influenza, three antiviral medications are used: zanamivir (Relenza), oseltamivir (Tamiflu), and peramivir (Rapivab).[16] Zanamivir is administered using an inhaler, oseltamivir is available as an oral capsule, and peramivir is given IV.

These antiviral drugs are neuraminidase inhibitors that prevent the virus from being released and spreading to other cells. These drugs shorten the duration of influenza symptoms and reduce the risk of complications. Treatment should be initiated as soon as possible in patients who are hospitalized with influenza, have severe or complicated illness, or are at high risk for complications. For maximum benefit in the treatment of influenza, therapy should begin within 2 days of the onset of symptoms, but it can be started later (based on clinical judgment).

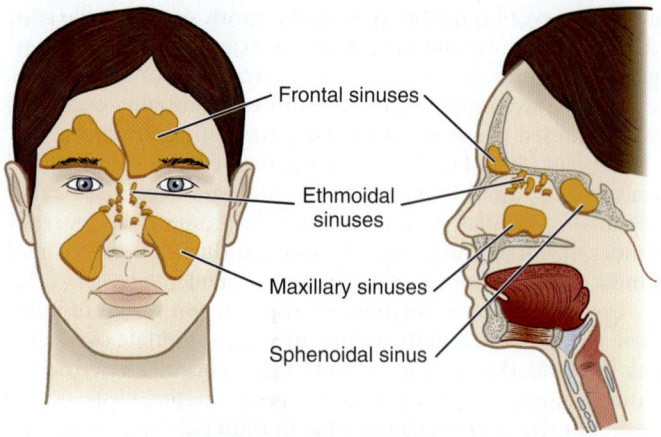

FIG. 26-2 Location of the sinuses.

COMPLEMENTARY & ALTERNATIVE THERAPIES

Zinc

Scientific Evidence

- Zinc is available in two forms: oral zinc (e.g., lozenges, tablets, syrup) and intranasal zinc (e.g., swabs, gels).
- When administered within 24 hr of onset of symptoms, zinc reduces the duration and severity of cold symptoms.
- When zinc supplementation is taken in low doses for at least 5 mo, the incidence of colds is reduced.

Nursing Implications

- Intranasal zinc has been linked to a severe side effect (irreversible loss of the sense of smell) and should not be used.
- Zinc is regarded as relatively safe when taken at recommended doses.
- Zinc lozenges are more apt to cause adverse effects (bad taste, nausea) than syrup or tablets.
- Oral zinc should not be taken with foods that will reduce its absorption, such as caffeine and dairy products.
- Zinc may interact with drugs, including antibiotics and penicillamine.

Source: *https://nccih.nih.gov/health/tips/flucold.htm.*

SINUSITIS

Sinusitis affects one out of every seven adults. It develops when inflammation or hypertrophy (swelling) of the mucosa blocks the openings (ostia) in the sinuses, through which mucus drains into the nose (Fig. 26-2). *Rhinosinusitis,* which may accompany sinusitis, is concurrent inflammation or infection of the nasal mucosa. Obstruction of mucus drainage can also be caused by nasal polyps, foreign bodies, deviated septa, or tumors. The secretions that accumulate behind the blocked ostia provide a rich medium for growth of bacteria, viruses, and fungi, all of which may cause infection.

Viral sinusitis typically follows an upper respiratory tract infection in which the virus penetrates the mucous membrane and decreases ciliary function. Viral infections usually resolve without treatment in less than 14 days. If symptoms worsen after 3 to 5 days or persist for longer than 10 days, a secondary bacterial infection may be present. Only 5% to 10% of patients with viral sinusitis develop a bacterial infection requiring antibiotic therapy.

Streptococcus pneumoniae, Haemophilus influenzae, and *Moraxella catarrhalis* are the most common causes of bacterial sinusitis. Fungal sinusitis is uncommon, usually occurring in patients who are debilitated or immunocompromised.

Sinusitis can be classified as acute, subacute, or chronic.[17] *Acute sinusitis* typically begins within 1 week of an upper respiratory tract infection and lasts less than 4 weeks. *Subacute sinusitis* is present when symptoms progress over 4 to 8 weeks. *Chronic sinusitis* (lasting longer than 8 weeks) is a persistent infection usually associated with allergies and nasal polyps. Chronic sinusitis generally results from repeated episodes of acute sinusitis that result in irreversible loss of the normal ciliated epithelium lining the sinus cavity.

Clinical Manifestations

Acute sinusitis causes significant pain over the affected sinus, purulent nasal drainage, nasal obstruction, congestion, fever, and malaise. The patient may appear acutely ill. Assessment involves inspection of the nasal mucosa and palpation of the sinus pressure points for pain. Findings that indicate acute sinusitis include edematous mucosa, discolored purulent nasal drainage, enlarged turbinates, tenderness over the involved frontal and/or maxillary sinuses, and *halitosis* (bad breath). Recurrent headaches that change in intensity with position changes or when secretions drain are not uncommon.

Chronic sinusitis is difficult to diagnose because symptoms are often nonspecific. The patient is rarely febrile. The patient may experience facial or dental pain, nasal congestion, and increased drainage, but severe pain and purulent drainage are often absent. Some symptoms mimic those seen with allergies. X-rays or CT scan of the sinuses may help confirm the diagnosis. CT scans may show the sinuses to be filled with fluid or a thickened mucous membrane. Nasal endoscopy with a flexible scope may be used to examine the sinuses, obtain a specimen for culture, and restore normal drainage.

As many as 50% of patients with moderate to severe asthma have chronic sinusitis. The exact link between these diseases is unclear. Postnasal drip associated with sinusitis may trigger asthma by stimulating bronchoconstriction. Gastroesophageal reflux disease (GERD) and smoking may increase the risk of a person with asthma developing sinusitis. Appropriate treatment of sinusitis often causes a reduction in asthma symptoms.

❖ NURSING AND INTERPROFESSIONAL MANAGEMENT: SINUSITIS

If allergies are the precipitating cause of sinusitis, instruct the patient about ways to reduce sinus inflammation and infection, including environmental control of allergens and appropriate drug therapy (see allergic rhinitis presented earlier in this chapter).

Initial treatment for acute sinusitis focuses on symptom relief. Medications include oral or topical decongestants to promote drainage, intranasal corticosteroids to decrease inflammation, analgesics to relieve pain, and saline nasal spray to relieve congestion. A clinical response to treatment should be observed within 72 hours.[18] Instruct patients using topical decongestants to use the medication for no longer than 4 to 5 days to prevent rebound congestion caused by vasodilation.

TABLE 26-5 Patient & Caregiver Teaching

Acute or Chronic Sinusitis

Include the following instructions when teaching the patient and caregiver about management of sinusitis.

1. Get plenty of rest to help body fight infection and promote recovery.
2. Keep well hydrated by drinking six to eight glasses of water to loosen secretions.
3. Take hot showers twice daily. Use a steam inhaler (15-min vaporization of boiled water), bedside humidifier, or nasal saline spray to promote secretion drainage.
4. Apply warm, damp towels around nose, cheeks, and eyes to ease facial pain.
5. Sleep with head elevated to help sinuses drain and reduce congestion.
6. Report a temperature of 100.4° F (38° C) or higher, which indicates infection.
7. Follow prescribed medication regimen:
   - Take analgesics to relieve pain.
   - Take decongestants/expectorants to relieve swelling.
   - Take antibiotics (as prescribed) for infection. Be sure to take entire prescription and report continued symptoms or a change in symptoms.
   - Administer nasal sprays correctly.
8. Perform nasal saline washes once or twice a day to wash sinuses.
9. Do not smoke, and avoid exposure to smoke. Smoke is an irritant and will worsen symptoms.
10. If allergies predispose to sinusitis, follow instructions regarding environmental control, drug therapy, and immunotherapy to reduce the inflammation and prevent sinus infection.

Saline irrigation of the nasal cavity can be used to rinse nasal passages, facilitate drainage, and decrease inflammation. Saline nasal spray is available over the counter.

If symptoms worsen or persist for longer than 1 week, antibiotic therapy may be prescribed. Amoxicillin is the first-line drug of choice and is continued for 10 to 14 days to prevent the formation of antibiotic-resistant organisms.[19] If symptoms do not resolve, the antibiotic should be changed to a fluoroquinolone or broader-spectrum cephalosporin antibiotic.

With chronic sinusitis, mixed bacterial flora is often present and infections are difficult to eliminate. Broad-spectrum antibiotics may be used for 4 to 6 weeks. Patient and caregiver teaching for acute and chronic sinusitis is presented in Table 26-5.

Medical therapy may not relieve the symptoms of some patients with persistent, recurrent, or chronic sinus illnesses. They may require nasal endoscopic surgery to relieve blockage caused by hypertrophy or septal deviation. This is usually performed as an outpatient procedure using local anesthesia. Propel, a self-expanding implant, can be placed directly in the sinus during surgery. Propel helps to maintain postoperative patency to the sinus cavity and provide localized corticosteroid delivery directly to the sinus lining before dissolving after 30 days.

OBSTRUCTION OF NOSE AND SINUSES

Nasal Polyps

Nasal polyps are soft, painless, benign (noncancerous) growths that form slowly in response to repeated inflammation of the sinus or nasal mucosa. They are most common in adults over age 40 and are twice as likely to occur in men than women.[20]

Polyps, which appear as chronic yellow, gray, or pink semitransparent projections in the naris, can exceed the size of a grape.

Small polyps are typically asymptomatic. Clinical manifestations of larger polyps include nasal obstruction, nasal discharge (usually clear mucus), and speech distortion. Topical and systemic corticosteroids are the primary medical therapy used to shrink nasal polyps. Endoscopic or laser surgery can remove nasal polyps, but recurrence is common.

Foreign Bodies

A variety of foreign bodies may potentially lodge in the upper respiratory tract of adults, but these are rare occurrences. Some of these situations may be the result of trauma or found in patients with mental illness. Foreign bodies may be inorganic or organic. Inorganic foreign bodies may cause no symptoms and be incidentally discovered on routine examination. Organic foreign bodies may produce a local inflammatory reaction and nasal discharge, which may become purulent and foul smelling if the object remains in the nasal cavity for an extended time. Foreign bodies can also cause pain, difficulty breathing, and nasal bleeding.

Foreign bodies should be removed from the nose through the route of entry. Sneezing or blowing the nose with the opposite nostril closed may be effective in removing the foreign object. Avoid irrigating the nose or pushing the object backward, since either could cause aspiration and airway obstruction. If sneezing or blowing the nose does not remove the object, an HCP should be consulted.

PROBLEMS OF PHARYNX

ACUTE PHARYNGITIS

Acute pharyngitis is an acute inflammation of the pharyngeal walls. It may include the tonsils, palate, and uvula. It can be caused by a viral, bacterial, or fungal infection. Viral pharyngitis accounts for approximately 90% of cases. Bacterial pharyngitis ("strep throat") usually results from group A β-hemolytic streptococci and accounts for 5% to 10% of cases.[21]

Fungal pharyngitis, such as candidiasis, can develop with the prolonged use of antibiotics or inhaled corticosteroids. It can also occur in immunosuppressed patients, especially those with human immunodeficiency virus (HIV) infection. Other causes of pharyngitis include dry air, smoking, GERD, allergy and postnasal drip, endotracheal (ET) intubation, chemicals, and cancer.

Clinical Manifestations

Symptoms of acute pharyngitis range in severity from a "scratchy" throat to pain so severe that swallowing is difficult. Because both viral and streptococcal infections appear as a red and edematous pharynx (with or without patchy exudates), it may be difficult to distinguish between the two types.

Four classic manifestations present in bacterial pharyngitis include fever greater than 100.4° F (38° C), anterior cervical lymph node enlargement, tonsillar or pharyngeal exudate, and the absence of cough.[22] However, appearance is not always diagnostic. When two or three of the above criteria are present, a rapid antigen detection test and/or a throat culture is done to establish the cause and direct appropriate management. White, irregular patches on the oropharynx suggest fungal infection with *Candida albicans.*

❖ NURSING AND INTERPROFESSIONAL MANAGEMENT: ACUTE PHARYNGITIS

The goals of nursing management are infection control, symptom relief, and prevention of secondary complications. For viral pharyngitis, antibiotics are not recommended. Instruct patients to use ibuprofen or acetaminophen for pain relief. Encourage the patient to increase fluid intake.

For symptom relief, instruct the patient to gargle with warm salt water (½ tsp of salt in 8 oz of water); drink warm or cold liquids; and suck on popsicles, hard candies, or throat lozenges. Cool, bland liquids and gelatin will not irritate the pharynx; citrus juices are often irritating. Encourage the patient to use a cool mist vaporizer or humidifier.

For bacterial pharyngitis caused by group A β-hemolytic streptococci, penicillin is the drug of choice. This antibiotic must be taken several times a day for a full 10 days to prevent complications such as rheumatic fever. For patients allergic to penicillin, erythromycin or clindamycin may be appropriate substitutes.[23] Other antibiotics (amoxicillin, azithromycin [Zithromax], cephalosporins) may also be used. Most people with streptococcal infections are contagious until they have been on antibiotics for 24 to 48 hours. Repeat throat cultures after antibiotic therapy are not required.

Candida infections are treated with nystatin, an antifungal antibiotic. Instruct patients to swish the preparation in their mouths for as long as possible before swallowing it. Treatment should continue until symptoms are gone. Patients taking inhaled corticosteroids are at risk for infection with *Candida* organisms. Thoroughly rinsing the mouth with water after using corticosteroids can prevent this infection.

PERITONSILLAR ABSCESS

Peritonsillar abscess is a complication of tonsillitis and is most often caused by group A β-hemolytic streptococci. The abscess causes pain, swelling, and blockage of the throat (when severe), threatening airway patency. The patient also experiences a high fever, chills, leukocytosis, difficulty swallowing, and a muffled voice. Treatment consists of IV antibiotic therapy and needle aspiration or incision and drainage of the abscess. In some cases an emergency tonsillectomy is performed, or an elective tonsillectomy is scheduled after the infection has subsided.

PROBLEMS OF TRACHEA AND LARYNX

AIRWAY OBSTRUCTION

Acute airway obstruction is a medical emergency. Airway obstruction can be caused by aspiration of food or a foreign body, allergic reactions, edema and inflammation caused by infections or burns, peritonsillar or retropharyngeal abscesses, malignancy, laryngeal or tracheal stenosis, and trauma.

Airway obstruction may be partial or complete. Clinical presentation of an airway obstruction often depends on the cause of the obstruction and/or location of the blockage due to an aspirated object such as food.[24] For example, objects lodged within the larynx may produce voice hoarseness or complete airway obstruction. Tracheal obstruction may produce wheezing, whereas objects lodged within the lower respiratory system (e.g., bronchus) may produce a cough or decreased air entry on the affected side.

Manifestations include choking, stridor, use of accessory muscles, suprasternal and intercostal retractions, flaring nostrils, wheezing, restlessness, tachycardia, cyanosis, and change in level of consciousness. Prompt assessment and treatment are essential because partial obstruction may quickly progress to complete obstruction. Complete airway obstruction can result in permanent brain damage or death if not corrected within 3 to 5 minutes.

Your immediate priority is to ensure the patient has a patent airway. Interventions to reestablish a patent airway include the obstructed airway (Heimlich) maneuver (see Appendix A), cricothyroidotomy, ET intubation, and tracheostomy. Unexplained partial airway obstruction or recurrent symptoms indicate the need for additional tests, such as a chest x-ray, laryngoscopy, and rigid bronchoscopy.

TRACHEOSTOMY

A **tracheostomy** is a surgically created stoma (opening) in the anterior portion of the trachea (Fig. 26-3, *A*). A tracheostomy may be undertaken to (1) establish a patent airway, (2) bypass an upper airway obstruction, (3) facilitate removal of secretions, (4) permit long-term mechanical ventilation, and (5) facilitate weaning from mechanical ventilation.[25]

The tracheostomy tube is shorter in length and slightly wider in diameter than an ET tube, thereby making it easier to keep the tube clean and facilitate better oral and bronchial hygiene. With the use of a tracheostomy (compared to an ET tube), patient comfort may be increased, because no tube is present in the mouth. There is also less risk of long-term damage to vocal cords.

A variety of tracheostomy tubes are available to meet individual patient needs (Table 26-6). All tracheostomy tubes contain a faceplate, or *flange,* which rests on the neck. In addition, all tracheostomy tubes come with an *obturator,* which is used to help insert the tube. Tracheostomy tubes have an *outer cannula* (which keeps the airway patent), and an *inner cannula* (which can be disposable or nondisposable and removed for cleaning) (Fig. 26-3).

Cuffed and *uncuffed* tracheostomy tubes are available. A tracheostomy tube with an inflated cuff (balloon) is most commonly used, particularly if the patient needs mechanical ventilation or is at risk of aspiration. The cuff, inflated via the *balloon inflation port* on the tracheostomy tube, helps keep the tracheostomy tube in place. Cuffless tubes are primarily used for the patient with a long-term tracheostomy, making eating and talking possible.

The outer and/or inner cannula may be *fenestrated* or *nonfenestrated.* A *fenestrated tube* has an opening (a hole) on the surface of the tube. A fenestrated tube allows the patient to breathe spontaneously. For example, with the use of a cuffed, fenestrated tracheostomy tube, when the cuff is deflated and the inner cannula removed, air can pass from the lungs up through the opening in the tracheostomy tube through the vocal cords and larynx, into the upper airway, and out the mouth and nose. This permits the patient to speak with the tracheostomy tube in place. When the cuff is reinflated and the inner cannula reinserted, air is prevented from passing from the lungs through the vocal cords.

Most patients who require mechanical ventilation are initially managed with an ET tube, which can be quickly inserted in an emergency. (The care of the patient with an ET tube is discussed in Chapter 65.) When swelling, trauma, or upper airway obstruction prevents ET intubation, an emergent *surgical tracheostomy* is required.

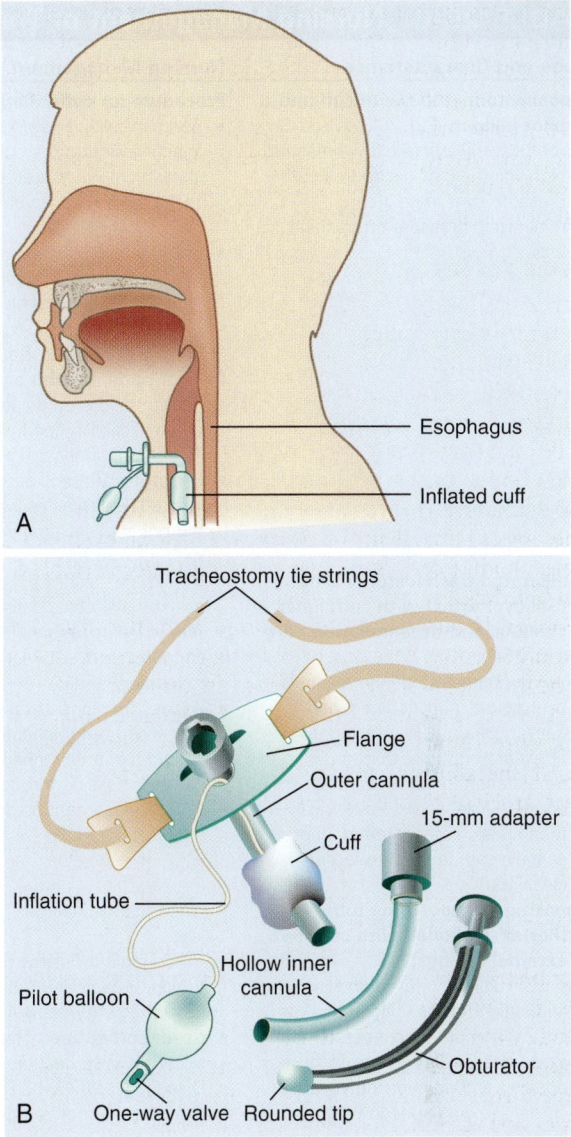

FIG. 26-3 Tracheostomy tube. **A,** Tracheostomy tube inserted in airway with inflated cuff. (See Table 26-6 and eNursing Care Plan 26-1 [on the website for this chapter] for related nursing management.) **B,** Parts of a tracheostomy tube.

Most surgical tracheostomies are performed in the operating room using general anesthesia. These may be undertaken electively on patients who are already intubated but require prolonged mechanical ventilation. A vertical incision is made on the anterior portion of the trachea. The tracheostomy tube is inserted, the incision is sutured, and a sterile dressing is applied.

A newer surgical technique is the *percutaneous tracheostomy.* Using local anesthesia, sedation, and under video-assisted guidance, a needle is placed into the middle of the trachea. A dilator is placed over the top of the needle. The opening is progressively made larger (with increasingly larger dilators) until the hole is big enough for insertion of the tracheostomy tube. Percutaneous tracheostomy approaches have less risk of bleeding and fewer postoperative complications.[26]

TABLE 26-6 Nursing Management of Tracheostomies

Tube and Characteristics	Nursing Management
Tracheostomy tube with cuff and pilot balloon (Fig. 26-3, *A* and *B*) When properly inflated, low-pressure, high-volume cuff distributes cuff pressure over large area, minimizing pressure on tracheal wall.	**Procedure for cuff inflation** • *Mechanically ventilated patient:* Inflate the cuff using *minimal occlusion volume (MOV) technique* by slowly injecting air into the cuff until no leak (sound) is heard at peak inspiratory pressure (end of ventilator inspiration) when a stethoscope is placed over the trachea. An alternative approach, termed *minimal leak technique* (MLT), involves inflating the cuff to minimal occlusion pressure and then withdrawing 0.1 mL of air. • *Spontaneously breathing patient:* Inflate cuff using MOV by slowly injecting air into the cuff until no sound is heard after deep breath or during inhalation with bag-valve-mask. If using MLT, remove 0.1 mL of air while maintaining seal. MLT should not be used if there is risk of aspiration. • *Immediately after cuff inflation (both groups):* Verify pressure is within accepted range (20 to 25 cm H_2O) with a manometer. Record cuff pressure and volume of air used for cuff inflation in chart. **Care of patients with an inflated cuff** • Monitor and record cuff pressure q8hr. Cuff pressure should be 20 to 25 cm H_2O to allow adequate tracheal capillary perfusion. If needed, remove or add air to the pilot tubing using a syringe and stopcock. Afterward, verify cuff pressure is within accepted range with manometer. • Report inability to keep the cuff inflated or need to use progressively larger volumes of air to keep cuff inflated. Potential causes include tracheal dilation at the cuff site or a crack or slow leak in the housing of the one-way inflation valve. If the leak is due to tracheal dilation, the physician may intubate the patient with a larger tube.
Fenestrated tracheostomy tube (Shiley, Portex) with cuff, inner cannula, and decannulation plug (Fig. 26-6) When nonfenestrated inner cannula is removed, cuff deflated, and decannulation plug inserted, air flows around tube, through fenestration in outer cannula, and up over vocal cords. Patient can then speak. A fenestrated inner cannula can be used to facilitate cleaning.	• If possible, assess risk of aspiration before removing inner cannula. A speech pathologist may be able to assist if available. Deflate cuff. Note coughing. • ***Never*** insert decannulation plug in tracheostomy tube until cuff is deflated and nonfenestrated inner cannula removed. Prior insertion will prevent patient from breathing (no air inflow). This may precipitate a respiratory arrest. • Assess for signs of respiratory distress when a fenestrated cannula is first used. If this occurs, remove the cap, insert a nonfenestrated inner cannula, and reinflate the cuff. • A nonfenestrated inner cannula must be used to suction patient to prevent tracheal damage from suction catheter passing through fenestrated openings. • Cuff management as described above.
Speaking tracheostomy tube (Portex, National) with cuff, two external tubings Has two tubings, one leading to cuff and second to opening above the cuff. When port is connected to air source, air flows out of opening and up over the vocal cords, allowing speech with cuff inflated.	• Once tube is inserted, wait 2 days before use so that the stoma can close around the tube and prevent leaks. • When patient desires to speak, connect port to compressed air (or O_2). Be certain to identify correct tubing. If gas enters the cuff, it will overinflate and rupture, requiring an emergency tube change. Use lowest flow (typically 4-6 L/min) that results in speech. High flows dehydrate mucosa. • Cover port adapter. This will cause the air to flow upward. Instruct patient to speak in short sentences because voice becomes a whisper with long sentences. • Disconnect flow when patient does not want to speak to prevent mucosal dehydration. • Cuff management as described above.
Tracheostomy tube (Bivona Fome-Cuf) with foam-filled cuff Cuff is filled with plastic foam. Before insertion, cuff is deflated. After insertion, cuff is allowed to fill passively with air. Pilot tubing is not capped, and no cuff pressure monitoring is required.	• Before insertion, withdraw all air from the cuff using a 20-mL syringe. Cap pilot balloon tubing to prevent reentry of air. After tracheostomy is inserted, remove cap from pilot tubing, allowing cuff to passively reinflate. • Do not inject air into tubing or cap pilot balloon tubing while it is in patient. Air will flow in and out in response to pressure changes (head turning). Place tag on tubing to alert staff not to cap or inflate cuff. • Deflate cuff daily via pilot balloon to evaluate integrity of cuff. Also assess ability to easily deflate cuff. Difficulty deflating cuff indicates a need for tube change. If aspirate returns with air, cuff is no longer intact. • Tube can be used for up to 1 mo in patients on home mechanical ventilation. • Good choice for patients who require inflated cuff at home, since teaching about cuff pressure is simplified.

The choice of tracheostomy often depends on the surgeon's personal preference. Both surgical and percutaneous tracheostomies may also be performed at the patient's bedside in the emergency department or ICU.

❖ NURSING MANAGEMENT: TRACHEOSTOMY

◆ Acute Care

Before the tracheostomy procedure (and time permitting), explain the purpose of the procedure to both the patient and caregiver. If the patient is having the tracheostomy in the operating room, follow all hospital policies and procedures for preparing the patient for surgery. (Care of the preoperative patient is discussed in Chapter 17.)

If the procedure is being done at the patient's bedside, ensure all appropriate personnel, including respiratory therapy, have been notified. Emergency resuscitation equipment, including a bag-valve-mask (BVM), should be readily available.

Record vital signs, including heart rate, respiratory rate and rhythm, BP, and SpO_2. Ensure an existing IV line is patent and that bedside suction is working. Help assemble and set up all necessary equipment. Position the patient supine. Administer

TABLE 26-7 Complications of Tracheostomy

Closely monitor patients with a tracheostomy for the following potential complications:

- Air leak
- Airway obstruction
- Altered body image
- Aspiration
- Bleeding
- Fistula formation
- Impaired cough
- Infection: wound or respiratory tract
- Subcutaneous emphysema
- Tracheal necrosis
- Tracheal stenosis
- Tube displacement

analgesia and sedation as ordered by the surgeon, and monitor patient response to analgesia and/or sedatives. Observe patient's tolerance to the procedure.

If you are asked to help during the procedure, ensure you place the obturator inside the outer cannula with its rounded tip protruding from the end of the tube to ease insertion. After insertion, immediately remove the obturator so that air can flow through the tube. Keep the obturator in an easily accessible place at the bedside so that it can be used quickly in case of accidental decannulation (removal of the tracheostomy).

Immediately after the procedure, the cuff (balloon) is inflated. The patient's chest is auscultated for air entry. Air entry should be heard in all lung fields. When placement is confirmed, the ET tube (if present) is removed. The tracheostomy tube is sutured and secured in place with cotton tracheostomy ties, tracheostomy tapes, or Velcro straps.

Many different complications can occur as a result of tracheostomy (Table 26-7). You must be aware of them, especially airway obstruction, bleeding, and infection.

Monitor and record the patient's heart rate, respiratory rate, BP, and SpO_2. SpO_2 readings should remain stable. Note and record the mechanical ventilator settings, including mode, FIO_2, and positive end expiratory pressure (PEEP). Observe the amount of blood at the tracheostomy insertion site. Notify the surgeon or most appropriate personnel if the bleeding persists. A chest x-ray should be taken after the procedure. (Care of the patient receiving mechanical ventilation is discussed in Chapter 65.)

Considerable variation in practice exists with regard to the care of a patient with a new tracheostomy. In some centers, it is a shared responsibility between nursing and respiratory therapy. You need to be familiar with your hospital's policies and procedures. The following discussion highlights general guidelines when caring for a patient with a tracheostomy in the first few days after the procedure.

The tracheostomy site must be assessed every shift (at a minimum). Observe the site for any redness, inflammation, edema, ulceration, or signs of infection. Clean around the stoma with normal saline. Apply a sterile pre-cut dressing around the tracheostomy tube site at least once per shift or more frequently based upon your nursing assessment.

Because an inflated cuff exerts pressure on the tracheal mucosa, it is important to inflate the cuff with the minimum volume of air required to obtain an airway seal. Cuff inflation pressure can be measured with a hand-held cuff manometer. The pressure should be monitored at least every 8 hours. Cuff inflation pressure should not exceed 20 to 25 cm H_2O because higher pressures may compress tracheal capillaries, limit blood flow, and predispose the patient to tracheal necrosis. The minimal leak technique (MLT) and the minimal occlusion volume (MOV) are two commonly used methods to inflate the tracheostomy cuff (Table 26-6). Routine cuff deflation is no longer recommended.[27]

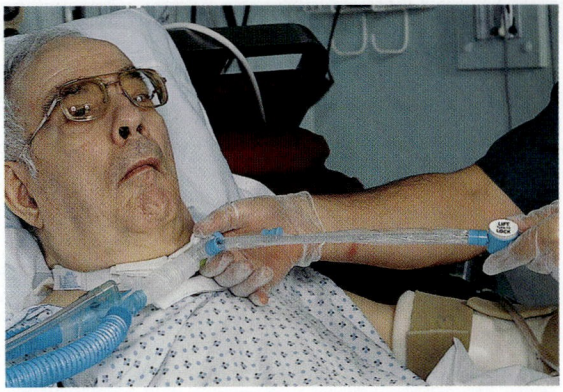

FIG. 26-4 Suctioning tracheostomy with closed system suction catheter. (From Potter PA, Perry AG: *Basic nursing: essentials for practice,* ed 7, St Louis, 2011, Mosby.)

Suction the airway via the tracheostomy tube as needed (Fig. 26-4 and Table 26-8). Try to avoid suctioning through the newly created tracheostomy in the first few hours after the procedure, as this may aggravate discomfort and promote bleeding. Initially, patients should receive humidified air to compensate for the loss of the upper airway to warm and moisturize secretions. Humidification is essential to prevent retention of tenacious secretions and formation of mucous plugs.

If the inner cannula is disposable, replace as per manufacturer and institutional guidelines. If nondisposable, clean the inner cannula at least every shift. Cleaning removes mucus from the inside of the tube to prevent airway obstruction (Table 26-9).

Change the tracheostomy tapes after the first 24 hours and then as required (Fig. 26-5 and Table 26-9). A two-person technique, one person to stabilize the tracheostomy and one to change the tapes, is best practice to ensure that the tracheostomy does not become accidentally dislodged during the procedure. At the end of the procedure, place two fingers underneath the tapes to ensure they are not too tight around the neck.

When turning and repositioning the patient, take care not to dislodge the tracheostomy tube. Because tube replacement is difficult, several precautions are required, including (1) keep a replacement tube of equal or smaller size at the bedside, readily available for emergency reinsertion; (2) do not change tracheostomy tapes for at least 24 hours after the insertion procedure; and (3) if necessary, an HCP performs the first tube change usually no sooner than 7 days after the tracheostomy.

CHECK YOUR PRACTICE

You are caring for a patient who had a surgically created tracheostomy 6 hours ago. While suctioning the patient, he coughs and the tracheostomy tube is dislodged.

- What should you do?

If the tube is accidentally dislodged, immediately call for help. While waiting for the HCP, a respiratory therapist, or other designated individual to arrive, several options may be used (depending on nursing scope of practice and hospital policies and procedures). One option is to quickly obtain a hemostat to spread the opening where the tube was displaced. Insert the obturator in the replacement (spare) tracheostomy tube,

TABLE 26-8 Suctioning a Tracheostomy

1. Assess the need for suctioning hourly. Indications include visible coughing, coarse crackles or wheezes over large airways, moist cough, increase in peak inspiratory pressure on mechanical ventilator, and restlessness or agitation. May be accompanied by decrease in SpO_2. Do not suction routinely.
2. If suctioning is indicated, explain procedure to patient.
3. Collect necessary sterile equipment: suction catheter (no larger than half the lumen of the tracheostomy tube), gloves, sterile water, cup, and drape. If a closed tracheal suction system is used, the catheter is enclosed in a plastic sleeve and reused (Fig. 26-4). No additional equipment is needed.
4. Check suction source and regulator. Adjust suction pressure to no greater than 125 mm Hg pressure with tubing occluded.
5. Assess heart rate and rhythm and SpO_2 to provide baseline for detecting change during suctioning.
6. Wash hands and put on personal protective equipment (eye goggles).
7. Use sterile technique to open package, fill cup with sterile water, put on sterile gloves, and connect catheter to suction tubing. Designate one hand as contaminated for (1) connecting and disconnecting the tubing at the suction catheter, (2) using the manual resuscitation bag (MRB), and (3) operating the suction control. Suction sterile water through the catheter to test the system.
8. Provide preoxygenation for a minimum of 30 seconds by (1) adjusting ventilator to deliver 100% O_2; or (2) using a reservoir-equipped bag-valve-mask connected to 100% O_2. The method chosen depends on whether the patient is attached to a mechanical ventilator or has a tracheostomy tube in place but is spontaneously breathing and receiving supplemental O_2. The patient who has had a tracheostomy for an extended period and is not acutely ill may be able to tolerate suctioning without use of an MRB or the ventilator.
9. Gently insert catheter *without suction* to minimize the amount of O_2 removed from the lungs. Insert the catheter to the point where the patient coughs. Do NOT insert the catheter until you meet resistance (this is the carina, and repeated trauma with suction catheter can promote bleeding). Apply suction as you slowly begin to withdraw the catheter.
10. Continuous suction should be applied for no more than 10 to 15 seconds.
11. Discontinue suctioning and immediately remove the suction catheter from the patient's trachea if heart rate decreases from baseline by 20 beats/min, increases from baseline by 40 beats/min, a dysrhythmia occurs, or SpO_2 decreases to less than 90%. A vagal response may have occurred.
12. After each suction pass, wait at least 30 seconds before suctioning again. Always hyperoxygenate for at least 30 sec (via mechanical ventilator or MRB with 5-6 breaths) in between each suctioning pass.
13. Repeat procedure until airway is clear. Limit insertions of suction catheter to as few as possible. If airway is not clear after three suction passes, allow the patient to rest before additional suctioning.
14. Return O_2 concentration to prior setting.
15. Rinse catheter. If using the in-line suction catheter (via mechanical ventilation), ensure that normal saline used to flush out the suction catheter does not enter the patient's airway. For disposable suction catheters, dispose of catheter by wrapping it around fingers of gloved hand and pulling glove over catheter. Discard equipment in proper waste container.
16. Suction the oropharynx or use mouth suction.
17. Reassess heart rate and rhythm and SpO_2. Auscultate to assess changes in lung sounds. Record time, amount, and character of secretions and patient response to suctioning.

lubricate with saline, and insert the tube into the stoma. Once the tube is inserted, remove the obturator immediately so that air can flow through the tube.

Another option is to insert a suction catheter to allow passage of air and to serve as a guide for insertion. Thread the tracheostomy tube over the catheter and remove the suction catheter.

If the tube cannot be replaced, immediately and quickly assess the patient's level of respiratory distress and position the patient in semi-Fowler's position to alleviate dyspnea until assistance arrives. Severe dyspnea may progress to respiratory arrest. If respiratory arrest occurs, cover the stoma with a sterile dressing and ventilate the patient with the BVM over the nose

TABLE 26-9 Tracheostomy Care

The following are general guidelines for basic tracheostomy care. Become familiar with the specific policies and/or procedures in your institution.

1. Explain procedure to patient.
2. Use tracheostomy care kit or collect necessary sterile equipment (e.g., suction catheter, gloves, water basin, drape, tracheostomy ties, tube brush or pipe cleaners, 4 × 4-inch gauze pads, sterile water or normal saline, and tracheostomy dressing [optional]). NOTE: Clean rather than sterile technique is used at home.
3. Position patient in semi-Fowler's position.
4. Assemble needed materials on bedside table next to patient.
5. Wash hands. Put on personal protective equipment (goggles and clean gloves).
6. Auscultate chest sounds. If wheezes or coarse crackles are present, suction the patient if unable to cough up secretions (Table 26-8). Remove soiled dressing and clean gloves.
7. Open sterile equipment, pour sterile H_2O or normal saline into two compartments of sterile container or two basins, and put on sterile gloves. NOTE: Hydrogen peroxide (3%) is no longer recommended unless an infection is present. If it is used, rinse the inner cannula and skin with sterile H_2O or normal saline afterward to prevent trauma to tissue.
8. Unlock and remove inner cannula, if present. Many tracheostomy tubes do not have inner cannulas. Care for these tubes includes all steps except for inner cannula care.
9. If disposable inner cannula is used, replace with new cannula. If a nondisposable cannula is used:
   - Immerse inner cannula in sterile solution and clean inside and outside of cannula using tube brush or pipe cleaners.
   - Rinse cannula in sterile solution. Remove from solution and shake to dry.
   - Insert inner cannula into outer cannula with the curved part downward, and lock in place.
10. Remove dried secretions from stoma using 4 × 4-inch gauze pad soaked in sterile water or saline. Gently pat area around the stoma dry. Be sure to clean under the tracheostomy flange (faceplate), using cotton swabs to reach this area.
11. Change tracheostomy tapes. Use two-person change technique or secure new tapes to flanges before removing the old ones. Tie tracheostomy tapes securely with room for two fingers between tapes and skin (Fig. 26-5). To prevent accidental tube removal, secure the tracheostomy tube by gently applying pressure to the flange of the tube during the tape changes. *Do not change tracheostomy tapes for 24 hours after the tracheostomy procedure.*
13. As an alternative, some patients prefer tracheostomy tapes made of Velcro, which are easier to adjust.
14. If drainage is excessive, place dressing around tube (Fig. 26-5). A pre-cut tracheostomy dressing or unlined gauze should be used. Do not cut the gauze because threads may be inhaled or wrap around the tracheostomy tube. Change the dressing as required. Wet dressings promote infection and stoma irritation.
15. Repeat care three times/day and as needed.

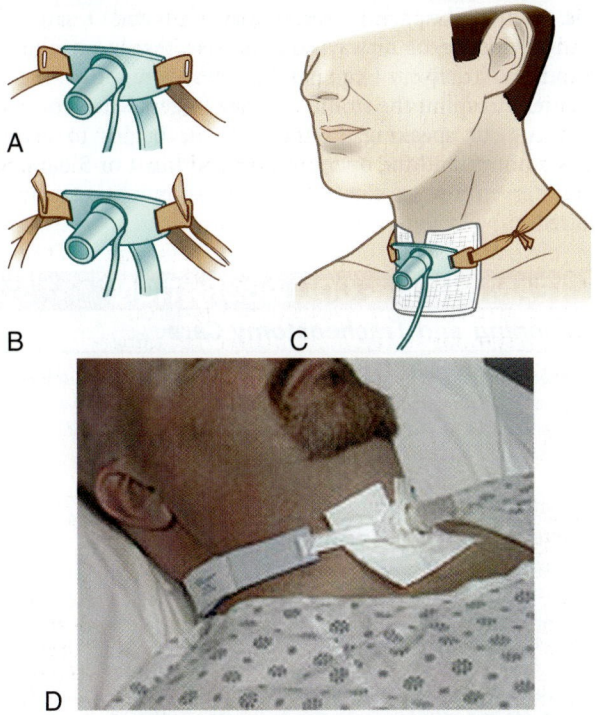

FIG. 26-5 Changing tracheostomy tapes. **A,** A slit is cut about 1 inch (2.5 cm) from the end. The slit end is put into the opening of the cannula. **B,** A loop is made with the other end of the tape. **C,** The tapes are tied together with a double knot on the side of the neck. **D,** A Velcro tracheostomy tube holder can be used instead of twill ties to make tracheostomy tube stabilization more secure. (*D,* Courtesy Dale Medical Products, Inc, Plainville, Mass.)

and mouth. If a patient has had a total laryngectomy, there will be complete separation between the upper airway and trachea. Ventilate this patient through the tracheostomy stoma.

Chronic Care

Some patients will never be able to be weaned from mechanical ventilation and will require a tracheostomy for life. Care of the patient with a long-term tracheostomy includes all of the same care as patients with a new tracheostomy, including observing the tracheostomy site, cleaning the inner cannula, suctioning, and changing tracheostomy tapes.

The tracheostomy tube should be changed approximately 1 month after the first tube change and monthly thereafter. When a tracheostomy has been in place for several months, the healed tract should be well formed. Changing the tracheostomy tube may be undertaken for two main reasons. First, it permits assessment of the stoma and cleaning of the tube. The patient may be taught to change the tube at home using a clean technique. Second, exchanging the tracheostomy tube for one of a different size (smaller internal diameter) will increase airway resistance and work of breathing for the patient. This will strengthen the respiratory muscles and help promote weaning from mechanical ventilation.

Swallowing Dysfunction

The patient with a tracheostomy who cannot protect the airway from aspiration requires an inflated cuff. However, an inflated cuff may result in swallowing dysfunction by interfering with the normal function of muscles used to swallow.

For long-term tracheostomy patients, it is important to evaluate the patient's swallowing ability and risk for aspiration.

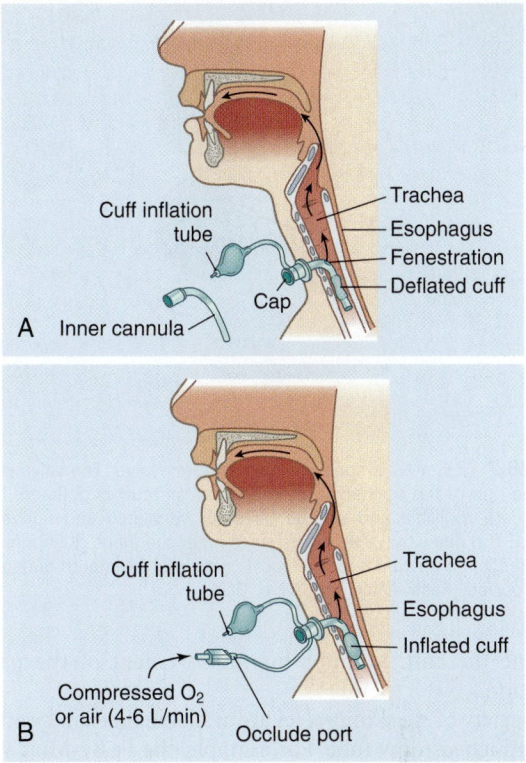

FIG. 26-6 Speaking tracheostomy tubes. **A,** Fenestrated tracheostomy tube with cuff deflated, inner cannula removed, and tracheostomy tube capped to allow air to pass over the vocal cords. **B,** Speaking tracheostomy tube. One tube is used for cuff inflation. The second tube is connected to a source of compressed air or O_2. When the port on the second tube is occluded, air flows up over the vocal cords, allowing speech with an inflated cuff. (See Table 26-6 and eNursing Care Plan 26-1 for related nursing management.)

Assessment of the patient's ability to swallow is most often done by a speech therapist. The patient is evaluated for aspiration and/or microaspiration using different consistencies of thickened fluids and under videofluoroscopy or with a fiberoptic endoscopy. If the patient is able to swallow without aspiration when the cuff is deflated, the cuff may be left deflated or a cuffless tube substituted. At this time, patients may also be permitted varying levels of thickened fluids and soft foods.

Speech With a Tracheostomy Tube

A number of techniques promote speech in the patient with a tracheostomy. When the patient initially requires attachment to a mechanical ventilator, provide the patient with a paper and pencil, a white board, or Magic Slate. A communication board with pictures of common needs is convenient for patients who may speak other languages. A visual alphabet for spelling words is useful for patients who are weak or have difficulty writing.

The spontaneously breathing patient may be able to talk with a tracheostomy. Several options are available depending upon the type of tracheostomy. For example, if it has been determined that the patient is at low risk for aspiration, (1) remove the inner cannula (if nonfenestrated), (2) deflate the cuff, and (3) place the decannulation cap in the tube (Fig. 26-6).

When the tracheostomy cuff is deflated, exhaled air is allowed to flow upward over the vocal cords. When a fenestrated cannula is first used, frequently assess the patient for signs of respiratory distress. If the patient is not able to tolerate the procedure, remove the cap, insert a nonfenestrated inner cannula, and

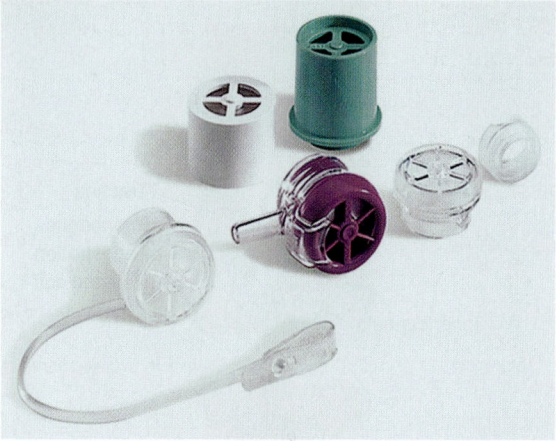

FIG. 26-7 Passy-Muir speaking tracheostomy valve. The valve is placed over the hub of the tracheostomy tube after the cuff is deflated. Multiple options are available and can be used for ventilated and nonventilated patients. The one-way valve allows air to enter the lungs during inspiration and redirects air upward over the vocal cords into the mouth during expiration. (Courtesy Passy-Muir, Inc, Irvine, Calif.)

reinflate the cuff. Monitor for improvement of the patient's condition.

A variety of speaking valves are available that can be attached to the tracheostomy tube. For example, the Passy-Muir valve is a simple device that attaches to the hub of the tracheostomy tube (Fig. 26-7). With the cuff deflated, the valve redirects air flow through the vocal cords. On inspiration, the valve on the device opens, allowing the patient to inhale. When the patient exhales, the valve closes, air flows upward around the tracheostomy, and through the vocal cords. The patient exhales through the nose and mouth instead of through the tracheostomy, allowing speech. The patient may initially only be able to tolerate short periods of use until he or she becomes accustomed to exhaling through the mouth. Remove the valve immediately if there are any signs and symptoms of respiratory distress. Advocating for the use of alternative speaking devices may help improve self-care and increase self-esteem for the patient with a tracheostomy.

◆ Decannulation

Removal of the tracheostomy from the trachea is known as **decannulation**. Removal is possible when the primary condition for which the patient initially received a tracheostomy has been resolved. In addition, the patient needs to (1) be hemodynamically stable; (2) have a stable, intact respiratory drive; and (3) be able to adequately exchange air and expectorate secretions.

Immediately prior to decannulation, explain to the patient what will occur. Monitor and record the vital signs. Suction the patient prior to decannulation through the tracheostomy. Clear the mouth of any oral secretions. Loosen and/or cut the tracheostomy tapes, and remove any visible sutures holding the tracheostomy in place. Most importantly, ensure that the tracheostomy cuff is deflated. Pull the tracheostomy tube outwards in one smooth motion. Stop if you meet any resistance and notify the appropriate personnel.

Once the tracheostomy tube is removed, post-decannulation care involves application of a sterile occlusive dressing and monitoring the site for bleeding. The dressing must be changed if it gets soiled or wet. If necessary, close the stoma with tape strips. Monitor the patient's respiratory status and O_2 saturation for any evidence of airway compromise. Apply an alternate method of O_2 delivery (e.g., nasal prongs) if required. Instruct the patient to splint the stoma with the fingers when coughing, swallowing, or speaking. Epithelial tissue begins to form in 24 to 48 hours, and the opening closes within 4 or 5 days. Surgical intervention to close the tracheostomy is usually not required.

TEAMWORK & COLLABORATION

Suctioning and Tracheostomy Care

Licensed practical nurses (LPNs) may do suctioning and give tracheostomy care to stable patients. In patients who have acute airway problems requiring an ET or tracheostomy tube, these interventions should be done by the registered nurse (RN).

Role of Nursing Personnel

Registered Nurse (RN)

For unstable patients:

- Assess for the need for suctioning.
- Suction the ET or tracheostomy tube.
- Evaluate for adverse effects of suctioning such as dysrhythmias.
- Evaluate whether patient status is improved after suctioning.
- Maintain appropriate cuff inflation pressure at 20 to 25 cm H_2O, or use minimal leak technique to maintain cuff pressure.
- Assess tracheostomy and any retention sutures for evidence of complications (e.g., infection).
- Replace the tracheostomy tube after accidental dislodgment.
- Ventilate the patient with a bag-valve-mask device after accidental tracheostomy dislodgment if needed.
- Assess swallowing ability and risk for aspiration.
- Develop plan to avoid aspiration in a patient with a tracheostomy.
- Teach patient and caregiver about home tracheostomy care.

Licensed Practical/Vocational Nurse (LPN/LVN)

For stable patients:

- Determine the need for suctioning.
- Suction the tracheostomy.
- Evaluate whether patient status is improved after suctioning.
- Provide tracheostomy care using sterile technique.

Unlicensed Assistive Personnel (UAP)

- Provide oral care to patient with a tracheostomy.
- Suction patient's oropharynx (after being trained and evaluated in this procedure).
- Report increased need for oropharyngeal suctioning to the RN.

Role of Other Team Members

Respiratory Therapist

- Ensures proper equipment is available for suctioning and tracheotomy care
- Has similar role to that of RN (see above)

LARYNGEAL POLYPS

Laryngeal polyps develop on the vocal cords from vocal abuse (e.g., excessive talking, singing) or irritation (e.g., intubation, cigarette smoking). The most common symptom is hoarseness. Polyps are treated conservatively with voice rest and adequate hydration. Surgical removal may be indicated for large polyps, which may cause dysphagia, dyspnea, and stridor. Polyps are usually benign but may be removed because they can become malignant.

HEAD AND NECK CANCER

Head and neck cancer is classified according to the area where it occurs. These cancers may involve the nasal cavity and paranasal sinuses, nasopharynx, oropharynx, larynx, oral cavity, and/or salivary gland. (Cancer of the oral cavity is discussed in Chapter 41.) Most head and neck cancers arise from squamous cells that line the mucosal surfaces of the head and neck.

More than 52,000 new cases of head and neck cancer are diagnosed each year in the United States. Eighty-five percent of head and neck cancers are caused by tobacco (including smokeless tobacco). Excessive alcohol consumption is also a major risk factor. Head and neck cancer most frequently occurs in people over age 50 and twice as often in men (compared to women). Head and neck cancers in patients younger than 50 years are often associated with human papillomavirus (HPV) infection. Other risk factors include sun exposure, radiation therapy to the head and neck, exposure to asbestos and other industrial carcinogens, and poor oral hygiene.[28]

Unfortunately, most people have locally advanced disease at the time of diagnosis. Disability from both the disease and subsequent treatment is significant because of the potential loss of voice, adverse effects from chemotherapy and/or radiation, disfigurement, and social concerns.

Clinical Manifestations

Early clinical manifestations of head and neck cancer vary with the location of the tumor. For example, cancer of the oral cavity may initially be seen as a white or red patch in the mouth, an ulcer that does not heal, or a change in the fit of dentures. Some patients experience what feels like a lump in the throat or a change in the quality of the voice. Hoarseness that lasts more than 2 weeks may be a symptom of early laryngeal cancer.

Other clinical manifestations may include a sore throat that does not get better with treatment, a unilateral sore throat or otalgia (ear pain), swelling or lumps in the neck, and coughing up blood. Unintentional weight loss and difficulty with chewing, swallowing, moving the tongue or jaw, and breathing are typically late symptoms. A partially or fully obstructed airway is also often a late manifestation of head and neck cancer.

Diagnostic Studies

Early detection is key to patient survival. Physical assessment involves thoroughly examining the oral cavity, including the area under the tongue and dentures, with a flashlight. There may be thickening of the normally soft and pliable oral mucosa. Inspect the floor of the mouth and tongue, and bimanually palpate the lymph nodes in the neck. *Leukoplakia* (white patch) or *erythroplakia* (fiery red patch) may be found. Both leukoplakia and carcinoma in situ (localized to a defined area) may precede invasive carcinoma by many years.

If lesions are suspected, the upper airways may be examined using indirect pharyngoscopy and laryngoscopy (which involves using a laryngeal mirror). The larynx and vocal cords are visually inspected for lesions and tissue mobility. Typically, multiple biopsy specimens are obtained to help determine the extent of the disease. A CT scan or MRI may be performed to detect local and regional spread. Positron emission tomography (PET) scanning is also used in diagnosis. (Interprofessional care of head and neck cancer is presented in Table 26-10.)

TABLE 26-10 Interprofessional Care

Head and Neck Cancer

Diagnostic Assessment	Management

• History and physical examination
• Indirect pharyngoscopy and laryngoscopy
• Endoscopy
• Biopsy
• Chest x-ray
• Barium swallow
	• Surgery
	  • Vocal cord stripping
	  • Laser surgery
	  • Cordectomy
	  • Partial or total laryngectomy
	  • Pharyngectomy
	  • Lymph node removal with neck dissection
	  • Tracheostomy
	  • Reconstructive procedures
	• Radiation therapy
	• Chemotherapy
	• Targeted therapy
	• Physical therapy
	• Occupational therapy
	• Speech therapy

Staging of Head and Neck Cancer

Head and neck cancer is staged based on the size of the tumor (T), number and location of involved lymph nodes (N), and extent of metastasis (M). This is referred to as *TNM staging.*[29] TNM staging classifies head and neck cancers as Stage 0 (carcinoma in situ) through Stage IV (spread to distant organs and tissues). (TNM staging is discussed in Chapter 15 on p. 241.)

Interprofessional Care

The choice of treatment for head and neck cancer is based on many factors, including the location of tumor, TNM stage, patient's age and overall general health, urgency of treatment, cosmetic and functional considerations (e.g., ability to talk, swallow, and chew), and patient choice. Treatment options may include surgery, radiation therapy, chemotherapy, targeted therapy, or any combination of these modalities.[30]

Surgical Therapy. Surgery is often the first-line treatment option for head and neck cancers. Some patients may be treated with surgery alone. For other patients, combining surgery with radiation therapy and/or chemotherapy may be appropriate. Depending on the location and stage of cancer, the following surgical procedures may be done:

- *Vocal cord stripping:* Removal of outer layers of tissue on the vocal cords. This approach may be used for a biopsy or to treat some stage 0 cancers confined to the vocal cords. Vocal cord stripping rarely affects speech.
- *Laser surgery:* An endoscope with a laser is inserted down the throat and the tumor can be vaporized or removed.
- *Cordectomy:* Part or all of the vocal cords are removed. Patients may experience changes in speech. Removing part of a vocal cord may lead to a hoarse voice. If both vocal cords are removed, speech will no longer be possible.
- *Partial or total laryngectomy:* A surgical procedure in which part or all of the larynx is removed. For the patient with a total laryngectomy, airflow in and out of the lungs will be altered as a result of surgery and normal voice production will not be possible (Fig. 26-8).
- *Pharyngectomy:* Part or all of the throat is removed.
- *Tracheostomy:* A tracheostomy is done to create an alternate pathway for breathing by creating a stoma in the trachea. (Tracheostomy was previously discussed on pp. 485-490.)

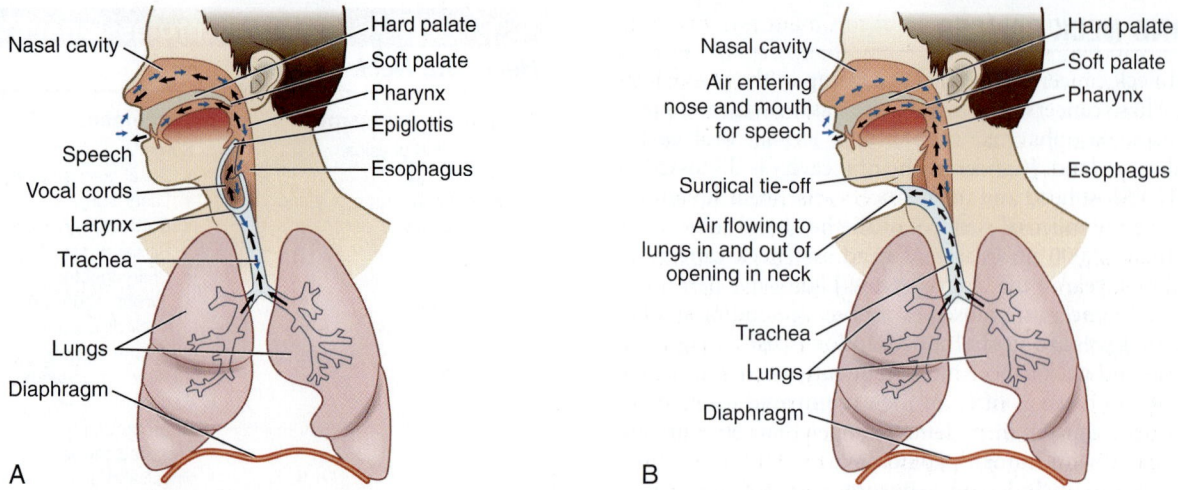

FIG. 26-8 **A,** Normal airflow in and out of the lungs. **B,** Airflow in and out of the lungs after total laryngectomy.

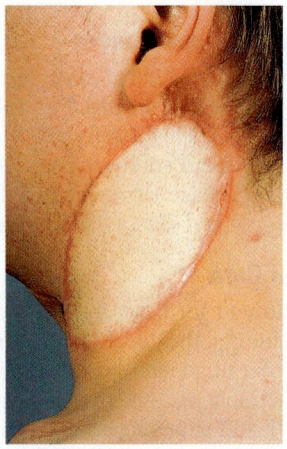

FIG. 26-9 Reconstructive surgery involving skin grafts and skin flaps may be needed after a radical neck dissection. (From Eggers G, Flechtenmacher C, Kurzen J, Hassfeld S: Infiltrating basal cell carcinoma of the neck 34 years after irradiation of an haemangioma in early childhood. A case-report, *J Craniomaxillofac Surg* 33:199, 2005.)

- *Lymph node removal:* Head and neck cancer sometimes spreads to the lymph nodes. The amount of tissue and number of lymph nodes that are removed depend on how far the cancer has spread.
- *Neck dissection surgery:* Three main types include:
  - *Radical neck dissection:* All the tissue on the side of the neck from the mandible to the clavicle is removed. The muscle, nerve, salivary gland, and major blood vessels in this area are removed.
  - *Modified radical neck dissection:* This is the most common type of neck dissection. All lymph nodes are removed. Less neck tissue is taken out than in radical dissection. This surgery may also spare the nerves in the neck and, sometimes, the blood vessels or muscle.
  - *Selective neck dissection:* If cancer has not spread far, fewer lymph nodes have to be removed. The muscle, nerve, and blood vessels in the neck may also be saved.

Following extensive surgery to remove head and neck cancer, reconstructive operations can help restore both the structure and function of the affected areas (Fig. 26-9).

Radiation Therapy. Radiation therapy can be delivered by either external-beam therapy or internal implants (brachytherapy). Brachytherapy is a concentrated and localized method of delivering radiation that involves placing a radioactive source into or near the tumor. The goal is to deliver high doses of radiation to the target area while limiting exposure of surrounding tissues. Thin, hollow, plastic needles are inserted into the tumor area, and radioactive seeds are placed in the needles. The seeds emit continuous radiation. (Radiation therapy and brachytherapy are discussed in Chapter 15.)

Radiation therapy is often preferred for patients with early head and neck cancer because it offers the patient good results with voice preservation. Some patients refuse surgical intervention for advanced lesions because of the extent of the procedure and potential risks involved. In this situation, radiation therapy is used as the sole treatment or in combination with chemotherapy. Other patients may opt for surgery and a combination of either radiation and/or chemotherapy treatments.

Chemotherapy and Targeted Therapy. Chemotherapy is used in combination with radiation therapy for patients with stage III or IV cancers. Chemotherapy agents include cisplatin, methotrexate, 5-fluorouracil (5-FU), docetaxel (Taxotere), ifosfamide (Ifex), and bleomycin.

Cetuximab (Erbitux), a targeted therapy, is used with chemotherapy to treat patients with late-stage head and neck cancer. The drug targets epidermal growth factor receptor (EGFR), a specific protein within cancer cells, and stops the cells from growing. (Targeted therapy is discussed in Chapter 15 and Table 15-13.)

Nutritional Therapy. Many patients with head and neck cancer are malnourished even before treatment begins. Treatment modalities increase the risk of malnutrition. For example, after radical neck surgery the patient may be unable to take in nutrients orally because of swelling, the location of sutures, or difficulty with swallowing. Side effects from chemotherapy and radiation therapy can impair the patient's ability to maintain adequate nutrition. Painful oral mucositis frequently leads to breaks in treatment if the patient is relying solely on oral intake for nutrition.

A thorough nutritional assessment and prophylactic placement of a gastrostomy tube in high-risk patients are vital to maintaining adequate nutrition. Enteral nutrition may be started before initiation of treatment to obtain and maintain optimal nutritional status needed for tissue repair. (Enteral nutrition is described in Chapter 39.) Observe for tolerance of the feedings and adjust the amount, time, and formula if nausea, vomiting, diarrhea, or distention occurs. Instruct the patient and caregiver about the tube feedings.

Patients who are not candidates for or who refuse tube feedings need to be monitored closely for weight loss. Antiemetics or analgesics may be given before meals to reduce nausea and mouth pain. Bland foods are easier for patients to tolerate. Patients can increase caloric intake by adding dry milk to foods during preparation, selecting foods high in calories, and using oral supplements. It is helpful to add mild sauces and gravies to food, which adds calories and moistens food so that it is more easily swallowed. Elevate the head of the bed while the patient is eating.

Anticipate swallowing problems when the patient resumes eating after surgery. The type and degree of difficulty varies depending on the surgical procedure. Videofluoroscopic swallowing studies may be used to evaluate the safety of the patient's swallowing. When the patient can successfully swallow with low or no risk of aspiration, small amounts of thickened liquids or pureed foods may be given with the patient in high Fowler's position. Avoid thin, watery fluids because they are difficult to swallow and increase the risk of aspiration. Closely observe for choking. Suctioning may be necessary to prevent aspiration.

Physical Therapy. After surgery for head and neck cancer, the physical therapist will help teach the patient how to use the upper extremities to assist with support and movement of the head. In the immediate postoperative period, the patient should begin an exercise program to maintain strength and movement in the shoulders and neck. Without exercise, the patient will be left with a "frozen" shoulder and limited range of neck motion. The patient should continue his or her exercise program after discharge to prevent future functional disabilities.

Speech Therapy. Preoperatively a speech therapist should meet with the patient and caregiver to discuss any effect that surgery will have on the voice and potential voice restoration options. The International Association of Laryngectomees, an association of laryngectomy patients, focuses on helping patients reestablish speech. Local groups, called "Lost Chord" or "New Voice" Clubs, often provide volunteers to visit the patient preoperatively.

There are three major approaches used to restore oral communication: (1) electrolarynx, (2) tracheoesophageal puncture (TEP) voice restoration, and (3) esophageal speech. An *electrolarynx* is a hand-held, battery-powered device that creates speech with the use of sound waves (Fig. 26-10, *A*). This option allows for speech immediately after surgery, is easy to learn, and requires little maintenance. The primary disadvantage of the electrolarynx is the mechanical sound quality, which many patients find unacceptable.

In *transesophageal puncture (TEP)* a fistula is created in the tracheoesophageal wall that diverts pulmonary air across the pharyngoesophageal mucosa for phonation when the tracheostoma is occluded. A one-way valve prosthesis is placed in the tract. The valve prevents aspiration of food or saliva from the esophagus into the tracheostomy. To speak, the patient manually blocks the stoma with the finger. Air moves from the lungs, through the prosthesis, into the esophagus, and out the mouth. Speech is produced by the air vibrating against the esophagus and is formed into words by moving the tongue and lips. A commonly used voice prosthesis is the Blom-Singer prosthesis

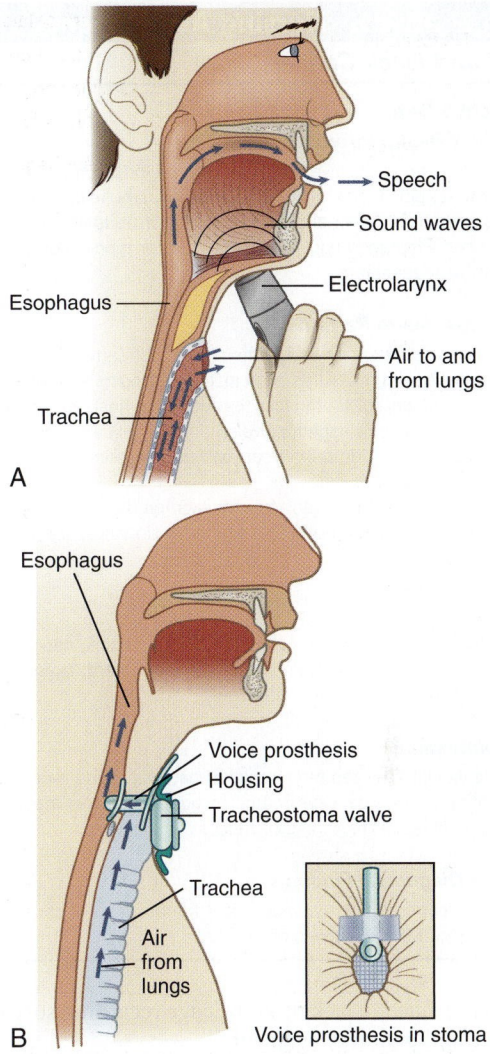

FIG. 26-10 **A,** The sound waves created by the electrolarynx allow the person to speak. **B,** The Blom-Singer voice prosthesis and valve.

(Fig. 26-10, *B*). TEP offers the best speech quality with the highest patient satisfaction.

Esophageal speech production depends upon air that is introduced into the esophagus and is then expelled past the pharyngoesophageal segment, the vibratory source for sound production. The primary disadvantages of developing esophageal speech are the length of time required to learn the technique and the reduction in voice quality.

❖ NURSING MANAGEMENT: HEAD AND NECK CANCER

◆ Nursing Assessment

Table 26-11 presents subjective and objective data to obtain from a person with head and neck cancer.

◆ Nursing Diagnoses

Nursing diagnoses for the patient with head and neck cancer include, but are not limited to, the following:

- Ineffective airway clearance *related to* presence of artificial airway and excessive mucus
- Risk for aspiration *related to* presence of tracheostomy tube and impaired swallowing

TABLE 26-11 Nursing Assessment

Head and Neck Cancer

Subjective Data

Important Health Information

Past health history: Positive family history; prolonged tobacco use (cigarettes, pipes, cigars, chewing tobacco, smokeless tobacco); prolonged, heavy alcohol use; poor intake of fruits and vegetables

Medications: Prolonged use of over-the-counter medication for sore throat, decongestants

Functional Health Patterns

Health perception–health management: Does not participate in preventive health measures, long history of alcohol and tobacco use

Nutritional-metabolic: Mouth ulcer that does not heal, change in fit of dentures, change in appetite, weight loss, swallowing difficulty (e.g., sensation of lump in throat, pain with swallowing, aspiration when swallowing)

Activity-exercise: Fatigue with minimal exertion

Cognitive-perceptual: Sore throat, pain on swallowing, referred ear pain

Objective Data

Respiratory

Hoarseness, change in voice quality, chronic laryngitis, nasal voice, palpable neck mass and lymph nodes (tender, hard, fixed), tracheal deviation; dyspnea, stridor (late sign)

Gastrointestinal

White (leukoplakia) or red (erythroplakia) patches inside mouth, ulceration of mucosa, asymmetric tongue, exudate in mouth or pharynx, mass or thickening of mucosa

Possible Diagnostic Findings

Mass on direct or indirect laryngoscopy; tumor on soft tissue x-ray, CT scan, or MRI; positive biopsy

- Anxiety *related to* lack of knowledge regarding surgical procedure and pain management
- Acute pain *related to* tissue injury from surgery
- Impaired verbal communication *related to* removal of vocal cords

Additional information on nursing diagnoses for the patient with head and neck cancer is presented in eNursing Care Plan 26-2 on the website for this chapter.

Planning

The overall goals are that the patient will have (1) a patent airway, (2) no spread of cancer, (3) no complications related to therapy, (4) adequate nutritional intake, (5) minimal to no pain, (6) the ability to communicate, and (7) an acceptable body image.

Nursing Implementation

Health Promotion. Most head and neck cancer can be prevented. The development of head and neck cancer is closely related to personal habits, primarily tobacco use and excessive alcohol ingestion. Poor oral hygiene and HPV infection are also risk factors for head and neck cancer.

Include information about risk factors in health teaching. Encourage good oral hygiene. Teach patients about safe sex practices to prevent HPV infection (e.g., use condoms for every sex act, be in a monogamous relationship, choose a partner who has had no or few previous partners). If cancer has been diagnosed, tobacco and alcohol cessation is still important. The likelihood of a cure, by any treatment modality, for a patient with head and neck cancer who continues to smoke and ingest alcoholic beverages is decreased. Additionally, the risk of a second primary cancer is significantly increased. Give patients information about smoking cessation programs and techniques for success. If necessary, refer to an alcohol treatment program. (Smoking cessation and treatment of alcohol abuse are discussed in Chapter 10.)

Acute Care. Teach the patient and caregiver about the type of treatment to be performed and care required. Help prepare them to deal with the psychologic impact of the diagnosis of cancer, alteration of physical appearance, possible need for enteral feedings, and potential for altered methods of communication because of the loss of a voice.

The care plan should include assessment of the patient's support system. The patient may not have someone to provide assistance after discharge, may be unemployed, or may have a job that cannot be continued.

Surgical Therapy. Preoperatively assess the patient's physical and psychosocial needs. Physical preparation is the same as for any major surgery, with an emphasis on oral hygiene. Assess knowledge and understanding of the planned surgical procedure, and clarify information as needed. Include the caregiver in preoperative teaching.

Tailor teaching to the planned surgical procedure. For example, include information about expected changes in speech following a laryngectomy. Magic Slates, alphabet boards, writing materials, pictorial guides, or hand signals are useful methods for communicating. Programmable speech-generating devices allow use of recorded messages that are matched with a graphic representing each message. Integration of this technology into patient care enhances the patient's ability to communicate basic needs postoperatively.

INFORMATICS IN PRACTICE

Communication Devices for Patient With Laryngectomy

- Assisting with communication will improve a patient's quality of life after a laryngectomy.
- Use an iPad or iPhone and download a text-to-speech application. These applications allow the patient to type in text, and then a computer voice says the text aloud.
- You can also teach the patient how to use a keyboard-based communication program. The patient types on a traditional keyboard and generates speech that is transmitted through hand-held speakers.

Immediately after surgery, focus your nursing care on airway management, wound care, nutrition, communication, and psychosocial issues related to body image changes. Maintenance of a patent airway is essential. The inflammation in the surgical area may compress the trachea. Keep the patient in a semi-Fowler's position to decrease edema and limit tension on the suture lines. The patient with a laryngectomy requires frequent suctioning via the tracheostomy tube. (Care of a patient with a tracheostomy was discussed earlier in this chapter on pp. 486-490.) Secretions typically change in amount and consistency over time. The patient may initially have copious blood-tinged secretions that diminish and thicken. Maintain adequate fluid intake (IV, enteral, and oral when allowed) and humidification of inspired gases to keep secretions liquid and mucous membranes moist. Encourage deep breathing and coughing.

Administer analgesic drugs as needed for pain control. Because patients may not be able to speak, have them nonverbally rate their pain (e.g., visual pain scale such as FACES) to help assess the effectiveness of the medication. (Pain management is discussed in Chapter 8.)

Monitor vital signs frequently because of the risk of hemorrhage. Many of the structures in the head and neck area are very vascular.

Pressure dressings, packing, or drainage tubes may be used for wound management, depending on the type of surgical procedure. Do not change the dressing unless you have a specific order from the surgeon. If skin flaps are used, dressings are typically not used. This allows better visualization of the flap and avoids excessive pressure on tissue (Fig. 26-9). Skin flaps must initially be checked hourly for color and any change in size or edema. Doppler ultrasound may be used to determine the presence of a pulse, depending upon the location of the skin flap. Hemovac, Jackson-Pratt, and Penrose are some of the drainage tubes that may be used.

Drainage may initially be bloody, then serosanguineous, and gradually decrease in volume over 24 hours. Monitor patency of drainage tubes every 4 hours to ensure proper functioning. If the tubing becomes obstructed, fluid will accumulate under the skin flap and predispose the patient to formation of hematomas or seromas, impair wound healing, and increase the risk for infection. After drainage tubes are removed, closely monitor the area to detect any swelling. Closely monitor incision sites for signs of infection.

The patient may have a nasogastric tube inserted during surgery to remove gastric contents via intermittent suction for the first 24 to 48 hours until peristalsis returns. Because the nasogastric tube lies close to internal incision lines, do not manipulate or move the tube. When bowel sounds return, enteral feedings may be started slowly and advanced to meet nutritional needs.

◆ ***Radiation Therapy.*** Dry mouth *(xerostomia)*, a frequent and annoying problem, typically begins within a few weeks of treatment. The patient's saliva decreases in volume and becomes thick. The change may be temporary or permanent. Pilocarpine hydrochloride (Salagen) is often effective in increasing saliva production.

CHECK YOUR PRACTICE

Your 64-yr-old male patient with oral cancer has been receiving radiation therapy for 3 weeks. He has developed xerostomia and oral mucositis. He asks if you have any suggestions to help relieve his symptoms.

- How would you respond?

Once patients are permitted to have foods or fluids by mouth, they can get symptom relief by increasing fluid intake, chewing sugarless gum or sugarless candy, using nonalcoholic mouth rinses (baking soda or glycerin solutions), and using artificial saliva. Instruct patients to always carry a water bottle with them. Fluoride gels or treatments can help prevent dental deterioration caused by xerostomia.

Oral mucositis can cause irritation, ulceration, and pain. Instruct the patient on oral care basics, including the use of a soft toothbrush and regular flossing. Empty fluoride gel trays, along with bite blocks, athletic mouth guards, or gauze pads, can be worn during radiation treatments. This prevents radiation scatter to the tongue and cheek from metal work in the mouth. Warm bland rinses such as those with salt and baking soda four to six times daily may be helpful. Sucking on ice chips can also help with the pain. Patients should avoid commercial mouthwashes and hot, spicy, or acidic foods because they are irritating.

Skin over the irradiated area often becomes reddened and sensitive to touch. Instruct patients to use only prescribed lotions and skin products while undergoing radiation therapy and to not use any lotions within 2 hours before treatment. (Skin care for patients having radiation therapy is discussed in Chapter 15.)

Fatigue is a common side effect of radiation therapy as well as chemotherapy. Encourage patients to walk 15 to 30 minutes each day, since regular exercise can give them more energy. Instruct patients to do activities that are most important to them and to rest during periods of low energy. Identify support systems and encourage patients to ask for help.

◆ ***Stoma Care.*** Should the patient have a stoma created as a result of surgery, instruct the patient before discharge in the proper care of the stoma. The patient should wash the area around the stoma daily with a moist cloth. A nasal wash spray (e.g., Alkalol) can be used every 1 to 2 hours to keep the stoma moist and prevent crusting. Dried secretions can be removed with tweezers. If a laryngectomy tube is in place, the patient must remove the entire tube at least daily and clean it in the same manner as a tracheostomy tube. The inner cannula may have to be removed and cleaned more frequently. A scarf or loose shirt can be used to hide the stoma.

The patient should cover the stoma when coughing (because mucus may be expectorated) and during any activity (e.g., shaving, applying makeup) that may lead to inhalation of foreign materials. Because water can easily enter the stoma, the patient should wear a plastic collar when taking a shower. Swimming is contraindicated. Initially, humidification is administered via a mechanical ventilation or, after extubation, with a tracheostomy mask. After discharge, the patient can use a bedside humidifier.

◆ ***Psychosocial Needs.*** Psychosocial care of the patient with head and neck cancer is very important. Issues concerning depression, change in body image, and sexuality are very common. Although changes are discussed before surgery, the patient may not be psychologically prepared for the extent of these changes.

Depression may occur for many reasons: inability to speak because of surgical procedure and/or presence of ET or tracheostomy tube, altered physical appearance due to the surgery and edema, loss of independence and reliance upon others, and feelings of helplessness and hopelessness. Depression may also be related to concern about the prognosis.

Allow the patient and caregiver to express their feelings and emotions, verbally or nonverbally. Convey acceptance to help patients regain positive feelings about their body image and self-concept. Encourage participation in support groups. Information about available groups can be obtained through the local branch of the American Cancer Society. A psychiatric referral may be appropriate for the patient who is experiencing prolonged or severe depression.

Surgery and foreign attachments such as tracheostomy and gastrostomy tubes may dramatically affect body image. Xerostomia and fatigue can physically affect sexuality. It may be difficult for the patient to talk about sexual problems because of the alteration in communication. Assist the patient and partner by allowing them to talk about their sexuality, and how surgery and treatment may affect their relationship. Helping the patient see that sexuality involves much more than appearance may relieve some anxiety.

◆ **Ambulatory Care.** The patient may be discharged with a tracheostomy and a nasogastric or gastrostomy feeding tube. Some patients initially need home health care to evaluate the patient's or caregiver's ability to perform self-care activities. The patient and caregiver need to learn how to manage tubes and whom to call if there are problems. Provide pictorial instructions for tracheostomy care, suctioning, stoma and skin care, and enteral feeding as appropriate. Encouraging the patient to participate in self-care is an important part of rehabilitation.

Inform the patient about the importance of wearing a Medic Alert bracelet or other identification that alerts emergency personnel of the possible alterations in breathing status as a result of surgery. Because the patient no longer breathes through the nose, the ability to smell smoke and food is often lost. Advise the patient to install smoke and carbon monoxide detectors in the home. Encourage preparation of food that is colorful, attractive, and nutritious because taste may also be diminished secondary to the loss of smell and radiation therapy.

The patient can resume exercise, recreation, and sexual activity when able. Most patients can return to work 1 to 2 months after surgery. However, many never return to full-time employment. The changes that follow a total laryngectomy can be upsetting. Loss of speech, loss of the ability to taste and smell, inability to produce audible sounds (including laughing and weeping), and the presence of a permanent tracheal stoma that produces undesirable mucus are often overwhelming to the patient. Although changes are discussed before surgery, the patient may not be prepared for the extent of these changes. If the patient has a significant other, this person's reaction to the patient's altered appearance is important. Acceptance by another person can promote an improved self-image.

◆ Evaluation

Expected outcomes for the patient with head and neck cancer who is treated surgically are that the patient will

- Demonstrate effective coughing and secretion clearance
- Demonstrate the ability to swallow oral foods without aspiration
- Report satisfaction with pain relief
- Use written and nonverbal techniques to effectively communicate with others

Other outcomes for the patient with head and neck cancer who is treated surgically are addressed in eNursing Care Plans 26-1 and 26-2 on the website for this chapter.

CASE STUDY

Laryngeal Cancer

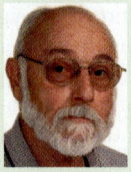

(©iStockphoto/Thinkstock)

Patient Profile

M.R., a 60-yr-old baker, was admitted to the hospital for influenza. He explained to his HCP that he has also experienced "a cough that just won't go away," some pain and difficulty swallowing, and "a sore throat that really hasn't gotten better" over the past year. His wife passed away 6 years ago. He has three children; one daughter lives in the same city. He has a history of hypertension, smoking, alcohol use, and type 2 diabetes mellitus.

Subjective Data

- States that his symptoms worsened in the past 3 months
- Has used various cough and cold remedies over the past 6 months to relieve symptoms without relief
- Has lost weight because of decrease in appetite and difficulty swallowing
- Has smoked three packs of cigarettes a day for 40 yr
- Consumes 4 to 6 cans of beer a day

Objective Data

Physical Examination

- *Vital signs:* Temperature 102.4° F (39.1° C), heart rate 99 beats/minute (pulse strong, regular), respiratory rate 24 breaths/minute (short, shallow, slightly labored), BP 176/84 (cuff), SpO_2 87% on room air
- *Inspection:* Awake and alert, appears gray, malnourished, dehydrated. Small, irregular white patches on the sides of oral cavity
- *Palpation:* Enlarged cervical nodes bilaterally (nontender)
- *Auscultation:* Adequate and clear air entry to upper lung fields; slightly decreased air entry to bases with occasional fine crackles on expiration

Diagnostic Studies

- Chest x-ray: Lung fields clear
- Laryngoscopy: Mass in subglottic area (requires further evaluation)
- CT scan: Subglottic lesion with lymph node involvement
- Diagnosis: Laryngeal cancer

Interprofessional Care

- *Surgery:* Suggests a total laryngectomy
- *Oncology:* Suggests radiation and chemotherapy postoperatively
- *ICU:* Preoperative consult (ICU admission for 24 hours postoperatively)
- *Gastroenterology:* Percutaneous gastrostomy tube preoperatively for enteral tube feeding
- *Dietary:* Explain nutritional options with/without ET tube/tracheostomy.
- *Physical therapy:* Visit pre-surgery to explain postoperative exercise routine.
- *Social worker:* Determine social supports available postoperatively.

Discussion Questions

1. What information in the assessment suggests that M.R. is at risk for cancer of the larynx?
2. ***Priority Decision:*** What are your priority teaching strategies for M.R. before and after total laryngectomy?
3. How would you explain the gastrostomy tube to M.R.?
4. Discuss methods that can be used to facilitate communication in the postoperative period.
5. Is there anything in his history that may affect wound healing after surgery?
6. ***Priority Decision:*** In the recovery room, M.R.'s heart rate is 138 (tachycardia), BP is 84/32, and SpO_2 is 91%. What are your priority nursing interventions?
7. ***Teamwork and Collaboration:*** M.R. is discharged from the ICU after 24 hours. What information would you want to know from the ICU nurse who has just transported M.R. to the clinical unit?

Progression of Case

M.R. is awake and alert. Vital signs are stable. BP 168/94. Large surgical dressing on neck with three Jackson-Pratt drains. Tracheostomy tube in place. Receiving O_2 via tracheal mask. Tube feeding @ 60 mL/hour via gastrostomy tube. Voiding independently. M.R. nonverbally indicating to you that he "wants to get out of bed."

8. ***Priority Decision:*** Based on the assessment data presented, what are your priority nursing diagnoses? Are there any collaborative problems?
9. ***Teamwork and Collaboration:*** M.R. has a tracheostomy. What role can unlicensed assistive personnel (UAP) have in relation to the tracheostomy?
10. ***Evidence-Based Practice:*** How could you best meet M.R.'s communication needs during the first few postoperative days?
11. Shortly after transfer to the clinical unit, M.R. is tearful and is staring at the wall. What should you do?
12. ***Patient-Centered Care:*** What teaching is required to help this patient assume self-care after his surgery? What precautions should the patient take because of his stoma?

Answers available at *http://evolve.elsevier.com/Lewis/medsurg.*

BRIDGE TO NCLEX EXAMINATION

The number of the question corresponds to the same-numbered outcome at the beginning of the chapter.

1. A patient was seen in the clinic for an episode of epistaxis, which was controlled by placement of anterior nasal packing. During discharge teaching, the nurse instructs the patient to
   a. use aspirin for pain relief.
   b. remove the packing later that day.
   c. skip the next dose of antihypertensive medication.
   d. avoid vigorous nose blowing and strenuous activity.
2. A patient with allergic rhinitis reports severe nasal congestion; sneezing; and watery, itchy eyes and nose at various times of the year. To teach the patient to control these symptoms, the nurse advises the patient to
   a. avoid all intranasal sprays and oral antihistamines.
   b. limit the usage of nasal decongestant spray to 10 days.
   c. use oral decongestants at bedtime to prevent symptoms during the night.
   d. keep a diary of when the allergic reaction occurs and what precipitates it.
3. A patient is seen at the clinic with fever, muscle aches, sore throat with yellowish exudate, and headache. The nurse anticipates that the interprofessional management will include *(select all that apply)*
   a. antiviral agents to treat influenza.
   b. treatment with antibiotics starting ASAP.
   c. a throat culture or rapid strep antigen test.
   d. supportive care, including cool, bland liquids.
   e. comprehensive history to determine possible etiology.
4. The *best* method for determining the risk of aspiration in a patient with a tracheostomy is to
   a. consult a speech therapist for swallowing assessment.
   b. have the patient drink plain water and assess for coughing.
   c. assess for change of sputum color 48 hours after patient drinks small amount of blue dye.
   d. suction above the cuff after the patient eats or drinks to determine presence of food in trachea.
5. Which nursing action would be of *highest priority* when suctioning a patient with a tracheostomy?
   a. Auscultating lung sounds after suctioning is complete
   b. Providing a means of communication for the patient during the procedure
   c. Assessing the patient's oxygenation saturation before, during, and after suctioning
   d. Administering pain and/or antianxiety medication 30 minutes before suctioning
6. When planning health care teaching to prevent or detect early head and neck cancer, which people would be the *priority* to target *(select all that apply)*?
   a. 65-year-old man who has used chewing tobacco most of his life
   b. 45-year-old rancher who uses snuff to stay awake while driving his herds of cattle
   c. 21-year-old college student who drinks beer on weekends with his fraternity brothers
   d. 78-year-old woman who has been drinking hard liquor since her husband died 15 years ago
   e. 22-year-old woman who has been diagnosed with human papilloma virus (HPV) of the cervix
7. While in the recovery room, a patient with a total laryngectomy is suctioned and has bloody mucus with some clots. Which nursing interventions would apply?
   a. Notify the physician immediately.
   b. Place the patient in the prone position to facilitate drainage.
   c. Instill 3 mL of normal saline into the tracheostomy tube to loosen secretions.
   d. Continue your assessment of the patient, including O_2 saturation, respiratory rate, and breath sounds.
8. Appropriate discharge teaching for the patient with a permanent tracheostomy after a total laryngectomy for cancer would include *(select all that apply)*
   a. encouraging regular exercise such as swimming.
   b. washing around the stoma daily with a moist washcloth.
   c. encouraging participation in postlaryngectomy support group.
   d. providing pictures and "hands-on" instruction for tracheostomy care.
   e. teaching how to hold breath and trying to gag to promote swallowing reflex.

1. d, 2. d, 3. c, d, e, 4. a, 5. c, 6. a, b, d, e, 7. d, 8. b, c, d

For rationales to these answers and even more NCLEX review questions, visit *http://evolve.elsevier.com/Lewis/medsurg.*

EVOLVE WEBSITE

http://evolve.elsevier.com/Lewis/medsurg

Review Questions (Online Only)
Key Points
Answer Keys for Questions
- Rationales for Bridge to NCLEX Examination Questions
- Answer Guidelines for Case Study on p. 496

Student Case Study
- Patient With Head and Neck Cancer/Laryngectomy With Tracheostomy

Nursing Care Plans
- eNursing Care Plan 26-1: Patient With a Tracheostomy
- eNursing Care Plan 26-2: Patient Having Total Laryngectomy and/or Radical Neck Surgery

Conceptual Care Map Creator

Supporting Media
- Animation
  - Tracheotomy

Audio Glossary
Content Updates

REFERENCES

1. American Academy of Otolaryngology–Head and Neck Surgery: Deviated septum. Retrieved from *www.entnet.org/content/deviated-septum.*
2. Patton KT, Thibodeau GA: *Human body in health and disease*, ed 6, St Louis, 2014, Elsevier Mosby.
3. Becker DG: Nasal and septal fractures. Retrieved from *http://emedicine.medscape.com/article/878595-overview#a03.*

4. Urden LD, Stacy KM, Lough ME: *Critical care nursing: diagnosis and management*, ed 7, St Louis, 2014, Mosby.
5. Haraldson SJ: Nasal fracture treatment and management. Retrieved from: *http://emedicine.medscape.com/article/84829-treatment.*
6. Pribitkin EA, Lavasani LS, Shindle C et al: Sonic rhinoplasty: Sculpting with the ultrasound bone aspirator. In Schiffman MA, Di Giuseppe A, editors: *Advanced aesthetic rhinoplasty: art, science, and new clinical techniques*, New York, 2013, Springer.
7. Fried MP: Epistaxis. Retrieved from *www.merckmanuals.com.*
8. Newson L: Nosebleed (epistaxis). Retrieved from *www.patient.co.uk/doctor/nosebleed-epistaxis-pro.*
9. deSchazo RD, Kemp SF: Patient information: allergic rhinitis (seasonal allergies). Retrieved from *www.uptodate.com/contents/allergic-rhinitis-seasonal-allergies-beyond-the-basics.*
10. Henochowicz SI: Allergic rhinitis. Retrieved from *www.nlm.nih.gov/medlineplus/ency/article/000813.htm.*
11. Sheikh J: Allergic rhinitis medication summary. Retrieved from *http://emedicine.medscape.com/article/134825-medication#1.*
12. New York Department of Health: Influenza (flu) fact sheet. Retrieved from *www.health.ny.gov/diseases/communicable/influenza/fact_sheet.htm.*
13. Centers for Disease Control and Prevention: Key facts about influenza (flu) & flu vaccine. Retrieved from *www.cdc.gov/flu/keyfacts.htm.*
14. Blanco EM: Diagnostic influenza tests. Retrieved from *http://emedicine.medscape.com/article/2053517-overview#aw2aab6b2.*
15. Centers for Disease Control and Prevention: Rapid Diagnostic Testing for Influenza: Information for Health Care Professionals. Retrieved from *www.cdc.gov/flu/professionals/diagnosis/rapidclin.htm.*
16. U.S. Food and Drug Administration (FDA): Influenza (Flu) Antiviral Drugs and Related Information. Retrieved from *www.fda.gov/Drugs/DrugSafety/InformationbyDrugClass/ucm100228.htm.*
17. Nazario B: Sinus infection: An overview of sinusitis. Retrieved from *www.webmd.com/allergies/sinusitis-and-sinus-infection.*
18. Kaplan A: Canadian guidelines for acute bacterial rhinosinusitis, *Canadian Family Physician* 60:227, 2014.
19. Hwang PH, Patel ZM: Acute sinusitis and rhinosinusitis in adults: treatment. Retrieved from *www.uptodate.com/contents/acute-sinusitis-and-rhinosinusitis-in-adults-treatment.*
20. Seidu L: Nasal polyps. Retrieved from *www.webmd.com/allergies/guide/nasal-polyps-symptoms-and-treatments.*
21. Carrillo-Marquez MA: Bacterial pharyngitis. Retrieved from *http://emedicine.medscape.com/article/225243-overview.*
22. Acerra JR: Pharyngitis clinical presentation. Retrieved from *http://emedicine.medscape.com/article/764304-clinical.*
23. Chow AW, Doron S: Evaluation of acute pharyngitis in adults. Retrieved from *www.uptodate.com/contents/evaluation-of-acute-pharyngitis-in-adults#H1.*
24. Murray AD: Foreign bodies of the airway. Retrieved from *http://emedicine.medscape.com/article/872498-overview.*
25. Morris L, Whitmer A, McIntosh E: Tracheostomy care and complications in the intensive care unit, *Critical Care Nurse* 33:18, 2013.
26. Batuwitage B, Webber S, Glossop A: Percutaneous tracheostomy. Continuing Education in Anesthesia, Critical Care, and Pain. Retrieved from *http://ceaccp.oxfordjournals.org/content/early/2014/01/02/bjaceaccp.mkt068.full.pdf+html.*
27. Agency for Clinical Innovation: Care of adult patients in acute care facilities with tracheostomy – clinical practice guidelines. Retrieved from *www.aci.health.nsw.gov.au/__data/assets/pdf_file/0005/181454/ACI_Tracheostomy_CPG.pdf.*
28. American Cancer Society: Retrieved from *www.cancer.org/research/cancerfactsstatistics/cancerfactsfigures2015/index.*
29. American Society of Clinical Oncology: Stages of cancer. Retrieved from *www.cancer.net/navigating-cancer-care/diagnosing-cancer/stages-cancer.*
30. American Society of Clinical Oncology: Head and neck cancer: treatment options. Retrieved from *www.cancer.net/cancer-types/head-and-neck-cancer/treatment-options.*

27

Lower Respiratory Problems

Eugene E. Mondor

What oxygen is to the lungs, such is hope to the meaning of life.

Emil Brunner

http://evolve.elsevier.com/Lewis/medsurg/

LEARNING OUTCOMES

1. Compare and contrast the clinical manifestations and nursing and interprofessional management of patients with acute bronchitis and pertussis.
2. Differentiate among the types of pneumonia and their etiology.
3. Describe the pathophysiology, clinical manifestations, diagnostic studies, interprofessional care, and nursing management of patients with pneumonia.
4. Describe the pathogenesis, classification, clinical manifestations, complications, diagnostic abnormalities, interprofessional care, and nursing management of patients with tuberculosis.
5. Describe the causes, clinical manifestations, and nursing and interprofessional management of patients with pulmonary fungal infections.
6. Explain the pathophysiology, clinical manifestations, and nursing and interprofessional management of a patient with a lung abscess.
7. Identify the causative factors, clinical manifestations, and nursing and interprofessional management of patients with environmental lung diseases.
8. Describe the etiology, risk factors, pathophysiology, clinical manifestations, interprofessional care, and nursing management of lung cancer.
9. Compare and contrast the pathophysiology, clinical manifestations, and nursing and interprofessional management of pneumothorax, fractured ribs, and flail chest.
10. Describe the purpose, function, and nursing responsibilities related to chest tubes and various chest drainage systems.
11. Explain the types of chest surgery and appropriate preoperative and postoperative care.
12. Describe the etiology, clinical manifestations, and nursing and interprofessional management of patients with restrictive lung disorders such as pleural effusion, pleurisy, and atelectasis.
13. Describe the pathophysiology, clinical manifestations, and nursing and interprofessional management of pulmonary embolism, pulmonary hypertension, and cor pulmonale.
14. Discuss the use of lung transplantation as a treatment for pulmonary disorders, emphasizing nursing and interprofessional management of the postoperative lung transplant patient.

KEY TERMS

acute bronchitis, p. 499
community-acquired pneumonia (CAP), p. 501
cor pulmonale, p. 533
empyema, p. 527
flail chest, p. 521
hemothorax, p. 520
hospital-acquired pneumonia (HAP), p. 501
lung abscess, p. 512
pertussis, p. 500
pleural effusion, p. 527
pleurisy (pleuritis), p. 528
pneumoconiosis, p. 513
pneumonia, p. 500
pneumothorax, p. 519
pulmonary edema, p. 529
pulmonary embolism (PE), p. 529
pulmonary hypertension, p. 531
tension pneumothorax, p. 520
thoracentesis, p. 527
thoracotomy, p. 524
tuberculosis (TB), p. 506

A variety of problems affect the lower respiratory system. Lung diseases that are characterized primarily by an obstructive disorder, such as asthma, chronic obstructive pulmonary disease (COPD), and cystic fibrosis, are discussed in Chapter 28. This chapter discusses other lower respiratory tract diseases, including infectious, oncologic, traumatic, restrictive, and vascular disorders.

LOWER RESPIRATORY TRACT INFECTIONS

Lower respiratory tract infection is both a common and serious occurrence. It is responsible for thousands of clinic and emergency department visits and hospital admissions each year. In the United States, pneumonia and influenza are responsible for more than 56,000 deaths annually.[1,2]

ACUTE BRONCHITIS

Acute bronchitis is a self-limiting inflammation of the bronchi in the lower respiratory tract and a common reason for seeking medical care. Most acute bronchial infections are caused by viruses. Air pollution, dust, inhalation of chemicals, smoking, chronic sinusitis, and asthma are other triggers of acute bronchitis.

Reviewed by Donna C. Bond, RN, DNP, CCNS, AE-C, CTTS, Pulmonary Clinical Nurse Specialist, Carilion Clinic, Roanoke, Virginia; Marylee Bressie, RN, DNP, CCRN, CCNS, CEN, Core Faculty/Nurse Planner, School of Public Service Leadership, Capella University, Minneapolis, Minnesota; Deborah Cline, RN, MS, Nursing Faculty, Carrington College, Reno, Nevada; and Cynthia M. Steinwedel, RN, PhD, CNE, Assistant Professor, Department of Nursing, Bradley University, Peoria, Illinois; and Beth D. Strauss, RN, DNP, ACNS-BC, Associate Professor, Edgewood College, Henry Predolin School of Nursing, Madison, Wisconsin.

HEALTHY PEOPLE

Prevention of Respiratory Diseases

- Avoid cigarette smoking and exposure to environmental smoke.
- Wash hands frequently to prevent and avoid spreading infections.
- Avoid exposure to allergens, indoor pollutants, and ambient air pollutants.
- Get a pneumococcal vaccine and yearly flu vaccine as directed by HCP.
- Wear proper personal protective equipment when working in an occupation with prolonged exposure to dust, fumes, or gases.

Cough, which is the most common symptom, lasts for up to 3 weeks. Clear, mucoid secretions are often present, although some patients produce purulent sputum. The presence of colored (e.g., green) sputum is not a reliable indicator of bacterial infection. Associated symptoms may include headache, fever, malaise, hoarseness, myalgias, dyspnea, and chest pain.

Diagnosis of acute bronchitis is based on clinical assessment. Assessment may reveal normal breath sounds or crackles or wheezes, usually on expiration and with exertion. *Consolidation* (occurs when fluid accumulates in the lungs), suggestive of pneumonia, is absent with bronchitis. Chest x-rays would be normal and are therefore not indicated unless pneumonia is suspected. (Chronic bronchitis is discussed in Chapter 28.)

The goal in acute bronchitis is to relieve symptoms and prevent pneumonia. Treatment is supportive, including cough suppressants, encouraging oral fluid intake, and using a humidifier. β_2-agonist (bronchodilator) inhalers are useful for patients with wheezes. Generally antibiotics are not prescribed for treating a viral infection, as they may cause side effects and promote antibiotic resistance. However, antibiotics may be prescribed for patients with underlying chronic conditions and who have a prolonged infection associated with systemic symptoms.

Patients should be encouraged not to smoke, avoid secondhand smoke, and to frequently wash their hands. If the acute bronchitis is due to an influenza virus, treatment with antiviral drugs, either zanamivir (Relenza) or oseltamivir (Tamiflu), can be started. These drugs should be initiated within 48 hours of the onset of symptoms.

PERTUSSIS

Pertussis is a highly contagious infection of the respiratory tract caused by a gram-negative bacillus, *Bordetella pertussis*. The bacteria attach to the cilia of the respiratory tract and release toxins that damage the cilia, causing inflammation and swelling. The incidence of pertussis has been steadily increasing in the United States since the 1980s, with the largest increase noted in adults. It is thought that immunity resulting from childhood vaccination with DPT (diphtheria, pertussis, tetanus) may diminish over time, allowing a milder (but still contagious) infection. The Centers for Disease Control and Prevention (CDC) currently recommends that all adults age 19 years and older who have not received a dose of Tdap (tetanus, diphtheria, and pertussis) receive a one-time vaccination as soon as possible.[3]

Clinical manifestations of pertussis occur in stages. The first (catarrhal) stage, occurring within the first 2 weeks of infection, manifests as a mild upper respiratory tract infection (URI) with a low-grade or no fever, runny nose, watery eyes, and mild, nonproductive cough. The second (paroxysmal) stage, from the second to tenth week of infection, is characterized by paroxysms of cough. The final (convalescent) stage lasts 2 to 3 weeks and is characterized by less severe cough and weakness.

The hallmark characteristic of pertussis is uncontrollable, violent coughing. Inspiration after each cough produces the typical "whooping" sound as the patient tries to breathe in air against an obstructed glottis. The "whoop" is often not present in teens and adults (especially those who have been vaccinated). Like acute bronchitis, the coughing is more frequent at night. Vomiting may also occur with the coughing. Unlike bronchitis, the cough with pertussis may last from 6 to 10 weeks.

The primary treatment for pertussis is antibiotics, usually macrolides (erythromycin, azithromycin [Zithromax]), to minimize symptoms and prevent spread of the disease. The patient is infectious from the beginning of the catarrhal stage through the third week after onset of symptoms or until 5 days after antibiotic therapy has been initiated. Cough suppressants and antihistamines should not be used, since they are ineffective and may induce coughing episodes. Corticosteroids and bronchodilators are also not useful.

PNEUMONIA

Pneumonia is an acute infection of the lung parenchyma. Until 1936, pneumonia was the leading cause of death in the United States.[4] The discovery of sulfa drugs and penicillin was pivotal in the treatment of pneumonia. Since that time, remarkable progress has been made in the development of antibiotics to treat pneumonia. However, despite newer antimicrobial agents, pneumonia is still associated with significant morbidity and mortality rates. The CDC reports that pneumonia and influenza are the eighth leading cause of death in the United States.[5]

Etiology

Normally, the airway distal to the larynx is protected from infection by various defense mechanisms. Mechanisms that create a mechanical barrier to microorganisms entering the tracheobronchial tree include air filtration, epiglottis closure over the trachea, cough reflex, mucociliary escalator mechanism, and reflex bronchoconstriction (see Chapter 25). Immune defense mechanisms include secretion of immunoglobulins A and G and alveolar macrophages.

Pneumonia is more likely to occur when defense mechanisms become incompetent or are overwhelmed by the virulence or quantity of infectious agents. Decreased consciousness weakens the cough and epiglottal reflexes, which may allow aspiration of oropharyngeal contents into the lungs. Tracheal intubation bypasses normal filtration processes and interferes with the cough reflex and mucociliary escalator mechanism. Air pollution, cigarette smoking, viral URIs, and normal changes that occur with aging can also impair the mucociliary mechanism. Chronic diseases can suppress the immune system's ability to inhibit bacterial growth. The risk factors for pneumonia are listed in Table 27-1.

Organisms that cause pneumonia reach the lung by three ways:

1. *Aspiration* of normal flora from the nasopharynx or oropharynx. Many organisms that cause pneumonia are normal inhabitants of the pharynx in healthy adults.
2. *Inhalation* of microbes present in the air. Examples include *Mycoplasma pneumoniae* and fungal pneumonias.
3. *Hematogenous spread* from a primary infection elsewhere in the body. Examples are streptococci and *Staphylococcus aureus* from infective endocarditis.

TABLE 27-1 Risk Factors for Pneumonia

- Abdominal or thoracic surgery
- Age >65 yr
- Air pollution
- Altered consciousness: alcoholism, head injury, seizures, anesthesia, drug overdose, stroke
- Bed rest and prolonged immobility
- Chronic diseases: chronic lung and liver disease, diabetes mellitus, heart disease, cancer, chronic kidney disease
- Debilitating illness
- Exposure to bats, birds, rabbits, farm animals
- Immunosuppressive disease and/or therapy (corticosteroids, cancer chemotherapy, human immunodeficiency virus [HIV] infection, immunosuppressive therapy after organ transplant)
- Inhalation or aspiration of noxious substances
- Intestinal and gastric feedings via nasogastric or nasointestinal tubes
- IV drug use
- Malnutrition
- Recent antibiotic therapy
- Resident of a long-term care facility
- Smoking
- Tracheal intubation (endotracheal intubation, tracheostomy)
- Upper respiratory tract infection

TABLE 27-2 Organisms Causing Pneumonia

Community-Acquired Pneumonia	Hospital-Acquired Pneumonia
*Streptococcus pneumoniae**	*Pseudomonas aeruginosa*†
Mycoplasma pneumoniae	*Escherichia coli*†
Haemophilus influenzae	*Klebsiella pneumoniae*†
Respiratory viruses	*Acinetobacter* species†
Chlamydophila pneumoniae	*Haemophilus influenzae*
Chlamydophila psittaci	*Staphylococcus aureus*
Coxiella burnettii	*Streptococcus pneumoniae*
Legionella pneumophila	*Proteus* species
Oral anaerobes	*Enterobacter* species
Moraxella catarrhalis	Oral anaerobes
Staphylococcus aureus	
Pseudomonas aeruginosa	
Enteric aerobic gram-negative bacteria (e.g., *Klebsiella* species)	
Fungi	
Mycobacterium tuberculosis	

*Most common cause of community-acquired pneumonia (CAP).
†Most common causes of hospital-acquired pneumonia (HAP).

Types of Pneumonia

Bacteria, viruses, *Mycoplasma* organisms, fungi, parasites, and chemicals are potential causes of pneumonia. Although pneumonia can be classified many different ways (e.g., according to the causative organism), the most widely recognized and clinically effective way is to classify pneumonia as *community-acquired* or *hospital-acquired* pneumonia. Classifying pneumonia is important because of the differences in the likely causative organisms (Table 27-2) and the selection of appropriate antimicrobial therapy.

Community-Acquired Pneumonia. Community-acquired pneumonia (CAP) is an acute infection of the lung occurring in patients who have not been hospitalized or resided in a long-term care facility within 14 days of the onset of symptoms. The decision to treat the patient at home or admit him or her to the hospital is based on several factors such as the patient's age, vital signs, mental status, presence of co-morbid conditions, and current physiologic condition. Clinicians can use tools such as the CURB-65 scale (Table 27-3) to supplement clinical judgment.

TABLE 27-3 Assessing Pneumonia Using CURB-65

The CURB-65 scale may be used as a supplement to clinical judgment to determine the severity of pneumonia and if patients need to be hospitalized.

Identifying the Level of Risk

Patients receive 1 point for each of the following indicators:

- **C:** Confusion (compared to baseline)
- **U:** BUN >20 mg/dL
- **R:** Respiratory rate ≥30 breaths/min
- **B:** Systolic blood pressure <90 mm Hg or diastolic blood pressure ≤60 mm Hg
- **65:** ≥Age 65 yr

Scoring and Decision Making

Score	Decision
0	Treat at home
1-2	Consider hospital admission
3 or more	Hospital admission
4-5	Consider admission to intensive care unit

Source: Lim WS, van der Eerden MM, Laing R, et al: Defining community acquired pneumonia severity on presentation to hospital: an international derivation and validation study, *Thorax* 58(5):377, 2003.

Empiric antibiotic therapy should be started as soon as possible. *Empiric antibiotic therapy,* the initiation of treatment before a definitive diagnosis or causative agent is confirmed, should be started as soon as CAP is suspected. Empiric antibiotic administration is based on experience and knowledge of drugs known to be effective for the most likely causative agent.

Hospital-Acquired Pneumonia. Hospital-acquired pneumonia (HAP), also known as *nosocomial pneumonia*, is a pneumonia in a nonintubated patient that begins 48 hours or longer after admission to hospital and was not present at the time of admission. *Ventilator-associated pneumonia* (VAP), also a type of HAP, refers to pneumonia that occurs more than 48 hours after endotracheal intubation.[6] (VAP is discussed in Chapter 65.) Once the diagnosis of HAP or VAP is made, treatment of pneumonia is initiated based on known risk factors, early versus late onset, and probable organism. Antibiotic therapy can be adjusted once the results of sputum cultures identify the exact pathogen. Both HAP and VAP are associated with longer hospital stays, increased associated costs, sicker patients, and increased risk of morbidity and mortality.

A major problem in treating pneumonia today is the development of multidrug-resistant (MDR) organisms. Primary culprits include methicillin-resistant *Staphylococcus aureus* and gram-negative bacilli. Risk factors for development of MDR pneumonia include advanced age, immunosuppression, history of antibiotic use, and prolonged mechanical ventilation. Antibiotic susceptibility tests can identify MDR organisms. The virulence of these organisms can severely limit the available and appropriate antimicrobial therapy. MDR organisms also increase the morbidity and mortality risks associated with pneumonia. (Chapter 14 discusses MDR organisms.)

Aspiration Pneumonia. *Aspiration pneumonia* results from the abnormal entry of material from the mouth or stomach into the trachea and lungs. Conditions that increase the risk of aspiration include decreased level of consciousness (e.g., seizure, anesthesia, head injury, stroke, alcohol intake), difficulty swallowing, and insertion of nasogastric tubes with or without tube feeding. With loss of consciousness, the gag and cough reflexes are depressed, and aspiration is more likely to occur.

The aspirated material (food, water, vomitus, or oropharyngeal secretions) triggers an inflammatory response. The most common form of aspiration pneumonia is a primary bacterial infection. Typically, more than one organism is identified on sputum culture, including aerobes and anaerobes, since they both make up the flora of the oropharynx.

Until cultures are completed and results obtained, initial antibiotic therapy is based on an assessment of probable causative organism, severity of illness, patient factors (e.g., malnutrition, current use of antibiotic therapy), and ability to treat common community-acquired organisms. For patients who aspirate in hospitals, appropriate antibiotics should include coverage for both gram-negative organisms and MRSA. In contrast, aspiration of acidic gastric contents causes *chemical (noninfectious) pneumonitis,* which may not require antibiotic therapy. However, secondary bacterial infection can occur 48 to 72 hours later.

Necrotizing Pneumonia. *Necrotizing pneumonia* is a rare complication of bacterial lung infection. It is characterized by liquefaction and, in some situations, cavitation of lung tissue. This often occurs as a result of community-acquired pneumonia (CAP). Although the exact pathophysiologic mechanisms involved are controversial, causative organisms include *Staphylococcus, Klebsiella,* and *Streptococcus.* Lung abscesses commonly occur. Signs and symptoms of necrotizing pneumonia include immediate respiratory insufficiency and/or failure, leukopenia, and bleeding into the airways.[7] Treatment often includes long-term antibiotic therapy and possible surgery.

Opportunistic Pneumonia. *Opportunistic pneumonia* is inflammation and infection of the lower respiratory tract in immunocompromised patients. Individuals at risk for opportunistic pneumonia include those with altered immune responses. This can include people with severe protein-calorie malnutrition or immunodeficiencies (e.g., human immunodeficiency virus [HIV] infection) and those receiving radiation therapy, chemotherapy, and any immunosuppressive therapy, including long-term corticosteroid therapy. In addition to the risk of bacterial and viral pneumonia, the immunocompromised person may develop an infection from microorganisms that do not normally cause disease, such as *Pneumocystis jiroveci* (formerly *carinii*) and cytomegalovirus (CMV).

P. jiroveci pneumonia (PJP) rarely occurs in the healthy individual but is the most common form of pneumonia in people with HIV disease. The onset is slow and subtle with symptoms of fever, tachypnea, tachycardia, dyspnea, nonproductive cough, and hypoxemia. The chest x-ray usually shows diffuse bilateral infiltrates. In widespread disease, the lungs have massive consolidation. PJP can be life-threatening, causing acute respiratory failure and death. Infection can also spread to other organs, including the liver, bone marrow, lymph nodes, spleen, and thyroid. Bacterial and viral pneumonias must first be ruled out because of the vague presentation of PJP. Although the causative agent is fungal, PJP does not respond to antifungal agents. Treatment consists of a course of trimethoprim/sulfamethoxazole (Bactrim, Septra) either IV or orally depending on the severity of disease and the patient's response.

CMV, a herpesvirus, can cause viral pneumonia. Most CMV infections are asymptomatic or mild, but severe disease can occur in people with an impaired immune response. CMV is the most common life-threatening infectious complication after hematopoietic stem cell transplantation.[8] Antiviral medications (e.g., ganciclovir [Cytovene], foscarnet [Foscavir], cidofovir) and high-dose immunoglobulin are used for treatment.

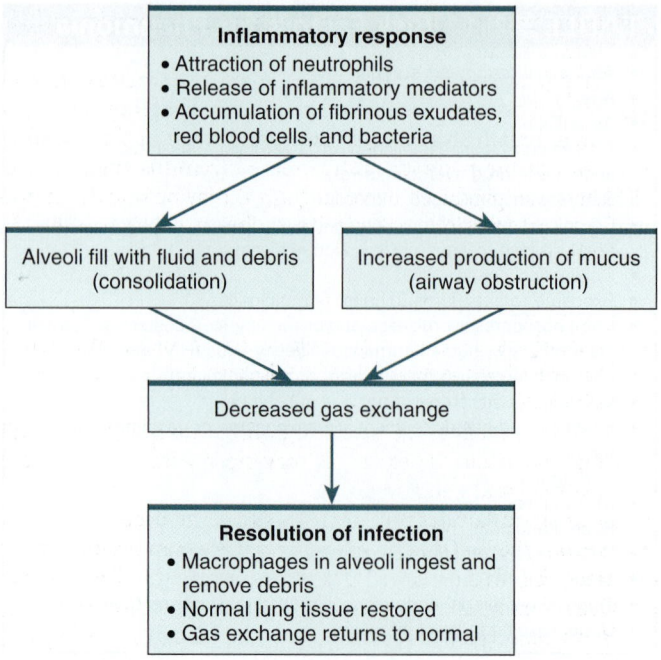

FIG. 27-1 Pathophysiologic course of pneumonia.

Pathophysiology

Specific pathophysiologic changes related to pneumonia vary according to the offending organism, but the majority of organisms trigger an inflammatory response in the lungs (Fig. 27-1). Inflammation, characterized by an increase in blood flow and vascular permeability, activates neutrophils to engulf and kill the offending organisms. As a result, the inflammatory process attracts more neutrophils, edema of the airways occurs, and fluid leaks from the capillaries and tissues into alveoli. Normal O_2 transport is affected, leading to clinical manifestations of hypoxia (e.g., tachypnea, dyspnea, tachycardia). *Consolidation,* a feature typical of bacterial pneumonia, occurs when the normally air-filled alveoli become filled with fluid and debris. Mucus production also increases, which can potentially obstruct airflow and impair gas exchange even further. Over time and with appropriate antibiotic therapy, macrophages lyse and process the debris, lung tissue is allowed to recover, and gas exchange returns to normal. Resolution and healing occur if there are no complications.

Clinical Manifestations

The most common presenting symptoms of pneumonia are cough, fever, chills, dyspnea, tachypnea, and pleuritic chest pain. The cough may or may not be productive. Sputum may appear green, yellow, or even rust colored (bloody). Viral pneumonia may initially be seen as influenza, with respiratory symptoms appearing and/or worsening 12 to 36 hours after onset.

The older or debilitated patient may not have classic symptoms of pneumonia. Confusion or stupor (possibly related to hypoxia) may be the only finding. Hypothermia, rather than fever, may also be noted with the older patient. Nonspecific clinical manifestations include diaphoresis, anorexia, fatigue, myalgias, and headache.

On physical examination, fine or coarse crackles may be auscultated over the affected region. If consolidation is present, bronchial breath sounds, egophony (a change in the sound of the voice of the patient), and increased fremitus (vibration of the chest wall produced by vocalization) may be noted. Patients with pleural effusion may exhibit dullness to percussion over the affected area.

Complications

Complications develop more frequently in older individuals and those with underlying chronic diseases. Potential complications include the following:

- *Atelectasis* (collapsed, airless alveoli) of one or part of one lobe may occur. These areas may clear with effective deep breathing and coughing.
- *Pleurisy* (inflammation of the pleura) may occur.
- *Pleural effusion* (fluid in the pleural space) can occur. In most cases, the effusion is sterile and is reabsorbed in 1 to 2 weeks. Occasionally, effusions require aspiration by thoracentesis.
- *Bacteremia* (bacterial infection in the blood) is more likely to occur in infections with *Streptococcus pneumoniae* and *Haemophilus influenzae.*
- *Pneumothorax* can occur when air collects in the pleural space, causing the lungs to collapse.
- *Meningitis* can be caused by *Streptococcus pneumoniae.* The patient with pneumonia who is disoriented, confused, or drowsy may have a lumbar puncture to evaluate the possibility of meningitis.
- *Acute respiratory failure* is one of the leading causes of death in patients with severe pneumonia. Failure occurs when pneumonia damages the lungs' ability to facilitate the exchange of O_2 and CO_2 across the alveolar-capillary membrane.
- *Sepsis/septic shock* can occur when bacteria within alveoli enter the bloodstream. Severe sepsis can lead to shock and multisystem organ dysfunction syndrome (MODS) (see Chapter 66).

Lung abscess is not a common complication of pneumonia. However, it may occur with pneumonia caused by *S. aureus* and gram-negative organisms. *Empyema,* the accumulation of purulent exudate in the pleural cavity, occurs in less than 5% of cases and requires antibiotic therapy and drainage of the exudate by a chest tube or open surgical drainage.[9] Pleurisy, pleural effusion, atelectasis, lung abscess, and pneumothorax are discussed later in this chapter.

Diagnostic Studies

The common diagnostic measures for pneumonia are presented in Table 27-4. History, physical examination, and chest x-ray often provide enough clinical information to make decisions about early treatment. Chest x-ray often shows a typical pattern characteristic of the infecting organism and is important in the diagnosis of pneumonia. X-ray may also show pleural effusions. A thoracentesis and/or bronchoscopy with washings may be used to obtain fluid samples from patients not responding to initial therapy.

Ideally, a sputum specimen for culture and Gram stain to identify the organism are obtained before beginning antibiotic therapy. However, antibiotic administration should not be delayed if a specimen cannot be readily obtained. Delays in antibiotic therapy can increase the risk of morbidity and mortality. Blood cultures are done for patients who are seriously ill. Arterial blood gases (ABGs) may be obtained to assess for hypoxemia (partial pressure of O_2 in arterial blood [PaO_2] less than 80 mm Hg), hypercapnia (partial pressure of carbon dioxide in arterial blood [$PaCO_2$] greater than 45 mm Hg), and acidosis (pH <7.35). Leukocytosis occurs in the majority of patients with bacterial pneumonia; the white blood cell (WBC) count is usually greater than 15,000/μL (15×10^9/L) with the presence of bands (immature neutrophils).

The use of biologic markers of infection to guide clinical decisions for treatment of pneumonia is under investigation. Serum levels of C-reactive protein (CRP) and procalcitonin are currently being explored as possible sources of information to help guide clinicians in distinguishing pneumonia from other types of cardiac and respiratory failure.[10-12]

TABLE 27-4 Interprofessional Care

Pneumonia

Diagnostic Assessment	Management
• History and physical examination • Chest x-ray • Gram stain of sputum • Sputum culture and sensitivity test • Pulse oximetry or ABGs (if indicated) • Complete blood count, WBC differential, and routine blood chemistries (if indicated) • Blood cultures (if indicated)	• Increased fluid intake (at least 3 L/day) • Balance between activity and rest • O_2 therapy (if indicated) ***Drug Therapy*** • Appropriate antibiotic therapy (Table 27-6) • Antipyretics • Analgesics

Interprofessional Care

Pneumococcal vaccine is used to prevent *Streptococcus pneumoniae* (Table 27-5). Prompt treatment with the appropriate antibiotic is essential. Antibiotics are highly effective for both bacterial and mycoplasma pneumonia. In uncomplicated cases, the patient responds to drug therapy within 48 to 72 hours. Indications of improvement include decreased temperature, improved breathing, and reduced chest discomfort. Abnormal physical findings can last more than 7 days. A repeat chest x-ray may be obtained in 6 to 8 weeks to assess for resolution.

In addition to antibiotic therapy, supportive measures are individualized to the patient's needs. These may include O_2 therapy to treat hypoxemia, analgesics to relieve chest pain, and antipyretics (e.g., aspirin, acetaminophen) for elevated temperature. Although cough suppressants, mucolytics, bronchodilators, and corticosteroids are often prescribed as adjunctive therapy, the use of these drugs is controversial. However, they may be prescribed for patients with underlying chronic conditions.

Individualize rest and activity to each patient's tolerance. Benefits of mobility include improved diaphragm movement and chest expansion, mobilization of secretions, and prevention of venous stasis.

Currently, no definitive treatment exists for the majority of viral pneumonias. As identified earlier, care is generally supportive. In most circumstances, viral pneumonia is self-limiting and will often resolve in 3 to 4 days. Antiviral therapy may be used to treat pneumonia caused by influenza (e.g., oseltamivir, zanamivir) and a few other viruses (e.g., acyclovir [Zovirax] for herpes simplex virus).[13]

Drug Therapy. Once the pneumonia is classified, the HCP selects empiric therapy on the likely infecting organism (Table 27-2). Table 27-6 presents the drug therapy for bacterial CAP.

For all types of pneumonia, empiric antibiotic therapy is based on whether the patient has risk factors for MDR organisms. The prevalence and resistance patterns of MDR pathogens vary among localities and institutions. Therefore the antibiotic regimen must be adapted to local patterns of antibiotic resistance. Multiple regimens exist, but all should initially include antibiotics that are effective against both resistant gram-negative and resistant gram-positive organisms.

Clinical improvement usually occurs in 3 to 5 days. Patients who deteriorate or fail to respond to therapy require aggressive reevaluation to assess for noninfectious etiologies, complications, coexisting infectious processes, or pneumonia caused by a drug-resistant pathogen.

IV antibiotic therapy should be switched to oral therapy as soon as the patient is hemodynamically stable, is improving clinically, is able to ingest oral medication, and has a functioning gastrointestinal tract. Stable patients do not need to be observed in the hospital and can be discharged to home on oral antibiotics. Total treatment time for patients with CAP should be a minimum of 5 days, and the patient should be afebrile for 48 to 72 hours before stopping treatment. However, you need to emphasize the importance of completing the full course of antibiotic treatment. Longer treatment time may be needed if initial therapy was not active against the identified pathogen or complications occur.

TABLE 27-5 Pneumococcal Vaccines

Vaccine*	Recommendations for Use
Pneumococcal conjugate vaccine (PCV13, Prevnar 13)†	• All children <5 yr • All adults ≥65 yr • Anyone 2-64 yr old with certain medical conditions (e.g., sickle cell disease, asplenia, immunodeficiencies, HIV infection, chronic renal failure, leukemia, generalized malignancy, long-term immunosuppressive therapy, cerebrospinal fluid leaks, cochlear implant[s])
Pneumococcal polysaccharide vaccine (PPSV23, Pneumovax 23)†	• All adults ≥65 yr • Anyone 2-64 yr old with certain long-term health problems (e.g., heart disease, lung disease, diabetes mellitus, alcoholism, cirrhosis, sickle cell disease, leaks of cerebrospinal fluid, cochlear implant) • Anyone 2-64 yr with a disease or condition that weakens the immune system or taking drugs that lowers body's resistance to infection (e.g., HIV infection; lymphoma or leukemia; kidney failure; damaged or no spleen; multiple myeloma; receiving immunosuppressive chemotherapy, radiation therapy, or long-term corticosteroids; after organ or bone marrow transplantation) • Adults 19-64 yr who smoke cigarettes or have asthma

*For additional details on scheduling of pneumococcal vaccinations, see *www.cdc.gov/mmwr/preview/mmwrhtml/mm6434a4.htm?s_cid=mm6434a4_w.*
†As their names imply, PCV13 and Prevnar 13 protect against 13 types of pneumococcal bacteria, and PPSV23 and Pneumovax 23 protect against 23 types of pneumococcal bacteria. The vaccinations have different mechanisms of action.

Nutritional Therapy. Hydration is important in the supportive treatment of pneumonia to prevent dehydration and to thin and loosen secretions. Individualize and carefully monitor fluid intake. If the patient is an older adult, has heart failure, or has a known preexisting respiratory condition, IV administration of fluids and electrolytes may be necessary.

TABLE 27-6 Drug Therapy
Bacterial Community-Acquired Pneumonia

Patient Variable	Treatment Options
Outpatient	
Previously healthy	
No recent antibiotic therapy in past 3 mo and no risk for drug-resistant *Staphylococcus pneumoniae* (DRSP)	Macrolide OR doxycycline
Co-morbidities (e.g., COPD; diabetes; chronic heart, liver, lung, or renal disease; malignancy; use of antibiotics in past 3 mo)	Respiratory fluoroquinolone OR β-Lactam plus macrolide (doxycycline may be substituted for macrolide)
Regions with ≥25% macrolide-resistant *S. pneumoniae*	Respiratory fluoroquinolone OR β-Lactam plus macrolide
Inpatient	
Medical unit	Respiratory fluoroquinolone OR β-Lactam plus macrolide
ICU	β-Lactam plus either azithromycin or respiratory fluoroquinolone
Special conditions	
• *Pseudomonas* infection	Antipneumococcal, antipseudomonal β-lactam plus either ciprofloxacin or levofloxacin OR Antipneumococcal, antipseudomonal β-lactam plus aminoglycoside and azithromycin OR Antipneumococcal, antipseudomonal β-lactam plus an aminoglycoside and an antipneumococcal fluoroquinolone
• *Pseudomonas* infection but patient has penicillin allergy	Substitute aztreonam for the above β-lactam
• Community-acquired methicillin-resistant *Staphylococcus aureus* (CA-MRSA)	Add vancomycin or linezolid (Zyvox)
Types of Antibiotics	
Macrolides	erythromycin, azithromycin (Zithromax), clarithromycin (Biaxin)
Fluoroquinolones	moxifloxacin (Avelox, Vigamox), levofloxacin (Levaquin), gemifloxacin (Factive)
β-Lactams	High-dose amoxicillin, amoxicillin/clavulanate (Augmentin), cefpodoxime, ceftriaxone (Rocephin), cefuroxime (Ceftin)
Antipneumococcal, antipseudomonal β-lactams	imipenem/cilastatin (Primaxin), meropenem (Merrem), cefepime (Maxipime), piperacillin/tazobactam (Zosyn)

Source: Adapted from the Infectious Diseases Society of America Practice Guidelines for CAP. Retrieved from *www.idsociety.org/Organ_System/#CommunityAcquired PneumoniaCAP*. For updated guidelines, check website.

Weight loss may occur in patients with pneumonia because of increased metabolic needs and difficulty eating due to nonspecific abdominal complaints or shortness of breath. Small, frequent meals are easier for dyspneic patients to tolerate. Offer foods high in calories and nutrients.

NURSING MANAGEMENT: PNEUMONIA

Nursing Assessment

Table 27-7 presents subjective and objective data to obtain from a patient with pneumonia.

Nursing Diagnoses

Nursing diagnoses for the patient with pneumonia may include, but are not limited to, the following:

- Impaired gas exchange *related to* fluid and exudate accumulation within the alveoli and surrounding lung tissue
- Ineffective breathing pattern *related to* inflammation and chest discomfort
- Acute pain (chest) *related to* inflammation and ineffective pain management and/or comfort measures
- Activity intolerance *related to* chest discomfort, inflammation, shortness of breath, generalized weakness

Additional information on nursing diagnoses for the patient with pneumonia is presented in eNursing Care Plan 27-1 on the website for this chapter.

TABLE 27-7 Nursing Assessment

Pneumonia

Subjective Data

Important Health Information

Past health history: Lung cancer, COPD, diabetes mellitus, chronic debilitating disease, malnutrition, altered consciousness, immunosuppression, exposure to chemical toxins, dust, or allergens

Medications: Antibiotics, corticosteroids, chemotherapy, or any immunosuppressants

Surgery or other treatments: Recent abdominal or thoracic surgery, splenectomy, endotracheal intubation, or any surgery with general anesthesia. Tube feedings

Functional Health Patterns

Health perception–health management: Cigarette smoking, alcoholism; recent upper respiratory tract infection, malaise

Nutritional-metabolic: Anorexia, nausea, vomiting. Chills

Activity-exercise: Prolonged bed rest or immobility. Fatigue, weakness. Dyspnea, cough (productive or nonproductive). Nasal congestion

Cognitive-perceptual: Pain with breathing, chest pain, sore throat, headache, abdominal pain, muscle aches

Objective Data

General

Fever, restlessness or lethargy. Splinting of affected area

Respiratory

Tachypnea, pharyngitis, asymmetric chest movements or retraction, decreased excursion, nasal flaring. Use of accessory muscles (neck, abdomen). Crackles, friction rub on auscultation, dullness on percussion over consolidated areas, increased tactile fremitus on palpation. Pink, rusty, purulent, green, yellow, or white sputum (amount may be scant to copious)

Cardiovascular

Tachycardia

Neurologic

Changes in mental status, ranging from confusion to delirium

Possible Diagnostic Findings

Leukocytosis. Abnormal ABGs with ↓ or normal PaO_2, ↓ or normal $PaCO_2$, and ↑ or normal pH initially, and later ↓ PaO_2, ↑ $PaCO_2$, and ↓ pH. Positive sputum on Gram stain and culture. Patchy or diffuse infiltrates, abscesses, pleural effusion, or pneumothorax on chest x-ray

Planning

The overall goals are that the patient with pneumonia will have (1) clear breath sounds, (2) normal breathing patterns, (3) no signs of hypoxia, (4) normal chest x-ray, (5) normal white blood cell (WBC) count, and (6) absence of complications related to pneumonia.

Nursing Implementation

Health Promotion. To reduce the risk of pneumonia, teach individuals to practice good health habits, such as frequent hand washing, proper nutrition, adequate rest, regular exercise, and coughing or sneezing into the elbow rather than hands. Avoidance of cigarette smoke is one of the most important health-promoting behaviors. If possible, avoid exposure to people with URIs. If a URI occurs, it requires prompt attention with supportive measures (e.g., rest, fluids). If symptoms persist for longer than 7 days, the person should seek medical care. Encourage those at risk for pneumonia (e.g., chronically ill, older adult) to obtain both influenza and pneumococcal vaccines (Table 27-5). Identifying patients at risk (Table 27-1) and taking measures to prevent pneumonia are priority interventions.

In the acute care setting, place the patient with altered consciousness in positions (e.g., side-lying, upright) that will prevent or minimize the risk of aspiration. Turn and reposition the patient at least every 2 hours to facilitate adequate lung expansion and mobilization of secretions. Encourage and assist with ambulation and positioning into a chair. In the ICU, strict adherence to all aspects of the ventilator bundle (see Table 67-8), a group of interventions aimed at reducing the risk of VAP, has been shown to significantly reduce VAP.

For the patient who has difficulty swallowing and needs assistance in eating, drinking, and taking medication to prevent aspiration, elevate the patient's head-of-bed to at least 30 degrees and have the patient sit up for all meals. Assess for a gag reflex before giving food or fluids. Patients who have orogastric or nasogastric tubes are at risk for aspiration pneumonia (see Chapter 39). Although feeding tubes are small, any interruption in the integrity of the lower esophageal sphincter can allow reflux of gastric contents. To prevent aspiration, elevate the head of the bed to at least 30 degrees and monitor gastric residual volumes (see Table 39-12).

Patients with impaired mobility from any cause need assistance with turning and moving as well as encouragement to breathe deeply at frequent intervals. Observe the patient's skin and all pressure points for any evidence of redness or breakdown, especially the sacrum and coccyx. Early mobilization, the use of an incentive spirometer, and twice-daily oral hygiene with chlorhexidine swabs have been shown to significantly reduce the incidence of pneumonia in postoperative patients.[14] Treat pain to a comfort level that permits the patient to deep breathe and cough but yet remain awake and alert and achieve optimum mobility.

Practice strict medical asepsis and adherence to infection control guidelines to reduce the incidence of health care–associated infection (HAI). Staff and visitors should wash their hands on entering and leaving the patient's room. Staff must wash or use sanitizing hand gel before and after providing care and on removing gloves. Use strict sterile aseptic technique when suctioning the patient's trachea, and use caution when handling ventilator circuits, tracheostomy tubing, and nebulizer circuits that can become contaminated from patient secretions. Avoid inappropriate use of antibiotics to prevent the development of drug-resistant organisms.

- **Acute Care.** Although many patients with pneumonia are treated on an outpatient basis, the nursing care plan for a patient with pneumonia (see eNursing Care Plan 27-1) applies to both individuals at home and in-hospital patients. Essential nursing care for patients with pneumonia includes monitoring physical assessment parameters, providing treatment, and monitoring the patient's response to treatment. Along with physical assessment (including pulse oximetry monitoring), prompt collection of specimens and initiation of antibiotics are critical. O_2 therapy, hydration, nutritional support, breathing exercises, early ambulation, and therapeutic positioning are part of nursing management. Collaborate with respiratory therapists for assistance in monitoring the patient's condition and with physical therapy for postural drainage and chest percussion.
- **Ambulatory Care.** Teach the patient about the importance of taking every dose of the prescribed antibiotic, any drug-drug and food-drug interactions for the prescribed antibiotic, and the need for adequate rest to facilitate recovery. Instruct the patient to drink plenty of liquids (at least 6 to 10 glasses/day, unless contraindicated) and to avoid alcohol and smoking. A cool mist humidifier or warm bath may help the patient breathe easier. Tell patients that it may be several weeks before their usual vigor and sense of well-being return. Explain that a follow-up chest x-ray may be done in 6 to 8 weeks to evaluate resolution of pneumonia. A prolonged period of convalescence may be necessary for the older adult or chronically ill patient.

Teaching should also include information about available influenza and pneumococcal vaccines. Patients can receive the pneumococcal vaccine and influenza vaccine at the same time but not in the exact same location, and the vaccines cannot be mixed into one injection.

Evaluation

The expected outcomes are that the patient with pneumonia will have

- Effective respiratory rate, rhythm, and depth of respirations
- Lungs clear to auscultation

Additional information on expected outcomes for the patient with pneumonia is presented in eNursing Care Plan 27-1 available on the website for this chapter.

TUBERCULOSIS

Tuberculosis (TB) is an infectious disease caused by *Mycobacterium tuberculosis*. It usually involves the lungs, but any organ can be infected, including brain, kidneys, and bones. The CDC reports that more than 2 billion people (one third of the world's population) are infected with TB. It is the leading cause of mortality in patients with HIV infection. The incidence of TB worldwide declined until the mid-1980s when HIV disease emerged. The major factors contributing to the resurgence of TB were (1) high rates of TB among patients with HIV infection and (2) the emergence of MDR strains of *M. tuberculosis*. Although the prevalence of TB has increased in Europe, it has steadily declined in the United States since reaching a resurgence peak in 1992.[15]

TB occurs disproportionately in the poor, underserved, and minorities. People most at risk include the homeless, residents of inner-city neighborhoods, foreign-born people, those living or working in institutions (long-term care facilities, prisons, shelters, hospitals), IV injecting drug users, poor people, and those with poor access to health care. Immunosuppression from any etiology (e.g., HIV infection, malignancy, long-term corticosteroid use) increases the risk of active TB infection.

CULTURAL & ETHNIC HEALTH DISPARITIES

Tuberculosis

- Of the reported tuberculosis (TB) cases in the United States, most occur in racial and ethnic minorities.
- Asians have the highest TB rate of any ethnic group in the United States. Native Hawaiian and other Pacific Islanders have the second-highest TB rate.
- Of all the TB cases in the United States, 65% occur in foreign-born people. This rate is 13 times higher than in U.S.-born people.
- The percentage of foreign-born people with multidrug-resistant TB has increased from 31% in 1993 to 90% in 2013.

Source: Centers for Disease Control and Prevention: Trends in tuberculosis—United States 2013. Retrieved from *www.cdc.gov/tb/statistics/reports/2013/pdf/report2013.pdf*.

Once a strain of *M. tuberculosis* develops resistance to two of the most potent first-line antituberculous drugs (e.g., isoniazid [INH], rifampin [Rifadin]), it is defined as *multidrug-resistant tuberculosis* (MDR-TB).[16] Extensively drug-resistant TB (XDR-TB) occurs when the organism is also resistant to any of the fluoroquinolones plus any injectable antibiotic agent. Resistance results from several problems, including incorrect prescribing, lack of public health case management, and patient nonadherence to the prescribed regimen.

Etiology and Pathophysiology

M. tuberculosis is a gram-positive, acid-fast bacillus (AFB) that is usually spread from person to person via airborne particles expectorated when breathing, talking, singing, sneezing, and coughing. A process of evaporation leaves small droplet nuclei, 1 to 5 μm in size, suspended in the air for minutes to hours. These bacteria are then inhaled by another person. TB is not highly infectious, as transmission usually requires close, frequent, or prolonged exposure. The disease cannot be spread by touching, sharing food utensils, kissing, or any other type of physical contact.

Factors that influence the likelihood of transmission include the (1) number of organisms expelled into the air, (2) concentration of organisms (small spaces with limited ventilation would mean higher concentration), (3) length of time of exposure, and (4) immune system of the exposed person. Once inhaled, these small particles lodge in bronchioles and alveoli. A local inflammatory reaction occurs, and the focus of infection is established. This is called the *Ghon lesion* or *focus*, which represents a calcified TB granuloma, the hallmark of a primary TB infection. The formation of a granuloma is a defense mechanism aimed at walling off the infection and preventing further spread. Replication of the bacillus is inhibited and the infection is stopped.

Most immunocompetent adults infected with TB are able to completely kill the mycobacteria. Some people contain the mycobacteria in a nonreplicating dormant state. Of these individuals, 5% to 10% develop active TB infection when the bacteria begin to multiply months or years later. *M. tuberculosis* is aerophilic (O_2 loving) and thus has an affinity for the lungs. However, the infection can spread via the lymphatic system and find favorable environments for growth in other organs, including the cerebral cortex, spine, epiphyses of the bone, and adrenal glands.

Classification

Several systems can be used to classify TB. The American Thoracic Society classifies TB based on development of the disease (Table 27-8). TB can also be classified according to (1) its presentation (primary, latent, or reactivated) and (2) whether it is pulmonary or extrapulmonary.

Primary TB infection occurs when the bacteria are inhaled and initiate an inflammatory reaction. The majority of people mount effective immune responses to encapsulate these organisms for the rest of their lives, preventing primary infection from progressing to disease.

Latent TB infection (LTBI) occurs in a person who does not have active TB disease (Table 27-9). People with LTBI have a positive skin test but are asymptomatic (Table 27-9). These individuals cannot transmit the TB bacteria to others but can develop active TB disease at some point. Immunosuppression, diabetes mellitus, poor nutrition, aging, pregnancy, stress, and chronic disease can precipitate the reactivation of LTBI. Consequently, treatment of LTBI is important (discussed later in this chapter).

If the initial immune response is not adequate, the body cannot contain the organisms. As a result, the bacteria replicate and *active TB disease* results. When active disease develops within the first 2 years of infection, it is termed *primary TB*. Individuals co-infected with HIV are at greatest risk for developing active TB. Post-primary TB, or *reactivation TB*, is defined as TB disease occurring 2 or more years after the initial infection. If the site of TB is pulmonary or laryngeal, the individual is considered infectious and can transmit the disease to others.

TABLE 27-8 Classification of Tuberculosis

Class	Exposure or Infection	Description
0	No TB exposure	No TB exposure, not infected (no history of exposure, negative tuberculin skin test)
1	TB exposure, no infection	TB exposure, no evidence of infection (history of exposure, negative tuberculin skin test)
2	Latent TB infection, no disease	TB infection without disease (significant reaction to tuberculin skin test, negative bacteriologic studies, no x-ray findings compatible with TB, no clinical evidence of TB)
3	TB, clinically active	TB infection with clinically active disease (positive bacteriologic studies or both a significant reaction to tuberculin skin test and clinical or x-ray evidence of current disease)
4	TB, but not clinically active	No current disease (history of previous episode of TB or abnormal, stable x-ray findings in a person with a significant reaction to tuberculin skin test. Negative bacteriologic studies if done. No clinical or x-ray evidence of current disease)
5	TB suspect	TB suspect (diagnosis pending). Individual should not be in this classification for >3 mo

Source: American Thoracic Society.

Clinical Manifestations

Symptoms of pulmonary TB usually do not develop until 2 to 3 weeks after infection or reactivation. The characteristic pulmonary manifestation is an initial dry cough that frequently becomes productive with mucoid or mucopurulent sputum. Active TB disease may initially manifest with constitutional symptoms such as fatigue, malaise, anorexia, unexplained weight loss, low-grade fevers, and night sweats. Dyspnea is a late symptom that may signify considerable pulmonary disease or a pleural effusion. Hemoptysis, which occurs in less than 10% of patients with TB, is also a late symptom.

Sometimes TB has a more acute, sudden presentation. The patient may have a high fever, chills, generalized flu-like symptoms, pleuritic pain, and a productive cough. Auscultation of the lungs may be normal or reveal crackles, and/or adventitious (such as bronchial) breath sounds.

Immunosuppressed (e.g., HIV-infected) people and older adults are less likely to have fever and other signs of an infection. In patients with HIV, classic manifestations of TB such as fever, cough, and weight loss may be wrongly attributed to *P. jiroveci* pneumonia (PJP) or other HIV-associated opportunistic diseases. Clinical manifestations of respiratory problems in patients with HIV must be carefully investigated to determine the cause. A change in cognitive function may be the only initial presenting sign of TB in an older person.

The clinical manifestations of extrapulmonary TB depend on the organs infected. For example, renal TB can cause dysuria and hematuria. Bone and joint TB may cause severe pain.

TABLE 27-9 Latent Tuberculosis Infection (LTBI) Compared to TB Disease

Latent TB Infection (LTBI)	TB Disease
Has no symptoms	Has symptoms that may include the following: • Bad cough that lasts ≥3 wk • Pain in the chest • Coughing up blood or sputum • Weakness or fatigue • Weight loss • No appetite • Chills • Fever • Sweating at night
Does not feel sick	Usually feels sick
Cannot spread TB bacteria to others	May spread TB bacteria to others
Usually has a skin test or blood test result indicating TB infection	Usually has a skin test or blood test result indicating TB infection
Has a normal chest x-ray and a negative sputum smear	May have an abnormal chest x-ray or positive sputum smear or culture
Needs treatment for latent TB infection to prevent active TB disease	Needs treatment for active TB disease

Source: Centers for Disease Control and Prevention: Latent tuberculosis infection: a guide for primary health care providers (2013). Retrieved from *www.cdc.gov/tb/publications/ltbi/pdf/TargetedLTBI.pdf*.

Headaches, vomiting, and lymphadenopathy may be present with TB meningitis.

Complications

Appropriately treated pulmonary TB typically heals without complications, except for scarring and residual cavitation within the lung. Significant pulmonary damage, although rare, can occur in patients who are poorly treated or who do not respond to TB treatment.

Miliary TB is the widespread dissemination of the mycobacterium. The bacteria are spread via the bloodstream to several distant organs. The infection is characterized by a large amount of TB bacilli and may be fatal if left untreated. It can occur as a result of primary disease or reactivation of latent infection. Clinical manifestations of miliary TB slowly progress over a period of days, weeks, or even months. Symptoms vary depending on the organs that are affected. Fever, cough, and lymphadenopathy are present. Hepatomegaly and splenomegaly may also occur.

Pleural TB, a specific type of extrapulmonary TB, can result from either primary disease or reactivation of a latent infection. Chest pain, fever, cough, and presence of a unilateral pleural effusion are common. A pleural effusion is caused by bacteria in the pleural space, which trigger an inflammatory reaction and a pleural exudate of protein-rich fluid. Empyema is less common than effusion but may occur from large numbers of tubercular organisms in the pleural space. Diagnosis is confirmed by AFB cultures and a pleural biopsy.

Because TB can infect organs throughout the body, various acute and long-term complications can result. TB in the spine (Pott's disease) can lead to destruction of the intervertebral disc and adjacent vertebrae. Central nervous system TB can cause severe bacterial meningitis. Abdominal TB can lead to peritonitis, especially in HIV-positive patients. The kidneys, adrenal glands, lymph nodes, and urogenital tract may also be affected.

Diagnostic Studies

Tuberculin Skin Test. The tuberculin skin test (TST) (Mantoux test) using purified protein derivative (PPD) is the standard method to screen people for *M. tuberculosis*. The test is administered by injecting 0.1 mL of PPD intradermally on the ventral surface of the forearm. The test is read by inspection and palpation 48 to 72 hours later for the presence or absence of induration. Induration, a palpable, raised, hardened area or swelling (not redness) at the injection site means the person has been exposed to TB and has developed antibodies.[17] (Antibody formation occurs 2 to 12 weeks after initial exposure to the bacteria.) The indurated area (if present) is measured and recorded in millimeters. Based on the size of the induration and the risk factors, an interpretation is made according to standards for determining a positive test reaction. Because the immunocompromised patient may have a decreased response to TST, smaller induration reactions (5 mm or larger) are considered positive. (See Table 25-11 for guidelines in interpreting responses to the TST.)

Some people who were previously infected with TB may have a waning immune response to the TST, resulting in a false negative result. However, repeating the TST may stimulate (boost) the body's ability to react to tuberculin in future tests. A positive reaction to a subsequent test could then be misinterpreted as a new infection, rather than the result of the boosted reaction to an old infection. To prevent misinterpretation in future testing, a two-step testing process is recommended for initial testing for health care workers (who get repeated testing) and for individuals who have a decreased response to allergens. A previously negative two-step TST ensures that any future positive results can be accurately interpreted as being caused by a new infection.

Interferon-γ Release Assays. Interferon-γ (INF-gamma) release assays (IGRAs) provide another screening tool for TB. IGRAs are blood tests that detect INF-gamma release from T cells in response to *Mycobacterium tuberculosis.* Examples of IGRAs include QuantiFERON-TB test and the T-SPOT.TB test. Test results are available in a few hours.

IGRAs offer several advantages over the TST in that they require only one patient visit, are not subject to reader bias, have no booster phenomenon, and are not affected by prior bacillus Calmette-Guérin (BCG) vaccination. The cost of an IGRA is substantially higher than the TST. Current guidelines suggest that both tests are viable options and that selection should be based on context and reasons for testing. Neither IGRAs nor TST can distinguish between LTBI and active TB infection. LTBI can only be diagnosed by excluding active TB.

Chest X-ray. Although the findings on chest x-ray examination are important, it is not possible to make a diagnosis of TB solely on chest x-ray findings. The chest x-ray may appear normal in a patient with TB. Findings suggestive of TB include upper lobe infiltrates, cavitary infiltrates, lymph node involvement, and pleural and/or pericardial effusion. Other diseases, such as sarcoidosis, can mimic the appearance of TB.

Bacteriologic Studies. Three consecutive sputum specimens obtained on different days are sent for smear and culture. The initial testing involves a microscopic examination of stained sputum smears for AFB. However, the definitive diagnosis of TB requires the demonstration of tubercle bacilli bacteriologically by sputum culture, which can take up to 8 weeks. Treatment is warranted pending the culture results for patients in whom clinical suspicion of TB is high. Samples for other suspected TB sites can be collected from gastric washings, cerebrospinal fluid (CSF), or fluid from an effusion or abscess.

Interprofessional Care

Most patients with TB are treated on an outpatient basis (Table 27-10). Many people can continue to work and maintain their lifestyles with few changes. Patients with sputum smear–positive TB are generally considered infectious for the first 2 weeks after starting treatment. Advise these patients to restrict visitors and avoid travel on public transportation and trips to public places. Remind them of the importance of good handwashing and oral hygiene. Hospitalization may be needed for the severely ill or debilitated. The mainstay of TB treatment is drug therapy

TABLE 27-10 Interprofessional Care

Pulmonary Tuberculosis

Diagnostic Assessment	Management
• History and physical examination • Tuberculin skin test (TST) • QuantiFERON-TB test • Chest x-ray • Bacteriologic studies • Sputum smear for acid-fast bacilli (AFB) • Sputum culture	• Long-term treatment with antimicrobial drugs (Tables 27-11 and 27-12) • Follow-up AFB smears, cultures, and chest x-rays • Follow-up care involving community health care workers and social workers

TABLE 27-11 Drug Therapy

Tuberculosis (TB)

Drug	Side Effects*
isoniazid	Hepatitis, asymptomatic elevation of aminotransferases (ALT, AST) Monitor liver function tests monthly
rifampin (Rifadin)	Hepatitis, thrombocytopenia, orange discoloration of bodily fluids (sputum, urine, sweat, tears)
pyrazinamide	Hepatitis, arthralgias, hyperuricemia
ethambutol (Myambutol)	Ocular toxicity (decreased red-green color discrimination) Monitor visual acuity and color discrimination regularly
rifabutin (Mycobutin)	Hepatitis, thrombocytopenia, neutropenia, orange discoloration of bodily fluids (sputum, urine, sweat, tears)
rifapentine (Priftin)	Similar to those of rifampin
streptomycin	Ototoxicity, neurotoxicity, nephrotoxicity
bedaquiline (Sirturo)	Dysrhythmias
aminoglycosides	Ototoxicity, nephrotoxicity
• capreomycin (Capastat) • amikacin	Used in selected cases for treatment of resistant strains
fluoroquinolones	GI disturbance, neurologic effects (dizziness, headache), rash
• levofloxacin (Levaquin) • moxifloxacin (Avelox, Vigamox)	Used in drug-resistant TB

ALT, Alanine transaminase; *AST,* aspartate aminotransferase.
*Only common side effects are listed.

TABLE 27-12 Drug Therapy

Tuberculosis Disease Regimens

Initial Phase	Continuation Phase
Option 1	
4-drug regimen consisting of isoniazid, rifampin, pyrazinamide, ethambutol Given daily for 56 doses (8 wk) OR 5 days/wk DOT for 40 doses (8 wk)	isoniazid, rifampin daily for 126 doses (18 wk) OR 5 days/wk DOT for 90 doses (18 wk)
Option 2	
4-drug regimen consisting of isoniazid, rifampin, pyrazinamide, ethambutol Given daily for 14 doses (2 wk), followed by twice weekly for 12 doses (6 wk) OR 5 days/wk DOT for 10 doses (2 wk), then twice weekly for 12 doses (6 wk)	isoniazid, rifampin twice weekly for 36 doses (18 wk) OR once weekly for 18 doses (18 wk)
Option 3	
4-drug regimen consisting of isoniazid, rifampin, pyrazinamide, ethambutol Given three times weekly for 24 doses (8 wk)	isoniazid, rifampin three times weekly for 54 doses (18 wk)
Option 4	
3-drug regimen consisting of isoniazid, rifampin, ethambutol Given daily for 56 doses (8 wk) OR 5 days/wk DOT for 40 doses (8 wk)	isoniazid, rifampin daily for 217 doses (31 wk) OR 5 days/wk DOT for 155 doses (31 wk) OR twice weekly for 62 doses (31 wk)

DOT, Directly observed therapy.
Source: American Thoracic Society, Centers for Disease Control and Prevention, and Infectious Diseases Society of America: Treatment of tuberculosis. Retrieved from *www.cdc.gov/mmwr/PDF/rr/rr5211.pdf.*

(Table 27-11). Promoting and monitoring adherence are critical for treatment to be successful.

Drug Therapy

Active TB Disease. Because of the growing prevalence of MDR-TB, it is important to manage the patient with active TB aggressively. Drug therapy is divided into two phases: initial and continuation (Table 27-12). In most circumstances the treatment regimen for patients with previously untreated TB consists of a 2-month initial phase with four drugs (isoniazid, rifampin, pyrazinamide, and ethambutol). If drug susceptibility test results indicate that the bacteria are susceptible to all drugs, ethambutol may be discontinued. If pyrazinamide cannot be included in the initial phase (because of liver disease, pregnancy, etc.), the remaining three drugs are used for the initial phase.

DRUG ALERT Isoniazid

- Alcohol may increase hepatotoxicity of the drug.
- Instruct patient to avoid drinking alcohol during treatment.
- Monitor for signs of hepatitis before and while taking drug.

If the patient develops a toxic reaction to the primary drugs, other drugs can be used, including rifabutin and rifapentine (Priftin). Treatment for drug-resistant TB is guided by sensitivity testing. MDR-TB therapy typically includes a fluoroquinolone and an injectable antibiotic (Table 27-11). Bedaquiline (Sirturo), a relatively new drug, is used in combination with other drugs to treat MDR-TB. It works by inhibiting an enzyme needed for *M. tuberculosis* to replicate.

Directly observed therapy (DOT) involves providing the antituberculosis drugs directly to patients and watching as they swallow the medications. To ensure adherence, it is the preferred strategy for all patients with TB, especially for those at risk for nonadherence.[18] Nonadherence is a major factor in the emergence of multidrug resistance and treatment failures. Many individuals do not adhere to the treatment program in spite of understanding the disease process and value of treatment. DOT is an expensive but essential public health measure. The risk for reactivation of TB and MDR-TB is increased in patients who do not complete the full course of therapy. In many areas, the public health nurse administers DOT at a clinic site.

When DOT is not used, fixed-dose combination drugs may enhance adherence. Combinations of isoniazid and rifampin (Rifamate) and of isoniazid, rifampin, and pyrazinamide (Rifater) are available to simplify therapy. The therapy for people with HIV follows the same therapy options outlined in Table 27-12. However, alternative regimens that include once-weekly isoniazid plus rifapentine continuation dosing in any HIV-infected patient and twice-weekly isoniazid plus rifampin or rifabutin should not be used if $CD4^+$ counts are less than 100/μL. HCPs must also be alert for possible drug interactions between antiretrovirals (used to treat HIV) and rifamycins.

Teaching patients about the adverse effects of these drugs and when to seek prompt medical attention is critical. The major side effect of isoniazid, rifampin, and pyrazinamide is nonviral hepatitis. Baseline liver function tests (LFTs) are done at the start of treatment and monitored closely (e.g., every 2 to 4 weeks), if results are abnormal.

Latent Tuberculosis Infection. In people with LTBI, drug therapy helps prevent a TB infection from developing into active TB disease. Because a person with LTBI has fewer bacteria, treatment is much easier. Usually only one drug is needed. Drug therapy regimens for LTBI are presented in Table 27-13.

TABLE 27-13 Drug Therapy

Latent Tuberculosis Infection Regimens

Drugs	Duration	Interval	Minimum Doses
isoniazid	9 mo	Daily	270
		Twice weekly*	76
isoniazid	6 mo	Daily	180
		Twice weekly*	52
isoniazid and rifapentine	3 mo	Once weekly*	12
rifampin	4 mo	Daily	120

Source: Centers for Disease Control and Prevention: Latent tuberculosis infection: a guide for primary health care providers (2013). Retrieved from *www.cdc.gov/tb/publications/ltbi/pdf/TargetedLTBI.pdf*
*Use directly observed therapy (DOT).

ETHICAL/LEGAL DILEMMAS

Patient Adherence

Situation

A health clinic at a homeless shelter discovers that F.C., a 64-yr-old male with tuberculosis (TB), has not been taking his prescribed medication. He tells you that it is hard for him to get to the clinic to obtain the medication, much less to keep on a schedule. You are concerned not only about this patient but also about the risks for the other people at the shelter, in the park, and at the meal sites.

Ethical/Legal Points for Consideration

- Adherence is a complex issue involving a person's culture and values, perceived risk of disease, availability of resources, access to treatment, and perceived consequences of available choices.
- Advocacy for the patient and the community obliges you to involve other members of the health care team, such as social services, to assist in obtaining the necessary resources or support for the patient to complete a course of treatment.
- Some cities and states have instituted a stepwise legal process for managing nonadherent TB patients.[1]
- Legally the constitutionally granted right to control one's own body may be limited by the state and federal obligation to protect public health and safety. Most of these laws have provisions for the protection of constitutional rights such as right to counsel, right to least restrictive alternative in terms of confinement setting, and right to prompt judicial review.
- The federal government and many states have provisions for quarantine, detention, and treatment. With the threats of bioterrorism and the globalization of exposure to highly lethal infectious diseases, it seems unlikely that the government's power to detain will be removed.

Discussion Questions

1. What alternatives of care can be offered to F.C.?
2. Under what circumstances are HCPs justified in overriding a patient's autonomy or decision making?

Reference

1. Guidelines for the Civil Detention of Persistently Non-Adherent Tuberculosis Patients in California. Retrieved from *http://ctca.org/fileLibrary/file_50.pdf.*

The standard treatment regimen for LTBI is 9 months of daily isoniazid. It is an effective and inexpensive drug that the patient can take orally. The 9-month regimen is more effective, but adherence issues may make a 6-month regimen preferable. For HIV patients and those with fibrotic lesions on chest x-ray, isoniazid is given for 9 months. An alternative 3-month regimen of isoniazid and rifapentine may be used for otherwise healthy patients who are not presumed to be infected with drug-resistant bacilli. Four-month therapy with rifampin may be indicated if the patient is resistant to isoniazid. Because of severe liver injury and deaths, the CDC does not recommend the combination of rifampin and pyrazinamide for treatment of LTBI.[19]

EVIDENCE-BASED PRACTICE

Applying the Evidence

Adherence to Tuberculosis Treatment Program

You are a nurse working in an outpatient health clinic with C.J., a 42-year-old male diagnosed 3 months ago with active tuberculosis (TB). You notice C.J. frequently misses or is late for his clinic appointments. He tells you he forgets when his appointments are scheduled and asks if he needs to continue with his visits because he is feeling much better.

Making Clinical Decisions

Best Available Evidence. TB clinic attendance and treatment completion rates are higher when patients receive pre-appointment reminder phone calls or letters. When appointments are missed, phone calls, letters, or home visits re-engage patients, resulting in improved clinic attendance and treatment completion.

Clinician Expertise. You know patients may stop attending clinics and taking their medications when feeling well again, which can lead to treatment failure and multidrug resistance.

Patient Preferences and Values. C.J. tells you that he has a busy lifestyle and that he does not remember his appointment dates or consider them important since he is feeling better.

Implications for Nursing Practice

1. What information would you provide C.J. regarding the importance of his clinic visits?
2. Your clinic indicates interest in starting a reminder system for clinic appointments. How will you support these efforts, and what system will you recommend?
3. How will you determine if C.J. is adhering to the recommended drug treatment program?

Reference for Evidence

Liu Q, Abba K, Alejandria MM, et al: Reminder systems to improve patient adherence to tuberculosis clinic appointments for diagnosis and treatment, *Cochrane Database Syst Rev* 11:CD006594, 2014.

Bacille-Calmette-Guerin Vaccine. Bacille-Calmette-Guerin (BCG) vaccine is a live, attenuated strain of *Mycobacterium bovis.* The vaccine is given to infants in parts of the world with a high prevalence of TB. In the United States it is typically not recommended because of the low risk of infection, the vaccine's variable effectiveness against adult pulmonary TB, and potential interference with TB skin test reactivity. The BCG vaccination can result in a false-positive TST. IGRA results are not affected. The BCG vaccine should be considered only for select individuals who meet specific criteria (e.g., health care workers who are continually exposed to patients with MDR-TB and when infection control precautions are not successful).

❖ NURSING MANAGEMENT: TUBERCULOSIS

◆ Nursing Assessment

Ask the patient about a previous history of TB, chronic illness, or any immunosuppressive medications. Obtain a social and occupational history to determine risk factors for transmission of TB. Assess the patient for productive cough, night sweats, temperature elevation, weight loss, pleuritic chest pain, and abnormal lung sounds. If the patient has a productive cough, early morning is the ideal time to collect sputum specimens for an AFB smear.

Nursing Diagnoses

Nursing diagnoses for the patient with TB may include, but are not limited to, the following:

- Ineffective breathing pattern *related to* decreased lung capacity
- Ineffective airway clearance *related to* increased secretions, fatigue, and decreased lung capacity
- Risk for infection (spread of infection to others) *related to* cough and sputum production, lack of knowledge of disease process, and social/economic circumstances
- Noncompliance and ineffective health management *related to* lack of knowledge of disease process, lack of motivation, long-term nature of treatment, and lack of resources

Planning

The overall goals are that the patient with TB will (1) comply with the therapeutic regimen, (2) have no recurrence of disease, (3) have normal pulmonary function, and (4) take appropriate measures to prevent the spread of the disease.

Nursing Implementation

Health Promotion. The ultimate goal is to eradicate TB worldwide. Screening programs in known risk groups are of value in detecting individuals with TB. Treatment of LTBI reduces the number of TB carriers in the community. The person with a positive TST should have a chest x-ray to assess for active TB disease. Individuals with a diagnosis of TB must be reported to the public health authorities for identification and assessment of contacts and risk to the community.

Programs to address the social determinants of TB are necessary to decrease transmission of TB. Reducing HIV infection, poverty, overcrowded living conditions, malnutrition, smoking, and drug and alcohol abuse can help minimize TB infection rates. Improving access to health care and education is also important.

Acute Care. Patients admitted to the emergency department or directly to the nursing unit with respiratory symptoms should be assessed for the possibility of TB. Those strongly suspected of having TB should (1) be placed on airborne isolation; (2) receive a medical workup, including chest x-ray, sputum smear, and culture; and (3) receive appropriate drug therapy. Airborne infection isolation is indicated for the patient with pulmonary or laryngeal TB until the patient is noninfectious. *Airborne infection isolation* refers to isolation of patients infected with organisms spread by the airborne route. It requires a single-occupancy room with negative pressure and airflow of 6 to 12 exchanges per hour.

High-efficiency particulate air (HEPA) masks are worn whenever entering the patient's room. These masks are highly effective at protecting from small particles 5 μm or less in diameter. Because there are many different types of HEPA masks currently available, health care professionals should be "fit tested" each time a different brand or model of mask is used to ensure proper mask size. Otherwise, the CDC recommends that yearly mask "fit testing" is acceptable.[20] To be effective, the mask must be molded to fit tightly around the nose and mouth.

Teach patients to cover the nose and mouth with paper tissues every time they cough, sneeze, or produce sputum. The tissues should be thrown into a paper bag and disposed of with the trash or flushed down the toilet. Emphasize careful hand washing after handling sputum and soiled tissues. If patients need to be out of the negative-pressure room, they must wear a standard isolation mask to prevent exposure to others. Minimize prolonged visitation to other parts of the hospital.

Identify and screen close contacts of the person with TB. Anyone testing positive for TB infection will undergo further evaluation and needs to be treated for either LTBI or active TB disease.

Ambulatory Care. Patients who respond clinically are discharged home (even with positive cultures) if their household contacts have already been exposed and the patient is not posing a risk to others. A sputum specimen for AFB smear and culture should be obtained at a minimum of monthly intervals until two consecutive specimens are negative on culture. More frequent AFB smears may be useful to assess the early response to treatment and provide an indication of infectiousness. Negative cultures are needed to declare the patient not infectious.

Teach the patient how to minimize exposure to close contacts and household members. Homes should be well ventilated, especially the areas where the infected person spends a lot of time. While still infectious, the patient should sleep alone, spend as much time as possible outdoors, and minimize time in congregate settings or on public transportation.

Teach the patient and caregiver about adherence with the prescribed regimen. This is important, since most treatment failures occur because the patient neglects to take the drug, discontinues it prematurely, or takes it irregularly. Strategies to improve adherence to drug therapy include teaching and counseling, reminder systems, incentives or rewards, contracts, and DOT.

Notification of the public health department is required. The public health nurse is responsible for follow-up on household contacts and assessment of the patient for adherence. If adherence is an issue, the public health agency may be responsible for DOT. Most individuals can be considered adequately treated when the therapy regimen has been completed and there is evidence of negative cultures, clinical improvement, and improvement on chest x-ray.

Because about 5% of individuals experience relapses, teach the patient to recognize the symptoms that indicate recurrence of TB. If these symptoms occur, the patient should seek immediate medical attention. Instruct the patient about certain factors that could reactivate TB, such as immunosuppressive therapy, malignancy, and prolonged debilitating illness. If the patient experiences any of these events, the HCP must be told so that TB can be closely monitored for reactivation. In some situations it is necessary to put the patient on anti-TB therapy. Because smoking is associated with poor outcomes in TB, patients should be encouraged to quit. Provide patients with teaching and resources to help them stop smoking.

Evaluation. The expected outcomes are that the patient with TB will have

- Resolution of the disease
- Normal pulmonary function
- Absence of any complications
- No further transmission of TB

ATYPICAL MYCOBACTERIA

There are more than 30 varieties of acid-fast mycobacteria that do not cause TB but can cause pulmonary disease, lymphadenitis,

TABLE 27-14 Fungal Infections of the Lung

Infection	Organism
Endemic Fungal Infections	
Histoplasmosis	*Histoplasma capsulatum*
Coccidioidomycosis	*Coccidioides immitis*
Blastomycosis	*Blastomyces dermatitidis*
Opportunistic Fungal Infections	
Candidiasis	*Candida albicans*
Aspergillosis	*Aspergillus niger* or *Aspergillus fumigatus*
Cryptococcosis	*Cryptococcus neoformans*

skin or soft tissue disease, or disseminated disease. Pulmonary disease is indistinguishable from TB clinically and radiologically but can be differentiated by bacteriologic culture. Atypical mycobacteria are not airborne and not transmitted by droplets. They can be found in tap water, soil, bird feces, and house dust.

Mycobacterium avium complex (MAC), found in aerosols generated from baths, hot spas, and swimming pools, is one cause of atypical mycobacteria pulmonary infection. Only a small number of people exposed to the organism actually develop MAC lung disease. People who are immunosuppressed (e.g., HIV/AIDS) or have chronic pulmonary disease are most susceptible. Treatment is similar to that for TB.

PULMONARY FUNGAL INFECTIONS

Pulmonary fungal pneumonia is an infectious process in the lungs caused by endemic (native and common) or opportunistic fungi (Table 27-14). *Endemic* fungal pathogens cause infection in healthy people and in immunocompromised people in certain geographic locations in the United States. For example, *Coccidioides*, which causes coccidioidomycosis, is a fungus found in the soil of dry, low-rainfall areas.[21] It is endemic in many areas of the southwestern United States. *Opportunistic* fungal infections occur in immunocompromised patients (e.g., those being treated with corticosteroids, chemotherapy, and immunosuppressive drugs) and in patients with HIV and cystic fibrosis. These infections can be very serious.

Fungal infections are acquired by inhalation of spores. These infections are not transmitted from person to person, and the patient does not have to be placed in isolation. The clinical manifestations are similar to those of bacterial pneumonia. Skin testing, serology, and biopsy methods assist in identifying the infecting organism.

Amphotericin B remains the standard therapy for treating serious systemic fungal infections. It must be given IV to achieve adequate blood and tissue levels because the GI tract does not absorb it well. Less serious infections can be treated with oral antifungals such as ketoconazole (Nizoral), fluconazole (Diflucan), voriconazole (Vfend), and itraconazole (Sporanox). Effectiveness of therapy can be monitored with fungal serology titers.

LUNG ABSCESS

Etiology and Pathophysiology

A **lung abscess** is necrosis of lung tissue typically resulting from bacteria aspirated from the oral cavity in patients with periodontal disease. Because oral secretions can contain large amounts of bacteria, even small amounts *(microaspiration)* can cause infection. The abscess usually develops slowly, beginning with an enlarging area of infection that becomes necrotic and eventually forms a cavity filled with purulent material. Lung abscesses can also result from IV drug use, malignancy, pulmonary emboli, TB, and various parasitic and fungal diseases. Abscesses usually contain more than one type of microbe, most commonly reflecting the anaerobic flora of the mouth.

The area of the lung most often affected due to aspiration is the posterior segment of the upper lobes. The abscess may erode into the bronchial system, causing the production of foul-smelling or sour-tasting sputum. It may grow toward the pleura and cause pleuritic pain. Multiple small abscesses, sometimes referred to as *necrotizing pneumonia,* can occur within the lung.

Clinical Manifestations and Complications

Clinical manifestations usually occur slowly over a period of weeks to months, especially if anaerobic organisms are the primary cause. Symptoms of abscess caused by aerobic bacteria develop more acutely and resemble bacterial pneumonia. The most common manifestation is cough-producing purulent sputum (often dark brown) that is foul smelling and foul tasting. Hemoptysis is common, especially when an abscess ruptures into a bronchus. Other common manifestations are fever, chills, prostration, night sweats, pleuritic pain, dyspnea, anorexia, and weight loss.

Physical examination of the lungs indicates dullness to percussion and decreased breath sounds on auscultation over the involved segment of lung. Bronchial breath sounds may be transmitted to the periphery if the communicating bronchus becomes patent and the segment begins to drain. Crackles may also be present in the later stages as the abscess drains.

The infection can also spread via the bloodstream and produce a number of other possible complications. Pulmonary abscess, bronchopleural fistula, bronchiectasis, and empyema from perforation of the abscess into the pleural cavity, have been reported.

Diagnostic Studies

A chest x-ray is often the only test needed for diagnosis of lung abscess. The presence of a solitary cavitary lesion with an air-fluid level and local infiltrate can confirm the diagnosis. CT scanning may be helpful if the cavitation is not clear on chest x-ray. As long as there is drainage via the bronchus, sputum will contain the microorganisms that are present in the abscess. However, expectorated sputum samples are contaminated with oral flora, making it difficult to determine the offending organisms.

Bronchoscopy may be used to (1) avoid oropharyngeal contamination, (2) collect a specimen if drainage is delayed, or (3) investigate if there is a possibility of an underlying malignancy. Pleural fluid and blood cultures may be useful to identify the offending organisms. Although nonspecific, an elevated neutrophil count from a complete blood count (CBC) may indicate an infectious process.

❖ NURSING AND INTERPROFESSIONAL MANAGEMENT: LUNG ABSCESS

Monitor the patient's vital signs, level of consciousness, and respiratory status for any signs of hypoxia. Note any cyanosis or clubbing of the fingers. Administer O_2 as needed. IV antibiotic therapy should be started as soon as possible. Clindamycin is first-line therapy. Parenteral antibiotics are switched to oral antibiotics once the patient shows clinical and x-ray evidence of improvement.

Because of the need for prolonged antibiotic therapy, the patient must be aware of the importance of continuing the medication for the prescribed period. To avoid the risk of a secondary or worsening infection, all antibiotics should be taken, as directed, for the entire prescribed period. Sometimes the patient is asked to return periodically during the course of antibiotic therapy for repeat cultures and sensitivity tests to ensure that the infecting organism is not becoming resistant to the antibiotic. When antibiotic therapy is completed, the patient is reevaluated.

Teach the patient how to cough effectively (see Table 28-23). Chest physiotherapy and postural drainage are not recommended because they may facilitate movement of microorganisms into other bronchi, extending infection. Rest, good nutrition, and adequate fluid intake are supportive measures to facilitate recovery. If dentition is poor and dental hygiene is not adequate, encourage the patient to obtain dental care. Consider collaboration with the social worker to evaluate available options for dental care if the patient has limited resources.

Percutaneous drainage of the abscess may be necessary if the patient does not adequately respond to antibiotic treatment. A small catheter, guided by CT or ultrasound, may be placed to drain the abscess. Surgery is rarely indicated but occasionally necessary when reinfection of a large cavitary lesion occurs or to establish a diagnosis when there is evidence of an underlying problem such as a neoplasm. The usual procedure in such cases is a lobectomy. A pneumonectomy may be necessary for multiple abscesses.

ENVIRONMENTAL LUNG DISEASES

Environmental or occupational lung diseases result from inhaled dust or chemicals. The extent of lung damage is influenced by the toxicity of the inhaled substance, amount and duration of exposure, and individual susceptibility. Environmentally induced lung disease includes pneumoconiosis, chemical pneumonitis, and hypersensitivity pneumonitis.

Pneumoconiosis is a general term for a group of lung diseases caused by inhalation and retention of mineral or metal dust particles. The literal meaning of *pneumoconiosis* is "dust in the lungs." These diseases are classified according to the origin of the dust (e.g., silicosis, asbestosis, berylliosis). Coal worker's pneumoconiosis (CWP), also known as *black lung,* is caused by inhalation of large amounts of coal dust, an occupational hazard for underground coal miners. The inhaled substance is ingested by macrophages, which releases substances that cause cell injury and death. Fibrosis occurs as a result of tissue repair after inflammation. Breathing problems become evident after many years of repeated exposure, resulting in diffuse *pulmonary fibrosis* (excess connective tissue).

Chemical pneumonitis results from exposures to toxic chemical fumes. Acutely, there is diffuse lung injury characterized as pulmonary edema. Chronically, the clinical picture is that of *bronchiolitis obliterans* (obstruction of the bronchioles due to inflammation and fibrosis), which is usually associated with a normal chest x-ray or one that shows hyperinflation. An example is silo filler's disease.

Hypersensitivity pneumonitis, or extrinsic allergic alveolitis, is a form of parenchymal lung disease seen when an individual inhales antigens to which he or she is allergic. Examples include bird fancier's lung and farmer's lung.

Asbestos is a group of minerals composed of microscopic fibers. For many years, asbestos was primarily used for insulation and to help fireproof buildings. When disturbed, asbestos releases tiny filament particles into the air. Once inhaled, the tiny fibers become deposited within the lung. Asbestosis is chronic inflammation of the lung, and people with repeated exposure are at a greater risk of disease. Lung cancer, either squamous cell carcinoma or adenocarcinoma, is the most frequent cancer associated with asbestos exposure. There is a minimum lapse of 15 to 19 years between first exposure and development of lung cancer. Mesothelioma, both pleural and peritoneal, is associated with asbestos exposure.

Clinical Manifestations

Symptoms of many environmental lung diseases may not occur until at least 10 to 15 years after the initial exposure to the inhaled irritant. Clinical manifestations common to all pneumoconioses include dyspnea, cough, wheezing, and weight loss. Pulmonary function studies often show reduced vital capacity. A chest x-ray often reveals lung involvement specific to the primary problem. CT scans have been useful in detecting early lung involvement.

Cor pulmonale, a condition in which the right side of the heart fails, is a late complication, especially in conditions characterized by diffuse pulmonary fibrosis. COPD is the most common complication of environmental lung disease. Other associated disorders include lung cancer, mesothelioma, and TB. Manifestations of these complications are often the reason the patient seeks health care.

Signs of acute hypersensitivity pneumonitis occur 4 to 6 hours after exposure and include chills, fever, cough, shortness of breath, and malaise. Symptoms of chronic hypersensitivity pneumonitis include cough, anorexia, and weight loss. Acute pulmonary edema may occur after exposure to chemical fumes.

Interprofessional Care

The best approach to management of environmental lung diseases is to prevent or decrease environmental and occupational exposure. Teach the public about the risk and the appropriate protective equipment. Using well-designed, effective ventilation systems and wearing masks are appropriate for some occupations and household activities. Inhalation of smoke by nonsmokers has led to regulations requiring a smoke-free workplace. Periodic inspections and monitoring of workplaces by agencies such as the Occupational Safety and Health Administration (OSHA) and the National Institute for Occupational Safety and Health (NIOSH) reinforce employers' obligations to provide a safe work environment. NIOSH is responsible for workplace safety and health regulations in the United States.

Early diagnosis is essential to halting the disease process. Strategies are directed toward preventing disease progression and improving or controlling respiratory symptoms. Strategies include O_2 therapy, inhaled bronchodilators, percussion therapy, and pulmonary rehabilitation. Patients should also be immunized against pneumococcal pneumonia and influenza. Discontinuation of exposure to the offending inhalant and smoking cessation may or may not be effective in stopping disease progression.

LUNG CANCER

Lung cancer is the leading cause of cancer-related deaths in the United States.[22] Lung cancer accounts for 28% of all cancer deaths, more than those caused by breast, prostate, and colon cancer combined. Annually about 221,000 new cases of lung cancer are diagnosed and 158,000 Americans die. Although lung cancer is associated with a high mortality and low cure rate, advances in medical treatment are improving the response to treatment.[23]

Etiology

Smoking is responsible for 80% to 90% of all lung cancers.[23] Tobacco smoke contains 60 carcinogens in addition to substances (carbon monoxide, nicotine) that interfere with normal cell development. Exposure to tobacco smoke causes changes in the bronchial epithelium, which usually returns to normal when smoking is discontinued. The risk of lung cancer gradually decreases with smoking cessation, reaching that of nonsmokers within 10 to 15 years of quitting.

The risk of developing lung cancer is directly related to total exposure to tobacco smoke, measured by total number of cigarettes smoked in a lifetime, age of smoking onset, depth of inhalation, tar and nicotine content, and the use of unfiltered cigarettes. Both smokers and nonsmokers can develop lung cancer. Sidestream smoke (smoke from burning cigarettes, cigars) contains the same carcinogens found in mainstream smoke (smoke inhaled and exhaled by the smoker). This exposure to secondhand smoke creates a health risk for nonsmoking adults and children.

Other common causes of lung cancer include high levels of pollution, radiation (especially radon exposure), and asbestos. Heavy or prolonged exposure to industrial agents such as ionizing radiation, coal dust, nickel, uranium, chromium, formaldehyde, and arsenic can also increase the risk of lung cancer, especially in smokers.[24]

Marked variations exist in a person's propensity to develop lung cancer. Differences in lung cancer incidence, risk factors, and survival exist between men and women (see Gender Differences box). Genetic, hormonal, and molecular influences may contribute to these differences.

Pathophysiology

Most primary lung tumors are believed to arise from mutated epithelial cells. The development of mutations, which are caused by carcinogens, is also influenced by various genetic factors. Once underway, tumor development is promoted by epidermal growth factor. These cells grow slowly, taking 8 to 10 years for a tumor to reach 1 cm in size, the smallest lesion detectable on x-ray. Lung cancers occur primarily in the segmental bronchi or beyond and usually occur in the upper lobes of the lungs (Figs. 27-2 and 27-3).

Primary lung cancers are categorized into two broad subtypes (Table 27-15): non–lung cancer (NSCLC) (80%) and small cell lung cancer (SCLC) (20%).[25] Lung cancers metastasize primarily by direct extension and via the blood and lymph system. The common sites for metastasis are the lymph nodes, liver, brain, bones, and adrenal glands.

Paraneoplastic Syndrome. Lung cancers can cause *paraneoplastic syndrome.* Paraneoplastic syndrome may be caused by hormones, cytokines, or enzymes (secreted by tumor cells) or by

GENDER DIFFERENCES

Lung Cancer

Men

- More men than women are diagnosed with lung cancer.
- More men than women die from lung cancer.
- Male smokers are 10 times more likely to develop lung cancer than nonsmokers.
- Men with lung cancer have a worse prognosis than women.
- Lung cancer incidence and deaths are decreasing in men.

Women

- Lung cancer incidence and deaths are increasing in women.
- Women develop lung cancer after fewer years of smoking than men do.
- Women develop lung cancer at a younger age than men.
- Nonsmoking women are at greater risk of developing lung cancer than men.
- Women with lung cancer live, on the average, 12 months longer than men.

CULTURAL & ETHNIC HEALTH DISPARITIES

Lung Cancer

African Americans

- Have the highest incidence of lung cancer
- Are more likely to die from lung cancer than any other ethnic group
- Have a higher rate of lung cancer among men than in other ethnic groups

Whites

- Have the second-highest death rate from lung cancer
- Have a higher rate of lung cancer among women than in other ethnic groups

Asian/Pacific Islanders and Hispanics

- Have the lowest rates of lung cancer in both men and women

Other

- Regional variations among ethnic groups may be due to smoking prevalence, exposure to cancer-causing substances, and other factors.
- Cigarette consumption has decreased dramatically in developed countries such as the United States and Canada.
- Cigarette smoking is increasing in developing countries (e.g., nations in Africa, Asia, Latin America).

Source: Centers for Disease Control and Prevention: Racial/ethnic disparities and geographic differences in lung cancer incidence—38 states and the District of Columbia, 1998-2006. Retrieved from *www.cdc.gov/mmwr/PDF/wk/mm5944.pdf.*

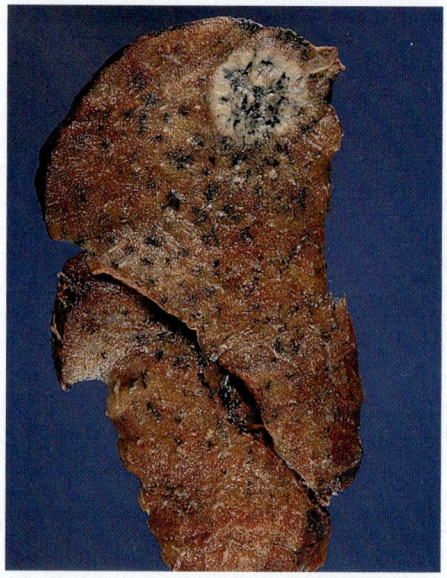

FIG. 27-2 Lung cancer (peripheral adenocarcinoma). The tumor shows prominent black pigmentation, suggestive of having evolved from anthracosis (coal dust in the lungs). (From Damjanov I, Linder J: *Anderson's pathology,* ed 10, St Louis, 1996, Mosby.)

TABLE 27-15 Types of Primary Lung Cancer

Type	Growth Rate	Characteristics	Response to Therapy
Non–Small Cell Lung Cancer (NSCLC)			
Squamous cell carcinoma	Slow	• Accounts for 20%-30% of lung cancers • Centrally located, producing early symptoms of nonproductive cough and hemoptysis • Does not have a strong tendency to metastasize	• Surgical resection may be attempted. • Adjuvant chemotherapy and radiation • Depending on the staging, life expectancy is better than for small cell lung cancer.
Adenocarcinoma	Moderate	• Accounts for 30%-40% of lung cancers • Most common lung cancer in people who have not smoked • Peripherally located • Often has no clinical manifestations until widespread metastasis is present	• Surgical resection may be attempted depending on staging. • Does not respond well to chemotherapy
Large cell (undifferentiated) carcinoma	Rapid	• Accounts for 10% of lung cancers • Composed of large cells that are anaplastic and often arise in bronchi • Is highly metastatic via lymphatics and blood	• Surgery is not usually attempted because of high rate of metastases. • Tumor may be radiosensitive but often recurs.
Small Cell Lung Cancer (SCLC)			
Small cell carcinoma	Very rapid	• Accounts for about 20% of lung cancers • Most malignant form of lung cancer • Spreads early via lymphatics and bloodstream • Frequent metastasis to brain • Associated with endocrine disturbances	• Chemotherapy mainstay of treatment but overall poor prognosis • Radiation is used as adjuvant therapy and palliative measure.

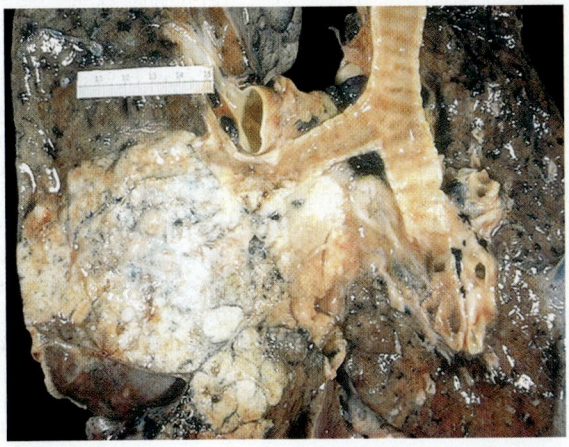

FIG. 27-3 Lung carcinoma. The gray-white tumor tissue is infiltrating the lung. Histologically this tumor is identified as a squamous cell carcinoma. (From Kumar V, Abbas AK, Aster JC, Fausto N: *Robbins and Cotran pathologic basis of disease*, ed 8, Philadelphia, 2010, Saunders.)

antibodies (produced by the body in response to the tumor) that destroy healthy cells. Sometimes the symptoms of paraneoplastic syndrome manifest even before the malignancy is diagnosed.

Examples of paraneoplastic syndrome include hypercalcemia, syndrome of inappropriate antidiuretic hormone secretion (SIADH), adrenal hypersecretion, polycythemia, and Cushing syndrome. SCLCs are most often associated with the paraneoplastic syndrome. These conditions may stabilize with treatment of the underlying neoplasm. (These effects of paraneoplastic syndrome are discussed in the section on metabolic emergencies in Chapter 15 on pp. 264.)

Clinical Manifestations

The clinical manifestations of lung cancer are usually nonspecific and appear late in the disease process. Symptoms may be masked by a chronic cough attributed to smoking or smoking-related lung disease. Manifestations depend on the type of primary lung cancer, its location, and metastatic spread. Lung cancer frequently manifests as a lobar pneumonia that does not respond to treatment.

One of the most common symptoms of lung cancer, and often the one reported first, is a persistent cough. Blood-tinged sputum may be produced because of bleeding caused by the cancer. The patient may complain of dyspnea or wheezing. Chest pain, if present, may be localized or unilateral, ranging from mild to severe.

Later manifestations include nonspecific systemic symptoms such as anorexia, fatigue, weight loss, and nausea and vomiting. Hoarseness may be present as a result of laryngeal nerve involvement. Unilateral paralysis of the diaphragm, dysphagia, and superior vena cava obstruction may occur because of intrathoracic spread of the malignancy. Sometimes there are palpable lymph nodes in the neck or axillae. Mediastinal involvement may lead to pericardial effusion, cardiac tamponade, and dysrhythmias.

Diagnostic Studies

A chest x-ray is the initial diagnostic test used for patients with suspected lung cancer. The x-ray may initially be normal or identify a lung mass or infiltrate. Evidence of metastasis to the ribs or vertebrae and a pleural effusion may also be seen on chest x-ray. CT scanning is used to further evaluate the lung mass. CT scans can identify the location and extent of masses in the chest, any mediastinal involvement, and lymph node enlargement.

Sputum cytologic studies can identify malignant cells, but sputum samples are rarely used in diagnosing lung cancer because malignant cells are not always present in the sputum. Biopsy is required for a definitive diagnosis. Cells for biopsy can be obtained by CT-guided needle aspiration, bronchoscopy, mediastinoscopy, or video-assisted thoracoscopic surgery (VATS). If a thoracentesis is performed to relieve a pleural effusion, the fluid is also analyzed for malignant cells.

Accurate assessment of lung cancer is critical for staging and determining appropriate treatment. Bone scans and CT scans of the brain, pelvis, and abdomen are used to determine if metastatic disease is present. A complete history and physical examination, CBC with differential, chemistry panel, liver function tests, renal function tests, and pulmonary function tests are necessary. MRI and/or positron emission tomography (PET)

TABLE 27-16 Interprofessional Care

Lung Cancer

Diagnostic Assessment	Management
• History and physical examination • Chest x-ray • Bronchoscopy • Cytologic study of bronchial washings or pleural space fluid • CT scan, MRI • Positron emission tomography (PET) • Mediastinoscopy • Video-assisted thoracoscopic surgery (VATS) • Transbronchial or percutaneous fine-needle aspiration	• Surgery • Radiation therapy • Chemotherapy • Targeted therapy and immunotherapy • Prophylactic cranial radiation • Bronchoscopic laser therapy • Photodynamic therapy • Airway stenting • Radiofrequency ablation

TABLE 27-17 Staging of Non–Small Cell Lung Cancer

Stages		Characteristics
I		Tumor is small and localized to lung. No lymph node involvement
	A	Tumor <3 cm
	B	Tumor 3-5 cm and invading surrounding local areas.
II		Increased tumor size, some lymph node involvement
	A	Tumor 3-5 cm with invasion of lymph nodes on same side of chest OR Tumor 5-7 cm without lymph node involvement
	B	Tumor 5-7 cm involving the bronchus and lymph nodes on same side of chest and tissue of other local organs OR Tumor >7 cm without lymph node involvement
III		Increased spread of tumor
	A	Tumor spread to the nearby structures (chest wall, pleura, pericardium) and regional lymph nodes
	B	Extensive tumor involving heart, trachea, esophagus, mediastinum, malignant pleural effusion, contralateral lymph nodes, scalene or supraclavicular lymph nodes
IV		Distant metastasis

may also be used to evaluate and stage lung cancer. Table 27-16 summarizes the diagnostic assessment of lung cancer.

Staging. Staging of NSCLC is performed according to the TNM staging system (see Table 15-5). Under the TNM system, the tumor is grouped into four stages with A or B subtypes. A simplified version of staging of NSCLC is presented in Table 27-17. Patients with stages I, II, and IIIA disease may be surgical candidates. However, stage IIIB or IV disease is usually inoperable and has a poor prognosis.

Staging of SCLC by TNM has not been useful because this cancer is aggressive and is always considered systemic. The stages of SCLC are *limited* and *extensive*. *Limited* means that the tumor is confined to one side of the chest and regional lymph nodes. *Extensive* SCLC means that the cancer extends beyond the limited stage. Most patients with SCLC have extensive disease at time of diagnosis.

Screening for Lung Cancer. Screening for high-risk patients is recommended by the U.S. Preventive Services Task Force (USPSTF).[26] Recommendations include annual screening for lung cancer in adults ages 55 to 80 with a history of smoking (30-pack year smoking history or currently smoke) or quit smoking but less than 15 years ago. Screening is done using low-dose CT. These guidelines have been endorsed by several other groups, including the American Cancer Society.[27]

Interprofessional Care

Surgical Therapy. Surgical resection is the treatment of choice in NSCLC stages I to IIIA without mediastinal involvement, since resection provides the best chance for a cure. Factors that affect survival include the size of the primary tumor and co-morbidities. For other NSCLC stages, patients may require surgery in conjunction with radiation therapy, chemotherapy, and targeted therapy. Many NSCLCs are not resectable at the time of diagnosis.

Surgical procedures that may be performed include pneumonectomy (removal of one entire lung), lobectomy (removal of one or more lobes of the lung), or segmental or wedge resection procedures. VATS may be used to treat lung cancers near the outside of the lung. Surgery is generally not indicated for SCLC because of its rapid growth and dissemination at the time of diagnosis.

When the tumor is considered operable, the patient's cardiopulmonary status must be evaluated to determine the ability to have surgery. Pulmonary function studies, ABGs, and an anesthesia consult are often completed preoperatively to assess the patient's cardiopulmonary status.

Radiation Therapy. Radiation therapy may be used as treatment for both NSCLC and SCLC. Radiation therapy may be given as curative therapy, palliative therapy (to relieve symptoms), or adjuvant therapy in combination with surgery, chemotherapy, or targeted therapy.

Radiation therapy may be used as primary therapy in the individual who is unable to tolerate surgical resection because of co-morbidities. Radiation therapy also relieves symptoms of dyspnea and hemoptysis resulting from bronchial obstructive tumors and treats superior vena cava syndrome. It can also be used to treat pain that is caused by metastatic bone lesions or cerebral metastasis. Sometimes radiation is used preoperatively to reduce the tumor mass before surgical resection. Complications of radiation therapy include esophagitis, skin irritation, nausea and vomiting, anorexia, and radiation pneumonitis (see Chapter 15).

Stereotactic Body Radiotherapy. Stereotactic body radiotherapy (SBRT), also called *stereotactic surgery* or *radiosurgery,* is a new lung cancer treatment. It is a type of radiation therapy that uses high doses of radiation delivered accurately to tumors outside the CNS. SBRT uses special positioning procedures and radiology techniques so that a higher dose of radiation can be delivered to the tumor and only a small part of the healthy lung is exposed. Therapy is given over 1 to 3 days. SBRT provides an option for patients with early stage lung cancers who are not surgical candidates for other medical reasons.

Chemotherapy. Chemotherapy is the primary treatment for SCLC. In NSCLC, chemotherapy may be used in the treatment of nonresectable tumors or as adjuvant therapy to surgery. A variety of chemotherapy drugs and multidrug regimens (i.e., protocols) are used. Chemotherapy for lung cancer typically consists of combinations of two or more of the following drugs: etoposide, carboplatin, cisplatin, paclitaxel (Taxol), vinorelbine (Navelbine), cyclophosphamide, ifosfamide (Ifex), docetaxel (Taxotere), gemcitabine (Gemzar), and pemetrexed (Alimta).

Targeted Therapy. Targeted therapy uses drugs that block the growth of molecules involved in specific aspects of tumor growth (see Chapter 15). Because this type of therapy inhibits growth rather than directly killing cancer cells, targeted therapy may be less toxic than chemotherapy. One type of targeted therapy for patients with NSCLC inhibits tyrosine kinase, an enzyme associated with speeding up molecular reactions. Tyrosine kinase inhibitors, which block signals for growth in the cancer cells, include cetuximab (Erbitux), erlotinib (Tarceva), afatinib (Gilotrif), gefitinib (Iressa), osimertinib (Tagrisso), and necitumumab (Portrazza).

Another type of kinase inhibitor is used to treat patients with NSCLC who have an abnormal anaplastic lymphoma kinase *(ALK)* gene. Drugs in this class include crizotinib (Xalkori) and ceritinib (Zykadia). These drugs directly inhibit the kinase protein produced by the *ALK* gene that is responsible for cancer development and growth.

Another type of targeted therapy used to treat lung cancer inhibits the growth of new blood vessels (angiogenesis) by targeting vascular endothelial growth factor. Bevacizumab (Avastin) is an angiogenesis inhibitor.

Immunotherapy. Nivolumab (Opdivo) and pembrolizumab (Keytruda) are drugs that target PD-1, a protein on T cells that normally helps keep these cells from attacking other cells in the body. By blocking PD-1, these drugs boost the immune response against cancer cells. This can shrink some tumors or slow their growth. Nivolumab and pembrolizumab can be used in people with metastatic NSCLC whose cancer has progressed after other treatments and with tumors that express PD-1.

Other Therapies

Prophylactic Cranial Radiation. Patients with SCLC have early metastases, especially to the central nervous system. Most chemotherapy does not penetrate the blood-brain barrier. Therefore after successful systemic treatment, the patient is at risk for cerebral metastases. Prophylactic radiation has been shown to decrease the incidence of cerebral metastases and improve the survival rate in patients with limited SCLC.[28]

Bronchoscopic Laser Therapy. Bronchoscopic laser therapy makes it possible to remove obstructing bronchial lesions. The laser's thermal energy is transmitted to the target tissue. It is a safe and effective treatment of endobronchial obstructions from tumors. Symptoms of airway obstruction are relieved as a result of thermal necrosis and shrinkage of the tumor. The procedure may be repeated as needed.

Photodynamic Therapy. Photodynamic therapy (PDT) is a form of treatment for early stage lung cancers that uses a combination of a drug and a specific type of light. Cancer cells are killed when the drug, known as a photosynthesizer, is exposed to a specific wavelength of light. Porfimer (Photofrin) is the most commonly used photosynthesizer. It is injected IV and selectively concentrates in tumor cells in the esophagus and outer layers of the airways. After a set time (usually 48 hours), the tumor is exposed to laser light via bronchoscopy, activating the drug and causing cell death. Necrotic tissue is removed with bronchoscopy a few days later. This process can also be repeated as required. PDT can also affect nutrient delivery to cancer cells and stimulate the immune system to attack the cancer cells.

Airway Stenting. Stents are used alone or in combination with other techniques for relief of dyspnea, cough, or respiratory insufficiency. The advantage of an airway stent is that it supports the airway wall against collapse or external compression and can delay extension of tumor into the airway lumen.

Radiofrequency Ablation. Radiofrequency ablation therapy is used to treat small NSCLC lung tumors that are near the outer edge of the lungs. This therapy is an alternative to surgery in patients who cannot or elect not to have surgery. A thin, needle-like probe is inserted through the skin into the tumor. CT scans are used to guide placement. An electric current is then passed through the probe, which heats and destroys tumor cells. Local anesthesia is used for this outpatient procedure.

NURSING MANAGEMENT: LUNG CANCER

Nursing Assessment

It is important to determine the patient and caregiver's understanding of diagnostic tests (those completed as well as those planned), the diagnosis or potential diagnosis, the treatment options, and the prognosis. At the same time, assess the patient's level of anxiety and support provided by the patient's significant others. Subjective and objective data that should be obtained from a patient with lung cancer are presented in Table 27-18.

Nursing Diagnoses

Nursing diagnoses for the patient with lung cancer may include, but are not limited to, the following:

- Ineffective airway clearance *related to* increased tracheobronchial secretions and presence of tumor
- Ineffective breathing pattern *related to* decreased lung capacity and presence of space-occupying lesion
- Impaired gas exchange *related to* tumor obstructing airflow
- Anxiety *related to* lack of knowledge of diagnosis or unknown prognosis and treatments
- Grieving *related to* new cancer diagnosis, lack of knowledge about the disease process, and therapeutic regimen

Planning

The overall goals are that the patient with lung cancer will have (1) effective breathing patterns, (2) adequate airway clearance, (3) adequate oxygenation of tissues, (4) minimal to no discomfort, and (5) a realistic attitude about treatment and prognosis.

Nursing Implementation

Health Promotion. The best way to halt the epidemic of lung cancer is to prevent people from smoking, help smokers stop smoking, and decrease exposure to environmental pollutants. Because most smokers start in the teenage years, prevention of teen smoking has the most significant role in reducing the incidence of lung cancer. A wealth of material is available to the smoker who is interested in smoking cessation. (Smoking cessation is discussed in Chapter 10.)

Modeling healthy behavior by not smoking, promoting smoking cessation programs, and actively supporting education and policy changes related to smoking are important nursing activities. Many changes have occurred as a result of the recognition that passive smoke is a health hazard. Laws prohibit smoking in most public places and limit public smoking to designated areas. Most hospital environments are now completely smoke free, prohibiting smoking by employees and patients. A new trend is for hospitals to refuse employment to anyone testing positive for nicotine. This includes not only smokers but also nonsmokers who are routinely exposed to secondhand smoke.

Acute Care. Care of the patient with lung cancer initially involves support and reassurance during the diagnostic evaluation. It is important to recognize the multiple stressors that

TABLE 27-18 Nursing Assessment

Lung Cancer

Subjective Data

Important Health Information

Past health history: Exposure to secondhand smoke, airborne carcinogens (e.g., asbestos, radon, hydrocarbons), or other pollutants. Urban living environment. Chronic lung disease (e.g., TB, COPD, bronchiectasis)

Medications: Cough medicines or other respiratory medications

Functional Health Patterns

Health perception–health management: Smoking history, including amount per day and number of years. Family history of lung cancer. Frequent respiratory tract infections

Nutritional-metabolic: Anorexia, nausea, vomiting, dysphagia (late). Weight loss. Chills

Activity-exercise: Fatigue. Persistent cough (productive or nonproductive). Dyspnea at rest or with exertion, hemoptysis (late symptom)

Cognitive-perceptual: Chest pain or tightness, shoulder and arm pain, headache, bone pain (late symptom)

Objective Data

General

Fever, neck and axillary lymphadenopathy, paraneoplastic syndrome (e.g., syndrome of inappropriate ADH secretion)

Integumentary

Jaundice (liver metastasis). Edema of neck and face (superior vena cava syndrome), digital clubbing

Respiratory

Wheezing, hoarseness, stridor, unilateral diaphragm paralysis, pleural effusions (late signs)

Cardiovascular

Pericardial effusion, cardiac tamponade, dysrhythmias (late signs)

Neurologic

Confusion, disorientation, unsteady gait (brain metastasis)

Musculoskeletal

Pathologic fractures, muscle wasting (late)

Possible Diagnostic Findings

Observance of lesion on chest x-ray, CT scan, or PET scan. MRI findings of vertebral, spinal cord, or mediastinal invasion. Positive sputum or bronchial washings for cytologic studies. Positive fiberoptic bronchoscopy and biopsy findings

ADH, Antidiuretic hormone.

occur when someone is diagnosed with lung cancer. The stress response is a normal and adaptive response but can become detrimental when stress is overwhelming and intense. Patients suffer the stress of their symptoms, including dyspnea and cough. Diagnostic and therapeutic procedures provide additional stress by placing patients in unfamiliar environments with unusual and perhaps painful results. Emotional stressors include the knowledge of the high mortality rate of lung cancer and the causal effect of cigarette smoking. Worries about role performance and ability to care for their family while undergoing cancer treatment provide further stress. Carefully assess each individual, since he or she will experience unique stressors. The insight gained will help the patient and caregiver cope with the stress of the illness and treatment.

Care of the patient undergoing thoracic surgery is discussed later in this chapter on pp. 524-527. Care of the patient undergoing radiation therapy and chemotherapy is discussed in Chapter 15. Individualized care depends on the plan for treatment. Assessment and intervention in symptom management are pivotal, as is teaching the patient to recognize signs and symptoms that may indicate progression or recurrence of disease. Provide patient comfort, teach methods to reduce pain, monitor for side effects of prescribed medications, foster appropriate coping strategies for both the patient and caregiver, assess smoking cessation readiness, and help patient access resources to deal with the illness.

◆ **Ambulatory Care.** Teach signs and symptoms to report, such as hemoptysis, dysphagia, chest pain, and hoarseness.

CHECK YOUR PRACTICE

You are doing discharge teaching with a 72-yr-old woman who had a lobectomy for NSCLC. She tells you, "I'm not going to give up smoking my cigarettes because I am just going to die anyhow. I might as well enjoy smoking while I still can."

- How would you respond?

Counseling patients on smoking cessation and prevention is essential in decreasing morbidity and mortality risks associated with lung cancer. Encourage the patient and family to provide a smoke-free environment. This may include smoking cessation for multiple family members. If the treatment plan includes home O_2, the teaching plan must include the safe use of O_2.

For many individuals who have lung cancer, little can be done to significantly prolong their lives. Radiation therapy and chemotherapy can provide palliative relief from distressing symptoms. Constant pain may become a major problem. (Measures used to relieve pain are discussed in Chapter 8. Care of the patient with cancer is discussed in Chapter 15.) The palliative care team should be involved as the patient and family move toward the end of life (see Chapter 9). The team can provide information about disability, financial planning, and community resources for end-of-life care such as hospice and home care.

◆ Evaluation

The expected outcomes are that the patient with lung cancer will

- Have adequate breathing patterns
- Have adequate oxygenation
- Experience minimal to no pain
- Convey feelings openly and honestly, with a realistic attitude about prognosis

OTHER TYPES OF LUNG TUMORS

SCLC and NSCLC account for 95% of lung tumors. The other 5% include the following:

- *Hamartomas,* the most common benign tumor, is a slow-growing congenital tumor composed of fibrous tissue, fat, and blood vessels.
- *Mucous gland adenoma* is a benign tumor arising in the bronchi that consists of columnar cystic spaces.
- *Mesotheliomas* are either malignant or benign and originate from the visceral pleura. Malignant mesotheliomas are associated with exposure to asbestos. Benign mesotheliomas are localized lesions.

Secondary metastases from other malignancies can occur. Malignant cells from another part of the body reach the lungs via the pulmonary capillaries or the lymphatic network. The primary malignancies that spread to the lungs often originate in the GI or genitourinary tract and in the breast. General symptoms of lung metastases are chest pain and nonproductive cough.

CHEST TRAUMA AND THORACIC INJURIES

Traumatic injuries to the chest contribute to the majority of all traumatic deaths. Thoracic injuries range from simple rib fractures to complex life-threatening rupture of organs. The mechanisms of injuries causing chest trauma are separated into two categories: blunt trauma and penetrating trauma.

Blunt trauma occurs when the chest strikes or is struck by an object. The impact can cause shearing and compression of thoracic structures. The external injury may appear minor, but internally the organs may have severe injuries. Rib and sternal fractures can lacerate lung tissue. In a high-velocity impact, shearing forces can result in laceration or tearing of the aorta. Compression of the chest may result in contusion, crush injury, and organ rupture.

Penetrating trauma is an injury in which a foreign object impales or passes through the body tissues, creating an open wound. Examples include knife wounds, gunshot wounds, and injuries with other sharp objects. Emergency care of the patient with a chest injury is presented in Table 27-19. The most common thoracic emergencies and their management are described in Table 27-20.

PNEUMOTHORAX

A **pneumothorax** is caused by air entering the pleural cavity. Normally, negative (subatmospheric) pressure exists between the visceral pleura (surrounding the lung) and parietal pleura (lining the thoracic cavity), known as the *pleural space.* The pleural space contains a few milliliters of lubricating fluid to reduce friction when the tissues move. When air enters this space, the change to positive pressure causes a partial or complete lung collapse (Fig. 27-4). As the volume of air in the pleural space increases, the lung volume decreases. This condition should be suspected after any trauma to the chest wall.

If a pneumothorax is small, mild tachycardia and dyspnea may be the only manifestations. If the pneumothorax occupies a large area, respiratory distress may be present, including shallow, rapid respirations; dyspnea; air hunger; and O_2 desaturation. On auscultation, no breath sounds are detected over the affected area. A chest x-ray shows air or fluid in the pleural space and reduction in lung volume.

Types of Pneumothorax

Spontaneous Pneumothorax. A spontaneous pneumothorax typically occurs due to the rupture of small blebs (air-filled sacs) located on the surface of the lung. These blebs can occur in healthy, young individuals or as a result of lung disease such

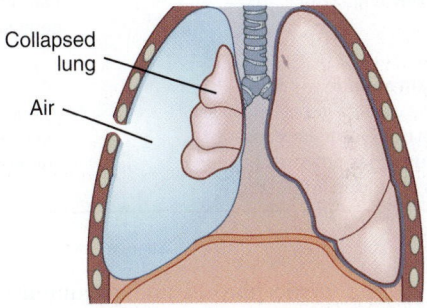

FIG. 27-4 Open pneumothorax resulting from collapse of lung due to disruption of chest wall and outside air entering.

TABLE 27-19 Emergency Management

Chest Trauma

Etiology	Assessment Findings	Interventions
Blunt • Motor vehicle accident • Pedestrian accident • Fall • Assault with blunt object • Crush injury • Explosion **Penetrating** • Knife • Gunshot • Stick • Arrow • Other missiles	**Respiratory** • Dyspnea, respiratory distress • Cough with or without hemoptysis • Cyanosis of mouth, face, nail beds, mucous membranes • Tracheal deviation • Audible air escaping from chest wound • Decreased breath sounds on side of injury • Decreased O_2 saturation • Frothy secretions **Cardiovascular** • Rapid, thready pulse • Decreased BP • Narrowed pulse pressure • Asymmetric BP values in arms • Distended neck veins • Muffled heart sounds • Chest pain • Dysrhythmias **Surface Findings** • Bruising • Abrasions • Open chest wound • Asymmetric chest movement • Subcutaneous emphysema	**Initial** • If unresponsive, assess circulation, airway, and breathing. • If responsive, monitor airway, breathing, and circulation. • Administer high-flow O_2 to keep SpO_2 >90%. • Establish IV access with two large-bore catheters. Begin fluid resuscitation as appropriate. • Remove clothing to assess injury. • Cover sucking chest wound with nonporous dressing taped on three sides. • Stabilize impaled objects with bulky dressings. *Do not remove object.* • Assess for other significant injuries and treat appropriately. • Place patient in a semi-Fowler's position if breathing is easier *after* cervical spine injury has been ruled out. • Administer small amounts of analgesia as necessary for pain and to help with breathing. • Prepare for emergency needle decompression if tension pneumothorax or cardiac tamponade present. **Ongoing Monitoring** • Monitor vital signs, level of consciousness, O_2 saturation, cardiac rhythm, respiratory status, and urine output. • Anticipate intubation for respiratory distress. • Release dressing if tension pneumothorax develops after sucking chest wound is covered.

TABLE 27-20 Emergency Management

Thoracic Injuries

Injury and Description	Manifestations	Intervention
Pneumothorax Air in pleural space (Fig. 27-4).	Dyspnea, decreased movement of involved chest wall, diminished or absent breath sounds on the affected side, hyperresonance to percussion	Chest tube insertion with chest drainage system.
Hemothorax Blood in the pleural space, may or may not occur in conjunction with pneumothorax.	Dyspnea, diminished or absent breath sounds, dullness to percussion, decreased Hgb, shock depending on blood volume lost	Chest tube insertion with chest drainage system. Autotransfusion of collected blood, treatment of hypovolemia as necessary.
Tension Pneumothorax Air in pleural space that does not escape Increased air in the pleural space shifts organs and increases intrathoracic pressure (Fig. 27-5).	Cyanosis, air hunger, extreme agitation, tracheal deviation away from affected side, subcutaneous emphysema, neck vein distention, hyperresonance to percussion	Medical emergency: needle decompression followed by chest tube insertion with chest drainage system.
Flail Chest Fracture of two or more adjacent ribs in two or more places with loss of chest wall stability (Fig. 27-6).	Paradoxical movement of chest wall, respiratory distress. May be associated hemothorax, pneumothorax, pulmonary contusion	O_2 as needed to maintain O_2 saturation, analgesia. Stabilize flail segment with positive pressure ventilation (intubation and mechanical ventilation). Treat associated injuries. Surgical fixation.
Cardiac Tamponade Blood rapidly collects in pericardial sac, compresses myocardium because pericardium does not stretch, and prevents ventricles from filling.	Muffled, distant heart sounds, hypotension, neck vein distention, increased central venous pressure	Medical emergency: pericardiocentesis with surgical repair as appropriate.

as COPD, asthma, cystic fibrosis, and pneumonia. Smoking increases the risk for bleb formation. Other risk factors include being tall and thin, male gender, family history, and previous spontaneous pneumothorax.

Iatrogenic Pneumothorax. *Iatrogenic pneumothorax* can occur due to laceration or puncture of the lung during medical procedures. For example, transthoracic needle aspiration, subclavian catheter insertion, pleural biopsy, and transbronchial lung biopsy all have the potential to injure the lung. Barotrauma from excessive ventilatory pressure during manual or mechanical ventilation can rupture alveoli or bronchioles. Esophageal procedures may also be involved in the development of a pneumothorax. Tearing during insertion of a gastric tube can allow air from the esophagus to enter the mediastinum and pleural space.

Tension Pneumothorax. Tension pneumothorax occurs when air enters the pleural space but cannot escape. The continued accumulation of air in the pleural space causes increasingly elevated intrapleural pressures. This results in compression of the lung on the affected side and pressure on the heart and great vessels, pushing them away from the affected side (Fig. 27-5). The mediastinum shifts toward the unaffected side, compressing the "good" lung, which further compromises oxygenation. As the pressure increases, venous return is decreased and cardiac output falls.

Tension pneumothorax may result from either an open or a closed pneumothorax. In an open chest wound, a flap may act as a one-way valve. Thus air can enter on inspiration but cannot escape. Tension pneumothorax can occur with mechanical ventilation and resuscitative efforts. It can also occur if chest tubes are clamped or become blocked in a patient with a pneumothorax. Unclamping the tube or relieving the obstruction may correct this situation.

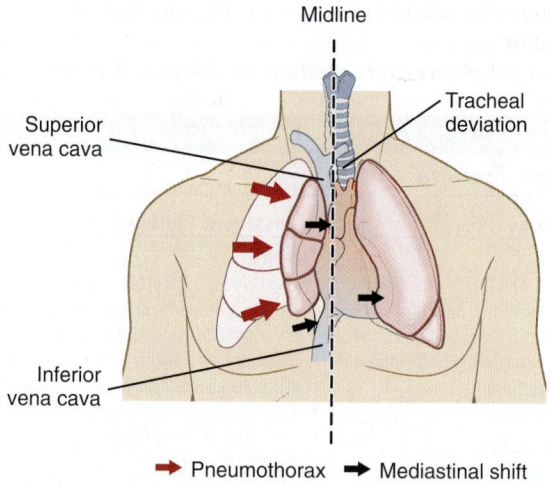

FIG. 27-5 Tension pneumothorax. As pleural pressure on the affected side increases, mediastinal displacement ensues with resultant respiratory and cardiovascular compromise. Tracheal deviation is an external (but late) manifestation of the mediastinal shift.

Tension pneumothorax is a medical emergency, with both the respiratory and cardiovascular systems affected. Manifestations include dyspnea, marked tachycardia, tracheal deviation, decreased or absent breath sounds on the affected side, neck vein distention, cyanosis, and profuse diaphoresis. If the tension in the pleural space is not relieved, the patient is likely to die from inadequate cardiac output or severe hypoxemia.

Hemothorax. Hemothorax is an accumulation of blood in the pleural space resulting from injury to the chest wall, diaphragm, lung, blood vessels, or mediastinum.[29] When it occurs with pneumothorax, it is called a *hemopneumothorax*. The patient with a traumatic hemothorax requires immediate insertion of a chest tube for evacuation of the blood, which can be recovered and reinfused for a short time after the injury. (Autotransfusion is discussed in Chapter 30.)

Chylothorax. *Chylothorax* is the presence of lymphatic fluid in the pleural space. The thoracic duct is disrupted either traumatically or from a malignancy, and the lymphatic fluid fills the pleural space.[30] This milky white fluid is high in lipids. Normal lymphatic flow through the thoracic duct is 1500 to 2500 mL/day. This amount can be increased up to tenfold after ingestion of fats. Some cases heal with conservative treatment (chest drainage, bowel rest, and dietary modifications). Octreotide has been used with some success to reduce the flow of lymphatic fluid. Surgery (thoracic duct ligation) and pleurodesis (the artificial production of adhesions between the parietal and visceral pleura) may be considered for refractory cases.

Interprofessional Care

Treatment of a pneumothorax depends on its severity and the underlying cause. If the patient is stable and has minimal air and/or fluid accumulated in the intrapleural space, no treatment may be necessary, since the condition may resolve spontaneously.

Pneumothorax can be classified as *open* (air entering through an opening in the chest wall) or *closed* (no external wound). Penetrating trauma allows air to enter the pleural space through an opening in the chest wall (Fig. 27-4). Examples include stab or gunshot wounds and surgical thoracotomy. A penetrating chest wound may be referred to as a *sucking chest wound,* since air enters the pleural space through the chest wall during inspiration.

Emergency treatment consists of covering the wound with an occlusive dressing that is secured on three sides (vent dressing). During inspiration, as negative pressure is created in the chest, the dressing pulls against the wound, preventing air from entering the pleural space. During expiration, as the pressure rises in the pleural space, the dressing is pushed out and air escapes through the wound and from under the dressing. If the object that caused the open chest wound is still in place, do not remove it until an HCP is present. Stabilize the impaled object with a bulky dressing.

The most definitive and common treatment of pneumothorax and hemothorax is to insert a chest tube and connect it to water-seal drainage. Repeated spontaneous pneumothorax may have to be treated surgically by a partial pleurectomy, stapling, or pleurodesis to promote adherence of the pleurae to one another. Tension pneumothorax is a medical emergency, requiring urgent needle decompression followed by chest tube insertion to water-seal drainage.

FRACTURED RIBS

Rib fractures are the most common type of chest injury resulting from blunt trauma. Ribs 5 through 9 are most frequently fractured because they are the least protected by chest muscles. If the fractured rib is splintered or displaced, it may damage the pleura, lungs, and other internal organs.

Clinical manifestations of fractured ribs include pain at the site of injury, especially during inspiration and with coughing. The patient splints the affected area and takes shallow breaths to try to decrease the pain. Atelectasis and pneumonia may develop because of decreased chest wall movement and retained secretions.

The goal of treatment is to decrease pain so that the patient can breathe adequately and clear secretions. Strapping the chest with tape or using a thoracic binder is not recommended, since it limits chest expansion and predisposes the individual to atelectasis. Nonsteroidal antiinflammatory drugs (NSAIDs), opioids, and thoracic nerve blocks can be used to reduce pain and aid with deep breathing and coughing. Patient teaching should emphasize deep breathing, coughing, incentive spirometry, and appropriate use of pain medications.

FLAIL CHEST

Flail chest results from the fracture of several consecutive ribs, in two or more separate places, causing an unstable segment (Fig. 27-6). It can also be caused by fracture of the sternum and several consecutive ribs. The resultant instability of the chest wall causes paradoxical movement during breathing. The affected (flail) area moves in the opposite direction with respect to the intact portion of the chest. During inspiration, the affected portion is sucked in, and during expiration, it bulges out. This paradoxical chest movement not only prevents adequate ventilation but also increases the work of breathing. The underlying lung may have a pulmonary contusion aggravating hypoxemia.

A flail chest is usually apparent on visual examination. The patient manifests rapid, shallow respirations and tachycardia. The patient moves air poorly, and movement of the thorax is asymmetric and uncoordinated. The patient may

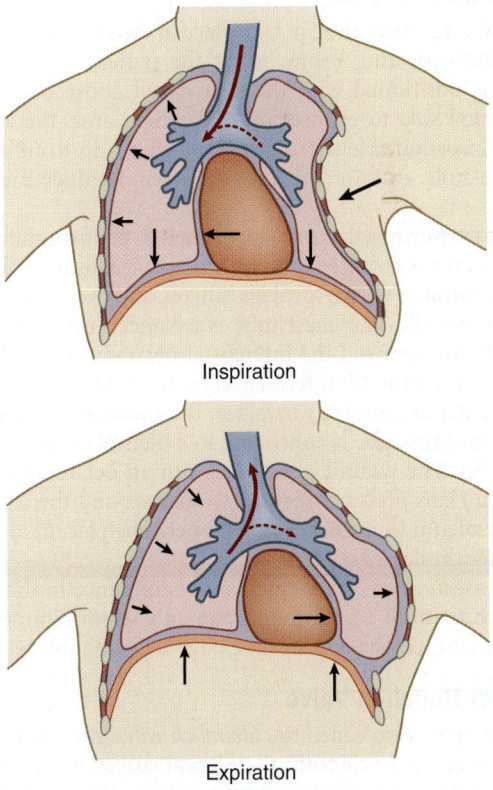

FIG. 27-6 Flail chest produces paradoxical respiration. On inspiration, the flail section moves inward with mediastinal shift to the uninjured side. On expiration, the flail section bulges outward with mediastinal shift to the injured side.

also attempt to splint the chest to assist with breathing. Observation of abnormal thoracic cavity movement, palpation for crepitus near the rib fractures, and chest x-ray all assist in the diagnosis.

Initial therapy consists of ensuring adequate ventilation and supplemental O_2 therapy. The goal is to facilitate lung expansion and ensure adequate oxygenation. Analgesia is necessary to help promote adequate respiration. Although many patients can be managed without mechanical ventilation, intubation and ventilation may be necessary. Surgical fixation of the flail segment may be done. The lung parenchyma and fractured ribs heal with time. Some patients continue to experience intercostal pain after the flail chest has resolved.

CHEST TUBES AND PLEURAL DRAINAGE

If enough fluid or air accumulates in the pleural space, the negative pressure becomes positive and the lungs collapse. As a result, chest tubes are inserted to drain the pleural space, reestablish negative pressure, and allow for proper lung expansion. Tubes may also be inserted in the mediastinal space to drain air and fluid postoperatively.

Chest tubes are approximately 20 inches (51 cm) long and vary in size from 12F to 40F. The size inserted is determined by the patient's condition. Large (36F to 40F) tubes are used to drain blood, medium (24F to 36F) tubes are used to drain fluid, and small (12F to 24F) tubes are used to drain air. Pigtail tubes are very small (10F to 14F) tubes with a curly end designed to keep them in place. They are a safe and effective alternative to larger-bore chest tubes for treatment of pneumothorax.

Chest Tube Insertion

Insertion of a chest tube can take place in the emergency department, the operating room, or at the patient's bedside. The patient is positioned with the arm raised above the head on the affected side to expose the midaxillary area, the standard site for insertion. Elevate the patient's head 30 to 60 degrees, when possible, to lower the diaphragm and reduce the risk of injury.

Time permitting, a chest x-ray is used to confirm the affected side. The area is cleansed with an antiseptic solution. The chest wall is infiltrated with a local anesthetic, and a small incision is made over a rib. The chest tube is advanced up and over the top of the rib to avoid the intercostal nerves and blood vessels that are behind the rib inferiorly (Fig. 27-7). Once inserted, the tube is secured (sutured) in place, the incision is closed with sutures, and the tube is connected to a pleural drainage system (Fig. 27-8). The wound is covered with an occlusive dressing. Most clinicians prefer to seal the wound around the chest tube with petroleum (airtight) gauze. Proper tube placement is confirmed by chest x-ray.

The insertion of a chest tube and its presence in the pleural space are painful. Monitor the patient's comfort at frequent intervals and use the appropriate pain-relieving interventions.

Flutter or Heimlich Valve

A flutter valve (also called the *Heimlich valve* after its inventor) is used to evacuate air from the pleural space (Fig. 27-9). This device consists of a one-way rubber valve within a rigid plastic tube. It is attached to the external end of the chest tube. During inspiration, when pressure in the chest is greater than atmospheric pressure, the valve opens. During expiration, when intrathoracic pressure is less than atmospheric pressure, the valve closes.

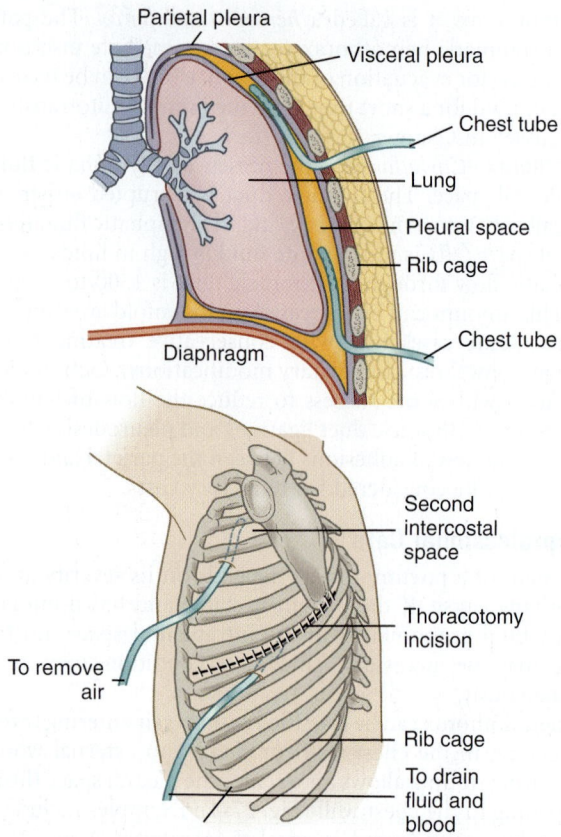

FIG. 27-7 Placement of chest tubes.

The flutter valve can be used for small to moderate-sized pneumothorax. It also allows for patient mobility, since the smaller drainage bag can be hidden under the clothes while the patient ambulates. Drainage bags attached to the flutter valve must have a vent to the atmosphere to prevent a potential tension pneumothorax. This can be accomplished by simply cutting a small slit in the top of any drainage bag that does not have a built-in vent. Patients may go home with a flutter valve in place.

Pleural Drainage

Insertion of a chest tube often requires attachment to a drainage device or chamber to collect fluid, air, and/or blood from the thoracic cavity. Several different disposable chest drainage units are currently available, but common to all drainage units are three basic compartments (Fig. 27-8).

The *first compartment,* or collection chamber, receives fluid and air from the pleural or mediastinal space. The drained fluid stays in this chamber while expelled air vents to the second compartment. The *second compartment,* the water-seal chamber, contains 2 cm of water, which acts as a one-way valve. Incoming air enters from the collection chamber and bubbles up through the water. The water prevents backflow of air into the patient. Brisk bubbling of air often occurs in this chamber when a pneumothorax is initially evacuated. Intermittent bubbling during exhalation, coughing, or sneezing (when the patient's intrathoracic pressure is increased) may be observed as long as there is air in the pleural space. Eventually, as the air leak resolves and the lung becomes more fully expanded, bubbling ceases.

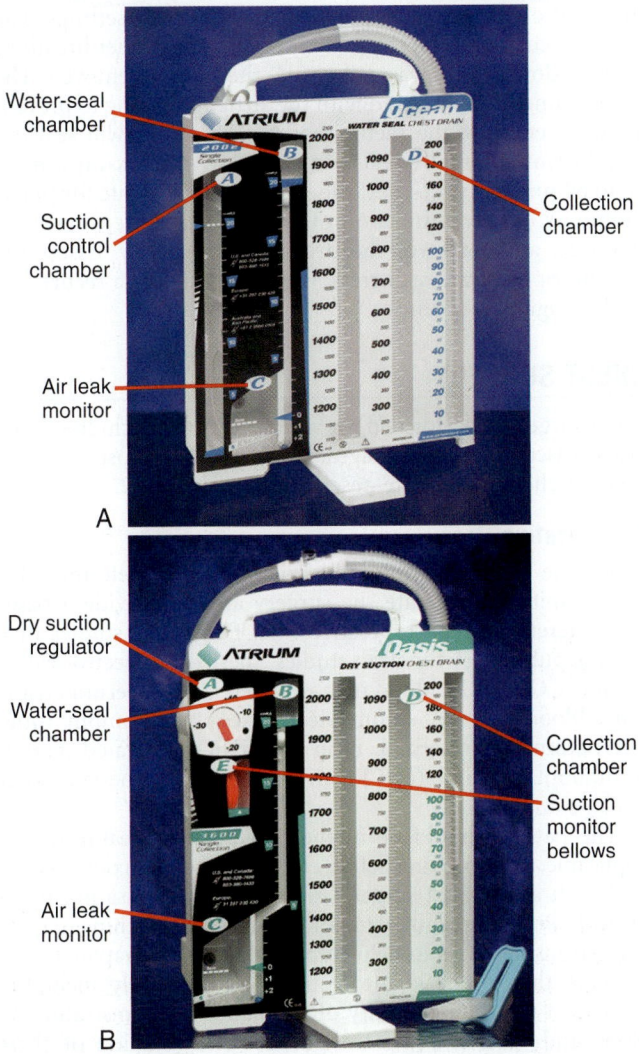

FIG. 27-8 Chest drainage unit. Both units have three chambers: (1) collection chamber; (2) water-seal chamber; and (3) suction control chamber. Suction control chamber requires a connection to a wall suction source that is dialed up higher than the prescribed suction for the suction to work. **A,** Water suction. This unit uses water in the suction control chamber to control the wall suction pressure. **B,** Dry suction. This unit controls wall suction by using a regulator control dial. (From Atrium Medical Corporation, Hudson, N.H.)

Normal fluctuation of the water within the water-seal chamber is called *tidaling.* This up and down movement of water in concert with respiration reflects intrapleural pressure changes during inspiration and expiration. Investigate any sudden cessation of tidaling, since this may signify an occluded chest tube. Gradual reduction and eventual cessation of tidaling are expected as the lung reexpands.

The *third compartment,* the suction control chamber, applies suction to the chest drainage system. There are two main types of suction control: water and dry. The water suction control chamber uses a column of water to control the amount of suction from the wall regulator. The chamber is typically filled with 20 cm of water. When the negative pressure generated by the suction source exceeds the set 20 cm, air from the atmosphere enters the chamber through a vent on top of the chest drainage unit and the air bubbles up through the water, causing a suction-breaker effect. As a result, excess pressure is relieved.

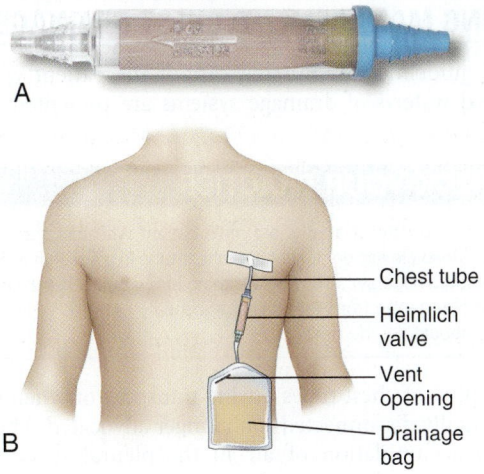

FIG. 27-9 **A,** Heimlich chest drain valve is a specially designed flutter valve that is used in place of a chest drainage unit for small uncomplicated pneumothorax with little or no drainage and no need for suction. The valve allows for escape of air but prevents the reentry of air into the pleural space. (*A,* Courtesy and © Copyright Becton, Dickinson and Company.) **B,** Placement of valve between chest tube and vented drainage bag, which can be worn under a person's clothes.

The amount of suction applied is regulated by the amount of water in this chamber and not by the amount of suction applied to the system. An increase in suction does not result in an increase in negative pressure to the system because any excess suction merely draws in air through the vent on top of the third chamber. The suction pressure is usually ordered to be –20 cm H_2O, although higher pressures (–40 cm H_2O) are sometimes necessary to evacuate the pleural space; lower pressure (–10 cm H_2O) may be used for frail and older patients at risk for tissue damage with higher pressures.

To initiate suction, adjust (increase) the vacuum source until gentle bubbling is present in the third chamber. Excessive bubbling does not increase the amount of suction but does increase the rate of evaporation of the water and the amount of noise made by the device.

The dry suction chest drainage system contains no water. It has a visual alert that indicates if the suction is working. It uses either a restrictive device or a regulator to dial the desired negative pressure; this is internal in the chest drainage system. To increase the suction pressures, turn the dial on the drainage system. Increasing the vacuum source does not increase the pressure. When decreasing suction, depress the manual vent to reduce excess vacuum to the lower prescribed level.

A variety of commercially disposable plastic chest drainage systems are available. Manufacturers include directions for set-up and use with each unit. Atrium Medical Corporation offers online educational videos of the principles of chest drainage and products at *www.atriummed.com/Products/Chest_Drains/education.asp.*

INFORMATICS IN PRACTICE

Chest Drainage System

- You find yourself in a situation in which you need to set up a chest drainage system. You have not done this since simulation lab in nursing school.
- On the Internet, find a procedure manual or watch a video or podcast on this procedure.

❖ NURSING MANAGEMENT: CHEST DRAINAGE

General guidelines for nursing care of the patient with chest tubes and water-seal drainage systems are presented in Table 27-21.

CHECK YOUR PRACTICE

You are taking care of a 26-yr-old male patient who has chest injuries from a motorcycle accident. He has a chest tube in place that is attached to a chest drainage system. While turning him, you accidentally disconnect the chest tube from the drainage system.

- What should you do next?

Clamping of chest tubes during transport or when the tube is accidentally disconnected is no longer advocated. The danger of rapid accumulation of air in the pleural space, causing tension pneumothorax, is far greater than that of a small amount of atmospheric air that enters the pleural space. If a chest tube becomes disconnected, the immediate priority is to reestablish the water-seal system. In some hospitals, when disconnection occurs, the chest tube is immersed in sterile water (about 2 cm) until the system can be reestablished. It is important to know the unit protocol, individual clinical situation (whether an air leak exists), and HCP preference before any chest tube clamping occurs.

Chest tubes may be momentarily clamped to change the drainage apparatus or to check for air leaks. Appearance of a new air leak warrants assessment of the drainage system to identify whether the air leak is coming from the patient or the system. Once again, you are encouraged to become familiar with the policies and procedures of their workplace regarding specific clinical situations and circumstances when chest tubes may be clamped.

Closely monitor the patient for complications associated with chest tube placement and drainage. If volumes from 1 to 1.5 L of fluid and/or blood are removed rapidly, reexpansion pulmonary edema or severe, symptomatic hypotension can occur. Subcutaneous emphysema can occur from air leaking into the tissue surrounding the chest tube insertion site. A "crackling" sensation will be felt when palpating the skin. A small amount of subcutaneous air is harmless and will be reabsorbed. However, severe subcutaneous emphysema can cause drastic swelling of the head and neck with potential airway compromise.

Meticulous sterile technique during dressing changes can reduce the incidence of infected sites. Nursing care and patient teaching can minimize the risk of atelectasis and shoulder stiffness. Encourage coughing, deep breathing, incentive spirometer use, and range-of-motion exercises. Monitor integrity of the chest tube system. Monitor the color and amount of drainage hourly in the first few hours post-chest tube insertion. Drainage greater than 200 mL in the first hour, development of subcutaneous emphysema, or any signs and symptoms of respiratory distress should be reported to the appropriate HCP at once.

◆ Chest Tube Removal

The chest tubes are removed when the lungs are reexpanded and fluid drainage has ceased or is minimal. In some centers, suction is discontinued and the chest drain is on gravity drainage for 24 hours before the tube is removed. Give the patient pain medication about 30 to 60 minutes before tube removal.

Gather dressing supplies and petroleum jelly dressing. Explain the procedure to the patient. The tube is removed by the HCP or an advanced practice nurse in most settings. The suture is cut, and with the patient holding his or her breath or bearing down (Valsalva maneuver), the tube is removed. The site is immediately covered with the airtight dressing to prevent air from entering the pleural space. The pleura will seal off, and the wound usually heals in a few days. A chest x-ray is done 30 to 60 minutes post-chest tube removal to evaluate for pneumothorax or reaccumulation of fluid. Observe the wound for drainage, and reinforce the dressing if necessary. Assess the patient for respiratory distress, which may signify a recurrence of the original problem.

CHEST SURGERY

Chest surgery is performed for various reasons, including lung, heart, vascular, and esophageal disorders. The most common types of chest surgery are described in Table 27-22.

Preoperative Care

Assess the patient's cardiopulmonary status to determine his or her ability to tolerate the surgery and to provide a baseline reference for postoperative care. Diagnostic studies may include pulmonary function studies, chest x-ray, electrocardiogram (ECG), ABGs, blood urea nitrogen (BUN), serum creatinine, blood glucose, serum electrolytes, prothrombin time/international normalized ratio (PT/INR), activated partial thromboplastin time (aPTT), and CBC. An anesthesia consult is also completed.

The patient should be in the best possible health and, if applicable, stop smoking before elective surgery. Anxiety associated with anticipated surgery makes smoking cessation more difficult. Provide encouragement, support, and teaching regarding various methods to help stop smoking (see Chapter 10).

Teach the patient what to expect postoperatively, including the use of O_2, the possibility of intubation, administration of blood and IV fluids, and the purpose and function of chest tubes. Reassure the patient that adequate medication will be used to reduce pain. Explain how to use patient-controlled analgesia (PCA), if planned. Preoperative teaching should always include exercises for effective deep breathing and use of incentive spirometry. If the patient practices these techniques before surgery, they will be easier to perform postoperatively. Show the patient how to splint the incision with a pillow to facilitate deep breathing. Teach and have the patient provide a return demonstration of range-of-motion exercises on the surgical side (similar to those for the mastectomy patient [see Fig. 51-9]).

The thought of losing part of a vital organ is frequently frightening. Reassure the patient that the lungs have a large degree of functional reserve. Even after the removal of one lung, enough lung tissue is left to maintain adequate oxygenation. Be available to answer the patient and caregiver's questions. Answer questions openly and honestly. Try to facilitate the expression of concerns, feelings, and questions. (General preoperative care and teaching are discussed in Chapter 17.)

Surgical Procedures

Thoracotomy. A **thoracotomy** is a surgical incision into the chest to gain access to the heart, lungs, esophagus, thoracic aorta, or anterior spine. Two common approaches to a thoracotomy are the median sternotomy and lateral thoracotomy. The median sternotomy involves splitting the sternum and is primarily used for surgery involving the heart. The lateral

TABLE 27-21 Chest Tubes and Water-Seal Drainage

Set-Up and Insertion

1. Make sure patient is aware of the procedure and informed consent is obtained.
2. Gather equipment.
   - Thoracotomy tray
   - Chest drainage unit (CDU)
   - Chest tube
   - Bottle of sterile water
   - 1% lidocaine
   - Suction tubing and collection container
   - Occlusive dressing
3. Prepare CDU.
   - *Wet suction:* add sterile water to 2-cm mark in water-seal chamber and to 20-cm mark (or as ordered) in suction control chamber.
   - *Dry suction:* add sterile water to the fill line of the air leak meter. Attach suction tubing and increase suction until the bellows-like float moves across the display window.
4. Position and support the patient to minimize movement during procedure.

Drainage System

1. Keep all tubing loosely coiled below chest level. Tubing should drop straight from bed or chair to drainage unit. Do not let it be compressed.
2. Keep all connections between chest tubes, drainage tubing, and the drainage collector tight, and tape at connections.
3. Observe for air fluctuations (tidaling) and bubbling in the water-seal chamber.
   - If tidaling (rising with inspiration and falling with expiration in the spontaneously breathing patient) is not observed, the drainage system is blocked, the lungs are reexpanded, or the system is attached to suction.
   - If bubbling increases, there may be an air leak in the drainage system or a leak from the patient (bronchopleural leak).
4. If the chest tube is connected to suction, disconnect from wall suction to check for tidaling.
5. Suspect a system leak when bubbling is continuous.
   - Retape tubing connections.
   - Ensure that dressing is air occlusive.
   - If leak persists, briefly clamp the chest tube at the patient's chest. If the leak stops, then the air is coming from the patient.*
   - If the air leak persists, briefly and methodically move the clamps down the tubing away from the patient until the air leak stops. The leak will then be present between the last two clamp points. If the air leak persists all the way to the drainage unit, replace the unit.*
6. High fluid levels in the water seal indicate residual negative pressure.
   - The chest system may have to be vented by using the high-negativity release valve available on the drainage system to release residual pressure from the system.
   - Do not lower water-seal column when wall suction is not operating or when patient is on gravity drainage.

Patient's Clinical Status

1. Monitor the patient's clinical status. Assess vital signs, lung sounds, and pain.
2. Assess for manifestations of reaccumulation of air and fluid in the chest (↓ or absent breath sounds), significant bleeding (>100 mL/hr), chest drainage site infection (drainage, erythema, fever, ↑ WBC), or poor wound healing. Notify HCP for management plan.
3. Evaluate for subcutaneous emphysema at chest tube site.
4. Encourage the patient to breathe deeply periodically to facilitate lung expansion and encourage range-of-motion exercises to the shoulder on the affected side. Encourage use of incentive spirometry every hour while awake to prevent atelectasis or pneumonia.

Chest Drainage

1. Never elevate the drainage system to the level of the patient's chest because this will cause fluid to drain back into the lungs. Secure the unit to the drainage stand. Change the unit if the collection chamber is full. Do not try to empty it.
2. Mark the time of measurement and the fluid level on the drainage unit according to the unit standards. Report any change in the quantity or characteristics of drainage (e.g., clear yellow to bloody) to the HCP and record the change. Notify HCP if >100 mL/hr drainage.
3. Check the position of the chest drainage container. If the drainage system is overturned and the water seal is disrupted, return it to an upright position and encourage the patient to take a few deep breaths, followed by forced exhalations and cough maneuvers.
4. If the drainage system breaks, place the distal end of the chest tubing connection in a sterile water container at a 2-cm level as an emergency water seal.
5. Milking or stripping chest tubes is no longer recommended, since these practices can dangerously increase intrapleural pressures and damage lung tissues. Position tubing so that drainage flows freely to negate need for milking or stripping.

Monitoring Wet Vs. Dry Suction Chest Drainage Systems

Suction Control Chamber in Wet Suction System

1. Keep the suction control chamber at the appropriate water level by adding sterile water as needed to replace water lost to evaporation.
2. Keep the cover over the suction control chamber in place to prevent more rapid evaporation of water and to decrease the noise of the bubbling.
3. After filling the suction control chamber to the ordered suction amount (generally 20 cm H_2O suction), connect the suction tubing to the wall suction.
4. Dial the wall suction regulator until continuous gentle bubbling is seen in the suction control chamber (generally 80-120 mm Hg). Vigorous bubbling is not necessary and will increase the rate of evaporation.
5. If no bubbling is seen in the suction control chamber, (1) there is no suction, (2) suction is not high enough, or (3) the pleural air leak is so large that suction is not high enough to evacuate it.

Suction Control Chamber in Dry Suction System

(see manufacturer's directions)

1. After connecting patient to system, turn the dial on the chest drainage system to amount ordered (generally –20 cm H_2O pressure), connect suction tubing to wall suction source, and increase the suction until the float appears in the window of the CDU.
2. If ordered to decrease suction, turn the dial down, depress the high-negativity vent, and assess for a rise in the water level of the water-seal chamber.

Chest Tube Dressings

1. Change dressing according to unit protocol and HCP preference.
2. Remove old dressing carefully. Assess the site for any evidence of inflammation or infection and culture site as indicated.
3. Cleanse the site according to protocol, maintaining strict sterile asepsis.
4. Redress with occlusive dressing. Some HCPs prefer the use of petroleum gauze dressing around the tube to prevent air leak. Date the dressing and document dressing change.

*As per institutional policy and procedures.

TABLE 27-22 Chest Surgeries

Type	Description	Indications
Lobectomy Removal of one lobe of lung	• Most common lung surgery • Need chest tubes postoperatively • Lung tissue expands to fill up space left by resected lobe	Lung cancer, bronchiectasis, TB, emphysematous bullae, benign lung tumors, fungal infections
Pneumonectomy Removal of entire lung	• Done only when lobectomy or segmental resection will not remove all diseased lung • May have chest tube postoperatively • Fluid will gradually fill space where lung has been removed • Position patient on operative side to facilitate expansion of remaining lung	Lung cancer (most common)
Segmental Resection Removal of one or more lung segments	• Done to remove bronchovascular lung segment • Need chest tubes postoperatively • Remaining lung tissue expands to fill space • Indicated for a patient unable to handle more extensive surgery	Lung cancer, bronchiectasis
Wedge Resection Removal of small, localized lesion that occupies only part of a segment	• Most conservative approach • Need chest tubes postoperatively • Done to remove small peripheral nodules or for patients unable to handle more extensive surgery	Lung biopsy, excision of small nodules
Decortication Removal or stripping of thick, fibrous membrane from visceral pleura	• Need chest tubes postoperatively	Empyema or other inflammatory process unresponsive to conservative management
Exploratory Thoracotomy Incision into thorax to look for injured or bleeding tissues	• Need chest tubes postoperatively	Chest trauma
Thoracotomy (Not Involving Lungs) Incision into thorax for surgery on other organs	• Postoperative care related to thoracotomy and primary reason for surgical procedure • Need chest tubes postoperatively	Hiatal hernia repair, open heart surgery, esophageal surgery, tracheal resection, thoracic aorta repair
Video-Assisted Thoracoscopic Surgery (VATS) Video-assisted technique with a rigid scope with a distal lens inserted into pleura and image shown on a monitor screen	• Allows surgeon to manipulate instruments passed into pleural space through separate small intercostal incisions • VATS done under general anesthesia in operating room • May require chest tube postoperatively	Procedures performed using VATS include lung biopsy, lobectomy, resection of nodules, repair of fistulas
Lung Volume Reduction Surgery (LVRS) **Open surgical procedure** **Bronchoscopic procedure**	• Involves reducing lung volume by multiple wedge excisions or VATS • Removes most diseased lung tissue • Used to place one-way valves in airways leading to the diseased parts of the lung • Valves let air out, but not in, thus collapsing a certain segment of lungs	Advanced bullous emphysema, α_1-antitrypsin emphysema

thoracotomy incision can be done using a posterolateral or anterolateral incision. The *posterolateral incision* is used for most surgeries involving the lung. The incision is made from front to back at the level of the fourth, fifth, or sixth intercostal space. Strong mechanical retractors are used to separate the ribs and gain access to the lung. The *anterolateral incision* is made in the fourth or fifth intercostal space from the sternal border to the midaxillary line. This procedure is commonly used for surgery or trauma victims, mediastinal operations, and wedge resections of the upper and middle lobes of the lung.

Video-Assisted Thoracic Surgery. *Video-assisted thoracoscopic surgery* (VATS) is a widely used, minimally invasive surgical approach. It provides a real-time two-dimensional video image of the inside of the chest cavity. It is used for diagnosis and treatment of diseases of the pleura, pulmonary masses and nodules, mediastinal masses, and interstitial lung disease. Through incisions just large enough to insert the instruments, the surgeon can inspect the chest cavity, biopsy suspicious areas, obtain samples of fluids for analysis, and remove tissue. VATS is increasingly being used for patients with thoracic trauma. The surgeon can examine, diagnose, and manage intrathoracic injuries in both blunt and penetrating trauma, including injuries to the diaphragm. A chest tube is placed in the pleural space through one or more of the incisions at the end of the procedure, secured with sutures, and connected to a drainage unit in the usual manner.

The advantages of VATS include less discomfort, faster return to normal activity level, reduced length of hospital stay, lower postoperative morbidity risk, and fewer complications.[31] Patients who have marginal respiratory reserve or are too debilitated to tolerate an open thoracotomy approach may benefit from the VATS procedure.

Postoperative Care

The thoracotomy incision is the most painful surgical incision for patients and one of the most difficult for medical-surgical nurses to manage. Postoperative pain after a thoracotomy is typically intense because respiratory muscles are cut during surgery. For most chest surgeries, chest tubes are placed in the pleural space to allow for lung reexpansion. In a pneumonectomy, chest tubes may or may not be placed in the space from which the lung was removed. Adequate pain management is a priority to prevent respiratory compromise. The use of PCA, epidural infusions, and intercostal nerve blocks enables patients to breathe deeply, cough, and move the arm and shoulder on the operative side.

Nursing care priorities in the postoperative period include assessment of respiratory function, including observation of respiratory rate and effort, sputum volume and color, breath sounds, and chest tube function and drainage. Daily chest x-rays are often ordered. Assessment of pain, monitoring of temperature, and observation of the surgical site are similar to care provided for other postoperative patients (see Chapter 19). Care after thoracotomy is presented in eNursing Care Plan 27-2 (available on the website for this chapter).

RESTRICTIVE RESPIRATORY DISORDERS

Disorders that impair the ability of the chest wall and diaphragm to move with respiration are called *restrictive respiratory disorders.* There are two categories: *extrapulmonary conditions,* in which the lung tissue is normal, and *intrapulmonary conditions,* in which the cause is the lung or pleura. Examples of extrapulmonary conditions that alter respirations are listed in Table 27-23. These disorders are further described in their respective chapters.

Examples of intrapulmonary causes are listed in Table 27-24. Lung damage can be caused by inflammation and scarring of lung tissue (interstitial lung disease), air spaces (pneumonitis), or pleura (empyema).

Pulmonary function tests are the best means of differentiating between restrictive and obstructive respiratory disorders. The hallmark characteristic of a restrictive lung disorder is a reduced total lung capacity (TLC), whereas the hallmark characteristic of an obstructive disorder is reduced forced expiratory volume (FEV_1). Mixed obstructive and restrictive disorders sometimes occur together. For example, a patient may have both asthma (an obstructive problem) and pulmonary fibrosis (a restrictive problem).

TABLE 27-23 Extrapulmonary Causes of Restrictive Lung Disease

Central Nervous System	Chest Wall
• Head injury, CNS lesion (e.g., tumor, stroke) • Opioid and barbiturate use	• Chest wall trauma (e.g., flail chest, fractured rib) • Obesity-hypoventilation syndrome (Pickwickian syndrome) • Kyphoscoliosis
Neuromuscular System	
• Spinal cord injury • Guillain-Barré syndrome • Amyotrophic lateral sclerosis • Myasthenia gravis • Muscular dystrophy	

PLEURAL EFFUSION

Types

The pleural space normally contains 5 to 15 mL of fluid that acts as a lubricant between the chest wall (parietal pleura) and lungs (visceral pleura). **Pleural effusion** is an abnormal collection of fluid in this space. It is not a disease but rather an indication of disease. A balance between hydrostatic pressure, oncotic pressure, and capillary membrane permeability governs movement of fluid in and out of the pleural space. Fluid accumulation can be a result of increased pulmonary capillary pressure, decreased oncotic pressure, increased pleural membrane permeability, or obstruction of lymphatic flow.

Pleural effusion is classified as transudative or exudative according to the protein content. A *transudate* occurs primarily in noninflammatory conditions and is an accumulation of protein-poor, cell-poor fluid. Transudative pleural effusions are clear, pale yellow, and caused by (1) increased hydrostatic pressure found in heart failure or (2) decreased oncotic pressure (from hypoalbuminemia) found in chronic liver or renal disease. An *exudative effusion* results from increased capillary permeability characteristic of an inflammatory reaction. It is most commonly associated with infections and malignancies.

An **empyema** is the collection of purulent fluid in the pleural space. It is caused by conditions such as pneumonia, TB, lung abscess, and infection of surgical wounds of the chest. Therapeutic treatment options for empyema include appropriate antibiotic therapy (necessary to eradicate the causative organism), percutaneous drainage, tube thoracostomy, VATS, intrapleural fibrinolytic therapy (instilled via the chest tube) to dissolve fibrous adhesions, decortication, and open window thoracostomy.

Clinical Manifestations

Common clinical manifestations of pleural effusion are dyspnea; cough; and occasional sharp, nonradiating chest pain that is worse on inhalation. Physical examination of the chest may indicate decreased movement of the chest on the affected side, dullness to percussion, and diminished breath sounds over the affected area. A chest x-ray and CT reveal the volume and location of the effusion. Indication of a possible empyema include the manifestations of pleural effusion as well as fever, night sweats, cough, and weight loss.

Thoracentesis

Thoracentesis is aspiration of intrapleural fluid for diagnostic and therapeutic purposes. For a thoracentesis, the patient may sit on the edge of a bed and lean forward over a bedside table. A chest x-ray or ultrasound images are used to determine the optimal puncture site. The skin is cleansed with an antiseptic solution and injected with a local anesthetic. The thoracentesis

TABLE 27-24 Intrapulmonary Causes of Restrictive Lung Disease

Pleural Disorders	Parenchymal Disorders
• Pleural effusion • Pleurisy (pleuritis) • Pneumothorax	• Acute respiratory distress syndrome (ARDS) • Atelectasis • Interstitial lung diseases • Pneumonia

needle is inserted into the intercostal space (see Fig. 25-13). Fluid is aspirated with a syringe, or tubing is connected to the needle to allow fluid to drain into a sterile container. After the fluid is removed, the needle is withdrawn, and a bandage is applied over the insertion site.

Usually only 1000 to 1200 mL of pleural fluid is removed at one time. Rapid removal of a large volume can result in hypotension, hypoxemia, or reexpansion pulmonary edema. A chest x-ray may be done after the procedure to assess for possible complications such as pneumothorax. During and after the procedure, monitor vital signs and pulse oximetry, and observe the patient for any manifestations of respiratory distress.

Interprofessional Care

The management of pleural effusions is to treat the underlying cause. For example, adequate treatment of heart failure with diuretics and sodium restriction may result in a decreased incidence of pleural effusion. The treatment of pleural effusions secondary to malignant disease represents a more difficult problem. These types of pleural effusions are frequently recurrent and reaccumulate quickly after thoracentesis.

Chemical pleurodesis is performed to obliterate the pleural space and prevent reaccumulation of effusion fluid in both malignant and nonmalignant pleural effusions. This procedure first requires chest tube drainage of the effusion. Once the fluid is drained, a chemical slurry is instilled into the pleural space. Talc is the most effective agent for pleurodesis. Other agents such as doxycycline and bleomycin can also be used. The chest tube is clamped for 8 hours while the patient is turned in different positions to allow the chemical to contact the entire pleural space. After 8 hours the chest tube is unclamped and attached to a drainage unit. Fever and chest pain are the most common side effects associated with pleurodesis. Chest tubes are left in place until fluid drainage is less than 150 mL/day and no air leaks are noted.

PLEURISY

Pleurisy (pleuritis) is an inflammation of the pleura. Inflammation can be caused by infectious diseases, neoplasms, autoimmune disorders, chest trauma, GI disease, and certain medications. The inflammation usually subsides with adequate treatment of the primary disease. The pain of pleurisy is typically abrupt, sharp in onset, and aggravated by inspiration. The patient's breathing is shallow and rapid to avoid unnecessary movement of the pleura and chest wall. A pleural friction rub may occur, which is the sound heard over areas where inflamed visceral pleura and parietal pleura rub over one another during inspiration. This sound, like a squeaking door, is usually loudest at peak inspiration but may be heard during exhalation as well.

Treatment of pleurisy is aimed at treating the underlying disease and providing pain relief. NSAIDs or analgesics and lying on or splinting the affected side may provide some relief. Teach the patient to splint the rib cage when coughing. If the pain is severe, intercostal nerve blocks may be considered.

ATELECTASIS

Atelectasis is a lung condition characterized by collapsed, airless alveoli. There may be diminished or absent breath sounds and dullness to percussion over the affected area. The most common cause of atelectasis is obstruction of the small airways with secretions. This is common in bedridden patients and in postoperative abdominal and thoracic surgery patients. Normally the pores of Kohn (see Fig. 25-1) provide collateral passage of air from one alveolus to another. Deep inspiration is necessary to open the pores effectively. For this reason, deep-breathing exercises, coughing, incentive spirometry, and early mobility are important to prevent atelectasis and treat the patient at risk. (The prevention and treatment of atelectasis are discussed in Chapter 19.)

INTERSTITIAL LUNG DISEASES

Interstitial lung disease (ILD), also called *diffuse parenchymal lung disease,* refers to more than 200 lung disorders in which the tissue between the air sacs of the lungs (the interstitium) is affected by inflammation or scarring (fibrosis).[32] ILDs can be caused by inhalation of occupational and environmental toxins, certain medications, radiation therapy, connective tissue disorders, malignancy, and infection. Treatment is aimed at reducing exposure to the causative agent and/or treating the underlying disease process. Although scarring is irreversible, treatment with corticosteroids and immunosuppressant drugs can minimize progression. A lung transplant may be an option for some patients.

Most of the ILDs are extremely rare. Many times the cause of ILD is unknown. The most common ILDs of unknown etiology are idiopathic pulmonary fibrosis and sarcoidosis.

IDIOPATHIC PULMONARY FIBROSIS

Idiopathic pulmonary fibrosis (IPF) is a chronic, progressive disorder characterized by chronic inflammation and formation of scar tissue in the connective tissue. Risk factors for IPF include a history of cigarette smoking and exposure to wood and metal dust. IPF affects more men than women and typically first appears between the ages of 50 and 70 years. There is no known cure for IPF.

Clinical manifestations of IPF include exertional dyspnea; dry, nonproductive cough; clubbing of the fingers; and inspiratory crackles. Fatigue, weakness, anorexia, and weight loss may occur as the disease progresses. Chest x-ray findings are generally nonspecific. Pulmonary function tests may be abnormal with evidence of restriction (reduced vital capacity) and impaired gas exchange. Open lung biopsy using VATS often helps to confirm the pathology and is considered the "gold standard" for diagnosis.

The clinical course of IPF is variable and the prognosis is poor, with a 5-year survival rate of 30% to 50% after diagnosis. Many people diagnosed with IPF are initially treated with a corticosteroid (prednisone), sometimes in combination with other drugs that suppress the immune system (e.g., methotrexate, cyclosporine). Kinase inhibitor drugs, which block multiple pathways that are involved in scarring, include nintedanib (Ofev) and pirfenidone (Esbriet).

O_2 therapy and pulmonary rehabilitation should be prescribed for all patients. Lung transplantation may be an option for those who meet the criteria.[33] (Lung transplantation is discussed later in this chapter on p. 533.)

SARCOIDOSIS

Sarcoidosis is a chronic, multisystem granulomatous disease of unknown cause that primarily affects the lungs. The disease may also involve the skin, eyes, liver, kidney, heart, and lymph nodes. African Americans and those with a family history of sarcoidosis are at higher risk for developing sarcoidosis.

Signs and symptoms vary depending on what organs are affected. Pulmonary symptoms include dyspnea, cough, and chest pain. Many patients do not have symptoms.

The disease is staged and treatment decisions are based on pulmonary function and progression of the disease. Some patients have a spontaneous remission. Treatment is aimed at suppression of the inflammatory response. Patients are followed every 3 to 6 months with pulmonary function tests, chest x-ray, and CT scan to monitor disease progression.

VASCULAR LUNG DISORDERS

PULMONARY EDEMA

Pulmonary edema is an abnormal accumulation of fluid in the alveoli and interstitial spaces of the lungs. It is a complication of various heart and lung diseases (Table 27-25). In severe circumstances, pulmonary edema can be a life-threatening medical emergency.

The most common cause of pulmonary edema is left-sided heart failure. (Pathophysiology, clinical manifestations, and management of pulmonary edema are described in Chapter 34.)

PULMONARY EMBOLISM

Etiology and Pathophysiology

Pulmonary embolism (PE) is the blockage of one or more pulmonary arteries by a thrombus, fat or air embolus, or tumor tissue. The word *embolus* derives from a Greek word meaning "plug" or "stopper." *Emboli* are mobile clots that generally do not stop moving until they lodge at a narrowed part of the circulatory system. A pulmonary embolus consists of material that gains access to the venous system and then to the pulmonary circulation. The embolus travels with blood flow through ever-smaller blood vessels until it lodges and obstructs perfusion of the alveoli (Fig. 27-10). The lower lobes of the lung are most commonly affected. Approximately 10% of patients with massive PE die within the first hour. Treatment with anticoagulants significantly reduces mortality.

Most pulmonary emboli arise from deep vein thrombosis (DVT) in the deep veins of the legs. *Venous thromboembolism* (VTE) is the preferred term to describe the spectrum of pathologic conditions from DVT to PE (see Table 37-7). Other sites of origin of PE include femoral or iliac veins, right side of the heart (atrial fibrillation), and pelvic veins (especially after surgery or childbirth). Upper extremity DVT occasionally occurs in the presence of central venous catheters or arterial lines. These cases may resolve with the removal of the catheter. A *saddle embolus* refers to a large thrombus lodged at an arterial bifurcation.

In addition to dislodged thrombi, less common causes of PE include fat emboli (from fractured long bones), air emboli (from improperly administered IV therapy), bacterial vegetation on heart valves, amniotic fluid, and tumors. Risk factors for PE include immobility or reduced mobility, surgery within the last 3 months (especially pelvic and lower extremity surgery), history of DVT, malignancy, obesity, oral contraceptives, hormone therapy, cigarette smoking, prolonged air travel, heart failure, pregnancy, and clotting disorders.

Clinical Manifestations

The signs and symptoms of PE are varied and nonspecific, making diagnosis difficult. Clinical manifestations depend on the size and extent of emboli. Small emboli may go undetected or produce vague, transient symptoms. Symptoms may begin slowly or suddenly. Dyspnea is the most common presenting symptom, occurring in 85% of patients with PE. A mild to moderate hypoxemia may be observed. Other manifestations may include tachypnea, cough, chest pain, hemoptysis, crackles, wheezing, fever, accentuation of the pulmonic heart sound, tachycardia, and syncope. Massive emboli may produce a sudden change in mental status, hypotension, and feelings of impending doom.

Complications

Complications of pulmonary emboli include pulmonary infarction and pulmonary hypertension. *Pulmonary infarction* (death of lung tissue) is most likely when the following factors are present: (1) occlusion of a large or medium-sized pulmonary vessel (more than 2 mm in diameter), (2) insufficient collateral blood flow from the bronchial circulation, or (3) preexisting lung disease. Infarction results in alveolar necrosis and hemorrhage. Occasionally the necrotic tissue becomes infected, and an abscess may develop. Concomitant pleural effusion is frequent.

Pulmonary hypertension results from hypoxemia or from involvement of more than 50% of the area of the normal pulmonary bed. As a single event, an embolus rarely causes pulmonary hypertension. Recurrent pulmonary emboli gradually cause a reduction in the capillary bed and eventual pulmonary hypertension. Dilation and hypertrophy of the right

TABLE 27-25 Causes of Pulmonary Edema

- Heart failure
- Overhydration with IV fluids
- Hypoalbuminemia: nephrotic syndrome, hepatic disease, nutritional disorders
- Altered capillary permeability of lungs: inhaled toxins, inflammation (e.g., pneumonia), severe hypoxia, near-drowning
- Malignancies of the lymph system (e.g., non-Hodgkin's lymphoma)
- O_2 toxicity
- Acute respiratory distress syndrome (ARDS)
- Unknown causes: neurogenic condition, opioid overdose, reexpansion pulmonary edema, high altitude

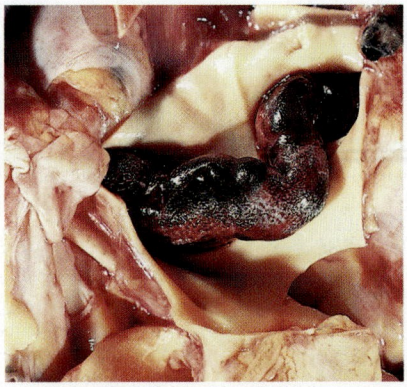

FIG. 27-10 Large embolus from the femoral vein lying in the main left and right pulmonary arteries. (From the teaching collection of the Department of Pathology, University of Texas Southwestern Medical School, Dallas, Tex. In Kumar V, Abbas AK, Aster JC, Fausto N, editors: *Robbins and Cotran pathologic basis of disease,* ed 8, Philadelphia, 2010, Saunders.)

ventricle can develop secondary to pulmonary hypertension. Depending on the degree of pulmonary hypertension and its rate of development, outcomes can vary, with some patients dying within months of the diagnosis and others living for decades.

Diagnostic Studies

D-dimer is a laboratory test that measures the amount of cross-linked fibrin fragments. These fragments are the result of clot degradation and are rarely found in healthy individuals. The disadvantage of D-dimer testing is that it is neither specific (many other conditions cause elevation) nor sensitive, because up to 50% of patients with small pulmonary emboli have normal results. Patients with suspected PE and an elevated D-dimer level but normal venous ultrasound may need a spiral CT or lung scan.

A *spiral (helical) CT scan* (also known as CT angiography or CTA) is the most frequently used test to diagnose PE (Table 27-26). An IV injection of contrast media is required to view the pulmonary blood vessels. The scanner continuously rotates around the patient while obtaining views (slices) of the pulmonary vasculature. This allows visualization of all anatomic regions of the lungs. Computer software reconstructs the data to provide a three-dimensional picture and assist in emboli visualization.

If a patient cannot have contrast media, a ventilation-perfusion (V/Q) scan is done. The V/Q scan has two components and is most accurate when both are performed:

1. *Perfusion scanning* involves IV injection of a radioisotope. A scanning device images the pulmonary circulation.
2. *Ventilation scanning* involves inhalation of a radioactive gas such as xenon. Scanning reflects the distribution of gas through the lung. The ventilation component requires the patient's cooperation and may be impossible to perform in the critically ill patient, particularly if the patient is intubated.

Pulmonary angiography is the most sensitive and specific test for PE. However, it is an expensive and invasive procedure that involves insertion of a catheter through the antecubital or femoral vein, advancement of the catheter to the pulmonary artery, and injection of contrast medium. The accessibility and accuracy of the spiral CT have greatly diminished the need for pulmonary angiography.

ABG analysis is important but not diagnostic. The PaO_2 may be low because of inadequate oxygenation secondary to occluded pulmonary vasculature preventing matching of perfusion to ventilation. The pH is often normal unless respiratory alkalosis develops as a result of prolonged hyperventilation or to compensate for lactic acidosis caused by shock. Abnormal findings are usually identified on the chest x-ray (atelectasis, pleural effusion) and the ECG (ST segment and T wave changes), but they are not diagnostic for PE. Serum troponin levels and b-type natriuretic peptide (BNP) levels are frequently elevated but not diagnostic.

TABLE 27-26 Interprofessional Care

Acute Pulmonary Embolism

Diagnostic Assessment	Management
• History and physical examination • Chest x-ray • Continuous ECG monitoring • ABGs • Spiral (helical) CT scan • Ventilation-perfusion (V/Q) lung scan • D-dimer level • Troponin level, BNP level • Pulmonary angiography	• Supplemental O_2, intubation if necessary • Monitor aPTT and INR levels • Balance activity and rest • Inferior vena cava filter • Pulmonary embolectomy in life-threatening situation ***Drug Therapy*** • Fibrinolytic agent • Unfractionated heparin IV • Low-molecular-weight heparin (e.g., enoxaparin [Lovenox]) • Warfarin (Coumadin) for long-term therapy • Opioids for pain relief

ABGs, Arterial blood gases; *aPTT,* activated partial thromboplastin time; *BNP,* b-type natriuretic peptide; *INR,* international normalized ratio.

Interprofessional Care

Prevention of PE begins with prevention of DVT. DVT prophylaxis includes the use of sequential compression devices, early ambulation, and anticoagulant medications.

To reduce mortality risk, treatment is begun as soon as PE is suspected (Table 27-26). The objectives are to (1) prevent further growth or extension of thrombi in the lower extremities, (2) prevent embolization from the upper or lower extremities to the pulmonary vascular system, and (3) provide cardiopulmonary support if indicated.

Supportive therapy for the patient's cardiopulmonary status varies according to the severity of the PE. O_2 can be given via mask or cannula, and the concentration of FIO_2 is determined by ABG analysis. In some situations, endotracheal intubation and mechanical ventilation are necessary to maintain adequate oxygenation. Respiratory measures such as turning, coughing, deep breathing, and incentive spirometry are important to help prevent or treat atelectasis. If manifestations of shock are present, IV fluids are administered followed by vasopressor agents as needed to support perfusion (see Chapter 66). If heart failure is present, diuretics are used (see Chapter 34). Pain resulting from pleural irritation or reduced coronary blood flow is treated with opioids.

Drug Therapy. Immediate anticoagulation is required for patients with PE. Subcutaneous administration of low-molecular-weight heparin (LMWH) (e.g., enoxaparin [Lovenox]) or fondaparinux has been found to be safer and more effective than use of unfractionated heparin.[34] It is the recommended treatment for patients with acute PE, administered once daily. Advantages of LMWH over unfractionated heparin include greater bioavailability, subcutaneous administration, and longer duration of therapeutic effect; furthermore, monitoring the aPTT is not necessary or useful with LMWH. Unfractionated IV heparin can be as effective but is more difficult to titrate to therapeutic levels.

Warfarin (Coumadin), an oral anticoagulant, should also be initiated at the time of diagnosis.[34] Warfarin should be administered for at least 3 months and then reevaluated. Alternatives to warfarin include apixaban (Eliquis), dabigitran (Pradaxa), and edoxaban (Savaysa). Anticoagulant therapy may be contraindicated if the patient has complicating factors such as blood dyscrasias, hepatic dysfunction causing alterations in the clotting, overt bleeding, a history of hemorrhagic stroke, or heparin-induced thrombocytopenia (HIT).

Although not common, some HCPs use direct thrombin inhibitors (see Table 37-10) in the treatment of PE. Similarly, fibrinolytic agents, such as tissue plasminogen activator (tPA) or alteplase (Activase), may help dissolve the pulmonary embolus and the source of the thrombus in the pelvis or deep leg veins, thereby decreasing the likelihood of recurrent emboli. Fibrinolytic therapy is discussed in Chapter 33.

Surgical Therapy. Hemodynamically unstable patients with massive PE in whom thrombolytic therapy is contraindicated may be candidates for immediate pulmonary embolectomy. Embolectomy, removal of emboli to help decrease right ventricular afterload, can be achieved via a vascular (catheter) or surgical approach. Surgical outcomes have improved in recent years, in part due to rapid diagnosis and enhanced surgical procedures, with mortality rates decreasing from 30% to 19%.[35]

To prevent further emboli, an inferior vena cava (IVC) filter may be the treatment of choice in patients who remain at high risk and patients for whom anticoagulation is contraindicated. This device, inserted percutaneously via the femoral vein, is placed at the level of the diaphragm in the inferior vena cava. Once inserted, the filter expands and prevents migration of large clots into the pulmonary system. Complications associated with this device are rare but include misplacement, migration, and perforation.

❖ NURSING MANAGEMENT: PULMONARY EMBOLISM

◆ Nursing Implementation

Nursing measures aimed at prevention of PE are similar to those for prophylaxis of VTE (see Chapter 37, pp. 818-819).

The prognosis of a patient with PE is good if therapy is promptly instituted. Keep the patient on bed rest in a semi-Fowler's position to facilitate breathing. Administer O_2 therapy as ordered. Assess the patient's cardiopulmonary status with careful monitoring of vital signs, cardiac rhythm, pulse oximetry, ABGs, and lung sounds. Maintain an IV line for medications and fluid therapy. Monitor laboratory results to ensure therapeutic ranges of INR (for warfarin) and aPTT (for IV heparin). Monitor the patient for complications of anticoagulant and fibrinolytic therapy (e.g., bleeding, hematomas, bruising). Provide appropriate interventions related to immobility and fall precautions, once the patient is permitted out of bed.

The patient is usually anxious because of pain, inability to breathe, and fear of death. Carefully explain the situation, the medications, and provide emotional support and reassurance to help relieve the patient's anxiety.

Patient teaching regarding long-term anticoagulant therapy is critical. Anticoagulant therapy continues for at least 3 months. Patients with recurrent emboli may be treated indefinitely with anticoagulants. INR levels are drawn at intervals and warfarin dosage is adjusted. Some patients are monitored by nurses in an anticoagulation clinic.

Long-term management of PE is similar to that for the patient with VTE (see discussion of VTE in Chapter 37 on pp. 818-819). Discharge planning is aimed at preventing worsening of the condition and avoiding complications and recurrence. Reinforce the need for the patient to return to the HCP for regular follow-up examinations.

◆ Evaluation

The expected outcomes are that the patient who has a PE will have

- Adequate tissue perfusion and respiratory function
- Adequate cardiac output
- Increased level of comfort
- Prevention of further recurrence of PE

PULMONARY HYPERTENSION

Pulmonary hypertension is characterized by elevated pulmonary artery pressure resulting from an increase in resistance to blood flow through the pulmonary circulation. Normally the pulmonary circulation is characterized by low resistance and low pressure. In pulmonary hypertension the pulmonary pressures are elevated with the mean pulmonary artery pressure greater than 25 mm Hg at rest (normal is 12 to 16 mm Hg) or greater than 30 mm Hg with exercise.

The World Health Organization (WHO) has identified five categories (groups) of pulmonary hypertension. Each group is based on etiology of the disorder.

Group 1: Pulmonary arterial hypertension attributable to medication, specific diseases, genetic (inherited) link, or idiopathic

Group 2: Related to left-sided heart failure

Group 3: Related to the lungs and hypoxemia

Group 4: Related to the cardiovascular system and thromboembolic occlusion

Group 5: Multifactorial (and often unclear) origins with hematologic or metabolic involvement

The disease commonly manifests with shortness of breath and fatigue. Pulmonary hypertension can occur as a primary disease *(idiopathic pulmonary arterial hypertension)* or as a secondary complication of a respiratory, cardiac, autoimmune, hepatic, or connective tissue disorder *(secondary pulmonary arterial hypertension)*.

IDIOPATHIC PULMONARY ARTERIAL HYPERTENSION

Idiopathic pulmonary arterial hypertension (IPAH) is pulmonary hypertension that occurs without an apparent cause. (It was previously known as *primary pulmonary hypertension* [PPH].) If untreated, this disorder can be rapidly progressive, causing right-sided heart failure and death within a few years. Although new drug therapy has greatly improved survival, the disease remains incurable.

Etiology and Pathophysiology

The etiology of IPAH is unknown. It has been associated with connective tissue diseases, cirrhosis, and HIV, but the exact relationship between these disorders and IPAH remains unclear. Similarly, the pathophysiology of IPAH is poorly understood. It has been suggested that some type of insult (e.g., hormonal, mechanical) to the pulmonary endothelium may occur, causing a cascade of events leading to vascular scarring, endothelial dysfunction, and smooth muscle proliferation (Fig. 27-11). IPAH affects females more than males.

Clinical Manifestations and Diagnostic Studies

Classic symptoms of pulmonary hypertension are dyspnea on exertion and fatigue. Exertional chest pain, dizziness, and syncope are other symptoms. These symptoms are related to the inability of cardiac output to increase in response to increased O_2 demand. Abnormal heart sounds may also be auscultated, including an S3. Eventually, as the disease progresses, dyspnea occurs at rest. Pulmonary hypertension increases the workload of the right ventricle and causes right ventricular hypertrophy (a condition called *cor pulmonale*) and eventually heart failure.

Right-sided cardiac catheterization is the definitive test to diagnose any type of pulmonary hypertension. In addition to providing an accurate measurement of pulmonary artery pressures, it also determines cardiac output and pulmonary vascular resistance. Confirmation of IPAH requires a thorough workup to exclude conditions that may cause secondary pulmonary hypertension. Diagnostic evaluation often includes ECG, chest x-ray, pulmonary function tests, echocardiogram, and CT scan.

The mean time between onset of symptoms and the diagnosis is about 2 years. By the time patients become symptomatic, the disease is already in the advanced stages and the pulmonary artery pressure is two to three times normal.

PATHOPHYSIOLOGY MAP

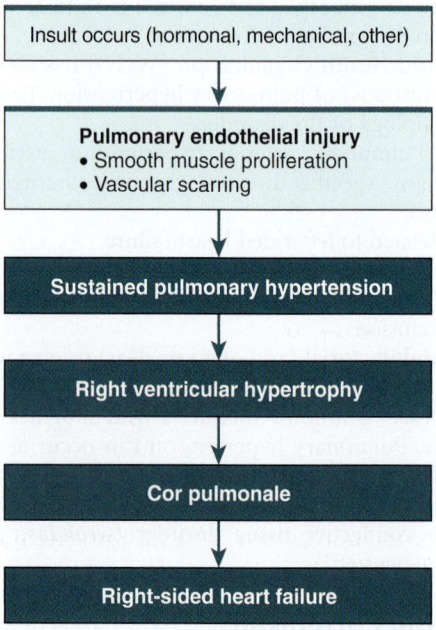

FIG. 27-11 Pathogenesis of pulmonary hypertension and cor pulmonale.

❖ NURSING AND INTERPROFESSIONAL MANAGEMENT: PULMONARY HYPERTENSION

Early recognition of pulmonary hypertension is essential to interrupt the vicious cycle responsible for progression of the disease. Encourage patients to report unexplained shortness of breath, syncope, chest discomfort, and edema of the feet and ankles to their primary care provider.[36]

Although IPAH has no cure, treatment can relieve symptoms, improve quality of life, and prolong life. Drug therapy consists of several drug classifications that promote vasodilation of the pulmonary blood vessels, reduce right ventricular overload, and reverse remodeling (Table 27-27). Diuretics are used to manage peripheral edema. The use of anticoagulants is also beneficial in pulmonary complications related to thrombus formation. Because hypoxia is a potent pulmonary vasoconstrictor, low-flow O_2 provides symptomatic relief. The goal is to keep O_2 saturation 90% or greater.

Surgical interventions for pulmonary hypertension include atrial septostomy (AS) and lung transplantation. AS is a palliative procedure that involves the creation of an intraatrial right-to-left shunt to decompress the right ventricle. It is used for a select group of patients awaiting lung transplantation.

TABLE 27-27 Drug Therapy

Pulmonary Hypertension

Drug	Mechanism of Action	Considerations
Calcium Channel Blockers		
nifedipine (Adalat CC, Procardia) diltiazem (Cardizem, Cardizem LA, Cartia XT, Tiazac)	• Act on vascular smooth muscle, causing dilation • Lower pulmonary artery pressure	• Can only be used in patients who do not have right-sided heart failure • Used at high doses in comparison to other uses of calcium channel blockers
Phosphodiesterase (Type 5) Enzyme Inhibitors		
sildenafil (Revatio) tadalafil (Adcirca)	• Promote selective smooth muscle relaxation in lung vasculature	• Given orally • Contraindicated in patients taking nitroglycerin, since may cause refractory hypotension
Vasodilators (Parenteral)		
epoprostenol (Flolan, Veletri) treprostinil (Remodulin) adenosine (Adenocard)	• Prostacyclin analog • Promote pulmonary vasodilation and reduce pulmonary vascular resistance	• Given IV to patients who do not respond to calcium channel blockers or have New York Heart Association (NYHA) class III or IV right-sided heart failure • Given by continuous IV (central line) or continuous subcutaneous route. Half-life of epoprostenol is short. Potential clinical deterioration from abrupt withdrawal if infusion disrupted
Vasodilators (Inhaled)		
iloprost (Ventavis) treprostinil (inhaled) (Tyvaso)	Synthetic analogs of prostacyclin (PGI_2) Dilate systemic and pulmonary arterial vasculature	• Indicated for patients with NYHA class III or IV heart failure • Administered 6-9 times a day using a disk inserted into a nebulizer • Can cause orthostatic hypotension. Do not give to patients with systolic BP <85 mm Hg.
Endothelin Receptor Antagonists		
bosentan (Tracleer) ambrisentan (Letairis) macitentan (Opsumit)	• Binds to endothelin-1 receptors and blocks the constriction of pulmonary arteries • Promote relaxation of pulmonary arteries and decrease pulmonary artery pressure	• Given orally • Indicated for patients with NYHA class II to IV symptoms • Hepatotoxic • Monitor liver function tests monthly.

Lung transplantation is indicated for those patients who do not respond to drug therapy and progress to severe right-sided heart failure. Recurrence of the disease has not been reported in individuals who have undergone transplantation.

SECONDARY PULMONARY ARTERIAL HYPERTENSION

Secondary pulmonary arterial hypertension (SPAH) occurs when a primary disease causes a chronic increase in pulmonary artery pressures. SPAH can develop as a result of parenchymal lung disease, left ventricular dysfunction, intracardiac shunts, chronic pulmonary thromboembolism, or systemic connective tissue disease. The specific primary disease pathology can result in anatomic or vascular changes causing the pulmonary hypertension.

The symptoms can reflect the underlying disease, but some are directly attributable to SPAH, including dyspnea, fatigue, lethargy, and chest pain. The initial physical findings can include right ventricular hypertrophy and signs of right ventricular failure (increased pulmonic heart sound, right-sided fourth heart sound, peripheral edema, and hepatomegaly).

Diagnosis of SPAH is similar to that of IPAH. Treatment of SPAH consists mainly of treating the underlying primary disorder. When irreversible pulmonary vascular damage has occurred, therapies used for IPAH are initiated. A pulmonary thromboendarterectomy (PTE) may offer a cure for patients with chronic pulmonary hypertension caused by thromboembolism. It is a technically demanding procedure and is performed only at selected centers.

COR PULMONALE

Cor pulmonale is enlargement of the right ventricle caused by a primary disorder of the respiratory system. Pulmonary hypertension is usually a preexisting condition in cor pulmonale. Cor pulmonale may be present with or without overt cardiac failure. The most common cause of cor pulmonale is COPD. Almost any disorder that affects the respiratory system can cause cor pulmonale. Fig. 27-11 outlines the etiology and pathogenesis of pulmonary hypertension and cor pulmonale.

Clinical Manifestations and Diagnostic Studies

Clinical manifestations are subtle and often masked by the symptoms of the pulmonary condition. Common symptoms include exertional dyspnea, tachypnea, cough, and fatigue. Physical signs include evidence of right ventricular hypertrophy on ECG and an increase in intensity of the second heart sound. Chronic hypoxemia leads to polycythemia and increased total blood volume and viscosity of the blood. Polycythemia is often present in cor pulmonale secondary to COPD.

If heart failure accompanies cor pulmonale, additional manifestations such as peripheral edema, weight gain, distended neck veins, full, bounding pulse, and enlarged liver may also be found. (Heart failure is discussed in Chapter 34.) Various laboratory tests and imaging studies are used to confirm the diagnosis of cor pulmonale (Table 27-28).

❖ NURSING AND INTERPROFESSIONAL MANAGEMENT: COR PULMONALE

Early identification of cor pulmonale is essential before changes to the heart occur that may be irreversible. The primary management of cor pulmonale is difficult but often directed at investigating the cause and treating the underlying pulmonary problem (Table 27-28).

TABLE 27-28 Interprofessional Care

Cor Pulmonale

Diagnostic Assessment	Management
• History and physical examination • ABGs, SpO_2 • Serum and urine electrolytes • b-Type natriuretic peptide (BNP) • ECG • Chest x-ray • Echocardiography • CT scan • MRI • Cardiac catheterization	• O_2 therapy • Low-sodium diet ***Drug Therapy*** • Bronchodilators • Diuretics • Vasodilators (if indicated) • Calcium channel blockers (if indicated) • Inotropic agents

TABLE 27-29 Indications for Lung Transplantation*

- Chronic obstructive pulmonary disease
- Idiopathic pulmonary fibrosis
- Cystic fibrosis
- Idiopathic pulmonary arterial hypertension
- α_1-Antitrypsin deficiency

*These are the most common indications.

Long-term O_2 therapy, the mainstay of treatment to correct the hypoxemia, reduces vasoconstriction and pulmonary hypertension. All other strategies must be individualized for each patient but are often directed at treating pulmonary hypertension that can lead to cor pulmonale. If fluid, electrolyte, and acid-base imbalances are present, they must be corrected. Diuretics may help decrease the plasma volume and reduce the workload on the heart but must be used with extreme caution. In some cases, decreases in fluid volume from diuresis can worsen cardiac function. Bronchodilator therapy is indicated if the underlying respiratory problem is due to an obstructive disorder.

Other treatments may include vasodilator therapy, calcium channel blockers, anticoagulants, digitalis, and phlebotomy, all of which have varying degrees of success. Chronic management of cor pulmonale resulting from COPD is similar to that described for COPD (see Chapter 28).

LUNG TRANSPLANTATION

Lung transplantation has become an important mode of therapy for patients with end-stage lung disease. The limiting factor for this therapy is the availability of donors. A variety of pulmonary disorders are potentially treatable with lung transplantation (Table 27-29). Improved patient selection criteria, technical advances, and better methods of immunosuppression have resulted in improved survival rates.

Preoperative Care

Patients being considered for lung transplantation need to undergo extensive evaluation. Absolute contraindications for lung transplant include malignancy within past 2 years (some types of skin cancer are excluded), chronic active hepatitis B or C, HIV, untreatable advanced dysfunction of another major organ system (e.g., liver or renal failure), current smoker, poor nutritional status, poor rehabilitation potential, and significant psychosocial problems. The patient and family must be able to cope with a complex postoperative regimen (e.g., strict adherence to immunosuppressive therapy, continuous monitoring for early signs of infection, prompt reporting of manifestations of infection). Many transplant centers require preoperative outpatient pulmonary rehabilitation to maximize physical conditioning.

In the United States, the United Network for Organ Sharing (UNOS) is a private, non-profit organization that works with the federal government to manage organ transplantation. UNOS designates recipients of donor lungs based on a lung allocation score (LAS). The LAS helps to prioritize waiting list recipients based on the urgency of need and expected post-transplant survival expectations.

Patients who are accepted as transplant candidates must carry a pager with them at all times in case a donor organ becomes available. These patients must be prepared to move to the location of their chosen transplant center at a moment's notice. Such patients may be encouraged to limit their travel within a certain geographic region to facilitate rapid transportation to a transplant center.

Surgical Procedure

Four types of transplant procedures are available: single-lung transplantation, bilateral lung transplantation, heart-lung transplantation, and transplantation of lobes from a living-related donor.

Single-lung transplantation involves a thoracotomy incision on the side of the chest. The opposite lung is ventilated while the diseased lung is excised, and the donor lung implanted. Three anastomoses are done: bronchus, pulmonary artery, and pulmonary veins. In *bilateral lung transplantation,* the incision is made across the sternum and the donor lungs are implanted separately. A median sternotomy incision is used for a *heart-lung transplant* procedure. *Lobar transplantation* from living donors is reserved for candidates who urgently need transplantation and are unlikely to survive until a donor becomes available. The majority of these transplant recipients are patients with cystic fibrosis, and their parents or relatives are donors. Once anastomosis is complete, the lung is gently reinflated, perfusion is reestablished, chest tubes are inserted, and the surgical incision is closed.

Postoperative Care

Early postoperative care often includes admission to ICU and provision of ventilatory support, fluid and hemodynamic management, immunosuppression, nutritional support, detection of early rejection, and prevention or treatment of infection. Once hemodynamic stability has been achieved, the patient is often transferred to a high acuity observation or surgical unit. Maintenance of accurate fluid balance is vital in the postoperative phase.

Lung transplant recipients are at high risk for multiple complications after surgery. Noninfectious issues may include VTE, diaphragmatic dysfunction, and malignancy. Infectious complications may be caused by bacteria, viruses, fungi, or protozoa. Infections are the leading cause of death at all time points after lung transplant. Bacterial bronchitis and pneumonia are the most common infections, but cytomegalovirus (CMV), fungi, viruses, and mycobacteria are also etiologic factors.

Immunosuppressive therapy usually includes a three-drug regimen of tacrolimus, mycophenolate mofetil (CellCept), and prednisone. (The mechanisms of action of these drugs are discussed in Table 13-16 and Fig. 13-13.) Drug levels are monitored on a regular basis. Lung transplant recipients usually receive higher levels of immunosuppressive therapy than other organ recipients.

Acute rejection is fairly common in lung transplantation, typically occurring in the first 5 to 10 days after surgery. Low-grade fever, fatigue, dyspnea, dry cough, and O_2 desaturation are possible signs of rejection. Accurate diagnosis of rejection is by transtracheal biopsy. Treatment consists of high doses of IV corticosteroids administered for 3 days, followed by high doses of oral prednisone. In patients with persistent or recurrent acute rejection, antilymphocyte therapy may be useful.

Bronchiolitis obliterans (BOS) is a manifestation of chronic rejection in lung transplant patients. BOS is characterized by airflow obstruction that progresses over time. The onset is often subacute, with gradual development of exertional dyspnea, nonproductive cough, wheezing, and/or low-grade fever. Airway obstruction is not responsive to bronchodilators and corticosteroid therapy. Although not proven effective, additional immunosuppressive agents may be used in the treatment of chronic rejection. Because acute rejection is a major risk factor for BOS, prevention of acute rejection is key to decreasing the incidence of chronic rejection.

Before discharge, the patient needs to be able to perform self-care activities, including medication management and activities of daily living, and to accurately identify when to call the transplant team. Patients should be instructed on pulmonary clearance measures, including aerosolized bronchodilators, chest physiotherapy, and deep-breathing and coughing techniques, to help minimize any potential complication. Home spirometry is useful in monitoring trends in lung function. Teach patients to keep medication logs, laboratory results, and spirometry records. Patients are placed in an outpatient rehabilitation program to improve physical endurance.

After discharge, the transplant team follows patients for transplant-related issues. Patients return to their primary care team for health maintenance and routine illnesses. As transplant procedures become more frequent, transplant patients will return to hospitals for other routine procedures. Coordination of care between the transplant team, primary care team, and inpatient teams is essential for ongoing successful management of these patients. (Organ transplantation, histocompatibility, rejection, and immunosuppressive therapy are discussed in Chapter 13.)

CASE STUDY

Pneumonia and Lung Cancer

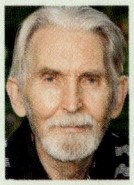

(©iStockphoto/Thinkstock)

Patient Profile

J.H. is a 52-year-old white man who comes to the emergency department complaining of shortness of breath. He has not seen an HCP for many years.

Subjective Data

- Has a 38 pack-year history of cigarette smoking
- States he has always been slender but has had 25-lb weight loss despite a normal appetite in the past few months
- Admits to a "smoker's cough" for the past 2 to 3 years; recently coughing up blood
- Is married and the father of three adult children

Objective Data

Physical Examination

- Thin, pale man, looking older than stated age
- Height 6 ft (182.9 cm); weight 135 lb (61.2 kg)
- Intermittently confused and anxious with rapid shallow respirations
- Vital signs: temperature 102.6° F (39.2° C), heart rate 120, respiratory rate 36
- Chest wall has limited excursion on right side; auscultation of left side reveals coarse crackles but clear with cough; right side has diminished breath sounds

Diagnostic Studies

- Arterial blood gases: pH 7.51, PaO_2 58 mm Hg, $PaCO_2$ 30 mm Hg, HCO_3^- 22 mEq/L, O_2 saturation 84% (room air)
- Chest x-ray: consolidation of the right lung, especially in the base with possible mass in the area of right bronchus; pleural effusion on the right side
- Bronchoscopy with biopsy of mass: small cell lung carcinoma

Interprofessional Care

- Diagnosis: pneumonia with small cell lung cancer
- Follow-up with patient and family to consider treatment options

Discussion Questions

1. How would you classify J.H.'s pneumonia? Why is this important?
2. What is your analysis of J.H.'s arterial blood gas results?
3. ***Priority Decision:*** Based on the assessment data presented, what are the priority nursing diagnoses? Are there any collaborative problems?
4. ***Priority Decision:*** What are the priority nursing interventions for J.H.?
5. ***Teamwork and Collaboration:*** Identify activities that can be delegated to unlicensed assistive personnel (UAP).
6. ***Patient-Centered Care:*** You are planning a meeting with J.H. and his family to discuss their needs. The physician tells you that J.H. is terminally ill. Who will you include in this meeting?
7. ***Evidence-Based Practice:*** J.H.'s children tell you that they are worried they will get lung cancer, since their father has it and they grew up around his secondhand smoke. They want to know what kind of screening is available for them. How will you respond?
8. What is the goal if radiation therapy is used for J.H.?
9. ***Patient-Centered Care:*** What issues should be addressed in your teaching of J.H. and his wife as you prepare him for discharge and care at home?

Answers available at *http://evolve.elsevier.com/Lewis/medsurg.*

BRIDGE TO NCLEX EXAMINATION

The number of the question corresponds to the same-numbered outcome at the beginning of the chapter.

1. When caring for a patient with acute bronchitis, the nurse will *prioritize*
   a. auscultating lung sounds.
   b. encouraging fluid restriction.
   c. administering antibiotic therapy.
   d. teaching the patient to avoid cough suppressants.
2. For which patients with pneumonia would the nurse suspect aspiration as the likely cause of pneumonia *(select all that apply)*?
   a. Patient with seizures
   b. Patient with head injury
   c. Patient who had thoracic surgery
   d. Patient who had a myocardial infarction
   e. Patient who is receiving nasogastric tube feeding
3. An appropriate nursing intervention for a patient with pneumonia with the nursing diagnosis of ineffective airway clearance related to thick secretions and fatigue would be to
   a. perform postural drainage every hour.
   b. provide analgesics as ordered to promote patient comfort.
   c. administer O_2 as prescribed to maintain optimal O_2 levels.
   d. teach the patient how to cough effectively to bring secretions to the mouth.
4. A patient with TB has been admitted to the hospital and is placed in an airborne infection isolation room. What should the patient be taught *(select all that apply)*?
   a. Expect routine TST to evaluate infection.
   b. Visitors will not be allowed while in airborne isolation.
   c. Take all medications for full length of time to prevent multidrug-resistant TB.
   d. Wear a standard isolation mask if leaving the airborne infection isolation room.
   e. Maintain precautions in airborne infection isolation room by coughing into a paper tissue.
5. A patient has been receiving high-dose corticosteroids and broad-spectrum antibiotics for treatment secondary to a traumatic injury and infection. The nurse plans care for the patient knowing that the patient is most susceptible to
   a. candidiasis.
   b. aspergillosis.
   c. histoplasmosis.
   d. coccidioidomycosis.
6. When caring for a patient with a lung abscess, what is the nurse's *priority* intervention?
   a. Postural drainage
   b. Antibiotic administration
   c. Obtaining a sputum specimen
   d. Patient teaching regarding home care

7. The emergency department nurse is caring for patients exposed to a chlorine leak from a local factory. The nurse would closely monitor these patients for
   a. pulmonary edema.
   b. anaphylactic shock.
   c. respiratory alkalosis.
   d. acute tubular necrosis.
8. The nurse receives an order for a patient with lung cancer to receive influenza vaccine and pneumococcal vaccines. The nurse will
   a. call the health care provider to question the order.
   b. administer both vaccines at the same time in different arms.
   c. administer the flu shot and tell the patient to come back 1 week later to receive the pneumococcal vaccine.
   d. administer the pneumococcal vaccine and suggest FluMist (nasal vaccine) instead of the influenza injection.
9. The nurse identifies a flail chest in a trauma patient when
   a. multiple rib fractures are determined by x-ray.
   b. a tracheal deviation to the unaffected side is present.
   c. paradoxical chest movement occurs during respiration.
   d. there is decreased movement of the involved chest wall.
10. The nurse notes tidaling of the water level in the tube submerged in the water-seal chamber in a patient with closed chest tube drainage. The nurse should
   a. continue to monitor the patient.
   b. check all connections for a leak in the system.
   c. lower the drainage collector further from the chest.
   d. clamp the tubing at progressively distal points away from the patient until the tidaling stops.
11. Following a pneumonectomy, an appropriate nursing intervention is
   a. monitoring chest tube drainage and functioning.
   b. positioning the patient on the unaffected side or back.
   c. doing range-of-motion exercises on the affected upper limb.
   d. auscultating frequently for lung sounds on the affected side.
12. A *priority* nursing intervention for a patient who has just undergone a chemical pleurodesis for recurrent pleural effusion is
   a. administering ordered analgesia.
   b. monitoring chest tube drainage.
   c. sending pleural fluid for laboratory analysis.
   d. monitoring the patient's level of consciousness.
13. When planning care for a patient at risk for pulmonary embolism, the nurse *prioritizes*
   a. maintaining the patient on bed rest.
   b. using sequential compression devices.
   c. encouraging the patient to cough and deep breathe.
   d. teaching the patient how to use the incentive spirometer.
14. Which statement(s) describe(s) the management of a patient following lung transplantation *(select all that apply)*?
   a. High doses of O_2 are administered around the clock.
   b. The use of a home spirometer will help to monitor lung function.
   c. Immunosuppressant therapy usually involves a three-drug regimen.
   d. Most patients experience an acute rejection episode in the first 2 days.
   e. The lung is biopsied using a transtracheal method if rejection is suspected.

1. a, 2. a, b, e, 3. d, 4. c, d, e, 5. a, 6. b, 7. a, 8. b, 9. c, 10. a, 11. c, 12. a, 13. b, 14. b, c, e

For rationales to these answers and even more NCLEX review questions, visit *http://evolve.elsevier.com/Lewis/medsurg.*

EVOLVE WEBSITE

http://evolve.elsevier.com/Lewis/medsurg

Review Questions (Online Only)
Key Points
Answer Keys for Questions
- Rationales for Bridge to NCLEX Examination Questions
- Answer Guidelines for Case Study on p. 355

Student Case Studies
- Patient With Lung Cancer
- Patient With Pulmonary Embolism and Respiratory Failure

Nursing Care Plans
- eNursing Care Plan 27-1: Patient With Pneumonia
- eNursing Care Plan 27-2: Patient After Thoracotomy

Conceptual Care Map Creator
Audio Glossary
Content Updates

REFERENCES

1. Centers for Disease Control and Prevention: Pneumonia deaths. Retrieved from *www.cdc.gov/nchs/fastats/pneumonia.htm.*
2. Centers for Disease Control and Prevention: Influenza deaths. Retrieved from *www.cdc.gov/nchs/fastats/flu.htm.*
3. Centers for Disease Control and Prevention: Pertussis (whooping cough): causes and transmission. Retrieved from *www.cdc.gov/pertussis/about/causes-transmission.html.*
4. American Lung Association: Influenza and pneumonia. Retrieved from *www.lung.org/assets/documents/publications/solddc-chapters/i-p.pdf.*
5. Centers for Disease Control and Prevention: Leading causes of death. Retrieved from *www.cdc.gov/nchs/fastats/leading-causes-of-death.htm.*
6. Kalanuria AA, Zai W, Mirski M: Ventilator-associated pneumonia in the ICU, *Crit Care* 18:208, 2014.
7. Löffler B, Niemann S, Ehrhardt C, et al: Pathogenesis of *Staphylococcus aureus* necrotizing pneumonia, *Expert Rev Anti Infect Ther* 11:1041, 2013.
8. Elborai Y: Management of cytomegalovirus (CMV) in hematopoietic stem cell transplant (HSCT), *J Pediatr Neonatal Care* 1:23, 2014.
9. Burgos J, Falcó V, Pahissa A: The increasing incidence of empyema, *Curr Opin Pulmonary Med* 19:350, 2013.
10. van Vugt SF, Broekhuizen BD, Lammens C, et al: Use of serum C reactive protein and procalcitonin concentrations in addition to symptoms and signs to predict pneumonia in patients presenting to primary care with acute cough: diagnostic study, *Br Med J* 346:f2450, 2013.

*11. Niu WY, Wan YG, Li MY, et al: The diagnostic value of serum procalcitonin, IL-10 and C-reactive protein in community-acquired pneumonia and tuberculosis, *Eur Rev Med Pharmacol Sci* 17:3329, 2013.

12. Joseph GG: Prognostic value of serum procalcitonin and C-reactive protein levels in critically ill patients who developed ventilator-associated pneumonia, *Ann Thorac Med* 10:137, 2015.
13. U.S. Food and Drug Administration: Influenza (flu) antiviral drugs and related information. Retrieved from *www.fda.gov/Drugs/DrugSafety/InformationbyDrugClass/ucm100228.htm#AntiviralMedications.*

*14. Keyt H, Faverio P, Restrepo MI: Prevention of ventilator-associated pneumonia in the intensive care unit: a review of clinically relevant recent advancements, *Indian J Med Res* 139:814, 2014.
15. Centers for Disease Control and Prevention: TB incidence in the United States, 1953-2013. Retrieved from *www.cdc.gov/tb/statistics/tbcases.htm.*
16. World Health Organization. Multidrug-resistant tuberculosis (MDR-TB): 2013 update. Retrieved from *www.who.int/tb/challenges/mdr/mdr_tb_factsheet.pdf?ua=1.*
17. Centers for Disease Control and Prevention: Tuberculosis (TB) fact sheets: skin testing. Retrieved from *www.cdc.gov/tb/publications/factsheets/testing/skintesting.htm.*
18. Joseph MR, Thomas RA, Nair S, et al: Directly observed treatment short course for tuberculosis. What happens to them in the long term? *Indian J Tuberc* 62:29, 2015.
19. Centers for Disease Control and Prevention: Tuberculosis (TB): treatment for latent TB infection. Retrieved from *www.cdc.gov/tb/topic/treatment/ltbi.htm.*
20. Centers for Disease Control and Prevention: The national personal protective technology laboratory (NPPTL): respirator trusted-source information. Section 3: Ancillary respirator information. Retrieved from *www.cdc.gov/niosh/npptl/topics/respirators/disp_part/RespSource3fittest.html#fith.*
21. Centers for Disease Control and Prevention: Fungal diseases: Valley fever (coccidioidomycosis). Retrieved from *www.cdc.gov/fungal/diseases/coccidioidomycosis.*
22. Centers for Disease Control and Prevention: Lung cancer. Retrieved from *www.cdc.gov/cancer/lung.*
23. American Lung Association: Lung cancer fact sheet. Retrieved from *www.lung.org/lung-disease/lung-cancer/resources/facts-figures/lung-cancer-fact-sheet.html.*
24. American Lung Association: Causes of cancer. Retrieved from *www.lung.org/associations/states/colorado/lung-disease/lung-cancer.html.*
25. Lung Cancer.Org: Lung cancer 101-Types and staging of lung cancer. Retrieved from *www.lungcancer.org/find_information/publications/163-lung_cancer_101/268-types_and_staging.*
*26. Blackmon SH, Feinglass SR: The United States Preventive Services Task Force Recommendations for Lung Cancer Screening, *Thorac Surg Clin* 25(2):199, 2015.
*27. Smith RA, Manassaram-Baptiste D, Brooks D, et al: Cancer screening in the United States, 2014: a review of current American Cancer Society guidelines and current issues in cancer screening, *CA Cancer J Clin* 64:30, 2014.
*28. Zhang W, Jiang W, Luan L, et al: Prophylactic cranial irradiation for patients with small-cell lung cancer: a systematic review of the literature with meta-analysis, *BMC Cancer* 14:793, 2014.
29. Mancini MC: Hemothorax. Retrieved from *emedicine.medscape.com/article/2047916-overview.*
30. Adams SD: Chylothorax. Retrieved from *emedicine.medscape.com/article/172527-overview.*
31. Hennon MW, Demmy TL: Video-assisted thoracoscopic surgery (VATS) for locally advanced lung cancer. Retrieved from *www.annalscts.com/article/view/476/608.*
32. British Lung Foundation: What is interstitial lung disease? Retrieved from *www.blf.org.uk/Page/What-is-interstitial-lung-disease.*
*33. Kistler KD, Nalysnyk L, Rotella P, et al: Lung transplantation in idiopathic pulmonary fibrosis: a systematic review of the literature, *BMC Pulm Med* 14:139, 2014.
*34. Guyatt GH, Akl EA, Crowther M, et al for the American College of Chest Physicians Antithrombotic Therapy and Prevention of Thrombosis Panel: Executive summary: Antithrombotic therapy and prevention of thrombosis, 9th ed: American College of Chest Physicians evidence-based clinical practice guidelines, *Chest* 141 (2 Suppl):7S, 2012.
35. Weinberg I, Jaff MR: Treating large pulmonary emboli: Do the guidelines guide us? *Curr Opin Pulmonary Med* 19:413, 2013.
36. Healthline Networks, Inc: The symptoms of pulmonary arterial hypertension. Retrieved from *www.healthline.com/health-slideshow/symptoms-pulmonary-arterial-hypertension#9.*

*Evidence-based information for clinical practice.

28

Obstructive Pulmonary Diseases

Susan Collazo

A nation that destroys its soils destroys itself. Forests are the lungs of our land, purifying the air and giving fresh strength to our people.

Franklin D. Roosevelt

http://evolve.elsevier.com/Lewis/medsurg/

LEARNING OUTCOMES

1. Describe the etiology, pathophysiology, clinical manifestations, and interprofessional care of asthma.
2. Describe the nursing management of the patient with asthma.
3. Describe the etiology, pathophysiology, clinical manifestations, and interprofessional care of the patient with chronic obstructive pulmonary disease (COPD).
4. Describe the effects of cigarette smoking on the lungs.
5. Identify the indications for O_2 therapy, methods of delivery, and complications of O_2 administration.
6. Explain the nursing management of the patient with COPD.
7. Describe the pathophysiology, clinical manifestations, interprofessional care, and nursing management of the patient with cystic fibrosis.
8. Describe the pathophysiology, clinical manifestations, interprofessional care, and nursing management of the patient with bronchiectasis.

KEY TERMS

α_1-antitrypsin (AAT) deficiency, p. 558
asthma, p. 539
bronchiectasis, p. 580
chest physiotherapy (CPT), p. 569
chronic bronchitis, p. 557
chronic obstructive pulmonary disease (COPD), p. 557
cor pulmonale, p. 560
cystic fibrosis (CF), p. 576
emphysema, p. 557
O_2 toxicity, p. 565
postural drainage, p. 570
pursed-lip breathing (PLB), p. 569

Imagine needing to consciously think about every breath that you take for minutes, hours, or even days. Many individuals with obstructive lung disease have this experience.

Approximately 31.5 million adult Americans are living with asthma or chronic obstructive pulmonary disease (COPD).[1,2]

Obstructive pulmonary disease, the most common chronic lung disease, is characterized by increased resistance to airflow as a result of airway obstruction or airway narrowing. Types of obstructive lung diseases include asthma, COPD, cystic fibrosis (CF), and bronchiectasis. *Asthma* is a lung disease that causes inflammation with variable episodes of airflow obstruction, but it is usually reversible. *COPD* is an obstructive pulmonary disease with progressive limitation in airflow that is not fully reversible. The patient with asthma has variations in airflow over time, usually with normal lung function between exacerbations. In contrast, the limitation in expiratory airflow in the patient with COPD is generally more constant. The pathophysiology of asthma and the response to therapy differ from those associated with COPD. However, the patient with a diagnosis of obstructive pulmonary disease may have features of both asthma and COPD. Patients with asthma who have less responsive reversible airflow obstruction are difficult to distinguish from COPD patients.

Cystic fibrosis, another form of obstructive pulmonary disease, is a genetic disorder. It produces airway obstruction because of changes in exocrine glandular secretions, resulting in increased mucus production.

Bronchiectasis is an obstructive disease characterized by dilated bronchioles, making it difficult to clear secretions. It most frequently results from untreated or poorly treated pulmonary infections, immune system problems, or genetic factors.

Acknowledgment: We would like to acknowledge the contributions of Jane Kaufman, MS, CRNP, ANP-BC, Advanced Senior Lecturer, University of Pennsylvania School of Nursing, Philadelphia, Pennsylvania, to this chapter over the past four editions of the book.
Reviewed by Marilyn Borkgren, APN, MS, CCNS, Pulmonary APN, Suburban Lung Associates, Elk Grove Village, Illinois; Kim Clevenger, RN, EdD, BC, Associate Professor of Nursing, BSN Program Coordinator, Morehead State University, Morehead, Kentucky; Deborah Cline, RN, MS, Nursing Faculty, Carrington College, Reno, Nevada; Marianne Ferrin, MSN, ACNP-BC, Coordinator Penn Lung Center, Adult Cystic Fibrosis Program, Philadelphia, Pennsylvania; Jane Kaufman, MS, CRNP, ANP-BC, Advanced Senior Lecturer, University of Pennsylvania School of Nursing, Philadelphia, Pennsylvania; Eugene E. Mondor, RN, MN, CNCC(C), Clinical Nurse Educator–Adult Critical Care, Royal Alexandra Hospital, Edmonton, Alberta, Canada; Cynthia M. Steinwedel, RN, PhD, CNE, Assistant Professor, Department of Nursing, Bradley University, Peoria, Illinois; and Kenneth Wysocki, PhD, FNP-BC, FAANP, Family Nurse Practitioner, Asthma and Genetics Researcher, Clinical Services, Matrix Medical Network, Scottsdale, Arizona.

GENDER DIFFERENCES

Asthma

Men

- Before puberty, more boys are affected than girls.

Women

- After puberty and into adulthood, more women are affected than men.
- Women who are admitted to the emergency department are more likely to need hospitalization than men.
- Death rate from asthma is greater in women than in men.

CULTURAL & ETHNIC HEALTH DISPARITIES

Obstructive Pulmonary Diseases

Asthma

- Asthma prevalence rates are more than 38% higher among African Americans than whites.
- Puerto Ricans have higher asthma prevalence rates and age-adjusted death rates than all other racial and ethnic subgroups.
- Female African Americans have the highest mortality rates from asthma among all ethnic/gender groups.

Chronic Obstructive Pulmonary Disease (COPD)

- Whites have the highest incidence of COPD despite higher rates of smoking among other ethnic groups.
- Hispanics have lower death rates related to COPD than other ethnic groups.

Cystic Fibrosis

- Whites have the highest incidence of cystic fibrosis.
- Cystic fibrosis is uncommon among African Americans, Hispanics, and Asian Americans.

ASTHMA

Asthma is a heterogenous disease characterized by a combination of clinical manifestations along with reversible expiratory airflow limitation or bronchial hyperresponsiveness. The variability of signs and symptoms can include episodes of wheezing, breathlessness, chest tightness, and cough, particularly at night or in the early morning. These episodes are associated with widespread but variable airflow obstruction that is usually reversible, either spontaneously or with treatment. The clinical course of asthma is unpredictable, ranging from periods of adequate control to exacerbations with poor control of symptoms.[3]

Asthma affects an estimated 18.8 million adult Americans. Among adults, women are 62% more likely to have asthma than men. Asthma is a public health concern, with more than 14.2 million lost workdays in adults. However, the good news is that after a long period of an increasing incidence of asthma, the mortality and use of health care services for asthma are continuing to plateau and/or decrease. Despite the decline in the number of deaths from asthma over the past 10 years, more than 3300 people yearly still die from asthma.[1]

Risk Factors for Asthma and Triggers of Asthma Attacks

Risk factors for asthma and triggers of asthma attacks can be related to the patient (e.g., genetic factors) or the environment (e.g., pollen) (Table 28-1). Male gender is a risk factor for asthma in children, but not adults. Obesity is also a risk factor for asthma.[4] Other factors and triggers are discussed in this section.

Genetics. Asthma has a component that is inherited, but the genetics are complex. Numerous genes may be involved in the development of asthma and a person's response to various asthma medications.[3,4] *Atopy,* the genetic predisposition to develop an allergic (immunoglobulin E [IgE]–mediated) response to common allergens, is a major risk factor for asthma.

Immune Response. The *hygiene hypothesis* suggests that a newborn baby's immune system must be conditioned so that it will function properly during infancy and the rest of life. People who have a lower incidence of asthma are exposed to certain infections early in life, use few antibiotics, are exposed to other children (e.g., siblings, day care), or live in rural settings or with pets. People for whom these factors are not present in childhood have a higher incidence of asthma.[3]

Allergens. Indoor and outdoor allergens, such as cockroaches, furry animals, fungi, pollen, and molds, can trigger asthma attacks. However, their role in the actual development of asthma is not as clear.[3,4]

Exercise. Asthma that is induced or exacerbated during physical exertion is called *exercise-induced asthma* (EIA) or *exercise-induced bronchospasm* (EIB). Typically, EIB occurs after vigorous exercise, not during it (e.g., jogging, aerobics, walking briskly, climbing stairs). Symptoms of EIA are pronounced during activities where there is exposure to cold, dry air. For example, swimming in an indoor heated pool is less likely to produce symptoms than downhill skiing. Airway obstruction may occur due to changes in the airway mucosa caused by hyperventilation during exercise, with either cooling or rewarming of air and capillary leakage in the airway wall.

Air Pollutants. Various air pollutants, such as cigarette or wood smoke or vehicle exhaust, can trigger asthma attacks. In heavily industrialized or densely populated areas, climatic conditions often lead to concentrated pollution in the atmosphere,

TABLE 28-1 Triggers of Asthma Attacks

Allergen Inhalation

- Animal dander (e.g., cats, mice, guinea pigs)
- Cockroaches
- House dust mite
- Molds
- Pollens

Air Pollutants

- Aerosol sprays
- Cigarette smoke
- Exhaust fumes
- Oxidants
- Perfumes
- Sulfur dioxides

Viral or Bacterial Infection

- Sinusitis, allergic rhinitis
- Viral upper respiratory tract infection

Drugs

- β-Adrenergic blockers
- Aspirin
- Nonsteroidal antiinflammatory drugs

Occupational Exposure

- Agriculture, farming
- Industrial chemicals and plastics
- Laundry detergents
- Metal salts
- Paints, solvents
- Pharmaceutical agents
- Wood and vegetable dusts

Food Additives

- Beer, wine, dried fruit, shrimp, processed potatoes
- Monosodium glutamate
- Sulfites (bisulfites and metabisulfites)
- Tartrazine

Other Factors

- Exercise and cold, dry air
- Gastroesophageal reflux disease (GERD)
- Hormones, menses
- Stress

especially with thermal inversions and stagnant air masses. Ozone alert days are regularly noted on the news reports, and patients should minimize outdoor activity during these times. Cigarette smoking is associated with an accelerated decline of lung functioning in a person with asthma, increases the severity of the disease, may cause the patient to be less responsive to treatment, and reduces the chance of the asthma being controlled. Despite the relationship of pollutants in triggering asthma attacks, the role of outdoor air pollution as a cause of asthma development remains controversial.[4]

Occupational Factors. *Occupational asthma* is the most common occupational respiratory disorder, with up to 15% of new asthma cases arising from job-related exposures to more than 300 agents.[4,5] Irritants cause a change in the responsiveness of the airways. However, the development of symptoms from this alteration may not occur until the patient has had months to years of exposure. Occupations with a high risk of occupational asthma include agricultural worker, baker, hospital worker, plastics manufacturer, and beautician. Characteristically people with occupational asthma give a history of arriving at work feeling well but gradually develop symptoms by the end of the day.

Respiratory Tract Infections. Respiratory tract infections (i.e., viral and not bacterial) are often the major precipitating factor of an acute asthma attack. Acute infection can increase airway narrowing and airway hyperresponsiveness. Viral-induced alterations of epithelial cells, increased inflammatory cell accumulation, edema of airway walls, and exposure of airway nerve endings contribute to altered airway function. These alterations in airway function may exacerbate asthma.

Nose and Sinus Problems. Most patients with asthma have a history of allergic rhinitis. Treatment of allergic rhinitis usually improves the symptoms of asthma. Additional information on the relationship of rhinitis and asthma can be found at *www.whiar.org.*

Acute and chronic sinusitis, especially allergic rhinosinusitis, may worsen asthma. Some patients with asthma have chronic sinus problems that cause inflammation of the mucous membranes. Sinusitis must be treated and large nasal polyps removed for an asthma patient to have good control. (Sinusitis is discussed in Chapter 26.)

Drugs and Food Additives. Sensitivity to specific drugs may occur in some people, especially those with nasal polyps and sinusitis. Some people with asthma have what is termed the *asthma triad:* nasal polyps, asthma, and sensitivity to aspirin and nonsteroidal antiinflammatory drugs (NSAIDs). Salicylic acid can be found in many over-the-counter (OTC) drugs and some foods, beverages, and flavorings. Some asthmatics who use aspirin or NSAIDs (e.g., ibuprofen [Motrin]) develop wheezing within 2 hours. In addition, there is usually profound rhinorrhea, congestion, tearing, and even angioedema. Avoidance of aspirin and NSAIDs is required. However, patients with aspirin sensitivity under the care of an allergist can be desensitized by daily administration of the drug.

β-Adrenergic blockers in oral form (e.g., metoprolol [Toprol XL]) or topical eye drops (e.g., timolol [Timoptic]) may trigger asthma because they can cause bronchospasm. Angiotensin-converting enzyme (ACE) inhibitors (e.g., lisinopril [Prinivil]) may produce cough in susceptible individuals, thus making asthma symptoms worse.

Other agents that may precipitate asthma in the susceptible patient are tartrazine (yellow dye no. 5, found in many foods) and sulfiting agents widely used in the food and pharmaceutical industries as preservatives and sanitizing agents. Sulfiting agents are commonly found in fruits, beer, and wine and used extensively in salad bars to protect vegetables from oxidation. Asthma exacerbations can occur after the use of sulfite-containing preservatives found in topical ophthalmic solutions, IV corticosteroids, and some inhaled bronchodilator solutions.

Food allergies triggering asthma reactions in adults are rare. Avoidance diets are not recommended until an allergy has been demonstrated, usually by oral challenges performed by a specialized HCP provider, such as an allergist.

Gastroesophageal Reflux Disease. Gastroesophageal reflux disease (GERD) is more common in people with asthma than in the general population. GERD may worsen asthma symptoms because reflux may trigger bronchoconstriction and cause aspiration. Asthma medications may worsen GERD symptoms. β_2-Agonists (especially given orally), which are used to treat asthma, relax the lower esophageal sphincter, thus allowing stomach contents to reflux into the esophagus and possibly be aspirated into the lungs. Effective treatment for GERD in an asthma patient can improve nocturnal asthma control, quality of life, and possibly exacerbations in these patients.[4,6] (GERD is discussed in Chapter 41.)

Psychologic Factors. Asthma is not a psychosomatic disease. However, many people with asthma report that symptoms worsen with stress. Certainly psychologic factors cause bronchoconstriction via stimulation of the cholinergic reflex pathways. Extreme emotional expressions (e.g., crying, laughing, anger, fear) can lead to hyperventilation and hypocapnia, which can cause airway narrowing.[4]

An asthma attack caused by any triggering event can produce panic, stress, and anxiety. However, it varies from patient to patient and in the same patient from episode to episode.

Pathophysiology

The primary pathophysiologic process in asthma is persistent but variable inflammation of the airways. The airflow is limited because the inflammation results in bronchoconstriction, airway hyperresponsiveness (hyperreactivity), and edema of the airways. Exposure to allergens or irritants initiates the inflammatory cascade (Fig. 28-1). A variety of inflammatory cells are involved, including mast cells, macrophages, eosinophils, neutrophils, T and B lymphocytes, and epithelial cells of the airways.

As the inflammatory process begins, mast cells (found beneath the basement membrane of the bronchial wall) degranulate and release multiple inflammatory mediators (Fig. 28-2). IgE antibodies are linked to mast cells, and the allergen cross-links the IgE. Then inflammatory mediators such as leukotrienes, histamine, cytokines, prostaglandins, and nitric oxide are released. Some inflammatory mediators have effects on the (1) blood vessels, causing vasodilation and increasing capillary permeability (runny nose), (2) nerve cells causing itching, (3) smooth muscle cells causing bronchial spasms and airway narrowing, and (4) goblet cells causing mucus production (Fig. 28-3). This whole process is sometimes referred to as the *early-phase response* in asthma. Clinically it can occur within 30 to 60 minutes after exposure to an allergen or irritant.

Symptoms can recur 4 to 6 hours after the early response because of the influx of many inflammatory cells, which are set in motion by the initial response. At this later time the patient may develop symptoms again or worsening of symptoms. This

PATHOPHYSIOLOGY MAP

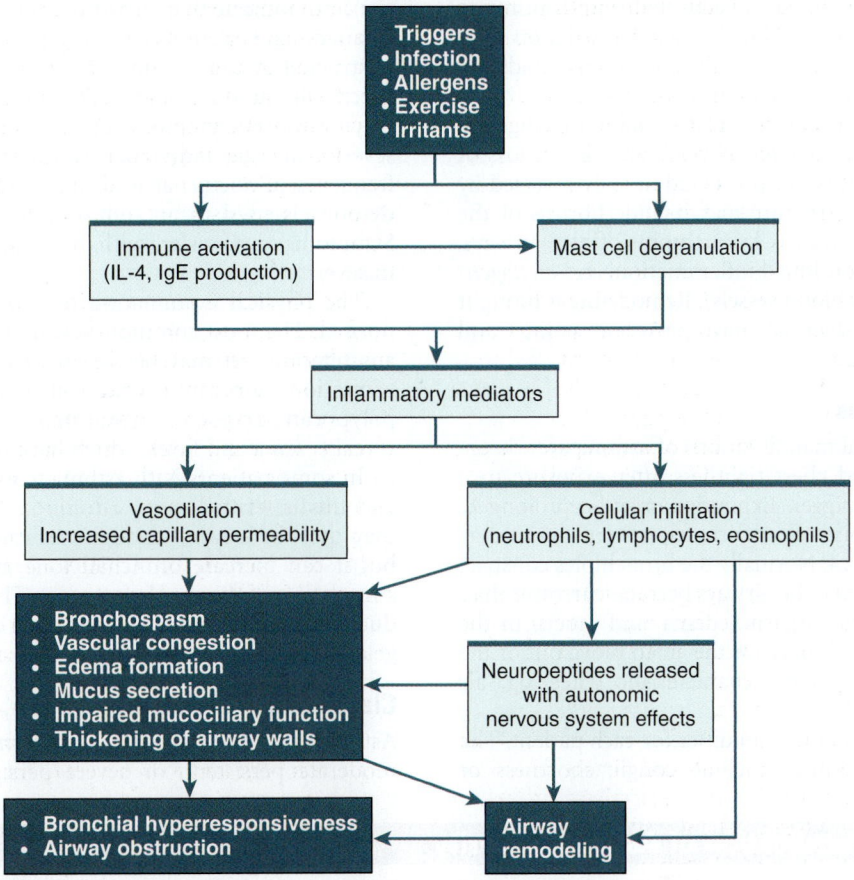

FIG. 28-1 Pathophysiology of asthma. *IL,* Interleukin. (Adapted from McCance KL, Huether SE, editors: *Pathophysiology: the biologic basis for disease in adults and children,* ed 6, St Louis, 2010, Mosby.)

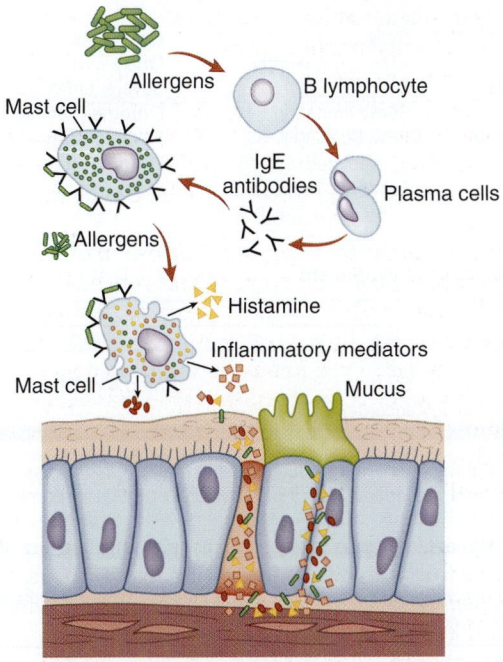

FIG. 28-2 Allergic asthma is triggered when an allergen cross-links IgE receptors on mast cells, which are then activated to release histamine and other inflammatory mediators (early-phase response). A late-phase response may occur due to further inflammation.

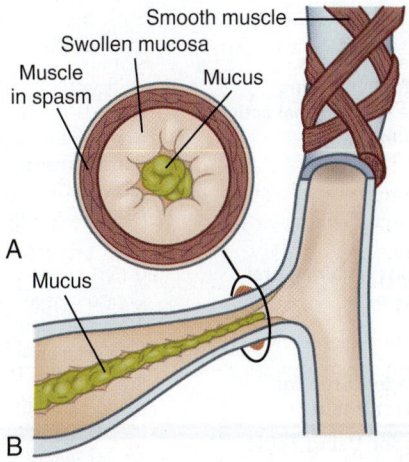

FIG. 28-3 Factors causing obstruction (especially expiratory obstruction) in asthma. **A,** Cross section of a bronchiole occluded by muscle spasm, swollen mucosa, and mucus in the lumen. **B,** Longitudinal section of a bronchiole. (Redrawn from Price SA, Wilson LM: *Pathophysiology: clinical concepts of disease processes,* ed 6, St Louis, 2003, Mosby.)

is called the *late-phase response,* which occurs in about 50% of individuals with asthma. In this late-phase response, more inflammatory cells are recruited and activated, with continuing inflammation of the airways. Thus bronchoconstriction with symptoms persists for 24 hours or more. Corticosteroids are effective in treating this inflammation.

Chronic inflammation may result in structural changes in the bronchial wall known as *remodeling.* A progressive loss of lung function occurs that is not prevented or fully reversed by therapy. The changes in structure may include fibrosis of the subepithelium, smooth muscle hypertrophy of the airways, mucus hypersecretion, continued inflammation, and *angiogenesis* (proliferation of new blood vessels). Remodeling is thought to explain why some individuals have persistent asthma and limited response to therapy.[3,4]

Clinical Manifestations

The characteristic clinical manifestations of asthma are wheezing, cough, dyspnea, and chest tightness after exposure to a precipitating factor or trigger. Expiration may be prolonged. Instead of a normal inspiratory-expiratory ratio of 1:2, it may be prolonged to 1:3 or 1:4. Normally the bronchioles constrict during expiration. However, the airways become narrower than usual as a result of bronchospasm, edema, and mucus in the bronchioles. Thus it takes longer for the air to move out of the bronchioles. This produces the characteristic wheezing, air trapping, and hyperinflation.

Asthma signs and symptoms can differ for each patient. The most common manifestations include cough, shortness of breath (dyspnea), wheezing, chest tightness, and variable airflow obstruction. The presence of any of these (usually in combination) can indicate that an asthma episode or attack is occurring. Changes have taken place to trigger the airways, and airflow is obstructed. A cough, either dry or productive, may be present specifically at night and early morning or after laughing or playing sports. Symptoms are variable both in frequency and severity in each individual asthma patient at any time. The frequency of nocturnal awakenings due to cough, wheezing, or dyspnea is used as an indicator for the severity of asthma. Symptoms can interfere with the patient's ADLs as they increase in severity.

The physical examination in people with asthma is often normal. The most common finding is expiratory wheezing on auscultation but may be absent or only heard during forced expiration. A runny nose, swollen nasal passages, and nasal polyps can be present. An examination of the patient's skin may reveal eczema and hives, which have been linked to asthma.

In some patients with asthma, cough is the only symptom, and this is termed *cough variant asthma.* The bronchospasm may not be severe enough to cause airflow obstruction, but it can increase bronchial tone and cause irritation with stimulation of the cough receptors. The cough may be nonproductive or with secretions, which may be thick, tenacious, white, gelatinous mucus, which makes their removal difficult.

Classification of Asthma

Asthma can be classified as intermittent, mild persistent, moderate persistent, or severe persistent (Table 28-2). The

TABLE 28-2 Classification of Asthma Severity

	ASTHMA SEVERITY			
		PERSISTENT		
Components of Severity	**Intermittent**	**Mild**	**Moderate**	**Severe**
Impairment				
Symptoms	≤2 days/wk	>2 days/wk, not daily	Daily	Continuous
Nighttime awakenings	≤2/mo	3-4/mo	>1/wk, not nightly	Often 7/wk
SABA use for symptoms	≤2 days/wk	>2 days/wk, not daily	Daily	Several times per day
Interference with normal activity	None	Minor limitation	Some limitation	Extremely limited
Lung function*	Normal FEV_1 between exacerbations FEV_1 >80% FEV_1/FVC normal	FEV_1 >80% predicted FEV_1/FVC normal	FEV_1 60%-80% predicted FEV_1/FVC reduced by 5%	FEV_1 <60% predicted FEV_1/FVC reduced by 5%
Risk				
Exacerbations requiring oral corticosteroids	0-1/yr	≥2/yr even in the absence of impairment.		
	Consider severity and interval since last exacerbation. →			
	Frequency and severity may fluctuate over time. →			
	Relative annual risk of exacerbation may be related to FEV_1. →			
Recommended Step for Initiating Treatment	Step 1	Step 2	Step 3†	Step 4 or 5†
	Reevaluate asthma control in 2-6 wk and adjust therapy accordingly.			

Guidelines for Using Table

- Patients should be assigned to the most severe step in which any feature occurs. Clinical features for individual patients may overlap across steps. Determine level of severity by assessment of both impairment and risk. Assess impairment by patient's recall of previous 2- to 4-wk spirometry results.
- An individual's classification should change over time as treatment is initiated. After treatment, the focus switches to the level of control, not the classification of severity.
- Patients at any level of severity of chronic asthma can have mild, moderate, or severe exacerbations of asthma. Some patients with intermittent asthma experience severe and life-threatening exacerbations separated by long periods of normal lung function and no symptoms.

Source: Adapted from National Asthma Education and Prevention Program, National Heart, Lung, and Blood Institute: *Expert Panel Report 3: guidelines for the diagnosis and management of asthma,* NIH pub no 08-4051, Bethesda, Md, 2007, National Institutes of Health. Retrieved from *www.nhlbi.nih.gov/guidelines.*

FEV_1, Forced expiratory volume in 1 sec; *FVC,* forced vital capacity; *SABA,* short-acting β_2-adrenergic agonist.

*Percent predicted values for FEV_1 or ratio of FEV_1/FVC. Normal FEV_1/FVC: 8-19 yr, 85%; 20-39 yr, 80%; 40-59 yr, 75%; 60-80 yr, 70%.

†Consider short-term corticosteroid therapy.

classification system is used to determine the treatment. Patients may move to different asthma classifications over the course of their disease.

Complications

Asthma exacerbations may occur and are classified as mild, moderate, severe, or life-threatening. Asthma is characterized by an unpredictable and variable course, with a person's asthma attacks ranging from seemingly minor interferences in breathing to life-threatening episodes. Depending on an individual's response, asthma can rapidly progress from normal breathing to acute severe or life-threatening asthma.

An attack of asthma may have an abrupt onset, but usually symptoms occur more gradually. Attacks may last for a few minutes to several hours. Between attacks, the patient may be asymptomatic with normal or near-normal spirometry, depending on the severity of disease. However, in some people, compromised pulmonary function (indicated by abnormal spirometry results) may lead to a state of continuous symptoms and chronic debilitation characterized by irreversible airway disease. Acute exacerbations of asthma are discussed in Table 28-7 later in this chapter in the section on Interprofessional Care on p. 546.

Diagnostic Studies

Underdiagnosis of asthma is common. A detailed history is important to determine if a person has had similar attacks, which are often precipitated by a known trigger. (Triggers are discussed on pp. 539-540.) Because wheezing and cough are seen with a variety of disorders (e.g., COPD, GERD, vocal cord dysfunction, heart failure), it is important to determine if asthma is the cause of these problems. (A comparison of asthma and COPD is presented in Table 28-3.)

Numerous tests that are used to diagnose asthma are presented in Table 28-4. In general, the HCP should consider the diagnosis of asthma if various indicators (i.e., clinical manifestations, health history, peak flow variability or spirometry) are positive.

The peak expiratory flow rate (PEFR) measured by the peak flow meter (at home or in a health care setting) is an aid to diagnose and monitor asthma. However, PEFR measurements are not interchangeable with other lung measurements of lung function (e.g., forced expiratory volume in 1 second [FEV_1]). Since types of peak flow meters vary, PEFR should be compared with the patient's own previous best measurements using their own meter.

Spirometry (measured in a health care setting) is usually normal between asthma attacks if the patient has no other underlying pulmonary disease. However, the patient with asthma may show an obstructive pattern including a decrease in forced vital capacity (FVC), FEV_1, PEFR, and FEV_1 to FVC ratio (FEV_1/FVC). (The normal values for spirometry and pulmonary function tests are discussed in Table 25-13 and Chapter 25.)

When spirometry is scheduled, ask the patient to stop taking any bronchodilator medications for 6 to 12 hours before the tests. Spirometry can be done before and after the administration of a bronchodilator to determine the degree of the response. This may help determine reversibility of airway obstruction, which is critical information for diagnosing asthma. A positive response to the bronchodilator is an increase of more than 200 mL and an increase of more than 12% between preadministration and postadministration values.

TABLE 28-3 Comparison of Asthma and COPD*

	Asthma	COPD
Clinical Features		
Age	Usually <40 yr (onset).	Usually 40-50 yr (onset).
Smoking history	Not causal.	Often long history (>10-20 pack-years).
Health and family history	Presence of allergy, rhinitis, eczema. Family history of asthma.	Infrequent allergies. May have exposure to environmental pollutants. With α_1-antitrypsin deficiency, family history of lung or liver disease without smoking history.
Clinical symptoms	Intermittent, vary day to day, worse at night or early morning.	Slowly progressive and persistent.
Dyspnea	Absent except in exacerbations or poor control.	Dyspnea during exercise.
Sputum	Infrequent.	Often.
Disease course	Stable (with exacerbations).	Progressive worsening (with exacerbations).
Diagnostic Study Results		
ABGs	Normal between or during exacerbations.	Between exacerbations in advanced COPD • Often low-normal pH and PaO_2 • High-normal $PaCO_2$ with high HCO_3^- (compensated respiratory acidosis)
pH	↑ Early in exacerbation, then ↓ if prolonged or severe exacerbation.	N→↓
PaO_2	↓	N→↓
$PaCO_2$	↓ Early in exacerbation, then ↑ if prolonged or severe exacerbation.	N→↑
Chest x-ray	May reveal hyperinflation.	Hyperinflation. May have cardiac enlargement, flattened diaphragm.
Lung volumes	Often normalizes.	Never normalizes.
• Total lung capacity	Increased.	Increased.
• Residual volume	Increased.	Increased.
• FEV_1	Decreased or normal.	Decreased.
• FEV_1/FVC	Normal to decreased.	Decreased (<70%).

ABGs, Arterial blood gases; *FEV_1,* forced expiratory volume in 1 sec; *FVC,* forced vital capacity.
*Individuals may have features of both asthma and COPD.

Some patients with symptoms of asthma have normal lung function. During an exacerbation of asthma, lung function parameters fall from their baseline levels.

An elevated serum eosinophil count and elevated serum IgE levels are highly suggestive of *atopy* (genetic predisposition to develop an allergic response), which may be a risk factor for asthma. Allergy skin testing may be of some value to determine sensitivity to specific allergens. However, a positive skin test does not necessarily mean that the allergen is causing the asthma attack. On the other hand, a negative allergy test does not mean that the asthma is not allergy related. (Allergy testing is discussed in Chapter 13.)

A chest x-ray in an asymptomatic patient with asthma is usually normal but can tell if something else (i.e., pneumonia, foreign body in the airway) could be causing symptoms similar to asthma. A routine chest x-ray in a patient with asthma is usually not done unless additional manifestations are present such as fever, chills, or upper airway stridor.

TABLE 28-4 Interprofessional Care

Asthma

Diagnostic Assessment

- History and physical examination
- Spirometry, including response to bronchodilator therapy
- Peak expiratory flow rate (PEFR)
- Chest x-ray
- Measurement of oximetry
- Allergy skin testing (if indicated)
- Blood level of eosinophils and IgE (if indicated)

Management

Intermittent or Persistent Asthma

- Identification and avoidance or elimination of triggers
- Patient and caregiver teaching
- Drug therapy (Tables 28-6 and 28-8 and Fig. 28-4)
- Asthma action plan (Fig. 28-8)
- Desensitization (immunotherapy) if indicated
- Assess for control (e.g., Asthma Control Test [ACT])*

Acute Exacerbations *(Table 28-7)*

- SaO_2 monitoring
- ABGs
- Inhaled β_2-adrenergic agonists
- Inhaled anticholinergics
- O_2 by nasal cannula or mask
- IV or oral corticosteroids
- IV fluids
- IV magnesium
- Intubation and assisted ventilation

ABGs, Arterial blood gases; *IgE,* immunoglobulin E; *SaO_2,* O_2 saturation.
*See *www.asthmacontroltest.com.*

Interprofessional Care

The goal of asthma treatment is to achieve and maintain control of the disease. Once the patient is diagnosed, guidelines provide direction on classification of asthma severity (Table 28-2) and which medications (based on steps 1 through 6) the patient requires (Table 28-5 and Fig. 28-4). The current guidelines focus on (1) assessing the severity of the disease at diagnosis and initial treatment and then (2) monitoring periodically to control the disease.[3,4]

At the initial diagnosis, a patient may have severe asthma and require steps 4 through 6 asthma medication. After treatment, the patient's level of control is assessed (i.e., well controlled, not well controlled, or very poorly controlled; Table 28-5). The HCP steps down the medication as the patient achieves control of the symptoms or steps it up if the symptoms worsen. Achieving rapid control of the symptoms is the goal to return the patient to his or her daily functioning at the best possible level (Fig. 28-4).

Validated questionnaires (e.g., Asthma Control Test [ACT] available at *www.asthmacontroltest.com*) can be used to assess quality-of-life issues in asthma patients. The level of control is determined by the patient's current peak flow or FEV_1. In addition, any exacerbations or adverse effects of treatment will determine the level of control.

Intermittent and Persistent Asthma. The classification of severity of asthma at initial diagnosis helps determine which types of drugs are best suited to control the asthma symptoms (Tables 28-2 and 28-5). Patients in all classifications of asthma require a short-term (rescue or reliever) medication. Short-acting β_2-adrenergic agonists (SABAs) (e.g., albuterol [ProAir HFA, Proventil HFA, Ventolin HFA]) are the most effective class of drugs used as rescue or reliever medications. Patients with persistent asthma must also be on a long-term or controller medication (Table 28-6). Inhaled corticosteroids (ICSs) (e.g., fluticasone [Flovent Diskus or HFA]) are the most effective class of drugs to treat the inflammation. (See later section on drug therapy in this chapter.)

TABLE 28-5 Components of Asthma Control

	CLASSIFICATION OF ASTHMA CONTROL		
Components of Control	**Well Controlled**	**Not Well Controlled**	**Very Poorly Controlled**
Impairment			
Symptoms	≤2 days/wk	>2 days/wk	Throughout the day
Nighttime awakenings	≤2/mo	1-3/wk	≥4/wk
Interference with normal activity	None	Some limitation	Extremely limited
SABA use	≤2 days/wk	>2 days/wk	Several times/day
FEV_1 or peak flow	>80% predicted/personal best	60%-80% predicted/personal best	<60% predicted/personal best
Risk			
Exacerbations requiring oral corticosteroids	0-1/yr	≥2/yr	≥2/yr
Progressive loss of lung function	Consider severity and interval since last exacerbation. →		
Treatment-related adverse effects	Evaluation requires long-term follow-up. →		
	Can vary in intensity from none to very troublesome and worrisome. Level of intensity does not correlate to specific levels of control but should be considered in the overall assessment of risk. →		
Recommended Action for Treatment (Based on assessment of control)	• Maintain current step. • Regular follow-up every 1-6 mo to maintain control • Consider step down if well controlled for at least 3 mo.	• Step up one step. • Reevaluate in 2-6 wk. • For side effects, consider alternative treatment options.	• Consider oral corticosteroids. • Step up one or two steps and reevaluate in 2 wk. • For side effects, consider alternative treatment options.

Source: Adapted from National Asthma Education and Prevention Program, National Heart, Lung, and Blood Institute: *Expert Panel Report 3: guidelines for the diagnosis and management of asthma,* NIH pub no 08-4051, Bethesda, Md, 2007, National Institutes of Health. Retrieved from *www.nhlbi.nih.gov/guidelines.*
FEV_1, Forced expiratory volume in 1 sec; *SABA,* short-acting β_2-adrenergic agonist.

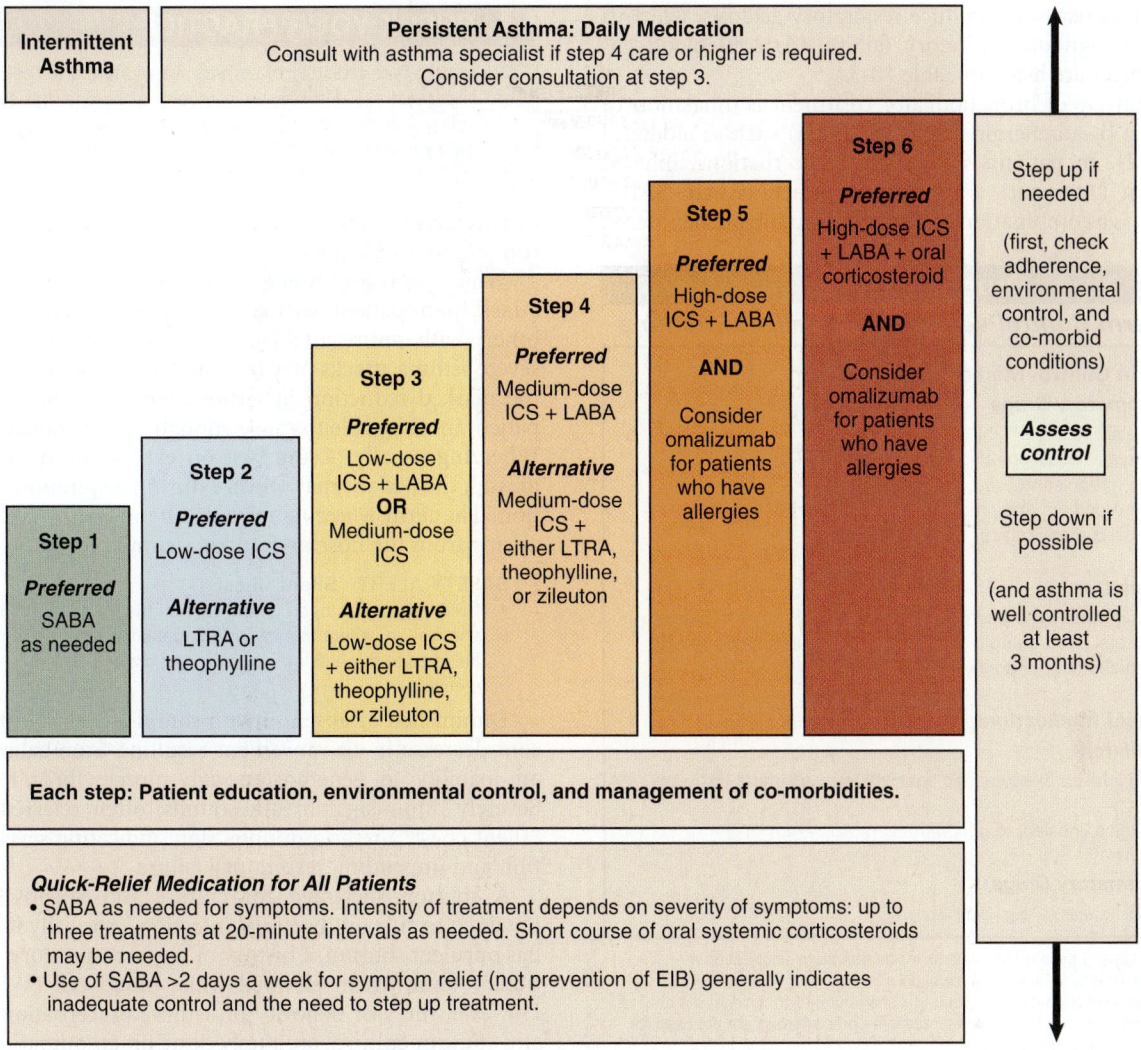

EIB, Exercise-induced bronchospasm; *ICS*, inhaled corticosteroid; *LABA*, long-acting inhaled β_2-agonist; *LTRA*, leukotriene receptor antagonist; *SABA*, short-acting inhaled β_2-agonist.

FIG. 28-4 Drug therapy: stepwise approach for managing asthma. (Modified from *Expert Panel Report 3: Guidelines for the Diagnosis and Management of Asthma.* Bethesda, Md, 2007, National Asthma Education and Prevention Program, National Heart, Lung, and Blood Institute.)

Acute Asthma Exacerbations. Acute asthma exacerbations can be classified as mild, moderate, severe, or life-threatening (Table 28-7). During an acute attack, the person sits forward to maximize the diaphragmatic movement with prominent wheezing, a respiratory rate higher than 30 breaths/minute, and pulse greater than 120 beats/minute. Accessory muscles in the neck are straining to lift the chest wall, and the patient is often agitated (from hypoxemia). Percussion of the lungs indicates hyperresonance. Auscultation of the lungs indicates inspiratory or expiratory wheezing. As the episode resolves, coughing produces thick, stringy mucus.

If a patient has wheezing and acute distress, it is not feasible to obtain a detailed health history (although a family member may supply some pertinent information). Continuous monitoring of the patient is critical. During an acute attack of asthma, bedside PEFR may be used to monitor airflow obstruction. Serial PEFR results, oximetry, and measurement of ABGs provide information about the severity of the attack and the response to therapy. These objective measures more reliably indicate the severity of the exacerbation than symptoms do. A few patients perceive asthma symptoms poorly and may have a significant decrease in lung function without any change in symptoms. Obtaining a PEFR during a severe asthma attack is usually not possible. However, if it can be obtained, and it is less than 200 L/min, it indicates severe obstruction in all but very small adults.

Management of the patient with acute exacerbations focuses on correcting hypoxemia and improving ventilation. O_2 monitoring should be continuous with pulse oximetry. Supplemental O_2 is given by nasal cannula or mask to achieve a PaO_2 of at least 60 mm Hg or O_2 saturation greater than 90%.

Hyperventilation occurs during an asthma attack as lung receptors respond to increased lung volume from trapped air and airflow limitation. Decreased perfusion and ventilation of the alveoli and increased alveolar gas pressure lead to ventilation-perfusion abnormalities in the lungs. The patient is hypoxemic early on with decreased $PaCO_2$ and increased pH (respiratory alkalosis) because he or she is hyperventilating. As the airflow limitation worsens with air trapping, the patient works much harder to breathe. The $PaCO_2$ normalizes as the patient tires, and then it increases to produce respiratory acidosis, which is an ominous sign of respiratory failure. (Arterial blood gas [ABG] changes are listed in Table 28-3.)

The mainstay of bronchodilator treatment is inhalation of short-acting β_2-adrenergic agonists (SABAs) such as albuterol (Table 28-2). In patients with severe exacerbations, inhaled ipratropium (Atrovent) is used in conjunction with SABA. Combivent is a combination of both ipratropium and albuterol.

TABLE 28-6 Drug Therapy

Long-Term Control versus Quick Relief of Asthma

Long-Term Control Medications

Antiinflammatory Drugs

Corticosteroids
- Inhaled (e.g., fluticasone [Flovent Diskus or HFA])
- Oral (e.g., prednisone)

Leukotriene modifiers (e.g., montelukast [Singulair])
Anti-IgE (omalizumab [Xolair])

Bronchodilators

Long-acting inhaled β_2-adrenergic agonists (e.g., salmeterol [Serevent])
Long-acting oral β_2-adrenergic agonists (e.g., albuterol [VoSpire ER])
Methylxanthines (e.g., theophylline [Theo-24])

Quick-Relief Medications

Bronchodilators

Short-acting inhaled β_2-adrenergic agonists (e.g., albuterol [Proventil HFA])
Anticholinergics (inhaled) (e.g., ipratropium [Atrovent HFA])*

Antiinflammatory Drugs

Corticosteroids (systemic) (e.g., prednisone)†

*Used as alternative if patient has intolerable side effects to albuterol or in emergency department for severe exacerbations.
†Considered quick-relief drugs when used in a short burst (3-10 days) at the start of therapy or during a period of gradual deterioration. Corticosteroids are not used for immediate relief of an ongoing attack.

CHECK YOUR PRACTICE

Your patient with a history of asthma was admitted to the ED in acute respiratory distress. He has been receiving therapy and seems to be responding. You notice he is no longer wheezing.
- Should you consider this finding an indication that he is doing better?

Corticosteroids are used for patients who do not initially respond to SABA alone.

Wheezing is an unreliable sign to gauge the severity of an attack. Many patients with minor attacks wheeze loudly, whereas others with severe attacks do not wheeze. The patient with severe asthma attacks may have no audible wheezing because of the marked reduction in airflow. For wheezing to occur, the patient must be able to move enough air to produce the sound. Wheezing usually occurs first on exhalation. As asthma progresses, the patient may wheeze during inspiration and expiration. The term *wheezing* may also be used to describe sounds arising from the nose and upper airways.

SAFETY ALERT Silent Chest
- If the patient has been wheezing and then there is an absence of a wheeze (i.e., silent chest) and the patient is obviously struggling, this is a life-threatening situation that may require mechanical ventilation.

Diminished or absent breath sounds may indicate a significant decrease in air movement resulting from exhaustion and an inability to generate enough muscle force to ventilate. Severely diminished breath sounds, often referred to as the "silent chest," are an ominous sign, indicating severe obstruction and impending respiratory failure.

A sputum specimen for culture and sensitivity may be obtained to rule out bacterial infection, especially if the patient has purulent sputum, a history of upper respiratory tract infection, a fever, or an elevated white blood cell (WBC) count. However, the vast majority of asthma exacerbations are viral, and sputum cultures are rarely done on an outpatient basis.

TABLE 28-7 Classification of Acute Asthma Exacerbations

Degree of Severity	Manifestations	Initial PEF (or FEV_1)	Clinical Course
Mild	Dyspnea occurs with activity and patient may feel that he or she "can't get enough air."	PEF ≥70% of predicted or personal best	• Usually treated at home • Prompt relief with inhaled SABA such as albuterol (delivered via a nebulizer or MDI with a spacer) • Patients instructed to take 2 to 4 puffs albuterol every 20 min three times to gain rapid control of symptoms • Occasionally short course of oral corticosteroids is needed.
Moderate	Dyspnea interferes with or limits usual activities.	PEF 40%-69% of predicted or personal best	• Usually requires office or ED visit • Relief is provided with frequent inhaled SABA. • Oral systemic corticosteroids. (Symptoms may persist for several days even after corticosteroids are started.)
Severe	Dyspnea at rest. Speaks in words, not sentences, because of difficulty of breathing. Feeling of suffocation.	PEF <40% of predicted or personal best	• Usually requires ED visit and likely hospitalization • Partial relief from frequent inhaled SABA • Oral systemic corticosteroids. Some symptoms last for >3 days after treatment is begun. • Adjunctive therapy: ipratropium, IV magnesium
Life-threatening*	Too dyspneic to speak. May be drowsy or confused. Perspiring	PEF <25% predicted or personal best	• Requires ED visit/hospitalization. Possible ICU • Minimal or no relief from frequent inhaled SABA • IV corticosteroids • Adjunctive therapy: ipratropium, IV magnesium

Source: Adapted from National Asthma Education and Prevention Program, National Heart, Lung, and Blood Institute: *Expert Panel Report 3: guidelines for the diagnosis and management of asthma*, NIH pub no 08-4051, Bethesda, Md, 2007, National Institutes of Health. Retrieved from *www.nhlbi.nih.gov/guidelines.*
ED, Emergency department, *FEV_1*, forced expiratory volume; *PEF*, peak expiratory flow.
*May be considered a subset of severe exacerbations

A hand-held, point-of-care device measuring fractional exhaled nitric oxide (FENO) can be used to measure airway inflammation related to asthma. Nitric oxide levels are increased in the breath of people with asthma associated with eosinophilic-induced airway inflammation. FENO may be a used to predict loss of asthma control and exacerbations, to assess a patient's adherence to therapy or to determine if he or she needs more inhaled or oral antiinflammatory medication.[7]

In severe and life-threatening asthma, adjunctive medications such as IV magnesium sulfate may be administered to patients with a very low FEV_1 or peak flow (less than 40% of predicted or personal best) or those who fail to respond to initial treatment. IV magnesium has a bronchodilator effect.

Occasionally, asthma exacerbations are life-threatening, and respiratory arrest is pending or actually occurring. The patient requires intubation and mechanical ventilation if there is no response to treatment. The patient is provided with 100% O_2, hourly or continuously nebulized SABA, IV corticosteroids, and possibly other adjunctive therapies as noted previously.

Antibiotics are not recommended for asthma treatment unless there are signs of pneumonia, fever, and purulent sputum, suggesting bacterial infections. Chest physiotherapy is generally not recommended for asthma because it is too stressful for the breathless patient.

Epinephrine is not routinely indicated for treatment in asthma exacerbations. However, a subcutaneous or IM injection of epinephrine may be indicated for acute treatment of anaphylaxis. If epinephrine is administered, patients need their BP and electrocardiogram (ECG) monitored closely.

Bronchial thermoplasty is a novel approach that may be used in severe asthma along with conventional therapy. A catheter is introduced via fiberoptic bronchoscopy and directly applies heat and reduces the muscle mass in the bronchial wall. This benefits the patient by reversing the accumulation of excessive tissue that is part of the remodeling process that causes narrowing of the airway size and adds to bronchoconstriction.[8]

Drug Therapy

A stepwise approach to drug therapy is based initially on the asthma severity and then on the level of control. Persistent asthma requires daily long-term therapy in addition to appropriate medications to manage acute symptoms. Medications are divided into two general classifications: (1) *quick-relief* or *rescue medications* to treat symptoms and exacerbations, such as SABAs and (2) *long-term control medications* to achieve and maintain control of persistent asthma, such as ICSs (Table 28-6). Some of the controllers are used in combination with long-acting bronchodilators (LABA) to gain better asthma control (Table 28-8).

Antiinflammatory Drugs

Corticosteroids. Chronic inflammation is a primary component of asthma. Corticosteroids are antiinflammatory medications that reduce bronchial hyperresponsiveness, block the late-phase response, and inhibit migration of inflammatory cells. Corticosteroids are more effective in improving asthma control than any other long-term drug. ICSs are first-line therapy for patients with persistent asthma requiring step 2 through 6 therapies (Fig. 28-4). Usually, ICSs must be administered for 1 to 2 weeks before maximum therapeutic effects can be seen. Some ICSs (e.g., fluticasone, budesonide [Pulmicort Flexhaler]) begin to have a therapeutic effect in 24 hours. ICSs must be administered on a fixed schedule.

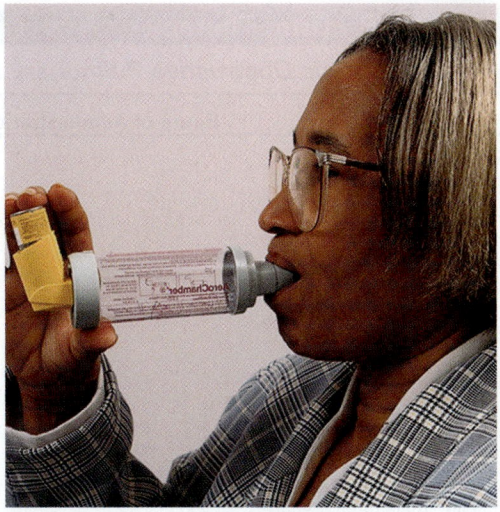

FIG. 28-5 Example of an AeroChamber spacer used with a metered-dose inhaler. (From Potter PA, Perry AG, Stockert P, et al: *Basic nursing: essentials for practice,* ed 7, St. Louis, 2011, Mosby.)

When ICSs are administered, asthma can usually be controlled without significant systemic side effects, since little systemic drug absorption occurs from these drugs. However, ICSs at the highest dosage levels have been associated with side effects (e.g., easy bruising, decreased bone mineral density).[4] Oropharyngeal candidiasis, hoarseness, and dry cough are local side effects caused by inhalation of corticosteroids. These problems can be reduced or prevented by using a spacer (Fig. 28-5) with the MDI and by gargling with water or mouthwash after each use. Using a spacer or holding device for inhalation of corticosteroids can be helpful in getting more medication into the lungs. However, drugs that are activated in the lungs (not the pharynx) (e.g., ciclesonide [Alvesco]) appear to minimize these side effects without the need for a spacer or mouth rinsing.[4]

To gain prompt control, orally administered corticosteroids are used for acute exacerbations of asthma. Maintenance doses of oral corticosteroids may be necessary to control asthma in patients with severe chronic asthma when long-term therapy is required. These patients should be under the care of a specialized pulmonary HCP. (Side effects of long-term corticosteroid therapy are discussed in Chapter 49.)

Women, especially postmenopausal women, who have asthma and who use corticosteroids should take adequate amounts of calcium and vitamin D and participate in regular weight-bearing exercise. (Osteoporosis is discussed in Chapter 63.)

Leukotriene Modifiers. Leukotriene modifiers include leukotriene receptor blockers (antagonists) (zafirlukast [Accolate], montelukast [Singulair]) and leukotriene synthesis inhibitors (zileuton [Zyflo CR]). These drugs interfere with the synthesis or block the action of leukotrienes. Leukotrienes are inflammatory mediators produced from arachidonic acid metabolism (see Fig. 11-2). Leukotrienes are potent bronchoconstrictors, and some also cause airway edema and inflammation, thus contributing to the symptoms of asthma. Because these drugs block the release of some substances from mast cells and eosinophils, they have both bronchodilator and antiinflammatory effects.

These drugs are not indicated for use in the reversal of bronchospasm in acute asthma attacks. They are used for

TABLE 28-8 Drug Therapy

Asthma and Chronic Obstructive Pulmonary Disease (COPD)

Drug	Route of Administration	Comments†
Corticosteroids		
hydrocortisone (Solu-Cortef)	IV	Alternate-day therapy minimizes side effects. Oral dose should be taken in morning with food or milk. When given in high dosages, observe for epigastric distress. Long-term corticosteroid therapy requires supplementation with vitamin D and calcium to prevent osteoporosis. Discontinue gradually over time to prevent adrenal insufficiency. If symptoms recur during tapering, notify HCP.
methylprednisolone (Medrol, Solu-Medrol)	Oral, IV	
prednisone	Oral	
fluticasone (Flovent HFA, Flovent Diskus, Arnuity Ellipta)	MDI, DPI	Not recommended for acute asthma attack. Rinse mouth with water or mouthwash after use to prevent oral fungal infections. Use of spacer device with MDI may decrease incidence of oral candidiasis. With ICSs, may not see effects until after at least 2 wk of regular treatment
beclomethasone (Qvar)	MDI	Same as fluticasone except less oral candidiasis because of very small particle size, which is deposited deeper in the airways
budesonide (Pulmicort Flexhaler)	DPI	Same as above
mometasone (Asmanex Twisthaler)	DPI	Same as above
ciclesonide (Alvesco)	MDI	Oral candidiasis and other localized oropharyngeal effects (e.g., hoarseness). Fewer side effects than other ICSs because of small particle size with minimal activation in oropharynx
Phosphodiesterase Inhibitor Type 4 (PDE-4)		
roflumilast (Daliresp)	Oral	Only used in severe COPD to reduce exacerbation frequency. Not to be used for acute bronchospasm. GI symptoms occur within 6 mo of initiating medication. Patients to report any psychiatric symptoms (e.g., anxiety, depression, suicidal thoughts). Not to be used with theophylline
Anticholinergics		
Short Acting (SAMA)*		
ipratropium (Atrovent HFA)	Nebulizer, MDI	Approved for COPD. May provide additive benefit to SABA in moderate to severe asthma exacerbations (used in emergency department with no benefit beyond that). Use in asthma as alternative for patients with intolerable side effects with SABA. Temporary blurred vision if sprayed in eyes. Use cautiously in patients with narrow-angle glaucoma or prostatic enlargement.
Long Acting (LAMA)*		
tiotropium (Spiriva HandiHaler)	DPI	Only approved for COPD. Blurred vision if powder comes in contact with eyes. Must discontinue use of ipratropium while on tiotropium. Patients with COPD must use SABA or short-acting anticholinergics for quick-relief medication. Maximum effect 1 wk after initiation of drug. Dosed once daily
aclidinium bromide (Tudorza, Pressair)	DPI	Only approved for COPD. Do not administer with other anticholinergics. Not for acute relief of bronchospasm. Dosed twice daily
umeclidinium (Incruse Ellipta)	DPI	Only approved for COPD. Used once daily as maintenance treatment of airflow obstruction
Monoclonal Antibodies		
Anti-IgE		
omalizumab (Xolair)	Subcutaneous	Only for moderate to severe, persistent, allergic asthma with symptoms not adequately controlled by ICSs. Not for acute bronchospasm. Administer only under direct medical supervision biweekly or monthly, depending on IgE levels and weight, and observe patient for a minimum of 2 hr after administration because anaphylaxis has been reported with use.
Anti-Interleukin 5		
mepolizumab (Nucala)	Subcutaneous	Only used for maintenance in patients with severe asthma attacks despite receiving current asthma medications. Administered once every 4 wk by health care professional
reslizumab (Cinqair)	IV only	
Leukotriene Modifiers		
Leukotriene Receptor Blocker		
zafirlukast (Accolate)	Oral tablets	Take at least 1 hr before or 2 hr after meals. Affects metabolism of erythromycin and theophylline. Not used to treat acute asthma episodes
montelukast (Singulair)	Oral tablets, chewable tablets, oral granules	Not used to treat acute asthma episodes
Leukotriene Inhibitor		
zileuton (Zyflo, Zyflo CR)	Oral tablets	Monitor liver enzymes. May interfere with metabolism of warfarin (Coumadin) and theophylline. Not used to treat acute asthma episodes

*Anticholinergics are muscarinic antagonists. Thus the abbreviations short-acting muscarinic antagonist (SAMA) and long-acting muscarinic antagonist (LAMA).

TABLE 28-8 Drug Therapy

Asthma and Chronic Obstructive Pulmonary Disease (COPD)—cont'd

Drug	Route of Administration	Comments†
β_2-Adrenergic Agonists		
Inhaled: Short Acting (SABA)		
albuterol (Proventil HFA, Ventolin HFA, ProAir HFA, AccuNeb, VoSpire ER [oral only])	Nebulizer, MDI, oral tablets, including extended release NOTE: Oral tablets not for acute use, only long acting	Use with caution in patients with cardiac disorders because β-agonists may cause ↑ BP and heart rate, CNS stimulation/excitation, and ↑ risk of dysrhythmias. Has rapid onset of action (1-3 min). Duration of action is 4-8 hr. Ventolin HFA is the only albuterol MDI with a counter.
levalbuterol (Xopenex, Xopenex HFA)	Nebulizer, MDI	Too frequent use can result in loss of effectiveness. Efficacy no better than other SABA
Inhaled: Long Acting (LABA)	*In asthma:* Never use as monotherapy. Use in combination with ICSs. *In COPD:* Can be used as monotherapy. Not used for rapid relief of dyspnea	
salmeterol (Serevent Diskus)	DPI	Not to exceed 2 puffs q12hr. Not used for acute exacerbations. Has a counter
formoterol (Foradil Aerolizer, Perforomist)	DPI, nebulizer (Perforomist)	Can affect blood glucose levels. Use with caution in patients with diabetes.
arformoterol (Brovana)	Nebulizer	See formoterol. For chronic COPD use
indacaterol (Arcapta Neohaler)	DPI	Only once-daily LABA. For chronic COPD use. Not intended to treat asthma
olodaterol (Striverdi Respimat)	MDI	2 puffs daily. Less expensive than other LABAs
Methylxanthines		
IV agent: aminophylline (second-line therapy) *Oral:* theophylline	Oral tablets, IV, elixir, sustained-release tablets	Wide variety of response to drug metabolism exists. Half-life is ↓ by smoking and ↑ by heart failure and liver disease. Cimetidine, ciprofloxacin, erythromycin, and other drugs may rapidly ↑ theophylline levels. Taking drug with food or antacids may help GI effects. Use usually limited to situations when other long-term bronchodilation not available or not affordable
Combination Agents		**Also see each component of medications for SE.**
SAMA/SABA		
ipratropium/albuterol (Combivent Respimat, DuoNeb)	Nebulizer (DuoNeb), inhalation spray (Combivent Respimat)	Patients must be careful not to overuse. Respimat is an inhaler, but propellant free, unlike an MDI. Respimat is independent of inspiratory flow. Has dose indicator
ICS/LABA		
fluticasone/salmeterol (Advair Diskus or HFA)	DPI, MDI	See salmeterol and fluticasone. Has a counter. Comes in three different strengths
budesonide/formoterol (Symbicort)	MDI	See budesonide and formoterol. Has a counter
mometasone furoate/formoterol fumarate (Dulera)	MDI	Not for relief of acute bronchospasm
fluticasone/vilanterol (Breo Ellipta)	DPI	Dose once daily.
LAMA/LABA		
umeclidinium/vilanterol (Anoro Ellipta)	DPI	Anticholinergic/LABA for COPD. Not for relief of acute bronchospasm

DPI, Dry powder inhaler; *HFA,* hydrofluoroalkane (propellant); *ICSs,* inhaled corticosteroids; *MDI,* metered-dose inhaler.
†For patient instructions in English and Spanish for the devices, see *www.chestnet.org/accp/patient-guides/patient-instructions-inhaled-devices-english-and-spanish.*

prophylactic and maintenance therapy. One advantage of leukotriene modifiers is that they are administered orally.

Anti-IgE. Omalizumab (Xolair) is a monoclonal antibody to IgE that decreases circulating free IgE levels. Omalizumab prevents IgE from attaching to mast cells, thus preventing the release of chemical mediators. This drug is indicated for patients with moderate to severe persistent, allergic asthma, or those requiring step 5 or 6 care with persistent asthma that cannot be controlled with ICSs. Omalizumab is administered subcutaneously every 2 to 4 weeks. The drug has a risk of anaphylaxis, and patients must receive the medication in an HCP's office, where this potential emergency problem can be handled.

Anti-Interleukin 5. Mepolizumab (Nucala) and reslizumab (Cinqair) are monoclonal antibodies to interleukin-5 (IL-5). IL-5 is a major cytokine involved in the inflammatory response in asthma by promoting eosinophil activity. By inhibiting IL-5, these drugs inhibit the production and survival of eosinophils. They are used for patients who have a history of severe asthma attacks despite using current asthma medication.

Bronchodilators. Three classes of bronchodilator drugs currently used in asthma therapy are β_2-adrenergic agonists (also referred to as β_2-agonists), methylxanthines and derivatives, and anticholinergics (Table 28-8).

β_2-Adrenergic Agonist Drugs. These drugs may be short-acting β_2-adrenergic agonists (SABAs) or long-acting β_2-adrenergic agonists (LABAs). Because inhaled SABAs are the most effective drugs for relieving acute bronchospasm (as seen in acute exacerbations of asthma), they are known as *rescue medications.* These drugs have an onset of action within minutes and are effective for 4 to 8 hours. These drugs act by stimulating β-adrenergic receptors in the bronchioles, thus producing bronchodilation. They also increase mucociliary clearance.

DRUG ALERT β_2-Adrenergic Agonists

- Use with caution in patients with cardiac disorders, since both SABAs and LABAs may cause elevated BP and heart rate, central nervous system stimulation or excitation, and increased risk of dysrhythmias.
- Any MDI is only effective if taken properly. Review MDI technique during each visit as a standard component of care (Fig. 28-6).

β_2-Adrenergic agonists are also useful in preventing bronchospasm precipitated by exercise and other stimuli because they prevent the release of inflammatory mediators from mast

Using an inhaler seems simple, but most patients do not use it the right way. When you use your inhaler the wrong way, less medicine gets to your lungs. (Your physician may give you other types of inhalers.)

For the next 2 weeks, read these steps aloud as you do them or ask someone to read them to you. Ask your physician or nurse to check how well you are using your inhaler.

Use your inhaler in one of the three ways pictured below (**A** or **B** is best, but **C** can be used if you have trouble with **A** or **B**).

Steps for Using Your Inhaler

Getting ready
1. Take off the cap and shake the inhaler.
2. Breathe out all the way.
3. Hold your inhaler the way your doctor said (**A, B,** or **C** below).

Breathe in slowly
4. As you start breathing in **slowly** through your mouth, press down on the inhaler **one** time. (If you use a holding chamber, first press down on the inhaler. Within 5 seconds, begin to breathe in slowly.)
5. Keep breathing in **slowly,** as deeply as you can.

Hold your breath
6. Hold your breath as you count to 10 slowly, if you can.
7. For inhaled quick-relief medicine (β_2-agonists), wait about 1 minute between puffs. There is no need to wait between puffs for other medicines.

A. Hold inhaler 1 to 2 inches in front of your mouth (about the width of two fingers).

B. Use a spacer/holding chamber. These come in many shapes and can be useful to any patient.

C. Put the inhaler in your mouth.

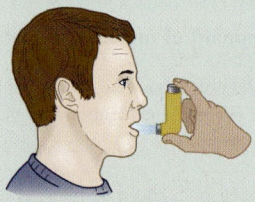

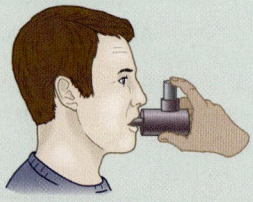

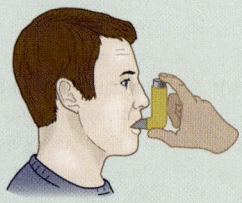

Clean Your Inhaler as Needed

Look at the hole where the medicine sprays out from your inhaler. If you see "powder" in or around the hole, clean the inhaler. Remove the metal canister from the L-shaped plastic mouthpiece. Rinse only the mouthpiece and cap in warm water. Let them dry overnight. In the morning, put the canister back inside. Put the cap on.

Know When to Replace Your Inhaler

For medicines you take each day (an example): Say your new canister has 200 puffs (number of puffs is listed on canister) and you are told to take 8 puffs per day.

$$8 \text{ puffs per day} \overline{)\,200 \text{ puffs in canister}} \quad 25 \text{ days}$$

So this canister will last 25 days. If you started using this inhaler on May 1, replace it on or before May 25. You can write the date on your canister.

For **quick-relief medicine take as needed** and count each puff.

Do not put your canister in water to see if it is empty as water may enter MDI and impair inhaler.

FIG. 28-6 How to use your metered-dose inhaler correctly.

cells. They do not inhibit the late-phase response of asthma or have antiinflammatory effects. If used frequently, inhaled β_2-adrenergic agonists may produce tremors, anxiety, tachycardia, palpitations, and nausea.

Too frequent use of β_2-adrenergic agonists indicates poor asthma control, may mask asthma severity, and may lead to reduced drug effectiveness. The use of SABAs should be limited to less than two times weekly. In other words, regularly scheduled, daily, or chronic use of inhaled SABA is not recommended for long-term control of asthma. SABA inhalers should last for months. Use of long-term bronchodilators with inhaled corticosteroids or other medications can achieve this goal if prescribed and used properly. In summary, SABAs are not used for long-term control, and they should not be used alone for persistent asthma.

LABAs, including salmeterol (Serevent Diskus) and formoterol (Foradil), are effective for 12 hours. LABAs are added to a daily dose of ICSs for long-term control of moderate to severe persistent asthma (i.e., step 3 or higher for long-term control; see Fig. 28-4) and prevention of symptoms, particularly at night. When LABAs are added to a patient's daily regimen of corticosteroids, they decrease the need for SABAs and allow patients to achieve better asthma control with a lower dosage of ICSs.

LABAs should never be used as monotherapy for asthma and should only be used if the patient is on ICS. Tell patients that these drugs should not be used to treat acute symptoms or to obtain quick relief from bronchospasm. Teach the patient that these drugs are used only once every 12 hours.

DRUG ALERT Long-Acting β_2-Adrenergic Agonists (LABAs)

- Should not be the first medicine used to treat asthma
- Should never be used as the only medication to treat asthma but should be added to the treatment plan only if other controller medicines do not control asthma
- Should not be used to treat wheezing that is getting worse
- Always use an SABA to treat sudden wheezing.

Combination therapy using an ICS and LABA is available in several inhalers (e.g., fluticasone/salmeterol [Advair] and budesonide/formoterol [Symbicort]). The combinations are more convenient, improve adherence, and ensure that patients receive the LABA together with an ICS.

Methylxanthines. Sustained-release methylxanthine (theophylline) preparations are not a first-line controller medication. They are used only as an alternative therapy for step 2 care in mild persistent asthma. Methylxanthine is a bronchodilator with mild antiinflammatory effects, but the exact mechanism of action is unknown.

DRUG ALERT Theophylline

- Instruct patient to report signs of toxicity: nausea, vomiting, seizures, insomnia.
- Avoid caffeine to prevent intensifying adverse effects.

The main problems with theophylline are the relatively high incidence of interaction with other drugs and the side effects, which include nausea, headache, insomnia, gastrointestinal distress, tachycardia, dysrhythmias, and seizures. Because theophylline has a narrow margin of safety, monitor serum blood levels regularly to determine if the drug is within therapeutic range.

Anticholinergic Drugs. Anticholinergic drugs are another group of bronchodilators that are different from SABA. β-agonists affect the bronchioles (small airways), whereas anticholinergics affect the muscles around the bronchi (large airways). When the lungs are irritated, these bands of muscle can tighten, causing bronchoconstriction via the parasympathetic nervous system. Anticholinergics work by preventing these muscles from tightening. Thus these drugs promote bronchodilation.

Anticholinergic drugs are less effective than equivalent doses of SABAs in asthma. However, they are more effective in COPD patients. Therefore short-acting anticholinergic drugs are not used in the routine management of asthma, except for the management of severe acute asthma exacerbations.

Inhalation Devices for Drug Delivery. The multiple devices for asthma drug administration can be confusing. The majority of asthma drugs are administered only or preferably by inhalation because systemic side effects are reduced and the onset of action is faster. Inhalation devices include metered-dose inhalers (MDIs), dry powder inhalers (DPIs), and nebulizers.

Inhalers. MDIs are small, hand-held, pressurized devices that deliver a measured dose of drug with each activation. Dosing is usually accomplished with one or two puffs. Depending on the specific MDI, a spacer or holding chamber (e.g., AeroChamber or InspirEase [Fig. 28-5]) is used to reduce the amount of drug delivered to the oropharynx and improve the amount of drug delivered to the lungs. In addition, spacers assist people who have hand-breath coordination problems.

All MDIs are mandated by international law to have an ozone-friendly propellant, which is a hydrofluoroalkane (HFA). This propellant is nontoxic, evaporates almost instantly once it forces medicine out of the MDI canister, and is not harmful to the patient. The number of times an MDI must be primed and the frequency of priming vary widely, so read the package insert with the patient.

The MDI should be cleaned by removing the dust cap and rinsing the holder (not the medication chamber) in warm water at least two times per week (Fig. 28-6). The patient who needs to use several MDIs is often unclear about the order in which to take the medications. Historically it had been recommended that SABAs should be used first to open up the airway and improve the delivery of subsequent medications. However, this technique is not evidence based. It is a potential source of confusion to patients because the SABAs are usually used on an as-needed (PRN) basis.

One of the major problems with metered-dose drugs is the potential for overuse (more than two canisters per month) rather than seeking needed medical care (Table 28-9). As a patient develops additional asthmatic symptoms, he or she may use the β_2-adrenergic agonist MDI repeatedly. β_2-Adrenergic agonists help by relieving bronchospasm. They do not treat the inflammatory response. Therefore teach the patient the correct therapeutic use of these drugs. The patient also needs to know the correct way to determine whether the MDI is empty (Fig. 28-6).

DPIs are simpler to use than MDIs (Fig. 28-7 and Table 28-10). The DPI contains dry, powdered medication and is breath activated. No propellant is used. Instead, an aerosol is created when the patient inhales through a reservoir containing a dose of powder. The convenient-to-carry diskus has several advantages over MDIs: (1) less manual dexterity is needed, (2) there is no need to coordinate device puffs with inhalation, and (3) no spacer is required. Disadvantages are that some commonly prescribed drugs are not yet available in DPIs, and the medication may clump if exposed to humidity. Since the medicine is delivered only by the patient's inspiratory effort, patients with a low FEV_1 (less than 1 L) may not be able to inspire the medication adequately.

Differences between MDIs and DPIs are presented in Table 28-11. Aerosolized medication delivery systems, when used with comparable drug doses, provide equivalent efficacy. Therefore patients should use the device best suited to their needs.

Nebulizers. Nebulizers are small machines used to convert drug solutions into mists. The mist can be inhaled through a face mask or mouthpiece held between the teeth. Nebulizers are

INFORMATICS IN PRACTICE

Home Monitoring of Asthma

- To reduce the rate of readmission to hospital, the patient with asthma may be discharged with a home monitoring system. These systems provide an easy and inexpensive approach to remotely monitoring patients' lung functions.
- Asthma home monitoring usually consists of peak flow rate, pulse oximetry, vital signs, and lung sounds. This information is sent to the HCP so that problems are quickly detected.
- As part of your discharge planning, assist the patient with receiving a system and reviewing its proper use.

TABLE 28-9 Problems Using a Metered-Dose Inhaler (MDI)

- Failing to coordinate activation with inspiration
- Activating MDI in the mouth while breathing through nose
- Inspiring too rapidly
- Not holding the breath for 10 sec (or as close to 10 sec as possible)
- Holding MDI upside down or sideways
- Inhaling more than 1 puff with each inspiration
- Not shaking MDI before use (if indicated)
- Not waiting a sufficient amount of time between each puff
- Not opening mouth wide enough (if using open mouth technique), causing medication to bounce off teeth, tongue, or palate
- Not having adequate strength to activate MDI
- Being unable to understand and follow directions

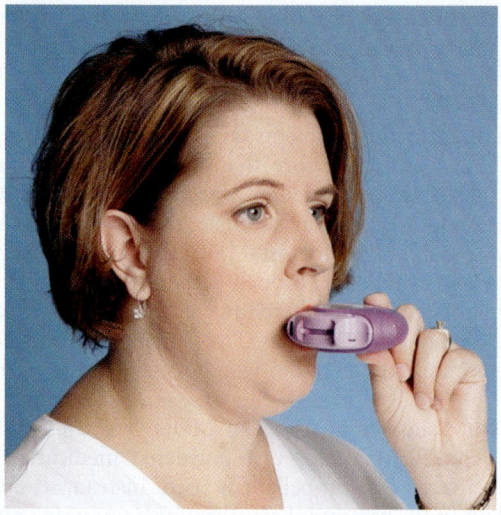

FIG. 28-7 Example of a dry powder inhaler (DPI). (From Potter PA, Perry AG, Stockert P, et al: *Basic nursing: essentials for practice,* ed 7, St. Louis, 2011, Mosby.)

TABLE 28-10 Patient Teaching

How to Use a Dry Powder Inhaler (DPI)

Include the following instructions when teaching a patient to use a DPI.

1. Remove mouthpiece cap or open the device according to manufacturer's instructions. Check for dust or dirt. If there is an external counter, note the number of doses remaining.
2. Load the medicine into the inhaler or engage the lever to allow the medicine to become available. Some DPIs should be held upright while loading. Others should be held sideways or in a horizontal position.
3. Do not shake your medicine.
4. Tilt your head back slightly and breathe out, getting as much air out of your lungs as you can. Do not breathe into your inhaler because this could affect the dose.
5. Close your lips tightly around the mouthpiece of the inhaler.
6. Breathe in deeply and quickly. This will ensure that the medicine moves down deeply into your lungs. You may not taste or sense the medicine going into your lungs.
7. Hold your breath for 10 seconds or as long as you can to disperse the medicine into your lungs.
8. If there is an external counter, note the number of doses remaining. It should be one less than the number in step 1 above.
9. Do not keep your DPI in a humid place such as a shower room because the medicine may clump.

usually used for individuals who have severe asthma or difficulty with the MDI inhalation since they do not provide better delivery of medication than a spacer with an inhaler.

Nebulizers are usually powered by a compressed air or O_2 generator. At home, the patient may have an air-powered compressor. In the hospital, wall O_2 or compressed air is used to power the nebulizer.

Aerosolized medication orders must include the medication, dose, diluent, and whether it is to be nebulized with O_2 or compressed air. The advantage of nebulization therapy is that it is easy to use. Medications that are routinely nebulized include albuterol and ipratropium.

The patient is placed in an upright position that allows for most efficient breathing to ensure adequate penetration and deposition of the aerosolized medication. The patient must breathe slowly and deeply through the mouth and hold

TABLE 28-11 Comparison of Metered-Dose and Dry Powder Inhalers

	Metered-Dose Inhaler (MDI)*	Dry Powder Inhaler (DPI)
Shake before use	May be needed for some (e.g., albuterol), but not for others (Read package insert)	No
Inspiration	Slow	Rapid
Spacer	May be used with inhaled corticosteroids or for more effective delivery (Read package insert)	None permitted
Counting device	Many have an external device, but some do not	Most preloaded forms include counter
Inhalations/dose	Often 2/dose	Often 1/dose
Cleaning	Use water for plastic case	Avoid moisture

For additional information, see National Jewish Hospital: *Instructions for Inhaler and Spacer Use Videos for various devices.* Available at *www.nationaljewish.org/healthinfo/medications/lung-diseases/devices/instructional-videos.*
*MDIs use hydrofluoroalkane (HFA) as a propellant.

inspirations for 2 or 3 seconds. Deep diaphragmatic breathing helps ensure deposition of the medication. Instruct the patient to breathe normally in between these large forced breaths to prevent alveolar hypoventilation and dizziness. After the treatment instruct the patient to cough effectively.

A disadvantage of nebulizer equipment use is the potential for bacterial growth. Review cleaning procedures for home respiratory equipment with the patient. A frequently used, effective home-cleaning method is to wash the nebulizer daily in soap and water, rinse it with water, and soak it for 20 to 30 minutes in a 1:1 white vinegar–water solution, followed by a water rinse and air drying.

Patient Teaching Related to Drug Therapy. When teaching patients about their medications, include the name, purpose, dosage, method of administration, and schedule. Take into consideration the patient's activities of daily living (ADLs) that require energy expenditure and thus O_2 (e.g., bathing). Teach about side effects, appropriate action if side effects occur, how to properly use and clean devices, how to prime and the frequency, and consequences of not taking medications as prescribed. One of the major factors determining success in asthma management is the correct administration of drugs.

Several factors can affect the correct use of inhalation devices. These include advanced age, alterations in physical dexterity (e.g., arthritis in hands, coordination), psychologic state (e.g., cognition), affordability, convenience, and administration time and preference.[7]

Poor adherence with asthma therapy is a major challenge in the long-term management of chronic asthma. Lack of adherence often occurs in chronic asthma because the patient is symptom free and does not use the long-term therapy (e.g., ICS) regularly because no immediate benefit is felt. The patient does not realize that ICSs are needed to treat the ongoing inflammatory process.

Explain the importance and purpose of taking the long-term therapy regularly, emphasizing that maximum improvement may take longer than 1 week. Tell the patient that, without regular use, the swelling in the airways may progress and the asthma will likely worsen over time. Become familiar with the vast array of compassionate-use programs offered by pharmaceutical companies to help lower-income patients obtain medications (e.g., *www.needymeds.com*).

Make sure that patients understand exactly how to use their inhaler device, and give them printed instructions. At every clinic visit or hospitalization, reassess the patient's inhaler technique. If package inserts are available, you can review them before teaching the patient. Drug company websites have numerous excellent teaching videos available.

Nonprescription Combination Drugs. Several nonprescription combination drugs are available OTC. They are usually combinations of a bronchodilator (ephedrine) and an expectorant (guaifenesin). Inhalers containing epinephrine may be available.[9] These agents are advertised as medications to relieve bronchospasm. Often patients seek OTC drugs because they are less expensive than prescription medication. Many people consider these drugs safe because they can be obtained without a prescription. In general, they should be avoided due to their potential side effects.

Drugs containing ephedrine and epinephrine are dangerous because they stimulate the central nervous and cardiovascular systems, causing nervousness, heart palpitations and dysrhythmias, tremors, insomnia, and increases in BP. Many respiratory products containing ephedrine are located behind the counter at pharmacies or require a prescription. This limited access is to prevent the diversion of ephedrine to the production of methamphetamine. Also many of the OTC products have been reformulated with phenylephrine, instead of ephedrine, which works well topically but has modest effects in the oral form.

An important teaching responsibility is to warn patients about the dangers associated with nonprescription combination drugs. These drugs are especially dangerous to a patient with underlying cardiac problems because elevated BP and tachycardia often occur. Caution the patient who persists in taking these medications to read and follow the directions on the label.

❖ NURSING MANAGEMENT: ASTHMA

◆ Nursing Assessment

If a patient is not in acute distress, take a detailed health history, including information about precipitating factors and what has helped alleviate asthma attacks in the past. When completing the health history, ask about specific herbs or supplements that a patient may be using.

Subjective and objective data that should be obtained from a patient with asthma are presented in Table 28-12. You may also assess the patient's asthma control using one of the validated self-administered questionnaires (e.g., ACT).

◆ Nursing Diagnoses

Nursing diagnoses for the patient with asthma may include, but are not limited to, the following:

- Ineffective airway clearance *related to* bronchospasm, excessive mucus production, tenacious secretions, and fatigue
- Anxiety *related to* difficulty breathing, perceived or actual loss of control, and fear of suffocation
- Deficient knowledge *related to* lack of information and education about asthma and its treatment

Additional information on nursing diagnoses is presented in eNursing Care Plan 28-1 on the website for this chapter.

TABLE 28-12 Nursing Assessment

Asthma

Subjective Data

Important Health Information

Past health history: Allergic rhinitis, sinusitis, or skin allergies. Previous asthma attack and hospitalization or intubation. Symptoms worsened by triggers in the environment. Gastroesophageal reflux disease (GERD). Occupational exposure to chemical irritants (e.g., paints, dust)

Medications: Adherence to medication, inhaler technique. Use of antibiotics. Pattern and amount of short-acting β_2-adrenergic agonist used per week. Medications that may precipitate an attack in susceptible asthmatics such as aspirin, nonsteroidal antiinflammatory drugs, β-adrenergic blockers

Functional Health Patterns

Health perception–health management: Family history of allergies or asthma. Recent upper respiratory tract or sinus infection

Activity-exercise: Fatigue, decreased or absent exercise tolerance. Dyspnea, cough (especially at night), productive cough with yellow or green sputum or sticky sputum. Chest tightness, feelings of suffocation, air hunger, talking in short sentences or words or phrases, sitting upright to breathe

Sleep-rest: Awakened from sleep because of cough or breathing difficulties, insomnia

Coping–stress tolerance: Emotional distress, stress in work environment or home

Objective Data

General

Restlessness or exhaustion, confusion, upright or forward-leaning body position

Integumentary

Diaphoresis, cyanosis (circumoral, nail bed), eczema

Respiratory

Nasal discharge, nasal polyps, mucosal swelling. Crackles, diminished or absent breath sounds, and wheezes on auscultation. Hyperresonance on percussion. Sputum (thick, white, tenacious), ↑ work of breathing with use of accessory muscles. Intercostal and supraclavicular retractions. Tachypnea with hyperventilation. Prolonged expiration

Cardiovascular

Tachycardia, pulsus paradoxus, jugular venous distention, hypertension or hypotension, premature ventricular contractions

Possible Diagnostic Findings

Abnormal ABGs during attacks, ↓ O_2 saturation, serum and sputum eosinophilia, ↑ serum IgE, positive skin tests for allergens, chest x-ray demonstrating hyperinflation with attacks, abnormal pulmonary function tests showing ↓ flow rates; FVC, FEV_1, PEFR, and FEV_1/FVC ratio that improve between attacks and with bronchodilators

ABGs, Arterial blood gases; *FEV_1,* forced expiratory volume in 1 sec; *FVC,* forced vital capacity; *IgE,* immunoglobulin E; *PEFR,* peak expiratory flow rate.

◆ Planning

The overall goals are that the patient with asthma will have asthma control as evidenced by (1) minimal symptoms during the day and night, (2) acceptable activity levels (including exercise and other physical activity), (3) maintenance of greater than 80% of personal best PEFR, (4) few or no adverse effects of therapy, (5) no acute exacerbations of asthma, and

(6) adequate knowledge to participate in and carry out the plan of care.

Nursing Implementation

Health Promotion. Your role in preventing asthma attacks or decreasing their severity focuses primarily on teaching the patient and caregiver. Teach the patient to identify and avoid known personal triggers for asthma (e.g., cigarette smoke, pet dander) and irritants (e.g., cold air, aspirin, foods, cats, indoor air pollution) (Table 28-1). Washing bedclothes in hot water or cooler water with detergent and bleach has some effect on allergen levels. Avoidance of furred animals is suggested, but pet allergens are nearly impossible to avoid. Pet allergens can be found in many public areas for months even after removal of the animal. Many people are allergic to cockroach remains and the dried droppings, so measures to avoid or control cockroaches are partly effective in removing allergens.

If cold air cannot be avoided, dressing properly with scarves or using a mask helps reduce the risk of an asthma attack. Aspirin and NSAIDs should be avoided if they are known to precipitate an attack. Many OTC drugs contain aspirin. Therefore teach the patient to read the labels carefully. Nonselective β-blockers (e.g., propranolol [Inderal]) are contraindicated because they inhibit bronchodilation. Selective β-blockers (e.g., atenolol [Tenormin]) should be used with caution. Desensitization (immunotherapy) may be partially effective in decreasing the patient's sensitivity to known allergens (see Chapter 13).

Prompt diagnosis and treatment of upper respiratory tract infections and sinusitis may prevent an asthma exacerbation. If occupational irritants are involved as etiologic factors of asthma, the patient may need to consider changing jobs. Individuals who are obese often find that weight loss improves control of asthma. Encourage the patient to maintain a fluid intake of 2 to 3 L/day, good nutrition, and adequate rest. If exercise is planned or if the patient has asthma only with exercise, the HCP can suggest a medication regimen for pretreatment or long-term control of symptoms to prevent bronchospasm.

Acute Care. A goal in asthma care is to maximize the patient's ability to safely manage acute asthma using an asthma action plan developed in conjunction with the HCP (Fig. 28-8). Action plans are particularly important for individuals with moderate to severe persistent asthma or acute exacerbations. The action plan dictates what symptoms or peak flow reading necessitates a change in asthma care to gain control.

The patient can take 2 to 4 puffs of an SABA every 20 minutes three times as a rescue plan. Depending on the response (e.g., alleviation of symptoms or improved peak flow), continued SABA use and/or oral corticosteroids may be a part of the home management plan at this point. If symptoms persist or if the patient's peak flow is less than 50% of the personal best, the HCP or emergency medical services (EMS) must be immediately contacted.

When the patient is in the health care facility with an acute exacerbation, it is important to monitor the patient's respiratory and cardiovascular systems. This includes (1) auscultating lung sounds; (2) taking the heart and respiratory rates and BP; and (3) monitoring pulse oximetry, peak expiratory flow rates, and ABGs.

Louder wheezing may actually occur in airways that are responding to the therapy as airflow increases. As improvement continues and airflow increases, breath sounds increase and wheezing decreases. Remember that, despite the disappearance of most of the bronchospasms, the edema and cellular infiltration of the airway mucosa and the viscous mucous plugs may take several days to improve. Thus intensive therapy must be continued even after clinical improvement.

TABLE 28-13 Patient Teaching

Pursed-Lip Breathing (PLB)

Teach the patient how to do PLB using the following guidelines.

1. Use PLB before, during, and after any activity causing you to be short of breath.
2. Inhale slowly and deeply through the nose.
3. Exhale slowly through pursed lips, almost as if whistling.
4. Relax your facial muscles without puffing your cheeks—like whistling—while you are exhaling.
5. Make breathing out (exhalation) three times as long as breathing in (inhalation).
6. The following activities can help you get the "feel" of PLB:
   - Blow through a straw in a glass of water with the intent of forming small bubbles.
   - Blow a lit candle enough to bend the flame without blowing it out.
   - Steadily blow a table-tennis ball across a table.
   - Blow a tissue held in the hand until it gently flaps.
7. Practice 8-10 repetitions of PLB three or four times a day.

An important nursing goal during an acute attack is to decrease the patient's anxiety and sense of panic. A calm, quiet, reassuring attitude may help the patient relax. Position the patient comfortably (usually sitting) to maximize chest expansion. Stay with the patient and be available to provide additional comfort. A technique called "talking down" can help the patient remain calm. In talking down, you gain eye contact with the patient. In a firm, calm voice coach the patient to use pursed-lip breathing, which keeps the airways open by maintaining positive pressure (Table 28-13), and abdominal breathing, which slows the respiratory rate and encourages deeper breaths (see Table 6-6). You or the caregiver should stay with the patient until the respiratory rate (with the assistance of the medications) has slowed.

When the acute attack subsides, provide rest and a quiet, calm environment for the patient. When the patient has recovered from exhaustion, try to obtain a health history and do a physical assessment. If the caregiver and other family members are present, they may be able to provide information about the patient's health history (Table 28-12). This information is important in planning an individualized nursing care plan.

Ambulatory Care. Control of symptoms can also be achieved by teaching the patient about medications. However, the drug regimen itself can be confusing and complex. Teach patients the importance of monitoring their response to medication. It is easy to undermedicate or overmedicate unless careful monitoring is ongoing. Some patients may benefit from keeping a diary to record medication use, wheezing or coughing, peak flow, side effects of drugs, and activity level. This information will help the HCP adjust the medication if needed.

Good nutrition is important. Physical exercise (e.g., swimming, walking, stationary cycling) within the patient's limit of tolerance is also beneficial and may require pretreatment with an SABA (as noted previously). Sleep that is uninterrupted by asthma symptoms is an important goal. If patients with asthma wake up because of asthma symptoms, their asthma is not under good control and their therapeutic plan should be reevaluated.

Together with the patient and caregiver, develop a written asthma action plan (Fig. 28-8). Base these plans on the patient's asthma symptoms and PEFR. To follow the management plan,

Asthma Action Plan

For: _____ Doctor: _____ Date: _____

Doctor's Phone Number _____ Hospital/Emergency Department Phone Number _____

GREEN ZONE

Doing Well

- No cough, wheeze, chest tightness, or shortness of breath during the day or night
- Can do usual activities

And, if a peak flow meter is used,

Peak flow: more than _____ (80 percent or more of my best peak flow)

My best peak flow is: _____

Take these long-term control medicines each day (include an antiinflammatory).

Medicine	How much to take	When to take it
_____	_____	_____
_____	_____	_____
_____	_____	_____
_____	_____	_____
_____	_____	_____
Before exercise ❒ _____	❒ 2 or ❒ 4 puffs _____	5 minutes before exercise

YELLOW ZONE

Asthma Is Getting Worse

- Cough, wheeze, chest tightness, or shortness of breath, or
- Waking at night due to asthma, or
- Can do some, but not all, usual activities

-Or-

Peak flow: _____ to _____ (50 to 79 percent of my best peak flow)

First — **Add: quick-relief medicine—and keep taking your GREEN ZONE medicine.**

_____ (short-acting beta$_2$-agonist) ❒ 2 or ❒ 4 puffs, every 20 minutes for up to 1 hour

❒ Nebulizer, once

Second — **If your symptoms (and peak flow, if used) return to GREEN ZONE after 1 hour of above treatment:**

❒ Continue monitoring to be sure you stay in the green zone.

-Or- _____

If your symptoms (and peak flow, if used) do not return to GREEN ZONE after 1 hour of above treatment:

❒ Take: _____ (short-acting beta$_2$-agonist) ❒ 2 or ❒ 4 puffs or ❒ Nebulizer

❒ Add: _____ (oral steroid) mg per day For _____ (3–10) days

❒ Call the doctor ❒ before/ ❒ within ____ hours after taking the oral steroid.

RED ZONE

Medical Alert!

- Very short of breath, or
- Quick-relief medicines have not helped, or
- Cannot do usual activities, or
- Symptoms are same or get worse after 24 hours in Yellow Zone

-Or-

Peak flow: less than _____ (50 percent of my best peak flow)

Take this medicine:

❒ _____ (short-acting beta$_2$-agonist) ❒ 4 or ❒ 6 puffs or ❒ Nebulizer

❒ _____ (oral steroid) mg

Then call your doctor NOW. Go to the hospital or call an ambulance if:

- You are still in the red zone after 15 minutes AND
- You have not reached your doctor.

DANGER SIGNS

- **Trouble walking and talking due to shortness of breath**
- **Lips or fingernails are blue**

- **Take ❒ 4 or ❒ 6 puffs of your quick-relief medicine AND**
- **Go to the hospital or call for an ambulance _____ NOW!** (phone)

FIG. 28-8 Asthma action plan. (Source: National Heart, Lung, and Blood Institute.)

the patient must measure his or her peak flow at least daily. Some patients may want to just monitor symptoms for self-management. Patients with asthma frequently do not perceive changes in their breathing. Therefore peak flow monitoring, when done correctly, can be a reliable, objective measurement of asthma control (Table 28-14).

If a patient's PEFR is within the green zone (usually 80% to 100% of the individual's personal best), the patient should remain on her or his usual medications. If the PEFR is within the yellow zone (usually 50% to 80% of personal best), it indicates caution. Something is triggering the patient's asthma (e.g., viral infection).

The patient should have a written asthma action plan that prescribes a step increase in medications during the acute phase of an infection (usually viral). The dose is stepped down once the viral infection symptoms subside. Based on the asthma

TABLE 28-14 Patient Teaching

How to Use Your Peak Flow Meter

Include the following instructions when teaching the patient to use a peak flow meter.

Why Use a Peak Flow Meter?

- Peak flow meters are used to check your asthma the way that BP cuffs are used to check BP. A peak flow meter is a device that measures how well air moves out of your lungs.
- During an asthma episode, the airways of the lungs usually begin to narrow slowly. The peak flow meter may tell you if there is narrowing in the airways hours, sometimes even days, before you have any asthma symptoms.
- By taking your medicines early (before symptoms), you may be able to stop the episode quickly and avoid a severe asthma episode.
- The peak flow meter also can be used to help you and your HCP:
  - Learn what makes your asthma worse.
  - Decide if your treatment plan is working well.
  - Decide when to add or stop medicine.
  - Decide when to seek emergency care.

How to Use Your Peak Flow Meter

Do the following five steps with your peak flow meter:

1. Move the indicator to the bottom of the numbered scale.
2. Stand up.
3. Take a deep breath, filling your lungs completely.
4. Place the mouthpiece in your mouth and close your lips around it. Do not put your tongue inside the hole.
5. Blow out as hard and fast as you can in a single blow.
   - Write down the number you get. But if you cough or make a mistake, do not write down the number. Do it over again.
   - Repeat steps 1 through 5 two more times, and write down the best of the three blows in your asthma diary.

Find Your Personal Best Peak Flow Number

- Your personal best peak flow number is the highest peak flow number you can achieve over a 2-week period when your asthma is under good control. Good control is when you feel good and do not have any asthma symptoms.
- Each patient's asthma is different, and your best peak expiratory flow (PEF) may be higher or lower than the peak flow of someone of your height, weight, and gender. This means that it is important for you to find your own personal best peak flow number, which is the basis for your treatment plan.
- To find your personal best peak flow number, take peak flow readings:
  - At least twice a day for 2-3 wk, between 12 noon and 2 PM when your peak flow is the highest
  - 15-20 min after taking inhaled short-acting β_2-agonist (SABA) for quick relief
  - As instructed by your HCP

The Peak Flow Zone System

Once you know your personal best peak flow number, your HCP will put the peak flow numbers into zones that are set up like a traffic light. This will help you know what to do when your peak flow number changes. For example:

Green Zone (more than __L/min [80% of your personal best number]) signals good control. No asthma symptoms are present. Take your medicines as usual.

Yellow Zone (between __ and __L/min [50% to <80% of your personal best number]) signals caution. If you remain in the yellow zone after several measures of peak flow, take an inhaled SABA. If you continue to register peak flow readings in the yellow zone, your asthma may not be under good control. Ask your HCP if you need to change or increase your daily medicines.

Red Zone (<__L/min [<50% of your personal best number]) signals a medical alert. Take an inhaled SABA (quick-relief medicine) right away. Call your HCP or the emergency department and ask what to do, or go directly to the emergency department.

Use the Diary to Keep Track of Your Peak Flow

- Record your personal best peak flow number and peak flow zones in your asthma diary.
- Measure your peak flow when you wake up, *before* taking medicine. Write down your peak flow number in the diary every day, or as instructed by your HCP.

Actions to Take When Peak Flow Numbers Change

- PEF goes between __ and __L/min (50% to <80% of personal best, yellow zone).

ACTION: Take an inhaled SABA (quick-relief medicine) as prescribed by your HCP.

- PEF increases ≥20% when measured before and after taking an inhaled SABA (quick-relief medicine).

ACTION: Talk to your HCP about adding more medicine to control your asthma better (e.g., an antiinflammatory medication).

Source: Adapted from National Asthma Education and Prevention Program, National Heart, Lung, and Blood Institute: *Expert Panel Report 3: guidelines for the diagnosis and management of asthma*, NIH pub no 08-4051, Bethesda, Md, 2007, National Institutes of Health. Retrieved from *www.nhlbi.nih.gov/guidelines*.

management plan, the patient can use different strategies, such as using the SABA more frequently.

If the PEFR is in the red zone (50% or less of personal best), it indicates a serious problem. A rescue plan should be a part of the asthma action plan. Teach the patient and caregiver to take definitive action. Emphasize to the patient the need to monitor PEFR daily or several times a day to have an objective measure that can be correlated with symptoms. Although it may happen, it is unusual for a patient's PEFR to drop from the green zone to the red zone quickly. Usually the patient has time to make changes in medications, avoid triggers, and notify the HCP.

It is important to involve the patient's caregiver or family. They should know where the patient's inhalers, oral medications, and emergency phone numbers are located. Instruct the caregiver or family on how to decrease the patient's anxiety if an asthma attack occurs. When the patient is stabilized or controlled, the caregiver can gently remind the patient about doing daily PEFR by asking questions such as, "What zone are you in? How's your peak flow today?" A patient and caregiver teaching guide for the patient with asthma is presented in Table 28-15.

CHECK YOUR PRACTICE

A 32-yr-old man is admitted to the emergency department for an acute exacerbation of asthma. It is his third admission in the past 2 months. He had been watching his 6-yr-old son play soccer when his attack started. He says to you, "I am just not a good father. My son is going to think I am just a 'sicky.' I cannot participate in his sports. I cannot even watch them without something happening."

- How would you respond to this man?

An increased number of older adults are diagnosed with asthma. This is a special concern because they have more complicated health issues than younger patients with asthma. Issues that face older adults are costly medications, nonadherence to medical regimen, and difficulty accessing the health care system.

TABLE 28-15 Patient & Caregiver Teaching

Asthma

Include the following information in a teaching plan for the patient with asthma and the caregiver. It will help to improve the patient's quality of life and promote lifestyle changes that support successful living with asthma.

What is Asthma?
- Basic anatomy and physiology of lung
- Pathophysiology of asthma
- Relationship of pathophysiology to signs and symptoms
- Measurement and correlation of spirometry and peak expiratory flow rate

What Is Good Asthma Control?
- Personal ideas of good control
- Use Asthma Control Test available at *www.asthmacontroltest.com*

Hindrances to Asthma Treatment and Control
- Discuss with patient and caregiver about possible hindrances (e.g., denial, poor perception of asthma severity by patient)

Environmental and Trigger Control
- Identifications of possible triggers and possible preventive measures (use trigger diary)
- Avoidance of allergens and other triggers
- Need to maintain good hydration

Medications
- Types (include mechanism of action)
- β_2-Agonists
- Corticosteroids
- Methylxanthines
- Anti-IgE
- Leukotriene modifiers
- Combination drugs
- Use of preventive and maintenance (e.g., antiinflammatory) agents
- Write out medication list and schedule
- Asthma Action Plan (Fig. 28-8)

Correct Use of Inhalers, Spacer, and Nebulizer
- Demonstration–return demonstration with placebo devices (Figs. 28-5 to 28-7 and Tables 28-9 to 28-11)

Breathing Techniques
- Pursed-lip breathing (Table 28-13)

Correct Use of Peak Flow Meter

See Table 28-14.

Asthma Action Plan (Fig. 28-8)
- Peak flow zones
- Individualize plan
- Patient completes asthma action plan and discusses it with HCP.
- Early recognition of infection
- Building a partnership with your HCP
- Questions patients may have about asthma, but patient cannot reach the HCP

For additional information, see the American Lung Association at *http://www.lung.org/lung-disease/asthma.*

Keep these factors in mind when implementing a management plan for older adults.

A variety of factors may contribute to why African Americans and Hispanics (especially those from Puerto Rico) have higher rates of poorly controlled asthma and deaths compared with whites. Some factors may be disparities in socioeconomic status and access to proper health care, cultural beliefs about the management of asthma, and underutilization of the long-term controller medications because of high costs.[10] Seek to explore and eliminate any barriers to health care. Also seek out culturally appropriate resources and educational material in languages other than English to improve asthma control for these individuals.

Relaxation therapies (e.g., yoga, meditation, relaxation techniques, breathing techniques) may help a patient relax respiratory muscles and decrease the respiratory rate. (Chapter 6 discusses relaxation breathing and other relaxation strategies.) A healthy emotional outlook is also important in preventing asthma attacks. Some communities have asthma support groups.

◆ Evaluation

The expected outcomes are that the patient with asthma will
- Maintain clear airway with removal of excessive secretions
- Have normal (for the individual) breath sounds and respiratory rate
- Report decreased anxiety with increased control of respirations
- Describe the disease process and treatment regimen
- Demonstrate correct administration of inhaled drugs
- Express confidence in ability for long-term management of asthma

Additional information on expected outcomes for the patient with asthma is presented in eNursing Care Plan 28-1 available on the website for this chapter.

CHRONIC OBSTRUCTIVE PULMONARY DISEASE

Chronic obstructive pulmonary disease (COPD) is a preventable and treatable disease characterized by persistent airflow limitation that is usually progressive. COPD is associated with an enhanced chronic inflammatory response in the airways and lungs, primarily caused by cigarette smoking and other noxious particles and gases. COPD exacerbations and other coexisting illnesses or co-morbidities contribute to the overall severity of the disease.[11]

Previous definitions of COPD have included such terms as *chronic bronchitis* and *emphysema,* but neither term is part of the current definition of COPD. **Chronic bronchitis,** the presence of cough and sputum production for at least 3 months in each of 2 consecutive years, is an independent disease that may precede or follow the development of airflow limitation. **Emphysema** is the destruction of the alveoli and is a pathologic term that explains only one of several structural abnormalities in COPD patients.

An estimated 12.7 million adults in the United States over age 18 have COPD.[2] An additional 24 million people have evidence of impaired lung function. The number of people with COPD is greatly underestimated because the disease is usually not diagnosed until it is moderately advanced. COPD is the third leading cause of death in the United States, resulting in more than 133,000 deaths in Americans each year.[12]

GENDER DIFFERENCES

Chronic Obstructive Pulmonary Disease (COPD)

Men

- COPD is more common in men than in women, but the incidence is not increasing in men.
- Fewer men die from COPD than women.

Women

- The number of women with COPD is increasing.
- Increase is probably due to increased number of women smoking cigarettes and increased susceptibility (e.g., smaller lungs and airways, lower elastic recoil).
- Women with COPD have lower quality of life, more exacerbations, increased dyspnea, and better response to O_2 therapy compared with men.

Etiology

Many factors can influence the development and progression of COPD. The following discussion addresses these numerous factors.

Cigarette Smoking. The major risk factor for developing COPD is cigarette smoking.[12,13] COPD affects about 15% of smokers.[14] An intriguing question is why some smokers develop COPD and others do not. COPD should be considered in any person who is over the age of 40 with a smoking history of 10 or more pack-years.

Cigarette smoke has several direct effects on the respiratory tract (Table 28-16). The irritating effect of the smoke causes hyperplasia of cells, including goblet cells, thereby increasing the production of mucus. Hyperplasia reduces airway diameter and increases the difficulty in clearing secretions. Smoking reduces the ciliary activity and may cause actual loss of cilia. Smoking also produces abnormal dilation of the distal air space with destruction of alveolar walls. Many cells develop large, atypical nuclei, which are considered a precancerous condition.

TABLE 28-16 Effects of Tobacco Smoke on Respiratory System

Area of Defect	Acute Effects	Long-Term Effects
Respiratory mucosa		
• Nasopharyngeal	↓ Sense of smell	Cancer
• Tongue	↓ Sense of taste	Cancer
• Vocal cords	Hoarseness	Chronic cough, cancer
• Bronchus and bronchioles	Bronchospasm, cough	Chronic bronchitis, asthma, cancer
Cilia	Paralysis, sputum accumulation, cough	Chronic bronchitis, cancer
Mucous glands	↑ Secretions, ↑ cough	Hyperplasia and hypertrophy of glands, chronic bronchitis
Alveolar macrophages	↓ Function	↑ Incidence of infection
Elastin and collagen fibers	↑ Destruction by proteases ↓ Function of antiproteases (α_1-antitrypsin) ↓ Synthesis and repair of elastin	Emphysema

Smoking causes chronic, enhanced inflammation of various parts of the lung with structural changes and repair (called *remodeling*). The reasons for the inflammatory response are not clearly understood but may be genetically determined, since patients who have never smoked can develop COPD.

Cigarette smoking causes oxidative stress, as well as an imbalance between proteases that break down connective tissue in the lung and antiproteases that protect the lungs. These changes resulting from cigarette smoking increase with more severe disease and persist even after smoking cessation. (See Chapter 10 for more details about cigarette smoking.)

Passive smoking is the exposure of nonsmokers to cigarette smoke, also known as *environmental tobacco smoke* (ETS) or secondhand smoke. In adults, involuntary smoke exposure is associated with decreased pulmonary function, increased respiratory symptoms, and severe lower respiratory tract infections (e.g., pneumonia). ETS is also associated with increased risk for lung cancer and nasal sinus cancer.

Occupational Chemicals and Dusts. If a person has intense or prolonged exposure to various dusts, vapors, irritants, or fumes in the workplace, symptoms of lung impairment consistent with COPD can develop. If a person has occupational exposure and smokes, the risk of COPD increases.[11]

Air Pollution. High levels of urban air pollution are harmful to people with existing lung disease. However, the effect of outdoor air pollution as a risk factor for the development of COPD is unclear. Another risk factor for COPD development is coal and other biomass fuels that are used for indoor heating and cooking. Many people who have never smoked are at significant risk for developing COPD because of cooking with these fuels in poorly ventilated areas.[11]

Infection. Infections are a risk factor for developing COPD. Severe recurring respiratory tract infections in childhood have been associated with reduced lung function and increased respiratory symptoms in adulthood. It is unclear whether the development of COPD can be related to recurrent infections in adults. People who smoke and also have human immunodeficiency virus (HIV) infection have an accelerated development of COPD. Tuberculosis is also a risk factor for COPD development.

Genetics. The fact that a relatively small percentage of smokers get COPD strongly suggests that genetic factors influence which smokers get the disease. Because of the genetic-environmental interaction, two people may have the same smoking history, but only one develops COPD. To date, one genetic factor has been clearly identified (see next section).

α_1-Antitrypsin (AAT) Deficiency. α_1-Antitrypsin (AAT) deficiency is an autosomal recessive disorder that may affect the lungs or liver. AAT deficiency is a genetic risk factor for COPD. Approximately 3% of all people diagnosed with COPD may have undetected AAT deficiency. AAT is a serum protein produced by the liver and normally found in the lungs. The main function of AAT, an α_1-protease inhibitor, is to protect normal lung tissue from attack by proteases during inflammation related to cigarette smoking and infections. Severe AAT deficiency leads to premature bullous emphysema in the lungs found on x-ray. Smoking greatly exacerbates the disease process in these patients.

Genetic Link

AAT deficiency is an autosomal recessive disorder (see Figs. 12-4 and 12-5 and the Genetics in Clinical Practice box on p. 184).

The severity of AAT deficiency depends on which forms of the gene are inherited. The most common abnormal genes are the S and Z alleles. The normal genotype is MM. The most common genotype associated with AAT disease is ZZ (also referred to as *PI-ZZ*). Other variations include MZ (slightly increased risk of poor lung function) and SZ (higher risk of lung and liver problems in smokers). Some individuals with MZ and SZ genotypes may never seek health care because they have minimal manifestations of the disorder.[15]

GENETICS IN CLINICAL PRACTICE

α_1-Antitrypsin (AAT) Deficiency

Genetic Basis

- Autosomal recessive disorder
- Mutations in *SERPINA1* gene (located on chromosome 14) cause AAT deficiency.
- Gene provides instructions for the liver to make the protein AAT, which protects the lungs and liver from powerful proteolytic enzymes.
- Without enough functional AAT, proteolytic enzymes destroy alveoli and cause lung disease.

Incidence

- Occurs in 1 in 1700 to 3500 live births in the United States
- People of northern European descent most affected

Genetic Testing

- DNA testing is available.
- Screening of siblings is useful.
- Serum assay is available to measure the amount of AAT.

Clinical Implications

- AAT deficiency can cause lung and liver disease.
- Onset of disease is between ages 20 and 40 yr.
- Treatment includes AAT replacement (Prolastin).
- Disease predisposes to early-onset emphysema.

Although 100,000 people in the United States are suspected of having the ZZ phenotype, fewer than 10% have been detected. Clues to AAT deficiencies are the onset of symptoms often occurring by age 40, minimal to no tobacco use, and family history of COPD and/or liver disease. Chronic liver disease as an infant or adult with increased liver enzyme levels may also be seen. Individuals with this type of COPD are primarily of northern European origin.[15]

A simple blood test can determine low levels of AAT. Those with borderline or low levels can then be genetically tested.

IV-administered AAT (e.g., Prolastin-C) augmentation therapy is used for people with AAT deficiency. The infusions are usually administered weekly. Its effectiveness in slowing the progression of the disease and the results of this treatment continue to be evaluated.

Aging. Although aging is often considered a risk factor for COPD, the evidence is unclear. Does the aging process lead to COPD, or is COPD a result of the cumulative exposures that occur over a long life? Normal aging results in loss of elastic recoil, stiffening of the chest wall, gas exchange alteration, and decrease in exercise tolerance. As people age, the lungs gradually lose their elastic recoil. Thoracic cage changes result from osteoporosis and calcification of the costal cartilages. The thoracic cage becomes stiff and rigid, and the ribs are less mobile. The shape of the rib cage gradually changes because of the increased residual volume (RV), causing it to expand and become rounded. Decreased chest compliance and elastic recoil of the lungs caused by aging affect the mechanical aspects of ventilation and increase the work of breathing.

As one ages, the number of functional alveoli decreases as peripheral airways lose supporting tissues. The surface area for gas exchange decreases, and the PaO_2 decreases. Changes in the elasticity of the lungs reduce the ventilatory reserve. These changes are similar to those seen in the patient with COPD.

Asthma. Patients with COPD may have asthma. Asthma may be a risk factor for the development of COPD. There is a considerable pathologic and functional overlap between these disorders, particularly among older adults, who may have components of both diseases. Recently this disorder has been called *asthma-COPD overlap syndrome.*

Gender. In the past, COPD prevalence and mortality were greater in men than women. Now the prevalence is almost equal, reflecting the changing patterns of cigarette smoking. Women may be more susceptible to the adverse effects of smoking.[16]

Pathophysiology

COPD is characterized by chronic inflammation of the airways, lung parenchyma (respiratory bronchioles and alveoli), and pulmonary blood vessels (Fig. 28-9). The pathogenesis of COPD is complex and involves many mechanisms. The defining feature of COPD is not fully reversible airflow limitation during forced exhalation. This is caused by loss of elastic recoil and airflow obstruction caused by mucus hypersecretion, mucosal edema, and bronchospasm.

In COPD, various processes occur, such as airflow limitation, air trapping, gas exchange abnormalities, and mucus hypersecretion. In severe disease, pulmonary hypertension and systemic manifestations occur (Fig. 28-9). COPD has an uneven distribution of pathologic changes, with severely destroyed lung areas existing together with areas of relatively normal lung.

The inflammatory process starts with inhalation of noxious particles and gases (e.g., cigarette smoke) but is magnified in the person with COPD. The abnormal inflammatory process causes tissue destruction and disrupts the normal defense mechanisms and repair process of the lung. The mechanisms for the enhanced inflammatory response are not clearly understood but may be genetically determined.

The predominant inflammatory cells in COPD are neutrophils, macrophages, and lymphocytes. This pattern of inflammatory cells is different from that in asthma. (In asthma, the inflammatory cells are eosinophils, mast cells, neutrophils, lymphocytes, and macrophages.) These inflammatory cells attract other inflammatory mediators (e.g., leukotrienes) and proinflammatory cytokines (e.g., tumor necrosis factor). The end result of the inflammatory process is structural changes in the lungs.

The inflammatory process may also be magnified by oxidants, which are produced by cigarette smoke and other inhaled particles and released from the inflammatory cells. The oxidants adversely affect the lungs as they inactivate antiproteases (which prevent the natural destruction of the lungs), stimulate mucus secretion, and increase fluid in the lungs.

After the inhalation of oxidants in tobacco or air pollution, the activity of proteases (which break down the connective tissue of the lungs) increases and the antiproteases (which protect against the breakdown) are inhibited. Therefore the natural balance of protease/antiprotease is tipped in favor

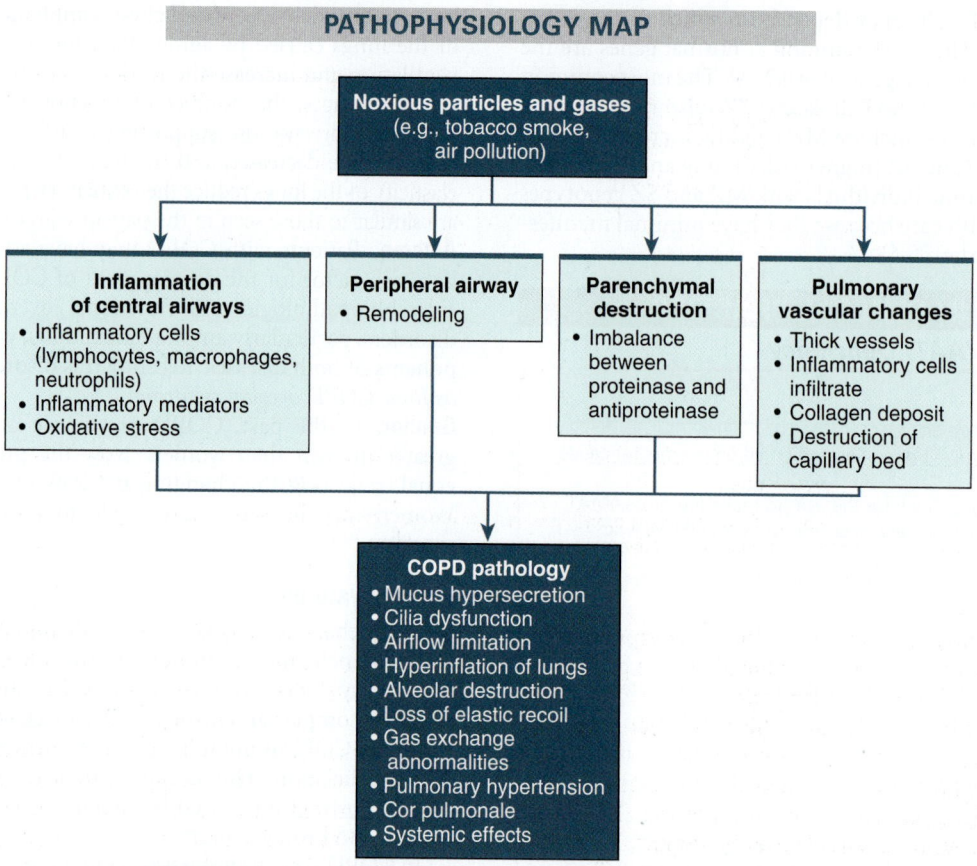

FIG. 28-9 Pathophysiology of chronic obstructive pulmonary disease *(COPD)*.

of destruction of the alveoli and loss of the lungs' elastic recoil.

Inability to expire air is a main characteristic of COPD. The primary site of the airflow limitation is in the smaller airways. As the peripheral airways become obstructed, air is progressively trapped during expiration. The volume of residual air becomes greatly increased in severe disease as alveolar attachments (similar to rubber bands) to small airways are destroyed. The residual air, combined with the loss of elastic recoil, makes passive expiration of air difficult. As air is trapped in the lungs, the chest hyperexpands and becomes barrel shaped because the respiratory muscles are not able to function effectively. The functional residual capacity is increased. The patient is now trying to breathe in when the lungs are in an "overinflated" state. Thus the patient appears dyspneic and exercise capacity is limited.

Gas exchange abnormalities result in hypoxemia and hypercapnia (increased CO_2) as the disease worsens. As the air trapping increases, walls of alveoli are destroyed (Fig. 28-10), and bullae (large air spaces in the parenchyma) and blebs (air spaces adjacent to pleurae) can form.

Bullae and blebs are not effective in gas exchange because they do not contain the capillary bed that normally surrounds each alveolus. Therefore a significant ventilation-perfusion (V/Q) mismatch and hypoxemia result. Peripheral airway obstruction also results in V/Q imbalance and, combined with the respiratory muscle impairment, can lead to CO_2 retention, particularly in severe disease.

Excess mucus production, resulting in a chronic productive cough, is a feature of individuals with predominant chronic bronchitis. However, not all COPD patients have sputum production. When present, excess mucus production is multifactorial, including (1) an increased number of mucus-secreting goblet cells, (2) enlarged submucosal glands, (3) dysfunction of cilia, and (4) stimulation from inflammatory mediators.

Pulmonary vascular changes resulting in mild to moderate pulmonary hypertension may occur late in the course of COPD. The small pulmonary arteries vasoconstrict due to hypoxia. As the disease advances, the structure of the pulmonary arteries changes, resulting in thickening of the vascular smooth muscle. Because of the loss of alveolar walls and the capillaries surrounding them, pressure in the pulmonary circulation increases.

Typically, the patient does not have difficulty with hypoxemia at rest until late in the disease. However, hypoxemia may develop during exercise, and the patient may benefit from supplemental O_2. Pulmonary hypertension may progress and lead to hypertrophy of the right ventricle of the heart (**cor pulmonale**). The right ventricle dilates and may eventually lead to right-sided heart failure.

In addition to lung disease, COPD is a systemic disease. Chronic inflammation is an underlying etiology for these systemic effects. Cardiovascular diseases commonly exist in COPD (smoking is a primary risk factor for both of them). Other common systemic diseases include cachexia (skeletal muscle wasting), osteoporosis, diabetes, and metabolic syndrome, which cannot be readily related to smoking.

Clinical Manifestations

Clinical manifestations of COPD typically develop slowly. A clinical diagnosis of COPD should be considered in any patient

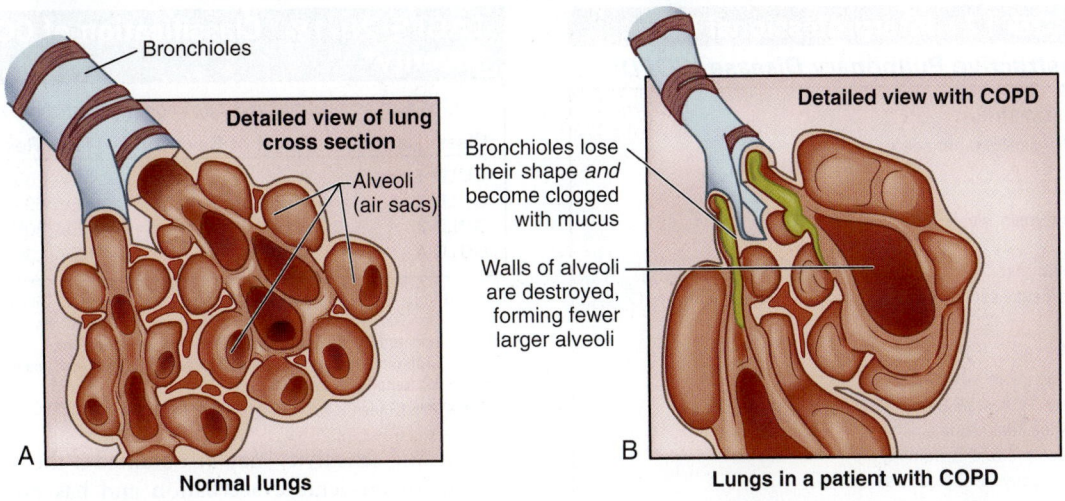

FIG. 28-10 **A,** Normal lungs showing bronchioles and alveoli. **B,** Changes in the bronchioles and alveoli in the lungs of a patient with chronic obstructive pulmonary disease *(COPD)*.

who has chronic cough or sputum production, dyspnea, and a history of exposure to risk factors for the disease (e.g., tobacco smoke, occupational dusts, and chemicals).

A chronic intermittent cough, which is often the first symptom to develop, may be present every day as the disease progresses. The cough is often dismissed by patients as they expect it with smoking or environmental exposures. The cough may be unproductive of mucus. However, significant airflow limitation may exist without sputum or cough. Typically dyspnea is progressive, usually occurs with exertion, and is present every day.

Patients may complain of not being able to take a deep breath, heaviness in the chest, gasping, increased effort to breathe, and air hunger. Patients usually ignore the symptoms and rationalize that "I'm getting older" and "I'm out of shape." They change behaviors to avoid dyspnea, such as taking the elevator instead of the stairs. Gradually the dyspnea interferes with daily activities, such as carrying grocery bags. They cannot walk as fast as their partners or peers. However, as symptoms worsen and interfere with daily activity or they have their first COPD exacerbation, patients usually seek medical care.

In late stages of COPD, dyspnea may be present at rest. As more alveoli become overdistended, increasing amounts of air are trapped. This causes the diaphragm to flatten, and the patient must breathe from partially inflated lungs. Effective abdominal breathing is decreased because of the flattened diaphragm from the overinflated lungs. The person becomes more of a chest breather, relying on the intercostal and accessory muscles. However, chest breathing is not efficient.

Wheezing and chest tightness may be present but may vary by time of the day or from day to day, especially in patients with more severe disease. Wheezes may arise from the laryngeal area, or wheezes may not be present on auscultation. Chest tightness, which often follows activity, may feel similar to muscular contraction.

The person with advanced COPD frequently experiences fatigue, weight loss, and anorexia. Even with adequate caloric intake, the patient still loses weight. Fatigue is a highly prevalent symptom that affects the patient's activities of daily living.[17] Paroxysms of coughing may be so severe that the patient faints or fractures a rib.

During physical examination a prolonged expiratory respiratory phase, wheezes, or decreased breath sounds are noted in all lung fields. The patient may need to breathe louder than normal for auscultated breath sounds to be heard. The anteroposterior diameter of the chest is increased ("barrel chest") from the chronic air trapping. The patient may sit upright with arms supported on a fixed surface such as an overbed table *(tripod position)*. The patient may naturally purse lips on expiration (pursed-lip breathing) and use accessory muscles, such as those in the neck, to aid with inspiration. Edema in the ankles may be the only clue to right-sided heart involvement (cor pulmonale).

Over time, hypoxemia (PaO_2 less than 60 mm Hg or O_2 saturation less than 88%) may develop with hypercapnia ($PaCO_2$ over 45 mm Hg). The bluish-red color of the skin results from polycythemia and cyanosis. Polycythemia develops as a result of increased production of red blood cells as the body attempts to compensate for chronic hypoxemia. Hemoglobin concentrations may reach 20 g/dL (200 g/L) or more. However, the person may also have lowered hemoglobin and hematocrit because of chronic anemia.

It is sometimes difficult to distinguish COPD from asthma, especially if the individual has a history of cigarette smoking. However, some clinical features are different (Table 28-3).

Complications

Complications that can occur in patients with COPD include cor pulmonale, acute exacerbations, and acute respiratory failure. These complications and their causes and treatment are discussed in the section on Interprofessional Care on p. 563.

Diagnostic Studies

A history and physical examination are extremely important in a diagnostic workup. Spirometry is required to confirm the diagnosis in individuals suspected of having COPD. Spirometry confirms the presence of airflow obstruction and determines the severity of COPD.

In spirometry, the patient is given a short-acting bronchodilator, and postbronchodilator values are compared with a normal reference value. A diagnosis of COPD is made when the FEV_1/FVC ratio is less than 70%. The value of FEV_1 provides

TABLE 28-17 Interprofessional Care

Chronic Obstructive Pulmonary Disease (COPD)

Diagnostic Assessment

- History and physical examination
- Spirometry
- Chest x-ray
- Serum α_1-antitrypsin levels
- ABGs
- Six-minute walk test
- COPD Assessment Test (CAT)* or Clinical COPD Questionnaire (CCQ)†

Management

- Cessation of cigarette smoking
- Drug therapies (Tables 28-8 and 28-19)
- Airway clearance techniques
- Breathing exercises and retraining
- Hydration of 3 L/day (if not contraindicated)
- Immunizations
  - Influenza yearly
  - Pneumococcal vaccine (see Table 27-5 for guidelines)
- Long-term O_2 (if indicated)
- Progressive plan of exercise, especially walking and upper body strengthening
- Pulmonary rehabilitation program
- Nutritional supplementation if low BMI
- Treatment of complications
  - Cor pulmonale
  - Acute exacerbations
  - Acute respiratory failure
- Surgical therapy
  - Lung volume reduction
  - Bullectomy
  - Lung transplantation

ABGs, Arterial blood gases; *BMI*, body mass index.
*See *www.catestonline.org*.
†See *www.ccq.nl*.

a guideline for the degree of severity of COPD. FEV_1 can be expressed as a percentage compared with a normal reference value (percent predicted). The lower the FEV_1, the more obstructed are the airways.

In addition to spirometry, other diagnostic studies may be performed (Table 28-17). Chest x-rays are not diagnostic but may show a flat diaphragm because of the hyperinflated lungs. Patients often have exercise-induced hypoxemia, and a 6-minute walk test may be done by a physical or respiratory therapist, with pulse oximetry readings taken when the patient is walking and at rest. If values of O_2 saturation are 88% or lower when at rest and the patient is breathing room air, he or she qualifies for supplemental O_2.

Validated questionnaires such as the COPD Assessment Test (CAT) *(www.catestonline.org)* and Clinical COPD Questionnaire (CCQ) *(www.ccq.nl)* are recommended for a comprehensive assessment of symptoms.

ABGs are usually assessed in the severe stages (FEV_1 less than 50%) and monitored in patients hospitalized with acute exacerbations. In the later stages of COPD, typical findings are low PaO_2, elevated $PaCO_2$, decreased or low-normal pH, and increased HCO_3^- levels (Table 28-3). In early stages, there may be a normal or only slightly decreased PaO_2 and a normal $PaCO_2$. An ECG may be normal or show signs of right ventricular failure.

An echocardiogram or multigated acquisition (MUGA) (cardiac blood pool) scan (see Table 31-6) can be used to evaluate right- and left-sided ventricular function. Sputum for culture and sensitivity may be obtained if the patient is hospitalized for an acute exacerbation and has not responded to antibiotic therapy.

TABLE 28-18 Classification of COPD Severity*

The following classification is based on postbronchodilator FEV_1.

Classification	Level of Severity	FEV_1 Results
GOLD 1	Mild	FEV_1 ≥80% predicted
GOLD 2	Moderate	FEV_1 50%-80% predicted
GOLD 3	Severe	FEV_1 30%-50% predicted
GOLD 4	Very severe	FEV_1 <30% predicted

Adapted from Global Initiative for Chronic Obstructive Lung Disease: Global strategy for the diagnosis, management, and prevention of chronic obstructive pulmonary disease (updated 2015). Retrieved from *www.goldcopd.org*.
COPD, Chronic obstructive pulmonary disease; *FEV_1*, forced expiratory volume in 1 sec; *FVC*, forced vital capacity.
*A diagnosis of COPD is made when a patient has a FEV_1/FVC <70%.

Classification of COPD

COPD can be classified as mild, moderate, severe, and very severe (Table 28-18). An FEV_1/FVC ratio of less than 70% establishes the diagnosis of COPD, and the severity of obstruction (as indicated by FEV_1) determines the stage of COPD. The management of COPD is based on the patient's symptoms, classification, and exacerbation history.

Interprofessional Care: Stable COPD

Most patients with COPD are treated as outpatients. They are hospitalized for complications such as acute exacerbations and acute respiratory failure.

Evaluate the patient's exposure to environmental or occupational irritants, and determine ways to control or avoid them. For example, teach the patient to avoid aerosol hair sprays and smoke-filled rooms. The patient with COPD is extremely susceptible to pulmonary infections. The patient with COPD should receive an influenza immunization yearly. The pneumococcal vaccine is recommended for all smokers ages 19 or older and all patients with COPD. (The guidelines for pneumococcal vaccine are presented in Table 27-5.)

Smoking Cessation. Cessation of cigarette smoking in any person with COPD at any level of severity is the most important intervention that can affect the natural history of COPD. After a person discontinues smoking, the accelerated decline in pulmonary function found with smoking slows to almost nonsmoking levels. Thus the sooner the smoker stops, the less pulmonary function is lost and the sooner the symptoms decrease, especially cough and sputum production. (Smoking cessation techniques are discussed in Chapter 10 and in Tables 10-4 to 10-6.)

Drug Therapy. Medications for COPD can reduce symptoms, increase exercise capacity, improve overall health, and reduce the number and severity of exacerbations. Bronchodilator drug therapy relaxes smooth muscles in the airway and improves the ventilation of the lungs, thus reducing the degree of breathlessness. Patients with COPD do not respond as dramatically to bronchodilator therapy as those with asthma. However, bronchodilator therapy reduces dyspnea and increases FEV_1. The inhaled route of medication is preferred and given on a PRN or regular basis.

Patients commonly do not properly administer inhaled medications. Therefore it is important for you to demonstrate

TABLE 28-19 Drug Therapy

Medication Guidelines for Stable COPD

The treatment guidelines are based on the FEV_1 results.

FEV_1 Results	Treatment Guidelines*
FEV_1 60%-80% predicted (with respiratory symptoms)	Treatment with inhaled bronchodilators may be used.
FEV_1 <60% predicted (with respiratory symptoms)	Treat with inhaled bronchodilators: anticholinergics or long-acting β_2–agonist OR Monotherapy with long-acting inhaled anticholinergics or long-acting β_2-agonist OR Combination therapy with long-acting inhaled anticholinergics, long-acting β_2-agonist, or inhaled corticosteroids

Source: Qaseem A, Wilt T, Weinberger S, et al: Diagnosis and management of stable chronic obstructive pulmonary disease: a clinical practice guideline update from the American College of Physicians, American College of Chest Physicians, American Thoracic Society, and European Respiratory Society, *Ann Intern Med* 155:179, 2011.
FEV_1, Forced expiratory volume in 1 sec.
*NOTE: Occasional use of short-acting inhaled bronchodilator for acute symptoms is not addressed in these recommendations.

and talk with patients about inhaler use. Give the patient clear, readable instructions.

Medications are given in a stepwise fashion according to the level of airflow obstruction determined from spirometry (FEV_1) and symptoms. Medications are stepped up but usually not stepped down, as in asthma, because in COPD continual symptoms are probably present (Table 28-19).

Bronchodilator medications commonly used are β_2-adrenergic agonists; anticholinergic agents; and, to a much lesser extent, methylxanthines (Table 28-8). The choice of a bronchodilator depends on the patient's response. These medications are given on a PRN or scheduled basis. When the patient has mild COPD or fewer symptoms, a short-acting bronchodilator is used. Albuterol or ipratropium may be used as single agents, but combining bronchodilators improves their effect and decreases the risk of adverse effects. Albuterol and ipratropium can be nebulized together (DuoNeb) or delivered by inhalation spray (Combivent Respimat).

In the moderate stage of COPD (FEV_1 less than 60%), a long-acting bronchodilator may be used (Tables 28-8 and 28-19). A short-acting bronchodilator may still be used PRN as a "rescue" for dyspnea. Salmeterol and formoterol are widely used LABAs, and they can be used in COPD as monotherapy (unlike drug therapy for asthma).

In COPD patients with FEV_1 of less than 60%, regular treatment with ICS is often prescribed and used in addition to LABA. Examples of combinations of ICSs with LABAs are fluticasone/salmeterol (Advair) and budesonide/formoterol (Symbicort).

Inhaled long-acting anticholinergics, LABAs, and ICSs all reduce COPD exacerbations. However, in COPD, unlike asthma, ICSs are not used as monotherapy because of the concerns about side effects. Some patients are on triple therapy with Advair and tiotropium. Oral corticosteroids should not be used for long-term therapy in COPD but are effective for short-term use to treat exacerbations.

The use of long-acting theophylline in the treatment of COPD is controversial because it interacts with many drugs. A low dose of theophylline with an ICS may benefit a few patients with COPD who do not respond to other inhaled medications.

Roflumilast (Daliresp) is an oral medication used to decrease the frequency of exacerbations in patients with severe COPD and the presence of chronic bronchitis. This drug is a phosphodiesterase inhibitor, which is an antiinflammatory drug that suppresses the release of cytokines and other inflammatory mediators and inhibits the production of reactive O_2 radicals.

New drug delivery devices are becoming available at a rapid pace. One example is Respimat, which is an easy-to-use, handheld device that provides a high deposition of drug to the lungs and low mouth and throat deposition. Respimat simplifies coordination between activation of the medication and inhalation without propellant, and it is independent of inspiratory flow. It also has a dose indicator. Combivent Respimat (ipratropium and albuterol) inhalation aerosol is available.

Interprofessional Care: COPD Complications

Cor Pulmonale. *Cor pulmonale* results from pulmonary hypertension, which is caused by diseases affecting the lungs or pulmonary blood vessels (Fig. 28-11). Cor pulmonale is a late manifestation of COPD, yet not all patients with COPD develop cor pulmonale. Once the patient develops cor pulmonale, the prognosis worsens.

In COPD, pulmonary hypertension is caused primarily by constriction of the pulmonary vessels in response to alveolar hypoxia. Chronic hypoxia also stimulates erythropoiesis, which causes polycythemia. This results in increased viscosity of the blood. These patients have increased pulmonary vascular resistance and thus develop pulmonary hypertension.

Normally the right ventricle and pulmonary circulatory system are low-pressure systems compared with the left ventricle and systemic circulation. When pulmonary hypertension develops, the pressures on the right side of the heart must increase to push blood into the lungs. Eventually, right-sided heart failure develops.

Dyspnea is the most common symptom of chronic cor pulmonale. Lung sounds are normal, or crackles may be heard in the bases of the lungs bilaterally. Heart sound changes occur but are usually masked by the underlying lung disease. Other manifestations of right-sided heart failure may develop, including distended neck veins (jugular venous distention), hepatomegaly with right upper quadrant tenderness, peripheral edema, and weight gain.

Typically the patient has large pulmonary vessels on chest x-ray and increased pressure on a right-sided heart cardiac catheterization. Echocardiogram may reflect right-sided heart enlargement. B-type natriuretic peptide (BNP) levels, which are used to diagnose heart failure, may be elevated in cor pulmonale secondary to the stretching of the right ventricle. Normally BNP levels are used to distinguish cardiac from respiratory causes of dyspnea, but in cor pulmonale the cause of the heart failure is the lung disease.

Treatment of cor pulmonale is initially targeted at managing the COPD, including bronchodilator and continuous low-flow, long-term O_2 therapy (for more than 15 hr/day), which improves survival.[18] Diuretics are generally administered, similar to their use with chronic heart failure. (Cor pulmonale is also discussed in Chapter 27.)

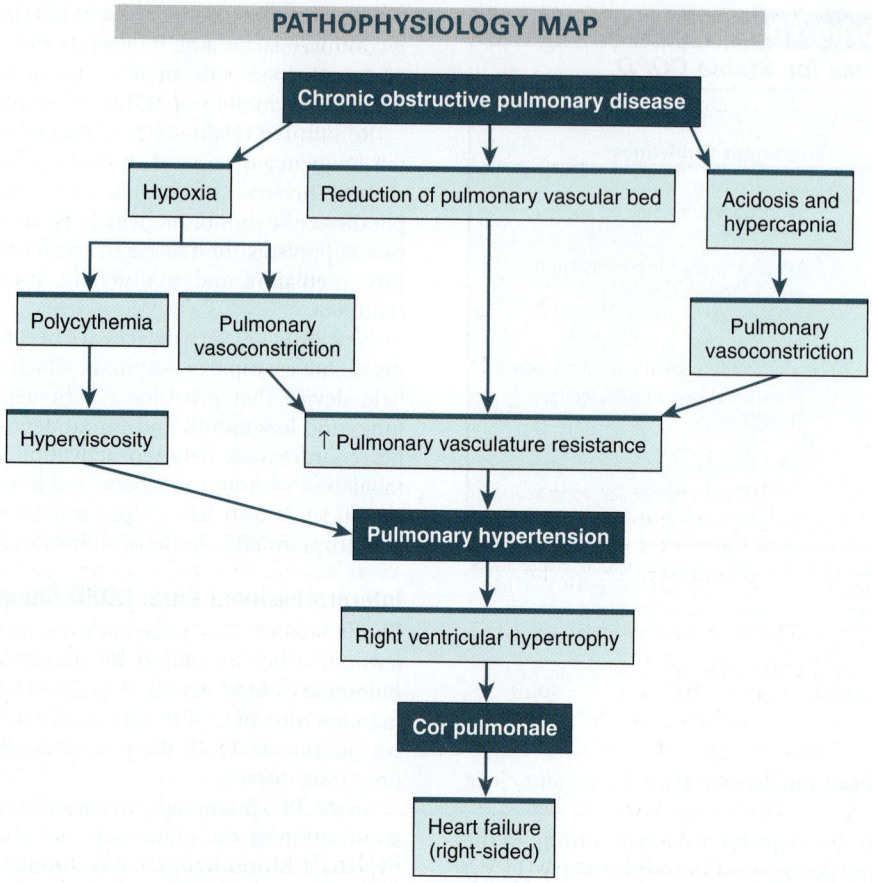

FIG. 28-11 Mechanisms involved in the pathophysiology of pulmonary hypertension and cor pulmonale secondary to chronic obstructive pulmonary disease.

Acute Exacerbations. An exacerbation of COPD is an acute event characterized by a worsening of the patient's respiratory symptoms. Exacerbations are signaled by an acute change in the patient's usual dyspnea, cough, and/or sputum (i.e., something different from the usual daily patterns). The primary causes of exacerbations are bacterial or viral infections.[11] Exacerbations of COPD are typical and increase in frequency (average one or two a year) as the disease progresses.

Assess patients for the classic manifestations of exacerbation: increased dyspnea, increased sputum volume, or increased sputum purulence. They may also have nonspecific complaints of malaise, insomnia, fatigue, depression, confusion, decreased exercise tolerance, increased wheezing, or fever without other causes.

As the severity of COPD increases, exacerbations of COPD are associated with poorer outcomes. Exacerbations may be treated at home or in the hospital, depending on the severity. The severity is determined by the patient's medical history before the exacerbation, the presence of other diseases, current symptoms, ABGs, and other laboratory tests. Typically in the later stages of COPD the patient has a low-normal pH, high-normal or above-normal $PaCO_2$, and high-normal bicarbonate (HCO_3^-). This indicates compensated respiratory acidosis as the patient has chronically retained CO_2 and the kidneys have conserved HCO_3^- to increase the pH to within the normal range (Table 28-3).

Carefully assess the patient's ABGs for any movement toward respiratory acidosis and further hypoxemia, indicating respiratory failure. Also assess the patient's medical history for the stage of COPD as noted by the level of FEV_1. Assess for new symptoms or worsening of usual symptoms. Determine the number of previous exacerbations per year and if treatment occurred in the home or hospital. The presence of other co-morbid conditions complicates the exacerbation. In addition, the current treatment affects its management. Be alert for signs of severity such as use of accessory muscles, central cyanosis, edema in the lower extremities, unstable BP, right-sided heart failure, and altered alertness. These manifestations affect whether the patient is treated as an inpatient or outpatient.

Short-acting bronchodilators, oral systemic corticosteroids, and antibiotics are the typical therapies for exacerbations. SABAs with or without short-acting anticholinergics are preferred for those who are breathless. Drug administration via MDI or nebulizer works equally well, although sicker patients often prefer the nebulizer. Antibiotics are used for the treatment of exacerbations caused by bacterial infections.[19]

Therapies used to treat exacerbations of COPD in the hospital are similar to home management, except supplemental O_2 therapy titrated by ABG measurement may be used. Attempts are made to use noninvasive mechanical methods (e.g., continuous positive airway pressure [CPAP] or bi-level positive airway pressure [Bi-Pap] to support ventilation rather than invasive ventilatory support [e.g., intubation and mechanical ventilation]).

Teach the patient and caregiver early recognition of the three cardinal manifestations of exacerbations (increased dyspnea, increased sputum volume, or increased sputum purulence) to promote early treatment. This may prevent hospitalization and possible respiratory failure.

Acute Respiratory Failure. Patients with severe COPD who have exacerbations are at risk for acute respiratory failure. Frequently, COPD patients wait too long to contact their HCP when they first develop symptoms suggestive of an exacerbation. Discontinuing bronchodilator or corticosteroid medication may also precipitate respiratory failure.[20] (Respiratory failure is discussed in Chapter 67.)

Interprofessional Care: Other COPD Treatments

Oxygen Therapy. O_2 therapy is frequently used in the treatment of COPD and other problems associated with hypoxemia. O_2 is a colorless, odorless, tasteless gas that constitutes 21% of the atmosphere. Administering supplemental O_2 increases the partial pressure of O_2 (PO_2) in inspired air. Used clinically, it is considered a prescribed medication and the only one that has been proven to improve survival of COPD patients.

O_2 is usually administered to treat hypoxemia caused by a variety of problems such as COPD, shock, pulmonary emboli, and many others. Goals for O_2 therapy are to keep the SaO_2 greater than 90% during rest, sleep, and exertion or the PaO_2 greater than 60 mm Hg.

Methods of Administration. There are various methods of O_2 administration (Table 28-20 and Fig. 28-12). The method selected depends on factors such as the fraction of inspired O_2 (FIO_2) required by the patient and delivered by the device, the patient's mobility, humidification required, patient cooperation, comfort, cost, and financial resources.

O_2 delivery systems are classified as low- or high-flow systems. Most methods of O_2 administration are low-flow devices that deliver O_2 in concentrations that vary with the person's respiratory pattern. In contrast, the Venturi mask is a high-flow device that delivers fixed concentrations of O_2 (e.g., 24%, 28%) independent of the patient's respiratory pattern. Mechanical ventilators are another example of a high-flow O_2 delivery system. Because room air is mixed with O_2 in low-flow systems, the percentage of O_2 delivered to the patient is not as precise as with high-flow systems.

Humidification and Nebulization. O_2 obtained from cylinders or wall systems is dry. Dry O_2 has an irritating effect on mucous membranes and dries secretions. Therefore it is important that a high liter flow of O_2, delivering more than 35% to 50% O_2, be humidified, either by humidification or nebulization. A common device used for humidification when the patient has a cannula or a mask is a small plastic jar filled with distilled water called a *bubble-through humidifier.* It is attached to the O_2 source by means of a flowmeter.

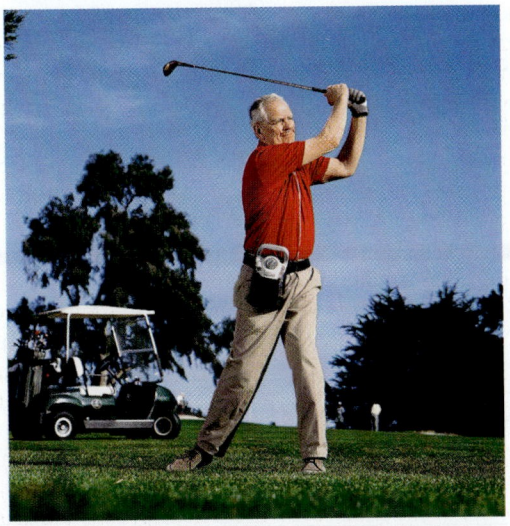

FIG. 28-12 Golfer uses Helios liquid portable O_2 system. (Courtesy Nellcor Puritan Bennett, Inc, Pleasanton, Calif.)

Complications

Combustion. O_2 supports combustion and increases the rate of burning, so it is important to prohibit smoking or have open flames in the area in which O_2 is being used. A "No Smoking" sign should be prominently displayed on the patient's door. Also caution the patient against smoking cigarettes with an O_2 cannula in place as it can cause significant burns.

CO_2 narcosis. The chemoreceptors in the respiratory center that control the drive to breathe respond to CO_2 and O_2. Normally, CO_2 accumulation is a major stimulant of the respiratory center. Over time some COPD patients with hypercapnia develop a tolerance for high CO_2 levels (the respiratory center loses its sensitivity to the elevated CO_2 levels). Theoretically, for these individuals a major "drive" to breathe is hypoxemia. Thus there has been concern regarding the dangers of administering O_2 to COPD patients and reducing their drive to breathe. However, the "hypoxic drive" is complex and involves other factors, including ventilation and perfusion. In addition, not all patients with COPD retain CO_2.

Pulse oximetry and/or ABGs are used as a guide to determine what FIO_2 level is sufficient and can be tolerated. Safe administration of O_2 can be achieved by gradually increasing the concentration of O_2 with close monitoring of both PaO_2 and $PaCO_2$. Venturi masks may be used to have tighter regulation of the maximal FIO_2 that is administered. With nasal cannulas, the O_2 flow rate is generally increased by 1 L per minute at a time. The goal is a pulse O_2 saturation (SpO_2) of at least 90% or a PaO_2 of at least 60 mmHg. Always remember to assess the patient's mental status and vital signs before starting O_2 therapy and frequently thereafter.

O_2 toxicity. Pulmonary **O_2 toxicity** may result from prolonged exposure to a high level of O_2 (PaO_2). High concentrations of O_2 can result in a severe inflammatory response because of O_2 radicals and damage to alveolar-capillary membranes resulting in severe pulmonary edema, shunting of blood, and hypoxemia. Although rare, these individuals can develop acute respiratory distress syndrome (ARDS) (see Chapter 67).

Prevention of O_2 toxicity is important for the patient who is receiving O_2. The amount of O_2 administered should be just enough to maintain the PaO_2 within a normal or acceptable range for the patient. Monitor ABGs frequently to evaluate the effectiveness of therapy and guide the tapering of supplemental O_2. A safe limit of O_2 concentrations has not yet been established. All levels above 60% and O_2 used for longer than 24 hours should be considered potentially toxic. Levels of 40% and below used for short periods may be regarded as relatively nontoxic and probably will not result in significant O_2 toxicity.

Infection. Infection can be a major hazard of O_2 administration. Heated nebulizers present the highest risk. The constant use of humidity supports bacterial growth, with the most common organism being *Pseudomonas aeruginosa.* Disposable equipment that operates as a closed system, such as the Ballard closed suctioning system, should be used. Each hospital has a policy on the required frequency of equipment changes based on the type of equipment used.

TABLE 28-20 Methods of Oxygen Administration

Description	Nursing Interventions
Low-Flow Delivery Devices	
Nasal Cannula	
• Most commonly used device • O_2 delivered via plastic nasal prongs • Safe and simple method that allows some freedom of movement. Patient can eat, talk, or cough while wearing device. • Useful for a patient requiring low O_2 concentrations • O_2 concentrations of 24% (at 1 L/min) to 44% (at 6 L/min) can be obtained.	• Stabilize nasal cannula when caring for a restless patient. • Amount of O_2 inhaled depends on room air and patient's breathing pattern. • Most patients with COPD can tolerate 2 L/min via cannula. • Assess patient's nares and ears for skin breakdown. May need to pad cannula where it sits on ears • If flow rates are >5 L/min, nasal membranes may dry and may cause pain in frontal sinuses.
Simple Face Mask	
• Covers patient's nose and mouth • Used only for short periods, especially when transporting patients • Longer use is typically not tolerated because of tight seal and heat generated around nose and mouth from mask. • O_2 concentrations of 35%-50% can be achieved with flow rates of 6-12 L/min. • Mask provides adequate humidification of inspired air.	• Wash and dry under mask q2hr. • Mask must fit snugly. • Nasal cannula may be provided while patient is eating. • Watch for pressure necrosis at top of ears from elastic straps if patient wears for a longer time. (Gauze or other padding may alleviate this problem.)
Partial and Non-Rebreather Masks	
• Useful for short-term (24 hr) therapy for patients needing higher O_2 concentrations (60%-90% at 10-15 L/min) • O_2 flows into reservoir bag and mask during inhalation. • This bag allows patient to rebreathe about first third of exhaled air (rich in O_2) in conjunction with flowing O_2. • Vents remain open on partial mask only. Some facilities prefer this over non-rebreather as a safety issue.	• O_2 flow rate must be sufficient to keep bag from collapsing during inspiration to avoid CO_2 buildup. • If deflation occurs, increase liter flow to keep bag inflated. • Mask should fit snugly. • With non-rebreather masks, make sure valves are open during expiration and closed during inhalation to prevent drastic decrease in FIO_2. • Monitor patient closely, since more advanced interventions may be required such as CPAP, BiPAP, or intubation with mechanical ventilation.
Oxygen-Conserving Cannula	
• Generally indicated for long-term O_2 therapy at home vs. during hospitalization (e.g., pulmonary fibrosis, pulmonary hypertension) • May be "moustache" (Oxymizer) or "pendant" type • Cannula has a built-in reservoir that ↑ O_2 concentration and allows patient to use lower flow, usually 30%-50%, which increases comfort, lowers cost, and can be increased with activities. • Can deliver O_2 up to 8L/min.	• May cause necrosis over tops of ears. Can be padded • Cannula cannot be cleaned. Manufacturer recommends changing cannula every week. • It is more expensive than standard cannulas and requires evaluation with ABGs and oximetry to determine correct flow for patient. • Cannula is highly visible.

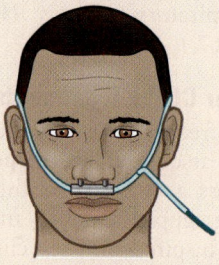

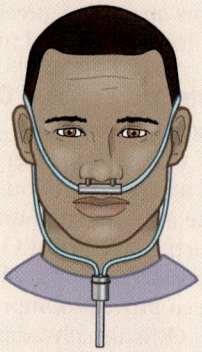

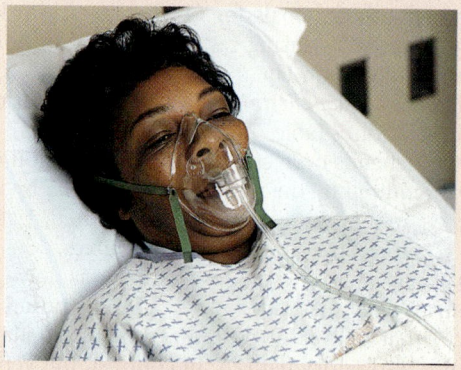

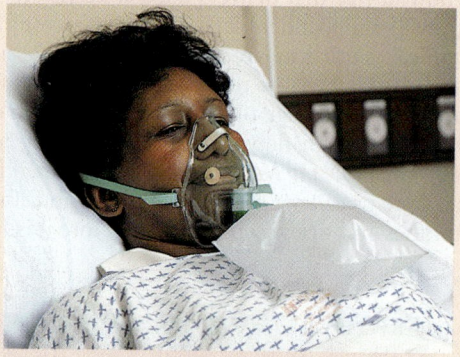

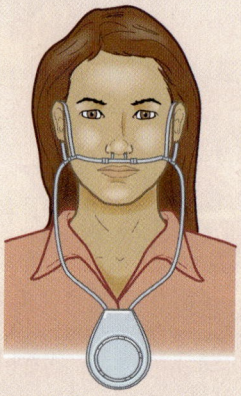

Pendant-type O_2-conserving cannula.

ABGs, Arterial blood gases; *BiPAP,* biphasic positive airway pressure; *CPAP,* continuous positive airway pressure;

TABLE 28-20 Methods of Oxygen Administration—cont'd

Description	Nursing Interventions
High-Flow Delivery Devices	
Tracheostomy Collar	
• Collar attaches to neck with elastic strap and can deliver high humidity and O_2 via tracheostomy. • O_2 concentration is lost into atmosphere because collar does not fit tightly. • Venturi device can be attached to flowmeter and thus can deliver exact amounts of O_2 via collar.	• Secretions collect inside collar and around tracheostomy. Remove collar and clean at least q4hr to prevent aspiration of fluid and infection. • Because condensation occurs in tubing, periodically drain distally to tracheostomy.
Tracheostomy T Bar	
• Almost identical to tracheostomy collar, but it has a vent and a T connector that allow an inline catheter (e.g., Ballard catheter) to be connected for suctioning. • Tight fit allows better O_2 and humidity delivery than tracheostomy collar.	• Empty as necessary. • Because T bars disconnect easily, monitor closely. • T bar may pull on a patient's tracheostomy tube, causing irritation and potential tissue damage. Monitor this closely. • See tracheostomy collar above.
Venturi Mask	
• Mask can deliver precise, high-flow rates of O_2. • Lightweight plastic, cone-shaped device is fitted to face. • Masks are available for delivery of 24%, 28%, 31%, 35%, 40%, and 50% O_2. • Method is especially helpful for administering low, constant O_2 concentrations to patients with COPD. • Adaptors can be applied to increase humidification.	• Entrainment device on mask must be changed to deliver higher concentrations of O_2. • Air entrainment ports must not be occluded. • Mask is uncomfortable. Remove when patient eats. • Patient can talk but voice may be muffled. • See other applicable nursing interventions under simple face mask above.
High-Flow Nasal Cannula	
• Blends O_2 with compressed air to generate FIO_2 up to 1.0 at flow rate of up to 60 L/min and PEEP 7.4 cm H_2O • Active heated humidifier capable of providing 100% body humidity • Soft and flexible nasal prongs. More comfortable than mask	• Nasal cannula must be smaller than 50% of nares to allow flow during exhalation and flush out end-expiratory CO_2. • Patients can eat and drink with device in place. • PEEP drops about 2 cm H_2O when patient's mouth is open.

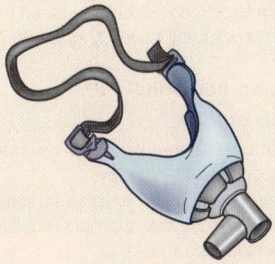

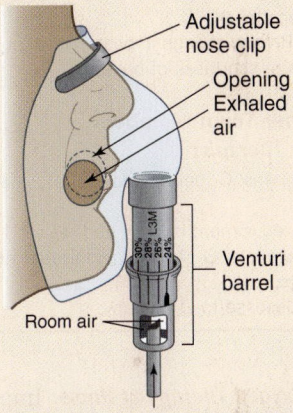

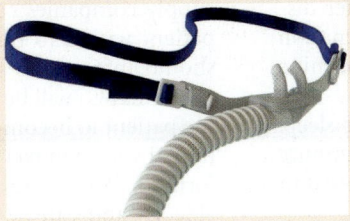

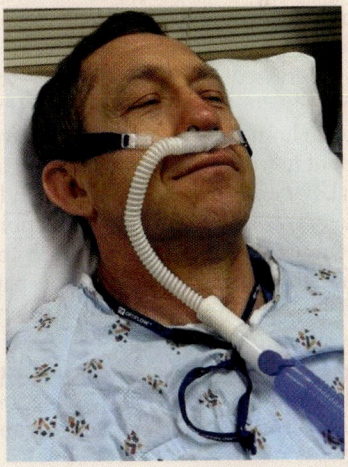

FIO_2, Fraction of inspired O_2.

TEAMWORK & COLLABORATION

Oxygen Administration

All members of the health care team should be alert to possible problems with gas exchange in patients who are receiving oxygenation. Patients who are hypoxemic should be cared for by the registered nurse (RN) until they consistently have O_2 saturations ≥90%.

Role of Nursing Personnel

Registered Nurse (RN)

- Assess need for adjustments in O_2 flow rate.
- Evaluate response to O_2 therapy.
- Monitor patient for signs of adverse effects of O_2 therapy.
- In many cases, choose the optimal O_2 delivery device (e.g., a nasal cannula or simple face mask).
- Teach patient and caregivers about home O_2 use.

Licensed Practical/Vocational Nurse (LPN/LVN)

- For stable patients, adjust O_2 flow rate depending on desired O_2 saturation level.

Unlicensed Assistive Personnel (UAP)

- Use pulse oximetry to measure O_2 saturation.
- Report O_2 saturation level to RN.
- Assist patient with adjustment of O_2 delivery devices (e.g., nasal cannula, face mask).
- Report to RN any change in patient level of consciousness or complaints of shortness of breath.

Role of Other Team Members

Respiratory Therapist

- Assist in optimal O_2 delivery device (e.g., nasal cannula or simple face mask).
- Make sure equipment is clean and replaced as needed.
- Check accuracy of O_2 delivery and assess need for adjustments in O_2 flow rate.
- Evaluate response to O_2 therapy.

Chronic Oxygen Therapy at Home. Improved survival occurs in patients with COPD who receive long-term O_2 therapy (LTOT) (more than 15 hr/day) to treat hypoxemia. The benefits of LTOT include improved mental status, sleep, and exercise tolerance; decreased hematocrit; and reduced pulmonary hypertension.[11]

Short-term home O_2 therapy (7 to 30 days) may be indicated for the patient in whom hypoxemia persists after discharge from the hospital. For example, a patient with underlying COPD who develops a serious respiratory tract infection may need continued O_2 therapy to treat hypoxemia for 4 to 6 weeks after discharge from the hospital. Measure the patient's oxygenation status by SpO_2 2 to 4 weeks after an acute episode to determine if the O_2 is still needed.

Patients may only receive O_2 during exercise and/or sleep. Evaluate the need for O_2 during these periods with a 6-minute walk test or overnight oximetry. (Pulse oximetry is discussed in Chapter 25.)

Periodic reevaluations are necessary for the patient who is using chronic supplemental O_2. Generally, the patient should be reevaluated every 30 to 90 days during the first year of therapy and annually after that, as long as the patient remains stable.

Nasal cannulas, either regular or the O_2-conserving type (Table 28-20), are usually used to deliver O_2 from a central source in the home. The source may be a liquid O_2 storage system, compressed O_2 in tanks, or an O_2 concentrator or extractor, depending on the patient's home environment, insurance coverage, activity level, and proximity to an O_2 supply company (Table 28-21). To increase mobility in the home, the patient can use extension tubing (up to 50 ft) without adversely affecting the O_2 flow delivery. Small, portable systems, such as liquid O_2, may be provided for the patient who remains active outside the home (Fig. 28-12).

TABLE 28-21 Home Oxygen Delivery Systems

- Liquid O_2
- Compressed O_2 cylinders
- Concentrator or extractor
- Portable O_2 concentrator
- O_2 conserving or pulsed devices

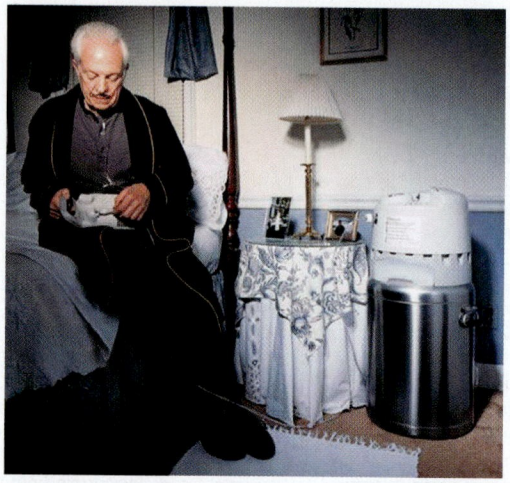

FIG. 28-13 A portable liquid O_2 unit can be refilled from a liquid O_2 reservoir unit. (Courtesy Nellcor Puritan Bennett, Inc, Pleasanton, Calif.)

Home O_2 systems are usually rented from a company that sends a respiratory therapist to the patient's home (Fig. 28-13). The therapist teaches the patient and caregiver how to use the O_2 system, how to care for it, and how to recognize when the supply is running low and must be reordered. A patient and caregiver teaching guide for the use of O_2 at home is presented in Table 28-22.

Encourage the patient who uses home O_2 to remain active and travel normally. If travel is by automobile, arrangements can be made for O_2 to be available at the destination point. O_2 supply companies can often assist in these arrangements. If a patient wishes to travel by bus, train, or airplane, the patient should inform the appropriate people when reservations are made that O_2 will be needed for travel. If there is a potential for the patient to become hypoxic, O_2 needs for flying can be determined via a hypoxia inhalation test or through a mathematical formula. Portable O_2 concentrators are a ready source of renewable O_2 and can be available by recharging at home or with a DC (e.g., auto) power supply. These systems are widely approved by airlines for in-flight use. The patient should contact the airline to determine the particular accommodations and policies for in-flight O_2.

Breathing Retraining. The patient with COPD has dyspnea with an increased respiratory rate. In addition, the accessory muscles of breathing in the neck and upper part of the chest are used excessively to promote chest wall movement. These

TABLE 28-22 Patient & Caregiver Teaching

Home Oxygen Use

The company that provides the prescribed O_2 therapy equipment will instruct the patient on equipment care. The following are some general instructions that you may include when teaching the patient and caregiver about the use of home O_2.

Decreasing Risk for Infection

- Brush teeth or use mouthwash several times a day.
- Wash nasal cannula (prongs) with a liquid soap and thoroughly rinse once or twice a week.
- Replace cannula every 2-4 wk.
- If you have a cold, replace the cannula after your symptoms pass.
- Always remove secretions that are coughed out.
- If you use an O_2 concentrator, every day unplug the unit and wipe down the cabinet with a damp cloth and dry it.
- Ask the company providing the equipment how often to change the filter.

Safety Issues

- Post "No Smoking" warning signs outside the home.
- O_2 will not "blow up," but it will increase the rate of burning, since it is a fuel for the fire.
- Do not allow smoking in the home, and do not smoke yourself while wearing O_2. Nasal cannulas and masks can catch fire and cause serious burns to face and airways.
- Do not use flammable liquids such as paint thinners, cleaning fluids, gasoline, kerosene, oil-based paints, or aerosol sprays while using O_2.
- Do not use blankets or fabrics that carry a static charge, such as wool or synthetics.
- Inform the staff at your electric company if you are using a concentrator. In case of a power failure, they will know the medical urgency of restoring your power.

Adapted from *www.YourLungHealth.org.*

muscles are not designed for long-term use, and as a result, the patient experiences increased fatigue.

The main types of breathing retraining exercises are (1) pursed-lip breathing and (2) diaphragmatic breathing. The purpose of **pursed-lip breathing (PLB)** is to prolong exhalation and thereby prevent bronchiolar collapse and air trapping. PLB is simple and easy to teach and learn, and it gives the patient more control over breathing, especially during exercise and periods of dyspnea (Table 28-13). Patients should be taught to use "just enough" positive pressure with the pursed lips because excessive resistance may increase the work of breathing.

Diaphragmatic (abdominal) breathing focuses on using the diaphragm instead of the accessory muscles of the chest to (1) achieve maximum inhalation and (2) slow the respiratory rate. However, the use of diaphragmatic breathing in patients with COPD may increase the work of breathing and dyspnea. Patients with moderate to severe COPD with marked hyperinflation may be poor candidates for diaphragmatic breathing.[21]

PLB slows the respiratory rate and is easier to learn than diaphragmatic breathing. In the setting of extreme acute dyspnea, it is most important to focus on helping the patient slow the respiratory rate by using the principles of PLB. Other techniques that decrease breathing frequency, such as yoga, may also be used to reduce dyspnea.

Airway Clearance Techniques. Many patients with COPD or other conditions (e.g., cystic fibrosis, bronchiectasis) who retain secretions require help to adequately clear their airways. Airway clearance techniques (ACTs) loosen mucus and secretions so they can be cleared by coughing. A variety of techniques can be used to achieve airway clearance.

TABLE 28-23 Patient & Caregiver Teaching

Effective Huff Coughing

When teaching effective huff coughing:

1. Help the patient assume a sitting position with head slightly flexed, shoulders relaxed, knees flexed, forearms supported by pillow, and, if possible, feet on the floor.

Then you should instruct the patient to:

2. Inhale slowly through the mouth while breathing deeply from the diaphragm.
3. Hold the breath for 2-3 seconds.
4. Forcefully exhale quickly as if one is fogging up a mirror with one's breath (thus creating a "huff"). (This moves the secretions to larger airways.)
5. Repeat the "huff" one or two more times while refraining from a "regular" cough.
6. Cough when mucus is felt in the breathing tubes.
7. Rest for five to ten regular breaths.
8. Repeat the huffs (three to five cycles) until you feel you have cleared mucus or you become tired.

ACTs are especially beneficial in patients who have a COPD exacerbation. Respiratory therapists, physical therapists, and nurses are involved in performing these techniques. ACTs are often used with other treatments. Typically the patient receives bronchodilator therapy via an inhaled device (e.g., nebulization) before ACT. Then the ACT is used, followed by effective coughing (e.g., huff coughing). ACTs include effective coughing, chest physiotherapy, airway clearance devices, and high-frequency chest ventilation.

Effective Coughing. Many patients with COPD have developed ineffective coughing patterns that do not adequately clear their airways of sputum. They also fear developing spastic coughing, resulting in increased dyspnea. Although other techniques (e.g., chest physiotherapy) are used to loosen secretions and mucus, the patient must cough effectively to bring the secretions to the central airways to expectorate them.

Huff coughing is an effective forced expiratory technique that you can easily teach the patient. Before starting, ensure that the patient is breathing deeply from the diaphragm. Place the patient's hands on the lower lateral chest wall and then ask the patient to breathe deeply through the nose. You should feel the patient's hands move outward, which represents a breath from the diaphragm. Guidelines for effective huff coughing are presented in Table 28-23.

Chest Physiotherapy. **Chest physiotherapy (CPT)** is primarily used for patients with excessive bronchial secretions who have difficulty clearing them (e.g., cystic fibrosis, bronchiectasis). CPT consists of postural drainage, percussion, and vibration. CPT should be performed by an individual who has been properly trained.

Percussion and *vibration* are manual or mechanical techniques used to augment postural drainage. These techniques are used after the patient has assumed a postural drainage position to assist in loosening the mobilized secretions. Percussion, vibration, and postural drainage assist in bringing secretions into larger, more central airways. Effective coughing (huff coughing) is then necessary to help raise these secretions.

Complications associated with improperly performed CPT include fractured ribs, bruising, hypoxemia, and discomfort.

CPT may be stressful for some patients, and some may develop hypoxemia and bronchospasms.

Postural drainage. Postural drainage is the use of positioning techniques that drain secretions from specific segments of the lungs and bronchi into the trachea. The postural drainage positions used depend on the areas of lung that are involved. This is determined by patient assessment (including the patient's preference), chest x-rays, and chest auscultation. For example, some patients with left lower lobe involvement require postural drainage of only the affected region, whereas a person with cystic fibrosis may require postural drainage of all segments.

The purpose of various positions in postural drainage is to drain each segment toward the larger airways. A side-lying position can be used for the patient who cannot tolerate a head-down position. Aerosolized bronchodilators and hydration therapy are usually administered before postural drainage. The chosen postural drainage position is maintained for about 5 minutes during percussion and vibration. A common order is two to four times a day. In acute situations, postural drainage may be performed as frequently as every 4 hours. Schedule the procedure to be completed at least 1 hour before meals or 3 hours after meals.

Beds are available that can rotate and percuss in various postural drainage positions, and these are quite effective. Some positions for postural drainage (e.g., Trendelenburg) should not be performed on the patient with chest trauma, hemoptysis, heart disease, pulmonary embolus, or head injury, and in other situations in which the patient's condition is not stable.

Percussion. *Percussion* is performed in the appropriate postural drainage position with the hands in a cuplike position, with the fingers and thumbs closed (Fig. 28-14). The cupped hand should create an air pocket between the patient's chest and the hand. Both hands are cupped and used in an alternating rhythmic fashion. If it is performed correctly, a hollow sound should be heard. The air-cushion impact facilitates the movement of thick mucus. Place a thin towel over the area to be percussed, or the patient may choose to wear a T-shirt or hospital gown.

Vibration. *Vibration* is accomplished by tensing the hand and arm muscles repeatedly and pressing mildly with the flat of the hand on the affected area while the patient slowly exhales a deep breath. The vibrations facilitate movement of secretions to larger airways. Commercial mechanical vibrators are available for hospital and home use.

Airway Clearance Devices. Various *airway clearance devices* are available to mobilize secretions, are easier to tolerate than CPT, and take less time than conventional CPT sessions. These devices include the Flutter, Acapella, and TheraPEP Therapy System. These devices use the principle of positive expiratory pressure (PEP) and may provide greater benefit to patients with COPD than other ACTs.

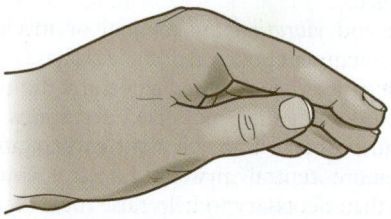

FIG. 28-14 Cupped-hand position for percussion. The hand should be cupped as though scooping up water.

The Flutter mucus clearance device is a hand-held device that is shaped like a small, fat pipe. It provides PEP treatment for patients with mucus-producing conditions. The Flutter has a mouthpiece, a high-density stainless steel ball, and a cone that holds the ball. When the patient exhales through the Flutter, the steel ball moves, which causes oscillations (vibrations) in the airways and loosens mucus to allow improved expectoration. The patient must be upright, and the angle at which the Flutter is held is critical.

The Acapella is another small hand-held device (Fig. 28-15) that combines the benefits of both PEP therapy and airway vibrations to mobilize pulmonary secretions. It can be used in virtually any setting, since patients are free to sit, stand, or recline.

TheraPEP Therapy System can also provide sustained PEP and can simultaneously deliver aerosols so that the patient can inhale and exhale through it. TheraPEP has a mouthpiece attached to tubing connected to a small cylindric resistor and a pressure indicator. The pressure indicator provides visual feedback about the pressure that the patient needs to hold in an exhalation to receive the PEP. (A description and photo of this system are available at *www.smiths-medical.com/catalog/bronchial-hygiene/therapep/therapep-system.html.*)

High-Frequency Chest Wall Oscillation. High-frequency chest wall oscillation uses an inflatable vest (e.g., the Vest Airway system or the SmartVest) with hoses connected to a high-frequency pulse generator. (A description and photo are available at *www.thevest.com/products.*) The pulse generator delivers air to the vest, which vibrates the chest. The high-frequency airwaves dislodge mucus from the airways, mobilize the mucus, and move it toward larger airways. The vest can be used without the aid of another person. The units weigh 23 to 30 lb and are quiet. They come in a suitcase and are portable.

Nutritional Therapy for COPD. Many COPD patients in the advanced stages are underweight with loss of muscle mass and cachexia. Weight loss is a predictor of a poor prognosis and increased frequency of COPD exacerbations. Malnutrition in COPD patients is multifactorial, including increased inflammatory mediators, increased metabolic rate due to the ventilatory effort, and lack of appetite. Other factors that contribute to malnutrition in COPD include altered taste caused by chronic mouth breathing, excessive sputum, fatigue, anxiety, depression, increased energy needs, numerous infections, and side effects of polypharmacy.

To decrease dyspnea and conserve energy, the patient should rest for at least 30 minutes before eating and use a bronchodilator before meals. Teach the patient to avoid exercise and treatments for at least 1 hour before and after eating. If a patient has O_2 therapy prescribed, use of supplemental O_2 by nasal cannula while eating may be beneficial. Assess the patient's dentition because broken or missing teeth or loose dentures make eating more difficult. Activity such as walking or getting out of bed during the day can stimulate the appetite and promote weight

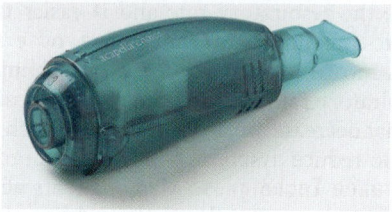

FIG. 28-15 Acapella airway clearance device. (Courtesy Smiths Medical North America.)

TABLE 28-24 Nutritional Therapy

Maximizing Food Intake in COPD

Sometimes it is difficult for patients with COPD to consume adequate amounts of nutrients. Teach the patients to make mealtimes easier and more nutritious by increasing calories and protein without increasing the amount of food eaten.

- Eat high-calorie foods first.
- Limit liquids at mealtimes.
- Rest before meals.
- Try more frequent meals and snacks.
- Increase calories by adding margarine, butter, mayonnaise, sauces, gravies, and peanut butter to foods.
- Keep favorite foods and snacks on hand.
- Try cold foods, which can make you feel less full than hot foods.
- Keep ready-prepared meals available for times when you have increased shortness of breath.
- Eat larger meals when you are not as tired.
- Avoid foods that you know cause gas (e.g., cabbage, beans, cauliflower).
- Add skim milk powder (2 Tbsp) to regular milk (8 oz) to add protein and calories.
- Use milk or half-and-half instead of water when making soups, cereals, instant puddings, cocoa, or canned soups.
- Add grated cheese to sauces, vegetables, soups, and casseroles.
- Choose dessert recipes that contain egg (e.g., sponge cake, angel food cake, egg custard, bread pudding, rice pudding).

Source: Grodner M, Roth S, Walkingshaw B: *Nutritional foundations and clinical applications: a nursing approach*, ed 5, St Louis, 2011, Mosby.

gain. Sensations of bloating and early satiety when eating can be attributed to swallowing air while eating, side effects of medication (especially corticosteroids and theophylline), and the abnormal position of the diaphragm relative to the stomach in association with hyperinflation of the lungs.

Getting the patient to eat adequate amounts of nutritionally sound foods may be difficult even though well-balanced meals are available. Give the patient or meal preparer printed information that can make mealtime easier and more nutritious (Table 28-24).

Underweight patients with COPD need extra protein and calories. They may need 25 to 45 kcal/kg body weight and more than 1.5 g of protein/kg body weight to maintain their weight. The patient with excessive malnutrition may need up to 2.5 g of protein/kg of body weight to restore muscle mass.

A diet high in calories and protein, moderate in carbohydrate, and moderate to high in fat is recommended and can be divided into five or six small meals a day.[22] High-protein, high-calorie nutritional supplements can be offered between meals (Table 28-24). The dietitian is the best resource to determine what combination of nutrients and what supplements are best for the patient. (Nutritional supplements are discussed in Chapter 39.)

Surgical Therapy for COPD. Four different surgical procedures are being used to treat severe COPD. One type of surgery is *lung volume reduction surgery* (LVRS). The goal of this surgery is to reduce the size of the lungs by removing the most diseased lung tissue so that the remaining healthy lung tissue can perform better. Reducing the size of the hyperinflated lungs results in decreased airway obstruction and increased room for the remaining normal alveoli (very small air sacs at the end of each bronchiole) to expand and function. The procedure reduces lung volume and improves lung and chest wall mechanics. LVRS can also allow the diaphragm (the strong wall of muscle that separates the chest cavity from the abdominal cavity; by moving downward, it creates suction in the chest to draw in air and expand the lungs) to return to its normal shape, allowing the patient to breathe more efficiently.

The second type of surgical procedure is *bronchoscopic lung volume reduction surgery* that works by placing one-way valves in the airways leading to the diseased parts of the lung. The valves let air out, but not in. This collapses a certain segment of the lung and produces a result similar to LVRS.[23]

The third surgical procedure is *bullectomy.* In this procedure, one or more very large bullae (large air sacs that form from destroyed alveoli) are removed. These air spaces can become so large that they interfere with breathing.

A fourth surgical procedure is *lung transplantation,* which benefits carefully selected patients with advanced COPD. Although single-lung transplant is the most commonly used technique because of a shortage of donors, bilateral transplantation can be performed. (Lung transplantation is discussed in Chapter 27.)

Gerontologic Considerations: COPD

Older adults have physiologic changes, including reduced lean body mass and decreased respiratory muscle strength that may increase the burden of disease from COPD, including more dyspnea and lower exercise tolerance. This causes a poorer ADL status and a higher incidence of acute exacerbations, which require hospitalization.[24] Smoking cessation is a key intervention but can be difficult to achieve.

COPD is frequently complicated by the presence of co-morbidities such as cardiovascular disease, serious infections, osteoporosis, psychologic problems (depression, anxiety), impaired cognition, and lung cancer.[25] The presence of co-morbidities can make it difficult for patients to cope with the stress of an exacerbation. Thus assessment of co-morbidities can assist in ensuring comprehensive and safe management, especially during an exacerbation.

Older patients may have difficulty in handling the increased secretions during an acute COPD exacerbation. The use of additional medications to manage the acute exacerbation can complicate disease management and increase the likelihood of adverse events. Assess for potential drug-drug interactions, especially in patients being treated for co-morbidities.

Some medications used to treat common disorders in older adults, such as hypertension, can worsen COPD symptoms. Nonspecific β-blockers should be avoided since they can also block the β_2 receptors in the airway and cause bronchoconstriction. Angiotensin-converting enzyme (ACE) inhibitors may cause a dry cough or worsen a present cough.

Older adults may not be adherent to drug therapies due to cognitive impairment and complexity of the polypharmacy prescribed. Arthritis in the hands can hinder the person from using proper technique for MDIs. It is important to review MDI technique during clinic visits and have DPI or spacers prescribed (if possible) because they are easier to use. An attempt to simplify the medication regimen with written large font action plans can be an important intervention in patients with poor memory and visual impairment. Long-term use of ICSs has the potential of causing local and systemic side effects, including cataracts, glaucoma, and osteoporosis. Monitoring of ocular pressures, bone densitometry, and using the lowest possible ICS dose should be recommended.[26]

Older patients with COPD generally have impaired QOL.[27] An important role for you is to focus on things that will improve these patients' quality of life. Psychologic and emotional support becomes imperative to help them achieve successful outcomes. In the later stages of COPD, get palliative and hospice care involved to help manage symptoms and improve the quality of the remainder of their lives.[28]

NURSING MANAGEMENT: CHRONIC OBSTRUCTIVE PULMONARY DISEASE

Nursing Assessment

Subjective and objective data that should be obtained from a person with COPD are presented in Table 28-25.

Nursing Diagnoses

The nursing diagnoses for the patient with COPD may include, but are not limited to, the following:

- Ineffective breathing pattern *related to* alveolar hypoventilation, anxiety, chest wall alterations, and hyperventilation
- Ineffective airway clearance *related to* expiratory airflow obstruction, ineffective cough, decreased airway humidity, and tenacious secretions
- Impaired gas exchange *related to* alveolar hypoventilation

Additional information on nursing diagnoses is presented in eNursing Care Plan 28-2 available on the website for this chapter.

Planning

The overall goals are that the patient with COPD will have (1) prevention of disease progression, (2) ability to perform ADLs and improved exercise tolerance, (3) relief from symptoms, (4) no complications related to COPD, (5) knowledge and ability to implement a long-term treatment regimen, and (6) overall improved quality of life.

Nursing Implementation

Health Promotion. The incidence of COPD would decrease dramatically if people would not begin smoking or would stop smoking. (Techniques to help patients stop smoking are discussed in Chapter 10 and Tables 10-4 to 10-6.) Avoiding or controlling exposure to occupational and environmental pollutants and irritants is another preventive measure to maintain healthy lungs. (These factors are discussed in the section on nursing management of lung cancer in Chapter 27.)

Counseling the patient in smoking cessation is vital, because it is the only way to slow the progression of COPD. As health care professionals, nurses who smoke should reevaluate their own smoking behavior and its relationship to their health. Nurses and other HCPs who smoke should be aware that the odor of smoke is obvious on their clothes, and it can be offensive or tempting to patients.

Early diagnosis and treatment of respiratory tract infections and exacerbations of COPD help prevent progression of the disease. People with COPD should avoid others who are sick, practice good hand-washing techniques, take medications as prescribed, exercise regularly, and maintain a healthy weight. Influenza and pneumococcal pneumonia vaccines are recommended for patients with COPD.

TABLE 28-25 Nursing Assessment

Chronic Obstructive Pulmonary Disease

Subjective Data

Important Health Information

Past health history: Long-term exposure to chemical pollutants, respiratory irritants, occupational fumes, dust; recurrent respiratory tract infections; previous hospitalizations

Medications: Use of O_2 and duration of O_2 use, bronchodilators, corticosteroids, antibiotics, anticholinergics, OTC drugs, herbs, medications purchased outside United States

Functional Health Patterns

Health perception–health management: Smoking (pack-years, including passive smoking, willingness to stop smoking, and previous attempts); family history of respiratory disease (especially α_1-antitrypsin deficiency)

Nutritional-metabolic: Anorexia, weight loss or gain

Activity-exercise: Increasing dyspnea and/or increase in sputum volume or purulence (to detect exacerbation); fatigue, ability to perform ADLs; swelling of feet; progressive dyspnea, especially on exertion; ability to walk up one flight of stairs without stopping; wheezing; recurrent cough; sputum production (especially in the morning); orthopnea

Elimination: Constipation, gas, bloating

Sleep-rest: Insomnia; sitting up position for sleeping, paroxysmal nocturnal dyspnea

Cognitive-perceptual: Headache, chest or abdominal soreness

Coping–stress tolerance: Anxiety, depression

Objective Data

General

Debilitation, restlessness, assumption of upright position

Integumentary

Cyanosis (bronchitis), pallor or ruddy color, poor skin turgor, thin skin, digital clubbing, easy bruising; peripheral edema (cor pulmonale)

Respiratory

Rapid, shallow breathing; inability to speak; prolonged expiratory phase; pursed-lip breathing; wheezing; crackles, diminished or bronchial breath sounds; ↓ chest excursion and diaphragm movement; use of accessory muscles; hyperresonant or dull chest sounds on percussion

Cardiovascular

Tachycardia, dysrhythmias, jugular venous distention, distant heart tones, right-sided S_3 (cor pulmonale), edema (especially in feet)

Gastrointestinal

Ascites, hepatomegaly (cor pulmonale)

Musculoskeletal

Muscle atrophy, ↑ anteroposterior diameter (barrel chest)

Possible Diagnostic Findings

Abnormal ABGs (compensated respiratory acidosis, ↓ PaO_2 or SaO_2, ↑ $PaCO_2$), polycythemia, pulmonary function tests showing expiratory airflow obstruction (e.g., low FEV_1, low FEV_1/FVC, large RV), chest x-ray showing flattened diaphragm and hyperinflation or infiltrates

ABGs, Arterial blood gases; *FEV_1,* forced expiratory volume in 1 sec; *FVC,* forced vital capacity; *RV,* residual volume.

Families with a history of COPD, as well as AAT deficiency, should be aware of the genetic nature of the disease. These individuals should consult a pulmonologist about regular spirometry screening, even though they do not have symptoms. Genetic counseling is appropriate for the patient with AAT deficiency who is planning to have children.

◆ **Acute Care.** The patient with COPD requires acute care for complications such as acute exacerbations of COPD, pneumonia, cor pulmonale, and acute respiratory failure. (The nursing care for these conditions is discussed in Chapters 27 and 67.) Once the crisis in these situations has been resolved, assess the degree and severity of the underlying respiratory problem. The information obtained will help in planning the nursing care.

◆ **Ambulatory Care.** By far the most important aspect in the long-term care of the patient with COPD is teaching. (A patient and caregiver teaching guide is presented in Table 28-26.)

◆ ***Pulmonary Rehabilitation.*** Pulmonary rehabilitation (PR) can be done in an inpatient or outpatient setting or in the home. Components of PR vary but usually include exercise training, smoking cessation, nutrition counseling, and education. A mandatory component of any PR program is exercise that focuses on the muscles used in ambulation, but upper limb exercises may be included also. Smoking cessation is critical to the patient's success. In PR an interprofessional team works together to individualize the treatment plan for COPD patients. Physical therapists or nurses who have experience in pulmonary care are often responsible for the management of pulmonary rehabilitation centers. A large part of your role is to teach patients self-management of their disease.

PR should not be viewed as a "last ditch" effort for patients with severe COPD since it is indicated for any degree of airway obstruction or GOLD classification. PR works best if the patient starts it when COPD is in a moderate stage. However, even people who have advanced COPD can benefit from PR. PR relieves dyspnea and fatigue, improves emotional function, and enhances the sense of control that individuals have over their COPD.[29,30]

PR may be inaccessible to some because of cost, disability, transportation, or geographic location. One alternative program to PR uses the Internet or gaming technology to deliver daily motivational messages and provide cardiopulmonary benefits.[31] However, these types of programs must be approved by the HCP to ensure safety.

INFORMATICS IN PRACTICE

Texting for Chronic Obstructive Pulmonary Disease (COPD) Patients

- Sometimes patients with COPD or those requiring O_2 therapy experience difficulty speaking because of shortness of breath.
- Encourage your patient to use typed messages displayed on a monitor to communicate.
- Texting and instant messaging family and friends are good alternatives to having phone conversations.

◆ ***Activity Considerations.*** Exercise training leads to energy conservation, which is an important component in COPD rehabilitation. The patient with severe COPD typically uses upper thoracic and neck muscles to breathe rather than the diaphragm. Thus the patient has difficulty performing upper-extremity activities, particularly those that require raising the arm above the head. Exercise training of the upper extremities may improve muscle function and help to reduce dyspnea.

TABLE 28-26 Patient & Caregiver Teaching

Chronic Obstructive Pulmonary Disease

Include the following information in the teaching plan to assist the patient with COPD and the caregiver to improve quality of life through teaching and promotion of lifestyle practices that support successful living with chronic obstructive pulmonary disease (COPD).

What is COPD?
- Basic anatomy and physiology of lung
- Basic pathophysiology of COPD
- Signs and symptoms of COPD, exacerbation, cold, flu, pneumonia
- Tests to assess breathing

Breathing and Airway Clearance Exercises
- Pursed-lip breathing (Table 28-13)
- Airway clearance technique: huff cough (Table 28-23)

Energy Conservation Techniques
- Daily activities (e.g., waking up, bathing, grooming, shopping, traveling)
- Consult with physical therapist and occupational therapist

Medications

Types (include mechanism of action and types of devices)
- Methylxanthines
- β_2-Adrenergic agonists
- Corticosteroids
- Anticholinergics
- Antibiotics
- Other medications

Establishing medication schedule

Correct Use of Inhalers, Spacer, and Nebulizer
- Demonstration–return demonstration with placebo devices (Figs. 28-5 to 28-7 and Tables 28-9 to 28-11)

Home Oxygen
- Explanation of rationale for use
- Guide for home O_2 use and equipment

Psychosocial/Emotional Issues

Open discussion (sharing with patient, caregiver, and family)
- Concerns about interpersonal relationships (e.g., intimacy)
- Problems with emotions (e.g., depression, anxiety, panic)
- Dependency

Treatment decisions
- Support and rehabilitation groups

End-of-life issues

COPD Management Plan

Nurse and patient develop and write up COPD management plan that meets individual needs.
- Focus on self-management
- Need to report changes
- Cause of flare-ups or exacerbation
- Recognition of signs and symptoms of respiratory infection, heart failure
- Reduce risk factors, especially smoking cessation
- Exercise program of walking and arm strengthening
- Yearly follow-up

Healthy Nutrition (Table 28-24)
- Strategies to lose weight (if overweight)
- Strategies to gain weight (if underweight)
- Consultation with dietitian

For additional information, see American Lung Association at *www.lung.org/lung-disease/copd.*

Frequently the patient has already adapted alternative energy-saving practices for ADLs. Alternative methods of hair care, shaving, showering, and reaching may have to be explored. An occupational therapist may help with ideas in these areas. Assuming a tripod posture (elbows supported on a table, chest in fixed position) and placing a mirror on the table while using an electric razor or hair dryer conserve much more energy than when the patient stands in front of a mirror to shave or blow-dry hair.

If the patient uses home O_2 therapy, O_2 should be used during activities of hygiene because these are energy consuming. Encourage the patient to make a schedule and plan daily and weekly activities to leave plenty of time for rest periods. The patient should also try to sit as much as possible when performing activities. Another energy-saving tip is to exhale when pushing, pulling, or exerting effort during an activity and inhale during rest.

Regular physical exercise is important for patients with COPD. To ensure long-term adherence, the exercise must be individualized and easy to perform. Walking or other endurance exercises (e.g., cycling) combined with strength training are the best interventions to strengthen muscles and improve the patient's endurance. Teach the patient coordinated walking with slow, pursed-lip breathing (Table 28-13). Many patients with moderate or severe COPD are anxious and fearful of walking or performing exercise. These patients and their caregivers require support while they build the confidence they need to walk or perform daily exercises.

Developing a patient's exercise endurance is very important. If it takes longer than 5 minutes to return to baseline, the patient most likely has overdone it and should proceed at a slower pace during the next exercise period. The patient may benefit from keeping a diary or log of the exercise program. Stationary cycling can also be used either alone or with walking. Cycles and treadmills are particularly good when weather prevents walking outside.

Fatigue, sleep disturbances, and dyspnea are common complaints of patients with COPD. Of these symptoms, dyspnea appears to be the one that affects the patient's ability to carry out daily activities. Therefore you and other members of the interprofessional team should focus your interventions on improving dyspnea, which would then improve the patient's functional performance.

Patients frequently ask whether moving to a warmer or drier climate will help. In general, such a move is not significantly beneficial. Discourage moves to places with an elevation of 4000 ft or more because of the lower partial pressure of O_2 found in the air at higher elevations. A disadvantage of moving may be that a person leaves a job, friends, and familiar environment, which could be psychologically stressful. Any advantage gained from a different climate may be outweighed by the psychologic effects of the move.

◆ ***Psychosocial Considerations.*** Healthy coping is a challenge for the COPD patient and family. People with COPD frequently have to deal with many lifestyle changes that may involve decreased ability to care for themselves, decreased energy for social activities, and loss or change in a job.

When a patient with COPD is first diagnosed or has complications that require hospitalization, expect a variety of emotional responses. Emotions frequently encountered include guilt, loneliness from social isolation, denial, and frustration from increased dependence. Guilt may result from the knowledge that the disease was caused primarily by cigarette smoking.

EVIDENCE-BASED PRACTICE

Applying the Evidence

Physical Activity and COPD

You are working as a nurse in the pulmonary clinic with R.P., a 65-yr-old man who has been recently discharged from the hospital after being newly diagnosed with COPD. He tells you he has been mostly inactive for the past few months because his breathing seems to worsen with activity.

Making Clinical Decisions

Best Available Evidence. Patients with COPD who participate in regular moderate physical activity (e.g., brisk walking) have fewer severe flare-ups and are less likely to be readmitted to the hospital.

Clinician Expertise. Physical inactivity is common in patients with COPD. You know that persistent inactivity may place a patient at greater risk for hospital readmissions.

Patient Preference and Values. R.P. tells you that he misses taking walks every day with his wife and is wondering if he would be able to resume this activity at a slow pace.

Implications for Practice

1. What important factors will you discuss with R.P. about physical activity and COPD?
2. How would you assess R.P.'s willingness and motivation to engage in physical activity?
3. How would you involve the interprofessional team members to assist R.P. in regular physical activity?

Reference for Evidence

Nguyen H, Chu L, Liu I, et al: Associations between physical activity and 30-day readmission risk in chronic obstructive pulmonary disease, *Ann Amer Thorac Soc* 11:695, 2014.

Patients with COPD experience many losses as the disease progresses. Because many patients with COPD experience depression and anxiety, assess for both. Ask patients if they "feel down or blue" most of the time. Do they appear anxious about being able to control their breathlessness or know what to do if they have an exacerbation? Are they exhibiting concern over more difficulty in self-care activities such as bathing? How is the family coping with the patient's disease?

It is important to convey a sense of understanding and caring to the patient. The patient with COPD may benefit from stress management techniques (e.g., massage, muscle relaxation [see Chapter 6]). In addition, teach patients about the treatment and disease, which can give them a sense of control of their disease and complex treatment regimens. It is important to include the patient's caregiver in the teaching so that he or she can help the patient cope physically and emotionally. Support groups at local American Lung Association chapters (such as the Better Breathers Club), hospitals, and clinics can also be helpful.

A consultation with a therapist may be needed for proper screening and diagnosis of depression or other mental health problems. Cognitive and behavioral therapy along with COPD teaching may improve the quality of life. Medications may be used to treat both depression and anxiety. Buspirone (BuSpar), which is used to treat anxiety, has few if any respiratory depression effects. Benzodiazepines should be avoided because they may depress the respiratory drive and may be habit forming. When the patient becomes anxious because of dyspnea, the use of pursed-lip breathing (Table 28-13) and short-acting bronchodilators may be appropriate.

◆ ***Sexuality and Sexual Activity.*** Modifying but not abstaining from sexual activity can also contribute to healthy psychologic well-being. Most patients with COPD are older. Assess and reflect on your own attitudes and feelings about sexuality, sexual functioning, and aging before exploring sexual issues with the older COPD patient. First assess the patient's concerns related to sexuality and functioning. Ask open-ended questions to determine if the patient wants to discuss any of these concerns. You could ask, "How has your breathing problem affected how you see yourself as a woman or man?" Another question could be, "How does your shortness of breath affect your desire for intimacy with your partner?" These types of questions give the person an opening to discuss concerns. Much of the sexual performance issues experienced by the patient with COPD are changes related to aging, and if you are aware of these changes, you can teach the patient the "normalcy" of the changes.

Dyspnea, the predominant symptom in COPD, should not be a major problem with success in sexual functioning, except for those patients in severe stages. If the patient can walk up two flights of stairs or walk briskly, he or she likely has sufficient energy for sexual activity. Erectile dysfunction can occur with COPD as with many chronic diseases. Using an inhaled bronchodilator before sexual activity can help ventilation. The patient with COPD may also find these suggestions helpful: (1) plan sexual activity during the part of the day when breathing is best, which is usually late morning or early afternoon (plus older men often achieve an erection more easily in the morning); (2) use slow pursed-lip breathing; (3) refrain from sexual activity after eating or drinking alcohol; (4) choose less stressful positions during intercourse (missionary position for men is the worst); (5) use O_2 if prescribed; and (6) understand that cigarettes can increase male impotence. Often the patient has coexisting cardiac disease and should obtain advice from a or an HCP related to appropriate levels of activity. These aspects of sexual activity require open communication between partners regarding their needs and expectations and the changes that may be necessary as the result of a chronic disease (e.g., changes in body image, role reversal).[32]

◆ ***Sleep.*** Adequate sleep is extremely important to maintain quality of life and productivity. Patients with COPD have an increased prevalence of sleep disorders. The hyperinflation of the lungs and reduction in ventilation can result in severe drops in O_2 saturation (down to 60% or less) during sleep. This leads to a strain on the heart. In addition, hypercapnia may develop with more frequent awakening. The net result is sleeping poorly and awakening unrefreshed and fatigued.

Current tobacco use, depression, and anxiety are all common in COPD and lead to more trouble sleeping. β_2-Agonists may cause restlessness and insomnia. Many patients with COPD have postnasal drip or nasal congestion that may cause coughing and wheezing at night. Nasal saline sprays or rinses before sleep and in the morning may help. If the patient is prescribed O_2 therapy, using it at night will decrease insomnia. If the patient is a restless sleeper, snores, stops breathing while asleep, and has a tendency to fall asleep during the day, the patient may need to be tested for sleep apnea (see Chapter 7).

◆ ***End-of-Life Considerations.*** The trajectory of COPD is a gradual decline in health characterized by increasing exacerbations that are associated with an increased risk of death. Palliative, end-of-life, and hospice care are important components of care for the patient with advanced COPD.[33]

Patients need to know that symptoms can be managed, but COPD cannot be cured. End-of-life issues and advance directives are important topics for discussion in the terminal stages of COPD. However, this may be difficult for the patient and family to consider because of the uncertainty of the disease. (Palliative care and end-of-life care are discussed in Chapter 9.)

ETHICAL/LEGAL DILEMMAS

Advance Directives

Situation

L.H., a 79-yr-old man with COPD, is in respiratory failure when he is admitted to the hospital. He is placed on a ventilator and responds occasionally by opening his eyes. His advance directives (ADs) were drawn up 5 years ago, and copies were given to his wife and HCP at that time. The patient's wife brings the documents to the intensive care unit and tells you that the hospital must stop treating her husband and allow him to die as he requested. However, the patient's oldest son is threatening the hospital with a lawsuit if the staff does not provide full care to his father.

Ethical/Legal Points for Consideration

- A Living Will, one form of AD, permits individuals to state their own preferences and refusals should the individual become terminally ill or be in a situation in which there is no hope of recovery, and the person is not able to speak for himself or herself.*
- The Durable Power Attorney for Health Care, another form of AD, permits individuals to identify a proxy to make health care decisions in the event the individual is incapacitated.
- The National POLST Paradigm is an approach to end-of-life planning that emphasizes patients' wishes about the care they receive. The POLST Paradigm is an approach to end-of-life planning emphasizing the medical orders and includes coverage, regardless of location (e.g., hospital, home, assisted living).[1]
- AD laws vary from state to state concerning the need for witnesses and who the proxy is.
- You have an obligation to check your state requirements.[2]
- Some families are deeply divided about decisions for their loved ones, and conflicts often arise when money and property are involved. This conflict situation requires the nurse to call for a consult from the ethics committee in the organization.
- HCPs are obligated to follow the patient's ADs when a patient is no longer able to speak for himself or herself.
- In your scope of nursing practice, you need to (1) be informed about the decision-making laws and regulations in your state, (2) make AD documents available to patients, (3) teach patients and their families about ADs, (4) determine if all involved health care providers are aware of the existence of ADs, (5) assist the patient and family in communicating with the health care providers when a "no code" order is requested, and (6) assist the conflicted family in obtaining appropriate counseling whenever necessary.

Discussion Questions

1. What should you do next with the information provided by L.H.'s wife?
2. How should you address the needs of each member of this family in L.H.'s plan of care?
3. What resources can you use to facilitate decision making in this situation?

References

1. Physician Orders for Life Sustaining Treatment (POLST) Program. *www.polst.org.*
2. *www.caringinfo.org/i4a/pages/index.cfm?pageid=3289.*

*Advance directives are listed in Table 9-6.

Evaluation

The expected outcomes are that the patient with COPD will

- Return to pre-exacerbation baseline respiratory function
- Demonstrate an effective rate, rhythm, and depth of respirations
- Experience clear breath sounds
- Maintain clear airway by effectively coughing
- Have $PaCO_2$ and PaO_2 values that return to normal for patient

Additional information on expected outcomes for the patient with COPD is presented in eNursing Care Plan 28-2 available on the website for this chapter.

CYSTIC FIBROSIS

Cystic fibrosis (CF) is an autosomal recessive, multisystem disease characterized by altered transport of sodium and chloride ions in and out of epithelial cells. This defect primarily affects the lungs, gastrointestinal tract (pancreas and biliary tract), and reproductive tract.

CF was first described in 1938 when autopsies of young children revealed multiple cysts in the pancreas, so the disease was called "cystic fibrosis of the pancreas."[34] Once advances in care allowed children to live into later childhood, the lung disease became the more significant problem.

Approximately 30,000 children and adults in the United States have CF. About 10 million (about 1 in every 31) Americans are carriers of the CF gene but do not have the disease. Of the CF patients in the Cystic Fibrosis Patient Registry, over 49% are 18 years of age or older.

The first signs and symptoms typically occur in children, but some patients are not diagnosed until they are adults; some live to over 80 years old. The severity and progression of the disease vary. With early diagnosis and improvements in therapy, the prognosis of patients with CF has significantly improved. The median predicted survival was 16 years in 1970 but has increased to more than 41 years.[35]

Etiology and Pathophysiology

Genetic Link. CF is an autosomal recessive disorder (see Figs. 12-4 and 12-5 and the Genetics in Clinical Practice box on this page). The CF gene is located on chromosome 7 and produces a protein called *CF transmembrane conductance regulator (CFTR)*. The CFTR protein localizes to the epithelial surface of the airways, gastrointestinal tract, and ducts of the liver, pancreas, and sweat glands. CFTR regulates sodium and chloride movement in and out of epithelial cells. Mutations in the *CFTR* gene alter this protein in such a way that the channels are blocked. As a result, cells that line the passageways of the lungs, pancreas, intestines, and other organs produce secretions that are low in sodium chloride content (thus low in water content), making mucus abnormally thick and sticky (Fig. 28-16). This mucus plugs up the ducts in these organs, thus causing scarring in the organs, ultimately resulting in organ failure. The high concentrations of sodium and chloride in the sweat of the patient with CF result from decreased chloride reabsorption in the sweat duct.

In the respiratory system, both the upper and lower respiratory tracts can be affected. Upper respiratory tract manifestations may include chronic sinusitis and nasal polyposis. The hallmark of respiratory involvement in CF is its effect on the airways. The disease progresses from being a disease of the

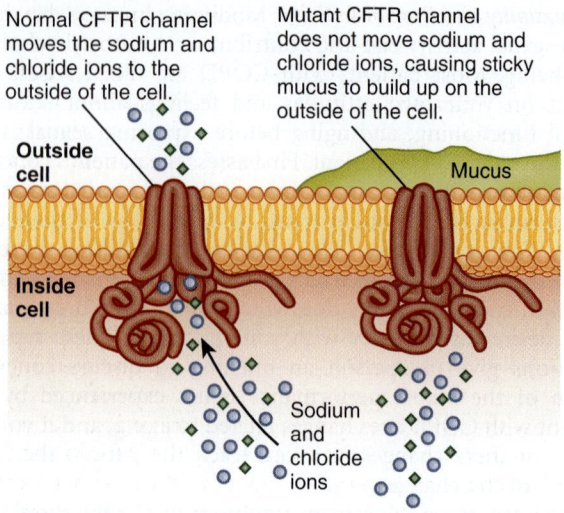

FIG. 28-16 People with cystic fibrosis inherit a defective gene on chromosome 7 called *cystic fibrosis transmembrane conductance regulator (CFTR)*. The protein produced by this gene normally helps sodium and chloride move in and out of cells. If the protein does not work correctly, then the movement of sodium and chloride is blocked and an abnormally thick sticky mucus is produced on the outside of the cell.

GENETICS IN CLINICAL PRACTICE

Cystic Fibrosis (CF)

Genetic Basis

- Autosomal recessive disorder
- Caused by mutations in CF transmembrane regulator *(CFTR)* gene on chromosome 7
- Many different mutations of *CFTR* gene have been identified.
- *CFTR* gene provides instructions for making protein that controls the channel that transports sodium and chloride.
- Mutations in the *CFTR* gene disrupt the function of the channels, preventing them from regulating the flow of sodium, chloride, and water across cell membranes.

Incidence

- In the United States 1 in 3000 white births
- Less common in other ethnic populations (1 in 17,000 African Americans and 1 in 31,000 Asian Americans)
- One in 20 to 25 whites are carriers of the gene.
- If both parents carry the affected gene, there is a 25% chance each offspring will have the disease (see Figs. 12-4 and 12-5).

Genetic Testing

- Blood-based DNA testing is available for disease and carrier states.
- All 50 states have passed legislation requiring that all newborns be screened for CF.
- Testing is usually done in children if CF is suspected or if parents are possible carriers.
- In parents who are known carriers, amniocentesis or chorionic villus sampling in pregnant women may be useful for prenatal testing.

Clinical Implications

- CF is the most common autosomal recessive disease in whites.
- CF has a wide range of clinical expression of disease.
- CF requires long-term medical management.
- Advances in medical care have improved life expectancy.
- Most people who have a child with CF are not aware of a family history of disease.
- CF screening should be offered to all individuals of reproductive age regardless of family history.

small airways *(chronic bronchiolitis)* to involvement of the larger airways and finally causes destruction of lung tissue. The mucus becomes dehydrated and tenacious due to the defect in the chloride secretion and excess sodium absorption. Cilia motility is decreased, thus allowing mucus to adhere to the airways. The bronchioles become obstructed with thick mucus, leading to scarring of the airways (bronchiectasis), air trapping, and hyperinflation of the lungs.

CF is characterized by chronic airway infection that cannot be eradicated. Organisms commonly cultured from the sputum of a patient with CF are *Staphylococcus aureus, Haemophilus influenzae,* and *Pseudomonas aeruginosa,* and less commonly but more seriously, *Burkholderia cepacia. Pseudomonas* is by far the most common organism in adults. Antibiotic resistance develops after multiple exposure to antibiotics. Pulmonary inflammation is associated with the chronic infection and can cause a decrease in respiratory function, thus further narrowing the lumen of the airways. Inflammatory mediators (e.g., interleukins, oxidants, proteases released by neutrophils) are increased and contribute to the progression of lung disease.

Lung disorders that initially occur are chronic bronchiolitis and bronchitis. However, after months or years, changes in the bronchial walls lead to bronchiectasis (Fig. 28-17). Over a long period, pulmonary vascular remodeling occurs because of local hypoxia and arteriolar vasoconstriction. Pulmonary hypertension, enlarged pulmonary arteries, and cor pulmonale occur in the later phases of the disease. Blebs and large cysts in the lung are also severe manifestations of lung destruction, and pneumothorax may develop. Other pulmonary complications include hemoptysis, which is caused by proliferation of capillaries in response to chronic infection. During exacerbations, erosion of these capillaries occurs. Hemoptysis may range from scant streaking to major bleeding, which can sometimes be fatal.

Pancreatic insufficiency is caused primarily by mucous plugging of the pancreatic exocrine ducts, which results in atrophy of the gland and progressive fibrotic cyst formation. The pancreas's exocrine function may be completely lost. Because of the exocrine dysfunction, pancreatic enzymes such as lipase, amylase, and proteases (trypsin, chemotrypsin) are not made in sufficient amounts to allow for absorption of nutrients. Malabsorption of fat, protein, and fat-soluble vitamins (A, D, E, and K) occurs. Fat malabsorption results in steatorrhea, and protein malabsorption results in failure to grow and gain weight.

CF-related diabetes mellitus (CFRD) is thought to be caused by underdevelopment of pancreatic islet cells (in utero) as well as destruction of islet cells over the individual's lifetime. CFRD is a unique type of diabetes with characteristics of both type 1 and type 2 diabetes. The pancreas in people with CF produces insulin but too late to fully respond to carbohydrate intake.

Other common disorders that develop in CF include osteopenia and osteoporosis. These disorders are related to malnutrition, malabsorption of vitamin D, insufficient testosterone levels, and chronically elevated inflammatory cytokines.

Individuals with CF often have other gastrointestinal problems, including GERD, which is often related to excessive coughing. The liver and gallbladder can be damaged by mucus deposits in the ducts. The liver enzymes may become chronically elevated, with cirrhosis developing over time. Gallstones, pancreatitis, and portal hypertension can also occur. Distal intestinal obstruction syndrome (DIOS) results from intermittent obstruction commonly occurring in the terminal ileum at the point of the ileocecal junction. It is caused by thickened,

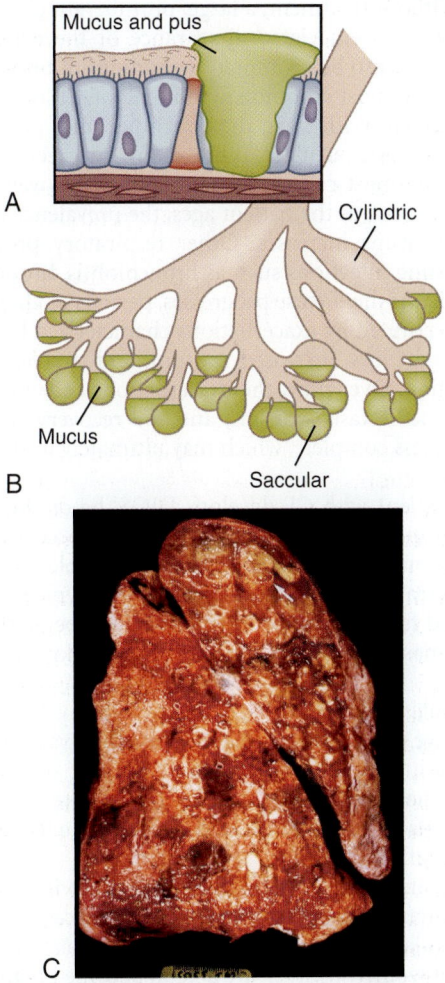

FIG. 28-17 Pathologic changes in bronchiectasis. **A,** Longitudinal section of bronchial wall where chronic infection has caused damage. **B,** Collection of purulent material in dilated bronchioles, leading to persistent infection. **C,** Bronchiectasis in a patient with cystic fibrosis who underwent lung transplantation. Cut surfaces of lung show markedly distended peripheral bronchi filled with mucopurulent secretions. (***C,*** From Kumar V, Abbas AK, Aster JC, et al: *Robbins and Cotran pathologic basis of disease,* ed 8, Philadelphia, 2010, Saunders.)

dehydrated stool and mucus. The patient may appear to have a small bowel obstruction. DIOS develops because of chronic malabsorption related to exocrine dysfunction, under- or overdosing of pancreatic replacement enzyme supplementation, dehydration, swallowing of mucus, and use of opioids.

Clinical Manifestations

The clinical manifestations of CF vary depending on the severity of the disease. Carriers are not affected by the mutation. The disease severity may vary greatly, both within families and among different families.

The median age at diagnosis of CF is 5 months of age; 72% are diagnosed in the first year of life.[35] Currently every state has mandatory newborn screening for CF, which has allowed for early intervention. An initial finding of meconium ileus in the newborn infant prompts the diagnosis in 20% of people with CF. Other signs that suggest a CF diagnosis are acute or persistent respiratory symptoms (wheezing, coughing, frequent pneumonia), failure to thrive or malnutrition, steatorrhea (large, oily, frequent bowel movements), and family history. Without treatment, a large, protuberant abdomen may develop with an emaciated appearance of the extremities. A diagnosis may also be prompted by findings of bronchiectasis.

One of the most common symptoms of CF in the adult is frequent cough. With time, the cough becomes persistent and produces viscous, purulent, often yellow or greenish sputum. Although the most common bacteria in the airways in childhood is *S. aureus*, as the patient ages, the prevalence of *Pseudomonas* organisms increases. Other respiratory problems are recurring lung infections such as bronchiolitis, bronchitis, and pneumonia. As the disease progresses, periods of clinical stability are interrupted by exacerbations characterized by increased cough, weight loss, increased sputum, and decreased pulmonary function. Over time, the exacerbations become more frequent, bronchiectasis worsens, and the recovery of lost lung function is less complete, which may ultimately lead to respiratory failure.

If the patient with CF develops DIOS, he or she may have right lower quadrant pain (the area of the ileocecal valve), loss of appetite, nausea, emesis, and often a palpable mass. Insufficient pancreatic enzyme release causes the typical pattern of protein and fat malabsorption with a person being thin with a low body mass index (BMI) and frequent, bulky, foul-smelling stools.

Both males and females have delayed puberty. Nearly all men with CF have reproductive issues because their vas deferens fails to develop in utero, so there is no transport of sperm from storage in the testes to the penile urethra. However, they make sperm normally, and with assisted reproductive technology are capable of fathering a child.

Some women with CF have difficulty conceiving; the cervical mucus is thought to be thickened. During exacerbations, menstrual irregularities and secondary amenorrhea are common. A majority of women with CF are able to become pregnant. Most pregnancies result in viable infants.

Complications

Complications in CF include CFRD, bone disease, sinus disease, and liver disease. Pneumothorax, a relatively uncommon but serious complication, is caused by the formation of bullae and blebs. A small amount of blood in sputum is common in the CF patient because of chronic lung infection. Massive hemoptysis, which is relatively uncommon, can be life-threatening. With advanced lung disease, digital clubbing occurs. Respiratory failure and cor pulmonale caused by pulmonary hypertension are late complications of CF.

Diagnostic Studies

The diagnostic criteria for CF include a combination of clinical presentation, family history, laboratory testing, and genetic testing. The sweat glands of CF patients secrete normal volumes of sweat, but sodium chloride cannot be absorbed from sweat as it moves through the sweat duct. Therefore four times the normal amount of sodium and chloride is excreted in sweat. This abnormality usually does not directly affect the person's general health, but it is the main diagnostic test for CF.

The sweat chloride test is considered the gold standard for the diagnosis of CF and is performed with the pilocarpine iontophoresis method. Pilocarpine is placed on the skin and carried by a small electric current to stimulate sweat production. This part of the process takes about 5 minutes, and the patient feels a slight tingling or warmth. The sweat is collected on filter paper or gauze and then analyzed for sweat chloride concentrations. The test takes approximately 1 hour. Sweat chloride values above 60 mmol/L are considered positive for the diagnosis of CF. A second sweat chloride test is obtained at the same time (one test in each arm) to confirm the diagnosis.

A genetic test is often used if the results from a sweat chloride test are unclear. A blood sample or cells taken inside the cheek (buccal smear) are sent to a laboratory that specializes in genetic testing. Most laboratories test for only the most common mutations of the CF gene. Because more than 1700 mutations cause CF, screening for all mutations is difficult and is performed in a specialty laboratory.

Interprofessional Care

An interprofessional team should be involved in the care of a patient with CF. The Cystic Fibrosis Foundation provides funding for and accredits more than 100 CF care centers nationwide. The high quality of specialized care available throughout the care center network has led to the improved length and quality of life for people with CF. These care centers offer the best care, treatments, and support for those with CF (see *www.cff.org/LivingWithCF/CareCenterNetwork/CFFoundation-accreditedCareCenters*). The teams at these care centers include a nurse, physician, respiratory therapist, physical therapist, dietitian, social worker, and often a nurse practitioner.

Management of pulmonary problems in CF aims at relieving airway obstruction and controlling infection. Drainage of thick bronchial mucus is assisted by aerosol and nebulization treatments of medications used to dilate the airways, liquefy mucus, and facilitate clearance. The abnormal viscosity of CF secretions is increased by concentrated deoxyribonucleic acid (DNA) from neutrophils involved in chronic infection. Agents that degrade the DNA in CF sputum (e.g., dornase alfa [Pulmozyme]) increase airflow and reduce the number of acute pulmonary exacerbations. Inhaled hypertonic saline (7%) is effective in clearing mucus and also decreases the frequency of exacerbations. Hypertonic saline is safe, but some patients require concomitant bronchodilators to avoid bronchospasm. Bronchodilators (e.g., β_2-adrenergic agonists) may be used to control bronchospasm, but the long-term benefit is not proven.

Airway clearance techniques are critical, since the normal ciliary motion in CF airways is impaired. CPT (including postural drainage with percussion and vibration) and high-frequency chest wall oscillation loosen mucus. Clearance is achieved by the specialized expiratory techniques aimed at using airflow to remove the loosened secretions. Examples of clearance techniques and devices are PEP devices (e.g., Flutter device, Acapella [Fig. 28-15]), breathing exercises (autogenic drainage [*http://hospitals.unm.edu/cf/autogenic_drainage.shtml*]), pursed-lip breathing (Table 28-13), and huff coughing (Table 28-23). Individuals with CF may prefer a certain technique or device that works well for them in a daily routine. No clear evidence exists that any of the airway clearance techniques are superior to the others. (Airway clearance techniques are discussed on p. 569.)

Most patients with CF die of complications from lung infection. Standard treatment of infections includes antibiotics for exacerbations and may include chronic suppressive therapy in conjunction with airway clearance. The use of antibiotics should be carefully guided by sputum culture results. Early intervention with antibiotics is useful, and long courses of antibiotics are the usual treatment. Prolonged high-dose therapy may be necessary because many drugs are abnormally metabolized and rapidly excreted in the patient with CF.

Most patients have *Pseudomonas* infection, which can be difficult to treat because over time the organism develops resistance to antibiotics. The organism also has the ability to form a biofilm that must be penetrated to kill it. One commonly used antibiotic to treat patients who are chronically infected with *Pseudomonas* is aerosolized tobramycin (TOBI) given every other month, twice a day. Tobramycin inhalation powder is also available for treatment of *Pseudomonas*.[36]

Oral agents commonly used for mild exacerbations (i.e., increased cough and sputum) are oral antibiotics such as a semisynthetic penicillin or trimethoprim/sulfamethoxazole (to treat *S. aureus*) or oral quinolones, especially ciprofloxacin (Cipro) (to treat *P. aeruginosa*). The quinolones are used judiciously because of the rapid development of resistant strains. Azithromycin, used chronically (longer than 6 months), decreases the frequency of pulmonary exacerbations in CF, especially in those infected with *Pseudomonas*. It is thought that it acts as an antiinflammatory.

If home support and resources are adequate, the CF patient and caregiver may choose to continue IV antibiotic therapy at home after hospital discharge.[37] The usual treatment is two antibiotics with different mechanisms of action (e.g., cephalosporin and an aminoglycoside). The patient with cor pulmonale or hypoxemia may require home O_2 therapy. (O_2 therapy is discussed on p. 565.) Patients with a large pneumothorax require chest tube drainage, perhaps repeatedly. Sclerosing of the pleural space or partial pleural stripping and pleural abrasion performed surgically may be indicated for recurrent episodes of pneumothorax. With massive hemoptysis, bronchial artery embolization is performed. CF has become a leading indication for lung transplantation. (Lung transplants are discussed in Chapter 27.)

The management of pancreatic insufficiency includes pancreatic enzyme replacement of lipase, protease, and amylase (e.g., pancrelipase [Pancreaze, Creon, Ultresa, Viokace, Zenpep, Pertzye]) administered before each meal and snack. Adequate intake of fat, calories, protein, and vitamins is important. Fat-soluble vitamins (A, D, E, and K) must be supplemented, since they are malabsorbed. Use of caloric supplements improves nutritional status. Added dietary salt is indicated whenever sweating is excessive, such as during hot weather, when fever is present, or from intense physical activity. Hyperglycemia may require insulin treatment.

If the patient develops DIOS with complete bowel obstruction, gastric decompression may be needed. This complication is most often managed medically. If DIOS does not resolve with medical treatment, surgery may be needed to prevent the development of ischemic bowel. Partial and uncomplicated episodes of DIOS are treated with ingestion of a balanced polyethylene glycol (PEG) electrolyte solution (MiraLax, GoLYTELY) used to hydrate bowel contents. In addition, water-soluble contrast enemas may be used. Careful monitoring of bowel habits and patterns is essential for CF patients.

Ivacaftor (Kalydeco) is used to treat patients who have mutations in the *CFTR* gene.[38] Ivacaftor, rather than treating the effects of the basic chloride ion channel defect (e.g., pancreatic insufficiency), targets the function of the gene itself, assisting this mutation to open the chloride channel. This drug proves that it is possible to alter the function of a mutation.

Ivacaftor is not effective in patients with CF who have two copies (homozygous) of the *F508* mutation in the *CFTR* gene, which is the most common mutation that results in CF. If a patient's genotype is unknown, a CF mutation test should be performed to detect the presence of a CFTR mutation. Ivacaftor/lumicaftor (Orkambi) is a combination drug used to treat patients who have *F508* mutations.

Aerobic exercise is effective in clearing the airways. Important needs to consider when planning an aerobic exercise program for the patient with CF are (1) meeting increased nutritional demands of exercise, (2) observing for dehydration, and (3) drinking large amounts of fluid and replacing salt losses.

There is a higher incidence of depression among individuals with CF than their unaffected peers. CF imposes a significant burden on the individual and family. Issues related to fertility, decreased life expectancy, costs of health care, burden of self-care, and career choices may lead to depression.

❖ NURSING MANAGEMENT: CYSTIC FIBROSIS

◆ Nursing Assessment

Subjective and objective data that should be obtained from the patient with CF are presented in Table 28-27.

◆ Nursing Diagnoses

Nursing diagnoses for the patient with CF may include, but are not limited to, the following:

- Ineffective airway clearance *related to* abundant, thick bronchial mucus, weakness, and fatigue
- Ineffective breathing pattern *related to* bronchoconstriction, anxiety, and airway obstruction
- Impaired gas exchange *related to* recurring lung infections
- Imbalanced nutrition: less than body requirements *related to* dietary intolerances, intestinal gas, and altered pancreatic enzyme production
- Ineffective coping *related to* multiple life stressors such as decreased life expectancy, cost of treatment, and limitation on career choices

◆ Planning

The overall goals are that the patient with CF will have (1) adequate airway clearance, (2) reduced risk factors associated with respiratory infections, (3) adequate nutritional support to maintain appropriate BMI, (4) ability to perform ADLs, (5) recognition and treatment of complications related to CF, and (6) active participation in planning and implementing a therapeutic regimen.

◆ Nursing Implementation

Assist young adults in gaining independence by helping them assume responsibility for their care and vocational or school goals. An important issue to discuss is sexuality. Delayed or irregular menstruation is not uncommon. There may be delayed development of secondary sex characteristics, such as breasts in girls. The person with CF may use the illness to avoid certain events or relationships. Other crises and life transitions that must be dealt with in the young adult include building confidence and self-respect on the basis of achievements, persevering with employment goals, developing motivation to achieve, learning to cope with the treatment program, and adjusting to the need for dependence if health fails. Disclosing the CF diagnosis to friends, potential spouses, or employers may pose emotional and financial challenges.

The issue of marrying and having children is difficult. Genetic counseling is an appropriate suggestion for the couple considering having children. Another concern is the uncertainty surrounding the shortened life span of the parent with CF. In

TABLE 28-27 Nursing Assessment

Cystic Fibrosis

Subjective Data

Important Health Information

Past health history: Recurrent respiratory and sinus infections, persistent cough with excessive sputum production

Medications: Use of and compliance with bronchodilators, antibiotics, herbs

Functional Health Patterns

Health perception–health maintenance: Family history of cystic fibrosis, diagnosis of cystic fibrosis in childhood, genetic testing in offspring

Nutritional-metabolic: Dietary intolerances, voracious appetite, weight loss, heartburn

Elimination: Intestinal gas. Large, frequent bowel movements, constipation

Activity-exercise: Fatigue, ↓ exercise tolerance, amount and type of exercise. Dyspnea, cough, excessive mucus or sputum production, coughing up blood, airway clearance techniques

Cognitive-perceptual: Abdominal pain

Sexuality-reproductive: Delayed menarche, menstrual irregularities, problems conceiving or fathering a child

Coping–stress tolerance: Anxiety, depression, problems adapting to diagnosis

Objective Data

General

Restlessness; failure to thrive

Integumentary

Cyanosis (circumoral, nail bed), digital clubbing; salty skin

Eyes

Scleral icterus

Respiratory

Sinus congestion, postnasal drip, persistent runny nose. Diminished breath sounds, adventitious breath sounds (crackles, wheezes). Sputum (thick, light or dark, tenacious), hemoptysis, ↑ work of breathing, use of accessory muscles of respiration, barrel chest

Cardiovascular

Tachycardia

Gastrointestinal

Protuberant abdomen; abdominal distention; foul, fatty stools

Possible Diagnostic Findings

Abnormal ABGs and pulmonary function tests; abnormal sweat chloride test, chest x-ray, fecal fat analysis

ABGs, Arterial blood gases.

addition, the parent's ability to care for the child must be taken into consideration.

Acute care for the patient with CF includes relief of bronchoconstriction, airway obstruction, and airflow limitation. Interventions include aggressive CPT, antibiotics, and O_2 therapy in severe disease. Good nutrition is important. Advances in long-term vascular access (e.g., implanted ports) and inhaled antibiotics have made administration of medication much easier. This has also eased the transition for treatment at home.

The family and person with CF have a great financial and emotional burden. The cost of drugs, special equipment, and health care is often a financial hardship. The burden of living with a chronic disease at a young age can be emotionally overwhelming. Community resources are often available to help the family. In addition, the Cystic Fibrosis Foundation can be of assistance. As the person continues toward and into adulthood, you and other skilled health professionals should be available to help the patient and the family cope with complications resulting from the disease.

BRONCHIECTASIS

Etiology and Pathophysiology

Bronchiectasis is characterized by permanent, abnormal dilation of medium-sized bronchi that is a result of inflammatory changes that destroy elastic and muscular structures supporting the bronchial wall. Infection is the primary reason for the continuing cycle of inflammation, airway damage, and remodeling. Bronchiectasis can follow a single episode of severe pneumonia, with a wide variety of infectious agents initiating the condition. Airways can become colonized with microorganisms (e.g., *Pseudomonas*), which causes the bronchial walls to weaken and pockets of infection begin to form (Fig. 28-17).

When the walls of the bronchial system are injured, the mucociliary mechanism is damaged, allowing bacteria and mucus to accumulate within the pockets. Stasis of thickened mucus occurs due to impaired clearance of mucus by the cilia. This results in a reduced ability to clear mucus from the lungs and decreased expiratory airflow. Thus bronchiectasis is classified as an obstructive lung disease. Large connections (anastomoses) develop between the blood vessels in the lungs, and hemoptysis is often the result.

A variety of pathophysiologic processes can result in bronchiectasis. CF is the main cause of bronchiectasis in children. In adults, the main cause is bacterial infections of the lungs that are either not treated or receive delayed treatment. Other causes of bronchiectasis are obstruction of an airway with mucus plugs or generalized impairment of pulmonary defenses. A number of systemic diseases such as inflammatory bowel disease, rheumatoid arthritis, or immune disorders (e.g., acquired immunodeficiency syndrome [AIDS]) may be associated with bronchiectasis.

Clinical Manifestations

The hallmark of bronchiectasis is persistent cough with consistent production of thick, tenacious, purulent sputum. However, some patients with severe disease and upper lobe involvement may have no sputum production and little cough. Recurrent infections injure blood vessels, and hemoptysis occurs. In severe cases it may be life-threatening. The other manifestations of bronchiectasis are pleuritic chest pain, dyspnea, wheezing, clubbing of digits, weight loss, and anemia. On auscultation of the lungs, a variety of adventitious sounds can be heard (e.g., crackles, wheezes).

Diagnostic Studies

An individual with a chronic productive cough with copious purulent sputum (which may be blood streaked) should be suspected of having bronchiectasis. Chest x-rays may show some nonspecific abnormalities. A high-resolution CT scan of the chest is the preferred method for diagnosing bronchiectasis.

Sputum may provide additional information regarding the severity of impairment and the presence of active infection.

Patients frequently have *H. influenzae, S. aureus,* or *P. aeruginosa,* with the latter leading to more frequent exacerbations and rapid decline in lung function. Spirometry usually shows an obstructive pattern, including a decrease in FEV_1 and FEV_1/FVC.

Interprofessional Care

Bronchiectasis is difficult to treat. Therapy is aimed at treating acute flare-ups and preventing a decline in lung function. Antibiotics are the mainstay of treatment and are often given empirically, but attempts are made to culture the sputum. Long-term suppressive therapy with antibiotics is reserved for those patients who have symptoms that recur a few days after stopping antibiotics. Antibiotics may be given orally, IV, or inhaled.

Concurrent bronchodilator therapy with LABAs, SABAs, or anticholinergics is given to prevent bronchospasm and stimulate mucociliary clearance. Hyperosmolar agents (e.g., hypertonic saline) may be given via a nebulizer to liquefy secretions. In addition, oral and inhaled corticosteroids may be used.

Maintaining good hydration is important to liquefy secretions. CPT and other airway clearance techniques are important to facilitate expectoration of sputum. Teach the patient to reduce exposure to excessive air pollutants and irritants, avoid cigarette smoking, and obtain pneumococcal and influenza vaccinations.

Surgical resection of parts of the lungs, which was common in the past, has largely been replaced by more effective supportive and antibiotic therapy. For selected patients who are disabled in spite of maximal therapy, lung transplantation is an option. Massive hemoptysis may require surgical resection or embolization of the bronchial artery.

❖ NURSING MANAGEMENT: BRONCHIECTASIS

Early detection and treatment of lower respiratory tract infections help prevent complications such as bronchiectasis. Any obstructing lesion or foreign body should be removed promptly.

An important nursing goal is to promote drainage and removal of mucus. Various airway clearance techniques can be effectively used to facilitate secretion removal. CPT with postural drainage is widely used.

Administration of the prescribed medications is important. The patient needs to understand the importance of taking the prescribed regimen of drugs to obtain maximum effectiveness. Rest is important to prevent overexertion.

If hemoptysis occurs, patients should be given explicit instructions on when they should contact the HCP. Some patients may periodically expectorate a "spot" of blood that is usual for them. In the acute care setting, if the patient has hemoptysis, contact the HCP immediately, elevate the head of the bed, and place the patient in a side-lying position with the suspected bleeding side down.

Good nutrition is important and may be difficult to maintain because the patient is often anorexic. Oral hygiene to cleanse the mouth and remove dried sputum crusts may improve the patient's appetite. Offer foods that are appealing, since they may increase the patient's desire to eat.

Adequate hydration to help liquefy secretions and thus make it easier to remove them is extremely important. Unless there are contraindications, instruct the patient to drink at least 3 L of fluid daily. To accomplish this, advise the patient to increase fluid consumption by increasing intake by one glass per day until the goal is reached. Generally, the patient should be counseled to use low-sodium fluids to avoid systemic fluid retention.

Direct hydration of the respiratory system may also prove beneficial in the expectoration of secretions. Often nebulized hypertonic saline may be ordered for a more aggressive effect. At home, a steamy shower can prove effective. Expensive equipment that requires frequent cleaning is usually unnecessary. Teach the patient and caregiver to recognize significant clinical manifestations to report to the HCP. These manifestations include increased sputum production, bloody sputum, increasing dyspnea, fever, chills, and chest pain.

BECOMING A NURSE LEADER

Coaching in Nursing

Situation

You are a new graduate nurse on a busy pulmonary medical unit. You learn from Mr. Boyd, your patient, that he is to be discharged this morning. You are upset because discharge planning would go so much better if Dr. Gooding, his pulmonary physician, would include the nurses when he makes rounds on patients. Your nurse manager coaches you about how you could approach Dr. Gooding about including the nurses in patient rounds. She helps you refocus this scenario as a patient safety issue and develop a plan to discuss it with the physician. You find an opportunity to talk with Dr. Gooding, and he agrees that it would help communication all around if nurses could round with him. You are pleased and you tell your nurse manager of your success.

Points for Consideration

- Often when the word *coaching* is mentioned in the workplace, it has negative connotations related to dealing with a problem. Coaching is not about disciplinary action.
- Coaching is a leadership style in which managers provide individualized feedback and assistance to improve an employee's performance and development. It is a technique that can be used by nurse managers to get the best from their staff and thus the best results for the whole organization.[1]
- Coaches can help new nurses identify areas for improvement and work with them to set personal and career goals.
- Coaches ideally focus on professional development, teamwork, leadership, and preparation for increased responsibility. They encourage growth and risk taking.[2]
- Coaches need to be nurturing, have a firm commitment to finding special talents in young nurses, and encourage the growth of every nurse.[3]

Discussion Questions

1. What have you learned from the coaching that you have received from your nurse manager? From your teachers?
2. How can you help others learn from your success related to dealing with Dr. Gooding?

References

1. Routson J: Coaching—an essential skill for nursing leaders. Retrieved from *www.healthecareers.com/article/coaching-an-essential-skill-for -nursing-leaders/158373.*
2. Hancock B: Developing new nurse leaders, *AJN* 114:59, 2014.
3. Hess V: Coaching communication: tips for nurse managers. Retrieved from *www.americannursetoday.com/coaching -communication-tips-for-nurse-managers.*

CASE STUDY

Chronic Obstructive Pulmonary Disease

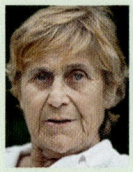

(©iStockphoto/Thinkstock)

Patient Profile

H.M. is a 68-year-old white, married, female, retired traffic police officer. She has been in the hospital for 3 days with an acute COPD exacerbation and will be discharged tomorrow.

Subjective Data

- Before admission had 7 days of exceptional shortness of breath and increased volume of sputum, which turned greenish
- Had increased Ventolin HFA use at home to five or six times a day for dyspnea
- Had jitters and racing heart
- Had three or four bouts of exacerbations of COPD in the past year that she treated at home
- Thirty pack-year history of smoking; smokes half a pack per day now to "clear out lungs" in the morning
- Eats a regular diet but "gets full fast"
- Cannot climb one flight of stairs without stopping; walks down the flat driveway 10 yards without difficulty
- Awakens two or three times per night coughing and short of breath

Objective Data

Physical Examination

- Weight 129 lb, height 5 ft 8 in, BMI 20 kg/m^2
- BP 136/76 mm Hg, pulse 86, respiratory rate 28
- Increased anteroposterior diameter of chest (barrel shaped)
- Slight use of accessory (neck) muscles with breathing
- Distant breath sounds with occasional wheezes
- No peripheral edema

Diagnostic Studies

- Last spirometry: decreased FEV_1 (48%) and FEV_1/FVC (62%)
- ABGs on admission: pH 7.34, $PaCO_2$ 49 mm Hg, HCO_3^- 27 mEq/L, PaO_2 70 mm Hg
- WBC: 14,000/μL on admission
- Chest x-ray: hyperinflation, flat diaphragm, no sign of pneumonia
- Sputum: negative for *Pseudomonas*

Interprofessional Care

- GOLD 3 (severe) COPD with acute exacerbation
- O_2 2 L via nasal catheter while in hospital
- Prednisone 40 mg daily PO for 5 days
- Levofloxacin 750 mg PO
- Ipratropium HFA MDI 2 puffs four times a day
- At discharge: Advair Diskus 250/50 one inhalation q12hr

Discussion Questions

1. What classic manifestations indicate the patient had a COPD exacerbation?
2. What are some likely causes of her COPD?
3. What symptoms indicate the overuse of inhalers, and which drug would cause the symptoms described?
4. ***Patient-Centered Care:*** What is the only way H.M. can halt the progression of her lung disease?
5. Why would H.M. "feel full fast" when eating? What could you do to minimize this issue?
6. Interpret the ABGs. What pattern do you see?
7. ***Priority Decision:*** What are nursing priorities for discharge planning and teaching?
8. ***Priority Decision:*** Based on the assessment data presented, what are the priority nursing diagnoses? Are there any collaborative problems?
9. ***Evidence-Based Practice:*** H.M.'s son has been trying to convince his mother to quit smoking for many years without success. He asks you to tell his mother the results of her spirometry to convince her it is time to quit. Will this approach work?

Answers available at *http://evolve.elsevier.com/Lewis/medsurg.*

BRIDGE TO NCLEX EXAMINATION

The number of the question corresponds to the same-numbered outcome at the beginning of the chapter.

1. A patient is concerned that he may have asthma. Of the symptoms that he relates to the nurse, which ones suggest asthma or risk factors for asthma *(select all that apply)*?
   a. Allergic rhinitis
   b. Prolonged inhalation
   c. History of skin allergies
   d. Cough, especially at night
   e. Gastric reflux or heartburn
2. In evaluating an asthmatic patient's knowledge of self-care, the nurse recognizes that additional instruction is needed when the patient says,
   a. "I use my corticosteroid inhaler when I feel short of breath."
   b. "I get a flu shot every year and see my HCP if I have an upper respiratory tract infection."
   c. "I use my inhaler before I visit my aunt who has a cat, but I only visit for a few minutes because of my allergies."
   d. "I walk 30 minutes every day but sometimes I have to use my bronchodilator inhaler before walking to prevent me from getting short of breath."
3. A plan of care for the patient with COPD could include *(select all that apply)*
   a. exercise such as walking.
   b. high flow rate of O_2 administration.
   c. low-dose chronic oral corticosteroid therapy.
   d. use of peak flow meter to monitor the progression of COPD.
   e. breathing exercises such as pursed-lip breathing that focus on exhalation.
4. The effects of cigarette smoking on the respiratory system include
   a. hypertrophy of capillaries causing hemoptysis.
   b. hyperplasia of goblet cells and increased production of mucus.
   c. increased proliferation of cilia and decreased clearance of mucus.
   d. proliferation of alveolar macrophages to decrease the risk for infection.
5. The major advantage of a Venturi mask is that it can
   a. deliver up to 80% O_2.
   b. provide continuous 100% humidity.
   c. deliver a precise concentration of O_2.
   d. be used while a patient eats and sleeps.

6. Which guideline would be a part of teaching patients how to use a metered-dose inhaler (MDI)?
   a. After activating the MDI, breathe in as quickly as you can.
   b. Estimate the amount of remaining medicine in the MDI by floating the canister in water.
   c. Disassemble the plastic canister from the inhaler and rinse both pieces under running water every week.
   d. To determine how long the canister will last, divide the total number of puffs in the canister by the puffs needed per day.
7. Which treatments in CF would the nurse expect to implement in the management plan of patients with CF *(select all that apply)*?
   a. Sperm banking
   b. IV corticosteroids on a chronic basis
   c. Airway clearance techniques (e.g., Acapella)
   d. GoLYTELY given PRN for severe constipation
   e. Inhaled tobramycin to combat *Pseudomonas* infection
8. A patient who has bronchiectasis asks the nurse, "What conditions would warrant a call to the clinic?"
   a. Blood clots in the sputum
   b. Sticky sputum on a hot day
   c. Increased shortness of breath after eating a large meal
   d. Production of large amounts of sputum on a daily basis

1. a, c, d, e, 2. a, 3. a, e, 4. b, 5. c, 6. d, 7. a, c, d, e, 8. a

For rationales to these answers and even more NCLEX review questions, visit *http://evolve.elsevier.com/Lewis/medsurg.*

EVOLVE WEBSITE

http://evolve.elsevier.com/Lewis/medsurg

Review Questions (Online Only)

Key Points

Answer Keys for Questions

- Rationales for Bridge to NCLEX Examination Questions
- Answer Guidelines for Case Study on p. 582
- Answer Guidelines for Managing Care of Multiple Patients Case Study (Section 5) on p. 585

Student Case Studies

- Patient With Asthma
- Patient With Chronic Obstructive Pulmonary Disease (COPD)
- Patient With Cystic Fibrosis

Nursing Care Plans

- eNursing Care Plan 28-1: Patient With Asthma
- eNursing Care Plan 28-2: Patient With Chronic Obstructive Pulmonary Disease

Conceptual Care Map Creator

- Conceptual Care Map for Case Study on p. 582

Audio Glossary

Content Updates

REFERENCES

1. American Lung Association: Trends in asthma morbidity and mortality, Epidemiology and Statistics Unit, Research and Health Education Division. Retrieved from *www.lungusa.org.*
2. American Lung Association: Trends in COPD (chronic bronchitis and emphysema): morbidity and mortality, Epidemiology and Statistics Unit, Research and Health Education Division. Retrieved from *www.lungusa.org.*

*3. National Heart, Lung, and Blood Institute and National Asthma Education and Prevention Program: Expert Panel Report 3: guidelines for the diagnosis and management of asthma, NIH pub no 08-4051, Bethesda, Md, 2007, National Institutes of Health. Retrieved from *www.nhlbi.nih.gov/guidelines.*

*4. Global Initiative for Asthma: Global strategy for asthma management and prevention, 2015. Retrieved from *www.ginasthma.org.*

5. Baur X, Sigsgaard T, Aasen TB, et al: Guidelines for management of work-related asthma, *Eur Respir J* 39:529, 2012.
6. Sandur V, Murugesh M, Banait V, et al: Prevalence of gastroesophageal reflux in patients with difficult to control asthma and effect of proton pump inhibitor therapy on asthma symptoms, reflux symptoms, pulmonary function and requirement for asthma medications, *J Postgrad Med* 60(3):282, 2014.
7. Lareau SC, Hodder R: Teaching inhaler use in chronic obstructive pulmonary disease patients, *J Am Acad Nurs Pract* 24:113, 2012.
8. Kane B, Fowler SJ, Niven R: Refractory asthma—beyond step 5, the role of new and emerging adjuvant therapies, *Chron Respir Dis* 12(1):69, 2015.
9. US Food and Drug Administration: Epinephrine CFC metered-dose inhalers: questions and answers. Retrieved from *www.fda.gov/Drugs/DrugSafety.informationbydrugclass/ucm080427.htm.*
10. Rosser FJ, Forno E, Cooper PJ, et al: Asthma in Hispanics: An 8-year update, *Am J Respir Crit Care Med* 189(11):1316, 2014.

*11. Global Initiative for Chronic Obstructive Lung Disease: Global strategy for the diagnosis, management, and prevention of chronic obstructive pulmonary disease (updated 2015). Retrieved from *www.goldcopd.org.*

12. National Heart, Lung, and Blood Institute: COPD: are you at risk? Retrieved from *www.nhlbi.nih.gov/health/public/lung/copd/campaign-materials/html/copd-atrisk.htm.*
13. National Institute on Drug Abuse: Info facts: cigarettes and other tobacco products. Retrieved from *www.drugabuse.gov/publications/infofacts/cigarettes-other-tobacco-products.*
14. Health 24: How many smokers develop COPD? Retrieved from *www.health24.com/medical/Condition_centres/777-792-805-1535,28674.asp.*
15. Alpha-1 Foundation: Healthcare providers: what is alpha-1? Retrieved from *www.alphaone.org.*
16. Rycroft CE, Heyes A, Lanza L, et al: Epidemiology of chronic obstructive pulmonary disease: a literature review, *Int J Chron Obstruct Pulmon Dis* 7:457, 2012.
17. Evans RA, Morgan MD: The systemic nature of chronic lung disease, *Clin Chest Med* 35(2): 283, 2014.
18. McDonald CF. Oxygen therapy for COPD, *J Thorac Dis* 6(11):1632, 2014.
19. Miravitlles M, Anzueto A: Antibiotics for acute and chronic respiratory infection in patients with chronic obstructive pulmonary disease, *Am J Respir Crit Care Med* 188(9):1052, 2013.
20. Farland MZ, Peters CJ, Williams JD, et al: β-Blocker use and incidence of chronic obstructive pulmonary disease exacerbations, *Ann Pharmacother* 47(5):651, 2013.

*21. Borge CR, Hagen KB, Mengshoel AM, et al: Effects of controlled breathing exercises and respiratory muscle training in people with chronic obstructive pulmonary disease: results from evaluating the quality of evidence in systematic reviews, *BMC Pulm Med* 14:184, 2014.

22. Seo SH: Medical nutrition therapy based on nutrition intervention for a patient with chronic obstructive pulmonary disease, *Clin Nutr Res* 3(2):150, 2014.
23. Taneja A: Bronchoscopic interventions in the management of chronic obstructive pulmonary disease, *Curr Opin Pulm Med* 19(2):145, 2013.
24. Kobayashi S, Yanai M, Hanagmana M, et al: The burden of chronic obstructive pulmonary disease in the elderly population, *Resp Investig* 52(5):296, 2014.
25. Areias V, Carreira S, Anciaes M, et al: Co-morbidities in patients with Gold stage 4 chronic obstructive lung disease, *Rev Port Pneumol* 20(1):5, 2014.

26. Battaglia S, Cardillo I, Lavorini F, et al: Safety considerations of inhaled corticosteroids in the elderly, *Drugs Aging* 31(11):787, 2014.
27. Rinaudo M, Ferrer M, Terraneo S, et al: Impact of chronic obstructive pulmonary disease in the outcome of intensive care unit-acquired pneumonia with and without previous intubation, *Chest* 147(6):1530, 2015.
28. Batzlaff CM, Karpman C, Afessa B, et al: Predicting 1-year mortality rate for patients admitted with an acute exacerbation of chronic obstructive pulmonary disease to an intensive care unit: an opportunity for palliative care, *Mayo Clin Proc* 85(9):638, 2014.
*29. McCarthy B, Casey D, Devane D: Pulmonary rehabilitation for chronic obstructive pulmonary disease, *Cochrane Database Syst Rev* 2:CD003793, 2015.
30. Who needs pulmonary rehabilitation? Retrieved from *www.nhlbi.nih.gov/health/health-topics/topics/pulreh/whoneeds.*
31. LeGear T, LeGear M, Preradovic D, et al: Does a Nintendo Wii exercise program provide similar exercise demands as a traditional pulmonary rehabilitation program in adults with COPD? *Clin Respir J* 10(3):303, 2016.
32. Theander K, Hasselgren M, Luhr K: Symptoms and impact of symptoms on function and health in patients with chronic obstructive pulmonary disease and chronic heart failure in primary health care, *Int J Chron Obstruct Pulmon Dis* 9:785, 2014.
33. Schroedl C, Yount S, Szmuilowicz E, et al: Outpatient palliative care for chronic obstructive pulmonary disease: a case series, *J Palliat Med* 17(11):1256, 2014.
34. Andersen D: Cystic fibrosis of the pancreas and its relation to celiac disease, *Am J Dis Child* 56:344, 1938. (Classic)
35. Cystic Fibrosis Foundation Patient Registry: *2013 annual data report*, Bethesda, Md, 2014, Cystic Fibrosis Foundation. Retrieved from *www.cff.org.*
36. Somayaji R, Parkins MD: Tobramycin inhalation powder: an efficient and efficacious therapy for the treatment of *Pseudomonas aeruginosa* infection in cystic fibrosis, *Ther Deliv* 6(2):12, 2015.
*37. Langton Hewer SC, Smyth AR: Antibiotic strategies for eradicating *Pseudomonas aeruginosa* in people with cystic fibrosis, *Cochrane Database Syst Rev* 10:11, 2014.
*38. Whiting P, Al M, Burgers L, et al: Ivacaftor for the treatment of patients with cystic fibrosis and the G551D mutation: a systematic review and cost-effectiveness analysis, *Health Technol Assess* 18(18):1, 2014.

*Evidence-based guidelines for clinical practice.

CASE STUDY

Managing Care of Multiple Patients

You are assigned to care for the following four patients on a medical-surgical unit. You are sharing one unlicensed assistive personnel (UAP) with another RN.

Patients

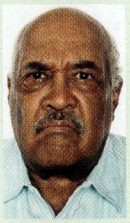

(©Fuse/ Thinkstock)

F.T. is a 70-yr-old man with a history of COPD who was admitted yesterday with bilateral lower lobe pneumonia. He is receiving O_2 at 2 L/min via nasal cannula and IV antibiotics. His last pulse oximetry reading was 92%.

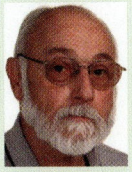

(©iStockphoto/ Thinkstock)

M.R. is a 60-yr-old man who is 3 days postoperative following a total laryngectomy with tracheostomy for treatment of laryngeal cancer. He is receiving intermittent tube feeding via a percutaneous endoscopic gastrostomy (PEG) tube and last received pain medication 4 hours ago.

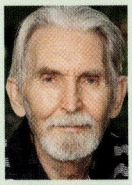

(©iStockphoto/ Thinkstock)

J.H. is a 52-yr-old man admitted with right lower lobe pneumonia. A bronchoscopy with biopsy revealed small cell lung carcinoma. He is intermittently confused and anxious with rapid, shallow respirations. He and his family are currently considering his treatment options.

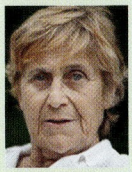

(©iStockphoto/ Thinkstock)

H.M. is a 68-yr-old white woman admitted 3 days ago with a COPD exacerbation. She has not been able to ambulate much because of her shortness of breath. She is on oral prednisone and ipratropium. She is anticipating discharge later today. She is to start Advair Diskus and chronic O_2 therapy at home after discharge.

Discussion Questions

1. ***Priority Decision:*** After receiving report, which patient should you see first? Provide a rationale for your decision.
2. ***Teamwork and Collaboration:*** Which morning tasks can you delegate to the UAP *(select all that apply)*?
   a. Take a pulse oximetry reading on F.T.
   b. Assess M.R.'s pain level and show him how to administer his tube feeding.
   c. Assist H.M. with AM care and gather belongings in anticipation of discharge.
   d. Teach F.T. how to use the incentive spirometer and titrate O_2 to obtain pulse oximetry >95%.
   e. Provide coffee and emotional support for J.H.'s family as they await a family meeting with the physician.
3. ***Priority Decision and Teamwork and Collaboration:*** While you are assessing J.H., the UAP tells you that H.M. is complaining of chest pain and worsening shortness of breath. M.R. is also requesting pain medication. What should you do *first*?
   a. Ask the UAP to get H.M.'s vital signs while you give M.R. pain medication.
   b. Ask the UAP to increase H.M.'s O_2 to 4 L/min while you assess M.R.'s pain.
   c. Ask the UAP to obtain a stat 12-lead ECG on H.M. while you perform a focused assessment.
   d. Ask the UAP to have another RN give M.R. his pain medication while you go directly to H.M.'s room.

Case Study Progression

After assessing H.M., you notify her HCP. A stat 12-lead ECG is obtained and a blood sample is drawn to check cardiac enzymes. H.M.'s chest pain is not relieved by sublingual nitroglycerin. You then administer 4 mg IV morphine. H.M. states that her pain is "a little better" but continues to complain of dyspnea. The 12-lead ECG and cardiac enzyme results are all within normal limits.

4. Because of H.M.'s reduced mobility, you recognize that she is at risk for _____ and anticipate the HCP will order which tests to determine the cause of her current symptoms?
   a. BNP and echocardiogram
   b. D-dimer and spiral CT scan
   c. CBC and abdominal flat-plate x-ray
   d. Serum electrolytes and renal ultrasound
5. While the charge nurse accompanies H.M. to radiology, you turn your attention back to your remaining three patients. Prior to administering M.R.'s 8 AM tube feeding, you aspirate 300 mL of gastric contents from his PEG tube. Which action should you take *next*?
   a. Discard the aspirated contents and administer the tube feeding as ordered.
   b. Replace the aspirated contents and administer half of ordered tube feeding volume.
   c. Discard the aspirated contents and withhold the next two scheduled tube feedings.
   d. Replace the aspirated contents and notify the HCP prior to administering any further tube feedings.
6. When preparing F.T.'s AM medications, you note that he is scheduled to receive the following antibiotics at 8 AM: levofloxacin (Levaquin) 750 mg in 150 mL normal saline over 90 minutes (give once q24hr) and cefazolin (Kefzol) 1 g in 100 mL normal saline over 30 minutes (give q8hr). He has only one IV site. Which action is *most* appropriate?
   a. Obtain a second peripheral IV site.
   b. Call the HCP to change the administration times.
   c. Check with pharmacy to see if they can be mixed together in the same IV bag.
   d. Administer the cefazolin first because it takes the least amount of time to infuse.
7. ***Management Decision:*** J.H.'s son calls you on the telephone to inquire about his father's current condition and long-term prognosis. Which initial response would be *most* appropriate?
   a. Ask the person calling what the code word is to identify himself or herself as family.
   b. Tell the caller that you are not allowed to discuss any information over the telephone.
   c. Empathize with the son's need to know his father's prognosis while acknowledging that no one really knows.
   d. Ask J.H.'s son what the physician has explained to him in order to clarify his current understanding of the situation.

Answers available at *http://evolve.elsevier.com/Lewis/medsurg.*

SECTION 6

Problems of Oxygenation: Transport

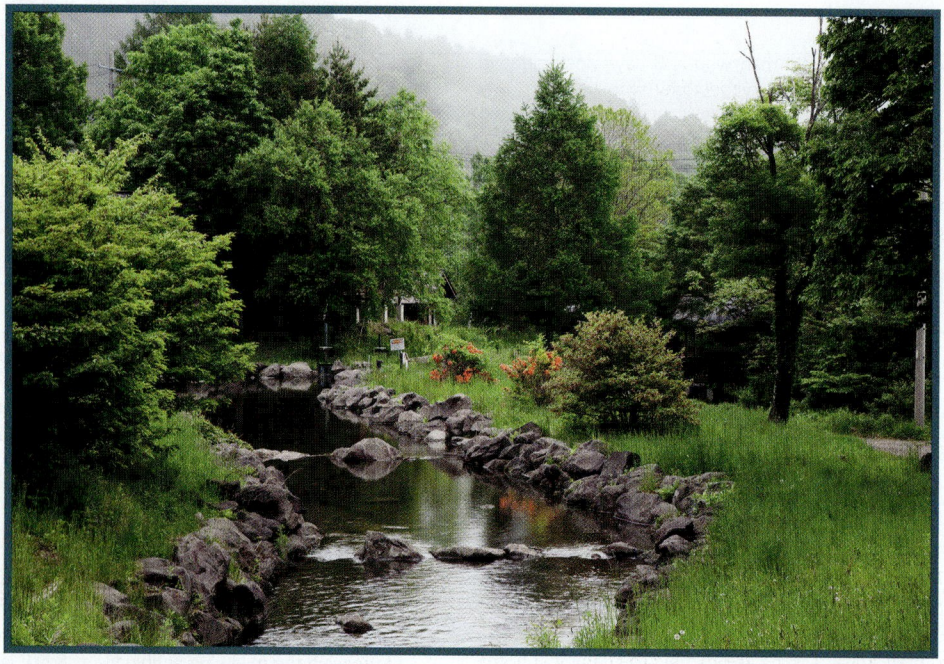

©KEITA SAWAKI/a.collectionRF/Thinkstock

What makes a river so restful to people is that it doesn't have any doubt—it is sure to get where it is going, and it doesn't want to go anywhere else.

Hal Boyle

Chapter 29 Assessment of Hematologic System, 587

Chapter 30 Hematologic Problems, 606

29

Assessment of Hematologic System

Sandra Irene Rome

There's a lot of blood, sweat, and guts between dreams and success.

Paul Bryant

http://evolve.elsevier.com/Lewis/medsurg/

LEARNING OUTCOMES

1. Describe the structures and functions of the hematologic system.
2. Differentiate among the different types of blood cells and their functions.
3. Explain the process of hemostasis.
4. Link the age-related changes in the hematologic system to differences in findings of hematologic studies.
5. Obtain significant subjective and objective assessment data related to the hematologic system from a patient.
6. Perform a physical assessment of the hematologic system using the appropriate techniques.
7. Differentiate normal from common abnormal findings of a physical assessment of the hematologic system.
8. Describe the purpose, significance of results, and nursing responsibilities related to diagnostic studies of the hematologic system.

KEY TERMS

ecchymoses, p. 598
erythropoiesis, p. 588
fibrinolysis, p. 591
hematopoiesis, p. 587
hemolysis, p. 589
leukopenia, p. 599
neutropenia, p. 600
pancytopenia, p. 599
petechiae, p. 598
reticulocyte, p. 589
thrombocytopenia, p. 600
thrombocytosis, p. 600

Hematology is the study of blood and blood-forming tissues. This includes the bone marrow, blood, spleen, and lymph system. A basic knowledge of hematology is useful in clinical settings to evaluate the patient's ability to transport O_2 and CO_2, maintain intravascular volume, coagulate blood, and combat infections. Assessment of the hematologic system is based on the patient's health history, physical examination, and results of diagnostic studies.

STRUCTURES AND FUNCTIONS OF HEMATOLOGIC SYSTEM

Bone Marrow

Blood cell production (**hematopoiesis**) occurs within the bone marrow. *Bone marrow* is the soft material that fills the central core of bones. Although there are two types of bone marrow (yellow [adipose] and red [hematopoietic]), the red marrow actively produces blood cells. In the adult, the red marrow is found primarily in the flat and irregular bones, such as the ends of long bones, pelvic bones, vertebrae, sacrum, sternum, ribs, flat cranial bones, and scapulae.

All three types of blood cells (red blood cells [RBCs], white blood cells [WBCs], and platelets) develop from a common hematopoietic stem cell within the bone marrow. The hematopoietic *stem cell* is best described as an immature blood cell that is able to self-renew and differentiate into hematopoietic progenitor cells. As the cells mature and differentiate, several different types of blood cells are formed (Fig. 29-1). The marrow responds to increased demands for various types of blood cells by increasing production via a negative feedback system. The bone marrow is stimulated by various factors or cytokines (e.g., erythropoietin, granulocyte colony-stimulating factor [G-CSF], stem cell factor, thrombopoietin) that cause differentiation of the stem cells into one of the committed hematopoietic cells (e.g., RBC). For example, when tissue hypoxia occurs, erythropoietin is secreted by the kidney and liver. It circulates to the bone marrow and causes differentiation of proerythroblasts in the bone marrow.[1]

Blood

Blood is a type of connective tissue that performs three major functions: transportation, regulation, and protection (Table 29-1). Blood has two major components: plasma and blood cells. In an adult weighing between 150 and 180 lb, the volume of blood is usually between 4.7 and 5.5 L (5 to 6 quarts).

Plasma. Approximately 55% of blood is plasma[1] (Fig. 29-2). Plasma is composed primarily of water, but it also contains proteins, electrolytes, gases, nutrients (e.g., glucose, amino acids, lipids), and waste. The term *serum* refers to plasma minus its clotting factors. Plasma proteins include albumin, globulin, and clotting factors (mostly fibrinogen). Most plasma proteins

Reviewed by Judy Carlyle, RN, MNSc, Faculty/Clinical Liaison, Arkansas Rural Nursing Education Consortium (ARNEC), Nashville, Arkansas; and Allison J. Terry, RN, PhD, Associate Professor of Nursing, Assistant Dean of Clinical Practice, School of Nursing, Auburn University Montgomery, Montgomery, Alabama.

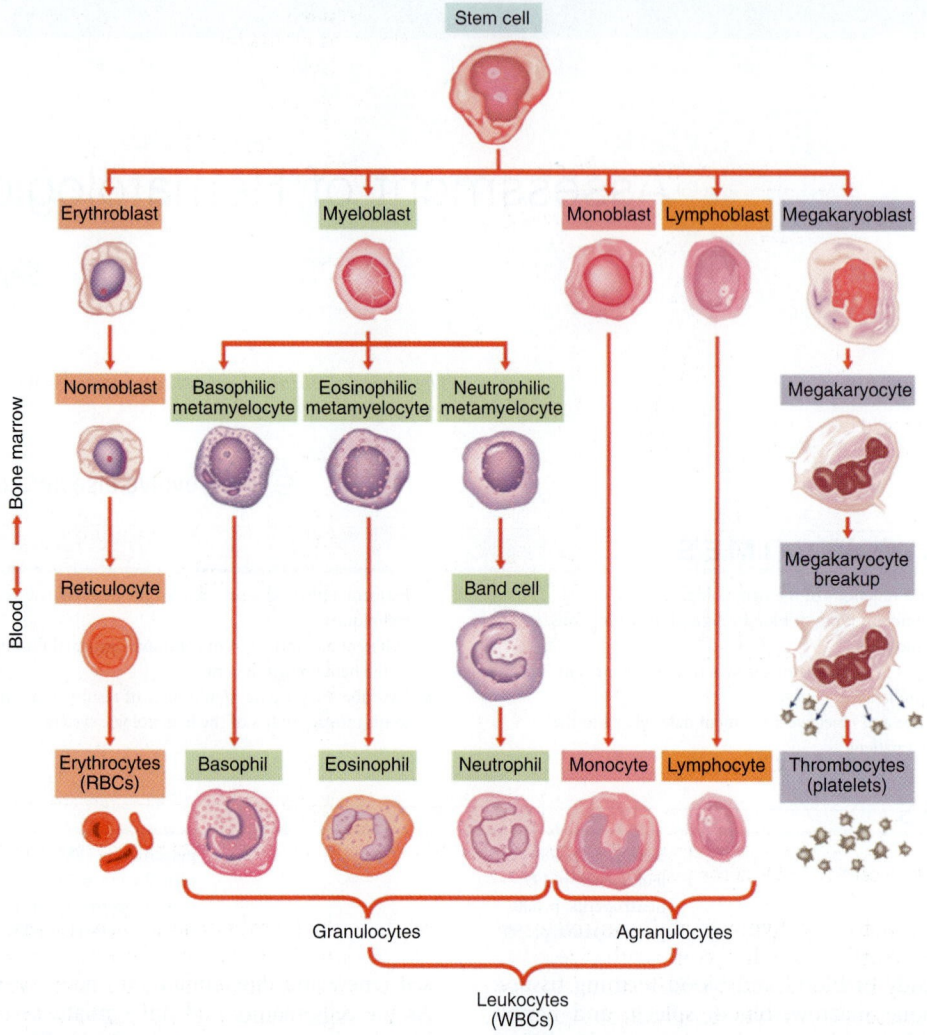

FIG. 29-1 Development of blood cells. *RBCs,* Red blood cells; *WBCs,* white blood cells.

are produced by the liver, except for antibodies (immunoglobulins), which are produced by plasma cells. Albumin is a protein that helps maintain oncotic pressure in the blood.[1]

Blood Cells. About 45% of the blood (Fig. 29-2) is composed of formed elements, or blood cells. The three types of blood cells are *erythrocytes* (RBCs), *leukocytes* (WBCs), and *thrombocytes* (platelets). The primary function of erythrocytes is O_2 transportation, whereas the leukocytes are involved in protecting the body from infection. Platelets promote blood coagulation.

Erythrocytes. The primary functions of RBCs include transport of gases (both O_2 and CO_2) and assistance in maintaining acid-base balance. RBCs are flexible cells with a unique biconcave shape. Flexibility enables the cell to alter its shape so that it can easily pass through tiny capillaries. The cell membrane is thin to facilitate diffusion of gases.

Erythrocytes are primarily composed of a large molecule called *hemoglobin*. Hemoglobin, a complex protein-iron compound composed of heme (an iron compound) and globin (a simple protein), binds with O_2 and CO_2. As RBCs circulate through the capillaries surrounding alveoli within the lung, O_2 attaches to iron on the hemoglobin. The O_2-bound hemoglobin is referred to as *oxyhemoglobin* and is responsible for giving arterial blood its bright red appearance. As RBCs flow to body tissues, O_2 detaches from the hemoglobin and diffuses from the capillary into tissue cells. CO_2 diffuses from tissue cells into the capillary, attaches to the globin portion of hemoglobin, and is transported to the lungs for removal. Hemoglobin also acts as a buffer and plays a role in maintaining acid-base balance. This buffering function is described further in Chapter 16.

Erythropoiesis (the process of RBC production) is regulated by cellular O_2 requirements and general metabolic activity.

TABLE 29-1 Functions of Blood

Function	Examples
Transportation	• O_2 from lungs to cells • Nutrients from GI tract to cells • Hormones from endocrine glands to tissues and cells • Metabolic waste products (e.g., CO_2, NH_3, urea) from cells to lungs, liver, and kidneys
Regulation	• Fluid and electrolyte balance • Acid-base balance • Body temperature • Maintaining intravascular oncotic pressure
Protection	• Maintaining homeostasis of blood coagulation • Combating invasion of pathogens and other foreign substances

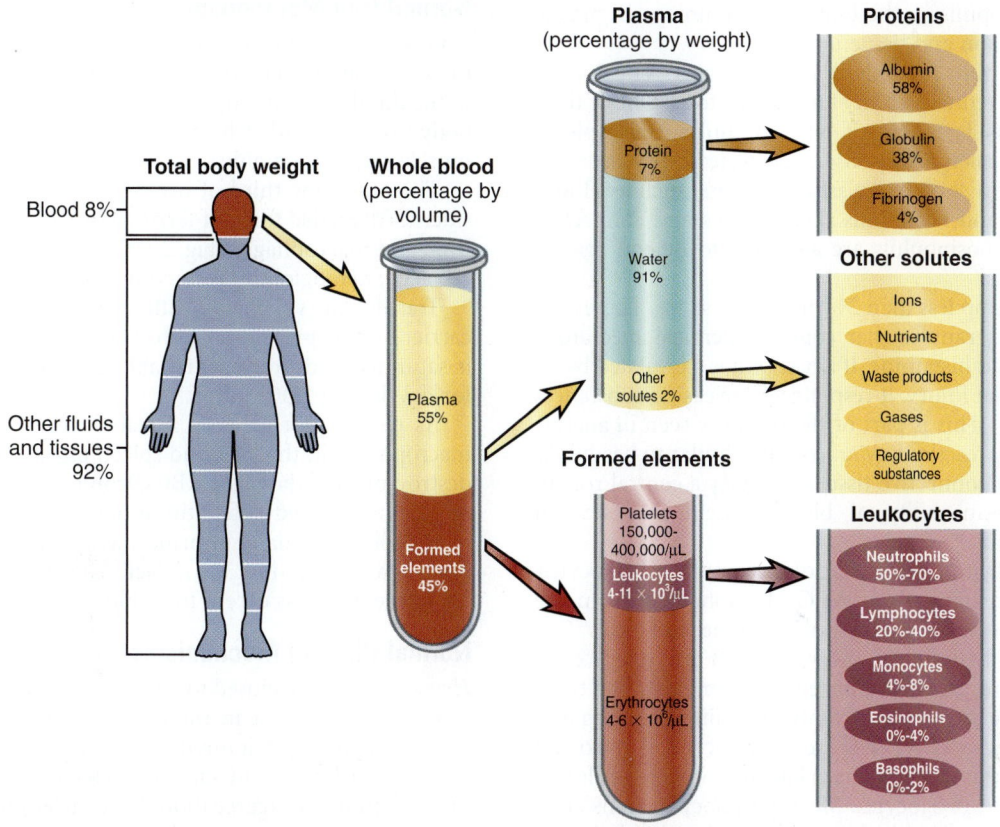

FIG. 29-2 Approximate values for the components of blood in the adult. Normally, 45% of the blood is composed of blood cells and 55% is composed of plasma.

Erythropoiesis is stimulated by hypoxia and controlled by *erythropoietin,* a glycoprotein growth factor synthesized and released primarily by the kidney. Erythropoietin stimulates the bone marrow to increase erythrocyte production. Approximately 2.5 million erythrocytes are produced per second. The normal life span of an erythrocyte is about 120 days. Erythropoiesis is also influenced by the availability of nutrients. Many essential nutrients are necessary for erythropoiesis, including protein, iron, folate (folic acid), cobalamin (vitamin B_{12}), riboflavin (vitamin B_2), pyridoxine (vitamin B_6), pantothenic acid, niacin, ascorbic acid (vitamin C), and vitamin E. Erythrocyte production is also affected by endocrine hormones, such as thyroxine, corticosteroids, and testosterone. For example, hypothyroidism is often associated with anemia.[1]

Several distinct cell types evolve during erythrocyte maturation (Fig. 29-1). The **reticulocyte** is an immature erythrocyte. Reticulocytes can develop into mature RBCs within 48 hours of release into the circulation. Therefore assessing the number of reticulocytes is a useful means of evaluating the rate and adequacy of erythrocyte production.

Hemolysis (destruction of RBCs) by monocytes and macrophages removes abnormal, defective, damaged, and old RBCs from circulation. Hemolysis normally occurs in the bone marrow, liver, and spleen. Because one of the components of RBCs is bilirubin, hemolysis of these cells results in increased bilirubin to be processed by the body. When hemolysis occurs via normal mechanisms, the liver is able to conjugate and excrete all bilirubin that is released (Fig. 30-2).

Leukocytes. *Leukocytes* (WBCs) appear white when separated from blood. Like the RBCs, leukocytes originate from stem cells within the bone marrow (Fig. 29-1) but may eventually reside in the thymus or secondary lymphoid tissues, such as the spleen, lymph nodes, and Peyer patches. There are different types of leukocytes, each with a different function. Leukocytes containing granules within the cytoplasm are called *granulocytes* (also known as *polymorphonuclear leukocytes*). Granulocytes include three types: neutrophils, basophils, and eosinophils.

Leukocytes that do not have granules within the cytoplasm are called *agranulocytes* and include lymphocytes and monocytes. Lymphocytes and monocytes are also referred to as *mononuclear cells* because they have only one discrete nucleus. Leukocytes have a widely variable life span. Granulocytes may only live for hours, yet some T lymphocytes may live for years.

Granulocytes. The primary function of the granulocytes is *phagocytosis,* a process by which WBCs engulf any unwanted organism and then digest and kill it. They can migrate through vessel walls and to the sites where they are needed. The *neutrophil* is the most common type of granulocyte, accounting for 50% to 70% of all WBCs. Neutrophils are the primary phagocytic cells involved in acute inflammatory responses. Once they engulf the pathogen, they die in 1 to 2 days. Neutrophil production and maturation are stimulated by hematopoietic growth factors (e.g., G-CSF, granulocyte-macrophage colony-stimulating factor [GM-CSF]) (see Table 13-3).

A mature neutrophil is called a *segmented neutrophil,* or "seg" or "polysegmented neutrophil," because the nucleus is segmented into two to five lobes connected by strands. An immature neutrophil is called a *band* (for the band appearance of the nucleus). Although band cells are sometimes found in the peripheral circulation of normal people and are capable of phagocytosis, the mature neutrophil is much more effective. An increase in neutrophils in the blood is a common diagnostic indicator of infection and tissue injury.

Eosinophils account for only 0% to 4% of all WBCs. They have a similar but reduced ability for phagocytosis. One of their primary functions is to engulf antigen-antibody complexes formed during an allergic response. An elevated level of eosinophils is also seen in some neoplastic disorders, such as Hodgkin's lymphoma, and in various skin diseases and connective tissue disorders.[2] Eosinophils are also able to defend against parasitic infections.

Basophils make up less than 2% of all leukocytes. These cells have cytoplasmic granules that contain chemical mediators, such as heparin and histamine. If a basophil is stimulated by an antigen or by tissue injury, it responds by releasing substances from the granules. This is part of the response seen in allergic and inflammatory reactions. *Mast cells* are similar to basophils, but they reside in connective tissues and play a central role in inflammation, permeability of blood vessels, and smooth muscle contraction.

Lymphocytes. Lymphocytes, one of the agranular leukocytes, constitute 20% to 40% of the WBCs. Lymphocytes form the basis of the cellular and humoral immune responses (see Chapter 13). Two lymphocyte subtypes are B cells and T cells. Although T cell precursors originate in the bone marrow, these cells migrate to the thymus gland for further differentiation into T cells. *Natural killer (NK) cells* are lymphocytes that do not require prior exposure to antigens to kill virus-infected cells and activate T cells and phagocytes. Most lymphocytes transiently circulate in the blood and also reside in lymphoid tissues. (Details of lymphocyte function are presented in Chapter 13.)

Monocytes. Monocytes, the other type of agranular leukocytes, account for approximately 4% to 8% of the total WBCs. Monocytes are potent phagocytic cells that ingest small or large masses of matter, such as bacteria, dead cells, tissue debris, and old or defective RBCs. These cells are only present in the blood for a short time before they migrate into the tissues and become macrophages (see Chapter 13). In addition to macrophages that have differentiated from monocytes, tissues also contain resident macrophages. These resident macrophages are given special names (e.g., Kupffer cells in the liver, osteoclasts in the bone, alveolar macrophages in the lung). These macrophages protect the body from pathogens at these entry points and are more phagocytic than monocytes. Macrophages also interact with lymphocytes to facilitate the humoral and cellular immune responses (see Chapter 13).

Thrombocytes. The primary function of thrombocytes, or *platelets,* is to initiate the clotting process by producing an initial platelet plug at a site of injury. Platelets must be available in sufficient numbers and must be structurally and metabolically sound for blood clotting to occur. At the site of any capillary damage, platelet activation is initiated. Increasing numbers of platelets accumulate to form an initial platelet plug that is stabilized with clotting factors. Platelets are also important in the process of clot shrinkage and retraction.

Platelets also originate from stem cells within the bone marrow (Fig. 29-1). The stem cell undergoes differentiation by transforming into a *megakaryocyte,* which fragments into platelets. About one third of the platelets in the body reside in the spleen.

Platelet production is partly regulated by *thrombopoietin,* a growth factor that acts on bone marrow to stimulate platelet production. It is produced in the liver, kidneys, smooth muscle, and bone marrow. Typically, platelets have a life span of only 8 to 10 days.

Normal Iron Metabolism

Iron is obtained from food and dietary supplements. Approximately 1 mg of every 10 to 20 mg of iron ingested is absorbed in the duodenum and upper jejunum. About two thirds of total body iron is bound to heme in erythrocytes (hemoglobin) and muscle cells (myoglobin).

The other one third of iron is stored as ferritin and hemosiderin (degraded form of ferritin) in the bone marrow, spleen, liver, and macrophages (Fig. 29-3). When the stored iron is not replaced, hemoglobin production is reduced.

Transferrin, which is synthesized in the liver, serves as a carrier plasma protein for iron. The degree to which transferrin is saturated with iron is a reliable indicator of the iron supply for developing RBCs.

As part of normal iron metabolism, iron is recycled after macrophages in the liver and spleen phagocytize, or ingest and destroy, old and damaged RBCs. Iron binds to transferrin in the plasma or is stored as ferritin or hemosiderin (Fig. 29-3). Only about 3% is lost daily in urine, sweat, bile, and epithelial cells in the gastrointestinal (GI) tract. Therefore there is normally very little iron loss except from blood loss.

Normal Clotting Mechanisms

Hemostasis is a term used to describe the arrest of bleeding. This process is important in minimizing blood loss when various body structures are injured. The sequence of events includes (1) vascular injury and subendothelial exposure, (2) adhesion, (3) activation, (4) aggregation, (5) platelet plug formation, and (6) clot retraction and dissolution.

Vascular Injury and Subendothelial Exposure. When a blood vessel is injured, an immediate local vasoconstrictive response occurs. Vasoconstriction reduces the leakage of blood from the vessel not only by restricting the vessel size but also by pressing the endothelial surfaces together. The latter reaction enhances vessel wall stickiness and maintains closure of the vessel even after vasoconstriction subsides. Vascular spasm may last for 20

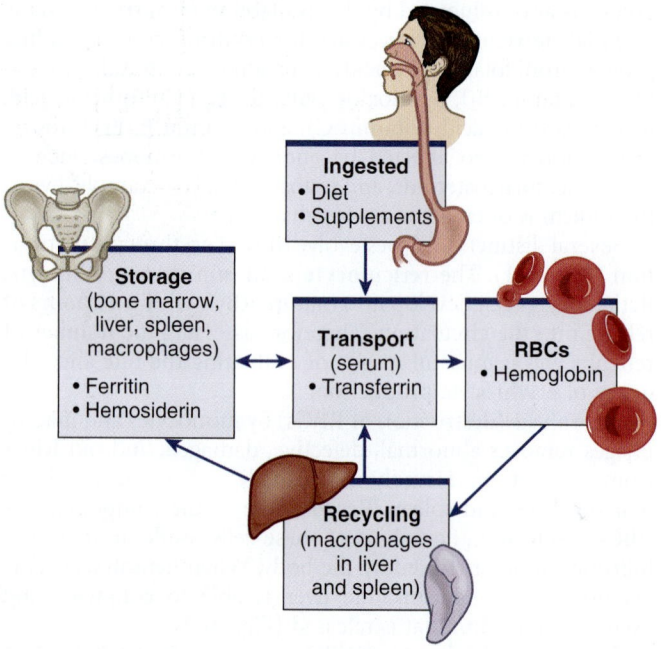

FIG. 29-3 Normal iron metabolism. Iron is ingested in the diet or from supplements. Macrophages break down ingested red blood cells *(RBCs).* Iron is returned to blood bound to transferrin or stored as ferritin or hemosiderin.

to 30 minutes, allowing time for the platelet response and plasma clotting factors to be activated. The platelet response and plasma clotting factors are triggered by endothelial injury and the release of substances such as thromboxane A_2 (TXA_2).

Platelet Adhesion. The loss of endothelial cells exposes adhesive glycoproteins such as collagen and von Willebrand factor (vWF), to which the platelets adhere. The stickiness is termed *adhesiveness,* and the formation of clumps is termed *aggregation* or *agglutination.*

Platelet Activation. The interaction above causes the platelets to undergo an activation process. This leads to changes in platelet shape. The platelets then have the ability to bind adhesive proteins, including fibrinogen and von Willebrand factor. Release of various platelet granules (including adenosine phosphate [ADP]) also recruits and activates other platelets, clotting factors, and growth factors. As Fig. 29-4 shows, platelet lipoproteins stimulate necessary conversions in the clotting process.

Platelet Aggregation. Platelet aggregation is stimulated by TXA_2 and ADP, which induce fibrinogen receptors on the platelet. The formation of a visible fibrin clot on the platelet plug is the conclusion of a complex series of reactions involving different clotting (coagulation) factors. The plasma clotting factors are labeled with both names and Roman numerals (Table 29-2).

Plasma proteins circulate in inactive forms until stimulated to initiate clotting through one of two pathways, intrinsic or extrinsic (Fig. 29-4). The *intrinsic pathway* is activated by collagen exposure from endothelial injury when the blood vessel is damaged. The *extrinsic pathway* is initiated when tissue factor or tissue thromboplastin is released extravascularly from injured tissues.

Regardless of whether clotting is initiated by substances internal or external to the blood vessel, coagulation ultimately follows the same final common pathway of the clotting cascade. Thrombin, in the common pathway, is the most powerful enzyme in the coagulation process (Fig. 29-4). It converts fibrinogen to fibrin, which is an essential component of a blood clot.

Platelet Plug Formation. The final blood clot is a meshwork of protein strands that stabilizes the platelet plug and traps other cells, such as erythrocytes, phagocytes, and microorganisms.

Clot Retraction and Dissolution. Just as some blood elements foster coagulation *(procoagulants),* others interfere with clotting *(anticoagulants).* This counter mechanism to blood clotting keeps blood in its fluid state.

Anticoagulation may be achieved by antithrombin activity, vessel and platelet activity, and fibrinolysis. As the name implies, antithrombins keep blood in a fluid state by antagonizing thrombin, a powerful coagulant. Endogenous heparin, antithrombin III, protein C, and protein S are examples of anticoagulants.

The second means of maintaining blood in its fluid form is **fibrinolysis**, a process resulting in the dissolution of the fibrin

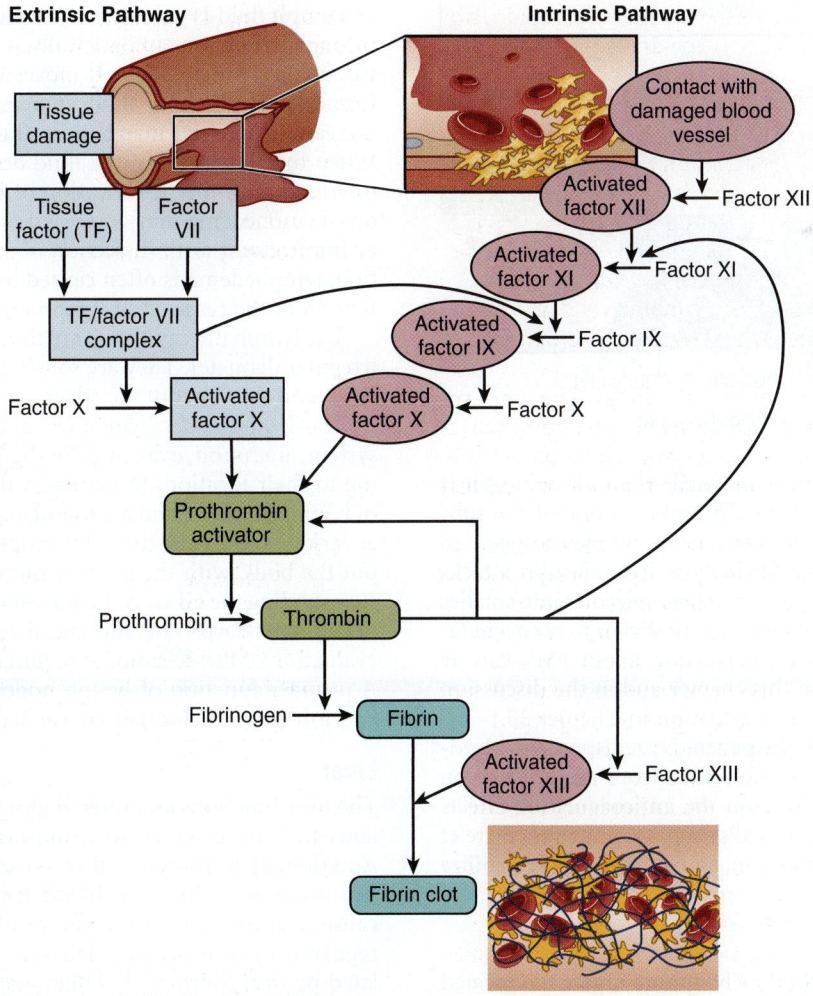

FIG. 29-4 Coagulation mechanism showing steps in the intrinsic pathway and extrinsic pathway as they would occur in the test tube.

TABLE 29-2 Coagulation Factors

Coagulation Factor	Action
I Fibrinogen	Source of fibrin to form a clot. Made in liver
II Prothrombin	Converted to thrombin, which then activates fibrinogen into fibrin as well as factors V, VII, VIII, XI, XIII, protein C, platelets
III Tissue factor, tissue thromboplastin	Released from damaged endothelial cells and activates the extrinsic pathway by reacting with factor VII
IV Calcium	Required cofactor at several points in the coagulation cascade
V Labile factor	Binds with factor X to activate prothrombin
VI	Not in use (now obsolete)
VII Stable factor, proconvertin	Forms a complex with factor III and activates factors IX and X
VIII Antihemophilic factor	Works with factor IX and calcium to activate factor X
IX Christmas factor	Together with factor VIII, activates factor X
X Stuart-Prower factor	Activates conversion of factor II (prothrombin) to thrombin
XI Plasma thromboplastin antecedent	Activates factor IX when calcium is present
XII Hageman factor	Activates factor XI, which starts the intrinsic pathway
XIII Fibrin-stabilizing factor	Cross-links fibrin strands and stabilizes fibrin clot

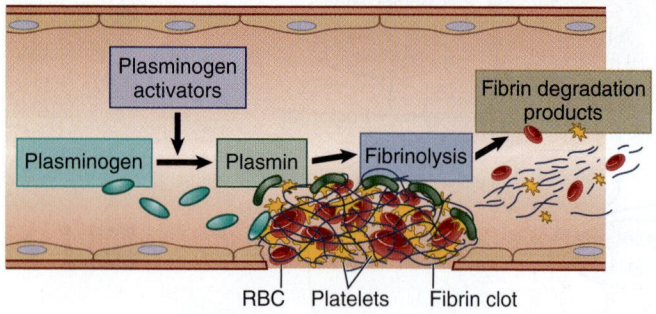

FIG. 29-5 Fibrinolytic system.

clot. The fibrinolytic system is initiated when plasminogen is activated to plasmin (Fig. 29-5). Thrombin is one of the substances that can activate the conversion of plasminogen to plasmin, thereby promoting fibrinolysis. The plasmin attacks either fibrin or fibrinogen by splitting the molecules into smaller elements known as *fibrin split products* (FSPs) or *fibrin degradation products* (FDPs). (More information about FSPs can be found in Table 29-7 later in this chapter and in the discussion of disseminated intravascular coagulation in Chapter 30.)

If fibrinolysis is excessive, the patient is predisposed to bleeding. In such a situation, bleeding results from the destruction of fibrin in platelet plugs or from the anticoagulation effects of increased FSPs. Increased FSPs lead to impaired platelet aggregation, reduced prothrombin, and an inability to stabilize fibrin.

Spleen

The spleen is the largest secondary lymphoid organ. It is located in the upper left quadrant of the abdomen. The spleen has four major functions: hematopoietic, filtration, immunologic, and storage. *Hematopoietic function* is manifested by the spleen's ability to produce RBCs during fetal development. The *filtration function* is demonstrated by the spleen's ability to remove old and defective RBCs from the circulation by the mononuclear phagocyte system. Filtration also involves the reuse of iron. The spleen is able to catabolize hemoglobin released by hemolysis and return the iron component of the hemoglobin to the bone marrow for reuse. The spleen also plays an important role in filtering circulating bacteria, especially encapsulated organisms such as gram-positive cocci. The *immunologic function* is demonstrated by the spleen's rich supply of lymphocytes, monocytes, and stored immunoglobulins. The *storage function* is reflected in its role as a storage site for RBCs and platelets. More than 300 mL of blood can be stored. About one third of platelets are stored in the spleen. A person who has had a splenectomy has higher circulating levels of platelets than a person who still has a spleen.

Lymph System

The lymph system, consisting of lymph fluid, lymphatic capillaries, ducts, and lymph nodes, carries fluid from the interstitial spaces to the blood. It is by means of the lymph that proteins and fat from the gastrointestinal (GI) tract and certain hormones are able to return to the circulatory system. The lymph system also returns excess interstitial fluid to the blood, which is important in preventing edema.

Lymph fluid is pale yellow interstitial fluid that has diffused through lymphatic capillary walls. It circulates through a special vasculature, much as blood moves through blood vessels. The formation of lymph fluid increases when interstitial fluid increases, thereby forcing more fluid into the lymph system. When too much interstitial fluid develops or when something interferes with the reabsorption of lymph, *lymphedema* develops. Lymphedema may occur as a complication of mastectomy or lumpectomy with dissection of axillary nodes. In this situation, lymphedema is often caused by the obstruction of lymph flow from the removal of lymph nodes.

The lymphatic capillaries are thin-walled vessels that have an irregular diameter. They are somewhat larger than blood capillaries and do not contain valves.

The *lymph nodes,* which are also a part of the lymphatic system, are round, oval, or bean shaped and vary in size according to their location. Structurally, the nodes are small clumps of lymphatic tissue and are found in groups along lymph vessels at various sites. More than 200 lymph nodes are found throughout the body, with the greatest number being in the abdomen surrounding the GI tract. Lymph nodes are situated both superficially and deep. The superficial nodes can be palpated, but evaluation of the deep nodes requires radiologic examination.[3,4] A primary function of lymph nodes is filtration of pathogens and foreign particles that are carried by lymph to the nodes.

Liver

The liver functions as a filter. It also produces all the procoagulants that are essential to hemostasis and blood coagulation. Additionally, it stores iron that is in excess of tissue needs, which can occur with frequent blood transfusions or diseases that cause iron overload. *Hepcidin*, produced by the liver, is a key regulator of iron balance. The synthesis of hepcidin is stimulated by iron overload or inflammation. Hepcidin inhibits the release of stored iron from enterocytes (in the intestines) and macrophages. Thus when iron is deficient, hepatocytes produce less hepcidin. This results in the release of stored iron and an increase in dietary absorption. Other functions of the liver are described in Chapters 38 and 43.

Gerontologic Considerations: Effects of Aging on Hematologic System

Physiologic aging is a gradual process that involves cell loss and organ atrophy. Aging leads to a decrease in bone marrow mass and cellularity and an increase in bone marrow fat. However, peripheral blood cell concentrations in healthy older adults are similar to those of younger adults. Although the older adult is still capable of maintaining adequate blood cell levels, the reserve capacity leaves the older adult more vulnerable to possible problems with clotting, transporting O_2, and fighting infection, especially during periods of increased demand. This results in a diminished ability of an older adult to compensate for an acute or chronic illness.

Hemoglobin levels begin to decrease in both men and women after middle age, with the low-normal levels seen in most older people. Total serum iron, total iron-binding capacity, and intestinal iron absorption are all decreased in older adults. Iron deficiency is usually responsible for the low hemoglobin levels. Healthy older patients are not able to produce reticulocytes in response to hemorrhage or hypoxemia as well as younger adults.

The RBC plasma membranes are more fragile in the older person. This may account for a slight increase in mean corpuscular volume (MCV) and a slight decrease in mean corpuscular hemoglobin concentration (MCHC) of RBCs in some older individuals. It is essential to assess for signs of disease processes such as GI bleeding before concluding that decreased hemoglobin levels are caused solely by aging. Thus iron deficiency anemia is a diagnosis that should be made after other causes have been ruled out.

The total WBC count and differential are generally not affected by aging. However, decreases in lymphocyte function occurs. During an infection, the older adult may have only a minimal elevation in the total WBC count. These laboratory findings suggest a diminished bone marrow reserve of granulocytes in older adults and reflect the possible impaired stimulation of hematopoiesis. The number of platelets is unaffected by the aging process, but functionally they may have increased adhesiveness. Changes in vascular integrity related to aging can manifest as easy bruising.

The effects of aging on hematologic studies are presented in Table 29-3. Immune changes related to aging are presented in Chapter 13.

TABLE 29-3 Gerontologic Assessment Differences

Effects of Aging on Hematologic Studies

Study	Changes
CBC Studies	
Hgb	Normal; possibly slight decrease
MCV	May be slightly increased
MCHC	May be slightly decreased
WBC count	Diminished response to infection
Platelets	Unchanged but possible increase in adhesiveness
Clotting Studies	
Partial thromboplastin time	Decreased
Fibrinogen	May be elevated
Factors V, VII, IX	May be elevated
ESR	Increased significantly
D-dimers	Increased
Iron Studies	
Serum iron	Decreased
Total iron-binding capacity	Decreased
Ferritin	Increased
Erythropoietin	May be decreased

ESR, Erythrocyte sedimentation rate; *MCHC,* mean corpuscular hemoglobin concentration; *MCV,* mean corpuscular volume.

CASE STUDY

Patient Introduction

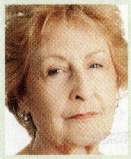

(©Lisa F. Young/iStock)

A.J. is a 63-year-old white woman who is brought to the emergency department by her husband. He came home from work and found his wife at home, weak and lying in bed after she returned from work. She says she has been slowly getting more and more "cold and tired" but "that is what happens when you continue to work at this age." Her husband states that she has become more and more tired over the last couple of weeks and has been having difficulty working all day and even gets short of breath when doing simple errands. She also recently had a "bad cold and sinus infection" that only improved after two courses of antibiotics. A.J. also states, "I've noticed I've had a lot of bruising lately."

Discussion Questions

1. What are the possible causes of A.J.'s weakness, pallor, and shortness of breath?
2. Is her condition stable or an emergency?

You will learn more about A.J. and her condition as you read through this assessment chapter. (See p. 596 for more information on A.J.)

Answers available at *http://evolve.elsevier.com/Lewis/medsurg.*

ASSESSMENT OF HEMATOLOGIC SYSTEM

Much of the evaluation of the hematologic system is based on a thorough health history. You need to be knowledgeable about what to include in the health history so that you can phrase questions to elicit the most information.[5]

Subjective Data

Important Health Information

Past Health History. Determine if the patient has had prior hematologic problems. Ask about previous problems with anemia, bleeding disorders, and blood diseases such as leukemia. Document other related medical conditions such as malabsorption or liver (e.g., hepatitis, cirrhosis), kidney, or spleen disorders. Patients may have received a kidney transplant, may have lost a spleen to traumatic injury, or may have a history of IV drug or alcohol use that affects their risk for hematologic disorders. A history of recent or recurrent infections or problems with blood clotting is also important to note.

Medications. A complete medication history of prescription and over-the-counter drugs is an important component of a hematologic assessment. Inquire about the use of vitamins, herbal products, or dietary supplements because many patients may not consider them to be drugs. Many drugs may interfere with normal hematologic function.[6,7] Herbs can interfere with clotting (see Complementary & Alternative Therapies box in

Chapter 37 on p. 820). Chemotherapy drugs used to treat cancer (see Chapter 15) and antiretroviral agents used to treat human immunodeficiency virus (HIV) infection (see Chapter 14) may cause bone marrow depression. A patient previously treated with chemotherapy agents, particularly alkylating agents, has a higher risk of developing a secondary malignancy of leukemia or lymphoma. A patient on long-term anticoagulant therapy such as warfarin (Coumadin) could be at risk for bleeding problems.

Surgery or Other Treatments. Ask the patient about specific past surgical procedures, including splenectomy, tumor removal, prosthetic heart valve placement, surgical excision of the duodenum (where iron absorption occurs), partial or total gastrectomy (which removes parietal cells, thus reducing intrinsic factor needed for the absorption of cobalamin [vitamin B_{12}]), gastric bypass (where the duodenum may be bypassed and parietal cell surface area decreased), and ileal resection (where cobalamin absorption takes place). Also assess how wound healing progressed postoperatively and if and when any bleeding problems occurred in relation to the surgery. Discuss wound healing and bleeding as responses to past injuries (including minor trauma) and dental extractions. Also determine the number of previous blood transfusions and possible complications during administration, since the risk of transfusion reactions and iron overload increases with the number of blood transfusions.

Functional Health Patterns. Key questions to ask a patient with a hematologic problem are presented in Table 29-4.

Health Perception–Health Management Pattern. Ask the patient to describe the usual and present state of health. Gather complete demographic data, including age, gender, race, and ethnic background. Ask if there is any family history of hematologic problems.

GENETIC RISK ALERT

- Hematologic problems that have a strong genetic link include sickle cell anemia, hemophilia, thalassemia, and hemochromatosis.
- People with a family history of these hematologic problems have a much greater risk of developing them.
- Other hematologic problems, such as leukemia, pernicious anemia, and clotting disorders, may have a genetic predisposition.

When taking a family health history, explore the following health problems: jaundice, anemia, malignancies, RBC disorders such as sickle cell disease, bleeding disorders such as hemophilia, and clotting disorders.

Assess risk factors such as alcohol and cigarette use that may disrupt the hematologic system. Alcohol is a caustic agent to the GI mucosa and can cause damage that results in GI bleeding, esophageal varices, and decreased absorption of cobalamin and other nutrients.

Chronic alcohol users frequently have vitamin deficiencies. Alcohol also exerts a damaging effect on platelet function and the liver, where clotting factors are produced. Consequently, bleeding problems can develop and should be anticipated in cases of known chronic alcohol use. Illicit drug use is also important to document, since many of these drugs may affect hematopoiesis.

Cigarette smoking increases low-density lipoprotein (LDL) cholesterol and levels of CO_2, leading to hypoxia and altering the anticoagulant properties of the endothelium. Smoking increases platelet reactivity, plasma fibrinogen, hematocrit, and blood viscosity.

Nutritional-Metabolic Pattern. Obtain the patient's weight and determine if the patient has experienced anorexia, nausea, vomiting, or oral discomfort. A dietary history may provide clues about the cause of anemia. Iron, cobalamin, and folic acid are necessary for the development of RBCs. Iron and folic acid deficiencies are associated with inadequate intake of foods such as liver, meat, eggs, whole-grain and enriched breads and cereals, potatoes, leafy green vegetables, dried fruits, legumes, and citrus fruits. Folic acid deficiencies may be offset by a diet including foods that are also high in iron.[8]

Hematemesis (bright red, brown, or black vomitus) is a manifestation of an underlying problem and should always be investigated. Peptic ulcer disease is a common cause of hematemesis.

Explore any changes in the skin's texture, color, or temperature. Ask about bleeding of gum tissue or bleeding from anywhere on the body. Also ask about any lumps or swelling in the neck, armpits, or groin. Specifically, ask what the lumps feel like (i.e., hard or soft, tender or nontender) and if they are mobile or fixed. Primary lymph tumors are usually not painful. A nontender, consistently swollen lymph node may be a sign of a malignancy, such as Hodgkin's or non-Hodgkin's lymphoma. Lymph nodes that are enlarged and tender are usually associated with an acute infection.[3] Explore any reports of fever. Determine if the patient currently has a fever, recurring fevers, chills, or night sweats.

Ask patients if they have a history of cardiac or pulmonary diseases. Cardiovascular disorders such as valvular disease or hypertension may predispose patients to hemolysis. Many of the medications used to treat cardiovascular disease can also cause abnormalities in hematopoietic cell production or coagulation. Pulmonary disorders that lead to hypoxemia may cause chronic stimulation of erythropoietin and result in *polycythemia* (excessive RBCs).

Elimination Pattern. Ask if blood has been noted in the urine or stool or if black, tarry stools have occurred. Ask the patient if he or she has had a recent stool tested for occult blood or colonoscopy. Document any decrease in urine output or diarrhea.

Activity-Exercise Pattern. Because fatigue is a prominent symptom in many hematologic disorders, ask about feelings of tiredness. Also determine any weakness or complaints of heavy extremities. Document symptoms of apathy, malaise, dyspnea, or palpitations. Note any change in the patient's ability to perform regular exercise and/or activities of daily living (ADLs), especially as they relate to patient safety and a history of falling.

Sleep-Rest Pattern. Determine whether the patient feels rested after a night's sleep. Fatigue secondary to a hematologic problem often does not resolve after sleep.

Cognitive-Perceptual Pattern. *Arthralgia* (joint pain) may be caused by a hematologic problem and should be assessed. Pain in the joint may indicate an autoimmune disorder, such as rheumatoid arthritis, or may be caused by gout secondary to increased uric acid production as a result of a hematologic malignancy or hemolytic anemia. Aching bones may result from pressure of expanding bone marrow with diseases such as leukemia. *Hemarthrosis* (blood in a joint) occurs in the patient with bleeding disorders and can be painful.

Paresthesias, numbness, and tingling may be related to a hematologic disorder and should be noted. Also assess any changes in vision, hearing, taste, or mental status.

Self-Perception–Self-Concept Pattern. Determine the effect of the health problem on the patient's perception of self and personal abilities. Also assess the effect of certain problems,

TABLE 29-4 Health History

Hematologic System

Health Perception–Health Management

- Do you have any difficulty performing daily activities because of a lack of energy?*
- Do you smoke cigarettes or drink alcohol?*
- Do you take any prescribed or over-the-counter medications?*
- Are you taking any herbs?* Home remedies?*
- Have you in the past or are you currently consuming illegal drugs? What agents? What route? How frequently? When did you last use?
- Have you ever received a blood transfusion?*
- Is there any family history of anemia, cancer, bleeding, or clotting problems?*
- Have you had any surgeries?*

Nutritional-Metabolic

- Do you have any difficulties with eating, chewing, or swallowing?*
- Have you had any mouth sores, sore tongue, swollen or sore gums, excessive oral bleeding?*
- What kind of diet do you follow? If a vegetarian, do you eat eggs, milk products, fish?
- How has your appetite been?
- Have you had any changes in your weight in the past year?*
- Do you take any vitamins, nutritional supplements, or iron?*
- Is nausea and vomiting a problem for you?*
- Have you ever experienced any unusual bleeding or bruising?*
- Have there been recent changes in the condition or color of your skin?*
- Have you experienced night sweats or cold intolerance?*
- Have you noticed any swelling in your armpits, neck, or groin?*

Elimination

- Have you had black or tarry stools?* Have you had light, clay-colored stools?*
- Have you noticed any blood or dark "tea color" in your urine?*
- Has your urine had a foul odor or cloudiness?
- Have you had any decrease in urine output?*
- Do you ever have diarrhea or change in bowel patterns?*

Activity-Exercise

- Do you have any shortness of breath at rest? With activity?*
- Do you have any limitations in joint motion?* Have any of your joints been swollen?*
- Do you have a problem with unsteady gait? Have you fallen recently?*
- Do you exercise regularly? What type and how frequently?*
- After activity, do you ever notice bleeding or bruising?*

Sleep-Rest

- Have you experienced excessive fatigue recently?*
- Are you more fatigued than usual?*
- Do you feel rested on awakening? If no, explain.

Cognitive-Perceptual

- Have you experienced any numbness or tingling?*
- Have you had any problems with your vision, hearing, or taste?*
- Have you noticed any changes in your mental function?*
- Do you have any pain, such as bone, joint, or abdominal pain, or abdominal fullness?*
- Do you have pain when moving your joints?*
- Have your muscles been sore or achy recently?*

Self-Perception–Self-Concept

- Does your health problem make you feel differently about yourself?*
- Do you have any physical changes that cause you distress?*

Role-Relationship

- Does your occupation bring you into contact with hazardous substances?*
- Has your present illness caused a change in your roles and relationships?*

Sexuality-Reproductive

- Has your hematologic problem caused any sexual or intimacy problems that concern you?*
- *Women:* When was your last menses? Do you consider your cycle normal? How long does your bleeding usually last? Have you had any increase in cramping or clotting?* Have there been any changes in the amount of flow?*
- *Men:* Do you experience impotence?*
- Have you had unprotected sex in the past 6 months?* Was your partner someone new or a person with whom you have had a long-term sexual relationship?

Coping–Stress Tolerance

- Do you have a support system to assist you when needed?
- What coping strategies do you use during exacerbation of symptoms?
- Do you experience any specific symptoms when you feel stressed?*

Value-Belief

- Do you have any personal or religious objection to receiving blood or blood products?*
- Do you have any conflicts between your planned therapy and your value-belief system?*

*If yes, describe.

such as bruising, petechiae, and lymph node swelling, on the patient's personal appearance.

Role-Relationship Pattern. Question the patient about any past or present occupational or household exposures to radiation or chemicals. If such exposure has occurred, determine the type, amount, and duration of the exposure.

A person who has been exposed to radiation, as a treatment modality or by accident, has a higher incidence of certain hematologic problems. The same is true of a person who has been exposed to certain chemicals (e.g., benzene, lead, naphthalene, phenylbutazone). These chemicals are commonly used by potters, dry cleaners, and individuals involved with occupations that use adhesives. Ask the patient about a history in the military. Many Vietnam War veterans were exposed to a dioxin-containing defoliant (Agent Orange), which has been linked with leukemia and lymphoma. Also assess the effect of the present illness on the patient's usual roles and responsibilities.

Sexuality-Reproductive Pattern. Obtain a careful menstrual history from women, including the age at which menarche and menopause began, duration and amount of bleeding, incidence of clotting and cramping, and any associated problems. Ask men if they have any problems related to impotence, since this is common in men with hematologic problems. Also question the patient about sexual behavior because HIV infection is potentially a concern, particularly among high-risk groups.

Coping–Stress Tolerance Pattern. The patient with a hematologic problem often needs assistance with ADLs. Ask the patient if adequate support is available to meet daily needs. Determine the patient's usual methods of handling stress. In the patient with platelet disorders or hemophilia, the potential for hemorrhage can be so frightening that usual life patterns may be drastically curtailed, affecting the person's quality of life. Explore the patient's understanding of the problem and provide teaching.

Value-Belief Pattern. Some hematologic problems are treated with blood transfusions or a bone marrow transplant. Determine if these types of treatments conflict with the patient's value-belief system, including the patient's cultural and religious beliefs related to blood and blood transfusions. If conflicts are identified, notify the HCP.

CASE STUDY

Subjective Data

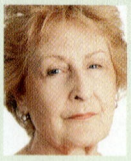

(©Lisa F. Young/iStock)

A focused subjective assessment of A.J. revealed the following information:

PMH: History of mild osteoarthritis. No surgical history. Prefers to take care of self with "natural therapy" and has not seen an HCP for 5 years, except for the recent sinus infection.

Medications: Metamucil 1 Tbsp PO daily; vitamins C, E, and D with calcium.

Health Perception–Health Management: A.J. denies family or personal history of anemia, cancer, or bleeding disorders. She believes she comes from a family with great genes for longevity because they "eat organic foods." She admits to drinking one glass of red wine with her evening meal "because it's good for your heart." She is a nonsmoker and just can't understand her gradual increase in shortness of breath with exertion. She states she really can't do anything anymore without having to stop and catch her breath. She says, "It's tough getting old."

Nutritional-Metabolic: A.J. and her husband eat a lot of pasta "because it is cheap." She uses a lot of garlic for flavoring and the "health benefit of it." Although not a vegetarian, she states that she eats little meat.

Elimination: Denies black or tarry stool. Occasional constipation. No problems with urination. Urine without odor.

Activity-Exercise: As noted above, A.J. is having difficulty performing ADLs without having to stop and catch her breath. Denies dyspnea at rest. States joints are stiff on arising in morning and after sitting but able to get around OK and work at her secretarial job. States her walking is steady but weak. No history of falling.

Sleep-Rest: Typically sleeps 8-9 hr/night with no difficulty falling asleep. However, she still feels tired and needs to nap during her lunch break and during her days off.

Cognitive-Perceptual: Denies any numbness or tingling. Admits to being a little hard-of-hearing but can still see "pretty good."

Value-Belief: Prefers natural therapies over traditional medication.

Discussion Questions

1. What type of assessment would be most appropriate for A.J.: comprehensive, focused, or emergency? On what basis did you make that decision? What would be your priority?
2. What assessment questions would you ask A.J.?
3. How will you individualize the physical assessment based on the information from A.J. and her husband?
4. What subjective assessment findings are of most concern to you?
5. Based on these subjective assessment findings, what type of physical assessment should be performed?

You will learn more about the physical examination of the hematologic system in the next section. (See p. 599 for more information on A.J.)

Answers available at *http://evolve.elsevier.com/Lewis/medsurg.*

Objective Data

Physical Examination. A complete physical examination is necessary to accurately examine all systems that affect or are affected by the hematologic system (see Chapter 3). Be aware that disorders of the hematologic system can manifest in various ways. Thus a patient's presenting symptoms may not immediately point to a hematologic problem (Table 29-5). For example, paresthesias of the lower extremities may not immediately appear to reflect a hematologic problem, but when combined with other clinical findings or risk factors, they may indicate cobalamin deficiency and resulting pernicious anemia. Although a full examination should be performed on patients suspected of a hematologic disorder, certain aspects of the physical examination are specifically relevant. These include skin, lymph nodes, spleen, and liver. Examination of the skin is discussed in Chapter 22; spleen and liver examination is found in Chapter 38.

Lymph Node Assessment. Lymph nodes are distributed throughout the body. Superficial lymph nodes can be evaluated by light palpation (Fig. 29-6). Deep lymph nodes cannot be palpated and are best evaluated by radiologic examination. Assess lymph nodes symmetrically and take note of location, size (in centimeters), degree of fixation (e.g., movable, fixed), tenderness, and texture. To assess superficial lymph nodes, lightly palpate the nodes using the pads of the fingers. Then gently roll the skin over the area and concentrate on feeling for possible lymph node enlargement.

Ordinarily, lymph nodes are not palpable in adults. If a node is palpable, it should be small (0.5 to 1 cm), mobile, firm, and nontender to be considered a normal finding. A node that is tender, hard, fixed, or enlarged (regardless if it is tender or not) is an abnormal finding and warrants further investigation. Tender nodes are usually a result of inflammation, whereas hard or fixed nodes suggest malignancy.[3]

Develop a sequence when examining the lymph nodes. A convenient sequence is to start at the head and neck. First,

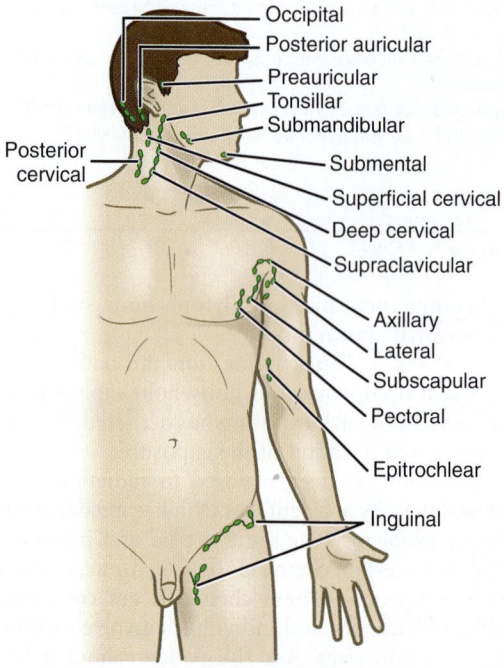

FIG. 29-6 Palpable superficial lymph nodes.

TABLE 29-5 Assessment Abnormalities

Hematologic System

Finding	Description	Possible Etiology and Significance
Skin		
Pallor of skin or nail beds	Paleness. Decreased or absence of skin coloration.	Low Hgb level (anemia).
Flushing	Transient, episodic redness of skin (usually around face and neck).	Increase in Hgb (polycythemia), congestion of capillaries. Flushing of palms of hands or soles of feet possible indication of anemia.
Jaundice	Yellow appearance of skin and mucous membranes.	Accumulation of bile pigment caused by rapid or excessive hemolysis or liver damage.
Cyanosis	Bluish discoloration of skin and mucous membranes	Reduced Hgb, excessive concentration of deoxyhemoglobin in blood.
Excoriation	Scratch or abrasion of skin.	Scratching from intense pruritus.
Pruritus	Unpleasant cutaneous sensation that provokes the desire to rub or scratch skin.	Hodgkin's lymphoma, cutaneous lymphomas, infiltrative leukemias, increased bilirubin.
Leg ulcers	Prominent on the malleoli on the ankles.	Sickle cell disease.
Angioma	Benign tumor consisting of blood or lymph vessels.	Most are congenital. Some may disappear spontaneously.
Telangiectasia	Small angioma with tendency to bleed. Focal red lesions, coarse or fine red lines.	Dilation of small vessels.
Spider nevus	Form of telangiectasia characterized by a round red central portion and branching radiations resembling profile of a spider. Usually develop on face, neck, or chest.	Elevated estrogen levels as in pregnancy or liver disease.
Purpura	Any of a small group of conditions characterized by ecchymosis or other small hemorrhages in skin and mucous membranes.	Decreased platelets or clotting factors resulting in hemorrhage into skin. Vascular abnormalities. Break in blood vessel walls resulting from trauma.
Petechiae	Pinpoint, nonraised, perfectly round area >2 mm. Purple, dark red, or brown.	Same as above
Ecchymosis (bruise)	Small hemorrhagic spot, larger than petechiae. Nonelevated. Round or irregular.	Same as above.
Hematoma	A localized collection of blood, usually clotted.	Same as above.
Chloroma	A tumor arising from myeloid tissue and containing a pale green pigment.	Acute myelogenous leukemia that has infiltrated the skin.
Plasmacytoma	Tumor arising from abnormal plasma cells.	Multiple myeloma that has infiltrated tissue.
Eyes		
Jaundiced sclera	Yellow appearance of sclera.	Accumulation of bile pigment resulting from rapid or excessive hemolysis or liver disease or infiltration.
Conjunctival pallor	Paleness. Decreased or absence of coloration in the conjunctiva.	Low Hgb level (anemia).
Blurred vision, diplopia, visual field cuts	Decreased visual acuity or areas of blindness (field cuts).	Anemia, extreme leukocytosis, polycythemia may cause visual abnormalities. Thrombocytopenia may cause intraocular hemorrhage with visual abnormalities. Excessive clotting may cause thromboses in circulation to the brain that cause visual field cuts.
Nose		
Epistaxis	Spontaneous bleeding from nares.	May occur with low platelet counts, especially if patient bends down for a long time, tries to lift a heavy item, or performs an intense Valsalva maneuver.
Mouth		
Gingival and mucous membrane changes	Pallor.	Low Hgb level (anemia).
	Gingival and mucosal ulceration, swelling, or bleeding.	Neutropenia. Inability of impaired leukocytes to combat oral infections. Thrombocytopenia. Gingival hyperplasia may be present with some types of leukemia.
Smooth tongue	Tongue surface smooth and shiny. Mucosa thin and red from decreased papillae.	Pernicious anemia, iron-deficiency anemia.
Musculoskeletal System		
Bone pain	Pain in pelvis, ribs, spine, sternum.	Multiple myeloma related to enlarged tumors that stretch periosteum. Bone invasion by leukemia cells. Bone demineralization resulting from various malignancies. Sickle cell disease.
Joint swelling	Fluid-filled spaces surrounding joints.	Occurs with hemophilia and sickle cell anemia as bleeding occurs into joint (hemarthrosis), causing inflammation.
Arthralgia	Joint pain.	Sickle cell disease from hemarthrosis.
Lymph Nodes		
Lymphadenopathy	Lymph nodes enlarged (>1 cm). May be tender to touch.	Infection; foreign infiltrations. Systemic disease such as leukemia, lymphoma, Hodgkin's lymphoma, and metastatic cancer.

Continued

TABLE 29-5 Assessment Abnormalities

Hematologic System—cont'd

Finding	Description	Possible Etiology and Significance
Heart and Chest		
Tachycardia	Heart rate >100 beats/min.	Compensatory mechanism in anemia to increase cardiac output.
Palpitations	Feeling the heartbeat, flutter, or pound in chest.	Anemia, fluid volume overload, hypotension with impending syncope, hypertension, dysrhythmias.
Altered blood pressure	*Orthostasis:* heart rate >20 beats/min increase or blood pressure >20 mm Hg decrease from baseline when moving from a lying position to either sitting or standing.	Orthostasis is a common manifestation in anemia, especially if also accompanied by low blood volume.
	Hypotension: <90 mm Hg systolic or >40 mm Hg drop from baseline.	Hypotension may indicate an infectious process, blood loss, or compromised cardiovascular compensatory mechanisms.
	Hypertension: >140/90 mm Hg.	Hypertension may occur initially as a compensatory mechanism for anemia.
Sternal tenderness	Abnormal sensitivity to touch or pressure on sternum.	Leukemia resulting from increased bone marrow cellularity, causing increase in pressure and bone erosion. Multiple myeloma as a result of stretching of periosteum
Low O_2 saturation	O_2-carrying capacity as reflected by O_2 saturation by pulse oximetry.	O_2 saturation may be decreased in cases of severe anemia.
Abdomen		
Hepatomegaly	Palpable liver.	Leukemia, cirrhosis, or fibrosis secondary to iron overload from sickle cell disease or thalassemia.
Splenomegaly	Palpable spleen.	Anemia, thrombocytopenia, leukemia, lymphomas, leukopenia, mononucleosis, malaria, cirrhosis, trauma, portal hypertension.
Distended abdomen	A larger than normal abdominal profile. May be soft or firm, tender or nontender, and accompanied by other symptoms such as nausea, vomiting, or rebound tenderness.	Lymphoma may manifest as abdominal adenopathy, mass(es), or bowel obstruction.
Nervous System		
Paresthesias of feet and hands, ataxia	Numbness sensation and extreme sensitivity experienced in central and peripheral nerves. Impaired muscle movement.	Cobalamin (vitamin B_{12}) deficiency or folate deficiency.
Weakness	Lacking physical strength or energy.	Low Hgb level (anemia).
Headache, nuchal rigidity	Pain in the cranium, potentially involving one area or extending from frontal area to back of neck.	Generalized headache is a common manifestation of mild to moderate anemia. Severe headache with or without visual disturbances may signal intracranial hemorrhage due to thrombocytopenia.

palpate the preauricular, posterior auricular, occipital, tonsillar, submandibular, submental, superficial cervical, posterior cervical chain, deep cervical chain, and supraclavicular nodes. Next, palpate the axillary lymph nodes and pectoral, subscapular, and lateral groups of nodes. Then examine the epitrochlear nodes, located in the antecubital fossa between the biceps and triceps muscles. Last, palpate the inguinal lymph nodes, found in the groin.

Palpation of Liver or Spleen. Both the liver and spleen are normally not detectable by palpating the abdomen. When they are enlarged, they may be detectable by percussion or palpation. Measure the degree of enlargement of the liver by the number of fingerbreadths it extends below the rib border. The spleen may be more difficult to detect because of its deep location in the left abdomen. Specific techniques for palpating the liver and spleen are described in Chapter 38.

Skin Assessment. In hematologic disorders, assessment of the skin may be a valuable source of information about the hematologic system. Examine the skin over the entire body in a systematic manner (e.g., starting with the face and oral cavity and moving downward over the body). In patients with RBC disorders the skin may be pale or pasty, or it may have a cyanotic tinge in severe anemia. Erythrocytosis often produces small vessel occlusions causing a purple, mottled appearance of the face, nose, fingers, or toes. *Clubbing of the fingers* (discussed in Chapter 25) can be seen with chronic anemia such as in patients with sickle cell disease.

Leukocyte disorders may cause infectious skin lesions or malignant nodular lesions. These may occur anywhere and have a variable distribution pattern. During the physical assessment of the skin, look carefully for **petechiae** (small purplish red pinpoint lesions), **ecchymoses** (bruising), and *spider nevus* (a form of *telangiectasia*) (Table 29-5), because these findings can indicate bleeding disorders. The location of petechiae can indicate an accumulation of blood in the skin or mucous membranes. Small vessels leak under pressure, and the platelet numbers are insufficient to stop the bleeding. Petechiae are more likely to occur where clothing constricts the circulation. In general, skin and mucosal bleeding indicates a platelet disorder, whereas spontaneous bleeding into joints or muscles indicates a coagulation factor problem.

A *focused assessment* is used to evaluate the status of previously identified hematologic problems and to monitor for signs of new problems (see Table 3-6). A focused assessment of the hematologic system is presented in the box on p. 599.

CASE STUDY

Objective Data: Physical Examination

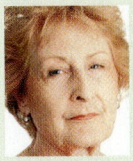

(©Lisa F. Young/iStock)

Physical examination findings of A.J. are as follows: BP 100/70 (lying), 88/60 (standing); apical pulse 110 (lying), 124 (standing), but regular in rhythm. Respiratory rate 26, temperature 96.8° F (36° C), O_2 saturation 90% on room air. No jugular venous distention. Weight: 106 lb (48 kg). Height: 5 ft 1 in. Skin pale and two ecchymoses on her arms and one on her left lower leg. A few scattered petechiae on both ankles. No jaundice noted. Conjunctivae pale. Tongue smooth and shiny. Lungs clear but diminished breath sounds in the bases bilaterally. No visible bleeding. No enlarged lymph nodes, spleen, or liver noted. General weakness with dyspnea on exertion. No numbness or tingling or peripheral edema.

Discussion Questions

1. What should be included in the physical assessment? For what would you be looking?
2. Which physical assessment findings are of most concern to you?
3. Based on the results of the subjective and physical assessment findings, what diagnostic studies do you think may be ordered for A.J.?

You will learn more about diagnostic studies in relation to the hematologic system in the next section. (See p. 605 for more information on A.J.)

Answers available at *http://evolve.elsevier.com/Lewis/medsurg.*

FOCUSED ASSESSMENT

Hematologic System

Use this checklist to make sure the key assessment steps have been done.

Subjective

Ask the patient about any of the following and note responses.

Unusual bleeding or bruising	Y	N
Black, tarry stool	Y	N
Blood in vomitus	Y	N
Swelling in neck, armpits, or groin	Y	N
Dark-colored urine	Y	N
Fatigue	Y	N
Heart palpitations	Y	N

Objective: Diagnostic

Check the following laboratory results for critical values.

CBC	✓
WBC count with differential	✓
Clotting: PT, INR, aPTT, platelets	✓
Hgb, Hct	✓

Objective: Physical Examination

Inspect

Skin for lesions or color changes	✓

Auscultate

BP for alteration or orthostasis	✓

Palpate

Pulse for tachycardia	✓
Liver and spleen for enlargement	✓
Lymph nodes for lymphadenopathy	✓

aPTT, Activated partial thromboplastin time; *INR,* international normalized ratio; *PT,* prothrombin time.

DIAGNOSTIC STUDIES OF HEMATOLOGIC SYSTEM

The most direct means of evaluating the hematologic system is through laboratory analysis (Tables 29-6, 29-7, 29-9) and other diagnostic studies (Table 29-10).

Laboratory Studies

Complete Blood Count. The complete blood count (CBC) involves several laboratory tests (Table 29-6). In addition to the CBC, a *peripheral smear* may be ordered. The smear is used to look at the *morphology* (shape and appearance) of the blood cells and may assist with the diagnosis. For example, a large number of immature *blast* WBCs may indicate acute leukemia.

Although the status of each cell type is important, the entire system may be disrupted by diseases or by treatment of diseases. When the entire CBC is suppressed, a condition termed **pancytopenia** (marked decrease in the number of RBCs, WBCs, and platelets) exists.

Red Blood Cells. Normal values of some RBC tests are reported separately for men and women because normal values are based on body mass, and men usually have a larger body mass than women.

The *hemoglobin (Hgb) value* is reduced in cases of anemia, hemorrhage, and hemodilution, such as that occurring when the fluid volume is excessive. Increases in hemoglobin are found in polycythemia or in states of hemoconcentration, which can develop from volume depletion (dehydration).

The *hematocrit (Hct) value* is determined by spinning blood in a centrifuge, which causes RBCs and plasma to separate. The RBCs, being the heavier elements, settle to the bottom (Fig. 29-2). The hematocrit value represents the percentage of RBCs compared with the total blood volume. Reductions and elevations of the hematocrit value are seen in the same conditions that raise and lower the hemoglobin value. The hematocrit value generally is three times the hemoglobin value.

The total RBC count is reported as RBC $\times 10^6/\mu L$. However, the total RBC count is not always reliable in determining the adequacy of RBC function. Consequently, other data, such as hemoglobin, hematocrit, and RBC indices, must also be evaluated. The RBC count is altered by the same conditions that raise and lower the hemoglobin and hematocrit values.

RBC indices are special indicators that reflect RBC volume, color, and hemoglobin saturation (Table 29-6). These parameters may provide insight into the cause of anemia. (The significance of these parameters is discussed further in Chapter 30.)

White Blood Cells. The WBC count provides two different sets of information. The first is a total count of WBCs in 1 μL of peripheral blood. Elevations in WBC count over 11,000/μL are associated with infection, inflammation, tissue injury or death, and malignancies (e.g., leukemia, lymphoma). Although the degree of WBC elevation does not necessarily predict the severity of illness, it can provide clues to the etiology. Certain types of leukemias are more likely to produce extremely high WBC counts (e.g., greater than 25,000/μL). A WBC count less than 4000/μL (**leukopenia**) is associated with bone marrow depression, severe or chronic illness, and some types of leukemia.

The second aspect of the WBC count, the *differential count,* measures the percentage of each type of leukocyte. The WBC differential provides valuable clues in determining the cause of illness. When infections are severe, more granulocytes are released from the bone marrow as a compensatory mechanism. To meet the increased demand, many young, immature polymorphonuclear neutrophils *(bands)* are released into circulation. More

TABLE 29-6 Diagnostic Studies

Complete Blood Count Studies

Study	Description and Purpose	Reference Intervals
Hemoglobin (Hgb)	Measurement of gas-carrying capacity of RBC	*Female:* 11.7-15.5 g/dL (117-155 g/L) *Male:* 13.2-17.3 g/dL (132-173 g/L)
Hematocrit (Hct)	Measure of packed cell volume of RBCs expressed as a percentage of the total blood volume	*Female:* 35%-47% (0.35-0.47) *Male:* 39%-50% (0.39-0.50)
Total RBC count	Number of circulating RBCs	*Female:* 3.8-5.1 × 10^6/μL (3.8-5.1 × 10^{12}/L) *Male:* 4.3-5.7 × 10^6/μL (4.3-5.7 × 10^{12}/L)
Red cell indices		
$MCV = \frac{Hct \times 10}{RBC \times 10^6}$	Determination of relative size of RBCs. Low MCV reflection of microcytosis, high MCV reflection of macrocytosis	80-100 fL
$MCH = \frac{Hgb \times 10}{RBC \times 10^6}$	Measurement of average weight of Hgb/RBCs. Low MCH indication of microcytosis or hypochromia, high MCH indication of macrocytosis	27-34 pg
$MCHC = \frac{Hgb \times 100}{Hct}$	Evaluation of RBC saturation with Hgb. Low MCHC indication of hypochromia, high MCHC evident in spherocytosis	32%-37% (0.32-0.37)
RBC morphology	Examination of shape and size of RBCs	No variation in RBC morphology
WBC count	Measurement of total number of WBCs	4000-11,000/μL (4-11 × 10^9/L)
WBC differential	Determination of whether each kind of WBC is present in proper proportion Absolute value of each type of WBC can be determined by multiplying the percentage of cell type by total WBC count and dividing by 100.	*Neutrophils:* 50%-70% (0.50-0.70) *Eosinophils:* 0%-4% (0-0.04) *Basophils:* 0%-2% (0-0.02) *Lymphocytes:* 20%-40% (0.20-0.40) *Monocytes:* 4%-8% (0.04-0.08)
Platelet count	Number of platelets available to maintain platelet clotting functions (not measurement of quality of platelet function)	150,000-400,000/μL (150-400 × 10^9/L)

MCH, Mean corpuscular hemoglobin; *MCHC,* mean corpuscular hemoglobin concentration; *MCV,* mean corpuscular volume.

mature neutrophils are called *polymorphonuclear segmented neutrophils (segs)*. Together bands and segs make up the *absolute neutrophil count* (ANC). The usual laboratory procedure is to report the WBCs in order of maturity, with the less mature forms on the left side of the written report. Consequently, the existence of many immature cells is termed a *"shift to the left."*

The WBC differential is of considerable significance because it is possible for the total WBC count to remain essentially normal despite a marked change in one type of leukocyte. For example, a patient may have a normal WBC count of 8800/μL, but the differential count may show that the proportion of lymphocytes is reduced to 10%. This is an abnormal finding that warrants further investigation.

When the bone marrow does not produce enough neutrophils, neutropenia occurs. **Neutropenia** is a condition in which the ANC is less than 1000 cells/μL; severe neutropenia is associated with an ANC of less than 500 cells/μL. The ANC is determined by multiplying the total WBC count by the percentage of neutrophils. Neutropenia results from a number of disease processes, such as leukemia, or from bone marrow depression (see Chapter 30), and is associated with a high risk of infection and death from sepsis.

Platelet Count. The platelet count is the number of platelets per microliter of blood. Normal platelet counts are between 150,000 and 400,000/μL. Counts below 100,000/μL signify a condition termed **thrombocytopenia**. Bleeding may occur with thrombocytopenia. Spontaneous hemorrhage is possible once platelet counts fall below 10,000/μL.[2] A more extensive description of clotting studies is presented in Table 29-7.

Thrombocytosis is defined as excessive platelets, a disorder that occurs with inflammation and some malignant disorders (see Chapter 30). The most likely complication related to thrombocytosis is excessive clotting.

Blood Typing and Rh Factor. Blood group antigens (A and B) are found only on RBC membranes and form the basis for the ABO blood typing system. The presence or absence of one or both of the two inherited antigens is the basis for the four blood groups: A, B, AB, and O. Blood group A has A antigens, group B has B antigens, group AB has both antigens, and group O has neither A nor B antigens. Each person has antibodies in the serum termed *anti-A* and *anti-B* that react with A or B antigens. These antibodies are found when the corresponding antigen is absent from the RBC surface. For example, B antibodies are found in the serum of people with blood group A (Table 29-8).

Blood reactions based on ABO incompatibilities result from intravascular hemolysis of the RBCs. RBCs *agglutinate* (or clump) when a serum antibody is present to react with the antigens on the RBC membrane. For example, agglutination would occur in the blood of a person with type A blood when he or she receives blood transfused from a person with B antigens (i.e., type B or AB). The anti-B antibodies in the type A blood would react with the B antigens, thus initiating the process that results in RBC hemolysis. (Blood component compatibilities for transfusions are presented in Table 30-32.)

The *Rh system* is based on a third antigen, D, which is also on the RBC membrane. Rh-positive people have the D antigen, whereas Rh-negative people do not. Rh-positive blood is indicated with a "+" after the ABO group (e.g., AB+). A Coombs test is used to evaluate the person's Rh status (Table 29-9).

As a result of transfusion therapy or during childbirth, an Rh-negative person may be exposed to Rh-positive blood. After exposure during childbirth, the mother forms an antibody, anti-D, which acts against Rh antigens. (Rh-positive people normally have no anti-D.) In subsequent pregnancies the mother's anti-D antibodies can cross the placenta and attack the RBCs of a fetus who is Rh-positive, thus causing hemolysis of the RBCs. A pregnant Rh-negative woman should receive Rho(D) immune globulin (RhoGAM) injections to prevent anti-D antibodies from forming.

TABLE 29-7 Diagnostic Studies

Clotting Studies

Study	Description and Purpose	Reference Intervals
Activated clotting time (ACT)	Evaluation of intrinsic coagulation status. More accurate than aPTT. Used during dialysis, coronary artery bypass procedure, arteriograms	70-120 sec
Activated partial thromboplastin time (aPTT)	Assessment of intrinsic coagulation by measuring factors I, II, V, VIII, IX, X, XI, XII. Longer in patients using heparin	25-35 sec
Antithrombin	Naturally occurring protein synthesized by liver that inhibits coagulation through inactivation of thrombin and other factors. Depleted in DIC and hypercoagulable disorders	21-30 mg/dL (210-300 mg/L) or 80%-120% of standard
Capillary fragility test (tourniquet test, Rumpel-Leede test)	Reflection of capillary integrity when positive or negative pressure is applied to various areas of the body. Positive test indication of thrombocytopenia, toxic vascular reactions	No petechiae or negative
D-dimer	Assay to measure a fragment of fibrin that is formed as a result of fibrin degradation and clot lysis. Used as an adjunctive measure in diagnosis of hypercoagulable conditions (e.g., DIC, pulmonary embolism)	<250 ng/mL (<250 mcg/L)
Fibrin split products (FSPs) or fibrin degradation products (FDPs)	Reflection of degree of fibrinolysis and predisposition to bleed (if present). Screening test for DIC. Elevated levels associated with DIC, advanced malignancy, severe inflammation	<10 mcg/mL (<10 mg/L)
Fibrinogen (Factor I)	Reflection of level of fibrinogen. Increase in fibrinogen possible indication of enhancement of fibrin formation, making patient hypercoagulable. Decrease in fibrinogen indicates that patient possibly predisposed to bleeding.	200-400 mg/dL (2-4 g/L)
International normalized ratio (INR)	Standardized system of reporting PT based on a reference calibration model and calculated by comparing patient's PT with a control value	2-3*
Plasminogen	Assessment of adequacy of plasminogen in patients who have multiple thromboembolic episodes	2.4-4.4 units/mL
Platelet count	Number of circulating platelets	150,000-400,000/μL
Prothrombin time (PT)	Assessment of extrinsic coagulation by measurement of factors I, II, V, VII, X	11-16 sec
Thrombin time	Reflection of adequacy of thrombin. Prolonged thrombin time indicates that coagulation is inadequate secondary to decreased thrombin activity.	17-23 sec

DIC, Disseminated intravascular coagulation.
*Desired therapeutic level with warfarin (Coumadin).

TABLE 29-8 ABO and Rh Blood Groups

	ANTIGENS PRESENT ON RBC		ANTIBODIES POSSIBLY PRESENT IN PLASMA		
Blood Type	**A or B**	**Rh (D)**	**A or B**	**Rh (D)**	**Percent of General Population**
O*	—	—	A, B	Rh†	35
O+	—	Rh	A, B	—	7
A	A	—	B	Rh†	35
A+	A	Rh	B	—	7
B	B	—	A	Rh†	8
B+	B	Rh	A	—	2
AB‡	A, B	—	—	Rh†	4
AB+	A, B	Rh	—	—	2

*Blood type O is considered universal donor.
†Rh (D) antibodies may develop if Rh– person has been exposed to Rh+ blood.
‡Blood type AB is considered universal recipient.

Iron Metabolism. The laboratory tests used to evaluate iron metabolism include serum iron, total iron-binding capacity (TIBC), serum ferritin, and transferrin saturation. Additional tests for nutritional deficiencies leading to defective RBC production may also be done (Table 29-9).

Serum iron is a measurement of the amount of protein-bound iron circulating in the serum. TIBC provides a measurement of all proteins that act to bind or transport iron between the tissues and bone marrow. Although this indirect measurement is a general reflection of the amount of transferrin present in the circulation, it overestimates transferrin levels by 16% to 20% because it also measures other proteins that can bind iron. These alternative proteins bind iron only when transferrin is more than half saturated. Also, TIBC varies inversely with tissue iron stores; it is higher when iron stores are low and lower when iron stores are high.

Transferrin saturation is a better indicator of the availability of iron for erythropoiesis than serum iron because, unlike serum iron, the iron bound to transferrin is readily available for the body to use. Transferrin saturation is calculated by dividing serum iron by TIBC and multiplying by 100. For example, a patient with a serum iron level of 100 mcg/dL and a TIBC of 300 mcg/dL would have a transferrin saturation of about 33%.

TABLE 29-9 Diagnostic Studies

Miscellaneous Blood Studies

Study	Description and Purpose	Normal Values
Bilirubin	Measurement of degree of RBC hemolysis or liver's inability to excrete normal quantities of bilirubin. Increase in indirect bilirubin with hemolytic problems. Increase in direct bilirubin with obstructive problems (e.g., gallstones, liver tumor, etc.)	*Total:* 0.2-1.2 mg/dL (3.0-21.0 μmol/L) *Direct:* 0.1-0.3 mg/dL (1.7-5.1 μmol/L) *Indirect:* 0.1-1.0 mg/dL (1.7-17.0 μmol/L)
Blood smear (peripheral blood smear)	Reviews color, size, shape, quantity of cells in peripheral blood. Can provide significant amount of information regarding disorders affecting RBCs, WBCs, or platelets	Normal quantity of each cell type, normal size, shape and color of RBCs, normal WBC differential count
Coombs test	Differentiation among types of hemolytic anemias. Detection of immune antibodies and Rh factor	Negative
• Direct	Detection of antibodies that are attached to RBCs	Negative
• Indirect	Detection of circulating antibodies against red cells in serum	Negative
Cobalamin (vitamin B_{12})	Level of cobalamin available for production of new RBCs	200-835 pg/mL (148-616 pmol/L)
Erythrocyte sedimentation rate (ESR)	Measurement of sedimentation or settling of RBCs in 1 hr. Inflammatory process causes an alteration in plasma proteins, resulting in aggregation of RBCs and making them heavier. The faster the sedimentation rate, the higher the ESR	<30 mm/hr (some gender variation)
Erythropoietin	Measurement of degree of hormonal stimulation to bone marrow to stimulate the release of RBCs	5-35 mU/mL (5-30 U/L)
Ferritin	Major iron storage protein. Is normally present in blood in concentrations directly related to iron storage	10-250 ng/mL (10-250 mcg/L)
Folic acid (folate)	Amount of folic acid (folate) available for RBC production	3-16 ng/mL (7-36 nmol/L)
Hemoglobin (Hgb) electrophoresis	Proteins involved in development of Hgb molecule have a definitive pattern of separation on electrophoresis. This pattern is altered with abnormal Hgb synthesis (e.g., thalassemia) or sickle cell anemia (where Hgb S is increased).	*Normal Hb A1:* >95% *Hb A2:* 1.5%-3.7% *Hb F:* <2% *Hb S:* 0 *Hb C:* 0
Homocysteine	Amino acid formed from methionine. Rapidly metabolized through pathways that require cobalamin (vitamin B_{12}) and folic acid. Increased in cobalamin and folic acid deficiency	*Male:* 5.2-12.9 μmol/L *Female:* 3.7-10.4 μmol/L
Iron		
• Serum iron	Reflection of amount of iron combined with proteins in serum. Accurate indication of status of iron storage and use	50-175 mcg/dL (9-31.3 μmol/L)
• Total iron-binding capacity (TIBC)	Measurement of all proteins available for binding iron. Transferrin represents the largest quantity of iron-binding proteins. Therefore TIBC is an indirect measure of transferrin, an evaluation of amount of extra iron that can be carried.	250-425 mcg/dL (45-76 μmol/L)
Lactic dehydrogenase (LDH)	Intracellular enzyme that is present in almost all body tissues. Levels rise in response to cell damage. Increased levels confirm diagnosis of injury or disease. May be used as a nonspecific marker of hematologic malignancy growth and response to treatment	140-280 U/L (0.83-2.5 μkat/L)
Methylmalonic acid (MMA)	Indirect test for cobalamin (Vitamin B_{12}). MMA metabolism requires cobalamin. Decreased levels with cobalamin deficiency. Helps differentiate cobalamin deficiency from folic acid deficiency	<0.2 μmol/L (<2.4 mcg/dL)
Microglobulin (Beta$_2$ microglobulin)	Protein that is found on the surface of all cells. It is increased in patients with malignancies such as lymphoma, leukemia, or multiple myeloma and may be used as a tumor marker.	Blood: 0.7-1.8 mcg/mL Urine: ≤300 mcg/L Spinal fluid: ≤2.4 mg/L
Reticulocyte count	Measurement of immature RBCs, a reflection of bone marrow activity in producing RBCs	0.5%-1.5% of RBC count (0.005-0.015 of RBC count)
Serum protein electrophoresis (SPEP)	Separates proteins in blood on basis of electric charge. Helps detect hyperglobulinemic states, such as in multiple myeloma or some lymphomas	Normal banding pattern of albumin and globulins. Increase in any protein *(protein spike)* is abnormal.
Transferrin	Largest of proteins that bind to iron. Increased in most people with iron-deficiency anemia	190-380 mg/dL (1.9-3.8 g/L)
Transferrin saturation (%)	Decreased in iron-deficiency anemia and increased in hemolytic and megaloblastic anemia	15%-50%

Under normal conditions, the serum ferritin concentration correlates closely with body iron stores. In normal patients, 1 ng/mL of ferritin corresponds to 8 to 10 mg of stored iron.

Biopsies

Biopsy procedures specific to hematologic assessment are bone marrow examination and lymph node biopsy. In general, these procedures are done because a peripheral blood smear is nonspecific and usually a diagnosis cannot be established from a peripheral blood smear. Furthermore, a biopsy provides additional information about a hematologic problem that is needed for diagnosis and treatment planning.

Bone Marrow Examination. Bone marrow examination is important in the evaluation of many hematologic disorders.

TABLE 29-10 Diagnostic Studies

Hematologic System

Study	Description and Purpose	Nursing Responsibility
Blood Studies	See Tables 29-6, 29-7, and 29-9.	
Urine Studies		
Bence Jones protein	An electrophoretic measurement is used to detect Bence Jones protein, which is found in most cases of multiple myeloma. Negative finding is considered normal.	*During:* Acquire random urine specimen early in the morning. If a 24-hr urine collection is ordered, discard first specimen and collect all urine voided during the 24 hr, keeping on ice or refrigerated. Remind patient not to put toilet paper in urine collection container.
Radioisotope Studies		
Bone scan	Same procedure as for spleen scan except used for evaluating structure of bones	*During:* Patient needs to lie still during imaging. Patient may be asked to drink 4-6 glasses of water and then void before imaging (to see pelvic bones).
SPECT scan (single-photon emission computed tomography)	Radioactive isotope is injected IV. Images from radioactive emissions are used to evaluate the structures such as spleen, liver, and bone and possible tumors. Patient is not a source of radioactivity.	No specific nursing responsibilities.
Radiologic Studies		
Skeletal x-ray	X-rays done as a bone survey to detect lytic lesions associated with multiple myeloma. Bone scans do not identify lesions in this condition because there is no uptake of radioactive isotopes due to lack of blood supply.	No specific nursing responsibilities.
Liver, spleen, or abdominal ultrasound	Noninvasive probe is lubricated and slid across the abdomen to detect density and borders of the abdominal organs. Can detect irregular borders, masses, vascular structure, fluid collections, and biliary tree	*During:* Patients must be comfortable lying flat and having probe compress abdomen.
Positron emission tomography (PET)	Nuclear tracer substance is injected and is taken up by metabolically active cells. Follow-up scan shows different-colored tissues based on metabolic rate. "Hot spots" reflect increased glucose consumption indicating presence of tumor. Valuable diagnostic tool to detect active malignancy because it highlights areas with increased metabolism. CT scanning may also be done in conjunction or images fused.	*Before:* IV access is required for injection of the tracer substance. Patients should be NPO, except for water and medications, for at least 4 hr before the test. IV solutions containing glucose should be held or changed to normal saline. Patients who are glucose intolerant or diabetic may need adjustments in their medications. Bowel preparation may also be needed, depending on area being studied.
Computed tomography (CT) scan	Noninvasive radiologic examination using computer-assisted x-ray evaluates the lymph nodes. Contrast medium often is used in abdominal studies of liver or spleen. Spiral (helical) CT scans are used to evaluate lymph nodes.	*Before:* Investigate iodine sensitivity if contrast medium used. IV and/or oral contrast may be given prior to procedure, depending on the area being studied. Patient may need to be NPO 4 hr prior to study. *After:* Encourage patient to drink fluids to avoid renal problems with contrast, if ordered.
Magnetic resonance imaging (MRI)	Noninvasive procedure produces sensitive images of soft tissue without using contrast media. No ionizing radiation is required. Technique is used to evaluate central nervous system, neck and back, bones and joints, heart, breasts. Provides a better contrast between normal tissue and pathologic tissue than CT.	*Before:* Instruct patient to remove all metal objects and ask about any history of surgical insertion of staples, plates, or other metal appliances. Inform patient of need to lie still in small chamber.
Biopsies/Procedures		
Bone marrow (Fig. 29-7)	Technique involves removal of bone marrow through a locally anesthetized site to evaluate status of blood-forming tissue. Used to diagnose and monitor multiple myeloma, myelodysplastic syndromes, leukemia, and some lymphomas and to stage some solid tumors (e.g., breast cancer).	*Before:* Explain procedure to patient. Obtain signed consent form. Ensure that a *time-out** is done before procedure. Analgesic administration may be done to enhance patient comfort and cooperation. *After:* Apply pressure dressing after procedure. Assess biopsy site for bleeding and apply pressure as needed.
Lumbar puncture (LP)	Purpose is to obtain cerebrospinal fluid for testing for malignancy or infection. It may also be used to administer chemotherapy to central nervous system.	*During:* Assist in positioning patient and provide support. *After:* Observe site for bleeding and signs of infection. Spinal headaches may occur but are not minimized by patient lying flat afterwards.
Lymph node biopsy	Purpose is to obtain lymph tissue for histologic examination to determine diagnosis and therapy.	*Before:* Explain procedure to patient. Obtain signed consent form.
• Open	Performed in operating room or procedure area using either local or general anesthesia. An incision is made, and the lymph node and surrounding tissue are dissected (excised) whenever possible.	*After:* Observe site for bleeding and monitor vital signs, especially if platelet count is low. Sterile dressing should be changed as ordered, and wound should be inspected for healing and infection.
• Closed (needle) or fine needle	Performed by a physician at bedside or in an outpatient area. An extremely small needle is used to reduce risk of tracking malignant cells through normal subcutaneous tissue.	
Molecular, Cytogenetic, and Gene Analysis Studies		
Fluorescence in situ hybridization (FISH) **Comparative genomic hybridization (CGH)** **Spectral karyotyping (SKY)**	Tests are performed on malignant cells, either peripheral blood (e.g., leukemia) or biopsy specimen (bone marrow, lymph node), or cerebrospinal fluid. Used to assess genetic or chromosomal abnormalities of cancer cells. May be useful in confirming diagnosis and determining treatment modalities and prognosis	*Before:* Explain purpose of testing to patient.

*Time-out is done just before the procedure starts to verify patient identification, surgical procedure, and surgical site.

The examination of the marrow may involve aspiration only or aspiration with biopsy. The benefits gained from bone marrow examination are (1) a full evaluation of hematopoiesis and (2) the ability to obtain specimens for cytopathologic and chromosomal abnormalities. The preferred site for both aspiration and biopsy of bone marrow is the posterior iliac crest. Bone marrow aspiration and biopsy are performed by a physician or specially credentialed nurse. Local anesthesia and sedation may be used to minimize anxiety and pain that the patient may experience.

For bone marrow aspiration, the skin over the puncture site is cleansed with a bactericidal agent. The skin, subcutaneous tissue, and periosteum are infiltrated with a local anesthetic agent. The patient may be uncomfortable when the periosteum is penetrated. Once the area is anesthetized, a bone marrow needle is inserted through the cortex of the bone. The stylet of the needle is then removed, the hub is attached to a 10-mL syringe, and 0.2 to 0.5 mL of the fluid marrow is aspirated (Fig. 29-7). The patient experiences pain with aspiration. Although it lasts only a few seconds, the pain may be quite uncomfortable. After the marrow aspiration, the needle is removed. Pressure is applied over the aspiration site to ensure hemostasis.

Although complications of bone marrow aspiration are minimal, there is a possibility of damaging underlying structures. Other complications include hemorrhage (especially if the patient is thrombocytopenic) and infection (especially if the patient is leukopenic).

The needle aspiration or biopsy site is covered with a sterile pressure dressing. Monitor the patient's vital signs until stable, and assess the site for excess drainage or bleeding. If bleeding is present, advise the patient to lie on the side for 30 to 60 minutes to maintain pressure on the site. If the bed is too soft, have the patient lie on a rolled towel to provide additional pressure.

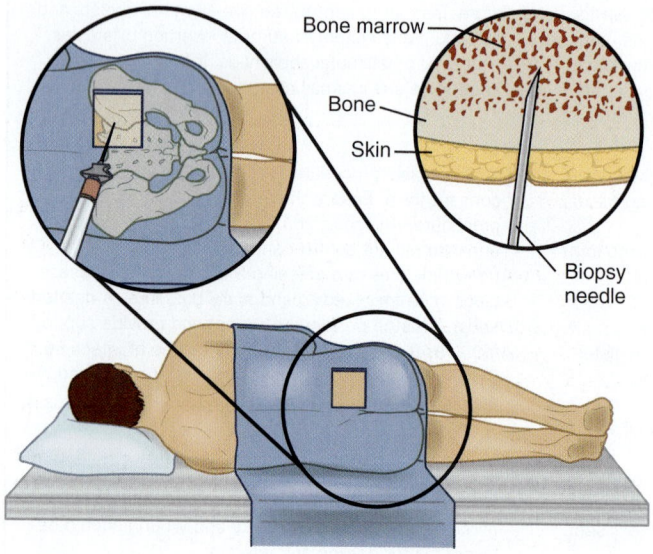

FIG. 29-7 Bone marrow aspiration from the posterior iliac crest.

Analgesics for postprocedure pain may be administered. Soreness over the puncture site for 3 to 4 days after the procedure is normal.

Lymph Node Biopsy. Lymph node biopsy involves obtaining lymph tissue for histologic examination to determine the diagnosis and help plan therapy. This may be accomplished by either an open biopsy or a closed (needle) biopsy.

If the results from a needle biopsy are negative, it may only indicate that the cancer cells were not part of the tissue in the biopsy specimen. However, a positive finding is sufficient evidence for confirming a diagnosis. This technique is rarely used to confirm an initial diagnosis because larger specimens are usually required to perform cytopathologic tests, but it may be used to validate disease recurrence or a new site of disease.

Molecular Cytogenetics and Gene Analysis

Testing for specific genetic or chromosomal variations in hematologic conditions is often helpful in diagnosis and staging. These results also help determine the treatment options and prognosis. If a large number of abnormal cells are circulating in the blood, such as in acute leukemia, these tests may be done by obtaining peripheral blood. However, testing is usually done on samples from bone marrow, lymph node biopsies, and sometimes cerebrospinal fluid. For example, fluorescence in situ hybridization (FISH) can identify specific areas by attaching a probe to a targeted region of deoxyribonucleic acid (DNA). It may be used to illuminate an abnormal extra chromosome 8, which is common in certain leukemias. Spectral karyotyping (SKY) allows each set of chromosomes to be painted different colors. It can be used to identify the translocation of chromosome 22 to 9 in the Philadelphia chromosome of chronic myelogenous leukemia. More information on genetics is in Chapter 12.

CASE STUDY

Objective Data: Diagnostic Studies

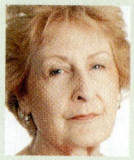

(©Lisa F. Young/iStock)

The HCP orders the following initial diagnostic studies for A.J.:

- CBC, basic metabolic panel (electrolytes, BUN, creatinine), PT/PTT
- Arterial blood gases
- Chest x-ray

A.J.'s CBC reveals a Hgb of 5.9 g/dL, Hct of 18.2%, WBC of 2600/μL (2.6×10^9/L), platelet count of 72,000/μL, PT = 18 sec, aPTT = 37. The arterial blood gases are normal as well as the chest x-ray. The HCP orders more blood work, including a WBC differential, RBC indices, and admits her to the hospital for further evaluation.

Discussion Questions

1. Are these the diagnostic studies that you expected to be ordered?
2. Which diagnostic study results are abnormal?
3. Which diagnostic study results are of most concern to you? What additional studies may be ordered on admission?

This case study is continued in Chapter 30 on p. 652.

Answers available at *http://evolve.elsevier.com/Lewis/medsurg.*

BRIDGE TO NCLEX EXAMINATION

The number of the question corresponds to the same-numbered outcome at the beginning of the chapter.

1. An individual who lives at a high altitude may normally have an increased Hgb and RBC count because
   a. high altitudes cause vascular fluid loss, leading to hemoconcentration.
   b. hypoxia caused by decreased atmospheric O_2 stimulates erythropoiesis.
   c. the function of the spleen in removing old RBCs is impaired at high altitudes.
   d. impaired production of leukocytes and platelets leads to proportionally higher red cell counts.
2. Malignant disorders that arise from granulocytic cells in the bone marrow will have the primary effect of causing
   a. risk for hemorrhage.
   b. altered oxygenation.
   c. decreased production of antibodies.
   d. decreased phagocytosis of bacteria.
3. An anticoagulant such as warfarin (Coumadin) that interferes with prothrombin production will alter the clotting mechanism during
   a. platelet aggregation.
   b. activation of thrombin.
   c. the release of tissue thromboplastin.
   d. stimulation of factor activation complex.
4. When reviewing laboratory results of an older patient with an infection, the nurse would expect to find
   a. minimal leukocytosis.
   b. decreased platelet count.
   c. increased hemoglobin and hematocrit levels.
   d. decreased erythrocyte sedimentation rate (ESR).
5. Significant information obtained from the patient's health history that relates to the hematologic system includes
   a. jaundice.
   b. bladder surgery.
   c. early menopause.
   d. multiple pregnancies.
6. While assessing the lymph nodes, the nurse should
   a. apply gentle, firm pressure to deep lymph nodes.
   b. palpate the deep cervical and supraclavicular nodes last.
   c. lightly palpate superficial lymph nodes with the pads of the fingers.
   d. use the tips of the second, third, and fourth fingers to apply deep palpation.
7. If a lymph node is palpated, what is a normal finding?
   a. Hard, fixed nodes
   b. Firm, mobile nodes
   c. Enlarged, tender nodes
   d. Hard, nontender nodes
8. Nursing care for a patient immediately after a bone marrow biopsy and aspiration includes *(select all that apply)*
   a. administering analgesics as necessary.
   b. preparing to administer a blood transfusion.
   c. instructing on need to lie still with a sterile pressure dressing intact.
   d. monitoring vital signs and assessing the site for excess drainage or bleeding.
   e. instructing on the need for preprocedure and postprocedure antibiotic medications.
9. You are taking care of a male patient who has the following laboratory values from his CBC: WBC $6.5 \times 10^3/\mu L$, Hgb 13.4 g/dL, Hct 40%, platelets $50 \times 10^3/\mu L$. What are you *most* concerned about?
   a. Your patient is neutropenic.
   b. Your patient has an infection.
   c. Your patient is at risk for bleeding.
   d. Your patient is at fall risk due to his anemia.

1. b, 2. d, 3. b, 4. a, 5. a, 6. c, 7. b, 8. a, c, d, 9. c

For rationales to these answers and even more NCLEX review questions, visit *http://evolve.elsevier.com/Lewis/medsurg.*

EVOLVE WEBSITE

http://evolve.elsevier.com/Lewis/medsurg

Review Questions (Online Only)

Key Points

Answer Keys for Questions

- Rationales for Bridge to NCLEX Examination Questions
- Answer Guidelines for Case Studies on pp. 593, 596, 599, and 604

Conceptual Care Map Creator

Audio Glossary

Content Updates

REFERENCES

1. McCance KL, Huether SE: *Pathophysiology: the biologic basis for disease in adults and children*, ed 6, St Louis, 2014, Mosby.
2. Hoffman R, Benz EJ, Silberstein LE, et al: *Hematology: basic principles and practice*, ed 6, Philadelphia, 2013, Elsevier.
3. Ball JW, Dains JE, Flynn JA, et al: *Seidel's physical examination handbook*, ed 8, St Louis, 2014, Mosby.
4. Pagana KD, Pagana TJ: *Mosby's manual of diagnostic and laboratory tests*, ed 5, St Louis, 2014, Mosby.
5. Rosenzweig MQ, Gardner D, Griffith B: The history and physical in cancer care: a primer for the oncology advanced practitioner, *J Adv Pract Onc* 5:262, 2014.
6. Rodgers GP, Young NS: *The Bethesda handbook of clinical hematology*, ed 3, Philadelphia, 2013, Lippincott Williams & Wilkins.
7. Micromedex 2.0. Truven Health Analytics, Inc. Retrieved from *www.microedexsolutions.com.*
8. American Dietetic Association: Food and Nutrition Topics. Retrieved from *www.eatright.org.*

30

Hematologic Problems

Sandra Irene Rome

We must let go of the life we have planned, so as to accept the one that is waiting for us.

Joseph Campbell

http://evolve.elsevier.com/Lewis/medsurg/

LEARNING OUTCOMES

1. Describe the general clinical manifestations and complications of anemia.
2. Differentiate the etiologies, clinical manifestations, diagnostic findings, and nursing and interprofessional management of iron-deficiency, megaloblastic, and aplastic anemias and anemia of chronic disease.
3. Explain the nursing management of anemia secondary to blood loss.
4. Describe the pathophysiology, clinical manifestations, and nursing and interprofessional management of anemia caused by increased erythrocyte destruction, including sickle cell disease and acquired hemolytic anemias.
5. Describe the pathophysiology and nursing and interprofessional management of polycythemia.
6. Explain the pathophysiology, clinical manifestations, and nursing and interprofessional management of various types of thrombocytopenia.
7. Describe the types, clinical manifestations, diagnostic findings, and nursing and interprofessional management of hemophilia and von Willebrand disease.
8. Explain the pathophysiology, diagnostic findings, and nursing and interprofessional management of disseminated intravascular coagulation.
9. Describe the etiology, clinical manifestations, and nursing and interprofessional management of neutropenia.
10. Describe the pathophysiology, clinical manifestations, and nursing and interprofessional management of myelodysplastic syndrome.
11. Compare and contrast the major types of leukemia regarding distinguishing clinical and laboratory findings.
12. Explain the nursing and interprofessional management of acute and chronic leukemias.
13. Compare Hodgkin's lymphoma and non-Hodgkin's lymphomas in terms of clinical manifestations, staging, and nursing and interprofessional management.
14. Describe the pathophysiology, clinical manifestations, and nursing and interprofessional management of multiple myeloma.
15. Describe the spleen disorders and related interprofessional care.
16. Describe the nursing management of the patient receiving transfusions of blood and blood components.

KEY TERMS

anemia, p. 606
aplastic anemia, p. 614
disseminated intravascular coagulation (DIC), p. 629
hemochromatosis, p. 619
hemolytic anemia, p. 615
hemophilia, p. 626
Hodgkin's lymphoma, p. 640
iron-deficiency anemia, p. 609
leukemia, p. 635
lymphomas, p. 640
megaloblastic anemias, p. 612
multiple myeloma, p. 645
myelodysplastic syndrome (MDS), p. 634
neutropenia, p. 632
non-Hodgkin's lymphomas (NHLs), p. 642
pernicious anemia, p. 612
polycythemia, p. 620
sickle cell disease (SCD), p. 616
thalassemia, p. 611
thrombocytopenia, p. 622

ANEMIA

Definition and Classification

Anemia is a deficiency in the number of erythrocytes (red blood cells [RBCs]), the quantity or quality of hemoglobin, and/or volume of packed RBCs (hematocrit). It is a prevalent condition with many diverse causes, such as blood loss, impaired production of erythrocytes, or increased destruction of erythrocytes (Fig. 30-1). Because RBCs transport O_2, erythrocyte disorders can lead to tissue hypoxia. This hypoxia accounts for many of the signs and symptoms of anemia. Anemia is not a specific disease. It is a manifestation of a pathologic process.

Anemia is diagnosed based on a complete blood count (CBC), reticulocyte count, and peripheral blood smear. Once anemia is identified, further investigation is done to determine its specific cause.[1]

Anemia can result from primary hematologic problems or can develop as a secondary consequence of diseases or disorders of other body systems. The various types of anemia can be classified according to either *morphology* (cellular characteristic) or *etiology* (cause). Morphologic classification is based on RBC size and color (Table 30-1). Etiologic classification is related to the clinical conditions causing the anemia[2] (Table 30-2). Although the morphologic system is the most accurate means of classifying anemias, it is easier to discuss patient care by focusing on the etiology of the anemia.

Reviewed by Judy Carlyle, RN, MNSc, Faculty/Clinical Liaison, Arkansas Rural Nursing Education Consortium (ARNEC), Nashville, Arkansas; and Allison J. Terry, RN, PhD, Associate Professor of Nursing, Assistant Dean of Clinical Practice, School of Nursing, Auburn University Montgomery, Montgomery, Alabama.

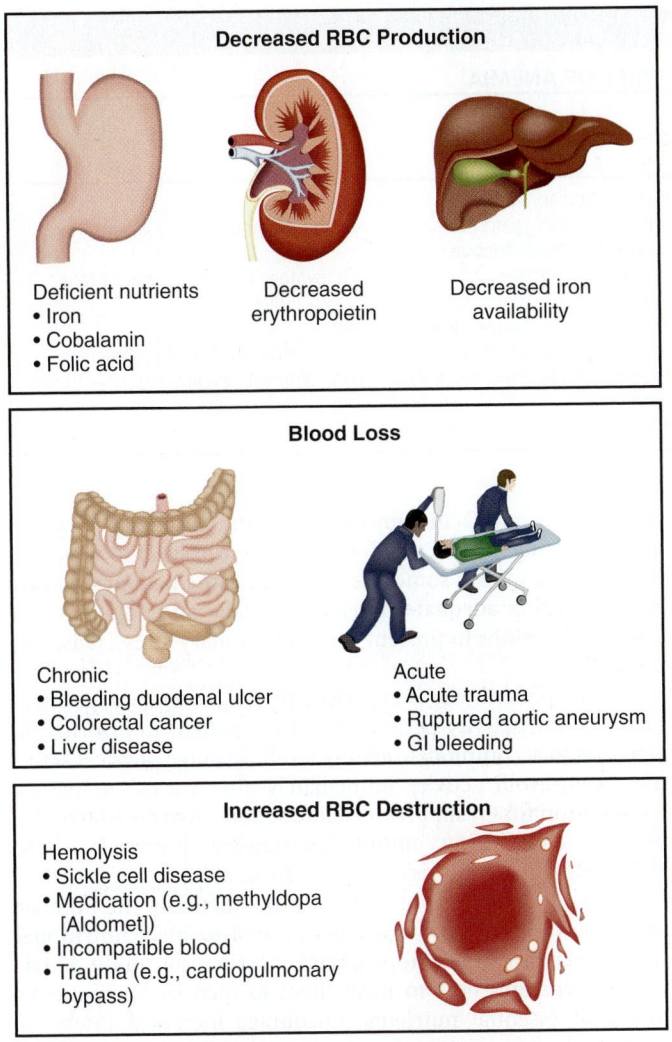

FIG. 30-1 Causes of anemia.

CULTURAL & ETHNIC HEALTH DISPARITIES

Hematologic Problems

- Sickle cell disease has a high incidence among African Americans.
- Thalassemia has a high incidence among African Americans and people of Mediterranean origin.
- Tay-Sachs disease has the highest incidence in families of Eastern European Jewish origin, especially the Ashkenazi Jews.
- Pernicious anemia has a high incidence among Scandinavians and African Americans.

Clinical Manifestations

The clinical manifestations of anemia are caused by the body's response to tissue hypoxia. Specific manifestations vary depending on the rate at which the anemia has evolved, its severity, and any coexisting disease. Hemoglobin (Hgb) levels are often used to determine the severity of anemia.

Mild states of anemia (Hgb 10 to 12 g/dL [100 to 120 g/L]) may exist without causing symptoms. If symptoms develop, it is because the patient has an underlying disease or is experiencing a compensatory response to heavy exercise. Symptoms include palpitations, dyspnea, and mild fatigue.

In moderate anemia (Hgb 6 to 10 g/dL [60 to 100 g/L]) the above cardiopulmonary symptoms are increased. The patient may experience them while resting, as well as with activity.

TABLE 30-1 Morphologic Classification of Anemia

Morphology	Etiology
Normocytic, normochromic (normal size and color) MCV 80-100 fL, MCH 27-34 pg	Acute blood loss, hemolysis, chronic kidney disease, chronic disease, cancers, sideroblastic anemia, endocrine disorders, starvation, aplastic anemia, sickle cell anemia, pregnancy
Microcytic, hypochromic (small size, pale color) MCV <80 fL, MCH <27 pg	Iron-deficiency anemia, vitamin B_6 deficiency, copper deficiency, thalassemia, lead poisoning
Macrocytic (megaloblastic), normochromic (large size, normal color) MCV >100 fL, MCH >34 pg	Cobalamin (vitamin B_{12}) deficiency, folic acid deficiency, liver disease (including effects of alcohol abuse)

MCH, Mean corpuscular hemoglobin; *MCV,* mean corpuscular volume.

TABLE 30-2 Etiologic Classification of Anemia

Decreased RBC Production

Decreased Hemoglobin Synthesis
- Iron deficiency
- Thalassemias (decreased globin synthesis)
- Sideroblastic anemia (decreased porphyrin)

Defective DNA Synthesis
- Cobalamin (vitamin B_{12}) deficiency
- Folic acid deficiency

Decreased Number of RBC Precursors
- Aplastic anemia and inherited disorders (e.g., Fanconi syndrome)
- Anemia of myeloproliferative diseases (e.g., leukemia) and myelodysplasia
- Chronic diseases or disorders
- Medications and chemicals (e.g., chemotherapy, lead)
- Radiation

Blood Loss

Acute
- Trauma
- Blood vessel rupture
- Splenic sequestration crisis

Chronic
- Gastritis
- Menstrual flow
- Hemorrhoids

Increased RBC Destruction (Hemolytic Anemias)

Hereditary (Intrinsic)
- Abnormal hemoglobin (sickle cell disease)
- Enzyme deficiency (G6PD)
- Membrane abnormalities (paroxysmal nocturnal hemoglobinuria, hereditary spherocytosis)

Acquired (Extrinsic)
- Physical destruction
  - Prosthetic heart valves
  - Extracorporeal circulation
  - Disseminated intravascular coagulopathy (DIC)
  - Thrombotic thrombocytopenic purpura (TTP)
- Antibodies against RBCs
- Infectious agents (e.g., malaria) and toxins

G6PD, Glucose-6-phosphate dehydrogenase.

In severe anemia (Hgb less than 6 g/dL [60 g/L]) the patient has many clinical manifestations involving multiple body systems (Table 30-3).

Integumentary Manifestations. Integumentary manifestations include pallor, jaundice, and pruritus. Pallor results from reduced amounts of hemoglobin and reduced blood flow to the skin. Jaundice occurs when hemolysis of RBCs results in an increased concentration of serum bilirubin. Pruritus occurs because of increased serum and skin bile salt concentrations. In addition to the skin, the sclera of the eyes and mucous

TABLE 30-3 Manifestations of Anemia

Body System	SEVERITY OF ANEMIA: Mild (Hgb 10-12 g/dL [100-120 g/L])	Moderate (Hgb 6-10 g/dL [60-100 g/L])	Severe (Hgb <6 g/dL [<60 g/L])
Integument	None	None	Pallor, jaundice,* pruritus*
Eyes	None	None	Icteric conjunctiva and sclera,* retinal hemorrhage, blurred vision
Mouth	None	None	Glossitis, smooth tongue
Cardiovascular	Palpitations	Increased palpitations, "bounding pulse"	Tachycardia, increased pulse pressure, systolic murmurs, intermittent claudication, angina, heart failure, myocardial infarction
Pulmonary	Exertional dyspnea	Dyspnea	Tachypnea, orthopnea, dyspnea at rest
Neurologic	None	"Roaring in the ears"	Headache, vertigo, irritability, depression, impaired thought processes
Gastrointestinal	None	None	Anorexia, hepatomegaly, splenomegaly, difficulty swallowing, sore mouth
Musculoskeletal	None	None	Bone pain
General	None or mild fatigue	Fatigue	Sensitivity to cold, weight loss, lethargy

*Caused by hemolysis.

membranes should be evaluated for jaundice because they reflect the integumentary changes more accurately, especially in a dark-skinned individual.

Cardiopulmonary Manifestations. Cardiopulmonary manifestations of severe anemia result from additional attempts by the heart and lungs to provide adequate amounts of O_2 to the tissues. Cardiac output is maintained by increasing the heart rate and stroke volume. The low viscosity of the blood contributes to the development of systolic murmurs and bruits. In extreme cases or when concomitant heart disease is present, angina pectoris and myocardial infarction (MI) may occur if myocardial O_2 needs cannot be met. Heart failure (HF), cardiomegaly, pulmonary and systemic congestion, ascites, and peripheral edema may develop if the heart is overworked for an extended period.

❖ NURSING AND INTERPROFESSIONAL MANAGEMENT: ANEMIA

This section discusses general management of anemia. Specific care related to various types of anemia is discussed later in this chapter.

◆ Nursing Assessment

Subjective and objective data that should be obtained from a patient with anemia are presented in Table 30-4.

◆ Nursing Diagnoses

Nursing diagnoses for the patient with anemia include, but are not limited to, the following:

- Fatigue *related to* inadequate oxygenation of the blood
- Imbalanced nutrition: less than body requirements *related to* inadequate nutritional intake and anorexia
- Ineffective health management *related to* lack of knowledge about appropriate nutrition and medication regimen

Additional information on nursing diagnoses are presented in eNursing Care Plan 30-1.

◆ Planning

The overall goals are that the patient with anemia will (1) assume normal activities of daily living, (2) maintain adequate nutrition, and (3) develop no complications related to anemia.

◆ Nursing Implementation

Correcting the cause of the anemia is ultimately the goal of therapy. Acute interventions may include blood transfusions, drug therapy (e.g., erythropoietin, vitamin supplements), RBC replacement, and O_2 therapy to stabilize the patient. Dietary and lifestyle changes (described in sections on specific types of anemia) can reverse some anemias. Assess the patient's knowledge regarding adequate nutritional intake and adherence to safety precautions to prevent cardiopulmonary stress, falls, and injury.

For the patient who is experiencing fatigue, encourage alternate rest and activity periods. Assist the patient in prioritizing activities to accommodate energy levels. Arrange physical activities (e.g., avoid activity immediately after meals) to reduce competition for O_2 supply to vital functions. Assist with regular physical activities (e.g., ambulation, transfers, personal care) to minimize fatigue and risk of injury from falls.

Determine, in collaboration with the dietitian, the number of calories and type of nutrients needed to meet nutritional requirements. Provide appropriate information about nutritional needs and how to meet them to increase the patient's intake of essential nutrients. Encourage increased intake of foods high in iron.

The numerous causes of anemia necessitate different nursing interventions specific to the patient's needs. General nursing interventions for patients with anemia are presented in eNursing Care Plan 30-1 (available on the website for this chapter).

Gerontologic Considerations: Anemia

Modest changes in RBC mass occur in older adults. Healthy older men have a modest decline in hemoglobin of about 1 g/dL between ages 70 and 88 years, in part because of the decreased production of testosterone. Only a minimal decrease in hemoglobin (about 0.2 g/dL) occurs between these ages in healthy women.[1]

Anemia is not a normal finding in older adults. However, the prevalence increases starting from the seventh decade of life. For the majority, anemia is related to an underlying cause such as iron deficiency, bleeding, chronic disease/inflammation, renal insufficiency, or a hematologic cancer. For many patients with anemia, there is no identifiable cause.[3]

Clinical manifestations of anemia in older adults may include pallor, confusion, ataxia, fatigue, and worsening cardiovascular and respiratory problems. Unfortunately, anemia may go unrecognized in older adults because these manifestations may be mistaken for normal aging changes or overlooked because of another health problem. By recognizing signs of anemia, you can play a pivotal role in health assessment and related interventions for older adults.

TABLE 30-4 Nursing Assessment

Anemia

Subjective Data

Important Health Information

Past health history: Recent blood loss or trauma; chronic liver, endocrine, or renal disease (including dialysis); GI disease (malabsorption syndrome, ulcers, gastritis, or hemorrhoids); inflammatory disorders (especially Crohn's disease); smoking, exposure to radiation or chemical toxins (arsenic, lead, benzenes, copper); infectious diseases (HIV) or recent travel with possible exposure to infection; angina, myocardial infarction; history of falling

Medications: Use of vitamin and iron supplements; aspirin, anticoagulants, oral contraceptives, phenobarbital, penicillins, nonsteroidal antiinflammatory drugs, omeprazole, phenacetin, phenytoin (Dilantin), sulfonamides, herbal products

Surgery or other treatments: Recent surgery, small bowel resection, gastrectomy, prosthetic heart valves, chemotherapy, radiation therapy

Dietary history: General dietary patterns, consumption of alcohol

Functional Health Patterns

Health perception–health management: Family history of anemia; malaise

Nutritional-metabolic: Nausea, vomiting, anorexia, weight loss; dysphagia, dyspepsia, heartburn; night sweats, cold intolerance

Elimination: Hematuria, decreased urine output; diarrhea, constipation, flatulence, tarry stools, bloody stools

Activity-exercise: Fatigue, muscle weakness and decreased strength; dyspnea, orthopnea, cough, hemoptysis; palpitations; shortness of breath with activity

Cognitive-perceptual: Headache; abdominal, chest, and bone pain; painful tongue; paresthesias of feet and hands; pruritus; disturbances in vision, taste, or hearing; vertigo; hypersensitivity to cold; dizziness

Sexuality-reproductive: Menorrhagia, metrorrhagia; recent or current pregnancy; male impotence

Objective Data

General

Lethargy, apathy, general lymphadenopathy, fever

Integumentary

Pale skin and mucous membranes; blue, pale white, or icteric sclera; cheilitis (inflammation of the lips); poor skin turgor; brittle, spoon-shaped fingernails; jaundice; petechiae; ecchymoses; nose or gingival bleeding; poor healing; dry, brittle, thinning hair

Respiratory

Tachypnea

Cardiovascular

Tachycardia, systolic murmur, dysrhythmias; postural hypotension, widened pulse pressure, bruits (especially carotid); intermittent claudication, ankle edema

Gastrointestinal

Hepatosplenomegaly; glossitis; beefy, red tongue; stomatitis; abdominal distention; anorexia

Neurologic

Headache, roaring in the ears, confusion, impaired judgment, irritability, ataxia, unsteady gait, paralysis, loss of vibration sense

Possible Diagnostic Findings

↓ RBCs, ↓ Hgb; ↓ Hct; ↑ or ↓ reticulocytes, ↑ or ↓ MCV; possible ↓ serum iron, ferritin, folate, or cobalamin (vitamin B_{12}); heme (guaiac)–positive stools; ↓ serum erythropoietin level; ↑ or ↓ LDH, bilirubin, transferrin (Table 30-6)

LDH, Lactate dehydrogenase; *MCV,* mean corpuscular volume.

ANEMIA CAUSED BY DECREASED ERYTHROCYTE PRODUCTION

Normally RBC production (termed *erythropoiesis*) is in equilibrium with RBC destruction and loss. This balance ensures that an adequate number of erythrocytes is available at all times. The normal life span of an RBC is 120 days. Three alterations in erythropoiesis may occur that decrease RBC production: (1) decreased hemoglobin synthesis may lead to iron-deficiency anemia, thalassemia, and sideroblastic anemia; (2) defective deoxyribonucleic acid (DNA) synthesis in RBCs (e.g., cobalamin deficiency, folic acid deficiency) may lead to megaloblastic anemias; and (3) diminished availability of erythrocyte precursors may result in aplastic anemia and anemia of chronic disease (Table 30-2).

IRON-DEFICIENCY ANEMIA

Iron-deficiency anemia is the most common nutritional disorder in the world. Those most susceptible to iron-deficiency anemia are the very young, those on poor diets, and women in their reproductive years.[4] Normally 1 mg of iron is lost daily in urine, bile, sweat, sloughing of epithelial cells from the skin and intestinal mucosa, and minor bleeding.[5]

Etiology

Iron-deficiency anemia may develop as a result of inadequate dietary intake, malabsorption, blood loss, or hemolysis. (Normal iron metabolism is discussed in Chapter 29 on pp. 590-592.) Normal dietary iron intake is usually sufficient to meet the needs of men and older women, but it may be inadequate for individuals with higher iron needs (e.g., menstruating or pregnant women). Table 30-5 lists nutrients needed for erythropoiesis.[6,7]

Malabsorption of iron may occur after certain types of gastrointestinal (GI) surgery and in malabsorption syndromes. Surgical procedures may involve removal or bypass of the duodenum. As iron absorption occurs in the duodenum, malabsorption syndromes may involve disease of the duodenum in which the absorption surface is altered or destroyed.

Blood loss is a major cause of iron deficiency in adults. Two milliliters of whole blood contain 1 mg of iron. The major sources of chronic blood loss are from the GI and genitourinary (GU) systems. GI bleeding is often not apparent and therefore may exist for a considerable time before the problem is identified. Loss of 50 to 75 mL of blood from the upper GI tract is required for stools to appear black *(melena).* The black color results from the iron in the RBCs.

Common causes of GI blood loss are peptic ulcer, gastritis, esophagitis, diverticula, hemorrhoids, and neoplasia. GU blood loss occurs primarily from menstrual bleeding. The average monthly menstrual blood loss is about 45 mL and causes the loss of about 22 mg of iron. Postmenopausal bleeding can contribute to anemia in a susceptible older woman. In addition to anemia of chronic kidney disease, dialysis treatment may cause iron-deficiency anemia because of the blood lost in the dialysis equipment and frequent blood sampling.

TABLE 30-5 Nutritional Therapy

Nutrients for Erythropoiesis

Role in Erythropoiesis	Food Sources
Cobalamin (Vitamin B_{12})	
RBC maturation	Red meats, especially liver, eggs, enriched grain products, milk and dairy foods, fish
Copper	
Mobilization of iron from tissues to plasma*	Shellfish, whole grains, beans, nuts, potatoes, organ meats
Folic Acid	
RBC maturation	Green leafy vegetables, liver, meat, fish, legumes, whole grains, orange juice, peanuts, avocado
Iron	
Hemoglobin synthesis	Liver and muscle meats, dried fruits, legumes, dark green leafy vegetables, whole-grain and enriched bread and cereals, beans
Niacin	
RBC maturation	Peanut butter, beans, meats, avocado; enriched and fortified grains
Pantothenic Acid (Vitamin B_5)	
Heme synthesis	Meats, vegetables, cereal grains, legumes, eggs, milk
Pyridoxine (Vitamin B_6)	
Heme synthesis	Meats, fortified cereals, whole grains, legumes, potatoes, cornmeal, bananas, nuts
Riboflavin (Vitamin B_2)	
Oxidative reactions	Milk and dairy foods, enriched bread and other grain products, salmon, chicken, eggs, green leafy vegetables
Vitamin E	
Heme synthesis. Protection against oxidative damage to RBCs	Vegetable oils, meat, eggs, wheat germ, whole-grain products, seeds, nuts, peanut butter
Amino Acids	
Heme and plasma membrane synthesis	Eggs, meat, milk and milk products (cheese, ice cream), poultry, fish, legumes, nuts, tofu
Ascorbic Acid (Vitamin C)	
Conversion of folic acid to its active forms, aids in iron absorption	Citrus fruits, green leafy vegetables, strawberries, potatoes, kiwi fruit

*Supplementation rarely needed and large amounts of copper are poisonous.

Clinical Manifestations

In the early course of iron-deficiency anemia, the patient may not have any symptoms. As the disease becomes chronic, any of the general manifestations of anemia may develop (Table 30-3). In addition, specific clinical manifestations may occur related to iron-deficiency anemia. Pallor is the most common finding, and *glossitis* (inflammation of the tongue) is the second most common. Another finding is *cheilitis* (inflammation of the lips). In addition, the patient may report headache, paresthesias, and a burning sensation of the tongue, all of which are caused by lack of iron in the tissues.

Diagnostic Studies

Laboratory abnormalities characteristic of iron-deficiency anemia are presented in Table 30-6. Other diagnostic studies (e.g., stool occult blood test) are done to determine the cause of the iron deficiency. Endoscopy and colonoscopy may be used to detect GI bleeding. A bone marrow biopsy may be done if other tests are inconclusive.

Interprofessional Care

The main goal is to treat the underlying disease that is causing reduced intake (e.g., malnutrition, alcoholism) or absorption of iron. In addition, efforts are directed toward replacing iron (Table 30-7). Teach the patient which foods are good sources of iron (Table 30-5). If nutrition is already adequate, increasing iron intake by dietary means may not be practical. Consequently, oral or occasionally parenteral iron supplements are used. If the iron deficiency is from acute blood loss, the patient may require a transfusion of packed RBCs.

Drug Therapy. Oral iron should be used whenever possible because it is inexpensive and convenient. Many iron preparations are available. When administering iron, consider the following five factors:

1. Iron is absorbed best from the duodenum and proximal jejunum. Therefore enteric-coated or sustained-release capsules, which release iron farther down in the GI tract, are counterproductive and expensive.
2. The daily dose should provide 150 to 200 mg of elemental iron. This can be ingested in three or four daily doses, with each tablet or capsule of the iron preparation containing between 50 and 100 mg of iron (e.g., a 300-mg tablet of ferrous sulfate contains 60 mg of elemental iron).
3. Iron is best absorbed as ferrous sulfate (Fe^{2+}) in an acidic environment. For this reason and to avoid binding the iron with food, iron should be taken about an hour before meals,

TABLE 30-6 Laboratory Results in Anemia

Etiology of Anemia	Hgb/Hct	MCV	Reticulocytes	Serum Iron	TIBC	Transferrin	Ferritin	Bilirubin	Serum B_{12}	Folate
Iron deficiency	↓	↓	N or slight ↓ or ↑	↓	↑	N or ↓	↓	N or ↓	N	N
Thalassemia major	↓	N or ↓	↑	↑	↓	↓	N or ↑	↑	N	↓
Cobalamin deficiency	↓	↑	N or ↓	N or ↑	N	Slight ↑	↑	N or slight ↑	↓	N
Folic acid deficiency	↓	↑	N or ↓	N or ↑	N	Slight ↑	↑	N or slight ↑	N	↓
Aplastic anemia	↓	N or slight ↑	↓	N or ↑	N or ↑	N	N	N	N	N
Chronic disease	↓	N or ↓	N or ↓	N or ↓	↓	N or ↓	N or ↑	N	N	N
Acute blood loss	↓	N or ↓	N or ↑	N	N	N	N	N	N	N
Chronic blood loss	↓	↓	N or ↑	↓	↓	N	N	N or ↓	N	N
Sickle cell anemia	↓	N	↓	N or ↑	N or ↓	N	N	↑	N	↓
Hemolytic anemia	↓	N or ↑	↑	N or ↑	N or ↓	N	N or ↑	↑	N	N

MCV, Mean corpuscular volume; *N,* normal; *TIBC,* total iron-binding capacity.

TABLE 30-7 Interprofessional Care

Iron-Deficiency Anemia

Diagnostic Assessment	Management

• History and physical examination
• Hct and Hgb levels
• RBC count, including morphology
• Reticulocyte count
• Serum iron
• Serum ferritin
• Serum transferrin
• Total iron-binding capacity (TIBC)
• Stool examination for occult blood
	• Identification and treatment of underlying cause
	• Drug therapy
	  • Oral: Ferrous sulfate or ferrous gluconate
	  • IM or IV: Iron dextran, sodium ferrous gluconate, iron sucrose
	• Nutritional therapy (Table 30-5)
	• Transfusion of packed RBCs

when the duodenal mucosa is most acidic. Taking iron with vitamin C (ascorbic acid) or orange juice, which contains ascorbic acid, enhances iron absorption. Gastric side effects, however, may necessitate ingesting iron with meals.

4. Undiluted liquid iron may stain the patient's teeth. Therefore it should be diluted and ingested through a straw.
5. GI side effects of iron administration may occur, including heartburn, constipation, and diarrhea. If side effects develop, the dose and type of iron supplement may be adjusted. For example, many individuals who need supplemental iron cannot tolerate ferrous sulfate because of the effects of the sulfate base. However, ferrous gluconate may be an acceptable substitute. Tell patients that the use of iron preparations will cause their stools to become black because the GI tract excretes excess iron. Constipation is common, and the patient should be started on stool softeners and laxatives, if needed, when started on iron.

DRUG ALERT Iron

- Some preparations of IV iron have a risk of an allergic reaction, and the patient should be monitored accordingly.
- Oral iron should be taken about 1 hr before meals.
- Vitamin C (ascorbic acid) enhances iron absorption.

In some situations it may be necessary to administer iron parenterally. Parenteral use of iron is indicated for malabsorption, intolerance of oral iron, a need for iron beyond oral limits, or poor patient adherence in taking the oral preparations of iron. Parenteral iron can be given IM or IV. An iron-dextran complex (INFeD) contains 50 mg/mL of elemental iron available in 2-mL single-dose vials. Sodium ferrous gluconate and iron sucrose are alternatives and may carry less risk of life-threatening anaphylaxis.[8]

Because IM iron solutions may stain the skin, separate needles should be used for withdrawing the solution and for injecting the medication. Use a Z-track injection technique.

❖ NURSING MANAGEMENT: IRON-DEFICIENCY ANEMIA

Certain groups of individuals are at an increased risk for the development of iron-deficiency anemia. These include premenopausal and pregnant women, persons from low socioeconomic backgrounds, older adults, and individuals experiencing blood loss. Diet teaching, with an emphasis on foods high in iron and ways to maximize absorption, is important for these groups.

Discuss with the patient the need for diagnostic studies to identify the cause. Reassess the hemoglobin and RBC counts to evaluate the response to therapy. Emphasize adherence with dietary and drug therapy. To replenish the body's iron stores, the patient needs to take iron therapy for 2 to 3 months after the hemoglobin level returns to normal. Patients who require lifelong iron supplementation should be monitored for potential liver problems related to the iron storage. (Nursing measures for anemia are presented in eNursing Care Plan 30-1.)

THALASSEMIA

Etiology

Thalassemia is a group of diseases involving inadequate production of normal hemoglobin, and therefore decreased erythrocyte production. Thalassemia is due to an absent or reduced globulin protein. α-Globin chains are absent or reduced in α-thalassemia, and β-globin chains are absent or reduced in β-thalassemia. Hemolysis also occurs in thalassemia, but insufficient production of normal hemoglobin is the predominant problem. Thalassemia is commonly found in members of ethnic groups whose origins are near the Mediterranean Sea and equatorial or near-equatorial regions of Asia, the Middle East, and Africa.

Genetic Link. Thalassemia has an autosomal recessive genetic basis (see Fig. 12-4 and Table 12-2). An individual with thalassemia may have a heterozygous or homozygous form of the disease. A person who is heterozygous has one thalassemic gene and one normal gene and has *thalassemia minor* (or thalassemic trait), which is a mild form of the disease. A homozygous person has two thalassemic genes, causing a severe condition known as *thalassemia major.*[9]

Clinical Manifestations

The patient with thalassemia minor is frequently asymptomatic. The patient has mild to moderate anemia with *microcytosis* (small cells) and *hypochromia* (pale cells).

Thalassemia major is a life-threatening disease in which growth, both physical and mental, is often retarded. The person who has thalassemia major is pale and displays other general symptoms of anemia (Table 30-3). The symptoms develop in childhood by 2 years of age and can cause growth and developmental deficits. Jaundice from the hemolysis of RBCs is prominent. In addition, the person has pronounced splenomegaly, since the spleen continuously tries to remove the damaged red cells. Hepatomegaly and cardiomyopathy may occur from iron deposition.

As the bone marrow responds to the reduced O_2-carrying capacity of the blood, RBC production is stimulated and the marrow becomes packed with immature erythroid precursors that die. This stimulates further erythropoiesis, leading to chronic bone marrow hyperplasia and expansion of the marrow space. This may cause thickening of the cranium and maxillary cavity. Thrombocytosis after spleen dysfunction and/or removal may occur.

Patients with thalassemia may have hepatitis C because of having received blood transfusions before donated blood was screened for hepatitis C virus (screening started in 1992). Hepatitis C may result in cirrhosis and hepatocellular carcinoma.

Cardiac complications from iron overload, pulmonary disease, and hypertension also contribute to early death. Endocrinopathies (hypogonadotrophic hypogonadism) and thrombosis may also be complications of the disease.

Interprofessional Care

The laboratory abnormalities of thalassemia major are summarized in Table 30-6. No specific drug or diet therapies are effective in treating thalassemia. Thalassemia minor requires no treatment because the body adapts to the reduction of normal hemoglobin.

Thalassemia major is managed with blood transfusions or exchange transfusions in conjunction with chelating agents that bind to iron: oral deferasirox (Exjade) or deferiprone (Ferriprox) or IV or subcutaneous deferoxamine (Desferal). These agents reduce the iron overloading (hemochromatosis) that occurs with chronic transfusion therapy.[10] Folic acid is given if there is evidence of hemolysis. Transfusions are administered to keep the hemoglobin level at approximately 10 g/dL (100 g/L) to maintain the patient's own erythropoiesis without causing the spleen to enlarge. Zinc supplementation may be needed since zinc is reduced with chelation therapy. Ascorbic acid supplementation may be needed during chelation therapy, since it increases urine excretion of iron. Other than during chelation therapy, ascorbic acid should not be taken because it increases the absorption of dietary iron. Iron supplements should not be given.

Because RBCs are sequestered in the enlarged spleen, thalassemia major may be treated by splenectomy. Hepatic, cardiac, and pulmonary organ function should be monitored and treated as appropriate.

Although hematopoietic stem cell transplantation (HSCT) remains the only cure for patients with thalassemia, the risk of this procedure may outweigh its benefits. With proper iron chelation therapy, patients are living longer.

MEGALOBLASTIC ANEMIAS

Megaloblastic anemias are a group of disorders caused by impaired DNA synthesis and characterized by the presence of large RBCs. When DNA synthesis is impaired, defective RBC maturation results. The RBCs are large *(macrocytic)* and abnormal and are referred to as *megaloblasts.* Macrocytic RBCs are easily destroyed because they have fragile cell membranes. Although the overwhelming majority of megaloblastic anemias result from cobalamin and folic acid deficiencies, this type of RBC deformity can also occur from suppression of DNA synthesis by drugs, inborn errors of cobalamin and folic acid metabolism, and *erythroleukemia* (malignant blood disorder characterized by a proliferation of erythropoietic cells in bone marrow) (Table 30-8).

TABLE 30-8 Classification of Megaloblastic Anemia

Cobalamin (Vitamin B_{12}) Deficiency
- Dietary deficiency
- Deficiency of gastric intrinsic factor
  - Pernicious anemia
  - Gastrectomy
  - Gastric bypass
  - Celiac disease
  - *Helicobacter pylori*
- Intestinal malabsorption
- Increased requirement (pregnancy)
- Chronic alcoholism

Folic Acid Deficiency
- Dietary deficiency (e.g., leafy green vegetables, citrus fruits)
- Malabsorption syndromes
  - Celiac disease
  - Crohn's disease
  - Small bowel resection
- Drugs interfering with absorption or use of folic acid
  - Methotrexate
  - Antiseizure drugs (e.g., phenobarbital, phenytoin [Dilantin])
- Increased requirement (pregnancy)
- Chronic alcoholism
- Chronic hemodialysis (folic acid lost during dialysis)

Drug-Induced Suppression of DNA Synthesis
- Folate antagonists
- Metabolic inhibitors
- Alkylating agents

Inborn Errors
- Defective folate metabolism
- Defective transport of cobalamin

Erythroleukemia

Megaloblastic Anemia: Cobalamin (Vitamin B_{12}) Deficiency

Normally, a protein termed *intrinsic factor* (IF) is secreted by the parietal cells of the gastric mucosa. IF is required for cobalamin (extrinsic factor) absorption. (Cobalamin is normally absorbed in the distal ileum.) Therefore if IF is not secreted, cobalamin will not be absorbed.

Etiology

Pernicious Anemia. The most common cause of cobalamin deficiency is **pernicious anemia,** which is caused by an absence of IF. In pernicious anemia the gastric mucosa is not secreting IF because of either gastric mucosal atrophy or autoimmune destruction of parietal cells. In the autoimmune process antibodies are directed against the gastric parietal cells and/or IF itself. Because parietal cells also secrete hydrochloric (HCl) acid, in pernicious anemia there is a decrease in HCl in the stomach. An acid environment in the stomach is required for the secretion of IF.

Pernicious anemia is a disease of insidious onset that begins in middle age or later (usually after age 40), with 60 years being the most common age at diagnosis. Pernicious anemia occurs frequently in persons of Northern European ancestry (particularly Scandinavians) and African Americans. In African Americans the disease tends to begin early, occurs with higher frequency in women, and is often severe.

Other Causes of Cobalamin Deficiency. Cobalamin deficiency can also occur in patients who have had GI surgery (e.g., gastrectomy, gastric bypass); patients who have had a small bowel resection involving the ileum; and patients with Crohn's disease, ileitis, celiac disease, diverticula of the small intestine, or chronic atrophic gastritis (Table 30-8). In these cases, cobalamin deficiency results from the loss of IF-secreting gastric mucosal cells or impaired absorption of cobalamin in the distal ileum. Cobalamin deficiency is also found in excessive alcohol or hot tea ingestion, smoking, long-term users of H_2-histamine receptor blockers and proton pump inhibitors, and those who are strict vegetarians.[11]

Clinical Manifestations

General manifestations of anemia related to cobalamin deficiency develop because of tissue hypoxia (Table 30-3). GI manifestations include a sore, red, beefy, and shiny tongue; anorexia, nausea, and vomiting; and abdominal pain. Typical neuromuscular manifestations include weakness, paresthesias of the feet and hands, reduced vibratory and position senses, ataxia, muscle weakness, and impaired thought processes ranging from confusion to dementia. Because cobalamin deficiency–related anemia has an insidious onset, it may take several months for these manifestations to develop.

Diagnostic Studies

Laboratory data reflective of cobalamin deficiency anemia are presented in Table 30-6. The RBCs appear large (macrocytic) and have abnormal shapes. This structure contributes to erythrocyte destruction because the cell membrane is fragile. Serum cobalamin levels are reduced.

Serum folate levels are also obtained. If they are normal and cobalamin levels are low, it suggests that megaloblastic anemia is due to a cobalamin deficiency. A serum test for anti-IF antibodies may be done that is specific for pernicious anemia. Because the potential for gastric cancer is increased in patients with pernicious anemia, an upper GI endoscopy and biopsy of the gastric mucosa may also be done.

Testing of serum methylmalonic acid (MMA) (elevated mainly in cobalamin deficiency) and serum homocysteine (elevated in both cobalamin and folic acid deficiencies) helps determine the cause of this type of anemia.

Interprofessional Care

Regardless of how much is ingested, the patient is not able to absorb cobalamin if IF is lacking or if absorption in the ileum is impaired. For this reason, increasing dietary cobalamin does not correct this anemia. However, instruct the patient on adequate dietary intake to maintain good nutrition (Table 30-5).

Parenteral vitamin B_{12} (cyanocobalamin or hydroxocobalamin) or intranasal cyanocobalamin (Nascobal, CaloMist) is the treatment of choice. Without cobalamin administration, these individuals will die in 1 to 3 years. A typical treatment schedule consists of 1000 mcg/day of cobalamin IM for 2 weeks and then weekly until the hemoglobin is normal, and then monthly for life. High-dose oral cobalamin and sublingual cobalamin are also available for those in whom GI absorption is intact. As long as supplemental cobalamin is used, the anemia can be reversed. However, if the person has had long-standing neuromuscular complications that may not be reversible, physical therapy may be warranted.

Megaloblastic Anemia: Folic Acid Deficiency

Folic acid (folate) deficiency also causes megaloblastic anemia. Folic acid is required for DNA synthesis leading to RBC formation and maturation. Common causes of folic acid deficiency are listed in Table 30-8.

The clinical manifestations of folic acid deficiency are similar to those of cobalamin deficiency. The disease develops insidiously, and the patient's symptoms may be attributed to other coexisting problems (e.g., cirrhosis, esophageal varices). GI disturbances include dyspepsia and a smooth, beefy red tongue. The absence of neurologic problems is an important diagnostic finding and differentiates folic acid deficiency from cobalamin deficiency.

The diagnostic findings for folic acid deficiency are presented in Table 30-6. In addition, the serum folate level is low (normal is 3 to 16 ng/mL [7 to 36 nmol/L]) and the serum cobalamin level is normal.

Folic acid deficiency is treated by replacement therapy. The usual dosage is 1 mg/day by mouth. In malabsorption states or with chronic alcoholism, up to 5 mg/day may be required. The duration of treatment depends on the reason for the deficiency. Encourage the patient to eat foods containing large amounts of folic acid (Table 30-5).

❖ NURSING MANAGEMENT: MEGALOBLASTIC ANEMIA

Because of the familial predisposition for pernicious anemia, the most common type of cobalamin deficiency, patients who have a positive family history of pernicious anemia should be evaluated for symptoms. Although the disease cannot be prevented, early detection and treatment can lead to reversal of symptoms. Also consider signs and symptoms of other possible megaloblastic anemias and bring them to the attention of the HCP. Ongoing care focuses on ensuring good patient adherence with treatment. Carefully assess for neurologic difficulties that were not fully corrected by replacement therapy. Because the potential for gastric cancer may be increased in patients with atrophic gastritis-related pernicious anemia, the patient should have frequent and careful appropriate screenings.

The nursing measures presented in eNursing Care Plan 30-1 for the patient with anemia are appropriate for the patient with cobalamin or folic acid deficiency anemia. In addition to these measures, ensure that injuries are not sustained because of the diminished sensitivity to heat and pain resulting from the neurologic impairment. Protect the patient from falling, burns, and trauma. If heat therapy is required, evaluate the patient's skin at frequent intervals to detect redness.

ANEMIA OF CHRONIC DISEASE

Anemia of chronic disease (also called *anemia of inflammation*) can be caused by chronic inflammation, autoimmune and infectious disorders (human immunodeficiency virus [HIV], hepatitis, malaria), HF, or malignant diseases. Bleeding episodes can also contribute to anemia of chronic disease.

Anemia of chronic disease is associated with an underproduction of RBCs and mild shortening of RBC survival. The RBCs are usually normocytic, normochromic, and hypoproliferative. The anemia is usually mild, but it can become more severe if the underlying disorder is not treated.

This type of anemia, which usually develops after 1 to 2 months of disease activity, has an immune basis. The cytokines released in these conditions, particularly interleukin 6 (IL-6), cause an increased uptake and retention of iron within macrophages (see Fig. 29-3). This leads to a diversion of iron from circulation into storage sites with subsequent limited iron available for erythropoiesis. There is also reduced RBC life span, suppressed production of erythropoietin, and an ineffective bone marrow response to erythropoietin.

For any chronic disease, additional factors may contribute to the anemia. For example, with renal disease, the primary factor causing anemia is decreased erythropoietin, a hormone made in the kidneys that stimulates erythropoiesis. With impaired renal function, erythropoietin production is decreased (see Chapter 46).

Anemia of chronic disease must first be recognized and differentiated from anemia of other etiologies. Findings of elevated serum ferritin and increased iron stores distinguish it from iron-deficiency anemia. Normal folate and cobalamin blood levels distinguish it from megaloblastic anemias secondary to folate and cobalamin deficiencies.

The best treatment of anemia of chronic disease is correction of the underlying disorder. If the anemia is severe, blood transfusions may be indicated, but they are not recommended for long-term treatment. Erythropoietin therapy is used for anemia related to renal disease (see Chapter 46) and may be used for anemia related to cancer and its therapies (see Chapter 15 and Table 15-15). However, erythropoietin therapy must be used conservatively because of the increased risk of thromboembolism and death in some patients.

APLASTIC ANEMIA

Aplastic anemia is a disease in which the patient has peripheral blood *pancytopenia* (decrease of all blood cell types—RBCs, white blood cells [WBCs], and platelets) and hypocellular bone marrow. The spectrum of the anemia can range from a chronic condition managed with erythropoietin or blood transfusions to a critical condition with hemorrhage and sepsis. The incidence of aplastic anemia is rare with an annual rate of 2 to 5 new cases per million per year.[2]

Etiology

Aplastic anemias, which are usually acquired, are idiopathic and thought to have an autoimmune basis[12] (Table 30-9).

Clinical Manifestations

Aplastic anemia can manifest abruptly (over days) or insidiously over weeks to months and can vary from mild to severe. Clinically the patient may have symptoms caused by suppression of any or all bone marrow elements. General manifestations of anemia such as fatigue and dyspnea, as well as cardiovascular and cerebral responses, may be seen (Table 30-3). The patient with neutropenia (low neutrophil count) is susceptible to infection and is at risk for septic shock and death. Even a low-grade fever (above 100.4°F [38°C]) should be considered a medical emergency. Thrombocytopenia is manifested by a predisposition to bleeding (e.g., petechiae, ecchymosis, epistaxis).

Diagnostic Studies

The diagnosis is confirmed by laboratory studies. Because all marrow elements are affected, hemoglobin, WBC, and platelet values are often decreased in aplastic anemia. Other RBC indices are generally normal (Table 30-6). The condition is therefore classified as a normocytic, normochromic anemia. The reticulocyte count is low.

Aplastic anemia can be further evaluated by assessing various iron studies. The serum iron and total iron-binding capacity (TIBC) may be elevated as initial signs of erythropoiesis suppression. Bone marrow biopsy, aspiration, and pathologic examination may be done for any anemic state. However, the findings are especially important in aplastic anemia because the marrow is hypocellular with increased yellow marrow (fat content).

TABLE 30-9 Causes of Acquired Aplastic Anemia

- Idiopathic or autoimmune
- Chemical agents and toxins (e.g., benzene, insecticides, arsenic, alcohol)
- Drugs (e.g., alkylating agents, antiseizure drugs, antimetabolites, antimicrobials, gold, nonsteroidal antiinflammatory drugs, antithyroid medications, allopurinol)
- Radiation
- Viral and bacterial infections

❖ NURSING AND INTERPROFESSIONAL MANAGEMENT: APLASTIC ANEMIA

Management of aplastic anemia is based on identifying and removing the causative agent (when possible) and providing supportive care until the pancytopenia reverses. Nursing interventions appropriate for the patient with pancytopenia from aplastic anemia are presented in eNursing Care Plan 30-1 for anemia and eNursing Care Plan 30-2 for thrombocytopenia and eNursing Care Plan 30-3 for neutropenia (available on the website for this chapter). Nursing actions are directed at preventing complications from infection and hemorrhage.

The prognosis of severe untreated aplastic anemia is poor. However, advances in medical management, including HSCT and immunosuppressive therapy with antithymocyte globulin (ATG) and cyclosporine or high-dose cyclophosphamide, have improved outcomes significantly. ATG is a horse serum that contains polyclonal antibodies against human T cells. It can cause anaphylaxis and serum sickness. The rationale for this therapy is that idiopathic aplastic anemia is considered an autoimmune disorder resulting from activated cytotoxic T cells that target and destroy the patient's own hematopoietic stem cells. (ATG and cyclosporine are discussed in Chapter 13 and Table 13-16.) Alemtuzumab (Campath) (a monoclonal antibody) and eltrombopag (Promacta) (an oral thrombopoietin receptor agonist) are also options for select patients who do not respond to other therapies.[13]

The treatment of choice for adults younger than 55 years of age who do not respond to the immunosuppressive therapy and who have a human leukocyte antigen (HLA)–matched donor is an HSCT. The best results occur in younger patients who have not had previous blood transfusions. Prior transfusions increase the risk of graft rejection. (HSCT is discussed in Chapter 15.)

For older adults without an HLA-matched donor, the treatment of choice is immunosuppression with ATG or cyclosporine or high-dose cyclophosphamide. High-dose corticosteroids may also be used. However, this therapy may be only partially beneficial. Patients who need ongoing supportive blood transfusion should be on an iron-binding agent to prevent iron overload.

ANEMIA CAUSED BY BLOOD LOSS

Anemia resulting from blood loss may be caused by either acute or chronic problems.

ACUTE BLOOD LOSS

Acute blood loss occurs as a result of sudden hemorrhage. Causes of acute blood loss include trauma, complications of surgery, and conditions or diseases that disrupt vascular integrity. There are two clinical concerns in such situations. First, a sudden reduction in the total blood volume can lead to hypovolemic shock. Second, if the acute loss is more gradual, the body maintains its blood volume by slowly increasing the plasma volume. Although the circulating fluid volume is preserved, the number of RBCs available to carry O_2 is significantly diminished.

Clinical Manifestations

The clinical manifestations of anemia from acute blood loss are caused by the body's attempts to maintain an adequate blood volume and meet O_2 requirements. Table 30-10 summarizes the clinical manifestations of patients with varying degrees of blood volume loss. It is essential to understand that the clinical signs and symptoms the patient is experiencing are more important than the laboratory values. For example, an adult with a bleeding peptic ulcer who had a 750-mL hematemesis (15% of a normal total blood volume) within the past 30 minutes may have postural hypotension but have normal values for hemoglobin and hematocrit. Over the next 36 to 48 hours, most of the blood volume deficit will be replaced by the movement of fluid from the extravascular into the intravascular space. Only then will the hemoglobin and hematocrit reflect the blood loss.

Assess the patient's expression of pain. Internal hemorrhage may cause pain because of tissue distention, organ displacement, and nerve compression. Pain may be localized or referred. In the case of retroperitoneal bleeding, the patient may not experience abdominal pain. Instead the patient may have numbness and pain in a lower extremity secondary to compression of the lateral cutaneous nerve, which is located in the region of the first to third lumbar vertebrae. The major complication of acute blood loss is shock (see Chapter 66).

Diagnostic Studies

When blood volume loss is sudden, plasma volume has not yet had a chance to increase, the loss of RBCs is not reflected in laboratory data, and values may seem normal or high for 2 to 3 days. However, once the plasma volume is replaced, the RBC mass is less concentrated. At this time, RBC, hemoglobin, and hematocrit levels are low and reflect the actual blood loss.

Interprofessional Care

Interprofessional care is initially concerned with (1) replacing blood volume to prevent shock and (2) identifying the source of the hemorrhage and stopping the blood loss. IV fluids used in emergencies include dextran, hetastarch, albumin, and crystalloid electrolyte solutions such as lactated Ringer's solution. The amount of infusion varies with the solution used. (Management of shock is discussed in Chapter 66.)

Once volume replacement is established, attention can be directed to correcting the RBC loss. The body needs 2 to 5 days to manufacture more RBCs in response to increased erythropoietin. Consequently, blood transfusions (packed RBCs) may be needed if the blood loss is significant. In addition, if the bleeding is related to a platelet or clotting disorder, replacement of that deficiency is addressed. If a large volume of blood is lost, platelets, plasma, and possibly cryoprecipitate will also be infused, because large volumes of RBCs would dilute the patient's own coagulation system.

The patient may also need supplemental iron because the availability of iron affects the marrow production of erythrocytes. When anemia exists after acute blood loss, dietary sources of iron will probably not be adequate to maintain iron stores. Therefore oral or parenteral iron preparations are administered.

TABLE 30-10 Manifestations of Acute Blood Loss

VOLUME LOST*		
%	mL	Manifestations
10	500	None or rare vasovagal syncope
20	1000	No detectable signs or symptoms at rest. Tachycardia with exercise and slight postural hypotension
30	1500	Normal supine blood pressure and pulse at rest. Postural hypotension and tachycardia with exercise
40	2000	Blood pressure, central venous pressure, and cardiac output below normal at rest; air hunger; rapid, thready pulse and cold, clammy skin
50	2500	Shock, lactic acidosis, and potential death

*Based on an adult with a total blood volume of 5 L.

❖ NURSING MANAGEMENT: ACUTE BLOOD LOSS

In the case of trauma, it may be impossible to prevent the loss of blood. For the postoperative patient, carefully monitor the blood loss from various drainage tubes and dressings and implement appropriate actions. The nursing care for the patient with anemia resulting from acute blood loss most likely includes administration of blood products (described at the end of this chapter on pp. 647-652).

The anemia should begin to correct itself once the source of hemorrhage is identified, blood loss is controlled, and fluid and blood volumes are replaced. There should be no need for long-term treatment of this type of anemia.

CHRONIC BLOOD LOSS

The sources of chronic blood loss are similar to those of iron-deficiency anemia (e.g., bleeding ulcer, hemorrhoids, menstrual and postmenopausal blood loss). The effects of chronic blood loss are usually related to the depletion of iron stores and considered as iron-deficiency anemia. Management of chronic blood loss anemia involves identifying the source and stopping the bleeding. Supplemental iron may be required.

ANEMIA CAUSED BY INCREASED ERYTHROCYTE DESTRUCTION

The third major cause of anemia is termed **hemolytic anemia**, a condition caused by the destruction or hemolysis of RBCs at a rate that exceeds production. Hemolysis can occur because of problems intrinsic or extrinsic to the RBCs. *Intrinsic hemolytic anemias,* which are usually hereditary, result from defects in the RBCs themselves (Table 30-2).

More common are the *acquired hemolytic anemias.* In this type of anemia the RBCs are normal, but damage is caused by external factors (Table 30-2). The spleen is the primary site of the destruction of RBCs that are old, defective, or moderately damaged. Fig. 30-2 indicates the sequence of events involved in extravascular hemolysis.

The patient with hemolytic anemia has the general manifestations of anemia and specific manifestations related to this type of anemia (Table 30-3). Jaundice is likely because the increased

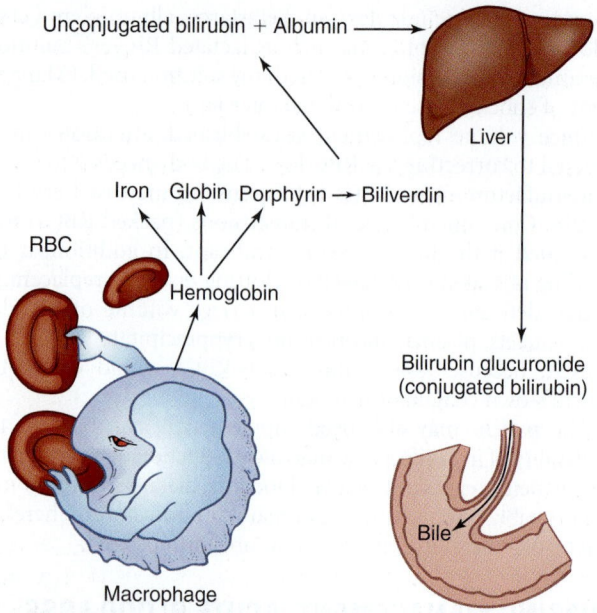

FIG. 30-2 Sequence of events in extravascular hemolysis.

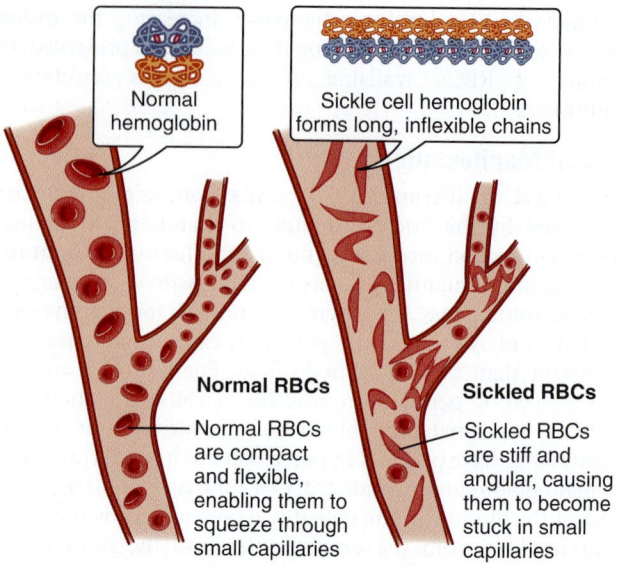

FIG. 30-3 In sickle cell, the hemoglobin forms long inflexible chains and alters the shape of the red blood cells (RBCs). The sickled RBCs can become stuck in the capillaries and occlude the blood flow.

destruction of RBCs causes an elevation in bilirubin levels. The spleen and liver may enlarge because of their hyperactivity, which is related to macrophage phagocytosis of the defective erythrocytes.

In all causes of hemolysis, a major focus of treatment is to maintain renal function. When RBCs are hemolyzed, the hemoglobin molecule is released and filtered by the kidneys. The accumulation of hemoglobin molecules can obstruct the renal tubules and lead to acute tubular necrosis (see Chapter 46).

SICKLE CELL DISEASE

Sickle cell disease (SCD) is a group of inherited, autosomal recessive disorders characterized by an abnormal form of hemoglobin in the RBC. (Autosomal recessive genetic disorders are discussed in Chapter 12.) Because this is a genetic disorder, SCD is usually identified during routine neonatal screening. It is an incurable disease that is often fatal by middle age because of renal failure, infection, pulmonary failure, and/or stroke.[9]

Etiology and Pathophysiology

Genetic Link. In SCD the abnormal hemoglobin, *hemoglobin S* (Hgb S), results from the substitution of valine for glutamic acid on the β-globin chain of hemoglobin (see Fig. 12-3). Hgb S causes the erythrocyte to stiffen and elongate, taking on a sickle shape in response to low O_2 levels (Fig. 30-3).

Types of SCD disorders include sickle cell anemia, sickle cell–thalassemia, sickle cell Hgb C disease, and sickle cell trait. *Sickle cell anemia,* the most severe of the SCD syndromes, occurs when a person is homozygous for hemoglobin S (Hgb SS); the person has inherited Hgb S from both parents. *Sickle cell–thalassemia* and *sickle cell Hgb C* occur when a person inherits Hgb S from one parent and another type of abnormal hemoglobin (such as thalassemia or hemoglobin C) from the other parent. Both of these forms of SCD are less common and less severe than sickle cell anemia. *Sickle cell trait* occurs when a person is heterozygous for hemoglobin S (Hgb AS); the person has inherited hemoglobin S from one parent and normal hemoglobin (Hgb A) from the other parent. Sickle cell trait is typically a mild to asymptomatic condition.

GENETICS IN CLINICAL PRACTICE

Sickle Cell Disease

Genetic Basis
- Autosomal recessive disorder.
- Mutation in β-globin *(HBB)* gene located on chromosome 11.
- Various versions of β-globin result from different mutations in the *HBB* gene.
- Hgb S variant involves substitution of valine for glutamic acid in the β-globin gene in sickle cell anemia.

Incidence
- Most common inherited blood disorder in the United States.
- Affects 8 of every 100,000 people.
- Affects 1 in 350 to 500 African Americans.
- Affects 1 in 1000 to 1400 Hispanic Americans.
- Also affects people of Mediterranean, Caribbean, Arabian, and East Indian descent.

Genetic Testing
- DNA testing is available.
- Electrophoresis of hemoglobin and sickling screening test are more commonly used.

Clinical Implications
- Requires ongoing continuity of care and extensive patient teaching.
- Sickle cell trait is the carrier state for sickle cell disease and represents a mild type of sickle cell disease; 1 in 10 to 12 African Americans and 1 in 25 Hispanics have sickle cell trait.
- If both parents have the trait, there is a 1 in 4 chance that their baby will have sickle cell disease.
- Management of sickle cell disease should focus on the prevention of sickle cell crisis (e.g., prevention of dehydration and infection).
- Genetic counseling is recommended for individuals with a family history of sickle cell disease. Individuals should understand the risks of transmitting the genetic mutation.

Sickling Episodes. The major pathophysiologic event of SCD is the sickling of RBCs (Fig. 30-3). Sickling episodes are most commonly triggered by low O_2 tension in the blood. Hypoxia or deoxygenation of the RBCs can be caused by viral or bacterial infection, high altitude, emotional or physical stress, surgery, and blood loss. Infection is the most common precipitating factor. Other events that can trigger or sustain a sickling episode include dehydration, increased hydrogen ion concentration (acidosis), increased plasma osmolality, decreased plasma volume, and low body temperature. A sickling episode can also occur without an obvious cause.

Sickled RBCs become rigid and take on an elongated, crescent shape (Fig. 30-3). Sickled cells cannot easily pass through capillaries or other small vessels and can cause vascular occlusion, leading to acute or chronic tissue injury. The resulting hemostasis promotes a self-perpetuating cycle of local hypoxia, deoxygenation of more erythrocytes, and more sickling. Circulating sickled cells are hemolyzed by the spleen, leading to anemia. Initially the sickling of cells is reversible with reoxygenation, but it eventually becomes irreversible because of cell membrane damage from recurrent sickling. Thus vaso-occlusive phenomena and hemolysis are the clinical hallmarks of SCD.

Sickle cell crisis is a severe, painful, acute exacerbation of RBC sickling, causing a vaso-occlusive crisis. As blood flow is impaired by sickled cells, vasospasm occurs, further restricting blood flow. Severe capillary hypoxia causes changes in membrane permeability, leading to plasma loss, hemoconcentration, thrombi, and further circulatory stagnation. Tissue ischemia, infarction, and necrosis eventually occur from lack of O_2. Shock is a possibly life-threatening consequence of sickle cell crisis because of severe O_2 depletion of the tissues and a reduction of the circulating fluid volume. Sickle cell crisis can begin suddenly and persist for days to weeks.

The frequency, extent, and severity of sickling episodes are highly variable and unpredictable but largely depend on the percentage of Hgb S present. Individuals with sickle cell anemia have the most severe form because the erythrocytes contain a high percentage of Hgb S.

Clinical Manifestations

The effects of SCD vary greatly from person to person, the severity of which may be due to genetic polymorphisms. Many people with sickle cell anemia are in reasonably good health the majority of the time. However, they may have chronic health problems and pain because of organ tissue hypoxia and damage (e.g., involving the kidneys or liver).

The typical patient is anemic but asymptomatic except during sickling episodes. Because most individuals with sickle cell anemia have dark skin, pallor is more readily detected by examining the mucous membranes. The skin may have a grayish cast. Because of the hemolysis, jaundice is common and patients are prone to gallstones (cholelithiasis).

The primary symptom associated with sickling is pain. The pain severity can range from trivial to excruciating. During sickle cell crisis the pain is severe because of ischemia of tissue. The episodes can affect any area of the body or several sites simultaneously, with the back, chest, extremities, and abdomen being most commonly affected. Pain episodes are often accompanied by clinical manifestations such as fever, swelling, tenderness, tachypnea, hypertension, nausea, and vomiting.

Complications

With repeated episodes of sickling, there is gradual involvement of all body systems, especially the spleen, lungs, kidneys, and brain. Organs that have a need for large amounts of O_2 are most often affected and form the basis for many of the complications of SCD (Fig. 30-4). Infection is a major cause of morbidity and mortality in patients with SCD. One reason for this is the failure of the spleen to phagocytize foreign substances as it becomes infarcted and dysfunctional (usually by 2 to 4 years of age) from the sickled RBCs. The spleen becomes small because of repeated scarring, a phenomenon termed *autosplenectomy.*

Pneumonia is the most common infection and often is of pneumococcal origin. Infections can be so severe that they cause an aplastic and hemolytic crisis and gallstones. *Aplastic crisis* can be so severe that it causes a temporary shutdown of RBC production in the bone marrow.

Acute chest syndrome is a term used to describe acute pulmonary complications that include pneumonia, tissue infarction, and fat embolism. It is characterized by fever, chest pain, cough, pulmonary infiltrates, and dyspnea. Pulmonary infarctions may cause pulmonary hypertension, MI, HF, and ultimately cor pulmonale. The heart may become ischemic and enlarged, leading to HF. Retinal vessel obstruction may result in hemorrhage, scarring, retinal detachment, and blindness. The kidneys may be injured from the increased blood viscosity and the lack of O_2, and renal failure may occur. Pulmonary embolism or stroke can result from thrombosis and infarction of cerebral blood vessels. Bone changes may include osteoporosis and osteosclerosis after infarction. Chronic leg ulcers can result from the hypoxia and are especially prevalent around the ankles. *Priapism* (persistent penile erection) may occur if penile veins become occluded.

Diagnostic Studies

A peripheral blood smear may reveal sickled cells and abnormal reticulocytes. The presence of Hgb S can be diagnosed by the sickling test, which uses RBCs (in vitro) and exposes them to a deoxygenation agent.

As a result of the accelerated RBC breakdown, the patient has characteristic clinical findings of hemolysis (jaundice, elevated serum bilirubin levels) and abnormal laboratory test results (Table 30-6). Hemoglobin electrophoresis may be done to determine the amount of hemoglobin S. Skeletal x-rays demonstrate bone and joint deformities and flattening. MRI may be used to diagnose a stroke caused by blocked cerebral vessels from sickled cells. Doppler studies may be used to assess for deep vein thromboses. Other tests may be indicated, such as a chest x-ray, to diagnose infection or organ malfunction.

❖ NURSING AND INTERPROFESSIONAL MANAGEMENT: SICKLE CELL DISEASE

Interprofessional care for a patient with SCD is directed toward (1) prevention of sequelae from the disease; (2) alleviating the manifestations from the complications of the disease; (3) minimizing end-organ damage; and (4) promptly treating serious sequelae, such as acute chest syndrome, that can lead to immediate death.[14] Teach patients with SCD to avoid high altitudes, maintain adequate fluid intake, and treat infections promptly. Screening for retinopathy should begin at age 10. Immunizations such as pneumococcal, *Haemophilus influenzae,* influenza, and hepatitis should be administered. Sickle cell crises may require hospitalization. O_2 may be administered to treat hypoxia and control sickling. Because respiratory failure is a most common cause of death, vigilantly assess for any changes in respiratory status. Rest may be instituted to reduce metabolic

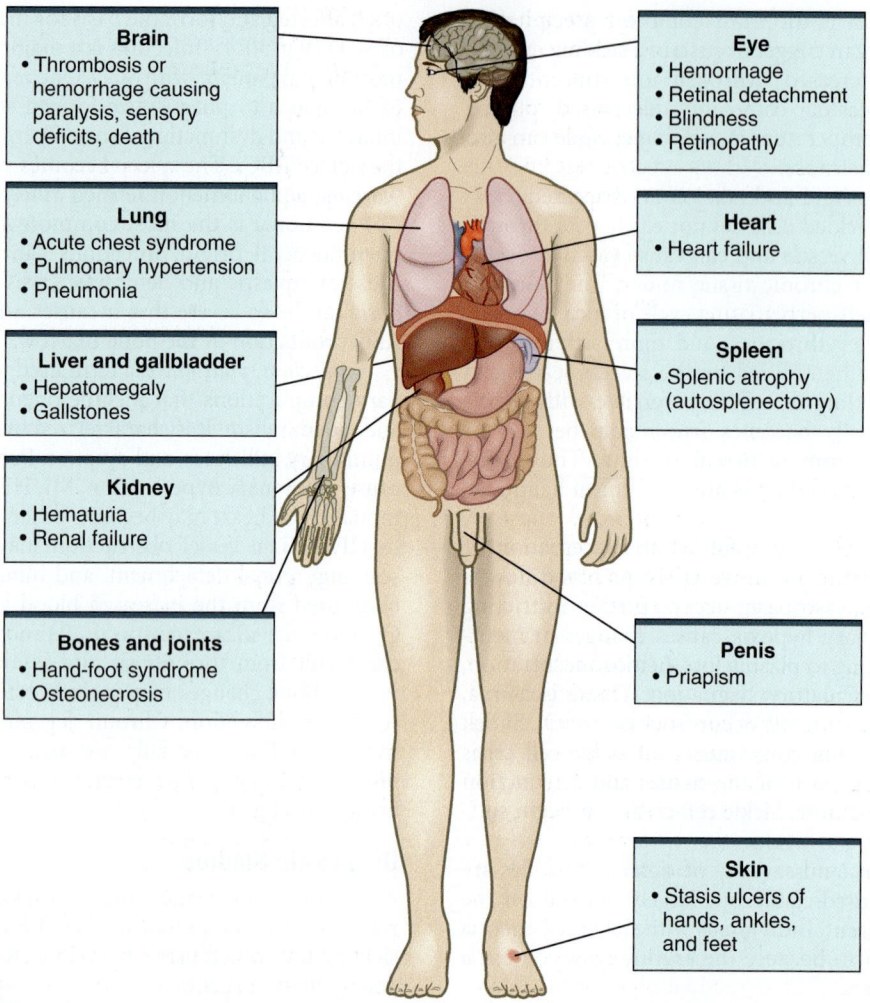

FIG. 30-4 Clinical manifestations and complications of sickle cell disease. (Modified from McCance KL, Huether SE: *Pathophysiology: the biologic basis for disease in adults and children,* ed 7, St Louis, 2014, Mosby.)

requirements, and deep vein thrombosis prophylaxis (using anticoagulants) should be prescribed. Fluids and electrolytes are administered to reduce blood viscosity and maintain renal function. Priapism is managed with pain medication, fluids, and nifedipine (Procardia). If it does not resolve within a few hours, a urologist can be called to inject the corpus cavernosum with a dilute solution of epinephrine to preserve penile function.

Transfusion therapy is indicated when an aplastic crisis occurs. Aggressive total RBC exchange transfusion programs may be implemented for patients who have frequent crises or serious complications, such as acute chest syndrome. These patients, like those with thalassemia major, may require iron chelation therapy to reduce transfusion-produced iron overload.

Undertreatment of sickle cell pain is a major problem. Lack of understanding can lead HCPs to underestimate how much pain these patients suffer. Patients, because of their prior opioid treatment, may be tolerant, and thus large doses may be needed to reduce the pain to a tolerable level. During an acute crisis, optimal pain control usually includes large doses of continuous (rather than as-needed [PRN]) opioid analgesics along with breakthrough analgesia, often in the form of patient-controlled analgesia (PCA). (PCA is discussed in Chapter 8.) Morphine and hydromorphone are the drugs of choice.

Because patients may be experiencing different types and sites of pain, as well as acute and chronic pain, a holistic approach should be used that addresses the pain and its impact on the patient's psychologic, social, and spiritual well-being[15] (see Chapter 8). In addition to opioids, adjunctive measures, such as nonsteroidal antiinflammatory agents, antineuropathic pain medications (e.g., tricyclic antidepressants, antiseizure medications), local anesthetics, or nerve blocks may be used. Occupational and physical therapy can optimize functioning. Referral to social and chaplain services can assist in addressing social, emotional, and spiritual needs.

Although pain is the most common symptom of patients with SCD, infection is a frequent complication and must be treated. Infections, such as chronic leg ulcers, may be treated with rest, antibiotics, warm saline soaks, mechanical or enzyme debridement, and grafting if necessary. Patients with acute chest syndrome are treated with broad-spectrum antibiotics, O_2 therapy, fluid therapy, and possibly exchange transfusion. Blood transfusions have little if any role in the treatment between crises, since patients develop antibodies to RBCs and iron overload. However, because chronic hemolysis results in increased use of folic acid stores, routine oral folic acid should be taken.

Although many antisickling agents have been tried, hydroxyurea (Hydrea) is the only one that has been shown to be clinically beneficial. This drug increases the production of hemoglobin F (fetal hemoglobin) and alters the adhesion of sickled RBCs to the endothelium. The increase in Hgb F is accompanied by a reduction in hemolysis, an increase in hemoglobin concentration, and a decrease in sickled cells and painful crises.[14]

HSCT is the only available treatment that can cure some patients with SCD. The selection of appropriate recipients, scarcity of appropriate donors, risk, and cost-effectiveness limit the use of HSCT for SCD. (HSCT is discussed in Chapter 15.)

CHECK YOUR PRACTICE

A 21-year-old African American graduate student was just admitted to the ED following a ski trip to Colorado. She is in excruciating pain in her chest and abdomen. She is also short of breath and her O_2 saturation is 86%. Your examination reveals that her heart rate is 110 bpm and respiratory rate 28/minute. She has crackles in the lungs. She has a history of six previous ED admissions for sickle cell crises.

- What are your priorities for her nursing care?

Patient teaching and support are important in the long-term care of the patient with SCD. The patient and caregiver must understand the basis of the disease and the reasons for supportive care and ongoing pertinent screening tailored to SCD manifestations, such as eye examinations. Teach the patient ways to avoid crises, including taking steps to avoid dehydration and hypoxia, such as avoiding high altitudes and seeking medical attention quickly to counteract problems such as upper respiratory tract infections. Teaching about pain control is also needed because the pain during a crisis may be severe and often requires considerable analgesia. Minor pain episodes that are not associated with infection or other symptoms warranting medical attention can sometimes be managed at home.

ETHICAL/LEGAL DILEMMAS

Pain Management

Situation

N.C., a 21-year-old African American man, is admitted to the emergency department (ED) in sickle cell crisis with complaints of excruciating pain. He is known to several of the nurses and HCPs in the ED. One of the nurses remarks to you that it must be time for his "fix" of pain drugs.

Ethical/Legal Points for Consideration

- The standard of care for pain requires that (1) a pain assessment is done based on the patient's self-report, (2) the best possible relief of pain is provided under the circumstances, and (3) competent and compassionate care is provided to all patients.
- The pain assessment also includes reviewing the patient's medical record to determine if there are health care issues or conditions (e.g., frequent ED visits to request pain medication) that may affect the patient's response to pain and pain management.
- As a nurse, you have a duty to notify the HCP of those issues or conditions. You also need to document behaviors exhibited by the patient related to pain management. Make sure that the documentation is objective (factual observations) rather than labeling (the patient was in withdrawal).
- When pain relief is inadequate, as a nurse, you are responsible for notifying the HCP. Efforts to notify must continue and be appropriately documented until the managing HCP has assessed the patient and made a plan of care based on that assessment.

Discussion Questions

1. How can you educate your colleagues regarding pain assessment and management?
2. What important factors would need to be included in your assessment and management of N.C.?

ACQUIRED HEMOLYTIC ANEMIA

Acquired hemolytic anemia results from hemolysis of RBCs from extrinsic factors. These factors include (1) physical destruction, (2) antibody reactions, and (3) infectious agents and toxins (Table 30-2).

Physical destruction of RBCs results from the exertion of extreme force on the cells. Traumatic events causing disruption of the RBC membrane include hemodialysis, extracorporeal circulation used in cardiopulmonary bypass, and prosthetic heart valves. In addition, the force needed to push blood through abnormal vessels, such as those that have been burned, irradiated, or affected by vascular disease (e.g., diabetes mellitus), may also physically damage RBCs.

RBCs can also be fragmented and destroyed as they try to pass through abnormal arterial or venous microcirculation. The RBCs are sheared as they try to pass by excessive platelet aggregation and/or fibrin polymer formation, such as is seen in thrombotic thrombocytopenic purpura (TTP) and disseminated intravascular coagulation (DIC) (discussed later in this chapter).

Antibodies may destroy RBCs by the mechanisms involved in antigen-antibody reactions. In blood transfusion reactions, the recipient's antibodies attack and hemolyze donor cells. Autoimmune antibody reactions occur when individuals develop antibodies against their own RBCs. This can be an idiopathic (no prior hemolytic history) or secondary to other autoimmune diseases (e.g., systemic lupus erythematosus), leukemia, lymphoma, or medications (penicillin, ibuprofen, metformin, chlorpromazine, procainamide).

Infectious agents cause hemolysis in three ways: (1) by invading the RBC and destroying its contents (e.g., parasites such as in malaria), (2) by releasing hemolytic substances (e.g., *Clostridium perfringens*), and (3) by generating an antigen-antibody reaction (e.g., *Mycoplasma pneumoniae*). Various agents may be toxic to RBCs and cause hemolysis. These hemolytic toxins involve chemicals such as oxidative drugs, arsenic, lead, copper, and bee stings or spider bites.

Laboratory findings in hemolytic anemia are presented in Table 30-6. Treatment and management of acquired hemolytic anemias involve general supportive care until the causative agent can be eliminated or at least made less injurious to the RBCs. Because a hemolytic crisis is a potential consequence, be ready to institute appropriate emergency therapy. This includes aggressive hydration and electrolyte replacement to reduce the risk of kidney injury caused by hemoglobin (from RBC lysis) clogging the kidney tubules and subsequent shock. Additional supportive care may include administering corticosteroids and blood products or removing the spleen.

For chronic hemolytic anemia, folate may have to be replaced. To suppress the RBC destruction, immunosuppressive agents may be used, such as rituximab (Rituxan) (monoclonal antibody to B-cell CD20) and eculizumab (Soliris) (monoclonal antibody to complement protein C5).

OTHER RED BLOOD CELL DISORDERS

HEMOCHROMATOSIS

Hemochromatosis is an iron overload disorder. Although it is caused primarily by a genetic defect, hemochromatosis may occur secondary to diseases such as sideroblastic anemia. It may also be caused by liver disease and chronic blood transfusions that are used to treat thalassemia and SCD.

Genetic Link. The genetic disorder *(hereditary hemochromatosis)* is an autosomal recessive disorder characterized by increased intestinal iron absorption and, as a result, increased tissue iron deposition. (Autosomal recessive disorders are discussed in Chapter 12 and Table 12-2.)

GENETICS IN CLINICAL PRACTICE

Hemochromatosis

Genetic Basis

- Autosomal recessive disorder
- Caused by mutations in the *HAMP, HFE, HFE2, SLC40A1,* and *TFR2* genes
- These genes play an important role in regulating the absorption, transport, and storage of iron.
- Mutations in these genes impair the control of iron absorption during digestion and alter the distribution of iron to other parts of the body. As a result, iron accumulates in tissues and organs.

Incidence

- Most common genetic disease in people of European ancestry
- One in 8 are carriers of the single HH gene mutation.
- Affects 1 in 200 to 500 in the United States
- Very low prevalence in other ethnic populations

Genetic Testing

- DNA testing is available and recommended for all first-degree relatives of people with the disease.
- American Hemochromatosis Society recommends genetic testing regardless of family history.
- Useful diagnostic tests include serum iron concentration, total iron-binding capacity, and transferrin saturation.

Clinical Implications

- Most of the 33 million Americans who have the gene mutation do not know it.
- Clinical expression is variable depending on dietary iron, blood loss, and other modifying factors.
- Early treatment can prevent serious complications.
- If untreated, progressive iron deposits can lead to multiple organ failure.

The normal range for total body iron is 2 to 6 g. Individuals with hemochromatosis accumulate iron at a rate of 0.5 to 1.0 g/yr and may exceed total iron concentrations of 50 g. Symptoms of hemochromatosis usually develop between 40 and 60 years of age.

Early symptoms are nonspecific and include fatigue, arthralgia, impotence, abdominal pain, and weight loss. Later, the excess iron accumulates in the liver and causes liver enlargement and eventually cirrhosis. Excess iron is deposited in the liver, pancreas, heart, joints, and endocrine glands, resulting in diabetes mellitus, skin pigment changes (bronzing), cardiac changes (e.g., cardiomyopathy), arthritis, and testicular atrophy. Physical examination reveals an enlarged liver and spleen and pigmentation changes in the skin.

Laboratory values demonstrate an elevated serum iron, TIBC, and serum ferritin. Testing for known genetic mutations confirms the diagnosis. Liver biopsy can quantify the amount of iron and establish the degree of organ damage.

The goal of treatment is to remove excess iron from the body and minimize any symptoms the patient may have. Iron removal is achieved by removing 500 mL of blood each week for 2 to 3 years until the iron stores in the body are depleted. Then blood is removed less frequently to maintain iron levels within normal limits.

Iron chelating agents may be used. Deferoxamine, which chelates and removes accumulated iron via the kidneys, can be administered IV or subcutaneously. Deferasirox and deferiprone are oral agents that chelate iron. Chelating agents form a complex with iron and promote its excretion from the body.[8]

Management of organ involvement (e.g., diabetes mellitus, HF) is the same as conventional treatment for these problems. Iron accumulation can also be reduced by dietary modifications such as avoidance of vitamin C and iron supplements, uncooked seafood, and iron-rich foods. The most common causes of death are cirrhosis, liver failure, hepatocellular cancer, and cardiac failure. With early diagnosis and treatment, life expectancy is normal. However, many cases go undetected and untreated.

POLYCYTHEMIA

Polycythemia is the production and presence of increased numbers of RBCs. The increase in RBCs can be so great that blood circulation is impaired as a result of the increased blood viscosity *(hyperviscosity)* and volume *(hypervolemia)*.

Etiology and Pathophysiology

The two types of polycythemia are primary polycythemia, or polycythemia vera, and secondary polycythemia (Fig. 30-5). Their etiologies and pathogenesis differ, although their complications and clinical manifestations are similar.

Primary Polycythemia. *Polycythemia vera* is a chronic myeloproliferative disorder. Therefore not only RBCs are involved but also WBCs and platelets, leading to increased production of each of these blood cells. The disease develops insidiously and follows a chronic, vacillating course. The median age at diagnosis is 60 years old, with a slight male predominance. In polycythemia vera there is enhanced blood viscosity and blood volume and congestion of organs and tissues with blood. Splenomegaly (which occurs in 90% of patients) and hepatomegaly are common. These patients have hypercoagulopathies that predispose them to clotting.

Genetic Link. Polycythemia vera is associated with mutations in the *Janus kinase-2 (JAK2)* gene. The *JAK2* gene provides instructions for making a protein that promotes proliferation of cells, especially blood cells from hematopoietic stem cells. Polycythemia vera begins with one or more DNA mutations of a single hematopoietic stem cell. Most cases of polycythemia vera are not inherited. This condition is associated with genetic changes that are somatic, which means they are acquired during a person's lifetime and are present only in certain cells.

Secondary Polycythemia. *Secondary polycythemia* can be either hypoxia driven or hypoxia independent. In hypoxia-driven secondary polycythemia, hypoxia stimulates erythropoietin (EPO) production in the kidney, which in turn stimulates RBC production. The need for O_2 may result from high altitude, pulmonary disease, cardiovascular disease, alveolar hypoventilation, defective O_2 transport, or tissue hypoxia.

EPO levels may return to normal once the hemoglobin is stabilized at a higher level. In this situation, secondary polycythemia is a physiologic response in which the body tries to compensate for a problem, rather than a pathologic response. (Hypoxia-driven secondary polycythemia is discussed

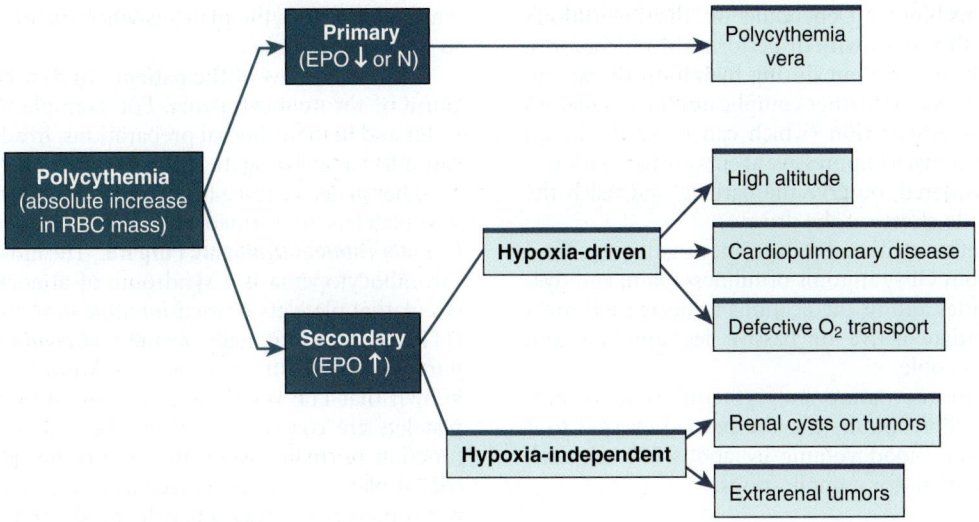

FIG. 30-5 Differentiating between primary and secondary polycythemia. *EPO,* Erythropoietin; *N,* normal.

in the section on chronic obstructive pulmonary disease in Chapter 28.)

In hypoxia-independent secondary polycythemia, EPO is produced by a malignant or benign tumor tissue. Serum EPO levels often remain elevated in these situations. Splenomegaly does not accompany secondary polycythemia.

Clinical Manifestations and Complications

Circulatory manifestations of polycythemia vera occur because of the hypertension caused by hypervolemia and hyperviscosity. They are often the first manifestations and include subjective complaints of headache, vertigo, dizziness, tinnitus, and visual disturbances. Generalized pruritus (often exacerbated by a hot bath) may be a striking symptom and is related to histamine release from an increased number of basophils. Paresthesias and *erythromelalgia* (painful burning and redness of the hands and feet) may also be present. In addition, the patient may experience angina, HF, intermittent claudication, and thrombophlebitis, which may be complicated by embolization. These manifestations are caused by blood vessel distention, impaired blood flow, circulatory stasis, thrombosis, and tissue hypoxia caused by the hypervolemia and hyperviscosity. The most common serious acute complication is stroke secondary to thrombosis.

Hemorrhagic phenomena caused by either vessel rupture from overdistention or inadequate platelet function may result in petechiae, ecchymoses, epistaxis, or GI bleeding. Hemorrhage can be acute and catastrophic. Hepatomegaly and splenomegaly from organ engorgement may contribute to patient complaints of satiety and fullness. The patient may also experience pain from peptic ulcer caused either by increased gastric secretions or by liver and spleen engorgement. *Plethora* (ruddy complexion) may also be present. Hyperuricemia is caused by the increase in RBC destruction that accompanies excessive RBC production. Uric acid is one of the products of cell destruction. As RBC destruction increases, uric acid production also increases, thus leading to hyperuricemia and possible gout.

Although the incidence is low, myelofibrosis and leukemia develop in some patients with polycythemia vera. These disorders may be caused by the chemotherapeutic drugs used to treat the disease, or they may be secondary to a disorder in the stem cells that progresses to erythroleukemia. The major cause of morbidity and mortality from polycythemia vera is related to thrombosis (e.g., stroke).

Diagnostic Studies

The following laboratory manifestations are seen in a patient with polycythemia vera: (1) elevated hemoglobin and RBC count with microcytosis; (2) low to normal EPO level (secondary polycythemia has a high level); (3) elevated WBC count with basophilia; (4) elevated platelet count (thrombocytosis) and platelet dysfunction; (5) elevated leukocyte alkaline phosphatase, uric acid, and cobalamin levels; and (6) elevated histamine levels. Bone marrow examination in polycythemia vera shows hypercellularity of RBCs, WBCs, and platelets.

Interprofessional Care

Treatment is directed toward reducing blood volume and viscosity and bone marrow activity. Phlebotomy is the mainstay of treatment. The aim of phlebotomy is to reduce the hematocrit and keep it less than 45% in men and 42% in women. Generally, at the time of diagnosis 300 to 500 mL of blood may be removed every other day until the hematocrit is reduced to normal levels. An individual managed with repeated phlebotomies eventually becomes deficient in iron, although this effect is rarely symptomatic. Avoid iron supplementation. Hydration therapy is used to reduce the blood's viscosity. Myelosuppressive agents such as hydroxyurea (Hydrea), busulfan (Myleran), and chlorambucil (Leukeran) are used.

Ruxolitinib (Jakafi), which inhibits the expression of the *JAK2* mutation, is used for patients who have not responded to hydroxyurea.[16] Low-dose aspirin is used to prevent clotting. α-Interferon (α-IFN) is of particular use in women of childbearing age or those with intractable pruritus. Anagrelide (Agrylin) may be used to reduce the platelet count and inhibit platelet aggregation. Allopurinol (Zyloprim) may reduce the number of acute gouty attacks.[17] (Gout may occur because of increased uric acid levels from the destruction of cells.)

❖ NURSING MANAGEMENT: POLYCYTHEMIA VERA

Primary polycythemia (polycythemia vera) is not preventable. When acute exacerbations of polycythemia vera develop, you have several responsibilities. Depending on the institution's policies, you may either assist with or perform the phlebotomy. Evaluate fluid intake and output during hydration therapy to avoid fluid overload (which further complicates the circulatory congestion) and underhydration (which can make the blood even more viscous). If myelosuppressive agents are used, administer the drugs as ordered, observe the patient, and teach the patient about the side effects of the drugs.

Assess the patient's nutritional status, since inadequate food intake can result from GI symptoms of fullness, pain, and dyspepsia. Begin activities and/or medications to decrease thrombus formation. Initiate active or passive leg exercises and ambulation when possible.

Because of its chronic nature, polycythemia vera requires ongoing evaluation. Phlebotomy may be needed every 2 to 3 months, reducing the blood volume by about 500 mL each time. Evaluate the patient for complications.

PROBLEMS OF HEMOSTASIS

Hemostasis involves the vascular endothelium, platelets, and coagulation factors, which normally function together to stop hemorrhage and repair vascular injury. (These mechanisms are described in Chapter 29.) Disruption in any of these components may result in bleeding or thrombotic disorders.

Three major disorders of hemostasis discussed in this section are (1) thrombocytopenia (low platelet count), (2) hemophilia and von Willebrand disease (inherited disorders of specific clotting factors), and (3) disseminated intravascular coagulation (DIC).

THROMBOCYTOPENIA

Etiology and Pathophysiology

Thrombocytopenia is a reduction of platelets below 150,000/μL (150×10^9/L). Acute, severe, or prolonged decreases from this normal range can result in abnormal hemostasis that manifests as prolonged bleeding from minor trauma or spontaneous bleeding without injury.

Platelet disorders can be inherited (e.g., Wiskott-Aldrich syndrome), but the majority are acquired (Table 30-11). A common cause of acquired disorders is the ingestion of certain drugs, often in high doses.[18,19] Although some agents are directly myelosuppressive (e.g., chemotherapy, ganciclovir [Cytovene]), the usual mechanism of thrombocytopenia caused by drugs is accelerated platelet destruction caused by antibodies. Antibodies attack the platelets when the offending agent binds to the platelet surface.

TABLE 30-11 Causes of Acquired Thrombocytopenia

- Immune thrombocytopenic purpura (ITP)
- Thrombotic thrombocytopenic purpura (TTP)
- Heparin-induced thrombocytopenia (HIT)
- Disseminated intravascular coagulation (DIC)
- Drugs
  - Chemotherapy drugs
  - Aspirin
- Quinine
- Infections
  - Viral infection (hepatitis C virus, HIV, cytomegalovirus)
  - Bacterial infection
- Hematologic malignancy (leukemia, lymphoma, myeloma)

A careful review of the patient's history helps to identify the cause of thrombocytopenia. For example, quinine is in tonic water and in many herbal preparations. In addition, some drugs can affect platelet aggregation. Aspirin doses as low as 81 mg can alter platelet aggregation. Normal function is restored when new platelets are formed.

Immune Thrombocytopenic Purpura. The most common acquired thrombocytopenia is a syndrome of abnormal destruction of circulating platelets termed *immune thrombocytopenic purpura* (ITP). It was originally termed *idiopathic thrombocytopenic purpura* because its cause was unknown. However, it is now known that ITP is primarily an autoimmune disease. In ITP, platelets are coated with antibodies. Although these platelets function normally, when they reach the spleen the antibody-coated platelets are recognized as foreign and are destroyed by macrophages. Decreased platelet production contributes to ITP. Sometimes infection, such as *Helicobacter pylori* or viral infection, contributes to this disorder.[18]

Platelets normally survive 8 to 10 days. However, in ITP survival of platelets is shortened. Generally, the clinical syndrome manifests as an acute condition in children and a chronic condition in adults.

Thrombotic Thrombocytopenic Purpura. *Thrombotic thrombocytopenic purpura* (TTP) is an uncommon syndrome characterized by hemolytic anemia, thrombocytopenia, neurologic abnormalities, fever (in the absence of infection), and renal abnormalities; not all features are present in all patients. Because it is almost always associated with hemolytic-uremic syndrome (HUS), it is often referred to as *TTP-HUS*. The disease is associated with enhanced aggregation of platelets, which form microthrombi that deposit in arterioles and capillaries.

In most cases the syndrome is caused by the deficiency of a plasma enzyme (ADAMTS13) that usually breaks down the von Willebrand clotting factor (vWF) into normal size. (vWF is the most important protein-mediating platelet adhesion to damaged endothelial cells.) Without the enzyme, unusually large amounts of vWF attach to activated platelets, thereby promoting platelet aggregation.

TTP is seen primarily in previously healthy adults, with a slight female predominance. The syndrome may be idiopathic (thought to be due to an autoimmune disorder against ADAMTS13), but it may be due to certain drug toxicities (e.g., chemotherapy, cyclosporine, quinine, oral contraceptives, valacyclovir [Valtrex], clopidogrel [Plavix]), pregnancy or preeclampsia, infection, or a known autoimmune disorder such as systemic lupus erythematosus or scleroderma.[20] TTP is a medical emergency because bleeding and clotting occur simultaneously.

Heparin-Induced Thrombocytopenia. One of the risks associated with the broad and increasing use of heparin is the development of the life-threatening condition called *heparin-induced thrombocytopenia* (HIT), also called *heparin-induced thrombocytopenia and thrombosis syndrome* (HITTS). Typically, patients develop thrombocytopenia 5 to 10 days after the onset of heparin therapy. HIT should be suspected if the platelet count falls by more than 50% or falls to below 150,000/μL. As many as 3% of patients on heparin therapy develop HIT.[21]

Although the major clinical problem of HIT is venous thrombosis, arterial thrombosis can also develop. Deep vein thromboses and pulmonary emboli most commonly result as a complication of the thromboses. Additional complications may include arterial vascular infarcts, resulting in skin necrosis, stroke, and end-organ damage (e.g., kidneys). Symptoms of bleeding are unusual because the platelet count rarely drops below 20,000/μL.

In HIT, platelet destruction and vascular endothelial injury are the two major responses to an immune-mediated response to heparin. Platelet factor 4 (PF4) (protein made and released by platelets) binds to heparin. This PF4-heparin complex then binds to the platelet surface, leading to further platelet activation and release of more PF4, thus creating a positive feedback loop. Antibodies are created against the PF4-heparin-platelet complex, and they are removed prematurely from circulation, leading to thrombocytopenia and platelet-fibrin thrombi. Platelet aggregation also induces heparin to be neutralized.

Clinical Manifestations

Many patients with thrombocytopenia are asymptomatic. The most common symptom is bleeding, usually mucosal or cutaneous. Mucosal bleeding may manifest as epistaxis and gingival bleeding, and large bullous hemorrhages may appear on the buccal mucosa because of the lack of vessel protection by the submucosal tissue.

Bleeding into the skin is manifested as petechiae, purpura, or superficial ecchymoses (Fig. 30-6). *Petechiae* are small, flat, pinpoint, red or reddish brown microhemorrhages. When the platelet count is low, RBCs may leak out of the blood vessels and into the skin to cause petechiae. When petechiae are numerous, the resulting reddish skin bruise is called *purpura.* Larger purplish lesions caused by hemorrhage are termed *ecchymoses.* Ecchymoses may be flat or raised; pain and tenderness sometimes are present.

Prolonged bleeding after routine procedures such as venipuncture or IM injection may indicate thrombocytopenia. Because the bleeding may be internal, be aware of manifestations that reflect this type of blood loss, including weakness, fainting, dizziness, tachycardia, abdominal pain, and hypotension.

The major complication of thrombocytopenia is hemorrhage. The hemorrhage may be insidious or acute, and internal or external. It may occur in any area of the body, including the joints, retina, and brain. Cerebral hemorrhage may be fatal. Insidious hemorrhage may first be detected by discovering the anemia that accompanies blood loss.

Because thrombocytopenia can be accompanied by vascular thromboses, signs and symptoms of vascular ischemic problems can manifest (see Chapter 37). For example, subtle confusion, headache, or even serious manifestations such as seizures and coma due to TTP-related thrombosis may be seen. Because signs and symptoms may be subtle, astute and thorough assessment of the patient is essential.

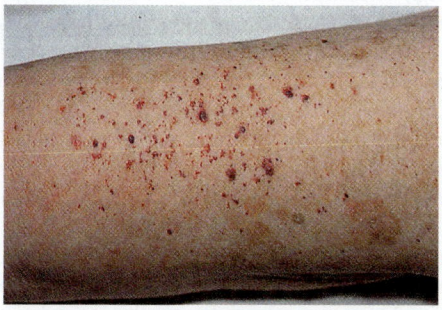

FIG. 30-6 Acute immune thrombocytopenic purpura commonly manifests with purpuric lesions of this kind, although they may often be widespread by the time medical attention is sought. (From Forbes CD, Jackson WF: *Colour atlas and text of clinical medicine,* ed 3, London, 2003, Mosby.)

Diagnostic Studies

The platelet count is decreased in thrombocytopenia. Any reduction below 150,000/μL (150×10^9/L) may be termed *thrombocytopenia.* However, prolonged bleeding from trauma or injury does not usually occur until platelet counts are less than 50,000/μL (50×10^9/L). When the count drops below 20,000/μL (20×10^9/L), spontaneous, life-threatening hemorrhages (e.g., intracranial bleeding) can occur. Platelet transfusions are generally not recommended until the count is below 10,000/μL (10×10^9/L), unless the patient is actively bleeding.

The patient's medical history and clinical examination, along with comparisons of laboratory parameters, help to determine the etiology of the thrombocytopenia. Table 30-12 compares the types of thrombocytopenia.[18]

Laboratory tests that assess secondary hemostasis or coagulation, such as the prothrombin time (PT) and aPTT, can be normal even in severe thrombocytopenia. If they are elevated, this may point toward DIC. Bone marrow examination is done to rule out production problems as the cause of thrombocytopenia (e.g., leukemia, aplastic anemia, other myeloproliferative disorders).

Specific assays, such as ITP antigen-specific assay, platelet activation/function assay, or PF4-heparin complex for HIT, can be done to assist with the diagnosis. In TTP, testing for deficiency of ADAMTS13 is not always diagnostic, so an increase of lactate dehydrogenase (LDH) may help establish the diagnosis. When thrombocytopenia occurs with anemia characterized by altered RBC morphology, including *spherocytes* (small, globular, completely hemoglobinated erythrocytes), fragmented cells (schistocytes), and pronounced reticulocytosis, a diagnosis of TTP should be suspected. These findings are partially a result

TABLE 30-12 Laboratory Results in Thrombocytopenia and DIC

Laboratory Test	ITP	TTP	HIT	DIC
Platelets	↓↓↓	↓↓↓	↓↓	↓↓↓
Hemolysis				
Hgb	N	↓↓	N	N or ↓
LDH	N	↑↑↑	N	↑
Reticulocytes	N	↑	N	N or ↑
Haptoglobin	N	↓	N	↓
Indirect bilirubin	N	↑	N	N or ↑
Schistocytes	N	↑↑↑	N or ↑	N or ↑
Coagulopathy				
PT	N	N	N	↑
aPTT	N	N	N	↑
D-dimer	N	N or ↑	↑	↑↑
Other tests	ITP antigen-specific assay, platelet activation/function assay, *Helicobacter pylori,* bone marrow biopsy	ADAMTS13	Platelet activation/function assay, PF4-heparin complex	

aPTT, Activated partial thromboplastin time; *LDH,* lactate dehydrogenase; *N,* normal; *PF4,* platelet factor 4; *PT,* prothrombin time.

of intravascular fibrin deposition causing a "slicing" of RBCs. In TTP, thrombocytopenia may be severe, but coagulation studies are normal.

Bone marrow analysis is performed if other test results are inconclusive. When destruction of circulating platelets is the cause, bone marrow analysis shows *megakaryocytes* (precursors of platelets) to be normal or increased, even though circulating platelets are reduced. The absence or decreased number of megakaryocytes on bone marrow biopsy is consistent with thrombocytopenia caused by decreased bone marrow production (e.g., aplastic anemia).

Interprofessional Care

Interprofessional care of thrombocytopenia differs based on the etiology. Removal or treatment of the underlying cause or disorder is sometimes sufficient. The patient with thrombocytopenia should avoid aspirin and other medications that affect platelet function or production. The following sections discuss management strategies for the different causes of thrombocytopenia (Table 30-13).

Immune Thrombocytopenic Purpura. Multiple therapies are used to manage the patient with ITP. If the patient is asymptomatic, therapy may not be used unless the patient's platelet count is below 10,000/μL. Corticosteroids (e.g., prednisone, methylprednisolone) are used initially to treat ITP because of their ability to suppress the phagocytic response of splenic macrophages. This alters the spleen's recognition of platelets and increases the life span of the platelets. In addition, corticosteroids depress antibody formation and reduce capillary leakage.

High doses of IV immunoglobulin (IVIG) and a component of IVIG, anti-Rh_o(D) (anti-D, WinRho), may be used in the patient who is unresponsive to corticosteroids or splenectomy, or for whom splenectomy is not an option. It is believed that one way these agents work is by competing with the antiplatelet antibodies for macrophage receptors in the spleen. Rituximab (Rituxan) may be used for its ability to lyse activated B cells, thereby reducing the immune recognition of platelets.

Splenectomy may be indicated if the patient does not respond to the above treatments. Splenectomy can usually be done laparoscopically, and 60% to 70% of patients benefit from splenectomy, resulting in a complete or partial remission.[18] The effectiveness of splenectomy is based on four factors. First, the spleen contains an abundance of the macrophages that sequester and destroy platelets. Second, structural features of the spleen enhance the interaction between antibody-coated platelets and macrophages. Third, some antibody synthesis occurs in the spleen; thus antiplatelet antibodies decrease after splenectomy. Fourth, the spleen normally sequesters approximately one third of the platelets, so its removal increases the number of platelets in circulation.

Romiplostim (Nplate) and eltrombopag (Promacta) are used for patients with chronic ITP who have had an insufficient response to the other treatments or who have a contraindication to splenectomy. These drugs are thrombopoietin receptor agonists, thus increasing platelet production. Danazol, an androgen, may be used along with corticosteroids in some patients. Although the mechanism is not totally understood, danazol reduces the ability of the body to remove antibody-coated platelets from the blood. Immunosuppressive therapy may be used in refractory cases[18] (Table 30-14).

Platelet transfusions may be used to increase platelet counts in cases of life-threatening hemorrhage. Platelets should not be administered prophylactically because of the possibility of antibody formation. The usual indication for administering platelets is for a platelet count less than 10,000/μL or if there is anticipated bleeding before a procedure. Epsilon-aminocaproic acid (EACA, Amicar), an antifibrinolytic agent, may be used for severe bleeding.

Thrombotic Thrombocytopenic Purpura. TTP may be treated in a variety of ways. The first step is to treat the underlying disorder (e.g., infection) or remove the causative agent, if identified. If untreated, TTP usually results in irreversible renal failure and death. Plasma exchange (plasmapheresis) (see Chapter 13) is used to aggressively reverse platelet consumption by supplying the appropriate vWF and enzyme (ADAMTS13) and removing the large vWF molecules that bind with platelets. Treatment should be continued daily until the patient's platelet counts normalize and hemolysis has ceased. Corticosteroids may be added to this treatment.

Rituximab is used for patients refractory to plasma exchange; it decreases the level of inhibitory ADAMTS13 IgG antibodies. Other immunosuppressants such as cyclosporine or cyclophosphamide may also be used. Splenectomy may be considered in patients who are refractory to plasma exchange or immunosuppression. The administration of platelets is generally

TABLE 30-13 Nursing Assessment

Thrombocytopenia

Subjective Data

Important Health Information

Past health history: Recent hemorrhage, excessive bleeding, or viral illness; HIV infection; cancer (especially leukemia or lymphoma); aplastic anemia; systemic lupus erythematosus; cirrhosis; exposure to radiation or toxic chemicals; disseminated intravascular coagulation

Medications: Many medications including chemotherapy agents, valproic acid (Depakote), furosemide (Lasix), gold, nonsteroidal antiinflammatory drugs, penicillin

Functional Health Patterns

Health perception–health management: Family history of bleeding problems; malaise

Nutritional-metabolic: Bleeding gingiva; coffee-ground or bloody vomitus; easy bruising

Elimination: Hematuria, dark or bloody stools

Activity-exercise: Fatigue, weakness, fainting; epistaxis, hemoptysis; dyspnea

Cognitive-perceptual: Pain and tenderness in bleeding areas (e.g., abdomen, head, extremities); headache

Sexuality-reproductive: Menorrhagia, metrorrhagia

Objective Data

General

Fever, lethargy

Integumentary

Petechiae, ecchymoses, purpura

Gastrointestinal

Splenomegaly, abdominal distention; guaiac-positive stools

Possible Diagnostic Findings

Platelet count <150,000/μL (150×10^9/L), prolonged bleeding time, ↓ hemoglobin and hematocrit; normal or ↑ megakaryocytes in bone marrow examination

TABLE 30-14 Interprofessional Care

Thrombocytopenia

Diagnostic Assessment
- History and physical examination
- Bone marrow aspiration and biopsy
- CBC, including platelet count
- Specific laboratory studies (Table 30-12)

Management

Immune Thrombocytopenic Purpura
- Corticosteroids
- IV immunoglobulin (IVIG)
- Anti-Rh_0(D)
- Rituximab (Rituxan)
- Splenectomy
- Romiplostim (Nplate)
- Eltrombopag (Promacta)
- Danazol
- Immunosuppressives (e.g., cyclosporine, cyclophosphamide, azathioprine [Imuran], mycophenolate mofetil [CellCept])
- Platelet transfusions

Thrombotic Thrombocytopenic Purpura
- Identification and treatment of cause
- Plasmapheresis (plasma exchange)
- Corticosteroids
- Rituximab (Rituxan)
- Immunosuppressives (e.g., cyclophosphamide)
- Chemotherapy (vincristine, vinblastine)
- Splenectomy

Heparin-Induced Thrombocytopenia
- Direct thrombin inhibitor (lepirudin [Refludan], argatroban [Acova])
- Indirect thrombin inhibitor (fondaparinux [Arixtra])
- Warfarin (Coumadin)
- Plasmapheresis (plasma exchange)
- Thrombolytic agents

Decreased Platelet Production
- Identification and treatment or removal of cause
- Corticosteroids
- Platelet transfusions

contraindicated because this may lead to new vWF-platelet complexes and increased clotting.

Heparin-Induced Thrombocytopenia. Heparin must be discontinued when HIT is first recognized. Heparin flushes for vascular catheters should also be stopped.

To maintain anticoagulation, the patient should be started on a direct thrombin inhibitor, such as lepirudin (Refludan) or argatroban (Acova). Fondaparinux (Arixtra), a factor Xa inhibitor (indirect thrombin inhibitor), may be used. Warfarin should be started only when the platelet count has reached 150,000/μL. If the clotting is severe, the most commonly used treatment modalities are plasmapheresis to clear the platelet-aggregating IgG from the blood, protamine sulfate to interrupt the circulating heparin, thrombolytic agents to treat the thromboembolic events, and surgery to remove clots. Platelet transfusions are not effective because they may enhance thromboembolic events.[21]

Patients who have had HIT should never be given heparin or low-molecular-weight heparin (LMWH). This should be clearly marked in the patient's medical record.

Thrombocytopenia From Decreased Platelet Production. The management of acquired thrombocytopenia is based on identifying the cause and treating the disease or removing the causative agent. If the precipitating factor is unknown, the patient may receive corticosteroids. Platelet transfusions are given if life-threatening hemorrhage develops.

Often acquired thrombocytopenia is caused by another underlying condition (e.g., aplastic anemia, leukemia) or therapy used to treat another problem. For example, in acute leukemia all blood cell types may be depressed. Additionally, the patient may receive chemotherapeutic drugs that cause bone marrow suppression. If the patient can be adequately supported throughout the course of chemotherapy-induced thrombocytopenia, the thrombocytopenia will also resolve.

❖ NURSING MANAGEMENT: THROMBOCYTOPENIA

◆ Nursing Assessment

Subjective and objective data that should be obtained from a patient with thrombocytopenia are presented in Table 30-13.

◆ Nursing Diagnoses

Nursing diagnoses for the patient with thrombocytopenia may include, but are not limited to, the following.
- Impaired oral mucous membrane *related to* low platelet counts and/or effects of pathologic conditions and treatment
- Risk for bleeding *related to* decreased platelets
- Deficient knowledge *related to* lack of information regarding the disease process and treatment

◆ Planning

The overall goals are that the patient with thrombocytopenia will (1) have no gross or occult bleeding, (2) maintain vascular integrity, and (3) manage home care to prevent any complications related to an increased risk for bleeding.

◆ Nursing Implementation

◆ **Health Promotion.** Discourage excessive use of over-the-counter (OTC) medications known to be possible causes of acquired thrombocytopenia. Many medications contain aspirin as an ingredient. Aspirin reduces platelet adhesiveness, thus contributing to bleeding.

Encourage persons to have a complete medical evaluation if manifestations of bleeding tendencies (e.g., prolonged epistaxis, petechiae) develop. Observe for early signs of thrombocytopenia in the patient receiving cancer chemotherapy drugs.

◆ **Acute Care.** The goal during acute episodes of thrombocytopenia is to prevent or control hemorrhage (see eNursing Care Plan 30-2 on the website for this chapter). In the patient with thrombocytopenia, bleeding is usually from superficial sites. Deep bleeding (into muscles, joints, and abdomen) usually occurs only when clotting factors are diminished. Emphasize that a seemingly minor nosebleed or new petechiae may indicate potential hemorrhage and the HCP should be notified.

Bleeding from the posterior nasopharynx may be difficult to detect because the blood may be swallowed. If a subcutaneous injection is unavoidable, the use of a small-gauge needle and application of direct pressure for at least 5 to 10 minutes after injection is indicated, or application of an ice pack may be helpful. Avoid IM injections. Help the patient understand the importance of adherence to self-care measures that reduce the risk of bleeding (Table 30-15).

Note that many of these disorders may be accompanied by vascular clotting, and appropriate assessment and management should be taken (see Chapter 37). As bleeding occurs, RBC and coagulation factors are consumed along with platelets, so it is important to monitor all blood cell and coagulation studies.

In a woman with thrombocytopenia, menstrual blood loss may exceed the usual amount and duration. Counting sanitary napkins used during menses is another important intervention to detect excess blood loss. Blood loss of 50 mL will completely soak a sanitary napkin. Suppression of menses with hormonal agents may be indicated during predictable periods of thrombocytopenia (e.g., during chemotherapy and HSCT) to reduce blood loss from menses.

Closely monitor the platelet count, coagulation studies, hemoglobin, and hematocrit. Together these provide important information regarding potential or actual bleeding.

The proper administration of platelet transfusions is an important nursing responsibility. This is discussed under Blood Component Therapy later in this chapter.

◆ **Ambulatory Care.** Monitor the patient with ITP who is receiving treatment for the response to therapy. Teach the person with acquired thrombocytopenia to avoid causative agents when possible (Table 30-11). If the causative agents cannot be avoided (e.g., chemotherapy), teach the patient to avoid injury or trauma during these periods and to be aware of the clinical signs and symptoms of bleeding caused by thrombocytopenia (Table 30-15).

TABLE 30-15 Patient & Caregiver Teaching

Thrombocytopenia

Include the following instructions when teaching a patient or caregiver the precautions to take when the platelet count is low.

1. Notify your HCP of any manifestations of bleeding. These include the following:
   - Black, tarry, or bloody bowel movements
   - Black or bloody vomit, sputum, or urine
   - Bruising or small red or purple spots on the skin
   - Bleeding from the mouth or anywhere in the body
   - Headache or changes in how well you can see
   - Difficulty talking, sudden weakness of an arm or leg, confusion
2. Ask your HCP regarding restrictions in your normal activities, such as vigorous exercise or lifting weights. Generally, walking can be done safely and should be done with sturdy shoes or slippers. If you are weak and at risk for falling, get help or supervision when getting out of bed or chair.
3. Do not blow your nose forcefully; gently pat it with a tissue if needed. For a nosebleed, keep your head up and apply firm pressure to the nostrils and bridge of your nose. If bleeding continues, place an ice bag over the bridge of your nose and the nape of your neck. If you are unable to stop a nosebleed after 10 min, call your HCP.
4. Do not bend down with your head lower than your waist.
5. Prevent constipation by drinking plenty of fluids. Do not strain when having a bowel movement. Your HCP may prescribe a stool softener. Do not use a suppository, an enema, or a rectal thermometer without the permission of your HCP.
6. Shave only with an electric razor. Do not use blades.
7. Do not tweeze your eyebrows or other body hair.
8. Do not puncture your skin, such as getting tattoos or body piercing.
9. Avoid using any medication that can prolong bleeding, such as aspirin. Other medications and herbs can have similar effects. If you are unsure about any medication, ask your HCP or pharmacist about it in relation to your thrombocytopenia.
10. Use a soft-bristle toothbrush to prevent injuring the gums. Flossing is usually safe if it is done gently using the thin tape floss. Do not use alcohol-based mouthwashes, since they can dry your gums and increase bleeding.
11. Women who are menstruating should keep track of the number of pads that are used per day. When you start using more pads per day than usual or bleed more days, notify your HCP. Do not use tampons; only use sanitary pads.
12. Ask your HCP before you have any invasive procedures done, such as a dental cleaning, manicure, or pedicure.

Patients with either ITP or acquired thrombocytopenia should have planned periodic medical evaluations to assess their status. These regular evaluations can be used to assess and treat situations in which exacerbations and bleeding are likely to occur. The impact of either an acute or a chronic condition on the patient's quality of life should also be addressed appropriately.

◆ Evaluation

The expected outcomes are that the patient with thrombocytopenia will

- Have no evidence of bleeding or bruising
- Verbalize required knowledge and skills to manage disease process at home

HEMOPHILIA AND VON WILLEBRAND DISEASE

Hemophilia is an X-linked recessive genetic disorder caused by a defective or deficient coagulation factor. The two major types of hemophilia, which can occur in mild to severe forms, are *hemophilia A* (classic hemophilia, factor VIII deficiency) and *hemophilia B* (Christmas disease, factor IX deficiency). *von Willebrand disease* is a related disorder involving a deficiency of the von Willebrand coagulation protein. Factor VIII is synthesized in the liver and circulates as a complex with von Willebrand factor (vWF).

Hemophilia A is the most common form of hemophilia, accounting for about 80% to 85% of all hemophilia cases. Although rare, there are cases of *acquired hemophilia A*, which is due to the development of antibodies against the body's own factor VIII. von Willebrand disease is considered the most common congenital bleeding disorder.[22]

Genetic Link. The inheritance patterns of hemophilia and von Willebrand disease are compared in Table 30-16. (X-linked genetic disorders are discussed in Chapter 12 and Table 12-2.)

Clinical Manifestations and Complications

All clinical manifestations relate to bleeding, and any bleeding episode in persons with hemophilia may lead to a life-threatening hemorrhage. Clinical manifestations and complications related to hemophilia include (1) slow, persistent, prolonged bleeding from minor trauma and small cuts; (2) delayed bleeding after minor injuries (the delay may be several hours or days); (3) uncontrollable hemorrhage after dental extractions or irritation of the gingiva with a hard-bristle toothbrush; (4) epistaxis,

TABLE 30-16 Types of Hemophilia

Type	Inheritance Pattern
Hemophilia A	
Factor VIII	Recessive sex-linked (transmitted by female carriers, displayed almost exclusively in men)
Hemophilia B	
Factor IX	Recessive sex-linked (transmitted by female carriers, displayed almost exclusively in men)
von Willebrand Disease	
vWF, variable factor VIII deficiencies and platelet dysfunction	Autosomal dominant, seen in both genders Recessive (in severe forms of the disease)

vWF, von Willebrand factor.

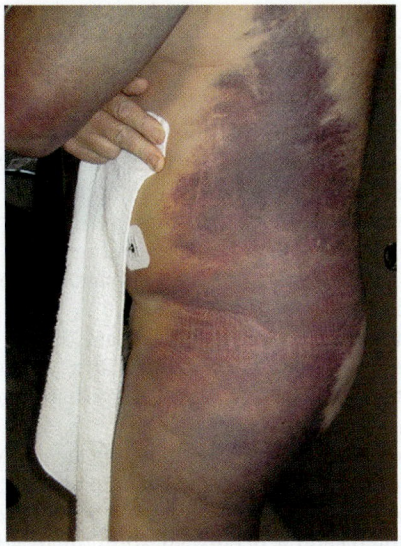

FIG. 30-7 Severe ecchymoses in a person with hemophilia after a fall. (Courtesy Peter Bonner.)

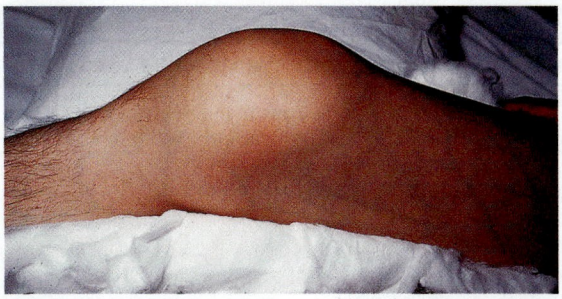

FIG. 30-8 Acute hemarthrosis of the knee is a common complication of hemophilia. (From Forbes CD, Jackson WF: *Colour atlas and text of clinical medicine,* ed 3, London, 2003, Mosby.)

GENETICS IN CLINICAL PRACTICE

Hemophilia A and B

Genetic Basis

- X-linked recessive disorder
- *Hemophilia A:* Caused by mutations in the *F8* gene that provides instructions for making coagulation factor VIII
- *Hemophilia B:* Caused by mutations in the *F9* gene that provides instructions for making coagulation factor IX
- Mutations in the *F8* or *F9* gene lead to the production of an abnormal version or reduced amounts of these coagulation factors.

Incidence

- *Hemophilia A:* 1 in 5000 to 10,000 male births
- *Hemophilia B:* 1 in 30,000 to 50,000 male births

Genetic Testing

- DNA testing is available.

Clinical Implications

- Female carriers transmit the genetic defect to 50% of their sons, and 50% of their daughters are carriers.
- Males with hemophilia do not transmit the genetic defect to their sons, but all of their daughters are carriers.
- Female hemophilia can occur if a male with hemophilia mates with a female carrier. However, this is a rare situation.
- Clinical manifestations of hemophilia A and B are similar.
- Replacement therapy is available for factors VIII and IX (Table 30-19).

especially after a blow to the face; (5) GI bleeding from ulcers and gastritis; (6) hematuria and potential renal failure from GU trauma and splenic rupture resulting from falls or abdominal trauma; (7) ecchymoses and subcutaneous hematomas (Fig. 30-7) and possible compartment syndrome; (8) neurologic signs, such as pain, anesthesia, and paralysis, which may develop from nerve compression caused by hematoma formation; and (9) hemarthrosis (bleeding into the joints) (Fig. 30-8), which may lead to joint injury and deformity severe enough to cause crippling (most commonly in knees, elbows, shoulders, hips, and ankles).[23]

In children these manifestations may lead to the diagnosis. In adults these developments may be the first sign of a newly diagnosed mild form of the disease that escaped detection through a childhood free of major injuries, dental procedures, or surgeries.

TABLE 30-17 Laboratory Results in Hemophilia

Test	Results
Prothrombin time	Normal. No involvement of extrinsic system
Thrombin time	Normal. No impairment of thrombin-fibrinogen reaction
Platelet count	Normal. Adequate platelet production
Partial thromboplastin time	Prolonged because of deficiency in intrinsic clotting system factor
Bleeding time	Prolonged in von Willebrand disease because of structurally defective platelets. Normal in hemophilia A and B because platelets not affected
Factor assays	Reductions of factor VIII in hemophilia A, factor IX in hemophilia B, vWF in von Willebrand disease

vWF, von Willebrand factor.

Diagnostic Studies

Laboratory studies are used to determine the type of hemophilia present. Any factor deficiency within the intrinsic system (factor VIII, IX, XI, or XII or vWF) will yield the laboratory results presented in Table 30-17.

Interprofessional Care

The goals of interprofessional care are to prevent and treat bleeding. Care for persons with hemophilia or von Willebrand disease requires (1) preventive care, (2) the use of replacement therapy during acute bleeding episodes and as prophylaxis, and (3) the treatment of the complications of the disease and its therapy. Today most patients can expect almost normal life spans free of bloodborne illnesses because of improved preparation of replacement products, improved screening of blood donor populations, and use of recombinant replacement factors.[23]

Replacement of deficient clotting factors is the primary means of supporting a patient with hemophilia. In addition to treating acute crises, replacement therapy may be given before surgery and dental care as a prophylactic measure.[24] Examples of replacement therapy[25] are listed in Table 30-18. Fresh frozen plasma, once commonly used for replacement therapy, is rarely used today.

TABLE 30-18 Drug Therapy

Replacement Factors for Hemophilia*

Factor VIII	Factor IX	Von Willebrand	For Patients Who Have Inhibitors
Advate	Alphanine SD	Vonvendi	NovoSeven (factor VIIa)
Alphanate	Alprolix		Autoplex T
Eloctate	Bebulin VH		FEIBA (factor VIII inhibitor bypassing activity)
Helixate FS	BeneFIX		
Hemofil M	Mononine		
Humate-P	Profilnine SD		
Koate-DVI	ProplexT		
Kogenate FS			
Monoclate P			
Obizur†			
Recombinate			
Xyntha			

*List is not all inclusive.
†For acquired hemophilia A.

For mild hemophilia A and certain subtypes of von Willebrand disease, desmopressin acetate (also known as *DDAVP*), a synthetic analog of vasopressin, may be used to stimulate an increase in factor VIII and vWF. This drug acts on platelets and endothelial cells to cause the release of vWF, which subsequently binds with factor VIII, thus increasing its concentration. It can be administered IV, subcutaneously, or by intranasal spray. Beneficial effects (e.g., decreased bleeding time) of DDAVP, when administered IV, are seen within 30 minutes and can last for more than 12 hours. Because the effect of DDAVP is relatively short lived, the patient must be closely monitored and repeated doses may be necessary. It is an appropriate therapy for minor bleeding episodes and dental procedures. The intranasal form may be indicated for home therapy for some patients with mild to moderate forms of the disease.

Antifibrinolytic therapy (tranexamic acid [Cyklokapron] and epsilon-aminocaproic acid) inhibits fibrinolysis by inhibiting plasminogen activation in the fibrin clot, thereby enhancing clot stability. These agents are used to stabilize clots in areas of increased fibrinolysis, such as the oral cavity, and in patients with difficult episodes of epistaxis and menorrhagia. Topical thrombin and fibrin sealants may also be used for mucosal bleeding.

Complications of the treatment of hemophilia include development of inhibitors to factors VIII or IX, transfusion-transmitted infectious disorders (hepatitis, HIV), allergic reactions, and thrombotic complications with the use of factor IX because it contains activated coagulation factors. Patients with vWF may also develop antibodies against vWF concentrates, the infusion of which could cause life-threatening anaphylaxis. Thus replacement factors for these patients should not contain vWF.

The most common difficulties with acute management are starting factor replacement therapy too late and stopping it too soon. Generally, minor bleeding episodes should be treated for at least 72 hours. Surgery and traumatic injuries may require more prolonged therapy. Chronically, development of inhibitors to the factor products has occurred and requires individualized expert patient management. Designated treatment centers in the United States and many other countries provide interprofessional care of hemophilia and related disorders. Gene therapy has been used on an experimental basis to treat hemophilia.[23]

NURSING MANAGEMENT: HEMOPHILIA

Nursing Implementation

- **Health Promotion.** Because of the hereditary nature of hemophilia, referral of affected persons for genetic counseling before reproduction is an important measure. This is especially important because many persons with hemophilia live into adulthood. Reproductive concerns and long-term effects are issues that you should include in the patient's care plan.
- **Acute Care.** Interventions are related primarily to controlling bleeding and include the following:
  1. Stop the topical bleeding as quickly as possible by applying direct pressure or ice, packing the area with Gelfoam or fibrin foam, and applying topical hemostatic agents such as thrombin.
  2. Administer the specific coagulation factor to raise the patient's level of the deficient coagulation factor. Monitor the patient for signs and symptoms, such as hypersensitivity.
  3. When joint bleeding occurs, in addition to administering replacement factors, it is important to totally rest the involved joint to prevent crippling deformities from hemarthrosis. Pack the joint in ice. Give analgesics (e.g., acetaminophen, codeine) to reduce severe pain. Aspirin and aspirin-containing compounds should never be used. As soon as bleeding ceases, encourage mobilization of the affected area through range-of-motion exercises and physical therapy. Weight bearing is avoided until all swelling has resolved and muscle strength has returned.
  4. Manage any life-threatening complications that may develop as a result of hemorrhage or side effects from coagulation factors. Examples include nursing interventions to prevent or treat airway obstruction from hemorrhage into the neck and pharynx, recognition of compartment syndrome in an extremity, and early assessment and treatment of intracranial bleeding.
- **Ambulatory Care.** Home management is a primary consideration for the patient with hemophilia because the disease follows a progressive, chronic course. The quality and length of life may be significantly affected by the patient's knowledge of the illness and how to live with it. The patient and caregiver can be referred to a local chapter of the Hemophilia Federation of America to encourage associations with other individuals who are dealing with the problems of hemophilia. Provide ongoing assessment of the patient's adaptation to the illness. Psychosocial support and assistance should be readily available as needed.

  Most of the long-term care measures are related to patient teaching. Teach the patient to recognize disease-related problems and to learn which problems can be resolved at home and which require hospitalization. Immediate medical attention is required for severe pain or swelling of a muscle or joint that restricts movement or inhibits sleep and for a head injury, swelling in the neck or mouth, abdominal pain, hematuria, melena, and skin wounds in need of suturing.

  Teach the patient to perform daily oral hygiene without causing trauma. Understanding how to prevent injuries is another consideration. Advise the patient to participate only in noncontact sports (e.g., golf) and to wear gloves when doing household chores to prevent cuts or abrasions from knives, hammers, and other tools. The patient should wear a Medic Alert tag to ensure that HCPs know about the hemophilia in case of an accident. Many patients or their caregivers can be taught to self-administer the factor replacement therapies at home.

Evaluation

The overall expected outcomes are similar to those for the patient with thrombocytopenia (see p. 626).

DISSEMINATED INTRAVASCULAR COAGULATION

Disseminated intravascular coagulation (DIC) is a serious bleeding and thrombotic disorder that results from abnormally initiated and accelerated clotting. Subsequent decreases in clotting factors and platelets ensue, which may lead to uncontrollable hemorrhage. The term *disseminated intravascular coagulation* can be misleading, because it suggests that blood is clotting. However, this condition is characterized by the profuse bleeding that results from the depletion of platelets and clotting factors. DIC is always caused by an underlying disease or condition. The underlying problem must be treated for the DIC to resolve.

Etiology and Pathophysiology

DIC is not a disease. It is an abnormal response of the normal clotting cascade stimulated by a disease process or disorder.[26,27] The diseases and disorders known to predispose a patient to DIC are listed in Table 30-19. DIC can occur as an acute, catastrophic condition or it may exist at a subacute or chronic level. Each condition may have one or multiple triggering mechanisms to start the clotting cascade. For example, tumors and traumatized or necrotic tissue release tissue factors into circulation. Endotoxin from gram-negative bacteria activates several steps in the coagulation cascade.

Tissue factor is released at the site of tissue injury and by some malignancies, such as leukemia, and enhances normal coagulation mechanisms. Abundant intravascular thrombin, the most powerful coagulant, is produced (Fig. 30-9). It catalyzes the conversion of fibrinogen to fibrin and enhances platelet aggregation. There is widespread fibrin and platelet deposition in capillaries and arterioles, resulting in thrombosis. This process can lead to multiorgan failure.

In addition, clotting inhibitory mechanisms, such as antithrombin III (AT III) and protein C, are depressed. Excessive clotting activates the fibrinolytic system, which in turn breaks down the newly formed clot, creating fibrin split products (FSPs). These products have anticoagulant properties and inhibit normal blood clotting. Ultimately, as FSPs accumulate and clotting factors are depleted, the blood loses its ability to clot. Therefore a stable clot cannot be formed at injury sites, which predisposes the patient to hemorrhage.

Chronic and subacute DIC is most commonly seen in patients with long-standing illnesses such as malignant disorders or autoimmune diseases. Occasionally these patients have

TABLE 30-19 Risk Factors for DIC

Acute DIC

Shock
- Hemorrhagic
- Cardiogenic
- Anaphylactic

Septicemia (bacterial, viral, fungal, parasitic)

Hemolytic processes
- Transfusion of mismatched blood
- Acute hemolysis from infection or immunologic disorders

Obstetric conditions
- Abruptio placentae
- Amniotic fluid embolism
- Septic abortion
- HELLP syndrome

Malignancies
- Acute leukemia
- Metastatic solid tumors

Tissue damage
- Extensive burns and trauma
- Heatstroke
- Severe head injury
- Transplant rejections
- Postoperative damage, especially after extracorporeal membrane oxygenation
- Fat and pulmonary emboli
- Snakebites
- Glomerulonephritis
- Acute anoxia (e.g., after cardiac arrest)
- Prosthetic devices
- Fulminant hepatitis

Subacute DIC

Malignancy
- Myeloproliferative/lymphoproliferative malignancies
- Metastatic cancer

Obstetric
- Retained dead fetus

Chronic DIC

Liver disease

Systemic lupus erythematosus

Malignancy

DIC, Disseminated intravascular coagulation; *HELLP syndrome,* a life-threatening liver disorder thought to be a type of severe preeclampsia, it is characterized by **H**emolysis (destruction of red blood cells), **E**levated **L**iver enzymes (which indicate liver damage), and **L**ow **P**latelet count.

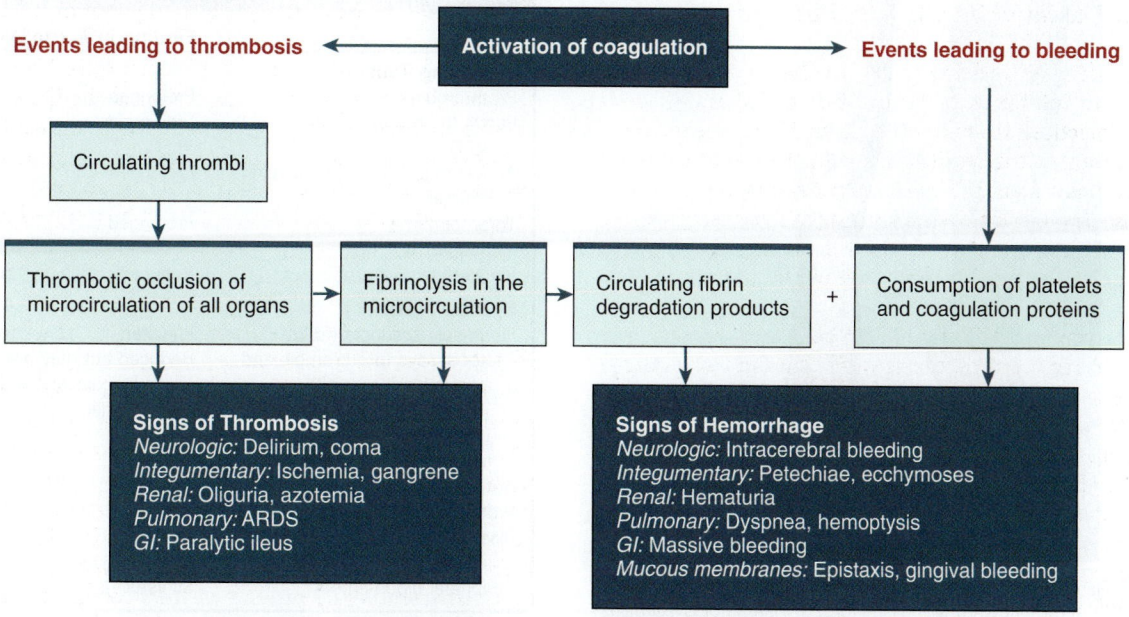

FIG. 30-9 Sequence of events that occur during disseminated intravascular coagulation (DIC).

subclinical disease manifested only by laboratory abnormalities. However, the clinical spectrum ranges from easy bruising to hemorrhage, and from hypercoagulability to thrombosis.

Clinical Manifestations

DIC has both bleeding and thrombotic manifestations. Multiple factors cause bleeding manifestations of DIC (Fig. 30-9) and result from consumption and depletion of platelets and coagulation factors, as well as clot lysis and formation of FSPs that have anticoagulant properties. Bleeding in a person with no previous history or obvious cause should be questioned because it may be one of the first manifestations of acute DIC.

Bleeding manifestations include (1) integumentary manifestations such as pallor, petechiae, purpura (Fig. 30-10), oozing blood, venipuncture site bleeding, hematomas, and occult hemorrhage; (2) respiratory manifestations such as tachypnea, hemoptysis, and orthopnea; (3) cardiovascular manifestations such as tachycardia and hypotension; (4) GI manifestations such as upper and lower GI bleeding, abdominal distention, and bloody stools; (5) urinary manifestations such as hematuria; (6) neurologic manifestations such as vision changes, dizziness, headache, changes in mental status, and irritability; and (7) musculoskeletal complaints such as bone and joint pain.

Thrombotic manifestations are a result of fibrin or platelet deposition in the microvasculature (Fig. 30-9). They include (1) integumentary manifestations, such as cyanosis, ischemic tissue necrosis (e.g., gangrene), and hemorrhagic necrosis; (2) respiratory manifestations, such as tachypnea, dyspnea, pulmonary emboli, and acute respiratory distress syndrome (ARDS); (3) cardiovascular manifestations, such as electrocardiogram (ECG) changes and venous distention; (4) GI manifestations, such as abdominal pain and paralytic ileus; and (5) kidney damage and oliguria, leading to failure.

Diagnostic Studies

Tests to diagnose acute DIC are listed in Table 30-20. As more clots are made in the body, more breakdown products from fibrinogen and fibrin are also formed. These are termed *fibrin split products* (FSPs), and they interfere with blood coagulation by (1) coating the platelets and interfering with platelet function; (2) interfering with thrombin and thus disrupting coagulation; and (3) attaching to fibrinogen, which interferes with the polymerization process necessary to form a stable clot. D-dimer, a polymer resulting from the breakdown of fibrin (and not fibrinogen), is a specific marker for the degree of fibrinolysis. In general, tests that measure raw materials needed for coagulation (e.g., platelets, fibrinogen) are reduced, and values that measure clotting times are prolonged. Fragmented erythrocytes (schistocytes), indicative of partial occlusion of small vessels by fibrin thrombi, may be found on blood smears.

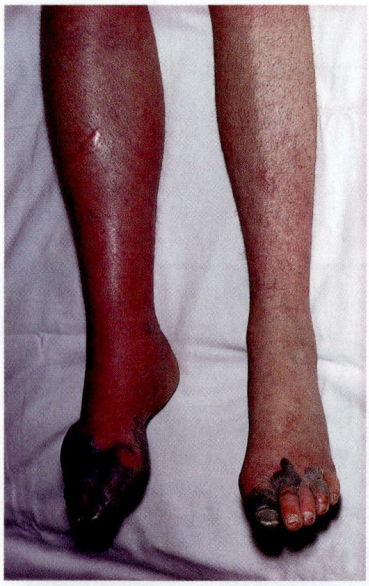

FIG. 30-10 Gangrene resulting from severe disseminated intravascular coagulation (DIC). (From Howard MR, Hamilton PJ: *Haematology: an illustrated colour atlas,* ed 4, London, 2013, Churchill Livingston.)

Interprofessional Care

It is important to diagnose DIC quickly, stabilize the patient (e.g., oxygenation, volume replacement), treat the underlying causative disease or problem, and control the ongoing thrombosis and bleeding. Depending on its severity, a variety of different methods are used to manage DIC (Fig. 30-11). First, if chronic DIC is diagnosed in a patient who is not bleeding, no therapy for DIC is necessary. Treatment of the underlying disease may be sufficient to reverse the DIC (e.g., chemotherapy when DIC is caused by malignancy). Second, when the patient with DIC is bleeding, therapy is directed toward providing support with necessary blood products while treating the primary disorder.

The blood products are administered cautiously based on specific component deficiencies to patients who have serious bleeding, are at high risk for bleeding (e.g., surgery), or require invasive procedures. Blood product support with platelets, cryoprecipitate, and fresh frozen plasma (FFP) is usually reserved for a patient with life-threatening hemorrhage. Therapy stabilizes a patient, prevents exsanguination or massive thrombosis, and permits institution of definitive therapy to treat the underlying cause. Cryoprecipitate replaces factor VIII and fibrinogen and is given if the fibrinogen level is below 80 to 100 mg/dL.[22] Fresh frozen plasma is given only to patients with

TABLE 30-20 Laboratory Results in Acute DIC

Test	Finding in Acute DIC
Screening Tests	
Prothrombin time (PT)	Prolonged
Partial thromboplastin time (PTT)	Prolonged
Activated partial thromboplastin time (aPTT)	Prolonged
Thrombin time	Prolonged
Fibrinogen	Reduced
Platelets	Reduced
Special Tests	
Fibrin split products (FSPs)	Elevated
Factor assays (prothrombin and factors V, VIII, X, XIII)	Reduced but may give misleading results, since V and VIII rise with inflammation
D-dimers (cross-linked fibrin fragments)	Elevated
Antithrombin III (AT III)	Reduced
Proteins C and S	Reduced
Plasminogen, tissue plasminogen activator	Reduced
Peripheral blood smear	Schistocytes present

DIC, Disseminated intravascular coagulation.

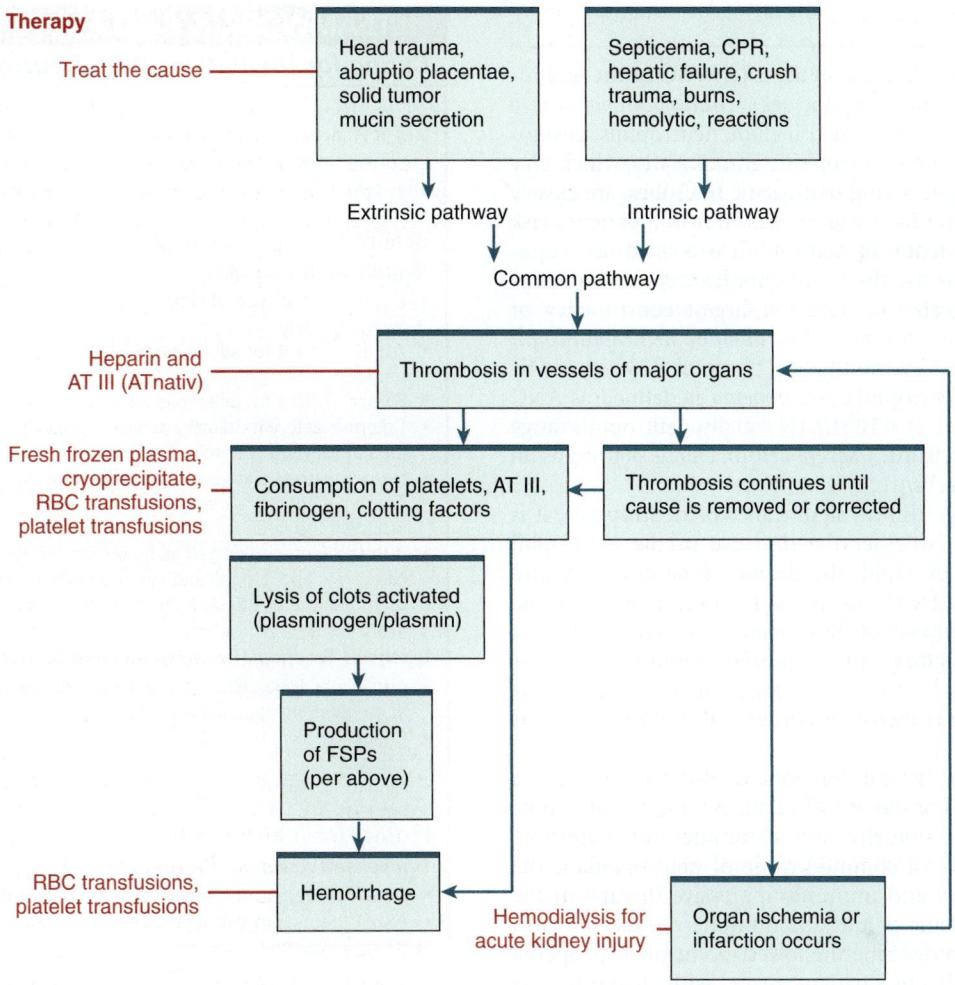

FIG. 30-11 Sites of action for therapies in disseminated intravascular coagulation (DIC). *AT III,* Antithrombin III; *FSPs,* fibrin split products.

significant bleeding and a prolonged PT and aPTT. It replaces all clotting factors except platelets and provides a source of antithrombin.

A patient with manifestations of thrombosis is often treated by anticoagulation with heparin or low-molecular-weight heparin. Heparin is used in the treatment of DIC only when the benefit (reduce clotting) outweighs the risk (further bleeding). Antithrombin III (ATnativ) may be useful in fulminant DIC, although it increases the risk of bleeding. Chronic DIC does not respond to oral anticoagulants, but it can be controlled with long-term use of heparin.

❖ NURSING MANAGEMENT: DISSEMINATED INTRAVASCULAR COAGULATION

◆ Nursing Diagnoses

Nursing diagnoses for the patient with DIC may include, but are not limited to, the following:

- Ineffective peripheral tissue perfusion *related to* bleeding and sluggish or diminished blood flow secondary to thrombosis
- Acute pain *related to* bleeding into tissues and diagnostic procedures
- Decreased cardiac output *related to* fluid volume deficit
- Anxiety *related to* fear of the unknown, disease process, diagnostic procedures, and therapy

◆ Nursing Implementation

Be alert to the possible development of DIC and especially to the precipitating factors listed in Table 30-19. Remember that because DIC is secondary to an underlying disease, the causative problem must be managed while providing supportive care for the manifestations of DIC.

Appropriate nursing interventions are essential to the survival of a patient with acute DIC. Astute ongoing assessment, active attention to manifestations of DIC, and prompt administration of prescribed therapies are crucial. Table 30-14 and eNursing Care Plan 30-2 (available on the website for this chapter) provide assessments and interventions appropriate for the patient with DIC.

Early detection of bleeding and clotting, both occult and overt, must be a primary goal. Assess for signs of external bleeding (e.g., petechiae, oozing at IV or injection sites), signs of internal bleeding (e.g., increased heart rate, changes in mental status, increasing abdominal girth, pain), and any indications that microthrombi may be causing clinically significant organ damage (e.g., decreased renal output). Minimize tissue damage and protect the patient from additional sources of bleeding.

An additional nursing responsibility is to administer blood products and medications correctly. (Blood product transfusion is discussed later in this chapter on pp. 647-652.)

NEUTROPENIA

Leukopenia refers to a decrease in the total WBC count (granulocytes, monocytes, and lymphocytes). *Granulocytopenia* is a deficiency of granulocytes, which include neutrophils, eosinophils, and basophils. The neutrophilic granulocytes, which play a major role in phagocytizing pathogenic microbes, are closely monitored in clinical practice as an indicator of a patient's risk for infection. A reduction in neutrophils is termed **neutropenia.** (Some clinicians use the terms *granulocytopenia* and *neutropenia* interchangeably because the largest constituency of granulocytes is the neutrophils.) The *absolute neutrophil count* (ANC) is determined by multiplying the total WBC count by the percentage of neutrophils. *Neutropenia* is defined as ANC less than 1000 cells/μL (1×10^9/L). (Normally, neutrophils range from 2200 to 7700 cells/μL.) *Severe neutropenia* is defined as an ANC less than 500 cells/μL.

In considering the clinical significance of neutropenia, it is important to know whether the decrease in the neutrophil count was gradual or rapid, the degree of neutropenia, and the duration. The faster the drop and the longer the duration, the greater the likelihood of life-threatening infection, sepsis, and death. Other factors and co-morbid conditions, such as being older than 60, having an existing infection, being in the hospital, and having diabetes, can increase the risk of a serious infection.

Neutropenia is a clinical consequence that occurs with a variety of conditions or disease[28,29] (Table 30-21). It can also be an expected effect, a side effect, or an unintentional effect of certain drugs. The most common cause of neutropenia is the use of chemotherapy and immunosuppressive therapy in the treatment of malignancies and autoimmune diseases. A term that is often used to describe the lowest point of neutropenia (and other blood cells) in a patient treated with chemotherapy is *nadir.*

Clinical Manifestations

The patient with neutropenia is predisposed to infection with opportunistic pathogens and nonpathogenic organisms from the normal body flora. When the WBC count is depressed or immature WBCs are present, normal phagocytic mechanisms are impaired. Also the classic manifestations of inflammation—redness, heat, and swelling—may not occur. WBCs are the major component of pus. Therefore in the patient with neutropenia, pus formation (e.g., as a visible skin lesion or as pulmonary infiltrates on a chest x-ray) is also absent.

SAFETY ALERT Neutropenia

- A low-grade fever in neutropenic patients is of great significance because it may indicate infection and lead to septic shock and death unless treated promptly.
- Neutropenic fever (≥100.4° F [38° C] and a neutrophil count <500/μL) is a medical emergency.
- Blood cultures should be drawn STAT and antibiotics started within 1 hr.

When fever occurs in a neutropenic patient, it is assumed to be caused by infection and requires immediate attention. The immunocompromised, neutropenic patient has little or no ability to fight infection. Thus minor infections can lead rapidly to sepsis. The mucous membranes of the throat and mouth, skin, perineal area, and pulmonary system are common entry points for pathogenic organisms in susceptible hosts.

Clinical manifestations related to infection at these sites include complaints of sore throat and dysphagia, ulcerative lesions of the pharyngeal and buccal mucosa, diarrhea, rectal tenderness, vaginal itching or discharge, shortness of breath, and nonproductive cough. Any minor complaint of pain or any other symptom by the patient may be significant and should be reported to the HCP immediately. These seemingly minor complaints can progress to fever, chills, sepsis, septic shock, and death if not recognized and treated early.

Systemic infections caused by bacterial, fungal, and viral organisms are common in patients with neutropenia. The patient's own flora (normally nonpathogenic) contributes significantly to life-threatening infections such as pneumonia. Organisms known to be common sources of infection include gram-positive coagulase-negative staphylococci and *Staphylococcus aureus* and gram-negative organisms such as *Escherichia coli* and *Pseudomonas aeruginosa.*[30] Fungi involved include *Candida* (usually *C. albicans*) and *Aspergillus* organisms. Viral infections caused by reactivation of herpes simplex and zoster are common after prolonged periods of neutropenia, such as in HSCT patients.

Diagnostic Studies

The primary diagnostic tests for assessing neutropenia are the peripheral WBC count and bone marrow aspiration and biopsy (Table 30-22). A total WBC count of less than 4000/μL (4×10^9/L) reflects leukopenia. However, only a differential count can confirm the presence of neutropenia (neutrophil count less than 1000/μL [1×10^9/L]). If the differential WBC count reflects an absolute neutropenia of 500 to 1000/μL (0.5 to 1.0×10^9/L),

TEAMWORK & COLLABORATION

Caring for the Patient With Neutropenia

All members of the health care team have important roles in preventing infection in the patient with neutropenia. Careful hand washing is an important preventive measure and should be done before, during, and after patient care by everyone caring for the patient.

Role of Nursing Personnel

Registered Nurse (RN)

- Determine the type of isolation precautions that need to be initiated, if any.
- Assess patient for subtle signs of infection such as confusion or fatigue.
- Screen visitors for infectious diseases.
- Communicate with dietary services to eliminate undercooked meats from the patient's diet.
- Instruct patient and visitors about hand washing.
- Teach patient and caregivers about how to avoid infection, including the need for skin care and oral hygiene.
- If the patient is managed as an outpatient, teach the patient and caregivers about signs and symptoms of infection and to report promptly to a health care facility if they occur.

Licensed Practical/Vocational Nurse (LPN/LVN)

- Administer antibiotics and hematopoietic growth factors (consider state nurse practice act and agency policy for IV medications).
- Check the skin, oral mucosa, and perineal area for signs of infection.
- Monitor for signs and symptoms of infection and report them to the RN.

Unlicensed Assistive Personnel (UAP)

- Obtain vital signs and report changes to the RN.
- Assist the patient with oral care and personal hygiene.

TABLE 30-21 Causes of Neutropenia

Drugs*
- Antitumor antibiotics (daunorubicin [Cerubidine], doxorubicin [Adriamycin])
- Alkylating agents (nitrogen mustard, busulfan [Myleran])
- Antimetabolites (methotrexate, 6-mercaptopurine [6-MP], cytarabine)
- Antiinflammatory drugs (phenylbutazone)
- Cardiovascular drugs (captopril [Capoten], procainamide [Pronestyl])
- Diuretics (furosemide [Lasix])
- Miscellaneous (gold, penicillamine)
- Antimicrobial agents (ganciclovir, penicillin G, trimethoprim/sulfamethoxazole [Bactrim])

Hematologic Disorders
- Idiopathic neutropenia
- Congenital (cyclic neutropenia)
- Aplastic anemia
- Fanconi syndrome
- Leukemia
- Myelodysplastic syndrome

Autoimmune Disorders
- Systemic lupus erythematosus
- Felty syndrome
- Rheumatoid arthritis

Infections
- Viral (e.g., hepatitis, influenza, HIV, measles)
- Fulminant bacterial infection (e.g., typhoid fever, miliary tuberculosis)
- Parasitic
- Rickettsial

Others
- Severe sepsis
- Bone marrow infiltration (e.g., carcinoma, tuberculosis, lymphoma)
- Hypersplenism (e.g., portal hypertension, storage diseases [e.g., Gaucher disease])
- Nutritional deficiencies (cobalamin, folic acid)
- Transfusion reaction
- Hemodialysis

*Not all inclusive.

TABLE 30-22 Interprofessional Care

Neutropenia

Diagnostic Assessment
- History and physical examination
- Risk assessment for severity and duration of neutropenia
- WBC count with differential count
- WBC morphology
- Hct and Hgb
- Reticulocyte and platelet count
- Bone marrow aspiration or biopsy
- Cultures of nose, throat, sputum, urine, stool, obvious lesions, blood (as indicated)
- Chest x-ray or other diagnostic tests

Management
- Identification and removal of cause of neutropenia (if possible)
- Identification of site of infection (if present) and causative organism
- Antimicrobial therapy (prophylactically or empiric)*
- Blood cultures drawn STAT, immediately before antibiotics
- Prophylactic hematopoietic growth factors (G-CSF, GM-CSF, pegfilgrastim [Neulasta]) after myelosuppressive chemotherapy
- Strict hand washing
- Patient hygiene (daily skin and frequent oral care; chlorhexidine bathing should be done in the inpatient setting if the patient has a central venous catheter)
- Single-patient room, positive-pressure or high-efficiency particulate air (HEPA) filtration, depending on risk
- Community isolation and home precautions (if outpatient)
  - Nutritional therapy (dietary instruction) on foods to avoid and safe food handling
  - Safe activity and ambulation to maintain physical and pulmonary function

G-CSF, Granulocyte colony-stimulating factor; *GM-CSF*, granulocyte-macrophage colony-stimulating factor.
*Prompt initiation of empiric broad-spectrum antibiotic therapy at any sign of infection, even a low-grade fever (100.4°F [38°C]), is essential.

the patient is at moderate risk for a bacterial infection. An absolute neutropenia of less than 500/μL (0.5×10^9/L) places the patient at severe risk. Note that patients with acute leukemia who present with a high WBC may in fact have neutropenia, because the majority of the WBCs are ineffective leukemia blasts cells.

A peripheral blood smear is used to assess for immature forms of WBCs (e.g., bands). The hematocrit level, reticulocyte count, and platelet count are done to evaluate bone marrow function. Also review the patient's recent past and current drug history. If the cause of neutropenia is unknown, bone marrow aspirations and biopsies are done to examine cellularity and cell morphology. Additional studies may be done as indicated to assess spleen and liver function.

❖ NURSING AND INTERPROFESSIONAL MANAGEMENT: NEUTROPENIA

The factors involved in the nursing and interprofessional care of neutropenia include (1) determining the cause of the neutropenia, (2) instituting antibiotic therapy promptly, (3) identifying the offending organisms if an infection has developed, (4) administering hematopoietic growth factors prophylactically after chemotherapy, and (5) implementing protective practices (e.g., strict hand washing, skin and oral hygiene)[30-32] (Table 30-22).

Occasionally the cause of the neutropenia can be easily treated (e.g., nutritional deficiencies). However, neutropenia can also be a side effect that must be tolerated as a necessary step in therapy (e.g., chemotherapy, radiation therapy). In some situations the neutropenia resolves when the primary disease or disorder is treated.

Monitor the neutropenic patient for signs and symptoms of infection (e.g., any fever 100.4°F [38°C] or greater) and early septic shock. Early identification of a potentially infective organism depends on acquiring cultures from various sites. Serial blood cultures (at least two) or one from a peripheral site and one from a venous access device should be done promptly and antibiotics started immediately (within 1 hour).

Administration of broad-spectrum antibiotics is usually by the IV route because of the rapidly lethal effects of infection. However, some oral antibiotics are highly effective and routinely used for prophylaxis against infection in some neutropenic patients. The use of a third- or fourth-generation cephalosporin with broad microorganism coverage (e.g., cefepime [Maxipime], ceftazidime [Ceptaz]), a carbapenem (e.g., imipenem/cilastatin [Primaxin]), will be initiated and augmented depending on the patient's response and/or results of the diagnostic tests.[30,33]

Regardless of the combination, initiate therapy promptly and observe the patient for side effects of antimicrobial agents. Additionally, ongoing febrile episodes or a change in the patient's assessment requires a call to the HCP for assessment, additional cultures, diagnostic tests, or additional antimicrobial therapies. The longer the neutropenia, the greater the risk of a fungal infection. Antifungal therapy is initiated whenever a culture is positive, or in patients who do not become afebrile with broad-spectrum antibiotic coverage.

Cultures of sputum, throat, lesions, wounds, urine, and feces may also be ordered in the surveillance of the patient. Depending on the clinical situation, it may also be necessary to do CT scans, bronchoscopy with bronchial brushings, or lung biopsy to diagnose the cause of pneumonic infiltrates. Invasive diagnostic studies are often contraindicated because of the concern of introducing infection and the fact that these patients are also often thrombocytopenic. Despite these many tests, the causative organism is identified in only approximately one half of neutropenic patients. Thus the priority is to obtain the blood cultures and administer the antibiotic STAT.

Granulocyte colony-stimulating factor (G-CSF) (filgrastim [Neupogen], pegfilgrastim [Neulasta]), and granulocyte-macrophage colony-stimulating factor (GM-CSF) (sargramostim [Leukine, Prokine]) (see Table 15-15) can be used to prevent neutropenia or to reduce its severity and duration.[34] Once neutropenia has occurred, these agents are generally not as effective. G-CSF stimulates the production and function of neutrophils. GM-CSF stimulates the production and function of neutrophils and monocytes. These agents can be given IV or subcutaneously. Keratinocyte growth factor (palifermin [Kepivance]) may also be used to reduce the duration and severity of mucositis that may contribute to infection. (G-CSF, GM-CSF, and palifermin are discussed in Chapter 15.)

Keep the following care principles in mind: (1) the patient's normal flora is the most common source of microbial colonization and infection; (2) transmission of organisms from humans most commonly occurs by direct contact with the hands; (3) air, food, water, and equipment provide additional opportunities for infection transmission; and (4) HCPs with transmissible illnesses and other patients with infections can also be sources of infection transmission under certain conditions.

Hand washing is the single most important preventive measure to minimize the risk of infection in the neutropenic patient. Strict hand washing by staff and visitors using an antiseptic hand wash, before and after contact, is the major method to prevent transmission of harmful pathogens.

Separate immunocompromised patients from those who are infected or have conditions that increase the probability of transmitting infections (e.g., poor hygiene caused by lack of understanding or cognitive dysfunction). Often patients can be managed on an outpatient basis if the patient and caregiver can astutely monitor for fever and other signs of infection and then report promptly to a nearby health care facility (Table 30-23). If the patient is hospitalized, a private room should be used. High-efficiency particulate air (HEPA) filtration is an air-handling method with a high-flow filtering system that can reduce or eliminate the number of aerosolized pathogens in the environment used for hematopoietic stem cell transplant patients. Care routines in a HEPA environment are essentially the same as care in any other private room. Additional neutropenic precaution guidelines may also be employed, such as prophylactic antibiotics and antifungals. The patient and caregiver should be instructed on a diet that restricts potentially hazardous foods, such as raw and undercooked meats and eggs and soft cheeses with molds. The nursing measures presented in eNursing Care Plan 30-3 (available on the website for this chapter) are important in the treatment of the patient with neutropenia.

Quality-of-life issues for the patient with neutropenia should not be overlooked. Fatigue, malaise, a decrease in functioning, and social isolation require coaching on safe activity.

TABLE 30-23 Patient & Caregiver Teaching

Neutropenia

Include the following instructions when teaching a patient or caregiver the precautions to take when the neutrophil count is low.

1. WASH YOUR HANDS frequently and make sure those around you wash their hands frequently, particularly if they help with your care. An antibacterial hand gel may also be used.
2. Notify your nurse or HCP if you have any of the following:
   - Fever ≥100.4°F (38°C)*
   - Chills or feeling hot
   - Redness, swelling, discharge, or new pain on or in your body
   - Changes in urination or bowel movements
   - Cough, sore throat, mouth sores, or blisters
3. If you are at home, take your temperature as directed and follow instructions on what to do if you have a fever.
4. Avoid crowds and people with colds, flu, or infections. If you are in a public area, wear a mask and use hand sanitizing gel frequently.
5. Avoid uncooked meats, seafood, or eggs and unwashed fruits and vegetables. Ask your HCP about specific dietary guidelines for you.
6. Bathe or shower daily. A moisturizer may be used to prevent skin from drying and cracking.
7. Maintain some daily activity as instructed by your health care team. This may include walking and moderate exercise while avoiding crowds.
8. Brush your teeth with a soft toothbrush four times daily. You may floss once daily if it does not cause excessive pain or bleeding. Avoid alcohol-based mouthwashes.
9. Do not perform gardening or clean up after pets. Feeding and petting your dog or cat are fine as long as you wash your hands well after handling.

*Need to verify cut-off temperature with HCP.

MYELODYSPLASTIC SYNDROME

Myelodysplastic syndrome (MDS) is a group of related hematologic disorders characterized by peripheral blood cytopenias (from ineffective blood cell production) and changes in the cellularity of the bone marrow with dysplastic changes. In MDS, *hematopoiesis* is disorderly and ineffective. It is estimated that the incidence is 4.5 per 100,000 people per year in the United States. Although it can occur in all age groups, the highest prevalence is in people over 80 years of age, at which point the rate increases to 51.5 per 100,000.[35]

Etiology and Pathophysiology

The etiology of MDS is unknown. People who have received radiation therapy, had chemotherapy with alkylating agents (e.g., chlorambucil, cyclophosphamide, melphalan), or have been exposed to industrial solvents (e.g., benzene) have a higher risk of developing MDS than people who have not had these exposures. Rarely, genetic disorders are responsible for the disease. Nevertheless, in 85% of MDS patients, no specific cause can be identified.[36]

INFORMATICS IN PRACTICE

Use of Internet to Access Information on Unfamiliar Diseases

- If you are assigned to take care of a patient with a disease or disorder that you are not familiar with, such as thalassemia, access the Internet and perform a quick search.
- Within minutes, you can learn the pathophysiology of thalassemia, treatment options, possible complications that you will need to monitor, and recommended medical and nursing interventions.
- Using this readily available information will help you deliver high-quality, evidence-based care.

MDS is referred to as a *clonal disorder,* because some bone marrow stem cells continue to function normally, whereas others (a specific clone) do not. The abnormal clone of the stem cells is usually found in the bone marrow but eventually may be found in the circulation.

Occasionally one type of MDS transforms into another. Depending on the subtype, MDS may progress to acute myelogenous leukemia (AML).[36] In contrast to AML, in which the leukemic cells show little normal maturation, the clonal cells in MDS always display some degree of maturity. Disease progression is slower than in AML, and sometimes treatment is not required.

Clinical Manifestations

Manifestations result from neoplastic transformation of the pluripotent hematopoietic stem cells in the bone marrow. MDS commonly manifests as infection and bleeding caused by inadequate numbers of ineffectively functioning circulating granulocytes or platelets. MDS is often discovered in the older adult during testing for the symptoms of anemia, thrombocytopenia, or neutropenia. It may also be diagnosed incidentally from a routine CBC. During the advanced stage of MDS, life-threatening anemia, thrombocytopenia, and neutropenia occur.

Diagnostic Studies

Bone marrow biopsy with aspirate analysis is essential for both the diagnosis and classification of the specific type of myelodysplasia. In MDS the patient has peripheral cytopenia and changes in the bone marrow (hypocellular or hypercellular). Laboratory data and bone marrow studies help rule out other causes of the dysplasia, such as nonmalignant disorders, cobalamin and folate deficiencies, and infections.

❖ NURSING AND INTERPROFESSIONAL MANAGEMENT: MYELODYSPLASTIC SYNDROME

Supportive treatment of MDS is based on the premise that the aggressiveness of treatment should match the aggressiveness of the disease. This is based on the amount and type of dysplasia in the bone marrow as well as genetic mutations.[35] Supportive treatment consists of hematologic monitoring (serial bone marrow and peripheral blood examinations); antibiotic therapy; or transfusions with blood products, along with iron chelators to prevent iron overload.

Low-risk patients can often be treated with erythropoietin and G-CSF. Only about one third of high-risk patients are treated with intensive chemotherapy and/or HSCT. Azacitidine (Vidaza) and decitabine (Dacogen) are drugs that help restore normal growth control and differentiation of hematopoietic cells and reduce the frequency of transformation of MDS to acute leukemia. Side effects include myelosuppression, nausea, vomiting, constipation or diarrhea, renal dysfunction, and injection site erythema.

Lenalidomide (Revlimid) or thalidomide may also be used. Other treatments for MDS include cytarabine (Cytosar, Ara-C) with or without antitumor antibiotics (anthracyclines), antithymocyte globulin, and cyclosporine. Nonmyeloablative (does not suppress bone marrow) chemotherapy and allogeneic HSCT have been used in patients with high-risk features to treat bone marrow dysfunction of MDS and restore it with normal hematopoiesis.

Nursing care of a patient with MDS is similar to that of a patient with manifestations of anemia, thrombocytopenia, and neutropenia. (See eNursing Care Plan 30-1 for the patient with anemia, eNursing Care Plan 30-2 for the patient with thrombocytopenia, and eNursing Care Plan 30-3 for the patient with neutropenia. The eNursing Care Plans are available on the website for this chapter.)

LEUKEMIA

Leukemia is the general term used to describe a group of malignant disorders affecting the blood and blood-forming tissues of the bone marrow, lymph system, and spleen. Leukemia occurs in all age groups. It results in an accumulation of dysfunctional cells because of a loss of regulation in cell division. It follows a progressive course that is eventually fatal if untreated. An estimated 52,380 new cases are diagnosed each year. Although often thought of as a disease of children, leukemia affects approximately 9 times more adults than children.[37]

Etiology and Pathophysiology

Regardless of the specific type, leukemia has no single cause. It is now known that all cancers, including leukemia, begin as a mutation in the DNA of certain cells. Most leukemias result from a combination of factors, including genetic and environmental influences. Abnormal genes *(oncogenes)* are capable of causing many types of cancers, including leukemias (see Chapter 15). Chemical agents (e.g., benzene), chemotherapeutic agents (e.g., alkylating agents), viruses, radiation, and immunologic deficiencies have all been associated with the development of leukemia. The incidence of leukemia is increased in radiologists, persons who have lived near nuclear bomb test sites or nuclear reactor accidents (e.g., Chernobyl), and persons previously treated with radiation therapy or chemotherapy.

Although ribonucleic acid (RNA) retroviruses cause a number of leukemias in animals, a viral cause for a human leukemia has been established only for some patients with adult T-cell leukemia. This form of leukemia is endemic in southwestern Japan and parts of the Caribbean and is caused by the human T-cell leukemia virus type 1 (HTLV-1).[37]

Classification

Leukemia can be classified based on acute versus chronic disease and on the type of WBC involved. The terms *acute* and *chronic* refer to cell maturity and nature of disease onset. Acute leukemia is characterized by the clonal proliferation of immature hematopoietic cells. The leukemia develops after malignant transformation of a single type of immature hematopoietic cell, followed by cellular replication and expansion of that malignant clone. Chronic leukemias involve more mature forms of the WBC, and the disease onset is more gradual.

Leukemia can also be classified by identifying the type of leukocyte involved, whether it is of myelogenous or lymphocytic origin. By combining the acute and chronic categories with the cell type involved, one can identify four major types of leukemia: acute lymphocytic leukemia (ALL), acute myelogenous leukemia (AML), chronic myelogenous (granulocytic) leukemia (CML), and chronic lymphocytic leukemia (CLL).[38-41] Other defining features of these leukemic subtypes are presented in Table 30-24.

Acute Myelogenous Leukemia. AML represents only one fourth of all leukemias, but it makes up approximately 80% of the acute leukemias in adults.[37] Its onset is often abrupt and dramatic. A patient may have serious infections and abnormal bleeding from the onset of the disease.

AML is characterized by uncontrolled proliferation of myeloblasts, the precursors of granulocytes. There is hyperplasia of the bone marrow. The clinical manifestations are usually related to replacement of normal hematopoietic cells in the marrow by leukemic myeloblasts and, to a lesser extent, to infiltration of other organs and tissue (Table 30-24).

Acute Lymphocytic Leukemia. ALL is the most common type of leukemia in children and accounts for about 20% of acute leukemia cases in adults.[37] In ALL, immature small lymphocytes proliferate in the bone marrow; most are of B-cell origin. The majority of patients have fever at the time of diagnosis. Signs and symptoms may appear abruptly with bleeding or fever, or they may be insidious with progressive weakness, fatigue, bone and/or joint pain, and bleeding tendencies.

Central nervous system (CNS) manifestations are especially common in ALL and represent a serious problem. Leukemic meningitis caused by arachnoid infiltration occurs in many patients with ALL.

Chronic Myelogenous Leukemia. CML is caused by excessive development of mature neoplastic granulocytes in the bone marrow. The excess neoplastic granulocytes move into the peripheral blood in massive numbers and ultimately infiltrate the liver and spleen.

The natural history of CML is a chronic stable phase, followed by the development of a more acute, aggressive phase referred to as the *blastic phase.* The chronic phase of CML can last for several years and can usually be well controlled with treatment. Even with treatment, the chronic phase of the disease eventually progresses to the accelerated phase, ending in a blastic phase. Once CML transforms to an acute or blastic phase, it must be treated more aggressively, similar to an acute leukemia.

Genetic Link. The *Philadelphia chromosome* originates from the translocation between the *BCR* gene on chromosome 22 and the *ABL* gene on chromosome 9. The protein that is encoded by the newly created *BCR-ABL* gene on the Philadelphia chromosome interferes with normal cell cycle events, such as the regulation of cell proliferation.

The Philadelphia chromosome, which is present in 90% to 95% of patients with CML, is a diagnostic hallmark of CML. In addition, its presence is an important indicator of residual disease or relapse after treatment. However, the presence of the Philadelphia chromosome is not specific to diagnose CML, since it is also found in ALL and occasionally in AML.

Chronic Lymphocytic Leukemia. CLL is the most common leukemia in adults.[37] CLL is characterized by the production and

TABLE 30-24 Types of Leukemia

Age of Onset	Clinical Manifestations	Diagnostic Findings
Acute Myelogenous Leukemia (AML)		
Accounts for 15%-20% of acute leukemia in children and 80% in adults. Increase in incidence with advancing age after 60 yr	Fatigue and weakness, headache, mouth sores, anemia, bleeding, fever, infection, sternal tenderness, gingival hyperplasia, mild hepatosplenomegaly (one third of patients)	Low RBC count, Hgb, Hct, platelet count. Low to high WBC count with myeloblasts. High LDH. Hypercellular bone marrow with myeloblasts
Acute Lymphocytic Leukemia (ALL)		
Peak prevalence occurs between ages 2 and 5 and after age 50.	Fever, pallor, bleeding, anorexia, fatigue, and weakness. Bone, joint, and abdominal pain. Generalized lymphadenopathy, infections, weight loss, hepatosplenomegaly, headache, mouth sores, neurologic manifestations: CNS involvement, increased intracranial pressure (nausea, vomiting, lethargy, cranial nerve dysfunction) secondary to meningeal infiltration	Low RBC count, Hgb, Hct, platelet count. Low, normal, or high WBC count. High LDH. Transverse lines of rarefaction at ends of metaphysis of long bones on x-ray. Hypercellular bone marrow with lymphoblasts. Lymphoblasts also possible in cerebrospinal fluid. Presence of Philadelphia chromosome (20%-25% of patients)
Chronic Myelogenous Leukemia (CML)		
Increase in incidence with advancing age with median age at diagnosis of 65. Rare in children	No symptoms early in disease. Fatigue and weakness, fever, sternal tenderness, weight loss, joint pain, bone pain, massive splenomegaly, increase in sweating	Low RBC count, Hgb, Hct. High platelet count early, lower count later. ↑ banded neutrophils and myeloblasts and often basophils, normal number of lymphocytes, and normal or low number of monocytes. Nucleated red cells are common. Low leukocyte alkaline phosphatase. Presence of Philadelphia chromosome in 90% of patients
Chronic Lymphocytic Leukemia (CLL)		
Increase in incidence with advancing age after 65 yr, with predominance in men	Frequently no symptoms. Detection of disease often during examination for unrelated condition, chronic fatigue, anorexia, splenomegaly and lymphadenopathy, hepatomegaly. May progress to fever, night sweats, weight loss, fatigue, and frequent infections	Mild anemia and thrombocytopenia with disease progression. Total WBC count >100,000/μL. Increase in peripheral lymphocytes and lymphocytes in bone marrow. May have autoimmune hemolytic anemia, idiopathic thrombocytopenic purpura, and hypogammaglobulinemia

LDH, Lactate dehydrogenase.

accumulation of functionally inactive but long-lived, small, mature-appearing lymphocytes. B cells are usually involved. The lymphocytes infiltrate the bone marrow, spleen, and liver. Lymph node enlargement (lymphadenopathy) is present throughout the body.

Complications are rare in early stage CLL but may develop as the disease advances. Pressure on nerves from enlarged lymph nodes causes pain and even paralysis. Mediastinal node enlargement leads to pulmonary symptoms. Because CLL is usually a disease of older adults, treatment decisions must be made by considering the progression of the disease and the side effects of treatment. Many individuals in the early stages of CLL require no treatment. Others may be followed closely and receive treatment only when the disease progresses. Approximately one third require immediate intervention at the time of diagnosis.

Other Leukemias. Occasionally the subtype of leukemia cannot be identified. The malignant leukemic cells may have lymphoid, myeloid, or mixed characteristics. Frequently these patients do not respond to treatment and have a poor prognosis. Other rare types include hairy cell and biphenotypic (both abnormal myeloid and lymphoid clones) leukemias.

Overlap Between Leukemia and Lymphoma. Overlap exists between leukemia and non-Hodgkin's lymphoma (NHL) because both involve proliferation of lymphocytes or their precursors. A leukemia-like picture with peripheral lymphocytosis and bone marrow involvement may be present in about 20% of adults with some types of NHL. Although differentiation can be difficult, generally patients with more extensive nodal involvement (especially mediastinal), fewer circulating abnormal cells, and fewer blast forms in the marrow are considered to have lymphoma. A prominent leukemic phase is less common in aggressive lymphomas, except Burkitt's and lymphoblastic lymphomas.[42]

Clinical Manifestations

Although the clinical manifestations of leukemia are varied (Table 30-24), they relate to problems caused by bone marrow failure and the formation of leukemic infiltrates (Fig. 30-12). Bone marrow failure results from (1) bone marrow overcrowding by abnormal cells and (2) inadequate production of normal marrow elements. The patient is predisposed to anemia, thrombocytopenia, and decreased number and function of WBCs.

As leukemia progresses, fewer normal blood cells are produced. The abnormal WBCs continue to accumulate because they do not go through the normal cell life cycle to death *(apoptosis)*. The leukemic cells may infiltrate the patient's organs, leading to problems such as splenomegaly, hepatomegaly, lymphadenopathy, bone pain, meningeal irritation, and oral lesions. Solid masses resulting from collections of leukemic cells called *chloromas* can also occur. A high leukemic white count in the peripheral blood (more than 100,000 cells/μL) can cause the blood to thicken and potentially block circulatory pathways. This is called *leukostasis* and can be life threatening.

Diagnostic Studies

Peripheral blood evaluation and bone marrow examination are the primary methods of diagnosing and classifying the types of leukemia. Morphologic, histochemical, immunologic, and cytogenetic methods are all used to identify leukemic cell types and stage of development. Identifying the type of leukemia is important because the various types have different prognoses and

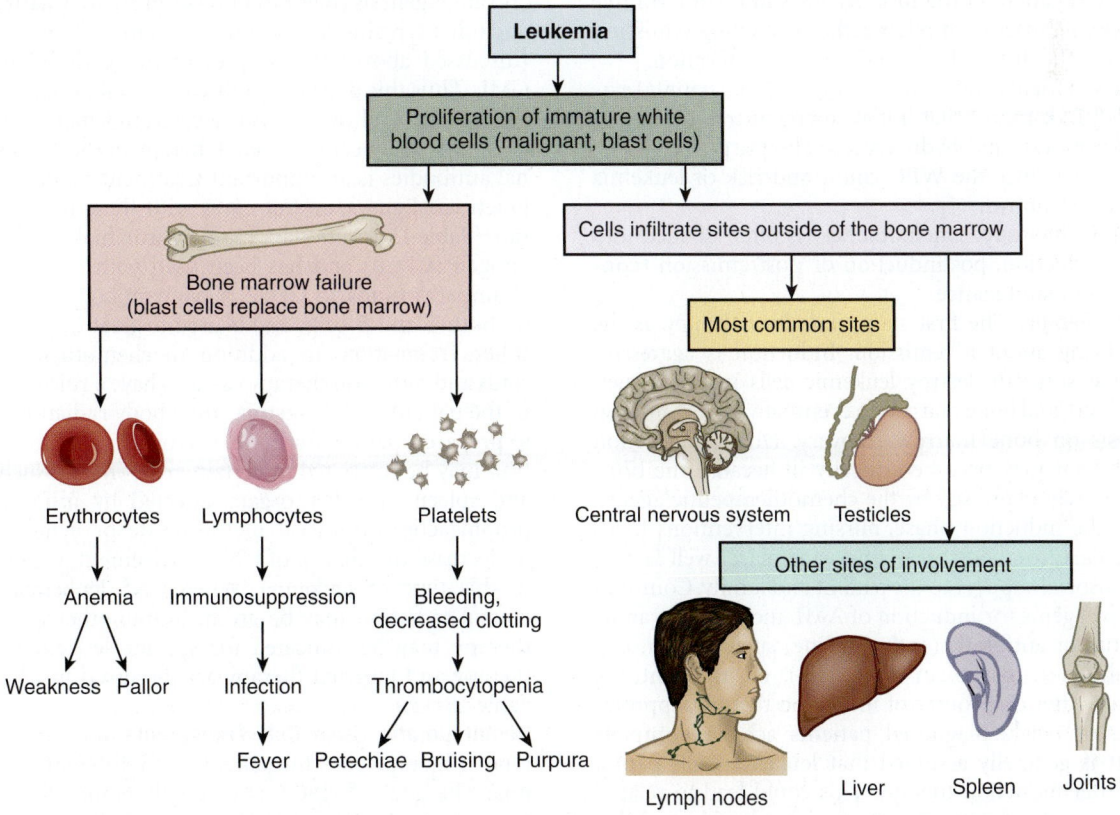

FIG. 30-12 Pathophysiology of leukemia. (Modified from McKinney ES, James SR, Murray SS, Nelson K: *Maternal-child nursing,* Philadelphia, 2000, Saunders.)

chemotherapeutic regimens. Other studies such as lumbar puncture and CT scan can detect leukemic cells outside of the blood and bone marrow.

The malignant cells in most patients with leukemia have specific cytogenetic abnormalities that are associated with distinct subsets of the disease. These cytogenetic abnormalities have diagnostic, prognostic, and therapeutic importance. For example, in CML, the finding of the Philadelphia chromosome is an important diagnostic indicator.

Interprofessional Care

Once a diagnosis of leukemia has been made, care is focused on the initial goal of attaining remission. Age and cytogenetic analysis often help form the basis of important treatment decisions. Because chemotherapy is the mainstay of the treatment, you need to understand the principles of cancer chemotherapy. (See the section on chemotherapy in Chapter 15.)

In some cases, such as nonsymptomatic patients with CLL, watchful waiting with active supportive care may be appropriate. Although a patient may not be cured, attaining remission or disease control is a realistic option for the majority of patients. In some cases, cure is a realistic goal. In *complete remission* there is no evidence of overt disease on physical examination, and the bone marrow and peripheral blood appear normal. A lesser state of control is known as partial remission. *Minimal residual disease* is defined as tumor cells that cannot be detected by morphologic examination but can be identified by molecular testing. *Partial remission* is characterized by a lack of symptoms and a normal peripheral blood smear but still evidence of disease in the bone marrow. *Molecular remission* indicates that all molecular studies are negative for residual leukemia. The patient's prognosis is directly related to the ability to maintain a remission. The patient's prognosis becomes more unfavorable with each relapse. After each relapse, the succeeding remission may be more difficult to achieve and shorter in duration.

Sometimes patients have such a high WBC count (e.g., 100,000 cells/μL or more) that initial emergent treatment may include leukapheresis and hydroxyurea. The purpose of these treatments is to reduce the WBC count and risk of leukemia cell–induced thrombosis.

Stages of Chemotherapy. Chemotherapy is often divided into three stages: induction, postinduction or postremission (consolidation), and maintenance.

Induction Therapy. The first stage, *induction therapy,* is the attempt to bring about a remission. Induction is aggressive treatment that seeks to destroy leukemic cells in the tissues, peripheral blood, and bone marrow to eventually restore normal hematopoiesis on bone marrow recovery. During induction therapy, a patient may become critically ill because the bone marrow is severely depressed by the chemotherapeutic agents. Throughout the induction phase, nursing interventions focus on neutropenia, thrombocytopenia, and anemia, as well as providing psychosocial support to the patient and family. Common chemotherapy agents for induction of AML include cytarabine and an antitumor antibiotic (anthracycline) such as daunorubicin (Cerubidine), idarubicin (Idamycin), or mitoxantrone (Novantrone). After one course of induction therapy, approximately 70% of newly diagnosed patients achieve complete remission. It is generally assumed that leukemic cells persist undetected after induction therapy. This could lead to relapse within a few months if no further therapy is administered.[38]

Postinduction or Postremission Therapy. Terms used to describe postinduction or postremission chemotherapy include *intensification* and *consolidation. Intensification therapy,* or high-dose therapy, may be given immediately after induction therapy for several months. Other drugs that target the cell in a different way than those administered during induction may also be added.

Consolidation therapy is started after a remission is achieved. It may consist of one or two additional courses of the same drugs given during induction or involve high-dose therapy (intensive consolidation). The purpose of consolidation therapy is to eliminate remaining leukemic cells that may not be clinically or pathologically evident.

Maintenance Therapy. *Maintenance therapy* is treatment with lower doses of the same drugs used in induction or other drugs given every 3 to 4 weeks for a prolonged period. Like consolidation or intensification, the goal is to keep the body free of leukemic cells. Each type of leukemia requires different maintenance therapy. In AML, maintenance therapy is rarely effective and therefore rarely administered.

Drug Therapy Regimens. The therapeutic agents used to treat leukemia vary. Table 30-25 gives examples of treatment regimens used in various types of leukemia.[16,42-45]

Combination therapy is the mainstay of treatment for leukemia. The three purposes for using multiple drugs are to (1) decrease drug resistance, (2) minimize the drug toxicity to the patient by using multiple drugs with varying toxicities, and (3) interrupt cell growth at multiple points in the cell cycle.

Some therapeutic drugs are aimed at small molecules that promote the growth and differentiation of leukemic cells. For example, arsenic trioxide (Trisenox), which is used to treat acute promyelocytic leukemia (a type of AML), causes DNA fragmentation and cell death. In addition, it inhibits cell proliferation and angiogenesis (new blood vessel growth). Imatinib (Gleevec) and other tyrosine-kinase inhibitors target the *BCR-ABL* protein (discussed above) that is present in nearly all patients with CML. Thus this drug kills only cancer cells, leaving healthy cells alone. (Targeted therapy is discussed in Chapter 15.)

The use of specific targeted therapy in the form of monoclonal antibodies is an important treatment modality in hematopoietic malignancies, but cures with these therapies alone are rare (Table 15-13 and Fig. 15-16). Rituximab binds to the B-cell antigen (CD20) and has been used with CLL. Alemtuzumab (Campath) binds to CD52, a panlymphocyte antigen present on both T and B cells, and is used to treat CLL.

Other Treatments. In addition to chemotherapy, corticosteroids and radiation therapy can also have a role in the treatment of the patient with leukemia. Total body radiation may be used to prepare a patient for bone marrow transplantation, or radiation may be restricted to certain areas (fields) such as the liver and spleen or other organs affected by infiltrates. In ALL, prophylactic intrathecal methotrexate or cytarabine is given to decrease the chance of CNS involvement, which is common in this type of leukemia. When CNS leukemia does occur, cranial radiation may be given. Immunotherapy and targeted therapy may be indicated for specific leukemias. (Immunotherapy and targeted therapy are discussed in Chapter 15 and Table 15-13.)

Hematopoietic Stem Cell Transplantation. HSCT is another type of therapy used for patients with different forms of leukemia. The goal of HSCT is to totally eliminate leukemic cells from the body using combinations of chemotherapy with or without total body irradiation. This treatment also eradicates the patient's hematopoietic stem cells, which are then replaced with those of an HLA-matched sibling or volunteer donor *(allogeneic)* or an identical twin *(syngeneic)*, or with the patient's own *(autologous)* stem cells that were removed (harvested) before the intensive therapy. (HSCT is discussed in Chapter 15.)

The primary complications for patients with allogeneic HSCT are graft-versus-host disease (GVHD), relapse of leukemia (especially ALL), and infection (especially interstitial pneumonia). GVHD is discussed in Chapter 13. Because HSCT has serious associated risks, the patient must weigh the significant risks of treatment-related death or treatment failure (relapse) with the hope of cure.

TABLE 30-25 Drug Therapy

Leukemia*

Drug Therapy	Other Therapy
Acute Myelogenous Leukemia	
cytarabine (Cytosar),† daunorubicin (Cerubidine),† idarubicin, mitoxantrone, arsenic trioxide (Trisenox),† tretinoin,† clofarabine (Clolar), decitabine (Dacogen), fludarabine, azacitidine (Vidaza) Combination chemotherapy of cytarabine and antitumor antibiotic (most common)	Autologous or allogeneic hematopoietic stem cell transplant (HSCT) (see Chapter 15)
Acute Lymphocytic Leukemia	
daunorubicin, doxorubicin, vincristine, prednisone, dexamethasone, L-asparaginase (Elspar), ponatinib (Iclusig), pegaspargase (Oncaspar), dasatinib (Sprycel), cyclophosphamide, methotrexate, 6-mercaptopurine, cytarabine, nelarabine (Arranon), imatinib (Gleevec), clofarabine (Clolar), blinatumomab (Blincyto), rituximab (Rituxan) Combination chemotherapy of several agents is common over a prolonged time	Cranial radiation therapy, intrathecal methotrexate or cytarabine, allogeneic HSCT (see Chapter 15)
Chronic Myelogenous Leukemia	
bosutinib (Bosulif), imatinib (Gleevec), dasatinib (Sprycel), nilotinib (Tasigna), omacetaxine (Synribo), ponatinib (Iclusig), hydroxyurea (Hydrea) Combination chemotherapy including any of the following: cytarabine, daunorubicin, methotrexate, prednisone, vincristine, L-asparaginase, 6-mercaptopurine, busulfan (Myleran)	Radiation, HSCT, α-interferon, leukapheresis
Chronic Lymphocytic Leukemia	
chlorambucil (Leukeran), cyclophosphamide, prednisone, vincristine, fludarabine, rituximab (Rituxan), alemtuzumab (Campath), pentostatin (Nipent), bendamustine (Treanda), oxaliplatin (Eloxatin), methotrexate, ofatumumab (Arzerra), idelalisib (Zydelig), obinutuzumab (Gazyva), ibrutinib (Imbruvica), lenalidomide (Revlimid), venetoclax (Venclexta)	Radiation, splenectomy, colony-stimulating factors, allogeneic HSCT

*The classification and mechanisms of action of these drugs are presented in Table 15-7.
†Used for acute promyelocytic leukemia.

❖ NURSING MANAGEMENT: LEUKEMIA

◆ Nursing Assessment

Subjective and objective data that should be obtained from a patient with leukemia are presented in Table 30-26.

TABLE 30-26 Nursing Assessment

Leukemia

Subjective Data

Important Health Information

Past health history: Exposure to chemical toxins (e.g., benzene, arsenic), radiation, or viruses (Epstein-Barr, HTLV-1); chromosome abnormalities (Down syndrome, Klinefelter syndrome, Fanconi syndrome), immunologic deficiencies; organ transplantation; frequent infections; bleeding tendencies
Medications: Chemotherapy
Surgery or other treatments: Radiation exposure; prior radiation and chemotherapy for cancer

Functional Health Patterns

Health perception–health management: Family history of leukemia; malaise
Nutritional-metabolic: Mouth sores, weight loss; chills, night sweats; nausea, vomiting, anorexia, dysphagia, early satiety; easy bruising
Elimination: Hematuria, decreased urine output; diarrhea, dark or bloody stools
Activity-exercise: Fatigue with progressive weakness; dyspnea, epistaxis, cough
Cognitive-perceptual: Headache; muscle cramps; sore throat; generalized sternal tenderness, bone, joint, abdominal pain; paresthesias, numbness, tingling, visual disturbances
Sexuality-reproductive: Prolonged menses, menorrhagia, metrorrhagia, impotence

Objective Data

General

Fever, generalized lymphadenopathy, lethargy

Integumentary

Pallor or jaundice; petechiae, ecchymoses, purpura, reddish brown to purple cutaneous infiltrates, macules, and papules

Cardiovascular

Tachycardia, systolic murmurs

Gastrointestinal

Gingival bleeding and hyperplasia; oral ulcerations, herpes and *Candida* infections; perirectal irritation and infection; hepatomegaly, splenomegaly

Neurologic

Seizures, disorientation, confusion, decreased coordination, cranial nerve palsies, papilledema

Musculoskeletal

Muscle wasting, bone pain, joint pain

Possible Diagnostic Findings

Low, normal, or high WBC count with shift to the left (↑ blast cells) and neutropenia; anemia, ↓ hematocrit and hemoglobin, thrombocytopenia, Philadelphia chromosome; hypercellular bone marrow aspirate or biopsy with myeloblasts, lymphoblasts, and markedly ↓ normal cells

HTLV-1, Human T-cell leukemia virus, type 1.

Nursing Diagnoses

Nursing diagnoses for the patient with leukemia include those for anemia (see p. 608), thrombocytopenia (see p. 625), and neutropenia (see eNursing Care Plan 30-3, available on the website).

Planning

The overall goals are that the patient with leukemia will (1) understand and adhere to the treatment plan; (2) experience minimal side effects and complications associated with both the disease and its treatment; and (3) establish realistic hope and goals, feeling supported during periods of treatment, relapse, or remission.

Nursing Implementation

Acute Care. The nursing role during acute phases of leukemia is extremely challenging because the patient has many physical and psychosocial needs. As with other forms of cancer, the diagnosis of leukemia can evoke great fear and be equated with death. It may be viewed as a hopeless, horrible disease with many painful and undesirable consequences. The treatment and prognosis of each patient with leukemia are driven by many factors, such as age and type of leukemia. Therefore you must understand the patient's type of leukemia, prognosis, treatment plan, and goals. By doing this, you can help the patient realize that, although the future may be uncertain, one can have a meaningful quality of life while in remission or with disease control, and that, in some cases, there is reasonable hope for cure.

The family also needs help adjusting to the stress of this abrupt onset of serious illness and the losses imposed by the sick role (e.g., dependence, withdrawal, changes in role responsibilities, alterations in body image). The diagnosis of leukemia often brings with it the need to make difficult decisions at a time of profound stress for the patient and family.

Patients may have co-morbid conditions that affect treatment decisions. Important nursing interventions include (1) maximizing the patient's physical functioning, (2) teaching patients that acute side effects of treatment are usually temporary, and (3) encouraging patients to discuss their quality-of-life issues. You are an important advocate in helping the patient and family understand the complexities of treatment decisions and manage the side effects and toxicities. A patient may require a long hospitalization or may need to temporarily relocate to an appropriate treatment center. This situation can lead a patient to feel deserted and isolated at a time when support is most needed. You have contact with a patient many hours a day and can help reverse feelings of abandonment and loneliness by balancing the demanding technical needs with a humanistic, caring approach. The needs of the patient with leukemia are best met by an interprofessional team (e.g., psychiatric and oncology clinical nurse specialists, case managers, dietitians, chaplains, and social workers).

From a physical care perspective, you are challenged to make astute assessments and plan care to help the patient manage the severe side effects of chemotherapy. The life-threatening results of bone marrow suppression (neutropenia, thrombocytopenia, and anemia) require aggressive nursing interventions. These patients may be at risk for oncologic emergencies such as tumor lysis syndrome, DIC, and leukostasis. Additional complications of chemotherapy may affect the patient's GI tract, nutritional status, skin and mucosa, cardiopulmonary status, liver, kidneys, and neurologic system. (Nursing interventions related to chemotherapy are discussed in Chapter 15.)

Review all drugs being administered, including the mechanism of action, purpose, routes of administration, usual doses, potential side effects, safe handling considerations, and toxic effects. Assess laboratory data reflecting the effects of the drugs and sequelae of the disease. Unlike treatments for solid tumors, chemotherapy is administered to patients with leukemia even if they have severe myelosuppression, since the underlying disorder is causing the problem and will not resolve unless treated. Patient survival and comfort during aggressive chemotherapy are significantly affected by the quality of nursing care.

Ambulatory Care. Ongoing care for the patient with leukemia is necessary to monitor for signs and symptoms of disease control or relapse. For a patient requiring long-term or maintenance chemotherapy, the fatigue of long-term chronic disease management can become discouraging. Therefore teach the patient and caregiver the importance of continued diligence in disease management and the need for follow-up care. Also teach them about the drugs, self-care measures, and when to seek medical attention.

The goals of rehabilitation for long-term survivors of leukemia are to manage the physical, psychologic, social, and spiritual consequences and delayed effects from the disease and its treatment. (Delayed effects are discussed in Chapter 15.) Assistance may be needed to reestablish the various relationships that are a part of the patient's life. Involving the patient in survivor networks and support groups or services may help the patient adapt to living after a life-threatening illness. Exploring resources in the community (e.g., American Cancer Society, Leukemia & Lymphoma Society) may reduce the financial burden and the feelings of dependence. Also provide the resources for spiritual support.

Vigilant follow-up care helps to ensure that the cancer survivor's unique needs are recognized and treated. Often these needs may require a referral or consultation. For example, physical therapy personnel may be asked to develop an exercise program to prevent posttreatment deficits caused by drug-induced peripheral neuropathy. Most patients should receive a pneumococcal vaccine and an annual influenza vaccine.[30] These needs can also include other concerns such as vocational retraining and reproductive concerns for a patient of childbearing age.

Evaluation

The expected outcomes are that the patient with leukemia will

- Cope effectively with the diagnosis, treatment regimen, and prognosis
- Experience no complications related to the disease or its treatment
- Feel comfortable and supported throughout treatment

LYMPHOMAS

Lymphomas are malignant neoplasms originating in the bone marrow and lymphatic structures resulting in the proliferation of lymphocytes. Lymphomas make up 4% of all cancers in the United States.[37] Two major types of lymphoma are Hodgkin's lymphoma and non-Hodgkin's lymphoma (NHL). A comparison of these two types of lymphoma is presented in Table 30-27.

HODGKIN'S LYMPHOMA

Hodgkin's lymphoma, also called *Hodgkin's disease*, makes up about 11% of all lymphomas. It is a malignant condition

TABLE 30-27 Comparison of Hodgkin's and Non-Hodgkin's Lymphoma

	Hodgkin's Lymphoma	Non-Hodgkin's Lymphoma
Cellular origin	B lymphocytes	B lymphocytes (88%) T or natural killer lymphocytes (12%)
Extent of disease	Localized to regional, but may be more widespread	Disseminated
B symptoms*	Common	Uncommon
Extranodal involvement	Rare	Common

*B symptoms include fever (>100.4°F [38°C]), drenching night sweats, and weight loss (>10% from baseline within 6 mo).

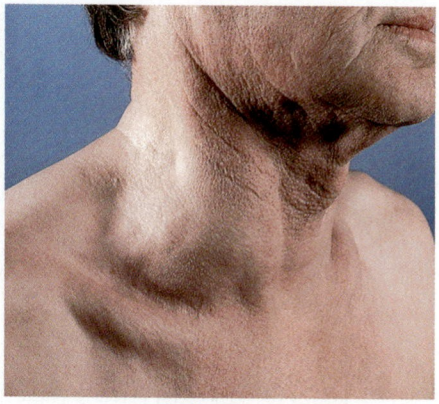

FIG. 30-13 Enlarged cervical lymph node in the neck of a man with Hodgkin lymphoma. (From Howard MR, Hamilton PJ: *Haematology: an illustrated colour atlas,* ed 4, London, 2013, Churchill Livingston.)

characterized by proliferation of abnormal giant, multinucleated cells, called *Reed-Sternberg cells,* which are located in lymph nodes. The disease has a bimodal age-specific incidence, occurring most frequently in persons from 15 to 30 years of age and above 55 years of age.[46] In adults, it is twice as prevalent in men as in women. Each year, approximately 9190 new cases of Hodgkin's lymphoma are diagnosed and approximately 1100 deaths occur. However, long-term survival exceeds 80% for all stages.[47]

Etiology and Pathophysiology

Although the cause of Hodgkin's lymphoma remains unknown, several key factors are thought to play a role in its development. The main interacting factors include infection with Epstein-Barr virus (EBV), genetic predisposition, and exposure to occupational toxins. The incidence of Hodgkin's lymphoma is increased in patients who have HIV infection.

Normally, the lymph nodes are composed of connective tissues that surround a fine mesh of reticular fibers and cells. In Hodgkin's lymphoma the normal structure of lymph nodes is destroyed by hyperplasia of monocytes and macrophages. The main diagnostic feature of Hodgkin's lymphoma is the presence of Reed-Sternberg cells in lymph node biopsy specimens. The disease is believed to arise in a single location (it originates in cervical lymph nodes in 80% of patients) and then spreads along adjacent lymphatics. However, in recurrent disease, it may be more diffuse and not necessarily contiguous. It eventually infiltrates other organs, especially lungs, spleen, and liver. When the disease begins above the diaphragm, it remains confined to lymph nodes for a variable time. Disease originating below the diaphragm frequently spreads to extralymphoid sites such as the liver.

Clinical Manifestations

The onset of symptoms in Hodgkin's lymphoma is usually insidious. The initial development is most often enlargement of cervical, axillary, or inguinal lymph nodes (Fig. 30-13); a mediastinal node mass is the second most common location. This lymphadenopathy affects discrete nodes that remain movable and nontender. The enlarged nodes are not painful unless they exert pressure on adjacent nerves.

The patient may notice weight loss, fatigue, weakness, fever, chills, tachycardia, or night sweats. A group of initial findings including fever (in excess of 100.4°F [38°C]), drenching night sweats, and weight loss (exceeding 10% in 6 months) are termed *B symptoms* and correlate with a worse prognosis. After the ingestion of even small amounts of alcohol, individuals with Hodgkin's lymphoma may complain of a rapid onset of pain at the site of disease. The cause for the alcohol-induced pain is unknown. Generalized pruritus without skin lesions may develop. Cough, dyspnea, stridor, and dysphagia may all reflect mediastinal node involvement.

In more advanced disease, there may be hepatomegaly and splenomegaly. Anemia results from increased destruction and decreased production of erythrocytes. Other physical signs vary depending on where the disease is located. For example, intrathoracic involvement may lead to superior vena cava syndrome, enlarged retroperitoneal nodes may cause palpable abdominal masses or interfere with renal function, jaundice may occur from liver involvement, spinal cord compression leading to paraplegia may occur with extradural involvement, and bone pain occurs as a result of bone involvement.

Diagnostic and Staging Studies

Peripheral blood analysis, excisional lymph node biopsy, bone marrow examination, and radiologic studies are important means of evaluating Hodgkin's lymphoma. Abnormalities in the CBC, such as a microcytic hypochromic anemia, are variable and not diagnostic. Leukopenia and thrombocytopenia may develop, but they are usually a consequence of treatment, advanced disease, or superimposed hypersplenism. Other blood studies may show elevated erythrocyte sedimentation rate, elevated leukocyte alkaline phosphatase from liver and bone involvement, hypercalcemia from bone involvement, and hypoalbuminemia from liver involvement.

Radiologic evaluation can help define all sites and determine the clinical stage of the disease. Positron emission tomography (PET) with CT scan is used to stage and then assess the response to therapy and to differentiate residual tumor from fibrotic masses after treatment. These scans may show increased uptake (by PET) and masses (by CT) such as mediastinal lymphadenopathy; renal displacement caused by retroperitoneal node enlargement; abdominal lymph node enlargement; and liver, spleen, bone, and brain infiltration.

❖ NURSING AND INTERPROFESSIONAL MANAGEMENT: HODGKIN'S LYMPHOMA

Using all of the information from the various diagnostic studies, one can determine a clinical stage of disease (Fig. 30-14). The

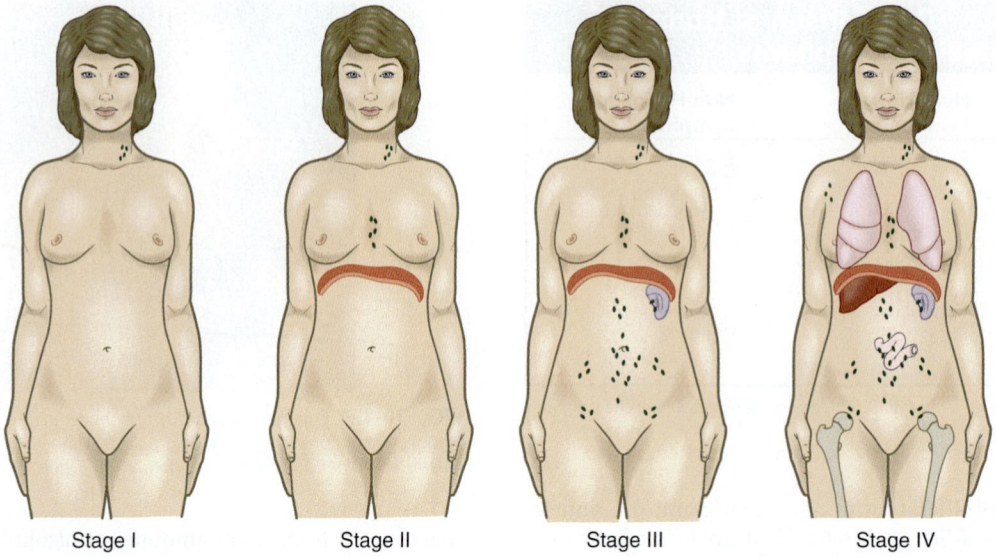

FIG. 30-14 Staging system for Hodgkin's lymphoma and non-Hodgkin's lymphoma. *Stage I,* involvement of single lymph node (e.g., cervical node). *Stage II,* involvement of two or more lymph nodes on one side of diaphragm. *Stage III,* lymph node involvement above and below the diaphragm. *Stage IV,* involvement outside of diaphragm (e.g., liver, bone marrow). The stage is followed by the letter *A* (absence) or *B* (presence) to indicate significant systemic symptoms (e.g., fever, night sweats, weight loss).

final staging is based on the clinical stage (extent of the disease), presence of B symptom, and other unfavorable prognostic features. Treatment depends on the nature and extent of the disease. The nomenclature used in staging involves an A or B classification, depending on whether symptoms are present when the disease is found, and a Roman numeral (I to IV) that reflects the location and extent of the disease.[46,47]

Once the stage of Hodgkin's lymphoma is established, management focuses on selecting a treatment plan. The standard for chemotherapy is the ABVD regimen: doxorubicin (**A**driamycin), **b**leomycin, **v**inblastine, and **d**acarbazine. Patients with favorable early stage disease receive two to four cycles of chemotherapy. Patients with early stage disease but unfavorable prognostic features (e.g., B symptoms) or intermediate-stage disease are treated with four to six cycles of chemotherapy. Advanced-stage Hodgkin's lymphoma is treated more aggressively using six to eight cycles of chemotherapy. A common regimen is BEACOPP (**b**leomycin, **e**toposide, doxorubicin (**A**driamycin), **c**yclophosphamide, vincristine (**O**ncovin), **p**rocarbazine, and **p**rednisone).[46,47] The role of radiation as a supplement to chemotherapy varies depending on sites of disease and the presence of resistant disease after chemotherapy. Response to therapy is determined by PET and CT scans and other diagnostic tests (e.g., bone marrow biopsy).

A variety of chemotherapy regimens and newer agents, such as brentuximab vedotin (Adcetris), are used to treat patients who have relapsed or refractory disease. Ideally, once remission is obtained, a hope for curative option may be intensive chemotherapy with the use of autologous or allogeneic HSCT.[46] HSCT has allowed patients to receive higher, potentially curative doses of chemotherapy while reducing life-threatening leukopenia (see Chapter 15). Combination chemotherapy works well because, as in leukemia, the drugs used have an additive antitumor effect without increasing side effects. As with leukemia, therapy must be aggressive. Therefore potentially life-threatening problems are encountered in an attempt to achieve a remission.

Maintenance chemotherapy does not contribute to increased survival once a complete remission is achieved. Occasionally, single drugs may be administered palliatively to patients who cannot tolerate intensive combination therapy. A serious consequence of the treatment for Hodgkin's lymphoma is the later development of secondary malignancies (see Chapter 15), as well as potential long-term toxicities from the treatment, such as endocrine, cardiac, and pulmonary dysfunction.[47] Secondary cancers occur 10 years after treatment for Hodgkin's lymphoma. The most common secondary malignancies are lung and breast cancer. Patients should have close follow-up and screening for early detection of these problems.[46]

The nursing care for Hodgkin's lymphoma is largely based on managing problems related to the disease (e.g., pain caused by a tumor, superior vena cava syndrome), pancytopenia, and other side effects of therapy. Because the survival of patients with Hodgkin's lymphoma depends on their response to treatment, supporting the patient through the consequences of treatment is extremely important.

Psychosocial considerations are as important as they are with leukemia. However, the prognosis for Hodgkin's lymphoma is better than that for many forms of cancer. The physical, psychologic, social, and spiritual consequences of the patient's disease must be addressed. Fertility issues may be of particular concern because this disease is frequently seen in adolescents and young adults. Help to ensure that these issues have been addressed soon after diagnosis. Evaluation of patients for long-term effects of therapy is important because delayed consequences of disease and treatment may not be apparent for many years. (Secondary malignancies and delayed effects are discussed in Chapter 15.)

NON-HODGKIN'S LYMPHOMA

Non-Hodgkin's lymphomas (NHLs) are a heterogeneous group of malignant neoplasms of primarily B-, T-, or natural killer (NK) cell origin affecting all ages. B-cell lymphomas

EVIDENCE-BASED PRACTICE

Applying the Evidence

Exercise and Hematologic Cancer

You are a nurse caring for G.R., a 59-year-old male patient with non-Hodgkin's lymphoma who is receiving chemotherapy. Due to a decrease in red blood cells and platelets, he was advised to rest and avoid the high level of physical exercise he once enjoyed. He misses his active lifestyle and now admits to you that he is "somewhat depressed."

Making Clinical Decisions

Best Available Evidence. Aerobic exercise, especially walking and stretching, to maintain mobility may improve physical functioning, fatigue, and depression in patients with hematologic cancers.

Clinician Expertise. You know recommendations to decrease intensive physical exercise may result in a diminished quality of life for many patients, especially for individuals who are used to being physically active.

Patient Preferences and Values. G.R. is considering joining a neighborhood bicycling club so that he can "feel better."

Implications for Nursing Practice

1. Why is intensive or extreme exercise contraindicated in someone who is getting chemotherapy or acutely ill?
2. What precautions would you discuss with G.R. before he increases his exercise level?
3. How would you involve G.R. in monitoring his fatigue?
4. As G.R. seeks ways to improve his quality of life, how would you support him?

Reference for Evidence

Bergenthal N, Will A, Streckmann F, et al: Aerobic physical exercise for adult patients with haematological malignancies, *Cochrane Database Syst Rev* 11:CD009075, 2014.

constitute about 88% of all NHLs. They are categorized by the level of differentiation, cell of origin, and rate of cellular proliferation.[42,48] A variety of clinical presentations and courses are recognized, from indolent (slowly developing) to rapidly progressive disease. NHL is the most commonly occurring hematologic cancer and is responsible for 3% of cancer-related deaths. Each year approximately 70,800 new cases of NHL are diagnosed and approximately 18,990 deaths occur.[37]

Etiology and Pathophysiology

As with Hodgkin's lymphoma, the cause of NHL is usually unknown. NHLs may result from chromosomal translocations, infections, environmental factors, and immunodeficiency states. Chromosomal translocations have an important role in the pathogenesis of many NHLs. Some viruses and bacteria are implicated in the pathogenesis of NHL, including HTLV-1, EBV, human herpesvirus 8, hepatitis B and C, *Helicobacter pylori*, *Chlamydophila psittaci*, *Campylobacter jejuni*, and *Borrelia burgdorferi*. Environmental factors linked to the development of NHL include chemicals (e.g., pesticides, herbicides, solvents, organic chemicals, wood preservatives). NHL is also more common in individuals who have inherited immunodeficiency syndromes and who have used immunosuppressive medications (e.g., to prevent rejection after an organ transplant or to treat autoimmune disorders) or received chemotherapy or radiation therapy.

NHL does not have a hallmark feature that parallels the Reed-Sternberg cell of Hodgkin's lymphoma. However, all NHLs involve lymphocytes arrested in various stages of

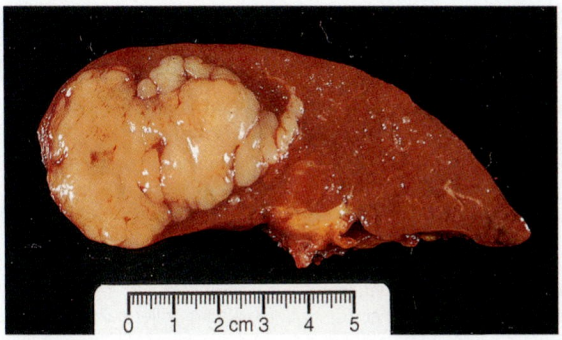

FIG. 30-15 Non-Hodgkin's lymphoma involving the spleen. The presence of an isolated mass is typical. (From Cotran RS, Kumar V, Abbas AK: *Robbins pathologic basis of disease*, ed 6, Philadelphia, 1999, Saunders.)

development and may mimic a leukemia. For example, small lymphocytic lymphoma (SLL) and chronic lymphocytic leukemia (CLL) result from malignant proliferation of small B lymphocytes, with CLL having the majority of disease within the bone marrow (versus the lymph nodes).[42] (The overlap among leukemia and NHLs is discussed on p. 637.)

Diffuse large B-cell lymphoma, the most common aggressive lymphoma, is a neoplasm that originates in the lymph nodes, usually in the neck or abdomen. Burkitt's lymphoma is the most highly aggressive disease and is thought to originate from B-cell blasts in the lymph nodes.

Clinical Manifestations

NHLs can originate outside the lymph nodes, the method of spread can be unpredictable, and the majority of patients have widely disseminated disease at the time of diagnosis (Fig. 30-15). The primary clinical manifestation is painless lymph node enlargement. The lymphadenopathy can wax and wane in indolent disease. Because the disease is usually disseminated when it is diagnosed, other symptoms are present depending on where the disease has spread (e.g., hepatomegaly with liver involvement, neurologic symptoms with CNS disease). NHL can also manifest in nonspecific ways, such as an airway obstruction, hyperuricemia and renal failure from tumor lysis syndrome, pericardial tamponade, and GI complaints.

Patients with high-grade lymphomas may have lymphadenopathy and constitutional symptoms (B symptoms) such as fever, night sweats, and weight loss. The peripheral blood is usually normal, but some lymphomas manifest in a "leukemic" phase.

Diagnostic and Staging Studies

Diagnostic studies used for NHL resemble those used for Hodgkin's lymphoma. However, because NHL is more often in extranodal sites, more diagnostic studies may be done, such as an MRI or lumbar puncture to rule out CNS disease, a bone marrow biopsy to determine bone marrow infiltration, or a barium enema, upper endoscopy, to visualize suspected GI involvement. Clinical staging, as described for Hodgkin's lymphoma, is used to help guide therapy (Fig. 30-14), but establishment of the precise histologic subtype is extremely important. Lymph node excisional biopsy establishes the cell type and pattern. NHL is classified based on morphologic, genetic, immunophenotypic (cell surface antigens, CD20, CD52), and clinical features.

The World Health Organization has categorized more than 60 unique types of NHL.[42] A simplified modification of the classification system is presented in Table 30-28.

TABLE 30-28 Classification of Non-Hodgkin's Lymphoma*

B-Cell Lymphomas	T-Cell and NK-Cell Lymphomas
• Diffuse large B-cell lymphoma (DBLCL) • Follicular lymphoma • Marginal zone B-cell lymphoma (MALT) • Small lymphocytic lymphoma/chronic lymphocytic leukemia • Mantle cell lymphoma • Burkitt's lymphoma • Plasmablastic lymphoma • AIDS-related B-cell lymphomas	• Lymphoblastic lymphoma • T-cell lymphoma • Mycosis fungoides and Sézary syndrome • Anaplastic large T-cell lymphoma • Natural killer cell lymphomas **Posttransplant Lymphoproliferative Disorders (PTLD)**

MALT, Mucosa-associated lymphoid tissue.
*This is only a partial list.

Treatment is guided by the cell type, cytogenetic studies, and clinical behavior: *indolent* (low grade), aggressive (high grade), or *highly aggressive* (very high grade). Additional factors, known as the International Prognostic Index (IPI), may be considered for each subtype to help select the appropriate treatment for these patients. Factors considered may include the clinical stage, number of extranodal sites, serum LDH, WBC count, hemoglobin, and patient's age and performance status.[48] Immunologic, cytogenetic, and molecular studies are also useful for making therapeutic decisions and assessing prognosis. Other studies might include blood tests for tumor lysis (see Chapter 15); screening for hepatitis, HIV, and *H. pylori*; skin biopsies; bone marrow biopsies; and lumbar punctures. The prognosis for NHL is based on the histopathology.

❖ NURSING AND INTERPROFESSIONAL MANAGEMENT: NON-HODGKIN'S LYMPHOMA

Treatment for NHL involves chemotherapy and sometimes radiation therapy[42,48] (Table 30-29). Ironically, more aggressive lymphomas (diffuse large B cell) are more responsive to treatment and more likely to be cured. In contrast, indolent lymphomas (e.g., follicular lymphomas have a naturally long course but are difficult to effectively treat).[48]

Patients with low-grade (indolent) lymphoma may live 10 years or more without treatment. However, some initial therapies can be well tolerated and have been shown to reduce the time to progression of the disease. Lymphomas that have an infectious basis, such as *H. pylori* gastric lymphomas, may be treated with antibiotic or antiviral therapy. HSCT may have some benefit in certain subtypes of aggressive or refractory lymphomas.

Rituximab, a monoclonal antibody against the CD20 antigen on the surface of normal and malignant B cells, is used to treat NHL. Once bound to the cells, rituximab causes lysis and cell death. Numerous chemotherapy combinations have been used to try to overcome the resistant nature of this disease (Table 30-29). Complete remissions are uncommon, but the majority of patients respond with improvement in symptoms.

DRUG ALERT Rituximab (Rituxan)

- Monitor patient for signs of severe hypersensitivity infusion reactions, especially with first infusion.
- Manifestations may include hypotension, bronchospasm, dysrhythmias, angioedema, and cardiogenic shock.
- Screen for history of hepatitis because the drug may reactivate hepatitis.

TABLE 30-29 Treatment of Non-Hodgkin's Lymphoma*†

Recommended Therapies	Common Chemotherapy Combinations
Indolent (Low Grade) (e.g., Follicular Lymphoma, Marginal Zone B-Cell Lymphoma [MALT])	
• Observation until disease progression for asymptomatic patients with low-volume tumors and normal blood counts • External beam irradiation for local, limited disease • Single-agent rituximab (Rituxan) • Single-agent chemotherapy (chlorambucil, cyclophosphamide, bendamustine) or idelalisib) • Rituximab with another agent (bendamustine, cyclophosphamide, fludarabine, cladribine, lenalidomide, chlorambucil) • Combination chemotherapy (R-CHOP or other) • Radioimmunotherapy • Hematopoietic stem cell transplant (HSCT)	**R-CHOP:** **r**ituximab, **c**yclophosphamide, doxorubicin **h**ydrochloride, vincristine (**O**ncovin), **p**rednisone **FCMR:** **f**ludarabine, **c**yclophosphamide **m**itoxantrone, **r**ituximab **R-CVP:** **r**ituximab, **c**yclophosphamide, **v**incristine, **p**rednisone **RFND:** **r**ituximab, **f**ludarabine, mitoxantrone (**N**ovantrone), **d**examethasone ± rituximab **FC:** **f**ludarabine, **c**yclophosphamide
Aggressive (Intermediate or High Grade) (e.g., Mantle Cell, Diffuse Large B-Cell, Peripheral T-Cell, Natural Killer Cell Lymphomas)	
• Combination chemotherapy with localized radiation if needed • Aggressive combination chemotherapy for 3-8 cycles with rituximab with local radiation if needed • Intrathecal chemotherapy if needed • Single agent or other combination treatment, depending on subtype and response (e.g., bendamustine, bortezomib, cladribine, ibrutinib, lenalidomide, belinostat, gemcitabine, alemtuzumab, oxaliplatin, belinostat, romidepsin) • HSCT	**R-CHOP** (see above) **ICE** (or "RICE" with rituximab): **i**fosfamide, **c**yclophosphamide, **e**toposide **R-EPOCH:** **r**ituximab, **e**toposide, **p**rednisone, vincristine (**O**ncovin), **c**yclophosphamide, doxorubicin **h**ydrochloride **ESHAP ± R:** **e**toposide, methylprednisolone (**S**olu-Medrol), **h**igh-dose cytarabine (**A**ra-C), cisplatin (**P**latinol), with or without **r**ituximab **Hyper-CVAD ± R:** hyperfractionated **c**yclophosphamide, **v**incristine, doxorubicin (**A**driamycin), **d**examethasone alternating with high-dose methotrexate and cytarabine with or without rituximab **DHAP ± R:** **d**examethasone, **h**igh-dose cytarabine (**A**ra-C), cisplatin (**P**latinol), with our without **r**ituximab **SMILE:** **s**teroids, **m**ethotrexate, **i**fosfamide, **L**-asparaginase, **e**toposide High-dose cytarabine and high-dose methotrexate with leucovorin rescue
Highly Aggressive (e.g., Burkitt's Lymphoma, AIDS-Related B-Cell Lymphomas)	
• Aggressive combination chemotherapy for 3-8 cycles • HSCT	**Hyper-CVAD ± R** (see above) **CODOX-M:** **c**yclophosphamide, vincristine (**O**ncovin), **dox**orubicin, high-dose **m**ethotrexate, with or without rituximab (includes intrathecal methotrexate)

MALT, Mucosa-associated lymphoid tissue.
*Not all inclusive.
†The acronym for some drug regimens use the trade name of chemotherapy agents. In some cases the trade name has been discontinued, and the drug currently used is the generic version.

Other therapies for some types of NHL include the monoclonal antibody ibritumomab tiuxetan (Zevalin). This antibody linked to a radioactive isotope (yttrium-90) (see Table 15-13). The monoclonal antibody targets the CD20 antigen, which is on the surface of mature B cells and B-cell tumors. This targeting allows for the delivery of radiation directly to the malignant cells. Side effects of this type of treatment include pancytopenia. Use radiation precautions in caring for these patients. Teach patients about safety issues and how to minimize the risk of radiation exposure to staff and others.

In general T-cell lymphomas are more difficult to treat and are often treated aggressively up front often followed by an HSCT. Cutaneous T-cell lymphomas may be treated with topical corticosteroids or topical chemotherapy for limited-stage disease. For more diffuse disease, treatment may include phototherapy, α-interferon, bexarotene (Targretin), vorinostat (Zolinza), or others.[42]

The nursing care for NHL is similar to that for Hodgkin's lymphoma. It is largely based on managing problems related to the disease (e.g., pain caused by the tumor, spinal cord compression, tumor lysis syndrome), pancytopenia, and other side effects of therapy. However, because NHL can be more extensive and involve specific organs (e.g., CNS, spleen, liver, GI tract, bone marrow), it is important to understand the subtype and extent of the disease. For example, a patient with known involvement of the colon may complain of acute abdominal pain. The patient most likely would have abdominal guarding and an enlarged and tympanic abdomen. This could indicate a bowel perforation and be considered a medical emergency. A patient with a Burkitt's NHL beginning chemotherapy would be at high risk for tumor lysis syndrome and would require frequent laboratory studies and monitoring, as well as strict documentation of intake and output. (Cancer-related therapies and side effects are discussed in Chapter 15.)

The patient undergoing external beam radiation therapy has special nursing needs. The skin in the radiation field requires attention. Concepts related to safety issues regarding radiation therapy are important to include in the plan of care (see Chapter 15).

Psychosocial considerations are important. Help the patient and family understand the disease, treatment, and expected and potential side effects. Some aggressive treatments require close follow-up and even inpatient admission. Fertility issues may be of concern in young patients. As in Hodgkin's lymphoma, evaluation of patients with NHL for long-term effects of therapy is important because the delayed consequences of disease and treatment may not become apparent for many years. (Secondary malignancies and delayed effects are discussed in Chapter 15.)

MULTIPLE MYELOMA

Multiple myeloma, or *plasma cell myeloma*, is a condition in which neoplastic plasma cells infiltrate the bone marrow and destroy bone. Multiple myeloma accounts for about 1% of all malignancies and for about 15% of all hematologic malignancies.[37] The disease is twice as common in men as in women and usually develops after 40 years of age, with an average age of 69 years. Multiple myeloma occurs in African Americans more commonly than in whites. Although it was previously not considered curable, the 5-year survival rate is close to 45% because of the variety of treatments that can be provided throughout the course of the disease.[49]

Etiology and Pathophysiology

The cause of multiple myeloma is unknown. It is possible that exposure to radiation, organic chemicals (such as benzene), metals, herbicides, and insecticides may play a role. Obesity and genetic factors and viral infection may also influence the risk of developing multiple myeloma.

The disease process involves excessive production of plasma cells. Plasma cells are activated B cells, which produce immunoglobulins (antibodies) that normally protect the body. However, in multiple myeloma instead of a variety of plasma cells producing antibodies to fight different infections, myeloma tumors produce monoclonal antibodies. *Monoclonal* means they are all of one kind, making them ineffective and even harmful. Not only do they not fight infections, but they also infiltrate the bone marrow. These monoclonal proteins (called *M proteins*) are made up of two light chains and two heavy chains. *Bence-Jones proteins* are the light chain part of these monoclonal antibodies. They show up in the urine in many patients with multiple myeloma.

Furthermore, plasma cell production of excessive and abnormal amounts of cytokines (interleukins [ILs]; IL-4, IL-5, and IL-6) also plays an important role in the pathologic process of bone destruction. As myeloma protein increases, normal plasma cells are reduced, which further compromises the body's normal immune response. Proliferation of malignant plasma cells and the overproduction of immunoglobulin and proteins result in the end-organ effects of myeloma on the bone marrow, bone, and kidneys and possibly the spleen, lymph nodes, liver, and even heart muscle.

Clinical Manifestations

Multiple myeloma develops slowly and insidiously. The patient often does not manifest symptoms until the disease is advanced, at which time skeletal pain is the major manifestation. Pain in the pelvis, spine, and ribs is particularly common and is triggered by movement. Diffuse osteoporosis develops as the myeloma protein destroys bone. Osteolytic lesions are seen in the skull, vertebrae, and ribs. Vertebral destruction can lead to collapse of vertebrae with ensuing compression of the spinal cord. Loss of bone integrity can lead to the development of pathologic fractures.

Bony degeneration also causes calcium to be lost from bones, eventually causing hypercalcemia. Hypercalcemia may cause renal, GI, or neurologic manifestations such as polyuria, anorexia, confusion, and ultimately seizures, coma, and cardiac problems. A serum *hyperviscosity syndrome* leading to cerebral, pulmonary, renal, and other organ dysfunction can occur in some patients. Even without hyperviscosity, high protein levels caused by the myeloma protein can result in renal tubular obstruction, interstitial nephritis, and renal failure. The patient may also display manifestations of anemia, thrombocytopenia, neutropenia, and immune dysfunction, all of which are related to the replacement of normal bone marrow with plasma cells. Neurologic abnormalities may be caused by regional myeloma cell growth compressing the spinal cord or cranial nerves, or by perineuronal or perivascular deposition.[50]

Diagnostic Studies

Evaluating multiple myeloma involves laboratory, radiologic, and bone marrow examination. M protein is found in the blood and urine. Possible findings include pancytopenia, hypercalcemia, Bence Jones protein in the urine, and an elevated serum creatinine.

Skeletal bone surveys, MRI, and/or PET and CT scans show distinct lytic areas of bone erosions; generalized thinning of the bones; or fractures, especially in the vertebrae, ribs, pelvis, and bones of the thigh and upper arms. Bone marrow analysis shows significantly increased numbers of plasma cells in the bone marrow. The simplest measure of staging and prognosis in multiple myeloma is based on blood levels of two markers: β_2-microglobulin and albumin. In general, higher levels of β_2-microglobulin and lower levels of albumin are associated with a poorer prognosis.

Interprofessional Care

Interprofessional care involves managing both the disease and its symptoms. The current treatment options include corticosteroids, chemotherapy, immunotherapy, and targeted therapy, and HSCT.[51] Multiple myeloma is seldom cured, but treatment can relieve symptoms, produce remission, and prolong life. Ambulation and adequate hydration are used to treat hypercalcemia, dehydration, and potential renal damage. Weight bearing helps the bones resorb some calcium, and fluids dilute calcium and prevent protein precipitates from causing renal tubular obstruction. Control of pain and prevention of pathologic fractures are other goals of management. Analgesics, orthopedic supports, and localized radiation help reduce the skeletal pain.

Kyphoplasty is sometimes used to control spine vertebral disease. *Kyphoplasty* is a minimally invasive procedure (usually done in an interventional radiology area) that injects cement to stabilize the vertebral compression.

Bisphosphonates, such as pamidronate (Aredia) and zoledronic acid (Zometa), inhibit bone breakdown and are used for the treatment of skeletal pain and hypercalcemia. They inhibit bone resorption without inhibiting bone formation and mineralization. They are given monthly by IV infusion.

DRUG ALERT Zoledronic Acid (Zometa)

- Patient should be adequately rehydrated before administering drug.
- Renal toxicity may occur if IV infusion of drug is administered in less than 15 min.

Chemotherapy with corticosteroids is usually the first treatment recommended for multiple myeloma. It is used to reduce the number of plasma cells. Initial treatment depends on whether the patient is a future bone marrow transplant candidate and anticipated tolerance of therapy. The treatment usually includes a corticosteroid (dexamethasone or prednisone) plus one or two chemotherapy agents, such as melphalan (Alkeran), vincristine (Oncovin), cyclophosphamide (Cytoxan), doxorubicin, and bendamustine (Treanda). High-dose chemotherapy followed by HSCT has evolved as the standard of care in eligible patients.[51]

Immunotherapy and targeted therapy are also used to treat multiple myeloma. Immunomodulator drugs (described in Chapter 15) include thalidomide (Thalidomide), lenalidomide (Revlimid), and pomalidomide (Pomalyst). Proteosome inhibitors include bortezomib (Velcade), carfilzomib (Kyprolis), and ixazomib (Ninlaro). Panobinostat (Farydak) is a drug that can affect which genes are active inside of cells. Daratumumab (Darzalex) is a monoclonal antibody against CD38, which is expressed on the surface of myeloma cells.

Drugs may also be used to treat complications of multiple myeloma. For example, allopurinol may be given to reduce hyperuricemia, and IV furosemide (Lasix) promotes renal excretion of calcium. In some patients, the levels of plasma proteins are so high that it causes a hyperviscosity syndrome leading to neurologic changes, renal insufficiency, and other problems related to lack of blood flow. In this instance plasmapheresis is used.

BECOMING A NURSE LEADER

Importance of Being a Leader

Situation

You are a senior nursing student who is doing a clinical rotation on a busy hematology unit. You are working with Gayla, who is an experienced RN. Gayla is a hardworking, dedicated, experienced nurse whom you greatly admire. You hear her discussing that she has just been appointed to the State Board of Nursing. Why, you wonder, is she getting involved in something like that when she is so busy at work and in her personal life?

Points for Consideration

- Leadership is needed from nurses at all levels and across all health care settings.
- The Institute of Medicine's Future of Nursing report recommends that opportunities be provided for nurses to assume leadership positions and serve as full partners in health care improvement.[1]
- Nurses must step up to be leaders to be full partners with HCPs and other health care professionals to assist in health care improvements.
- The Future of Nursing report states that nurses will need a leadership style that works in full partnership with others respectfully and collaboratively. This leadership style helps to improve patient outcomes, reduces errors, and results in less staff turnover.

Discussion Questions

1. What may be Gayla's motivation for getting involved with the State Board of Nursing?
2. What benefit will Gayla gain from her experience with the State Board of Nursing? How will her colleagues in her work setting benefit from her experience?
3. What leadership skills do you have? How can these leadership skills be used to promote improvements in health care?

Reference

1. Institute of Medicine. The future of nursing: leading change, advancing health. Retrieved from *http://thefutureofnursing.org/sites/default/files/Summary%20%281-14%29.pdf*

NURSING MANAGEMENT: MULTIPLE MYELOMA

A major focus of care relates to the bone involvement and sequelae from bone breakdown. Maintaining adequate hydration is a primary nursing consideration to minimize problems from hypercalcemia. IV fluids may be administered to attain a urine output of 1.5 to 2 L/day if the patient does not already have renal compromise. Although tumor lysis is rare, once chemotherapy is initiated, allopurinol may be given to prevent any renal damage from uric acid accumulation (from cell breakdown). Because of the myeloma proteins, the patient is at additional risk of renal dysfunction and electrolyte and fluid imbalances.

Because of the potential for pathologic fractures, use caution when moving and ambulating the patient. A slight twist or strain in the wrong area (e.g., a weak area in the patient's bones) may be sufficient to cause a fracture. In addition, the development of peripheral neuropathy is common with several therapies for multiple myeloma and can contribute to discomfort, the inability to perform basic activities of daily living, and the risk of injury from falling. Pain medications and therapies can also lead to severe constipation.

Pain management requires innovative and knowledgeable nursing interventions. Analgesics, such as nonsteroidal antiinflammatory drugs, acetaminophen, or an acetaminophen/opioid combination, may be more effective than opioids alone in diminishing bone pain. Braces, especially for the spine, may also help control pain. As in any pain management situation, assess the patient and implement necessary measures to alleviate the pain. (Pain management is discussed in Chapter 8.) Patients may also be at risk for deep vein thrombosis related to chemotherapy and immobility and should have appropriate preventive measures employed.[50]

Assessment and prompt treatment of infection are important in the care of patients with multiple myeloma. These recurrent infections may be due to a decrease in the production of normal immunoglobulins, the ineffectiveness of the overproduced and abnormal immunoglobulins, corticosteroids, and/or neutropenia as a result of the bone marrow infiltration or side effects of treatment.

The patient's psychosocial needs require sensitive, skilled management. Help the patient and significant others adapt to changes fostered by chronic illness and adjust to the losses related to the disease process, while helping to maximize functioning and quality of life. The patient with multiple myeloma may experience remissions and exacerbations. Patients may be on dialysis because of myeloma-induced renal failure. Consequently acute care is needed at various times during the course of the illness.

The final, acute phase is unresponsive to treatment and usually short in duration. The way in which patients and families confront death may be affected by the manner in which they have learned to accept and live with the chronic disease.

DISORDERS OF THE SPLEEN

The spleen can be affected by many illnesses, most of which can cause some degree of *splenomegaly* (enlarged spleen)[52] (Table 30-30). However, an enlarged spleen may be present in certain individuals without any evidence of disease. The term *hypersplenism* refers to the occurrence of splenomegaly and peripheral cytopenias (anemia, leukopenia, and thrombocytopenia).[26] The degree of splenic enlargement varies with the disease. For example, massive splenic enlargement occurs with infectious mononucleosis, chronic myelogenous leukemia, and thalassemia major. Mild splenic enlargement occurs with HF and systemic lupus erythematosus. The normal spleen contains 350 mL of blood, and about one third of the platelet mass is sequestered in the spleen.

When the spleen enlarges, its normal filtering and sequestering capacity increases. Consequently, there is often a reduction in the number of circulating blood cells as they engorge the spleen. In addition, there are unusual findings in the peripheral smear, such as pitted or pocked erythrocytes or Howell-Jolly bodies. These findings assist in diagnosing a malfunctioning spleen. A slight to moderate enlargement of the spleen is usually asymptomatic and found during routine examination of the abdomen. Even massive splenomegaly can be well tolerated, but the patient may complain of abdominal discomfort and early satiety. In addition to physical examination, other techniques to assess the size of the spleen include radionuclide colloid liver-spleen scan, CT or PET scan, MRI, and ultrasound scan.

Occasionally a splenectomy is done either via laparoscopy or open laparotomy as part of the evaluation or treatment of splenomegaly. Another major indication for splenectomy is splenic rupture. The spleen may rupture from trauma; inadvertent tearing during other surgical procedures; and diseases such as mononucleosis, malaria, and lymphoid neoplasms. After a splenectomy, there can be a dramatic increase in peripheral RBC, WBC, and platelet counts.

Nursing responsibilities for the patient with spleen disorders vary depending on the problem. Splenomegaly may be painful and may require analgesic administration; care in moving, turning, and positioning; and evaluation of lung expansion because spleen enlargement may impair diaphragmatic excursion. If anemia, thrombocytopenia, or leukopenia develops from splenic enlargement, institute nursing measures to support the patient and prevent life-threatening complications. If splenectomy is performed, observe the patient for hemorrhage and shock.

After splenectomy, immunologic deficiencies may develop, such as low IgG levels. Postsplenectomy patients have a lifelong risk for infection, especially from encapsulated organisms such as *Pneumococcus* species. This risk is reduced by immunization with pneumococcal vaccine.[52]

TABLE 30-30 Causes of Splenomegaly

Infections and Inflammations
- Bacterial infections: endocarditis, salmonella
- Mycobacterial infections: tuberculosis
- Spirochetes: syphilis, Lyme disease
- Viral infections: hepatitis, human immunodeficiency virus, cytomegalovirus, mononucleosis
- Parasitic infections: malaria, trypanosomiasis, schistosomiasis, leishmaniasis, toxoplasmosis
- Rickettsial infections: Rocky Mountain spotted fever, typhoid fever
- Fungal infections: histoplasmosis
- Autoimmune diseases: systemic lupus erythematosus, rheumatoid arthritis

Infiltrative Diseases and Tumors or Cysts
- Acute and chronic leukemia
- Lymphomas
- Polycythemia vera
- Multiple myeloma, amyloidosis
- Other primary or secondary neoplasms and cysts
- Sarcoidosis
- Gaucher disease

Congestion
- Cirrhosis of the liver
- Heart failure (portal hypertension)
- Portal or splenic vein thrombosis
- Sickle cell disease
- Thalassemia
- Acquired hemolytic anemia
- Immune thrombocytopenia

BLOOD COMPONENT THERAPY

Blood component therapy is frequently used to manage hematologic diseases. Many therapeutic and surgical procedures depend on blood product support. However, blood component therapy only temporarily supports the patient until the underlying problem is resolved. Because transfusions are not free from hazards, they should be used only if necessary.

Avoid developing a complacent attitude about this common but potentially dangerous therapy. Make sure that the HCP has

TABLE 30-31 Blood Products*

Description	Special Considerations	Indications for Use
Packed RBCs		
Packed RBCs are prepared from whole blood by sedimentation or centrifugation. One unit contains 250-350 mL. They can be stored up to 35 days depending on processing.	Use of RBCs for treatment allows remaining components of blood (e.g., platelets, albumin, plasma) to be used for other purposes. There is less danger of fluid overload. Packed RBCs are preferred RBC source because they are more component specific. Leukocyte depletion (leukoreduction) by filtration, washing, or freezing is frequently used. Decreases hemolytic febrile or mild allergic reactions in patients who receive frequent transfusions	Severe or symptomatic anemia, acute blood loss. One unit of RBCs can be expected to increase Hgb by 1 g/dL or Hct by 3% in a typical adult. One unit of RBCs can replace a blood loss of 500 mL.
Frozen RBCs		
Frozen RBCs are prepared from RBCs using glycerol for protection and frozen. They can be stored for 10 yr.	Must be used within 24 hr of thawing. Successive washings with saline solution remove majority of WBCs and plasma proteins.	Autotransfusion. Stockpiling or rare donors for patients with alloantibodies
Platelets		
Platelets are prepared from fresh whole blood. One donor unit contains 3×10^{11} platelets (from whole blood). Platelets may also be pooled from multiple donors. (One apheresed unit is roughly equivalent to 4-6 random donor-pooled platelets). An apheresed single donation is usually 200-400 mL in volume.	Multiple units of platelets can be obtained from one donor by plateletpheresis. They can be kept at room temperature for 1-5 days depending on type of collection and storage bag used. Bag should be agitated periodically. For patients who receive frequent transfusions and become refractory, may give leukocyte reduced, HLA, or type specific to prevent alloimmunization to HLA antigens	Bleeding caused by thrombocytopenia. May be contraindicated in thrombotic thrombocytopenic purpura and heparin-induced thrombocytopenia except in life-threatening hemorrhage Expected increase is 5,000/μL/U. Failure to have an increase may be due to fever, sepsis, splenomegaly, or DIC or development of antibodies *(refractory)*.
Fresh Frozen Plasma		
Liquid portion of whole blood is separated from cells and frozen. One unit contains approximately 250 mL. Plasma is rich in clotting factors but contains no platelets. May be stored for ≥1 yr, depending on storage. Must be used within 24 hr after thawing	Use of plasma in treating hypovolemic shock is being replaced by pure preparations such as albumin and plasma expanders.	Bleeding caused by deficiency in clotting factors (e.g., DIC, hemorrhage, massive transfusion, liver disease, vitamin K deficiency, excess warfarin)
Albumin		
Albumin is prepared from plasma. It can be stored for 5 yr. It is available in 5% or 25% solution.	Albumin 25 g/dL is osmotically equal to 500 mL of plasma. Hyperosmolar solution acts by moving water from extravascular to intravascular space. It is heat treated and does not transmit viruses.	Hypovolemic shock, hypoalbuminemia
Cryoprecipitates and Commercial Concentrates		
Cryoprecipitate is prepared from fresh frozen plasma, with 10-20 mL/bag. It can be stored for 1 yr. Once thawed, must be used within 5 days	Table 30-18	Replacement of clotting factors, especially factor VIII, von Willebrand factor, and fibrinogen

DIC, Disseminated intravascular coagulation; *HLA*, human leukocyte antigen.
*Component therapy has replaced the use of whole blood, which is infrequently used. Granulocyte transfusions are not included here because they are rarely used.

discussed the risks, benefits, and alternatives with the patient and that this is documented in the patient's medical record.

Traditionally, the term *blood transfusion* meant the administration of whole blood. Blood transfusion now has a broader meaning because of the ability to administer specific components of blood such as platelets, packed red blood cells (PRBCs), or plasma. Usually a specific component is ordered, although whole blood may be rarely used with massive hemorrhage or for an exchange transfusion[53,54] (Table 30-31).

Administration Procedure

Blood components may be administered with a 22-gauge IV needle, cannula, or catheter.[55] However, larger sizes (e.g., 18- or 16-gauge) may be preferred if rapid transfusions are given or if the infusion is sluggish. Smaller needles can be used for platelets, albumin, and clotting factor replacement. Whatever type of venous access is used, verify its patency before requesting the blood component from the blood bank. Most blood product administration tubing is of a "Y type" with a microaggregate filter (filters out particulate), with one arm of the Y for the isotonic saline solution and the other arm of the Y for the blood product. Infusion pumps may be used if approved for blood administration and according to institution policy.

! SAFETY ALERT Blood Transfusions

- Do not use dextrose solutions or lactated Ringer's solution for administering blood because they will cause RBC hemolysis.
- Do not give any additives (including medications) via the same tubing as the blood unless the tubing is first cleared with saline solution.

After obtaining the blood or blood components from the blood bank, make a positive identification of the donor blood and recipient. Improper product-to-patient identification is the most common cause of hemolytic transfusion reactions, thus placing a great responsibility on nurses to carry out the

ETHICAL/LEGAL DILEMMAS

Religious Beliefs

Situation

W.D., an 81-year-old woman with dementia, is transferred from a nursing home to a hospital because of gastrointestinal bleeding from an unknown cause. Some of her family members tell you that she is a Jehovah's Witness and must not receive blood products. If she does not have exploratory surgery and transfusions, the surgeon believes that she will die.

Ethical/Legal Points for Consideration

- Competent adults have the right to make health care decisions, including the right to refuse treatment, based on their religious beliefs.
- If the patient is determined to be incompetent and a guardian has been appointed, the guardian has the legal right to make the consent or refusal.
- If the HCP believes that the treatment is essential to preserve life and health and there is no legal decision maker, a request is made for a legal determination of whether the patient is incapable of consent or refusal. If the judge agrees, the patient is made a ward of the court for this issue. Usually the HCP is directed to make a decision based on the patient's best interests.
- Courts tend to defer to any past information coming directly from patients about their own personal desires, even if that information is not in valid advance directives.[1]

Discussion Questions

1. What resources do you have available to consult about religious practices?
2. How could you make a determination if the family were acting in W.D.'s best interest or their own?
3. What nonblood alternatives are available for Jehovah's Witnesses?

identification procedure appropriately. Follow the policy and procedures at your place of employment. Many institutions have implemented a dual-checking system with two licensed individuals checking the patient identification with the labeled blood component. The blood bank is responsible for typing and crossmatching the donor's blood with the recipient's blood. The result of the compatibility testing should be noted on the product bag or tag, if pertinent. Table 30-32 outlines blood component compatibilities for transfusions.[53,56]

ABO compatibility is not a prerequisite for platelet transfusions. However, after multiple platelet transfusions, a patient may develop anti-HLA antibodies to the transfused platelets. With the use of lymphocyte typing to match HLA types of the donor and recipient, multiple platelet transfusions can be given

TABLE 30-32 Blood Component Compatibilities for Transfusions

	DONOR PRODUCT			
Recipient's Type	**Packed Red Blood Cells**	**Plasma**	**Platelets**	**Cryo-precipitate**
O+	O+ , O–	All groups	O, B, A, AB	Any group is safe to transfuse
O–	O–			
A+	A+, A–, O+, O–	A, AB	A, AB, B, O	
A–	A–, O–			
B+	B+, B–, O+, O–	B, AB	B, AB, A, O	
B–	B–, O+			
AB+	All groups	Only AB	Any group	
AB–	AB–, B–, A–, O–			

TEAMWORK & COLLABORATION

Blood Transfusions

Role of Nursing Personnel

Registered Nurse (RN)

- Ensure that an IV line is being used with a large-bore needle, catheter, or cannula, preferably 19 gauge or larger.
- Double-check patient identification and blood product identification data with another licensed nurse (consider state nurse practice act and agency policy).
- Adjust infusion rate of transfusion according to patient needs.
- Evaluate patient for signs of transfusion reactions.
- Evaluate for therapeutic effect of blood product (improvement in complete blood count, increased blood pressure, improved patient color, decreased bleeding).
- Monitor for signs of circulatory overload (e.g., shortness of breath) if the transfusion must be given rapidly.

Licensed Practical/Vocational Nurse (LPN/LVN)

- Assist with checking patient identification and blood product identification data with the RN (consider state nurse practice act and agency policy).
- Monitor blood transfusion rate (consider state nurse practice act and agency policy).

Unlicensed Assistive Personnel (UAP)

- Obtain blood products from the blood bank as directed by the RN.
- Take vital signs before the transfusion and after the first 15 min.

Role of Other Team Members

Blood Bank Personnel

- Responsible for typing and crossmatching the donor's blood with the recipient's blood.
- Result of the compatibility testing should be noted on the product bag or tag.
- When handing off the blood or blood component to nursing personnel, ensure that a positive identification is made with product and patient's information.

with fewer complications to those who develop antibodies to platelets. The patient may be premedicated with an antihistamine (e.g., diphenhydramine [Benadryl]) and hydrocortisone to decrease the possibility of reacting to platelet transfusions if he or she has a history of reactions.[54,57]

Take the patient's vital signs before beginning the transfusion so that you have a baseline measure. If the patient has abnormal vital signs (e.g., high fever), call the HCP to clarify when the blood component may be administered. Administer the blood as soon as it is brought to the patient. Do not refrigerate it on the nursing unit. If the blood is not used within 30 minutes, return it to the blood bank. During the first 15 minutes or 50 mL of blood infusion, remain with the patient. If there are any untoward reactions, they are most likely to occur at this time. The rate of infusion during this period should be no more than 2 mL/minute. Do not infuse PRBCs quickly except in an emergency. Rapid infusion of cold blood may cause the patient to become chilled. If rapid replacement of large amounts of blood is necessary, a blood-warming device may be used. Other blood components, such as fresh frozen plasma and platelets, may be infused over 15 to 30 minutes. Refer to your institution's policy and procedure.

After the first 15 minutes, vital signs are usually retaken, and the rate of infusion is determined by the patient's clinical condition and the product being infused. Observe the patient periodically throughout the transfusion (e.g., every 30 minutes) and up to 1 hour after the transfusion. Most patients not in danger of fluid overload can tolerate the infusion of 1 unit of PRBCs over 2 hours. The transfusion should not take more than 4 hours to administer because of the increased risk of bacterial growth in the product once it is out of refrigeration. Never store blood components in unmonitored refrigerators in nursing units.

Blood Transfusion Reactions

A *blood transfusion reaction* is an adverse reaction to blood transfusion therapy that can range in severity from mild symptoms to a life-threatening condition. Because complications of transfusion therapy may be significant, judicious evaluation of the patient is required. Blood transfusion reactions can be classified as acute or delayed[53,57,58] (Tables 30-33 and 30-34).

If a transfusion reaction occurs, take the following steps: (1) stop the transfusion; (2) maintain a patent IV line with saline solution; (3) notify the blood bank and the HCP

CHECK YOUR PRACTICE

Your 82-yr-old male patient with severe iron deficiency anemia is receiving his second unit of packed RBCs. He received his first transfusions without any problems. He is now complaining of chills and feeling like his heart is racing.

- What should you do?

TABLE 30-33 Acute Transfusion Reactions

Cause	Manifestations	Management	Prevention
Acute Hemolytic Reaction			
Infusion of ABO-incompatible whole blood, RBCs, or components containing ≥10 mL of RBCs Antibodies in the recipient's plasma attach to antigens on transfused RBCs, causing RBC destruction.	Reactions usually develop in first 15 min. Fever with or without chills; low back, abdominal, chest or flank pain; flushing, tachycardia, dyspnea, tachypnea, hypotension, vascular collapse, hemoglobinuria, acute jaundice, dark urine, bleeding, acute kidney injury, shock, cardiac arrest, DIC, death	• Treat shock and DIC if present. • Draw blood samples for serologic testing slowly to avoid hemolysis from the procedure. Send urine specimen to the laboratory. • Maintain BP with IV colloid solutions. Give diuretics as prescribed to maintain urine flow. • Insert indwelling urinary catheter or measure voided amounts to monitor hourly urine output. Dialysis may be required if renal failure occurs. • Do not transfuse additional RBC-containing components until blood bank has provided newly crossmatched units.	Meticulously verify and document patient identification from sample collection to component infusion (e.g., visually compare label on sample collection and blood component with patient identification).
Febrile, Nonhemolytic Reaction (Most Common)			
Sensitization to donor WBCs (most common), platelets, or plasma proteins	Sudden chills, rigors, and fever (rise in temperature of >1°C), headache, flushing, anxiety, vomiting, muscle pain	• Give antipyretics as prescribed (acetaminophen). Avoid aspirin in thrombocytopenic patients. • Do not restart transfusion unless HCP orders.	Consider leukocyte-reduced blood products (filtered, washed, or frozen) for patients with a history of two or more such reactions. Give acetaminophen or diphenhydramine (Benadryl) 30 min before transfusion.
Mild Allergic Reaction			
Sensitivity to foreign plasma proteins More common in people with history of allergies	Flushing, itching, pruritus, urticaria (hives)	• Give antihistamine, corticosteroid, epinephrine, as ordered. • If symptoms are mild and transient, transfusion may be restarted slowly with HCP's order. • Do not restart transfusion if fever or pulmonary symptoms develop.	Treat prophylactically with antihistamines or steroids. Consider washed RBCs and platelets.
Anaphylactic and Severe Allergic Reaction			
Sensitivity to donor plasma proteins Infusion of IgA proteins to IgA-deficient recipient who has developed IgA antibody	Anxiety, urticaria, dyspnea, wheezing, progressing to cyanosis, bronchospasm, hypotension, shock, and possible cardiac arrest	• Initiate CPR, if indicated. Administer O_2. • Have epinephrine ready for injection. • Antihistamines, corticosteroids, β_2-agonists may also be prescribed. • Do not restart transfusion.	Transfuse extensively washed RBC products from which all plasma has been removed. Use blood from IgA-deficient donor. Use autologous components.
Circulatory Overload Reaction			
Fluid administered faster than the circulation can accommodate People with cardiac or renal disease at risk	Cough, dyspnea, pulmonary congestion, adventitious breath sounds, headache, hypertension, tachycardia, distended neck veins	• Place patient upright with feet in dependent position. • Obtain chest x-ray STAT if ordered. • Administer prescribed diuretics, O_2, morphine. • Phlebotomy may be indicated.	Adjust transfusion volume and flow rate based on patient size and clinical status. Have blood bank divide future units into smaller aliquots for better spacing of fluid infused.
Sepsis			
Transfusion of bacterially infected blood components	Rapid onset of chills, high fever, vomiting, diarrhea, marked hypotension, or shock	• Obtain culture of patient's blood. • Treat septicemia as directed—antibiotics, IV fluids, vasopressors.	Collect, process, store, and transfuse blood products according to blood banking standards and complete the transfusion within 4 hr of starting time.

TABLE 30-33 Acute Transfusion Reactions—cont'd

Cause	Manifestations	Management	Prevention
Transfusion-Related Acute Lung Injury (TRALI) Reaction			
Reaction between transfused antileukocyte antibodies and recipient's leukocytes, causing pulmonary inflammation and capillary leak	Fever, chills, hypotension, tachypnea, frothy sputum, dyspnea, hypoxemia, respiratory failure. Noncardiogenic pulmonary edema Leading cause of transfusion-related deaths. Arises within 1-6 hours of transfusion	• Draw blood for arterial blood gases and HLA or antileukocyte antibodies. Obtain chest x-ray STAT. • Provide O_2 and administer corticosteroids (diuretics of no value) as ordered. • Initiate CPR if needed and provide ventilatory and BP support if needed.	Provide leukocyte-reduced products. Identify donors who are implicated in TRALI reactions and do not allow them to donate.
Massive Blood Transfusion Reaction			
Can occur with replacement of 10 or more RBC units within 24 hr RBC transfusions do not contain clotting factors, albumin, and platelets.	Hypothermia and cardiac dysrhythmias (from rapid infusion of large quantities of cold blood) Citrate toxicity and hypocalcemia (from the use of citrate as a storage solution) Hypocalcemia (citrate binds calcium) manifested as muscle tremors and ECG changes Hyperkalemia (from potassium leaking from stored RBCs). Manifested as muscle weakness, diarrhea, paresthesias, paralysis of the cardiac or respiratory muscles, and cardiac arrest	• When patients receive massive transfusions of blood products, monitor clotting status and electrolyte levels.	Use blood-warming equipment. Infusion of 10% calcium gluconate (10 mL with every 1 L of citrated blood). Because of dilution effect on coagulation due to massive RBC transfusion, platelets and plasma will also be administered.

DIC, Disseminated intravascular coagulation; *HLA,* human leukocyte antigen; *IgA,* immunoglobulin A.

TABLE 30-34 Delayed Transfusion Reactions

Manifestations	Prevention and Management
Delayed Hemolytic	
Fever, mild jaundice, decreased hemoglobin. Occurs as early as 3 days or as late as several months posttransfusion as the result of destruction of transfused RBCs by alloantibodies not detected during crossmatch	Generally, no acute treatment is required. Hemolysis may be severe enough to warrant further transfusions.
Hepatitis B*	
Elevated liver enzymes (AST and ALT), anorexia, malaise, nausea and vomiting, fever, dark urine, jaundice Usually resolves spontaneously within 4-6 wk. Chronic carrier state can develop and result in permanent damage to the liver.	Hepatitis B virus can be detected in donated blood by the presence of hepatitis B surface antigen (HBsAg). Treat symptomatically.
Hepatitis C*	
Similar to hepatitis B, but symptoms are usually less severe. Chronic liver disease and cirrhosis may develop.	Before testing of anti-HCV in donated blood, accounted for 90%-95% of all posttransfusion hepatitis. Treat symptomatically.
Iron Overload	
Excess iron is deposited in heart, liver, pancreas, and joints, causing dysfunction. Heart failure, dysrhythmias, impaired thyroid and gonadal function, diabetes, arthritis, cirrhosis. Occurs in patients receiving >100 units for chronic anemia (e.g., sickle cell anemia, β-thalassemia) over time	Treat symptomatically. Deferoxamine (Desferal), which chelates and removes accumulated iron via the kidneys, administered IV or subcutaneously. Deferasirox (Exjade) and deferiprone (Ferriprox) are oral agents that chelate iron and should be started before more than 50 units of red cells are transfused.
Other	
Cytomegalovirus (CMV), HIV, human herpesvirus type 6 (HSV-6), Epstein-Barr virus (EBV), human T cell leukemia virus, HTLV-1, and malaria Most recent threats have been agents that primarily affect animals, but have been transmitted to the blood supply through the food supply, or vectors such as mosquitoes or ticks. These include *Plasmodium* species (malaria), dengue fever virus, West Nile virus, *Trypanosoma cruzi* (Chagas' disease), *Babesia* species (babesiosis), human herpesvirus 8 (KS virus), and variant Creutzfeldt-Jakob disease ("mad cow disease").	Treatment based on the cause Ways of detecting some of these agents are now available and required, such as the nucleic acid test for West Nile virus, HIV, and *T. cruzi.* Donor screening has been the only available method to reduce the risk of donor-contaminated blood for others.

ALT, Alanine aminotransferase; *AST,* aspartate aminotransferase; *HCV,* hepatitis C virus; *HTLV-1,* human T-cell leukemia virus, type 1; *KS,* Kaposi sarcoma.
*New cases of transfusion-related hepatitis B and C are not common.

immediately; (4) recheck identifying tags and numbers; (5) monitor vital signs and urine output; (6) treat symptoms per HCP order; (7) save the blood bag and tubing and send them to the blood bank for examination; (8) collect required blood and urine specimens at intervals based on the hospital policy to evaluate for hemolysis; and (9) document on transfusion reaction form and patient chart. The blood bank and laboratory are responsible for identifying the type of reaction.

A transfusion reaction is a *serious reportable event* (SRE) and a *sentinel event.* (These events are discussed in Chapter 1.)

Acute Transfusion Reactions. The most common cause of hemolytic reactions is transfusion of ABO-incompatible blood (Table 30-33). This is an example of a type II cytotoxic hypersensitivity reaction (see Chapter 13). Severe hemolytic reactions are rare. Mislabeling specimens and administering blood to the wrong individual cause most acute hemolytic reactions. This again points to the importance of using proper patient identifiers when drawing blood samples and when administering medications and blood products.

Delayed Transfusion Reactions. Delayed transfusion reactions include delayed hemolytic reactions (discussed previously), infections, and iron overload (Table 30-34).

Autotransfusion

Autotransfusion, or autologous transfusion, involves removing whole blood from a person and transfusing that blood back into the same person. The problems of incompatibility, allergic reactions, and transmission of disease can be avoided. Methods of autotransfusion include the following:

- *Autologous donation* or *elective phlebotomy* (predeposit transfusion). A person donates blood before a planned surgical procedure. The blood can be frozen and stored for up to 10 years. Usually the blood is stored without being frozen and is given to the person within a few weeks of donation. This technique is especially beneficial to the patient with a rare blood type or for any patient who may be expected to require limited blood product support during a major surgical procedure (e.g., elective orthopedic surgery).
- *Autotransfusion.* A newer method for replacing blood volume involves safely and aseptically collecting, filtering, and returning the patient's own blood lost during a major surgical procedure or from a traumatic injury. This system was originally developed in response to patients' concerns about the safety of blood from blood products. However, today it provides an important way to safely replace volume and stabilize bleeding patients. Collection devices are most often used during surgeries. Some systems allow blood to be automatically and continuously reinfused. Others require collecting the blood for a time (usually no longer than 4 hours) and then reinfusing it.

Drainage after the first 24 hours or drainage that is suspected to contain pathogens should not be reinfused. Anticoagulants may or may not be added before reinfusion. Development of clots after blood is filtered through the collection system can sometimes prevent reinfusion of the blood. Sometimes blood that has been collected has become depleted of its normal coagulation factors. Therefore monitoring coagulation studies in the patient receiving an autotransfusion is important.

CASE STUDY

Leukemia

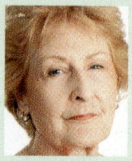

(©Lisa F. Young/iStock)

Patient Profile

A.J. is a 63-year-old white woman who is brought to the emergency department by her husband (see Chapter 29 case study on p. 593). She has become progressively weaker and was admitted for further evaluation.

Subjective Data

- Complains of progressive weakness over the last couple of weeks
- Has had a recent sinus infection that resolved after two courses of antibiotics
- Complains of shortness of breath
- Has noticed a lot of bruising lately

Objective Data

Physical Examination

- Has scattered petechiae on both ankles and two ecchymoses on her arms and one on her left lower leg
- Her skin is very pale
- BP 100/70 (lying), temperature 96.8°F (36°C), respiratory rate 26/min, pulse 110/min

Laboratory Results

- Hct 18.2%
- Hgb 5.9 g/dL, WBC count 2600/μL (2.6×10^9/L)
- Platelet count 72,000/μL (72×10^9/L)
- Peripheral blood smear indicates that 80% of the WBCs are blasts
- PT 18 sec, aPTT 37 sec
- LDH 560 units/L

Bone Marrow Biopsy

- Multiple myeloblasts (>50%)

Interprofessional Care

- Consultation with a hematologist-oncologist
- Two units of packed red blood cells
- *Diagnosis:* Acute myelogenous leukemia

Discussion Questions

1. What components of the laboratory test results and bone marrow biopsy suggest acute leukemia?
2. How is acute myelogenous leukemia treated?
3. What is A.J.'s prognosis?
4. What are the life-threatening problems that can occur as a result of this disease and treatment? How can you anticipate and assess for these problems?
5. ***Priority Decision:*** What are the priority nursing interventions for A.J.?
6. ***Patient-Centered Care:*** What are the priorities for patient teaching with a newly diagnosed adult with leukemia?
7. ***Priority Decision:*** Based on the assessment data presented, what are the priority nursing diagnoses? Are there any collaborative problems?
8. ***Teamwork and Collaboration:*** What nursing interventions can the registered nurse (RN) delegate to unlicensed assistive personnel (UAP) while A.J. is getting her blood transfusions?
9. ***Evidence-Based Practice:*** A.J. becomes fatigued after starting chemotherapy. She wants to know if she can still work and do household chores even if she is so fatigued. What is your best advice for her?

Answers available at *http://evolve.elsevier.com/Lewis/medsurg.*

BRIDGE TO NCLEX EXAMINATION

The number of the question corresponds to the same-numbered outcome at the beginning of the chapter.

1. In a severely anemic patient, the nurse would expect to find
   a. dyspnea and tachycardia.
   b. cyanosis and pulmonary edema.
   c. cardiomegaly and pulmonary fibrosis.
   d. ventricular dysrhythmias and wheezing.
2. When obtaining assessment data from a patient with a microcytic, hypochromic anemia, the nurse would question the patient about
   a. folic acid intake.
   b. dietary intake of iron.
   c. a history of gastric surgery.
   d. a history of sickle cell anemia.
3. Nursing interventions for a patient with severe anemia related to peptic ulcer disease include *(select all that apply)*
   a. instructions for high-iron diet.
   b. taking vital signs every 8 hours.
   c. monitoring stools for occult blood.
   d. teaching self-injection of erythropoietin.
   e. administration of cobalamin (vitamin B_{12}) injections.
4. The nursing management of a patient in sickle cell crisis includes *(select all that apply)*
   a. monitoring CBC.
   b. optimal pain management and O_2 therapy.
   c. blood transfusions if required and iron chelation.
   d. rest as needed and deep vein thrombosis prophylaxis.
   e. administration of IV iron and diet high in iron content.
5. A complication of the hyperviscosity of polycythemia is
   a. thrombosis.
   b. cardiomyopathy.
   c. pulmonary edema.
   d. disseminated intravascular coagulation (DIC).
6. When caring for a patient with thrombocytopenia, the nurse instructs the patient to
   a. dab his or her nose instead of blowing.
   b. be careful when shaving with a safety razor.
   c. continue with physical activities to stimulate thrombopoiesis.
   d. avoid aspirin because it may mask the fever that occurs with thrombocytopenia.
7. The nurse would anticipate that a patient with von Willebrand disease undergoing surgery would be treated with administration of vWF and
   a. thrombin.
   b. factor VI.
   c. factor VII.
   d. factor VIII.
8. DIC is a disorder in which
   a. the coagulation pathway is genetically altered, leading to thrombus formation in all major blood vessels.
   b. an underlying disease depletes hemolytic factors in the blood, leading to diffuse thrombotic episodes and infarcts.
   c. a disease process stimulates coagulation processes with resultant thrombosis, as well as depletion of clotting factors, leading to diffuse clotting and hemorrhage.
   d. an inherited predisposition causes a deficiency of clotting factors that leads to overstimulation of coagulation processes in the vasculature.
9. Priority nursing actions when caring for a hospitalized patient with a new-onset temperature of 102.2°F (39°C) and severe neutropenia include *(select all that apply)*
   a. administering the prescribed antibiotic STAT.
   b. drawing peripheral and central line blood cultures.
   c. ongoing monitoring of the patient's vital signs for septic shock.
   d. taking a full set of vital signs and notifying the physician immediately.
   e. administering transfusions of WBCs treated to decrease immunogenicity.
10. Because myelodysplastic syndrome arises from the pluripotent hematopoietic stem cell in the bone marrow, laboratory results the nurse would expect to find include a(n)
    a. excess of T cells.
    b. excess of platelets.
    c. deficiency of granulocytes.
    d. deficiency of all cellular blood components.
11. The most common type of leukemia in older adults is
    a. acute myelocytic leukemia.
    b. acute lymphocytic leukemia.
    c. chronic myelocytic leukemia.
    d. chronic lymphocytic leukemia.
12. Multiple drugs are often used in combinations to treat leukemia and lymphoma because
    a. there are fewer toxic and side effects.
    b. the chance that one drug will be effective is increased.
    c. the drugs are more effective without causing side effects.
    d. the drugs work by different mechanisms to maximize killing of malignant cells.
13. The nurse is aware that a major difference between Hodgkin's lymphoma and non-Hodgkin's lymphoma is that
    a. Hodgkin's lymphoma occurs only in young adults.
    b. Hodgkin's lymphoma is considered potentially curable.
    c. non-Hodgkin's lymphoma can manifest in multiple organs.
    d. non-Hodgkin's lymphoma is treated only with radiation therapy.
14. A patient with multiple myeloma becomes confused and lethargic. The nurse would expect that these clinical manifestations may be explained by diagnostic results that indicate
    a. hyperkalemia.
    b. hyperuricemia.
    c. hypercalcemia.
    d. CNS myeloma.
15. When reviewing the patient's hematologic laboratory values after a splenectomy, the nurse would expect to find
    a. leukopenia.
    b. RBC abnormalities.
    c. decreased hemoglobin.
    d. increased platelet count.
16. Complications of transfusions that can be decreased by the use of leukocyte depletion or reduction of RBC transfusion are
    a. chills and hemolysis.
    b. leukostasis and neutrophilia.
    c. fluid overload and pulmonary edema.
    d. transmission of cytomegalovirus and fever.

1. a, 2. b, 3. a, c, 4. a, b, c, d, 5. a, 6. a, 7. d, 8. c, 9. a, b, c, d, 10. d, 11. d, 12. d, 13. c, 14. c, 15. d, 16. d

For rationales to these answers and even more NCLEX review questions, visit *http://evolve.elsevier.com/Lewis/medsurg.*

EVOLVE WEBSITE

http://evolve.elsevier.com/Lewis/medsurg

Review Questions (Online Only)

Key Points

Answer Keys for Review Questions

- Rationales for Bridge to NCLEX Examination Questions
- Answer Guidelines for Case Study on p. 652
- Answer Guidelines for Managing Care of Multiple Patients Case Study (Section 6) on p. 656

Student Case Studies

- Patient With Chronic Myelogenous Leukemia Including End-of-life Care
- Patient With Sickle Cell Anemia

Nursing Care Plans

- eNursing Care Plan 30-1: Patient With Anemia
- eNursing Care Plan 30-2: Patient With Thrombocytopenia
- eNursing Care Plan 30-3: Patient With Neutropenia

Conceptual Care Map Creator

- Conceptual Care Map for Case Study on p. 652

Audio Glossary

Content Updates

REFERENCES

1. Marks PW: Approach to anemia in the adult and child. In Hoffman R, Benz EJ, Silberstein LE, et al, editors: *Hematology: basic principles and practice*, ed 6, Philadelphia, 2013, Saunders.
2. Rote NS, McCance KL: Alterations of erythrocyte function. In McCance KL, Huether SE, editors: *Pathophysiology: the biologic basis for disease in adults and children*, ed 7, St Louis, 2014, Mosby.
3. Artz AS, Ershler WB: Hematology in aging. In Hoffman R, Benz EJ, Silberstein LE, et al, editors: *Hematology: basic principles and practice*, ed 6, Philadelphia, 2013, Saunders.
4. World Health Organization. Retrieved from *www.who.int*.
5. Rote NS, McCane KL: Structure and function of the hematologic system. In McCance KL, Huether SE, editors: *Pathophysiology: the biologic basis for disease in adults and children*, ed 7, St Louis, 2014, Mosby.
6. American Dietetic Association. Retrieved from *www.eatright.org*.
7. WebMD. Retrieved from *www.webmd.com*.
8. Micromedex 2.0. Truven Analytics, Inc. Retrieved from *www.micromedexsolutions.com*.
9. Kline NE: Alterations of hematologic function in children. In McCance KL, Huether SE, editors: *Pathophysiology: the biologic basis for disease in adults and children*, ed 7, St Louis, 2014, Mosby.
10. Carson SM, Martin MB: Effective iron chelation practice for patients with β-thalassemia major, *Clin J Oncol Nurs* 18:102, 2014.
11. Townsley DM, Rodgers GP: Deficiencies of vitamin B_{12} and folate. In Rodgers GP, Young NS: *The Bethesda handbook of clinical hematology*, ed 3, Philadelphia, 2013, Lippincott.
12. Scheinberg P, Young NS, Liu JM: Bone marrow failure syndromes: aplastic anemia, acquired and constitutional; paroxysmal nocturnal hemoglobinuria; pure red blood cell aplasia; and agranulocytosis. In Rodgers GP, Young NS: *The Bethesda handbook of clinical hematology*, ed 3, Philadelphia, 2013, Lippincott.
13. Willis L, Rexwinkle A, Bryan J, et al: Recent developments in drug therapy for aplastic anemia, *Ann Pharmacother* 48:1469, 2014.

*14. Yawn BP, Buchanan GR, Afenyi-Annan AN, et al: Management of sickle cell disease: Summary of the 2014 evidence-based report by expert panel members, *J Am Med Assoc* 312:1033, 2014.

15. Taylor LV, Stotts NA, Humphreys J, et al: A biopsychosocial-spiritual model of chronic pain in adults with sickle cell disease, *Pain Manag Nurs* 14:287, 2013.
16. Food and Drug Administration. Retrieved from *www.FDA.gov*.
17. Parikh AR, Olnes MJ: The myeloproliferative neoplasms: polycythemia vera, essential thrombocythemia, and primary myelofibrosis. In Rodgers GP, Young NS: *The Bethesda handbook of clinical hematology*, ed 3, Philadelphia, 2013, Lippincott.
18. Fogarty PF, Dunbar CE: Thrombocytopenia. In Rodgers GP, Young NS: *The Bethesda handbook of clinical hematology*, ed 3, Philadelphia, 2013, Lippincott.
19. Diz-Kucukkaya R, Lopez JA: Acquired disorders of platelet function. In Hoffman R, Benz EJ, Silberstein LE, et al, editors: *Hematology: basic principles and practice*, ed 6, Philadelphia, 2013, Saunders.
20. McCrae KR, Sadler JE, Cines DB: Thrombotic thrombocytopenic purpura and the hemolytic uremic syndrome. In Hoffman R, Benz EJ, Silberstein LE, et al, editors: *Hematology: basic principles and practice*, ed 6, Philadelphia, 2013, Saunders.
21. Warkentin TE: Heparin-induced thrombocytopenia. In Hoffman R, Benz EJ, Silberstein LE, et al, editors: *Hematology: basic principles and practice*, ed 6, Philadelphia, 2013, Saunders.
22. Fogarty PF: Disorders of hemostasis II. In Rodgers GP, Young NS: *The Bethesda handbook of clinical hematology*, ed 3, Philadelphia, 2013, Lippincott.
23. Carcao M, Moorehead P, Lillicrap D: Hemophilia A and B. In Hoffman R, Benz EJ, Silberstein LE, et al, editors: *Hematology: basic principles and practice*, ed 6, Philadelphia, 2013, Saunders.

*24. Oldenburg J, Brackmann H: Prophylaxis in adult patients with severe haemophilia A, *Thromb Res* 134:S33, 2014.

25. Kempton CL, Meeks SL: Toward optimal therapy for inhibitors in hemophilia, *Blood* 124:3365, 2014.
26. Schwartz A, Rote NS: Alterations of leukocyte, lymphoid, and hemostatic function. In McCance KL, Huether SE. editors: *Pathophysiology: the biologic basis for disease in adults and children*, ed 7, St Louis, 2014, Mosby.
27. Levi M: Disseminated intravascular coagulation. In Hoffman R, Benz EJ, Silberstein LE, et al, editors: *Hematology: basic principles and practice*, ed 6, Philadelphia, 2013, Saunders.
28. Noel P, Jaben EA: Consultative hematology. In Rodgers GP, Young NS: *The Bethesda handbook of clinical hematology*, ed 3, Philadelphia, 2013, Lippincott.
29. Maciejewski JP, Tiu RV: Acquired disorders of red cell, white cell, and platelet production. In Hoffman R, Benz EJ, Silberstein LE, et al, editors: *Hematology: basic principles and practice*, ed 6, Philadelphia, 2013, Saunders.

*30. Baden LR, Bensinger W, Angarone M, et al: Prevention and treatment of cancer-related infections, NCCN Clinical Practice Guidelines, version 2, 2014. Retrieved from *www.nccn.org*.

*31. Boubekri A: Reducing central line-associated bloodstream infections in the blood and marrow transplantation population: a review of the literature, *Clin J Oncol Nurs* 17:297, 2013.

*32. Foster M: Re-evaluating the neutropenic diet: time to change, *Clin J Oncol Nurs* 18:239, 2014.

*33. Freifeld AG, Bow EJ, Sepkowitz KA: Clinical practice guideline for the use of antimicrobial agents in neutropenic patients with cancer: 2010 Update by the Infectious Diseases Society of America, *Clin Infect Dis* 52:e56, 2011. (Classic)

*34. Crawford J, Becker PS, Armitage J, et al: Myeloid growth factors, NCCN Clinical Practice Guidelines, version 2, 2014. Retrieved from *www.nccn.org*.

*35. Greenberg PL, Stone RM, Bejar R: Myelodysplastic Syndromes, NCCN Clinical Practice Guidelines, version 1, 2015. Retrieved from *www.nccn.org*.

36. Klotz J, Parikh AR, Battiwalla M: The myelodysplastic syndromes. In Rodgers GP, Young NS: *The Bethesda handbook of clinical hematology*, ed 3, Philadelphia, 2013, Lippincott.
37. American Cancer Society. *Cancer Facts and Figures 2014*. Atlanta: American Cancer Society, 2014. Retrieved from *www.cancer.org*.
38. Yin F, Malkovska V: Acute myeloid leukemia. In Rodgers GP, Young NS: *The Bethesda handbook of clinical hematology*, ed 3, Philadelphia, 2013, Lippincott.
39. Shah NN, Wayne AS: Acute lymphoblastic leukemia. In Rodgers GP, Young NS: *The Bethesda handbook of clinical hematology*, ed 3, Philadelphia, 2013, Lippincott.
40. Yong AS, Barrett AJ: Chronic myelogenous leukemia. In Rodgers GP, Young NS: *The Bethesda handbook of clinical hematology*, ed 3, Philadelphia, 2013, Lippincott.

41. Farooqui MZ, Wiestner A, Aue G: Chronic lymphocytic leukemia. In Rodgers GP, Young NS: *The Bethesda handbook of clinical hematology*, ed 3, Philadelphia, 2013, Lippincott.
*42. Zelenetz AD, Gordon LI, Wierda WG, et al: Non-Hodgkin's lymphomas, NCCN Clinical Practice Guidelines, version 5, 2014. Retrieved from *www.nccn.org*.
*43. O'Donnell MR, Tallman MS, Abboud CH, et al: Acute myeloid leukemia, NCCN Clinical Practice Guidelines, version 2, 2014. Retrieved from *www.nccn.org*.
*44. Alvarnas JC, Brown PA, Aoun P, et al: Acute lymphoblastic leukemia, NCCN Clinical Practice Guidelines, version 1, 2014. Retrieved from *www.nccn.org*.
*45. O'Brien S, Radich JP, Abboud CN, et al: Chronic myelogenous leukemia, NCCN Clinical Practice Guidelines, version 1, 2015. Retrieved from *www.nccn.org*.
*46. Hoppe RT, Advani RH, Ai WZ, et al: Hodgkin lymphoma, NCCN Clinical Practice Guidelines, version 2, 2014. Retrieved from *www.nccn.org*.
47. Kanate AS, Craig M, Abraham J, et al: Hodgkin lymphoma. In Rodgers GP, Young NS: *The Bethesda handbook of clinical hematology*, ed 3, Philadelphia, 2013, Lippincott.
48. Little RF, Wilson WH: Non-Hodgkin lymphomas. In Rodgers GP, Young NS: *The Bethesda handbook of clinical hematology*, ed 3, Philadelphia, 2013, Lippincott.
49. Surveillance, Epidemiology, and End Results Program (SEER): SEER Stat Fact Sheets: Myeloma. Retrieved from *www.seer.cancer.gov*.
50. Manasanch EE, Tageja N, Landgren CO: Multiple myeloma. In Rodgers GP, Young NS: *The Bethesda handbook of clinical hematology*, ed 3, Philadelphia, 2013, Lippincott.
*51. Anderson KC, Bensinger W, Alsina M, et al: Multiple myeloma, NCCN Clinical Practice Guidelines, version 2, 2015. Retrieved from *www.nccn.org*.
52. Connell NT, Shurin SB, Schiffman FJ: The spleen and its disorders. In Hoffman R, Benz EJ, Silberstein LE, et al, editors: *Hematology: basic principles and practice*, ed 6, Philadelphia, 2013, Saunders.
53. Desmond R, Klein HG: Blood transfusion. In Rodgers GP, Young NS: *The Bethesda handbook of clinical hematology*, ed 3, Philadelphia, 2013, Lippincott.
54. Maynard K: Administration of blood components. In Fung MK, Grossman BJ, Hillyer CD, et al, editors: *Technical manual: standards for blood banks and transfusion services*, ed 18, Bethesda, 2014, AABB.
*55. Stupnyckyj C, Smolarek S, Reeves C, et al: Changing blood transfusion policy and practice, *Am J Nurs* 114:50, 2014.
56. Pagana KD, Pagana TJ: *Mosby's manual of diagnostic and laboratory tests*, ed 5, St Louis, 2014, Mosby.
57. Mazzei CA, Popovsky MA, Kopko PM: Noninfectious complications of blood transfusion. In Fung MK, Grossman BJ, Hillyer CD, et al, editors: *Technical manual: standards for blood banks and transfusion services*, ed 18, Bethesda, 2014, AABB.
58. Galel SA: Infectious disease screening. In Fung MK, Grossman BJ, Hillyer CD, et al, editors: *Technical manual: standards for blood banks and transfusion services*, ed 18, Bethesda, 2014, AABB.

*Evidence-based information for clinical practice.

CASE STUDY

Managing Care of Multiple Patients

You are working on the oncology unit and have been assigned to care for the following four patients. You have one UAP who is assigned to help you, and there are two other RNs on your clinical unit.

Patients

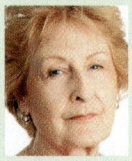

(©Lisa F. Young/iStock)

A.J. is a 63-yr-old white woman who is admitted with severe anemia (Hgb 5.9 g/dL and Hct 18.2%). Her WBC count is 2600/μL and platelet count is 72,000/μL. She prefers to take care of herself with "natural therapy" and has not seen an HCP for 5 years. A.J. is having difficulty performing ADLs without having to stop and catch her breath. She received 2 units of RBCs. After a further workup, she is diagnosed with acute myelocytic leukemia (AML). She remains hospitalized as she starts chemotherapy.

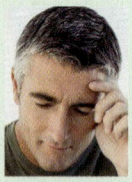

(©g-stockstudio/iStock/Thinkstock)

J.J. is a 52-yr-old white man newly diagnosed with acute lymphocytic leukemia (ALL). His most recent vital signs are BP 100/70, temperature 102.2°F (39°C), respiratory rate 26/min, pulse 110. Laboratory results reveal Hgb 6.9 g/dL, Hct 20%, WBC count 120,000/μL (120×10^9/L), and platelet count 25,000/μL (25×10^9/L). He is admitted for blood transfusions and induction therapy.

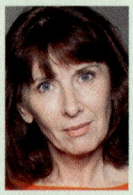

(©Studio Grand Ouest/iStock/Thinkstock)

P.H. is a 45-yr-old woman who is currently receiving chemotherapy for treatment of ovarian cancer. She is admitted with fever and chills. Her WBC count is 2200/μL (2.2×10^9/L) with an absolute neutrophil count (ANC) of 400/μL (0.4×10^9/L). She is admitted for IV antibiotic therapy and is in isolation. Her most recent vital signs are BP 118/60, temperature 99.2°F (37.3°C), respiratory rate 20/min, pulse 98.

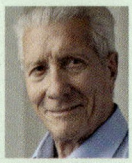

(©Ridofranz/iStock)

G.L. is a 67-yr-old man who came to the ED yesterday evening with complaints of abdominal pain. A CT scan of the abdomen revealed several masses in his lymphatic system. The HCP suspects non-Hodgkin's lymphoma and admits him for a diagnostic workup. He currently rates his pain as a 3 on a scale of 0 to 10.

Discussion Questions

1. ***Priority Decision:*** After receiving report, which patient should you see first? Provide a rationale for your decision.
2. ***Teamwork and Collaboration:*** Which task could you delegate to the UAP *(select all that apply)*?
   a. Assist A.J. to a chair after completing her AM care.
   b. Obtain the first unit of blood for J.J. from the blood bank.
   c. Explain the importance of isolation to P.H. and her family.
   d. Ask A.J. why she has not been willing to get any medical care for 5 years.
   e. Ask G.L. about the presence of additional clinical manifestations of non-Hodgkin's lymphoma.
3. ***Priority and Delegation Decision:*** When you enter J.J.'s room, you find him somewhat confused and lethargic. His family states he had just had a severe coughing episode. What initial action would be the *most* appropriate?
   a. Perform a focused neurologic examination.
   b. Call respiratory therapy to give him a breathing treatment.
   c. Ask his family members if they have a copy of his living will.
   d. Have the UAP stay with J.J. while you page the HCP stat.

Case Study Progression

J.J.'s HCP orders a repeat CBC and an emergency CT scan of the head. Your supervisor makes arrangements for another RN to accompany J.J. to the CT scan while you prepare to administer the first unit of RBCs.

4. The HCP orders ferrous sulfate 325 mg TID for A.J. You teach A.J. to take her iron *(select all that apply)*
   a. at breakfast time in the morning.
   b. with orange juice to increase absorption.
   c. 1 hour before meals to facilitate absorption.
   d. 2 hours after eating to minimize side effects.
   e. whenever she feels tired or is short of breath with activity.
5. When teaching P.H.'s family about neutropenic precautions, you emphasize that the *most* important intervention to prevent infection is
   a. hand washing.
   b. wearing a mask.
   c. keeping P.H. in a private room.
   d. limiting the number of visitors in her room.
6. G.L. asks you to explain the diagnostic testing he can expect to undergo related to the suspected lymphoma. Which tests will you explain to him *(select all that apply)*?
   a. PET scan
   b. Bone marrow biopsy
   c. Peripheral blood smear
   d. Excisional lymph node biopsy
   e. Lymphangiography of internal lymph nodes
7. ***Management Decision:*** An RN from the float pool arrives to accompany J.J. to CT scan at the same time the UAP arrives with his first unit of RBCs. Which intervention would be *most* appropriate?
   a. Put the unit of RBCs in the refrigerator to start when J.J. returns to the floor.
   b. Ask the RN to verify the correct unit of RBCs with you and start the infusion.
   c. Give the RN an SBAR report on J.J. and ask her to start the blood on the way to her CT scan.
   d. Ask the RN if she would prefer to give the blood or hold it for J.J.'s return to the unit.

Answers available at *http://evolve.elsevier.com/Lewis/medsurg.*

SECTION 7

Problems of Oxygenation: Perfusion

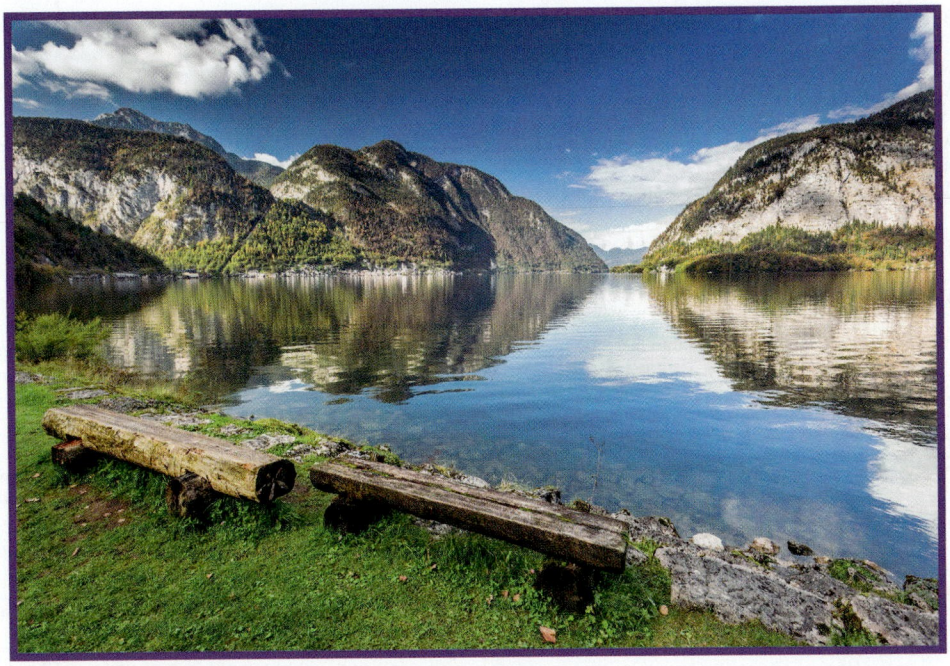

©Shaiith/iStock/Thinkstock

Sit by a river. Find peace and meaning in the rhythm of the lifeblood of the Earth.

Anonymous

Chapter 31 Assessment of Cardiovascular System, 658

Chapter 32 Hypertension, 681

Chapter 33 Coronary Artery Disease and Acute Coronary Syndrome, 702

Chapter 34 Heart Failure, 737

Chapter 35 Dysrhythmias, 757

Chapter 36 Inflammatory and Structural Heart Disorders, 780

Chapter 37 Vascular Disorders, 802

31

Assessment of Cardiovascular System

Angela DiSabatino Herman, Linda Bucher

The only way to do great work is to love what you do.

Steve Jobs

http://evolve.elsevier.com/Lewis/medsurg/

LEARNING OUTCOMES

1. Differentiate the anatomic location and function of the following structures of the heart: pericardial layers, atria, ventricles, and valves.
2. Relate the coronary circulation to the areas of heart muscle supplied by the major coronary arteries.
3. Differentiate the structure and function of arteries, veins, capillaries, and endothelium.
4. Describe the mechanisms involved in the regulation of blood pressure.
5. Relate the various waveforms on a normal electrocardiogram to the associated cardiac events.
6. Obtain significant subjective and objective assessment data related to the cardiovascular system from a patient and/or caregiver.
7. Perform a physical assessment of the cardiovascular system using the appropriate techniques.
8. Differentiate normal from abnormal findings of a physical assessment of the cardiovascular system.
9. Link the age-related changes of the cardiovascular system to the differences in assessment findings.
10. Describe the purpose, significance of results, and nursing responsibilities related to diagnostic studies of the cardiovascular system.

KEY TERMS

action potential, p. 659
afterload, p. 661
arterial blood pressure, p. 662
cardiac index (CI), p. 660
cardiac output (CO), p. 660
cardiac reserve, p. 661
coronary angiography, p. 678
diastole, p. 659
diastolic blood pressure (DBP), p. 662
ejection fraction (EF), p. 671
heaves, p. 667
Korotkoff sounds, p. 662
mean arterial pressure (MAP), p. 662
murmur, p. 662
point of maximal impulse (PMI), p. 667
preload, p. 660
pulse pressure, p. 662
systole, p. 660
systolic blood pressure (SBP), p. 662

STRUCTURES AND FUNCTIONS OF CARDIOVASCULAR SYSTEM

Heart

Structure. The heart is a four-chambered hollow muscular organ normally about the size of a fist. It lies within the thorax in the mediastinal space that separates the right and left pleural cavities. The heart is composed of three layers: a thin inner lining, the *endocardium;* a layer of muscle, the *myocardium;* and an outer layer, the *epicardium.* The heart is covered by a fibroserous sac called the *pericardium.* This sac consists of two layers: the inner *(visceral)* layer of the pericardium (part of the epicardium) and the outer *(parietal)* layer. A small amount of pericardial fluid (approximately 10 to 15 mL) lubricates the space between the pericardial layers *(pericardial space)* and prevents friction between the surfaces as the heart contracts.[1]

The heart is divided vertically by the septum. The interatrial septum creates a right and left atrium, and the interventricular septum creates a right and left ventricle. The thickness of the wall of each chamber is different. The atrial myocardium is thinner than that of the ventricles, and the left ventricular wall is two or three times thicker than the right ventricular wall.[1] The thickness of the left ventricle is necessary to produce the force needed to pump the blood into the systemic circulation.

Blood Flow Through Heart. The blood flow through the heart is illustrated in Fig. 31-1.

Heart Valves. The four valves of the heart keep blood flowing in a forward direction. The cusps of the mitral and tricuspid valves are attached to thin strands of fibrous tissue termed *chordae tendineae* (Fig. 31-2). Chordae are anchored in the papillary muscles of the ventricles. This support system prevents the eversion of the leaflets into the atria during ventricular contraction. The pulmonic and aortic valves (also known as *semilunar valves*) prevent blood from regurgitating into the ventricles at the end of each ventricular contraction.

Blood Supply to Myocardium. The myocardium has its own blood supply, the *coronary circulation* (Fig. 31-3). Blood flow

Reviewed by Janie Corbitt, RN, MLS, Retired Instructor of Nursing, Milledgeville, Georgia; Cynthia Hambach, RN, MSN, CCRN, Assistant Clinical Professor, Drexel University, Philadelphia, Pennsylvania; and Jennifer Saylor, RN, PhD, ACNS-BC, Assistant Professor, University of Delaware, Newark, Delaware.

into the two major coronary arteries occurs primarily during diastole (relaxation of the myocardium). The left coronary artery arises from the aorta and divides into two main branches: the left anterior descending artery and left circumflex artery. These arteries supply the left atrium, left ventricle, interventricular septum, and a portion of the right ventricle. The right coronary artery also arises from the aorta, and its branches supply the right atrium, right ventricle, and a portion of the posterior wall of the left ventricle. In 90% of people the atrioventricular (AV) node and the bundle of His receive blood supply from the right coronary artery. For this reason, blockage of this artery often causes serious defects in cardiac conduction.

The divisions of coronary veins parallel the coronary arteries. Most of the blood from the coronary system drains into the coronary sinus (a large channel), which empties into the right atrium near the entrance of the inferior vena cava.

Conduction System. The conduction system consists of specialized tissue responsible for creating and transporting the electrical impulse, or action potential. This impulse starts depolarization of the heart cells and subsequently heart contraction (Fig. 31-4, *A*). The electrical impulse normally begins in the sinoatrial (SA) node (pacemaker of the heart). Each impulse coming from the SA node travels through interatrial pathways to depolarize the atria, resulting in a contraction.

The electrical impulse travels from the atria to the AV node through internodal pathways. The signal then moves through

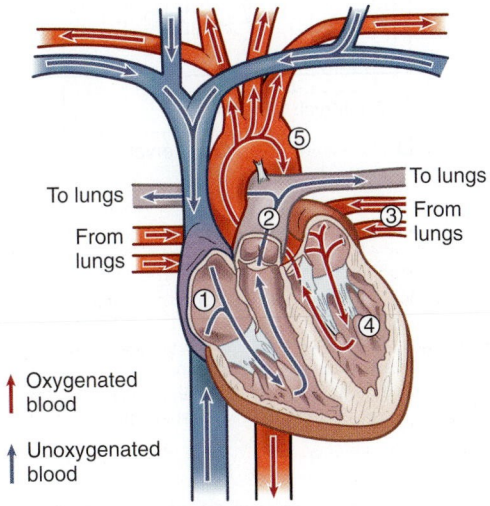

FIG. 31-1 Schematic representation of blood flow through the heart. *Arrows* indicate direction of flow. *1,* The right atrium receives venous blood from the inferior and superior venae cavae and the coronary sinus. The blood then passes through the tricuspid valve into the right ventricle. *2,* With each contraction, the right ventricle pumps blood through the pulmonic valve into the pulmonary artery and to the lungs. *3,* Oxygenated blood flows from the lungs to the left atrium by way of the pulmonary veins. *4,* It then passes through the mitral valve and into the left ventricle. *5,* As the heart contracts, blood is ejected through the aortic valve into the aorta and thus enters the systemic circulation.

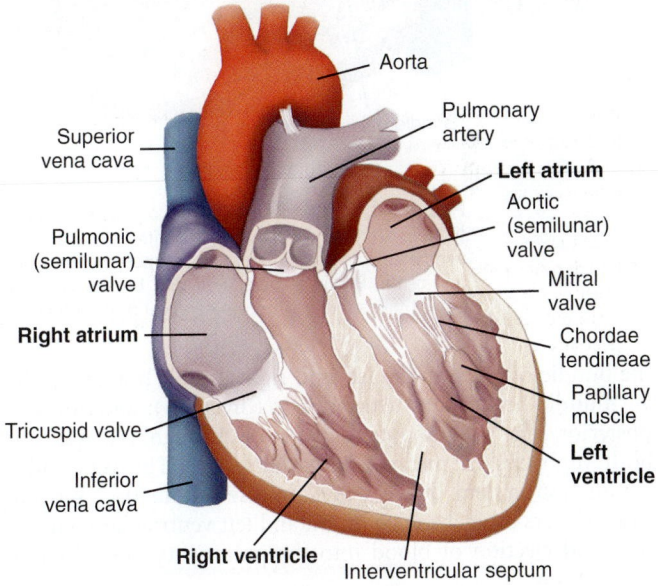

FIG. 31-2 Anatomic structures of the heart and heart valves.

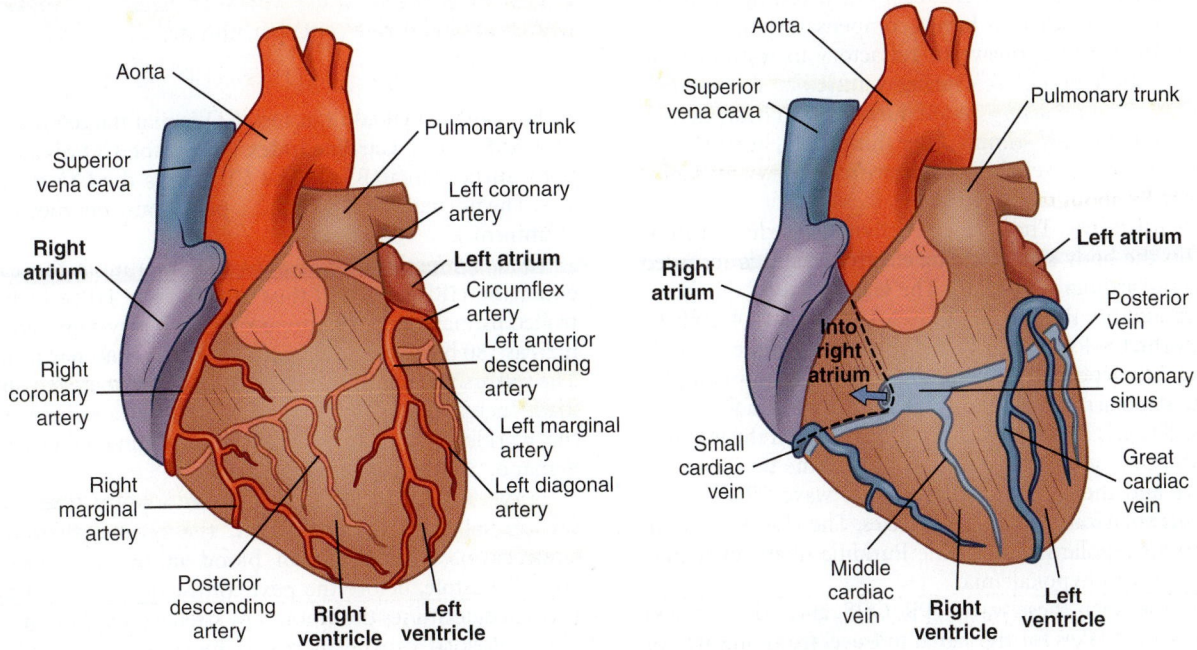

FIG. 31-3 Coronary arteries and veins.

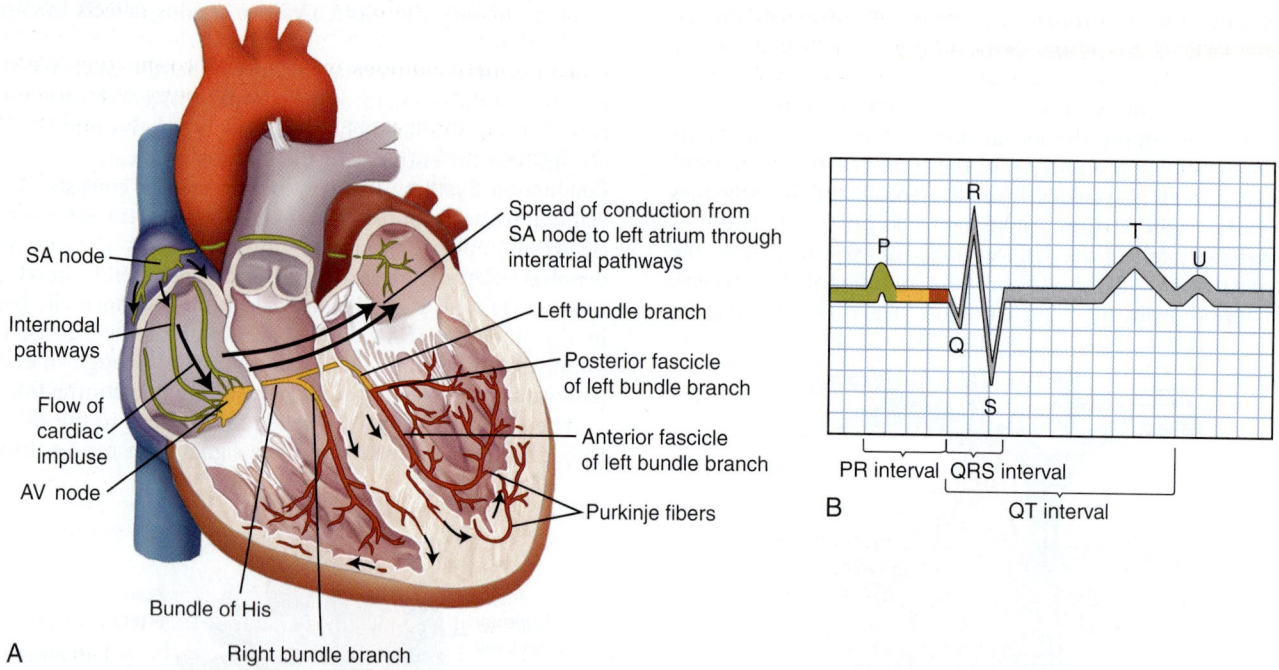

FIG. 31-4 **A,** Conduction system of the heart. *AV,* Atrioventricular; *SA,* sinoatrial. **B,** The normal electrocardiogram (ECG) pattern. The P wave represents depolarization of the atria. The QRS complex indicates depolarization of the ventricles. The T wave represents repolarization of the ventricles. The U wave, if present, may represent repolarization of the Purkinje fibers, or it may be associated with hypokalemia. The PR, QRS, and QT intervals reflect the time it takes for the impulse to travel from one area of the heart to another.

the bundle of His and the left and right bundle branches. The left bundle branch has two fascicles (divisions): anterior and posterior. The action potential moves through the walls of both ventricles by means of *Purkinje fibers.* The ventricular conduction system delivers the impulse within 0.12 second. This triggers a synchronized right and left ventricular contraction and ejection of blood into the pulmonary and systemic circulations.

Last, repolarization occurs when the contractile fiber cells and the conduction pathway cells regain their resting polarized condition. Heart muscle cells have a compensatory mechanism that makes them unresponsive or refractory to restimulation during the action potential. During ventricular contraction, there is an *absolute refractory period* during which heart muscle does not respond to any stimuli. After this period, heart muscle gradually recovers its excitability, and a *relative refractory period* occurs by early diastole.

Resting period

Electrocardiogram. The electrical activity of the heart can be detected on the body surface using electrodes and is recorded on an electrocardiogram (ECG). The letters *P, QRS, T,* and *U* are used to identify the separate waveforms (Fig. 31-4, *B*). The first waveform, the P wave, begins with the firing of the SA node and represents depolarization of the atria. The QRS complex represents depolarization from the AV node throughout the ventricles. There is a delay of impulse transmission through the AV node that accounts for the time between the beginning of the P wave and the beginning of the QRS wave. The T wave represents repolarization of the ventricles. The U wave, if seen, may represent repolarization of the Purkinje fibers, or it may be associated with hypokalemia.[2]

Intervals between these waves (PR, QRS, and QT intervals) reflect the time it takes for the signal to travel from one area of the heart to another. These time intervals are measured, and changes from these time references often indicate pathologic conditions. (See Chapter 35 for a complete discussion of ECG monitoring.)

Mechanical System. *Depolarization* triggers mechanical activity. **Systole**, contraction of the heart muscle, results in ejection of blood from the ventricles. Relaxation of the heart muscle, *diastole,* allows for filling of the ventricles. **Cardiac output (CO)**, the amount of blood pumped by each ventricle in 1 minute, is calculated by multiplying the amount of blood ejected from the ventricle with each heartbeat: *stroke volume* (SV) times heart rate (HR) per minute:

$$CO = SV \times HR$$

For the normal adult at rest, CO is maintained in the range of 4 to 8 L/min. **Cardiac index (CI)** is the CO divided by the body surface area (BSA). The CI adjusts the CO to the body size. The normal CI is 2.8 to 4.2 L per minute per meter squared ($L/min/m^2$).

Factors Affecting Cardiac Output. Numerous factors can affect either the HR or SV, and thus the CO. The HR, which is controlled primarily by the autonomic nervous system, can reach as high as 180 beats/min for short periods without harmful effects. The factors affecting the SV are preload, contractility, and afterload. Increasing preload, contractility, and afterload increases the workload of the heart muscle, resulting in increased O_2 demand.

Frank-Starling law states that, to a point, the more the myocardial fibers are stretched, the greater their force of contraction. The volume of blood in the ventricles at the end of diastole, before the next contraction, is called **preload.** Preload determines the amount of stretch placed on myocardial fibers. Preload can be increased by a number of conditions such as hypertension, aortic valve disease, and hypervolemia.[3]

Contractility can be increased by epinephrine and norepinephrine released by the sympathetic nervous system. Increasing contractility raises the SV by increasing ventricular emptying.

Afterload is the peripheral resistance against which the left ventricle must pump. Afterload is affected by the size of the ventricle, wall tension, and arterial blood pressure (BP). If the arterial BP is elevated, the ventricles meet increased resistance to ejection of blood, increasing the work demand. Eventually this results in *ventricular hypertrophy,* an enlargement of the heart muscle without an increase in CO or the size of chambers (Fig. 35-1, *B*).

Cardiac Reserve. The cardiovascular system must respond to numerous situations in health and illness (e.g., exercise, stress, hypovolemia). The ability to respond to these demands by altering CO is termed **cardiac reserve**.

Vascular System

Blood Vessels. The three major types of blood vessels in the vascular system are the arteries, veins, and capillaries. Arteries, except for the pulmonary artery, carry oxygenated blood away from the heart. Veins, except for the pulmonary veins, carry deoxygenated blood toward the heart. Small branches of arteries and veins are arterioles and venules, respectively. Blood circulates from the left side of the heart into arteries, arterioles, capillaries, venules, and veins, and then back to the right side of the heart.

Arteries and Arterioles. The arterial system differs from the venous system by the amount and type of tissue that make up arterial walls (Fig. 31-5). The large arteries have thick walls composed mainly of elastic tissue. This elastic property cushions the impact of the pressure created by ventricular contraction and provides recoil that propels blood forward into the circulation. Large arteries also contain some smooth muscle. Examples of large arteries are the aorta and pulmonary artery.

Arterioles have relatively little elastic tissue and more smooth muscle. Arterioles serve as the major control of arterial BP and distribution of blood flow. They respond readily to local conditions such as low O_2 and increasing levels of CO_2 by dilating or constricting.

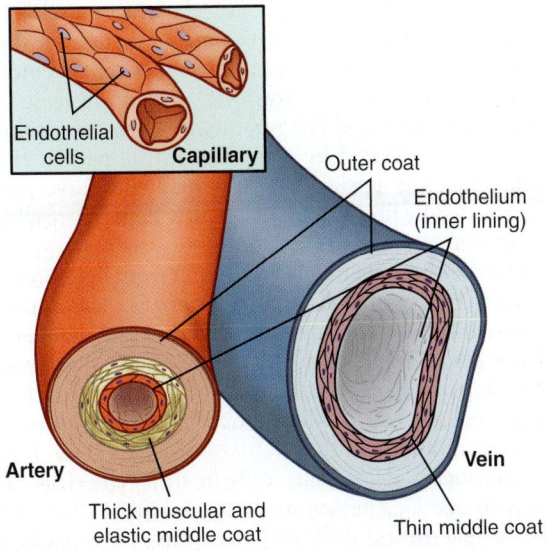

FIG. 31-5 Comparative thickness of layers of the artery, vein, and capillary.

The innermost lining of the arteries is the endothelium. The endothelium maintains hemostasis, promotes blood flow, and, under normal conditions, inhibits blood coagulation. When the endothelial surface is disrupted (e.g., rupture of an atherosclerotic plaque), the coagulation cascade is initiated and results in the formation of a fibrin clot.

Capillaries. The thin capillary wall, made up of endothelial cells, has no elastic or muscle tissue (Fig. 31-5). The exchange of cellular nutrients and metabolic end products takes place through these thin-walled vessels. Capillaries connect the arterioles and venules.

Veins and Venules. Veins are large-diameter, thin-walled vessels that return blood to the right atrium (Fig. 31-5). The venous system is a low-pressure, high-volume system. The larger veins contain semilunar valves at intervals to maintain the blood flow toward the heart and to prevent backward flow. The amount of blood in the venous system is affected by a number of factors, including arterial flow, compression of veins by skeletal muscles, alterations in thoracic and abdominal pressures, and right atrial pressure.

The largest veins are the *superior vena cava,* which returns blood to the heart from the head, neck, and arms, and the *inferior vena cava,* which returns blood to the heart from the lower part of the body. These large-diameter vessels are affected by the pressure in the right side of the heart. Elevated right atrial pressure can cause distended neck veins or liver engorgement as a result of resistance to blood flow.

Venules are relatively small vessels made up of a small amount of muscle and connective tissue. Venules collect blood from the capillary beds and channel it to the larger veins.

Regulation of Cardiovascular System

Autonomic Nervous System. The autonomic nervous system consists of the sympathetic nervous system and parasympathetic nervous system (see Chapter 55).

Effect on Heart. Stimulation of the sympathetic nervous system increases the HR, speed of impulse conduction through the AV node, and force of atrial and ventricular contractions. This effect is mediated by specific sites in the heart called *beta (β)-adrenergic receptors,* which are receptors for norepinephrine and epinephrine.

In contrast, stimulation of the parasympathetic system (mediated by the vagus nerve) slows the HR by decreasing the impulses from the SA node and thus conduction through the AV node.

Effect on Blood Vessels. The source of neural control of blood vessels is the sympathetic nervous system. The alpha$_1$ (α_1)-adrenergic receptors are located in vascular smooth muscles. Stimulation of α_1-adrenergic receptors results in vasoconstriction. Decreased stimulation to α_1-adrenergic receptors causes vasodilation. (Sympathetic nervous system receptors that influence BP are presented in Table 32-1.)

The parasympathetic nerves have selective distribution in the blood vessels. For example, blood vessels in skeletal muscle do not receive parasympathetic input.

Baroreceptors. *Baroreceptors* in the aortic arch and carotid sinus (at the origin of the internal carotid artery) are sensitive to stretch or pressure within the arterial system. Stimulation of these receptors (e.g., volume overload) sends information to the vasomotor center in the brainstem. This results in temporary inhibition of the sympathetic nervous system and enhancement of the parasympathetic influence, causing a decreased HR and peripheral vasodilation. Decreased arterial pressure causes the opposite effect.

Chemoreceptors. *Chemoreceptors* are located in the aortic and carotid bodies and the medulla. They are capable of causing changes in respiratory rate and BP in response to increased arterial CO_2 pressure (hypercapnia) and, to a lesser degree, decreased plasma pH (acidosis) and arterial O_2 pressure (hypoxia). When the chemoreceptors in the medulla are triggered, they stimulate the vasomotor center to increase BP.[3]

Blood Pressure

The **arterial blood pressure** is a measure of the pressure exerted by blood against the walls of the arterial system. The **systolic blood pressure (SBP)** is the peak pressure exerted against the arteries when the heart contracts. The **diastolic blood pressure (DBP)** is the residual pressure in the arterial system during ventricular relaxation (or filling).

The two main factors influencing BP are CO and *systemic vascular resistance* (SVR):

$$BP = CO \times SVR$$

SVR is the force opposing the movement of blood. This force is created primarily in small arteries and arterioles. Normal blood pressure is SBP <120 mm Hg and DBP <80 mm Hg[4] (see Chapter 32).

Measurement of Arterial Blood Pressure. BP can be measured by invasive and noninvasive techniques. The invasive technique consists of catheter insertion into an artery. The catheter is attached to a transducer, and the pressure is measured directly (see Chapter 65).

Noninvasive, indirect measurement of BP can be done with a sphygmomanometer and stethoscope. The sphygmomanometer consists of an inflatable cuff and a pressure gauge. The BP is measured by auscultating for sounds of turbulent blood flow through a compressed artery (termed **Korotkoff sounds**). The brachial artery is the recommended site for taking a BP.

After placing the appropriate size cuff on the upper arm, inflate the cuff to a pressure 20 to 30 mm Hg above the SBP. This causes blood flow in the artery to cease. If the SBP is not known, estimate the pressure by palpating the brachial pulse and inflating the cuff until the pulse ceases. The pressure noted at this time is the estimated SBP. Inflate the BP cuff 20 to 30 mm Hg above this number.

As the pressure in the cuff is lowered, auscultate the artery for Korotkoff sounds. There are five phases of Korotkoff sounds. The first phase is a tapping sound caused by the spurt of blood into the constricted artery as the pressure in the cuff is gradually deflated. This sound is noted as the SBP. The fifth phase occurs when the sound disappears, which is noted as the DBP.[5]

BP is recorded as the ratio of SBP to DBP (e.g., 120/80 mm Hg). Sometimes, an *auscultatory gap* occurs, which is a loss of sound between the SBP and DBP. Proper BP technique (e.g., using the correct cuff size, positioning arm at heart level) is essential for accurate readings (see Table 32-11).

Another noninvasive way to measure BP indirectly is an automated device that uses oscillometric measurements to assess BP. Though this method does not involve auscultation, the same attention to proper technique is essential for accuracy. SBP (and pulse) can be assessed using a Doppler ultrasonic flowmeter. The hand-held transducer is positioned over the artery (identified by audible, pulsatile sounds). The cuff is applied above the artery, inflated until the sounds disappear, and then another 20 to 30 mm Hg beyond that point. The cuff is then slowly deflated until sounds return. This point is the SBP.

Pulse Pressure and Mean Arterial Pressure. **Pulse pressure** is the difference between the SBP and DBP. It is normally about one third of the SBP. If the BP is 120/80 mm Hg, the pulse pressure is 40 mm Hg. An increased pulse pressure due to an increased SBP may occur during exercise or in individuals with atherosclerosis of the larger arteries. A decreased pulse pressure may be found in heart failure or hypovolemia.

Another measurement related to BP is **mean arterial pressure (MAP)**. The MAP refers to the average pressure within the arterial system that is felt by organs in the body. It is not the average of the DBP and SBP, because the length of diastole exceeds that of systole at normal HRs. MAP is calculated as follows:

$$MAP = (SBP + 2\,DBP) \div 3$$

A person with a BP of 120/60 mm Hg has an estimated MAP of 80 mm Hg. In patients with invasive BP monitoring, this value is automatically calculated and takes the patient's HR into consideration (see Chapter 65).

A MAP greater than 60 mm Hg is needed to adequately perfuse and sustain the vital organs of an average person under most conditions. When the MAP falls below this number for a period of time, vital organs are underperfused and will become ischemic.

Gerontologic Considerations: Effects of Aging on the Cardiovascular System

One of the greatest risk factors for cardiovascular disease (CVD) is age. CVD remains the leading cause of death in adults older than age 65. The most common cardiovascular problem is coronary artery disease (CAD) due to atherosclerosis. It is difficult to separate normal aging changes from the pathophysiologic changes of atherosclerosis. Many of the physiologic changes in the cardiovascular system of older adults are a result of the combined effects of the aging process, disease, environmental factors, and lifetime health behaviors rather than just age alone.[6]

Age-related changes in the cardiovascular system and differences in assessment findings are found in Table 31-1. With increased age, the amount of collagen in the heart increases and elastin decreases. These changes affect the heart muscle's ability to stretch and contract. One of the major changes in the cardiovascular system is the response to physical or emotional stress. In times of increased stress, CO and SV decrease due to reduced contractility and HR response. The resting supine HR is not markedly affected by aging. When the patient changes positions (e.g., sits upright), the sympathetic nerve pathway may be affected by fibrous tissue and fatty deposits, resulting in a blunted (reduced) HR response.[6]

Heart valves become thicker and stiffer from lipid accumulation, degeneration of collagen, and fibrosis. The aortic and mitral valves are most frequently affected. These changes result in either regurgitation of blood when the valve should be closed or narrowing of the orifice of the valve *(stenosis)* when the valve should be open. The turbulent blood flow across the affected valve results in a **murmur**.

The number of pacemaker cells in the SA node decreases with age. By age 75, a person may have only 10% of the normal number of pacemaker cells. Although this is compatible with adequate SA node function, it may account for the frequency of some sinus dysrhythmias in older adults. Similar decreases

TABLE 31-1 Gerontologic Assessment Differences

Cardiovascular System

Changes	Differences in Assessment Findings
Chest Wall	
Kyphosis	Altered chest landmarks for palpation, percussion, and auscultation. Distant heart sounds.
Heart	
Myocardial hypertrophy, ↑ collagen and scarring, ↓ elastin	↓ Cardiac reserve, heart failure.
Downward displacement	Difficulty in isolating apical pulse.
↓ CO, HR, SV in response to exercise or stress	↓ Response to exercise and stress. Slowed recovery from activity.
Cellular aging and fibrosis of conduction system	↓ Amplitude of QRS complex and slight lengthening of PR, QRS, and QT intervals. Irregular cardiac rhythms, ↓ maximal HR, ↓ HR variability.
Valvular rigidity from calcification, sclerosis, or fibrosis, impeding complete closure of valves	Systolic murmur (aortic or mitral) possible without an indication of cardiovascular disease.
Blood Vessels	
Arterial stiffening caused by loss of elastin in arterial walls, thickening of intima of arteries, and progressive fibrosis of media	↑ In SBP and possible ↑ or ↓ in DBP. Possible widened pulse pressure. Pedal pulses diminished. ↑ In intermittent claudication.
Venous tortuosity increased	Inflamed, painful, or cordlike varicosities. Dependent edema.

also occur in the number of conduction cells in the internodal tracts, bundle of His, and bundle branches. These changes contribute to the development of atrial dysrhythmias and heart blocks. About 50% of older adults have an abnormal resting ECG that shows increases in the PR, QRS, and/or QT intervals.[7]

The autonomic nervous system control of the cardiovascular system changes with aging. The number and function of β-adrenergic receptors in the heart decrease with age. So the older adult not only has a decreased response to physical and emotional stress but also is less sensitive to β-adrenergic agonist drugs. The lower maximum HR during exercise results in only a twofold increase in CO compared with the three or four times increase seen in younger adults.

Arterial and venous blood vessels thicken and become less elastic with age. Arteries increase their sensitivity to vasopressin (antidiuretic hormone). With aging both of these changes contribute to a progressive increase in SBP and a decrease or no change in DBP. Thus an increase in the pulse pressure is found. Valves in the large veins in the lower extremities have a reduced ability to return the blood to the heart, often resulting in dependent edema.

Orthostatic hypotension, which is estimated to be present in more than 30% of patients over age 70 with systolic hypertension, may be related to drugs and/or decreased baroreceptor function. *Postprandial hypotension* (decrease in BP of at least 20 mm Hg that occurs within 75 minutes after eating) may also occur in about a third of otherwise healthy older adults. Both orthostatic and postprandial hypotension may be related to falls in older adults. Despite the changes associated with aging, the heart is able to function adequately under most circumstances.

CASE STUDY

Patient Introduction

(©Jupiterimages/ Banana-Stock/ Thinkstock)

L.P., a 63-year-old Asian American male, is brought to the emergency department by ambulance at 6 AM with complaints of chest tightness, shortness of breath (SOB), and palpitations. The paramedics have started an IV and O_2 at 2 L/min via nasal cannula. They also administered four chewable baby ASA and a nitroglycerin tablet, and they obtained a 12-lead ECG. L.P. is pain free on arrival but still complains of palpitations.

Discussion Questions

1. What are the possible causes of L.P.'s chest tightness, SOB, and palpitations?
2. What would be your major priorities when assessing L.P.?
3. Is L.P.'s condition stable or unstable?

You will learn more about L.P. and his condition as you read through this assessment chapter.

(See p. 666 for more information on L.P.)

Answers available at *http://evolve.elsevier.com/Lewis/medsurg.*

ASSESSMENT OF CARDIOVASCULAR SYSTEM

Subjective Data

A careful health history and physical examination will help you distinguish symptoms that reflect a cardiovascular problem from problems of other body systems. Explore and record all cues that alert you to the possibility of underlying CVD.

Important Health Information

History of Present Illness. Ask the patient what problem has brought him or her to the health care facility or provider. Fully explore all symptoms the patient is experiencing (Table 31-1).

Past Health History. Many illnesses affect the cardiovascular system directly or indirectly. Ask the patient about a history of chest pain, shortness of breath, fatigue, alcohol and tobacco use, anemia, rheumatic fever, streptococcal throat infections, congenital heart disease, stroke, palpitations, dizziness with position changes, syncope, hypertension, thrombophlebitis, intermittent claudication, edema, and varicosities.

Medications. Assess the patient's current and past use of medications. This includes over-the-counter (OTC) drugs, herbal supplements, and prescription drugs. For example, aspirin prolongs the blood clotting time and is found in many drugs used to treat cold symptoms. List all of the patient's drugs. Include dose, time last taken, and the patient's understanding of the drug's purpose and side effects. Many noncardiac drugs can adversely affect the cardiovascular system and should be assessed (Table 31-2).

Surgery or Other Treatments. Ask the patient about specific treatments, past surgeries, or hospital admissions related to cardiovascular problems. Explore any admissions or procedures performed for cardiovascular symptoms. Note whether an ECG or a chest x-ray has been done for baseline data.

Functional Health Patterns. The strong correlation between components of a patient's lifestyle and cardiovascular health supports the need to review each functional health pattern. Key questions to ask a person with a cardiovascular problem are listed in Table 31-3.

TABLE 31-2 Cardiovascular Effects of Noncardiac Drugs*

Drug Classification	Examples	Cardiovascular Effects
Anticancer agents	daunorubicin (Cerubidine) doxorubicin	Dysrhythmias, cardiomyopathy
Antipsychotics	chlorpromazine haloperido	Dysrhythmias, orthostatic hypotension
Corticosteroids	cortisone prednisone	Hypotension, edema, potassium depletion
Hormone therapy, oral contraceptives	estrogen + progestin (Prempro)	Myocardial infarction, thromboembolism, stroke, hypertension
Nonsteroidal antiinflammatory drugs (NSAIDs)	ibuprofen celecoxib (Celebrex) diclofenac (Voltaren)	Myocardial infarction, stroke, hypertension, heart failure
Psychostimulants	cocaine amphetamines	Tachycardia, angina, myocardial infarction, hypertension, dysrhythmias
Tricyclic antidepressants	amitriptyline doxepin (Sinequan)	Dysrhythmias, orthostatic hypotension

*List is not all-inclusive.

Health Perception–Health Management Pattern. Ask the patient about the presence of major cardiovascular risk factors. These include abnormal serum lipids, hypertension, sedentary lifestyle, diabetes, obesity, and tobacco use. If a patient uses tobacco, estimate the number of pack-years of tobacco use (number of packs smoked per day multiplied by the number of years the patient has smoked). Record the patient's attitude about tobacco use and attempts and methods used to stop. Record any alcohol use. Include information about the type of alcohol, amount, frequency, and any changes in the reaction to it. Also note any use of habit-forming drugs, including recreational drugs.

Question the patient about any drug allergies, including food and environmental allergies. Determine whether the patient has ever experienced a drug reaction or an allergic or anaphylactic reaction. Ask specifically about any allergic reaction to contrast media.

GENETIC RISK ALERT

Coronary Artery Disease

- Specific genetic links, especially related to lipoprotein genes, have been identified for some families with CAD.
- The clustering of CAD in families is strong if there is early age of onset affecting several relatives.

Cardiomyopathy

- Hypertrophic cardiomyopathy can be caused by autosomal dominant mutations.
- Dilated cardiomyopathy can be caused by autosomal and X-linked dominant mutations.

Hypertension

- Hypertension results from a complex interplay between genetic and environmental factors.
- Lifestyle choices (e.g., smoking, lack of exercise) may trigger genetic tendencies to hypertension.

Confirmed illnesses of blood relatives can highlight any genetic or familial tendencies toward CAD, hypertension, bleeding, diabetes, atherosclerosis, and stroke. Note any family members who had heart disease at an early age (<50 years of age for men; <55 years of age for women). In addition, disorders affecting the vascular system, such as intermittent claudication and varicosities, may be familial. Last, assess any family health history of noncardiac problems such as lung, kidney, or liver disease and obesity, because they can affect the cardiovascular system.

Nutritional-Metabolic Pattern. Being underweight or overweight may indicate potential cardiovascular problems. It is important to assess the patient's weight history (e.g., over the past year) in relation to height. Determine the amount of salt and saturated fats in the patient's typical diet. In addition to actual food habits, which may be influenced by culture, explore the patient's attitudes and plans relative to diet and weight management.

Elimination Pattern. The patient on diuretics may report increased voiding and/or nocturia. Ask about any history of incontinence or constipation, including any use of drugs (prescribed and OTC) for constipation. Teach patients with heart problems to avoid straining during a bowel movement *(Valsalva maneuver)*. Ask patients if they have any swelling of the lower extremities and if it resolves when their feet are elevated or after an overnight sleep.

Activity-Exercise Pattern. The benefit of exercise for cardiovascular health is clear, with aerobic exercise being most beneficial. Record the types of exercise done and the duration, intensity, and frequency of each. Ask about and note the occurrence of any symptoms during exercise (e.g., chest pain, shortness of breath, claudication) that may indicate a cardiovascular problem.

Sleep-Rest Pattern. Cardiovascular problems often disrupt sleep. *Paroxysmal nocturnal dyspnea* (attacks of shortness of breath, especially at night that awaken the patient) and *Cheyne-Stokes respiration* (periods of very shallow breaths to alternating periods of apnea and deep, rapid breathing) are associated with heart failure. Many patients with heart failure need to sleep with several pillows or upright in a chair. Note the number of pillows needed to sleep or the need to sleep upright *(orthopnea)* and whether this has changed recently.

Sleep apnea has been associated with an increased risk of life-threatening dysrhythmias, especially in patients with heart failure. Nocturia, a common finding with cardiovascular patients, also interrupts normal sleep patterns. Fully explore both conditions.

Cognitive-Perceptual Pattern. It is important to ask both the patient and caregiver about cognitive-perceptual problems. Cardiovascular problems such as dysrhythmias, hypertension, and stroke may cause problems with syncope, language, and memory. Report any pain associated with the cardiovascular system (e.g., chest pain, claudication).

Self-Perception–Self-Concept Pattern. If a cardiovascular event is acute, the patient's self-perception may be affected. Invasive diagnostic procedures often lead to body image concerns for the patient. When CVD is chronic, the patient may not be able to identify the cause but can often describe the inability to "keep up" previous levels of activity. This may also affect the patient's quality of life, so ask about the effects of the illness on the patient.

Role-Relationship Pattern. The patient's gender, race, and age are all related to cardiovascular health. In addition, the patient's marital status, role in the household, employment status,

TABLE 31-3 Health History

Cardiovascular System

Health Perception–Health Management

- Do you practice any preventive measures to decrease risk factors for heart disease?*
- Have you noticed an increase in heart symptoms such as chest pain or dyspnea?*
- Does your heart problem cause you to be less able to care for yourself?*
- Do you foresee any potential self-care problems because of your heart problem?*
- Have you ever used tobacco? If yes, in what form, how much, and for how long? Have you tried to quit? If yes, what methods have you tried? Are you interested in more information about quitting?
- How often and how much alcohol do you drink?

Nutritional-Metabolic

- Describe your usual daily diet, including salt, fat, and liquid intake.
- What is your present weight? What was your weight 1 year ago? If different, explain.
- Does eating cause fatigue or shortness of breath?*

Elimination

- Do your feet or ankles ever swell?* If yes, how far up your legs? Does it go away after sleeping all night?
- Have you ever taken drugs to help you get rid of excess fluid or to relieve constipation?*
- Are you having any problems related to urination?*
- Do you ever strain to have a bowel movement?

Activity-Exercise

- Are your daily activities or exercise limited because of your heart problem?*
- When were you last able to comfortably perform your usual activities or exercise?
- Do you experience any discomfort or symptoms as a result of exercise or any activity?*
- Can you comfortably walk and talk at the same time?
- How often do you attend activities outside your home?
- What was your most strenuous activity in the last few weeks compared with 6 months ago?

Sleep-Rest

- How many pillows do you sleep on at night? Has this changed recently?*
- Do you ever wake up suddenly and feel as if you cannot catch your breath?*
- Do you have a history of sleep apnea?*
- Do you ever sleep in a chair at night? Is yes, how often?
- How many times a night do you awaken to urinate?

Cognitive-Perceptual

- Do you ever experience dizziness or fainting?*
- Do you ever find it difficult to express yourself or to remember things?*
- Do you experience any pain (e.g., chest pain, leg pain with activity) as a result of your heart problem?*

Self-Perception–Self-Concept

- Have your perceptions of yourself changed since you were diagnosed with heart disease?*
- How has your heart disease affected the quality of your life?

Role-Relationship

- Has this illness affected any of the roles that you play in your daily life?*
- How have your significant others been affected by your heart disease?

Sexuality-Reproductive

- Has your heart disease caused a change in your sexual activity?*
- Do you experience any heart-related symptoms during sexual activity?*
- Do any of your drugs affect your ability to participate in sexual activities?*
- Females: Are you currently taking oral contraceptives, hormonal therapy, or drug therapy for breast cancer?

Coping–Stress Tolerance

- Describe your normal coping mechanisms during times of stress or anxiety.
- To whom or where would you turn during a time of stress? Are these people or services helping you now?*
- Do you practice any stress reduction techniques?*
- Do you have a history of depression?*
- Do you feel capable of handling your present health situation?
- Do you experience any heart symptoms (e.g., chest pain, palpitations) during times of stress or anger?*

Values-Beliefs

- What influence have your values or beliefs had during your illness?
- Do you feel any conflicts between your values or beliefs and the plan of care?*
- Describe any cultural or religious beliefs that may influence the management of your heart problem.

*If yes, describe.

number of children and their ages, living environment, and caregivers help you to identify strengths and support systems in the patient's life. Assess the patient's level of satisfaction or dissatisfaction with life roles, since this may alert you to possible areas of stress or conflict.

Sexuality-Reproductive Pattern. Ask the patient about the effect of the cardiovascular problem on sexual activity. Because some patients often fear sudden death during sexual intercourse, it may lead to changes in their sexual behavior. Fatigue, chest pain, or shortness of breath may also limit sexual activity. Erectile dysfunction (ED) may be a symptom of peripheral vascular disease and/or a side effect of some drugs used to treat CVD (e.g., β-blockers, diuretics). Ask about the use of drugs for ED (e.g., sildenafil [Viagra]). These drugs are contraindicated if the patient is also taking a nitrate because the combination can cause significant hypotension.[8] Decide if counseling may be helpful.

Ask female patients if they use oral contraceptives, hormone therapy (HT) for symptoms of menopause, or drug therapy for breast cancer. Women who smoke tobacco and use oral contraceptives are at increased risk for blood clots (e.g., venous thromboembolism). Similarly, there is an increased risk for CVD with the use of HT and selective estrogen-receptor modulators (e.g., tamoxifen [Novaldex]).[9]

Coping–Stress Tolerance Pattern. Ask the patient to identify areas that cause stress and the usual methods of coping with stress. Potentially stressful areas include health concerns, marital relationships, family and friends, occupation, and finances.

Work-related stress, depression, and inadequate social support are risk factors for CVD and heart events. Ask the patient about each of these factors. Information about support systems such as family, extended family and friends, counselors, or religious groups can provide vital insight when planning care.

Values-Belief Pattern. Individual values and beliefs, which are greatly affected by culture, may play a major role in the real or potential conflict that a patient faces when dealing with CVD. Some patients may attribute their illness to punishment from God; others may think that a "higher power" can help them. Information about a patient's values and beliefs will help you intervene during periods of crisis.

CASE STUDY

Subjective Data

(@Jupiterimages/ Banana-Stock/ Thinkstock)

A focused subjective assessment of L.P. revealed the following information:

- ***PMH:*** History of hypertension, mitral valve prolapse with mild regurgitation, heart failure, and type 2 diabetes.
- ***Medications:*** Lisinopril (Prinivil) 10 mg/day PO, metoprolol (Lopressor) 50 mg PO BID, ASA 81 mg/day PO, furosemide (Lasix) 40 mg/day PO, and glipizide (Glucotrol) 5 mg/day PO.
- ***Health Perception–Health Management:*** L.P. denies any previous history of chest pain or CAD. He was feeling fine until this morning when he awoke and experienced SOB, chest tightness, and palpitations while walking to the bathroom. He became frightened that he was having a heart attack, so his wife called 911. Denies smoking or alcohol intake. SOB and chest tightness are now gone, but he continues to feel palpitations.
- ***Elimination:*** Denies any edema. States takes Lasix in the morning and typically "passes urine until lunchtime." Denies nocturia.

Discussion Questions

1. What type of assessment would be most appropriate for L.P.: emergency, focused, or comprehensive? On what basis did you make that decision?
2. What assessment questions will you ask him?
3. How will you individualize the assessment based on his age, ethnic/cultural background, and condition?
4. Is this an appropriate time to teach him about the proper use of nitroglycerin tablets? Why or why not?

You will learn more about the physical examination of the cardiovascular system in the next section.

(See p. 669 for more information on L.P.)

Answers available at *http://evolve.elsevier.com/Lewis/medsurg.*

Objective Data

Physical Examination

Vital Signs. After you observe the patient's general appearance, obtain vital signs. Measure BP bilaterally. These readings can vary from 5 to 15 mm Hg. Use the arm with the highest BP for subsequent measurements. Take orthostatic (postural) BPs and HRs while the patient is supine, sitting with legs dangling, and standing. SBP should not decrease more than 20 mm Hg from the supine to the standing position. HR should not increase more than 20 beats/minute from the supine to the standing position.

Peripheral Vascular System

Inspection. Inspect the skin for color, hair distribution, and venous pattern. Check the extremities for conditions such as edema, dependent rubor, clubbing of the nail beds, varicosities, and lesions such as stasis ulcers. Edema in the legs can be caused by gravity, varicosities, or right-sided heart failure.

Inspect the large veins in the neck (internal and external jugular) while the patient is gradually moved from a supine position to an upright (30 to 45 degrees) position. Distention and prominent pulsations of these neck veins, referred to as *jugular venous distention,* can be caused by right-sided heart failure.

Palpation. Palpate the upper and lower extremities for temperature, moisture, pulses, and edema bilaterally to assess for symmetry. Look for edema by depressing the skin over the tibia or medial malleolus for 5 seconds. Normally, there is no depression after releasing pressure. If pitting edema is present, grade it from 1+ (mild pitting, slight brief indentation) to 4+ (very deep pitting, indentation that lasts a long time).[5]

Palpate the pulses in the neck and extremities for information on arterial blood flow. Assess the rhythm (e.g., regular, irregular) and force. It is important to palpate each carotid pulse separately to avoid vagal stimulation and possible dysrhythmias. Compare the characteristics of the arteries on the right and left extremities simultaneously to determine symmetry.

When palpating the arteries identified in Fig. 31-6, rate the force of the pulse using the following scale:

0 = Absent
1+ = Weak
2+ = Normal
3+ = Increased, full, bounding

The rigidity (hardness) of the vessel should also be noted. The normal pulse feels like a tap, whereas a vessel wall that is narrowed or bulging vibrates. The term for a palpable vibration is *thrill.*

Capillary refill is used to assess arterial flow to the extremities. Position the patient's hands near the level of the heart and

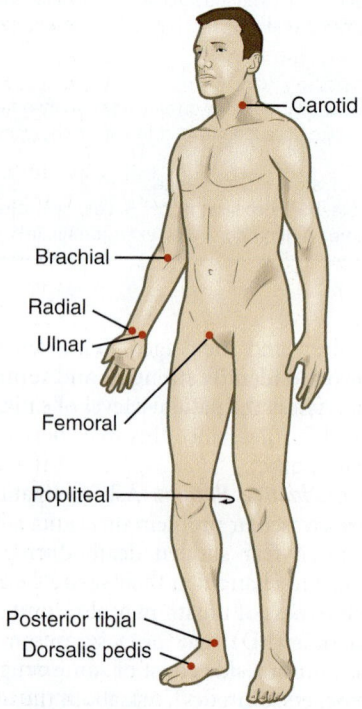

FIG. 31-6 Common sites for palpating arteries.

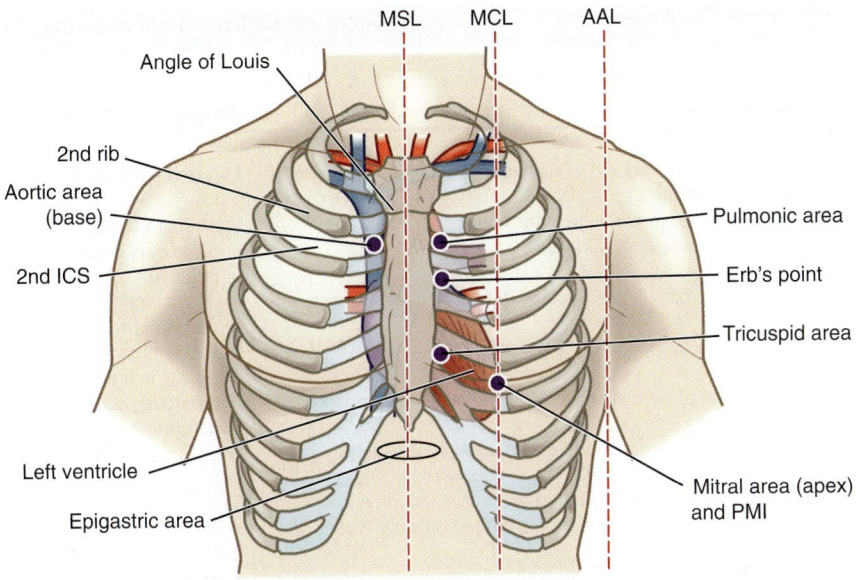

FIG. 31-7 Orientation of the heart within the thorax and cardiac auscultatory areas. *Red lines* indicate the midsternal line *(MSL)*, midclavicular line *(MCL)*, and anterior axillary line *(AAL)*. *ICS*, Intercostal space; *PMI*, point of maximal impulse.

squeeze a nail bed to produce blanching. Observe for the return of color. This should occur in less than 2 seconds with normal tissue perfusion and CO.

Auscultation. An artery that is narrowed or has a bulging wall may create turbulent blood flow. This abnormal flow can cause a buzzing or humming termed a *bruit*. This is heard with the bell of the stethoscope placed over the vessel. Auscultation of major arteries such as the carotid arteries, abdominal aorta, and femoral arteries should be part of the initial cardiovascular assessment. Abnormalities of the cardiovascular system are described in Table 31-4.

Thorax

Inspection and Palpation. An overall inspection and palpation of the thorax are the first steps in the examination. Next, inspect and palpate the areas where the heart valves project their sounds by identifying the intercostal spaces (ICSs). The raised notch, the *angle of Louis*, is where the manubrium and body of the sternum are joined. It is located at the level of the second rib. It is palpable in the midline of the sternum. It is used to count ICSs and locate specific auscultatory areas (Fig. 31-7).

Locate the following auscultatory areas: aortic area in the second ICS to the right of the sternum, pulmonic area in the second ICS to the left of the sternum, tricuspid area in the fifth left ICS close to the sternum, and mitral area in the left midclavicular line at the fifth ICS. A fifth auscultatory area is *Erb's point*, located at the third left ICS near the sternum. Normally, no pulsations are felt in these areas unless the patient has a thin chest wall.

A heart valve disorder may be suspected if abnormal pulsations or thrills are felt. Next, inspect and palpate the epigastric area, which lies on either side of the midline just below the xiphoid process. In a thin person, you may see the pulsation of the abdominal aorta. Normally, you can palpate it here. Next, inspect the precordium, which is located over the heart, for heaves. **Heaves** are sustained lifts of the chest wall in the precordial area that can be seen or palpated. They may be caused by left ventricular hypertrophy. Normally no pulsations are seen or felt here.

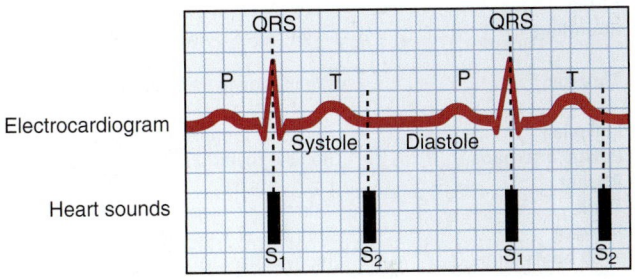

FIG. 31-8 Relationship of electrocardiogram, cardiac cycle, and heart sounds.

When the patient is supine, palpate the mitral valve area for the **point of maximal impulse (PMI)** (also called the *apical pulse*). This reflects the pulsation of the apex of the heart. The PMI lies medial to the midclavicular line in the fourth or fifth ICS. If you can palpate the PMI, record its position in relation to the midclavicular line and ICSs. When the PMI is below the fifth ICS and left of the midclavicular line, the heart may be enlarged.

Auscultation. Normal heart sounds are made by the movement of blood through the heart valves. These sounds can be heard through a stethoscope placed on the chest wall. The first heart sound (S_1) is associated with closure of the tricuspid and mitral valves. It has a soft lubb sound. The second heart sound (S_2) is associated with closure of the aortic and pulmonic valves. It has a sharp dupp sound. S_1 signals the beginning of systole. S_2 signals the beginning of diastole (Fig. 31-8). Listen to the auscultatory areas in sequence (Fig. 31-7).

S_1 and S_2 are heard best with the diaphragm of the stethoscope because they are high pitched. Extra heart sounds (S_3 or S_4), if present, are heard best with the bell of the stethoscope because they are low pitched. Have the patient lean forward while sitting to enhance the sounds from the second ICSs (aortic and pulmonic areas). Place the patient in a left side-lying position to enhance the sounds at the mitral area.

When auscultating the apical area, simultaneously palpate the radial pulse. Determine whether the rhythm is regular or

TABLE 31-4 Assessment Abnormalities

Cardiovascular System

Finding*	Description	Possible Etiology* and Significance
Inspection		
Jugular venous distention	Distended neck (jugular) veins with patient sitting at 30- to 45-degree angle	Elevated right atrial pressure, right-sided heart failure
Central cyanosis	Bluish or purplish tinge in central areas such as tongue, conjunctivae, inner surface of lips	Inadequate O_2 saturation of arterial blood because of pulmonary or cardiac disorders (e.g., congenital defects)
Peripheral cyanosis	Bluish or purplish tinge in extremities or in nose and ears	Reduced blood flow because of heart failure, vasoconstriction, cold environment
Splinter hemorrhages	Small red to black streaks under fingernails	Infective endocarditis (infection of endocardium, usually in area of cardiac valves)
Clubbing of nail beds	Obliteration of normal angle between base of nail and skin	Endocarditis, congenital defects, prolonged O_2 deficiency
Color changes in extremities with postural change	Pallor, cyanosis, mottling of skin after limb elevation. Dependent rubor (reddish blue discoloration). Glossy skin	Chronic decreased arterial perfusion
Ulcers	*Venous:* Necrotic crater-like lesion usually found on lower leg at medial malleolus. Characterized by slow wound healing	Poor venous return, varicose veins, incompetent venous valves.
	Arterial: Pale ischemic base, well-defined edges usually found on toes, heels, lateral malleoli	Arteriosclerosis, diabetes
Varicose veins	Visible dilated, discolored, tortuous vessels in lower extremities	Incompetent valves in vein
Palpation		
Pulse		
Bounding	Sharp, brisk, pounding pulse	Hyperkinetic states (e.g., anxiety, fever), anemia, hyperthyroidism
Thready	Weak, slowly rising pulse easily obliterated by pressure	Blood loss, decreased cardiac output, aortic valve disease, peripheral arterial disease
Irregular	Regularly irregular or irregularly irregular. Skipped beats	Cardiac dysrhythmias
Pulsus alternans	Regular rhythm, but strength of pulse varies with each beat	Heart failure, cardiac tamponade
Absent	Lack of pulse	Atherosclerosis, trauma, embolus
Thrill	Vibration of vessel or chest wall	Aneurysm, aortic regurgitation, arteriovenous fistula
Rigidity	Stiffness or inflexibility of vessel wall	Atherosclerosis
>100 beats/min	Tachycardia	Exercise, anxiety, shock, need for increased cardiac output, hyperthyroidism
<60 beats/min	Bradycardia	Rest or sleeping, SA or AV node damage, athletic conditioning, side effect of drugs (e.g., β-blockers), hypothyroidism
Displaced point of maximal impulse (apical pulse)	Point of maximal impulse is palpated (or auscultated) below the fifth ICS and to the left of the MCL	Cardiac enlargement as a result of coronary artery disease, heart failure, cardiomyopathy
Extremities		
Unusually warm extremities	Hands and feet warmer than normal	Possible thyrotoxicosis
Cold extremities	Hands and/or feet cold to touch. External covering necessary for comfort	Intermittent claudication, peripheral arterial disease, low cardiac output, severe anemia
Pitting edema of lower extremities or sacral area	Visible finger indentation after application of firm pressure, weight gain, tightening of clothing (including shoes), marks or indentations from constricting garments	Interruption of venous return to heart, right-sided heart failure
Abnormal capillary refill	Blanching of nail bed for ≥2 sec after release of pressure	Possible reduced arterial capillary perfusion, anemia
Asymmetry in limb circumference	Measurable swelling of involved limb	Venous thromboembolism, varicose veins, lymphedema
Auscultation		
Pulse deficit	Apical heart rate exceeding peripheral pulse rate	Cardiac dysrhythmias, most often atrial fibrillation/flutter or premature ventricular contractions
Arterial bruit	Turbulent flow sound in peripheral artery	Arterial obstruction or aneurysm
Third heart sound (S_3)	Extra heart sound, low pitched, heard in early diastole. Similar to sound of a gallop	Left ventricular failure. Volume overload. Mitral, aortic, or tricuspid regurgitation. Hypertension (possible)
Fourth heart sound (S_4)	Extra heart sound, low pitched, heard in late diastole. Similar to sound of a gallop	Forceful atrial contraction from resistance to ventricular filling (e.g., in left ventricular hypertrophy, aortic stenosis, hypertension, coronary artery disease)
Heart murmurs	Turbulent sounds occurring between normal heart sounds. Characterized by loudness, pitch, shape, quality, duration, timing	Heart valve disorder, abnormal blood flow patterns
Pericardial friction rub	High-pitched, scratchy sound heard during S_1 and/or S_2 at the apex. Heard best with patient sitting and leaning forward, and while holding breath at the end of expiration	Pericarditis

*Limited to common abnormal assessment findings and etiologic factors. (Further discussion of conditions listed may be found in Chapters 32 to 37, 65, and 66.)

irregular while listening and feeling. If the apical and radial pulses are not equivalent, count the apical pulse while a second person simultaneously counts the radial pulse for 1 full minute. The difference between the two numbers is called a *pulse deficit* and can indicate dysrhythmias.

Normally no sound is heard between S_1 and S_2. Sounds heard during these periods may represent abnormalities and should be described. An exception to this is a normal splitting of S_2, which is best heard at the pulmonic area during inspiration. Splitting of this heart sound can be abnormal if it is heard during expiration or if it is constant (fixed) during the respiratory cycle.

The S_3 heart sound is a low-intensity vibration of the ventricular walls usually associated with decreased compliance of the ventricles during filling. An S_3 heart sound may be normal (physiologic) in young adults. It is pathologic in patients with left-sided heart failure or mitral valve regurgitation. S_3 is heard closely after S_2 and is known as a *ventricular gallop.* The S_4 heart sound is a low-frequency vibration caused by atrial contraction. It precedes S_1 of the next cycle, and is known as an *atrial gallop.* An S_4 heart sound may be normal in older adults with no evidence of heart disease. It is pathologic in patients with CAD, cardiomyopathy, left ventricular hypertrophy, or aortic stenosis.

Murmurs, if heard, are graded on a six-point Roman numeral scale of loudness and recorded as a ratio. I/VI indicates a murmur that is barely audible with the stethoscope, heard only in a quiet room and then not easily. VI/VI indicates a murmur that can be heard with the stethoscope lifted just off the chest wall.

Pericardial friction rubs are sounds caused by friction that occurs when inflamed surfaces of the pericardium (pericarditis) move against each other. They are high-pitched, scratchy sounds that may be intermittent and may last several hours to days. Friction rubs are heard best at the apex, with patients upright and leaning forward, and while holding their breath following expiration.[5]

Record any abnormal sounds. This includes the timing (during systole or diastole), location (the anatomic site on the chest where it is heard the loudest), position (heard best when the patient is supine, sitting and leaning forward, or in the left side-lying position), and any other abnormal findings (irregular apical pulse or palpable chest wall heaves) associated with the sound.

Abnormal assessment findings are described in Table 31-4. A method of recording data from the cardiovascular assessment is presented in Table 31-5.

A *focused assessment* is used to evaluate the status of previously identified cardiovascular problems and to monitor for signs of new problems (see Table 3-7). A focused assessment of the cardiovascular system is presented in the box in right column.

CASE STUDY

Objective Data: Physical Examination

(©Jupiterimages/ Banana-Stock/ Thinkstock)

Physical examination findings of L.P. are as follows:

- BP 100/54, apical-radial pulse 154, pulse irregular, respiratory rate 20, temperature 98.2°F (36.8°C), O_2 saturation 94% on room air
- Awake, alert, and oriented ×3
- Lungs clear on auscultation; systolic murmur present
- Heart monitor shows atrial fibrillation with a rapid ventricular response
- +1 pedal pulses bilaterally
- No peripheral edema, jugular venous distention, or heaves noted

Discussion Questions

1. What should be included in the physical assessment?
2. Which physical assessment findings are of most concern to you?
3. Based on the results of the subjective and physical assessment findings, what diagnostic studies do you think will be ordered for L.P.?

You will learn more about diagnostic studies related to the cardiovascular system in the next section.

(See p. 679 for more information on L.P.)

Answers available at *http://evolve.elsevier.com/Lewis/medsurg.*

FOCUSED ASSESSMENT

Cardiovascular System

Use this checklist to make certain the key assessment steps have been done.

Subjective

Ask the patient about any of the following and note responses.

Chest pain, discomfort	Y	N
Palpitations	Y	N
Shortness of breath (especially when lying down or at rest)	Y	N
Edema in legs or any part of body	Y	N
Leg pain during exercise	Y	N
Excess urination at night	Y	N

Objective: Diagnostic

Check the following for critical values or changes.

Cardiac biomarkers	✓
Hematocrit, hemoglobin, platelets	✓
Glucose, electrolytes, BUN, creatinine	✓
Electrocardiogram	✓
Chest x-ray	✓

Objective: Physical Examination

Inspect and Palpate

Anterior chest wall for pulsations and heaves	✓
Pulses for symmetry, quality, and rhythm	✓

Auscultate

Bilateral blood pressures	✓
Heart for rate, rhythm, and sounds	✓

DIAGNOSTIC STUDIES OF CARDIOVASCULAR SYSTEM

Numerous diagnostic tests are available to assess the cardiovascular system. Table 31-6 identifies the most common studies. Select studies are described in more detail below.

Blood Studies

Many blood studies provide information about the cardiovascular system. For example, some reflect the O_2-carrying capacity (red blood cell count and hemoglobin) and coagulation properties (clotting times) of the blood. (See Chapter 29 and Tables 29-6, 29-7, and 26-9 for hematology studies.)

Cardiac Biomarkers. When cells are injured, they release their contents, including enzymes and other proteins, into the circulation. These *biomarkers* are useful in the diagnosis of acute coronary syndrome (ACS).

TABLE 31-5 Normal Physical Assessment of Cardiovascular System

Inspection	Skin warm, normal color. PMI not visible. No JVD with patient at 45-degree angle.
Palpation	Capillary refill <2 sec. PMI palpable in fourth ICS at left MCL. No thrills or heaves. Slight palpable pulsations of abdominal aorta in epigastric area. Carotid and extremity pulses 2+ and equal bilaterally. No pedal edema.
Auscultation	S_1 and S_2 heard. Apical-radial pulse rate equal, 72, and regular. No murmurs or extra heart sounds.

ICS, Intercostal space; *JVD,* jugular venous distention; *MCL,* midclavicular line; *PMI,* point of maximal impulse.

Cardiac-specific troponin is a heart muscle protein released into circulation after injury or infarction. Two subtypes, cardiac-specific troponin T (cTnT) and cardiac-specific troponin I (cTnI), are specific to heart muscle. Normally the level in the blood is very low, so a rise in level is diagnostic of myocardial infarction (MI) or injury. cTnT and cTnI are detectable within hours (on average 4 to 6 hours) of MI or injury, peak at 10 to 24 hours, and can be detected for up to 10 to 14 days (see Fig. 33-10). Troponin is the biomarker of choice in the diagnosis of ACS. High-sensitivity troponin (hs-cTnT, hs-cTnI) assays may provide even earlier detection of a heart event.[10]

Creatine kinase (CK) enzymes are found in a variety of organs and tissues and occur as three isoenzymes. These isoenzymes are specific to skeletal muscle (CK-MM), brain and nervous tissue (CK-BB), and the heart (CK-MB). CK-MB rise is specific for MI or injury. Levels begin to increase 3 to 6 hours after symptom onset, peak in 12 to 24 hours, and return to baseline within 12 to 48 hours after MI.[11] The peak level and return to normal can be delayed in a patient with a large MI. Levels drop more rapidly in patients who are quickly and successfully treated for an MI. (Fig. 33-10 depicts the changes in cardiac markers related to an MI.)

Copeptin, a substitute marker for arginine vasopressin (AVP), is an additional diagnostic test that can be used for patients presenting with signs of ACS. In patients with an acute MI, it can be detected immediately. A combination of troponin and copeptin provide increased sensitivity for diagnosing an acute MI.[12]

Myoglobin is a low-molecular-weight heme protein found in heart and skeletal muscle. Myoglobin elevation is a sensitive indicator of very early myocardial injury but lacks specificity for MI. Its usefulness in diagnosing MI is limited.[11]

Correct interpretation of diagnostic tests requires consideration of the time from onset of symptoms and the time of the expected presence and elevation of the biomarkers. Additional data (patient symptoms, history, and ECG changes) complete the diagnostic picture for the patient with suspected ACS.

C-Reactive Protein. C-reactive protein (CRP) is a protein produced by the liver during periods of acute inflammation. CRP can be measured using a high-sensitivity test (hs-CRP). An increased level of CRP has been linked with the presence of atherosclerosis and the first occurrence of a heart event. In addition, the level of CRP may predict the risk for future heart events in patients with MI. However, studies on the usefulness of assessing CRP have produced conflicting results, and measuring CRP routinely in patients with and without CVD is not done.[13]

Homocysteine. Homocysteine (Hcy) is an amino acid that is produced during protein catabolism. Elevated Hcy levels can be either hereditary or acquired from dietary deficiencies of vitamin B_6, vitamin B_{12}, or folate. Elevated levels of Hcy have been linked to a higher risk of CVD, peripheral vascular disease, and stroke. It is recommended that Hcy testing be done in patients with a familial predisposition for early CVD or a history of CVD in the absence of other common risk factors.[14]

Cardiac Natriuretic Peptide Markers. There are three natriuretic peptides: (1) atrial natriuretic peptide (ANP) from the atrium, (2) b-type natriuretic peptide (BNP) from the ventricles, and (3) c-type natriuretic peptide from endothelial and renal epithelial cells. BNP is the marker of choice for distinguishing a cardiac or respiratory cause of dyspnea. N-terminal pro-brain natriuretic peptide (NT-pro-BNP) is also secreted in the ventricles and is more sensitive but less specific than BNP as a diagnostic marker of heart failure.[11] When DBP increases (e.g., heart failure), BNP and NT-pro-BNP are released and increase natriuresis (excretion of sodium in the urine). (ANP and BNP are also discussed in Chapter 32 on p. 683 and in Chapter 34 on p. 740.)

Serum Lipids. Serum lipids consist of triglycerides, cholesterol, and phospholipids. They circulate in the blood bound to protein. Thus they are often referred to as *lipoproteins.*

Triglycerides are the main storage form of lipids and make up about 95% of fatty tissue. Cholesterol, a structural component of cell membranes and plasma lipoproteins, is a precursor of corticosteroids, sex hormones, and bile salts. In addition to being absorbed from food in the gastrointestinal tract, cholesterol can also be synthesized in the liver. Phospholipids contain glycerol, fatty acids, phosphates, and a nitrogenous compound. Although formed in most cells, phospholipids usually enter the circulation as lipoproteins synthesized by the liver. Apoproteins are water-soluble proteins that combine with most lipids to form lipoproteins.

Different classes of lipoproteins contain varying amounts of the naturally occurring lipids. These include the following:

1. *Chylomicrons:* primarily exogenous triglycerides from dietary fat
2. *Low-density lipoproteins (LDLs):* mostly cholesterol with moderate amounts of phospholipids
3. *High-density lipoproteins (HDLs):* about 50% protein and 50% phospholipids and cholesterol
4. *Very-low-density lipoproteins (VLDLs):* primarily endogenous triglycerides with moderate amounts of phospholipids and cholesterol

A lipid panel usually measures cholesterol, triglyceride, LDL, and HDL. Elevations in triglycerides and LDL are strongly associated with CAD. An increased HDL level is associated with a decreased risk of CAD. High levels of HDLs serve a protective role by mobilizing cholesterol from tissues.

Although an association exists between elevated serum cholesterol levels and CAD, a measure of total cholesterol alone is not sufficient for an assessment of CAD. A risk assessment is calculated by comparing the total cholesterol to HDL ratio over time. An increase in the ratio indicates increased risk. This provides more information than either value alone.

Plasma levels of apolipoprotein A-I (apo A-I) (the major HDL protein) and the ratio of apo A-I to apolipoprotein B (apo B) (the major LDL protein) are stronger predictors of CAD than the HDL cholesterol level alone. Measurements of these lipoproteins can be useful in identifying patients at risk for CAD.[11]

Lipoprotein (a), or Lp(a), has been studied for its role as a risk factor for CAD. Increased levels of Lp(a), especially with increased levels of lactate dehydrogenase (LDH), have been linked with the progression of atherosclerosis, especially in women.

Lipoprotein-Associated Phospholipase A_2. Lipoprotein-associated phospholipase A_2 (Lp-PLA_2) is an inflammatory enzyme expressed in atherosclerotic plaques. Elevated levels of Lp-PLA_2 are related to an increased risk of CAD, especially in African American women.[15]

Chest X-Ray

A radiographic picture of the chest can show heart shape and size, and anatomic changes in individual chambers (Fig. 31-9). The chest x-ray records any displacement or enlargement of the heart, extra fluid around the heart (pericardial effusion), and pulmonary congestion.

Electrocardiogram

The basic P, QRS, and T waveforms (Fig. 31-4, *B*) are used to assess heart activity. Deviations from the normal sinus rhythm can indicate problems in heart function. There are many types of ECG monitoring, including a resting 12-lead ECG, ambulatory ECG monitoring, and exercise or stress testing (Table 31-6). Continuous ambulatory ECG (Holter monitoring) provides diagnostic information over a period of time. (See Chapter 35 for a complete discussion of ECG monitoring.)

Event Monitor or Loop Recorder. An event monitor or loop recorder is used to record less frequent ECG events. An event monitor is a portable unit that uses electrodes to store ECG data once triggered by the patient. A disadvantage of this type of monitoring is that, if symptoms occur for only a brief time, they may be over before the patient puts on the device and triggers it to record. Likewise, if patients are extremely symptomatic (e.g., syncopal), they may not be physically able to trigger the ECG recording. These devices can be used for routine pacemaker checks over the phone to the HCP.[16]

An implantable loop recorder is used for patients who may have serious yet infrequent dysrhythmias. This small recorder is implanted though a small incision into the chest wall. It is activated to record either by the patient using a remote device or automatically if the HR exceeds or goes below a set rate. External loop recorders are worn for a month and require electrodes continuously placed on the skin. This device only records when activated by the patient when symptoms occur.

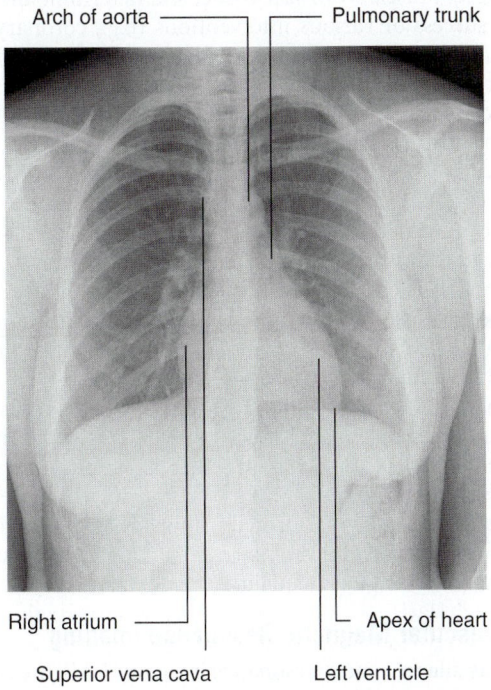

FIG. 31-9 Chest x-ray: standard posterior-anterior view. (From Drake RL, Vogl AW, Mitchell AWM: *Gray's anatomy for students*, ed 2, Philadelphia, 2010, Churchill Livingstone.)

Exercise or Stress Testing

Heart symptoms frequently occur only with activity because of the demand on the coronary arteries to provide more O_2. Exercise testing is used to evaluate the heart's response to physical stress. This helps to assess CVD and set limits for exercise programs. Exercise testing is used for persons who are able to walk unassisted or use a bicycle. It is also helpful for those with normal ECGs that limit diagnostic interpretation (e.g., pacemakers) (Table 31-6).

Echocardiogram

The echocardiogram uses ultrasound (US) waves to record the movement of the structures of the heart. In the normal heart, US waves directed at the heart are reflected back in typical patterns. *Contrast echocardiography* involves the addition of an IV contrast agent (e.g., agitated saline) to assist in defining the images, especially in technically difficult patients (e.g., obese).

The echocardiogram provides information about abnormalities of (1) valvular structures and motion, (2) heart chamber size and contents, (3) ventricular and septal motion and thickness, (4) pericardial sac, and (5) ascending aorta. The **ejection fraction (EF)**, or the percentage of end-diastolic blood volume that is ejected during systole, can also be measured. The EF provides information about the function of the left ventricle during systole.

Two commonly used types of echocardiograms are the *motion-mode (M-mode) echocardiogram* and the *two-dimensional (2-D) echocardiogram.* In the M-mode, a single US beam is directed toward the heart, recording the motion of the intracardiac structures and detecting wall thickness and chamber size. The 2-D echocardiogram sweeps the US beam through an arc, producing a cross-sectional view. This shows correct spatial relationships among the structures.

Doppler technology allows for sound evaluation of the flow or motion of the scanned object (heart valves, ventricular walls, blood flow). *Color-flow imaging (duplex)* is the combination of 2-D echocardiography and Doppler technology (Fig. 31-10). It uses color changes to demonstrate the speed and direction of blood flow. Pathologic conditions, such as valvular leaks and congenital defects, can be diagnosed more effectively.

Real-time three-dimensional (3-D) ultrasound is a technology that uses multiple 2-D echo images with computer technology to provide a reconstruction of the heart. This technique produces information about the structures of the heart and how these structures change during the cardiac cycle.

Stress echocardiography, a combination of treadmill test or pharmacologic test and US images, evaluates wall motion abnormalities. With the use of a digital computer to compare images before and after exercise, wall motion and function are revealed. This test combines the information from a stress test with the information from an echocardiogram. For those individuals unable to exercise, IV drugs are used. These include dobutamine [Dobutrex], which produces pharmacologic stress on the heart and dipyridamole (Persantine), which promotes vasodilation of healthy arteries. Unhealthy arteries do not respond as well, which is seen on the echocardiogram.

Transesophageal echocardiography (TEE) provides more precise echocardiography of the heart than surface 2-D

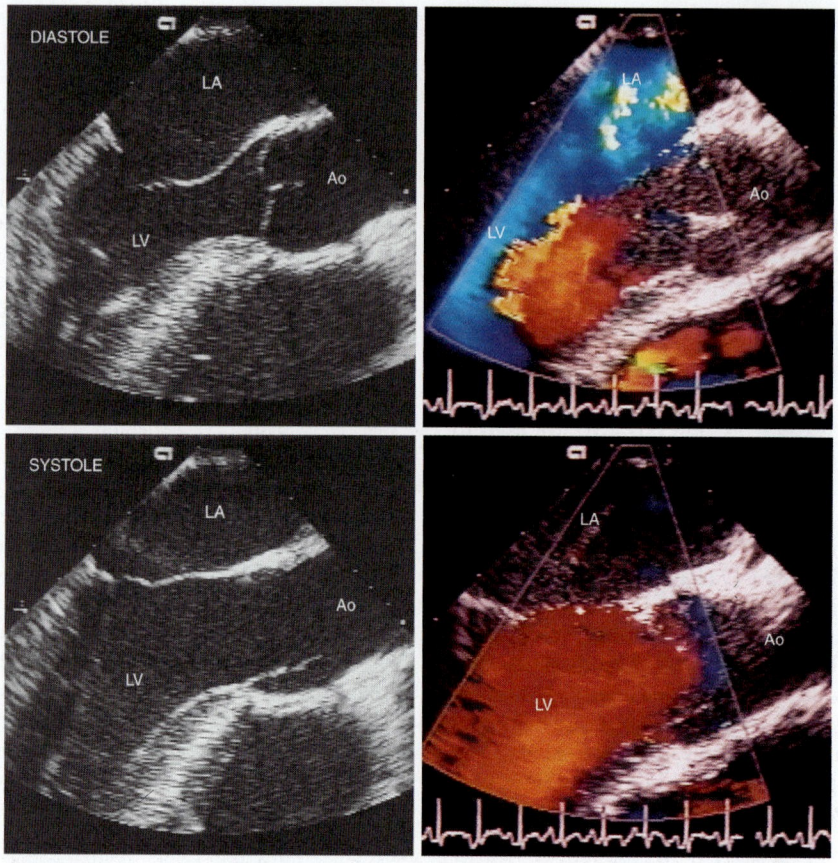

FIG. 31-10 Long-axis images of the aortic and mitral valve with the depth adjusted to optimize evaluation of valve anatomy and motion. The 2-D images *(left)* in diastole *(top)* and systole *(bottom)* show normal aortic and mitral opening and closure. The color flow images *(right)* show normal left ventricular inflow with no aortic regurgitation in diastole *(top)* and normal antegrade flow in the left ventricular outflow tract and no mitral regurgitation in systole *(bottom)*. (From Otto C: *Textbook of clinical echocardiography,* ed 3, St Louis, 2004, Saunders.)

echocardiography by removing interference from the chest wall and lungs. The TEE uses a flexible endoscope with an US transducer in the tip for imaging of the heart and great vessels. The scope is passed into the esophagus to the level of the heart, and M-mode, 2-D, Doppler, and color-flow imaging can be obtained.

TEE is used frequently in an outpatient setting for evaluation of mitral valve disease and for identification of endocarditis vegetation, thrombus before cardioversion, or the source of heart emboli. In addition, TEE is used in the operating room to assess intraoperative heart function and in the emergency department to detect suspected aortic dissection.

The risks of TEE are low. However, complications may include perforation or tearing of the esophagus, hemorrhage, dysrhythmias, vasovagal reactions, and transient hypoxemia. TEE is contraindicated if the patient has a history of esophageal disorders, dysphagia, or radiation therapy to the chest wall. Patients require sedation during a TEE.

Nuclear Cardiology

One of the most common nuclear imaging tests is the multigated acquisition (MUGA) or cardiac blood pool scan. This test provides information on wall motion during systole and diastole, heart valves, and EF (Table 31-6).

Perfusion imaging is also used with exercise testing to determine whether the coronary blood flow changes with increased activity. Stress perfusion imaging may show an abnormality even when a resting image is normal. This procedure is used to diagnose CAD, make a prognosis in existing CAD, differentiate viable heart muscle from scar tissue, and determine the potential for success of various interventions (e.g., coronary artery bypass surgery, percutaneous coronary intervention)[17] (see Chapter 33).

Exercise stress perfusion imaging is always preferred but, if a patient cannot exercise, IV regadenoson (Lexiscan), dipyridamole, or adenosine (Adenocard) can be given to dilate the coronary arteries and simulate the effect of exercise. After the drug takes effect, the isotope is injected and the imaging is done.

Single-photon emission computed tomography (SPECT) uses technetium, thallium, or sestamibi as an imaging agent (isotope). Both obese patients and women with large breasts can have attenuation artifacts, which can lead to false-positive results. Patients with severe multi-vessel coronary disease or blockages in their left main coronary artery may have false-negative results.

Positron emission tomography (PET) stress testing is increasingly being used due to its high sensitivity for revealing myocardial ischemia and viability. This type of myocardial perfusion imaging is commonly performed using ^{82}rubidium. This agent allows for quicker studies with lower radiation exposure and provides better diagnostic quality.[18]

Cardiovascular Magnetic Resonance Imaging

Cardiovascular magnetic resonance imaging (CMRI) can detect and find areas of MI in a 3-D view. It is sensitive enough to find

Text continued on p. 678

TABLE 31-6 Diagnostic Studies

Cardiovascular System

Study	Description and Purpose	Nursing Responsibility
Blood Studies*		
Troponin (cardiac)	Contractile proteins that are released after an MI. Both troponin T and troponin I are highly specific to cardiac tissue. *Reference intervals:* *Troponin I (cTnI)* Negative: <0.5 ng/mL (<0.5 mcg/L) Indeterminate or suspicious for injury to myocardium: 0.5-2.3 ng/mL (0.5-2.3 mcg/L) Positive for myocardial injury: >2.3 ng/mL (>2.3 mcg/L) *Troponin T (cTnT)* <0.1 ng/mL (<0.1 mcg/L)	*Before:* Explain purpose of serial sampling (e.g., q6hr × 3) in conjunction with CK-MB and serial ECGs. *During:* Rapid point-of-care (bedside) assays are available.
CK-MB	Cardiospecific isoenzyme that is released from cells when myocardial tissue is injured. Concentrations >4%-6% of total creatine kinase (CK) are highly indicative of MI. Serum levels increase within 4-6 hr after MI.	*Before:* Explain purpose of serial sampling that is often done in conjunction with troponin and ECGs.
Copeptin	Substitute for arginine vasopressin (AVP) that directly reflects AVP concentration. Can be used as a cardiac biomarker for detecting acute MI. Higher in men than women, increased after exercise and stress, and influenced by fasting and water load. *Reference interval:* <10 pmol/L	*Before:* Explain to patient that blood is drawn and sent to laboratory.
Myoglobin	Serum concentrations rise 30-60 min after MI and raidly cleared from circulation. Limited use in the diagnosis of cardiac injury/infarction. *Reference interval:* *Male:* 15.2-91.2 mcg/L *Female:* 11.1-57.5 mcg/L	*Before:* Explain to patient that blood is drawn and sent to laboratory.
C-reactive protein (CRP)	Marker of inflammation. May have value in predicting risk of cardiac disease and cardiac events. High-sensitivity (hs) CRP assay used. *Lowest risk:* <1 mg/L *Moderate risk:* 1-3 mg/L *High risk:* >3 mg/L	*Before:* Explain to patient that blood is drawn and sent to laboratory.
Homocysteine	Amino acid produced during protein catabolism that has been identified as a risk factor for cardiovascular disease. Homocysteine may cause damage to the endothelium or have a role in formation of thrombi. *Reference interval:* *Male:* 5.2-12.9 μmol/L *Female:* 3.7-10.4 μmol/L	*Before:* Explain to patient that blood is drawn and sent to laboratory.
b-Type natriuretic peptide (BNP)	Peptide that causes natriuresis. Elevation helps to distinguish cardiac vs. respiratory cause of dyspnea. Infusion of nesiritide (Natrecor) elevates levels temporarily. *Reference interval:* *BNP* (diagnostic for heart failure) >100 pg/mL (28.8 pmol/L)	*Before:* Explain to patient that blood is drawn and sent to laboratory.
NT-Pro-BNP	Aids in assessing the severity of heart failure in symptomatic and asymptomatic patients. In patients with renal insufficiency, concentrations may increase and may not correlate with New York Heart Association functional classification of heart failure. *Reference interval:* *≤74 yr:* 124 pg/mL *>75 yr:* 449 pg/mL	*Before:* Explain to patient that blood is drawn and sent to laboratory.
Serum Lipids		
Cholesterol	A blood lipid. Elevated cholesterol is considered a risk factor for cardiovascular heart disease. *Reference interval:* <200 mg/dL (<5.18 mmol/L) (varies with age and gender)	*Before:* Explain to patient that blood is drawn and sent to laboratory. *During:* Can be obtained in a nonfasting state.
Triglycerides	Mixtures of fatty acids. Elevations are associated with cardiovascular disease and diabetes. *Reference interval:* <150 mg/dL (<1.7 mmol/L) (varies with age)	*Before:* Explain to patient that blood is drawn and sent to laboratory. Alcohol should be withheld for 24 hr before testing. *During:* Can be obtained in a nonfasting state. Some protocols continue to recommend obtaining results in a fasting state.

*Reference ranges for the laboratory tests vary by institution because of differences in equipment and reagents used.

Continued

TABLE 31-6 Diagnostic Studies

Cardiovascular System—cont'd

Study	Description and Purpose	Nursing Responsibility
Serum Lipids—cont'd		
Lipoproteins (HDL, LDL)	Electrophoresis is done to separate lipoproteins into HDL and LDL. There are marked day-to-day fluctuations in serum lipid levels. More than one determination is needed for accurate diagnosis and treatment. *Reference intervals* (vary with age): HDL *Recommended* *Male:* >40 mg/dL (>1.04 mmol/L) *Female:* >50 mg/dL (>1.3 mmol/L) *Low risk for CAD:* ≥60 mg/dL (>1.55 mmol/L) *High risk for CAD:* <40 mg/dL (<1.04 mmol/L) LDL *Recommended:* <100 mg/dL (<2.6 mmol/L) *Near optimal:* 100-129 mg/dL (2.6-3.34 mmol/L) *Moderate risk for CAD:* 130-159 mg/dL (3.37-4.12 mmol/L) *High risk for CAD:* >160 mg/dL (>4.14 mmol/L)	*Before:* Explain to patient that blood is drawn and sent to laboratory. *During:* Can be obtained in a nonfasting state. Some protocols continue to recommend obtaining results in a fasting state. *After:* Risk for heart disease is assessed by dividing the total cholesterol level by the HDL level and obtaining a ratio. *Low risk:* Ratio <3 *Average risk:* Ratio 3-5 *Increased risk:* Ratio >5
Lipoprotein (a) (Lp[a])	Increased levels are associated with an increased risk of CAD and stroke. *Reference interval:* <30 mg/dL (<0.3 g/L)	*Before:* Explain to patient that blood is drawn and sent to laboratory. *During:* Can be obtained in a nonfasting state.
Lipoprotein-associated phospholipase A_2 (Lp-PLA_2)	Elevated levels of Lp-PLA_2 are associated with vascular inflammation and increased risk for CAD. Serum levels of Lp-PLA_2 are measured by the PLAC test. *Reference intervals:* *Low risk:* ≤151 ng/mL *Moderate risk:* 152-194 ng/mL *High risk:* ≥195 ng/mL	*Before:* Explain to patient that blood is drawn and sent to laboratory. *During:* Can be obtained in a nonfasting state.
Chest X-Ray	Patient is placed in two upright positions to examine lung fields and heart size. The two common positions are posteroanterior (PA) (Fig. 31-9) and lateral. Normal heart size and contour for the individual's age, sex, and size are noted.	*Before:* Ask about frequency of recent x-rays and possibility of pregnancy. Provide lead shielding to areas not being viewed. Remove any jewelry or metal objects that may obstruct the view of heart and lungs.
12-Lead ECG	Electrodes are placed on the chest and extremities, allowing the ECG machine to record cardiac electrical activity from 12 different views. A resting 12-lead ECG can identify conduction problems, dysrhythmias, position of heart, cardiac hypertrophy, pericarditis, myocardial ischemia or infarction, pacemaker activity, and effectiveness of drug therapy at one point in time.	*Before:* Prepare skin and apply electrodes and leads. Place patient supine (or with head of bed elevated, if short of breath). Tell patient that no discomfort is involved and to lie still to decrease motion artifact.
Signal-averaged ECG (SAECG)	A high-resolution ECG that can identify electrical activity called late potentials, indicating a patient is at risk for developing ventricular dysrhythmias (e.g., ventricular tachycardia).	Same as for 12-lead ECG.
Ambulatory ECG Monitoring		
Holter monitoring	Recording of ECG rhythm for 24-48 hr and then correlating rhythm changes with symptoms and activities recorded in diary. Normal patient activity is encouraged to simulate conditions that produce symptoms. Electrodes are placed on chest, and a recorder is used to store information until it is recalled, printed, and analyzed for any rhythm disturbance.	*Before:* Prepare skin and apply electrodes and leads. Explain importance of keeping an accurate diary of activities and symptoms. Tell patient that bathing and showering are prohibited during monitoring. Skin irritation may develop from electrodes.
Event monitor or loop recorder	Records rhythm disturbances that are not frequent enough to be recorded in one 24-hr period. It allows more freedom than a regular Holter monitor. Some units have electrodes that are attached to chest and have a loop of memory that captures the onset and end of an event. Other types are placed directly on patient's wrist, chest, or fingers and have no loop of memory but record the patient's ECG in real time. Recordings may be transmitted over the phone to a receiving unit.	*Before:* Instruct in the use of equipment for recording and transmitting (if appropriate) of events. Teach patient about skin preparation for lead placement or steady skin contact for units not requiring electrodes. This will ensure the best transmission of quality ECG tracings for analysis. Tell patient to start recording as soon as symptoms begin or as soon thereafter as possible.

TABLE 31-6 Diagnostic Studies

Cardiovascular System—cont'd

Study	Description and Purpose	Nursing Responsibility
Exercise or Stress Testing	Various protocols are used to evaluate the effect of exercise tolerance on cardiovascular function. A common protocol uses 3-min stages at set speeds and elevation of treadmill belt. The patient can exercise to either predicted peak HR (calculated by subtracting the person's age from 220) or to peak exercise tolerance, at which time the test is ended. The test is also ended for chest discomfort, significant changes in vital signs from baseline, or significant ECG changes (e.g., ischemia, dysrhythmias). Vital signs and ECG are monitored. The ECG is monitored after exercise for rhythm disturbances or, if ECG changes occurred with exercise, for return to baseline. Continual monitoring of vital signs and ECG for ischemic changes is important in the diagnosis of CAD. An exercise bike may be used if the patient is unable to walk on the treadmill.	*Before:* Tell patient to wear comfortable clothes and shoes that can be used for walking or running. Tell patient about procedure and importance of reporting any symptoms that occur. β-Blockers may be held 24 hr before the test because they blunt the HR and limit the patient's ability to achieve maximal HR. Caffeine-containing food and fluids are held for 24 hr. Patients must refrain from smoking and strenuous exercise for 3 hr before test. *During:* Monitor vital signs and obtain 12-lead ECG before exercise, during each stage of exercise, and after exercise until all vital signs and ECG changes have returned to normal or baseline. Monitor patient's response throughout procedure for any signs of distress (e.g., angina, shortness of breath).
6-Minute Walk Test	Distance patient is able to walk on a flat surface in 6 min. Used to measure response to treatments and determine functional capacity for activities of daily living. Useful in people who are unable to perform treadmill or exercise bike testing. May be a better measure of fitness for older adults than exercise testing.	*Before:* Tell patient to wear comfortable shoes. Inform patient to carry or pull O_2 if used routinely. *During:* Encourage patient to walk as quickly as possible.
Echocardiogram • Contrast • M-mode • Two-dimensional • Color-flow imaging (duplex) • Real-time three-dimensional	Transducer that emits and receives ultrasound waves is placed in four positions on the chest above the heart. Transducer records sound waves that are bounced off the heart. Also records direction and flow of blood through the heart and transforms it to audio and graphic data that measure valve abnormalities, congenital heart defects, wall motion, EF, and heart function. IV contrast agent may be used to enhance images (Fig. 31-10).	*Before:* Place patient in a left side-lying position. Tell patient about procedure and sensations (pressure and mechanical movement from head of transducer). No contraindications to procedure exist.
Stress echocardiogram	Combination of exercise test and echocardiogram. Resting images of the heart are taken with ultrasound, and then the patient exercises. Postexercise images are taken within 1 min of stopping exercise. Differences in left ventricular wall motion and thickening before and after exercise are evaluated.	*Before:* Prepare patient for treadmill or exercise bicycle. Tell patient of importance of timely return to examination table for imaging after exercise.
Pharmacologic echocardiogram	Used as a substitute for the exercise stress test in individuals unable to exercise. IV adenosine, dobutamine, or dipyridamole is given over several minutes or regadenoson (Lexiscan) is given as a single bolus over 10 sec while echocardiogram is performed to detect wall motion abnormalities.	*Before:* Explain procedure to patient. Obtain IV access for injection of drugs. *During:* Give drugs per protocol. Monitor vital signs before, during, and after test until baseline achieved. Monitor patient for signs and symptoms of distress during procedure. Observe patient for any side effects (e.g., shortness of breath, dizziness, nausea). Aminophylline may be given to prevent or reverse side effects of dipyridamole. Contraindications include any known allergies to the drugs.
Transesophageal echocardiogram (TEE)	A probe with an ultrasound transducer at the tip is swallowed while the physician controls angle and depth. As it passes down the esophagus, it sends back clear images of heart size, wall motion, valve abnormalities, endocarditis vegetation, and possible source of thrombi without interference from lungs or chest ribs. A contrast medium may be injected IV for evaluating direction of blood flow if an atrial or ventricular septal defect is suspected. Doppler ultrasound and color-flow imaging can also be used concurrently.	*Before:* Tell patient to fast for at least 6 hr before test. Remove dentures. *During:* IV sedation is given and throat locally anesthetized. A bite block is placed in the mouth. Monitor vital signs and O_2 saturation levels and perform suctioning as needed during procedure. Assist patient to relax. *After:* Patient may not eat or drink until gag reflex returns. Sore throat is temporary. A designated driver is needed if test is done in the outpatient department.
Nuclear Cardiology	Study involves IV injection of radioactive isotopes (^{99m}technetium-sestamibi [Cardiolite]). Radioactive uptake is counted over the heart by scintillation camera. It supplies information about heart contractility, myocardial perfusion, and acute injury.	*Before:* Explain procedure to patient. Women must remove bras to decrease breast attenuation. Obtain IV access for injection of isotopes. Explain that radioactive isotope used is a small, diagnostic amount and will lose most of its radioactivity in a few hours. Tell patient that he or she will be lying still on back with arms extended overhead for 20 min. *During:* Repeat scans are done within a few minutes to hours after the injection.

Continued

TABLE 31-6 Diagnostic Studies

Cardiovascular System—cont'd

Study	Description and Purpose	Nursing Responsibility
Nuclear Cardiology—cont'd		
Multigated acquisition (MUGA) (cardiac blood pool) scan	Small amount of the patient's blood is removed, mixed with a radioactive isotope (e.g., ^{99m}technetium-sestamibi), and reinjected IV. With the ECG used for timing, images are obtained during the cardiac cycle. Indicated for patients with MI, heart failure, or valve disease. Can be used to evaluate the effect of various cardiac or cardiotoxic drugs on the heart.	*Before:* Explain procedure to patient. Obtain IV access for removal of blood sample and reinjection of isotope. Start ECG monitoring. Tell patient that procedure involves little risk.
Single-photon emission computed tomography (SPECT)	Used to determine size or risk of infarction and to determine infarction size. Small amounts of a radioactive isotope (e.g., ^{99m}technetium-tetrofosmin [Myoview], thallium-201) are injected IV and recordings are made of the radioactivity emitted over a specific area of the body. Circulation of the isotope can be used to detect coronary artery blood flow, intracardiac shunts, motion of ventricles, EF, and size of the heart chambers.	*Before:* Explain procedure to patient. Obtain IV access for injection of isotope. Start ECG monitoring. Tell patient that procedure involves little risk.
Exercise (stress) nuclear imaging	Nuclear imaging images are taken at rest and after exercise. Injection is given at maximum HR (usually 85% of age-predicted maximum) on bicycle or treadmill. Patient is then required to continue exercise for 1 min to circulate the radioactive isotope. Scanning is done 15-60 min after exercise. A resting scan is performed 60-90 min after initial infusion or 24 hr later.	*Before:* Explain procedure to patient. Tell patient to eat only a light meal between scans. Certain drugs may need to be held for 1-2 days before the scan. Patients should not have caffeine 12 hr prior. Obtain IV access. *During:* If targeted maximum HR is not achieved with exercise, test may be changed to pharmacologic imaging.
Pharmacologic nuclear imaging	Regadenoson, dipyridamole, or adenosine is used to produce vasodilation when patients are unable to tolerate exercise. Vasodilation increases blood flow to well-perfused coronary arteries. Scanning procedure is same. Aminophylline may be given to prevent or reverse side effects of dipyridamole (e.g., shortness of breath, dizziness, nausea). Dobutamine is used if vasodilators are contraindicated.	*Before:* Explain procedure to patient. Tell patient to hold all caffeine products and theophylline (for regadenoson or dipyridamole testing) for 12 hr before procedure. Calcium channel blockers and β-blockers should be held 24 hr before the test. Obtain IV access. *During:* Observe patient for any side effects (e.g., shortness of breath, dizziness, nausea).
Positron emission tomography (PET)	Highly sensitive in distinguishing viable and nonviable heart tissue. Uses two radionuclides. Nitrogen-13-ammonia is injected IV first and scanned to evaluate myocardial perfusion. A second radioactive isotope, fluoro-18-deoxyglucose, is then injected and scanned to show myocardial metabolic function. In the normal heart, both scans match, but in an ischemic or damaged heart, they differ. The patient may or may not be stressed. A baseline resting scan is usually obtained for comparison.	*Before:* Explain that patient will be scanned by a machine and will need to stay still for a time. If exercise is included as part of testing, patient needs to fast and refrain from tobacco and caffeine for 24 hr before test. Obtain IV access. *During:* Patient's glucose level must be between 60-140 mg/dL (3.3-7.8 μmol/L) for accurate glucose metabolic activity.
Cardiovascular Magnetic Resonance Imaging (CMRI)	Noninvasive imaging technique obtains information about heart tissue, EF, aneurysms, cardiac output, and patency of proximal coronary arteries. It does not involve ionizing radiation and is an extremely safe procedure. Provides images in multiple planes with uniformly good resolution.	*Before:* Explain procedure to patient. Tell patient that the small diameter of the cylinder, along with loud noise of the procedure, may cause anxiety or panic. Antianxiety drugs and distraction strategies (e.g., music) may be provided. Patient must lie still during test. Contraindicated for persons with implanted metallic devices or other metal fragments unless noted to be MRI safe. Discuss any implants before scan.
Magnetic resonance angiography (MRA)	Used for imaging vascular occlusive disease and abdominal aortic aneurysms. Same as MRI but with use of gadolinium as IV contrast medium.	*Before:* Contraindications include any known allergies to contrast medium and persons with implanted metallic devices or other metal fragments unless noted to be MRA safe. Discuss any implants before scan. Obtain IV access.
Cardiac Computed Tomography (CT)	Cardiac CT is heart-specific CT imaging technology with or without IV contrast medium used to visualize heart anatomy, coronary circulation, and blood vessels.	*Before:* Explain procedure to patient.
Coronary CT angiography (CTA)	Use of CT with injected IV contrast medium to obtain images of blood vessels and diagnose CAD.	*Before:* Explain procedure to patient. Obtain IV access. Metal objects should be removed before examination. The patient may need to fast for several hours before the procedure. A β-blocker may be given before the test to control HR. *During:* Patients must have a regular heart rhythm for accurate testing.

TABLE 31-6 Diagnostic Studies

Cardiovascular System—cont'd

Study	Description and Purpose	Nursing Responsibility
Calcium-scoring CT scan • Electron beam computed tomography (EBCT)	EBCT, also known as *ultrafast CT,* uses a scanning electron beam to quantify calcification in coronary arteries and heart valves (Fig. 31-11). Primarily used for risk assessment in asymptomatic patients and to assess for heart disease in patients with atypical symptoms potentially related to cardiac causes.	*Before:* Explain procedure to patient. Tell patient that procedure is quick and involves little or no risk.
Cardiac Catheterization	Involves insertion of catheter into heart to obtain information about O_2 levels and pressure readings within heart chambers. Contrast medium is injected to assist in seeing structures and motion of heart. Procedure is done by insertion of catheter into a vein (for right side of heart) and/or an artery (for left side of heart).	*Before:* Check for sensitivity to contrast media. Withhold food and fluids for 6-12 hr before procedure. Explain the procedure to the patient including use of local anesthesia at insertion site, placement of catheter, flushed feeling when dye is injected, and possible fluttering sensation of heart as catheter is passed. Note that patient may be asked to cough or take a deep breath when dye is injected and that patient is monitored by ECG throughout procedure. Give sedative and other drugs, as ordered. *After:* Frequently assess circulation to extremity used for catheter insertion. Check peripheral pulses, color, and sensation of extremity per agency protocol. Observe insertion site for hematoma and bleeding. Place compression device over arterial site to achieve hemostasis, if indicated. Monitor vital signs and ECG. Assess for hypotension or hypertension, dysrhythmias, and signs of pulmonary emboli (e.g., respiratory difficulty).
Coronary angiography	During a cardiac catheterization, contrast medium is injected directly into coronary arteries. Used to evaluate patency of coronary arteries and collateral circulation.	Same as for cardiac catheterization.
Intravascular ultrasound (IVUS)	During cardiac catheterization a small ultrasound probe is introduced into coronary arteries. Used to assess size and consistency of plaque, arterial walls, and effectiveness of intracoronary artery treatment.	Same as for cardiac catheterization.
Fractional flow reserve (FFR)	During cardiac catheterization a specialized wire is inserted into coronary arteries to measure pressure and flow. Information is used to determine need for angioplasty or stenting on nonsignificant blockages.	Same as for cardiac catheterization.
Electrophysiology Study (EPS)	Invasive study used to record intracardiac electrical activity using catheters (with multiple electrodes) inserted via the femoral or jugular veins into right side of heart. Catheter electrodes record the electrical activity in different heart structures. In addition, dysrhythmias can be induced and terminated.	*Before:* Antidysrhythmic drugs may be stopped several days before study. Keep patient NPO 6-8 hr before test. Give premedication to promote relaxation if ordered. Obtain IV access. IV sedation often used during procedure. *After:* Assess vital signs frequently and monitor ECG continuously after the procedure per agency protocol.
Peripheral Arteriography and Venography	Peripheral vessel blood flow is assessed by injecting contrast media into appropriate arteries or veins (arteriography and venography). Serial x-ray studies done to detect and visualize any atherosclerotic plaques, occlusion, aneurysms, venous abnormalities, or traumatic injury. See Table 37-9 for additional peripheral vascular diagnostic studies.	*Before:* Check for allergy to contrast media. Give mild sedative, if ordered. *During:* Observe patient for allergic reactions to contrast media. *After:* Check extremity with puncture site for pulsation, warmth, color, and motion. Inspect insertion site for bleeding or swelling.
Hemodynamic Monitoring	Invasive and minimally invasive bedside hemodynamic monitoring is done using intraarterial, pulmonary artery, and central vein catheters to monitor arterial BP, stroke volume variation, pulmonary artery pressure, pulmonary artery wedge pressure, cardiac output, and central venous pressure. Used to evaluate cardiovascular status and response to treatment.	Patients requiring hemodynamic monitoring are critically ill and are monitored in intensive care units. See Chapter 65 for complete information on hemodynamic monitoring.

even small MIs that are not apparent with SPECT. CMRI aids in the final diagnosis of MI and the assessment of EF. It also plays a role in prediction of recovery from MI and in the diagnosis of congenital heart and aortic disorders and CAD.[19] One major advantage of CMRI is that it does not require any radiation to the patient.

Patients with coronary stents can undergo CMRI 6 weeks after stent placement.[20] In patients with older-model pacemakers and ICDs, CMRI is discouraged because the magnets can change the function of the devices. However, when there is a strong clinical need and the benefits outweigh the risks, CMRI should only be performed in these patients at centers experienced in this procedure.[19] Many newer models of pacemakers and ICDs are approved for use with MRI.

Cardiac Computed Tomography

Cardiac computed tomography (CT) is a heart-imaging test that uses CT technology with or without IV contrast (dye) to see the heart anatomy, coronary circulation, and great blood vessels (e.g., aorta, pulmonary veins, artery). This technology is often called *multidetector CT (MDCT) scanning*. Types of CT scans used to diagnose heart disease include coronary CT angiography (CTA) and calcium-scoring CT scan (Table 31-6).

Coronary CTA is a noninvasive test. It can be done faster than a cardiac catheterization with less risk and discomfort to the patient.[21] Patients must have a normal sinus rhythm for this test. Although the use of coronary CTA is increasing, cardiac catheterization (discussed in the next section) remains the gold standard to diagnose CAD. Further, when a cardiac catheterization is done, procedures (e.g., angioplasty, stent placement) can be done if coronary blockages are found. Last, the radiation exposure during a cardiac catheterization is less than the exposure during a CTA.

The calcium-scoring CT scan is used to find calcium deposits in plaque in the coronary arteries. The most common method used is the electron beam CT (EBCT) (Fig. 31-11). It can detect early coronary calcification before symptoms develop and confirm CAD in patients with suspected CAD. The amount of coronary calcium is a predictor of future cardiac events. The calcium score can be used in the risk analysis of patients without known CVD.[22]

Cardiac Catheterization

Cardiac catheterization is a common procedure. It provides information about CAD, coronary spasm, congenital and valvular heart disease, and ventricular function. Cardiac catheterization is also used to measure intracardiac pressures and O_2 levels, as well as CO and EF. With injection of contrast media and fluoroscopy, the coronary arteries can be seen, chambers of the heart can be outlined, and wall motion can be observed.

Cardiac catheterization is done by inserting a radiopaque catheter into the right and/or left side of the heart. For the right side of the heart, a catheter is inserted through an arm vein (basilic or cephalic) or a leg vein (femoral). Pressures are recorded as the catheter is moved into the vena cava, right atrium, right ventricle, and pulmonary artery. The catheter is then moved until it is wedged or lodged in position. This blocks the blood flow and pressure from the right side of the heart and looks ahead through the pulmonary capillary bed to the pressure in the left side of the heart *(pulmonary artery wedge pressure)*. This pressure is used to assess the function of the left side of the heart.

Left-sided heart catheterization is done by inserting a catheter into a radial, femoral, or brachial artery. The catheter is passed in a retrograde manner up to the aorta, across the aortic valve, and into the left ventricle.

Coronary angiography is done with a left-sided heart catheterization. The catheter is positioned at the origin of the coronary arteries (Fig. 31-3), and contrast medium is injected into the arteries. Patients often feel a temporary flushed sensation with dye injection. The images identify the location and severity of any coronary blockages (see Figs. 31-12 and 33-6). Complications of cardiac catheterization include bleeding or hematoma at the puncture site; allergic reactions to the contrast media; looping or kinking of the catheter; infection; thrombus formation; aortic dissection; dysrhythmias; MI; stroke; and puncture of the ventricles, septum, or lung tissue.

Intravascular Ultrasound. Intravascular ultrasound (IVUS), also known as intracoronary ultrasound (ICUS), is an invasive procedure performed in the catheterization laboratory with coronary angiography. The 2-D or 3-D US images provide a cross-sectional view of the arterial walls of the coronary arteries. In this procedure a miniature transducer attached to a small catheter is moved to the artery to be studied. Once it is

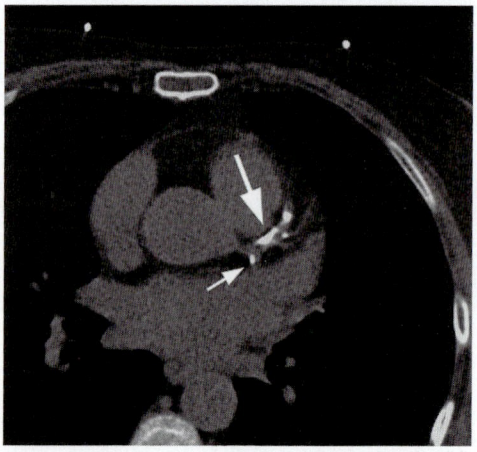

FIG. 31-11 Examples of coronary calcification of the left anterior descending coronary artery *(large arrow)* and left circumflex artery *(small arrow)* as seen on electron beam computed tomography. (From Libby P, Bonow R, Zipes D, et al: *Braunwald's heart disease: a textbook of cardiovascular medicine*, ed 8, St Louis, 2008, Saunders.)

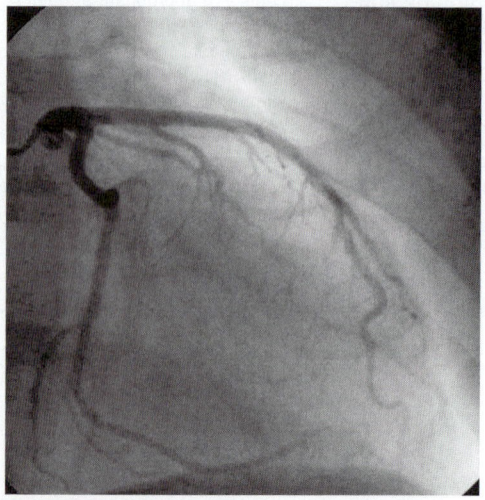

FIG. 31-12 Angiogram showing a normal left coronary and circumflex artery. (From Drake RL, Vogl AW, Mitchell AWM: *Gray's anatomy for students*, ed 2, Philadelphia, 2010, Churchill Livingstone.)

in the artery, US images are obtained. The health of the arterial layers is assessed, including the composition, location, and thickness of any plaque. IVUS can evaluate vessel response to treatments such as stent placement and atherectomy, as well as any complications that may have occurred during the procedure (see Chapter 33). Patients often have IVUS in addition to angiography or a coronary intervention. Thus nursing care is similar to that following cardiac catheterization (Table 31-6).

Fractional Flow Reserve. Fractional flow reserve (FFR) is a procedure that is done during a cardiac catheterization. It involves using a special wire that can measure pressure and flow in the coronary artery. FFR helps to determine the need to perform angioplasty or stenting on nonsignificant blockages.

Electrophysiology Study

The electrophysiology study (EPS) records and manipulates the heart's electrical activity using electrodes placed inside the heart chambers. It provides information on SA node, AV node, and ventricular conduction. It is particularly helpful in determining the source and treatment of dysrhythmias. Patients with symptomatic tachydysrhythmias are at risk for sudden cardiac death. Information from an EPS helps to make an accurate diagnosis and guides treatment decisions.

In EPS, catheters are inserted in a manner similar to that used in a right-sided heart catheterization. These catheters are placed at specific anatomic sites within the heart to record electrical activity. Nursing care for patients after EPS is similar to the care of patients after cardiac catheterization (Table 31-6).

CASE STUDY

Objective Data: Diagnostic Studies

(©Jupiterimages/ Banana-Stock/ Thinkstock)

The HCP orders the following initial diagnostic studies for L.P.:

- 12-lead ECG
- CBC, basic metabolic panel (glucose, electrolytes, BUN, creatinine)
- PTT, PT, INR
- Pro-BNP
- Troponin, CK-MB
- TSH, free T_4
- Chest x-ray

L.P.'s initial troponin and CK-MB levels are within normal limits. The ECG demonstrates atrial fibrillation with a rapid ventricular response. Chest x-ray, CBC, and coagulation studies are all within normal limits. The potassium level is 3.1 mEq/L and pro-BNP is elevated (1204 pg/mL). The HCP orders 250 mL NSS IV bolus; a po dose of potassium, a loading dose of IV diltiazem (Cardizem) followed by a continuous infusion, and weight-based heparin to be started in the emergency department. L.P. will be admitted to the progressive care unit and will have a consult with a cardiologist.

Discussion Questions

1. Are these the diagnostic studies that you expected to be ordered?
2. Which diagnostic study results are abnormal?
3. Which diagnostic study results are of most concern to you?

Answers available at *http://evolve.elsevier.com/Lewis/medsurg.*

BRIDGE TO NCLEX EXAMINATION

The number of the question corresponds to the same-numbered outcome at the beginning of the chapter.

1. A patient with a tricuspid valve disorder will have impaired blood flow between the
   a. vena cava and right atrium.
   b. left atrium and left ventricle.
   c. right atrium and right ventricle.
   d. right ventricle and pulmonary artery.
2. A patient has a severe blockage in his right coronary artery. Which heart structures are *most* likely to be affected by this blockage *(select all that apply)*?
   a. AV node
   b. Left ventricle
   c. Coronary sinus
   d. Right ventricle
   e. Pulmonic valve
3. The portion of the vascular system responsible for hemostasis is the
   a. thin capillary vessels.
   b. endothelial layer of the arteries.
   c. elastic middle layer of the veins.
   d. smooth muscle of the arterial wall.
4. When a person's blood pressure rises, the homeostatic mechanism to compensate for an elevation involves stimulation of
   a. baroreceptors that inhibit the sympathetic nervous system, causing vasodilation.
   b. chemoreceptors that inhibit the sympathetic nervous system, causing vasodilation.
   c. baroreceptors that inhibit the parasympathetic nervous system, causing vasodilation.
   d. chemoreceptors that stimulate the sympathetic nervous system, causing an increased heart rate.
5. A P wave on an ECG represents an impulse arising at the
   a. SA node and repolarizing the atria.
   b. SA node and depolarizing the atria.
   c. AV node and depolarizing the atria.
   d. AV node and spreading to the bundle of His.
6. When collecting subjective data related to the cardiovascular system, which information should be obtained from the patient *(select all that apply)*?
   a. Annual income
   b. Smoking history
   c. Religious preference
   d. Number of pillows used to sleep
   e. Blood for basic laboratory studies
7. The auscultatory area in the left midclavicular line at the level of the fifth ICS is the best location to hear sounds from which heart valve?
   a. Aortic
   b. Mitral
   c. Tricuspid
   d. Pulmonic
8. When assessing a patient, you note a pulse deficit of 23 beats. This finding may be caused by
   a. dysrhythmias.
   b. heart murmurs.
   c. gallop rhythms.
   d. pericardial friction rubs.
9. When assessing the cardiovascular system of a 79-year-old patient, you may expect to find
   a. a narrowed pulse pressure.
   b. diminished carotid artery pulses.
   c. difficulty in isolating the apical pulse.
   d. an increased heart rate in response to stress.

10. Which nursing responsibilities are priorities when caring for a patient returning from a cardiac catheterization *(select all that apply)*?
    a. Monitoring vital signs and ECG
    b. Checking the catheter insertion site and distal pulses
    c. Assisting the patient to ambulate to the bathroom to void
    d. Informing the patient that he will be sleepy from the general anesthesia
    e. Instructing the patient about the risks of the radioactive isotope injection

1. c, 2. a, b, d, 3. b, 4. a, 5. b, 6. b, c, d, 7. b, 8. a, 9. c, 10. a, b

For rationales to these answers and even more NCLEX review questions, visit *http://evolve.elsevier.com/Lewis/medsurg*.

EVOLVE WEBSITE

http://evolve.elsevier.com/Lewis/medsurg

Review Questions (Online Only)

Key Points

Answer Keys for Questions

- Rationales for Bridge to NCLEX Examination Questions
- Answer Guidelines for Case Studies on pp. 663, 666, 669, and 679

Conceptual Care Map Creator

Audio Glossary

Supporting Media

- Animations
  - Auscultation of Heart Valves
  - Blood Flow: Circulatory System
  - Cardiac Cycle During Systole and Diastole
  - Pulse Variations
- Audio
  - Diastolic Murmur
  - Fourth Heart Sound (S_4)
  - Murmurs: Blowing, Harsh or Rough, and Rumble
  - Murmurs: High, Medium, and Low
  - S_1 at Various Locations
  - S_2 at Various Locations
  - Single S_1
  - Single S_2
  - Systolic Murmur
  - Third Heart Sound (S_3)

Content Updates

REFERENCES

1. Patton KT, Thibodeau GA: *Anatomy and physiology*, ed 8, St Louis, 2013, Mosby.
2. Wesley K: *Huszar's basic dysrhythmias and acute coronary syndromes*, ed 4, St Louis, 2011, Mosby Jems.
3. McCance K, Huether S: *Pathophysiology: biologic basis for disease in adults and children*, ed 7, St Louis, 2014, Elsevier.
4. American Heart Association: Understanding blood pressure readings, 2014. Retrieved from *www.heart.org/HEARTORG/Conditions/HighBloodPressure/AboutHighBloodPressure/Understanding-Blood-Pressure-Readings_UCM_301764_Article.jsp*.
5. Ball JW, Dains JE, Flynn JA, et al: *Seidel's physical examination*, ed 8, St Louis, 2015, Elsevier.
6. North BJ, Sinclair DA: The intersection between aging and cardiovascular disease, *Circ Res* 110:1097, 2012.
7. National Institute on Aging: Aging heart and arteries: a scientific quest, 2014. Retrieved from *www.nia.nih.gov/health/publication/aging-hearts-and-arteries/preface*.
8. Skidmore-Roth L: *Mosby's 2015 nursing drug reference*, ed 28, St Louis, 2015, Elsevier.

*9. Mosca L, Benjamin EJ, Berry K, et al: Effectiveness-based guidelines for cardiovascular disease prevention in women: 2011 update, *Circulation* 123:1243, 2011.

10. Sherwood MW, Newby LK: High-sensitivity troponin assay: evidence, indications, and reasonable use, *J Am Heart Assoc* 3:1, 2014.
11. Pagana KD, Pagana TJ: *Mosby's manual of diagnostic and laboratory tests*, ed 5, St Louis, 2014, Elsevier.

*12. Lipenski LJ, Escarcego RO, D'Ascenzo F, et al: A systematic review and collaborative meta-analysis to determine the incremental value of copeptin for rapid rule-out of acute myocardial infarction, *Am J Cardiol* 113:1581, 2014.

13. Makrygiannis SS, Ampartzidou OS, Zairis MN, et al: Prognostic usefulness of serial C-reactive protein measurements in ST-elevation acute myocardial infarction, *Am J Cardiol* 111:26, 2013.
14. American Heart Association: Homocysteine, folic acid and cardiovascular disease. Retrieved from *www.heart.org/HEARTORG/GettingHealthy/NutritionCenter/Homocysteine-Folic-Acid-and-Cardiovascular-Disease_UCM_305997_Article.jsp*.
15. Ridker PM, Lüscher TF: Anti-inflammatory therapies for cardiovascular disease, *Eur Heart J* 35:1782, 2014.
16. American Heart Association: Cardiac event recorder, 2014. Retrieved from *http://www.heart.org/HEARTORG/Conditions/Arrhythmia/PreventionTreatmentofArrhythmia/Cardiac-Event-Recorder_UCM_447317_Article.jsp*.
17. Zaret BL, Beller GA: *Clinical nuclear cardiology*, ed 4, St Louis, 2010, Mosby.
18. Li Y, Zhang W, Wu H, et al: Advanced tracers in PET imaging of cardiovascular disease, *BioMed Res Intern* 2014:1, 2014.

*19. Hundley WG, Bluemke DA, Finn JP, et al: ACCF/ACR/AHA/NASCI/SCMR 2010 expert consensus document on cardiovascular magnetic resonance: a report of the American College of Cardiology Foundation Task Force on Expert Consensus Documents, *Circulation* 121:2462, 2010.

20. Ramos LM: Cardiac diagnostic testing: what bedside nurses need to know, *Crit Care Nurse* 34:16, 2014.

*21. Mark DB, Berman DS, Budoff MJ, et al: ACCF/ACR/AHA/NASCI/SAIP/SCAI/SCCT 2010 expert consensus document on coronary computed tomographic angiography: a report of the American College of Cardiology Foundation Task Force on Expert Consensus Documents, *Circulation* 121:2509, 2010.

*22. Mieres JH, Gulati M, Merz NB, et al: Role of noninvasive testing in the clinical evaluation of women with suspected ischemic heart disease: a consensus statement from the American Heart Association, *Circulation* 130:350, 2014.

*Evidence-based information for clinical practice.

32

Hypertension

Melissa L. Hutchinson

One way to get high blood pressure is to go mountain climbing over molehills.

Earl Wilson

http://evolve.elsevier.com/Lewis/medsurg/

LEARNING OUTCOMES

1. Relate the pathophysiologic mechanisms associated with primary hypertension to the clinical manifestations and complications.
2. Select appropriate strategies for the prevention of primary hypertension.
3. Describe the interprofessional care for primary hypertension, including drug therapy and lifestyle modifications.
4. Explain the interprofessional care of the older adult with primary hypertension.
5. Prioritize the nursing management of the patient with primary hypertension.
6. Describe the nursing and interprofessional care of a patient with a hypertensive crisis.

KEY TERMS

blood pressure (BP), p. 681
hypertension, p. 684
hypertensive crisis, p. 698
isolated systolic hypertension (ISH), p. 684
orthostatic hypotension, p. 695
prehypertension, p. 684
primary hypertension, p. 684
secondary hypertension, p. 684
systemic vascular resistance (SVR), p. 681

Hypertension, or high blood pressure (BP), is one of the most important modifiable risk factors that can lead to the development of cardiovascular disease (CVD). As BP increases, so does the risk of myocardial infarction (MI), heart failure, stroke, and renal disease. This chapter discusses the nursing and interprofessional care of patients at risk for or who have hypertension.

Hypertension affects one in three adults in the United States. Heart disease, often directly related to hypertension, accounts for 23.7% of all deaths each year in the United States.[1,2] *Healthy People 2020* lists the number of adults with hypertension whose BP is under control as one of the 26 high-priority, leading health indicators for the coming decade.[3] The National Health and Nutrition Examination Survey (NHANES) tracks prevention, treatment, and control of hypertension. Data from NHANES showed that 83% of people 20 years of age and older with hypertension were aware that they had high BP. Of these people, 76% were being treated. Of those aware of their hypertension, 48% did not currently have their BP well controlled.[4,5]

The American College of Cardiology Foundation and the American Heart Association (AHA) provide performance measures for hypertension management that address not only treatment but also control of BP to target goals. Target goals have been updated with new information from the evidence-based Guideline for the Management of High Blood Pressure in Adults report from the Eighth Joint National Committee (JNC 8) and the Systolic Blood Pressure Intervention Trial (SPRINT). Target goals take into consideration both age and co-morbidities when recommending treatment options.[6,7]

National guidelines are designed to apply to all racial and ethnic groups. However, certain groups have a higher incidence of risk factors[6-8] (see boxes on Cultural & Ethnic Health Disparities and Gender Differences on p. 682).

NORMAL REGULATION OF BLOOD PRESSURE

Blood pressure (BP) is the force exerted by the blood against the walls of the blood vessel. It must be adequate to maintain tissue perfusion during activity and rest. The maintenance of normal BP and tissue perfusion requires the integration of both systemic factors and local peripheral vascular effects. BP is primarily a function of cardiac output (CO) and systemic vascular resistance (SVR) (Fig. 32-1).

CO is the total blood flow through the systemic or pulmonary circulation per minute. It is described as the stroke volume (SV) or the amount of blood pumped out of the left ventricle per beat (approximately 70 mL) multiplied by the heart rate (HR).

Systemic vascular resistance (SVR) is the force opposing the movement of blood within the blood vessels. The radius of the small arteries and arterioles is the principal factor determining SVR. As arteries narrow, resistance to blood flow increases. As arteries dilate, resistance to blood flow decreases. A small change in the radius of the arterioles creates a major change in the SVR.

Reviewed by Elisabeth G. Bradley, MS, APN, ACNS-BC, AGPCNP-BC, Clinical Leader, Cardiovascular Prevention Program, Christiana Care Health System, Newark, Delaware; Janie Corbitt, RN, MLS, Retired Instructor of Nursing, Milledgeville, Georgia; and Susan J. Eisel, RN, MSEd, Associate Professor of Nursing, Mercy College of Ohio, Toledo, Ohio.

CULTURAL & ETHNIC HEALTH DISPARITIES

Hypertension

African Americans

- Have the highest prevalence of hypertension in the world
- Develop hypertension at a younger age than whites
- Have a higher incidence of hypertension among women than among men
- Demonstrate more nocturnal non-dipping BP than whites
- Hypertension is more aggressive and results in more severe end-organ damage.
- Have a higher death rate resulting from hypertension than whites
- Produce less renin and do not respond well to renin-inhibiting drugs
- Calcium channel blockers and diuretics provide better BP control, especially with monotherapy.
- Have a higher risk of angioedema with angiotensin-converting enzyme inhibitors than whites

Mexican Americans

- Are less likely to receive treatment for hypertension than whites and African Americans
- Have lower rates of BP control than whites and African Americans
- Have lower levels of awareness of hypertension and its treatment than whites and African Americans

GENDER DIFFERENCES

Hypertension

Men

- Before early middle age, hypertension is more common in men than in women.

Women

- Hypertension is two to three times more common in women who take oral contraceptives than in women who do not.
- A history of preeclampsia may be an early sign of risk for cardiovascular disease.
- After age 64, hypertension is more common in women than in men. Part of the rise in BP in women is attributed to menopause-related factors such as estrogen withdrawal, overproduction of pituitary hormones, and weight gain.
- It is more difficult to control hypertension in older women (ages 70-79) than in women ages 50-69, despite having similar rates of treatment.

If SVR is increased and CO remains constant or increases, arterial BP will increase.

The mechanisms that regulate BP can affect either CO or SVR, or both. Regulation of BP is a complex process involving both short-term (seconds to hours) and long-term (days to weeks) mechanisms. Short-term mechanisms, including the sympathetic nervous system (SNS) and vascular endothelium, are active within a few seconds. Long-term mechanisms include renal and hormonal processes that regulate arteriolar resistance and blood volume. In a healthy person these regulatory mechanisms function in response to the body's demands.

Sympathetic Nervous System

The nervous system, which reacts within seconds after a drop in BP, increases BP primarily by activating the SNS. Increased SNS activity increases HR and cardiac contractility, produces widespread vasoconstriction in the peripheral arterioles, and promotes the release of renin from the kidneys. The net effect of SNS activation is to increase BP by increasing both CO and SVR.

Specialized nerve cells called *baroreceptors (pressoreceptors)* are located in the carotid arteries and arch of the aorta. These cells sense changes in BP and transmit this information to the vasomotor centers in the brainstem. The brainstem sends this information through complex networks of neurons that excite or inhibit efferent nerves. SNS efferent nerves innervate cardiac and vascular smooth muscle cells. Under normal conditions, a low level of continuous SNS activity maintains vascular tone. BP may be reduced by withdrawal of SNS activity or by stimulation of the parasympathetic nervous system (PNS). The PNS decreases the HR (via the vagus nerve) and thereby decreases CO.

The neurotransmitter norepinephrine (NE) is released from SNS nerve endings. NE activates receptors located in the sinoatrial node, myocardium, and vascular smooth muscle. The response to NE depends on the type of receptors present. SNS receptors are classified as α_1, α_2, β_1, and β_2 (Table 32-1). The smooth muscle of the blood vessels has α-adrenergic and β_2-adrenergic receptors. α-Adrenergic receptors located in the peripheral vasculature cause vasoconstriction when stimulated by NE. β_1-Adrenergic receptors in the heart respond to NE and epinephrine with increased HR (chronotropic), increased force of contraction (inotropic), and increased speed of conduction (dromotropic). β_2-Adrenergic receptors are activated primarily

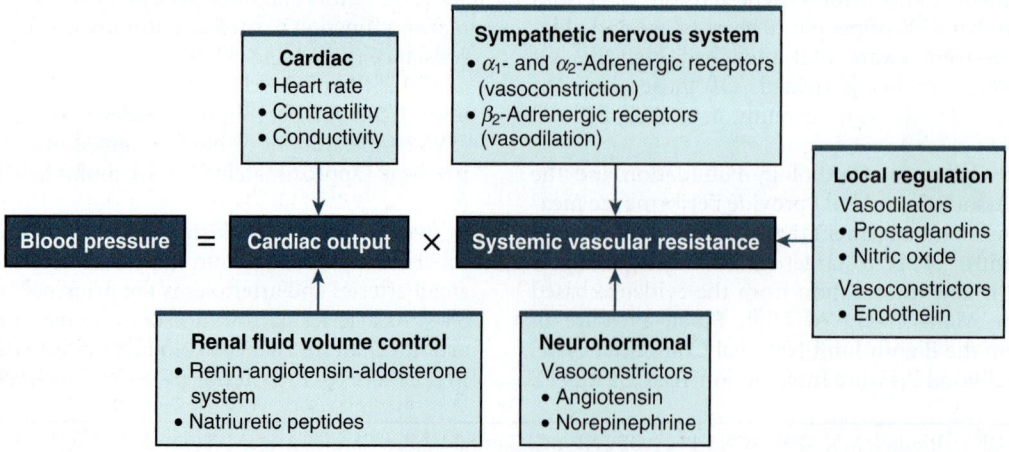

FIG. 32-1 Factors influencing blood pressure (BP). Hypertension develops when one or more of the BP-regulating mechanisms are defective.

TABLE 32-1 Sympathetic Nervous System Receptors Affecting BP

Receptor	Location	Response When Activated
α_1	Vascular smooth muscle	Vasoconstriction
	Heart	Increased contractility (positive inotropic effect)
α_2	Presynaptic nerve terminals	Inhibition of norepinephrine release
	Vascular smooth muscle	Vasoconstriction
β_1	Heart	Increased contractility (positive inotropic effect) Increased heart rate (positive chronotropic effect) Increased conduction (positive dromotropic effect)
	Juxtaglomerular cells of the kidney	Increased renin secretion
β_2	Smooth muscle of blood vessels in heart (e.g., coronary arteries), lungs (e.g., bronchi), and skeletal muscle	Vasodilation
Dopamine receptors	Primarily renal blood vessels	Vasodilation

by epinephrine released from the adrenal medulla and cause vasodilation (Fig. 32-1).

The sympathetic vasomotor center interacts with many areas of the brain to maintain normal BP under various conditions. It is activated during times of pain, stress, and exercise. The SNS response causes an appropriate increase in CO and BP to adjust to the body's increased O_2 demands. During postural change from lying to standing, there is a transient decrease in BP. The vasomotor center is stimulated, and the SNS response causes peripheral vasoconstriction and increased venous return to the heart. If this response did not occur, blood flow to the brain would be inadequate, resulting in dizziness or syncope.

Baroreceptors. *Baroreceptors* have an important role in the maintenance of BP stability during normal activities. They are sensitive to stretching and, when stimulated by an increase in BP, send inhibitory impulses to the sympathetic vasomotor center. Inhibition of the SNS results in decreased HR, decreased force of contraction, and vasodilation in peripheral arterioles.

When a fall in BP is sensed by the baroreceptors, the SNS is activated. The result is constriction of the peripheral arterioles, increased HR, and increased contractility of the heart. In long-standing hypertension, the baroreceptors become adjusted to elevated BP levels and recognize this level as their new "normal."

Vascular Endothelium

The vascular endothelium is a single-cell layer that lines the blood vessels. For years the endothelium was thought to be inert, serving only as a passive lining for the vessels. Now information shows that the endothelium is very active and responsible for a number of different critical functions. These include platelet adhesion, coagulation regulation, immune function, and regulation of fluid control within the vessel and extravascular space. The endothelium can also cause adhesion and aggregation of neutrophils and stimulate smooth muscle growth.

One of the most important findings was the discovery that the endothelium was essential to the regulation and maintenance of the vasodilating and vasoconstricting substances.[9] Endothelium-derived vasoactive substances include *nitric oxide* (NO) and *prostacyclin*, which are both vasodilators. Another product of the endothelium is *endothelin* (ET), which is a potent vasoconstrictor (Fig. 32-1). A disruption or dysfunction of arterial tone (either through excessive constriction or dilation) is an early warning signal of CVD.

Renal System

The kidneys contribute to BP regulation by controlling sodium excretion and extracellular fluid (ECF) volume (see Chapter 44). Sodium retention results in water retention, which causes an increase in ECF volume. This increases the venous return to the heart and stroke volume. Together these increase CO and BP.

The renin-angiotensin-aldosterone system (RAAS) also plays an important role in BP regulation (Fig. 32-1). The juxtaglomerular apparatus in the kidney secretes renin in response to SNS stimulation, decreased blood flow through the kidneys, or decreased serum sodium concentration. Renin is an enzyme that converts angiotensinogen to angiotensin I. Angiotensin I is then converted to angiotensin II (A-II) by angiotensin-converting enzyme (ACE). A-II increases BP by two different mechanisms (see Fig. 44-4). First, A-II is a potent vasoconstrictor and increases SVR. This results in an immediate increase in BP. Second, over a period of hours or days, A-II increases BP indirectly by stimulating the adrenal cortex to secrete aldosterone (discussed below).

A-II also acts at a local level within the heart and blood vessels. These effects include vasoconstriction and tissue growth that result in remodeling of the vessel walls, which can be due to or caused by endothelial dysfunction. These changes are linked to the development of primary hypertension and also the long-term effects of hypertension (e.g., atherosclerosis, renal disease, cardiac hypertrophy).

Prostaglandins (PGE_2 and PGI_2) secreted by the renal medulla have a vasodilator effect on the systemic circulation. This results in decreased SVR and lowering of BP. (Prostaglandins are discussed in Chapter 11.) The natriuretic peptides (atrial natriuretic peptide [ANP] and b-type natriuretic peptide [BNP]) are secreted by heart cells. They antagonize the effects of antidiuretic hormone (ADH) and aldosterone. This results in *natriuresis* (excretion of sodium in urine) and diuresis, resulting in reduced blood volume and BP.

Endocrine System

Stimulation of the SNS results in release of epinephrine along with a small fraction of NE by the adrenal medulla. Epinephrine increases the CO by increasing the HR and myocardial contractility. Epinephrine activates β_2-adrenergic receptors in peripheral arterioles of skeletal muscle, causing vasodilation. In peripheral arterioles with only α_1-adrenergic receptors (skin and kidneys), epinephrine causes vasoconstriction.

A-II stimulates the adrenal cortex to release aldosterone. (Release of aldosterone is also regulated by other factors [see Chapters 47 and 49].) Aldosterone stimulates the kidneys to retain sodium and water. This increases blood volume and CO (see Fig. 44-4).

An increased blood sodium and osmolarity level stimulates the release of ADH from the posterior pituitary gland. ADH increases the ECF volume by promoting the reabsorption of water in the distal and collecting tubules of the kidneys. The resulting increase in blood volume causes an increase in CO and BP.

HYPERTENSION

Classification of Hypertension

Hypertension is defined as a persistent systolic BP (SBP) of 140 mm Hg or more, diastolic BP (DBP) of 90 mm Hg or more, or current use of antihypertensive medication.[9] **Prehypertension** is defined as SBP of 120 to 139 mm Hg or DBP of 80 to 89 mm Hg.

Isolated systolic hypertension (ISH) is defined as an average SBP of 140 mm Hg or more, coupled with an average DBP of less than 90 mm Hg.[10] SBP increases with aging. DBP rises until approximately age 55 and then declines. Control of ISH decreases the incidence of stroke, heart failure, and death.

BP classification is based on the confirmation of office BP readings with ambulatory BP monitoring.[11] Table 32-2 presents the BP classification for people 18 years of age and older.

Etiology

Hypertension can result from either primary or secondary causes.

Primary Hypertension. **Primary** *(essential* or *idiopathic)* **hypertension** is elevated BP without an identified cause, and it accounts for 90% to 95% of all cases of hypertension. Although the exact cause of primary hypertension is unknown, there are several contributing factors. These include changes in endothelial function related to either vasoconstricting or vasodilating agents, increased SNS activity, overproduction of sodium-retaining hormones, increased sodium intake, greater-than-ideal body weight, diabetes, tobacco use, and excessive alcohol intake.

Secondary Hypertension. **Secondary hypertension** is elevated BP with a specific cause that often can be identified and corrected (Table 32-3). This type of hypertension accounts for 5% to 10% of hypertension in adults. Secondary hypertension should be suspected in people who suddenly develop high BP, especially if it is severe. Clinical findings that suggest secondary hypertension relate to the underlying cause. For example, an abdominal bruit heard over the renal arteries may indicate renal disease. Treatment of secondary hypertension is aimed at removing or treating the underlying cause. Secondary hypertension is a contributing factor to hypertensive crisis (discussed later in this chapter).

TABLE 32-2 Classification of Hypertension

Category	SBP (mm Hg)		DBP (mm Hg)
Normal	<120	and	<80
Prehypertension	120-139	or	80-89
Hypertension, stage 1	140-159	or	90-99
Hypertension, stage 2	≥160	or	≥100

From the National Heart, Lung, and Blood Institute: Seventh report of the Joint National Committee on Detection, Evaluation, and Treatment of High Blood Pressure (JNC-7), NIH Publication No. 04-5230, Bethesda, Md, 2004, The Institute. Retrieved from *www.nhlbi.nih.gov/guidelines/hypertension/jnc7full.pdf.*
DBP, Diastolic blood pressure; *SBP,* systolic blood pressure.

TABLE 32-3 Causes of Secondary Hypertension*

- Cirrhosis
- Coarctation or congenital narrowing of the aorta
- Drug-related: estrogen replacement therapy, oral contraceptives, corticosteroids, nonsteroidal antiinflammatory drugs (e.g., cyclooxygenase-2 inhibitors), sympathetic stimulants (e.g., cocaine, monoamine oxidase)
- Endocrine disorders (e.g., pheochromocytoma, Cushing syndrome, thyroid disease)
- Neurologic disorders (e.g., brain tumors, quadriplegia, traumatic brain injury)
- Pregnancy-induced hypertension
- Renal disease (e.g., renal artery stenosis, glomerulonephritis)
- Sleep apnea

*List is not all-inclusive.

Pathophysiology of Primary Hypertension

BP rises with any increase in CO or SVR. Increased CO is sometimes found in the person with prehypertension. Later in the course of hypertension, the SVR rises and CO returns to normal. The hemodynamic hallmark of hypertension is persistently increased SVR. This persistent elevation in SVR may occur in various ways. Table 32-4 presents factors that relate to the development of primary hypertension or contribute to its consequences. Abnormalities of any of the mechanisms involved in the maintenance of normal BP can result in hypertension (Fig. 32-1).

Genetic Link

Different sets of genes may regulate BP at different times throughout the life span.[2] Genetic variations are associated with the development of hypertension. For example, genetic abnormalities have been associated with a rare form of hypertension characterized by excess levels of potassium. Several genetic variants of substances on the endothelium affect BP and the development of hypertension by influencing the body's sensitivity to salt.[12] When endothelial surface proteins are activated, proinflammatory properties are stimulated. This impairs the endothelial cells' ability to activate vasodilatory effects, which leads to hypertension.

More research is needed to understand the connection among genetics, endothelial function, and hypertension. In practice, children and siblings of persons with hypertension should be screened and strongly advised to adopt healthy lifestyles to reduce their risk of hypertension.[12]

Water and Sodium Retention. Excessive sodium intake is linked to the development of hypertension. Although most people consume a high-sodium diet, only one in three will develop hypertension. When sodium is restricted in many people with hypertension, their BP falls. This suggests that some degree of sodium sensitivity may exist for high sodium intake to trigger the development of hypertension. A high sodium intake may activate a number of systemic mechanisms. Figure 32-2 shows the relationship among salt intake, BP, and changes in structure of the heart.

In clinical practice, there is not an easy or simple test to identify individuals whose BP will rise with even a small increase in salt intake *(salt sensitive)* versus those who can ingest large amounts of sodium without much change in BP *(salt resistant)*. Ongoing research may help to understand the most effective treatment options for people based on genetic predisposition. What is known is that the effect of sodium on BP has a strong genetic component. Additionally, the effect of sodium is greater in African Americans and in middle-aged and older adults.[13,14]

Altered Renin-Angiotensin-Aldosterone Mechanism. High plasma renin activity (PRA) increases the conversion of angiotensinogen to angiotensin I (see Fig. 44-4). This alteration in the RAAS may contribute to the development of hypertension. Any rise in BP inhibits the release of renin from the renal juxtaglomerular cells. Based on this feedback loop, low levels of PRA would be expected in patients with primary hypertension. However, only about 30% have low PRA, 50% have normal levels, and 20% have high PRA. These normal or high PRA levels may be related to excess renin secretion from ischemic nephrons.

Stress and Increased Sympathetic Nervous System Activity. It has long been recognized that BP is influenced by factors such as anger, fear, and pain. Physiologic responses to stress, which are normally protective, may persist to a pathologic degree, resulting in a prolonged increase in SNS activity. Increased SNS stimulation produces increased vasoconstriction, increased HR, and increased renin release. Increased renin activates the RAAS, leading to elevated BP. People exposed to high levels of repeated psychologic stress develop hypertension to a greater extent than those who experience less stress.

TABLE 32-4 Risk Factors for Primary Hypertension

Risk Factor	Description
Age	• SBP rises progressively with increasing age, although DBP may decrease with age. • After age 50, SBP >140 mm Hg is a more important cardiovascular risk factor than DBP.
Alcohol	• Excessive alcohol intake is strongly associated with hypertension. • Moderate intake of alcohol has cardioprotective properties; males with hypertension should limit their daily intake of alcohol to 2 drinks per day, and 1 drink per day for females with hypertension.
Tobacco use	• Smoking tobacco greatly ↑ risk of cardiovascular disease. • People with hypertension who smoke tobacco are at even greater risk for cardiovascular disease.
Diabetes mellitus	• Hypertension is more common in patients with diabetes. • When hypertension and diabetes coexist, complications (e.g., target organ disease) are more severe.
Elevated serum lipids	• ↑ Levels of cholesterol and triglycerides are primary risk factors in atherosclerosis. • Hyperlipidemia is more common in people with hypertension.

Excess dietary sodium	• High sodium intake can
	  • Contribute to hypertension in salt-sensitive patients.
	  • Decrease the effectiveness of certain antihypertensive medications.

Gender	• Hypertension is more prevalent in men in young adulthood and early middle age. • After age 64, hypertension is more prevalent in women. (See Gender Differences box on p. 682.)
Family history	• History of a close blood relative (e.g., parents, sibling) with hypertension is associated with an ↑ risk for developing hypertension.
Obesity	• Weight gain is associated with increased frequency of hypertension. • Risk increases with central abdominal obesity.
Ethnicity	• Incidence of hypertension is 2 times higher in African Americans than in whites. (See Cultural & Ethnic Health Disparities box on p. 682.)
Sedentary lifestyle	• Regular physical activity can help control weight and reduce cardiovascular risk. • Physical activity may ↓ BP.
Socioeconomic status	• Hypertension is more prevalent in lower socioeconomic groups and among the less educated.
Stress	• People exposed to repeated stress may develop hypertension more frequently than others. • People who develop hypertension may respond differently to stress than those who do not develop hypertension.

DBP, Diastolic blood pressure; *SBP,* systolic blood pressure.

Insulin Resistance and Hyperinsulinemia. Defects in glucose, insulin, and lipoprotein metabolism are common in primary hypertension. These defects are not present in secondary hypertension and do not improve when primary hypertension is treated. Insulin resistance is a risk factor in the development of hypertension and CVD. High insulin levels stimulate SNS activity and impair nitrous oxide–mediated vasodilation. Additional pressor effects of insulin include vascular hypertrophy and increased renal sodium reabsorption.

Endothelial Dysfunction. Endothelial dysfunction is recognized as a marker for CVD, including primary hypertension.[12] Hypertension can present as a prolonged vasoconstriction response or as a reduced vasodilator response. Prolonged vasoconstriction may be caused by high levels of ET. Vasodilation effects can be altered by oxygen free radicals, which impair the bioavailability of NO. This leads to cellular dysfunction and an imbalance of the vasodilation and vasoconstriction mechanisms in the endothelium.

Clinical Manifestations

Hypertension is often called the "silent killer" because it is frequently asymptomatic until it becomes severe and target organ disease occurs. A patient with severe hypertension may experience a variety of symptoms secondary to the effects on blood vessels in the various organs and tissues or to the increased workload of the heart. These secondary symptoms include fatigue, dizziness, palpitations, angina, and dyspnea.

In the past, symptoms of hypertension were thought to include headache and nosebleeds. Unless BP is very high, these symptoms are no more frequent in people with hypertension than in the general population. However, patients with hypertensive crisis (discussed later in the chapter) may experience severe headaches, dyspnea, anxiety, and nosebleeds.[15]

Complications

The most common complications of hypertension are *target organ diseases* occurring in the heart (hypertensive heart disease), brain (cerebrovascular disease), peripheral vessels (peripheral vascular disease), kidneys (nephrosclerosis), and eyes (retinal damage) (Table 32-5).

Hypertensive Heart Disease

Coronary Artery Disease. Hypertension is a major risk factor for coronary artery disease (CAD). The mechanisms by which hypertension contributes to the development of atherosclerosis are not fully known. The "response-to-injury" theory of atherogenesis suggests that hypertension disrupts the coronary artery endothelium (see Fig. 33-1). This results in a stiff arterial wall with a narrowed lumen, and accounts for a high rate of CAD, angina, and MI.

Left Ventricular Hypertrophy. Sustained high BP increases the cardiac workload and produces left ventricular hypertrophy (LVH) (Fig. 32-3). Initially, LVH is a compensatory mechanism that strengthens cardiac contraction and increases CO. However, increased contractility increases myocardial work and O_2

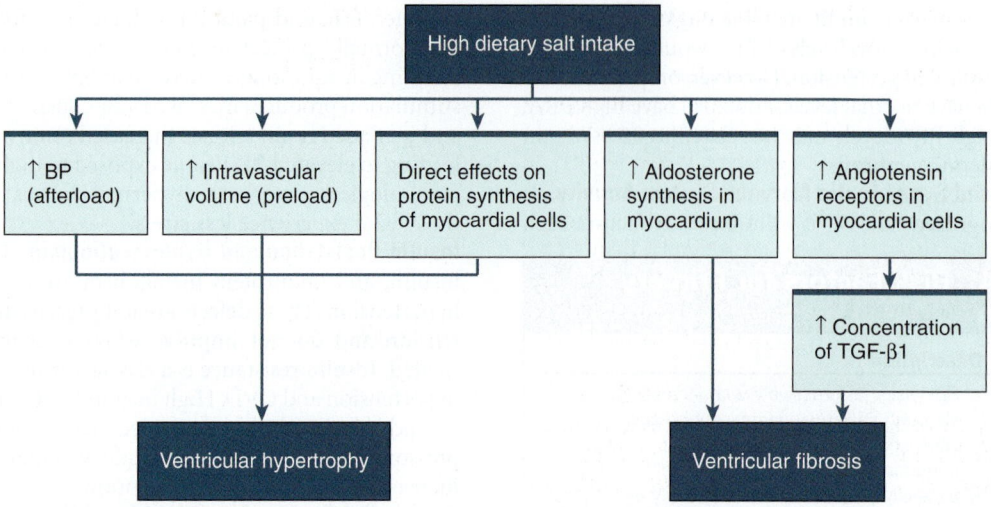

FIG. 32-2 Proposed link among salt intake, blood pressure, and changes in the heart. High dietary salt intake exerts hypertrophic effects on the left (and potentially also on right) ventricle. Ventricular fibrosis can also result from the high salt intake through mechanisms mediated by the renin-angiotensin-aldosterone system (RAAS). Transforming growth factor-β1 (TGF-β1) is a multifunctional cytokine with fibrogenic properties. Overproduction of TGF-β1 (in part mediated by angiotensin II) results in fibrosis and ventricular dysfunction. (Modified from Frisoli TM, Schmieder RE, Grodzicki T, et al: Salt and hypertension: Is salt dietary reduction worth the effort? *Am J Med* 125:433, 2012.)

TABLE 32-5 Manifestations of Target Organ Disease

Organ	Manifestations
Cardiac	• Clinical, electrocardiographic, or radiologic evidence of coronary artery disease (e.g., previous MI, coronary revascularization) • Left ventricular hypertrophy by ECG or echocardiography • Left ventricular dysfunction or heart failure
Cerebrovascular	• Transient ischemic attack • Stroke
Peripheral vascular	• One or more major pulses in the extremities (except for dorsalis pedis) faint or absent • Intermittent claudication • Abdominal or carotid bruits or thrills • Aneurysm
Renal	• Serum creatinine ≥1.5 mg/dL (130 μmol/L) • Proteinuria (≥1+) • Microalbuminuria
Retinopathy	• Generalized or focal narrowing of retinal arterioles • Arteriovenous nicking • Hemorrhages or exudates with or without papilledema

Source: National Heart, Lung, and Blood Institute: Seventh report of the Joint National Committee on Detection, Evaluation, and Treatment of High Blood Pressure (JNC-7), NIH Publication No. 04-5230, Bethesda, Md, 2004, The Institute. Retrieved from *www.nhlbi.nih.gov/guidelines/hypertension/jnc7full.pdf.*

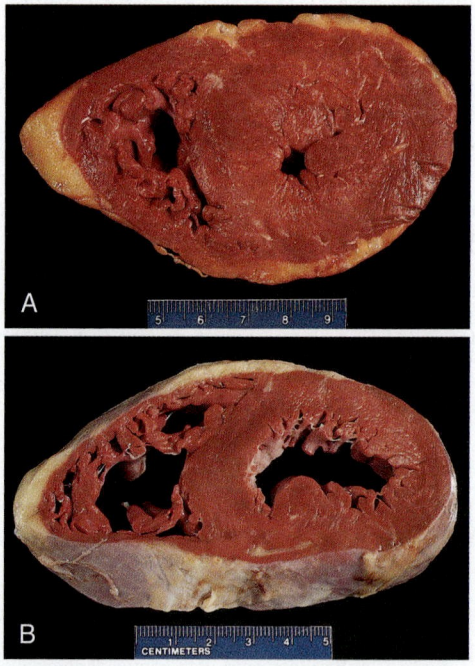

FIG. 32-3 **A,** Massively enlarged heart caused by hypertrophy of the muscle in the left ventricle. **B,** Compare with the thickness of the normal left ventricle. The patient suffered from severe hypertension. (From Kumar V, Cotran RS, Robbins SL: *Robbins basic pathology,* ed 8, Philadelphia, 2007, Saunders.)

demand. Progressive LVH, especially in the presence of CAD, is associated with the development of heart failure.

Heart Failure. Heart failure occurs when the heart's compensatory mechanisms are overwhelmed and the heart can no longer pump enough blood to meet the body's demands (see Chapter 34). Contractility is depressed, and stroke volume and CO are decreased. The patient may complain of shortness of breath on exertion, paroxysmal nocturnal dyspnea, and fatigue.

Cerebrovascular Disease. Atherosclerosis is the most common cause of cerebrovascular disease. Hypertension is a major risk factor for cerebral atherosclerosis and stroke. Even in mildly hypertensive people, the risk of stroke is four times higher than in normotensive people. Adequate control of BP diminishes the risk of stroke.

Atherosclerotic plaques are commonly found at the bifurcation of the common carotid artery and in the internal and external carotid arteries. Portions of the atherosclerotic plaque or the blood clot that forms with disruption of the plaque may break off and travel to cerebral vessels, producing a thromboembolism. The patient may experience transient ischemic attacks or a stroke. (These conditions are discussed in Chapter 57.)

Hypertensive encephalopathy may occur after a marked rise in BP if the cerebral blood flow is not decreased by autoregulation. *Autoregulation* is a physiologic process that maintains constant cerebral blood flow despite fluctuations in BP. Normally, as pressure in the cerebral blood vessels rises, the vessels constrict to maintain constant flow. When BP exceeds the body's ability to autoregulate, the cerebral vessels suddenly dilate, capillary permeability increases, and cerebral edema develops. This produces a rise in intracranial pressure. If left untreated, patients can die quickly from brain damage. (Chapter 56 discusses cerebral blood flow and autoregulation.)

Peripheral Vascular Disease. Hypertension speeds up the process of atherosclerosis in the peripheral blood vessels. This leads to the development of peripheral vascular disease, aortic aneurysm, and aortic dissection (see Chapter 37). *Intermittent claudication* (ischemic leg pain precipitated by activity and relieved with rest) is a classic symptom of peripheral vascular disease.

Nephrosclerosis. Hypertension is one of the leading causes of chronic kidney disease, especially among African Americans. Some degree of renal disease is usually present in the hypertensive patient, even those with minimally elevated BP. Renal disease results from ischemia caused by the narrowing of the renal blood vessels. This leads to atrophy of the tubules, destruction of the glomeruli, and eventual death of nephrons. Initially intact nephrons can compensate, but these changes may eventually lead to renal failure. Laboratory indications of renal disease are albuminuria, proteinuria, microscopic hematuria, and elevated serum creatinine and blood urea nitrogen (BUN) levels. An early manifestation of renal disease is usually nocturia (see Chapter 46).

Retinal Damage. The appearance of the retina provides important information about the severity and duration of hypertension. The blood vessels of the retina can be directly visualized with an ophthalmoscope. Damage to the retinal vessels provides an indication of related vessel damage in the heart, brain, and kidneys. Manifestations of severe retinal damage include blurring of vision, retinal hemorrhage, and loss of vision.

Diagnostic Studies

Measurement of BP is essential in assessing and monitoring hypertension. Chapter 31 (p. 662) and the Nursing Management section later in this chapter discuss BP measurement.

Some controversy exists over the diagnostic workup in the initial assessment of a person with hypertension. Most hypertension is classified as primary hypertension and testing for secondary causes is not routinely done. Basic laboratory studies are performed to (1) identify or rule out causes of secondary hypertension, (2) evaluate target organ disease, (3) determine overall cardiovascular risk, or (4) establish baseline levels before initiating therapy.

Table 32-6 lists basic diagnostic studies performed in a person with hypertension. Routine urinalysis, BUN, and serum creatinine levels are used to screen for renal involvement and provide baseline information about kidney function. Creatinine clearance reflects the glomerular filtration rate. Decreases in creatinine clearance indicate renal insufficiency. (Chapter 44 discusses serum creatinine and creatinine clearance.)

Measurement of serum electrolytes, especially potassium, is important to detect hyperaldosteronism, a cause of secondary hypertension. Blood glucose levels assist in the diagnosis of diabetes. A lipid profile provides information about additional risk factors related to atherosclerosis and CVD. Uric acid levels establish a baseline, since the levels often rise with diuretic therapy. An electrocardiogram (ECG) provides baseline information about heart status. It can identify the presence of LVH, cardiac ischemia, or previous MI. If LVH is suspected, echocardiography is often performed. If the patient's age, history, physical examination, or severity of hypertension points to a secondary cause, further diagnostic testing is indicated.

TABLE 32-6 Interprofessional Care

Hypertension

Diagnostic Assessment

- History and physical examination, including an ophthalmic examination
- Routine urinalysis
- Basic metabolic panel (serum glucose, sodium, potassium, chloride, carbon dioxide, BUN, and creatinine)
- Complete blood count
- Serum lipid profile (total lipids, triglycerides, HDL and LDL cholesterol, total-to-HDL cholesterol ratio)
- Serum uric acid, calcium, and magnesium
- 12-lead electrocardiogram (ECG)

Optional:

- 24-hr urinary creatinine clearance
- Echocardiography
- Liver function studies
- Serum thyroid-stimulating hormone (TSH)

Management

- Periodic monitoring of BP
  - Home BP monitoring
  - Ambulatory BP monitoring
  - Every 3-6 months by a HCP once goal BP is achieved and stabilized
- Nutritional therapy
  - Restrict salt and sodium
  - Restrict cholesterol and saturated fats
  - Maintain adequate intake of potassium, calcium, and magnesium
  - Weight management
- Regular, moderate physical activity
- Tobacco cessation (see Tables 10-4 through 10-6)
- Moderation of alcohol intake
- Stress management techniques (see Chapter 6)
- Antihypertensive drugs (Tables 32-7 and 32-8)
- Patient and caregiver teaching

HDL, High-density lipoprotein; *LDL,* low-density lipoprotein.

Ambulatory Blood Pressure Monitoring. Some patients have elevated BP readings in a clinical setting and normal readings when BP is measured elsewhere. This phenomenon is referred to as *"white coat"* hypertension. Ambulatory BP monitoring (ABPM) is the best method for diagnosing hypertension.[11] It is a noninvasive, fully automated system that measures BP at preset intervals over a 12-24-hour period. The equipment includes a BP cuff and a microprocessing unit that fits into a pouch worn on a shoulder strap or belt. Tell patients to hold their arm still by their side when the device is taking a reading. Also ask them to maintain a diary of activities that may affect BP. Other potential applications for ABPM include suspected antihypertensive drug resistance, hypotensive symptoms with antihypertensive drugs, episodic hypertension, or SNS dysfunction.

BP demonstrates diurnal variability expressed as sleep-wakefulness difference. For day-active people, BP is highest in the early morning, decreases during the day, and is lowest at night. BP at night (during sleep) usually drops by 10% or more from daytime (awake) BP.[10] The presence of diurnal variability is confirmed with ABPM.

Some patients with hypertension do not show a normal nocturnal dip in BP and are referred to as "nondippers." Patients at highest risk of CVD are "reverse dippers." These patients demonstrate an increase in nighttime systolic BP. Current research is focused on the use of drugs to optimize cardioprotective effects and convert non-dippers and reverse dippers to dippers.

EVIDENCE-BASED PRACTICE

Applying the Evidence

Lifestyle Changes and Uncontrolled Hypertension

You are caring for F.H., a 43-year-old female patient with a history of poorly controlled hypertension and chronic kidney disease (CKD). She is taking three antihypertensive drugs and tells you she no longer can tolerate the side effects of the drugs (e.g., fatigue, peripheral edema, dry mouth, frequent voiding). She wants to stop taking the drugs and control her hypertension by weight loss, exercise, and reducing her salt intake.

Making Clinical Decisions

Best Available Evidence. Antihypertensive drugs reduce the risk of cerebrovascular events, heart failure, and overall mortality in patients with concurrent risk for cardiovascular disease (e.g., diabetes, kidney disease). Most patients with hypertension will need to take two or more drugs on a long-term basis to achieve their goal BP in addition to lifestyle changes.

Clinician Expertise. You know lifestyle changes can help reduce and control BP in many patients. However, patients with poorly controlled hypertension and target organ disease require drugs to control BP and prevent further complications.

Patient Preferences and Values. F.H. wants to stop her antihypertensive drugs because of unacceptable side effects.

Implications for Nursing Practice

1. What important factors would you discuss with F.H. related to hypertension treatment and preventing further target organ disease?
2. Would you support F.H. in her desire to stop taking hypertensive drugs? Why or why not?
3. How can you help F.H. with her intentions to make lifestyle changes?

References for Evidence

Eckel RH, Jakicic JM, Ard JD, et al: 2013 AHA/ACC guideline on lifestyle management to reduce cardiovascular risk: a report of the American College of Cardiology/American Heart Association Task Force on Practice Guidelines, *J Am Coll Cardiol* 63:2960, 2014.

James PA, Oparil S, Carter BL, et al: 2014 Evidence-based guideline for the management of high blood pressure in adults: report from the panel members appointed to the Eighth Joint National Committee (JNC 8), *JAMA* 311:507, 2014.

Interprofessional Care

Table 32-6 summarizes the interprofessional care for a patient with hypertension. Goals include achieving and maintaining goal BP and reducing cardiovascular risk and target organ disease. Lifestyle modifications are indicated for all patients with prehypertension and hypertension.

Lifestyle Modifications. Lifestyle modifications are directed toward reducing the patient's BP and overall cardiovascular risk. Modifications include (1) weight reduction, (2) Dietary Approaches to Stop Hypertension (DASH) eating plan, (3) dietary sodium reduction, (4) moderation of alcohol intake, (5) regular physical activity, (6) avoidance of tobacco use (smoking and chewing), and (7) management of psychosocial risk factors.

Weight Reduction. Overweight persons have an increased incidence of hypertension and increased risk for CVD. Weight reduction has a significant effect on lowering BP in many people, and the effect is seen with even moderate weight loss. A weight loss of 22 lb (10 kg) may decrease SBP by approximately 5 to 20 mm Hg.[10] When a person decreases caloric intake, sodium and fat intake are usually also reduced. Although reducing the fat content of the diet has not been shown to produce sustained benefits in BP control, it may slow the progress of atherosclerosis and reduce overall CVD risk (see Chapter 33). Weight reduction through a combination of calorie restriction and moderate physical activity is recommended for overweight patients with hypertension (see Chapter 40).

DASH Eating Plan. The DASH eating plan emphasizes fruits, vegetables, fat-free or low-fat milk and milk products, whole grains, fish, poultry, beans, seeds, and nuts. Compared with the typical American diet, the plan contains less red meat, salt, sweets, added sugars, and sugar-containing beverages. The DASH eating plan significantly lowers BP, and these decreases compare with those achieved with BP-lowering medication. Additional benefits also include lowering of low-density lipoprotein (LDL) cholesterol.[13]

Dietary Sodium Reduction. Healthy adults should restrict sodium intake to less than or equal to 2300 mg/day. African Americans; people middle aged and older; and those with hypertension, diabetes, or chronic kidney disease should restrict sodium to less than or equal to 1500 mg/day.[13] This involves avoiding foods known to be high in sodium (e.g., canned soups, frozen dinners) and not adding salt in the preparation of foods or at meals (see Table 34-8).

Most adults exceed the recommended limits for sodium. Average sodium intake is approximately 4200 mg/day in men and 3300 mg/day in women.[13] The patient and caregiver, especially the person who prepares the meals, need to learn about sodium-restricted diets. Instruction should include reading labels of over-the-counter drugs, packaged foods, and health products (e.g., toothpaste containing baking soda) to identify hidden sources of sodium (see Fig. 34-6). Review the patient's normal diet to identify foods high in sodium.

Sodium restriction may be enough to control BP in some patients. If drug therapy is needed, a lower dosage may be effective if the patient also restricts sodium intake. Further, moderate sodium restriction lessens the risk of hypokalemia associated with diuretic therapy. However, the response differs between patients who are salt sensitive or salt resistant.

The significance of other dietary elements for the control of hypertension is not certain. Increased levels of dietary potassium, calcium, vitamin D, and omega-3 fatty acids are associated with lower BP in the general population and in those with hypertension. People with hypertension should maintain adequate potassium, calcium, and vitamin D intake from food sources. Calcium supplements are not recommended to lower BP. Omega-3 fatty acids found in certain fish oils can contribute to a reduction in BP and triglycerides (see Complementary & Alternative Therapies box).

Moderation of Alcohol Intake. Excessive alcohol intake is strongly associated with hypertension. Drinking three or more alcoholic drinks daily is also a risk factor for CVD and stroke. Men should limit their intake of alcohol to no more than two

COMPLEMENTARY & ALTERNATIVE THERAPIES

Fish Oil and Omega-3 Fatty Acids

Dietary sources of omega-3 fatty acids include fish oil and certain plant and nut oils. Fish oil contains both docosahexaenoic acid (DHA) and eicosapentaenoic acid (EPA). Some nuts and vegetable oils contain α-linolenic acid (ALA).

Scientific Evidence

- Reduce blood triglyceride levels
- May cause a small reduction in BP
- Although studies have not shown significant benefits of fish oil and omega-3 fatty acid supplementation to hypertension management, no studies have shown harm or adverse effects.
- May reduce the risk of heart attack, stroke, and death among people with cardiovascular disease. There is concern that omega-3 fatty acids in fish oil may be related to increases in prostate cancer.

Nursing Implications

- For healthy adults with no history of heart disease, the American Heart Association recommends eating fish at least two times per week. Fatty fish such as anchovies, bluefish, carp, catfish, halibut, lake trout, mackerel, pompano, salmon, striped sea bass, albacore tuna, and whitefish are recommended.
- Fish oil is generally safe in recommended dosages. Higher doses may result in increased risk of bleeding.
- There is no evidence to support the safety of fish oil consumption in persons with shellfish allergies.

Sources: *www.naturalstandard.com* and *http://nccam.nih.gov/health/providers/digest/omega3.*

drinks per day and women and lighter-weight men to no more than one drink per day. One drink is defined as 12 oz of regular beer, 5 oz of wine (12% alcohol), or 1.5 oz of 80-proof distilled spirits. Excessive alcohol intake that results in cirrhosis is the most frequent cause of secondary hypertension.

Physical Activity. A physically active lifestyle is essential to promote and maintain good health. The AHA and American College of Sports Medicine recommend that adults perform moderate-intensity aerobic physical activity for at least 30 minutes most days (i.e., more than 5 days per week) with a goal of at least 150 minutes per week. Exercise goals can be accomplished by performing shorter periods of exercise that last at least 10 minutes. Additionally, combinations of moderate and vigorous activity are acceptable (e.g., walking briskly for 30 minutes on 2 days of the week and jogging for 20 minutes on 2 other days).[16]

Differences in physical activity guidelines exist for adults age 18 to 65 years, adults over 65 years, and adults age 50 to 64 years with functional limitations. The differences relate to the definition of moderate and vigorous aerobic activity. For adults ages 18 to 65, walking briskly at a pace that noticeably increases the pulse defines moderate-intensity aerobic activity. Jogging at a pace that substantially increases the pulse and causes rapid breathing is an example of vigorous activity for this age group. For all other adults, individual fitness levels guide aerobic intensity.[16]

All adults should perform muscle-strengthening activities using the major muscles of the body at least twice a week. This helps to maintain or increase muscle strength and endurance. Additionally, flexibility and balance exercises are recommended at least twice a week for older adults, especially for those at risk for falls.[17] Moderate-intensity activities can lower BP, promote relaxation, and decrease or control body weight. Regular activity of this type can reduce SBP by approximately 4 to 9 mm Hg.[10]

Generally, physical activity is more likely to become a habit if it is safe and enjoyable, fits easily into one's daily schedule, and is inexpensive. Many shopping malls open early in the morning and provide a warm, safe, flat area for walking. Some health clubs offer special "off-peak" rates to encourage physical activity among older adults. Some health insurance carriers offer health club discounts as a benefit to encourage member fitness. Cardiac rehabilitation programs offer supervised exercise and education about cardiovascular risk factor reduction.

Help people with hypertension to increase their physical activity by explaining the need for physical activity, describing the different types of physical activities, and assisting in starting an exercise plan. Advise sedentary people to increase activity levels gradually. Individuals with CVD or other serious health problems need a thorough examination and possibly a stress test before beginning an exercise program.

Avoidance of Tobacco Products. Nicotine contained in tobacco causes vasoconstriction and increases BP, especially in people with hypertension. Smoking tobacco is also a major risk factor for CVD. The cardiovascular benefits of stopping tobacco use are seen within 1 year in all age-groups. Strongly encourage everyone, especially patients with hypertension, to avoid tobacco use. Advise those who continue to use tobacco products to monitor their BP during use. (Chapter 10 discusses tobacco use and smoking cessation.)

Management of Psychosocial Risk Factors. Psychosocial risk factors can contribute to the risk of developing CVD, and to a poorer prognosis and clinical course in patients with CVD. These risk factors include low socioeconomic status, social isolation and lack of support, stress at work and in family life, and negative emotions such as depression and hostility. Frequently, these risk factors are clustered together. For example, rates of depression tend to be higher in individuals with job stress.

Psychosocial risk factors have direct effects on the cardiovascular system by activating the SNS and stress hormones. This can cause a wide variety of pathophysiologic responses, including hypertension and tachycardia, inflammation, endothelial dysfunction, increased platelet aggregation, insulin resistance, and central obesity.[18]

Psychosocial risk factors can contribute to CVD indirectly as well, simply by their impact on lifestyle behaviors and choices. Screening for psychosocial risk factors is important. Make appropriate referrals (e.g., counseling), when indicated. Suggest behavioral interventions such as relaxation training, stress management courses, support groups, and exercise training for individuals who are not in acute psychologic distress.[18]

Drug Therapy. The following are recommendations for antihypertensive drug therapy from the JNC 8.[6]

- In patients 60 years or over, start drug treatment for BP greater than or equal to 150 mm Hg systolic or greater than or equal to 90 mm Hg diastolic and treat to goal BP less than those thresholds.
- In patients less than 60 years, treatment initiation and goals should be 140/90 mm Hg, the same threshold used in patients 18 years or older with either chronic kidney disease (CKD) or diabetes.

Findings from the SPRINT indicate that treatment of systolic BP to less than 120 mm Hg (rather than 140 mm Hg) reduced the rates of major cardiovascular events by almost one-third and the risk of death by almost one-fourth.[7] These data may result in changes to the JNC 8 guidelines.

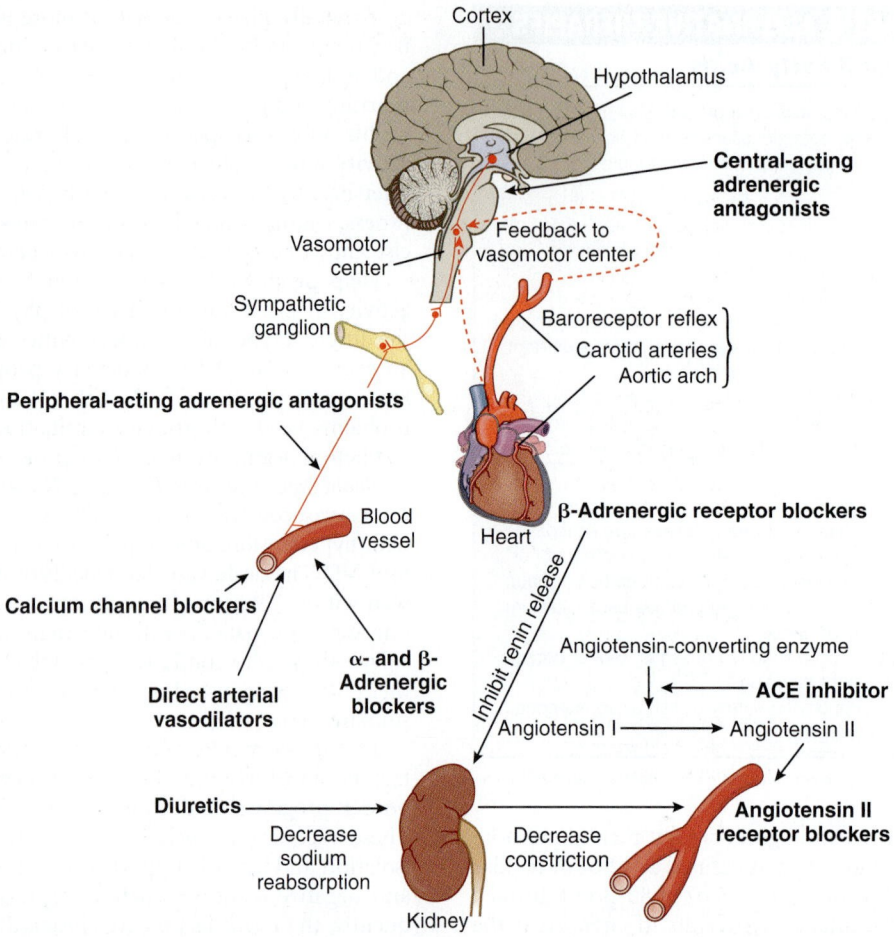

FIG. 32-4 Site and method of action of various antihypertensive drugs *(bold type). ACE,* Angiotensin-converting enzyme. (From US Department of Health and Human Services: *Seventh report of the Joint National Committee on Prevention, Detection, Evaluation, and Treatment of High Blood Pressure [JNC 7],* Washington, DC, 2003, National Institutes of Health.)

The drugs currently available for treating hypertension have two main actions: (1) decrease the volume of circulating blood and (2) reduce SVR[19,20] (Table 32-7). Fig. 32-4 presents the various sites and methods of action of antihypertensive drugs. The drugs used in the treatment of hypertension include the following:

- *Diuretics* promote sodium and water excretion, reduce plasma volume, and reduce the vascular response to catecholamines.
- *Adrenergic-inhibiting agents* act by diminishing the SNS effects that increase BP. Adrenergic inhibitors include drugs that act centrally on the vasomotor center and peripherally to inhibit norepinephrine release or to block the adrenergic receptors on blood vessels.
- *Direct vasodilators* decrease the BP by relaxing vascular smooth muscle and reducing SVR.
- *Calcium channel blockers* increase sodium excretion and cause arteriolar vasodilation by preventing the movement of extracellular calcium into cells.
- *Angiotensin-converting enzyme (ACE) inhibitors* prevent the conversion of angiotensin I to angiotensin II and reduce angiotensin II (A-II)–mediated vasoconstriction and sodium and water retention.
- *A-II receptor blockers (ARBs)* prevent angiotensin II from binding to its receptors in the walls of the blood vessels.

Most patients who are hypertensive require two or more antihypertensive drugs to achieve their goal BP. The addition of a second drug from a different class is started when use of a single drug in adequate doses fails to achieve the goal BP. These can be separate prescriptions or combination therapy (Table 32-8). If a drug is not tolerated or is contraindicated, then a drug from another class is used.

Once antihypertensive therapy is started, patients should return for follow-up and adjustment of drugs at monthly intervals until the goal BP is reached. More frequent visits are necessary for patients with stage 2 hypertension or with co-morbidities. After BP is at goal and stable, follow-up visits can usually be at 3- to 6-month intervals. Co-morbidities (e.g., heart failure), associated diseases (e.g., diabetes), and the need for ongoing monitoring (e.g., laboratory testing) influence the frequency of visits.

Patient and Caregiver Teaching Related to Drug Therapy. Side effects of antihypertensive drugs are common and may be so severe or undesirable that the patient does not adhere to the therapy[19,20] (Table 32-7). Patient and caregiver teaching related to drug therapy helps them to identify and minimize side effects. This may help the patient adhere to therapy. Side effects may be an initial response to a drug and may decrease over time. Telling the patient about side effects that may decrease with time may help the person to continue taking the drug. The

TABLE 32-7 Drug Therapy

Hypertension

Drug	Mechanism of Action	Nursing Considerations
Diuretics		
Thiazide and Related Diuretics		
chlorothiazide (Diuril) chlorthalidone hydrochlorothiazide indapamide metolazone (Zaroxolyn)	Inhibit NaCl reabsorption in the distal convoluted tubule. Increase excretion of Na^+ and Cl^-. Initial decrease in ECF. Sustained decrease in SVR. Lower BP moderately in 2-4 wk.	Monitor for orthostatic hypotension, hypokalemia, and alkalosis. Thiazides may potentiate cardiotoxicity of digoxin by producing hypokalemia. Dietary sodium restriction reduces the risk of hypokalemia. NSAIDs can decrease diuretic and antihypertensive effect of thiazide diuretics and potentially cause renal impairment. Advise patient to supplement with potassium-rich foods.
Loop Diuretics		
bumetanide (Bumex) furosemide (Lasix) torsemide (Demadex)	Inhibit NaCl reabsorption in the ascending limb of the loop of Henle. Increase excretion of Na^+ and Cl^-. More potent diuretic effect than thiazides, but shorter duration of action. Less effective for hypertension.	Monitor for orthostatic hypotension and electrolyte abnormalities. Loop diuretics remain effective despite renal insufficiency. Diuretic effect of drug increases at higher doses.
Potassium-Sparing Diuretics		
amiloride (Midamor) triamterene (Dyrenium)	Reduce K^+ and Na^+ exchange in the distal and collecting tubules. Reduce excretion of K^+, H^+, Ca^{++}, and Mg^{++}.	Monitor for orthostatic hypotension and hyperkalemia. Contraindicated in patients with renal failure. Use with caution in patients on ACE inhibitors or angiotensin II blockers. Avoid potassium supplements.
Aldosterone Receptor Blockers		
spironolactone (Aldactone) eplerenone (Inspra)	Inhibit the Na^+-retaining and K^+-excreting effects of aldosterone in the distal and collecting tubules.	Monitor for orthostatic hypotension and hyperkalemia. Do not combine with potassium-sparing diuretics or potassium supplements. Use with caution in patients on ACE inhibitors or angiotensin II blockers. These drugs are also classified as potassium-sparing diuretics.
Adrenergic Inhibitors		
Central-Acting α-Adrenergic Agonist		
clonidine (Catapres) clonidine patch (Catapres-TTS)	Reduce sympathetic outflow from CNS. Reduce peripheral sympathetic tone, produces vasodilation, decreases SVR and BP.	Sudden discontinuation may cause withdrawal syndrome, including rebound hypertension, tachycardia, headache, tremors, apprehension, sweating. Chewing gum or hard candy may relieve dry mouth. Alcohol and sedatives increase sedation. Transdermal patch may be related to fewer side effects and better adherence.
guanabenz guanfacine (Tenex)	Same as clonidine.	Same as clonidine, but not available in transdermal formulation.
methyldopa	Same as clonidine.	Instruct patient about daytime sedation and avoidance of hazardous activities. Taking a single daily dose at bedtime minimizes sedative effect.
Peripheral-Acting α-Adrenergic Agonist		
reserpine	Depletes central and peripheral stores of norepinephrine. Results in peripheral vasodilation (decreases SVR and BP).	Must be given twice daily. Contraindicated in patients with history of depression. Monitor mood and mental status regularly. Advise patient to avoid barbiturates, alcohol, opioids.
α_1-Adrenergic Blockers		
doxazosin (Cardura) prazosin (Minipress) terazosin	Block α_1-adrenergic effects, producing peripheral vasodilation (decreases SVR and BP). Beneficial effects on lipid profile.	Reduced resistance to the outflow of urine in benign prostatic hyperplasia. Taking drug at bedtime reduces risks associated with orthostatic hypotension.
phentolamine (Regitine)	Blocks α_1-adrenergic receptors, resulting in peripheral vasodilation (decreases SVR and BP).	Used in short-term management of pheochromocytoma. Also used locally to prevent necrosis of skin and subcutaneous tissue after extravasation of adrenergic drug. No oral formulation.
β-Adrenergic Blockers		
Cardioselective Blockers		
acebutolol (Sectral) atenolol (Tenormin) betaxolol bisoprolol (Zebeta) esmolol (Brevibloc) metoprolol (Lopressor) nebivolol (Bystolic)	Cardioselective agents block β_1-adrenergic receptors (Table 32-1). Reduce BP by blocking β-adrenergic effects. Decrease CO and reduce sympathetic vasoconstrictor tone. Decrease renin secretion by kidneys.	Monitor pulse and BP regularly. Use with caution in patients with diabetes because drug may depress the tachycardia associated with hypoglycemia and may adversely affect glucose metabolism. Drug of choice for patients with a history of an MI or heart failure. Less effective BP reduction in African American patients. Esmolol is for IV use only. Cardioselective agents lose cardioselectivity at higher doses.

Continued

TABLE 32-7 Drug Therapy

Hypertension—cont'd

Drug	Mechanism of Action	Nursing Considerations
Adrenergic Inhibitors—cont'd		
β-Adrenergic Blockers—cont'd		
Non-cardioselective Blockers		
nadolol (Corgard) pindolol propranolol (Inderal)	Nonselective agents block β_1- and β_2-adrenergic receptors (Table 32-1). Reduce BP by blocking β_1- and β_2-adrenergic effects.	Same as cardioselective, except nonselective agents may cause bronchospasm, especially in patients with a history of asthma.
Mixed α- and β-Blockers		
carvedilol (Coreg) labetalol	α_1-, β_1-, and β_2-adrenergic blocking properties producing peripheral vasodilation and decreased heart rate (Table 32-1). Reduce CO, SVR, and BP.	Same as β-blockers. IV form available for hypertensive crisis in hospitalized patients. Patients must be kept supine during IV administration. Assess patient tolerance of upright position (severe orthostatic hypotension) before allowing upright activities (e.g., commode).
Direct Vasodilators		
fenoldopam (Corlopam)	Activates dopamine receptors, resulting in systemic and renal vasodilation.	IV use only for hypertensive crisis in hospitalized patients. Use cautiously in patients with glaucoma. Patient should remain flat for 1 hr after administration.
hydralazine	Reduces SVR and BP by direct arterial vasodilation.	IV use for hypertensive crisis in hospitalized patients. Twice-daily oral dosage. Not used as monotherapy because of side effects. Contraindicated in patients with coronary artery disease.
minoxidil	Reduces SVR and BP by direct arterial vasodilation.	Reserved for treatment of severe hypertension associated with renal failure and resistant to other therapy. Once- or twice-daily dosage.
nitroglycerin	Relaxes arterial and venous smooth muscle, reducing preload and SVR. At low dose, venous dilation predominates; at higher dose, arterial dilation is present.	IV use for hypertensive crisis in hospitalized patients with myocardial ischemia. Given by continuous IV infusion with pump or control device.
sodium nitroprusside	Direct arterial vasodilation reduces SVR and BP.	IV use for hypertensive crisis in hospitalized patients. Given by continuous IV infusion with pump or control device. Arterial monitoring of BP recommended. Wrap IV solutions with an opaque material to protect from light. Stable for 24 hr. Metabolized to cyanide, then thiocyanate. Monitor thiocyanate levels with prolonged use (>3 days) or doses ≥4 mcg/kg/min.
Angiotensin Inhibitors		
Angiotensin-Converting Enzyme Inhibitors		
benazepril (Lotensin) captopril enalapril (Vasotec) fosinopril lisinopril (Zestril) moexipril (Univasc) perindopril (Aceon) quinapril (Accupril) ramipril (Altace) trandolapril (Mavik)	Inhibit ACE, reduce conversion of angiotensin I to angiotensin II (A-II). Inhibit A-II–mediated vasoconstriction.	Aspirin and NSAIDs may reduce drug effectiveness. Addition of diuretic enhances drug effect. Should not be used with potassium-sparing diuretics. Can cause increase in serum creatinine. Inhibit breakdown of bradykinin, which may cause a dry, hacking cough that can occur at any point during treatment, even years later. Captopril may be given orally for hypertensive crisis.
Angiotensin II Receptor Blockers		
azilsartan (Edarbi) candesartan (Atacand) eprosartan (Teveten) irbesartan (Avapro) losartan (Cozaar) olmesartan (Benicar) telmisartan (Micardis) valsartan (Diovan)	Prevent action of A-II and produce vasodilation and increased Na^+ and water excretion.	Full effect on BP may not be seen for 3-6 wk. Do not affect bradykinin levels, therefore acceptable alternative to ACE inhibitors in people who develop dry cough. In patients with kidney disease, ACE inhibitors and ARBs should not be used together due to adverse renal effects.
Renin Inhibitors		
aliskiren (Tekturna)	Directly inhibits renin, thus reducing conversion of angiotensinogen to angiotensin I.	May cause angioedema of the face, extremities, lips, tongue, glottis, and/or larynx. Not to be used in pregnancy.

TABLE 32-7 Drug Therapy

Hypertension—cont'd

Drug	Mechanism of Action	Nursing Considerations
Calcium Channel Blockers		
Non-Dihydropyridines		
diltiazem extended release (Cardizem LA) verapamil intermediate release (Calan) verapamil long-acting (Covera-HS) verapamil timed-release (Verelan PM)	Inhibit movement of Ca^{++} across cell membrane, resulting in vasodilation Cardioselective resulting in decrease in heart rate and slowing of AV conduction.	Use with caution in patients with heart failure. Serum concentrations and toxicity of certain calcium channel blockers may be increased by grapefruit juice; avoid concurrent use. Used for supraventricular tachydysrhythmias. Avoid in patients with second- or third-degree AV block or left ventricular systolic dysfunction.
Dihydropyridines		
amlodipine (Norvasc) clevidipine (Cleviprex) felodipine isradipine nicardipine sustained release nifedipine long acting (Procardia XL) nisoldipine (Sular)	Cause vascular smooth muscle relaxation resulting in decreased SVR and arterial BP.	More potent peripheral vasodilators. Clevidipine is for IV use only. Use of sublingual short-acting nifedipine in hypertensive emergencies is unsafe and not effective. Serious adverse events (e.g., stroke, acute MI) have been reported. IV nicardipine available for hypertensive crisis in hospitalized patients. Change peripheral IV infusion sites every 12 hr.

ACE, Angiotensin-converting enzyme; *AV,* atrioventricular; *CO,* cardiac output; *DBP,* diastolic blood pressure; *ECF,* extracellular fluid; *HDL,* high-density lipoprotein; *LDL,* low-density lipoprotein; *SBP,* systolic blood pressure; *SVR,* systemic vascular resistance.

number or severity of side effects may relate to the dose. It may be necessary to change the drug or decrease the dose. Advise the patient to report all side effects to the HCP.

A common side effect of several of the antihypertensive drugs is orthostatic hypotension. This condition results from an alteration of the autonomic nervous system's mechanisms for regulating BP, which are needed for position changes. Consequently, the patient may feel dizzy and faint when assuming an upright position after sitting or lying down. Table 32-12 (later in this chapter) presents specific measures to control or decrease orthostatic hypotension.

Sexual problems may occur with many of the antihypertensive drugs. This can be a major reason that patients do not adhere to the treatment plan. Problems can range from reduced libido to erectile dysfunction. Rather than discussing a sexual problem with an HCP, the patient may decide just to stop taking the drug. Approach the patient on this sensitive subject and encourage discussion of any sexual problem that may be experienced. The sexual problems may be easier for the patient to discuss once you explain that the drug may be the source of the problem.

Changing to another antihypertensive drug can decrease or remove these side effects. Encourage the patient to discuss sexual issues with the HCP. If the patient is reluctant to do so, offer to alert the HCP to the side effects that the patient is experiencing. There are many drug options for treating hypertension and a plan that is acceptable to the patient should be the goal.[20]

Some unpleasant side effects of drugs result from their therapeutic effect, but these can be decreased. For example, diuretics cause dry mouth and frequent voiding. Sugarless gum or hard candy may help ease the dry mouth. Taking diuretics earlier in the day may limit frequent voiding during the night and preserve sleep.

Resistant Hypertension. Carefully explore all reasons why a patient may not be at goal BP (Table 32-9). *Resistant hypertension* is the failure to reach goal BP in patients who are taking full doses of an appropriate three-drug therapy regimen that includes a diuretic. Overactive renal nerves can be one cause of resistant hypertension. Percutaneous catheter-based radiofrequency ablation of the renal nerves (known as *renal denervation*) lowers BP and sympathetic nerve activity in patients with resistant hypertension.[21]

❖ NURSING MANAGEMENT: PRIMARY HYPERTENSION

◆ Nursing Assessment

Table 32-10 presents subjective and objective data to obtain from a patient with hypertension.

◆ Nursing Diagnoses

Nursing diagnoses and collaborative problems for the patient with hypertension include, but are not limited to, the following.

- Ineffective health management *related to* lack of knowledge of pathology, complications, and management of hypertension
- Anxiety *related to* complexity of management regimen
- Sexual dysfunction *related to* side effects of antihypertensive medication
- Risk for decreased cardiac tissue perfusion
- Risk for ineffective cerebral tissue perfusion
- Risk for ineffective renal perfusion
- Potential complication: stroke, MI

◆ Planning

The overall goals for the patient with hypertension are that the patient will (1) achieve and maintain the goal BP; (2) follow the therapeutic plan, including appointments with the HCP; (3) experience minimal side effects of therapy; and (4) manage and cope with this condition.

◆ Nursing Implementation

◆ **Health Promotion.** Primary prevention of hypertension is a cost-effective approach. Current recommendations for primary

TABLE 32-8 Drug Therapy

*Combination Therapy for Hypertension**

Combinations	Trade Names
Angiotensin-Converting Enzyme Inhibitors and Diuretics	
benazepril/hydrochlorothiazide	Lotensin HCT
enalapril/hydrochlorothiazide	Vaseretic
lisinopril/hydrochlorothiazide	Zestoretic
Angiotensin II Receptor Blockers and Diuretics	
candesartan/hydrochlorothiazide	Atacand HCT
losartan/hydrochlorothiazide	Hyzaar
olmesartan medoxomil/ hydrochlorothiazide	Benicar HCT
valsartan/hydrochlorothiazide	Diovan HCT
β-Blockers and Diuretics	
metoprolol/hydrochlorothiazide	Lopressor HCT
nadolol/bendroflumethiazide	Corzide
Angiotensin-Converting Enzyme Inhibitors and Calcium Channel Blockers	
amlodipine/benazepril	Lotrel
Angiotensin II Receptor Blockers and Calcium Channel Blockers	
telmisartan/amlodipine	Twynsta
valsartan/amlodipine	Exforge
olmesartan/amlodipine	Azor
Diuretics and Diuretics	
spironolactone/hydrochlorothiazide	Aldactazide
triamterene/hydrochlorothiazide	Dyazide, Maxzide
Angiotensin II Receptor Blocker, Calcium Channel Blocker, and Diuretic	
olmesartan medoxomil/amlodipine/ hydrochlorothiazide	Tribenzor
amlodipine/hydrochlorothiazide/valsartan	Exforge HCT

*List is not all inclusive and only contains examples of the various categories.

EVIDENCE-BASED PRACTICE

Translating Research Into Practice

Can Home-Based Blood Pressure Monitoring Improve Hypertension Screening?

Clinical Question

In adults screened for hypertension (P), what is the effect of home-based blood pressure (BP) monitoring (I) on the validation of office-based BP results (O)?

Synthesis of Best Available Evidence

- Systematic review of randomized controlled trials (RCTs), diagnostic accuracy and cohort BP studies.
- More than 60 studies examining high BP screening among adults (n >150,000). Review summarized BP measurement methods including office-based and home-based (ambulatory) monitoring, diagnostic and predictive accuracy of BP methods on cardiovascular outcomes, and rescreening intervals.
- Home-based BP monitoring with multiple measurements over time in a nonmedical setting may reduce measurement error and the misdiagnosis and overtreatment of isolated clinic hypertension.
- Home-based BP monitoring predicted long-term cardiovascular outcomes independent of office monitoring.
- Rescreening intervals of up to 6 years found persons at higher risk for hypertension were older age, African Americans, and those with high-normal BP and/or above-normal body mass index.

Conclusions

- Unless immediate treatment is needed, hypertension detected by office-based measurements should be confirmed by home-based BP monitoring.
- Persons with identified risk factors should be screened more often for hypertension.

Implications for Nursing Practice

1. Why is it important for HCPs to be aware of the importance of home-based BP monitoring as an adjunct to office-based monitoring?
2. What information will you share with patients who are worried about a newly elevated BP detected in the office?
3. How will you determine if patients are accurately monitoring their BP at home?

Reference for Evidence

Piper MA, Evans CV, Burda BU, et al: Diagnostic and predictive accuracy of blood pressure screening methods with consideration of rescreening intervals: a systematic review for the U.S. Preventive Services Task Force, *Ann Intern Med* 162:192, 2015.

P, Patient population of interest; *I*, intervention or area of interest; *C*, comparison of interest or comparison group; *O*, outcomes of interest; *T*, timing (see p. 15).

prevention include lifestyle modifications that prevent or delay the rise in BP in at-risk people. Following the DASH diet and reducing sodium can lower BP. This diet is recommended for primary prevention in the general population. Dietary changes by the food industry (e.g., reducing the amount of salt in processed foods) may also be effective.

The National Heart, Lung, and Blood Institute provides web-based educational materials for HCPs, patients, and the public to raise awareness about the dangers of high BP. (See Your Guide to Lowering High Blood Pressure at *www.nhlbi.nih.gov/health/resources/heart/hbp-guide-to-lower.*)

◆ ***Individual Patient Evaluation.*** Hypertension is usually identified through routine screening for insurance, preemployment, and military physical examinations. You are in an ideal position to assess for the presence of hypertension, identify the risk factors for hypertension and CAD, and teach patients about these conditions. In addition to BP measurement, a health assessment should include such factors as age, gender, and race; diet history (including salt and alcohol intake); weight patterns; tobacco use; and family history of CVD, stroke, renal disease, and diabetes. Note all drugs taken, both prescribed and over-the-counter. Last, ask the patient about a previous history of high BP and the results of treatment (if any) (Table 32-10).

◆ ***Blood Pressure Measurement.*** BP can be measured using the oscillatory or auscultatory method.[22] First, take the BP in both arms to note any differences. Atherosclerosis in the subclavian artery can cause a falsely low reading on the side where the narrowing occurs. Use the arm with the highest BP and take at least two readings, a minimum of 1 minute apart (Table 32-11). Waiting for at least 1 minute between readings allows the blood to drain from the arm and prevents inaccurate readings. Record the average pressure as the value for that visit.

Proper size and correct placement of the BP cuff are critical for accurate measurement. Place the cuff snugly around the patient's bare upper arm with the midline of the bladder of the cuff (usually marked on the cuff by the manufacturer) placed in line with the brachial artery. Place the patient's arm at the level of the heart during BP measurement. For BP measurements taken in the sitting position, raise and support the arm at the level of the heart. For measurements taken in a supine position, raise and support (e.g., with a small pillow) the arm at heart level. If the arm is resting on the bed, it will be below heart level.

TABLE 32-9 Causes of Resistant Hypertension

- **Improper BP measurement**
- **Volume overload**
  - Excess salt intake
  - Volume retention from kidney disease
  - Inadequate diuretic therapy
- **Drug-induced or other causes**
  - Nonadherence (e.g., due to drug side effects, finances)
  - Illegal drugs (e.g., cocaine, amphetamines)
  - Inadequate drug dosages
  - Inappropriate combinations of drug therapy
  - Nonsteroidal antiinflammatory drugs
  - Sympathomimetics (e.g., decongestants, diet pills)
  - Oral contraceptives
  - Corticosteroids
  - Cyclosporine and tacrolimus (Prograf)
  - Erythropoietin
  - Licorice
  - Some chewing tobacco
  - Selected over-the-counter dietary or herbal supplements and drugs (e.g., ma huang, bitter orange)
- **Associated conditions**
  - Increasing obesity
  - Excess alcohol intake
- **Identifiable causes of secondary hypertension**

Source: National Heart, Lung, and Blood Institute: Seventh Report of the Joint National Committee on Detection, Evaluation, and Treatment of High Blood Pressure (JNC-7), NIH Publication No. 04-5230, Bethesda, Md, 2004, The Institute. Retrieved from *www.nhlbi.nih.gov/guidelines/hypertension/jnc7full.pdf.*

If neither upper arm can be used to measure the BP (e.g., presence of IV lines, fistula), or if a maximum size BP cuff does not fit the upper arm, use the forearm. In this case, position the proper size cuff midway between the elbow and the wrist. Auscultate Korotkoff sounds over the radial artery or use a Doppler device to note SBP. Use of an oscillometric device on the forearm is acceptable. Forearm and upper arm BPs are not interchangeable.[22]

SAFETY ALERT Blood Pressure Measurement

- If using the forearm for BP measurement, always document the site.
- BP cuffs that are too small or too large will result in readings that are falsely high or low, respectively.
- If bilateral BP measurements are not equal, document this finding and use the arm with the highest BP for all future measurements.

Assess for orthostatic (or postural) changes in BP and HR in older adults, in people taking antihypertensive drugs, and in patients who report symptoms consistent with reduced BP on standing (e.g., light-headedness, dizziness, syncope). Measure serial BP and HR with the patient in the supine, sitting, and standing positions. First, measure BP and HR with the patient in the supine position after at least 2 to 3 minutes of rest. Reposition the patient in the sitting position with legs dangling and measure BP and HR again within 1 to 2 minutes. Last, reposition the patient to the standing position and measure the BP and HR within 1 to 2 minutes. Usually the SBP decreases slightly (less than 10 mm Hg) on standing, whereas the DBP and pulse increase slightly. **Orthostatic hypotension** occurs when a patient moves from a supine to standing position, and there is a decrease of 20 mm Hg or more in SBP, a decrease of 10 mm Hg or more in DBP, and/or an increase in the HR of 20 beats/minute. Common causes of orthostatic hypotension include dehydration and inadequate vasoconstrictor mechanisms related to disease or drugs.

TABLE 32-10 Nursing Assessment
Hypertension

Subjective Data

Important Health Information

Past health history: Known duration and past workup of high BP; cardiovascular, cerebrovascular, renal, or thyroid disease; diabetes mellitus; pituitary disorders; obesity; dyslipidemia; menopause or hormone replacement status

Medications: Use of any prescription or over-the-counter, illicit, or herbal drugs or products; previous use of antihypertensive drug therapy

Functional Health Patterns

Health perception–health management: Family history of hypertension or cardiovascular disease; tobacco use, alcohol use; sedentary lifestyle; health literacy; readiness for change

Nutritional-metabolic: Usual salt and fat intake; weight gain or loss

Elimination: Nocturia

Activity-exercise: Fatigue; dyspnea on exertion, palpitations, exertional chest pain; intermittent claudication, muscle cramps; usual pattern and type of exercise

Cognitive-perceptual: Dizziness; blurred vision; paresthesias

Sexual-reproductive: Erectile dysfunction, decreased libido

Coping–stress tolerance: Stressful life events

Objective Data

Cardiovascular

SBP consistently >140 mm Hg or DBP >90 mm Hg for patients <60 yr old or >150 mm Hg or DBP >90 mm Hg for patients >60 years old. Orthostatic changes in BP and HR; bilateral BPs significantly different; abnormal heart sounds; laterally displaced apical pulse; diminished or absent peripheral pulses; carotid, renal, or femoral bruits; peripheral edema

Gastrointestinal

Obesity (BMI ≥30 kg/m^2); abnormal waist-hip ratio

Neurologic

Mental status changes

Possible Diagnostic Findings

Abnormal serum electrolytes (especially potassium); ↑ BUN, creatinine, glucose, cholesterol, and triglyceride levels; proteinuria, albuminuria, microscopic hematuria; evidence of ischemic heart disease and left ventricular hypertrophy on ECG; evidence of structural heart disease and left ventricular hypertrophy on echocardiogram; evidence of arteriovenous nicking, retinal hemorrhages, and papilledema on funduscopic examination

BMI, Body mass index; *DBP,* diastolic blood pressure; *HR,* heart rate; *SBP,* systolic blood pressure.

DRUG ALERT Doxazosin (Cardura)

- Use caution when giving the first dose. It is recommended to give the first dose at bedtime to reduce the first dose BP drop.
- Syncope occasionally occurs 30 to 90 min after the first dose, a too-rapid increase in dose, or addition of another antihypertensive agent to therapy.
- Drug interactions (severe low BP) can occur with patients taking phosphodiesterase inhibitors such as sildenafil (Viagra).

In acute care settings, BP measurement is usually done to evaluate vital signs, volume status, and effects of drugs, rather than to diagnose hypertension. Trends in BP are more important

TABLE 32-11 Blood Pressure Measurement

The patient should not have smoked, exercised, or ingested caffeine within 30 min before measurement.

1. Seat patient with legs uncrossed, feet on the floor, and back supported. Bare patient's arm and support it at heart level.
2. Begin measurement after patient has rested quietly for 5 min. Ask patient to relax as much as possible and not to talk during the measurement.
3. Measure and record BP in both arms initially.
4. Select the appropriate cuff size, following instructions for fit and placement according to manufacturer's recommendations.
5. Take the BP with a recently calibrated aneroid or mercury sphygmomanometer, or electronic oscillometric device. Accuracy of oscillometric devices may be limited if patients are hypertensive, hypotensive, or have heart dysrhythmias (e.g., atrial fibrillation).
6. For auscultatory measurement, estimate SBP by palpating the radial pulse and inflating the cuff until the pulse disappears. Inflate the cuff 20-30 mm Hg above this level.
7. Deflate the cuff at a rate of 2-3 mm Hg/sec.
8. Record the SBP and DBP. Note the SBP when the first of two or more Korotkoff sounds is heard and the DBP when sound disappears.
9. Average two or more readings (taken at intervals of at least 1 min). Obtain additional readings if the first two readings differ by more than 5 mm Hg.
10. Provide the patient (verbally and in writing) with the BP reading, BP goal, and recommendations for follow-up.
11. Clean BP cuffs between patients according to agency policy.

Sources: National Heart, Lung, and Blood Institute: Seventh report of the Joint National Committee on Detection, Evaluation, and Treatment of High Blood Pressure (JNC-7), NIH Publication No. 04-5230, Bethesda, Md, 2004, The Institute. Retrieved from *www.nhlbi.nih.gov/guidelines/hypertension/jnc7full.pdf* and Martin B: AACN practice alert: non-invasive blood pressure monitoring, 2010. Retrieved from *www.aacn.org/wd/practice/docs/practicealerts/non-invasive-bp-monitoring.pdf?menu=aboutus*

DBP, Diastolic blood pressure; *SBP,* systolic blood pressure.

than a single value. Inform the HCP of any patient with a persistent elevated BP. These patients should be evaluated for hypertension before discharge, if appropriate, or after discharge.[10]

◆ ***Screening Programs.*** Screening programs in the community are widely used to identify persons who have a high BP. At the time of the BP measurement, give each person a written, numeric value of the reading. Explain why further evaluation is needed.

Focus efforts on the following: (1) controlling BP in persons already identified as having hypertension; (2) identifying and controlling BP in at-risk groups such as African Americans, obese people, and blood relatives of people with hypertension; (3) screening those with limited access to health care; and (4) connecting persons with an HCP and/or health insurance (e.g., Marketplace at *www.healthcare.gov*) if needed.

◆ ***Cardiovascular Risk Factor Modification.*** Teaching regarding CVD risk factors is appropriate for all persons and during targeted screening programs. Modifiable CVD risk factors include hypertension, obesity, diabetes, tobacco use, and physical inactivity. Discuss lifestyle modifications based on identified risk factors. (Table 33-2 discusses health-promoting behaviors for risk factor reduction.)

◆ **Ambulatory Care.** Your primary roles in long-term management of hypertension are to assist the patient to reach the goal BP and adhere to the treatment plan. Your actions include evaluating therapeutic effectiveness, detecting and reporting any adverse treatment effects, assessing and enhancing adherence, and patient and caregiver teaching (Table 32-12).

◆ ***Home BP Monitoring.*** Most patients with known or suspected hypertension should monitor their BP at home. Home BP monitoring reduces the white coat effect of measurement by an HCP. The readings are often lower than those taken in the office setting and are a better predictor of CVD risk.

Patient teaching is critical to ensure accuracy. Tell patients to buy an oscillometric BP monitor that uses a cuff for the upper arm or wrist. The patient should bring the BP monitor to the office to verify proper cuff size, accuracy of the device, and the patient's technique.

TEAMWORK & COLLABORATION

Caring for the Patient With Hypertension

You will work with many members of the health care team to care for a patient with hypertension. You will need to collaborate with the team members to deliver, delegate, and coordinate care based on the patient's status.

Role of Nursing Personnel

Registered Nurse (RN)

- Develop and conduct hypertension screening programs.
- Assess patients for hypertension risk factors and develop risk modification plans.
- Teach patients about lifestyle management and drug use.
- Evaluate the effectiveness of lifestyle management and drugs in decreasing BP to acceptable levels.
- Teach about home BP monitoring, including the correct use of automatic BP monitors. Check that the device selected by the patient meets the Association for the Advancement of Medical Instrumentation standards (*www.dableducational.org/sphygmomanometers/devices_1_clinical.html#ClinTable*).
- Make appropriate referrals to other HCPs, such as dietitians or stress management programs.
- Monitor for complications of hypertension such as coronary artery disease, heart failure, cerebrovascular disease, peripheral vascular disease, and renal disease.
- Assess the patient with hypertensive crisis for evidence of target organ disease (e.g., encephalopathy, renal insufficiency, cardiac decompensation).
- Manage the patient with hypertensive urgency or emergency, including administration of drugs and evaluation for resolution of the crisis.

Licensed Practical/Vocational Nurse (LPN/LVN)

- Give antihypertensive drugs to stable patients.
- Monitor for adverse effects of antihypertensive drugs.
- Reinforce teaching about drugs and lifestyle management.

Unlicensed Assistive Personnel (UAP)

- Obtain accurate BP readings in outpatient and inpatient settings.
- Report high or low BP readings immediately to RN.
- Check for postural changes in BP as directed.

Role of Other Team Members

Dietitian

- Obtain a diet history from the patient.
- Teach the components of the DASH diet.
- Provide instructions for dietary changes as needed.

Physical Therapist

- Assess patient's current level of fitness.
- Develop an exercise plan with the patient.

TABLE 32-12 Patient & Caregiver Teaching

Hypertension

When teaching the patient and/or caregiver about hypertension, include the following information.

General Instructions

1. Provide the patient's BP reading and explain what it means (e.g., high, low, goal, borderline). Encourage patient to monitor BP at home and instruct the patient to call the HCP if BP exceeds high or low limits set by HCP.
2. Hypertension is usually asymptomatic and symptoms (e.g., nosebleeds) do not reliably indicate BP levels.
3. Hypertension means high BP and does not relate to a "hyper" personality.
4. Long-term therapy and follow-up care are necessary to treat hypertension. Therapy involves lifestyle changes (e.g., weight management, sodium reduction, smoking cessation, regular physical activity) and, in most cases, drugs.
5. Therapy will not cure, but should control, hypertension.
6. Controlled hypertension usually results in an excellent prognosis and a normal lifestyle.
7. Explain the potential dangers of uncontrolled hypertension (e.g., stroke, heart attack).

Instructions Related to Medications

1. Be specific about the names, actions, dosages, and side effects of prescribed drugs.
2. Help the patient plan regular and convenient times for taking drugs and measuring BP.
3. Do not stop drugs abruptly because withdrawal may cause a severe hypertensive reaction.
4. Do not double up on dose when a dose is missed.
5. If BP increases or decreases, do not adjust the drug dose without consulting the HCP.
6. Do not take any drugs belonging to someone else.
7. Supplement diet with foods high in potassium (e.g., citrus fruits, green leafy vegetables) if taking potassium-wasting diuretics.
8. Avoid hot baths, excessive amounts of alcohol, and strenuous exercise within 3 hours of taking drugs that promote vasodilation.
9. Many drugs cause orthostatic hypotension. Reduce the effects of orthostatic hypotension by rising slowly from bed, sitting on the side of the bed for a few minutes, standing slowly, and beginning to move if no symptoms develop (e.g., dizziness, light-headedness). Do not stand still for prolonged periods, do leg exercises to increase venous return, or sleep with the head of the bed raised. Do lie or sit down when dizziness occurs.
10. Some drugs cause sexual problems (e.g., erectile dysfunction, decreased libido). Consult with the HCP about changing drugs or dosages if sexual problems develop.
11. Some side effects of drug(s) may decrease with time (e.g., fatigue, diarrhea).
12. Be careful about taking potentially high-risk over-the-counter drugs, such as high-sodium antacids, NSAIDs, appetite suppressants, and cold and sinus medications. Read warning labels and consult with a pharmacist.

Teach the patient to obtain a BP according to the steps in Table 32-11. Tell the patient to measure BP in the nondominant arm, or arm with the higher BP if there is a known difference between arms. Tell the patient to measure BP first thing in the morning (if possible, before taking medications) and at night before going to bed. Have the patient record all BP measurements and bring the record to office visits.

For clinical decision making (e.g., changes in dosage, start of new drug), tell patients to take BP readings as described for 1 week. Stable, normotensive patients should measure morning and evening BP for at least 1 week every 3 months. Devices that have memory or printouts of the readings are recommended to ensure accurate reporting.[10]

Home BP readings may help achieve patient adherence by reinforcing the need to remain on therapy. However, some patients become overly concerned with the BP readings. Discourage too frequent checking of their BP. Generally, home BP monitoring should reassure the patient that the treatment is effective. It is also important for patients to know what their goal or target BP is.

◆ ***Patient Adherence.*** A major problem in the long-term management of the patient with hypertension is poor adherence with the treatment plan. The reasons for nonadherence are complex and can include inadequate patient teaching, low health literacy, unpleasant side effects of drugs, return of BP to normal range while on drugs, high cost of drugs, and lack of insurance.

It is important to determine the reasons why a patient is not adhering to treatment. Also assess the patient's diet, activity level, and lifestyle as additional indicators of adherence. Develop a plan with the patient and caregiver to improve adherence. The plan should be compatible with the patient's habits, cultural beliefs, and lifestyle. Active patient participation increases the chance of adherence to the plan. Measures include involving the patient in selecting drugs that are affordable and involving caregivers to help increase patient adherence.

Substituting combination drugs for multiple drugs once the BP is stable may also facilitate adherence. Combination drugs reduce the number of pills that the patient has to take each day and may reduce costs. (Combination drugs are presented in Table 32-8.)

It is important to help the patient and caregiver understand that hypertension is a chronic illness that cannot be cured. Emphasize that it can be controlled with drug therapy, diet

CHECK YOUR PRACTICE

You are making a home visit for a 78-year-old woman who is recovering from a hip replacement after she fractured her femur. She currently takes a combination of lisinopril/hydrochlorothiazide. The patient's daughter (her caregiver) tells you that her BP that morning was 150/88 and then she took it two more times and it was the same. They are both worried and anxious that something is wrong because they heard that BP over 120/80 is very bad.

- What should you do? What teaching would you provide?

INFORMATICS IN PRACTICE

Monitoring Blood Pressure

- Smartphones and computer applications can be used to help patients manage their care, including BP self-monitoring, drug history, and appointment tracking. Patients can enter a variety of variables including: SBP and DBP, HR, time of day, arm or wrist used, and position (e.g., lying, sitting).
- Remote BP monitoring using telehealth technology can also be used for patients who have limited access to health care services.
- Reports can be generated to evaluate how well the patient's BP has been controlled.

DBP, Diastolic BP; *HR,* heart rate; *SBP,* systolic BP.

changes, physical activity, periodic follow-up, and other relevant lifestyle modifications.

Evaluation

The overall expected outcomes are that the patient with hypertension will:

- Achieve and maintain goal BP as defined for the individual
- Understand, accept, and implement the treatment plan
- Report minimal side effects of drug therapy

Gerontologic Considerations: Hypertension

The prevalence of hypertension increases with age. The lifetime risk of developing hypertension is approximately 90% for middle-aged (ages 55 to 65) and older (over 65) normotensive men and women.[19] ISH is the most common form of hypertension in people over 50 years of age. Additionally, older adults are more likely to have white coat hypertension.[10]

The pathophysiology of hypertension in the older adult involves the following age-related physical changes: (1) loss of elasticity in large arteries from atherosclerosis, (2) increased collagen content and stiffness of the myocardium, (3) increased peripheral vascular resistance, (4) decreased adrenergic receptor sensitivity, (5) blunting of baroreceptor reflexes, (6) decreased renal function, and (7) decreased renin response to sodium and water depletion.

In the older adult who is taking antihypertensive drugs, absorption of some drugs may be altered as a result of decreased blood flow to the gut. Metabolism and excretion of drugs may also be prolonged.

Careful technique is important in assessing BP in older adults. Some older people have a wide gap between the first Korotkoff sound and subsequent beats. This is called the *auscultatory gap.* Failure to inflate the cuff high enough may result in underestimating SBP (Table 32-11).

Current recommendations for target BP goals in people older than 60 years of age are controversial and range from less than 120/80 mm Hg[7] to less than 150/90 mm Hg.[6] The preferred three first-line antihypertensive drugs are a thiazide diuretic, a calcium channel blocker, and an ACE inhibitor or ARB. A diuretic should always be the first or second drug ordered for most patients.[14]

Orthostatic hypotension often occurs in older adults because of varying degrees of impaired baroreceptor reflexes, especially in those with ISH. Orthostatic hypotension in this age group is often associated with volume depletion or chronic disease states, such as decreased renal and hepatic function or electrolyte imbalance.

Additionally, older adults experience postprandial drops in BP. The greatest decrease occurs approximately 1 hour after eating. BP returns to preprandial levels 3 to 4 hours after eating. To reduce the likelihood of orthostatic hypotension, antihypertensive drugs should be started at low doses and increased slowly. Measure BP and HR in the supine, sitting, and standing positions at every visit.

After CVD, arthritis is the second most prevalent disease in older adults. The most frequently taken drugs by older adults are nonsteroidal antiinflammatory drugs (NSAIDs), both prescription and over-the-counter. Nonselective NSAIDs (e.g., ibuprofen [Advil]) and selective NSAIDs (e.g., celecoxib [Celebrex]) cause loss of BP control and heart failure. Additionally, there is the potential for adverse renal effects and/or hyperkalemia when NSAIDs are used with ACE inhibitors, ARBs, or aldosterone antagonists.[20]

HYPERTENSIVE CRISIS

Hypertensive crisis is a term used to indicate either a hypertensive urgency or emergency. Hypertensive crisis occurs at systolic BP greater than 180 mm Hg and/or diastolic BP greater than 110 mm Hg. BPs can often be greater than 220/140 mm Hg. The difference between a hypertensive urgency and emergency is the absence or presence of target organ damage.

Hypertensive urgency develops over hours to days and does not have clinical evidence of target organ disease. It may not require hospitalization to correct.

Hypertensive emergencies have target organ disease and most often require hospitalization for prompt, controlled reduction of BP. If prompt treatment is not obtained, a hypertensive emergency can produce severe problems. These include encephalopathy, intracranial or subarachnoid hemorrhage, heart failure, MI, renal failure, dissecting aortic aneurysm, and retinopathy.[23]

The rate of increase of BP is more important than the absolute value in determining the need for emergency treatment. Patients with chronic hypertension can tolerate much higher BPs than normotensive people. Prompt recognition and management of a hypertensive crisis are essential to decrease the threat to organ function and life.

Hypertensive crisis occurs more often in patients with a history of hypertension who have not adhered to their drug regimens or who have been undermedicated. Rapidly increasing BP can cause shearing of the endothelial surface due to turbulent blood flow within the vessels. This can lead to further vascular damage and the release of additional vasoconstricting substances. A vicious cycle of BP elevation follows, leading to life-threatening damage to target organs.

Hypertensive crisis related to cocaine or crack use is a frequent problem. Other drugs, such as amphetamines, phencyclidine (PCP), and lysergic acid diethylamide (LSD), can also cause hypertensive crisis that may be complicated by drug-induced seizures, stroke, MI, or encephalopathy. Table 32-13 lists causes of hypertensive crisis.

Clinical Manifestations

A hypertensive emergency is often manifested as *hypertensive encephalopathy*, a syndrome in which a sudden rise in BP is associated with severe headache, nausea, vomiting, seizures, confusion, and coma. The manifestations of encephalopathy are the result of increased cerebral capillary permeability. This leads to cerebral edema and a disruption in cerebral function. On retinal examination, exudates, hemorrhages, and/or papilledema are found (Fig. 32-5).

Renal insufficiency ranging from minor injury to complete renal failure can occur. Rapid cardiac decompensation ranging

TABLE 32-13 Causes of Hypertensive Crisis

- Exacerbation of chronic hypertension
- Renovascular hypertension
- Preeclampsia, eclampsia
- Pheochromocytoma
- Drugs (cocaine, amphetamines)
- Monoamine oxidase inhibitors taken with tyramine-containing foods
- Rebound hypertension (from abrupt withdrawal of some antihypertensive drugs such as clonidine [Catapres] or β-blockers)
- Head injury
- Acute aortic dissection

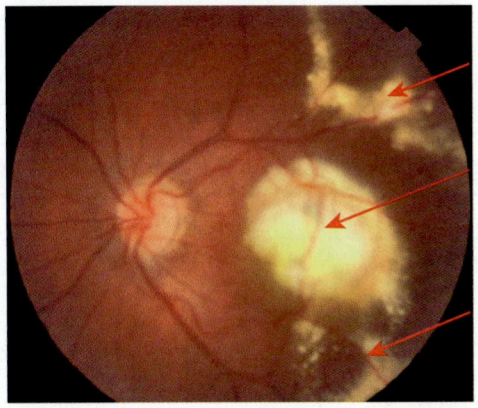

FIG. 32-5 Massive retinal exudates (indicated by *arrows*) from hypertensive retinopathy. To see what a normal retina looks like on ophthalmoscopic examination, see Fig. 20-5 on p. 359. (From Kliegman RM, Behrman RE, Jenson HB, Stanton B: *Nelson textbook of pediatrics,* ed 18, Philadelphia, 2011, Saunders.)

from unstable angina to MI and pulmonary edema is also possible. Patients can have chest pain and dyspnea. Aortic dissection can develop and will cause sudden, excruciating chest and back pain and possibly reduced or absent pulses in the extremities.

Patient assessment is extremely important. Monitor for signs of neurologic deficits, retinal damage, heart failure, pulmonary edema, and renal failure. The neurologic changes are often similar to those related to a stroke. However, a hypertensive crisis does not show focal or lateralizing signs often seen with a stroke. (In a stroke, focal impairments affect a specific region of the body [e.g., weakness in the left arm, right leg]. Lateralizing signs are restricted to one side of the body [e.g., weakness of an arm or leg].)

❖ NURSING AND INTERPROFESSIONAL MANAGEMENT: HYPERTENSIVE CRISIS

Hypertensive emergencies require hospitalization, IV administration of antihypertensive drugs, and intensive care monitoring.

BP level alone is a poor marker of the seriousness of the patient's condition. It is not the major factor in deciding the treatment for a hypertensive crisis. The link between elevated BP and signs of new or progressive target organ disease determines the seriousness of the situation.

When treating hypertensive emergencies, the mean arterial pressure (MAP) is often used instead of BP readings to guide and evaluate drug therapy. MAP is calculated as follows:

$$MAP = (SBP + 2\,DBP) \div 3$$

The initial goal is to decrease MAP by no more than 20% to 25%, or to decrease MAP to 110 to 115 mm Hg. If the patient is clinically stable, drugs can be titrated to gradually lower BP over the next 24 hours. Lowering the BP too quickly or too much may decrease cerebral, coronary, or renal perfusion. This could cause a stroke, MI, or renal failure.

Special circumstances include patients with aortic dissection. These patients should have their SBP lowered to less than 100 to 120 mm Hg as soon as possible (if tolerated). Another exception is patients with acute ischemic stroke, in whom BP is lowered to allow the use of thrombolytic agents. Last, an elevated BP in the immediate poststroke period may be a compensatory response to improve cerebral perfusion to ischemic brain tissue. There is no clear evidence supporting the use of antihypertensive drugs in these patients[10] (see Chapter 57).

CHECK YOUR PRACTICE

A 68-yr-old male patient is admitted to the emergency department with a BP 210/118 and complaining of a severe headache and vomiting. You know that his BP is dangerously high and must be lowered.

- Calculate his MAP.
- What treatments would you expect to be ordered for this patient?

IV drugs used for hypertensive emergencies include vasodilators (e.g., sodium nitroprusside, fenoldopam [Corlopam], nicardipine [Cardene]), adrenergic inhibitors (e.g., phentolamine [Regitine], labetalol, esmolol [Brevibloc]), and the calcium channel blocker clevidipine (Cleviprex)[24] (Table 32-7). Sodium nitroprusside is the most effective IV drug to treat hypertensive emergencies. Oral agents may be given along with IV drugs to help make an earlier transition to long-term therapy.

DRUG ALERT Labetalol

- Instruct patient not to discontinue drug abruptly.
- Abrupt cessation may precipitate angina or heart failure.

Antihypertensive drugs given IV have a rapid (within seconds to minutes) onset of action. Assess the patient's BP and HR every 2 to 3 minutes during the initial administration of these drugs. Use an arterial line (see Chapter 65) or an automated, noninvasive BP machine to monitor the BP. Titrate the drug according to MAP or BP as ordered. Monitor the ECG for dysrhythmias and signs of ischemia or MI. Use extreme caution in treating the patient with CAD or cerebrovascular disease. Measure urine output hourly to assess renal perfusion. Patients receiving IV antihypertensive drugs may be restricted to bed. Getting up (e.g., to use the commode) may cause severe cerebral ischemia and fainting.

Ongoing assessment is essential to evaluate the effectiveness of these drugs and the patient's response to therapy. Frequent neurologic checks, including level of consciousness, pupillary size and reaction, and movement of extremities, help detect any changes in the patient's condition. Monitor cardiac, pulmonary, and renal systems for decompensation caused by the severe elevation in BP (e.g., angina, pulmonary edema, renal failure).

Hypertensive urgencies usually do not require IV drugs but can be managed with oral agents. The patient with hypertensive urgency may not need hospitalization but will require follow-up. The oral drugs most frequently used for hypertensive urgencies are captopril, labetalol, clonidine (Catapres), and amlodipine (Norvasc)[24] (Table 32-7). The disadvantage of oral drugs is the inability to regulate the dosage moment to moment, as can be done with IV drugs. If a patient with hypertensive urgency is not hospitalized, outpatient follow-up care should be arranged within 24 hours.

Once the hypertensive crisis is resolved, it is important to determine the cause. The patient will need appropriate management and teaching to avoid future crises.

DRUG ALERT Clonidine (Catapres)

- Instruct patient to change positions slowly to limit orthostatic hypotension.
- Hazardous activities should be avoided since the drug may cause drowsiness.
- Drug should not be stopped abruptly as this may cause rebound hypertension.

Not every patient with an elevated BP and no target organ disease will require emergent drug therapy or hospitalization. Allowing the patient to sit for 20 or 30 minutes in a quiet environment may significantly reduce BP. Oral drugs may be started or adjusted. Additional nursing interventions include encouraging the patient to verbalize any concerns or fears, answering questions regarding hypertension, and eliminating any adverse stimuli (e.g., excess noise) in the patient's environment.

CASE STUDY

Primary Hypertension

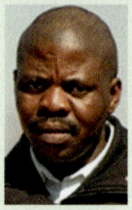

(©iStockphoto/Thinkstock)

Patient Profile

R.L. is a 45-year-old African American man with no previous history of hypertension. At a screening clinic 2 months ago, his BP was found to be 150/95 mm Hg. His HCP has followed him for the past month. During this time he has been taking hydrochlorothiazide 12.5 mg/day. He is here today for a follow-up visit.

Subjective Data

- Father died of stroke at age 60
- Mother is alive but has hypertension and a history of MI
- States that he feels fine and is not a "hyper" person
- Smokes one pack of cigarettes daily for the past 28 yr
- Drinks 1-2 six-packs of beer on most Friday and Saturday nights
- Has heard that BP drugs "make you impotent"

Objective Data

Physical Examination

- Mild retinopathy (retinal arteriolar narrowing on ophthalmoscopic examination)
- BP: 166/108 mm Hg (average of two readings, 2 min apart)
- Sustained apical impulse palpable in the fourth intercostal space just lateral to the midclavicular line

Diagnostic Studies

- ECG: mild left ventricular hypertrophy
- Urinalysis: protein 30 mg/dL (0.3 g/L)
- Serum creatinine level: 1.6 mg/dL (141 mmol/L)

Interprofessional Care

- Low-sodium, DASH diet
- Hydrochlorothiazide 25 mg/day PO (dose increase)
- Nicardipine (Cardene) sustained release 30 mg PO bid (second drug added)

Discussion Questions

1. What risk factors for hypertension does R.L. have?
2. What evidence of target organ disease is present?
3. ***Patient-Centered Care:*** What misconceptions about hypertension should be corrected?
4. ***Priority Decision:*** Based on the assessment data, what are the priority nursing diagnoses and interventions? What are the collaborative problems?
5. ***Evidence-Based Practice:*** R.L. wants to know the most effective nonpharmacologic strategies to lower his BP. What would you tell him?
6. ***Patient-Centered Care:*** What lifestyle preferences should be addressed in R.L's plan of care?
7. ***Teamwork and Collaboration:*** What referrals may be indicated for this patient?
8. ***Safety:*** What safety precautions should be considered when changing antihypertensive drugs for R.L.?
9. ***Quality Improvement:*** What outcomes would indicate that interprofessional care was successful?

Answers available at *http://evolve.elsevier.com/Lewis/medsurg.*

BRIDGE TO NCLEX EXAMINATION

The number of the question corresponds to the same-numbered outcome at the beginning of the chapter.

1. Which BP-regulating mechanism(s) can result in the development of hypertension if defective *(select all that apply)*?
   a. Release of norepinephrine
   b. Secretion of prostaglandins
   c. Stimulation of the sympathetic nervous system
   d. Stimulation of the parasympathetic nervous system
   e. Activation of the renin-angiotensin-aldosterone system
2. While obtaining subjective assessment data from a patient with hypertension, the nurse recognizes that a modifiable risk factor for the development of hypertension is
   a. a low-calcium diet.
   b. excessive alcohol intake.
   c. a family history of hypertension.
   d. consumption of a high-protein diet.
3. In teaching a patient with hypertension about controlling the illness, the nurse recognizes that
   a. all patients with elevated BP require medication.
   b. obese persons must achieve a normal weight to lower BP.
   c. it is not necessary to limit salt in the diet if taking a diuretic.
   d. lifestyle modifications are indicated for all persons with elevated BP.
4. A *priority* consideration in the management of the older adult with hypertension is to
   a. prevent primary hypertension from converting to secondary hypertension.
   b. recognize that the older adult is less likely to adhere to the drug therapy regimen than a younger adult.
   c. ensure that the patient receives larger initial doses of antihypertensive drugs because of impaired absorption.
   d. use careful technique in assessing the BP of the patient because of the possible presence of an auscultatory gap.
5. A patient with newly discovered high BP has an average reading of 158/98 mm Hg after 3 months of exercise and diet modifications. Which management strategy will be a *priority* for this patient?
   a. Medication will be required because the BP is still not at goal.
   b. BP monitoring should continue for another 3 months to confirm a diagnosis of hypertension.
   c. Lifestyle changes are less important, since they were not effective, and medications will be started.
   d. More vigorous changes in the patient's lifestyle are needed for a longer time before starting medications.

6. A patient is admitted to the hospital in hypertensive emergency (BP 244/142 mm Hg). Sodium nitroprusside is started to treat the elevated BP. Which management strategy(ies) would be *most* appropriate for this patient *(select all that apply)*?
   a. Measuring hourly urine output
   b. Decreasing the MAP by 50% within the first hour
   c. Continuous BP monitoring with an arterial line
   d. Maintaining bed rest and providing tranquilizers to lower the BP
   e. Assessing the patient for signs and symptoms of heart failure and changes in mental status

1. a, c, e, 2. b, 3. d, 4. d, 5. a, 6. a, c, e

For rationales to these answers and even more NCLEX review questions, visit *http://evolve.elsevier.com/Lewis/medsurg.*

EVOLVE WEBSITE

http://evolve.elsevier.com/Lewis/medsurg

Review Questions (Online Only)
Key Points
Answer Keys for Questions
- Rationales for Bridge to NCLEX Examination Questions
- Answer Guidelines for Case Study on p. 700

Student Case Study
- Patient With Hypertension and Stroke

Conceptual Care Map Creator
Audio Glossary
Content Updates

REFERENCES

1. Centers for Disease Control and Prevention: High blood pressure facts. Retrieved from *www.cdc.gov/bloodpressure/facts.htm.*
2. Go AS, Mozaffarian D, Roger VL, et al: Heart disease and stroke statistics—2014 update: a report from the American Heart Association, *Circulation* 129:e28, 2013.
3. US Department of Health and Human Services: Healthy People 2020. Retrieved from *www.healthypeople.gov.*
4. Nwankwo R, Yoon SS, Burt V, et al: *Hypertension among adults in the United States*, 2011–2012, NCHS Data Brief, 133, Hyattsville, Md: National Center for Health Statistics.
5. Johnson N, Hayes L, Hoo E, et al: CDC National Health Report: leading causes of morbidity and mortality and associated behavioral risk and protective factors—United States, 2005-2013, *MMWR Surveillance Summary*, 2014.

*6. James PA, Oparil S, Carter BL, et al: 2014 Evidence-based guideline for the management of high blood pressure in adults: report from the panel members appointed to the Eighth Joint National Committee (JNC 8), *JAMA* 311:507, 2014.

*7. National Heart, Lung, and Blood Institute. Landmark NIH study shows intensive blood pressure management may save lives. Retrieved from *www.nhlbi.nih.gov/news/press-releases/2015/landmark-nih-study-shows-intensive-blood-pressure-management-may-save-lives.*

*8. Mosca L, Benjamin EJ, Berra K, et al: Effectiveness-based guidelines for the prevention of cardiovascular disease in women—2011 update, *Circulation* 123:1243, 2011.

9. Flammer AJ, Anderson T, Celermajer DS, et al: The assessment of endothelial function: from research into clinical practice, *Circulation* 126:6, 2012.

*10. National Heart, Lung, and Blood Institute: *Seventh report of the Joint National Committee on Detection, Evaluation, and Treatment of High Blood Pressure (JNC-7), NIH Publication No. 04-5230*, Bethesda, Md, 2004, The Institute. Retrieved from *www.nhlbi.nih.gov/health-pro/guidelines/current/hypertension-jnc-7/complete-report.*

*11. Piper MA, Evans CV, Burda BU, et al: Diagnostic and predictive accuracy of blood pressure screening methods with consideration of rescreening intervals: a systematic review for the U.S. Preventive Services Task Force, *Ann Intern Med* 162:192, 2015.

12. Liu F, He J, Gu D, et al: Associations of endothelial system genes with blood pressure changes and hypertension incidence: the GenSalt study, *Am J Hypertens* 27:1370, 2014.

13. National Heart, Lung, and Blood Institute: *Your guide to lowering your blood pressure with DASH, NIH Pub No 06-5834*, Bethesda, Md, 2006. Retrieved from *http://catalog.nhlbi.nih.gov/catalog/product/In-Brief-Your-Guide-to-Lowering-Your-Blood-Pressure-With-DASH/06-5834.*

*14. Weber MA, Schiffrin EL, White WB, et al: Clinical practice guidelines for the management of hypertension in the community: a statement by the American Society of Hypertension and the International Society of Hypertension, *J Hypertens* 32:1, 2014.

15. American Heart Association: What are the symptoms of high blood pressure? Retrieved from *www.heart.org/HEARTORG/Conditions/HighBloodPressure/SymptomsDiagnosisMonitoringofHighBloodPressure/What-are-the-Symptoms-of-High-Blood-Pressure_UCM_301871_Article.jsp.*

*16. Haskell WL, Lee I-M, Pate RR, et al: Physical activity and public health: updated recommendations for adults from the American College of Sports Medicine and the American Heart Association, *Circulation* 116:1081, 2007.

*17. Nelson ME, Rejeski WJ, Blair SN, et al: Physical activity and public health in older adults: recommendation from the American College of Sports Medicine and the American Heart Association, *Circulation* 116:1094, 2007. (Classic)

18. Rozanski A, Blumenthal JA, Davidson KW, et al: The epidemiology, pathophysiology, and management of psychosocial risk factors in cardiac practice, *J Am Coll Cardiol* 45:637, 2005. (Classic)

*19. Aronow WS, Fleg JL, Pepine CJ, et al: ACCF/AHA 2011 expert consensus document on hypertension in the elderly, *J Am Coll Cardiol* 57:2037, 2011.

20. Lehne RA: *Pharmacology for nursing care*, ed 8, St Louis, 2013, Saunders.

*21. Krum H, Schlaich M, Sobotka P, et al: Percutaneous renal denervation in patients with treatment-resistant hypertension: final 3-year report of the Simplicity HTN-1 study, *Lancet* 383:9917, 2014.

*22. Martin B: AACN practice alert: non-invasive blood pressure monitoring, 2010. Retrieved from *www.aacn.org/wd/practice/docs/practicealerts/non-invasive-bp-monitoring.pdf?menu=aboutus.*

23. Rafey MA: Hypertension, Cleveland Clinic Center for Continuing Education. Retrieved from *www.clevelandclinicmeded.com/medicalpubs/diseasemanagement/nephrology/arterial-hypertension.*

24. Smithburger PL, Kane-Gill SL, Nestor BL, et al: Recent advances in the treatment of hypertensive emergencies, *Crit Care Nurse* 30:24, 2010.

*Evidence-based information for clinical practice.

33

Coronary Artery Disease and Acute Coronary Syndrome

Rose Shaffer and Linda Bucher

The best and most beautiful things in the world cannot be seen or even touched—they must be felt with the heart.

Helen Keller

http://evolve.elsevier.com/Lewis/medsurg/

LEARNING OUTCOMES

1. Relate the etiology and pathophysiology of coronary artery disease (CAD) and acute coronary syndrome (ACS) to the clinical manifestations of each disorder.
2. Describe the nursing role in the promotion of therapeutic lifestyle changes in patients at risk for CAD.
3. Differentiate the precipitating factors, clinical manifestations, interprofessional care, and nursing management of the patient with CAD and chronic stable angina.
4. Explain the clinical manifestations, diagnostic studies, complications, and interprofessional care of the patient with ACS.
5. Evaluate commonly used drug therapy in treating patients with CAD and ACS.
6. Prioritize key components to include in the rehabilitation of patients recovering from ACS and coronary revascularization procedures.
7. Differentiate the precipitating factors, clinical presentation, and interprofessional care of patients who are at risk for or have experienced sudden cardiac death.

KEY TERMS

acute coronary syndrome (ACS), p. 718
angina, p. 712
atherosclerosis, p. 702
chronic stable angina, p. 712
collateral circulation, p. 703
coronary artery disease (CAD), p. 702
coronary revascularization, p. 717
metabolic equivalent (MET), p. 731
myocardial infarction (MI), p. 719
percutaneous coronary intervention (PCI), p. 717
Prinzmetal's angina, p. 713
silent ischemia, p. 713
stent, p. 717
sudden cardiac death (SCD), p. 733
unstable angina (UA), p. 719

Cardiovascular disease (CVD) is the major cause of death in the United States. Coronary artery disease (CAD) is the most common type of CVD and accounts for approximately 1.1 million of these deaths.[1] Patients with CAD can be asymptomatic or develop chronic stable angina (or chest pain). CAD may also evolve to more serious conditions of unstable angina (UA) and myocardial infarction (MI), which are called acute coronary syndrome (ACS). This chapter discusses the care of patients with CAD and ACS.

CORONARY ARTERY DISEASE

Coronary artery disease (CAD) is a type of blood vessel disorder that is included in the general category of atherosclerosis. The term **atherosclerosis** comes from two Greek words: *athere,* meaning "fatty mush," and *skleros,* meaning "hard." This combination means that atherosclerosis begins as soft deposits of fat that harden with age. Consequently, atherosclerosis is commonly referred to as "hardening of the arteries." Although this disease can occur in any artery in the body, the *atheromas* (fatty deposits) prefer the coronary arteries. The terms *arteriosclerotic heart disease, cardiovascular heart disease, ischemic heart disease, coronary heart disease,* and *CAD* all describe this disease process.

Etiology and Pathophysiology

Atherosclerosis is the major cause of CAD. It is characterized by lipid deposits within the intima of the artery. Endothelial injury and inflammation play a central role in the development of atherosclerosis.

The endothelium (inner lining of the vessel wall) is normally nonreactive to platelets and leukocytes, as well as coagulation, fibrinolytic, and complement factors. However, the endothelial lining can be injured as a result of tobacco use, hyperlipidemia, hypertension, toxins, diabetes, hyperhomocysteinemia, and infection causing a local inflammatory response[2] (Fig. 33-1, *A*).

C-reactive protein (CRP), a protein produced by the liver, is a nonspecific marker of inflammation. It is increased in many patients with CAD[3] (see Table 31-6). CRP levels rise when there

Reviewed by Marylee Bressie, RN, DNP, CCRN, CCNS, CEN, Core Faculty/Nurse Planner, Department of Nursing, School of Public Service Leadership, Capella University, Minneapolis, Minnesota; Christina D. Keller, RN, MSN-Ed, Instructor, Clinical Simulation Center, Radford University, Radford, Virginia; and Bonnie Tong, MSN, ACNP-BC, Nurse Practitioner, Mount Sinai Hospital, New York, New York.

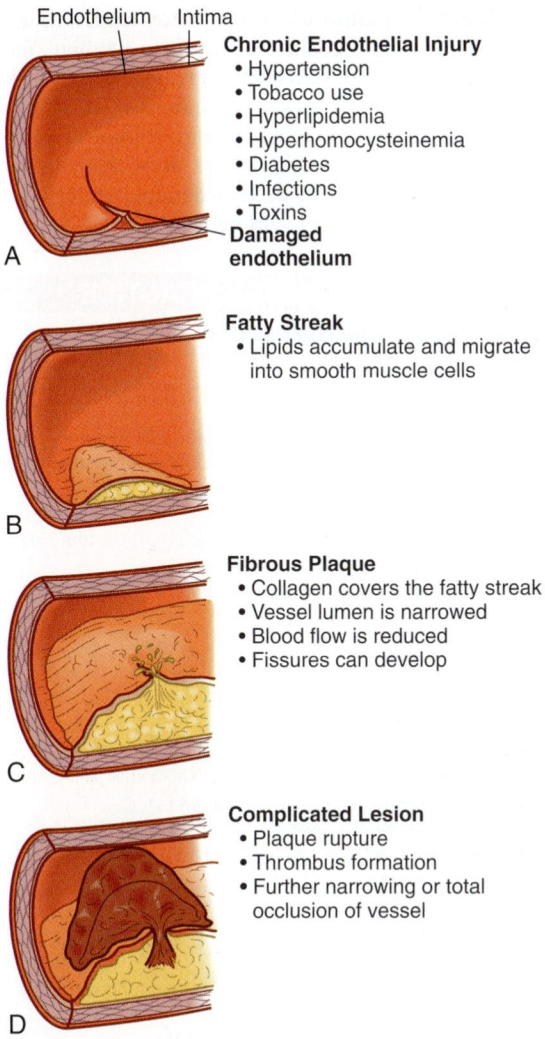

FIG. 33-1 Pathogenesis of atherosclerosis. **A,** Damaged endothelium. **B,** Fatty streak and lipid core formation. **C,** Fibrous plaque. Raised plaques are visible: some are yellow; others are white. **D,** Complicated lesion: thrombus is red; collagen is blue. Plaque is complicated by red thrombus deposition.

is systemic inflammation. Chronic elevations of CRP are linked with unstable plaques and the oxidation of low-density lipoprotein (LDL) cholesterol.

Developmental Stages. CAD is a progressive disease that develops over many years. When it becomes symptomatic, the disease process is usually well advanced. The stages of development in atherosclerosis are (1) fatty streak, (2) fibrous plaque, and (3) complicated lesion.

Fatty Streak. *Fatty streaks,* the earliest lesions of atherosclerosis, are characterized by lipid-filled smooth muscle cells. As streaks of fat develop within the smooth muscle cells, a yellow tinge appears. Fatty streaks can be seen in the coronary arteries by age 20 and involve an increasing amount of surface area as one ages. Treatment that lowers LDL cholesterol may reverse this process (Fig. 33-1, *B*).

Fibrous Plaque. The *fibrous plaque* stage is the beginning of progressive changes in the endothelium of the arterial wall. These changes can appear in the coronary arteries by age 30 and increase with age.

Normally the endothelium repairs itself immediately. This does not occur in the person with CAD. LDLs and growth factors from platelets stimulate smooth muscle proliferation

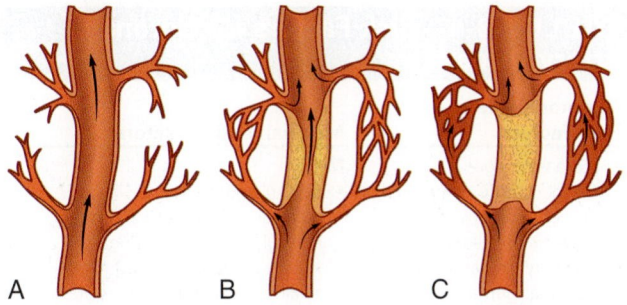

FIG. 33-2 Vessel occlusion with collateral circulation. **A,** Open, functioning coronary artery. **B,** Partial coronary artery closure with collateral circulation being established. **C,** Total coronary artery occlusion with collateral circulation bypassing the occlusion to supply blood to the myocardium.

and thickening of the arterial wall. Once endothelial injury has taken place, lipoproteins (carrier proteins within the bloodstream) transport cholesterol and other lipids into the arterial intima. Collagen covers the fatty streak and forms a fibrous plaque with a grayish or whitish appearance. These plaques can form on one portion of the artery or in a circular fashion involving the entire lumen. The borders can be smooth or irregular with rough, jagged edges. The result is a narrowing of the vessel lumen and a reduction in blood flow to the distal tissues (Fig. 33-1, *C*).

Complicated Lesion. The final stage in the development of the atherosclerotic lesion is the most dangerous. As the fibrous plaque grows, continued inflammation can result in plaque instability, ulceration, and rupture. Once the integrity of the artery's inner wall is compromised, platelets accumulate in large numbers, leading to a thrombus. The thrombus may adhere to the wall of the artery, leading to further narrowing or total occlusion of the artery. Activation of the exposed platelets causes expression of glycoprotein IIb/IIIa receptors that bind fibrinogen. This, in turn, leads to further platelet aggregation and adhesion, further enlarging the thrombus. At this stage the plaque is referred to as a *complicated lesion* (Fig. 33-1, *D*).

Collateral Circulation. Normally some arterial anastomoses or connections, called **collateral circulation**, exist within the coronary circulation. Two factors contribute to the growth and extent of collateral circulation: (1) inherited predisposition to develop new blood vessels *(angiogenesis)* and (2) presence of chronic ischemia. When plaque blocks the normal flow of blood through a coronary artery and the resulting *ischemia* is chronic, increased collateral circulation develops (Fig. 33-2). When blockages in coronary arteries occur slowly over a long period, there is a greater chance of collateral circulation developing, and the heart muscle may still receive an adequate amount of blood and O_2.

However, with rapid-onset CAD (e.g., familial hypercholesterolemia) or coronary spasm, time is inadequate for collateral development. Consequently, a reduced blood flow results in a more severe ischemia or infarction.

Risk Factors for Coronary Artery Disease

Risk factors are characteristics or conditions that are linked with a high incidence of a disease. Many risk factors have been associated with CAD. They are grouped as nonmodifiable and modifiable (Table 33-1). *Nonmodifiable risk factors* are age, gender, ethnicity, family history, and genetics. *Modifiable risk factors* include elevated serum lipids, elevated BP, tobacco use,

TABLE 33-1 Risk Factors for Coronary Artery Disease

Nonmodifiable Risk Factors	Modifiable Risk Factors

• Increasing age
• Gender (more common in men than in women until 75 yr of age)
• Ethnicity (more common in white men than in African Americans)
• Genetic predisposition and family history of heart disease
	Major
	• Serum lipids:
	  • Total cholesterol >200 mg/dL
	  • Triglycerides ≥150 mg/dL*
	  • LDL cholesterol >160 mg/dL
	  • HDL cholesterol <40 mg/dL in men or <50 mg/dL in women*
	• BP ≥140/90 mm Hg*
	• Diabetes
	• Tobacco use
	• Physical inactivity
	• Obesity: Waist circumference ≥102 cm (≥40 in) in men and ≥88 cm (≥35 in) in women*
	Contributing
	• Fasting blood glucose ≥100 mg/dL*
	• Psychosocial risk factors (e.g., depression, hostility, anger, stress)
	• Elevated homocysteine levels

*Three or more of these risk factors meet the criteria for metabolic syndrome (discussed in Chapter 40).

physical inactivity, obesity, diabetes, metabolic syndrome, psychologic states, and elevated homocysteine level.

Nonmodifiable Risk Factors

Age, Gender, and Ethnicity. The incidence of CAD is highest among middle-aged men. After age 75, the incidence of serious heart events in men and women equalizes, although CAD causes more deaths in women than men.[1] Additionally, CAD is present in African American women at rates higher than those of their white counterparts.[4] (See Cultural & Ethnic Health Disparities box for additional differences in CAD among ethnic groups.)

CULTURAL & ETHNIC HEALTH DISPARITIES

Coronary Artery Disease

Whites
- White men have the highest incidence of coronary artery disease (CAD).

African Americans
- African Americans have an early age of onset of CAD.
- Deaths from cardiovascular diseases (e.g., CAD, stroke) are higher for African Americans than for the overall population in the United States.
- African American women have a higher incidence and death rate related to CAD than white women.

Native Americans
- Native Americans die from heart disease earlier than expected. Mortality rates for those under 65 yr old are twice as high as those of other Americans.
- Major modifiable cardiovascular risk factors for Native Americans are tobacco use, hypertension, obesity, and diabetes.

Hispanics
- Hispanics have slightly lower rates of CAD than either non-Hispanic whites or African Americans.
- Hispanics have lower death rates from CAD than non-Hispanic whites.

Heart disease kills almost 10 times more women than breast cancer and is the leading cause of death in women. Yet most women do not consider CAD their greatest health risk.[4] On average, women with CAD are older than men who have CAD, and women are more likely to have co-morbidities (e.g., hypertension, diabetes). Most women have atypical symptoms of angina rather than symptoms of MI when they experience their first heart event[5] (see Gender Differences box).

GENETICS IN CLINICAL PRACTICE

Familial Hypercholesterolemia

Genetic Basis
- Autosomal dominant disorder
- Mutation in low-density lipoprotein receptor *(LDLR)* gene
- Gene codes for low-density lipoprotein (LDL) receptor that binds to LDLs.
- LDLs are the primary carriers of cholesterol in the blood. By removing LDLs from the bloodstream, the LDL receptors play a critical role in regulating cholesterol levels.
- Exists in both heterozygous (most common) and homozygous forms

Incidence
- Heterozygotes: 1 in 500
- Homozygotes: rare

Genetic Testing
- Disorder is characterized by elevated serum LDLs.
- Serum lipid profile can be used to measure total cholesterol, triglycerides, LDLs, and high-density lipoproteins (HDLs).
- DNA testing is available.

Clinical Implications
- Common genetic disease
- High cholesterol levels are a result of defective function of the LDL receptors.
- Elevated plasma levels of LDLs throughout life
- Develop severe atherosclerosis in early to middle years
- Develop xanthomas
- Treatment strategies include low-fat diet, exercise, and lipid-lowering drugs (e.g., PCSK9 inhibitors).*
- Homozygous familial hypercholesterolemia is much more severe than the heterozygous form. Cholesterol levels may exceed 600 mg/dL in these patients.

*See Table 33-5.

Genetic Link

Genetic predisposition is an important factor in the occurrence of CAD. Family history is a risk factor for CAD and MI. Often, patients with angina or MI can name a parent or sibling who died of CAD.

The genetic basis of CAD/MI is complex and poorly understood. It is estimated that the genetic contribution to CAD/MI is as high as 40% to 60%. This proportion relates mainly to genes that control known risk factors (e.g., lipid metabolism).[6] (See Genetics in Clinical Practice box.)

Major Modifiable Risk Factors

Elevated Serum Lipids. An elevated serum lipid level is one of the four most firmly established risk factors for CAD.[7] The risk of CAD is associated with a serum cholesterol level greater than 200 mg/dL (5.2 mmol/L) or a fasting triglyceride level greater than 150 mg/dL (3.7 mmol/L). (See Table 31-6 for normal serum lipid values.)

GENDER DIFFERENCES

Coronary Artery Disease and Acute Coronary Syndrome

Men	Women
Coronary Artery Disease	
• First heart event for men is more often MI than angina. • Men report more typical signs and symptoms of angina and MI. • Men receive more evidence-based therapies (e.g., aspirin, statins, diagnostic catheterization, PCI) when acutely ill from CAD (e.g., MI) than women. • Mortality rates from CAD have decreased more rapidly for men than women.	• Women experience the onset of heart disease approximately 10 yr later than men. • CAD is the leading cause of death for women, regardless of race or ethnicity. • More women with MI (compared to men with MI) die of sudden cardiac death before reaching the hospital. • Before menopause, women have higher HDL cholesterol levels and lower LDL cholesterol levels than men. After menopause LDL levels increase.
Acute Coronary Syndrome	
• After age 75, the incidence of MI in men and women equalizes. • Men present more frequently than women with an acute MI as the first manifestation of CAD. • Men develop greater collateral circulation than women. • Men have larger-diameter coronary arteries than women. Vessel diameter is inversely related to risk of restenosis after interventions. • Standard screening for risk of sudden cardiac death (e.g., EP studies) is more predictive in men.	• Women are older than men when seen with first MI and often have more co-morbidities. • Women seek medical care later in the CAD process and often are more ill on presentation than men. • First heart event for women is more often unstable angina than MI. • Once a woman reaches menopause, her risk for an MI quadruples. • Fewer women than men manifest the "classic" signs and symptoms of UA or MI. • Fatigue is often the first symptom of ACS in women. • Women experience more "silent" MIs compared with men. • Among those who have an MI, women are more likely to suffer a fatal heart event within 1 yr than men. • Women report more disability after a heart event than men. • Women who have coronary artery bypass graft surgery have a higher mortality rate and more complications after surgery than men.

ACS, Acute coronary syndrome; *CAD,* coronary artery disease; *EP,* electrophysiology; *HDL,* high-density lipoprotein; *LDL,* low-density lipoprotein; *PCI,* percutaneous coronary intervention, *UA,* unstable angina.

For lipids to be used and transported by the body, they must become soluble in blood by combining with proteins. Lipids combine with proteins to form lipoproteins. Lipoproteins are vehicles for fat mobilization and transport and vary in composition. Three major lipoproteins are high-density lipoproteins (HDLs), LDLs, and very-low-density lipoproteins (VLDLs).

HDLs contain more protein by weight and fewer lipids than any other lipoprotein. HDLs carry lipids away from arteries and to the liver for metabolism. This process of HDL transport prevents lipid accumulation within the arterial walls. Therefore high serum HDL levels are desirable and lower the risk of CAD.

There are several types of HDLs. They differ by their density and apolipoprotein composition. Apolipoproteins are found on lipoproteins and activate enzyme or receptor sites that promote the removal of fat from plasma. Several types of apolipoproteins exist (e.g., apo A-I, apo B-100, apo C-I). Women have more apo A-I than men, and premenopausal women have HDL levels approximately three times greater than men. This is thought to be related to the protective effects of natural estrogen. After menopause, women's HDL levels decrease and quickly near those of men. In general, HDL levels are higher in women, decrease with age, and are low in individuals with CAD. Physical activity and moderate alcohol intake increase HDL levels.

LDLs contain more cholesterol than any of the lipoproteins and have an attraction for arterial walls. VLDLs contain both cholesterol and triglycerides and may deposit cholesterol directly on the walls of arteries. Elevated LDL levels correlate closely with an increased incidence of atherosclerosis and CAD. Therefore low serum LDL levels are desirable.[7]

Certain diseases (e.g., type 2 diabetes, chronic kidney disease), drugs (e.g., corticosteroids, hormone therapy), and genetic disorders have been associated with elevated triglyceride levels. Lifestyle factors that can contribute to elevated triglycerides include high alcohol intake, high intake of refined carbohydrates and simple sugars, and physical inactivity. When a high triglyceride level is combined with a high LDL level, a smaller, denser LDL particle is formed, which favors deposition on arterial walls. People with insulin resistance often have this pattern.

Guidelines for treating elevated LDL cholesterol are based on a person's 10-year and lifetime risk for having heart disease or stroke. The following data generate a risk score: (1) age, (2) gender, (3) race, (4) use of tobacco, (5) diabetes, (6) systolic BP, (7) diastolic BP, (8) use of BP drugs, (9) total cholesterol level, and (10) HDL cholesterol level.[8] A 10-year risk calculator is available at *http://www.cvriskcalculator.com/* as well as for smartphones (e.g., ASCVD Risk Estimator app).

In general, individuals with no or only one risk factor are considered at low risk for the development of CAD, and their LDL goal is less than 160 mg/dL (4.14 mmol/L). Those at very high risk for developing CAD have multiple risk factors. They have an LDL goal of less than 70 mg/dL (1.8 mmol/L).[7]

Hypertension. The second major risk factor in CAD is hypertension, which is defined as a BP greater than 140/90 mm Hg. For people older than 60 years, a goal BP of less than 150/90 mm Hg has been recommended to prevent stroke, CVD, and heart failure.[9] Newer findings recommend a goal of less than 120/80 mm Hg.[10] Hypertension increases the risk of death from CAD 10-fold in all people. In postmenopausal women, hypertension is associated with a higher incidence of CAD than in men and premenopausal women.

BP is classified as (1) normal (BP less than 120/80 mm Hg), (2) *prehypertension* (BP of 120 to 139/80 to 89 mm Hg), (3) stage 1 hypertension (140 to 159/90 to 99 mm Hg), and (4) stage 2 hypertension (BP greater than or equal to 160/100 mm Hg).[11] The cause of hypertension in 90% of those affected is unknown, but it is usually controllable with drugs and/or diet. Therapeutic lifestyle changes should begin in people with prehypertension. Those with stage 1 or 2 hypertension often require more than one drug to reach therapeutic goals (see Table 32-7). Teach all people with elevated systolic or diastolic BP the importance of achieving and maintaining target BP goals.

The stress of an elevated BP increases the rate of atherosclerosis. This relates to the shearing stress that causes endothelial injury. Atherosclerosis, in turn, causes narrowed, thickened arterial walls and decreases the distensibility and elasticity of vessels. More force is required to pump blood through diseased arteries. This increased force is reflected in a higher BP. This added workload results in left ventricular (LV) hypertrophy and decreased stroke volume with each contraction. Salt intake positively correlates with elevated BP, adding volume and increasing systemic vascular resistance (SVR) to the heart's workload. (See Chapter 32 for a complete discussion of hypertension.)

Tobacco Use. A third major risk factor in CAD is tobacco use. The risk of developing CAD is two to six times higher in those who smoke tobacco or use smokeless tobacco than in those who do not. Further, tobacco smoking decreases estrogen levels, placing premenopausal women at greater risk for CAD. Risk is proportional to the number of cigarettes smoked.

Nicotine in tobacco smoke causes catecholamine (i.e., epinephrine, norepinephrine) release. These neurohormones cause an increased heart rate (HR), peripheral vasoconstriction, and increased BP. These changes increase the heart's workload. Tobacco smoke is also related to an increase in LDL level, a decrease in HDL level, and release of toxic O_2 radicals. All of these add to vessel inflammation and thrombosis.

Carbon monoxide, found in tobacco smoke, affects the O_2-carrying capacity of hemoglobin by reducing the sites available for O_2 transport. Thus the effects of an increased cardiac workload and the O_2-depleting effect of carbon monoxide significantly decrease the O_2 available to the heart muscle. There is also some indication that carbon monoxide is a chemical irritant and causes injury to the endothelium.

The benefits of smoking cessation are dramatic and almost immediate. CAD mortality rates drop to those of nonsmokers within 12 months. However, nicotine is highly addictive, and often intensive intervention is needed to assist people to quit. Individual and group counseling, nicotine replacement therapy, smoking cessation drugs (e.g., bupropion [Zyban], varenicline [Chantix]), and hypnosis are examples of smoking cessation strategies. (See Chapter 10, Tables 10-4 through 10-6 for information on smoking cessation.)

Chronic exposure to environmental tobacco (secondhand) smoke also increases the risk of CAD.[7] People who live in the same house as the person who smokes should encourage that person to quit. This reinforces the person's effort and decreases the risk of ongoing exposure to environmental smoke. Pipe and cigar smokers, who often do not inhale, have an increased risk of CAD similar to those exposed to secondhand smoke.

Physical Inactivity. Physical inactivity is the fourth major modifiable risk factor. Physical inactivity implies a lack of adequate physical exercise on a regular basis. An example of health-promoting regular physical activity is brisk walking (3 to 4 miles per hour) for at least 30 minutes five or more times a week.[12]

The mechanism by which physical inactivity predisposes a person to CAD is still unclear. Physically active people have increased HDL levels. Exercise improves thrombolytic activity, thus reducing the risk of clot formation. Exercise may also encourage the development of collateral circulation in the heart.

Exercise training for those who are physically inactive reduces the risk of CAD through more efficient lipid metabolism, increased HDL production, and more efficient O_2 extraction by the muscles, thereby decreasing the heart's workload. For individuals with CAD, regular physical activity reduces symptoms, improves functional capacity, and improves other risk factors such as insulin resistance and glucose intolerance.

Obesity. The death rate from CAD is higher in obese individuals. Obesity is defined as a body mass index (BMI) of greater than 30 kg/m^2 and a waist circumference more than 40 inches for men and more than 35 inches for women. BMI is a measure of body fat based on height and weight. It can be calculated online *(http://www.nhlbi.nih.gov/health/educational/lose_wt/BMI/bmicalc.htm)*.

The increased risk for CAD is proportional to the degree of obesity. Obese individuals may produce increased levels of LDLs and triglycerides, which are strongly related to atherosclerosis. Obesity is often linked with hypertension and insulin resistance. People who tend to store fat in the abdomen (an "apple" figure) rather than in the hips and buttocks (a "pear" figure) have a higher incidence of CAD (see Table 40-2).

Contributing Modifiable Risk Factors

Diabetes Mellitus. The incidence of CAD is two to four times greater among people who have diabetes, even those with well-controlled blood glucose levels, than the general population. The patient with diabetes manifests CAD not only more often but also at an earlier age. There is no age difference between male or female patients with diabetes in the onset of symptoms of CAD. Diabetes virtually eliminates the lower incidence of CAD in premenopausal women.

Undiagnosed diabetes is frequently discovered at the time a person has an MI. The person with diabetes has an increased tendency toward endothelial dysfunction. This may account for the development of fatty streaks in these patients. Patients with diabetes also have changes in lipid metabolism and tend to have high cholesterol and triglyceride levels. Management of diabetes should include lifestyle changes and drug therapy to achieve a glycosylated hemoglobin (A1C or Hb A1C) level of less than 7%.[7]

Metabolic Syndrome. *Metabolic syndrome* refers to a cluster of risk factors for CAD whose underlying pathophysiology may be related to insulin resistance. These risk factors include central obesity, hypertension, abnormal serum lipids, and an elevated fasting blood glucose (see Table 40-11). These interrelated risk factors appear to promote the development of CAD. (Chapter 40 discusses metabolic syndrome.)

Psychologic States. Certain behaviors and lifestyles may contribute to the development of CAD. One type of behavior, referred to as type A, includes perfectionism and a hardworking, driven personality. The type A person often suppresses anger and hostility, has a sense of time urgency, is impatient, and creates stress and tension. This person may be more prone to MIs than a type B person, who is more easygoing, takes upsets in stride, knows personal limitations, takes time to relax, and is not an overachiever. However, the relationship between behaviors and the risk for CAD/MI remains controversial and complex.

Psychologic risk factors thought to increase the risk of CAD include depression, acute and chronic stress (e.g., poverty, serving as a caregiver), anxiety, hostility and anger, and lack of social support.[13,14] In particular, depression is a risk factor for both the development and worsening of CAD. Depressed patients have elevated levels of circulating catecholamines. This may contribute to endothelial injury and inflammation and platelet activation. Higher levels of depression are also associated with an increased number of adverse heart events.[13]

Stressful states can contribute to the development of CAD.[14] Sympathetic nervous system (SNS) stimulation and its effect on the heart are the physiologic mechanisms by which stress predisposes a person to the development of CAD. SNS stimulation causes an increased release of catecholamines (i.e., epinephrine, norepinephrine). This stimulation increases HR and the force of myocardial contraction. Both results increase myocardial O_2 demand. Also, stress-induced mechanisms can cause elevated lipid and glucose levels and changes in blood coagulation, which can lead to increased atherosclerosis.

Homocysteine. High blood levels of homocysteine have been linked to an increased risk for CAD and other CVDs.[15] Homocysteine is produced by the breakdown of the essential amino acid methionine, which is found in dietary protein. High homocysteine levels may contribute to atherosclerosis by (1) damaging the inner lining of blood vessels, (2) promoting plaque buildup, and (3) altering the clotting mechanism to make clots more likely to occur.

Research to determine if a decline in homocysteine can reduce the risk of CVD is ongoing. B-complex vitamins (B_6, B_{12}, folic acid) have been shown to lower blood levels of homocysteine. Generally, a screening test for homocysteine is limited to those suspected of having elevated levels. These include older patients with pernicious anemia or people who develop CAD at an early age.

Substance Abuse. The use of illegal drugs, such as cocaine and methamphetamine, can produce coronary spasm resulting in myocardial ischemia and chest pain. Most patients seen in the emergency department (ED) with drug-induced chest pain are initially indistinguishable from those with CAD. Although MI can occur, these patients often have sinus tachycardia, high BP, angina, and anxiety.[16]

The U.S. Food and Drug Administration (FDA) prohibits the sale of dietary supplements containing ephedrine alkaloids. These compounds should be avoided because they can cause high BP, MI, and stroke.

❖ NURSING AND INTERPROFESSIONAL MANAGEMENT: CORONARY ARTERY DISEASE

◆ Health Promotion

The appropriate management of risk factors in CAD may prevent, modify, or slow the progression of the disease. In the United States, there has been a gradual decline in CVD-related deaths over the past 35 years. This relates to people's efforts to become generally healthier, as well as advances in the treatment of CAD. Prevention and early treatment of heart disease must involve a multifaceted approach and must be ongoing throughout the life span.

◆ **Identification of High-Risk Individuals.** Clinical signs of CAD are not apparent in the early stages of the disease. Therefore regardless of the health care setting, it is critical to identify people at risk for CAD. Risk screening involves obtaining a thorough health history. Ask the patient about a family history of heart disease in parents and siblings. Note the presence of any cardiovascular symptoms. Assess environmental factors, such as eating habits, type of diet, and level of exercise, to elicit lifestyle patterns. Include a psychosocial history to determine tobacco use, alcohol intake, recent stressful events (e.g., loss of a spouse), and any negative psychologic states (e.g., anxiety, depression, anger). The place and type of employment provide important information on the kind of activity performed, exposure to pollutants or toxins, and the degree of stress associated with work.

Identify the patient's attitudes and beliefs about health and illness. This information can give you insight to how disease and lifestyle changes may affect the patient. It also can reveal possible misconceptions about heart disease. Knowing the

EVIDENCE-BASED PRACTICE

Translating Research Into Practice

Do Cardiac Rehabilitation Programs Improve Outcomes?

Clinical Question

In patients with coronary artery disease (P), do cardiac rehabilitation programs (I) versus usual care (C) reduce readmissions, improve quality of life, and affect mortality rates (O)?

Synthesis of Best Available Evidence

- Six Cochrane reviews of randomized controlled trials (RCTs)
- 148 RCTs (n = 93,093) of patients with MI who underwent heart surgery or had chronic heart failure (HF). Cardiac rehabilitation programs may include exercise, healthy lifestyle education, and/or psychologic interventions such as stress reduction counseling. Programs were conducted in supervised centers or home-based. Outcomes included hospital readmission, health-related quality of life, and mortality. Program uptake (attendance or enrollment) and adherence were also determined.
- Participants in exercise-based programs compared to individuals receiving usual care had reduced hospital admissions, improved quality of life, and no increase in short-term mortality.
- Although programs with only education or psychologic interventions had minimal impact on readmissions or mortality, quality of life may be improved.
- Positive changes to program uptake were noted with structured nurse-led contacts, appointments made soon after discharge, and motivational letters.
- Adherence improved with self-monitoring and tailored counseling.
- Home-based and center-based programs were equally effective on outcomes measured with financial costs of the two programs similar.

Conclusions

- Patients with HF or after MI or PCI may safely engage in cardiac rehabilitation programs with no increased mortality.
- Cardiac rehabilitation programs may reduce hospital admissions and improve quality of life.

Implications for Nursing Practice

1. What strategies may be useful in motivating patients to stay engaged in a program?
2. Why is it important to reinforce the benefits of adhering to a recommended exercise program, and what actions would you take to positively affect adherence?
3. What would you suggest to patients who are not able to travel to a supervised center–based program?

Reference for Evidence

Anderson L, Taylor RS: Cardiac rehabilitation for people with heart disease: an overview of Cochrane systematic reviews, *Cochrane Database Syst Rev* 12:CD011273, 2014.

P, Patient population of interest; *I*, intervention or area of interest; *C*, comparison of interest or comparison group; *O*, outcomes of interest; *T*, timing (see p. 15).

patient's educational background and health literacy can help to identify teaching needs. If the patient has prescribed drugs, it is important to know the names and dosages and if the patient adheres to the drug regimen.

◆ **Management of High-Risk Individuals.** Recommend preventive measures for all individuals at risk for CAD. Risk factors such as age, gender, ethnicity, and genetics cannot be modified. However, the person with any of these risk factors can still reduce the risk of CAD by controlling the additive effects of modifiable risk factors. For example, a young man with a family history of heart disease can decrease the risk of CAD by maintaining an ideal body weight, getting adequate physical exercise, reducing intake of saturated fats, and avoiding tobacco and illicit drug use.

Encourage people who have modifiable risk factors to make lifestyle changes to reduce their risk of CAD. You can play a major role in teaching health-promoting behaviors (Table 33-2). For highly motivated individuals, knowing how to reduce this risk may be the information they need to get started.

For individuals who are less motivated to take charge of their health, the idea of reducing risk factors may be so remote that they are unable to perceive a threat of CAD. Few people desire to make lifestyle changes, especially in the absence of symptoms. First help these patients to clarify their personal values. Then, discuss risk factors and have them identify their individual risks. This can help patients set realistic goals and choose which risk factor(s) to change first. Some individuals are reluctant to change until they begin to have symptoms or actually suffer an MI. Others, having suffered an MI, may find the idea of changing lifelong habits still unacceptable. Help them identify their choices and respect their final decision.

◆ Physical Activity

A physical activity program should be designed to improve physical fitness by following the FITT formula: Frequency (how often), Intensity (how hard), Type (isotonic), and Time (how long). Everyone should aim for at least 30 minutes of moderate physical activity on most days of the week. In addition, adding weight training to an exercise program two days a week can help treat metabolic syndrome and improve muscle strength. Examples of moderate physical activity include brisk walking, hiking, biking, and swimming. Regular physical activity helps with weight reduction, reduces systolic BP, and, in some men more than women, increases HDL cholesterol. The AHA has developed a program to encourage people, especially women, to increase their daily physical activity (My Heart, My Life at *www.startwalkingnow.org*).

◆ Nutritional Therapy

Therapeutic lifestyle changes are recommended for all people to reduce the risk of CAD by lowering LDL cholesterol. These recommendations emphasize a decrease in saturated fat and cholesterol and an increase in complex carbohydrates (e.g., whole grains, fruit, vegetables) and fiber (Tables 33-3 and 33-4). Fat intake should be about 25% to 35% of total calories, with most coming from mono- and polyunsaturated fats. Red meat, egg yolks, and whole milk products are major sources of saturated fat and cholesterol and should be reduced or

TABLE 33-2 Patient & Caregiver Teaching

Reducing Risk Factors for Coronary Artery Disease

Include the following instructions when teaching risk reduction for coronary artery disease.

Risk Factor	Health-Promoting Behaviors
Hypertension	• Monitor home-based BP and obtain regular checkups. • Take prescribed drugs for BP control. • Reduce salt intake. • Stop tobacco use. Avoid exposure to environmental tobacco (secondhand) smoke. • Control or reduce weight. • Perform physical activity daily.
Elevated serum lipids	• Reduce total fat intake. • Reduce animal (saturated) fat intake. • Take prescribed drugs for lipid reduction. • Adjust total caloric intake to achieve and maintain ideal body weight. • Engage in daily physical activity. • Increase amount of complex carbohydrates, fiber, and vegetable proteins in diet.
Tobacco use*	• Begin a tobacco cessation program. • Change daily routines associated with tobacco use to reduce desire to smoke. • Substitute other activities for smoking. • Ask caregivers to support efforts to stop smoking. • Avoid exposure to environmental tobacco smoke.
Physical inactivity	• Develop and maintain at least 30 min of moderate physical activity daily (minimum 5 days a week). • Increase activities to a fitness level.
Psychologic state	• Increase awareness of behaviors that are harmful to health. • Alter patterns that add to stress (e.g., get up 30 min earlier so that breakfast is not eaten on way to work). • Set realistic goals for self. • Reassess priorities in light of identified risk factors. • Learn effective stress management strategies (see Chapter 6). • Seek professional help if feeling depressed, angry, anxious, etc. • Plan time for adequate rest and sleep (see Chapter 7).
Obesity†	• Change eating patterns and habits. • Reduce caloric intake to achieve body mass index of 18.5–24.9 kg/m^2. • Increase physical activity to increase caloric expenditure. • Avoid fad and crash diets, which are not effective over time. • Avoid large, heavy meals. Consider smaller, more frequent meals.
Diabetes‡	• Follow the recommended diet. • Control or reduce weight. • Take prescribed drugs for diabetes. • Monitor blood glucose levels regularly.

*Smoking cessation is discussed in Chapter 10 and Tables 10-4 through 10-6.
†See Chapter 40 for additional health-promoting behaviors.
‡See Chapter 48 for additional health-promoting behaviors.

TABLE 33-3 Nutritional Therapy

Therapeutic Lifestyle Changes Diet

Dietary Recommendations	Recommended Daily Intake
Combined total fat calories from: • *Saturated fats:* found in fats that are usually solid at room temperature (e.g., bacon, lard, butter, egg yolks) and should be limited) • *Trans fats:* found mainly in foods made with hydrogenated vegetable oils, such as many hard margarines and shortenings • *Monounsaturated fats:* found in greatest amounts in foods from plants including olive, canola, sunflower, and peanut oils • *Polyunsaturated fats:* found in greatest amounts in many kinds of nuts and in foods from plants including safflower, sunflower, corn, soybean, cottonseed oils	25%-35% of total daily calories (including <7% from saturated fat)
Cholesterol	<200 mg
Plant stanols or sterols (e.g., margarines, nuts, seeds, legumes, vegetable oils)*	2 g
Dietary fiber*	10-25 g of soluble fiber
Total calories	Only enough calories to reach or maintain a healthy weight

Physical Activity

In addition to diet, teach the patient to get at least 30 minutes of a moderate intensity physical activity, such as brisk walking, on most, and preferably all, days of the week.

Source: U.S. Department of Health and Human Services: Your Guide to Lowering Your Cholesterol with TLC. Retrieved from *www.nhlbi.nih.gov/health/public/heart/chol/chol_tlc.pdf.*
*Diet options for additional lowering of low-density lipoprotein (LDL).

eliminated from diets. If the serum triglyceride level is elevated, alcohol and simple sugars should be reduced or eliminated.

Omega-3 fatty acids reduce the risks associated with CAD when eaten regularly. For individuals without CAD, the AHA recommends eating fatty fish twice a week. Fatty fish such as salmon and tuna contain two types of omega-3 fatty acids: eicosapentaenoic acid (EPA) and docosahexaenoic acid (DHA). Patients with CAD are encouraged to take EPA and DHA supplements with their diet. The AHA also recommends eating tofu and other forms of soybean, canola, walnut, and flaxseed because these products contain alpha-linolenic acid, which becomes omega-3 fatty acid in the body.

Lifestyle changes such as a low-saturated-fat, high-fiber diet; avoidance of tobacco; and increase in physical activity can promote the reversal of CAD and reduce heart events.

◆ Lipid-Lowering Drug Therapy

An estimated 31.9 million American adults have cholesterol levels greater than or equal to 240 mg/dL (6.2 mmol/L).[1] Guidelines for treatment of high cholesterol focus on LDL cholesterol. A complete lipid profile is recommended every 5 years beginning at age 20. Guidelines recommend the following groups of people receive statin therapy: (1) patients with known CVD, (2) patients with primary elevations of LDL cholesterol levels greater than or equal to 190 mg/dL (e.g., familial hypercholesterolemia), (3) patients between 40 and 75 years old with diabetes and LDL cholesterol levels between 70 and 189 mg/dL, and (4) patients between 40 and 75 years old with LDL cholesterol levels between 70 and 189 mg/dL and a 10-year risk for CVD of at least 7.5%.[8]

TABLE 33-4 Nutritional Therapy

Tips to Make Diet and Lifestyle Changes

General Tips

1. Know your calorie needs to achieve and maintain a healthy weight.
2. Know the calorie content of the foods and beverages you eat.
3. Track your weight, physical activity, and calorie intake.
4. Prepare and eat smaller, more frequent meals.
5. Track your activities and, whenever possible, decrease sedentary activities (e.g., watching television, computer time).
6. Incorporate physical movement into daily activities (e.g., take stairs and extra steps whenever possible).
7. Do not smoke or use tobacco products.
8. If you drink alcohol, do so in moderation (i.e., no more than one drink for women or two drinks for men a day).

Tips Related to Food Choices and Preparation

1. Use the Nutrition Facts panel on food labels and ingredients list when choosing foods to buy.
2. Use fresh vegetables and fruits in place of canned vegetables and fruits.
3. Replace high-calorie foods with fresh fruits and vegetables.
4. Increase fiber intake by eating beans (legumes), whole-grain products, fruits, and vegetables.
5. Use liquid vegetable oils in place of solid fats.
6. Limit beverages and foods high in added sugars (e.g., sucrose, glucose, fructose, maltose, dextrose, corn syrups, concentrated fruit juice, honey).
7. Choose foods made with whole grains (e.g., whole wheat, oats, rye, barley, brown rice, wild rice, buckwheat).
8. Avoid pastries and high-calorie bakery products (e.g., muffins, doughnuts).
9. Select milk and dairy products that are either fat free or low fat.
10. Reduce salt intake by
    - Comparing the sodium content of similar products (e.g., different brands of tomato sauce) and choosing products with less sodium.
    - Choosing versions of processed foods that are reduced in salt, including cereals, canned products, and baked goods.
    - Limiting condiments (e.g., soy sauce, ketchup).
11. Use lean cuts of meat and remove skin from poultry before cooking or eating.
12. Avoid processed meats that are high in saturated fat and sodium (e.g., deli meats).
13. Grill, bake, or broil fish, meat, and poultry.
14. Incorporate plant-based meat substitutes into recipes (e.g., soy, tofu, quinoa).
15. Consume whole vegetables and fruits in place of juices.

Adapted from Gidding SS, Lichtenstein AH, Faith MS, et al: Implementing American Heart Association pediatric and adult nutrition guidelines, *Circulation* 119:1161, 2009.

Treatment also includes weight loss (if overweight), decreased dietary fat and cholesterol intake, and increased physical activity. Serum lipid levels should be reassessed after 6 weeks of therapy. If they remain elevated, changes in drug therapy (Table 33-5) and additional dietary options (see the Complementary & Alternative Therapies box on the following page) should be considered.

◆ Drugs That Restrict Lipoprotein Production

◆ ***HMG-CoA Reductase Inhibitors (Statins).*** The statin drugs are the most widely used lipid-lowering drugs. These drugs inhibit the synthesis of cholesterol in the liver. An unexplained result of the inhibition of cholesterol synthesis is an increase in hepatic LDL receptors. Consequently, the liver is able to remove more

COMPLEMENTARY & ALTERNATIVE THERAPIES

Lipid-Lowering Agents

Agent	Evidence for Use
Garlic	Inconsistent scientific evidence for reductions in total cholesterol and low-density lipoproteins (LDLs) over short periods
Flaxseed	Some evidence for reducing risk of heart disease, diabetes, and stroke
Niacin	Evidence for increased high-density lipoproteins. Less dramatic reduction of LDLs
Omega-3 fatty acids	Strong scientific evidence for reduction of triglyceride levels
Psyllium	Strong scientific evidence for modest reduction in total cholesterol and LDLs
Plant sterols	Strong scientific evidence for reduction of total cholesterol
Red yeast rice	Strong scientific evidence for reduction of total cholesterol, LDLs, and triglycerides
Soy	Strong scientific evidence for moderate reduction in total cholesterol and LDLs

Source: *www.naturalstandard.com.*

LDLs from the blood. In addition, statins produce a small increase in HDLs and lower CRP levels. Serious adverse effects of these drugs are rare and include liver damage and myopathy that can progress to rhabdomyolysis (breakdown of skeletal muscle). Liver enzymes (e.g., aspartate aminotransferase, alanine aminotransferase) are initially monitored and rechecked with any increase in dosage. Creatine kinase isoenzymes (e.g., CK-MM) should be assessed if symptoms of myopathy (e.g., muscle aches, weakness) occur.

DRUG ALERT Simvastatin (Zocor)
- Increased risk for rhabdomyolysis when also used with gemfibrozil (Lopid) or niacin (Niaspan)
- Signs of rhabdomyolysis: ↑ creatine kinase levels, muscle pain

◆ ***Niacin.*** Niacin, a water-soluble B vitamin, is highly effective in lowering LDL and triglyceride levels by interfering with their synthesis. Niacin also increases HDL levels better than many other lipid-lowering drugs. Unfortunately, side effects of this drug are common and may include severe flushing, pruritus, gastrointestinal (GI) symptoms, and orthostatic hypotension.

DRUG ALERT Niacin (Niaspan)
- Instruct patient that flushing (especially of face and neck) may occur within 20 minutes after taking drug and may last for 30 to 60 minutes.
- Patient can premedicate with aspirin 30 minutes before taking to reduce flushing.
- Use of extended-release niacin may decrease side effects.

◆ ***Fibric Acid Derivatives.*** The *fibric acid derivatives* (Table 33-5) work by aiding the removal of VLDLs and increasing the production of apolipoproteins A-I and A-II. They are the most effective drugs for lowering triglycerides and increasing HDL levels. They have no effect on LDLs. Although most patients tolerate the drugs well, complaints may include GI irritability. These drugs should be used with caution when combined with statin medications.

DRUG ALERT Gemfibrozil (Lopid)
- May increase the risk of bleeding in patients taking warfarin (Coumadin)
- May increase the effects of antihyperglycemic drugs (e.g., repaglinide [Prandin])

◆ Drugs That Increase Lipoprotein Removal

◆ ***Bile Acid Sequestrants.*** The major route of elimination of cholesterol is by conversion to bile acids in the liver. Bile-acid sequestrants increase conversion of cholesterol to bile acids and decrease hepatic cholesterol (Table 33-5). The primary effect is a decrease in total cholesterol and LDL levels.

These drugs have been associated with complaints related to taste and a variety of upper and lower GI symptoms. These include belching, heartburn, nausea, abdominal pain, and constipation. The bile-acid sequestrants interfere with absorption of many other drugs (e.g., warfarin, thiazides, thyroid hormones, β-adrenergic blockers [β-blockers]). Separating the time of administration of these drugs from that of other drugs decreases this adverse effect.[17]

◆ ***Proprotein Convertase Subtilisin/Kexin 9 (PCSK9) Inhibitors.*** PCSK9 inhibitors are a new class of cholesterol-lowering drugs (Table 33-5). PCSK9 reduces the number of receptors on the liver that remove LDL cholesterol from the blood. By blocking PCSK9's ability to work, more receptors are available and can get rid of LDL, thus decreasing circulating LDL levels. Evolocumab (Repatha) and alirocumab (Praluent) are two PCSK9 inhibitors. These drugs are used in addition to diet and maximum statin therapy in adults with familial hypercholesterolemia or clinical evidence of atherosclerotic heart disease who need increased lowering of LDL.[18]

◆ **Drugs That Decrease Cholesterol Absorption.** Ezetimibe (Zetia) selectively inhibits the absorption of dietary and biliary cholesterol across the intestinal wall (Table 33-5). It serves as an adjunct to dietary changes, especially in patients with primary hypercholesterolemia. When it is combined with a statin (e.g., ezetimibe and simvastatin [Vytorin]), even greater reductions in LDLs are found.

Drug therapy for hyperlipidemia often continues for a lifetime. New combination drug therapy (e.g., atorvastatin/ezetimibe [Liptruzet]) is available and may be considered. Concurrent diet modification is essential to reduce the need for drug therapy. The patient must fully understand the rationale and goals of treatment, as well as the safety and side effects of lipid-lowering drugs.

◆ Antiplatelet Therapy

Aspirin is recommended for most people at risk for CVD. Low-dose aspirin (81 mg) is recommended for adults 50 to 59 years old who have a calculated 10-year CVD risk of 10% or more, are not at increased risk for bleeding (e.g., history of GI bleeding), have a life expectancy of at least 10 years, and are willing to take low-dose aspirin for at least 10 years. For adults 60 to 69 years old who have a calculated 10-year CVD risk of 10% or more, the decision to take low-dose aspirin is an individual one. Adults who have no contraindications (e.g., history of stroke), have a life expectancy of at least 10 years, and are willing to take low-dose aspirin daily for at least 10 years are more likely to benefit. Currently there is insufficient evidence to recommend low-dose aspirin for those younger than 50 or older than 70.[19]

Gerontologic Considerations: Coronary Artery Disease

The incidence of heart disease is greatly increased in older adults and is the leading cause of death in older individuals.[1] In the older adult, CAD is often a result of the complex interaction of nonmodifiable risk factors (e.g., age) and lifelong modifiable risk behaviors (e.g., inactivity, tobacco use). Strategies to reduce CAD risk and to treat CAD are effective in this age group.

TABLE 33-5 Drug Therapy

Hyperlipidemia

Drug	Mechanism of Action	Side Effects	Nursing Considerations
Restrict Lipoprotein Production			
HMG-CoA Reductase Inhibitors (Statins)			
atorvastatin (Lipitor) fluvastatin (Lescol) lovastatin pravastatin (Pravachol) simvastatin (Zocor) rosuvastatin (Crestor)	Block synthesis of cholesterol and increase LDL receptors in liver ↓ LDL ↓ Triglycerides ↑ HDL	Rash, GI disturbances, elevated liver enzymes, myopathy, rhabdomyolysis	Well tolerated with few side effects. Monitor liver enzymes and creatine kinase (if muscle weakness or pain occurs).
Niacin			
niacin (Niaspan)	Inhibits synthesis and secretion of VLDL and LDL ↓ LDL ↓ Triglycerides ↑ HDL	Flushing and pruritus in upper torso and face, GI disturbances (e.g., nausea and vomiting, dyspepsia, diarrhea), orthostatic hypotension, elevated homocysteine levels	Most side effects subside with time. Decreased liver function may occur with high doses. Taking aspirin or NSAID 30 min before drug may prevent flushing. Take drug with food. Treat elevated homocysteine levels with folic acid.
Fibric Acid Derivatives			
fenofibrate (Tricor) gemfibrozil (Lopid)	Decrease hepatic synthesis and secretion of VLDL. Reduce triglycerides by ↓ VLDL ↓ LDL ↓ Triglycerides ↑ HDL	Rashes, mild GI disturbances (e.g., nausea, diarrhea), elevated liver enzymes	May ↑ effects of warfarin (Coumadin) and some antihyperglycemic drugs. When used in combination with statins, may increase adverse effects of statins, especially myopathy.
Omega-3 Fatty Acid			
icosapent ethyl (Vascepa)	Inhibits synthesis and/or secretion of triglycerides	Arthralgia	Used for patients with severe hypertriglyceridemia (levels ≥500 mg/dL)
Increase Lipoprotein Removal			
Bile-Acid Sequestrants			
cholestyramine (Prevalite) colesevelam (WelChol) colestipol (Colestid)	Bind with bile acids in intestine, forming insoluble complex and excreted in feces Binding results in removal of LDL and cholesterol ↓ LDL	Unpleasant quality to taste, GI disturbances (e.g., indigestion, constipation, bloating)	Effective and safe for long-term use. Side effects diminish with time. Interfere with absorption of many drugs (e.g., digoxin, thiazide diuretics, warfarin, some antibiotics [e.g., penicillins])
Proprotein Convertase Subtilisin/Kexin 9 (PCSK9) Inhibitors			
evolocumab (Repatha) alirocumab (Praluent)	Inactivate PCSK9 protein ↓ LDL	Injection-site reactions, muscle pain, limb pain, and fatigue	Used with diet and maximum statin therapy to treat familial hypercholesterolemia and for those who need LDL lowering and are statin intolerant Drugs are given by injection every 2-4 wk.
Decrease Cholesterol Absorption			
Cholesterol Absorption Inhibitor			
ezetimibe (Zetia)	Inhibits the intestinal absorption of cholesterol ↓ LDL ↑ HDL	Infrequent, but may include headache and mild GI distress	When used with a statin, LDL is further reduced. Should not be used by patients with liver impairment

Aggressive treatment of hypertension and hyperlipidemia stabilizes plaques in the coronary arteries of older adults, and cessation of tobacco use helps to decrease the risk for CAD at any age. Similarly, encourage the older patient to consider a planned program of physical activity. Activity performance, endurance, and ability to tolerate stress are improved in the older adult with physical training. Positive psychologic benefits from physical activity can include increased self-esteem and emotional well-being and improved body image. For the older adult who is obese, making modest dietary changes and slowly increasing physical activity (e.g., walking) results in more positive benefits than aiming for a significant weight loss.

When planning a physical activity program for the older adult, recommend the following: (1) longer warm-up periods, (2) longer periods of low-level activity, or (3) longer rest periods between sessions. Heat intolerance in the older adult results from a decreased ability to sweat efficiently. Teach the patient to avoid physical activity in extremes of temperature and to maintain a moderate pace. The older adult should exercise a minimum of 30 minutes on most days of the week as able.

Encouraging the older patient to adopt a healthy lifestyle may increase the quality of life and reduce the risk of CAD and fatal heart events. Older adults face many of the same challenges as younger individuals when it comes to making lifestyle changes. Older adults are more likely to consider change at two points in time: (1) when hospitalized and (2) when symptoms (e.g., chest pain) are the result of CAD and not normal aging (see Table 31-1). First, assess the older adult for readiness to change and health literacy. Then help the patient select the lifestyle changes most likely to produce the greatest reduction in risk for CAD.

CHRONIC STABLE ANGINA

CAD is a chronic and progressive disease. Patients may be asymptomatic for many years or may develop chronic stable chest pain. When the demand for myocardial O_2 exceeds the ability of the coronary arteries to supply the heart with O_2, *myocardial ischemia* occurs. Angina, or chest pain, is the clinical manifestation of myocardial ischemia. It is caused by either an increased demand for O_2 or a decreased supply of O_2 (Table 33-6). The most common reason for angina to develop is narrowing of one or more coronary arteries by atherosclerosis. This leads to insufficient blood flow to the heart muscle. For ischemia secondary to atherosclerotic plaque to occur, the artery is usually blocked (stenosed) 70% or more (50% or more for the left main coronary artery).[5,20]

Chronic stable angina refers to chest pain that occurs intermittently over a long period of time with a similar pattern of onset, duration, and intensity of symptoms. It is often provoked by physical exertion, stress, or emotional upset. When asked, some patients may deny feeling pain but describe a pressure, heaviness, or discomfort in the chest (Table 33-7). This discomfort is often described as a squeezing, heavy, tight, or suffocating sensation. It may be associated with other symptoms such as dyspnea or fatigue. Chronic angina pain usually does not change with position or breathing and is rarely described as sharp or stabbing.

Although most angina pain occurs substernally, it may radiate to other locations, including the jaw, neck, shoulders, and/or arms. Many people with angina complain of indigestion or a burning sensation in the epigastric region. The sensation may also be felt between the shoulder blades (Fig. 33-3). Often people who complain of pain between the shoulder blades or indigestion type pain dismiss it as not being heart related. Some patients, especially women and older adults, report atypical symptoms of angina including dyspnea, nausea, and/or fatigue.[4] This is referred to as *angina equivalent*.

The pain of chronic stable angina usually lasts for only a few minutes and commonly subsides when the precipitating factor is resolved (e.g., resting, calming down, using sublingual nitroglycerin (SL NTG) (Nitrostat) (Table 33-8). Pain at rest is unusual and often a symptom of UA. A 12-lead electrocardiogram (ECG) often shows ST segment depression and/or T wave

TABLE 33-6 Factors Influencing Myocardial O_2 Needs*

Decreased O_2 Supply	Increased O_2 Demand or Consumption
Cardiac	
• Coronary artery atherosclerosis	• Aortic stenosis
• Coronary artery spasm	• Cardiomyopathy
• Coronary artery thrombosis	• Dysrhythmias
• Dysrhythmias	• Left ventricular hypertrophy
• Heart failure	• Tachycardia
• Valve disorders	
Noncardiac	
• Anemia	• Anxiety
• Asthma	• Hypertension
• Chronic obstructive pulmonary disease	• Hyperthermia
• Hypovolemia	• Hyperthyroidism
• Hypoxemia	• Physical exertion
• Pneumonia	• Substance (stimulant) abuse (e.g., cocaine, amphetamines)
• Substance (stimulant) abuse (e.g., cocaine, amphetamines)	

*Lists are not all-inclusive.

TABLE 33-7 PQRST Assessment of Angina

Use the following memory aid to obtain information from the patient who has chest pain.

	Factor	Questions to Ask Patient
P	Precipitating events	What events or activities precipitated the pain or discomfort (e.g., argument, exercise, resting)?
Q	Quality of pain	What does the pain or discomfort feel like (e.g., pressure, dull, aching, tight, squeezing, heaviness)?
R	Region (location) and radiation of pain	Can you point to where the pain or discomfort is located? Does the pain or discomfort radiate to other areas (e.g., back, neck, arms, jaw, shoulder, elbow)?
S	Severity of pain	On a scale of 0 to 10, with 0 indicating no pain and 10 being the most severe pain you could imagine, what number would you give the pain or discomfort?
T	Timing	When did the pain or discomfort begin? Has it changed since this time? Have you had pain/discomfort like this before?

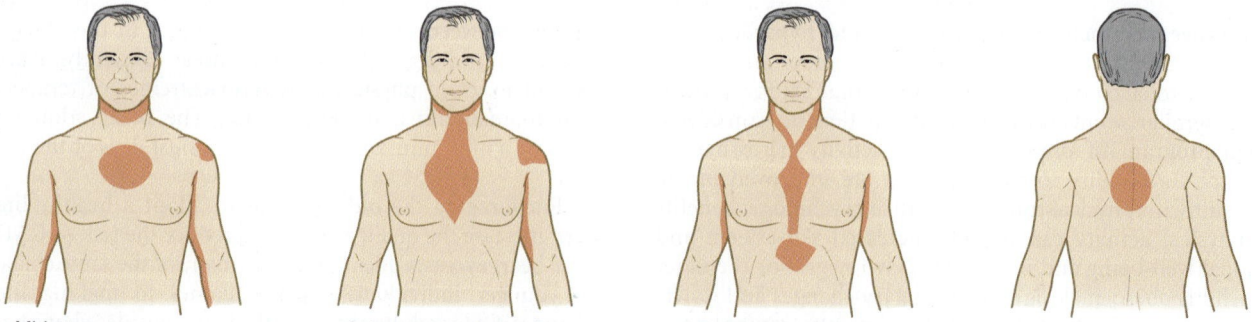

• Mid sternum
• Left shoulder and down both arms
• Neck and arms

• Substernal radiating to neck and jaw
• Substernal radiating down left arm

• Epigastric
• Epigastric radiating to neck, jaw, and arms

• Intrascapular

FIG. 33-3 Common locations and patterns of pain during angina or myocardial infarction.

TABLE 33-8 Precipitating Factors of Angina

Physical Exertion
- Increases HR, reducing the time the heart spends in diastole (the time of greatest coronary blood flow), resulting in an increase in myocardial O_2 demand.
- Isometric exercise of the arms (e.g., raking, lifting heavy objects, snow shoveling) can cause exertional angina.

Temperature Extremes
- Increase the workload of the heart.
- Blood vessels constrict in response to a cold stimulus.
- Blood vessels dilate and blood pools in the skin in response to a hot stimulus.

Strong Emotions
- Stimulate the sympathetic nervous system, activating the stress response.
- Increase the workload of the heart.

Consumption of Heavy Meal (e.g., holiday meals)
- Can increase the workload of the heart.
- During the digestive process, blood is diverted to the GI system, reducing blood flow in the coronary arteries.

Tobacco Use and Environmental Tobacco Smoke
- Diminish available O_2 by increasing the level of carbon monoxide.
- Nicotine stimulates catecholamine release, causing vasoconstriction and an increased HR.

Sexual Activity
- Increases the cardiac workload and sympathetic stimulation.
- In a person with CAD, the extra cardiac workload may precipitate angina.

Stimulants (e.g., cocaine, amphetamines)
- Increase HR and BP and subsequently increases myocardial O_2 demand.
- Stimulate vasoconstriction and subsequently decreases myocardial O_2 supply.
- May precipitate dysrhythmias

Circadian Rhythm Patterns
- Manifestations of CAD tend to occur in the early morning after awakening.

inversion indicating ischemia (see Chapter 35). The ECG returns to baseline when the pain is relieved.

Chronic stable angina is controlled with drugs on an outpatient basis. Because chronic stable angina is often predictable, drugs are timed to provide peak effects during the time of day when angina is likely to occur. For example, if angina occurs when rising, the patient can take medication as soon as awakening and wait 30 minutes to 1 hour before engaging in activity. (A comparison of the major types of angina is presented in Table 33-9.)

Silent ischemia refers to ischemia that occurs in the absence of any subjective symptoms. Patients with diabetes have an increased prevalence of silent ischemia. This is most likely due to diabetic neuropathy affecting the nerves that innervate the cardiovascular system. When patients are monitored (e.g., Holter monitor) and silent ischemia occurs, ECG changes are revealed. Ischemia with pain or without pain has the same prognosis.

TABLE 33-9 Comparison of Major Types of Angina

Type	Etiology	Characteristics
Chronic stable angina	Myocardial ischemia (usually secondary to CAD) caused by an O_2 supply/demand mismatch	• Episodic pain lasting a few minutes • Provoked by exertion or stress • Relieved by rest or nitroglycerin
Prinzmetal's angina	Coronary vasospasm	• Occurs primarily at rest • Triggered by smoking and increased levels of some substances (e.g., histamine, epinephrine, cocaine) • May occur in presence or absence of CAD
Microvascular angina	Myocardial ischemia secondary to microvascular disease affecting the small, distal branches of coronary arteries	• More common in women • Triggered by activities of daily living (e.g., shopping, work) vs. physical exercise (exertion) • Treatment may include nitroglycerin
Unstable angina	Rupture of unstable plaque, exposing thrombogenic surface	• New-onset angina • Chronic stable angina that increases in frequency, duration, or severity • Occurs at rest or with minimal exertion • Lasts more than 10 min

Prinzmetal's Angina

Prinzmetal's angina *(variant angina)* is a rare form of angina that often occurs at rest and not with increased physical demand. It is sometimes seen in patients with a history of migraine headaches, Raynaud's phenomenon, and heavy smoking. It is usually due to spasm of a major coronary artery. The spasm may occur in the presence or absence of CAD. Strong contraction (spasm) of smooth muscle in the coronary artery results from increased intracellular calcium.[21]

Factors contributing to coronary artery spasm include increased myocardial O_2 demand and increased levels of certain substances (e.g., tobacco smoke, alcohol, cocaine). When spasm occurs, the patient experiences angina and transient ST segment elevation (see Chapter 35). The pain may occur during rapid-eye-movement (REM) sleep when myocardial O_2 consumption increases or when exposed to cold temperatures. The pain may be relieved by moderate exercise, with SL NTG, or it may disappear spontaneously. Cyclic, short bursts of pain at a usual time each day may also occur with this type of angina. Calcium channel blockers and/or nitrates are used to control the pain, as well as stopping any offending substances.

Microvascular Angina

In *microvascular angina,* chest pain occurs in the absence of significant CAD or coronary spasm of a major coronary artery. In these patients, chest pain is related to myocardial ischemia associated with atherosclerosis or spasm of the small distal branch vessels of the coronary microcirculation. This is known as *coronary microvascular disease* (MVD). It is also referred to as *Syndrome X.*[4] It is more common in postmenopausal women. Often the angina in these patients is prolonged and brought on by physical exertion. These patients usually have positive stress test results and have an inconsistent response to nitrates. Prevention and treatment of coronary MVD follow the same recommendations as for CAD.[22]

INTERPROFESSIONAL CARE: CHRONIC STABLE ANGINA

The treatment of chronic stable angina aims to decrease O_2 demand and/or increase O_2 supply. The reduction of risk factors is a priority and should include those strategies discussed for patients with CAD (see pp. 707-712). In addition to antiplatelet and lipid-lowering drug therapy, the most common therapeutic interventions for the management of chronic stable angina are the use of nitrates, angiotensin-converting enzyme (ACE) inhibitors, β-blockers, and calcium channel blockers to optimize myocardial perfusion (Table 33-10 and Fig. 33-4).

Drug Therapy

Drug therapy for chronic stable angina aims to reduce symptoms and the risk of MI and death. Aspirin (previously discussed) is given in the absence of contraindications (Table 33-11).

Short-Acting Nitrates. Short-acting nitrates are first-line therapy for the treatment of angina. Nitrates produce their principal effects by the following mechanisms:

Dilating peripheral blood vessels: This results in decreased SVR, venous pooling, and decreased venous blood return to the

TABLE 33-10 Treatment of Chronic Stable Angina

*Strategies for the patient with chronic stable angina should address all the treatment elements and related patient teaching in the following mnemonic:**

Element	Treatment
A	Antiplatelet/anticoagulant therapy Antianginal therapy ACE inhibitor/angiotensin receptor blocker
B	β-blocker BP control
C	Cigarette smoking cessation Cholesterol (lipid) management Calcium channel blockers Cardiac rehabilitation
D	Diet (weight management) Diabetes management Depression screening
E	Education Exercise
F	Flu vaccination

*Modified from Smith SC, Benjamin EJ, Bonow RO, et al: AHA/ACCF secondary prevention and risk reduction therapy for patients with coronary and other atherosclerotic vascular disease: 2011 update, *J Am Coll Cardiol* 58:2432, 2011.

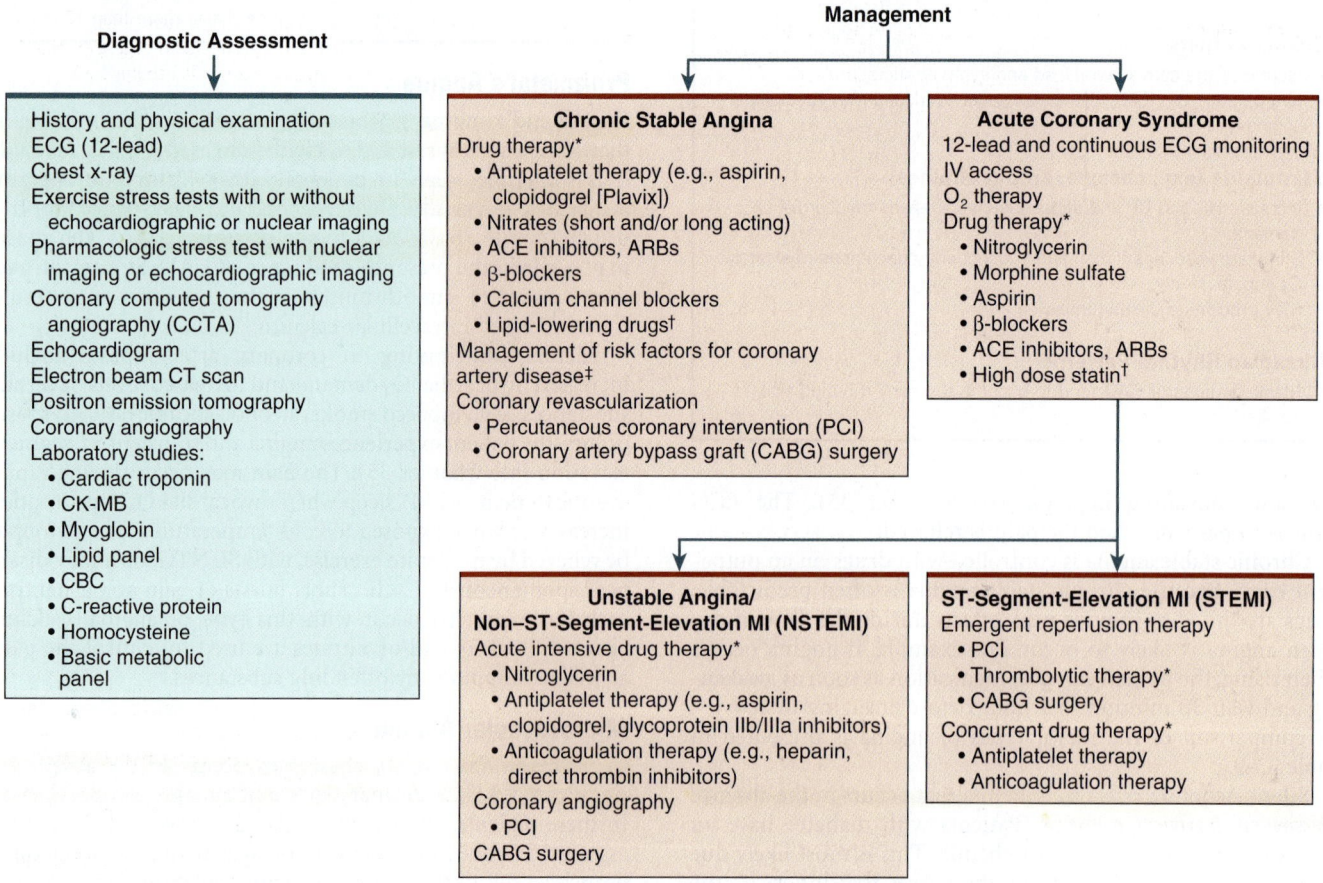

FIG. 33-4 Interprofessional care: chronic stable angina and acute coronary syndrome. *ACE,* Angiotensin-converting enzyme; *ARBs,* angiotensin II receptor blockers; *CK,* creatine kinase.
*Table 33-11.
†Table 33-5.
‡Tables 33-2, 33-3, and 33-4.

TABLE 33-11 Drug Therapy

Chronic Stable Angina and Acute Coronary Syndrome

Drug	Mechanism of Action and Comments
Antiplatelet Agents	
aspirin	• Inhibits cyclooxygenase, which in turn produces thromboxane A_2, a potent platelet activator • Should be administered as soon as ACS is suspected, unless truly allergic • Initial dose 162-325 mg, then 81-325 mg daily
cangrelor (Kengreal)	• Inhibits platelet aggregation • Given IV • Approved for use in patients having PCI
clopidogrel (Plavix)	• Inhibits platelet aggregation • Alternative for patients who cannot take aspirin • Used to treat ACS with medical therapy alone or used in combination with aspirin after PCI for chronic stable angina or ACS
prasugrel (Effient)	• Inhibits platelet aggregation • Used as an alternative to clopidogrel in combination with aspirin for patient with ACS who have PCI • Not indicated to treat ACS with medical therapy alone
ticagrelor (Brilinta)	• Inhibits platelet aggregation • Alternative for patient who cannot take aspirin • Used to treat ACS with medical therapy alone or used in combination with aspirin after PCI for ACS • If used in combination with aspirin, effectiveness may be decreased by aspirin dosages >100 mg/day (according to a boxed warning)
vorapaxar (Zontivity)	• Inhibits platelet aggregation • Increases risk of bleeding, including life-threatening and fatal bleeding (according to a boxed warning) • Must not be used in people who have had a stroke, transient ischemic attack (TIA), or bleeding in the head, because the risk of bleeding in the head is too great
Glycoprotein IIb/IIIa Inhibitors	
abciximab (ReoPro) eptifibatide (Integrilin) tirofiban (Aggrastat)	• Prevent the binding of fibrinogen to platelets, thereby blocking platelet aggregation • May be used in combination with aspirin for patients with ACS
Anticoagulant Agents	
Unfractionated Heparin*	
heparin	• Prevents conversion of fibrinogen to fibrin and prothrombin to thrombin
Low-Molecular-Weight Heparin*	
dalteparin (Fragmin) enoxaparin (Lovenox)	• Bind to antithrombin III, enhancing its effect • Heparin–antithrombin III complex inactivates activated factor X and thrombin. • Prevent conversion of fibrinogen to fibrin
Vitamin K Antagonist*	
warfarin (Coumadin)	• Interferes with hepatic synthesis of vitamin K–dependent clotting factors • Used for patients with atrial fibrillation or those who are risk for thromboembolism (large anterior wall infarctions or ventricular aneurysms) • Closely monitor for bleeding when taking with antiplatelet drugs.
Direct Thrombin Inhibitors	
bivalirudin (Angiomax) argatroban	• Direct inhibition of the clotting factor thrombin
Nitrates	
Sublingual nitroglycerin (Nitrostat) Translingual spray nitroglycerin (Nitrolingual) nitroglycerin ointment (Nitro-Bid) Transdermal nitroglycerin (Transderm-Nitro) isosorbide dinitrate (Isordil) Isosorbide mononitrate IV nitroglycerin	• Promote peripheral vasodilation, decreasing preload and afterload • Promote coronary artery vasodilation • May prevent or control coronary vasospasm
Angiotensin-Converting Enzyme (ACE) Inhibitors†	
captopril enalapril (Vasotec) lisinopril (Zestril)	• Prevent conversion of angiotensin I to angiotensin II, resulting in vasodilation • May prevent or limit ventricular remodeling • Decrease endothelial dysfunction • Useful with heart failure, decreased LV function, tachycardia, MI, hypertension, diabetes, and chronic kidney disease
Angiotensin II Receptor Blockers†	
losartan (Cozaar) valsartan (Diovan)	• Inhibit binding of angiotensin II to angiotensin I receptors, resulting in vasodilation • Used for patients intolerant of ACE inhibitors
β-Adrenergic Blockers†	
atenolol (Tenormin) carvedilol (Coreg) metoprolol (Lopressor) nadolol (Corgard)	• Inhibit sympathetic nervous stimulation of the heart • Reduce heart rate, contractility, and BP • Reduce ischemia • Decrease afterload
Calcium Channel Blockers†	
amlodipine (Norvasc) diltiazem (Cardizem) felodipine nicardipine (Cardene) verapamil (Calan) nifedipine (Procardia)	• Prevent calcium entry into vascular smooth muscle cells and myocytes (cardiac cells) • May prevent or control coronary vasospasm • Promote coronary and peripheral vasodilation • Reduce heart rate, contractility, and BP

*See Table 37-10.
†See Table 32-7.

Continued

TABLE 33-11 Drug Therapy

Chronic Stable Angina and Acute Coronary Syndrome—cont'd

Drug	Mechanism of Action and Comments
Opioid	
morphine	• Functions as an analgesic and sedative • Acts as a vasodilator to reduce preload and myocardial O_2 consumption
Thrombolytic Agents	
reteplase (Retavase) alteplase (Activase) tenecteplase (TNKase)	• Break up fibrin meshwork in clots • Used only in ST-segment–elevation MI when access to a hospital with PCI capability is not available
Lipid-Lowering Agents	
Drugs listed in Table 33-5	• Have been shown to reduce morbidity and mortality from CAD

PCI, Percutaneous coronary intervention.

heart (preload). Therefore myocardial O_2 demand is decreased because of the reduced cardiac workload.

Dilating coronary arteries and collateral vessels: This may increase blood flow to the ischemic areas of the heart. However, when the coronary arteries are severely atherosclerotic, coronary dilation is difficult to achieve.

Sublingual Nitroglycerin. SL NTG or translingual spray (Nitrolingual) usually relieves pain in about 5 minutes and lasts approximately 30 to 40 minutes. The recommended dose of NTG is one tablet taken sublingually (SL) or one metered spray on the tongue for symptoms of angina. If symptoms are unchanged or worse after 5 minutes, tell the patient or caregiver to repeat NTG every 5 minutes for a maximum of three doses and contact emergency response system (ERS) if symptoms have not resolved completely.

Instruct the patient in the proper use of NTG. It should be easily accessible to the patient at all times. The patient should store the tablets away from light and heat sources, including body heat, to protect them from degradation. Tablets are packaged in light-resistant bottles with metal caps. Once opened, the tablets lose potency, and should be replaced every 6 months.

Tell the patient to sit down and place a NTG tablet under the tongue and allow it to dissolve. If using the spray, the patient should direct it on the tongue, not inhale it. SL NTG should cause a tingling sensation when taken; otherwise it may be outdated. Warn the patient that a headache, dizziness, or flushing may occur. Caution the patient to change positions slowly after NTG use because orthostatic hypotension may occur.

Patients can use NTG prophylactically before starting an activity that is known to cause angina. In these cases the patient can take a tablet or spray 5 to 10 minutes before beginning the activity. Tell the patient to report to the HCP any changes in the usual pattern of pain, especially increasing frequency, nighttime angina, or angina at rest.

Long-Acting Nitrates. Nitrates, such as isosorbide dinitrate (Isordil) and isosorbide mononitrate, are longer acting than SL or translingual NTG. They are used to reduce the frequency of anginal attacks. The main side effect of all nitrates is headache from the dilation of cerebral blood vessels. Tell patients to take acetaminophen (Tylenol) to relieve the headache. Over time, the headaches may decrease, but the antianginal effects are still present.

Orthostatic hypotension is a complication of all nitrates. Monitor BP after the first dose, since the venous dilation that occurs may cause a drop in BP, especially in volume-depleted patients. Finally, tolerance to long-acting NTG can develop. To limit this, patients are often scheduled a 10- to 14-hour nitrate-free period every day. Remind patients that taking a long-acting NTG preparation should not keep them from using translingual or SL NTG if angina develops.

Nitroglycerin Ointment. Nitropaste is a 2% NTG topical ointment dosed by the inch. It is placed on the upper body or arm, over a flat muscular area that is free of hair and scars. Once absorbed, it produces anginal prophylaxis for 3 to 6 hours. It is especially useful for nighttime and UA. The ointment should be wiped off to allow for a 10- to 14-hour nitrate-free interval in order to prevent nitrate tolerance.

Transdermal Controlled-Release Nitrates. Currently two systems are available for transdermal NTG drug delivery: silicone gel and polymer matrix. These systems allow timed release of NTG over a 24-hour period. These preparations should also be removed in the evening to allow for a 10- to 14-hour nitrate-free interval.

DRUG ALERT Nitrates

- NTG tablets must be kept in a dark, airtight container to maintain potency.
- SL NTG must be placed under the tongue.
- Translingual NTG should be sprayed on the tongue, not under the tongue.
- Tell patient not to combine with drugs used for erectile dysfunction (e.g., sildenafil [Viagra]) as severe hypotension can occur.
- Monitor for orthostatic hypotension because it may occur after administration.
- Headaches are common after taking any NTG preparation.
- Use gloves to apply and remove NTG ointment or transdermal patches to avoid contact with drug.
- Never discharge a cardioverter-defibrillator over NTG ointment or transdermal patch.
- When using long-acting nitrates, provide a 10- to 14-hour nitrate-free period.

Angiotensin-Converting Enzyme (ACE) Inhibitors and Angiotensin Receptor Blockers (ARBs). Patients with chronic stable angina who have an ejection fraction (EF) of 40% or less, diabetes, hypertension, or chronic kidney disease should take an ACE inhibitor (e.g., lisinopril [Zestril]) indefinitely, unless contraindicated. Patients with chronic stable angina and a normal EF, diabetes, and one other CAD risk factor should also take an ACE inhibitor to decrease the risk of MI, stroke, and death.

These drugs result in vasodilation and reduced blood volume. Most important, they can prevent or reverse ventricular remodeling in patients who have had an MI (see pp. 725-726). For patients who are intolerant of ACE inhibitors (e.g., cough, angioedema), ARBs (e.g., losartan [Cozaar]) are used. (ACE inhibitors and ARBs are discussed later in the chapter and in Chapter 32 and Table 32-7).

β-Adrenergic Blockers. β-Blockers are ordered for relief of angina symptoms in patients with chronic stable angina. Patients who have LV dysfunction, elevated BP, or have had an MI should start and continue β-blockers indefinitely, unless contraindicated. These drugs decrease myocardial contractility, HR, SVR, and BP, all of which reduce the myocardial O_2 demand. β-Blockers that have been shown to reduce the risk of death in patients with LV dysfunction, heart failure (HF), or MI are carvedilol (Coreg), metoprolol (Lopressor, Toprol XL), and bisoprolol (Zebeta).[5]

β-Blockers have many side effects and can be poorly tolerated. Side effects may include bradycardia, hypotension, wheezing from bronchospasm, and GI complaints. Many patients also complain of weight gain, depression, fatigue, and sexual dysfunction. Absolute contraindications to using β-blockers include severe bradycardia and acute HF. Patients with asthma should avoid β-blockers. They are used cautiously in patients with diabetes, since they mask signs of hypoglycemia. β-Blockers should not be stopped abruptly without medical supervision, as this may result in an increase in the number and intensity of angina attacks.

Calcium Channel Blockers. If β-blockers are contraindicated, are poorly tolerated, or do not control anginal symptoms, calcium channel blockers are used. The primary effects of calcium channel blockers are (1) systemic vasodilation with decreased SVR, (2) decreased myocardial contractility, (3) coronary vasodilation, and (4) decreased HR.

There are two groups of calcium channel blockers. The dihydropyridines (e.g., amlodipine [Norvasc]), which have more vasodilatory effects, and the nondihydropyridines (e.g., verapamil [Calan], diltiazem [Cardizem]), which have more rate and contractility effects.

Calcium channel blockers enhance the action of digoxin by increasing serum digoxin levels (see Chapter 34). Therefore serum digoxin levels should be closely monitored after starting calcium channel blockers. Teach the patient the signs and symptoms of digoxin toxicity. Verapamil can cause severe constipation, especially in older adults.[5]

Lipid-Lowering Drugs. Although patients with chronic stable angina are encouraged to follow a diet low in saturated fat and cholesterol, a moderate or high dose of a lipid-lowering drug should be ordered, unless contraindicated.

Sodium Current Inhibitor. Ranolazine (Ranexa), a sodium current inhibitor, is used to treat chronic angina in patients who have not had an adequate response with other antianginals. It is not a first-line drug for chronic stable angina. Because ranolazine prolongs the QT interval, patients with a long QT interval or who are taking QT-prolonging drugs (e.g., fluoxetine [Prozac]) should not use it (see Chapter 35). Common side effects of ranolazine include dizziness, nausea, constipation, and headache.

Diagnostic Studies

When CAD is suspected in a patient or when a patient with chronic stable angina has a change in the anginal pattern, a variety of studies are completed (Fig. 33-4). After a detailed health history and physical examination, a chest x-ray is done to look for cardiac enlargement, aortic calcifications, and pulmonary congestion. A 12-lead ECG is done and compared with a previous ECG whenever possible to look for any changes. Laboratory tests (e.g., lipid profile, C-reactive protein) are done to identify specific risk factors for CAD. An echocardiogram may be done to look for resting LV wall motion abnormalities, which may suggest evidence of CAD. An exercise stress test with or without echocardiography or nuclear imaging may be ordered. For patients with physical limitations in walking, a pharmacologic (adenosine [Adenocard] or dipyridamole [Persantine]) stress test with nuclear imaging, or a pharmacologic (dobutamine [Dobutrex]) stress echocardiogram may be ordered. Coronary blockages less than 70% are not usually detected with stress testing.[5] (See Chapter 31 and Table 31-6 for a discussion of these studies, including nursing considerations.)

The electron beam computed tomography (EBCT) scan locates and measures coronary calcification (see Fig. 31-11). However, additional testing (e.g., stress testing or heart catheterization) is needed to further assess the impact of the lesion on coronary blood flow. Further studies are needed to determine the accuracy of the EBCT scan to diagnose high-grade blockages because many atherosclerotic plaques are not calcified.

Coronary computed tomography angiography (CCTA) may be considered. Using IV contrast and radiation, CCTA can detect calcified and noncalcified plaques in the artery, as well as other heart conditions. Limitations of using CCTA include patients with rapid HRs (greater than 90 beats per minute), extensive coronary artery calcifications, obesity, and a history of prior coronary artery stent. Patients allergic to IV contrast dye must be premedicated with corticosteroids. Patients with chronic kidney disease need hydration pre- and postprocedure. A baseline serum creatinine level should be obtained as the IV contrast dye can cause or worsen renal dysfunction.

Cardiac Catheterization. For patients with increasing angina symptoms, a cardiac catheterization is ordered. Cardiac catheterization and coronary angiography use radiation and IV contrast dye to provide images of the coronary circulation and identify the location and severity of any blockage. A patient who is allergic to IV contrast dye must be premedicated with corticosteroids. Patients with chronic kidney disease need hydration pre- and postprocedure. A baseline serum creatinine level is obtained because the IV contrast dye can cause or worsen renal dysfunction. Monitor renal function closely after the procedure. This procedure should only be done if the patient is a candidate for percutaneous or surgical coronary revascularization.

If a coronary blockage is amenable to treatment, **coronary revascularization** with an elective **percutaneous coronary intervention (PCI)** may be recommended. PCI may be done at the same time as the catheterization or at a later date. During PCI, a catheter with a deflated balloon tip is inserted into the appropriate coronary artery. The deflated balloon is positioned in the blockage and inflated. This compresses the plaque against the artery wall, resulting in vessel dilation and a larger vessel diameter. This procedure is called *balloon angioplasty.*

Intracoronary stents are usually placed along with balloon angioplasty. A **stent** is an expandable mesh-like structure designed to keep the vessel open after balloon angioplasty. It provides support to the arterial wall (Figs. 33-5 and 33-6). Because stents are thrombogenic, many different types of drugs are used to prevent platelet aggregation within the stent. Drugs commonly used during PCI are unfractionated heparin (UH) or low-molecular-weight heparin (LMWH), a direct thrombin inhibitor (e.g., bivalirudin [Angiomax]), and/or a glycoprotein IIb/IIIa inhibitor (e.g., eptifibatide [Integrilin]) (Table 33-11).

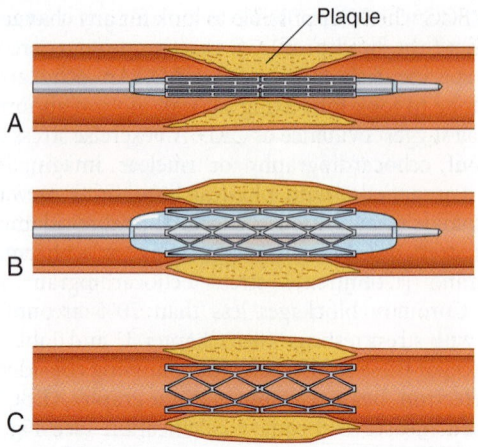

FIG. 33-5 Placement of a coronary artery stent. **A,** The stent is positioned at the site of the lesion. **B,** The balloon is inflated, expanding the stent. The balloon is then deflated and removed. **C,** The implanted stent is left in place.

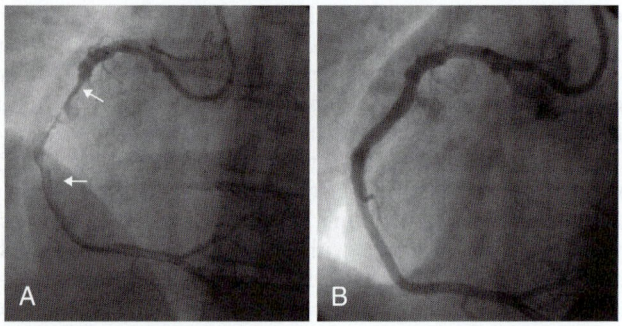

FIG. 33-6 **A,** A thrombotic occlusion of the right coronary artery is noted *(arrows).* **B,** Right coronary artery is opened and blood flow restored following angioplasty and placement of a 4-mm stent. (From Zipes DB, Libby P, Bonow RO, Braunwald E: *Braunwald's heart disease: a textbook of cardiovascular medicine,* ed 7, St Louis, 2005, Saunders.)

After PCI, the patient is treated with dual antiplatelet drugs (e.g., aspirin [indefinitely] and clopidogrel) up to 12 months or longer, until the intimal lining grows over the stent and provides a smooth vascular surface.

There are two types of stents: bare metal stents (BMS) and drug-eluting stents (DES). DESs are coated with a drug (e.g., paclitaxel, everolimus) to reduce the risk of overgrowth of the intimal lining *(neointimal hyperplasia)* within the stent. This is the primary cause of in-stent restenosis (ISR). Following DES placement, dual antiplatelet drugs are taken to prevent thrombus formation within the stent (stent thrombosis) for a minimum of 12 months or longer. The duration of dual antiplatelet drugs for patients with BMS is a minimum of 1 month but ideally 1 full year after PCI.[20] Some DES are gradually absorbed by the body in approximately 3 years.

Potential complications from cardiac catheterization with PCI include abrupt closure from coronary artery dissection, vascular injury at the artery access site (e.g., femoral, radial), acute MI, stent embolization, coronary spasm, dye allergy, renal compromise, bleeding (e.g., retroperitoneal), infection, stroke, and emergent coronary artery bypass graft (CABG) surgery. The possibility of dysrhythmias during and after the procedure is always present.

PCI may not be a feasible option for all patients (e.g., patients with three-vessel CAD [three different coronary arteries] and/or significant left main coronary artery disease). Coronary revascularization with CABG surgery may be recommended and is discussed later in the chapter.

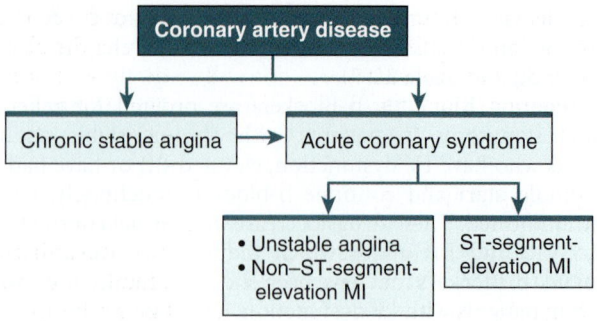

FIG. 33-7 Relationships among coronary artery disease, chronic stable angina, and acute coronary syndrome.

Alternative Therapies for Refractory Chronic Stable Angina

For patients with refractory stable angina, *enhanced external counterpulsation* (EECP) may be used. EECP consists of placing inflatable BP cuffs around the legs. The cuffs sequentially inflate during diastole and deflate during systole from the calves to the thighs. This action is thought to increase venous return and augment diastolic BP in order to increase coronary perfusion, improve LV diastolic filling, and help with collateral circulation. Patients get treatments 5 days a week for a total of 35 treatments. EECP is contraindicated in patients with decompensated HF, severe peripheral arterial disease, and severe aortic insufficiency.

Spinal cord stimulation may also help relieve symptoms in patients who are refractory to drugs or revascularization. The stimulation lead is placed in the epidural space between T1 and T2 and is connected to an implanted subcutaneous pulse generator. The mechanism by which angina is reduced is not well understood.

ACUTE CORONARY SYNDROME

When ischemia is prolonged and not immediately reversible, **acute coronary syndrome (ACS)** develops. ACS includes the spectrum of UA, *non–ST-segment-elevation myocardial infarction* (NSTEMI), and *ST-segment-elevation myocardial infarction* (STEMI) (Fig. 33-7). When patients first present with chest pain, ST-elevations on the 12-lead ECG are most likely indicative of a STEMI. The ECG should always be compared to a previous ECG whenever possible. For patients with chest pain who do not show ST segement elevation or ST-T wave changes on the ECG, it is difficult to distinguish between UA and NSTEMI until serum cardiac biomarkers are measured.[23]

On the cellular level, the heart muscle becomes hypoxic within the first 10 seconds of a total coronary occlusion. Heart cells are deprived of O_2 and glucose needed for aerobic metabolism and contractility. Anaerobic metabolism begins and lactic acid accumulates. In ischemic conditions, heart cells are viable for approximately 20 minutes. Irreversible heart damage starts after 20 minutes if there is no collateral circulation[21] (Fig. 33-2). With restoration of blood flow (reperfusion), aerobic metabolism resumes, contractility is restored, and cellular repair begins.

ACS is caused by the decline of a once-stable atherosclerotic plaque. The previously stable plaque ruptures, releasing substances into the vessel. This causes platelet aggregation and thrombus formation. The vessel may be partially blocked by a thrombus (manifesting as UA or NSTEMI) or totally blocked by a thrombus (manifesting as STEMI). What causes the plaque to suddenly become unstable is not well understood, but systemic inflammation (described earlier) is thought to play a role. Patients with suspected ACS need immediate hospitalization.

UNSTABLE ANGINA

Unstable angina (UA) is chest pain that is new in onset, occurs at rest, or occurs with increasing frequency, duration, or with less effort than the patient's chronic stable angina pattern. The pain usually lasts 10 minutes or more. Prompt treatment is needed for patients with suspected UA.

The patient with chronic stable angina may develop UA, or UA may be the first clinical sign of CAD. Unlike chronic stable angina, UA is unpredictable. The patient with previously diagnosed chronic stable angina describes a significant change in the pattern of angina. It occurs with increasing frequency and is easily provoked by minimal or no exertion, during sleep, or even at rest. The patient without previously diagnosed angina describes anginal pain that has progressed rapidly in the past few hours, days, or weeks, often ending in pain at rest.

Women seek medical attention for symptoms of UA more often than men. Despite efforts to increase awareness, women's symptoms continue to be underrecognized as heart related. These symptoms include fatigue, shortness of breath, indigestion, and anxiety. Fatigue is the most prominent symptom.[4] However, all these symptoms can relate to many different diseases and syndromes. Thus women often present with UA before CAD is diagnosed. (See Gender Differences box on p. 705 earlier in this chapter.)

MYOCARDIAL INFARCTION: ST-ELEVATION AND NON–ST-ELEVATION

A **myocardial infarction (MI)** occurs because of abrupt stoppage of blood flow through a coronary artery from a thrombus caused by platelet aggregation. This causes irreversible myocardial cell death (necrosis) in the heart muscle beyond the blockage (Figs. 33-8 and 33-9). Most MIs occur in the setting of preexisting CAD.[21]

A STEMI caused by an occlusive thrombus creates ST-elevation in the ECG leads facing the area of infarction (see Figs. 35-28 and 35-30). A STEMI is an emergency situation. In order to limit the infarct size, the artery must be opened within 90 minutes of presentation. This can be done either by PCI or thrombolytic (fibrinolytic) therapy. PCI is the first-line treatment if a hospital is capable of performing PCI.

NSTEMI, caused by a nonocclusive thrombus, does not cause ST segment elevation on the 12-lead ECG. Patients may or may not develop ST-T wave changes in the leads affected by the infarction. NSTEMI patients do not go to the catheterization laboratory emergently but usually undergo the procedure within 12 to 72 hours if there are no contraindications. Thrombolytic therapy is not indicated for NSTEMI patients.

With either a NSTEMI or STEMI, an echocardiogram may show *hypokinesis* (worsening myocardial contractility) or *akinesis* (absent myocardial contractility) in the necrotic area(s). The degree of LV dysfunction depends on the area of the heart involved and size of the infarction.

The acute MI process evolves over time. The earliest tissue to become ischemic is the subendocardium (the innermost layer of tissue in the heart muscle). If ischemia persists, it takes approximately 4 to 6 hours for the entire thickness of the heart muscle to become necrosed. If the thrombus is not completely blocking the artery, the time to complete necrosis may be as long as 12 hours.

The majority of MIs affect the LV and are usually described based on the location of damage (e.g., anterior, inferior, lateral, septal, or posterior wall infarction). The location of the MI and ECG changes correlate with the involved coronary artery (see Table 35-14). For example, in most people, the right coronary artery provides blood to the inferior and posterior LV walls. Blockage of the right coronary artery results in an inferior wall and/or posterior wall MI. Anterior wall infarctions result from blockages in the left anterior descending artery. Blockages in the left circumflex artery usually cause lateral LV wall MIs. Damage can occur in more than one location, especially if more than one coronary artery is involved (e.g., anterolateral MI). Right ventricular MIs are much less common and treated differently than LV MIs.

Not everyone develops collateral circulation, but if present, the degree of collateral circulation influences the severity of the MI (Fig. 33-2). A person with a long history of CAD may develop good collateral circulation to provide the area surrounding the infarction site with a blood supply. This is one

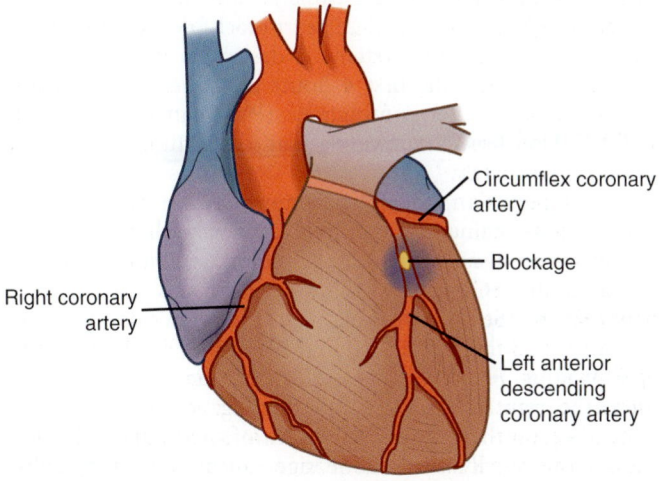

FIG. 33-8 Occlusion of the left anterior descending coronary artery, resulting in a myocardial infarction.

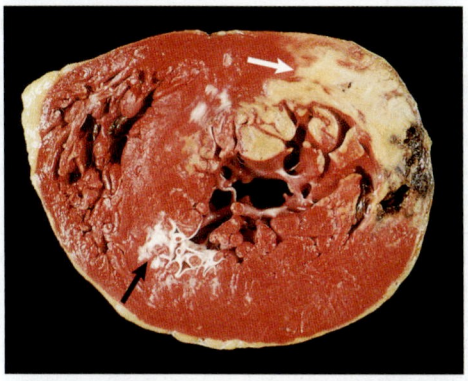

FIG. 33-9 Acute myocardial infarction in the posterolateral wall of the left ventricle. This is demonstrated by the absence of staining in the areas of necrosis *(white arrow)*. Note the scarring from a previous anterior wall myocardial infarction *(black arrow)*. (From Kumar V, Abbas AK, Aster JC, Fausto N: *Robbins and Cotran pathologic basis of disease*, ed 8, Philadelphia, 2010, Saunders.)

reason why a younger person may have a more serious first MI than an older person with the same degree of blockage.

Clinical Manifestations of Myocardial Infarction

Pain. Severe chest pain not relieved by rest, position change, or nitrate administration is the hallmark of an MI. Persistent and unlike any other pain, it is usually described as heavy, pressure, tight, burning, constricted, or crushing feeling. Common locations are substernal or epigastric areas. The pain may radiate to the neck, lower jaw, and arms or to the back (Fig. 33-3). When epigastric pain is present, the patient may relate it to indigestion and take antacids without relief. It may occur while the patient is active or at rest, asleep, or awake. However, it often occurs in the early morning hours. It usually lasts for 20 minutes or longer and is more severe than usual anginal pain.

Not everyone who has an MI has classic symptoms. Some patients may not experience pain but may have "discomfort," weakness, nausea, indigestion, or shortness of breath. Although women and men have more similarities than differences in their acute MI symptoms, some women may experience atypical discomfort, shortness of breath, or fatigue. Patients with diabetes may experience silent (asymptomatic) MIs because of cardiac neuropathy or may manifest atypical symptoms (e.g., dyspnea). An older patient may experience a change in mental status (e.g., confusion), shortness of breath, pulmonary edema, dizziness, or a dysrhythmia.

Sympathetic Nervous System Stimulation. During the initial phase of MI, the ischemic heart cells release catecholamines (norepinephrine and epinephrine) that are normally found in these cells. This results in release of glycogen, diaphoresis, increased HR and BP, and vasoconstriction of peripheral blood vessels. On physical examination, the patient's skin may be ashen, clammy, and cool to touch.

Cardiovascular Manifestations. In response to the release of catecholamines, BP and HR may be elevated initially. Later, the BP may drop because of decreased cardiac output (CO). If severe enough, this may result in decreased renal perfusion and urine output. Crackles, if present, may persist for several hours to several days, suggesting LV dysfunction. Jugular venous distention, hepatic engorgement, and peripheral edema may indicate right ventricular dysfunction.

Examination may reveal abnormal heart sounds that may seem distant. Other abnormal sounds suggesting LV dysfunction are S_3 and S_4. In addition, a loud holosystolic murmur may develop. This may indicate a ventricular septal defect, papillary muscle rupture, or valve dysfunction.

Nausea and Vomiting. The patient may experience nausea and vomiting. These symptoms can result from reflex stimulation of the vomiting center by the severe pain. They can also result from vasovagal reflexes initiated from the area of the infarcted heart muscle.

Fever. The temperature may increase to 100.4° F (38° C) within 24 to 48 hours. The temperature elevation may last for as long as 4 to 5 days. This increase in temperature is due to a systemic inflammatory process caused by the death of heart cells.

Healing Process

The body's response to cell death is the inflammatory process (see Chapter 11). Within 24 hours, leukocytes infiltrate the area. The dead heart cells release enzymes that are important diagnostic indicators of MI (see serum cardiac biomarkers later in this chapter). The proteolytic enzymes of the neutrophils and macrophages begin to remove necrotic tissue by the fourth day. During this time the necrotic muscle wall is thin. Once infarction takes place, catecholamine-mediated lipolysis and glycogenolysis occur. These processes allow the increased plasma glucose and free fatty acids to be used by the O_2-depleted myocardium for anaerobic metabolism. For this reason, serum glucose levels are frequently elevated after MI.

The necrotic zone of an STEMI is identified by ECG changes (e.g., lowering of the ST segments, T wave inversion plus a pathologic Q wave) within a day or two. At this point, the neutrophils and monocytes have cleared the necrotic debris from the injured area, and the collagen matrix that will eventually form scar tissue is laid down.

At 10 to 14 days after MI, the new scar tissue is still weak. The heart muscle is vulnerable to increased stress during this time because of the unstable state of the healing heart. At the same time the patient's activity level may be increasing, so special caution and assessment are necessary. By 6 weeks after MI, scar tissue has replaced necrotic tissue and the injured area is considered healed. Often the scarred area is less compliant than the surrounding area. This condition may be manifested by abnormal wall motion on an echocardiogram or nuclear imaging, LV dysfunction, altered conduction patterns, or HF.

These changes in the infarcted heart muscle also cause changes in the unaffected areas. In an attempt to compensate for the damaged muscle, the normal myocardium hypertrophies and dilates. This process is called *ventricular remodeling.* Remodeling of normal myocardium can lead to the development of late HF, especially in the person with atherosclerosis of other coronary arteries and/or an anterior MI. ACE inhibitors are given to limit ventricular remodeling.

Complications of Myocardial Infarction

Dysrhythmias. Any condition that affects the heart cells' sensitivity to nerve impulses (e.g., ischemia, electrolyte imbalances, SNS stimulation) can cause dysrhythmias that adversely affect the damaged heart muscle. Dysrhythmias are the most common complication after an MI. They occur in 80% to 90% of patients. Ventricular tachycardia (VT) and ventricular fibrillation (VF) are the most common cause of death in patients in the prehospital period. If a patient survives a cardiac arrest, start therapeutic hypothermia (also known as targeted temperature management) as soon as possible.[20] (See Chapter 68 for a discussion of therapeutic hypothermia.)

Bradycardias (e.g., complete heart block) develop when key areas of the conduction system are destroyed. VT or VF most often occur within the first 4 hours after the onset of pain. Premature ventricular contractions (PVCs) may precede VT and VF. Life-threatening ventricular dysrhythmias must be treated immediately.

With reperfusion, it is not uncommon to see PVCs, asymptomatic nonsustained VT, and idioventricular rhythms. These rhythms are not associated with an increased risk of sudden cardiac death (SCD) and are not treated unless the patient is symptomatic. (See Chapter 35 for a detailed description of dysrhythmias and their management.)

Heart Failure. *Heart failure* (HF) is a complication that occurs when the right or left heart's pumping action is reduced. Depending on the severity and extent of the injury, left-sided HF occurs initially with subtle signs such as mild dyspnea, restlessness, agitation, or slight tachycardia. Other signs indicating the onset of left-sided HF include pulmonary congestion on chest x-ray, S_3 or S_4 heart sounds on auscultation of the heart, crackles on auscultation of the lungs, paroxysmal nocturnal dyspnea (PND), and orthopnea. Signs of right-sided HF include jugular venous distention, hepatic congestion, or lower extremity edema. (The treatment of acute decompensated HF is discussed in Chapter 34.)

Cardiogenic Shock. *Cardiogenic shock* occurs when O_2 and nutrients supplied to the tissues are inadequate because of severe LV failure, papillary muscle rupture, ventricular septal rupture, LV free wall rupture, or right ventricular infarction. This occurs less often with the early and rapid treatment of STEMI with PCI or thrombolytic therapy. When cardiogenic shock does occur, it is associated with a high death rate. Cardiogenic shock requires aggressive management. This includes control of dysrhythmias, intraaortic balloon pump (IABP) therapy, and support of contractility with vasoactive drugs. Goals of therapy are to maximize O_2 delivery, reduce O_2 demand, and prevent complications (e.g., acute kidney injury). (Cardiogenic shock is discussed in Chapter 66.)

Papillary Muscle Dysfunction or Rupture. *Papillary muscle dysfunction* may occur if the infarcted area includes or is near the papillary muscle that attaches to the mitral valve (see Fig. 31-2). Suspect papillary muscle dysfunction if you hear a new murmur at the cardiac apex. An echocardiogram confirms the diagnosis.

Papillary muscle rupture is a rare and life-threatening complication. It causes immediate and massive mitral valve regurgitation with no time for the heart to compensate. This is not the case with mitral regurgitation, which has a gradual onset. Dyspnea, pulmonary edema, and decreased CO result from the backup of blood in the left atrium. This condition aggravates an already damaged LV by reducing CO even further. The patient undergoes rapid clinical decline. Treatment includes afterload reduction with nitroprusside (Nipride) and/or IABP therapy and immediate cardiac surgery with mitral valve repair or replacement. (See Chapter 36 for discussion of valve disorders.)

Left Ventricular Aneurysm. *Left ventricular aneurysm* results when the infarcted heart wall is thin and bulges out during contraction. This can develop within a few days, weeks, or months. It is more common with anterior MIs. The patient with a ventricular aneurysm may experience HF, dysrhythmias, and angina. Besides ventricular rupture, which is usually fatal, ventricular aneurysms can hide thrombi that can lead to an embolic stroke. Anticoagulation therapy is recommended for these patients if not contraindicated.

Ventricular Septal Wall Rupture and Left Ventricular Free Wall Rupture. A new loud systolic murmur heard in patients with acute MI may signal ventricular septal wall rupture. Depending on the size of the defect and degree of right and LV dysfunction, HF and cardiogenic shock may occur. The patient must receive emergency repair, either surgically or percutaneously. The defect can quickly expand and lead to hemodynamic compromise.

LV free wall rupture is an emergent clinical situation. Rapid hemodynamic compromise and death ensues if not treated immediately. Although this is a rare complication, death rates are high. Free wall rupture is seen more frequently in patients suffering their first MI, patients with anterior MIs, older adults, and women.[20]

Pericarditis. *Acute pericarditis,* an inflammation of the visceral and/or parietal pericardium, may occur 2 or 3 days after an acute MI. Pericarditis is characterized by mild to severe chest pain that increases with inspiration, coughing, and movement of the upper body. Sitting in a forward position often relieves the pain. The pain is usually different from pain associated with an MI.

Assess the patient with suspected pericarditis for the presence of a friction rub over the pericardium. The sound is best heard with the diaphragm of the stethoscope at the mid to lower left sternal border. It may be persistent or intermittent. Fever may also be present. The patient may have hypotension and/or a narrow pulse pressure if it is complicated by a pericardial effusion or cardiac tamponade.

Diagnosis of pericarditis can be made with serial 12-lead ECGs. Typical ECG changes include diffuse ST segment elevations. This reflects the inflammation of the pericardium. Treatment includes pain relief with high doses of aspirin (e.g., 650 mg every 4 to 6 hours). (Pericarditis is discussed in Chapter 36.)

Dressler Syndrome. *Dressler syndrome* is pericarditis and fever that develop 1 to 8 weeks after MI. Although the cause is unclear, it may be an autoimmune reaction to the necrotic heart muscle. The patient experiences chest pain, fever, malaise, a pericardial friction rub, and arthralgia. A pericardial effusion may be present. Laboratory findings include an elevated white blood cell count and sedimentation rate. High-dose aspirin is the treatment of choice. Nonsteroidal antiinflammatory drugs (NSAIDs) and corticosteroids are avoided in the first 4 weeks following MI because they can interfere with myocardial scar formation.

DIAGNOSTIC STUDIES: ACUTE CORONARY SYNDROME

In addition to the patient's history of pain, risk factors, and health history, the primary diagnostic studies used to determine whether a person has UA or an MI include an ECG and serum cardiac biomarkers (Fig. 33-4).

Electrocardiogram Findings

The ECG is one of the primary tools to diagnose UA or an MI (STEMI or NSTEMI). Whenever possible, it should be compared to a previous ECG. Changes in the QRS complex, ST segment, and T wave caused by ischemia and infarction can develop slowly or quickly with UA and MI.

The ECG must be read carefully, since changes can be absent or subtle at first. For this reason, serial 12-lead ECGs are done. For diagnostic and treatment purposes, it is important to distinguish between STEMI and NSTEMI/UA. STEMI patients usually have a complete coronary occlusion. ST elevation is first seen on the 12-lead ECG. Within a few hours to days, T wave inversion and pathologic Q waves develop. Patients with NSTEMI or UA usually have transient thrombosis or incomplete coronary occlusion. These patients often develop ST depression or T wave inversion on the initial ECG. They usually do not develop pathologic Q waves. Because MI is a dynamic process that evolves over time, serial ECGs are done to show the evolution of ischemia, injury, infarction, and resolution of the infarction. (See Chapter 35 for discussion of ECG changes associated with ischemia and MI and Fig. 35-29.)

Serum Cardiac Biomarkers

Serum cardiac biomarkers are proteins released into the blood from necrotic heart muscle after an MI (see Table 31-6). These

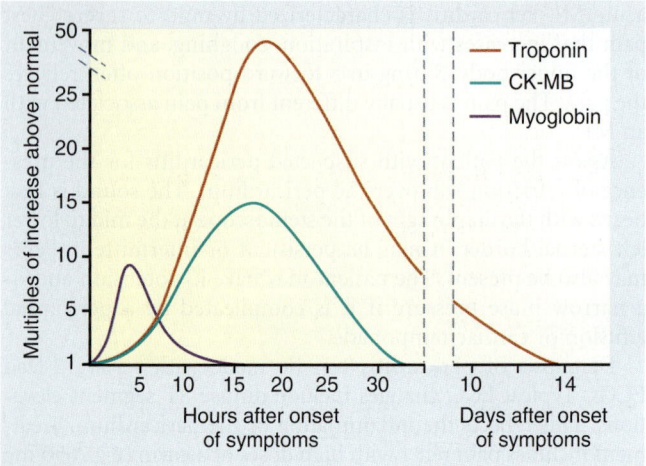

FIG. 33-10 Serum cardiac biomarkers found in the blood after myocardial infarction.

biomarkers are important in the diagnosis of MI. The onset, peak, and duration of levels of these biomarkers are shown in Fig. 33-10.

Cardiac-specific troponin has two subtypes: cardiac-specific troponin T (cTnT) and cardiac-specific troponin I (cTnI). These biomarkers are highly specific indicators of MI and have greater sensitivity and specificity for myocardial injury than creatine kinase MB (CK-MB). Serum levels of cTnI and cTnT increase 4 to 6 hours after the onset of MI, peak at 10 to 24 hours, and return to baseline over 10 to 14 days. Serial cardiac biomarkers are drawn over 24 hours (e.g., every 6 hours × 3). The presence of biomarkers helps to differentiate between a diagnosis of UA (negative biomarkers) and NSTEMI (positive biomarkers).

CK levels begin to rise about 6 hours after an MI, peak at about 18 hours, and return to normal within 24 to 36 hours. The CK enzymes are fractionated into bands. The CK-MB band is specific to heart muscle cells and helps to quantify myocardial damage.

Myoglobin is released into the circulation within 2 hours after an MI and peaks in 3 to 15 hours. Although it is one of the first serum cardiac biomarkers to appear after an MI, it lacks cardiac specificity. Its role in diagnosing MI is limited.

Coronary Angiography

The patient with a STEMI must undergo coronary angiography within 90 minutes of presentation or receive thrombolytic therapy within 30 minutes in agencies without PCI capability. This will open the totally occluded artery and limit the infarction size. The patient with UA or NSTEMI may or may not undergo coronary angiography to evaluate the extent of the disease. Guidelines suggest that it is reasonable to do coronary angiography on stable but high-risk patients with UA or NSTEMI within 12 to 72 hours after presentation. If appropriate, a PCI is performed at this time. Some patients may be treated only with conservative medical management.[23]

Other Measures

When the ECG and serum cardiac biomarkers do not confirm MI, other measures for diagnosing CAD are considered (see Table 31-6). To assess for ischemia or infarction, pharmacologic stress testing may be done when a patient has an abnormal but nondiagnostic ECG and negative biomarkers. (See Chapter 31 for additional information on cardiac assessment.)

INTERPROFESSIONAL CARE: ACUTE CORONARY SYNDROME

It is extremely important to quickly diagnose and treat a patient with ACS to preserve heart muscle. Initial management of the patient with chest pain most often occurs in the ED. Table 33-12 presents the emergency care of the patient with chest pain. Obtain a 12-lead ECG and start continuous ECG monitoring. Position the patient in an upright position unless contraindicated, and start O_2 by nasal cannula to keep O_2 saturation above 93%. Obtain IV access for drug administration. Give SL NTG and 162 to 325 mg of aspirin (chewable) if not given before arrival at the ED. A high-dose statin (atorvastatin [Lipitor]) is started if not already taking prior to the hospitalization. Morphine sulfate is given for pain unrelieved by NTG.

The patient is usually transferred to a critical care unit where ongoing care including continuous ECG monitoring is available. Dysrhythmias are treated according to agency protocols. Some patients are started on glycoprotein IIb/IIIa inhibitors (e.g., eptifibatide) either before catheterization or at the time of PCI. Fig. 33-4 on p. 714 presents the interprofessional care of ACS.

Monitor vital signs (including pulse oximetry) frequently (e.g., every hour) during the first few hours after admission and closely thereafter, according to agency protocol. Maintain bed rest and limit activity for 12 to 24 hours, with a gradual increase in activity unless contraindicated.

For patients with UA and NSTEMI, aspirin and heparin (UH or LMWH) are recommended. Dual antiplatelet therapy (e.g., aspirin and clopidogrel) (Table 33-11) and heparin are recommended for NSTEMI patients. Cardiac catheterization with possible PCI is considered for both UA and NSTEMI patients once the patient is stabilized and angina is controlled or if angina returns or increases in severity.

For patients with STEMI, reperfusion therapy is started (Figs. 33-6 and 33-7). *Reperfusion therapy* includes emergent PCI (preferred) or thrombolytic therapy for STEMI. The goal in the treatment of STEMI is to save as much heart muscle as possible. Dual antiplatelet therapy and heparin are also used.

Emergent PCI

Emergent PCI is the first line of treatment for patients with confirmed STEMI (i.e., ST-elevation on the ECG and/or positive cardiac biomarkers). The goal is to open the blocked artery within 90 minutes of arrival to a facility that has an interventional cardiac catheterization laboratory. In this case the patient undergoes a cardiac catheterization to locate and assess the severity of the blockage(s), determine the presence of collateral circulation, and evaluate LV function. During the procedure, a bare metal stent (BMS) or drug-eluting stent (DES) is inserted into the blocked coronary artery. Additional arteries may also be stented at this time if appropriate.[20] Patients with severe LV dysfunction may require the addition of IABP therapy and/or inotropes (e.g., dobutamine). A small percentage of patients may require emergent CABG surgery.

The advantages of PCI (compared to thrombolytic therapy) include the following: (1) it provides an alternative to surgical

TABLE 33-12 Emergency Management

Chest Pain

Etiology	Assessment Findings	Interventions
Cardiovascular • Myocardial ischemia • Myocardial infarction • Dysrhythmia • Pericarditis • Aortic aneurysm • Aortic valve disease **Respiratory** • Costochondritis • Pleurisy • Pneumonia • Pneumothorax, hemothorax • Pulmonary edema • Pulmonary embolus **Chest Trauma** • Rib/sternal fracture • Flail chest • Cardiac tamponade • Hemothorax • Pulmonary contusion • Great vessel injury **Gastrointestinal** • Esophagitis • GERD • Hiatal hernia • Peptic ulcer • Cholecystitis **Others** • Stress • Strenuous exercise • Drugs (e.g., cocaine) • Acute anxiety	• Pain in chest, neck, jaw, arm, or shoulder • Cold, clammy skin • Diaphoresis • Nausea and vomiting • Epigastric pain • Indigestion, heartburn • Dyspnea, tachypnea • Weakness • Anxiety • Feeling of impending doom • Tachycardia, bradycardia • Irregular HR, murmurs • Palpitations • Dysrhythmias • Decreased or increased BP • Narrowed pulse pressure • Unequal BP readings in upper extremities • Syncope, loss of consciousness • Decreased O_2 saturation • Decreased or absent breath sounds • Pericardial friction rub	**Initial** • If unresponsive, assess circulation, airway, and breathing. • If responsive, monitor airway, breathing, and circulation. • Position patient upright unless contraindicated and give O_2 by nasal cannula or non-rebreather mask. • Obtain baseline vital signs, including O_2 saturation. • Auscultate heart and breath sounds. • Obtain 12-lead ECG. • Insert two IV catheters. • Assess pain using PQRST mnemonic (Table 33-7). • Medicate for pain as ordered (e.g., nitroglycerin, morphine). • Start continuous ECG monitoring and identify underlying rhythm. • Obtain baseline blood work (e.g., cardiac biomarkers, CBC, basic metabolic panel, coagulation studies). • Obtain portable chest x-ray. • Assess for contraindications for antiplatelet, anticoagulant, or thrombolytic therapy, or PCI as appropriate. • Give aspirin for heart-related chest pain unless contraindicated. • Give a high-dose statin. • Give antidysrhythmic drugs for life-threatening dysrhythmias. **Ongoing Monitoring** • Monitor ABCs, vital signs, level of consciousness, heart and breath sounds, heart rhythm, and O_2 saturation. • Assess and record response to drugs (e.g., decrease in chest pain) and remedicate or titrate drugs (e.g., nitroglycerin) as needed. • Provide reassurance and emotional support to patient and caregiver. • Explain all interventions and procedures to patient and caregiver in simple terms. • Anticipate need for intubation if respiratory distress is evident. • Prepare for CPR and defibrillation if cardiac arrest is evident. • Anticipate need for transcutaneous pacing for symptomatic bradycardia or heart block.

GERD, Gastroesophageal reflux disease; *PCI,* percutaneous coronary intervention.

intervention; (2) it is performed with local anesthesia; (3) the patient is ambulatory shortly after the procedure; (4) the length of hospital stay is approximately 3 to 4 days after MI compared with the 4 to 6 days with CABG surgery, thus reducing hospital costs; and (5) the patient can return to work several weeks sooner after PCI, compared with a 6- to 8-week convalescence after CABG.

Advances in PCI techniques have significantly reduced the need for emergent CABG. More PCIs are performed in the U.S. than CABGs.[1] Complications of PCI that may lead to emergent CABG include dissection of the coronary artery, abrupt artery closure, coronary artery rupture, acute stent thrombosis, and failure to cross the blockage with a balloon or stent. There is a risk that the infarction could be extended should a part of the plaque dislodge and block the vessel distal to the catheter. Coronary spasm from the mechanical irritation of the catheter or balloon can occur, as well as renal dysfunction or an allergic reaction from the contrast dye used in the procedure. Other complications of PCI include vascular access-site bleeding or other vascular complications, stroke, and infection.

In-stent restenosis (ISR) is a potential problem whenever stents are placed in a coronary artery. ISR usually occurs within a few months to a year after stent placement. Nursing care of the patient following PCI is similar to that after cardiac catheterization (see Table 31-6).

Thrombolytic Therapy

Thrombolytic (fibrinolytic) therapy is indicated only for patients with a STEMI. Advantages include the availability and rapid administration in agencies that do not have an interventional cardiac catheterization laboratory or when one is too far away to transfer the patient safely. Treatment of STEMI with thrombolytic therapy aims to limit the infarction size by dissolving the thrombus in the coronary artery and reperfusing the heart muscle. The goal is to give the thrombolytic within 30 minutes of the patient's arrival to the ED. Patients who are taken to non–PCI-capable hospitals can be moved to a PCI capable hospital if the first medical contact to balloon inflation (PCI) time can be done within 120 minutes.[20]

Indications and Contraindications. All thrombolytics are given IV (Table 33-11). The cost, efficacy, and ease of administration guide the choice of a thrombolytic agent. Although these drugs have different pharmacokinetics, they all open the blocked artery by lysis of the thrombus. Because all thrombolytics lyse the pathologic clot, they may also lyse other clots (e.g., a postoperative site). Therefore patient selection is important because minor or major bleeding can be a complication of therapy.

Inclusion criteria for thrombolytic therapy are (1) chest pain less than 12 hours with 12-lead ECG findings consistent with acute STEMI and (2) no absolute contraindications (Table 33-13). Patients with chest pain lasting 12 to 24 hours with ECG

TABLE 33-13 Contraindications for Thrombolytic Therapy

Absolute Contraindications

- Any prior history of intracranial hemorrhage
- Known structural or vascular abnormality (e.g., arteriovenous malformation)
- Known intracranial neoplasm (primary or metastatic)
- Recent (within past 3 mo) ischemic stroke
- Significant closed-head or facial trauma within past 3 mo
- Intracranial or intraspinal surgery within 2 mo
- Severe uncontrolled hypertension
- Active internal bleeding or bleeding diathesis (excluding menstruation)
- Suspected aortic dissection
- For streptokinase, prior treatment within the past 6 months

Relative Contraindications

- Active peptic ulcer disease
- Current use of oral anticoagulants
- Pregnancy
- Prior ischemic stroke (>3 mo ago)
- Dementia
- Known intracranial pathology not covered in absolute contraindications
- Noncompressible vascular punctures
- Recent (within 2-4 wk) internal bleeding
- Major surgery (<3 wk)
- History of chronic, severe, poorly controlled hypertension
- Significant hypertension on presentation (SBP >180 mm/Hg or DBP >110 mm/Hg)
- Traumatic or prolonged (>10 min) cardiopulmonary resuscitation

Source: O'Gara PT, Kushner FG, Ascheim DD, et al: 2013 ACCF/AHA guideline for the management of ST-elevation myocardial infarction: a report of the American College of Cardiology Foundation/American Heart Association Task Force on Practice Guidelines, *Circulation* 127:e362, 2013.

changes supporting STEMI may be considered for thrombolytic therapy.[20]

Procedure. Each hospital has a protocol for giving thrombolytic therapy, but several factors are common. Draw blood to obtain baseline laboratory values and start two or three lines for IV therapy. All other invasive procedures are done before the thrombolytic agent is given to reduce the possibility of bleeding.

Depending on the drug selected, therapy is given in one IV bolus or over time (30 to 90 minutes). Note the time at which therapy begins, and monitor the patient during and after giving the thrombolytic. Assess heart rhythm, vital signs, and pulse oximetry. Assess the heart and lungs frequently to evaluate the patient's response to therapy. Regularly assess for changes in neurologic status, since this may indicate cerebral bleeding.

When reperfusion occurs (i.e., the coronary artery that was blocked is opened and blood flow is restored to the heart muscle), several clinical signs may be seen. The most reliable sign is the return of the ST segment to baseline on the ECG. Other signs include a resolution of chest pain and an early, rapid rise of the serum cardiac biomarkers within 3 hours of therapy, peaking within 12 hours. These levels increase as the necrotic heart cells release proteins into the circulation after perfusion is restored to the area. The presence of *reperfusion dysrhythmias* (e.g., accelerated idioventricular rhythm) is a less reliable sign of reperfusion. These dysrhythmias are generally self-limiting and do not require aggressive treatment. (See Chapter 35 for management of dysrhythmias.)

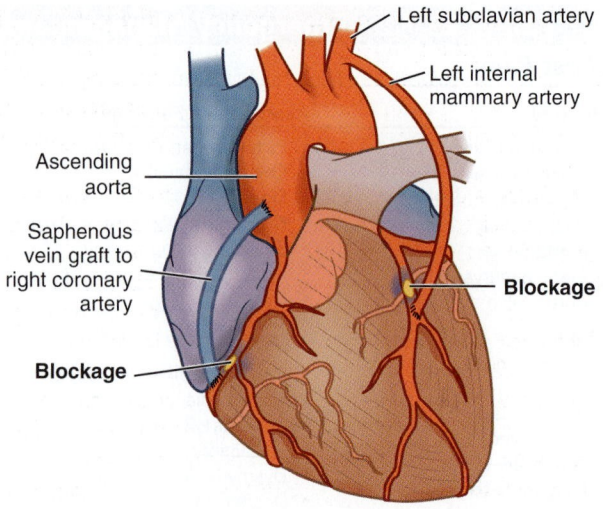

FIG. 33-11 Distal end of the left internal mammary artery is grafted below the area of blockage in the left anterior descending artery. Proximal end of the saphenous vein is grafted to the aorta, and the distal end is grafted below the area of blockage in the right coronary artery.

A major concern with thrombolytic therapy is reocclusion of the artery. The site of the thrombus is unstable, and formation of another clot or spasm of the artery may occur. Therefore IV heparin therapy is started. If another clot develops, the patient will have similar complaints of chest pain and ECG changes will return. Patients receiving thrombolytic therapy should be moved to a facility with PCI capabilities as soon as possible so PCI can be performed if thrombolytic therapy fails.

The major complication with thrombolytic therapy is bleeding. Ongoing nursing assessment is essential. Minor bleeding (e.g., surface bleeding from IV sites or gingival bleeding) is expected and controlled by applying a pressure dressing or ice packs.

! SAFETY ALERT Thrombolytic Therapy

- Minor or major bleeding can occur with thrombolytic drugs.
- Place two or three IV lines before thrombolytic therapy is started.
- If signs and symptoms of major bleeding occur (e.g., drop in BP, increase in HR, sudden change in the patient's mental status, blood in the urine or stool), stop the drug and notify the HCP.

Coronary Surgical Revascularization

Coronary revascularization with CABG surgery is recommended for patients who (1) fail medical management, (2) have left main coronary artery or three-vessel disease, (3) are not candidates for PCI (e.g., blockages are long or difficult to access), or (4) have failed PCI and continue to have chest pain. CABG may also be the option for patients with diabetes, LV dysfunction, or chronic kidney disease.[24] CABG surgery and PCI are considered palliative treatment for CAD and not a cure.

Traditional Coronary Artery Bypass Graft Surgery. CABG surgery consists of the placement of arterial or venous grafts to provide blood between the aorta or other major arteries and the heart muscle distal to the blocked coronary artery (or arteries). The procedure may involve one or more grafts using the internal mammary (thoracic) artery (IMA or ITA), saphenous vein, radial artery, gastroepiploic artery, and/or inferior epigastric artery (Fig. 33-11).

CABG surgery requires a sternotomy (opening of the chest cavity) and *cardiopulmonary bypass* (CPB). During CPB, blood is diverted from the patient's heart to a machine. Here it is oxygenated and returned (via a pump) to the patient. This allows the surgeon to operate on a quiet, nonbeating, bloodless heart while perfusion to vital organs is maintained. CPB is associated with postoperative neurologic dysfunction, renal dysfunction and systemic inflammatory response syndrome (SIRS).[24]

The IMA is the most common artery used for bypass graft. It is left attached to its origin (the subclavian artery) but then dissected from the chest wall. Next, it is *anastomosed* (connected with sutures) to the coronary artery distal to the blockage.

Saphenous veins are also used for bypass grafts. The surgeon endoscopically removes the saphenous vein from one or both legs. A section is sutured into the ascending aorta near the native coronary artery opening and then sutured to the coronary artery distal to the blockage. Saphenous vein grafts are more prone to develop diffuse intimal hyperplasia. This contributes to future stenosis and graft occlusion. The use of antiplatelet and statin therapy after surgery improves vein graft patency.

The radial artery, another potential graft, is a thick muscular artery that is prone to spasm. Perioperative calcium channel blockers and long-acting nitrates can control the spasms. Patency rates are not as good as the IMA but better than saphenous veins. Serious extremity complications (e.g., hand ischemia, wound infection) are rare after removal of the radial artery. Paresthesia and impaired sensation are common side effects after radial artery harvest.[25]

Other potential grafts include the gastroepiploic or inferior epigastric artery. Like the radial artery, these also are prone to spasms.

Women have higher periprocedural mortality and morbidity rates than men. This has been attributed to the late treatment of CAD in women because women first present with CAD at an older age and have more co-morbidities at the time of surgery. Other possible factors include smaller-diameter coronary vessels, smaller body surface area, and the fact that women are less likely to be referred for catheterization and PCI.[24]

Minimally Invasive Direct Coronary Artery Bypass. *Minimally invasive direct coronary artery bypass* (MIDCAB) offers patients with disease of the left anterior descending or right coronary artery an approach to surgical treatment that does not involve a sternotomy and CPB. The technique requires several small incisions between the ribs or a mini-thoracotomy. A thoracoscope or robotic assistance is used to dissect the IMA from the chest. A mechanical stabilizer immobilizes the operative site. The IMA is then sutured to the left anterior descending or right coronary artery. Some patients undergo hybrid procedures in which they have a MIDCAB for the left anterior descending artery and undergo a PCI of a second or third artery at a later time.

Off-Pump Coronary Artery Bypass. The *off-pump coronary artery bypass* (OPCAB) procedure uses a median sternotomy to access all coronary vessels. OPCAB is performed on a beating heart (no CPB) using mechanical stabilizers. OPCAB is associated with less blood loss, less renal dysfunction, less postoperative atrial fibrillation, and fewer neurologic complications. It is estimated that less than 20% of CABG procedures are OPCAB procedures. OPCAB is primarily used for patients with multiple co-morbidities who should avoid CPB.[25]

Robotic or Totally Endoscopic Coronary Artery Bypass (TECAB). This technique uses a robot in performing CABG surgery. This procedure is done without the use of CPB or with the use of CPB using femoral access. TECAB is used for limited bypass grafting. The benefits include increased precision, smaller incisions, decreased blood loss, less pain, and shorter recovery time.[25]

Transmyocardial Laser Revascularization. *Transmyocardial laser revascularization* is an indirect revascularization procedure. It is used for patients with advanced CAD who are not candidates for traditional CABG surgery and who have persistent angina despite maximum medical therapy. The procedure involves the use of a high-energy laser to create channels in the heart muscle to allow blood flow to ischemic areas. The procedure can be done using a left thoracotomy approach or in combination with CABG surgery. It is as an adjunctive therapy when bypass grafts cannot be placed.

Drug Therapy

When a patient presents with suspected ACS, dual antiplatelet therapy (e.g., chewable aspirin, clopidogrel), IV NTG, atorvastatin, and systemic anticoagulation with either subcutaneous LMWH or IV UH are drug treatments of choice. Glycoprotein IIb/IIIa inhibitors may also be used if PCI is anticipated. Oral β-blockers are given within the first 24 hours if there are no contraindications (e.g., HF, heart block, hypotension). ACE inhibitors are added for select patients following MI if there are no contraindications. Calcium channel blockers are added if the patient cannot tolerate β-blockers. These drugs must be used cautiously after MI because of their effect on contractility.[26] Nitrates may be used if the patient has persistent chest pain.

Table 33-11 and Fig. 33-4 present drug therapy for patients with ACS. These drugs are discussed on pp. 714-717. Drugs that are specifically used to treat ACS are discussed in this section.

IV Nitroglycerin. IV NTG is used in the initial treatment of the patient with ACS. The goal of therapy is to reduce anginal pain and improve coronary blood flow. IV NTG decreases preload and afterload while increasing the myocardial O_2 supply. The onset of action is immediate. Titrate NTG to control and stop chest pain. Because hypotension is a common side effect, closely monitor BP during this time. Patients who do become hypotensive are often volume depleted and can benefit from an IV fluid bolus.

Morphine. Morphine sulfate is the drug of choice for chest pain that is unrelieved by NTG. As a vasodilator, it decreases cardiac workload by lowering myocardial O_2 consumption, reducing contractility, and decreasing BP and HR. In addition, morphine can help reduce anxiety and fear. In rare situations, morphine can depress respirations. Monitor patients for signs of bradypnea or hypotension, which are conditions to avoid in myocardial ischemia and infarction.

β-Adrenergic Blockers. β-Blockers decrease myocardial O_2 demand by reducing HR, BP, and contractility. The use of these drugs in patients who are not at risk for complications of MI (e.g., cardiogenic shock, bradycardia, hypotension) reduces the risk of reinfarction and the development of HF. β-blockers are continued indefinitely. (See Table 33-11, Chapter 32 and Table 32-7 for a discussion of β-blockers.)

Angiotensin-Converting Enzyme Inhibitors and Angiotensin Receptor Blockers. ACE inhibitors should be started within the first 24 hours if the BP is stable and there are no contraindications. They are continued indefinitely in patients recovering from STEMI or NSTEMI, with heart failure, or an EF of 40% or less. The use of ACE inhibitors can help prevent ventricular remodeling and prevent or slow the progression of HF. For patients who cannot tolerate ACE inhibitors (e.g., angioedema, cough), ARBs should be considered. (See Tables 33-11 and 32-7.)

Antidysrhythmic Drugs. Dysrhythmias are the most common complications after an MI. In general, they are self-limiting and not treated aggressively unless they are life threatening (e.g., sustained ventricular tachycardia). (Chapter 35 discusses the drugs used in the treatment of dysrhythmias.)

Lipid-Lowering Drugs. A lipid panel is obtained on all patients with ACS. All patients with ACS or diagnosed with CAD should receive lipid-lowering drugs indefinitely, unless contraindicated (Table 33-5).

Stool Softeners. After an MI, the patient may be predisposed to constipation because of bed rest and use of opioid drugs. Stool softeners (e.g., docusate sodium [Colace]) are given to aid bowel movements. This prevents straining and the resultant vagal stimulation from the *Valsalva maneuver*. Vagal stimulation produces bradycardia and can provoke dysrhythmias.

Nutritional Therapy

Initially, patients may be NPO (nothing by mouth) except for water until stable (e.g., pain free, nausea resolved). Advance the diet as tolerated to a low-salt, low-saturated-fat, and low-cholesterol diet (Tables 33-3 and 33-4).

❖ NURSING MANAGEMENT: CHRONIC STABLE ANGINA AND ACUTE CORONARY SYNDROME

◆ Nursing Assessment

Table 33-14 presents the subjective and objective data to obtain from a patient with ACS.

◆ Nursing Diagnoses

Nursing diagnoses for the patient with ACS may include, but are not limited to, the following:

- Decreased cardiac output *related to* altered contractility and altered heart rate and rhythm
- Acute pain *related to* an imbalance between myocardial O_2 supply and demand
- Anxiety *related to* perceived or actual threat of death, pain, and/or possible lifestyle changes
- Activity intolerance *related to* general weakness secondary to decreased cardiac output and poor lung and tissue perfusion
- Ineffective health management *related to* lack of knowledge of disease process, risk factor reduction, rehabilitation, home activities, and medications

More information on nursing diagnoses of patients with ACS is presented in eNursing Care Plan 33-1 available on the website for this chapter.

◆ Planning

The overall goals for a patient with ACS include (1) relief of pain, (2) preservation of heart muscle, (3) immediate and appropriate treatment, (4) effective coping with illness-associated anxiety, (5) participation in a rehabilitation plan, and (6) reduction of risk factors. In addition, the Joint Commission has identified a core measure related to the timing of thrombolytics in the management of patients with an acute MI to reflect standards of evidence-based care (available at *www.jointcommission.org/acute_myocardial_infarction/default.aspx*).

TABLE 33-14 Nursing Assessment

Acute Coronary Syndrome

Subjective Data

Important Health Information

Past health history: Previous history of CAD, chest pain/angina, MI, valve disease (e.g., aortic stenosis), heart failure, or cardiomyopathy. Hypertension, diabetes, anemia, lung disease, hyperlipidemia

Medications: Use of antiplatelets or anticoagulants, nitrates, angiotensin-converting enzyme inhibitors, β-blockers, calcium channel blockers, antihypertensive drugs, lipid-lowering drugs, over-the-counter drugs (e.g., vitamin and herbal supplements)

History of present illness: Description of events related to current illness (Table 33-8), including any self-treatments and response

Functional Health Patterns

Health perception–health management: Family history of heart disease. Sedentary lifestyle, tobacco use, exposure to environmental smoke

Nutritional-metabolic: Indigestion, heartburn, nausea, belching, vomiting

Elimination: Urinary urgency or frequency, straining at stool

Activity-exercise: Palpitations, dyspnea, dizziness, weakness

Cognitive-perceptual: Substernal chest pain or pressure (squeezing, constricting, aching, sharp, tingling), possible radiation to jaw, neck, shoulders, back, or arms (Table 33-7)

Coping–stress tolerance: Stressful lifestyle, depression; anger, anxiety. Feeling of impending doom

Objective Data

General

Anxious, fearful, restless, distressed

Integumentary

Cool, clammy, pale skin

Cardiovascular

Tachycardia or bradycardia, pulsus alternans (alternating weak and strong heartbeats), pulse deficit, dysrhythmias (especially ventricular), S_3, S_4, ↑ or ↓ BP, murmur

Possible Diagnostic Findings

Positive serum cardiac biomarkers, ↑ serum lipids; ↑ WBC count. Positive exercise or pharmacologic stress test and thallium scans. Pathologic Q wave, ST segment elevation, and/or T wave abnormalities on ECG. Cardiac enlargement, calcifications, or pulmonary congestion on chest x-ray. Abnormal wall motion with stress echocardiogram. Positive coronary angiography.

◆ Nursing Implementation: Chronic Stable Angina

◆ **Health Promotion.** Behaviors to reduce the risk for CAD are presented in Table 33-2 and discussed on pp. 707-712.

◆ **Acute Care.** If your patient experiences angina, perform the following measures: (1) position patient upright unless contraindicated and apply supplemental O_2, (2) assess vital signs, (3) obtain a 12-lead ECG, (4) provide prompt pain relief first with NTG followed by an opioid analgesic if needed, and (5) assess heart and breath sounds. The patient will most likely be anxious and may have pale, cool, clammy skin. The BP and HR may be elevated. Auscultation of the heart may reveal an atrial (S_4) or a ventricular (S_3) gallop. A new murmur heard during an anginal attack may indicate ischemia of a papillary muscle of the mitral valve. The murmur is likely to be transient and disappear when symptoms stop.

Ask the patient to describe the pain and to rate it on a scale of 0 to 10 before and after treatment to evaluate the effectiveness of the interventions (Table 33-7). It is important to use the same words that patients use to describe their symptoms (e.g., tightness, pressure). Assess for other signs of pain, such as restlessness; ECG changes; elevated HR, respiratory rate, or BP; clutching of the bed linens; or other nonverbal cues. Support and reassure the patient. Use a calm approach to help reduce the patient's anxiety during an anginal attack.

CHECK YOUR PRACTICE

A visitor finds you in the hallway and tells you that her father is having chest pain. The patient is not assigned to you.

- How would you proceed?

◆ **Ambulatory Care.** Reassure the patient with a history of angina that a long, active life is possible. Prevention of angina is preferable to its treatment. This is why teaching is important. Give the patient information about CAD, angina, precipitating factors for angina, risk factor reduction, and drugs.

Patient teaching can be done in a variety of ways. One-on-one contact between you and the patient is often the most effective approach. Time spent providing daily care (e.g., giving drugs) offers many teachable moments. Teaching aids such as DVDs, heart models, and printed information are important parts of patient and caregiver teaching (see Chapter 4).

Help the patient to identify factors that precipitate angina (Table 33-8). Tell the patient how to avoid or control these factors. For example, teach the patient to avoid exposure to extremes of weather and eating large, heavy meals. If a heavy meal is eaten, tell the patient to rest for 1 to 2 hours after the meal because blood is shifted to the GI tract to aid digestion and absorption.

Help the patient to identify personal risk factors for CAD. Then discuss the various ways modifiable risk factors can be reduced (Table 33-2). Teach the patient and caregiver about diets that are low in salt and saturated fats (Tables 33-3 and 33-4). Maintaining ideal body weight is important in controlling angina because excess weight increases the heart's workload.

It is important that the patient has a regular, individualized program of physical activity that conditions rather than stresses the heart. For example, tell patients that walking briskly on a flat surface at least 30 minutes a day, most days of the week is recommended.

It is important to teach the patient and caregiver the proper use of NTG (see pp. 714 and 716). NTG may be used prophylactically before an emotionally stressful situation, sexual intercourse, or physical exertion (e.g., climbing a long flight of stairs).

If needed, arrange for counseling to assess the psychologic adjustment of the patient and caregiver to the diagnosis of CAD and the resulting angina. Many patients feel a threat to their identity and self-esteem and may be unable to fill their usual roles in society. These emotions are normal and real.

◆ Nursing Implementation: Acute Coronary Syndrome

◆ **Acute Care.** Priorities for nursing interventions in the initial phase of ACS include (1) pain assessment and relief, (2) physiologic monitoring, (3) promotion of rest and comfort, (4) alleviation of stress and anxiety, and (5) understanding of the patient's emotional and behavioral reactions. Patients with increased anxiety levels have a greater risk for adverse outcomes such as recurrent ischemic events and dysrhythmias. Proper management of these priorities decreases the O_2 needs of a compromised heart muscle and reduces the risk of complications. In addition, start measures to avoid the hazards of immobility while encouraging periods of rest.

◆ ***Pain.*** Provide NTG, morphine, and supplemental O_2 as needed to eliminate or reduce chest pain. Ongoing evaluation and documentation of the effectiveness of the interventions are important. Once pain is relieved, you may have to deal with denial in a patient who interprets the absence of pain as an absence of heart disease.

◆ ***Monitoring.*** Maintain continuous ECG monitoring while the patient is in the ED and ICU and after transfer to a step-down or general unit. Dysrhythmias must be identified quickly and treated. During the initial period after MI, ventricular fibrillation is the most common lethal dysrhythmia. In many patients, premature ventricular contractions or ventricular tachycardia precedes this dysrhythmia. Monitor the patient for reinfarction or ischemia by monitoring the ST segment for shifts above or below the baseline of the ECG. Silent ischemia can occur without subjective symptoms (e.g., chest pain). It is noted by ST segment changes only. Notify the HCP if you see ST segment changes without any clinical symptoms. (See Chapter 35 for a complete discussion of ECG monitoring.)

Perform a physical assessment to detect changes from the patient's baseline findings. Assess heart and breath sounds and any signs of early HF (e.g., dyspnea, tachycardia, pulmonary congestion, distended neck veins). In addition to routine vital signs, monitor intake and output at least once a shift.

Assessment of the patient's oxygenation status is important, especially if the patient is receiving O_2. If a nasal cannula is used to deliver O_2, check the nares for irritation or dryness, which can cause considerable discomfort.

◆ ***Rest and Comfort.*** It is important to promote rest and comfort with any degree of heart damage. Bed rest may be ordered for the first few days after an MI that involves a large portion of the LV. A patient with an uncomplicated MI (e.g., angina resolved, no signs of complications) may rest in a chair within 8 to 12 hours after the event. The use of a commode or bedpan is based on patient preference.

When sleeping or resting, the body requires less work from the heart than it does when active. It is important to plan nursing and other interventions to ensure adequate rest periods free from interruption. Comfort measures that can promote rest include a quiet environment, use of relaxation techniques (e.g., music therapy, guided imagery), and assurance that staff are nearby and responsive to the patient's needs.

It is important that the patient understand the reasons why activity is limited but not completely restricted. Gradually increase the patient's heart workload through more demanding physical tasks. It is important that the patient achieve a discharge activity level adequate for home care. Table 33-15 outlines the phases of cardiac rehabilitation.

◆ ***Anxiety.*** To some degree anxiety is present in all patients with ACS. Your role is to identify the source of anxiety and assist the patient in reducing it. If the patient is afraid of being alone, allow a caregiver to sit by quietly or check in with the patient frequently. If a source of anxiety is fear of the unknown, explore these concerns with the patient. For anxiety caused by lack of information, provide teaching based on the patient's stated need and level of understanding. Answer the patient's questions with clear, simple explanations.

TABLE 33-15 Phases of Rehabilitation After Acute Coronary Syndrome

Phase I: Hospital
- Occurs while the patient is still hospitalized
- Activity level depends on severity of angina or MI.
- Patient may first sit up in bed or chair, perform range-of-motion exercises and self-care (e.g., washing, shaving), and progress to walking in hallway and limited stair climbing.
- Attention focuses on management of chest pain, anxiety, dysrhythmias, and complications.

Phase II: Early Recovery
- Begins after the patient is discharged
- Usually lasts from 2-12 wk and is held in an outpatient facility
- Activity level is gradually increased under the supervision of the cardiac rehabilitation team and with ECG monitoring.
- Team may suggest that physical activity (e.g., walking) be started at home.
- Information regarding risk factor reduction is provided at this time.

Phase III: Late Recovery
- Long-term maintenance program
- Individual physical activity programs are designed and implemented at home, a local gym, or the rehabilitation center.
- Patient and caregiver possibly restructure lifestyles and roles.
- Therapeutic lifestyle changes should become lifelong habits.
- Medical supervision is still recommended.

CHECK YOUR PRACTICE

You are walking in the hallway with a 64-yr-old woman who had an MI 3 days ago. She is scheduled to be discharged tomorrow. She is visibly anxious and irritable, wringing her hands, and talking very fast. She tells you, "My heart is pounding." You do not know if she is anxious or about to have another MI.
- What should you do?

It is important to start teaching at the patient's level rather than to present a prepackaged program. For example, patients generally are not ready to learn about the pathology of CAD. The earliest questions usually relate to how the disease affects perceived control and independence. Examples include the following.
- When will I leave the intensive care unit?
- When can I be out of bed?
- When will I be discharged?
- When can I return to work?
- How many changes will I have to make in my life?
- Will this happen again?

Tell the patient that more complete teaching will begin once the patient is feeling stronger. Often the patient may not be able to ask the most serious concern of ACS patients: Am I going to die? Even if a patient denies this concern, it is helpful for you to start a conversation by remarking that fear of dying is a common concern among most patients who have experienced ACS. This gives the patient "permission" to talk about an uncomfortable and fearful topic.

◆ ***Emotional and Behavioral Reactions.*** Patients' emotional and behavioral reactions vary, but often follow a predictable response pattern (Table 33-16). Your role is to understand what the patient is currently experiencing and to support the use of constructive coping styles.

TABLE 33-16 Psychosocial Responses to Acute Coronary Syndrome

Denial
- May have history of ignoring signs and symptoms related to heart disease
- Minimizes severity of health condition
- Ignores activity restrictions
- Avoids discussing illness or its significance

Depression
- Mourns loss of health, altered body function, and changes in lifestyle
- Realizes seriousness of situation
- Begins to worry about future implications of health problem
- Shows manifestations of withdrawal, crying, apathy
- May be more evident after discharge

Anger and Hostility
- Is commonly expressed as, "Why did this happen to me?"
- May be directed at family, staff, or medical regimen

Anxiety and Fear
- Fears long-term disability and death
- Overtly displays apprehension, restlessness, insomnia, tachycardia
- Less overtly displays increased verbalization, projection of feelings to others, hypochondriasis
- Fears activity
- Fears recurrent chest pain, heart attacks, and sudden death

Dependency
- Is totally reliant on staff
- Is unwilling to perform tasks or activities unless approved by HCP
- Wants to be monitored by ECG at all times
- Is hesitant to leave the intensive care or telemetry unit or hospital

Realistic Acceptance
- Focuses on optimum rehabilitation
- Plans changes compatible with altered cardiac function
- Actively engages in lifestyle changes to address modifiable risk factors

Assess the support structure of the patient and caregiver. Determine how you can help maximize the support system. Often the patient is separated from the most significant support system at the time of hospitalization. Your role can include talking with the caregiver(s), informing them of the patient's progress, allowing the patient and caregivers to interact as necessary, and supporting the caregivers who will provide the necessary support to the patient. Open visitation is helpful in decreasing anxiety and increasing support for the patient with ACS.[27] It is important for you to help the patient identify additional support systems (e.g., spiritual care, Mended Hearts) that can assist after discharge.

◆ **Coronary Revascularization.** Patients with ACS may undergo coronary revascularization with PCI or CABG surgery. The major nursing responsibilities for patient care after PCI involve monitoring for signs of recurrent angina; frequent assessment of vital signs, including HR and rhythm; evaluation of the catheter insertion site for signs of bleeding; neurovascular assessment of the involved extremity; and maintenance of bed rest per agency policy.

For patients having CABG surgery, care is provided in the ICU for the first 24 to 36 hours. Ongoing and intensive monitoring of the patient's hemodynamic status is critical. The

TEAMWORK & COLLABORATION

Cardiac Catheterization and Percutaneous Coronary Intervention (PCI)

Before and after cardiac catheterization and PCI, patients require frequent interventions by RNs. The RN is responsible for assessing the patient, developing and implementing an individualized plan of care, evaluating the patient, and providing discharge teaching. Much of the care can be delegated to LPN/LVNs and UAP. Respiratory therapy may also have a role in the patient's care depending on the patient's past medical history.

Role of Nursing Personnel

Registered Nurse (RN)

Preprocedure

- Assess for allergies, especially to contrast dye. Perform baseline assessment, including vital signs, pulse oximetry, heart and breath sounds, neurovascular assessment of extremities (e.g., distal pulses, skin temperature, skin color, sensation).
- Assess baseline laboratory values (e.g., cardiac biomarkers, creatinine).
- Teach patient and caregiver about procedure and postprocedure care.

Postprocedure

- Perform assessment and compare to baseline: vital signs, pulse oximetry, heart and breath sounds, neurovascular assessment of extremity used for procedure, assessment of catheter insertion site for hematoma, bleeding, and bruit.
- Monitor ECG for dysrhythmias or other changes (e.g., ST segment elevation).
- Monitor patient for chest pain and other sources of pain or discomfort.
- Monitor IV infusions of anticoagulants, antiplatelets.
- Teach patient and caregiver about discharge drugs (e.g., aspirin, clopidogrel, antianginal drugs).
- Teach patient and caregiver about discharge care including signs and symptoms to report to HCP (e.g., site complications, return of chest pain).

Licensed Practical/Vocational Nurse (LPN/LVN)

- Give drugs before and after the procedure (consider state nurse practice act and agency policy).
- Assess neurovascular status of involved extremity every 15 min for the first hour, then according to agency policy (consider state nurse practice act and agency policy).
- Check for bleeding at catheter insertion site every 15 min for the first hour, then according to agency policy.
- Report changes in neurovascular status of involved extremity or any bleeding to the RN.

Unlicensed Assistive Personnel (UAP)

- Take vital signs and report increases or decreases in HR or BP to RN.
- Report decreases in pulse oximetry to the RN.
- Report patient complaints of chest pain, shortness of breath, and/or any other discomfort or distress to RN.
- Assist with oral hygiene and hydration, meals, and toileting.
- Record oral intake and urine output as ordered.
- Perform related skills as ordered (e.g., capillary blood glucose).

Role of Other Team Members

Respiratory Therapist

- Provide respiratory therapies (e.g., nebulizer treatments) as ordered and per agency policy.

patient will have numerous invasive lines for monitoring heart status and other vital organs (see Chapter 65). These include (1) a pulmonary artery catheter for hemodynamic monitoring (e.g., CO), (2) an arterial line for continuous BP monitoring, (3) pleural and mediastinal chest tubes for chest drainage, (4) continuous ECG monitoring, (5) an endotracheal tube connected to mechanical ventilation, (6) epicardial pacing wires for emergency pacing of the heart, (7) a urinary catheter to monitor urine output, and (8) a nasogastric tube for gastric decompression. Most patients are extubated within 6 hours and transferred to a step-down unit within 24 hours for continued monitoring of heart status.

Many of the postoperative complications that develop after CABG surgery relate to the use of cardiopulmonary bypass (CPB). Major consequences of CPB are systemic inflammation. This includes complications of bleeding and anemia from damage to red blood cells and platelets, fluid and electrolyte imbalances, hypothermia as blood is cooled as it passes through the CPB machine, and infections. Focus your care on assessing the patient for bleeding (e.g., chest tube drainage, incision sites), hemodynamic monitoring, checking fluid status, replacing blood and electrolytes as needed, and restoring temperature (e.g., warming blankets).

Postoperative dysrhythmias, especially atrial dysrhythmias (e.g., atrial fibrillation [AF]), are common in the first 3 days after CABG surgery.[24] β-Blockers should be restarted as soon as possible after surgery (unless contraindicated) to reduce the incidence of AF. Discharge is often delayed in these patients in order to begin anticoagulation therapy. (See Chapter 35 for information on treatment of AF.)

Nursing care for the patient with a CABG involves caring for the surgical sites (e.g., leg, chest, arm). Care of the leg incision is minimal since endoscopy is used to harvest the vein. Chest incisions are usually closed with Dermabond and do not require dressings. Management of the chest wound, which involves a sternotomy, is similar to that of other chest surgeries (see Chapter 27).

Care of the radial artery harvest site includes monitoring sensory and motor function of the hand. The patient with radial artery harvest should take a calcium channel blocker for approximately 3 months to reduce the incidence of arterial spasm at the arm or anastomosis site.

After CABG other interventions include strategies to manage pain and prevent venous thromboembolism (e.g., early ambulation, sequential compression device) and respiratory complications (e.g., use of incentive spirometer, splinting during coughing and deep-breathing exercises). (See Chapter 19 for care of the postoperative patient.)

Postoperatively, patients may experience some cognitive dysfunction. This includes impairment of memory, concentration, language comprehension, and social integration. Patients may cry or become teary. *Postoperative cognitive dysfunction* (POCD) can manifest days to weeks to months after surgery and may become a chronic disorder.[28] (POCD is discussed in Chapter 19.)

In the older patient, elective CABG is generally well tolerated. However, the incidence of postoperative complications (e.g., dysrhythmias, stroke, POCD, infection) is high. Although the benefits of treatment may outweigh risks in this group, complications are higher than in younger individuals.

Postoperative nursing care of the patient with a MIDCAB, OPCAB, or TECAB procedure is similar to that for CABG surgery patients. The recovery time is somewhat shorter with these procedures, and patients often resume routine activities sooner than patients who have CABG surgery. However, pain control is important regardless of the procedure. Patients have higher levels of pain with a thoracotomy incision than a sternotomy incision.

◆ **Ambulatory Care.** *Cardiac rehabilitation* is the restoration of a person to an optimal state of function in six areas: physiologic, psychologic, mental, spiritual, economic, and vocational. Many patients recover from ACS physically but do not attain psychologic well-being. All patients (e.g., those with ACS, chronic stable angina, heart surgery) need to be referred to a cardiac rehabilitation program. In considering rehabilitation, the patient must recognize that CAD is a chronic disease. It is not curable. Therefore basic changes in lifestyle must be made to promote recovery and future health. These changes often are needed when a person is middle aged or older. The patient must realize that recovery takes time. Tell patients that resuming physical activity after ACS or heart surgery is slow and gradual. However, with appropriate and adequate supportive care, recovery is more likely to occur.

◆ ***Patient Teaching.*** Patient teaching must occur at every stage of the patient's hospitalization and recovery (e.g., ED, telemetry unit, home care). The purpose of teaching is to give the patients and caregivers the tools they need to make informed decisions about their health. For teaching to be meaningful, the patient must be aware of the need to learn. Careful assessment of the patient's health literacy and learning needs helps you set goals that are realistic (see Chapter 4).

The timing of the teaching is important. When patients and caregivers are in crisis (either physiologic or psychologic), they may not be ready to learn new information. Answer the patient's questions in simple, brief terms. The answers often require repetition. When the shock accompanying a crisis subsides, the patient and caregiver are better able to focus on new and more detailed information.

EVIDENCE-BASED PRACTICE

Translating Research Into Practice

Do Behavioral Interventions Reduce Cardiovascular Risk Factors?

Clinical Question

In adults with cardiovascular risk factors (P), what is the effect of behavioral intervention (I) versus control group (C) on cardiovascular health outcomes (O) at 12 to 24 months (T)?

Synthesis of Best Available Evidence

- Systematic review of randomized controlled trials (RCTs) or controlled clinical trials
- 74 trials of adults (*n* >33,000) with at least one cardiovascular risk factor, including hypertension, dyslipidemia, impaired fasting glucose or glucose tolerance, metabolic syndrome, and cigarette smoking. Intervention was intensive behavioral counseling on diet or physical activity delivered alone or part of a multicomponent program with follow-up of at least 6 months. Control group was usual care, minimal intervention or attention. Physiologic outcomes included BP, weight, cholesterol and glucose levels, and diabetes incidence. Depression and quality of life were also measured.
- After 1 to 2 years, weight, systolic and diastolic BP, cholesterol and fasting glucose levels had decreased with lowered incidence of diabetes in the intervention group.
- Improvements in diet and physical activity were consistent with positive physiologic changes in the intervention group.
- Inconclusive if depression and quality of life significantly improved in the intervention group

Conclusions

- Intensive behavioral counseling for up to 2 years resulted in positive decreases in cardiovascular risk factors.

Implications for Nursing Practice

1. What would you advise an overweight patient with hypertension who asks if a lifestyle counseling program may be helpful to her?
2. What information would you offer a patient who after 3 weeks of counseling is discouraged that the test results did not show significant improvements in total cholesterol or fasting glucose levels?

Reference for Evidence

Lin JS, O'Connor E, Evans CV, et al: Behavioral counseling to promote a healthy lifestyle in individuals with cardiovascular risk factors: A systematic review for the U.S. Preventive Services Task Force, *Ann Intern Med* 161:568, 2014.

P, Patient population of interest; *I,* intervention or area of interest; *C,* comparison of interest or comparison group; *O,* outcomes of interest; *T,* timing (see p. 15).

BECOMING A NURSE LEADER

Bullying in the Workplace

Situation

Laura is a nursing student who is doing her cardiac rotation. Although sensitive about her inexperience, Laura was unprepared to deal with the negative attitude and disrespect of her preceptor. Laura's preceptor referred to her as "Hey, student!" and "Little newbie!" throughout her 3-day clinical rotation while continually rolling her eyes and acting perturbed when Laura asked her questions about the care of patients. Laura was very upset and felt bullied and put-down by her preceptor.

Points for Consideration

- Bullying is the use of force, threat, or coercion to abuse, intimidate, or aggressively dominate others. The behavior, which is often repeated and habitual, is used to gain control and power.
- This type of behavior may involve hidden or open acts of verbal and nonverbal aggression, such as verbal abuse, criticism, sarcasm, demeaning statements, false accusations, and gossiping.
- *Horizontal* or *lateral violence* refers to acts between peers or colleagues.
- *Bullying* is often described as acts perpetrated by one in a higher level of authority *(vertical violence).*
- Such demeaning behavior makes the work place stressful and unpleasant. These types of behavior also result in enough psychologic distress for nurses to cause them to leave the profession.
- Bullying ultimately places patient safety at risk.
- New standards address disruptive and inappropriate behaviors in health care workplaces.[1]

Discussion Questions

1. What would you do if you were Laura and were treated this way by your preceptor?
2. What damaging effects can bullying have on you? On your patients?
3. What strategies can you use to prevent and/or deal with bullying behavior?

Reference

1. American Nurses Association Position Statement on Incivility, Bullying, and Workplace Violence. Retrieved from *www.nursingworld.org/MainMenuCategories/Policy-Advocacy/Positions-and-Resolutions/ANAPositionStatements/Position-Statements-Alphabetically/Incivility-Bullying-and-Workplace-Violence.html.*

TABLE 33-17 Patient & Caregiver Teaching

Acute Coronary Syndrome

Include the following information in the teaching plan for the patient with acute coronary syndrome and the caregiver.

- Signs and symptoms of angina and MI and what to do should they occur (e.g., take nitroglycerin)*
- When and how to seek help (e.g., contact ERS)
- Anatomy and physiology of the heart and coronary arteries
- Cause and effect of CAD
- Definition of terms (e.g., CAD, angina, MI, sudden cardiac death, heart failure)
- Identification of and plan to decrease risk factors* (Tables 33-2, 33-3, and 33-4)
- Reasons for tests and treatments (e.g., ECG monitoring, lab work, angiography), activity limitations and rest, diet, and drugs*
- Appropriate expectations about recovery (anticipatory guidance)
- Resumption of work, physical activity, sexual activity
- Measures to promote recovery and health (e.g., cardiac rehabilitation)
- Importance of the gradual, progressive resumption of activity*

*Identified by patients as most important to learn before discharge.

TABLE 33-18 Energy Expenditure in Metabolic Equivalents

Low-Energy Activities (<3 METs or <3 cal/min)

Activities in Hospital

- Resting supine
- Eating
- Washing hands, face

Activities Outside Hospital

- Sweeping floor
- Painting, seated
- Driving a car
- Sewing by machine

Moderate-Energy Activities (3-6 METs or 3-5 cal/min)

Activities in Hospital

- Sitting on bedside commode
- Showering
- Using bedpan
- Walking at 3-4 mph

Activities Outside Hospital

- Ironing, standing
- Cycling at 5.5 mph on level ground
- Golfing
- General gardening
- Painting, standing
- Ascending a flight of stairs

High-Energy Activities (6-8 METs or 6-8 cal/min)

- Walking 5 mph
- Performing carpentry
- Mowing lawn using walking mower

Very-High-Energy Activities (>9 METs or >9 cal/min)

- Cross-country skiing
- Running at >6 mph
- Cycling at >13 mph
- Shoveling heavy snow

Limit your use of medical terms. For example, you are caring for a patient with unstable angina and he asks you why he has chest tightness when he climbs stairs. Begin by explaining that the heart is a muscle that works as a pump. Like all muscles, it needs O_2 to work (or pump) properly. When blood vessels supplying the heart muscle with O_2 are blocked by plaque, less O_2 is available to the muscle. As a result, the pump cannot work well. Tell the patient that the chest tightness (angina) is the heart's message that it is having trouble doing its work. Use a model of the heart to support what you are explaining to the patient. Provide an angina log for the patient to use that is available from the AHA.[29]

Anticipatory guidance involves preparing the patient and caregiver for what to expect in the course of recovery and rehabilitation. By learning what to expect during treatment and recovery, the patient gains a sense of control over his or her life.

The idea of perceived control is operationalized as the process by which the patient makes decisions by cutting back. Cutting back is one way of reducing the psychologic and physiologic losses after ACS (or any other life-changing event). For example, a middle-aged man who smokes two packs of cigarettes a day, is 20 pounds overweight, and gets no physical exercise has a seemingly overwhelming task. He may decide that he can live with a weight reduction plan and will get more exercise (although perhaps not daily) but that it is not possible for him to quit smoking. He believes that because he is changing two of his three risk factors, he will be healthier. Ideally, the tobacco risk factor should be a priority for this patient. If the information regarding risks and effects of tobacco use is not accepted, you must respect the patient's choices.

In addition to teaching the patient and caregiver what they wish to know, several types of information are essential in achieving optimal health. Table 33-17 presents a teaching guide for the patient with ACS and the caregiver.

◆ ***Physical Activity.*** Physical activity, an integral part of rehabilitation, is necessary for optimal physiologic functioning and psychologic well-being. It has a direct, positive effect on maximal O_2 uptake, increasing CO, decreasing blood lipids, decreasing BP, increasing blood flow through the coronary arteries, increasing muscle mass and flexibility, improving the psychologic state, and assisting in weight loss and control. A regular schedule of physical activity, even after many years of sedentary living, is beneficial.[12]

One method of identifying levels of physical activity is by using **metabolic equivalent (MET)** units: 1 MET is the amount of O_2 needed by the body at rest—3.5 mL of O_2 per kilogram per minute, or 1.4 cal/kg of body weight per minute. The MET determines the energy costs of various exercises (Table 33-18).

In the hospital, the activity level is gradually increased so that by the time of discharge the patient can tolerate moderate-energy activities of 3 to 6 METs. Many patients with UA that has resolved or an uncomplicated MI are in the hospital for approximately 3 or 4 days. By day 2, the patient can walk in the hallway and begin stair climbing (e.g., three or four steps). Many HCPs order low-level exercise stress tests before discharge to assess readiness for discharge, optimal HR for an exercise program, and potential for ischemia or reinfarction. If tests are positive (i.e., ischemia at a low level of energy expenditure), the patient is evaluated for cardiac catheterization before discharge. If the test is negative, a catheterization may still be done before discharge or several weeks after discharge. Because of the short hospital stay, it is critical to give the patient specific guidelines for physical activity so that overexertion will not occur. Tell the patient to always "listen to what your body is saying"—the most important aspect of recovery.

Teach patients to check their HR. The patient should know the limits within which to exercise. Tell the patient the maximum HR that should be present at any point. If the HR exceeds this level or does not return to the resting HR within a few minutes, tell the patient to stop and rest. Also tell the patient to stop exercising and rest if chest pain or shortness of breath occurs.

In a normal, healthy person the minimum goal for improving cardiopulmonary fitness is 60% of the age-predicted maximum HR (calculate by subtracting the person's age from 220). The ideal training target HR is 80% of maximum HR. The patient who has been physically inactive and is just starting an exercise program should do so under supervision whenever possible.

TABLE 33-19 Patient & Caregiver Teaching

FITT Activity Guidelines After Acute Coronary Syndrome

Include the following information in the teaching plan for the patient with acute coronary syndrome and the caregiver:

Warm-Up/Cool-Down

Perform mild stretching for 3-5 min before the physical activity and 5 min after the activity. Activity should not be started or stopped abruptly.

Frequency

Perform physical activity on most days of the week.

Intensity

Activity intensity is determined by the patient's HR. If an exercise stress test has not been performed, the HR of the patient recovering from an MI should not exceed 20 beats/min over the resting HR.

Type of Physical Activity

Select physical activity that is regular, rhythmic, and repetitive, using large muscles to build up endurance (e.g., walking, cycling, swimming, rowing).

Time

Physical activity sessions should be at least 30 min long. Begin slowly at personal tolerance (perhaps only 5-10 min) and build up to 30 min.

The more important factor is the patient's response to physical activity in terms of symptoms rather than absolute HR, especially since many patients are taking β-blockers and may not be able to reach a target HR. This point cannot be overstressed. Basic physical activity guidelines for patients after ACS follow the FITT formula (Table 33-19).

The basic categories of physical activity are isometric (static) and isotonic (dynamic). Most daily activities are a mixture of the two. *Isometric activities* involve the development of tension during muscular contraction but produce little or no change in muscle length or joint movement. Lifting, carrying, and pushing heavy objects are isometric activities. These activities are associated with the Valsalva maneuver and may cause a vasovagal response. Because the HR and BP change rapidly during isometric work, isometric exercises should be limited.

Isotonic activities involve changes in muscle length and joint movement with rhythmic contractions at relatively low muscular tension. Walking, jogging, swimming, bicycling, and jumping rope are examples of activities that are mostly isotonic. Isotonic exercise can put a safe, steady load on the heart and lungs and improve the circulation in many organs.

Discuss participation in an outpatient cardiac rehabilitation program with all patients (Table 33-15). These programs are helpful, but not all patients choose or are able to participate in them (e.g., location and travel limitations). Home-based cardiac rehabilitation programs can provide an alternative. Physical activity guidelines are developed for the patient, and staff maintains ongoing contact with the patient (e.g., telehealth, exercise logs, Internet). Maintaining contact with the patient is one key to the success of these programs.

Older women (65 years or older) who experience MI may frequently have poor adherence to a regular physical activity program. Often these women describe continued fatigue post-MI that is poorly understood. Another factor that has been linked to poor adherence to a physical activity program after MI is depression. Depression is common among patients with CAD, especially in women.[30] Routinely screen for depression in all patients with CAD and recommend treatment as appropriate.

◆ **Resumption of Sexual Activity.** It is important to include sexual counseling for heart patients and their partners. This often-neglected area of discussion may be difficult for both the patient and HCP to approach. However, the patient's concern about resumption of sexual activity after hospitalization for ACS often produces more stress than the physiologic act itself. Most patients change their sexual behavior not because of physical problems, but because they are concerned about sexual inadequacy, death during intercourse, and impotence. A concerned and knowledgeable HCP could clarify any misconceptions with specific counseling.

Before providing guidelines on resumption of sexual activity, it is important to know the patient's physiologic status, physiologic effects of sexual activity, and psychologic effects of having an MI. Sexual activity for most middle-aged men and women with their usual partners is considered a moderate-energy activity equivalent to climbing two flights of stairs.[31]

You may be uncertain of how and when to begin counseling about resumption of sex. It is helpful to consider sex as a physical activity and to discuss or explore feelings in this area when other physical activities are discussed. One helpful approach is, "Many people who have had a heart attack wonder when they will be able to resume sexual activity. Has this been of concern to you?" You may also state, "Sexual activity, like other forms of activity, should be gradually resumed after MI. If your ability to perform sexually is concerning you, the energy you use is no more than walking briskly." Facilitate discussion by providing the patient with reading material on resumption of sexual activity. Say something like, "If resuming sexual activity has been of concern to you, this information should be helpful." This type of nonthreatening statement brings up the topic, allows the patient to explore personal feelings, and gives the patient an opportunity to raise questions with you or another HCP. Common guidelines are presented in Table 33-20.

Tell the patient that the inability to perform sexually after MI is common and that sexual dysfunction usually disappears after several attempts. Reinforce the idea that patience and understanding usually solve the problem. However, many male patients may be interested in using drugs to correct erectile dysfunction. Warn the patient that these drugs are not to be used with nitrates because severe hypotension and even death have been reported. Tell patients to discuss the use of these drugs with their HCP.

It is common for a patient who experiences chest pain on physical exertion to have some angina during sexual stimulation or intercourse. The patient may be told to take NTG prophylactically. Tell the patient to delay sex after a heavy meal or excessive intake of alcohol, when extremely tired or stressed, or with unfamiliar partners. Patients should also avoid anal intercourse because of the likelihood of eliciting a vasovagal response.

Tell the patient that resumption of sex depends on the patient and his or her partner's emotional readiness and on the HCP's assessment of the extent of recovery. It is generally safe to resume sexual activity 7 to 10 days after an uncomplicated

TABLE 33-20 Patient & Partner Teaching

Sexual Activity After Acute Coronary Syndrome

Include the following information in the teaching plan for the patient and his/her partner after an acute coronary syndrome:

- Sexual activity should be resumed at a level that relates to sexual activity before experiencing ACS.
- Physical training may improve the physiologic response to intercourse. Encourage daily physical activity during recovery.
- Consumption of food and alcohol should be reduced before intercourse is anticipated (e.g., waiting 3-4 hr after ingesting a large meal before engaging in sexual activity).
- Familiar surroundings and a familiar partner reduce anxiety.
- Masturbation may be a useful sexual outlet and may reassure the patient that sexual activity is still possible.
- Hot or cold showers should be avoided just before and after intercourse.
- Foreplay is desirable because it allows a gradual increase in heart rate before orgasm.
- Positions during intercourse are a matter of individual choice.
- Orogenital sex places no undue strain on the heart.
- A relaxed atmosphere free of fatigue and stress is optimal.
- Prophylactic use of nitrates to decrease chest pain during sexual activity may be suggested.
- Use of erectile agents (e.g., sildenafil) is contraindicated if taking nitrates in any form.
- Anal intercourse should be avoided because of the possibility of inducing a vasovagal response.

MI. However, some HCPs believe that the patient should decide when he or she is ready to resume sex. Others believe patients must be asymptomatic when performing moderate-energy activities before resuming sexual activity.[31]

◆ Evaluation

The expected outcomes are that the patient with ACS will

- Maintain stable signs of adequate cardiac output
- Report relief of pain
- Report decreased anxiety and increased sense of self-control
- Achieve a realistic program of activity that balances physical activity with energy-conserving activities
- Describe the disease process, measures to reduce risk factors, and rehabilitation activities necessary to manage the therapeutic regimen

Additional information on expected outcomes for the patient with ACS is presented in eNursing Care Plan 33-1 available on the website for this chapter.

SUDDEN CARDIAC DEATH

Sudden cardiac death (SCD) is unexpected death resulting from a variety of cardiac causes. Almost 400,000 people experience SCD yearly.[1]

Etiology and Pathophysiology

In SCD a sudden disruption in heart function produces an abrupt loss of CO and cerebral blood flow. The affected person may or may not have a known history of heart disease. SCD is often the first sign of illness for 25% of those who die of heart disease.[32]

Acute ventricular dysrhythmias (e.g., ventricular tachycardia, ventricular fibrillation) cause the majority of cases of SCD. Structural heart disease accounts for 10% of the cases of SCD. Patients in this group include those with LV hypertrophy, myocarditis, and hypertrophic cardiomyopathy. Hypertrophic cardiomyopathy is a risk factor for SCD, especially in young, athletic people.

Some cases of SCD (especially in people less than age 45) occur in the absence of structural heart disease. These involve disturbances in the conduction system (e.g., prolonged QT syndrome, Wolff-Parkinson-White syndrome).

It is difficult to know who is at high risk for SCD. However, LV dysfunction (EF less than 30%) and ventricular dysrhythmias following MI have been found to be the strongest predictors.[32] Other risk factors include history of syncope, LV outflow tract obstruction (e.g., aortic stenosis), male gender (especially African American men), and family history of ventricular dysrhythmias.

Clinical Manifestations and Complications

Individuals who experience SCD because of CAD fall into two groups: (1) those who did not have an acute MI and (2) those who did have an acute MI. The first group accounts for the majority of cases of SCD.[32] These people usually have no warning signs or symptoms. Patients who survive SCD are at risk for another SCD event because of the continued electrical instability of the heart that caused the first event to occur.

The second, smaller group of patients includes those who have had an MI and have suffered SCD. Such patients usually have prodromal symptoms, such as chest pain, palpitations, and dyspnea. Death often occurs within 1 hour of the onset of acute symptoms.

❖ NURSING AND INTERPROFESSIONAL MANAGEMENT: SUDDEN CARDIAC DEATH

People who survive an episode of SCD require a diagnostic workup to determine whether they have had an MI. Serial analysis of cardiac biomarkers and ECGs are done, and the patient is treated accordingly. (See section on interprofessional care of ACS.) In addition, because most individuals with SCD have CAD, cardiac catheterization is done to determine the possible location and extent of coronary artery occlusion. PCI or CABG surgery may be indicated.

Most SCD patients have a lethal ventricular dysrhythmia that is associated with a high incidence of recurrence. It is useful to know when those individuals are most likely to have a recurrence and what drug therapy is the most effective treatment. Assessment of dysrhythmias in these patients includes 24-hour Holter monitoring or other type of event recorder, exercise stress testing, signal-averaged ECG, and electrophysiology study (EPS).

EPS is performed under fluoroscopy. Pacing electrodes are placed in various intracardiac areas, and stimuli are selectively used in an attempt to produce dysrhythmias. The patient's response to various antidysrhythmic drugs is determined and monitored in a controlled environment. (See Chapters 31 and 35 for a discussion of EPS.)

The most common approach to preventing a recurrence of SCD is the use of an implantable cardioverter-defibrillator (ICD). It has been shown that an ICD improves survival compared with drug therapy alone.[32] (See Chapter 35 for a discussion of ICDs.) Drug therapy with amiodarone (Cordarone) may be used with an ICD to decrease episodes of ventricular dysrhythmias.

Some patients at risk for SCD may consider using a LifeVest as a bridge to ICD or heart transplantation[33] (see Chapter 35). A LifeVest is a personal external defibrillator that has two main parts: a garment and monitor. The garment is worn under clothing and has electrodes that continuously record the patient's ECG. The monitor is worn around the waist or from a shoulder strap. If the patient has ventricular tachycardia or ventricular fibrillation, the device sounds an alarm to confirm that the patient is unresponsive. If the patient is conscious, the patient can press two buttons to stop the shock. If the patient does not respond, the device warns bystanders that a shock is about to be delivered. If the dysrhythmia continues and the patient still does not respond, a treatment shock is delivered through the electrodes.[33]

Teaching people about the symptoms of impending cardiac arrest and the actions to take can save lives. Rapid cardiopulmonary resuscitation (CPR) (see Appendix A) and defibrillation with an automatic external defibrillator (AED), combined with early advanced cardiac life support, have improved long-term survival rates for a witnessed arrest.

When caring for these patients, be alert to the patient's psychosocial adaptation to this sudden "brush with death." Many of these patients develop a "time bomb" mentality. They fear the recurrence of cardiac arrest and may become anxious, angry, and depressed. Their caregivers are likely to experience the same feelings. Patients and caregivers may also need to deal with additional issues such as possible driving restrictions, role reversal, and change in occupation. The grief response varies among patients and caregivers. Be attuned to the specific needs of the patient and caregiver. Teach them accordingly while providing appropriate emotional support.

CASE STUDY

Myocardial Infarction

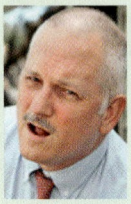

(©iStockphoto/Thinkstock)

Patient Profile

D.M., a 51-year-old, white, successful executive, is rushed to the hospital by ambulance after experiencing crushing, substernal chest pain that radiates down his left arm. He also complains of dizziness and nausea.

Subjective Data

- Has a history of chronic stable angina and hypertension
- States he is "borderline diabetic"
- Overweight but recently lost 10 pounds
- Rarely exercises
- Has three teenage children who are causing "problems"
- Recently experienced loss of best friend and business partner, who died from cancer

Objective Data

Physical Examination

- Diaphoretic, short of breath, nauseous
- BP 165/100 mm Hg, pulse rate 120/min, respiratory rate 26/min

Diagnostic Studies

- 12-lead ECG shows sinus tachycardia with occasional premature ventricular contractions and ST elevation in leads II, III, aVF, V_5, V_6 consistent with an inferolateral wall MI
- Cardiac-specific troponin I level elevated
- Total cholesterol 350 mg/dL (9.1 mmol/L)
- Hb A1C 9.0%

Interprofessional Care

Emergency Department: Notify the cardiac catheterization laboratory of patient with STEMI:

- O_2 2 L/min via nasal cannula, titrate to keep O_2 saturation above 93%
- Continuous ECG monitoring
- 2 IV access sites
- Aspirin 325 mg (chewable)
- Atorvastatin (Lipitor) 80 mg PO
- Eptifibatide (Integrilin) IV
- Weight-based heparin IV
- Nitroglycerin IV, titrate to relieve chest pain; hold for systolic BP below 100 mm Hg
- Morphine 2 mg IV q5-15 min PRN for chest pain unrelieved by nitroglycerin
- Vital signs (including pulse oximetry) every 10 minutes
- Prepare patient for transfer to cardiac catheterization laboratory for possible PCI

Discussion Questions

1. Which coronary artery(ies) is (are) most likely occluded in D.M.'s coronary circulation?
2. Explain the pathogenesis of CAD. What risk factors contribute to its development? What risk factors were present in D.M.'s life?
3. What is angina? How does chronic stable angina differ from angina associated with acute coronary syndrome?
4. Explain the pathophysiologic basis for the clinical manifestations that D.M. exhibited.
5. Explain the significance of the results of the laboratory tests and the 12-lead ECG findings.
6. Provide a rationale for each treatment measure ordered for D.M.
7. ***Priority Decision:*** Based on the assessment data presented, what are the priority nursing diagnoses? Identify any collaborative problems.
8. ***Priority Decision:*** What are the priority nursing interventions for D.M. before PCI? Immediately after his PCI?
9. ***Teamwork and Collaboration:*** Identify activities that can be delegated to unlicensed assistive personnel (UAP).
10. ***Evidence-Based Practice:*** Two days after an uncomplicated PCI and the placement of two stents, D.M. wants to know what the most effective strategies are to prevent another MI. Based on his clinical situation, what would you tell him?
11. ***Quality Improvement:*** What outcomes would indicate that the interdisciplinary care was successful?

Answers and a corresponding conceptual care map available at *http://evolve.elsevier.com/Lewis/medsurg.*

BRIDGE TO NCLEX EXAMINATION

The number of the question corresponds to the same-numbered outcome at the beginning of the chapter.

1. In teaching a patient about coronary artery disease, the nurse explains that the changes that occur in this disorder include *(select all that apply)*
   a. diffuse involvement of plaque formation in coronary veins.
   b. abnormal levels of cholesterol, especially low-density lipoproteins.
   c. accumulation of lipid and fibrous tissue within the coronary arteries.
   d. development of angina due to a decreased blood supply to the heart muscle.
   e. chronic vasoconstriction of coronary arteries leading to permanent vasospasm.
2. After teaching about ways to decrease risk factors for CAD, the nurse recognizes that additional instruction is needed when the patient says
   a. "I would like to add weight lifting to my exercise program."
   b. "I can only keep my blood pressure normal with medication."
   c. "I can change my diet to decrease my intake of saturated fats."
   d. "I will change my lifestyle to reduce activities that increase my stress."
3. A hospitalized patient with a history of chronic stable angina tells the nurse that she is having chest pain. The nurse bases his actions on the knowledge that ischemia
   a. will always progress to myocardial infarction.
   b. will be relieved by rest, nitroglycerin, or both.
   c. indicates that irreversible myocardial damage is occurring.
   d. is frequently associated with vomiting and extreme fatigue.
4. The nurse is caring for a patient who is 2 days post MI. The patient reports that she is experiencing chest pain. She states, "It hurts when I take a deep breath." Which action would be a *priority*?
   a. Notify the physician STAT and obtain a 12-lead ECG.
   b. Obtain vital signs and auscultate for a pericardial friction rub.
   c. Apply high-flow O_2 by face mask and auscultate breath sounds.
   d. Medicate the patient with PRN analgesic and reevaluate in 30 minutes.
5. A patient is admitted to the ICU with a diagnosis of unstable angina. Which drugs(s) would the nurse expect the patient to receive *(select all that apply)*?
   a. ACE inhibitor
   b. Antiplatelet therapy
   c. Thrombolytic therapy
   d. Prophylactic antibiotics
   e. Intravenous nitroglycerin
6. A patient is recovering from an uncomplicated MI. Which rehabilitation guideline is a *priority* to include in the teaching plan?
   a. Refrain from sexual activity for a minimum of 3 weeks.
   b. Plan a diet program that aims for a 1- to 2-pound weight loss per week.
   c. Begin an exercise program that aims for at least five 30-minute sessions per week.
   d. Consider the use of erectile agents and prophylactic NTG before engaging in sexual activity.
7. The most common finding in individuals at risk for sudden cardiac death is
   a. aortic valve disease.
   b. mitral valve disease.
   c. left ventricular dysfunction.
   d. atherosclerotic heart disease.

1. b, c, d, 2. a, 3. b, 4. b, 5. a, b, e, 6. c, 7. c

For rationales to these answers and even more NCLEX review questions, visit *http://evolve.elsevier.com/Lewis/medsurg*.

EVOLVE WEBSITE

http://evolve.elsevier.com/Lewis/medsurg

Review Questions (Online Only)
Key Points
Answer Keys for Questions
- Rationales for Bridge to NCLEX Examination Questions
- Answer Guidelines for Case Study on p. 734

Student Case Study
- Patient With Coronary Artery Disease and Acute Coronary Syndrome

Nursing Care Plan
- eNursing Care Plan 33-1: Patient With Acute Coronary Syndrome

Conceptual Care Map Creator
- Conceptual Care Map for Case Study on p. 734

Audio Glossary
Content Updates

REFERENCES

1. Go AS, Mozaffarian D, Roger VL, et al: Heart disease and stroke statistics: 2014 update: a report from the American Heart Association, *Circulation* 129:e28, 2014.
2. McCance KL, Huether SE: *Pathophysiology*, ed 7, St Louis, 2014, Mosby.
3. Strang F, Schunkert H: C-reactive protein and coronary heart disease: all said—is not it? *Mediators Inflamm* 2014:757123, 2014. doi: 10.1155/2014/757123.

*4. McSweeney JC, Rosenfeld AG, Abel WM, et al: Preventing and experiencing ischemic heart disease as a woman: state of the science a scientific statement from the American Heart Association, *Circulation* 133:00, 2016. DOI: 10.1161/CIR.0000000000000381.

*5. Fihn SD, Blankenship JC, Alexander KP, et al: 2014 CC/AHA/AATS/PCNA/SCAI/STS focused update of the guideline for the diagnosis and management of patients with stable ischemic heart disease: a report of the American College of Cardiology Foundation/American Heart Association Task Force on Practice Guidelines and the American College of Physicians, American Association for Thoracic Surgery, Preventive Cardiovascular Nurses Association, Society for Cardiovascular Angiography and Interventions, and Society of Thoracic Surgeons, *Circulation* 130:1749,2014.

6. Sasidhar MV, Reddy S, Naik A, et al: Genetics of coronary artery disease—a clinician's perspective, *Indian Heart J* 66(6):663, 2014.

*7. Eckel RH, Jakicic JM, Ard JD, et al: 2013 AHA/ACC guideline on lifestyle management to reduce cardiovascular risk - a report of the American College of Cardiology/American Heart Association Task Force on Practice Guidelines, *Circulation* 129(suppl 2):S76, 2014.

*8. Goff DC, Lloyd-Jones DM, Bennett G, et al: 2013 ACC/AHA guideline on the assessment of cardiovascular risk: a report of the American College of Cardiology/American Heart Association Task Force on Practice Guidelines, *Circulation* 12(suppl 2):S49, 2014.

*9. James PA, Oparil S, Carter BL, et al: 2014 evidence-based guideline for the management of high blood pressure in adults: report from the panel members appointed to the eighth Joint National Committee (JNC 8), *JAMA* 311:507, 2014.

*10. National Heart, Lung, and Blood Institute. Landmark NIH study shows intensive blood pressure management may save lives. Retrieved from *http://www.nhlbi.nih.gov/news/press-releases/2015/landmark-nih-study-shows-intensive-blood-pressure-management-may-save-lives.*

*11. National Institutes of Health: *Seventh report of the Joint National Committee on Prevention, Detection, Evaluation, and Treatment of High Blood Pressure (JNC 7), pub no 03-5233*, Bethesda, Md, 2003, US Department of Health and Human Services.

*12. Jhamnani S, Patel D, Heimlich L, et al: Meta-analysis of the effects of lifestyle modifications on coronary and carotid atherosclerotic burden, *Am J Cardiol* 115(2):268, 2015.

*13. Burg MM, Edmondson D, Shimbo D, et al: The "perfect storm" and acute coronary syndrome onset: do psychosocial factors play a role? *Prog Cardiovasc Dis* 55(6):601, 2013.

*14. Cohen BE, Edmondson D, Kronish IM: State of the art review: depression, stress, anxiety, and cardiovascular disease, *Am J Hypertens* 28(11):1295, 2015.

15. American Heart Association: Homocysteine, folic acid, and cardiovascular disease. Retrieved from *http://www.heart.org/HEARTORG/GettingHealthy/NutritionCenter/Homocysteine-Folic-Acid-and-Cardiovascular-Disease_UCM_305997_Article.jsp.*

16. National Institute on Drug Abuse: Drug facts: cocaine. Retrieved from *http://www.drugabuse.gov/publications/drugfacts/cocaine.*

17. Lehne RA: *Pharmacology for nursing care*, ed 8, St Louis, 2013, Saunders.

18. Pietrangelo A: PCSK9 inhibitors: what you need to know. Retrieved from *http://www.healthline.com/health/pcsk9-inhibitors-what-you-need-to-know#Overview1*

*19. Bibbins-Domingo K, Grossman DC, Curry SJ, et al: Aspirin use for the primary prevention of cardiovascular disease and colorectal cancer: U.S. preventive services task force recommendation statement, *Ann Intern Med* doi:10.7326/M16-0577 Retrieved from *http://annals.org/article.aspx?articleid=2513179*, 2016.

*20. Levine GN, O'Gara PT, Bates ER, et al: 2015 ACC/AHA/SCAI focused update on primary percutaneous coronary intervention for patients with ST-elevation myocardial infarction: an update of the 2011 ACCF/AHA/SCAI guideline for percutaneous coronary intervention and the 2013 ACCF/AHA guideline for the management of ST-elevation myocardial infarction, *Circulation* 133:1135, 2016.

21. Mann DL, Zipes DP, Libby P, et al: *Braunwald heart disease: a textbook of cardiovascular medicine*, ed 10, St Louis, 2015, Saunders.

22. Fiore DP, Beltrame JF: Chest pain in patients with 'normal angiography': could it be cardiac? *Int J Evid-Based Health* 11:56, 2013.

*23. Amsterdam EA, Wenger NK, Brindis RG, et al: 2014 AHA/ACC guideline for the management of patients with non-ST-elevation acute coronary syndromes: executive summary, *JACC* 64:2645, 2014.

*24. Hillis LD, Smith PK, Anderson JL, et al: 2011 ACCF/AHA guideline for coronary artery bypass graft surgery: a report of the American College of Cardiology Foundation/American Heart Association Task Force on Practice Guidelines, *Circulation* 124:e652, 2011.

25. Bojar RM: *Manual of perioperative care in adult cardiac surgery*, ed 5, Hoboken, NJ, 2011, Wiley-Blackwell.

*26. Jneid H, Anderson JL, Wright RS, et al: 2012 ACCF/AHA focused update of the guidelines for the management of patients with unstable angina/non-ST-elevation myocardial infarction (updating the 2007 guideline and replacing the 2011 focused update), *J Am Coll Cardiol* 126:875, 2012.

*27. American Association of Critical-Care Nurses: Family presence: visitation in the adult ICU (2011). Retrieved from *www.aacn.org/WD/practice/docs/practicealerts/family-visitation-adult-icu-practicealert.pdf.*

28. Rovai D, Giannessi D, Andreassi MG, et al: Mind injuries after cardiac surgery, *J Cardiovasc Med (Hagerstown)*. 16(12):844, 2015.

29. American Heart Association: Angina log. Retrieved from *https://www.heart.org/idc/groups/heart-public/@wcm/@hcm/documents/downloadable/ucm_307470.pdf.*

30. European Society of Cardiology: Women more likely to develop anxiety and depression after heart attack (2014). Retrieved from *www.escardio.org/about/press/press-releases/pr-14/Pages/women-develop-anxiety-post-infarction.aspx.*

*31. Levine GN, Steinke EE, Bakaeen FG, et al: Sexual activity and cardiovascular disease: a scientific statement from the American Heart Association, *Circulation* 125:1058, 2012.

32. Mitrani RD, Myerburg RJ: Ten advances defining sudden cardiac death, *Trends Cardiovasc Med* 26(1):23, 2016.

33. Cleveland Clinic: LifeVest. Retrieved from *http://my.clevelandclinic.org/services/heart/services/lifevest.*

*Evidence-based information for clinical practice.

34

Heart Failure

Carolyn Moffa

Wherever you go, go with all your heart.

Confucius

http://evolve.elsevier.com/Lewis/medsurg/

LEARNING OUTCOMES

1. Compare the pathophysiology of systolic and diastolic heart failure (HF).
2. Relate the compensatory mechanisms involved in HF to the development of acute decompensated heart failure (ADHF) and chronic HF.
3. Select appropriate nursing and interprofessional care to manage the patient with ADHF.
4. Select appropriate nursing and interprofessional care to manage the patient with chronic HF.
5. Describe the indications for heart transplantation and the nursing care of heart transplant recipients.

KEY TERMS

diastolic failure, p. 738
heart failure (HF), p. 737
heart transplantation, p. 753
paroxysmal nocturnal dyspnea (PND), p. 742
pulmonary edema, p. 741
systolic failure, p. 738

HEART FAILURE

Heart failure (HF) is a complex clinical syndrome that results in the inability of the heart to provide sufficient blood to meet the O_2 needs of tissues and organs. It is a major health problem in the United States. This chapter discusses the nursing and interprofessional care of patients experiencing this syndrome.

A defect in either ventricular filling (diastolic dysfunction) or ventricular ejection (systolic dysfunction) are the key manifestations of HF. The amount of blood pumped by the left ventricle with each heart beat is called the *ejection fraction* (EF). The American Academy of Cardiology Foundation (ACCF) has adopted the terms *heart failure with reduced EF* (HFrEF) and *heart failure with preserved EF* (HFpEF) to describe systolic and diastolic HF.[1]

HF is associated with numerous cardiovascular diseases (CVDs), particularly long-standing hypertension, coronary artery disease (CAD), and myocardial infarction (MI). Unlike other CVDs, HF is increasing in incidence and prevalence. This is in part due to better survival after cardiac events and the aging population. HF is primarily a disease of older adults. The incidence is similar in men and women.[2]

The American Heart Association (AHA) estimates that more than 650,000 new cases of HF are diagnosed each year.[2] It is the most common reason for hospital admission in adults over the age of 65. This places a significant economic burden on the health care system.[1] The complex, progressive nature of HF often results in poor outcomes, the most costly being hospital readmissions. Approximately 25% of patients discharged with a primary diagnosis of HF are readmitted within 30 days. The total cost of HF care in the United States exceeds $40 billion annually, with over half of these costs spent on hospitalizations.[2]

Etiology

Hypertension and CAD are the primary risk factors for HF. Hypertension is a modifiable risk factor that should be aggressively treated and managed. Long-term treatment of hypertension reduces the incidence of HF by 50%.[1] Other co-morbidities, such as diabetes, metabolic syndrome, advanced age, tobacco use, and vascular disease, also contribute to the development of HF. (Metabolic syndrome is discussed in Chapter 40.)

HF may be caused by any interference with the normal mechanisms regulating cardiac output (CO). CO depends on (1) preload, (2) afterload, (3) myocardial contractility, and (4) heart rate (HR). (Preload and afterload are discussed in Chapter 31.) Any changes in these factors can lead to decreased ventricular function and HF.

The major causes of HF may be divided into two subgroups: (1) primary causes (Table 34-1) and (2) precipitating causes

Reviewed by Vera Barton-Caro, RN, PhD, FNP-BC, CHFN, Assistant Professor of Nursing, Wheeling Jesuit University, Wheeling, West Virginia; Carla V. Hannon, MS, APRN, CCRN, CCNS, Clinical Nurse Specialist, Medical Intensive Care Unit, Yale–New Haven Hospital, New Haven, Connecticut; Patricia Lea, RN, DNP, CCRN, Assistant Professor, University of Texas Medical Branch School of Nursing, Galveston, Texas; and Rebecca Personett, RN, PhD, NEA-BC, Professor of Nursing, North Central Texas College, Gainesville, Texas and Brookhaven College, Dallas, Texas.

TABLE 34-1 Primary Causes of Heart Failure

- Hypertension, including hypertensive crisis
- Coronary artery disease, including myocardial infarction
- Rheumatic heart disease
- Congenital heart defects (e.g., ventricular septal defect)
- Pulmonary hypertension
- Cardiomyopathy (e.g., viral, postpartum, substance abuse)
- Hyperthyroidism
- Valvular disorders (e.g., mitral stenosis)
- Myocarditis

CULTURAL & ETHNIC HEALTH DISPARITIES

Heart Failure

- African Americans have a higher incidence of HF, develop HF at an earlier age, and experience higher mortality rates related to HF than whites.
- African Americans may experience more ACE inhibitor–related angioedema than whites.
- Isosorbide dinitrate/hydralazine (BiDil) is used for the treatment of HF in African Americans. This combination drug is approved for use only in this ethnic group.
- Asians have an extremely high risk (15%-50%) for ACE inhibitor–related cough.

ACE, Angiotensin-converting enzyme; *HF,* heart failure.

(Table 34-2). Precipitating causes often increase the workload of the heart, resulting in an acute condition and decreased heart function.

Genetic Link

Specific genes and gene mutations have been linked to the development of hypertension, CAD, and cardiomyopathy (weakening of the heart muscle) (see Chapters 32, 33, and 36). These CVDs are known risk factors for HF. Cardiomyopathy, a common cause of HF, may be attributed to as many as 40 different defective genes. The body's largest protein is a muscle protein called *titin,* which is found in cardiac sarcomeres (part of the heart muscle that contracts). Mutations in the titin gene are the most common known genetic cause of dilated cardiomyopathy.[3] More research into the effects of these gene mutations, as well as other genetic mutations, is needed.

Pathophysiology

Left-Sided Heart Failure. The most common form of HF is left-sided HF. Left-sided HF results either from the inability of the left ventricle (LV) to (1) empty adequately during systole or (2) fill adequately during diastole. Left-sided HF can be further classified as systolic, diastolic, or mixed systolic and diastolic failure.

Systolic Failure or Heart Failure with Reduced EF. **Systolic failure**, also known as HFrEF, results from an inability of the heart to pump blood effectively. The hallmark of systolic failure is a decrease in the EF. Normal EF is 55% to 60%. Patients with HFrEF generally have an EF less than 45%. It can be as low as 5% to 10%. HFrEF is caused by impaired contractile function (e.g., MI), increased afterload (e.g., hypertension), cardiomyopathy, and mechanical abnormalities (e.g., valvular heart disease).

TABLE 34-2 Precipitating Causes of Heart Failure*

Cause	Mechanism
Anemia	↓ O_2-carrying capacity of the blood stimulating ↑ in CO to meet tissue demands, leading to increase in cardiac workload and increase in size of LV
Infection	↑ O_2 demand of tissues, stimulating ↑ CO
Thyrotoxicosis	Changes the tissue metabolic rate, ↑ HR and workload of the heart
Hypothyroidism	Indirectly predisposes to ↑ atherosclerosis. Severe hypothyroidism decreases myocardial contractility.
Dysrhythmias	May ↓ CO and ↑ workload and O_2 requirements of myocardial tissue
Bacterial endocarditis	*Infection:* ↑ metabolic demands and O_2 requirements *Valvular dysfunction:* causes stenosis or regurgitation
Obstructive sleep apnea	Frequent nighttime apnea results in ↑ afterload, intermittent hypoxia, and ↑ sympathetic nervous system activity.
Pulmonary embolism	↑ Pulmonary pressure resulting from obstruction leads to pulmonary hypertension, ↓ CO.
Paget's disease	↑ Workload of the heart by ↑ vascular bed in the skeletal muscle
Nutritional deficiencies	May ↓ cardiac function by ↑ myocardial muscle mass and myocardial contractility
Hypervolemia	↑ Preload causing volume overload on the RV

CO, Cardiac output; *LV,* left ventricle; *RV,* right ventricle.
*List is not all inclusive.

The LV in systolic failure loses its ability to generate enough pressure to eject blood forward through the aorta. Over time, the LV becomes dilated and hypertrophied. The weakened heart muscle cannot generate adequate stroke volume, which affects CO. Because the LV cannot effectively push blood forward, end diastolic volumes and pressures in the LV increase. When the LV fails, blood backs up into the left atrium. This causes fluid accumulation in the lungs. The increased pulmonary hydrostatic pressure causes fluid leakage from the pulmonary capillary bed into the interstitium and then the alveoli. This results in pulmonary congestion and edema (Fig. 34-1, *A* through *D*).

Diastolic Failure or Heart Failure With Preserved EF. **Diastolic failure**, or HFpEF, is the inability of the ventricles to relax and fill during diastole. Approximately 50% of patients with HF have HFpEF. Hypertension is the most important cause of diastolic failure.[1] Other risk factors include older age, female gender, diabetes, and obesity (see Gender Differences box). In diastolic failure, the LV is generally stiff and noncompliant. Diastolic failure is characterized by high filling pressures because of stiff ventricles. Decreased filling of the ventricles results in decreased stroke volume and CO. The end result of diastolic failure is the same as systolic failure (e.g., pulmonary congestion). HFpEF is diagnosed by the following criteria: (1) signs and symptoms of HF, (2) normal EF, and (3) evidence of LV diastolic dysfunction by echocardiography or cardiac catheterization. Therapies for HFpEF are targeted at reducing underlying risk factors and treating co-morbidities.

Mixed Systolic and Diastolic Failure. Mixed systolic and diastolic failure is seen in disease states such as *dilated cardiomyopathy* (DCM). DCM is a condition in which poor systolic function is further compromised by a dilated LV that is unable

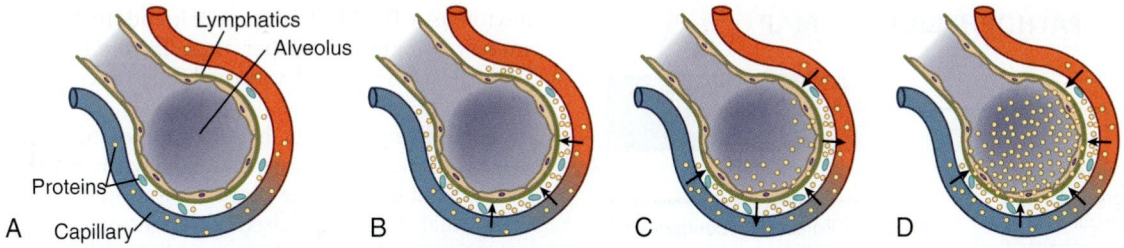

FIG. 34-1 As pulmonary edema progresses, it inhibits O_2 and CO_2 exchange at the alveolar-capillary interface. **A,** Normal relationship. **B,** Increased pulmonary capillary hydrostatic pressure causes fluid to move from the vascular space into the pulmonary interstitial space. **C,** Lymphatic flow increases in an attempt to pull fluid back into the vascular or lymphatic space. **D,** Failure of lymphatic flow and worsening of left-sided heart failure result in further movement of fluid into the interstitial space and into the alveoli. (Modified from Urden LD, Stacy KM, Lough ME: *Critical care nursing: diagnosis and management,* ed 6, St Louis, 2010, Mosby.)

GENDER DIFFERENCES

Heart Failure

Men	Women
• Men experience systolic failure more frequently than women. • Men with asymptomatic systolic failure experience greater mortality benefit from ACE inhibitor therapy than women.	• Women experience diastolic failure more frequently than men. • Women have a higher risk of ACE inhibitor–related cough than men. • Women experience more digitalis-related death than men. • Women with diabetes are more predisposed to HF than men.

ACE, Angiotensin-converting enzyme; *HF,* heart failure.

to relax (see Chapter 36). These patients often have extremely low EFs (less than 35%), high pulmonary pressures, and *biventricular failure* (both ventricles are dilated and have poor filling and emptying capacity).

The patient with ventricular failure of any type may have low BP, low CO, and poor renal perfusion. Poor exercise tolerance and heart dysrhythmias are also common. The patient may arrive at this point acutely from an MI or chronically from worsening cardiomyopathy or hypertension. In both acute and chronic causes of HF, the body's response to low CO is to mobilize its compensatory mechanisms to maintain CO and BP.

Right-Sided Heart Failure. Right-sided HF occurs when the right ventricle (RV) fails to pump effectively. When the RV fails, fluid backs up into the venous system. This causes movement of fluid into the tissues and organs (e.g., peripheral edema, abdominal ascites, hepatomegaly, jugular venous distention).

The most common cause of right-sided HF is left-sided HF (Fig. 34-2). As the LV fails, fluid backs up into the pulmonary system, causing increased pressures in the lungs. The RV has to work harder to push blood to the pulmonary system. Over time, this increased workload weakens the RV and gradually it fails. Other causes of right-sided HF (independent of the function of the LV) include RV infarction, pulmonary embolism, and *cor pulmonale* (RV dilation and hypertrophy caused by pulmonary disease) (see Chapter 27).

Compensatory Mechanisms. HF can have an abrupt onset as with acute MI, or it can be a subtle process resulting from slow, progressive changes. The overloaded heart uses compensatory mechanisms to try to maintain adequate CO. The main compensatory mechanisms include (1) neurohormonal responses: renin-angiotensin-aldosterone system (RAAS) and the sympathetic nervous system (SNS), (2) ventricular dilation, and (3) ventricular hypertrophy.

Neurohormonal Response

Renin-angiotensin-aldosterone system. The RAAS is a regulatory system that works to maintain normal homeostasis. The activation of the RAAS results in BP control and fluid and electrolyte balance. In response to stress, the role of the RAAS is to promote retention of fluid and sodium and cause vasoconstriction to raise BP. However, recurrent activation of the RAAS in HF is what is responsible for the signs and symptoms that develop.

As CO falls, blood flow to the kidneys decreases. This is sensed by the juxtaglomerular apparatus in the kidneys as decreased volume. In response, the kidneys release renin, which converts angiotensinogen to angiotensin I (see Chapter 44 and Fig. 44-4). Angiotensin I is next converted to angiotensin II by a converting enzyme made in the lungs. Angiotensin II causes (1) activation of the SNS to increase BP and HR; (2) release of aldosterone from the adrenal cortex, which results in sodium and water retention; (3) increased peripheral vasoconstriction, which increases BP; and (4) stimulation of the pituitary gland, which releases antidiuretic hormone (ADH), which results in water reabsorption. The outcome of the cascade results in further water and sodium retention in an already overloaded state and increased workload of the failing heart.

Other factors also contribute to the development of HF. The production of *endothelin,* a potent vasoconstrictor produced by the vascular endothelial cells, is stimulated by ADH, angiotensin II, and catecholamines. This results in further arterial vasoconstriction and an increase in cardiac contractility and hypertrophy.

Locally, proinflammatory cytokines are released by heart cells in response to various forms of heart injury (e.g., MI). Two cytokines, tumor necrosis factor (TNF) and interleukin-1 (IL-1), further depress heart function by causing hypertrophy, contractile dysfunction, and cell death. Over time, a systemic inflammatory response also occurs.

Sympathetic nervous system. In response to an inadequate stroke volume and CO, the SNS is activated, resulting in the release of catecholamines (epinephrine and norepinephrine). The circulating catecholamines enhance peripheral vasoconstriction and cause an increase in the HR *(chronotropy)* and

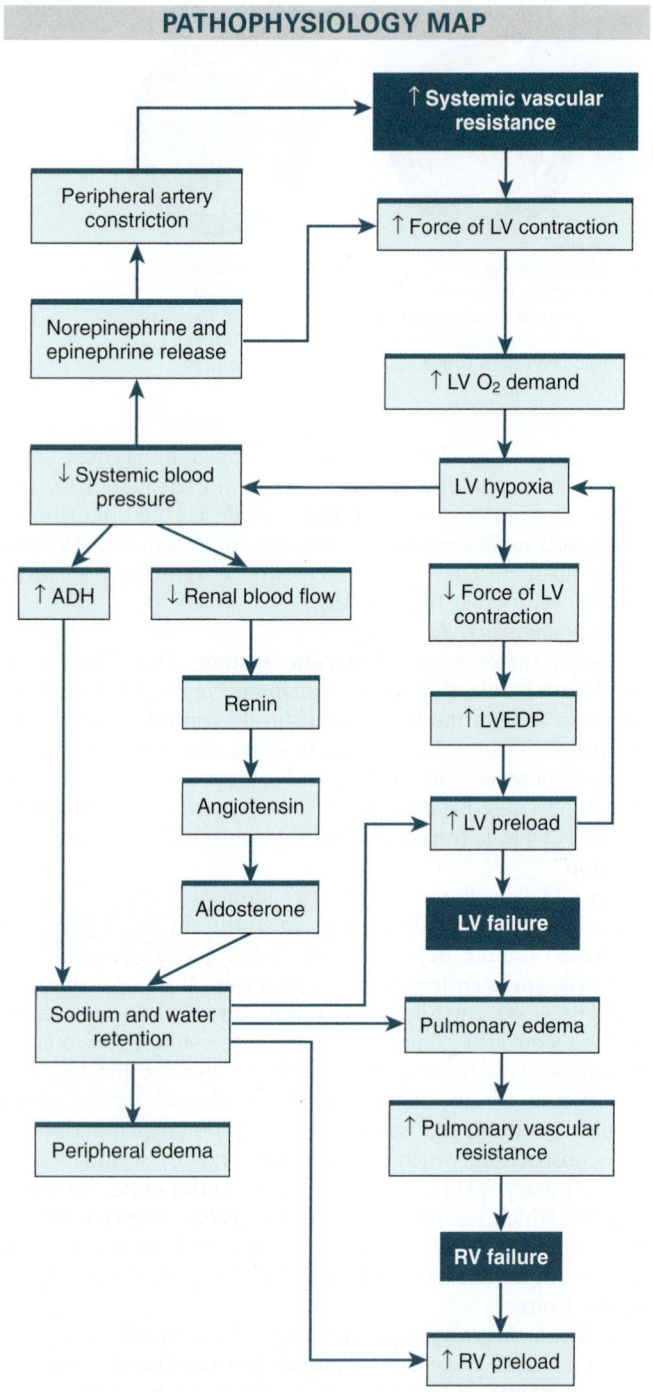

FIG. 34-2 Pathophysiology of heart failure. Elevated systemic vascular resistance results in left-sided heart failure that leads to right-sided heart failure. Systemic vascular resistance and preload are exacerbated by the renin-angiotensin-aldosterone system. *ADH,* Antidiuretic hormone; *LA,* left atrium; *LV,* left ventricle; *LVEDP,* left ventricular end-diastolic pressure; *RV,* right ventricle. (Modified from Huether SE, McCance KL: *Understanding pathophysiology,* ed 3, St Louis, 2004, Mosby.)

myocardial contractility *(inotropy)*. Initially, the compensatory mechanisms are beneficial with a result of increased CO. However, over time these factors become harmful and counterproductive, as they increase the workload, preload (volume), and O_2 requirement in an already failing heart.

In HF, continuous activation of the neurohormonal responses (RAAS and SNS) leads to elevated levels of norepinephrine, angiotensin II, aldosterone, ADH, endothelin, and proinflammatory cytokines. Together, these factors result in an increase in the heart's workload, ventricular dysfunction, and *ventricular remodeling.*

Remodeling involves hypertrophy of the ventricular myocytes. This results in large, abnormally shaped contractile cells. This altered shape of the ventricles eventually leads to increased ventricular mass, increased wall tension, increased O_2 consumption, and impaired contractility. Although the ventricles become larger, they become less effective pumps. Ventricular remodeling is a risk factor for life-threatening dysrhythmias and sudden cardiac death (SCD). Drug therapies to prevent or reverse remodeling and decrease mortality are recommended. These include ACE inhibitors, β-adrenergic blockers (β-blockers), and aldosterone antagonists.

Dilation. *Dilation* is an enlargement of the chambers of the heart (Fig. 34-3, *A*). It occurs when pressure in the heart chambers (usually the LV) is elevated over time. The heart muscle fibers stretch in response to the volume of blood in the heart at the end of diastole. The degree of stretch is directly related to the force of the contraction (systole) (this is the *Frank-Starling law*). This increased contraction initially leads to increased CO and maintenance of BP and perfusion. Dilation starts as an adaptive mechanism to cope with increasing blood volume. Eventually this mechanism becomes inadequate, because the elastic elements of the muscle fibers are overstretched and can no longer contract effectively, thereby decreasing the CO.

Hypertrophy. *Hypertrophy* is an increase in the muscle mass and heart wall thickness in response to overwork and strain (Fig. 34-3, *B*). It occurs slowly because it takes time for this increased muscle tissue to develop. Initially, the increased contractile power of the muscle fibers leads to an increase in CO and maintenance of tissue perfusion. Over time, hypertrophic heart muscle has poor contractility, requires more O_2 to perform work, has poor coronary artery circulation (tissue becomes ischemic more easily), and is prone to dysrhythmias.

Counterregulatory Mechanisms. The body's attempts to maintain balance are demonstrated by several counterregulatory processes. Natriuretic peptides (atrial natriuretic peptide [ANP] and brain [b-type] natriuretic peptide [BNP]) are hormones produced by the heart muscle. ANP is released from the atria, and BNP is released from the ventricles in response to increased blood volume in the heart.[4]

The natriuretic peptides have renal, cardiovascular, and hormonal effects. Renal effects include (1) increased glomerular filtration rate and diuresis and (2) excretion of sodium (natriuresis). Cardiovascular effects include vasodilation and decreased BP. Hormonal effects include (1) inhibition of aldosterone and renin secretion and (2) interference with ADH release. The combined effects of ANP and BNP help to counter the adverse effects of the SNS and RAAS in patients with HF.[4]

Nitric oxide (NO) and prostaglandin are counterregulatory substances released from the vascular endothelium in response to the compensatory mechanisms activated in HF. Like the natriuretic peptides, NO and prostaglandin work to relax the arterial smooth muscle, resulting in vasodilation and decreased afterload.

Compensated HF occurs when compensatory mechanisms succeed in maintaining an adequate CO that is needed for tissue perfusion. Decompensated HF occurs when these mechanisms can no longer maintain adequate CO and inadequate tissue perfusion results.

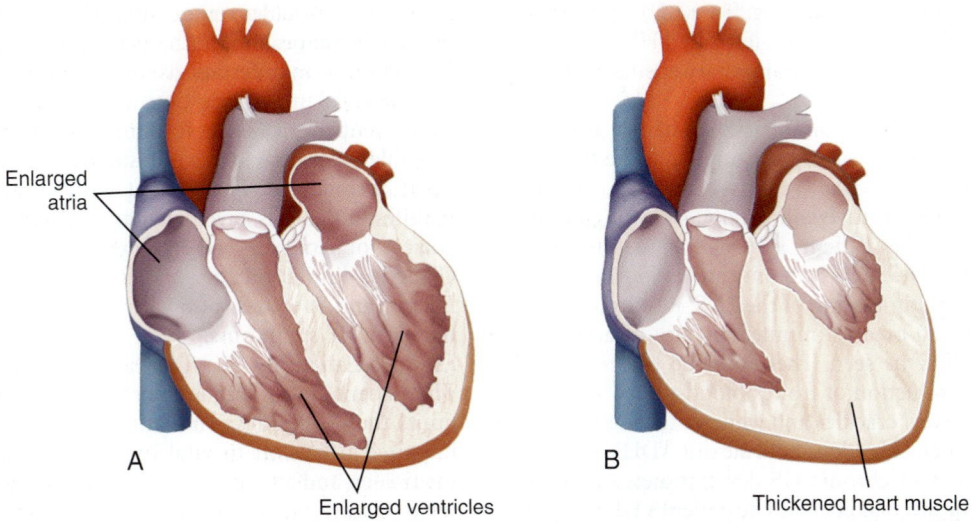

FIG. 34-3 **A,** Dilated heart chambers. **B,** Hypertrophied heart chambers.

Classification of Heart Failure

The New York Heart Association (NYHA) developed functional guidelines for classifying people with heart disease based on tolerance to physical activity. Because this system only reflected exercise capacity, the American College of Cardiology Foundation/AHA (ACCF/AHA) developed a staging system that identified disease progression and treatment strategies.[1] This system allows for identification of people at risk for developing HF but who do not currently have heart disease. The ACCF/AHA system encourages clinicians to actively address the patient's risk factors and treat any existing conditions to prevent further disease progression. This may help reduce the growing number of HF patients.

Patients may move between levels in the NYHA classification system based on worsening or improving symptoms. However, the ACCF/AHA staging system is progressive. Patients can only advance to a higher (worse) stage as the disease progresses (Table 34-3).

TABLE 34-3 Comparison of ACCF/AHA Stages of Heart Failure and NYHA Functional Classifications

ACCF/AHA Stages of Heart Failure (HF)	NYHA Functional Classifications
A At high risk for HF, but without structural heart disease or symptoms of HF	None
B Structural heart disease, but without signs or symptoms of HF	**I** No limitation of physical activity. Ordinary physical activity does not cause symptoms of HF.
C Structural heart disease with prior or current symptoms of HF	**I** No limitation of physical activity. Ordinary physical activity does not cause symptoms of HF.
	II Slight limitation of physical activity. Comfortable at rest, but ordinary physical activity results in symptoms of HF.
	III Marked limitation of physical activity. Comfortable at rest, but less than ordinary activity causes symptoms of HF.
	IV Unable to carry on any physical activity without symptoms of HF, or symptoms of HF at rest
D Refractory HF requiring specialized interventions	**IV** Unable to carry on any physical activity without symptoms of HF, or symptoms of HF at rest

Reprinted with permission. *Circulation* 128:e240-e327, 2013. ©2013 American Heart Association, Inc.
ACCF, American College of Cardiology Foundation; *AHA,* American Heart Association; *HF,* heart failure; *NYHA,* New York Heart Association.

Clinical Manifestations: Acute Decompensated Heart Failure

Acute decompensated HF (ADHF) is defined as the sudden onset of signs and symptoms of HF, requiring urgent medical care. The universal finding in ADHF is pulmonary and systemic congestion due to elevated left-sided and right-sided filling pressures. In ADHF, an increase in pulmonary venous pressure is caused by failure of the LV. This results in engorgement of the pulmonary vascular system (Fig. 34-1, *A* and *B*). As a result, the lungs become less compliant, and there is increased resistance in the small airways. To help compensate, the lymphatic system increases its flow to help maintain a constant volume of the pulmonary extravascular fluid. This early stage is clinically associated with a mild increase in the respiratory rate and a decrease in partial pressure of O_2 in arterial blood (PaO_2).

If pulmonary venous pressure continues to increase, the increase in intravascular pressure causes more fluid to move into the interstitial space than the lymphatics can remove. *Interstitial edema* occurs at this point (Fig. 34-1, *C*). Tachypnea develops, and the patient becomes symptomatic (e.g., short of breath). If the pulmonary venous pressure increases further, the alveoli lining cells are disrupted, and a fluid containing red blood cells (RBCs) moves into the alveoli *(alveolar edema)*. As the disruption becomes worse from further increases in the pulmonary venous pressure, the alveoli and airways are flooded with fluid. This is accompanied by a worsening of the arterial blood gas values (i.e., lower PaO_2 and possible increased partial pressure of CO_2 in arterial blood [$PaCO_2$] and progressive respiratory acidosis).

ADHF can manifest as **pulmonary edema.** This is an acute, life-threatening situation, in which the lung alveoli become filled with serosanguineous fluid (Fig. 34-1, *D*). The most common cause of pulmonary edema is left-sided HF secondary to CAD. (Other etiologic factors for pulmonary edema are listed in Table 27-25.)

Clinical manifestations of pulmonary edema are distinct. The patient has dyspnea and *orthopnea* (unable to lie flat due to shortness of breath). Jugular venous distention is often present and is the most sensitive and specific sign for elevated LV filling pressures. The patient is usually anxious, pale, and possibly cyanotic. The skin is clammy and cold from vasoconstriction caused by stimulation of the SNS. Respiratory rate is often greater than 30 breaths/minute, and use of accessory muscles to breathe may be seen. There may be wheezing and coughing with the production of frothy, blood-tinged sputum. Breath sounds may reveal crackles and wheezes throughout the lungs. The absence of crackles does not rule out ADHF as many patients with a history of chronic HF develop increased lymphatic drainage of the alveolar edema. The patient's HR is rapid, and an abnormal S_3 or S_4 heart sound may be auscultated (see Table 31-4). BP may be elevated or decreased depending on the severity of the HF.

CHECK YOUR PRACTICE

You are assigned to a patient with ADHF who has been admitted to the Heart Failure Unit. Your assessment reveals that the patient has bilateral crackles in the mid-lower lung fields and dyspnea on exertion (e.g., moving from the bed to the commode). The patient's skin is warm and pulses are present in all extremities. Your preceptor asks you to categorize your patient based on the classification system in Table 34-4.

- In what category would you put your patient?

Patients with ADHF can be categorized into one of four groups based on hemodynamic and clinical status: dry-warm, dry-cold, wet-warm, and wet-cold[1] (Table 34-4). The most common presentation in patients with ADHF is the wet and warm patient. A patient is "wet" due to volume overload (e.g., congestion, dyspnea) but "warm" due to adequate perfusion (warm skin, positive pulses).

Clinical Manifestations: Chronic Heart Failure

Chronic HF is characterized as a progressive worsening of ventricular function and chronic neurohormonal activation that results in ventricular remodeling. This process involves changes in the size, shape, and mechanical performance of the ventricle. The clinical manifestations of chronic HF depend on the patient's age, underlying type and extent of heart disease, and which ventricle is failing to pump effectively.

Table 34-5 lists the manifestations of right-sided and left-sided chronic HF. The patient with chronic HF usually has manifestations of biventricular failure. The Heart Failure Society of America (HFSA) developed the acronym *FACES* (*F*atigue, limitation of *A*ctivities, chest *C*ongestion/cough, *E*dema, and *S*hortness of breath) to help teach patients to identify early HF symptoms.[5]

Fatigue. Fatigue is one of the earliest symptoms of chronic HF. The patient notes fatigue after usual activities and eventually limits these activities. The fatigue is caused by decreased CO, impaired perfusion to vital organs, decreased oxygenation of the tissues, and anemia. Anemia can result from poor nutrition, renal disease, or drug therapy (e.g., angiotensin-converting enzyme [ACE] inhibitors).

Dyspnea. Dyspnea is a common manifestation of chronic HF. It is caused by increased pulmonary pressures secondary to interstitial and alveolar edema. Dyspnea can occur with mild exertion or at rest. Orthopnea often accompanies dyspnea. Careful questioning of patients often reveals adaptive behaviors such as sleeping with two or more pillows or in a chair to aid breathing.

Paroxysmal nocturnal dyspnea (PND) occurs when the patient is asleep. The patient awakens in a panic and has feelings of suffocation and a strong desire to sit or stand to aid breathing. PND is caused by the reabsorption of fluid from dependent body areas when the patient is flat. A cough is often associated

TABLE 34-4 Clinical Profile in Acute Decompensated Heart Failure

		CONGESTION (WET)	
		No	**Yes**
LOW PERFUSION (COLD)	**No**	**Dry-Warm** • PAWP normal • CO normal • Signs and symptoms: none	**Wet-Warm** • PAWP ↑ • CO normal • Possible signs and symptoms: dyspnea, edema, orthopnea
	Yes	**Dry-Cold** • PAWP ↓ or normal • CO ↓ • Possible signs and symptoms: edema, hypotension, cool extremities	**Wet-Cold** • PAWP ↑ • CO ↓ • Possible signs and symptoms: altered mental status, decreased O_2 saturation, reduced urine output, shock

CO, Cardiac output; *PAWP*, pulmonary artery wedge pressure.

TABLE 34-5 Manifestations of Heart Failure

Right-Sided Heart Failure	Left-Sided Heart Failure
Signs	
• RV heaves • Murmurs • Jugular venous distention • Edema (e.g., pedal, scrotum, sacrum) • Weight gain • ↑ HR • Ascites • Anasarca (massive generalized body edema) • Hepatomegaly (liver enlargement)	• LV heaves • Pulsus alternans (alternating pulses: strong, weak) • ↑ HR • PMI displaced inferiorly and left of the midclavicular line (LV hypertrophy) • ↓ PaO_2, slight ↑ $PaCO_2$ (poor O_2 exchange) • Crackles (pulmonary edema) • S_3 and S_4 heart sounds • Pleural effusion • Changes in mental status • Restlessness, confusion
Symptoms	
• Fatigue • Anxiety, depression • Dependent, bilateral edema • Right upper quadrant pain • Anorexia and GI bloating • Nausea	• Weakness, fatigue • Anxiety, depression • Dyspnea • Shallow respirations up to 32-40/min • Paroxysmal nocturnal dyspnea • Orthopnea • Dry, hacking cough • Nocturia • Frothy, pink-tinged sputum (advanced pulmonary edema)

LV, Left ventricle; *$PaCO_2$*, partial pressure of CO_2 in arterial blood; *PaO_2*, partial pressure of O_2 in arterial blood; *PMI*, point of maximal impulse; *RV*, right ventricle.

with HF and may be the first clinical symptom. It begins as a dry, nonproductive cough and may be misdiagnosed as asthma or other lung disease. The cough is not relieved by position change or over-the-counter cough medicine.

Tachycardia. Tachycardia is an early clinical sign of HF. One of the body's first responses to compensate for a failing heart is to increase the HR via activation of the SNS. This works to increase CO. Initially this response is favorable, but over time, persistent tachycardia is harmful and may exacerbate HF. Adequate HR control in patients with chronic HF has been associated with better clinical outcomes, including decreased hospitalizations and mortality.[6]

Edema. Edema is a common sign of HF. It may occur in dependent body areas (peripheral edema), liver (hepatomegaly), abdominal cavity (ascites), and lungs (pulmonary edema and pleural effusion). If the patient is in bed, sacral and scrotal edema may develop. Pressing the edematous skin with the finger may leave a depression *(pitting edema)*. The development of dependent edema or a sudden weight gain of more than 3 lb (1.4 kg) in 2 days is often a sign of ADHF. It is important to note that not all lower-extremity edema is a result of HF. Hypoproteinemia, immobility, venous insufficiency, and certain drugs can cause peripheral edema.

Nocturia. Nocturia is the tendency to urinate excessively during the night. Chronic HF is frequently associated with poor renal perfusion and function. Patients develop increased peripheral and systemic edema. At night when lying flat, extravascular fluid is reabsorbed from the interstitial spaces back into the circulatory system. This results in increased perfusion to the kidneys. The increased renal blood flow results in diuresis. The patient may complain of having to urinate frequently throughout the night.

Skin Changes. Because tissue capillary O_2 extraction is increased in a person with chronic HF, the skin may appear dusky. Often the lower extremities are shiny and swollen, with diminished or absent hair growth. Chronic swelling may result in pigment changes. This causes the skin to appear brown or brawny in areas covering the ankles and lower legs.

Behavioral Changes. Cerebral circulation may be reduced with chronic HF secondary to decreased CO. The patient or caregiver may report unusual behavior, including restlessness, confusion, and decreased attention span or memory. This may also be secondary to poor gas exchange and worsening HF. It is often seen in the late stages of HF. Coexisting psychologic disorders, especially depression and anxiety, contribute a twofold risk of mortality and higher readmission rates and health care costs in patients with HF. Approximately 1 in 5 patients with HF have clinical depression.[7] In addition, patients with psychologic disorders have poorer adherence to treatment plans. Assess patients with HF for depression and anxiety and, if needed, initiate appropriate consults.

Chest Pain. HF can precipitate chest pain (angina) because of decreased coronary artery perfusion from decreased CO and increased myocardial work. Chest pain may accompany either ADHF or chronic HF.

Weight Changes. Many factors contribute to weight changes. First, a progressive weight gain may occur because of fluid retention. Renal failure may also contribute to fluid retention. Abdominal fullness from ascites and hepatomegaly frequently causes anorexia and nausea. As HF advances, the patient may have cardiac *cachexia* with muscle wasting and fat loss. This can be masked by the patient's edematous condition and may not be seen until after the edema subsides.

Complications of Heart Failure

Pleural Effusion. *Pleural effusion* is a common complication in HF. There are two pleural layers or membranes: the visceral pleura lines the lungs, while the parietal pleura lines the chest cavity. Normally there is a small amount of fluid between the two layers for lubrication and to aid breathing. A pleural effusion occurs when excess fluid builds up in the pleural cavity of the lungs secondary to increasing pressure in the pleural capillaries. Fluid then moves from these capillaries into the pleural space. Pleural effusions may result in symptoms of dyspnea, cough, and chest pain. (Pleural effusion is discussed in Chapter 27.)

Dysrhythmias. Chronic HF causes enlargement of the chambers of the heart. This enlargement can cause changes in the normal electrical pathways. Patients with HF are at high risk for atrial dysrhythmias. The prevalence of atrial fibrillation in patients with HF increases as the severity of HF increases. Atrial fibrillation occurs when numerous sites in the atria fire spontaneously and rapidly, and the organized atrial depolarization (contraction) no longer occurs. Loss of "atrial kick" during systole may contribute to decreased CO and worsening HF symptoms.

Atrial fibrillation also promotes thrombus formation within the atria. Thrombi can break loose and form emboli. This places patients with atrial fibrillation at risk for stroke. Treatment with anticoagulation should be considered if there are no significant contraindications. Treatment with drugs to achieve HR control is a primary goal. Restoring normal sinus rhythm with cardioversion, ablation, and antidysrhythmic drugs may be considered.

Patients with HF are also at risk for ventricular dysrhythmias (e.g., ventricular tachycardia [VT], ventricular fibrillation [VF]). Sudden cardiac death (SCD) is a major cause of death in the HF population. Patients with decreased LV function are at the greatest risk for SCD. Guidelines recommend implantation of a prophylactic implantable cardioverter-defibrillator (ICD) for patients with an EF less than 35%, who are NYHA Class II or III.[8] (SCD is discussed in Chapter 33, and dysrhythmias are discussed in Chapter 35.)

Left Ventricular Thrombus. With ADHF or chronic HF, the enlarged LV and decreased CO combine to increase the risk of thrombus formation in the LV. Once a thrombus has formed, it may also decrease LV contractility, decrease CO, and worsen the patient's perfusion. The development of emboli from the thrombus also places the patient at risk for stroke.

Hepatomegaly. HF can lead to severe hepatomegaly, especially with RV failure. The liver becomes congested with venous blood. The hepatic congestion leads to impaired liver function. Eventually liver cells die, fibrosis occurs, and cirrhosis can develop (see Chapter 43).

Renal Failure. The decreased CO that accompanies chronic HF results in decreased perfusion to the kidneys and can lead to renal insufficiency or failure (see Chapter 46).

Diagnostic Studies

Diagnosing HF is often difficult. Patient signs and symptoms are not highly specific and may mimic those associated with many other medical conditions (e.g., anemia, lung disease). Diagnostic tests for ADHF and chronic HF are presented in Table 34-6. A primary goal in diagnosis is to find the underlying cause of HF.

An echocardiogram is a common diagnostic tool used in patients with HF. It provides information on the EF. This helps

TABLE 34-6 Interprofessional Care

Heart Failure

Both ADHF and Chronic HF	ADHF	Chronic HF
Diagnostic Assessment		
• History and physical examination • Determination of underlying cause • Serum chemistries, cardiac biomarkers, BNP or NT-proBNP level (see Table 31-6), liver function tests, thyroid function tests, CBC, lipid profile, kidney function tests, urinalysis • Chest x-ray • 12-lead ECG • 2-dimensional echocardiogram (see Table 31-6) • Nuclear imaging studies (see Table 31-6) • Cardiac catheterization (see Table 31-6)	• Measurement of LV function • Hemodynamic monitoring • Endomyocardial biopsy in select patients	• Cardiopulmonary exercise stress test • 6-minute walk test • Sleep studies in select patients
Management		
• Treatment of underlying cause • Circulatory assist devices (e.g., ventricular assist device) • Daily weights • Sodium- and possibly fluid-restricted diet	• High Fowler's position • O_2 by mask or nasal cannula • Noninvasive positive pressure ventilation • Circulatory assist device: intraaortic balloon pump • Endotracheal intubation and mechanical ventilation • Vital signs, urine output at least q1hr until stable • Continuous ECG and pulse oximetry monitoring • Hemodynamic monitoring (e.g., intraarterial BP, PAWP, CO) • Drug therapy (Table 34-7) • Possible cardioversion (e.g., atrial fibrillation) • Ultrafiltration	• O_2 therapy by nasal cannula if indicated • Drug therapy (Table 34-7) • Cardiac resynchronization therapy with biventricular pacing and internal cardioverter-defibrillator • LVAD • Heart transplantation • Rest-activity periods • Dietitian consult • Physical/occupational therapy consult • Cardiac rehabilitation • Home health nursing care (e.g., telehealth monitoring) • Palliative and end-of-life care

ADHF, Acute decompensated heart failure; *BNP,* b-type natriuretic peptide; *CO,* cardiac output; *HF,* heart failure; *LVAD,* left ventricular assist device; *NT-proBNP,* N-terminal prohormone of BNP; *PAWP,* pulmonary artery wedge pressure.

to differentiate between HFpEF and HFrEF. An echocardiogram also provides information on the structure and function of the heart valves. Heart chamber enlargement or stiffness can also be assessed. Other useful tests include electrocardiogram (ECG), chest x-ray, 6-minute walk test, multi-gated acquisition (MUGA) scan, cardiopulmonary exercise stress test, and heart catheterization. Studies for obstructive sleep apnea may be done in select patients. An endomyocardial biopsy (EMB) may be done as part of a heart catheterization in select acutely ill patients who develop unexplained, new-onset HF that is unresponsive to usual care.[9]

Laboratory studies also aid in the diagnosis of HF. In general, BNP levels correlate positively with the degree of LV failure. Many agencies routinely measure the N-terminal prohormone of BNP (NT-proBNP). This is a more precise test to aid in the diagnosis of HF. Levels are temporarily higher in patients receiving nesiritide (Natrecor) and may be high in patients with chronic, stable HF. Increases in BNP or NT-proBNP levels can be caused by conditions other than HF. These include pulmonary embolism, renal failure, and acute coronary syndrome.

Interprofessional Care: Acute Decompensated Heart Failure

Patients with ADHF need continuous monitoring and assessment. If unstable, these patients are managed in an intensive care unit (ICU). In the ICU, monitor heart rhythm and O_2 saturation continuously. Assess vital signs and urine output at least every hour. The patient may have hemodynamic monitoring, including arterial BP and pulmonary artery pressures. If a pulmonary artery catheter is placed, evaluate CO and pulmonary artery wedge pressure (PAWP). Therapy is titrated to maximize CO and reduce PAWP. A normal PAWP is generally between 8 and 12 mm Hg. Patients with ADHF may have a PAWP as high as 30 mm Hg. (Hemodynamic monitoring is discussed in Chapter 65.)

Provide supplemental O_2 to help increase the percentage of O_2 in inspired air. (O_2 therapy is discussed in Chapter 28.) In severe pulmonary edema, the patient may need noninvasive positive pressure ventilation (e.g., bilevel positive airway pressure [BiPAP]) or intubation and mechanical ventilation. BiPAP is also effective in decreasing preload. (Ventilatory support is discussed in Chapter 65.)

More stable patients with ADHF may require hospitalization but do not need to be in an ICU. They are often admitted to a telemetry or stepdown unit for treatment. Assess these patients every 4 hours (e.g., vital signs, pulse oximetry) for adequate oxygenation. Record intake and output and daily weights to evaluate fluid status.

If the patient has dyspnea, place in a high Fowler's position with the feet horizontal in the bed or dangling at the bedside. This position helps decrease venous return because of the pooling of blood in the extremities. This position also increases the thoracic capacity, allowing for improved breathing.

Ultrafiltration (UF), or *aquapheresis,* is an option for the patient with volume overload.[1] It is a process to remove excess salt and water from the patient's blood. UF can rapidly remove intravascular fluid volume while maintaining hemodynamic stability. The ideal patients for UF are those with major pulmonary or systemic volume overload who have shown resistance to diuretics and are hemodynamically stable. UF also may be an appropriate adjunctive therapy for patients with HF and coexisting renal failure. (UF is discussed in Chapter 46.)

In the ICU, circulatory assist devices are used to manage patients with worsening HF. The intraaortic balloon pump (IABP) is a device that increases coronary blood flow to the heart muscle and decreases the heart's workload through a process called *counterpulsation*. The IABP is useful in hemodynamically unstable patients because it decreases pulmonary artery pressures and systemic vascular resistance (SVR), leading to improved CO.

Ventricular assist devices (VADs) can be used to maintain the pumping action of a heart that cannot effectively pump. A VAD is a mechanical pump that is surgically implanted. (IABPs and VADs are discussed in Chapter 65.) Once the patient is more stable, determination of the cause of ADHF is important. Diagnosis of systolic or diastolic HF will then direct further treatment protocols.

Drug Therapy. Drug therapy is essential in treating ADHF (Table 34-7).

Diuretics. Diuretics are the mainstay of treatment in patients with volume overload. They decrease sodium reabsorption at various sites within the nephrons, thereby enhancing sodium and water loss. Decreasing intravascular volume with the use of diuretics reduces venous return (preload) and subsequently the volume returning to the LV. This allows the LV to pump more efficiently. CO is increased, pulmonary vascular pressures are decreased, and gas exchange is improved. Loop diuretics (e.g., furosemide [Lasix]) can be given by IV push and act rapidly in the kidneys.

Vasodilators. IV nitroglycerin is a vasodilator that reduces circulating blood volume. It also improves coronary artery blood flow by dilating the coronary arteries. Therefore nitroglycerin reduces preload, slightly reduces afterload (in high doses), and increases myocardial O_2 supply. When titrating IV nitroglycerin, monitor BP frequently (every 5 to 10 minutes) to avoid hypotension.

Sodium nitroprusside (Nitropress) is a potent IV vasodilator that reduces both preload and afterload, thus improving myocardial contraction, increasing CO, and reducing pulmonary congestion. Complications of IV sodium nitroprusside include hypotension and thiocyanate toxicity, which can develop after 48 hours of use. Sodium nitroprusside is given in an ICU, since symptomatic hypotension is the main adverse effect.

DRUG ALERT Sodium Nitroprusside (Nitropress)

- Arterial BP monitoring is recommended during drug infusion.
- Record baseline BP and continuously monitor during administration.
- Too rapid rate of IV infusion can reduce BP too quickly and cause hypotension.
- Headache, dizziness, nausea, agitation, and restlessness can occur.
- Monitor thiocyanate (drug by-product) levels if infusion is greater than 3 mcg/kg/min, as toxicity can occur.

Nesiritide, given IV, is a recombinant form of BNP. It causes both arterial and venous dilation. The main hemodynamic effects of nesiritide include a (1) reduction in PAWP and (2) decrease in systemic BP. Although classified as a vasodilator, nesiritide is also a neurohormonal blocking agent. It can be used for short-term treatment of ADHF. Nesiritide does not need titration after the initial IV bolus. It can be given in the emergency department (ED) and non-ICU setting. Because the

TABLE 34-7 Drug Therapy

Heart Failure

Drug	Mechanism of Action
Diuretics (see Table 32-7) ***Loop Diuretics*** furosemide (Lasix) bumetanide (Bumex) ***Thiazide Diuretics**** • hydrochlorothiazide • metolazone (Zaroxolyn) ***Potassium-Sparing Diuretics*** • spironolactone (Aldactone) • eplerenone (Inspra)	• Decrease fluid volume • Decrease preload • Decrease pulmonary venous pressure • Relieve symptoms of heart failure (e.g., edema)
Renin-Angiotensin-Aldosterone System Inhibitors (see Table 32-7) ***ACE Inhibitors*** • captopril • benazepril (Lotensin) • enalapril (Vasotec) ***Angiotensin II Receptor Blockers*** • losartan (Cozaar) • valsartan (Diovan) • valsartan/sacubitril (Entresto)	• Dilate venules and arterioles • Improve renal blood flow • Decrease fluid volume • Relieve symptoms of heart failure • Promote reverse remodeling • Decrease morbidity and mortality
Vasodilators • hydralazine* • isosorbide dinitrate/hydralazine (BiDil)* • nitrates (e.g., nitroglycerin [Nitro-Bid], isosorbide dinitrate [Isordil]) • nesiritide (Natrecor)† • nitroprusside (Nitropress)†	• Reduce cardiac afterload, leading to increased CO • Dilate the arterioles of the kidneys, leading to increased renal perfusion and fluid loss • Decrease BP • Decrease preload • Relieve symptoms of heart failure (e.g., dyspnea)
β-Adrenergic Blockers* (see Table 32-7) • metoprolol (Toprol XL) • bisoprolol (Zebeta) • carvedilol (Coreg)	• Promote reverse remodeling • Decrease afterload • Inhibit SNS • Decrease morbidity and mortality
Positive Inotropes ***β-Adrenergic Agonists†*** • dopamine • dobutamine ***Phosphodiesterase Inhibitor†*** • milrinone ***Digitalis Glycoside**** • digoxin	• Increase contractility (positive inotropic effect) • Increase CO • Increase heart rate (positive chronotropic effect) • Produce mild vasodilation • Increase stroke volume and CO • Promote vasodilation
Cardiac Sinus Node Inhibitor* • ivabradine (Corlanor)	• Decreases heart rate
Morphine†	• Decreases anxiety • Decreases preload and afterload
Antidysrhythmic Drugs (see Table 35-9)	• Prevent or treat dysrhythmias
Anticoagulants	• Prevent thromboembolism • Recommended for patients with an ejection fraction <20% and/or atrial fibrillation

ACE, Angiotensin-converting enzyme; *ADHF*, acute decompensated heart failure; *CO*, cardiac output; *SNS*, sympathetic nervous system.
*Used for chronic HF only.
†Used for ADHF only.

main adverse effect of nesiritide is symptomatic hypotension, monitor BP closely.

Morphine. Morphine sulfate reduces preload and afterload. It is frequently used in the treatment of HF and acute coronary syndrome (see Chapter 33). It dilates both pulmonary and systemic blood vessels. Results include a decrease in pulmonary pressures and myocardial O_2 needs and an improvement in gas exchange. When morphine is used, the patient often experiences relief from dyspnea and, consequently, the anxiety often associated with dyspnea.

Use morphine cautiously in patients with ADHF. Morphine is related to more adverse events, including a greater need for mechanical ventilation, more ICU admissions, prolonged hospitalization, and higher mortality rates in these patients.[10]

Positive Inotropes. Inotropic therapy increases myocardial contractility. Drugs include β-agonists (e.g., dopamine, dobutamine, norepinephrine [Levophed]), the phosphodiesterase inhibitor milrinone, and digitalis. The β-agonists are only used as a short-term treatment of ADHF. In addition to increasing myocardial contractility and SVR, dopamine dilates the renal blood vessels and enhances urine output. Unlike dopamine, dobutamine is a selective β-agonist and works mainly on the β_1-receptors in the heart. Dobutamine does not increase SVR and is preferred for short-term treatment of ADHF.[11]

DRUG ALERT Dopamine

- Monitor IV site for signs of extravasation.
- Tissue necrosis with sloughing can occur with drug extravasation.
- High dosages may produce ventricular dysrhythmias.

Milrinone is a phosphodiesterase inhibitor that has been called an inodilator. It increases myocardial contractility (inotropic effect) and promotes peripheral vasodilation. Inhibition of phosphodiesterase increases cyclic adenosine monophosphate (cAMP). This enhances calcium entry into the cell and improves myocardial contractility. Milrinone increases CO and reduces BP (decrease afterload). Like dopamine and dobutamine, this drug is available only for IV use. Adverse effects include dysrhythmias, thrombocytopenia, and hepatotoxicity.

Digitalis is a positive inotrope that improves LV function. Digitalis increases contractility but also increases myocardial O_2 consumption. Because digitalis requires a loading dose and time to work, it is not recommended for the initial treatment of ADHF.[11]

Currently, inotropic therapy is only recommended for use in the short-term management of patients with ADHF who have not responded to conventional drug therapy (e.g., diuretics, vasodilators, morphine).[1]

SAFETY ALERT Infusion Pumps

- To control the rate and assist with titration, use an infusion pump whenever you are giving IV vasodilators and inotropes.
- Ideally, pumps that contain drug libraries can help to avoid rates and dosages that are out of the safe range for the drug being given.

Interprofessional Care: Chronic Heart Failure

With the addition of new drugs and devices, the management of HF has dramatically changed in the past few years. Because of the large number of patients and the high cost of care related to hospital readmissions, strategies to improve outcomes have been developed. One example is the use of guideline-directed medical therapy as defined by the AACF/AHA.[1] Another example is specialized HF inpatient units with transitional programs to the outpatient setting to help manage these patients. These units are staffed with multidisciplinary HF teams, including nurses who are educated in the care of these patients (Table 34-6).

The main goals in the treatment of chronic HF are to treat the underlying cause and contributing factors, maximize CO, reduce symptoms, improve ventricular function, improve quality of life, preserve target organ function, and reduce mortality and morbidity. The management of hypertension is discussed in Chapter 32, CAD in Chapter 33, dysrhythmias in Chapter 35, and valvular disorders in Chapter 36.

In a person with HF, O_2 saturation of the blood can be reduced because the blood is not adequately oxygenated in the lungs. The use of supplemental O_2 improves saturation and assists in meeting tissue O_2 needs. This helps to relieve dyspnea and fatigue. Optimally pulse oximetry is used to monitor the need for and effectiveness of O_2 therapy.

Physical and emotional rest allows the patient to conserve energy and decreases the need for additional O_2. The degree of rest recommended depends on the severity of HF. A patient with severe HF may be on bed rest with limited activity. A patient with mild to moderate HF can be ambulatory with restriction of strenuous activity. Tell the patient to participate in prescribed activities with adequate recovery periods. A structured exercise program, such as cardiac rehabilitation (CR), should be considered for all patients with chronic HF. CR has been associated with decreased hospitalizations and reduced mortality. Patients enrolled in CR programs have also reported improved quality of life and less depression.[1,12]

The CardioMems system is a new device to help monitor patients' pulmonary pressures. It is implanted in a patient's distal pulmonary artery during a right heart catheterization. The permanent device is approved for patients with NYHA Class III HF symptoms. It allows for close monitoring of changes in pulmonary pressures. Data are sent wirelessly from the patient's home to a secure website. The data are reviewed by the HCP. Early interventions such as drug adjustments can be started. This may help prevent worsening of HF symptoms and possibly hospitalizations.[13]

Nonpharmacologic therapies are an integral part of the care of HF patients. Patients with an EF less than 35% are at an increased risk of SCD from VT or VF. An ICD is recommended for SCD prophylaxis. In HF, neurohormonal effects and cardiac remodeling can result in dyssynchrony of the LV and RV. This contributes to poor CO. In these patients, biventricular pacing, known as *cardiac resynchronization therapy (CRT)*, is recommended.[1] In CRT an extra pacing lead is placed through the coronary sinus to a coronary vein of the LV. This lead coordinates right and left ventricular contractions (Fig. 34-4). The ability to have normal electrical conduction (synchrony) between the RV and the LV increases left ventricular function and CO. At times, patients may need both CRT and an ICD. (Pacemakers and defibrillators are discussed in Chapter 35.)

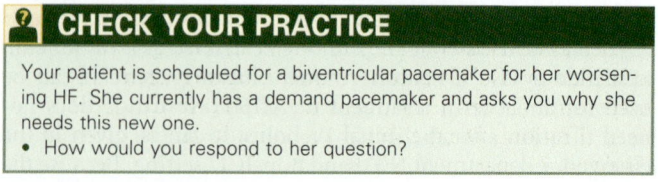

CHECK YOUR PRACTICE

Your patient is scheduled for a biventricular pacemaker for her worsening HF. She currently has a demand pacemaker and asks you why she needs this new one.

- How would you respond to her question?

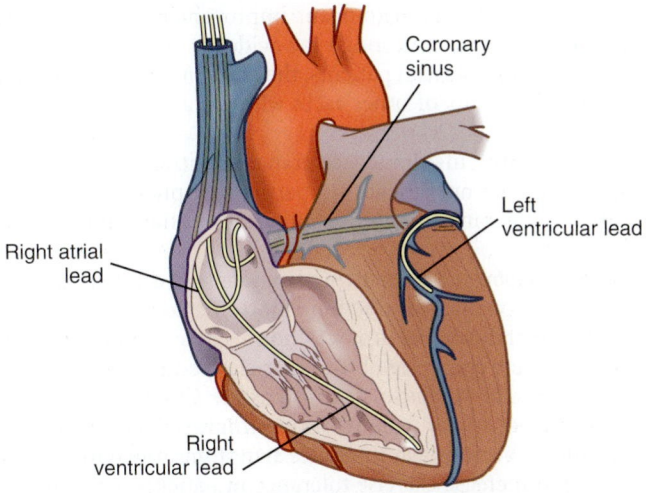

FIG. 34-4 Placement of pacing leads in cardiac resynchronization therapy.

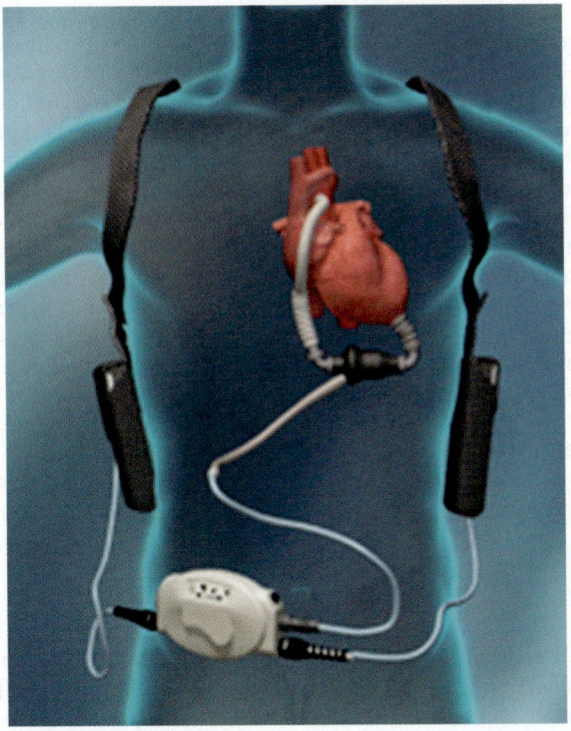

FIG. 34-5 Left ventricular assist device. (Reprinted with the permission of Thoratec Corporation.)

Several mechanical options are available to sustain HF patients with deteriorating conditions, especially those awaiting heart transplantation. These include the IABP and VADs. However, the limitations of bed rest and the risk of infection and vascular complications preclude long-term use of the IABP. VADs provide highly effective long-term support and have become standard care in many heart transplant centers. The heart pump is operated via a driveline that exits the abdominal wall and is attached to a system controller with patient specific settings. VADs operate on AC current or batteries (Fig. 34-5). They may be used as a bridge to transplant (BTT), or as destination therapy (DT) in patients who do not meet criteria for heart transplant. (IABPs and VADs are discussed in Chapter 65.)

Drug Therapy. Drug therapy for chronic HF is presented in Table 34-7.

Diuretics. Diuretics are used to reduce edema, pulmonary venous pressure, and preload (see Table 32-7). If excess extracellular fluid is removed, blood volume returning to the heart can be reduced and cardiac function improved.

Diuretics act on the kidney by promoting excretion of sodium and water. Many varieties of diuretics are available. Loop diuretics (e.g., bumetanide [Bumex]) are potent diuretics. These drugs act on the ascending loop of Henle to promote sodium, chloride, and water excretion. Problems in using loop diuretics include reduction in serum potassium levels, ototoxicity, and possible allergic reaction in patients sensitive to sulfa-type drugs.

Thiazide diuretics inhibit sodium reabsorption in the distal tubule, thus promoting excretion of sodium and water. They can be added to loop diuretics to obtain results if patients become resistant to loop diuretics. Thiazide diuretics also can cause severe reductions in potassium levels.

Diuretics are effective in relieving the congestive symptoms of HF. However, their use does activate the SNS and RAAS, which can exacerbate the HF syndrome. In chronic HF, the lowest effective dose of diuretic should be used.

Renin-Angiotensin-Aldosterone System Inhibitors

Angiotensin-converting enzyme inhibitors. ACE inhibitors are the primary drug of choice for blocking the RAAS system in HF patients with systolic failure.[1] Examples of ACE inhibitors are listed in Table 34-7. Other examples of ACE inhibitors are discussed in Chapter 32 and listed in Table 32-7.

The conversion of angiotensin I to the potent vasoconstrictor angiotensin II requires ACE. ACE inhibitors block this enzyme, resulting in reduced levels of angiotensin II. The end result of the neurohormonal blockade is decreased plasma aldosterone levels, decreased SNS activity, vasodilation, and sodium and water excretion. ACE inhibitors also decrease the development of ventricular remodeling by inhibiting ventricular hypertrophy.

DRUG ALERT Captopril

- Excessive hypotension and hyperkalemia may occur.
- Monitor patient for first-dose hypotension (first-dose syncope).
- Skipping doses or discontinuing the drug can result in rebound hypertension.
- Angioedema, a rare adverse effect, can develop suddenly and can be life-threatening.

Major side effects of ACE inhibitors include symptomatic hypotension, intractable cough, hyperkalemia, *angioedema* (allergic reaction involving edema of the face and airways), and renal insufficiency (when ACE inhibitors are used in high doses). Aging and renal insufficiency slow the metabolism of ACE inhibitors and may lead to increased serum drug levels. Carefully monitor patients taking ACE inhibitors for potential adverse effects. For example, a cough may be attributed to ACE inhibitors when, in fact, it is also a common symptom of an exacerbation of HF. It is critical that the exact cause of cough and other side effects be confirmed before stopping ACE inhibitor therapy.

Angiotensin II receptor blockers. For patients who are unable to tolerate ACE inhibitors, angiotensin II receptor blockers (ARBs) (see Table 32-7) are recommended.[14] These agents prevent the vasoconstrictor and aldosterone-secreting effects of angiotensin II by binding to the angiotensin II receptor sites.

Combination therapy. Combination therapy with valsartan/sacubitril (Entresto), an ARB/neprilysin inhibitor, is recommended for HF patients with reduced EF. Inhibition of neprilysin increases several endogenous vasoactive peptides, including natriuretic peptides, bradykinin, and adrenomedullin (vasodilator peptide hormone). The combination of these two drugs is used as an alternative to an ACE inhibitor (or single agent ARB) therapy in these patients.[15]

Aldosterone antagonists. Spironolactone (Aldactone) and eplerenone (Inspra) are aldosterone antagonists. They block the harmful neurohormonal effects of aldosterone on the heart blood vessels. Aldosterone antagonists may prolong survival in patients with HFrEF.[16] They are also potassium-sparing diuretics that promote sodium and water excretion while retaining potassium. These effects occur because these agents bind to receptors at the aldosterone-dependent sodium-potassium exchange site in the distal renal tubule.

DRUG ALERT Spironolactone (Aldactone)

- Monitor potassium levels during treatment.
- Use with caution in patients taking digoxin, since hyperkalemia may reduce the effects of digoxin.
- Instruct patient to avoid foods high in potassium (e.g., bananas, oranges, dried apricots).
- Assess male patients for gynecomastia, a common side effect of long-term use of spironolactone.

β-Adrenergic Blockers. β-Blockers directly block the negative effects of the SNS (e.g., increased HR) on the failing heart. Three β-blockers have been shown to decrease mortality in patients with HFrEF: metoprolol succinate (Toprol XL), bisoprolol (Zebeta), and carvedilol (Coreg). These β-blockers may also increase EF. The improvement in EF is dose-related, and therefore the highest tolerated dose should be given.[1,14] However, because β-blockers can reduce myocardial contractility, care must be taken to start at a low dose. Dosage is increased every 2 weeks as tolerated by the patient. Major adverse effects include edema, worsening of HF, hypotension, fatigue, and bradycardia.

DRUG ALERT Carvedilol (Coreg)

- Overdosage can produce profound bradycardia, hypotension, bronchospasm, and cardiogenic shock.
- Obtain standing BP 1 hr after dosing to assess tolerance.
- Abrupt withdrawal may result in sweating, palpitations, and headaches.

Vasodilators

Nitrates. Nitrates cause vasodilation by acting directly on the smooth muscle of the vessel wall. Nitrates can be used in combination with hydralazine for chronic HF management in patients who cannot tolerate ACE inhibitors or ARBs. Nitrates are of particular benefit in the management of myocardial ischemia related to HF because they promote vasodilation of the coronary arteries.

Long-term use of nitrates may result in tolerance to the drug, making it less effective. Nitrates are contraindicated in patients who take phosphodiesterase inhibitors (PDE5 inhibitors) (e.g., sildenafil [Viagra], tadalafil [Cialis]). These drugs are used to treat pulmonary artery hypertension and erectile dysfunction. The combined use of nitrates and PDE5 inhibitors may result in symptomatic hypotension.

Combination therapy. Combination therapy with hydralazine and isosorbide dinitrate (Bidil) may be helpful in African American patients with HF who are getting optimal therapy with ACE inhibitors and β-blockers. The same benefit is not found in white patients. The combination of the two drugs is also associated with a significant improvement in LV EF and exercise tolerance.[1,17] Although the evidence of benefit is stronger in African American patients, the combination therapy may be used in patients of other races who are already on optimal therapy.

As previously mentioned, tolerance to nitrates can develop. Hydralazine has antioxidant properties that prevent the development of tolerance to nitrates and preserves the helpful effects of nitrates.[17]

Positive Inotropes. Digitalis preparations (e.g., digoxin) increase the force of cardiac contraction (inotropic action). They also decrease the HR (chronotropic action). These actions allow for more complete emptying of the ventricles, reducing the volume remaining in the ventricles during diastole. CO increases due to the increased stroke volume from improved contractility.[11] Digoxin has been shown to reduce symptoms, improve quality of life, and increase exercise tolerance in patients with mild to moderate HF. It has not been shown to decrease mortality in patients with HF.[1]

Patients taking a digitalis preparation are at risk for digitalis toxicity. Hypokalemia, secondary to the use of potassium-depleting diuretics (e.g., thiazides, loop diuretics), is one of the most common causes of digitalis toxicity. Low serum potassium enhances the action of digitalis, causing a therapeutic dose to reach toxic levels. Similarly, hyperkalemia inhibits the action of digitalis, resulting in a subtherapeutic dose. Both hypokalemia and hyperkalemia can also cause dysrhythmias. Monitor serum potassium levels of all patients taking digitalis preparations and potassium-depleting and potassium-sparing diuretics. Other electrolyte imbalances, such as hypercalcemia and hypomagnesemia, can also trigger digitalis toxicity. (Manifestations of electrolyte imbalances are discussed in Chapter 16.)

DRUG ALERT Digoxin

- Monitor for signs of hypokalemia and hyperkalemia, since these can increase or decrease the effects of digoxin, respectively.
- Monitor for early signs of toxicity: anorexia, nausea and vomiting, fatigue, headache, depression, visual changes.
- Monitor for late signs of toxicity, such as dysrhythmias (e.g., bradycardia, atrioventricular block).

Diseases of the kidney and liver increase the risk of digitalis toxicity, because most preparations are metabolized and eliminated by these organs. An older adult is especially prone to digitalis toxicity. This is because digitalis accumulation occurs sooner with decreased liver and kidney function and slowed body metabolism.

The usual treatment of toxicity consists of withholding the drug until the symptoms subside. In the case of life-threatening toxicity, IV digoxin immune Fab (ovine) (DigiFab) is an antidote. The treatment of life-threatening dysrhythmias is started as needed (see Chapter 35).

Cardiac Sinus Node Inhibitor. Ivabradine (Corlanor) is a new category of oral drug that inhibits the sinus node and reduces HR. It is used for patients who have symptoms of chronic HF. They must be in sinus rhythm with a resting HR of at least 70 beats per minute and taking β-blockers at the highest dose tolerated. Ivabradine also reduces the risk of hospitalization for worsening HF.[18]

The most common side effects of ivabradine include symptomatic bradycardia, high BP, atrial fibrillation, and vision disturbance (i.e., flashes of light). Tell patients to call their HCP if they experience symptoms of an irregular HR, feel that their heart is pounding or racing, or have chest pressure or worsened dyspnea. Low HR is a common side effect of ivabradine and can be serious. Patients should tell their HCP if they experience dizziness, weakness, or fatigue.[18]

COMPLEMENTARY & ALTERNATIVE THERAPIES

Hawthorn

Scientific Evidence*

- Strong evidence for its use in mild to moderate HF
- May have a diuretic effect
- May inhibit angiotensin-converting enzyme
- May reduce incidence of sudden cardiac death in patients with ejection fractions >25%

Nursing Implications

- Potentially beneficial treatment for patients who cannot or will not take prescription drugs
- May add to the effects of established therapies (e.g., cardiac glycosides, antihypertensives, lipid-lowering drugs)

*Source: *www.naturalstandard.com.*

Nutritional Therapy

Poor adherence to a low-sodium diet and failure to take prescribed drugs as directed are the two most common reasons for readmissions of HF patients to the hospital. Therefore it is critical that you accurately assess a patient's diet and teach both the patient and caregiver about the importance of diet.

Diet teaching and weight management are essential to the patient's control of chronic HF. You or a dietitian should obtain a detailed diet history. Determine not only what foods the patient eats but also when, where, and how often the patient dines out. In addition, assess the cultural value of food. Use this information to assist the patient in making appropriate dietary choices when developing a diet plan. The National Heart, Lung, and Blood Institute provides helpful dietary guidelines for heart-healthy food preparation for people of various cultures (e.g., Hispanics, Asian Americans). These are available online at *www.nhlbi.nih.gov/health/educational/lose_wt/menuplanner.html.* Diet and weight management recommendations must be individualized and culturally sensitive if the necessary changes are to be made.

The edema associated with chronic HF is often treated by dietary restriction of sodium. Teach the patient what foods are low and high in sodium and ways to enhance food flavors without the use of salt (e.g., substituting lemon juice, various spices). The degree of sodium restriction depends on the severity of the HF and the effectiveness of diuretic therapy. The Dietary Approaches to Stop Hypertension (DASH) diet is effective as a first-line therapy for many individuals with hypertension. (The DASH diet is discussed in Chapter 32.) This diet is now also widely used for the patient with HF, with or without hypertension.

The average American adult's daily intake of sodium ranges from 7 to 15 g. A commonly ordered diet for a patient with HF is a 2-g sodium diet (Table 34-8). All foods high in sodium (more than 400 mg/serving) should be avoided. On this diet, processed meats, cheese, bread, cereals, canned soups, and canned vegetables must be limited. Teach the patient and caregiver how to read labels to look for sodium content (Fig. 34-6).

TABLE 34-8 Nutritional Therapy

Low-Sodium Diets

General Principles

Do not add salt or seasonings containing sodium when preparing foods.*
Do not use salt at the table.*
Avoid high-sodium foods (e.g., canned soups, processed meats, cheese, frozen meals).
Limit milk products to 2 cups daily.

Sample Menu Plans for 2400-mg Sodium Diet

Breakfast	*Sodium (mg)*
⅔ cup bran cereal	161
(⅔ cup Shredded Wheat cereal)†	3
1 slice whole-wheat bread	149
1 medium banana	1
6 oz fruit yogurt, fat free	85
1 cup fat-free milk	126
2 Tbsp jelly	5
Coffee, 8 oz	5
Lunch	
Chicken breast sandwich	
2 slices (3 oz) chicken breast, skinless	65
2 slices whole wheat bread	299
1 slice (¾ oz) American cheese	328
(1 slice [¾ oz] Swiss cheese, natural)†	54
Large-leaf romaine lettuce	1
2 slices tomato	90
1 Tbsp mayonnaise, low fat	90
1 medium peach	7
Dinner	
¾ cup vegetarian spaghetti sauce	459
(6 oz no-salt-added tomato paste)†	260
1 cup spaghetti	1
3 Tbsp parmesan cheese	349
Spinach salad	
1 cup fresh spinach leaves	24
¼ cup fresh carrots (grated)	10
¼ cup fresh mushrooms (sliced)	1
2 Tbsp vinaigrette dressing	0
½ cup canned pears, juice pack	4
½ cup corn, cooked from frozen	4
Snack	
⅓ cup almonds	4
¼ cup dried apricots	3
6 oz fruit yogurt, fat free	85

*1 tsp of salt equals 2.3 g of sodium.
†Substitutes to reduce to 1500-mg sodium diet.

The patient and caregiver should also be aware of the high sodium content of most restaurant foods.

Fluid restrictions are not commonly ordered for the patient with mild to moderate HF. However, in moderate to severe HF and renal insufficiency, fluids are limited to less than 2 L/day.[14] Helping patients deal with thirst as a side effect of the drugs is important. Suggest ice chips, gum, hard candy, or ice pops.

To monitor fluid status, tell patients to weigh themselves at the same time each day. Ideally this should be before breakfast, using the same scale, and wearing the same type of clothing. This helps ensure valid comparisons from day to day and helps identify early signs of fluid retention. For patients with visual limitations, suggest scales with larger numbers or an audible response. Tell patients to call the HCP if they see a weight gain of 3 lb (1.4 kg) over 2 days or a 3- to 5-lb (2.3-kg) gain over a week.[14]

Chicken Noodle Soup

Nutrition Facts

Serving Size 1/2 cup (120 mL) condensed soup
Servings Per Container about 2.5

Amount Per Serving			
Calories 60		Calories from Fat 15	
			% Daily Value*
Total Fat 1.5 g			2%
Saturated Fat 0.5 g			3%
Trans Fat 0 g			
Cholesterol 15 mg			
Sodium 890 mg			37%
Total Carbohydrate 8 g			3%
Dietary Fiber 1 g			4%
Sugars 1 g			
Protein 3 g			
Vitamin A 4%	**Calcium** 0%		
Vitamin C 0%	**Iron** 2%		

*Percent Daily Values are based on a 2,000 calorie diet Your Daily Values may be higher or lower depending on your calorie needs.

	Calories	2000	2500
Total Fat	Less than	65 g	80 g
Sat Fat	Less than	20 g	25 g
Cholesterol	Less than	300 g	300 g
Sodium	Less than	2400 mg	2400 mg
Total Carbohydrate		300 g	375 g
Dietary Fiber		25 g	30 g

FIG. 34-6 Typical nutrition label. Note that a single serving (½ cup) provides more than one third of the daily recommended intake of sodium.

NURSING MANAGEMENT: HEART FAILURE

Nursing Assessment

Subjective and objective data that you should obtain from a patient with HF are presented in Table 34-9. Carefully review the patient's current prescription and over-the-counter drugs. Assess for use of any nonsteroidal antiinflammatory drugs (NSAIDs), since they can contribute to sodium retention and an exacerbation of HF. In addition, review the patient's dietary habits to identify issues related to an exacerbation of HF.

Explore the patient's chronic health problems as they may act as exacerbating factors, affecting the plan of care and the timing and selection of therapies. For example, a patient with sleep apnea may not regularly use his or her continuous positive airway pressure device at night. This can worsen pulmonary or systemic hypertension and lead to an exacerbation of HF.

Nursing Diagnoses

Nursing diagnoses for the patient with HF include, but are not limited to, the following:

- Impaired gas exchange *related to* increased preload and alveolar-capillary membrane changes
- Decreased cardiac output *related to* altered contractility, altered preload, and/or altered stroke volume
- Excess fluid volume *related to* increased venous pressure and decreased renal perfusion secondary to heart failure
- Activity intolerance *related to* imbalance between O_2 supply and demand secondary to cardiac insufficiency and pulmonary congestion

Additional information on nursing diagnoses for the patient with HF is presented in eNursing Care Plan 34-1 on the website for this chapter.

TABLE 34-9 Nursing Assessment

Heart Failure

Subjective Data

Important Health Information

Past health history: CAD (including recent MI), hypertension, cardiomyopathy, valvular or congenital heart disease, diabetes mellitus, hyperlipidemia, renal disease, thyroid or lung disease, rapid or irregular heart rate

Medications: Use of and adherence with any heart drugs. Use of diuretics, estrogens, corticosteroids, nonsteroidal antiinflammatory drugs, over-the-counter drugs, herbal supplements

Functional Health Patterns

Health perception–health management: Fatigue, depression, anxiety

Nutritional-metabolic: Usual sodium intake. Nausea, vomiting, anorexia, stomach bloating. Weight gain, ankle swelling

Elimination: Nocturia, decreased daytime urine output, constipation

Activity-exercise: Dyspnea, orthopnea, cough (e.g., dry, productive). Palpitations, dizziness, fainting

Sleep-rest: Number of pillows used for sleeping. Paroxysmal nocturnal dyspnea, insomnia, sleep apnea

Cognitive-perceptual: Chest pain or heaviness. RUQ pain, abdominal discomfort. Behavioral changes, visual changes

Objective Data

Integumentary

Cool, diaphoretic skin. Cyanosis or pallor. Peripheral edema (right-sided heart failure)

Respiratory

Tachypnea, crackles, wheezes. Frothy, blood-tinged sputum

Cardiovascular

Tachycardia, S_3, S_4, murmurs. Pulsus alternans. PMI displaced inferiorly and posteriorly, lifts and heaves, jugular venous distention

Gastrointestinal

Abdominal distention, hepatosplenomegaly, ascites

Neurologic

Restlessness, confusion, decreased attention or memory

Possible Diagnostic Findings

Altered serum electrolytes (especially Na^+ and K^+), ↑ BUN, creatinine, or liver function tests. ↑ NT-proBNP or BNP. Chest x-ray demonstrating cardiomegaly, pulmonary congestion, and interstitial pulmonary edema. Echocardiogram showing increased chamber size, decreased wall motion, decreased EF or normal EF with evidence of diastolic failure. Atrial and ventricular enlargement on ECG. ↓ O_2 saturation

BNP, b-Type natriuretic peptide; *BUN,* blood urea nitrogen; *EF,* ejection fraction; *NT-proBNP,* N-terminal prohormone of BNP; *PMI,* point of maximal impulse; *RUQ,* right upper quadrant.

Planning

The overall goals for the patient with HF include (1) a decrease in symptoms (e.g., shortness of breath, fatigue), (2) a decrease in peripheral edema, (3) an increase in exercise tolerance, (4) adherence with the treatment regimen, and (5) no complications related to HF.

Nursing Implementation

Health Promotion. Communication and joint decision making among the patient, caregiver, and interprofessional team are integral to selection and delivery of high-quality, patient-centered care. Currently, the emphasis is on aggressively identifying and treating risk factors for HF to prevent or slow the progression of the disease.[19] For example, teach a patient with hypertension or hyperlipidemia ways to manage BP or cholesterol with drugs, diet, and exercise. Encourage patients to obtain the flu and pneumococcal vaccinations. Patients with valvular disease should be evaluated for valve replacement procedures if they are contributing to HF and symptoms. Coronary revascularization procedures should be considered in patients with CAD. The use of antidysrhythmic drugs or pacing therapy is indicated for patients with serious dysrhythmias or conduction disturbances.

◆ **Acute Care.** Many persons with HF experience one or more episodes of ADHF. When they do, they are usually admitted through the ED, first stabilized, and then cared for in an ICU, an intermediate care unit, or a specialized HF unit with continuous ECG monitoring capability.

Successful HF care depends on several important principles: (1) HF is a progressive disease, and treatment plans are established along with quality-of-life goals; (2) symptom management is controlled by the patient with self-management tools (e.g., daily weights, drug regimens, diet and exercise plans); (3) salt and, at times, water must be restricted; (4) energy must be conserved; and (5) support systems are essential to the success of the entire treatment plan.

Reduction of anxiety is an important nursing function, since anxiety may increase the SNS response and further increase myocardial workload. Reducing anxiety may be aided by a variety of nursing interventions (e.g., imagery) and the use of sedatives (e.g., benzodiazepines).

In the past, the Joint Commission had identified core measures in the management of patients with HF to reflect standards of evidence-based care.[20] Currently, the AHA has developed a program, Get With the Guidelines—Heart Failure, to improve adherence to standards of evidence-based care of patients hospitalized with HF.[21] These approaches work to ensure high-quality care for patients with HF.

◆ **Ambulatory Care.** HF is a chronic illness. When a patient is diagnosed with HF, care should focus on slowing the progression of the disease. Your important nursing responsibilities include (1) teaching the patient about the physiologic changes that have occurred, (2) helping the patient adapt to both physiologic and psychologic changes, and (3) including the patient and caregiver in the overall care plan. Review the signs and symptoms of HF exacerbations with the patient and caregiver. Give them a clear action plan to follow should symptoms occur.[14] Early detection of worsening HF may help prevent an acute episode requiring hospitalization. A patient and caregiver guide for the patient with HF is presented in Table 34-10 below.

TABLE 34-10 Patient & Caregiver Teaching

Heart Failure

Include the following instructions when teaching the patient and caregiver about the management of heart failure.

Dietary Therapy

- Consult the diet plan and list of permitted and restricted foods.
- Examine labels to determine sodium content. Also examine the labels of over-the-counter drugs such as laxatives, cough medicines, and antacids for sodium content.
- Avoid using salt when preparing foods or adding salt to foods.
- Weigh yourself at the same time each day, preferably in the morning, using the same scale and wearing similar clothes.
- Eat small, frequent meals.

Activity Program

- Increase walking and other activities gradually, provided they do not cause fatigue or dyspnea.
- Consider a cardiac rehabilitation program.
- Avoid extremes of heat and cold.

Ongoing Monitoring

- Know the signs and symptoms of worsening heart failure (Think *FACES*: *F*atigue, limitation of *A*ctivities, chest *C*ongestion/cough, *E*dema, and *S*hortness of breath).
- Recall the symptoms experienced when illness began. Reappearance of previous symptoms may indicate a recurrence.
- Report immediately any of the following to the HCP:
  - Weight gain of 3 lb (1.4 kg) in 2 days, or 3-5 lb (2.3 kg) in a wk
  - Difficulty breathing, especially with activity or when lying flat
  - Waking up breathless at night
  - Frequent dry, hacking cough, especially when lying down
  - Fatigue, weakness
  - Swelling of ankles, feet, or abdomen. Swelling of face or difficulty breathing (if taking ACE inhibitors)
  - Nausea with abdominal swelling, pain, and tenderness
  - Dizziness or fainting
- Follow up with HCP on regular basis.
- Consider joining a local support group with your family members and/or caregiver(s).

Health Promotion

- Obtain annual flu vaccination.
- Obtain pneumococcal vaccine (see Table 27-5 for guidelines on pneumococcal vaccination).
- Develop plan to reduce risk factors (e.g., BP control, tobacco cessation, weight reduction).

Rest

- Plan a regular daily rest and activity program.
- After exertion, such as exercise and ADLs, plan a rest period.
- Consider shorter working hours or schedule rest period during working hours
- Avoid emotional upsets. Share any concerns, fears, feelings of depression, etc. with HCP.

Drug Therapy

- Take each drug as ordered.
- Develop a system (e.g., daily chart, weekly pillbox) to ensure drugs have been taken.
- Count pulse rate each day before taking drugs (if appropriate). Know the limits that your HCP wants for your pulse rate.
- Take BP at determined intervals (if appropriate). Know your target BP limits.
- Know signs and symptoms of orthostatic hypotension and how to prevent them (see Table 32-12).
- If taking anticoagulants, know signs and symptoms of internal bleeding (bleeding gums, increased bruises, blood in stool or urine) and what to do.
- Know your INR and target range if taking warfarin (Coumadin) and how often to have blood checked.

ACE, Angiotensin-converting enzyme; *INR*, international normalized ratio.

Patients with HF are at risk for anxiety and depression.[7] Emphasize to the patient that it is possible to live a productive life with this chronic illness. Patients with HF usually need to take drugs for the rest of their lives. This often becomes difficult because a patient may be asymptomatic when HF is under control. You must stress that the disease is chronic, and that drugs must be continued to keep the HF under control.

Teach the patient the expected actions of the ordered drugs and the signs of drug toxicity. Also teach the patient and caregiver how to take a pulse rate. The pulse should always be taken for 1 full minute. A pulse less than 50 beats/minute may be a contraindication to taking a β-blocker or a digitalis preparation unless directed by the HCP. However, in the absence of symptoms (e.g., heart block, ventricular ectopy, syncope), a pulse less than 50 beats/minute may be acceptable. Include clear information about when a drug, especially β-blockers and digitalis, should be held and an HCP called.

Teach the patient the symptoms of hypokalemia and hyperkalemia if diuretics that deplete or spare potassium are ordered. Weakness, fatigue, constipation, and muscle cramping may occur, but often there are no physical signs of hypo- or hyperkalemia. Frequently the patient who takes thiazide or loop diuretics is given supplemental potassium. It may also be appropriate to teach patients home BP monitoring, especially those with hypertension.

The physical therapist, occupational therapist, or you can instruct the patient in energy-conserving and energy-efficient behaviors after an evaluation of daily activities has been done. For example, once you understand the patient's daily routine, make suggestions to simplify work or modify an activity.

Exercise training (e.g., cardiac rehabilitation) improves symptoms of chronic HF but is often underprescribed. Exercise for patients with HF has been found to be safe and to improve the overall sense of well-being. It has also been related to a decrease in mortality.[1,12]

Frequently the patient needs a prescription for rest after an activity. Many hard-driving persons need the "permission" to not feel "lazy." Sometimes the patient may need to stop an activity that he or she enjoys. In such cases, help the patient explore alternative activities that cause less physical stress. Changes may be needed if some situations produce an increased cardiac workload (e.g., frequent climbing of stairs). Help a patient identify areas where changes can be made and outside assistance obtained if needed.

Managing HF patients out of the hospital is a priority. Effective home health care can prevent or limit future hospitalizations by providing ongoing assessments (e.g., monitoring vital signs and weight, evaluating response to therapies).[21] Many agencies offer specialized programs designed to manage HF patients at home. For example, these programs may include the use of telehealth monitoring technology (e.g., electronic scale, BP cuff, pulse oximeter) to collect physiologic data (Fig. 34-7). The technology may also audibly ask the patient questions such as, "Are you short of breath today?" Results are transmitted via the telephone or computer to the HCP. After the data are reviewed, the patient may be called to further assess the situation or schedule a visit.

Home health nurses frequently work with protocols set up with the patient's HCP. The protocols enable you and the patient to identify problems, such as an increase in weight or dyspnea, as evidence of worsening HF. To prevent hospitalization, interventions can be started such as changing drugs or dosages and restricting fluids. Home health nursing care of HF patients is vital in reducing the number of hospitalizations, increasing functional capacity, and improving the quality of life.

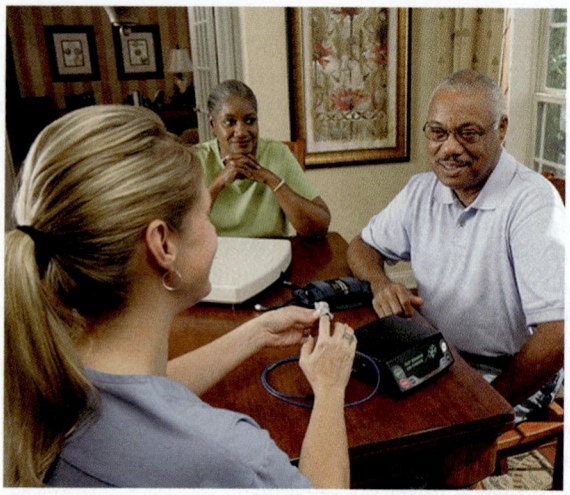

FIG. 34-7 Home-based telehealth monitoring unit. (Used with permission from Honeywell HomMed.)

EVIDENCE-BASED PRACTICE

Applying the Evidence

Home Care and Heart Failure

B.H. is a 68-yr-old Hispanic female with chronic heart failure (HF) who is being discharged home tomorrow. You have made arrangements for the interprofessional home health care team to resume visits. B.H. tells you that since her hospitalization she does not feel the home visits have been helpful and that she is now considering home care from "family" only. She also tells you her heart is not getting better. B.H.'s daughter is her caregiver and she wants to continue the home care visits.

Making Clinical Decisions

Best Available Evidence. In patients with HF, transitional home health care programs result in decreased readmissions and mortality compared to the usual care.

Clinician Expertise. You know it is important for patients to receive home visits to avoid preventable adverse outcomes after hospitalization (e.g., readmission). You also understand that HF is a progressive illness and is often not predictable.

Patient Preferences and Values. B.H. believes that continuation of home health care visits will not be beneficial.

Implications for Nursing Practice

1. What will you discuss with B.H. related to the purpose of the home visits?
2. Why is it important for you to determine B.H.'s understanding of HF?
3. How will you involve B.H.'s daughter if B.H. remains undecided about home health care visits?
4. How will you engage B.H. in her own care before she is discharged home?

Reference for Evidence

Feltner C, Jones CD, Cené CW, et al: Transitional care interventions to prevent readmissions for people with heart failure. AHRQ comparative effectiveness reviews, Rockville, Md, 2014, Agency for Healthcare Research and Quality (US).

◆ **Palliative and End-of-Life Care.** HCPs are often reluctant to refer patients with advanced HF for palliative or end-of-life care.

The unpredictable trajectory of HF during the last few months of life makes assessing the prognosis of the disease difficult.[22] In addition, patients and caregivers may have a poor understanding of the disease and may fail to recognize HF as a terminal illness.[23]

The ACCF/AHA provides guidelines for patients with end-stage HF (stage D).[1] HCPs in collaboration with the patient and caregiver can select either advanced treatment interventions (e.g., heart transplant, VAD), or palliative care for symptom management and hospice care. The guidelines recommend (1) ongoing patient and caregiver teaching regarding prognosis and survival, (2) patient and caregiver teaching about options for composing advance directives (e.g., deactivation of ICD), and (3) continuity of medical care (e.g., continuous infusion of inotropes for symptom control).[1]

Patients are eligible for hospice when an HCP certifies that they are likely to have a life expectancy of 6 months or less. Unfortunately, many eligible patients are not referred to hospice. There are a number of reasons for this. These include a lack of understanding of the role of hospice, lack of an identifiable terminal phase for HF, and concerns about meeting hospice referral criteria. African American and Hispanic patients with HF use hospice less than whites.[24]

The seriousness of the prognosis and the actual knowledge of the expected short life span are misunderstood by many HF patients and caregivers. Many HCPs and HF patients overestimate the life expectancy. When caring for these patients, attempt to identify those who may be eligible for hospice and initiate a discussion among the patient, caregiver, and HCP.

Because patients with end-stage HF have multiple symptoms, your care should involve ongoing assessment and evaluation of interventions for effectiveness. Strategies involve patient and caregiver support, drug therapies, and nondrug therapies. Drugs are continued unless they are not tolerated. The goals of providing comfort and relieving suffering remain priorities in the care of patients with end-stage HF. (Palliative and end-of-life care are discussed in Chapter 9.)

◆ Evaluation

The expected outcomes are that the patient with HF will

- Maintain adequate O_2/CO_2 exchange at the alveolar-capillary membrane to meet O_2 needs of the body
- Maintain adequate blood pumped by the heart to meet metabolic demands of the body
- Experience reduction or absence of edema and stable baseline weight
- Achieve a realistic program of activity that balances physical activity with energy-conserving activities

Additional information on expected outcomes for the patient with HF is presented in eNursing Care Plan 34-1 on the website for this chapter.

HEART TRANSPLANTATION

Heart transplantation is the transfer of a healthy donor heart to a patient with a diseased heart. This surgery is used to treat a variety of terminal or end-stage heart conditions (Table 34-11). Retransplantation (i.e., a second or third heart transplant) is also done. In the United States, approximately 3000 patients are listed for heart transplants. However, on average only 2000 hearts become available. The 1-year transplant survival rate is 85% to 90%, whereas the 3-year survival rate is approximately 75%.[25]

TABLE 34-11 Indications and Contraindications for Heart Transplantation*

Indications

- End-stage HF refractory to medical care
- Severe, decompensated, inoperable, valvular heart disease
- Recurrent life-threatening dysrhythmias not responsive to maximal interventions, including defibrillators
- Any other heart abnormalities that severely limit normal function and/or have a mortality risk of more than 50% at 2 yr

Absolute Contraindications

- Chronologic age over 70 yr or physiologic age over 65 yr
- Life-threatening illness (e.g., malignancy) that will limit survival to <5 yr despite therapy
- Advanced cerebral or peripheral vascular disease not amenable to correction
- Active infection, including HIV infection
- Severe pulmonary disease that will likely result in the patient being ventilator dependent after transplant

Relative Contraindications

- Severe obesity
- Psychologic impairment
- Active substance abuse (e.g., alcohol, drugs, tobacco)
- Uncontrolled diabetes with vascular and neurologic complications
- Irreversible liver or kidney dysfunction not explained by HF
- Evidence of noncompliance with accepted medical practices
- Lack of social support network that can make long-term commitment for patient's welfare
- Unrealistic expectations by the patient or caregiver regarding transplant, its risks, and its benefits

*These are representative examples from various heart transplant centers.

Criteria for Selection

A careful selection process ensures that hearts are distributed fairly and to those who will benefit most from the donor heart. The United Network for Organ Sharing (UNOS) is in charge of a system that gives organs fairly to people. (UNOS is discussed in Chapter 13.)

Indications and contraindications for heart transplantation are identified in Table 34-11. Once a person meets the criteria for heart transplantation, a complete physical examination and diagnostic workup are done. In addition, the patient and caregiver undergo a comprehensive psychologic evaluation. This includes assessing coping skills, support systems, and commitment to follow the rigorous regimen that is essential to a successful transplantation. The complexity of the transplant process may be overwhelming to a patient with inadequate support systems and a poor understanding of the lifestyle changes needed after transplant.

Donor and recipient matching is based on body and heart size and an immunologic evaluation. The immunologic assessment includes ABO blood type, antibody screen, panel of reactive antibody (PRA) level, and human leukocyte antigen typing (explained in Chapter 13).

Once a person is accepted as a transplant candidate (this may happen quickly during an acute illness or after a longer period), he or she is placed on a transplant list. Patients may wait at home and receive ongoing medical care if their condition is stable. If not, they may require hospitalization for more intensive therapy. Unfortunately, the overall waiting period for a new heart is long. Many patients die while waiting for a transplant.

Bridge to Transplantation

Several devices are available as a bridge to transplantation (BTT), but only two have received FDA approval for heart recovery after a life-threatening cardiac event. The AB5000 Circulatory Support System and the BVS 5000 Biventricular Support System provide temporary support for one or both sides of the heart in situations in which the heart has failed but has the potential to recover (e.g., reversible HF, myocarditis, acute MI). Patients with these devices are critically ill and require close observation in an ICU.

The Thoratec HeartMate II and the HeartWare LVAD are permanent pumps that support the heart. After the initial surgery and recovery period, patients do not require ongoing hospitalization. The HeartMate II is approved as a BTT or destination therapy (DT) for those patients who do not meet criteria for a heart transplant. The HeartWare device is currently only approved as a BTT.

Surgical Procedure

The surgical procedure actually involves two surgeries. First, the donor heart is retrieved. The donor is someone who has suffered irreversible brain injury *(brain death)*. A surgical team goes to the hospital of the donor to remove donated organs once brain death has been determined. The retrieved organs are transported on ice until they can be implanted. For the heart, this is optimally less than 4 hours. Often the donor heart is flown to the recipient's hospital.

Next, the donor heart is implanted into the recipient. Two different approaches are used in this surgery. In the biatrial approach, the recipient's damaged heart is removed at the midatrial level and the donor heart connected at the left atrium, pulmonary artery, aorta, and right atrium. In the bicaval approach, the right atrium of the recipient's heart (with the sinoatrial node and atrial conduction intact) is preserved, and then the donor heart is connected. Cardiopulmonary bypass is needed during the surgical procedure to maintain oxygenation and perfusion to vital organs.

Posttransplantation

After the transplant a variety of complications can occur, including a risk for SCD. Acute rejection is an immediate posttransplant complication, and immunosuppressive therapy is the key in posttransplant management. In the first year after transplantation, the major causes of death are acute rejection and infection. Later, malignancy (especially lymphoma) and cardiac vasculopathy (accelerated CAD) are major causes of death.[26]

Most immunosuppressive regimens include corticosteroids, calcineurin inhibitors (tacrolimus [Prograf]), and antiproliferative drugs (mycophenolate mofetil [CellCept]). (The mechanisms of action and side effects of these and other immunosuppressants are discussed in Chapter 13 and Table 13-16.) Because of the use of immunosuppressive therapy, infection is a primary complication after transplant surgery. On a long-term basis, immunosuppressive therapy increases the risk for cancer.[26]

To detect rejection, an EMB is obtained on a weekly basis for the first month, monthly for the following six months, and yearly thereafter. In this procedure, a catheter is inserted into the jugular vein and moved into the RV. The catheter uses a bioptome, a device with two small cups that can be closed, to remove small samples of heart muscle.[26]

Nursing management throughout the posttransplant period focuses on promoting patient adaptation to the transplant process, monitoring heart function, managing lifestyle changes, and providing ongoing teaching of the patient and caregiver.

ETHICAL/LEGAL DILEMMAS

Competence

Situation

M.T., a 60-yr-old man, has been awaiting heart transplantation for 6 months. He has been a patient in intensive care for 1 month, since he has required a ventricular assist device for his failing heart. He recently suffered a stroke, which is a complication of the device. It left him paralyzed on his right side. He is only able to answer yes/no questions by shaking his head. He has required mechanical ventilation since his stroke. For the past 2 weeks, he has needed hemodialysis because of renal failure. Recently, when you suction him, he turns his head away from you and bites down on the endotracheal tube. Although he does not have an advance directive, his wife and daughter tell you that, on numerous occasions before these events, he expressed that he would not want to live if he lost his independence. His wife and daughter request to have the mechanical ventilator withdrawn.

Ethical/Legal Points for Consideration

- Decisional capacity for informed consent related to treatment decisions involves four elements: (1) information provided about possible treatment options must be understandable to patients, (2) patients must have the capacity to deliberate about the treatment choices and their consequences, (3) patients' treatment decisions must be freely chosen and made without coercion, and (4) patients must be able to communicate their decisions.
- Legal competence, as determined by the courts, has a fairly low threshold. The ability to respond to questions by signaling a yes or no may be enough to demonstrate understanding of the questions, ability to discriminate between choices, and ability to communicate choices, providing that the answers make sense and are appropriate. You need to know how legal competence is defined in your state.
- Next of kin are the legal decision makers in the absence of advance directives if he is unable to make decisions for himself. However, decisional capacity should be tested without assuming it is absent.
- Some courts have accepted past assertions of preferences, past behavior, and assertions of their parties as evidence to support end-of-life preferences in the absence of advance directives.
- You must be knowledgeable of your agency's policies and about the local jurisdiction's laws and regulations regarding informed consent and end-of-life decision making.

Discussion Questions

1. What would you do next given M.T.'s behavior and the information you obtained from his wife?
2. What are your feelings and concerns about participating in the care of a patient for whom withdrawal of treatment will result in death?

CASE STUDY

Heart Failure

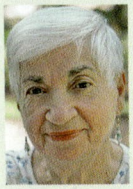

(©iStockphoto/ Thinkstock)

Patient Profile

J.E. is a 70-yr-old Hispanic woman who was admitted to the intermediate care unit with complaints of increasing shortness of breath, fatigue, and weight gain.

Subjective Data

- History of hypertension for 20 yr
- History of MI at 58 yr of age
- Has experienced increasing shortness of breath, fatigue, and an unexplained 11-lb weight gain during the past 2 wk
- Had a respiratory tract infection 2 wk ago; has persistent cough and edema in legs
- Cannot climb a flight of stairs without getting short of breath
- Sleeps with head elevated on three pillows
- Lives alone, does not always remember to take medication

Objective Data

Physical Examination

- Moderate respiratory distress, use of accessory muscles, respiratory rate 36 breaths/minute
- Systolic heart murmur
- Bilateral crackles in all lung fields
- Cyanotic lips and extremities
- Skin cool and diaphoretic

Diagnostic Studies

- Chest x-ray results: cardiomegaly with right and left ventricular hypertrophy; fluid in lower lung fields
- Echocardiogram results: EF 20%

Interprofessional Care

- Furosemide (Lasix) 40 mg IV bid
- Potassium 40 mEq PO bid
- Enalapril (Vasotec) 5 mg/day PO
- Nesiritide (Natrecor) 2 mcg/kg IV bolus followed by a continuous infusion of 0.01 mcg/kg/min
- Continuous ECG monitoring
- Diet: 2-g sodium diet
- Titrate O_2 to keep O_2 saturation >93%
- Monitor intake and output, and daily weights
- Serum electrolytes; cardiac biomarkers q8hr × 3

Discussion Questions

1. Explain the pathophysiology of J.E.'s heart disease and symptoms.
2. What clinical manifestations of ADHF did J.E. exhibit?
3. What is the significance of the findings of the diagnostic studies?
4. How would a serum NT-proBNP be beneficial in the diagnosis of ADHF?
5. Provide the rationale for each of the HCP's orders prescribed for J.E.
6. ***Priority Decision:*** Based on the assessment data presented, what are the priority nursing diagnoses? Identify any collaborative problems.
7. ***Priority Decision:*** What are your priority nursing interventions for J.E.?
8. ***Teamwork and Collaboration:*** Which interventions could be delegated to unlicensed assistive personnel (UAP) or other members of the interprofessional team?
9. ***Patient-Centered Care:*** What priority patient teaching measures should be instituted to prevent recurrence of ADHF and prepare J.E. for discharge?
10. ***Evidence-Based Practice:*** J.E. asks you why it is so important to "watch her salt." She tells you that food tastes better with salt. How would you respond to her?

Answers and a corresponding concept map available at *http://evolve.elsevier.com/Lewis/medsurg.*

BRIDGE TO NCLEX EXAMINATION

The number of the question corresponds to the same-numbered outcome at the beginning of the chapter.

1. The nurse recognizes that *primary* manifestations of systolic failure include
   - **a.** ↓ EF and ↑ PAWP.
   - **b.** ↓ PAWP and ↑ EF.
   - **c.** ↓ pulmonary hypertension associated with normal EF.
   - **d.** ↓ afterload and ↓ left ventricular end-diastolic pressure.
2. A compensatory mechanism involved in HF that leads to inappropriate fluid retention and additional workload of the heart is
   - **a.** ventricular dilation.
   - **b.** ventricular hypertrophy.
   - **c.** neurohormonal response.
   - **d.** sympathetic nervous system activation.
3. You are caring for a patient with ADHF who is receiving IV dobutamine (Dobutrex). You know that this drug is ordered because it *(select all that apply)*
   - **a.** increases SVR.
   - **b.** produces diuresis.
   - **c.** improves contractility.
   - **d.** dilates renal blood vessels.
   - **e.** works on the β_1-receptors in the heart.
4. A patient with chronic HF and atrial fibrillation is treated with a digitalis glycoside and a loop diuretic. To prevent possible complications of this combination of drugs, what does the nurse need to do *(select all that apply)*?
   - **a.** Monitor serum potassium levels.
   - **b.** Teach the patient how to take a pulse rate.
   - **c.** Keep an accurate measure of intake and output.
   - **d.** Teach the patient about dietary restriction of potassium.
   - **e.** Withhold digitalis and notify health care provider if pulse is irregular.
5. Patients with a heart transplantation are at risk for which complications in the first year after transplantation *(select all that apply)*?
   - **a.** Cancer
   - **b.** Infection
   - **c.** Rejection
   - **d.** Vasculopathy
   - **e.** Sudden cardiac death

1. a, 2. c, 3. c, e, 4. a, b, 5. b, c, e

For rationales to these answers and even more NCLEX review questions, visit *http://evolve.elsevier.com/Lewis/medsurg.*

EVOLVE WEBSITE

http://evolve.elsevier.com/Lewis/medsurg

Review Questions (Online Only)

Key Points

Answer Keys for Questions

- Rationales for Bridge to NCLEX Examination Questions
- Answer Guidelines for Case Study on p. 755

Student Case Study

- Patient With Heart Failure

Nursing Care Plan

- eNursing Care Plan 34-1: Patient With Heart Failure

Conceptual Care Map Creator

- Conceptual Care Map for Case Study on p. 755

Audio Glossary

Content Updates

REFERENCES

*1. Yancy CW, Jessup M, Bozkurt B, et al: 2013 ACCF/AHA guideline for the management of heart failure: executive summary: a report of the American College of Cardiology Foundation/American Heart Association Task Force on practice guidelines, *Circulation* 128:1810, 2013.

2. Go AS, Mozaffarian D, Roger VL, et al: Heart disease and stroke statistics—2014 update: a report from the American Heart Association, *Circulation* 129:e28, 2013.

3. LeWinter M, Granzier H: Titin is a major human disease gene, *Circulation* 127:938, 2013.

*4. Silver MA, Maisel A, Yancy CW, et al: BNP Consensus Panel 2004: a clinical approach for the diagnostic, prognostic, screening, treatment monitoring, and therapeutic roles of natriuretic peptides in cardiovascular diseases, *Congest Heart Fail* 10(5 Suppl 3):1, 2004. (Classic)

5. Heart Failure Society of America: Who is the patient with heart failure? Think FACES, 2002. Retrieved from *www.hfsa.org/hfsa-wp/content/uploads/2014/10/faces_card.pdf.* (Classic)

6. Nawarskas JJ, Bowman BN, Anderson JR: Ivabradine: a unique and intriguing medication for treating cardiovascular disease, *Cardiol Rev* 23(4):201, 2015.

7. Newhouse A, Jiang W: Heart failure and depression, *Heart Fail Clin* 10(2):295, 2014.

*8. Tracy CM, Epstein AE, Darbar D, et al: 2012 ACCF/AHA/HRS Focused update incorporated into the ACCF/AHA/HRS 2008 Guidelines for Device-Based Therapy of Cardiac Rhythm Abnormalities: a report of the American College of Cardiology Foundation/American Heart Association Task Force on Practice Guidelines and the Heart Rhythm Society, *J Am Coll Cardiol* 61(3):e6, 2013.

*9. Thiene G, Bruneval P, Veinot J, Leone O: Diagnostic use of the endomyocardial biopsy: a consensus statement, *Virchows Arch* 463(1):1, 2013.

10. Coons JC, McGraw M, Murali S: Pharmacotherapy for acute heart failure syndromes, *Am J Health Syst Pharm* 68(1):21, 2011.

11. Key JL, Hayes ER, McCuistion LE: *Pharmacology: a patient centered nursing process approach,* ed 8, St Louis, 2015, Elsevier.

12. Ades PA, Keteyian SJ, Balady GJ, et al: Cardiac rehabilitation exercise and self-care for chronic heart failure, *JCHF* 1(6):540, 2013.

*13. Abraham WT, Adamson PB, Bourge RC, et al: Wireless pulmonary artery haemodynamic monitoring in chronic heart failure: a randomised controlled trial, *Lancet* 377:658, 2011.

*14. Lindenfeld J, Albert NM, Boehmer JP, et al: Executive summary: HFSA 2010 comprehensive heart failure practice guidelines, *J Card Fail* 16:475, 2010.

15. O'Riordan M: FDA approves valsartan/sacubitril (Entresto) combination for heart failure. Retrieved from *www.medscape.com/viewarticle/847619.*

*16. Lee D, Wilson K, Akehurst R, et al: Eplerenone in Mild Patients Hospitalization and Survival Study in Heart Failure (EMPHASIS-HF) Study: cost-effectiveness of eplerenone in patients with systolic heart failure and mild symptoms, *Heart* 100(21):1681, 2014.

*17. Ferdinand KC, Elkayam U, Mancini D, et al: Use of isosorbide dinitrate and hydralazine in African-Americans with heart failure 9 years after the African-American Heart Failure Trial, *Am J Cardiol* 114(1):151, 2014.

18. U.S. Food and Drug Administration: FDA approves Corlanor. Retrieved from *www.drugs.com/history/corlanor.html.*

*19. Schocken DD, Benjamin EJ, Fonarow G, et al: Prevention of heart failure: a scientific statement from the American Heart Association councils on epidemiology and prevention, clinical cardiology, cardiovascular nursing, and high blood pressure research, *Circulation* 117:2544, 2008.

20. The Joint Commission: Advanced certification in heart failure: standardized performance measures. Retrieved from *www.jointcommission.org/adv_certification_heart_failure_standardized_performance_measures.*

21. American Heart Association: Get with the guidelines—heart failure: fact sheet. Retrieved from *www.heart.org/idc/groups/heart-public/@wcm/@private/@hcm/@gwtg/documents/downloadable/ucm_310967.pdf.*

*22. Huynh B, Rovner A, Rich M: Identification of older patients with heart failure who may be candidates for hospice care: development of a simple four-item risk score, *J Am Geriatr Soc* 56:1111, 2008. (Classic)

*23. Allen LA, Stevenson l, Grady KL, et al: Decision making in advanced heart failure: a scientific statement from the American Heart Association, *Circulation* 125:1928, 2012.

24. Givens JL, Tjia J, Zhou C, et al: Racial and ethnic differences in hospice use among patients with heart failure, *Arch Intern Med* 170:427, 2010.

25. Stehlik J, Edwards LB, Kucheryavaya AY, et al: The registry of the International Society of Heart and Lung Transplantation: Twenty eighth Adult Heart Transplant Report—2011, *J Heart Lung Transplant* 30(10):1078, 2011.

*26. Taylor D, Meiser B, Webber S, et al: The International Society of Heart and Lung Transplantation Guidelines for the Care of Heart Transplant Recipients: task force 2: immunosuppression and rejection, *J Heart Lung Transplant* 29(8):926, 2010.

*Evidence-based information for clinical practice.

35

Dysrhythmias

Linda Bucher

The greatest test of courage on earth is to bear defeat without losing heart.

Robert Green Ingersoll

http://evolve.elsevier.com/Lewis/medsurg/

LEARNING OUTCOMES

1. Examine the nursing care of patients needing continuous electrocardiographic (ECG) monitoring.
2. Distinguish the clinical characteristics and ECG patterns of normal sinus rhythm, common dysrhythmias, and acute coronary syndrome (ACS).
3. Compare the nursing and interprofessional management of patients with common dysrhythmias and ECG changes associated with ACS.
4. Differentiate between defibrillation and cardioversion, including indications for use and physiologic effects.
5. Describe the nursing and interprofessional management of patients with pacemakers and implantable cardioverter-defibrillators.
6. Select appropriate interventions for patients undergoing electrophysiologic testing and radiofrequency catheter ablation therapy.

KEY TERMS

asystole, p. 765
atrial fibrillation, p. 766
atrial flutter, p. 765
automatic external defibrillator (AED), p. 771
cardiac pacemaker, p. 773
complete heart block, p. 768
dysrhythmias, p. 757
premature atrial contraction (PAC), p. 764
premature ventricular contraction (PVC), p. 768
telemetry monitoring, p. 760
ventricular fibrillation (VF), p. 770
ventricular tachycardia (VT), p. 769

This chapter describes basic principles of electrocardiographic monitoring and recognition and treatment of common dysrhythmias. In addition, it presents ECG changes that are associated with acute coronary syndrome (ACS).

RHYTHM IDENTIFICATION AND TREATMENT

Your ability to recognize normal and abnormal heart rhythms, called **dysrhythmias**, is an essential nursing skill.[1] Prompt assessment of dysrhythmias and the patient's response to the rhythm is critical.

Conduction System

Four properties of heart cells allow the conduction system to start an electrical impulse, send it through the heart tissue, and stimulate muscle contraction (Table 35-1). The heart's conduction system consists of specialized neuromuscular tissue located throughout the heart (see Fig. 31-4, *A*). A normal impulse starts in the sinoatrial (SA) node in the upper right atrium near the entrance of the vena cava. It spreads over the atrial myocardium via interatrial and internodal pathways, causing atrial contraction. The impulse then travels to the atrioventricular (AV) node, through the bundle of His, and down the left and right bundle branches. It ends in the Purkinje fibers, which transmit the impulse to the ventricles.

Nervous Control of the Heart

The autonomic nervous system plays an important role in the rate of impulse formation, speed of conduction, and strength of cardiac contraction. The components of the autonomic nervous system that affect the heart are the vagus nerve fibers of the parasympathetic nervous system and nerve fibers of the sympathetic nervous system.

Stimulation of the vagus nerve causes a decreased rate of firing of the SA node and slowed impulse conduction of the AV node. Stimulation of the sympathetic nerves increases SA node firing, AV node impulse conduction, and cardiac contractility.[2]

Electrocardiographic Monitoring

The *electrocardiogram* (ECG) is a graphic tracing of the electrical impulses produced in the heart. The waveforms on the ECG represent electrical activity produced by the movement of ions across the membranes of heart cells, representing depolarization and repolarization (see Fig. 31-4, *B*).

The membrane of a heart cell is semipermeable. This allows it to maintain a high concentration of potassium and a low

Reviewed by Linda R. Lewis, MSN, RN-BC, Faculty Specialist, Nursing, University of Scranton, Scranton, Pennsylvania; and Tamekia L. Thomas, MSN, APN, PCCN, ACNS-BC, Critical Care Education Coordinator, Christiana Care Health System, Newark, Delaware.

TABLE 35-1 Properties of Heart Cells

Property	Definition
Automaticity	Ability to initiate an impulse spontaneously and continuously
Excitability	Ability to be electrically stimulated
Conductivity	Ability to transmit an impulse along a membrane in an orderly manner
Contractility	Ability to respond mechanically to an impulse

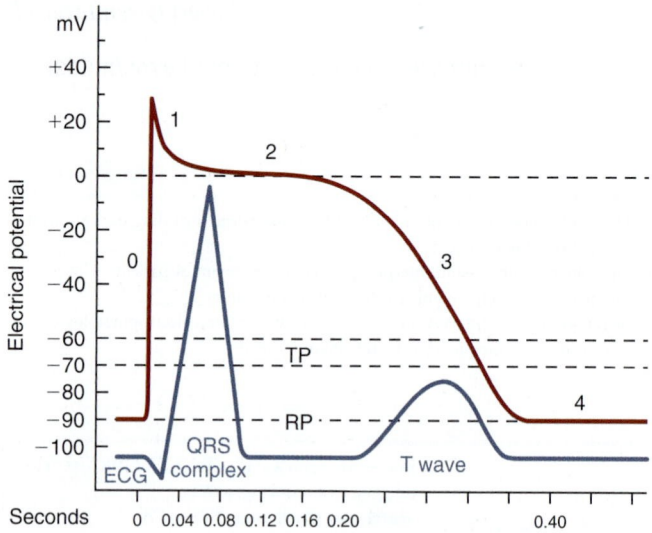

FIG. 35-1 Phases of the cardiac action potential. The electrical potential, measured in millivolts (mV), is indicated along the vertical axis of the graph. Time, measured in seconds (sec), is indicated along the horizontal axis. The action potential has five phases, labeled *0* through *4*. Each phase represents a particular electrical event or combination of electrical events. Phase 0 is the upstroke of rapid depolarization and corresponds with ventricular contraction. Phases 1, 2, and 3 represent repolarization. Phase 4 is known as complete repolarization (or the polarized state) and corresponds to diastole. *RP,* Resting membrane potential; *TP,* threshold membrane potential.

concentration of sodium inside the cell. Outside the cell a high concentration of sodium and a low concentration of potassium exist. The inside of the cell, when at rest, or in the polarized state, is negative compared with the outside. When a cell or groups of cells are stimulated, the cell membrane changes its permeability. This allows sodium to move rapidly into the cell, making the inside of the cell positive compared with the outside *(depolarization)*. A slower movement of ions across the membrane restores the cell to the polarized state, called *repolarization*. Fig. 35-1 describes the phases of the cardiac action potential.[2]

The ECG has 12 recording leads. Six of the leads measure electrical forces in the frontal plane. These are bipolar (positive and negative) leads I, II, and III and unipolar (positive) leads aVR, aVL, and aVF (Fig. 35-2, *A* and *B*). The remaining six unipolar leads (V_1 through V_6) measure the electrical forces in the horizontal plane (precordial leads) (Fig. 35-2, *C*). The 12-lead ECG may show changes suggesting structural changes, conduction disturbances, damage (e.g., ischemia, infarction), electrolyte imbalance, or drug toxicity. Obtaining 12-lead ECG views of the heart is also helpful in the assessment of dysrhythmias. Fig. 35-3 is an example of a normal 12-lead ECG.

One or more ECG leads can be used to continuously monitor a patient. The most common leads selected are leads II and V_1 (Fig. 35-4). A modified chest lead (MCL_1) is used when only three leads are available for monitoring. MCL_1 is similar to V_1. Accurate interpretation of an ECG depends on the correct placement of the leads on the patient. The monitoring leads selected are determined by the patient's clinical status.[3,4]

The monitor continuously displays the heart rhythm. ECG paper attached to the monitor records the ECG (i.e., rhythm strip). This provides a record of the patient's rhythm. It also allows for measurement of complexes and intervals, and for assessment of dysrhythmias.

To correctly interpret an ECG, measure time and voltage on the ECG paper. ECG paper consists of large (heavy lines) and small (light lines) squares (Fig. 35-5). Each large square consists of 25 smaller squares (five horizontal and five vertical). Horizontally, each small square (1 mm) represents 0.04 second. This means that one large square equals 0.20 second and that 300 large squares equal 1 minute. Vertically, each small square

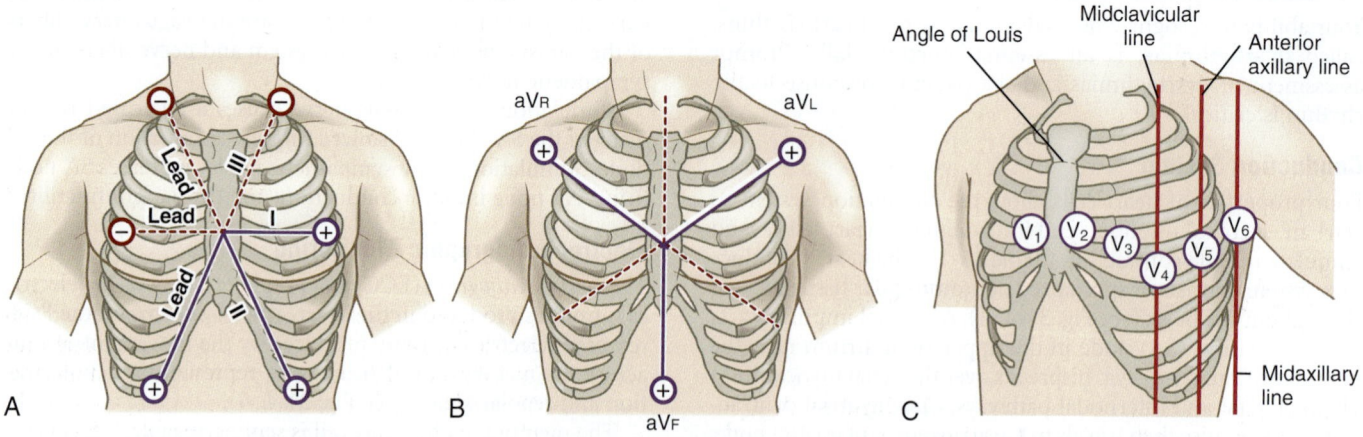

FIG. 35-2 **A,** Limb leads I, II, and III. These bipolar leads are located on the extremities. Illustrated are the angles from which these leads view the heart. **B,** Limb leads aVR, aVL, and aVF. These unipolar leads use the center of the heart as their negative electrode. **C,** Placement for the unipolar chest leads: V_1, fourth intercostal space at the right sternal border; V_2, fourth intercostal space at the left sternal border; V_3, halfway between V_2 and V_4; V_4, fifth intercostal space at the left midclavicular line; V_5, fifth intercostal space at the left anterior axillary line; V_6, fifth intercostal space at the left midaxillary line.

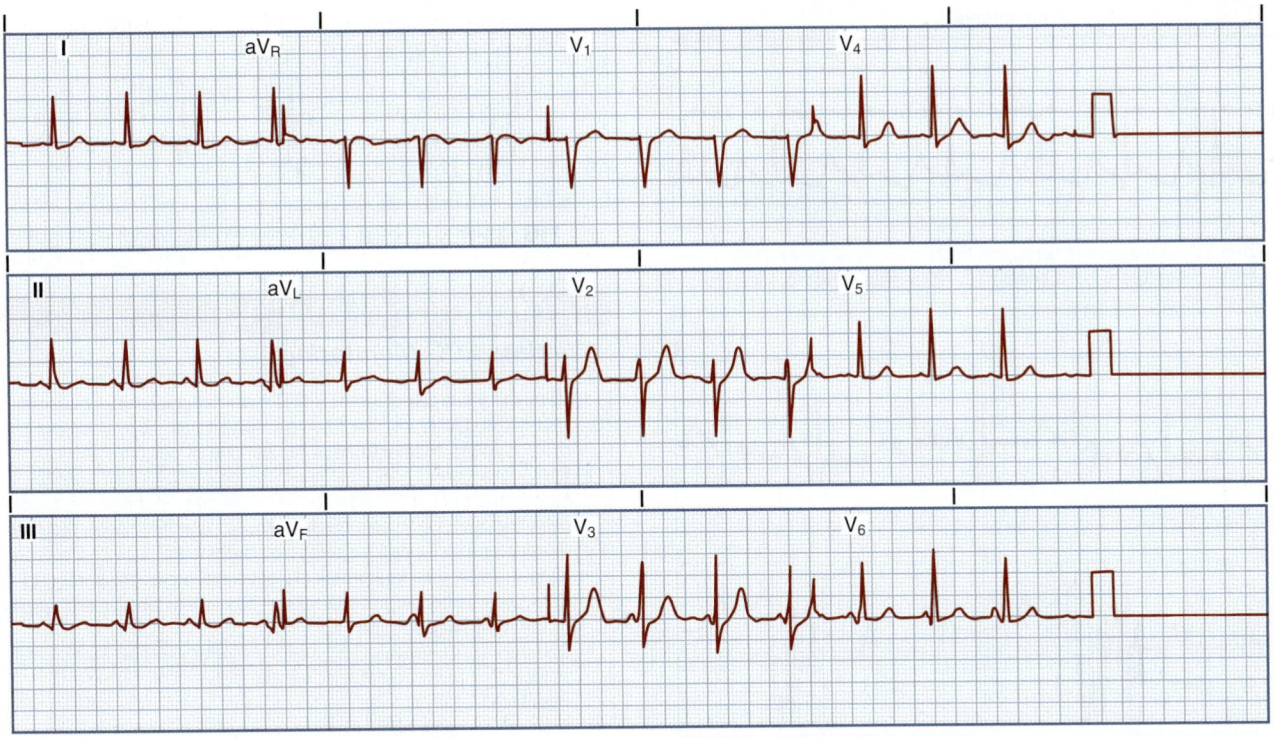

FIG. 35-3 Twelve-lead electrocardiogram showing a normal sinus rhythm.

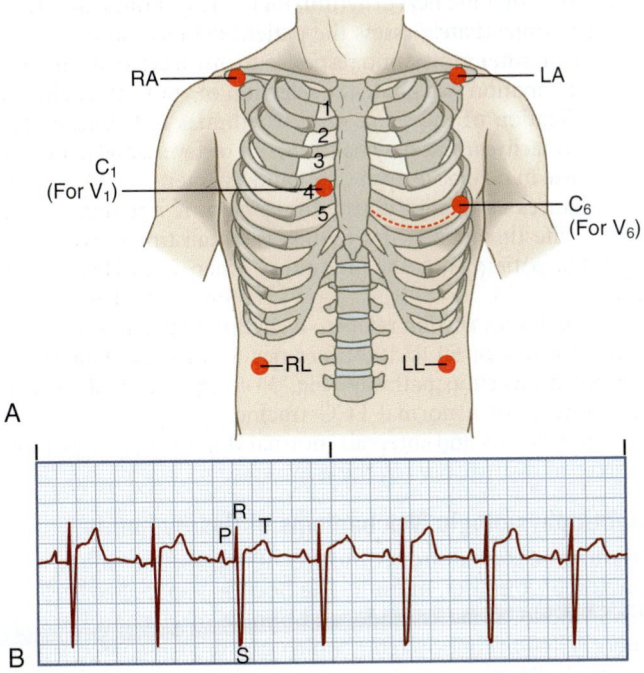

FIG. 35-4 A, Lead placement for V_1 or V_6 using a five-lead system. **B,** Typical ECG tracing in lead V_1. *C,* Chest; *LA,* left arm; *LL,* left leg; *RA,* right arm; *RL,* right leg.

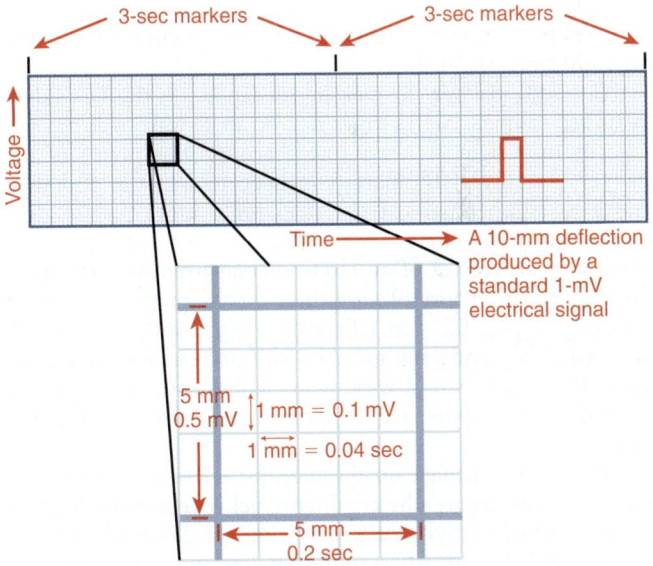

FIG. 35-5 Time and voltage on the electrocardiogram; 6-sec strip. (Modified from Wesley K: *Basic dysrhythmias and acute coronary syndromes,* ed 4, St Louis, 2011, Mosby JEMS.)

(1 mm) represents 0.1 millivolt (mV). This means that one large square equals 0.5 mV. Use these squares to calculate the heart rate (HR) and measure time intervals for the different ECG complexes.

You can use a variety of methods to calculate the HR from an ECG. The most accurate way is to count the number of QRS complexes in 1 minute. However, because this method is time consuming, a simpler process is used. Note that every 3 seconds a marker appears on the ECG paper (Fig. 35-5). Count the number of R-R intervals in 6 seconds and multiply that number by 10. (An R wave is the first upward [or positive] wave of the QRS complex.) This is the estimated number of beats per minute (Fig. 35-6).

Another method is to count the number of small squares between one R-R interval. Divide this number into 1500 to get the HR. Last, you can count the number of large squares between one R-R interval and divide this number into 300 to get the HR

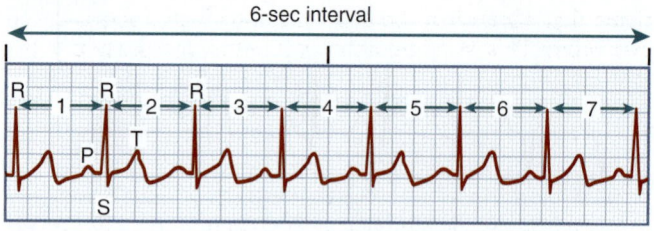

FIG. 35-6 When the rhythm is regular, heart rate can be easily determined. The estimated heart rate is 70 beats/min. NOTE: Recorded from lead II.

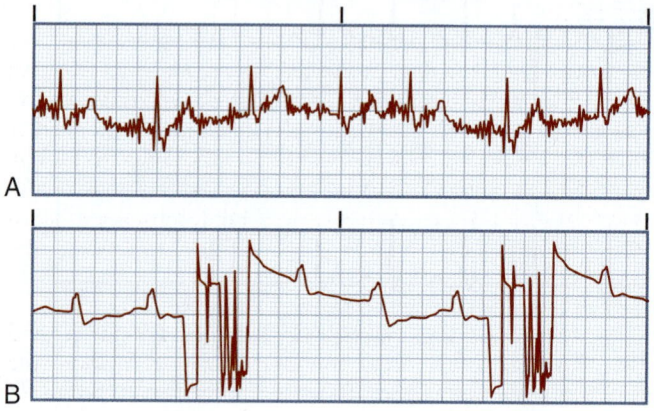

FIG. 35-7 Artifact. **A,** Muscle tremor. **B,** Loose electrodes.

(Fig. 35-6). All these methods are most accurate when the rhythm is regular.[1]

An additional way to measure distances on the ECG strip is to use calipers. Many times a P or an R wave will not fall directly on a light or heavy line. Place the fine points of the calipers exactly on the parts you need to measure and then move to another part of the strip for a more precise time measurement.

ECG leads consist of an electrode pad fixed with electrical conductive gel. Before placing these on the patient, you must properly prepare the skin. Clip excessive hair on the chest wall with scissors. Gently rub the skin with dry gauze until slightly pink. If the skin is oily, wipe with alcohol first. If the patient is diaphoretic, apply a skin protectant before placing the electrode.

You will see artifact on the monitor when leads and electrodes are not secure, the conductive gel is becoming dry, and there is muscle activity (e.g., shivering) or electrical interference. *Artifact* is a distortion of the baseline and waveforms seen on the ECG (Fig. 35-7). Accurate interpretation of heart rhythm is difficult when artifact is present. If artifact occurs, check the connections in the equipment. Replace the electrodes if the conductive gel has dried out.

Telemetry Monitoring. Telemetry monitoring is the observation of a patient's HR and rhythm at a site distant from the patient. The use of this technology can help rapidly identify dysrhythmias, ischemia, or infarction. Two types of systems are used for telemetry monitoring. The first type, a centralized monitoring system, requires you or a telemetry technician to continuously observe a group of patients' ECGs at a central location. The second system of telemetry monitoring does not require constant surveillance. These systems have the capability of detecting and storing data. Advanced alarm systems provide different levels of detection of dysrhythmias, ischemia, or infarction.

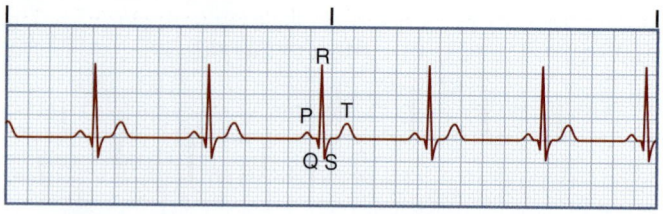

FIG. 35-8 Normal sinus rhythm. NOTE: Recorded from lead II.

INFORMATICS IN PRACTICE

Wireless ECG Monitoring

- Wireless electrocardiogram (ECG) monitoring systems continuously monitor and interpret the findings, sending an alert when patient rhythm and/or measurements fall outside of set parameters.
- Early detection of abnormal heart rhythms allows you time to assess the patient for signs of hemodynamic instability (e.g., chest pain, hypotension, palpitations, dyspnea) and determine the need to intervene (e.g., call the rapid response team).
- These systems can automatically save the pre-event portion of the ECG while continuing to record the post-event portion and send all of the information to the HCP.
- Computerized monitoring systems are not fail-proof. Frequently assess all monitored patients for any signs of hemodynamic instability.

Assessment of Heart Rhythm

When assessing the heart rhythm, make an accurate interpretation and immediately assess the patient's clinical status. Assess the patient's hemodynamic response to any change in rhythm. This information will guide the selection of your interventions. Determination of the cause of dysrhythmias is a priority. For example, tachycardias may be the result of fever and may cause a decrease in cardiac output (CO) and hypotension. Electrolyte disturbances can cause dysrhythmias and, if not treated, can lead to life-threatening dysrhythmias. At all times, assess and treat the patient, not the "monitor" when a dysrhythmia is noted.

Normal sinus rhythm refers to a rhythm that starts in the SA node at a rate of 60 to 100 times per minute and follows the normal conduction pathway (Fig. 35-8). Fig. 35-9 shows the components of a normal ECG tracing. Table 35-2 describes ECG waveforms and intervals, normal durations, and possible sources of disturbances in these features.

Electrophysiologic Mechanisms of Dysrhythmias

Dysrhythmias result from disorders of impulse formation, conduction of impulses, or both. The heart has specialized cells in the SA node, atria, AV node, and bundle of His and Purkinje fibers (His-Purkinje system), which can fire (discharge) spontaneously. This is termed *automaticity.* Normally, the SA node is the pacemaker of the heart. It spontaneously fires 60 to 100 times per minute (Table 35-3). A secondary pacemaker from another site may fire in two ways. If the SA node fires more slowly than a secondary pacemaker, the electrical signals from the secondary pacemaker may "escape." The secondary pacemaker will then fire automatically at its intrinsic rate. These secondary pacemakers may start from the AV node at a rate of 40 to 60 times per minute or the His-Purkinje system at a rate of 20 to 40 times per minute.

Another way that secondary pacemakers can start is when they fire more rapidly than the normal pacemaker of the SA node. *Triggered beats* (early or late) may come from an *ectopic focus* or *accessory pathway* (area outside the normal conduction pathway) in the atria, AV node, or ventricles. This results in a dysrhythmia, which replaces the normal sinus rhythm.

The impulse started by the SA node or an ectopic focus must be conducted to the entire heart. The property of myocardial tissue that allows it to be depolarized by a stimulus is called *excitability.* This is an important part of the transmission of the impulse from one cell to another. The level of excitability is determined by the length of time after depolarization that the tissues can be restimulated. The recovery period after stimulation is the *refractory phase* or period. The *absolute refractory phase* or period occurs when excitability is zero and the heart cannot be stimulated. The *relative refractory period* occurs slightly later in the cycle, and excitability is more likely. In states of *full excitability,* the heart is completely recovered. Fig. 35-10 shows the relationship between the refractory period and ECG.

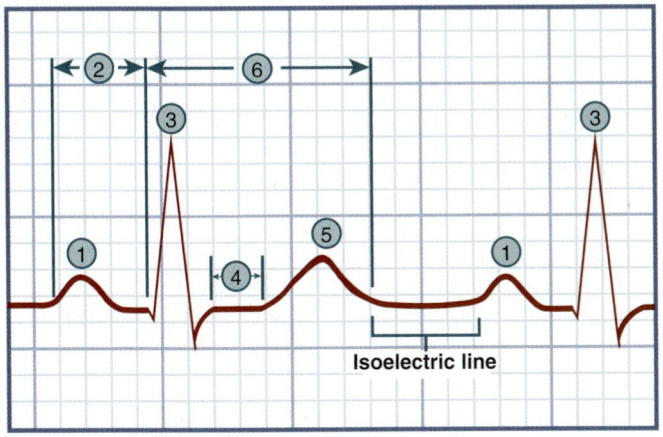

FIG. 35-9 The ECG tracing as seen in normal sinus rhythm. *1,* P wave; *2,* PR interval; *3,* QRS complex: Q wave, R wave, S wave; *4,* ST segment; *5,* T wave; *6,* QT interval. Isoelectric (flat) line or baseline represents the absence of electrical activity in the heart cells. (Table 35-2 for timing of intervals.)

If conduction is depressed and some areas of the heart are blocked (e.g., by infarction), the unblocked areas are activated earlier than the blocked areas. When the block is unidirectional, this uneven conduction may allow the initial impulse to reenter areas that were previously not excitable but have recovered. The reentering impulse may be able to depolarize the atria and ventricles, causing a premature beat. If the reentrant excitation continues, tachycardia occurs.

Evaluation of Dysrhythmias

Dysrhythmias occur as the result of various abnormalities and disease states. The cause of a dysrhythmia influences the patient's treatment. Table 35-4 presents common causes of

TABLE 35-2 ECG Waveforms and Intervals*

Description	Normal Duration (sec)	Source of Possible Variation
P Wave		
Represents time for the passage of the electrical impulse through the atrium causing atrial depolarization (contraction). Should be upright	0.06-0.12	Disturbance in conduction within atria
PR Interval		
Measured from beginning of P wave to beginning of QRS complex. Represents time taken for impulse to spread through the atria, AV node and bundle of His, bundle branches, and Purkinje fibers, to a point immediately before ventricular contraction	0.12-0.20	Disturbance in conduction usually in AV node, bundle of His, or bundle branches but can be in atria as well
QRS Complex		
Q wave: First negative (downward) deflection after the P wave, short and narrow, not present in several leads	<0.03	MI may result in development of a pathologic Q wave that is wide (≥0.03 sec) and deep (≥25% of the height of the R wave)
R wave: First positive (upward) deflection in the QRS complex	Not usually measured	
S wave: First negative (downward) deflection after the R wave	Not usually measured	
QRS Interval		
Measured from beginning to end of QRS complex. Represents time taken for depolarization (contraction) of both ventricles (systole)	<0.12	Disturbance in conduction in bundle branches or in ventricles
ST Segment		
Measured from the S wave of the QRS complex to the beginning of the T wave. Represents the time between ventricular depolarization and repolarization (diastole). Should be isoelectric (flat)	0.12	Disturbances (e.g., elevation, depression) usually caused by ischemia, injury, or infarction
T Wave		
Represents time for ventricular repolarization. Should be upright	0.16	Disturbances (e.g., tall, peaked; inverted) usually caused by electrolyte imbalances, ischemia, or infarction
QT Interval†		
Measured from beginning of QRS complex to end of T wave. Represents time taken for entire electrical depolarization and repolarization of the ventricles. Normal adult women have slightly longer QT intervals than men.	0.34-0.43	Disturbances usually affecting repolarization more than depolarization and caused by drugs, electrolyte imbalances, and changes in heart rate

AV, Atrioventricular.
*Heart rate influences the duration of these intervals, especially the PR and QT intervals (e.g., QT interval shortens in duration as heart rate increases).
†A corrected QT interval (QTc) is calculated to account for the influence of heart rate.

TABLE 35-3 Intrinsic Rates of the Conduction System

Part of Conduction System	Rate
SA node and atria	60-100 times/min
AV node and bundle of His	40-60 times/min
Bundle branches and Purkinje fibers	20-40 times/min

AV, Atrioventricular; *SA,* sinoatrial.

TABLE 35-4 Common Causes of Dysrhythmias*

Heart Conditions	Other Conditions
• Accessory pathways	• Acid-base imbalances
• Cardiomyopathy	• Alcohol
• Conduction defects	• Caffeine, tobacco
• Heart failure	• Connective tissue disorders
• Myocardial ischemia, infarction	• Drug effects (e.g., antidysrhythmia drugs, stimulants, β-blockers) or toxicity
• Valve disease	• Electric shock
	• Electrolyte imbalances (e.g., hyperkalemia, hypocalcemia)
	• Emotional crisis
	• Herbal supplements (e.g., areca nut, wahoo root bark, yerba maté)
	• Hypoxia
	• Metabolic conditions (e.g., thyroid dysfunction)
	• Drowning
	• Sepsis, shock
	• Toxins

*List is not all-inclusive.

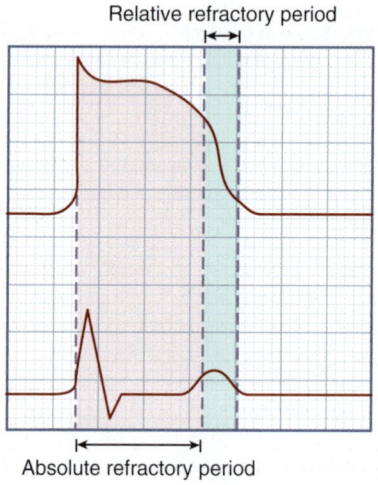

FIG. 35-10 Absolute and relative refractory periods correlated with the heart muscle's action potential and with an ECG tracing. (Modified from Urden LD, Stacy KM, Lough ME: *Critical care nursing: diagnosis and management,* ed 6, St Louis, 2010, Mosby.)

dysrhythmias. Table 35-5 presents a systematic approach to assessing a heart rhythm.

Dysrhythmias occurring in nonmonitored settings present management challenges. If the patient becomes symptomatic (e.g., chest pain, syncope), determination of the rhythm by heart monitoring is a high priority. Activate the emergency

TABLE 35-5 Approach to Assessing Heart Rhythm

When assessing a heart rhythm, use a consistent and systematic approach. One such approach includes the following:

1. Look for the P wave. Is it upright or inverted? Is there one for every QRS complex or more than one? Are atrial fibrillatory or flutter waves present?
2. Evaluate the atrial rhythm. Is it regular or irregular?
3. Calculate the atrial rate.
4. Measure the duration of the PR interval. Is it normal duration or prolonged? Is the duration consistent before each QRS?
5. Evaluate the ventricular rhythm. Is it regular or irregular?
6. Calculate the ventricular rate.
7. Measure the duration of the QRS complex. Is it normal duration or prolonged?
8. Assess the ST segment. Is it isoelectric (flat), elevated, or depressed?
9. Measure the duration of the QT interval. Correct for heart rate (cQT) to determine if it is normal or prolonged.*
10. Note the T wave. Is it upright or inverted?

Additional questions to consider include the following:

1. What is the dominant or underlying rhythm and/or dysrhythmia?
2. What is the clinical significance of your findings?
3. What is the treatment for the particular rhythm?

*A website for calculating the cQT interval for heart rate can be found at *www.mdcalc.com/corrected-qt-interval-qtc.*

response system (ERS). Table 35-6 outlines the emergency care of the patient with a dysrhythmia.

In addition to continuous ECG monitoring during hospitalization, several other tests can assess dysrhythmias and the effectiveness of antidysrhythmia drug therapy. An electrophysiologic study, Holter monitoring, event monitoring (or loop recorder), exercise treadmill testing, and signal-averaged ECG can be performed on an inpatient or outpatient basis (see Table 31-6 for nursing care related to these tests).

An *electrophysiologic study* (EPS) can identify the causes of heart blocks, tachydysrhythmias (dysrhythmias with rates greater than 100 beats/minute), bradydysrhythmias (dysrhythmias with rates less than 60 beats/minute), and syncope. An EPS study can also locate accessory pathways and determine the effectiveness of antidysrhythmia drugs.

The Holter monitor continuously records the ECG while the patient is ambulatory and performing daily activities. The patient keeps a diary and records activities and any symptoms. Events in the diary are correlated with any dysrhythmias seen on the ECG. Use of event monitors has improved the evaluation of dysrhythmias in outpatients. Event monitors are recorders that the patient activates only when he or she experiences symptoms. New technology using smart phone apps can obtain and save ECG recordings and even detect some dysrhythmias (e.g., AliveECG at *https://itunes.apple.com/us/app/aliveecg/id579769143?mt=8*).

Exercise treadmill testing evaluates the patient's heart rhythm during exercise. If exercise-induced dysrhythmias or ECG changes occur, they are reviewed. If needed, drug therapy can be started and evaluated.

The signal-averaged ECG identifies *late potentials,* strongly suggesting that the patient may be at risk for developing serious ventricular dysrhythmias. (See Chapter 31 for a discussion of diagnostic procedures for assessment of the cardiovascular system and related nursing care.)

TABLE 35-6 Emergency Management

Dysrhythmias

Etiology	Assessment Findings	Interventions
Table 35-4	• Irregular rate and rhythm; tachycardia, bradycardia • Decreased or increased BP • Decreased O_2 saturation • Chest, neck, shoulder, back, jaw, or arm pain • Dizziness, syncope • Dyspnea • Extreme restlessness, anxiety • Decreased level of consciousness, confusion • Feeling of impending doom • Numbness, tingling of arms • Weakness and fatigue • Cold, clammy skin • Diminished peripheral pulses • Diaphoresis • Pallor • Palpitations • Nausea and vomiting	**Initial** • If unresponsive, assess circulation, airway, and breathing (CAB). • If responsive, monitor airway, breathing, and circulation (ABC). • Apply O_2 via nasal cannula or non-rebreather mask. • Obtain baseline vital signs, including O_2 saturation. • Obtain 12-lead ECG. • Begin continuous ECG monitoring. • Identify underlying rate and rhythm. • Identify dysrhythmia. • Establish IV access. • Obtain baseline laboratory studies (e.g., CBC, electrolytes). **Ongoing Monitoring** • Monitor ABCs, vital signs, level of consciousness, O_2 saturation, and heart rhythm. • Anticipate need for antidysrhythmia drugs and analgesics. • Anticipate need for intubation if respiratory distress is evident. • Anticipate need to begin advanced cardiovascular life support (e.g., CPR, defibrillation, transcutaneous pacing).

Types of Dysrhythmias

Figs. 35-11 to 35-19 provide examples of the ECG tracings of common dysrhythmias. Table 35-7 presents the descriptive characteristics.

Sinus Bradycardia. In *sinus bradycardia* the conduction pathway is the same as that in sinus rhythm, but the SA node fires at a rate less than 60 beats/minute (Fig. 35-11, *A*). *Symptomatic bradycardia* refers to an HR that is less than 60 beats/minute and is inadequate for the patient's condition. This causes the patient to experience symptoms (e.g., fatigue, dizziness, chest pain, syncope).

Clinical Associations. Sinus bradycardia may be a normal sinus rhythm in aerobically trained athletes and in some people during sleep. It also occurs in response to carotid sinus massage, Valsalva maneuver, hypothermia, increased intraocular pressure, vagal stimulation, and certain drugs (e.g., β-blockers, calcium channel blockers). Common disease states associated with sinus bradycardia are hypothyroidism, increased intracranial pressure, and inferior myocardial infarction (MI).

ECG Characteristics. In sinus bradycardia, the HR is less than 60 beats/minute and rhythm is regular. The P wave precedes each QRS complex and has a normal shape and duration. The PR interval is normal and the QRS complex has a normal shape and duration.

Clinical Significance. The clinical significance of sinus bradycardia depends on how the patient tolerates it. Manifestations of symptomatic bradycardia include pale, cool skin; hypotension; weakness; angina; dizziness or syncope; confusion or disorientation; and shortness of breath.

Treatment. For the patient with symptoms, treatment consists of giving IV atropine (anticholinergic drug). If atropine is ineffective, transcutaneous pacing or a dopamine or epinephrine (Adrenalin) infusion is considered. Permanent pacemaker therapy may be needed. If bradycardia is due to drugs, these may have to be held, discontinued, or reduced.

Sinus Tachycardia. The conduction pathway is the same in *sinus tachycardia* as that in normal sinus rhythm. The discharge rate from the sinus node increases because of vagal inhibition or sympathetic stimulation. The sinus rate is 101 to 200 beats/minute (Fig. 35-11, *B*).

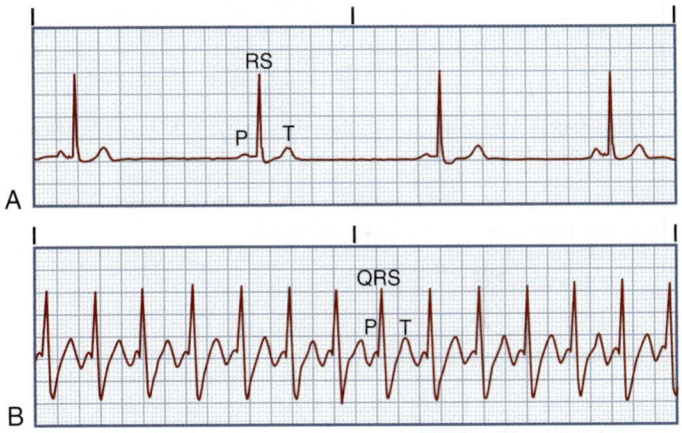

FIG. 35-11 **A,** Sinus bradycardia. **B,** Sinus tachycardia.

Clinical Associations. Sinus tachycardia is associated with physiologic and psychologic stressors such as exercise, fever, pain, hypotension, hypovolemia, anemia, hypoxia, hypoglycemia, myocardial ischemia, heart failure (HF), hyperthyroidism, anxiety, and fear. It can also be an effect of drugs such as epinephrine, norepinephrine (Levophed), atropine, caffeine, theophylline, or hydralazine. In addition, many over-the-counter cold remedies have active ingredients (e.g., pseudoephedrine [Sudafed]) that can cause tachycardia.

ECG Characteristics. In sinus tachycardia, the HR is 101 to 200 beats/minute and rhythm is regular. The P wave is normal, precedes each QRS complex, and has a normal shape and duration. The PR interval is normal and the QRS complex has a normal shape and duration.

Clinical Significance. The clinical significance of sinus tachycardia depends on the patient's tolerance of the increased HR. The patient may have dizziness, dyspnea, and hypotension because of decreased CO. Increased myocardial O_2 consumption is associated with an increased HR. Angina or an increase

TABLE 35-7 Characteristics of Common Dysrhythmias

Pattern	Rate and Rhythm	P Wave	PR Interval	QRS Complex
Normal sinus rhythm (NSR)	60-100 beats/min and regular	Normal	Normal	Normal
Sinus bradycardia	<60 beats/min and regular	Normal	Normal	Normal
Sinus tachycardia	101-200 beats/min and regular	Normal	Normal	Normal
Premature atrial contraction (PAC)	Usually 60-100 beats/min and irregular	Abnormal shape	Normal	Normal (usually)
Paroxysmal supraventricular tachycardia (PSVT)	150-220 beats/min and regular	Abnormal shape, may be hidden in the preceding T wave	Normal or shortened	Normal (usually)
Atrial flutter	*Atrial:* 200-350 beats/min and regular *Ventricular:* > or <100 beats/min and may be regular or irregular	Flutter (F) waves (sawtoothed pattern); more flutter waves than QRS complexes; may occur in a 2:1, 3:1, 4:1, etc., pattern	Not measurable	Normal (usually)
Atrial fibrillation	*Atrial:* 350-600 beats/min and irregular *Ventricular:* > or <100 beats/min and irregular	Fibrillatory (f) waves	Not measurable	Normal (usually)
Junctional dysrhythmias	40-180 beats/min and regular	Inverted, may be hidden in QRS complex	Shortened, if present	Normal (usually)
First-degree AV block	Normal and regular	Normal	>0.20 sec	Normal
Second-degree AV block				
• **Type I** (Mobitz I, Wenckebach heart block)	*Atrial:* Normal and regular *Ventricular:* Slower and irregular	Normal	Progressive lengthening	Normal QRS width, with pattern of one nonconducted (blocked) QRS complex
• **Type II** (Mobitz II heart block)	*Atrial:* Usually normal and regular *Ventricular:* Slower and regular or irregular	More P waves than QRS complexes (e.g., 2:1, 3:1)	Normal or prolonged but consistent for every QRS	Widened QRS, preceded by ≥2 P waves, with nonconducted (blocked) QRS complex
Third-degree AV block (complete heart block)	*Atrial:* Regular but may appear irregular due to P waves hidden in QRS complexes *Ventricular:* 20-60 beats/min and regular	Normal, but no connection with QRS complex	Inconsistent	Normal or widened, no relationship with P waves
Premature ventricular contraction (PVC)	Underlying rhythm can be any rate, regular or irregular rhythm, PVCs occur at variable rates	Not usually visible, hidden in the PVC	Not measurable	Wide and distorted
Ventricular tachycardia (VT)	150-250 beats/min and regular or irregular	Not usually visible	Not measurable	Wide and distorted
Accelerated idioventricular rhythm	40-100 beats/min and regular	Not usually visible	Not measurable	Wide and distorted
Ventricular fibrillation (VF)	Not measurable and irregular	Absent	Not measurable	Not measurable

AV, Atrioventricular.

in infarction size may accompany sinus tachycardia in patients with coronary artery disease (CAD) or an acute MI.

Treatment. The underlying cause of tachycardia guides the treatment. For example, if the patient is experiencing tachycardia from pain, effective pain management is important to treat the tachycardia. In clinically stable patients, vagal maneuvers can be attempted. In addition, IV β-blockers (e.g., metoprolol [Lopressor]), adenosine (Adenocard), or calcium channel blockers (e.g., diltiazem [Cardizem]) can be given to reduce HR and decrease myocardial O_2 consumption. In clinically unstable patients, synchronized cardioversion is used. (Cardioversion is discussed on p. 772.)

Premature Atrial Contraction. A **premature atrial contraction (PAC)** is a contraction starting from an ectopic focus in the atrium (i.e., a location other than the SA node) and coming sooner than the next expected sinus beat. The ectopic signal starts in the left or right atrium and travels across the atria by an abnormal pathway. This creates a distorted P wave (Fig. 35-12). At the AV node, it may be stopped (nonconducted PAC), delayed (lengthened PR interval), or conducted normally. If the signal moves through the AV node, in most cases it is conducted normally through the ventricles.

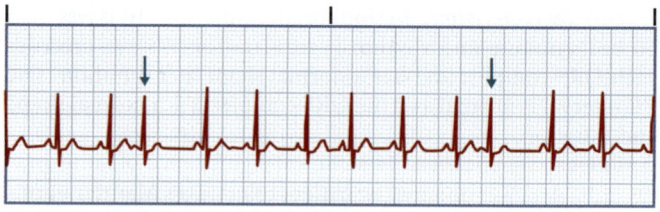

FIG. 35-12 Premature atrial contractions *(arrows).*

Clinical Associations. In a normal heart, a PAC can result from emotional stress or physical fatigue or from the use of caffeine, tobacco, or alcohol. A PAC can also result from hypoxia; electrolyte imbalances; and disease states such as hyperthyroidism, chronic obstructive pulmonary disease (COPD), and heart disease, including CAD and valvular disease.

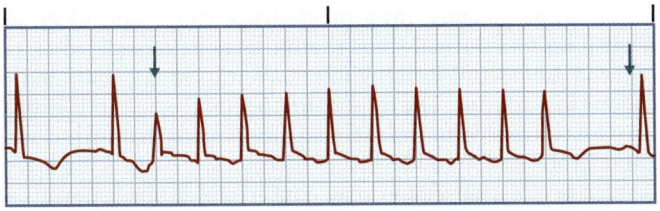

FIG. 35-13 Paroxysmal supraventricular tachycardia (PSVT). *Arrows* indicate beginning and ending of PSVT.

ECG Characteristics. HR varies with the underlying rate and frequency of the PAC. The rhythm is irregular. The P wave has a different shape from that of a P wave originating in the SA node, or it may be hidden in the preceding T wave. The PR interval may be shorter or longer than the PR interval coming from the SA node, but it is within normal limits. The QRS complex is usually normal. If the QRS interval is 0.12 second or more, abnormal conduction through the ventricles occurs.

Clinical Significance. In persons with healthy hearts, isolated PACs are not significant. Patients may report palpitations or a sense that their hearts "skipped a beat." In persons with heart disease, frequent PACs may indicate enhanced automaticity of the atria or a reentry mechanism. Such PACs may warn of or start more serious dysrhythmias (e.g., supraventricular tachycardia).

Treatment. Treatment depends on the patient's symptoms. Withdrawal of sources of stimulation such as caffeine or sympathomimetic drugs may be needed. β-Blockers may be used to decrease PACs.

Paroxysmal Supraventricular Tachycardia. *Paroxysmal supraventricular tachycardia* (PSVT) is a dysrhythmia starting in an ectopic focus anywhere above the bifurcation of the bundle of His (Fig. 35-13). Identification of the ectopic focus is often difficult even with a 12-lead ECG, since it requires recording the dysrhythmia as it starts.

PSVT occurs because of a reentrant phenomenon (reexcitation of the atria when there is a one-way block). Usually a PAC triggers a run of repeated premature beats. *Paroxysmal* refers to an abrupt onset and ending. Termination is sometimes followed by a brief period of **asystole** (absence of all cardiac electrical activity). Some degree of AV block may be present. PSVT can occur in the presence of Wolff-Parkinson-White (WPW) syndrome or "preexcitation." In this syndrome, there is extra conduction or accessory pathways.

Clinical Associations. In the normal heart, PSVT is associated with overexertion, emotional stress, deep inspiration, and stimulants such as caffeine and tobacco. PSVT is also associated with rheumatic heart disease, digitalis toxicity, CAD, and cor pulmonale.

ECG Characteristics. In PSVT, the HR is 150 to 220 beats/minute and rhythm is regular or slightly irregular. The P wave is often hidden in the preceding T wave. If seen, it may have an abnormal shape. The PR interval may be shortened or normal and the QRS complex is usually normal.

Clinical Significance. The clinical significance of PSVT depends on the associated symptoms. A prolonged episode and HR greater than 180 beats/minute will cause decreased CO because of reduced stroke volume. Manifestations include hypotension, palpitations, dyspnea, and angina.

Treatment. Treatment for PSVT includes vagal stimulation and drug therapy. Common vagal maneuvers include Valsalva, carotid massage, and coughing. IV adenosine is the drug of choice to convert PSVT to a normal sinus rhythm. This drug has a short half-life (10 seconds) and is well tolerated.[5] IV β-blockers and calcium channel blockers (diltiazem and verapamil [Calan]) can also be used. If vagal stimulation and drug therapy are ineffective and the patient becomes hemodynamically unstable, synchronized cardioversion is used.[6] (Cardioversion is discussed on p. 772.)

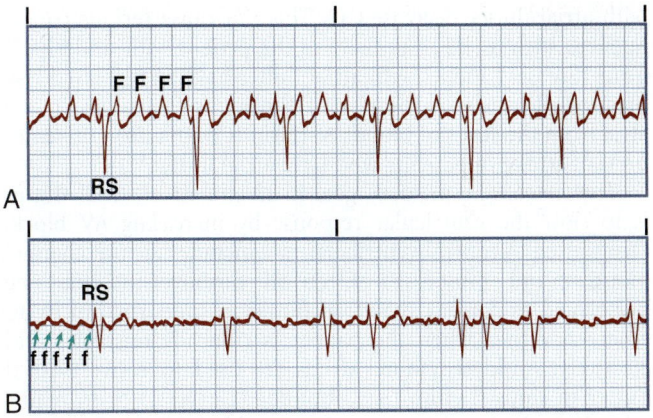

FIG. 35-14 **A,** Atrial flutter with a 4:1 conduction (four flutter *[F]* waves to each QRS complex). **B,** Atrial fibrillation with a controlled ventricular response. Note the chaotic fibrillatory *(f)* waves *(arrows)* between the RS complexes. NOTE: Recorded from lead V_1.

DRUG ALERT Adenosine (Adenocard)

- Injection site should be as close to the heart as possible (e.g., antecubital area).
- Give IV dose rapidly (over 1 to 2 sec) and follow with a rapid 20 mL normal saline flush.
- Monitor patient's ECG continuously. Brief period of asystole is common.
- Observe patient for flushing, dizziness, chest pain, or palpitations.

Ongoing treatment of recurring PSVT and PSVT in patients with WPW syndrome includes radiofrequency catheter ablation of the accessory pathway.[6] (Catheter ablation therapy is discussed on p. 775.)

Atrial Flutter. **Atrial flutter** is an atrial tachydysrhythmia identified by recurring, regular, sawtooth-shaped flutter waves that originate from a single ectopic focus in the right atrium or, less commonly, the left atrium (Fig. 35-14, *A*).

Clinical Associations. Atrial flutter rarely occurs in a healthy heart. It is associated with CAD, hypertension, mitral valve disorders, pulmonary embolus, chronic lung disease, cor pulmonale, cardiomyopathy, hyperthyroidism, and the use of drugs such as digoxin, quinidine, and epinephrine.

ECG Characteristics. Atrial rate is 200 to 350 beats/minute. The ventricular rate varies based on the conduction ratio. In 2:1 conduction, the ventricular rate is typically found to be approximately 150 beats/minute. Atrial rhythm is regular and ventricular rhythm is usually regular. The atrial flutter waves represent atrial depolarization followed by repolarization. The PR interval is variable and not measurable. The QRS complex is usually normal. Because the AV node can delay signals from the atria, there is usually some AV block in a fixed ratio of flutter waves to QRS complexes.

Clinical Significance. The high ventricular rates (greater than 100 beats/minute) and loss of the atrial "kick" (atrial contraction reflected by a sinus P wave) that are associated with atrial flutter decrease CO. This can cause serious consequences such as HF, especially in the patient with underlying heart disease. Patients with atrial flutter have an increased risk of stroke because of the risk of thrombus formation in the atria from the stasis of blood. Warfarin (Coumadin) is given to prevent stroke in patients who have atrial flutter.[6]

Treatment. The primary goal in treatment of atrial flutter is to slow the ventricular response by increasing AV block. Drugs used to control ventricular rate include calcium channel blockers and β-blockers. Electrical cardioversion may be performed to convert the atrial flutter to sinus rhythm in an emergency (i.e., when the patient is clinically unstable) and electively. Antidysrhythmia drugs are used to convert atrial flutter to sinus rhythm (e.g., ibutilide [Corvert]) or to maintain sinus rhythm (e.g., amiodarone, flecainide, dronedarone [Multaq]).[5]

Radiofrequency catheter ablation is the treatment of choice for atrial flutter.[7] The procedure is done in an EPS laboratory and involves placing a catheter in the right atrium. With the use of a low-voltage, high-frequency form of electrical energy, the ectopic foci are ablated (or destroyed), dysrhythmia is ended, and normal sinus rhythm is restored. (Catheter ablation is discussed on p. 775.)

Atrial Fibrillation. **Atrial fibrillation** is characterized by a total disorganization of atrial electrical activity because of multiple ectopic foci, resulting in loss of effective atrial contraction (Fig. 35-14, *B*). The dysrhythmia may be paroxysmal (i.e., beginning and ending spontaneously) or persistent (lasting more than 7 days).[1] Atrial fibrillation is the most common, clinically significant dysrhythmia with respect to morbidity and mortality rates and economic impact. Its prevalence increases with age.[8]

Clinical Associations. Atrial fibrillation usually occurs in a patient with underlying heart disease, such as CAD, valvular heart disease, cardiomyopathy, hypertensive heart disease, HF, and pericarditis. It often develops acutely with thyrotoxicosis, alcohol intoxication, caffeine use, electrolyte disturbances, stress, and heart surgery.

ECG Characteristics. During atrial fibrillation, the atrial rate may be as high as 350 to 600 beats/minute. P waves are replaced by chaotic, fibrillatory waves. Ventricular rate varies and the rhythm is usually irregular. When the ventricular rate is between 60 and 100 beats/minute, it is atrial fibrillation with a *controlled ventricular response.* Atrial fibrillation with a ventricular rate greater than 100 beats/minute is atrial fibrillation with a *rapid (or uncontrolled) ventricular response.* The PR interval is not measurable, and the QRS complex usually has a normal shape and duration. At times, atrial flutter and atrial fibrillation may coexist.[1]

Clinical Significance. Atrial fibrillation results in a decrease in CO because of ineffective atrial contractions (loss of atrial kick) and/or a rapid ventricular response. Thrombi (clots) form in the atria because of blood stasis. An embolized clot may develop and move to the brain, causing a stroke. Atrial fibrillation accounts for as many as 17% of all strokes.[9]

Treatment. The goals of treatment of atrial fibrillation include a decrease in ventricular response (to less than 100 beats/minute), prevention of stroke, and conversion to sinus rhythm, if possible. Ventricular rate control is a priority for patients with atrial fibrillation. Drugs used for rate control include calcium channel blockers (e.g., diltiazem), β-blockers (e.g., metoprolol), dronedarone, and digoxin (Lanoxin).

For some patients, drug or electrical conversion of atrial fibrillation to a normal sinus rhythm may be considered (e.g., reduced exercise tolerance with rate control drugs, contraindications to warfarin). The most common antidysrhythmia drugs used for conversion to and maintenance of sinus rhythm include amiodarone and ibutilide.[8]

Electrical cardioversion may convert atrial fibrillation to a normal sinus rhythm. If a patient is in atrial fibrillation for longer than 48 hours, anticoagulation therapy with warfarin is needed for 3 to 4 weeks before the cardioversion and for several weeks after successful cardioversion.[5] Anticoagulation therapy is necessary because the procedure can cause the clots to dislodge, placing the patient at risk for stroke. A transesophageal echocardiogram may be performed to rule out clots in the atria. If no clots are present, anticoagulation therapy may not be needed before the cardioversion.

If drugs or cardioversion does not convert atrial fibrillation to normal sinus rhythm, long-term anticoagulation therapy is needed (Table 35-8). Warfarin is the drug of choice, and patients are monitored for therapeutic levels (e.g., international normalized ratio [INR]). Alternatives to warfarin are available for anticoagulation therapy in patients with nonvalvular atrial fibrillation. Examples include dabigatran (Pradaxa), apixaban (Eliquis), and rivaroxaban (Xarelto). These drugs do not require routine laboratory testing.[8] (See Chapter 37 for discussion of anticoagulation therapy.)

For patients with drug-refractory atrial fibrillation or who do not respond to electrical conversion and remain symptomatic, radiofrequency catheter ablation (similar to procedure for atrial flutter), AV nodal ablation, and the Maze procedure are further options. AV nodal ablation involves the destruction of the AV node and insertion of a permanent ventricular pacemaker.[8]

The Maze procedure is a surgical intervention that stops atrial fibrillation by interrupting the ectopic foci that are

TABLE 35-8 Drug Therapy

Antithrombotic Therapy for Atrial Fibrillation*

Risk Category	Recommended Therapy
Mechanical heart valve	Warfarin (target INR 2.5-3.5)
CHA_2DS_2-VASc† score of 0	No therapy recommended
CHA_2DS_2-VASc score of 1	No therapy recommended or an oral anticoagulant or aspirin (e.g., 81-325 mg/day) may be considered
CHA_2DS_2-VASc score of ≥2	Warfarin Dabigatran (Pradaxa)‡ Apixaban (Eliquis)‡ Rivaroxaban (Xarelto)‡
CHA_2DS_2-VASc score of ≥2 and end-stage kidney disease or on hemodialysis	Warfarin

Source: January CT, Wann LS, Albert JS, et al: 2014 AHA/ACC/HRS guideline for the management of patients with atrial fibrillation: executive summary: a report of the American College of Cardiology/American Heart Association Task Force on Practice Guidelines and the Heart Rhythm Society, *J Am Coll Cardiol* 64(21):e1, 2014.

CHA_2DS_2-VASc, Congestive heart failure; hypertension; age ≥75 [doubled]; diabetes; prior stroke, transient ischemic attack, thromboembolism [doubled]; vascular disease; age 65-74; sex, *INR,* international normalized ratio.

*For atrial flutter, antithrombotic therapy is recommended as for atrial fibrillation.

†The CHA_2DS_2-VASc score for nonvalvular atrial fibrillation stroke risk can be calculated at *www.mdcalc.com/cha2ds2-vasc-score-for-atrial-fibrillation-stroke-risk/*

‡Renal function should be assessed prior to starting direct thrombin inhibitor (e.g., dabigatran) or factor Xa inhibitor (e.g., apixaban, rivaroxaban) and regularly thereafter.

responsible for the dysrhythmia. Incisions are made in both atria, and *cryoablation* (cold therapy) is used to stop the formation and conduction of these signals and restore normal sinus rhythm.

Left atrial appendage occlusion. The left atrial appendage (LAA) is a pouch that extends off the left atrium. The LAA is known to trigger atrial fibrillation and is a common source of blood clots in patients with atrial fibrillation. LAA occlusion is a treatment strategy to prevent blood clot formation in patients who have atrial fibrillation. By removing or occluding the LAA, the incidence of strokes can be decreased.

A special stapler can be used to remove the LAA or sutures can be used to manually occlude the LAA. In addition, LAA occlusion devices (e.g., AtriClip, Watchman) are available. These devices are positioned around the LAA and then closed, similar to a clamp that is used to shut off the blood supply. This prevents blood from flowing into and out of the LAA. LAA occlusion can be used as an alternative for patients who cannot use oral anticoagulants such as warfarin.[10]

CHECK YOUR PRACTICE

You are assigned to a 72-yr-old female patient who was admitted with chest pain. She has continuous EGG monitoring. You notice that her ECG tracing is difficult to interpret. Your preceptor tells you that there is a lot of artifact.

- How would you proceed to improve her tracing?

Junctional Dysrhythmias. *Junctional dysrhythmias* refer to dysrhythmias that start in the area of the AV node to the bundle of His known as the AV junction. They result because the SA node fails to fire or the signal is blocked. When this occurs, the AV node becomes the pacemaker of the heart. The impulse from the AV node usually moves in a retrograde (backward) fashion. This produces an abnormal P wave that occurs just before or after the QRS complex or that is hidden in the QRS complex. The impulse usually moves normally through the ventricles. Junctional premature beats may occur, and they are treated in a manner similar to that for PACs. Other junctional dysrhythmias include junctional escape rhythm (Fig. 35-15), accelerated junctional rhythm, and junctional tachycardia. These dysrhythmias are treated according to the patient's tolerance of the rhythm and the patient's clinical condition.

Clinical Associations. Junctional dysrhythmias are often associated with CAD, HF, cardiomyopathy, electrolyte imbalances, inferior MI, and rheumatic heart disease. Certain drugs (e.g., digoxin, nicotine, amphetamines, caffeine) can also cause junctional dysrhythmias.

ECG Characteristics. In junctional escape rhythm, the HR is 40 to 60 beats/minute. It is 61 to 100 beats/minute in accelerated junctional rhythm and 101 to 180 beats/minute in junctional tachycardia. Rhythm is regular. The P wave is abnormal in shape and inverted, or it may be hidden in the QRS complex (Fig. 35-15). The PR interval is less than 0.12 second when the P wave precedes the QRS complex. The QRS complex is usually normal.

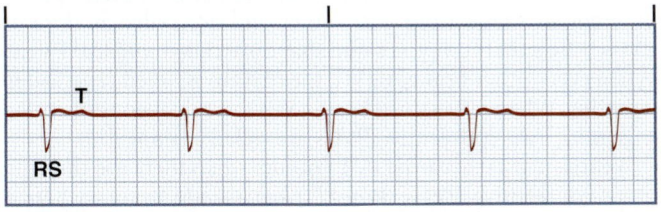

FIG. 35-15 Junctional escape rhythm. P wave is hidden in the RS complex. NOTE: Recorded from lead V_1.

Clinical Significance. Junctional escape rhythms serve as a safety mechanism when the SA node has not been effective. Escape rhythms such as this should not be suppressed. Accelerated junctional rhythm is due to sympathetic stimulation to improve CO. Junctional tachycardia indicates a more serious problem. This rhythm may reduce CO, causing the patient to become hemodynamically unstable (e.g., hypotensive).

Treatment. Treatment varies according to the type of junctional dysrhythmia. If a patient has symptoms with a junctional escape rhythm, atropine can be used. In accelerated junctional rhythm and junctional tachycardia caused by drug toxicity, the drug is stopped. In the absence of digitalis toxicity, β-blockers, calcium channel blockers, and amiodarone are used for rate control. Cardioversion should not be used.

First-Degree AV Block. *First-degree AV block* is a type of AV block in which every impulse is conducted to the ventricles but the time of AV conduction is prolonged (Fig. 35-16, *A*). After the impulse moves through the AV node, the ventricles usually respond normally.

Clinical Associations. First-degree AV block is associated with MI, CAD, rheumatic fever, hyperthyroidism, electrolyte

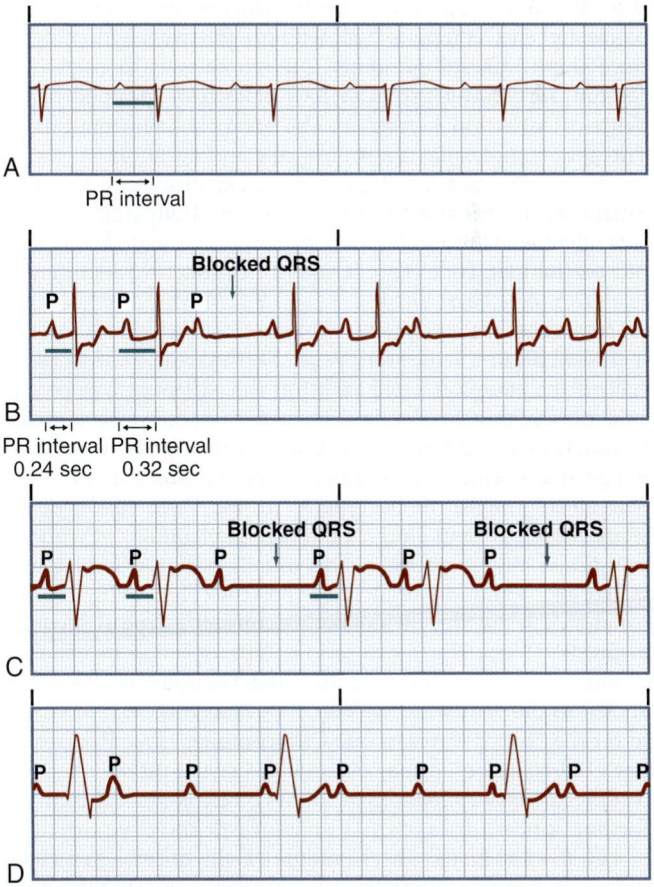

FIG. 35-16 Heart block. **A,** First-degree atrioventricular (AV) block with a PR interval of 0.40 sec. **B,** Second-degree AV block, type I, with progressive lengthening of the PR interval until a QRS complex is blocked. **C,** Second-degree AV block, type II, with constant PR intervals and variable blocked QRS complexes. **D,** Third-degree AV block. Note that there is no relationship between P waves and QRS complexes.

imbalances (e.g., hypokalemia), vagal stimulation, and drugs such as digoxin, β-blockers, calcium channel blockers, and flecainide.

ECG Characteristics. In first-degree AV block, the HR is normal and rhythm is regular. The P wave is normal, the PR interval is prolonged (greater than 0.20 second), and the QRS complex usually has a normal shape and duration.

Clinical Significance. First-degree AV block is usually not serious but can be a sign of higher degrees of AV block. Patients with first-degree AV block are asymptomatic.

Treatment. There is no treatment for first-degree AV block. Changes to potentially causative situations may be considered. Monitor patients for any new changes in heart rhythm (e.g., more serious AV block).

Second-Degree AV Block, Type I. *Type I second-degree AV block (Mobitz I* or *Wenckebach heart block)* includes a gradual lengthening of the PR interval. It occurs because of a prolonged AV conduction time until an atrial impulse is nonconducted and a QRS complex is blocked (missing) (Fig. 35-16, *B*). Type I AV block most commonly occurs in the AV node, but it can also occur in the His-Purkinje system.

Clinical Associations. Type I AV block may result from drugs such as digoxin or β-blockers. It may also be associated with CAD and other diseases that can slow AV conduction.

ECG Characteristics. Atrial rate is regular, but ventricular rate may be slower because of nonconducted or blocked QRS complexes resulting in bradycardia. Once a ventricular beat is blocked, the cycle repeats itself with progressive lengthening of the PR intervals until another QRS complex is blocked. The rhythm appears on the ECG in a pattern of grouped beats. Ventricular rhythm is irregular. The P wave has a normal shape. The QRS complex has a normal shape and duration.

Clinical Significance. Type I AV block is usually a result of myocardial ischemia or inferior MI. It is generally transient and well tolerated. However, in some patients (e.g., acute MI) it may be a warning sign of a more serious AV conduction disturbance (e.g., complete heart block).

Treatment. If the patient is symptomatic, atropine is used to increase HR, or a temporary pacemaker may be needed, especially if the patient has had an MI. If the patient is asymptomatic, the rhythm is closely observed with a transcutaneous pacemaker on standby. Bradycardia is more likely to become symptomatic when hypotension, HF, or shock is present.

Second-Degree AV Block, Type II. In *type II second-degree AV block (Mobitz II heart block),* a P wave is nonconducted without progressive PR lengthening. This usually occurs when a block in one of the bundle branches is present (Fig. 35-16, *C*). On conducted beats, the PR interval is constant. Type II second-degree AV block is a more serious type of block in which a certain number of impulses from the SA node are not conducted to the ventricles. This occurs in ratios of 2:1, 3:1, and so on (i.e., two P waves to one QRS complex, three P waves to one QRS complex). It may occur with varying ratios.

Clinical Associations. Type II AV block is associated with rheumatic heart disease, CAD, anterior MI, and drug toxicity.

ECG Characteristics. Atrial rate is usually normal. Ventricular rate depends on the degree of AV block. Atrial rhythm is regular, but ventricular rhythm may be irregular. The P wave has a normal shape. The PR interval may be normal or prolonged in duration and remains constant on conducted beats. The QRS complex is usually greater than 0.12 second because of bundle branch block.

Clinical Significance. Type II AV block often progresses to third-degree AV block and is associated with a poor prognosis. The reduced HR frequently results in decreased CO with subsequent hypotension and myocardial ischemia. Type II AV block is an indication for therapy with a permanent pacemaker.

Treatment. Transcutaneous pacing or the insertion of a temporary pacemaker may be necessary before the insertion of a permanent pacemaker if the patient becomes symptomatic (e.g., hypotension, angina).[11] (Temporary pacemakers are discussed on pp. 774 to 775.) Atropine is not an effective drug for this dysrhythmia.

Third-Degree AV Block. Third-degree AV block, or **complete heart block**, constitutes one form of AV dissociation in which no impulses from the atria are conducted to the ventricles (Fig. 35-16, *D*). The atria are stimulated and contract independently of the ventricles. The ventricular rhythm is an escape rhythm, and the ectopic pacemaker may be above or below the bifurcation of the bundle of His.

Clinical Associations. Third-degree AV block is associated with severe heart disease, including CAD, MI, myocarditis, cardiomyopathy, and some systemic diseases such as amyloidosis and progressive systemic sclerosis (scleroderma). Some drugs can also cause third-degree AV block, such as digoxin, β-blockers, and calcium channel blockers.

ECG Characteristics. The atrial rate is usually a sinus rate of 60 to 100 beats/minute. The ventricular rate depends on the site of the block. If it is in the AV node, the rate is 40 to 60 beats/minute, and if it is in the His-Purkinje system, it is 20 to 40 beats/minute. Atrial and ventricular rhythms are regular but unrelated to each other. The P wave has a normal shape. The PR interval is variable, and there is no relationship between the P wave and the QRS complex. The QRS complex is normal if an escape rhythm is initiated at the bundle of His or above. It is widened if an escape rhythm is initiated below the bundle of His.

Clinical Significance. Third-degree AV block usually results in reduced CO with subsequent ischemia, HF, and shock. Syncope from third-degree AV block may result from severe bradycardia or even periods of asystole.

Treatment. For symptomatic patients, a transcutaneous pacemaker is used until a temporary transvenous pacemaker can be inserted.[7] (Types of temporary pacemakers are discussed on pp. 774-775.) The use of drugs such as dopamine and epinephrine is a temporary measure to increase HR and support BP until temporary pacing is started.[11] Patients need a permanent pacemaker as soon as possible. Atropine is not an effective drug for this dysrhythmia.

Premature Ventricular Contractions. A **premature ventricular contraction (PVC)** is a contraction coming from an ectopic focus in the ventricles. It is the premature (early) occurrence of a QRS complex. A PVC is wide and distorted in shape compared with a QRS complex coming down the normal conduction pathway (Fig. 35-17). PVCs that arise from different foci appear different in shape from each other and are called *multifocal* PVCs. PVCs that have the same shape are called *unifocal* PVCs. When every other beat is a PVC, the rhythm is called *ventricular bigeminy.* When every third beat is a PVC, it is called *ventricular trigeminy.* Two consecutive PVCs are called a *couplet.*

Ventricular tachycardia (VT) occurs when there are three or more consecutive PVCs. *R-on-T phenomenon* occurs when a PVC falls on the T wave of a preceding beat. This is especially dangerous because the PVC is firing during the relative

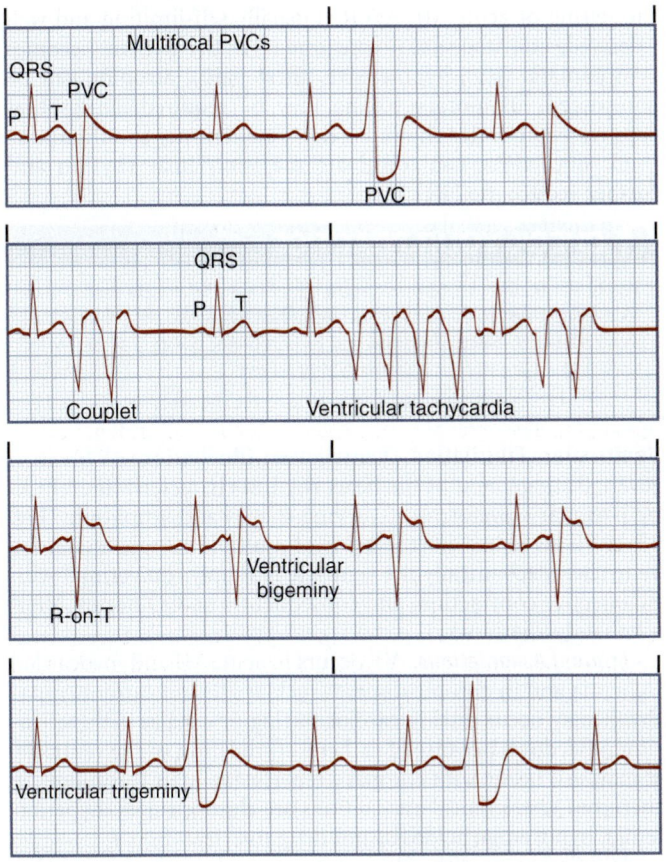

FIG. 35-17 Various types of premature ventricular contractions (PVCs).

refractory phase of ventricular repolarization. Excitability of the heart cells increases during this time, and the risk for the PVC to start VT or ventricular fibrillation (VF) is great.

Clinical Associations. PVCs are associated with stimulants such as caffeine, alcohol, nicotine, aminophylline, epinephrine, isoproterenol, and digoxin. They are also associated with electrolyte imbalances, hypoxia, fever, exercise, and emotional stress. Disease states associated with PVCs include MI, mitral valve prolapse, HF, cardiomyopathy, and CAD.

ECG Characteristics. HR varies according to intrinsic rate and number of PVCs. Rhythm is irregular because of premature beats. The P wave is rarely visible and is usually lost in the QRS complex of the PVC. Retrograde conduction may occur and the P wave may be seen after the ectopic beat. The PR interval is not measurable. The QRS complex is wide and distorted in shape, lasting more than 0.12 second. The T wave is generally large and opposite in direction to the major direction of the QRS complex.

Clinical Significance. PVCs are usually not harmful in a patient with a normal heart. In heart disease, PVCs may reduce the CO and lead to angina and HF depending on the frequency. Because PVCs in CAD or acute MI indicate ventricular irritability, assess the patient's physiologic response to PVCs. Obtain the patient's apical-radial pulse rate, since PVCs often do not generate a sufficient ventricular contraction to result in a peripheral pulse. This can lead to a pulse deficit.

Treatment. Treatment relates to the cause of the PVCs (e.g., O_2 therapy for hypoxia, electrolyte replacement). Assessment of the patient's hemodynamic status is important to

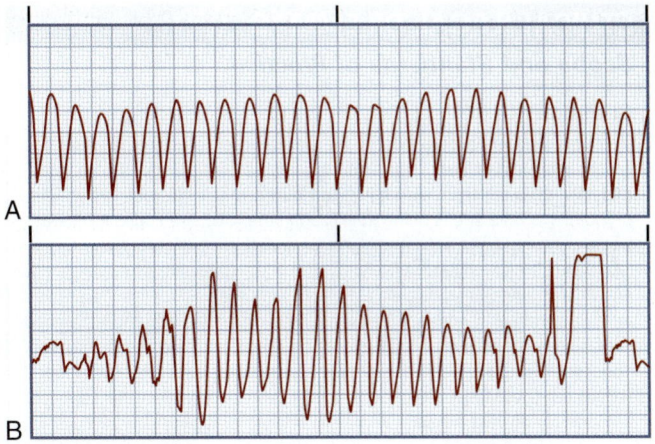

FIG. 35-18 Ventricular tachycardia. **A,** Monomorphic. **B,** Torsades de pointes (polymorphic).

determine if treatment with drug therapy is needed. Drug therapy includes β-blockers, procainamide, or amiodarone.

Ventricular Tachycardia. A run of three or more PVCs defines **ventricular tachycardia (VT)**. It occurs when an ectopic focus or foci fire repeatedly and the ventricle takes control as the pacemaker. Different forms of VT exist, depending on QRS configuration. *Monomorphic* VT (Fig. 35-18, *A*) has QRS complexes that are the same in shape, size, and direction. *Polymorphic* VT occurs when the QRS complexes gradually change back and forth from one shape, size, and direction to another over a series of beats. *Torsades de pointes* (French for "twisting of the points") is polymorphic VT associated with a prolonged QT interval of the underlying rhythm (Fig. 35-18, *B*).

VT may be sustained (longer than 30 seconds) or nonsustained (less than 30 seconds). The development of VT is an ominous sign. It is a life-threatening dysrhythmia because of decreased CO and the possibility of development of VF, which is lethal.

Clinical Associations. VT is associated with MI, CAD, significant electrolyte imbalances, cardiomyopathy, long QT syndrome, drug toxicity, and central nervous system disorders. This dysrhythmia can be seen in patients who have no evidence of heart disease.

ECG Characteristics. Ventricular rate is 150 to 250 beats/minute. Rhythm may be regular or irregular. AV dissociation may be present, with P waves occurring independently of the QRS complex. The atria may be depolarized by the ventricles in a retrograde fashion. The P wave is usually buried in the QRS complex, and the PR interval is not measurable. The QRS complex is distorted in appearance and wide (greater than 0.12 second in duration). The T wave is in the opposite direction of the QRS complex (Fig. 35-18).

Clinical Significance. VT can be stable (patient has a pulse) or unstable (patient is pulseless). Sustained VT causes a severe decrease in CO because of decreased ventricular diastolic filling times and loss of atrial contraction. This results in hypotension, pulmonary edema, decreased cerebral blood flow, and cardiopulmonary arrest. The dysrhythmia must be treated quickly, even if it occurs only briefly and stops abruptly. Episodes may recur if prophylactic treatment is not started. VF may also develop.

Treatment. Precipitating causes (e.g., electrolyte imbalances, ischemia) must be identified and treated. If the VT is monomorphic and the patient is clinically stable (i.e., pulse is present)

ETHICAL/LEGAL DILEMMAS

Scope and Standards of Practice

Situation

A young woman is admitted to the intensive care unit (ICU) from the emergency department after experiencing several episodes of nonsustained ventricular tachycardia (VT) attributed to a history of viral cardiomyopathy. While she is being stabilized in the ICU, she codes (pulseless VT) and intubation is indicated. A nurse anesthetist attempts to intubate her three times unsuccessfully. There is an unforeseen delay in the arrival of the anesthesiologist. P.F., an ICU nurse and former paramedic who is certified in advanced trauma life support (ATLS) and advanced cardiovascular life support (ACLS), attempts to intubate the patient and does so successfully. The next day the nursing supervisor questions P.F. about intubating the patient, since this is not within the scope of practice for an ICU nurse.

Ethical/Legal Points for Consideration

- The RN *Scope of Practice,* including rules and regulations that guide practice, are defined by individual state Boards of Nursing and can vary from state to state.
- Individual agencies also have policies and procedures that describe the scope of practice for nurses. These can be more restrictive than those of the state.
- *Scope and Standards of Practice* are also defined by professional nursing organizations (e.g., American Nurses Association, American Association of Critical-Care Nurses). These are authoritative statements that serve to define expected competent practice in various registered nurse (RN) roles (e.g., Scope and Standards for Nursing Administration).
- P.F. has had training, education, and certification beyond the usual nursing role.
- A life-threatening situation provides for extenuating circumstances.
- Negligence may have been a factor if P.F., who is a nurse with training and experience, had not acted.

Discussion Questions

1. What would you have done in this situation?
2. How would you respond to the nursing supervisor?
3. What are the legal ramifications for P.F. in this situation?
4. What are the ethical issues in this situation?

and has preserved left ventricular function, IV procainamide, sotalol, or amiodarone is used. These drugs can also be used if the VT is polymorphic with a normal baseline QT interval.

Polymorphic VT with a prolonged baseline QT interval is treated with IV magnesium, isoproterenol, phenytoin (Dilantin), or antitachycardia pacing (discussed later in this chapter). Drugs that prolong the QT interval (e.g., dofetilide [Tikosyn]) should be discontinued. Cardioversion is used if drug therapy is ineffective.

VT without a pulse is a life-threatening situation. It is treated in the same manner as VF. Cardiopulmonary resuscitation (CPR) and rapid defibrillation are the first lines of treatment, followed by the administration of vasopressors (e.g., epinephrine) and antidysrhythmics (e.g., amiodarone) if defibrillation is unsuccessful.[11]

An *accelerated idioventricular rhythm* (AIVR) can develop when the intrinsic pacemaker rate (SA node or AV node) becomes less than that of a ventricular ectopic pacemaker. The rate is between 40 and 100 beats/minute. It is most commonly associated with acute MI and reperfusion of the myocardium after thrombolytic therapy or percutaneous coronary interventions (e.g., angioplasty). It can be seen with digitalis toxicity. In the setting of acute MI, AIVR is usually self-limiting and well tolerated, and it needs no treatment. If the patient becomes symptomatic (e.g., hypotensive, chest pain), atropine can be considered. Temporary pacing may be required. Drugs that suppress ventricular rhythms (e.g., amiodarone) should not be used, since these can terminate the ventricular rhythm and further reduce the HR.

CHECK YOUR PRACTICE

You are assigned to a 69-yr-old male patient on a telemetry unit who is recovering from colon surgery. He has a history of two MIs and he has three stents in place. You hear his ECG monitor alarm and see what looks like ventricular tachycardia on the screen.

- What should you do?

Ventricular Fibrillation. Ventricular fibrillation (VF) is a severe derangement of the heart rhythm characterized on ECG by irregular waveforms of varying shapes and amplitude (Fig. 35-19). This represents the firing of multiple ectopic foci in the ventricle. Mechanically the ventricle is simply "quivering," with no effective contraction, and consequently no CO occurs. VF is a lethal dysrhythmia.

Clinical Associations. VF occurs in acute MI and myocardial ischemia and in chronic diseases such as HF and cardiomyopathy. It may occur during cardiac pacing or cardiac catheterization procedures because of catheter stimulation of the ventricle. It may also occur with coronary reperfusion after thrombolytic therapy. Other clinical associations are electric shock, hyperkalemia, hypoxemia, acidosis, and drug toxicity.

ECG Characteristics. HR is not measurable. Rhythm is irregular and chaotic. The P wave is not visible, and the PR interval and the QRS interval are not measurable.

Clinical Significance. VF results in an unresponsive, pulseless, and apneic state. If it is not rapidly treated, the patient will not recover.

Treatment. Treatment consists of immediate initiation of CPR and advanced cardiovascular life support (ACLS) with the use of defibrillation and definitive drug therapy (e.g., epinephrine, vasopressin). There should be no delay in starting chest compressions and using a defibrillator once available.

Asystole. Asystole represents the total absence of ventricular electrical activity. Occasionally, P waves are seen. No ventricular contraction occurs because depolarization does not occur. Patients are unresponsive, pulseless, and apneic. Asystole is a lethal dysrhythmia that requires immediate treatment. VF may masquerade as asystole. Always assess the rhythm in more than one lead. The prognosis of a patient with asystole is extremely poor.

Clinical Associations. Asystole is usually a result of advanced heart disease, a severe cardiac conduction system disturbance, or end-stage HF.

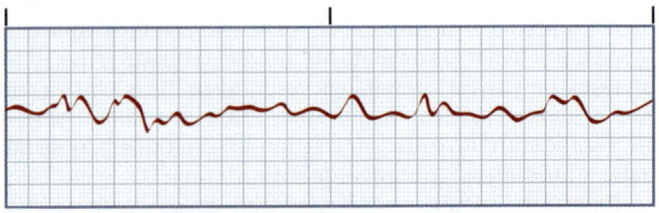

FIG. 35-19 Ventricular fibrillation.

Clinical Significance. Generally the patient with asystole has end-stage heart disease or has a prolonged arrest and cannot be resuscitated.

Treatment. Treatment consists of CPR with initiation of ACLS measures. These include definitive drug therapy with epinephrine and/or vasopressin, and intubation.

Pulseless Electrical Activity. *Pulseless electrical activity* (PEA) is a situation in which organized electrical activity is seen on the ECG, but there is no mechanical heart activity and the patient has no pulse. It is the most common dysrhythmia seen after defibrillation. Prognosis is poor unless the underlying cause is quickly identified and treated. The most common causes of PEA include hypovolemia, hypoxia, metabolic acidosis, hyperkalemia, hypokalemia, hypoglycemia, hypothermia, toxins (e.g., drug overdose), cardiac tamponade, thrombosis (e.g., MI, pulmonary embolus), tension pneumothorax, and trauma. Treatment begins with CPR followed by drug therapy (e.g., epinephrine) and intubation. Correcting the underlying cause is critical to prognosis.

Sudden Cardiac Death. The term *sudden cardiac death* (SCD) refers to death from a cardiac cause. Most SCDs result from ventricular dysrhythmias, specifically VT or VF. (SCD is discussed in Chapter 33.)

Prodysrhythmia. Antidysrhythmia drugs can cause life-threatening dysrhythmias similar to those for which they are given. This concept is termed *prodysrhythmia.* The patient who has severe left ventricular dysfunction is the most susceptible to prodysrhythmias. Digoxin and class IA, IC, and III antidysrhythmia drugs can cause a prodysrhythmic response.[5] The first several days of drug therapy are the vulnerable period for developing prodysrhythmias. For this reason, many oral antidysrhythmia drug regimens are started in a monitored hospital setting.

Antidysrhythmia Drugs

Table 35-9 categorizes antidysrhythmia drugs by their primary effects on the heart cells and the ECG.

Defibrillation

Defibrillation is the treatment of choice to end VF and pulseless VT. It is most effective when the myocardial cells are not anoxic or acidotic. Rapid defibrillation (within 2 minutes) is critical to a successful patient outcome. Defibrillation involves the passage of an electric shock through the heart to depolarize the myocardial cells. The goal is that the following repolarization of heart cells will allow the SA node to resume the role of pacemaker.

Defibrillators deliver energy using a monophasic or biphasic waveform. Monophasic defibrillators deliver energy in one direction, and biphasic defibrillators deliver energy in two directions (Fig. 35-20). Biphasic defibrillators deliver shocks at lower energies and with fewer postshock ECG dysrhythmias than monophasic defibrillators.

The output of a defibrillator is measured in *joules,* or watts per second. The recommended energy for initial shocks in defibrillation depends on the type of defibrillator. Biphasic defibrillators deliver the first and any successive shocks using 120 to 200 joules. Recommendations for monophasic defibrillators include an initial shock at 360 joules. After the first shock, start CPR immediately beginning with chest compressions. (CPR is discussed in Appendix A of this book.)

TABLE 35-9 Drug Therapy

Antidysrhythmia Drugs

Drug	Actions*	Effects on ECG
Class I: Sodium Channel Blockers	Decrease impulse conduction in the atria, ventricles, and His-Purkinje system	
Class IA disopyramide (Norpace) procainamide quinidine	Delay repolarization	Widened QRS and prolonged QT interval
Class IB mexiletine phenytoin (Dilantin)	Accelerate repolarization	Little or no effect on ECG
Class IC flecainide propafenone (Rythmol)	Decrease impulse conduction	Pronounced prodysrhythmic actions, widened QRS, prolonged QT interval
Class II: β-Adrenergic Blockers esmolol (Brevibloc) metoprolol (Lopressor) propranolol (Inderal)	Decrease automaticity of the SA node, slow impulse conduction in AV node, reduce atrial and ventricular contractility	Bradycardia, prolonged PR interval, AV block
Class III: Potassium Channel Blockers amiodarone (Cordarone) dofetilide (Tikosyn) ibutilide (Corvert) sotalol† (Betapace)	Delay repolarization, resulting in prolonged duration of action potential and refractory period	Prolonged PR and QT intervals, widened QRS, bradycardia
Class IV: Calcium Channel Blockers diltiazem (Cardizem) verapamil (Calan)	Decrease automaticity of SA node, delay AV node conduction; reduce myocardial contractility	Bradycardia, prolonged PR interval, AV block
Other Antidysrhythmia Drugs		
adenosine (Adenocard) digoxin (Lanoxin)	Decrease conduction through AV node, reduce automaticity of SA node	Prolonged PR interval, AV block
dronedarone (Multaq)‡	Suppresses atrial dysrhythmias though mechanism is unknown	Prolonged QT interval
magnesium	Decreases impulse conduction through AV node	AV block

AV, Atrioventricular; *SA,* sinoatrial.

*Antidysrhythmia drugs have a direct effect on the various phases of the action potential (Fig. 35-1).
†Sotalol has both class II and class III properties.
‡Dronedarone has class I through IV properties.

Rapid defibrillation can be performed using a manual or automatic device (Fig. 35-21). Manual defibrillators require you to interpret heart rhythms, determine the need for a shock, and deliver a shock. An **automatic external defibrillator (AED)** can detect heart rhythms and advise the user to deliver a shock using hands-free defibrillator pads. Proficiency in the use of the

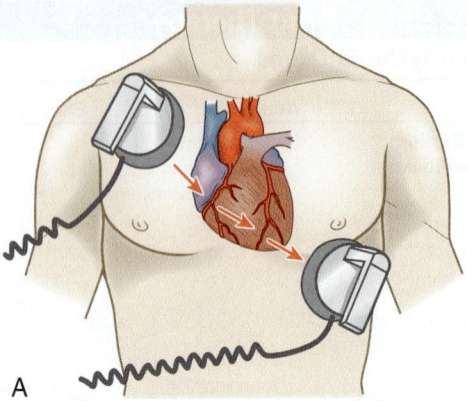

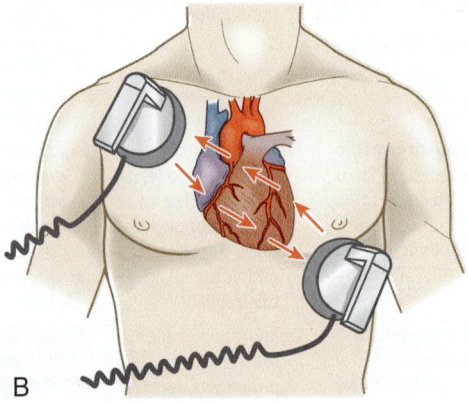

FIG. 35-20 Paddle placement and current flow in monophasic defibrillation **(A)** and biphasic defibrillation **(B)**.

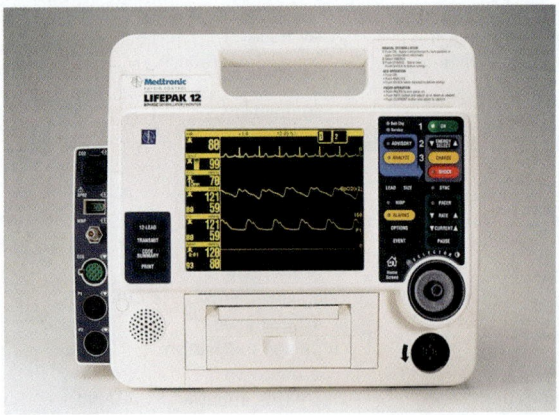

FIG. 35-21 LifePak contains a monitor, defibrillator, and transcutaneous pacemaker. (Courtesy Medtronic Physio-Control, Redmond, Wash.)

AED is part of the basic life support course for health care professionals. You must be familiar with the operation of the type of defibrillator used in your clinical setting.

The following general steps are taken for defibrillation: (1) CPR should be in progress until the defibrillator is available; (2) turn the defibrillator on, and select the proper energy level; (3) check to see that the synchronizer switch is turned off (discussed later); (4) apply conductive materials (e.g., defibrillator gel pads) to the chest, one to the right of the sternum just below the clavicle, and the other to the left of the apex; (5) charge the defibrillator using the button on the defibrillator or the paddles; (6) position the paddles firmly on the chest wall over the conductive material (Fig. 35-20); (7) call and look to see that everyone is "all clear" to ensure that staff are not touching the patient or the bed at the time of discharge; and (8) deliver the charge by depressing buttons on both paddles simultaneously.

Hands-free, multifunction defibrillator pads are available and are placed on the chest as described earlier. Connect the cables from the pads to the defibrillator. Charge and discharge the defibrillator using buttons on the defibrillator. It is still essential to ensure that all staff are clear before discharging the defibrillator.

Synchronized Cardioversion. *Synchronized cardioversion* is the therapy of choice for the patient with ventricular tachydysrhythmias (e.g., VT with a pulse) or supraventricular tachydysrhythmias (e.g., atrial flutter with a rapid ventricular response). A synchronized circuit in the defibrillator delivers a shock that is programmed to occur on the R wave of the QRS complex of the ECG. The synchronizer switch must be turned on when cardioversion is planned.

The procedure for synchronized cardioversion is the same as for defibrillation with the following exceptions. If synchronized cardioversion is done on a nonemergency basis (i.e., the patient is awake and hemodynamically stable), the patient is sedated (e.g., IV midazolam) before the procedure. Strict attention to maintaining the patient's airway is critical. If a patient with supraventricular tachycardia or VT with a pulse becomes hemodynamically unstable, synchronized cardioversion should be performed as quickly as possible. Start the initial energy for synchronized cardioversion at 50 to 100 joules (biphasic defibrillator) and 100 joules (monophasic defibrillator), and increase if needed. If the patient becomes pulseless or the rhythm changes to VF, turn the synchronizer switch off and perform defibrillation.

! SAFETY ALERT Defibrillation and Cardioversion

- Check that the synchronizer switch is OFF when defibrillation is planned.
- Turn the synchronizer switch ON when cardioversion is planned.
- Never apply the defibrillator pads over a pacemaker or implantable cardioverter-defibrillator.
- Be certain that personnel are "all clear" before discharging the device.

Implantable Cardioverter-Defibrillator. The *implantable cardioverter-defibrillator* (ICD) is an important technology for patients who (1) have survived SCD, (2) have spontaneous sustained VT, (3) have syncope with inducible VT or VF during EPS, or (4) are at high risk for future life-threatening dysrhythmias (e.g., have cardiomyopathy). The use of ICDs has significantly decreased mortality rates in these patients.[12]

The ICD consists of a lead system placed via a subclavian vein to the endocardium. A battery-powered pulse generator is implanted subcutaneously, usually over the pectoral muscle on the patient's nondominant side. The pulse generator is similar in size to a pacemaker. Most systems are single-lead systems (Fig. 35-22). The ICD sensing system monitors the HR and rhythm and identifies VT or VF. After the sensing system detects a lethal dysrhythmia, the device delivers a 25-joule or less shock to the patient's heart. If the first shock is unsuccessful, the device recycles and can continue to deliver shocks.

In addition to defibrillation capabilities, ICDs are equipped with *antitachycardia* and *antibradycardia pacing* capabilities.

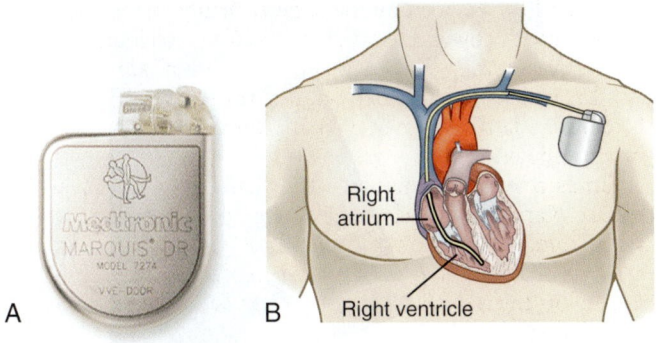

FIG. 35-22 **A,** The implantable cardioverter-defibrillator (ICD) pulse generator from Medtronic, Inc. (Courtesy Medtronic, Inc., Minneapolis, Minn.) **B,** The ICD is placed in a subcutaneous pocket over the pectoral muscle. A single-lead system is placed transvenously from the pulse generator to the endocardium. The single lead detects dysrhythmias and delivers an electric shock to the heart muscle.

These devices use algorithms that detect dysrhythmias and determine the appropriate response. They can initiate *overdrive pacing* of supraventricular tachycardia and VT, sparing the patient painful defibrillator shocks. They also provide backup pacing for bradydysrhythmias that may occur after defibrillation. Preprocedure and postprocedure nursing care of the patient undergoing ICD placement is similar to the care of a patient undergoing permanent pacemaker implantation (see p. 775).

Recent research has focused on a totally subcutaneous ICD (S-ICD). The S-ICD pulse generator is placed under the skin on the left side of the chest and the electrode is placed under the skin above the sternum. The system delivers a shock when VT or VF is detected. Since the S-ICD does not have any electrodes implanted in the heart, it has no pacing capability.[13]

Teaching the patient who is receiving an ICD and the caregiver is extremely important. Patients experience a variety of emotions, including fear of body image change, fear of recurrent dysrhythmias, expectation of pain with ICD discharge (described as a feeling of a blow to the chest), and anxiety about going home. Encourage patients and caregivers to participate in local or online ICD support groups[14] *(www.facebook.com/ICD.pacemaker)*. Table 35-10 presents a teaching guide for the patient with an ICD and the caregiver.

Pacemakers

The artificial **cardiac pacemaker** is an electronic device used to pace the heart when the normal conduction pathway is damaged. The basic pacing circuit consists of a power source (battery-powered pulse generator) with programmable circuitry, one or more pacing leads, and the myocardium. The electrical signal (stimulus) travels from the pulse generator, through the leads, to the wall of the myocardium. The heart muscle is "captured" and stimulated to contract (Fig. 35-23). Recently a leadless pacemaker that is fully implanted in the right ventricle has been approved by the FDA.

Current pacemakers are small, sophisticated, and physiologically precise. They pace the atrium and/or one or both of the ventricles. Most pacemakers are *demand pacemakers.* This means that they sense the heart's electrical activity and fire only when the HR drops below a preset rate. Demand pacemakers have two distinct features: (1) a sensing device that inhibits the pacemaker when the HR is adequate and (2) a pacing device that triggers the pacemaker when no QRS complexes occur within a preset time.[1]

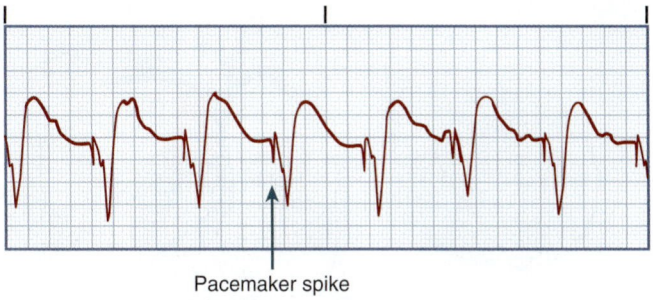

FIG. 35-23 Ventricular capture (depolarization) secondary to signal *(pacemaker spike)* from pacemaker lead in the right ventricle.

TABLE 35-10 Patient & Caregiver Teaching

Implantable Cardioverter-Defibrillator (ICD)

Include the following information in the teaching plan for a patient receiving an ICD and the patient's caregiver.

1. Follow up with an HCP for routine checks of the function of the ICD. This is often done by interrogating the device using a telephone.
2. Report any signs of infection at incision site (e.g., redness, swelling, drainage) or fever to your HCP immediately.
3. Keep incision dry for 4 days after insertion or as instructed.
4. Avoid lifting arm on ICD side above shoulder until approved.
5. Discuss resuming sexual activity with your HCP. It is usually safe to resume sexual activity once your incision is healed.
6. Avoid driving until cleared by your HCP. This decision is usually based on the ongoing presence of dysrhythmias, the frequency of ICD firings, your overall health, and state laws regarding drivers with ICDs.
7. Avoid direct blows to ICD site.
8. Avoid large magnets and strong electromagnetic fields because these may interfere with the device.
9. You should not have magnetic resonance imaging (MRI) unless the ICD is approved as MRI safe or there is a protocol in place for patient safety during the procedure.
10. Travel is not restricted. Inform security (e.g., airport, train station, public buildings) of presence of ICD because it may set off the metal detector. If hand-held screening wand is used, it should not be placed directly over the ICD. Manufacturer information may vary regarding the effect of metal detectors on the function of the ICD.
11. Avoid standing near antitheft devices in doorways of stores and public buildings. You should walk through them at a normal pace.
12. If your ICD fires, call your HCP immediately.
13. If your ICD fires and you feel sick, contact the emergency response system (ERS).
14. If your ICD fires more than once, contact ERS.
15. You should obtain and wear a Medic Alert ID device at all times.
16. Always carry the ICD identification card and a current list of your drugs.
17. Consider joining an ICD support group (e.g., *www.facebook.com/ICD.pacemaker*).
18. Caregivers should learn cardiopulmonary resuscitation (CPR).

In addition to antibradycardia pacing, devices now include antitachycardia and overdrive pacing. *Antitachycardia pacing* involves the delivery of a stimulus to the ventricle to end tachydysrhythmias (e.g., VT). Overdrive pacing involves pacing the atrium at rates of 200 to 500 impulses per minute in an attempt to terminate atrial tachycardias (e.g., atrial flutter with a rapid ventricular response). You can refer to textbooks on pacemaker therapy for more detailed information.[15]

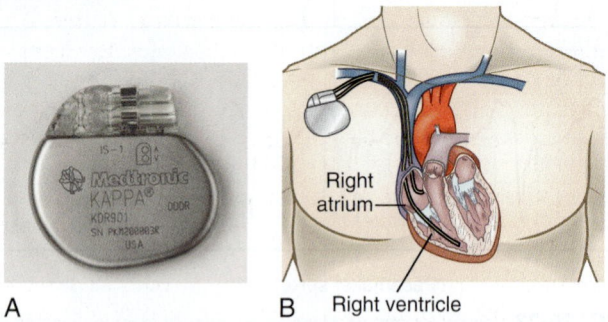

FIG. 35-24 **A,** A dual-chamber rate-responsive pacemaker from Medtronic, Inc., is designed to treat patients with chronic heart problems in which the heart beats too slowly to adequately support the body's circulation needs. (Courtesy Medtronic, Inc., Minneapolis, Minn.) **B,** Pacing leads in both the atrium and the ventricle enable a dual-chamber pacemaker to sense and pace in both heart chambers.

TABLE 35-11 Indications for Permanent Pacemakers

- Acquired AV block
- Second-degree AV block
- Third-degree AV block
- Atrial fibrillation with a slow ventricular response
- Bundle branch block
- Cardiomyopathy
  - Dilated
  - Hypertrophic
- Heart failure
- SA node dysfunction
- Tachydysrhythmias (e.g., ventricular tachycardia)

AV, Atrioventricular; *SA,* sinoatrial.

Permanent Pacemaker. A *permanent pacemaker* is implanted totally within the body (Fig. 35-24). The power source is placed subcutaneously, usually over the pectoral muscle on the patient's nondominant side. The pacing leads are placed transvenously to the right atrium and/or one or both ventricles and attached to the power source. Common reasons for insertion of a permanent pacemaker are found in Table 35-11.

New technology and research are focused on miniaturized, leadless permanent pacemakers. Most candidates for the new device are patients who need single-chamber pacing for atrial fibrillation with AV block. The device is placed in the right ventricle. The lack of a transvenous lead and subcutaneous pulse generator is a major shift in cardiac pacing.[16]

Cardiac Resynchronization Therapy. *Cardiac resynchronization therapy* (CRT) is a pacing technique that resynchronizes the heart cycle by pacing both ventricles *(biventricular pacing)*. This promotes improvement in ventricular function (Fig. 34-4). Most HF patients have intraventricular conduction delays causing abnormal ventricular contraction. This causes dyssynchrony between the right and left ventricles and results in reduced systolic function, pump inefficiency, and worsened HF. For patients with severe left ventricular dysfunction, CRT is combined with an ICD for maximum therapy.[17] (HF is discussed in Chapter 34.)

Temporary Pacemaker. A *temporary pacemaker* is one that has the power source outside the body (Fig. 35-25). There are three types of temporary pacemakers: transvenous, epicardial, and transcutaneous. Table 35-12 lists common reasons for temporary pacing.

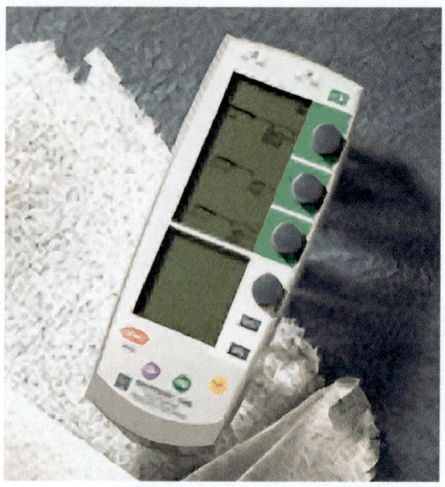

FIG. 35-25 Temporary external, dual-chamber demand pacemaker. (Courtesy Medtronic, Inc., Minneapolis, Minn.)

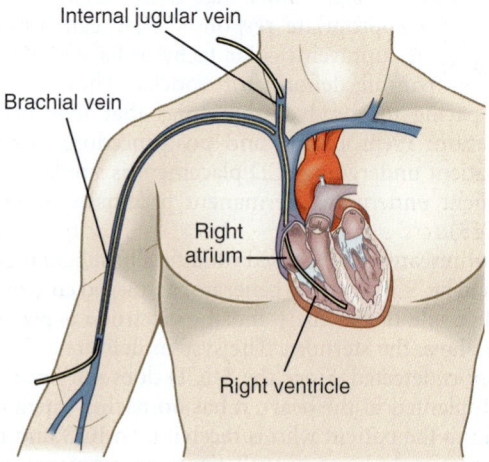

FIG. 35-26 Temporary transvenous pacemaker catheter insertion. A single lead is positioned in the right ventricle through the brachial, subclavian, jugular, or femoral vein.

TABLE 35-12 Indications for Temporary Pacemakers*

- Maintenance of adequate HR and rhythm during special circumstances such as surgery and postoperative recovery, during cardiac catheterization or coronary angioplasty, during drug therapy that may cause bradycardia, and before implantation of a permanent pacemaker
- As prophylaxis after open heart surgery
- Acute anterior MI with second- or third-degree AV block or bundle branch block
- Acute inferior MI with symptomatic bradycardia and AV block
- Electrophysiologic studies to evaluate patient with bradydysrhythmias and tachydysrhythmias

*List is not all-inclusive.
AV, Atrioventricular; *HR,* heart rate; *MI,* myocardial infarction.

A *transvenous pacemaker* consists of a lead or leads that are threaded transvenously to the right atrium and/or right ventricle and attached to the external power source (Fig. 35-26). Most temporary transvenous pacemakers are inserted in emergency departments and critical care units in emergency situations. They provide a bridge to insertion of a permanent

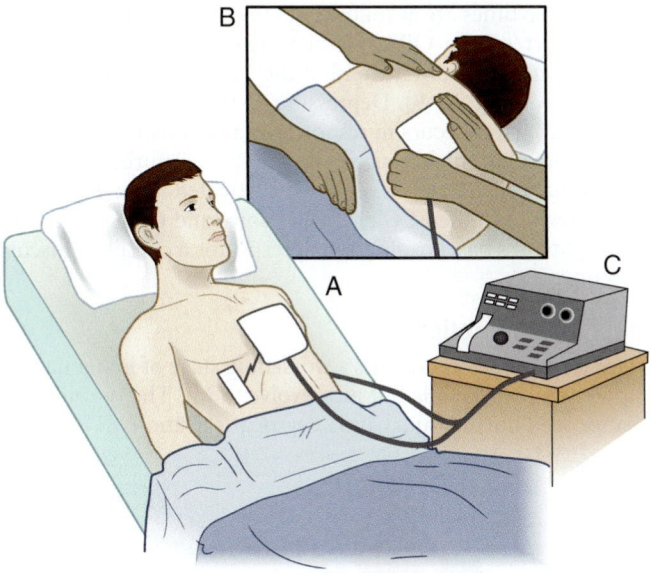

FIG. 35-27 Transcutaneous pacemaker. Pacing electrodes are placed on the patient's anterior *(A)* and posterior *(B)* chest walls and attached to an external pacing unit *(C)*.

pacemaker or until the underlying cause of the dysrhythmia is resolved.

Epicardial pacing involves attaching an atrial and ventricular pacing lead to the epicardium during heart surgery. The leads are passed through the chest wall and attached to the external power source. Epicardial pacing leads are placed prophylactically in case any bradydysrhythmias or tachydysrhythmias occur in the early postoperative period.[7]

A *transcutaneous pacemaker* (TCP) is used to provide adequate HR and rhythm to the patient in an emergency situation. Placement of the TCP is a noninvasive, temporary procedure used until a transvenous pacemaker is inserted or until more definitive therapy is available.[7]

The TCP consists of a power source and a rate- and voltage-control device that attaches to two large, multifunction electrode pads. Position one pad on the anterior part of the chest, usually on the V_4 lead position, and the other pad on the back between the spine and left scapula at the level of the heart (Fig. 35-27). When programming the TCP, always use the lowest current that results in a ventricular contraction (capture) to minimize patient discomfort.

Before starting TCP therapy, it is important to tell the patient what to expect. Explain that the muscle contractions created by the pacemaker when the current passes through the chest wall are uncomfortable. Reassure the patient that the TCP is temporary and that it will be replaced by a transvenous pacemaker as soon as possible. Whenever possible, provide analgesia and/or sedation while the TCP is in use.

Monitoring of Patients With Pacemakers. Patients with temporary or permanent pacemakers are ECG monitored to evaluate the status of the pacemaker. Pacemaker malfunction primarily involves a failure to sense or a failure to capture. *Failure to sense* occurs when the pacemaker fails to recognize spontaneous atrial or ventricular activity, and it fires inappropriately. This can result in the pacemaker firing during the excitable period of the cardiac cycle, resulting in VT. Failure to sense is caused by fibrosis around the tip of the pacing lead, battery failure, sensing set too high, or dislodgment of the electrode.

Failure to capture occurs when the electrical charge to the myocardium is insufficient to produce atrial or ventricular contraction. This can result in serious bradycardia or asystole. Failure to capture is caused by pacer lead damage, battery failure, dislodgment of the electrode, electrical charge set too low, or fibrosis at the electrode tip.

Complications of invasive temporary (i.e., transvenous) or permanent pacemaker insertion include infection and hematoma formation at the insertion site, pneumothorax, failure to sense or capture, perforation of the atrial or ventricular septum by the pacing lead, and appearance of "end-of-life" battery power on testing the pacemaker. Several measures can prevent or assess for complications. These include prophylactic IV antibiotic therapy before and after insertion, postinsertion chest x-ray to check lead placement and to rule out a pneumothorax, careful observation of insertion site, and continuous ECG monitoring of the patient's rhythm.

After the pacemaker has been inserted, the patient can be out of bed once stable. Have the patient limit arm and shoulder activity on the operative side to prevent dislodging the newly implanted pacing leads. Observe the insertion site for signs of bleeding, and check that the incision is intact. Note any temperature elevation or pain at the insertion site and treat as ordered. Most patients are discharged the next day if stable.

Provide teaching in addition to observing for complications after pacemaker insertion. The patient with a newly implanted pacemaker and the caregiver may have questions about activity restrictions and fears concerning body image after the procedure. The goals of pacemaker therapy include enhancing physiologic functioning and quality of life. Emphasize this to the patient and caregiver, and provide specific advice on activity restrictions. Table 35-13 outlines patient and caregiver teaching for the patient with a pacemaker.

After discharge, patients need to check pacemaker function on a regular basis. This can include outpatient visits to a pacemaker clinic or home monitoring using telephone transmitter devices. Another method to evaluate pacemaker performance is noninvasive program stimulation. This procedure is done on an outpatient basis in the EPS laboratory.

Radiofrequency Catheter Ablation Therapy

Radiofrequency catheter ablation therapy uses electrical energy to "burn" or ablate areas of the conduction system as definitive treatment of tachydysrhythmias. Ablation therapy is done after EPS has identified the source of the dysrhythmia. An electrode-tipped ablation catheter ablates accessory pathways or ectopic sites in the atria, AV node, and ventricles. Catheter ablation is considered the nonpharmacologic treatment of choice for atrial dysrhythmias resulting in rapid ventricular rates and AV nodal reentrant tachycardia refractory to drug therapy.[8]

The ablation procedure is an effective treatment with a low complication rate. Care of the patient after ablation therapy is similar to that of a patient undergoing cardiac catheterization (see Chapter 31 and Table 31-6).

ECG CHANGES ASSOCIATED WITH ACUTE CORONARY SYNDROME

The 12-lead ECG is a major diagnostic tool used to evaluate patients with ACS. ECG changes that occur with ACS direct many treatment decisions. The ECG changes are in response to ischemia, injury, or infarction (necrosis) of heart cells. The leads facing the area of involvement demonstrate the definitive ECG changes (Fig. 35-28). The leads facing opposite the area involved in ACS often demonstrate reciprocal (opposite) ECG changes. In addition, the pattern of ECG changes among the 12 leads provides information on the coronary artery involved in ACS (Table 35-14).

Ischemia

Typical ECG changes that are seen in myocardial ischemia include ST segment depression and/or T wave inversion (Fig. 35-29, *A*). ST segment depression is significant if it is at least 1 mm (one small box) below the isoelectric line in at least two contiguous (neighboring) leads (Fig. 35-5). The isoelectric line is flat and represents those normal times in the cardiac cycle when the ECG is not recording any electrical activity in the heart. These times are as follows: (1) from the end of the P wave to the start of the QRS complex, (2) during the entire ST segment, and (3) from the end of the T wave to the start of the next P wave (Fig. 35-9). Depression in the ST segment and/or T wave inversion occurs in response to an inadequate supply of blood and O_2, which causes an electrical disturbance in the myocardial cells.[6,7] Once the patient is treated (adequate blood flow is restored), the ECG changes resolve and the ECG returns to the patient's baseline. (See Chapter 33 for a complete discussion of ACS.)

Injury and Infarction

Myocardial injury represents a worsening stage of ischemia that is potentially reversible but may evolve to MI. The typical ECG change seen during injury is ST segment elevation. ST segment

TABLE 35-13 Patient & Caregiver Teaching

Pacemaker

Include the following information in the teaching plan for a patient with a pacemaker and the patient's caregiver.

1. Maintain follow-up care with your HCP to begin regular pacemaker function checks. This is often done by interrogating the device using a telephone.
2. Report any signs of infection at incision site (e.g., redness, swelling, drainage) or fever to your HCP immediately.
3. Keep incision dry for 4 days after implantation, or as ordered.
4. Avoid lifting arm on pacemaker side above shoulder until approved by your cardiologist.
5. Avoid direct blows to pacemaker site.
6. Avoid close proximity to high-output electric generators, since these can interfere with the function of the pacemaker.
7. You should not have magnetic resonance imaging (MRI) unless the pacemaker is approved as MRI safe or there is a protocol in place for patient safety during the procedure.
8. Microwave ovens are safe to use and do not interfere with pacemaker function.
9. Avoid standing near antitheft devices in doorways of department stores and public libraries. You should walk through them at a normal pace.
10. Travel is not restricted. Inform security (e.g., airport, train station, public buildings) of presence of pacemaker because it may set off the metal detector. If hand-held screening wand is used, it should not be placed directly over the pacemaker. Manufacturer information may vary regarding the effect of metal detectors on the function of the pacemaker.
11. Monitor pulse and inform HCP if heart rate drops below predetermined rate.
12. Carry pacemaker information card and a current list of your drugs at all times.
13. Obtain and wear a Medic Alert ID device at all times.
14. Consider joining a pacemaker support group (e.g., *www.facebook.com/ICD.pacemaker*).

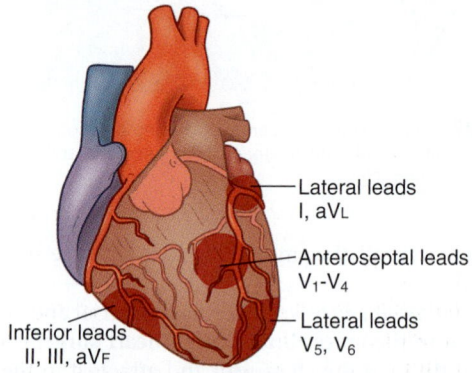

FIG. 35-28 Definitive ECG changes occur in leads that face the area of ischemia, injury, or infarction. Reciprocal changes may occur in leads facing opposite the area of ischemia, injury, or infarction.

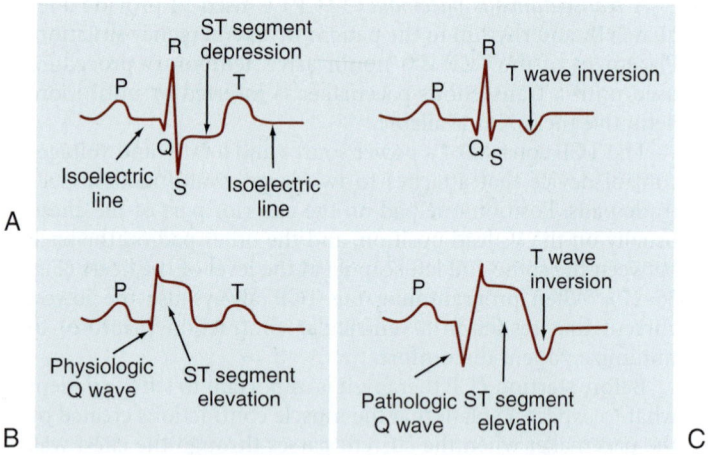

FIG. 35-29 ST segment, T wave, and Q wave changes associated with myocardial ischemia **(A)**, injury **(B)**, and infarction **(C)**. (From Bucher L, Melander S: *Critical care nursing*, Philadelphia, 1999, Saunders.)

TABLE 35-14 ECG Evidence in Acute Coronary Syndrome

	ECG EVIDENCE		
Left Ventricle Involvement	**Leads Facing Area**	**Leads Opposite Area (Reciprocal Changes)**	**Associated Coronary Artery**
Septal wall	V_1, V_2	II, III, aVF	Left anterior descending
Anterior wall	V_2-V_4	II, III, aVF	Left anterior descending
Lateral wall, low	V_5, V_6	II, III, aVF	Left anterior descending or circumflex
Lateral wall, high	I, aVL	II, III, aVF	Circumflex
Inferior wall	II, III, aVF	I, aVL, V_5, V_6	Right coronary artery, posterior descending coronary artery

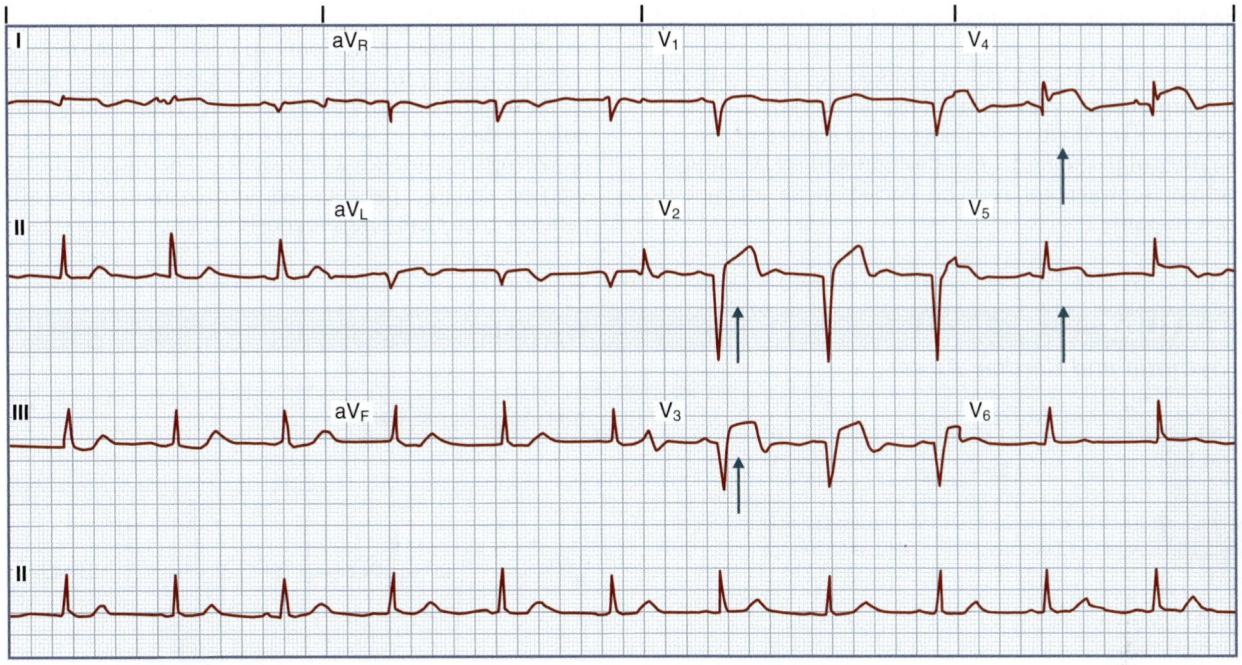

FIG. 35-30 ECG findings with anteroseptal lateral wall myocardial infarction. Normally, leads I, aVL, and V_1 to V_3 have a positive R wave. Note the pathologic Q waves in these leads and the ST segment elevation in leads V_2 to V_5 *(arrows)*.

elevation is significant if it is 1 mm or more above the isoelectric line in at least two contiguous leads (Fig. 35-29, *B*). If treatment is fast and effective, it is possible to restore O_2 to the heart muscle and avoid or limit infarction. The absence of serum cardiac biomarkers confirms this.

In addition to ST segment elevation, a pathologic Q wave may be seen on the ECG in patients with MI (Fig. 35-29, *C*). A physiologic Q wave is the first negative deflection (wave) following the P wave. It is normally very short and narrow (Fig. 35-9 and Table 35-2). A pathologic Q wave that develops during MI is wide (greater than 0.03 second in duration) and deep (greater than or equal to 25% of the height of the R wave).[1,7] This is referred to as a *Q wave MI.* The pathologic Q wave may remain on the ECG indefinitely.

T wave inversion related to MI occurs within hours following the event and may persist for months. The ECG changes seen in injury and MI reflect electrical disturbances in the heart cells caused by a prolonged lack of blood and O_2 leading to necrosis (Fig. 35-30).

Patient Monitoring

Monitoring guidelines for patients who are suspected of having ACS include continuous, multilead ECG and ST segment monitoring.[3] The leads selected for monitoring should minimally include the leads that reflect the area of ischemia, injury, or infarction.

SYNCOPE

Syncope, a brief lapse in consciousness accompanied by a loss in postural tone (fainting), is a common diagnosis of patients coming to the emergency department. The causes of syncope can be cardiovascular or noncardiovascular. The most common cause of syncope is cardioneurogenic syncope, or "vasovagal" syncope (e.g., carotid sinus sensitivity). Other cardiovascular causes relate to dysrhythmias (e.g., tachycardias, bradycardias), prosthetic valve malfunction, pulmonary emboli, and HF. Noncardiovascular causes vary and include stress, hypoglycemia, dehydration, stroke, and seizure.[17]

A diagnostic workup for a patient with syncope from a suspected heart cause begins with ruling out structural and ischemic heart disease. This is done with echocardiography and stress testing. In the older patient, who is more likely to have structural and ischemic heart disease, EPS is used to diagnose atrial and ventricular tachydysrhythmias and conduction disturbances causing bradydysrhythmias, all of which can cause syncope. These problems can be treated with antidysrhythmia drug therapy, pacemakers, ICDs, and/or catheter ablation therapy.

In patients without structural heart disease or in whom EPS testing is not diagnostic, the *head-up tilt-test* may be performed. Normally, an upright position results in gravity displacing 300 to 800 mL of blood to the lower extremities. Specialized nerve fibers called mechanoreceptors are located throughout the vascular system. These respond to the increased blood volume by starting a reflex increase in sympathetic stimulation and decrease in parasympathetic output. The end results are a slight increase in HR and diastolic BP, and a slight decrease in systolic BP.[18]

In cardioneurogenic syncope, the increase in venous pooling that occurs in the upright position reduces venous return to the heart. This results in a sudden, compensatory increase in ventricular contraction. This is mistaken by the brain as a hypertensive state, and consequently sympathetic stimulation is withdrawn. This produces a paradoxical vasodilation and bradycardia (vasovagal response). The end results are bradycardia, hypotension, cerebral hypoperfusion, and syncope.

In the head-up tilt-test the patient is placed on a table supported by a belt across the torso and feet. Baseline ECG, BP, and HR are obtained in the horizontal position. Next, the table is tilted 60 to 80 degrees and the patient is kept in this upright position for 20 to 60 minutes. ECG and HR are recorded continuously and BP is measured every 3 minutes throughout the test.

If the patient's BP and HR responses are abnormal and clinical symptoms are reproduced (e.g., faintness), the test is considered positive. If after 30 minutes there is no response, the table is returned to the horizontal position and an IV infusion of low-dose isoproterenol may be started in an attempt to provoke a response.

Additional diagnostic tests for syncope can include various recording devices (e.g., Holter monitor or event monitor/loop recorder, which are discussed in Chapter 31 and Table 31-6), blood volume determination, hemodynamic testing, and autonomic reflex testing. About 30% of those who have one episode of syncope experience a recurrence. The underlying cause of syncope and the patient's age and co-morbidities affect the patient's treatment and prognosis.[18]

CASE STUDY

Dysrhythmia and Cardiac Arrest

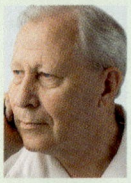

(©iStockphoto/Thinkstock)

Patient Profile

J.M., a 68-yr-old white, retired postal worker, was admitted to the telemetry unit with a diagnosis of acute decompensated heart failure (HF). He experienced a cardiac arrest (pulseless ventricular tachycardia [VT]) and was successfully defibrillated after one shock. He is transferred to the cardiac care unit. J.M. is awake but lethargic and responds appropriately to questions.

Subjective Data

- History of hypertension, coronary artery disease, two MIs, and chronic HF
- Reports shortness of breath at rest and even in an upright position

Objective Data

Physical Examination

- Appears weak, anxious
- BP 102/60 mm Hg, pulse 70/min, respirations 26/min
- Lungs: bilateral coarse crackles in the bases
- Heart: S_3 gallop at apex

Diagnostic Studies

- Echocardiogram: severe left ventricular dysfunction with ejection fraction of 24%
- Serum potassium: 2.9 mEq/L (2.9 mmol/L)
- Serum cardiac biomarkers: negative
- Serum b-type natriuretic peptide (BNP): 1852 pg/mL

Interprofessional Care

- Continuous ECG monitoring

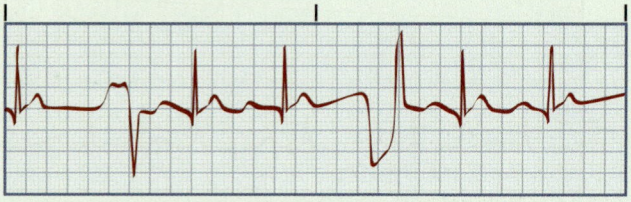

- Amiodarone infusion
- Cardiac rehabilitation consult
- Dietary consult

Discussion Questions

1. Why is J.M. at risk for sudden cardiac death?
2. Explain the rationale for using amiodarone after cardiac arrest.
3. What methods are used to assess the effectiveness of the antidysrhythmia therapy?
4. Interpret the rhythm strip.
5. Explain the significance of the diagnostic studies and other interprofessional care orders.
6. Why would J.M. be a candidate for CRT and an ICD?
7. ***Priority Decision:*** Based on the assessment data provided, what are the priority nursing diagnoses?
8. ***Priority Decision:*** Based on these nursing diagnoses, what are the priority nursing interventions for J.M.?
9. ***Teamwork and Collaboration:*** Which tasks could be delegated to unlicensed assistive personnel (UAP)?
10. ***Evidence-Based Practice:*** Once J.M. is stable, he is scheduled for the insertion of a CRT/ICD. On your rounds, he asks you why he needs two devices.

Answers available at *http://evolve.elsevier.com/Lewis/medsurg.*

BRIDGE TO NCLEX EXAMINATION

The number of the question corresponds to the same-numbered outcome at the beginning of the chapter.

1. A patient admitted with ACS has continuous ECG monitoring. An examination of the rhythm strip reveals the following characteristics: atrial rate 74 beats/min and regular; ventricular rate 62 beats/min and irregular; P wave normal shape; PR interval lengthens progressively until a P wave is not conducted; QRS normal shape. The *priority* nursing intervention would be to
   a. perform synchronized cardioversion.
   b. administer epinephrine 1 mg IV push.
   c. observe for symptoms of hypotension or angina.
   d. apply transcutaneous pacemaker pads on the patient.
2. The nurse is monitoring the ECG of a patient admitted with ACS. Which ECG characteristics would be *most* suggestive of myocardial ischemia?
   a. Sinus rhythm with a pathologic Q wave
   b. Sinus rhythm with an elevated ST segment
   c. Sinus rhythm with a depressed ST segment
   d. Sinus rhythm with premature atrial contractions
3. The ECG monitor of a patient in the cardiac care unit after an MI indicates ventricular bigeminy with a rate of 50 beats/min. The nurse would anticipate
   a. performing defibrillation.
   b. treating with IV amiodarone.
   c. inserting a temporary transvenous pacemaker.
   d. assessing the patient's response to the dysrhythmia.

4. The nurse prepares a patient for synchronized cardioversion knowing that cardioversion differs from defibrillation in that
   a. defibrillation requires a lower dose of electrical energy.
   b. cardioversion is indicated to treat atrial bradydysrhythmias.
   c. defibrillation is synchronized to deliver a shock during the QRS complex.
   d. patients should be sedated if cardioversion is done on a non-emergency basis.
5. Which patient teaching points should the nurse include when providing discharge instructions to a patient with a new permanent pacemaker and the caregiver *(select all that apply)*?
   a. Avoid or limit air travel.
   b. Take and record a daily pulse rate.
   c. Obtain and wear a Medic Alert ID device at all times.
   d. Avoid lifting arm on the side of the pacemaker above shoulder.
   e. Avoid microwave ovens because they interfere with pacemaker function.
6. Important teaching for the patient scheduled for a radiofrequency catheter ablation procedure includes explaining that
   a. ventricular bradycardia may be induced and treated during the procedure.
   b. a catheter will be placed in both femoral arteries to allow double-catheter use.
   c. the procedure will destroy areas of the conduction system that are causing rapid heart rhythms.
   d. a general anesthetic will be given to prevent the awareness of any "sudden cardiac death" experiences.

1. c, 2. c, 3. d, 4. d, 5. b, c, d, 6. c

For rationales to these answers and even more NCLEX review questions, visit *http://evolve.elsevier.com/Lewis/medsurg.*

EVOLVE WEBSITE

http://evolve.elsevier.com/Lewis/medsurg

Review Questions (Online Only)
Key Points
Answer Keys for Questions
- Rationales for Bridge to NCLEX Examination Questions
- Answer Guidelines for Case Study on p. 778

Case Study
- Patient With Atrial Fibrillation

Conceptual Care Map Creator
Audio Glossary
Content Updates

REFERENCES

1. Wesley K: *Huszar's basic dysrhythmias and acute coronary syndrome,* ed 4, St Louis, 2011, Mosby Jems.
2. Patton KT, Thibodeau GA: *Anatomy and physiology,* ed 8, St Louis, 2013, Mosby.
*3. American Association of Critical-Care Nurses: AACN practice alert: ST segment monitoring. Retrieved from *www.aacn.org/wd/practice/docs/practicealerts/st-segment-monitoring.pdf?menu=aboutus.*
*4. American Association of Critical-Care Nurses: AACN practice alert: dysrhythmia monitoring. Retrieved from *www.aacn.org/wd/practice/docs/practicealerts/dysrhythmia-monitoring.pdf?menu=aboutus.*
5. Lehne RA: *Pharmacology for nursing care,* ed 8, St Louis, 2013, Saunders.
*6. Page RL, Joglar JA, Caldwell MA, et al: 2015 ACC/AHA/HRS Guideline for the management of adult patients with supraventricular tachycardia: executive summary, *Circulation* 133:e471, 2016.
7. Alspach JG: *Core curriculum for critical care nursing,* ed 6, St Louis, 2011, Saunders.
*8. January CT, Wann LS, Albert JS, et al: 2014 AHA/ACC/HRS guideline for the management of patients with atrial fibrillation: executive summary: a report of the American College of Cardiology/American Heart Association Task Force on Practice Guidelines and the Heart Rhythm Society, *J Am Coll Cardiol* 64(21):e1, 2014.
9. Go AS, Mozaffarian D, Roger VL, et al: Heart disease and stroke statistics—2013 update: a report from the American Heart Association, *Circulation* 127:e6, 2013.
10. FDA U.S. Food and Drug Administration: WATCHMAN LAA Closure Technology—P130013. Retrieved from *www.fda.gov/MedicalDevices/ProductsandMedicalProcedures/DeviceApprovalsandClearances/Recently-ApprovedDevices/ucm440621.htm.*
11. Sinz E, Navarro K, Soderberg ES, editors: *Advanced cardiovascular life support: provider manual,* Dallas, 2011, American Heart Association.
*12. Tracy CM, Epstein AE, Darbar D, et al: 2012 ACCF/AHA/HRS focused update of the 2008 guidelines for device-based therapy of cardiac rhythm abnormalities: a report of the American College of Cardiology Foundation/American Heart Association Task Force on Practice Guidelines, *Circulation* 126:1784, 2012.
*13. Burke MC, Gold MR, Knight BP: Safety and efficacy of the totally subcutaneous implantable defibrillator: 2-year results from a pooled analysis of the IDE study and EFFORTLESS registry, *J Am Coll Cardiol* 65(16):1605, 2015.
*14. Dunbar SB, Dougherty CM, Sears SF, et al: Educational and psychological interventions to improve outcomes for recipients of implantable cardioverter defibrillators and their families: a scientific statement from the American Heart Association, *Circulation* 126:2146, 2012.
15. Burri H, Deharo J-C, Israel C: *The EHRA book of pacemaker, ICD, and CRT troubleshooting: case-based learning with multiple-choice questions,* Oxford, United Kingdom, 2015, Oxford University Press.
*16. Knops RE, Tjong FV, Neuzil P, et al: Chronic performance of a leadless cardiac pacemaker: 1-year follow-up of the LEADLESS trial, *J Am Coll Cardiol* 65(15):1497, 2015.
17. McAlister FA, Ezekowitz J, Dryden DM, et al: Cardiac resynchronization therapy and implantable cardiac defibrillators in left ventricular systolic dysfunction, AHRQ Pub No 07-E009. Retrieved from *http://archive.ahrq.gov/downloads/pub/evidence/pdf/defib/defib.pdf.* (Classic)
18. Cleveland Clinic: Syncope. Retrieved from *http://my.clevelandclinic.org/services/heart/disorders/syncope.*

*Evidence-based information for clinical practice.

36

Inflammatory and Structural Heart Disorders

Nancy Kupper, De Ann F. Mitchell

A kind heart is a fountain of gladness, making everything in its vicinity freshen into smiles.

Washington Irving

http://evolve.elsevier.com/Lewis/medsurg/

LEARNING OUTCOMES

1. Differentiate the etiology, pathophysiology, and clinical manifestations of infective endocarditis and pericarditis.
2. Describe the interprofessional care and nursing management of the patient with infective endocarditis and pericarditis.
3. Describe the etiology, pathophysiology, and clinical manifestations of myocarditis.
4. Describe the interprofessional care and nursing management of the patient with myocarditis.
5. Differentiate the etiology, pathophysiology, and clinical manifestations of rheumatic fever and rheumatic heart disease.
6. Describe the interprofessional care and nursing management of the patient with rheumatic fever and rheumatic heart disease.
7. Relate the pathophysiology to the clinical manifestations and diagnostic studies for the various types of valvular heart disease.
8. Describe the interprofessional care and nursing management of the patient with valvular heart disease.
9. Relate the pathophysiology to the clinical manifestations and diagnostic studies for the different types of cardiomyopathy.
10. Compare the nursing and interprofessional management of patients with different types of cardiomyopathy.

KEY TERMS

aortic regurgitation (AR), p. 792
aortic stenosis (AS), p. 792
cardiac tamponade, p. 785
cardiomyopathy (CMP), p. 796
chronic constrictive pericarditis, p. 787
dilated cardiomyopathy, p. 796
hypertrophic cardiomyopathy, p. 798
infective endocarditis (IE), p. 780
mitral valve prolapse (MVP), p. 791
myocarditis, p. 787
pericardiocentesis, p. 786
pericarditis, p. 784
regurgitation, p. 791
rheumatic fever (RF), p. 788
rheumatic heart disease, p. 788
stenosis, p. 791

This chapter describes the pathophysiology and management of patients experiencing select inflammatory and structural heart disorders. In addition, the interprofessional care and nursing management of these patients is presented.

INFLAMMATORY DISORDERS OF HEART

INFECTIVE ENDOCARDITIS

Infective endocarditis (IE) is an infection of the endocardial layer of the heart. The *endocardium* is the innermost layer of the heart (Fig. 36-1) and heart valves. Therefore IE affects the valves. Treatment of IE with antibiotic therapy has improved the prognosis of this disease. Although relatively uncommon, an estimated 10,000 to 15,000 new cases of IE are diagnosed in the United States each year.[1]

Classification

IE was traditionally classified as subacute or acute. The *subacute form* affects those with preexisting valve disease and has a clinical course that may extend over months. In contrast, the *acute form* affects those with healthy valves and manifests as a rapidly progressive illness. Today IE is more often classified based on the cause (e.g., IV drug abuse IE [IVDA IE], fungal endocarditis) or site of involvement (e.g., prosthetic valve endocarditis [PVE]).

Etiology and Pathophysiology

The most common causative organisms of IE, *Staphylococcus aureus* and *Streptococcus viridans,* are bacterial. Other possible pathogens include fungi and viruses.[2] IE occurs when blood flow within the heart allows the causative organism to infect previously damaged valves or other endothelial surfaces. IE can occur in persons with a variety of underlying cardiac and noncardiac conditions (Table 36-1).

Vegetations, the primary lesions of IE, consist of fibrin, leukocytes, platelets, and microbes that stick to the valve surface or endocardium (Fig. 36-2). The loss of parts of these fragile vegetations into the circulation results in *emboli.* Many persons with IE will develop systemic embolization. This occurs when left-sided heart vegetation moves to various organs (e.g., brain, kidneys, spleen) and to the extremities, causing limb infarction.

Reviewed by Vickie Lee Doscher, MSN, FNP-C, APRN, Family Nurse Practitioner, Chesapeake Regional Medical Center, Chesapeake, Virginia; Tracy H. Knoll, RN, MSN, Nursing Instructor, Chamberlain College of Nursing, St. Louis, Missouri; and Rebecca Personett, RN, PhD, NEA-BC, Professor of Nursing, North Central Texas College, Gainesville, Texas and Brookhaven College, Dallas, Texas.

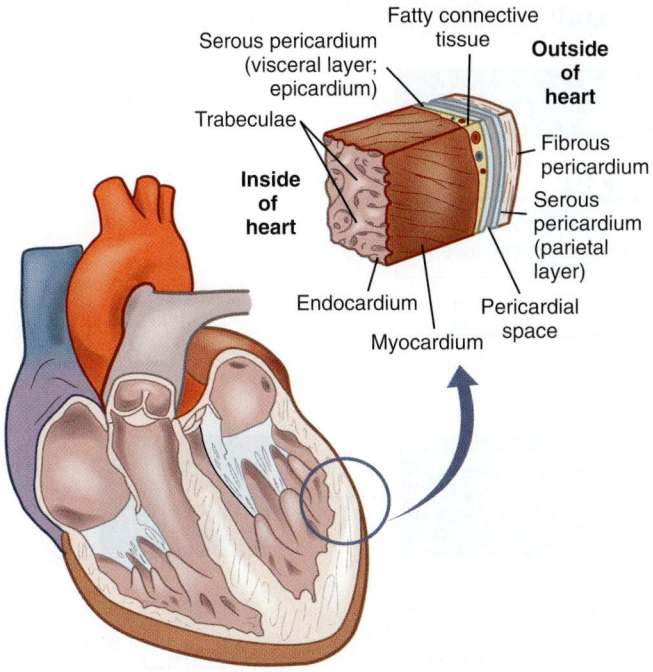

FIG. 36-1 Layers of the heart muscle and pericardium. The section of the heart wall shows the fibrous pericardium, the parietal and visceral layers of the serous pericardium (with the pericardial sac between them), the myocardium, and the endocardium. (Modified from Patton KT, Thibodeau GA: *The human body in health and disease,* ed 5, St Louis, 2010, Mosby.)

TABLE 36-1 Risk Factors for Endocarditis*

Cardiac Conditions
- Prior endocarditis
- Prosthetic heart valve(s)
- Acquired valve disease (e.g., mitral valve prolapse with regurgitation, calcified aortic stenosis)
- Heart lesions (e.g., ventricular septal defect, asymmetric septal hypertrophy)
- Rheumatic heart disease (e.g., mitral valve regurgitation)
- Congenital heart disease
- Pacemaker
- Marfan's syndrome
- Cardiomyopathy

Noncardiac Conditions
- Hospital-acquired bacteremia
- IV drug abuse

Procedure-Associated Risks
- Intravascular devices (e.g., central venous catheter)
- Procedures listed in Table 36-2

*List is not all-inclusive.

Right-sided heart lesions move to the lungs, resulting in pulmonary emboli.

The infection may spread locally and damage the valves or their supporting structures. This causes dysrhythmias, valve dysfunction, and eventual invasion of the myocardium, leading to heart failure (HF), sepsis, and heart block (Fig. 36-3).

At one time rheumatic heart disease was the most common cause of IE. Now it accounts for less than 20% of cases. The main contributing factors to IE include (1) aging (more than 50% of older people have calcified aortic stenosis [AS]), (2) IVDA, (3) use of prosthetic valves, (4) use of intravascular devices resulting in health care–associated infections (e.g., methicillin-resistant *S. aureus* [MRSA]), and (5) renal dialysis.[1]

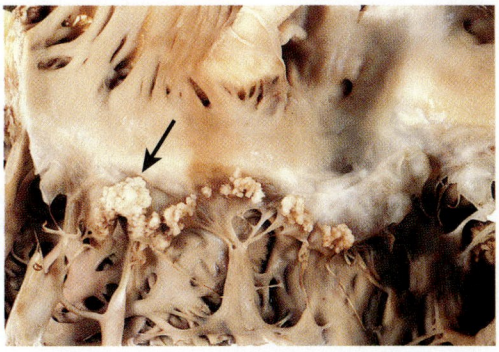

FIG. 36-2 Bacterial endocarditis of the mitral valve. The valve is covered with large, irregular vegetations *(arrow).* (From Damjanov I, Linder J: *Pathology: a color atlas,* St Louis, 2000, Mosby.)

Clinical Manifestations

The clinical manifestations of IE are nonspecific and can involve multiple organ systems. Symptoms include fever, chills, weakness, malaise, fatigue, and anorexia. Arthralgias, myalgias, back pain, abdominal discomfort, weight loss, headache, and clubbing of fingers may occur in subacute forms of IE. Fever may be absent in older adults or those who are immunocompromised.

Vascular signs of IE include *splinter hemorrhages* (black longitudinal streaks) that may occur in the nail beds. Petechiae may result from fragmentation and microembolization of vegetative lesions. They can occur on the conjunctivae, lips, buccal mucosa, and palate and over the ankles, feet, and antecubital and popliteal areas. *Osler's nodes* (painful, tender, red or purple, pea-size lesions) may be found on the fingertips or toes. *Janeway's lesions* (flat, painless, small, red spots) may be seen on the fingertips, palms, soles of feet, and toes. Eye examination may reveal hemorrhagic retinal lesions called *Roth's spots.*

The onset of a new or worsening systolic murmur is noted in most patients with IE. The aortic and mitral valves are most often affected. Murmurs are usually absent in tricuspid endocarditis because right-sided heart sounds are too low to be heard. HF occurs in up to 80% of patients with aortic valve endocarditis and approximately 50% of patients with mitral valve endocarditis.[3]

Clinical signs secondary to embolization may be present in various body organs. Embolization to the spleen may cause sharp, left upper quadrant pain and splenomegaly, local tenderness, and abdominal rigidity. Embolization to the kidneys may cause flank pain, hematuria, and renal failure. Emboli may lodge in small peripheral blood vessels of the arms and legs and may cause ischemia and gangrene. Embolization to the brain may cause neurologic damage, resulting in hemiplegia, ataxia, aphasia, visual changes, and change in mental status. Pulmonary emboli may occur in right-sided endocarditis and cause dyspnea, chest pain, hemoptysis, and respiratory arrest.

Diagnostic Studies

The patient's health history is important in assessing IE. Ask patients if they have had any recent (within the past 3 to 6 months) dental, urologic, surgical, or gynecologic procedures, including normal or abnormal obstetric delivery. Note any previous history of IVDA, heart disease, recent heart

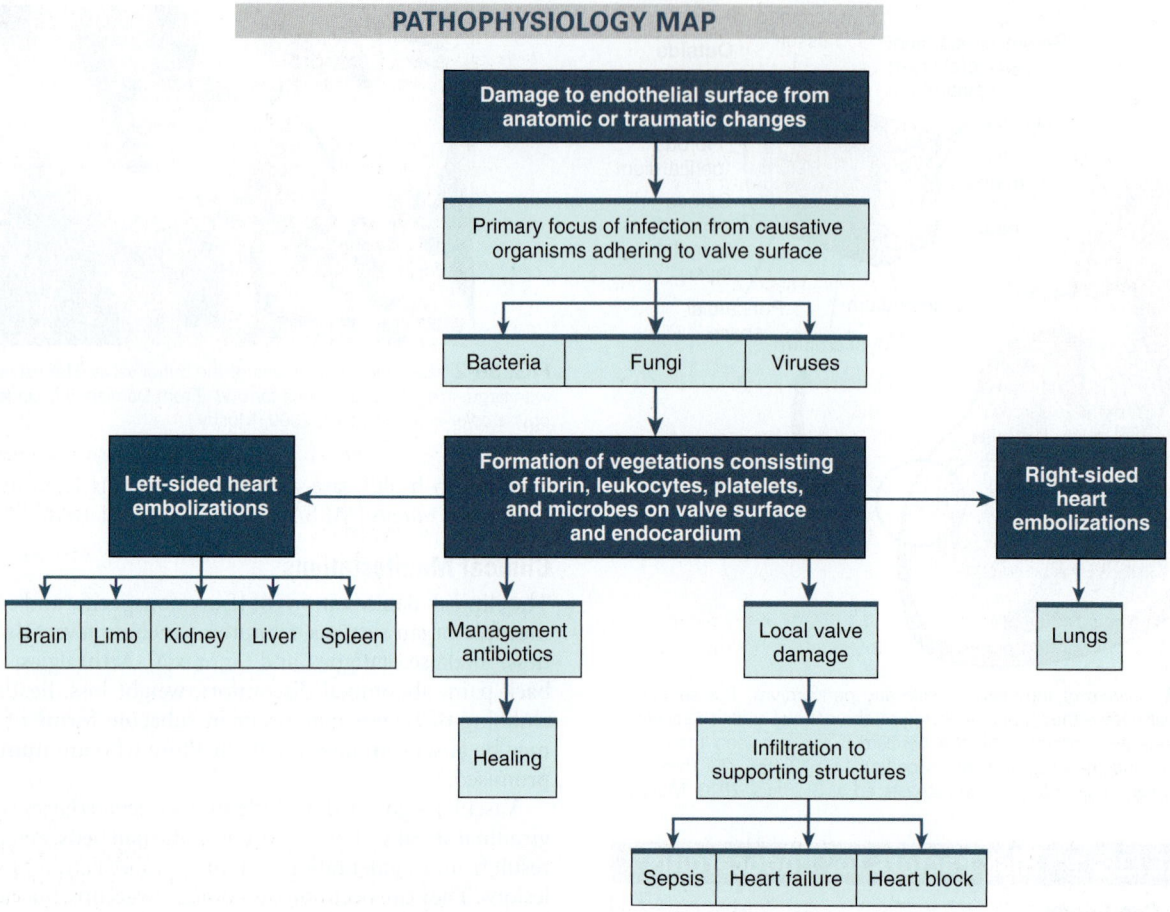

FIG. 36-3 Pathogenesis of infective endocarditis.

catheterization, heart surgery, intravascular device placement, renal dialysis, or infections (e.g., skin, respiratory, urinary tract).

Three blood cultures drawn over a period of 1 hour from three different sites will be positive in most patients.[3] Culture-negative endocarditis is often associated with antibiotic usage within the previous 2 weeks, or results from a pathogen not easily detected by standard culture tests. Cultures that are negative should be kept for 3 weeks if the clinical diagnosis remains IE because of the possibility of slow-growing organisms. A mild leukocytosis occurs in acute IE (uncommon in subacute). The erythrocyte sedimentation rate (ESR) and C-reactive protein (CRP) levels may also be elevated.

Major criteria to diagnose IE include at least two of the following: two positive blood cultures 12 hours apart, nonvalvular regurgitation, or intracardiac mass or vegetation noted on echocardiography.[3] Echocardiography (e.g., transesophageal echocardiogram, two- or three-dimensional [2-D or 3-D] transthoracic echocardiogram) is critical in the diagnostic workup of a patient suspected of having IE and should be done in a timely manner.[3]

A chest x-ray is done to detect *cardiomegaly* (an enlarged heart). An electrocardiogram (ECG) may show first- or second-degree atrioventricular (AV) block. Heart block occurs because the heart valves lie close to conductive tissue, especially the AV node. Heart catheterization may be used to assess valve function and the coronary arteries when surgery is being considered.[4]

Interprofessional Care

Prophylactic Treatment. The situations and conditions requiring antibiotic prophylaxis are presented in Table 36-2.

Drug Therapy. Accurate identification of the causative organism is the key to successful treatment of IE. Long-term treatment is necessary to kill dormant bacteria within the valvular vegetations. Complete removal of the organism generally takes weeks, and relapses are common.[3]

Patients are hospitalized and IV antibiotic therapy, based on blood cultures, is started. The effectiveness of therapy is assessed with subsequent blood cultures. Cultures that remain positive indicate inadequate or inappropriate selection of antibiotic, aortic root or myocardial abscess, or the wrong diagnosis (e.g., an infection elsewhere).

Fungal endocarditis and PVE respond poorly to antibiotic therapy alone. Early valve replacement followed by prolonged (6 weeks or more) antibiotics is needed in these situations. Valve replacement (discussed later in this chapter) has become an important adjunct procedure in the management of IE.[3]

Fever may persist for several days after treatment has been started. It can be treated with aspirin, acetaminophen (Tylenol), fluids, and rest. Complete bed rest is usually not needed unless the temperature remains elevated, or there are signs of HF. Endocarditis with HF responds poorly to drug therapy and valve replacement and is often life threatening.

! SAFETY ALERT Communicating Test Results

- The results of a blood culture on a patient diagnosed with IE indicate that the causative organism is not susceptible to the ordered antibiotic.
- Immediately share this information with the HCP.
- A National Patient Safety Goal stresses the importance of communicating critical test results to the right HCP in a timely manner.

TABLE 36-2 Antibiotic Prophylaxis to Prevent Endocarditis

Target Groups for Prophylactic Antibiotics

People with the following heart conditions should receive prophylactic antibiotics when they have the conditions or procedures listed below.

- Prosthetic heart valve or prosthetic material used to repair heart valve
- Previous history of infectious endocarditis
- Congenital heart disease (CHD)*
  - Unrepaired cyanotic CHD (including palliative shunts and conduits)
  - Repaired congenital heart defect with prosthetic material or device for 6 mo after the procedure
  - Repaired CHD with residual defects at the site or adjacent to the site of prosthetic patch or prosthetic device
- Heart transplantation recipients who develop heart valve disease

Conditions or Procedures Requiring Antibiotic Prophylaxis*

When the target groups have the following conditions or procedures, they need prophylactic antibiotics.

- Oral
  - Dental manipulation involving the gums or roots of the teeth
  - Dental manipulation involving puncture of the oral mucosa
- Respiratory
  - Respiratory tract incisions (e.g., biopsy)
  - Tonsillectomy and adenoidectomy
- Surgery
  - Procedures that involve infected skin, skin structures, or musculoskeletal tissue

Sources: Habib G, Hoen B, Tornos P, et al: Guidelines on the prevention, diagnosis and treatment of infective endocarditis (new version 2009): the Task Force on the Prevention, Diagnosis, and Treatment of Infective Endocarditis of the European Society of Cardiology, *Eur Heart J* 30:2369, 2009. Nishimura RA, Otto CM, Bonow RO, et al: 2014 AHA/ACC Guidelines for the management of patients with valvular heart disease: executive summary: a report of the American College of Cardiology/American Heart Association Task Force on Practice Guidelines, *Circulation* 129:2440, 2014.
*Except for the conditions listed above, prophylaxis is no longer recommended for any form of CHD or for patients undergoing gastrointestinal or genitourinary tract procedures.

❖ NURSING MANAGEMENT: INFECTIVE ENDOCARDITIS

◆ Nursing Assessment

Subjective and objective data that you should obtain from a patient with IE are found in Table 36-3. Assess vital signs together with heart sounds to detect a murmur, a change in a preexisting murmur, and extra sounds (e.g., S_3).

Arthralgia is common in IE. It may involve multiple joints and be accompanied by myalgias. Assess the patient for joint tenderness, decreased range of motion (ROM), and muscle tenderness. Examine the patient for petechiae, splinter hemorrhages, and Osler's nodes. Complete a general systems assessment to determine any hemodynamic or embolic complications.

◆ Nursing Diagnoses

Nursing diagnoses for the patient with IE may include, but are not limited to, the following:

- Decreased cardiac output *related to* altered heart rhythm, valvular insufficiency, and fluid overload
- Activity intolerance *related to* generalized weakness, arthralgia, and alteration in O_2 transport secondary to valvular dysfunction

Additional information on nursing diagnoses is presented in eNursing Care Plan 36-1 available on the website for this chapter.

TABLE 36-3 Nursing Assessment

Infective Endocarditis

Subjective Data

Important Health Information

Past health history: Valvular, congenital, or syphilitic heart disease, including valve repair or replacement. Previous endocarditis, childbirth, staphylococcal or streptococcal infections, hospital-acquired bacteremia

Medications: Immunosuppressive therapy

Surgery or other treatments: Recent obstetric or gynecologic procedures. Invasive procedures, including catheterization, cystoscopy. Recent dental or surgical procedures, GI procedures (e.g., endoscopy)

Functional Health Patterns

Health perception–health management: IV drug abuse, alcohol abuse. Malaise

Nutritional-metabolic: Weight gain or loss, anorexia. Chills, diaphoresis

Elimination: Bloody urine

Activity-exercise: Exercise intolerance, generalized weakness, fatigue. Cough, dyspnea on exertion, orthopnea, palpitations

Sleep-rest: Night sweats

Cognitive-perceptual: Chest, back, or abdominal pain. Headache, joint tenderness, muscle tenderness

Objective Data

General

Fever

Integumentary

Osler's nodes on extremities, splinter hemorrhages under nail beds, Janeway's lesions on fingertips, palms, soles of feet, and toes. Petechiae of skin, mucous membranes, or conjunctivae. Purpura, peripheral edema, finger clubbing

Respiratory

Tachypnea, crackles

Cardiovascular

Dysrhythmia, tachycardia, new murmurs, S_3, S_4. Retinal hemorrhages

Possible Diagnostic Findings

Leukocytosis, anemia, ↑ ESR, ↑ CRP and cardiac biomarkers. Positive blood cultures, hematuria. Echocardiogram showing chamber enlargement, valvular dysfunction, and vegetations. Chest x-ray showing cardiomegaly and pulmonary infiltrates. ECG demonstrating ischemia and conduction defects. Signs of systemic embolization or pulmonary embolism

CRP, C-reactive protein; *ESR*, erythrocyte sedimentation rate.

◆ Planning

The overall goals for the patient with IE include (1) normal or baseline heart function, (2) performance of activities of daily living (ADLs) without fatigue, and (3) knowledge of the therapeutic regimen to prevent recurrence of endocarditis.

◆ Nursing Implementation

◆ **Health Promotion.** The incidence of IE can be decreased by identifying individuals who are at risk for the disease (Tables 36-1 and 36-2). Assessment of the patient's history and an understanding of the disease are crucial for planning and implementing appropriate health promotion strategies.

Teaching the patient at high risk for IE helps to reduce the incidence and recurrence of the disease. Teaching is important for the patient's understanding of and adherence to the treatment regimen. Tell the patient to avoid people with infections, especially upper respiratory tract infections, and to report cold, flu, and cough symptoms. Stress the importance of avoiding excessive fatigue, and the need to plan rest periods before and after activity. Good oral hygiene, including daily care and regular dental visits, is critical.[3]

Tell the patient to inform HCPs performing certain invasive procedures of the history of IE. Be certain the patient understands the importance of prophylactic antibiotic therapy before certain invasive procedures. Refer the patient with a history of IVDA for drug rehabilitation.

◆ **Ambulatory Care.** A patient with IE has many problems that require nursing management (see eNursing Care Plan 36-1 on the website for this chapter). IE generally requires treatment with antibiotics for 4 to 6 weeks. After initial treatment in the hospital, the patient may continue treatment at home if hemodynamically stable and adherent. Assess the home setting for adequate support. Patients who receive outpatient IV antibiotics require vigilant home nursing care.

Assessment findings are often nonspecific (Table 36-3) but can help with the treatment plan. Fever, chronic or intermittent, is a common early sign. Tell the patient and caregiver about the importance of monitoring body temperature. Persistent temperature elevations may mean that the antibiotic is ineffective. Patients with IE are at risk for life-threatening complications, such as stroke, pulmonary edema, and HF. Teach patients and caregivers to recognize signs and symptoms of these complications (e.g., change in mental status, dyspnea, chest pain, unexplained weight gain).

The patient with IE needs adequate periods of physical and emotional rest. Bed rest may be necessary when the patient has fever or complications (e.g., heart damage). Otherwise the patient may walk and perform moderate activity. To prevent problems related to decreased mobility, teach the patient to wear elastic compression stockings, perform ROM exercises, and deep breathe and cough every 2 hours. The patient may experience anxiety and fear associated with the illness. You must recognize this and begin strategies to help the patient cope with the illness.

Monitor laboratory data to determine the effectiveness of the antibiotic therapy. Ongoing monitoring of the patient's blood cultures is necessary to ensure destruction of the infecting organism. Assess IV lines for patency and signs of complications (e.g., phlebitis). Give antibiotics as ordered, and monitor the patient for any adverse drug reactions.

Management also focuses on teaching the patient and caregiver the nature of the disease and on reducing the risk of reinfection. Explain to the patient the relationship of follow-up care, good nutrition and dental care, and early treatment of common infections (e.g., colds) to stay healthy. Teach the patient about symptoms that may indicate another infection (e.g., fever, fatigue, chills). Tell the patient to notify the HCP if any of these symptoms occur. Finally, tell the patient about the importance of prophylactic antibiotic therapy before certain invasive procedures (Table 36-2).

◆ Evaluation

The expected outcomes are that the patient with IE will

- Maintain adequate tissue and organ perfusion
- Maintain normal body temperature
- Report an increase in physical and emotional comfort

Additional information on expected outcomes for the patient with IE is presented in eNursing Care Plan 36-1 on the website for this chapter.

ACUTE PERICARDITIS

Pericarditis is a condition caused by inflammation of the pericardial sac (pericardium).The pericardium is composed of the inner serous membrane (visceral pericardium) and the outer fibrous (parietal) layer (Fig. 36-1). The pericardial space is the cavity between these two layers. Normally it contains 10 to 15 mL of serous fluid. The pericardium serves an anchoring function, provides lubrication to decrease friction between heart contractions, and helps to prevent excessive dilation of the heart during diastole. It may be congenitally absent or surgically removed.

Etiology and Pathophysiology

Common causes of acute pericarditis are listed in Table 36-4. Most often the cause of acute pericarditis is *idiopathic* (unknown), with a variety of suspected viral causes. The coxsackievirus B is the most commonly identified virus.[5]

Pericarditis in the patient with an MI may be described as two distinct syndromes. The first is *acute pericarditis,* which may occur within the first 48 to 72 hours after an MI. The second is *Dressler syndrome* (late pericarditis), which occurs 4 to 6 weeks after an MI (see Chapter 33). An inflammatory response is the characteristic pathologic finding in acute pericarditis. There is an influx of neutrophils, increased pericardial vascularity, and eventually fibrin deposition on the epicardium (Fig. 36-4).

TABLE 36-4 Common Causes of Pericarditis

Infectious

- Viral: Coxsackie A and B virus, echovirus, adenovirus, mumps, hepatitis, Epstein-Barr, varicella zoster, human immunodeficiency virus
- Bacterial: Pneumococci, staphylococci, streptococci, *Neisseria gonorrhoeae, Legionella pneumophila, Mycobacterium tuberculosis,* septicemia from gram-negative organisms
- Fungal: *Histoplasma, Candida* species
- Others: Toxoplasmosis, Lyme disease

Noninfectious

- Renal failure
- Acute myocardial infarction
- Neoplasms: Lung cancer, breast cancer, leukemia, Hodgkin's lymphoma, non-Hodgkin's lymphoma
- Trauma: Thoracic surgery, pacemaker insertion, cardiac diagnostic procedures
- Radiation
- Dissecting aortic aneurysm
- Myxedema

Hypersensitive or Autoimmune

- Dressler syndrome
- Postpericardiotomy syndrome
- Rheumatic fever
- Drug reactions (e.g., procainamide, hydralazine)
- Rheumatologic diseases: Rheumatoid arthritis, systemic lupus erythematosus, systemic sclerosis (scleroderma), ankylosing spondylitis

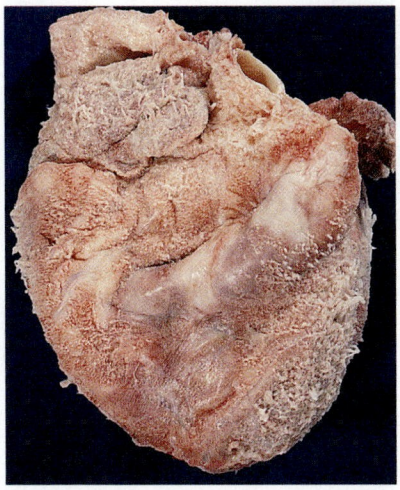

FIG. 36-4 Acute pericarditis. Note shaggy coat of fibers covering surface of heart. (From Damjanov I, Linder J: *Pathology: a color atlas,* St Louis, 2000, Mosby.)

Clinical Manifestations

In acute pericarditis, clinical symptoms include progressive, frequently severe, sharp chest pain. The pain is generally worse with deep inspiration and when lying flat. It is relieved by sitting up and leaning forward. The pain may radiate to the neck, arms, or left shoulder, making it difficult to differentiate from angina. One distinction is that the pain from pericarditis can be referred to the trapezius muscle (shoulder, upper back). The dyspnea that accompanies acute pericarditis is related to the patient's need to breathe in rapid, shallow breaths to avoid chest pain. Dyspnea may be aggravated by fever and anxiety.

The hallmark finding in acute pericarditis is the *pericardial friction rub.* The rub is a scratching, grating, high-pitched sound believed to result from friction between the roughened pericardial and epicardial surfaces. It is best heard with the stethoscope placed at the lower left sternal border of the chest with the patient leaning forward. Since it is difficult to tell a pericardial friction rub from a pleural friction rub, ask the patient to hold his or her breath. If you still hear the rub, then it is cardiac. Pericardial friction rubs may require frequent attempts to identify because they are often intermittent and short lived.

Complications

Two major complications that may result from acute pericarditis are pericardial effusion and cardiac tamponade. *Pericardial effusion* is a build-up of fluid in the pericardium. It can occur rapidly (e.g., chest trauma) or slowly (e.g., tuberculosis pericarditis). Large effusions may compress nearby structures. Pulmonary tissue compression can cause cough, dyspnea, and tachypnea. Phrenic nerve compression can cause hiccups, and compression of the laryngeal nerve may result in hoarseness. Heart sounds are generally distant and muffled, although BP is usually maintained.

Cardiac tamponade develops as the pericardial effusion increases in volume. This results in compression of the heart. The speed of fluid accumulation affects the severity of clinical manifestations. Cardiac tamponade can occur acutely (e.g., rupture of heart, trauma) or subacutely (e.g., secondary to renal failure, malignancy).

The patient with cardiac tamponade may report chest pain and is often confused, anxious, and restless. As the compression of the heart increases, there is decreased cardiac output (CO), muffled heart sounds, and narrowed pulse pressure. The patient develops tachypnea and tachycardia. Neck veins are usually markedly distended because of increased jugular venous pressure.

Pulsus paradoxus, which may be present, is a decrease in systolic BP during inspiration that is exaggerated in cardiac tamponade (Table 36-5). In a patient with a slow onset of a cardiac tamponade, dyspnea may be the only clinical manifestation.

TABLE 36-5 Measurement of Pulsus Paradoxus

1. Position the patient in a semirecumbent position.
2. Instruct patient to breathe normally.*
3. Using a manually operated BP cuff, determine systolic BP.
4. Inflate BP cuff at least 20 mm Hg above systolic BP.
5. Deflate cuff slowly until you hear sounds throughout the respiratory cycle (inspiration and expiration), and note the pressure.
6. Determine the difference between the measurements taken in steps 4 and 5. This will equal the amount of paradox:

Sounds heard on expiration at	110 mm Hg
Sounds heard throughout cycle at	–82 mm Hg
Amount of paradox	28 mm Hg

The difference is normally <10 mm Hg. If the difference is >10 mm Hg, cardiac tamponade may be present.

*Ask the patient to breathe slowly and deeply to reveal this finding when pulsus paradoxus is not severe.

Diagnostic Studies

The ECG is useful in the diagnosis of acute pericarditis, with changes noted in approximately 90% of cases. The most sensitive ECG changes include diffuse (widespread) ST segment elevations. This reflects the abnormal repolarization that develops secondary to the pericardial inflammation. You need to differentiate these changes from the ST changes seen in MI. (See Chapter 35 for more information on ECG monitoring.)

Echocardiographic findings are most useful in determining the presence of a pericardial effusion or cardiac tamponade. Methods such as Doppler imaging and color M-mode assess diastolic function and diagnose constrictive pericarditis (discussed later in the chapter). A CT scan and MRI provide for visualization of the pericardium and pericardial space. Chest x-ray findings are generally normal, but cardiomegaly may be seen in a patient who has a large pericardial effusion (Fig. 36-5).

Common laboratory findings include leukocytosis and elevation of CRP and ESR. Troponin levels may be elevated in patients with ST segment elevation and acute pericarditis, which could indicate concurrent heart damage. HIV and antinuclear antibody testing may be done. The fluid obtained during pericardiocentesis or the tissue from a pericardial biopsy may be studied to determine the cause of the pericarditis.

Interprofessional Care

Management of acute pericarditis is aimed at identifying and treating the underlying problem and symptoms (Table 36-6). Antibiotics treat bacterial pericarditis, and nonsteroidal antiinflammatory drugs (NSAIDs) (e.g., salicylates [aspirin], ibuprofen) control the pain and inflammation. Corticosteroids are generally reserved for patients with pericarditis secondary to systemic lupus erythematosus, patients already taking corticosteroids for rheumatologic or other autoimmune conditions, or patients who do not respond to NSAIDs. They are used

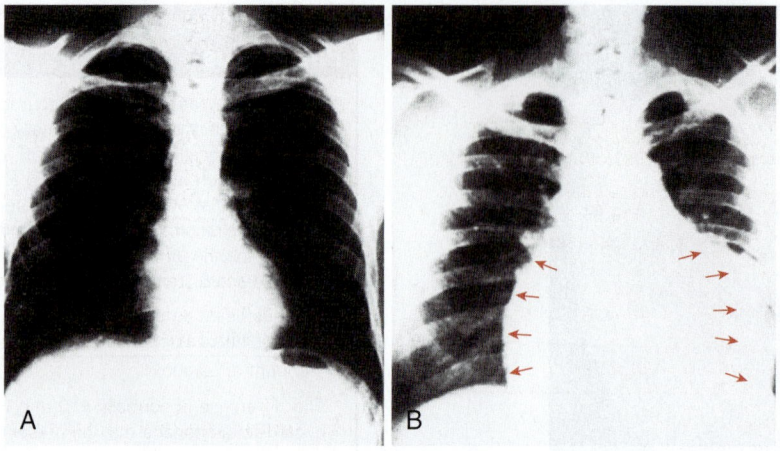

FIG. 36-5 **A,** X-ray of a normal chest. **B,** Pericardial effusion is present, and the cardiac silhouette is enlarged with a globular shape *(arrows)*. (From Guzzetta CE, Dossey BM: *Cardiovascular nursing: holistic practice,* St Louis, 1992, Mosby.)

TABLE 36-6 Interprofessional Care

Acute Pericarditis

Diagnostic Assessment	Management

• History and physical examination (assess for pericardial friction rub, pulsus paradoxus)
• Laboratory: CRP, ESR, white blood cell count
• Electrocardiogram
• Chest x-ray
• Echocardiogram
• CT scan
• MRI
• Pericardiocentesis, pericardial window
• Pericardial biopsy
	• Treatment of underlying disease
	• Bed rest
	• Drug therapy
	  • Nonsteroidal antiinflammatory drugs
	  • Corticosteroids
	• Pericardiocentesis (for tamponade)
	• Pericardial window (for tamponade or ongoing pericardial effusion)

CRP, C-reactive protein; *ESR,* erythrocyte sedimentation rate.

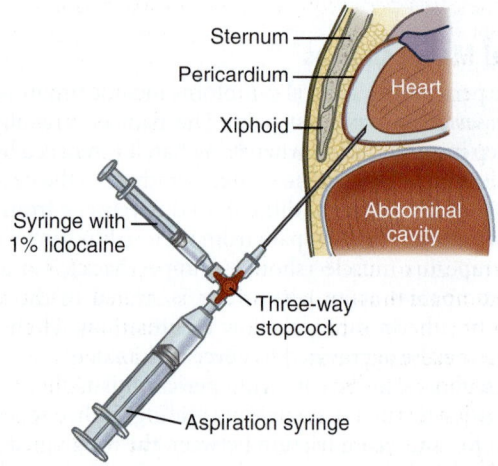

FIG. 36-6 Pericardiocentesis performed under sterile conditions in conjunction with electrocardiogram (ECG) and hemodynamic measurements.

cautiously because of their numerous side effects (see Chapter 49). Colchicine, an antiinflammatory drug used for gout, can be used for patients who have recurrent pericarditis.[5]

Pericardiocentesis is usually done for pericardial effusion with acute cardiac tamponade, purulent pericarditis, and suspected neoplasm. Hemodynamic support for the patient being prepared for the pericardiocentesis may include giving volume expanders and inotropic agents (e.g., dopamine) and discontinuing any anticoagulants. The procedure is done rapidly and safely using a percutaneous approach that is guided by echocardiography (Fig. 36-6). A needle is inserted into the pericardial space to remove fluid for analysis and to relieve heart pressure. Complications from pericardiocentesis include dysrhythmias, further cardiac tamponade, pneumomediastinum, pneumothorax, myocardial laceration, and coronary artery laceration.

A *pericardial window* can be used for diagnosis or for drainage of excess fluid. This involves cutting a "window" or portion of the pericardium. This allows the fluid to drain continuously into the peritoneum or chest.

❖ NURSING MANAGEMENT: ACUTE PERICARDITIS

The management of the patient's pain and anxiety during acute pericarditis is your primary nursing consideration. Assess the pain to distinguish angina (myocardial ischemia) (see Table 33-7) from the pain of pericarditis. Pericarditis pain is usually located in the precordium or left trapezius region and has a sharp, pleuritic quality that increases with inspiration. Pain is often relieved when the patient sits up or leans forward and is worse when lying flat.

An ECG can help to distinguish the cause of pain. In acute pericarditis, there are diffuse ST segment changes. In myocardial ischemia, there are usually localized ST segment changes. In addition, in acute pericarditis serial ECGs do not show evolving changes such as those with MI.

Pain relief measures include keeping the patient on bed rest with the head of the bed raised to 45 degrees and providing an overbed table for support. Antiinflammatory drugs can help control the pain. However, because of the risk of gastrointestinal (GI) bleeding, give these drugs with food or milk and tell the patient to avoid alcohol. Other drugs, such as a proton pump inhibitor (e.g., pantoprazole [Protonix]), may be given to reduce stomach acid.

Anxiety-reducing measures for the patient with acute pericarditis include providing simple, complete explanations of all procedures and possible causes of the pain. These explanations are particularly important for the patient whose diagnosis of acute pericarditis is being established and for the patient who has previously experienced angina or an MI.

The patient with acute pericarditis is at risk for cardiac tamponade and decreased CO. Monitor for manifestations of tamponade and prepare for possible pericardiocentesis.

CHECK YOUR PRACTICE

You are assigned to a 58-yr-old male patient who had an MI 3 days ago. He has now developed pericarditis. When you are making your rounds, you assess that the patient is slightly confused, has a rapid heart rate, and has prominent neck veins.

- What should you do next?

CHRONIC CONSTRICTIVE PERICARDITIS

Etiology and Pathophysiology

Chronic constrictive pericarditis results from scarring of the pericardium with consequent loss of elasticity of the pericardial sac. It usually begins with an initial episode of acute pericarditis. It is characterized by fibrin deposition with a clinically undetected pericardial effusion. Reabsorption of the effusion slowly follows, with progression toward the chronic stage. This involves fibrous scarring, thickening of the pericardium from calcium deposition, and eventual destruction of the pericardial space. The fibrotic, thickened, and adherent pericardium encases the heart. This impairs the ability of the atria and ventricles to stretch adequately.

Clinical Manifestations and Diagnostic Studies

Manifestations of chronic constrictive pericarditis occur over time and mimic those of HF and cor pulmonale. Decreased CO accounts for many of the clinical manifestations. These include dyspnea on exertion, peripheral edema, ascites, fatigue, anorexia, and weight loss. The most prominent finding on physical examination is jugular venous distention (JVD). Unlike with cardiac tamponade, the presence of pulsus paradoxus (greater than 10 mm Hg) is not common.

ECG changes are often nonspecific in chronic constrictive pericarditis. The heart on the chest x-ray may be normal or enlarged depending on the degree of pericardial thickening and the presence of a pericardial effusion. 2-D echocardiography findings may reveal a thickened pericardium but without a large pericardial effusion. CT and MRI provide measurement of pericardial thickness and assessment of diastolic filling patterns.

❖ NURSING AND INTERPROFESSIONAL MANAGEMENT: CHRONIC CONSTRICTIVE PERICARDITIS

Unless the patient is free of symptoms or the condition is inoperable, the treatment of choice for chronic constrictive pericarditis is a *pericardiectomy.* This involves complete resection of the pericardium through a median sternotomy with the use of cardiopulmonary bypass (see Chapter 33). Some patients show immediate improvement after, but others may take weeks. The prognosis improves when surgery is done before the patient becomes clinically unstable.

MYOCARDITIS

Etiology and Pathophysiology

Myocarditis is a focal or diffuse inflammation of the myocardium. Possible causes include viruses, bacteria, fungi, radiation therapy, and pharmacologic and chemical factors. Coxsackie A and B viruses are the most common causative agents. Autoimmune disorders (e.g., polymyositis) have been linked with the development of myocarditis. It may also be idiopathic. Myocarditis is one of the most common causes of dilated cardiomyopathy[6] (discussed later in this chapter).

When the myocardium becomes infected, the causative agent invades the myocytes and causes cellular damage and necrosis. The immune response is activated, and cytokines and O_2 free radicals are released. As the infection progresses, an autoimmune response is activated. This causes further destruction of myocytes. Myocarditis results in heart dysfunction.

Clinical Manifestations

The clinical features of myocarditis are variable, ranging from a benign course without any overt symptoms to severe heart involvement or sudden cardiac death (SCD). Fever, fatigue, malaise, myalgias, pharyngitis, dyspnea, lymphadenopathy, and nausea and vomiting are early manifestations of the viral illness.

Early cardiac signs appear 7 to 10 days after viral infection. These include pleuritic chest pain with a pericardial friction rub and effusion because pericarditis often accompanies myocarditis. Late cardiac signs relate to the development of HF and may include an S_3 heart sound, crackles, JVD, syncope, peripheral edema, and angina.

Diagnostic Studies and Interprofessional Care

The ECG changes for a patient with myocarditis are often nonspecific but may reflect associated pericardial involvement (e.g., diffuse ST segment changes). Dysrhythmias and conduction disturbances may be present. Laboratory findings are often inconclusive. They may include mild to moderate leukocytosis and atypical lymphocytes, increased ESR and CRP levels, elevated levels of cardiac biomarkers such as troponin, and elevated viral titers. The virus is generally present in tissue and pericardial fluid samples only during the initial 8 to 10 days of illness.

Histologic confirmation of myocarditis is through an *endomyocardial biopsy.* A biopsy done during the first 6 weeks of acute illness is most diagnostic. This is the period in which lymphocytic infiltration and myocyte damage are present. Nuclear scans, echocardiography, and MRI are used to assess heart function.

Treatment for myocarditis consists of managing associated heart symptoms. Angiotensin-converting enzyme (ACE) inhibitors and β-adrenergic blockers (β-blockers) are used if the heart is enlarged or to treat HF (see Chapter 34). Diuretics reduce fluid volume and decrease preload. If hypotension is not present, IV drugs such as nitroprusside (Nitropress) and milrinone reduce afterload and improve CO by decreasing systemic vascular resistance. Digoxin (Lanoxin) improves heart contractility and reduces heart rate. However, it is used cautiously in patients with myocarditis because of the heart's increased sensitivity to the adverse effects of this drug (e.g., dysrhythmias) and the potential toxicity. Anticoagulation therapy reduces the risk of clot formation from blood stasis in patients with a low ejection fraction (EF).

DRUG ALERT Digoxin (Lanoxin)

- Use cautiously in patients with myocarditis.
- Myocarditis predisposes to drug-related dysrhythmias and toxicity.

Some types of myocarditis have an autoimmune basis and are treated with immunosuppressive agents. These drugs reduce heart inflammation and prevent irreversible heart damage. However, the use of these drugs for the treatment of myocarditis remains controversial since they may also lead to recurrence.[6]

General supportive measures for management of myocarditis include O_2 therapy, bed rest, and restricted activity. In cases of severe HF, intraaortic balloon pump therapy and ventricular assist devices may be required (see Chapters 34 and 65).

❖ NURSING MANAGEMENT: MYOCARDITIS

Decreased CO is an ongoing problem in the care of the patient with myocarditis. Focus your interventions on managing the signs and symptoms of HF. Select nursing measures to decrease cardiac workload. These include placing the patient in a semi-Fowler's position, spacing activity and rest periods, and providing a quiet environment. Carefully monitor drugs that increase the heart's contractility and decrease preload, afterload, or both. Evaluate the effectiveness of your interventions on an ongoing basis.

The patient may be anxious about the diagnosis of myocarditis and recovery. Assess the level of anxiety, take measures to decrease anxiety, and keep the patient and caregiver informed about the therapeutic plan.

The patient who receives immunosuppressive therapy is at increased risk for infection. Monitor for complications and provide the patient with proper infection control procedures.

Although most patients with myocarditis recover spontaneously, some may develop dilated cardiomyopathy (discussed later in this chapter). If severe HF occurs, the patient may require heart transplantation.

RHEUMATIC FEVER AND RHEUMATIC HEART DISEASE

Rheumatic fever (RF) is an acute inflammatory disease of the heart potentially involving all layers (endocardium, myocardium, and pericardium). **Rheumatic heart disease** is a chronic condition resulting from RF that is characterized by scarring and deformity of the heart valves.

Etiology and Pathophysiology

RF is a complication that occurs as a delayed result (usually after 2 to 3 weeks) of a group A streptococcal pharyngitis. Manifestations of RF appear to be related to an abnormal immunologic response to group A streptococcal cell membrane antigens.[7] RF affects the heart, skin, joints, and central nervous system (CNS). Rheumatic heart disease, caused by RF, primarily affects young adults.

RF has declined in developed countries because of the effective use of antibiotics to treat streptococcal infections. However, it remains an important public health problem in developing countries.[7]

Cardiac Lesions and Valve Deformities. About 40% of RF episodes are marked by pancarditis, meaning that all layers of the heart (endocardium, myocardium, and pericardium) are involved (Fig. 36-1). This gives rise to the term *rheumatic pancarditis.*

Rheumatic endocarditis is found mainly in the valves, with swelling and erosion of the valve leaflets. Vegetation forms from deposits of fibrin and blood cells in areas of erosion. The lesions initially create thickening of the valve leaflets, fusion of commissures and chordae tendineae, and fibrosis of the papillary muscle. Valve leaflets may become calcified, resulting in stenosis. The less mobile valve leaflets may not close properly, resulting in regurgitation. The mitral and aortic valves are most commonly affected.

Nodules, called *Aschoff's bodies,* are formed by a reaction to inflammation with swelling and destruction of collagen fibers. As the Aschoff's bodies age, they become more fibrous, and scar tissue forms in the myocardium. Rheumatic pericarditis develops and affects both layers of the pericardium. The layers become thick and covered with a fibrinous exudate. A serosanguineous pericardial effusion may develop. When healing occurs, fibrosis and adhesions develop that partially or completely destroy the pericardial sac. These pathophysiologic changes in the heart can begin during an initial attack of RF. Recurrent infections cause further structural damage.

Extracardiac Lesions. The lesions of RF are systemic and involve the skin, joints, and CNS. Painless subcutaneous nodules, arthralgias or arthritis, and chorea may develop.

Clinical Manifestations

A cluster of signs and symptoms, including laboratory findings, leads to the diagnosis of acute RF. Established criteria provide a basis for diagnosis.[8] The presence of two major criteria or one major and two minor criteria plus evidence of a preceding group A streptococcal infection indicate a high probability of acute RF (Table 36-7).

Major Criteria. *Carditis* is the most important manifestation of RF and results in three signs: (1) heart murmur or murmurs of mitral or aortic regurgitation, or mitral stenosis; (2) heart enlargement and HF secondary to myocarditis; and (3) pericarditis resulting in muffled heart sounds, chest pain, pericardial friction rub, or signs of effusion.

Monoarthritis or *polyarthritis* is the most common finding in RF. The inflammatory process affects the synovial

TABLE 36-7 Revised Jones Criteria for Diagnosing Rheumatic Fever*

Major Criteria
- Carditis: clinical and/or subclinical†
- Arthritis
  - Monoarthritis or polyarthritis
  - Polyarthralgia
- Sydenham's chorea
- Erythema marginatum
- Subcutaneous nodules

Minor Criteria
- Monoarthralgia
- Fever
- Laboratory findings: ↑ ESR and/or ↑ CRP
- ECG findings: Prolonged PR interval after accounting for age variability (unless carditis is a major criterion)

Evidence of Group A Streptococcal Infection
- Laboratory findings
- ↑ Antistreptolysin-O titer, positive throat culture, or positive rapid antigen test for group A streptococci

Modified from Gewitz MH, Baltimore RS, Tani LY, et al: Revision of the Jones criteria for the diagnosis of acute rheumatic fever in the era of Doppler echocardiography: a scientific statement from the American Heart Association, *Circulation* 131:1806, 2015.
CRP, C-reactive protein; *ESR,* erythrocyte sedimentation rate.
*Criteria apply to initial episodes of rheumatic fever in moderate or high risk populations as defined by an all age prevalence of rheumatic heart disease of ≥1 per 1000 population per year.
†Subclinical carditis is defined by echocardiographic valvulitis.

membranes of the joints. This causes swelling, heat, redness, tenderness, and limitation of motion. The larger joints, particularly the knees, ankles, elbows, and wrists, are most frequently affected.

Sydenham's chorea is the major CNS manifestation of RF. It is often a delayed sign occurring several months after the initial infection. It is characterized by involuntary movements, especially of the face and limbs; muscle weakness; and disturbances of speech and gait.

Erythema marginatum lesions are a less common feature of RF. The bright pink, nonpruritic, maplike macular lesions occur mainly on the trunk and proximal extremities and may be exacerbated by heat (e.g., warm bath).

Subcutaneous nodules, usually associated with severe carditis, are firm, small, hard, painless swellings located over extensor surfaces of joints, particularly the knees, wrists, and elbows.

Minor Criteria. Minor clinical manifestations (Table 36-7) are frequently present and are helpful in diagnosing the disease. The minor criteria are used as supplemental information to confirm the presence of RF when only one major criterion is present.

Evidence of Infection. In addition to the major and minor criteria, there must also be evidence of a preceding group A streptococcal infection. Table 36-7 lists the various laboratory tests used to confirm evidence of infection.

Complications

A complication that can result from RF is *chronic rheumatic carditis.* It results from changes in valvular structure that may occur months to years after an episode of RF. Rheumatic endocarditis can result in fibrous tissue growth in valve leaflets and chordae tendineae with scarring and contractures. The mitral valve is most frequently involved. The aortic and tricuspid valves may also be affected.

Diagnostic Studies and Interprofessional Care

No single diagnostic test exists for RF. An echocardiogram may show valvular insufficiency and pericardial fluid or thickening.[9] A chest x-ray may show an enlarged heart if HF is present. The most consistent ECG change is delayed AV conduction as evidenced by a prolonged PR interval.

Treatment consists of drug therapy and supportive measures (Table 36-8). Antibiotic therapy does not change the course of the acute disease or the development of carditis. It does eliminate residual group A streptococci remaining in the tonsils and pharynx and prevents the spread of organisms to close contacts. Salicylates, NSAIDs, and corticosteroids are the anti-inflammatory agents most widely used in the management of RF. All are effective in controlling the fever and joint manifestations. Salicylates or NSAIDs are used when arthritis is the main manifestation, and corticosteroids are used if severe carditis is present.

TABLE 36-8 Interprofessional Care

Rheumatic Fever

Diagnostic Assessment	Management

• History and physical examination
• Laboratory studies (Table 36-7)
  • Chest x-ray
  • Echocardiogram
  • Electrocardiogram
	• Bed rest or limited activity
	• Drug therapy
	  • Antibiotics
	  • Nonsteroidal antiinflammatory drugs
	  • Salicylates
	  • Corticosteroids

❖ NURSING MANAGEMENT: RHEUMATIC FEVER AND RHEUMATIC HEART DISEASE

◆ Nursing Assessment

Table 36-9 presents the subjective and objective data that you should obtain from a patient with RF and rheumatic heart disease.

Inspect the patient's skin for subcutaneous nodules and erythema marginatum. This involves palpating for subcutaneous nodules over all bony surfaces and along extensor tendons of the hands and feet. The nodules range in size from 1 to 4 cm and are hard, painless, and freely movable. Erythema marginatum can occur on the trunk and inner aspects of the upper arm and thigh. The erythematous maculae do not itch and are flat. Assess for these bright pink maculae in good light because the rash is difficult to observe, especially in dark-skinned patients.

TABLE 36-9 Nursing Assessment

Rheumatic Fever and Rheumatic Heart Disease

Subjective Data

Important Health Information

Past health history: Recent streptococcal infection, previous history of rheumatic fever or rheumatic heart disease

Functional Health Patterns

Health perception–health management: Family history of rheumatic fever. Malaise

Nutritional-metabolic: Anorexia, weight loss

Activity-exercise: Palpitations, generalized weakness, fatigue, ataxia

Cognitive-perceptual: Chest pain, widespread joint pain and tenderness (especially large joints)

Objective Data

General

Fever

Integumentary

Subcutaneous nodules and erythema marginatum

Cardiovascular

Tachycardia, pericardial friction rub, muffled heart sounds, murmurs, peripheral edema

Neurologic

Chorea (involuntary, purposeless, rapid motions; facial grimaces)

Musculoskeletal

Signs of monoarthritis or polyarthritis, including swelling, heat, redness, limitation of motion (especially of knees, ankles, elbows, shoulders, wrists)

Possible Diagnostic Findings

Cardiomegaly on chest x-ray. Prolonged PR interval on ECG. Valve abnormalities, chamber dilation, and pericardial effusion on echocardiogram. ↑ antistreptolysin-O titer, positive throat culture, positive rapid antigen test for group A streptococci, ↑ ESR, ↑ CRP, leukocytosis

CRP, C-reactive protein; *ESR,* erythrocyte sedimentation rate.

Nursing Diagnoses

Nursing diagnoses for the patient with RF and rheumatic heart disease may include, but are not limited to, the following:

- Decreased CO *related to* valve dysfunction or HF
- Activity intolerance *related to* arthralgia or arthritis secondary to joint pain, pain from pericarditis, and HF
- Ineffective health management *related to* lack of knowledge concerning possible disease sequelae and the need for long-term prophylactic antibiotic therapy

Planning

The goals for a patient with RF and rheumatic heart disease include (1) normal or baseline heart function, (2) resumption of daily activities without joint pain, and (3) verbalization of the ability to manage the disease sequelae.

Nursing Implementation

Health Promotion. RF is a preventable heart disease. It involves early detection and immediate treatment of group A streptococcal pharyngitis. Adequate treatment of streptococcal pharyngitis prevents initial attacks of RF. Treatment with oral penicillin V (Penicillin VK) or amoxicillin (Moxatag) for 10 days is recommended. If the patient is allergic to penicillin, a narrow-spectrum cephalosporin (e.g., cephalexin [Keflex]), clindamycin (Cleocin), azithromycin (Zithromax) is used.[10] Therapy requires strict adherence to the full course of treatment. Your role is to teach people in the community to seek medical attention for symptoms of streptococcal pharyngitis and to emphasize the need for prompt and adequate treatment.

Acute Care. The primary goals of managing a patient with RF are to (1) control and remove the infecting organism; (2) prevent heart complications; and (3) relieve joint pain, fever, and other symptoms. Give antibiotics as ordered to treat the streptococcal infection. Teach the patient that completing the full course of antibiotics is vital to successful treatment. Give salicylates, NSAIDs, and corticosteroids as ordered and monitor fluid intake as appropriate.

Promoting optimal rest is essential to reduce cardiac workload and the body's metabolic needs. A priority nursing goal is relief of joint pain. Position painful joints for comfort and proper alignment. Apply heat and give drugs as ordered for joint pain.

After the acute symptoms have subsided, the patient without carditis can walk. If the patient has carditis with HF, bed rest restrictions may apply (see Chapter 34 for care of a patient with HF). Stress the importance of nonstrenuous activities once recovery has begun.

CHECK YOUR PRACTICE

Your 28-year-old male patient is recovering from carditis secondary to RF. You are preparing him for discharge from the hospital. When you walk into his room, you notice that he is pacing the floor and seems quite upset. You ask him to sit down so you can talk. He tells you, "I'm a cardiac cripple. I'll never be able to play ball with my sons or go skiing again. I might as well just go to bed and stay there."

- What are the key elements that you should include in your teaching plan?

Ambulatory Care. The aim of secondary prevention is to stop the recurrence of RF. Teach the patient with a history of RF about the disease process, possible sequelae, and the need for ongoing antibiotic prophylaxis.

Prior history of RF makes the patient more susceptible to a second attack after a streptococcal infection. The best prevention is treatment with prophylactic antibiotics. Patients with RF without carditis require prophylaxis until age 20 and for a minimum of 5 years. Patients with rheumatic carditis and residual heart disease (e.g., persistent valve disease) need longer-term and even lifelong prophylaxis.[10]

Teach the patient about good nutrition, hygienic practices, and adequate rest. Caution the patient about the possible development of heart valve disease. Tell the patient to seek medical attention if symptoms such as excessive fatigue, dizziness, palpitations, unexplained weight gain, or exertional dyspnea develop.[11]

Evaluation

The expected outcomes are that the patient with RF and rheumatic heart disease will

- Be able to perform ADLs with minimal fatigue and pain
- Adhere to treatment regimen
- Express confidence in managing disease
- Use measures to prevent complications

VALVULAR HEART DISEASE

The heart contains two AV valves (mitral and tricuspid) and two semilunar valves (aortic and pulmonic), which control blood flow through the heart (see Fig. 31-1). Valvular heart disease is defined according to the valve or valves affected and the type of dysfunction: stenosis or regurgitation (Fig. 36-7).

The pressure on either side of an open valve is normally equal. However, in a stenotic valve, the valve opening is smaller. The forward flow of blood is impaired. This creates a difference

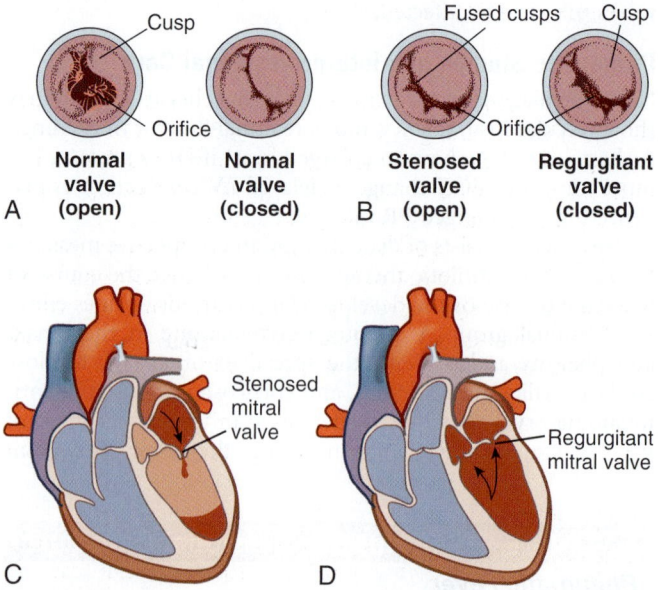

FIG. 36-7 Valvular stenosis and regurgitation. **A,** Normal position of the valve leaflets, or cusps, when the valve is open and closed. **B,** Open position of a stenosed valve *(left)* and closed position of regurgitant valve *(right)*. **C,** Hemodynamic effect of mitral stenosis. The stenosed valve is unable to open sufficiently during left atrial systole, inhibiting left ventricular filling. **D,** Hemodynamic effect of mitral regurgitation. The mitral valve does not close completely during left ventricular systole, permitting blood to reenter the left atrium. At the same time, blood is moving forward through the aortic valve. (From McCance KL, Huether SE: *Pathophysiology: the biologic basis for disease in adults and children*, ed 6, St Louis, 2010, Mosby.)

in pressure on the two sides of the open valve. The amount of **stenosis** (constriction or narrowing) is seen in the pressure differences (i.e., the higher the difference, the greater the stenosis). When **regurgitation** occurs (referred to as *incompetence* or *insufficiency*), there is incomplete closure of the valve. This results in the backward flow of blood.

Congenital heart conditions are the most common cause of valve disorders in children and adolescents. Valvular heart disease remains prevalent because of an increased number of older adults who have some form of heart disease. AS and mitral regurgitation (MR) are common valve disorders in older adults. Other causes of valve disease in adults include disorders related to acquired immunodeficiency syndrome and the use of some antiparkinsonian drugs.[12]

MITRAL VALVE STENOSIS

Etiology and Pathophysiology

Most cases of adult mitral valve stenosis result from rheumatic heart disease. Rheumatic mitral stenosis is widespread in developing countries. Less common causes are congenital mitral stenosis, rheumatoid arthritis, and systemic lupus erythematosus. Rheumatic endocarditis causes scarring of the valve leaflets and the chordae tendineae. Contractures and adhesions develop between the commissures (the junctional areas). The stenotic mitral valve takes on a "fish mouth" shape because of the thickening and shortening of the mitral valve structures.

These deformities block the blood flow and create a pressure difference between the left atrium and left ventricle during diastole. As a result, left atrial pressure and volume increase, causing higher pulmonary vasculature pressure. The overloaded left atrium places the patient at risk for atrial fibrillation. In chronic mitral stenosis, pressure overload occurs in the left atrium, pulmonary bed, and right ventricle.

Clinical Manifestations

The primary symptom of mitral stenosis is exertional dyspnea caused by reduced lung compliance (Table 36-10). Heart sounds include a loud first heart sound and a low-pitched, diastolic murmur (best heard at the apex with the stethoscope). Less often, patients may have hoarseness (from atrial enlargement pressing on the laryngeal nerve), hemoptysis (from pulmonary hypertension), and chest pain (from decreased CO and coronary perfusion). Emboli can form in the left atrium secondary to atrial fibrillation and cause a stroke.[12] Fatigue and palpitations from atrial fibrillation may also occur.

MITRAL VALVE REGURGITATION

Etiology and Pathophysiology

Mitral valve function depends on intact mitral leaflets, mitral annulus, chordae tendineae, papillary muscles, left atrium, and left ventricle. A defect in any of these structures can result in regurgitation. Most cases of mitral regurgitation (MR) are caused by MI, chronic rheumatic heart disease, mitral valve prolapse, ischemic papillary muscle dysfunction, and IE. MI with left ventricular failure increases the risk for rupture of the chordae tendineae and acute MR.

MR allows blood to flow backward from the left ventricle to the left atrium because of incomplete valve closure during systole. Both the left ventricle and left atrium must work harder to preserve an adequate CO. In acute MR the sudden increase in pressure and volume transmits to the pulmonary bed. This results in pulmonary edema and, if not treated, cardiogenic shock. In chronic MR the additional volume results in left atrial enlargement, left ventricular dilation and hypertrophy, and, finally, a decrease in CO.

TABLE 36-10 Manifestations of Valvular Heart Disease

Type	Manifestations
Mitral valve stenosis	Dyspnea on exertion, hemoptysis, fatigue. Atrial fibrillation on ECG. Palpitations. Loud, accentuated S_1. Low-pitched, diastolic murmur
Mitral valve regurgitation	*Acute:* Generally poorly tolerated. New systolic murmur with pulmonary edema and cardiogenic shock develop rapidly. *Chronic:* Weakness, fatigue, exertional dyspnea, palpitations, S_3 gallop, holosystolic murmur
Mitral valve prolapse	Palpitations, dyspnea, chest pain, activity intolerance, syncope, holosystolic murmur
Aortic valve stenosis	Angina, syncope, dyspnea on exertion, heart failure, normal or soft S_1, diminished or absent S_2, systolic murmur, prominent S_4
Aortic valve regurgitation	*Acute:* Abrupt onset of profound dyspnea, chest pain, left ventricular failure and cardiogenic shock *Chronic:* Fatigue, exertional dyspnea, orthopnea, PND. Water-hammer pulse, heaving precordial impulse, diminished or absent S_1, S_3, or S_4. Soft high-pitched diastolic murmur, Austin Flint murmur
Tricuspid and pulmonic stenosis	*Tricuspid:* Peripheral edema, ascites, hepatomegaly. Diastolic low-pitched murmur with increased intensity during inspiration *Pulmonic:* Fatigue, loud midsystolic murmur

PND, Paroxysmal nocturnal dyspnea.

Clinical Manifestations

The clinical course of MR is determined by the nature of its onset (Table 36-10). Patients with acute MR have thready, peripheral pulses and cool, clammy extremities. A low CO may mask a new systolic murmur. Rapid assessment (e.g., heart catheterization) and intervention (e.g., valve repair or replacement) are critical.

Patients with chronic MR may remain asymptomatic for many years. Early symptoms of left ventricular failure may include weakness, fatigue, palpitations, and dyspnea. These gradually progress to orthopnea, paroxysmal nocturnal dyspnea, and peripheral edema. Increased left ventricular volume leads to an audible third heart sound (S_3), even with normal left ventricular function. The murmur is a loud holosystolic murmur at the apex radiating to the left axilla. Patients with asymptomatic MR must be monitored carefully. Surgery (valve repair or replacement) should be considered before significant left ventricular failure or pulmonary hypertension develops.[12]

MITRAL VALVE PROLAPSE

Etiology and Pathophysiology

Mitral valve prolapse (MVP) is an abnormality of the mitral valve leaflets and the papillary muscles or chordae that allows the leaflets to prolapse, or buckle, back into the left atrium during systole (Fig. 36-8). It is the most common form of valvular heart disease in the United States. It affects both genders equally.[13]

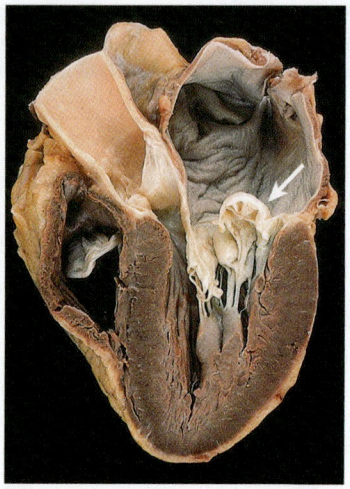

FIG. 36-8 Mitral valve prolapse. In this valvular abnormality, the mitral leaflets have prolapsed back into the left atrium. They also demonstrate hooding *(arrow)*. The left ventricle is on the right. (From Kumar V, Abbas AK, Aster JC, et al: *Robbins and Cotran pathologic basis of disease,* ed 8, Philadelphia, 2010, Saunders.)

The use of the term *prolapse* can be misleading because it is used even when the valve is working normally. MVP is usually benign, but serious complications can occur, including MR, IE, SCD, HF, and cerebral ischemia.

Genetic Link

Although the etiology of MVP is unknown, some patients have an increased familial incidence. The genetic inheritance is frequently autosomal dominant (see Chapter 12). MVP in this group results from a connective tissue defect affecting only the valve, or as part of Marfan's syndrome or other hereditary conditions that affect the structure of collagen in the body.

Clinical Manifestations

MVP covers a broad range of severity. Most patients are asymptomatic and remain so for their entire lives. About 10% of those with MVP become symptomatic. A characteristic of MVP is a murmur from regurgitation that is louder during systole. MVP does not alter S_1 or S_2 heart sounds. Severe MR is an uncommon but serious complication of MVP.

M-mode and 2-D echocardiography are used to confirm MVP. Dysrhythmias such as premature ventricular contractions, paroxysmal supraventricular tachycardia, and ventricular tachycardia may cause palpitations, light-headedness, and syncope. IE may occur in patients with MR associated with MVP.

Patients may or may not have chest pain. The cause of the chest pain is not known. It may be the result of abnormal tension on the papillary muscles. If chest pain occurs, episodes tend to occur in clusters, especially during periods of emotional stress. Dyspnea, palpitations, and syncope may occasionally accompany the chest pain and do not respond to antianginal treatment (e.g., nitrates). β-Blockers may be given to control palpitations and chest pain. Encourage the patient to stay hydrated, exercise regularly, and avoid caffeine.

The majority of patients with MVP generally have a benign, manageable course. For those who do develop symptomatic MR, no accepted medical therapy appears to delay the need for valve surgery.[13] A teaching plan for patients with MVP is presented in Table 36-11.

TABLE 36-11 Patient & Caregiver Teaching

Mitral Valve Prolapse

Include the following information in the teaching plan for a patient with mitral valve prolapse (MVP) and the patient's caregiver.

- Take drugs as prescribed (e.g., β-blockers to control palpitations, chest pain).
- Adopt healthy eating habits.
- Avoid caffeine because it is a stimulant and may exacerbate symptoms.
- If you use diet pills or other over-the-counter drugs, check for common ingredients that are stimulants (e.g., caffeine, ephedrine), since these can exacerbate symptoms.
- Begin (or maintain) an exercise program to achieve optimal health.
- Contact the HCP or emergency response system (ERS) if symptoms develop or worsen (e.g., palpitations, fatigue, shortness of breath, anxiety).

AORTIC VALVE STENOSIS

Etiology and Pathophysiology

Congenital **aortic stenosis (AS)** is generally found in childhood, adolescence, or young adulthood. In older adults, AS is a result of RF or degeneration that may have an etiology similar to that of coronary artery disease. It affects 3% of people over 65 years of age.[14] In rheumatic valve disease, fusion of the commissures and secondary calcification cause the valve leaflets to stiffen and retract, resulting in stenosis. AS due to rheumatic heart disease accompanies mitral valve disease. Isolated AS is usually nonrheumatic in origin. The incidence of rheumatic aortic valve disease has been decreasing, but degenerative stenosis is increasing as the population ages.

AS causes obstruction of blood flow from the left ventricle to the aorta during systole. The effect is left ventricular hypertrophy and increased myocardial O_2 consumption because of the increased myocardial mass. As the disease progresses and compensatory mechanisms fail, reduced CO leads to decreased tissue perfusion, pulmonary hypertension, and HF. Left untreated, severe AS has approximately a 50% mortality rate at 1 year.[14]

Clinical Manifestations

Manifestations of AS (Table 36-10) develop when the valve orifice becomes about one third its normal size. These manifestations include the classic triad of angina, syncope, and exertional dyspnea, reflecting left ventricular failure.[14]

The prognosis is poor for patients who exhibit manifestations and those whose valve obstruction is not fixed. Nitroglycerin is used cautiously to treat angina, since the drug can significantly reduce BP and worsen chest pain. Auscultation of AS often reveals a normal or soft S_1, a diminished or absent S_2, a systolic murmur, and a prominent S_4.

DRUG ALERT Nitroglycerin

- Use cautiously in patients with AS, since significant hypotension may occur.
- When the drug is used, chest pain can worsen due to a decrease in preload and drop in BP.

AORTIC VALVE REGURGITATION

Etiology and Pathophysiology

Aortic regurgitation (AR) may be the result of primary disease of the aortic valve leaflets, the aortic root, or both. Trauma, IE, or aortic dissection can cause acute AR, which constitutes a life-threatening emergency. Chronic AR is generally the result of rheumatic heart disease, a congenital bicuspid aortic valve, syphilis, or chronic rheumatic conditions, such as ankylosing spondylitis or reactive arthritis.

AR causes retrograde (backward) blood flow from the ascending aorta into the left ventricle during diastole. This results in volume overload. The left ventricle initially compensates for chronic AR by dilation and hypertrophy. Myocardial contractility eventually declines, and blood volume in the left atrium and pulmonary bed increases. This leads to pulmonary hypertension and right ventricular failure.

Clinical Manifestations

Patients with acute AR have sudden signs of cardiovascular collapse (Table 36-10). The left ventricle is exposed to aortic pressure during diastole. The patient develops severe dyspnea, chest pain, and hypotension indicating left ventricular failure and cardiogenic shock, a life-threatening emergency.

Patients with chronic, severe AR develop a *water-hammer pulse* (strong, quick beat that collapses immediately). Heart sounds may include a soft or absent S_1, S_3, or S_4 and a soft, high-pitched diastolic murmur.

The patient with chronic AR generally remains asymptomatic for years. Exertional dyspnea, orthopnea, and paroxysmal nocturnal dyspnea develop only after considerable heart dysfunction has occurred (Table 36-10). Angina occurs less frequently than in AS.

TRICUSPID AND PULMONIC VALVE DISEASE

Etiology and Pathophysiology

Diseases of the tricuspid and pulmonic valves are uncommon, with stenosis occurring more frequently than regurgitation. *Tricuspid stenosis* occurs almost exclusively in patients who have RF or who abuse IV drugs. Tricuspid stenosis results in right atrial enlargement and elevated systemic venous pressures. *Pulmonic stenosis* is almost always congenital and results in right ventricular hypertension and hypertrophy (Table 36-10).

DIAGNOSTIC STUDIES: VALVULAR HEART DISEASE

Diagnosis of valvular heart disease includes information from the patient's history and physical examination and a variety of tests (Table 36-12). A CT scan of the chest with contrast is the gold standard for evaluating aortic disorders. An echocardiogram reveals valve structure, function, and heart chamber size. Transesophageal echocardiography and Doppler color-flow imaging help diagnose and monitor valvular heart disease progression. Real-time 3-D echocardiography can help assess mitral valve and congenital heart disease.

Chest x-ray reveals the heart size, altered pulmonary circulation, and valve calcification. An ECG identifies heart rate, rhythm, and any ischemia or ventricular hypertrophy. Heart catheterization detects pressure changes in the heart chambers, records pressure differences across the valves, and measures the size of valve openings.

INTERPROFESSIONAL CARE: VALVULAR HEART DISEASE

Conservative Therapy

An important aspect of conservative management of valvular heart disease is prevention of recurrent RF and IE (Table 36-12). Treatment depends on the valve involved and disease severity.

TABLE 36-12 Interprofessional Care

Valvular Heart Disease

Diagnostic Assessment
- History and physical examination
- Chest x-ray
- CBC
- Electrocardiogram
- Echocardiography (Doppler and transesophageal)
- Heart catheterization

Management

Conservative Therapy
- Prophylactic antibiotic therapy (Table 36-2)
  - Rheumatic fever
  - Infective endocarditis
- Sodium restriction
- Drug therapy to treat or control HF
- Vasodilators* (e.g., nitrates, ACE inhibitors)
  - Positive inotropes (e.g., digoxin)
  - Diuretics
  - β-Blockers
- Anticoagulation therapy (see Table 37-10)
- Antidysrhythmic drugs
- Percutaneous transluminal balloon valvuloplasty
- Percutaneous valve replacement

Surgical Therapy
- Valve repair
  - Commissurotomy (valvulotomy)
  - Valvuloplasty
  - Annuloplasty
- Valve replacement

ACE, Angiotensin-converting enzyme; *HF*, heart failure.
*Use cautiously in patients with aortic stenosis.

It focuses on preventing exacerbations of HF, acute pulmonary edema, thromboembolism, and recurrent endocarditis. HF is treated with vasodilators, positive inotropes, β-blockers, diuretics, and a low-sodium diet (see Chapter 34).

Anticoagulant therapy prevents and treats systemic or pulmonary emboli. It is used prophylactically in patients with atrial fibrillation. Atrial dysrhythmias are common and treated with calcium channel blockers, β-blockers, antidysrhythmic drugs, or electrical cardioversion (see Chapter 35).

Percutaneous Transluminal Balloon Valvuloplasty. An alternative treatment for some patients with valvular heart disease is *percutaneous transluminal balloon valvuloplasty* (PTBV). During PTBV, the fused commissures are split open. Balloon valvuloplasty is used for mitral, tricuspid, and pulmonic stenosis, and less often for AS.

The procedure is done in the heart catheterization laboratory. It involves threading a balloon-tipped catheter from the femoral artery or vein to the stenotic valve. The balloon is inflated in an attempt to separate the valve leaflets. A single- or double-balloon technique may be used for the PTBV procedure. Currently, the use of a single Inoue balloon with hourglass shape allows sequential inflation (Fig. 36-9). This technique is the most popular because it is easy and has good results with few complications (e.g., left ventricular perforation). The PTBV procedure is generally indicated for older adults and for those who are poor surgery candidates. The long-term results of PTBV are similar to those of surgical commissurotomy.

Similar to PTBV, the Sapien Transcatheter Heart Valve (THV) is used for select patients with AS. The THV is inserted

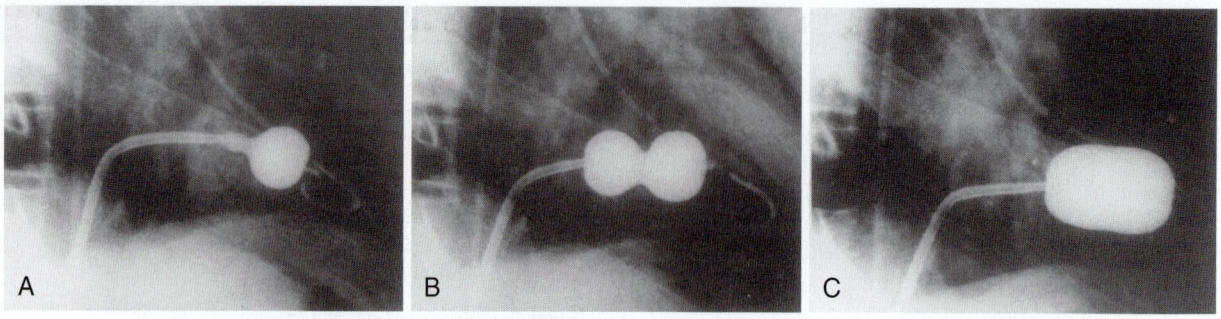

FIG. 36-9 Mitral valvuloplasty performed by the Inoue technique. The catheter is placed in the mitral valve and the distal part of the Inoue balloon inflated **(A).** The balloon is then pulled back in the mitral valve and inflated for 10 to 15 sec under fluoroscopic control **(B)** until the waist of the balloon is no longer visible **(C)** and the balloon falls back into the left atrium. (From Crawford MH, DiMarco JP, Paulus WJ: *Cardiology,* ed 3, Edinburgh, 2010, Mosby Ltd.)

through the femoral artery and moved to the heart. It is released and expanded with a balloon in the location of the aortic valve. This procedure is limited to patients who are eligible for surgery but who are at high risk for surgical complications (e.g., patients with multiple co-morbidities).

Surgical Therapy

The decision for surgical intervention depends on the patient's clinical state using the New York Heart Association classification system for functional disability (see Table 34-3). The type of surgery can be valve repair or valve replacement. The procedure that is used depends on the (1) valves involved, (2) pathology and severity of the disease, and (3) patient's clinical condition. All types of valve surgery are palliative, not curative, and patients require lifelong health care.

Valve Repair. Valve repair is usually the surgical procedure of choice. It has a lower operative mortality rate than valve replacement and is often used in mitral or tricuspid valvular heart disease.[14] Although valve repair avoids the risks of replacement, it may not restore total valve function.

Mitral *commissurotomy (valvulotomy)* is the procedure of choice for patients with pure mitral stenosis. The less precise closed method of commissurotomy has generally been replaced by the open method. In the *closed procedure* the surgeon inserts a transventricular dilator through the apex of the left ventricle into the opening of the mitral valve. The direct vision procedure, or *open procedure,* requires the use of cardiopulmonary bypass. The surgeon removes thrombi from the atrium and makes a commissure incision. Next, the fused chordae are separated by splitting the papillary muscle and debriding the calcified valve.

Open surgical *valvuloplasty* involves repair of the valve by suturing the torn leaflets, chordae tendineae, or papillary muscles. It is primarily used to treat mitral or tricuspid regurgitation.

Minimally invasive valvuloplasty surgery involves a ministernotomy or parasternal approach. It may include robotic and thoracoscopic surgical systems. Results compare with those of the open procedure. In addition, shorter lengths of stay, fewer blood transfusions, less pain, and lower risk of sternal infection and postoperative atrial fibrillation have been reported.[15]

For patients with mitral or tricuspid regurgitation, further valve repair or reconstruction using annuloplasty is an option. *Annuloplasty* involves reconstruction of the annulus, with or without the aid of prosthetic rings.

Valve Replacement. Valve replacement may be required for mitral, aortic, tricuspid, and occasionally pulmonic valve disease.

ETHICAL/LEGAL DILEMMAS

Do Not Resuscitate

Situation

J.L., a 68-yr-old man, is admitted for a second mitral valve surgery and coronary artery bypass graft surgery. He did not adhere to the treatment plan after his original surgery 7 years ago. You are worried about his future adherence with drugs, diet, and exercise. His kidneys are failing and he is on dialysis, making him a high-risk surgical patient. The patient and his caregiver want all possible treatment and refuse to discuss advance directives (ADs) or do not resuscitate (DNR) orders.

Ethical/Legal Points for Consideration

- Based on their expertise, HCPs have the right to refuse to provide treatment that offers no benefit to the patient.
- ADs do not include a DNR order. If the patient is unable to speak for himself or herself, a DNR order can be started only by the HCP after conversation with the health care proxy and/or nearest kin. The decision usually depends on evidence of the patient's preferences (substituted judgment standard) or what is in the best interest of the patient.
- If there is an AD refusing resuscitation, the HCP is required to act accordingly but is not compelled to enact a DNR without clear direction from the patient or proxy.
- Patient adherence with past treatment plans is not a factor that must be considered in DNR decisions. Many circumstances related to nonadherence are outside the patient's control, such as finances, transportation, availability of assistance, and declining physical and medical capabilities.
- If the involved parties disagree about the patient's treatment plan, a referral can be made to an ethics committee, they can seek treatment from another HCP, or they may seek legal intervention by way of a court order.

Discussion Questions

1. How can a lack of understanding or limited financial resources contribute to nonadherence with the plan of care?
2. What type of information should be provided to a patient and caregiver in discussions about ADs and DNR orders? Who should provide this information?
3. Who can initiate a referral to an ethics committee?

A wide variety of prosthetic valves are currently available. Desirable valves are nonthrombogenic and durable, and create minimal stenosis. Prosthetic valves are categorized as mechanical or biologic (tissue) valves (Fig. 36-10).

Mechanical valves are manufactured from artificial materials and consist of combinations of metal alloys, pyrolytic carbon, and Dacron. *Biologic valves* are constructed from bovine, porcine, and human (cadaver) heart tissue and usually contain

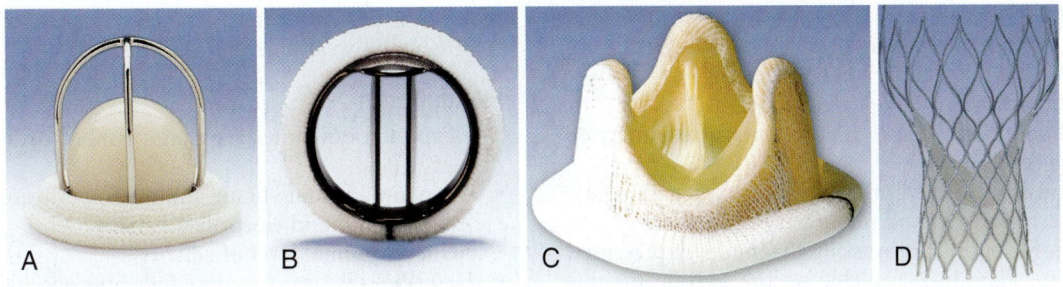

FIG. 36-10 Types of prosthetic heart valves. **A,** Starr-Edwards caged ball valve. **B,** St. Jude bi-leaflet valve. **C,** Carpentier-Edwards porcine valve. **D,** CoreValve transcatheter aortic valve (CV26 Hero), Medtronic 2015. (A through C, From Bonow RO, Mann DL, Zipes DP, et al: *Braunwald's heart disease: a textbook of cardiovascular medicine,* ed 9, Philadelphia, 2012, Saunders.)

INFORMATICS IN PRACTICE

Heart Surgery DVD/TV

- Many patients prefer to watch DVDs or the patient education channel of the hospital's TV system instead of reading educational pamphlets. For a patient facing heart surgery, these formats can be effective tools to teach the patient and caregiver what to expect before and after the procedure.
- Remember that the DVD or TV is not the teacher.
- Beforehand discuss what the DVD or TV will cover.
- Encourage the patient and caregiver to write down questions or note what they do not understand.
- After the patient and caregiver view the material, answer any questions they have. Reinforce important information.

some man-made materials. A "decellularizing" process removes the cadaver cells from the valve. This lowers the risk of immune response and tissue rejection. Biologic valves are asymmetric in shape and produce a more natural pattern of blood flow compared with mechanical valves. Asymmetric mechanical valve prototypes are being tested.

Mechanical prosthetic valves are more durable and last longer than biologic valves. However, they have an increased risk of thromboembolism and require long-term anticoagulation therapy.[13] The main risk of mechanical valves is bleeding from the use of anticoagulants. Biologic valves do not require anticoagulation therapy because of their low thrombogenicity. However, they are less durable and tend to cause early calcification, tissue degeneration, and stiffening of the leaflets. Either type of prosthetic valve can leak and cause endocarditis.

Minimally invasive aortic valve replacement uses a transcatheter or transapical approach and is the surgical choice for patients at high risk for traditional surgery.[16] The CoreValve transcatheter aortic valve is made of tissue obtained from the heart of a pig[17] (Fig. 36-10, *D*). Prolonged waiting time for aortic valve replacement is associated with greater mortality, and surgery should be done on a semi-urgent basis.[18]

Long-term anticoagulation is needed for those patients with biologic valves who have atrial fibrillation. Some patients with biologic valves or annuloplasty with prosthetic rings may need anticoagulation the first few months after surgery until the suture lines are covered by endothelial cells (endothelialized).

The choice of valves depends on many factors. For example, if a patient cannot take an anticoagulant (e.g., women of childbearing age), a biologic valve is considered. A mechanical valve may be best for a younger patient because it is more durable. For patients over age 65, durability is less important than the risks of bleeding from anticoagulants, so most receive a biologic valve.

TABLE 36-13 Nursing Assessment

Valvular Heart Disease

Subjective Data

Important Health Information

- *Past health history:* Rheumatic fever, infective endocarditis; congenital defects, heart attack, chest trauma, cardiomyopathy; syphilis, Marfan's syndrome, streptococcal infections

Functional Health Patterns

Health perception–health management: IV drug abuse, fatigue
Activity-exercise: Palpitations, generalized weakness, activity intolerance, dizziness, fainting, dyspnea on exertion, cough, hemoptysis, orthopnea
Sleep-rest: Paroxysmal nocturnal dyspnea
Cognitive-perceptual: Angina or atypical chest pain

Objective Data

General

Fever

Integumentary

Diaphoresis, flushing, cyanosis, clubbing, peripheral edema

Respiratory

Crackles, wheezes, hoarseness

Cardiovascular

Abnormal heart sounds, including murmurs, S_3, and S_4. Dysrhythmias, including atrial fibrillation, premature ventricular contractions. Tachycardia. ↑ or ↓ in pulse pressure, hypotension, water-hammer or thready peripheral pulses

Gastrointestinal

Ascites, hepatomegaly, unexplained weight gain

Possible Diagnostic Findings

Cardiomegaly on chest x-ray. ECG abnormalities specific to involved valve. Echocardiogram (valve disorders and chamber dilation), heart catheterization (abnormal valves, chamber pressures, cardiac output, and blood flow depending on involved valve)

❖ NURSING MANAGEMENT: VALVULAR DISORDERS

◆ Nursing Assessment

Table 36-13 presents the subjective and objective data to obtain from a patient with valve disease.

Nursing Diagnoses

Nursing diagnoses for the patient with valvular heart disease may include, but are not limited to, the following:

- Decreased CO *related to* valvular incompetence
- Excess fluid volume *related to* fluid retention secondary to valvular-induced HF
- Activity intolerance *related to* insufficient oxygenation secondary to decreased CO and pulmonary congestion

Additional information on nursing diagnoses is presented in eNursing Care Plan 36-2 available on the website for this chapter.

Planning

The overall goals for the patient with valve disease include (1) normal heart function, (2) improved activity tolerance, and (3) an understanding of the disease process and health maintenance measures.

Nursing Implementation

Health Promotion. Diagnosing and treating streptococcal infections and providing prophylactic antibiotics for patients with a history of RF are critical to prevent acquired rheumatic valve disease. The patient at risk for endocarditis and any patient with certain heart conditions must also receive prophylactic antibiotics (Table 36-2).

The patient must adhere to ordered therapies. The person with a history of RF, endocarditis, and congenital heart disease should know the symptoms of valvular heart disease so that early medical treatment may begin.

Acute Care and Ambulatory Care. A patient with progressive valvular heart disease may need outpatient care or hospitalization for management of HF, endocarditis, embolic disease, or dysrhythmias. HF is the most common reason for ongoing medical care.

Your role is to implement therapeutic interventions and evaluate their effects. Design activities considering the patient's limitations. An appropriate exercise plan can increase cardiac tolerance, but activities that cause fatigue and dyspnea should be limited. Discourage tobacco use. Tell the patient to avoid strenuous physical exercise because damaged valves may not handle the increased CO demand. Develop your patient's care plan to emphasize conserving energy, setting priorities, and taking planned rest periods. Consider a referral to a vocational counselor if the patient has a physically or emotionally demanding job.

Perform ongoing cardiac assessments to monitor the effectiveness of drugs. Teach the actions and side effects of drugs to increase adherence. The patient must understand the importance of prophylactic antibiotic therapy to prevent IE (Table 36-2). If the valve disease was caused by RF, ongoing prophylaxis to prevent recurrence is necessary.

When valvular heart disease can no longer be managed medically, surgery is necessary (see Chapter 33 for the care of a patient having heart surgery). The patient on anticoagulation therapy (e.g., warfarin [Coumadin]) after surgery for valve replacement must have the international normalized ratio (INR) checked regularly to determine proper dosage and adequacy of therapy. INR values of 2.5 to 3.5 are therapeutic for patients with mechanical valves.

A teaching guide related to anticoagulation therapy is found in Table 37-14. The patient must know that valve surgery is not a cure and that regular follow-up with an HCP is needed. Also, teach the patient when to seek medical care. Any signs of infection, HF, or bleeding and any planned invasive or dental work require the patient to notify the HCP. Last, encourage patients to obtain and wear a Medic Alert device.

Evaluation

The expected outcomes are that a patient with valvular heart disease will

- Maintain adequate tissue and organ perfusion
- Achieve fluid and electrolyte balance
- Achieve optimal level of activity
- Describe disease process and appropriate measures to prevent complications

Additional information on expected outcomes is presented in eNursing Care Plan 36-2 available on the website for this chapter.

CARDIOMYOPATHY

Cardiomyopathy (CMP) is a group of diseases that directly affect myocardial structure or function. A diagnosis of CMP is based on the patient's clinical manifestations and noninvasive and invasive diagnostic procedures.

CMP can be classified as primary or secondary. *Primary CMP* refers to those conditions in which the etiology of the disease is idiopathic. The heart muscle in this case is the only part of the heart involved, and other heart structures are unaffected. In *secondary CMP* the cause of the myocardial disease is known and is secondary to another disease process. Common causes of secondary CMP are listed in Table 36-14.

Three major types of CMP are dilated, hypertrophic, and restrictive. Each type has its own pathogenesis, clinical presentation, and treatment protocols (Tables 36-15 and 36-16). CMP can lead to cardiomegaly and HF. It is the primary reason that heart transplants are done.

Takotsubo cardiomyopathy (TCM) is a transient heart syndrome that mimics acute coronary syndrome. Patients often have chest pain, ST segment elevation on ECG, and elevated cardiac biomarkers consistent with an MI. However, when the patient undergoes heart catheterization, there is no significant coronary artery disease. TCM is an acute, stress-related syndrome that is more common in postmenopausal women. Normal heart function returns in days or weeks after supportive therapy.[19]

DILATED CARDIOMYOPATHY

Etiology and Pathophysiology

Dilated cardiomyopathy is the most common type of CMP, with a prevalence of 5 to 8 cases per 100,000 people in the

TABLE 36-14 Causes of Cardiomyopathy

Dilated	Hypertrophic
• Cardiotoxic agents: alcohol, cocaine, doxorubicin • Coronary artery disease • Genetic (autosomal dominant) • Hypertension • Metabolic disorders • Muscular dystrophy • Myocarditis • Pregnancy • Valve disease	• Aortic stenosis • Genetic (autosomal dominant) • Hypertension
Restrictive	
• Amyloidosis • Endomyocardial fibrosis • Neoplastic tumor • Post-radiation therapy • Sarcoidosis • Ventricular thrombus	

TABLE 36-15 Types of Cardiomyopathy

Dilated	Hypertrophic	Restrictive
Major Manifestations		
Fatigue, weakness, palpitations, dyspnea	Exertional dyspnea, fatigue, angina, syncope, palpitations	Dyspnea, fatigue
Cardiomegaly		
Moderate to severe	Mild to moderate	Mild
Contractility		
Decreased	Increased or decreased	Normal or decreased
Valvular Incompetence		
Atrioventricular (AV) valves, especially mitral	Mitral valve	AV valves
Dysrhythmias		
Sinus tachycardia, atrial and ventricular dysrhythmias	Atrial and ventricular dysrhythmias	Atrial and ventricular dysrhythmias
Cardiac Output		
Decreased	Normal or decreased	Normal or decreased
Outflow Tract Obstruction		
None	Increased	None

TABLE 36-16 Interprofessional Care

Cardiomyopathy

Diagnostic Assessment
- History and physical examination
- Electrocardiogram
- b-Type natriuretic peptide (BNP)
- Chest x-ray
- Echocardiogram
- Nuclear imaging studies
- Heart catheterization
- Endomyocardial biopsy

Management
- Drug therapy
  - Nitrates (except in hypertrophic CMP)
  - β-Blockers
  - Antidysrhythmics
  - ACE inhibitors
  - Diuretics
  - Digitalis (except in hypertrophic CMP unless used to treat atrial fibrillation)
  - Anticoagulants (if indicated)
- Ventricular assist device
- Cardiac resynchronization therapy
- Implantable cardioverter-defibrillator
- Surgical repair
- Heart transplantation
- Cardiac rehabilitation
- Palliative and hospice care

ACE, Angiotensin-converting enzyme; *CMP*, cardiomyopathy.

United States. It causes HF in 25% to 40% of cases, occurs more frequently in middle-aged African Americans and men, and has a genetic link in 30% of cases. Dilated CMP often follows an infectious myocarditis. Some evidence links dilated CMP with an autoimmune process.[20] Alcoholic dilated CMP is underrecognized and has a unique presentation, treatment, and outcomes.[21] Other common causes of dilated CMP are listed in Table 36-14.

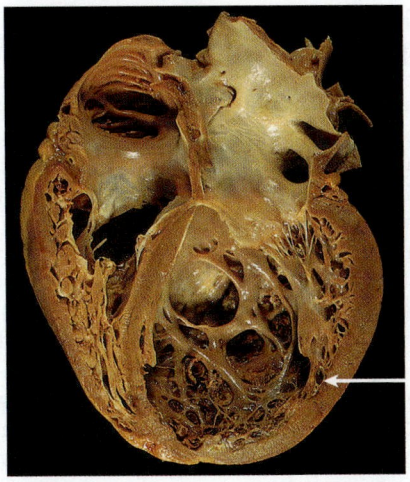

FIG. 36-11 Dilated cardiomyopathy. The dilated left ventricular wall has thinned *(arrow)*, and the chamber size and volume are increased. (From Kumar V, Abbas AK, Aster JC, et al: *Robbins and Cotran pathologic basis of disease*, ed 8, Philadelphia, 2010, Saunders.)

Dilated CMP is characterized by a diffuse inflammation and rapid degeneration of heart fibers. This results in ventricular dilation, impaired systolic function, atrial enlargement, and stasis of blood in the left ventricle. SCD from ventricular dysrhythmias is a leading cause of death in idiopathic dilated CMP.[22] *Cardiomegaly* results from ventricular dilation (Fig. 36-11). This causes contractile dysfunction in spite of an enlarged chamber size. In contrast to HF, the walls of the ventricles do not hypertrophy.

Clinical Manifestations

The signs and symptoms of dilated CMP may develop acutely after an infection or slowly over time. Most people eventually develop HF. Symptoms can include decreased exercise capacity, fatigue, dyspnea at rest, paroxysmal nocturnal dyspnea, and orthopnea. As the disease progresses, the patient may experience dry cough, palpitations, abdominal bloating, nausea, vomiting, and anorexia. Signs can include an abnormal S_3 and/or S_4, dysrhythmias, heart murmurs, pulmonary crackles, edema, weak peripheral pulses, pallor, hepatomegaly, and JVD. Decreased blood flow through an enlarged heart promotes stasis and blood clot formation and may lead to systemic embolization.

Diagnostic Studies

The diagnosis of dilated CMP is based on the patient's history and exclusion of other causes of HF. Doppler echocardiography is the basis for the diagnosis of dilated CMP in the majority of patients. The chest x-ray may show cardiomegaly with signs of pulmonary venous hypertension and pleural effusion. The ECG may reveal tachycardia, bradycardia, and dysrhythmias with conduction disturbances. Laboratory studies may show elevated serum levels of b-type natriuretic peptide (BNP) in the presence of HF.

Heart catheterization confirms or rules out coronary artery disease, and multiple gated acquisition (MUGA) nuclear scan determines EF. EF less than 20% is associated with a 50% mortality rate within 1 year. Endomyocardial biopsy is done at the time of the right-sided heart catheterization to identify any infectious organisms in heart tissue.

❖ NURSING AND INTERPROFESSIONAL MANAGEMENT: DILATED CARDIOMYOPATHY

Interventions focus on controlling HF by enhancing heart contractility and decreasing preload and afterload. This is similar to the management of chronic HF. Treatment guidelines are based on the specific stage of disease progression (see Table 34-3). Treatment of patients with Class IV (stage D) HF is more palliative than curative.

Several different types of drugs are available to manage HF (see Table 34-7). Nitrates (e.g., nitroglycerin [Nitrol]) and diuretics (e.g., furosemide [Lasix]) decrease preload, and ACE inhibitors (e.g., captopril [Capoten]) reduce afterload. β-Blockers (e.g., metoprolol [Lopressor]) and aldosterone antagonists (e.g., spironolactone [Aldactone]) control the neurohormonal stimulation that occurs in HF. Dysrhythmias are treated with antidysrhythmics (e.g., amiodarone) as indicated (see Chapter 35). Anticoagulation therapy reduces the risk of systemic embolization from clots. These may form in the heart chambers secondary to atrial fibrillation.

Drug and nutritional therapy and cardiac rehabilitation may help (1) alleviate symptoms of HF and (2) improve CO and quality of life. A patient with secondary dilated CMP must be treated for the underlying disease process. For example, the patient with alcohol-related dilated CMP must abstain from all alcohol. (See Chapter 10 for a discussion on addictive behaviors and Chapter 34 for a discussion on HF.)

Unfortunately, dilated CMP does not respond well to therapy, and patients experience multiple episodes of HF. Patients are often hospitalized for infusions of dobutamine (Dobutrex) or milrinone followed by aggressive diuresis. Sometimes these treatments are done in an outpatient setting or in the home under nursing supervision. After treatment, many patients experience an improvement in symptoms that lasts several weeks. The use of statins (e.g., atorvastatin [Lipitor]) in ischemic and idiopathic dilated CMP increases survival, improves heart function, and reduces inflammatory markers[23] (see Table 33-5).

Patients also may benefit from nondrug therapies. A ventricular assist device (VAD) allows the heart to rest and recover from acute HF. It may also serve as a bridge to heart transplantation. Additionally, cardiac resynchronization therapy and an implantable cardioverter-defibrillator are used in appropriate patients (see Chapter 34).

The patient with terminal or end-stage CMP may consider heart transplantation. The use of a permanent, implantable VAD, known as *destination therapy,* is an option for patients with advanced disease who are not candidates for heart transplantation (see Chapter 34). Currently, approximately 50% of heart transplantations that are performed are for treatment of CMP. Heart transplant recipients have a good prognosis. However, donor hearts are difficult to obtain, and many patients with dilated CMP die before receiving a heart.

Patients with dilated CMP are very ill and have a grave prognosis. Your expert nursing care is critical. Observe for signs and symptoms of worsening HF, dysrhythmias, embolus formation, and drug effectiveness. The goals of therapy are to keep the patient at an optimal level of functioning and out of the hospital. Always include caregivers when planning a patient's care. Encourage caregivers to learn cardiopulmonary resuscitation (CPR). Teach them when and how to access emergency care.

Home health and hospice nursing can provide the patient and caregiver with palliative care. This includes strategies to maximize and maintain functional status or end-of-life care to prepare for a peaceful death.

HYPERTROPHIC CARDIOMYOPATHY

Etiology and Pathophysiology

Hypertrophic cardiomyopathy is asymmetric left ventricular hypertrophy without ventricular dilation.[24] In one form of the disease the septum between the two ventricles becomes enlarged and blocks the blood flow from the left ventricle. It is termed *hypertrophic obstructive cardiomyopathy* (HOCMP) or *asymmetric septal hypertrophy* (ASH).

Although hypertrophic CMP can be idiopathic, about half of all cases have a genetic basis characterized by inappropriate myocardial hypertrophy. Early identification is important (Table 36-14). Hypertrophic CMP occurs less commonly than dilated CMP. It is more common in men than in women. It is usually diagnosed in young adults and, most often, in active, athletic individuals. Hypertrophic CMP is the most common cause of SCD in otherwise healthy young people. It accounts for 3% of deaths in young competitive athletes.[25]

The four main characteristics of hypertrophic CMP are (1) massive ventricular hypertrophy; (2) rapid, forceful contraction of the left ventricle; (3) impaired relaxation (diastole); and (4) obstruction to aortic outflow (not present in all patients). Ventricular hypertrophy is associated with a thickened intraventricular septum and ventricular wall (Fig. 36-12). The end result is impaired ventricular filling as the ventricle becomes noncompliant and unable to relax. The primary defect of hypertrophic CMP is diastolic dysfunction from left ventricular stiffness. Decreased ventricular filling and obstruction to outflow can result in decreased CO, especially during exertion.

Clinical Manifestations

Patients with hypertrophic CMP may be asymptomatic or may have exertional dyspnea, fatigue, angina, and syncope. The most common symptom is dyspnea, which is caused by an elevated left ventricular diastolic pressure. Fatigue occurs because of the resultant decrease in CO and in exercise-induced flow obstruction. Angina can occur and is most often caused by the increased left ventricular mass or compression of the small coronary arteries by the hypertrophic ventricular myocardium. The

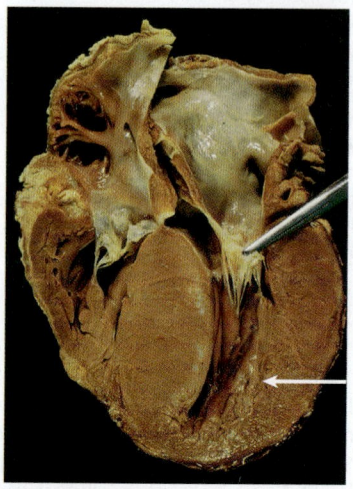

FIG. 36-12 Hypertrophic cardiomyopathy. There is marked left ventricular hypertrophy *(arrow),* and the chamber size and volume are decreased. (From Kumar V, Abbas AK, Aster JC, et al: *Robbins and Cotran pathologic basis of disease,* ed 8, Philadelphia, 2010, Saunders.)

patient may also have syncope, especially during exertion. Syncope is most often caused by an increase in obstruction to aortic outflow during increased activity. This results in decreased CO and cerebrovascular circulation. Syncope can also be caused by dysrhythmias. Common dysrhythmias include supraventricular tachycardia, atrial fibrillation, ventricular tachycardia, and ventricular fibrillation. Any of these dysrhythmias may lead to syncope or SCD (see Chapters 33 and 35).

Diagnostic Studies

Clinical findings on examination may be unremarkable. However, on palpation of the chest the apical impulse can be exaggerated and displaced to the left. Auscultation may reveal an S_4 and a systolic murmur between the apex and sternal border at the fourth intercostal space. ECG findings usually indicate ventricular hypertrophy, ST-T wave abnormalities, prominent Q waves in the inferior or precordial leads, and ventricular and atrial dysrhythmias (see Chapter 35).

The echocardiogram is the primary diagnostic tool used to confirm hypertrophic CMP. The echocardiogram may also demonstrate wall motion abnormalities and diastolic dysfunction. Heart catheterization and nuclear stress testing may also be helpful in diagnosing and guiding the treatment of hypertrophic CMP.

❖ NURSING AND INTERPROFESSIONAL MANAGEMENT: HYPERTROPHIC CARDIOMYOPATHY

Goals of care are to improve ventricular filling by reducing ventricular contractility and relieving left ventricular outflow obstruction. These can be done with the use of β-blockers (e.g., metoprolol) or calcium channel blockers (e.g., verapamil [Calan]). Digitalis is considered if needed to treat atrial fibrillation. Amiodarone or sotalol (Betapace) are effective antidysrhythmic drugs. However, their use does not prevent SCD. For patients at risk for SCD, a cardioverter-defibrillator is needed (see Chapter 35).

AV pacing is helpful for patients with hypertrophic CMP and outflow obstruction. When the ventricles are paced from the apex of the right ventricle, septal depolarization occurs first. This allows the septum to move away from the left ventricular wall and reduces the degree of obstruction of the outflow tract.

Some patients may be candidates for surgical treatment of their hypertrophied septum. The indications for surgery include severe symptoms unresponsive to therapy with marked obstruction to aortic outflow. The surgery is termed a *ventriculomyotomy and myectomy.* It involves cutting into the thickened septal muscle and removing some of the ventricular muscle. Most patients have an improvement in symptoms and exercise tolerance after surgery.

An alternative nonsurgical procedure to reduce symptoms and the left ventricular outflow obstruction is alcohol-induced, *percutaneous transluminal septal myocardial ablation* (PTSMA). This procedure consists of injecting alcohol into the first septal artery branching off the left anterior descending artery. This causes ischemia and septal wall infarction. Ablation of the septal wall decreases the obstruction to flow, and the patient's symptoms decrease. The procedure improves HF symptoms and exercise capacity 3 months after ablation.[26] Potential complications of PTSMA include conduction disturbances (e.g., heart block) and MI.

Nursing interventions for hypertrophic CMP focus on relieving symptoms, observing for and preventing complications, and providing emotional support. Focus your teaching on helping patients avoid strenuous activity and dehydration. Any activity that causes an increase in systemic vascular resistance (thus increasing the obstruction to forward flow) is dangerous and should be avoided. Rest and elevation of the feet to improve venous return to the heart can manage chest pain in these patients. Vasodilators such as nitroglycerin may worsen the chest pain by decreasing venous return and further increasing obstruction of blood flow from the heart.

RESTRICTIVE CARDIOMYOPATHY

Etiology and Pathophysiology

Restrictive cardiomyopathy is the least common type of CMP. It is a disease of the myocardium that impairs diastolic filling and stretch. Systolic function remains unchanged. Although the specific etiology of restrictive CMP is unknown, a number of pathologic processes may be involved in its development. Myocardial fibrosis, hypertrophy, and infiltration produce stiffness of the ventricular wall with loss of ventricular compliance. Secondary causes of restrictive CMP include amyloidosis, endocardial fibrosis, sarcoidosis, fibrosis of different etiology, and radiation to the thorax. With restrictive CMP, the ventricles are resistant to filling and therefore demand high diastolic filling pressures to maintain CO.

Clinical Manifestations and Diagnostic Studies

Classic manifestations of restrictive CMP are fatigue, exercise intolerance, and dyspnea. These occur because the heart cannot increase CO by increasing the heart rate without further compromising ventricular filling. Additional symptoms may include angina, orthopnea, syncope, and palpitations. The patient may have signs of HF, including dyspnea, peripheral edema, weight gain, ascites, hepatomegaly, and JVD.

The chest x-ray may be normal, or it may show cardiomegaly from right and left atrial enlargement. Pleural effusions and pulmonary congestion may be seen in the patient with progression to HF. The ECG may reveal a mild tachycardia at rest. The most common dysrhythmias are supraventricular (atrial fibrillation) or AV block. Echocardiography may reveal a left ventricle that is normal size with a thickened wall, slightly dilated right ventricle, and dilated atria. Endomyocardial biopsy, CT scan, and nuclear imaging may help in the diagnosis.

❖ NURSING AND INTERPROFESSIONAL MANAGEMENT: RESTRICTIVE CARDIOMYOPATHY

Currently, there is no specific treatment for restrictive CMP. Interventions are aimed at improving diastolic filling and the underlying disease process. Treatment includes conventional therapy for HF and dysrhythmias. Heart transplant may also be a consideration. Nursing care is similar to the care of a patient with HF. As in the treatment of patients with hypertrophic CMP, teach the patient to avoid situations that impair ventricular filling and increase systemic vascular resistance, such as strenuous activity and dehydration.

Nursing care of a patient with CMP includes individualized teaching based on the patient's clinical manifestations. All patients with CMP are at risk for IE from any procedure that may cause bacteremia. Instruct the patient on the need for prophylactic antibiotics (Table 36-2). A guide for patient and caregiver teaching is presented in Table 36-17.

TABLE 36-17 Patient & Caregiver Teaching

Cardiomyopathy

Include the following information in the teaching plan for a patient with cardiomyopathy and the patient's caregiver.

1. Take all drugs as prescribed and regularly follow up with HCP.
2. Follow a low-sodium diet (if ordered) and read all product labels (food and over-the-counter drugs) for sodium content.
3. Drink 6 to 8 glasses of water a day unless fluids are restricted.
4. Achieve and maintain a reasonable weight and avoid large meals.
5. Avoid alcohol, caffeine, diet pills, and over-the-counter cold medicines that may contain stimulants.
6. Balance activity and rest periods.
7. Avoid heavy lifting or vigorous isometric exercises, and check with HCP for exercise guidelines.
8. Use stress management techniques: relaxation breathing, guided imagery.
9. Report any signs of heart failure to HCP, including weight gain, edema, shortness of breath, and increased fatigue.
10. Encourage caregivers to learn CPR because of the potential for cardiac arrest (see Appendix A).
11. Access emergency response system (ERS) according to the HCP's instructions.

CPR, Cardiopulmonary resuscitation.

CASE STUDY

Valvular Heart Disease

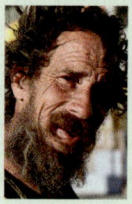

(©JennaDub/ iStock/ Thinkstock)

Patient Profile

R.B., a 50-yr-old white man, is admitted to the hospital for acute decompensated heart failure due to valvular heart disease.

Subjective Data

- Reports past history of IV drug abuse
- Reports current regular alcohol intake approximately 1 pint of whiskey per day
- Complains of chest pain with minimal exertion
- Recently unemployed
- States, "I'm short of breath all the time. I can't sleep when I lay down."
- States, "I'm always tired."
- States, "The drugs are too expensive. I can't afford them."
- Smokes a pack of cigarettes a day for past 35 years

Objective Data

Physical Examination

- Third heart sound (S_3)
- Loud holosystolic murmur of mitral regurgitation
- Edentulous (secondary to periodontal disease)
- Vital signs: temperature 99.0°F (37.2°C); apical-radial pulse equal at 110 beats per min, irregular; respirations 24; BP 104/58

Diagnostic Studies

- ECG shows atrial fibrillation with a rapid ventricular response
- Chest x-ray reveals pulmonary congestion and cardiomegaly
- Transesophageal echocardiography shows left atrial and ventricular hypertrophy and mitral and aortic regurgitation. Ejection fraction 30%

Discussion Questions

1. Identify the cause and course of R.B.'s disease based on his history and current examination.
2. Differentiate between mitral and aortic regurgitation.
3. What medical treatments or surgical procedures will R.B. probably require as his condition worsens?
4. ***Priority Decision:*** On the basis of the assessment data provided, what are the priority nursing diagnoses?
5. ***Priority Decision:*** Identify the priority nursing interventions for R.B.
6. ***Safety:*** What safety precautions should be initiated for R.B.?
7. ***Teamwork and Collaboration:*** Identify the tasks that you could delegate to unlicensed assistive personnel (UAP).
8. ***Evidence-Based Practice:*** R.B. asks you why he needs to be on "blood thinners" after his valves are replaced.

Answers are available at *http://evolve.elsevier.com/Lewis/medsurg.*

BRIDGE TO NCLEX EXAMINATION

The number of the question corresponds to the same-numbered outcome at the beginning of the chapter.

1. Assessment of an IV cocaine user with infective endocarditis should focus on which signs and symptoms *(select all that apply)*?
   a. Retinal hemorrhages
   b. Splinter hemorrhages
   c. Presence of Osler's nodes
   d. Painless nodules over bony prominences
   e. Painless erythematous macules on the palms and soles
2. The nurse is caring for a patient with chronic constrictive pericarditis. Which assessment finding reflects a *more* serious complication of this condition?
   a. Fatigue
   b. Peripheral edema
   c. Jugular venous distention
   d. Thickened pericardium on echocardiography
3. A patient is admitted with myocarditis. While performing the initial assessment, the nurse may find which clinical signs and symptoms *(select all that apply)*?
   a. Angina
   b. Pleuritic chest pain
   c. Splinter hemorrhages
   d. Pericardial friction rub
   e. Presence of Osler's nodes
4. *Priority* nursing management for a patient with myocarditis includes interventions related to
   a. meticulous skin care.
   b. antibiotic prophylaxis.
   c. tight glycemic control.
   d. oxygenation and ventilation.
5. When teaching a patient about the long-term consequences of rheumatic fever, the nurse should discuss the possibility of
   a. valvular heart disease.
   b. pulmonary hypertension.
   c. superior vena cava syndrome.
   d. hypertrophy of the right ventricle.

6. Which is a *priority* nursing intervention for a patient during the acute phase of rheumatic fever?
   a. Administration of antibiotics as ordered
   b. Management of pain with opioid analgesics
   c. Encouragement of fluid intake for hydration
   d. Performance of frequent active range-of-motion exercises
7. Which clinical finding would *most* likely indicate decreased cardiac output in a patient with aortic valve regurgitation?
   a. Reduction in peripheral edema and weight
   b. Carotid venous distention and new-onset atrial fibrillation
   c. Significant pulsus paradoxus and diminished peripheral pulses
   d. Shortness of breath on minimal exertion and a diastolic murmur
8. A patient is diagnosed with mitral stenosis and new-onset atrial fibrillation. Which interventions could the nurse delegate to unlicensed assistive personnel (UAP) *(select all that apply)*?
   a. Obtain and record daily weight.
   b. Determine apical-radial pulse rate.
   c. Observe for overt signs of bleeding.
   d. Obtain and record vital signs, including pulse oximetry.
   e. Teach the patient how to purchase a Medic Alert device.
9. Which diagnostic study *best* differentiates the various types of cardiomyopathy?
   a. Echocardiography
   b. Arterial blood gases
   c. Heart catheterization
   d. Endomyocardial biopsy
10. The nurse is caring for a patient newly admitted with heart failure secondary to dilated cardiomyopathy. Which intervention would be a *priority*?
   a. Encourage caregivers to learn CPR.
   b. Consider a consultation with hospice for palliative care.
   c. Monitor the patient's response to prescribed medications.
   d. Arrange for the patient to enter a cardiac rehabilitation program.

1. a, b, c, e, 2. c, 3. a, b, d, 4. d, 5. a, 6. a, 7. d, 8. a, c, d, 9. a, 10. c

For rationales to these answers and even more NCLEX review questions, visit *http://evolve.elsevier.com/Lewis/medsurg*.

EVOLVE WEBSITE

http://evolve.elsevier.com/Lewis/medsurg

Review Questions (Online Only)

Key Points

Answer Keys for Questions

- Rationales for Bridge to NCLEX Examination Questions
- Answer Guidelines for Case Study on p. 800

Student Case Study

- Patient With Rheumatic Fever and Heart Disease

Nursing Care Plans

- eNursing Care Plan 36-1: Patient With Infective Endocarditis
- eNursing Care Plan 36-2: Patient With Valvular Heart Disease

Conceptual Care Map Creator

Audio Glossary

Supporting Media

- Audio
  - Pericardial Friction Rub

Content Updates

REFERENCES

1. Keynan Y, Singal R, Kumar K, et al: Infective endocarditis in the intensive care unit, *Crit Care Clin* 29(4):923, 2013.
2. Josephson L: Infective endocarditis: a review for nurses, *Dimens Crit Care Nurs* 33(6):327, 2014.

*3. Baddour LM, Wilson WR, Bayer AS, et al: Infective endocarditis in adults: diagnosis, antimicrobial therapy, and management of complications. A scientific statement for healthcare professionals from the American Heart Association, *Circulation* 132:e215, 2015.

4. Gupta A, Gupta A, Kaul U, et al: Infective endocarditis in an Indian setup: are we entering the 'modern' era? *Indian J Crit Care Med* 17(3):140, 2013.
5. Eun J, Smith A: Safety and efficacy of colchicine therapy in the prevention of recurrent pericarditis, *Am J Health-Syst Pharm* 71(15):1277, 2014.
6. Kindermann I, Barth C, Mahfoud F, et al: Update on myocarditis, *J Am Coll Cardiol* 59(9):779, 2012.
7. Kumar RK, Tandon R: Rheumatic fever & rheumatic heart disease: the last 50 years, *Indian J Med Res* 137(4):643, 2013.

*8. Gewitz MH, Baltimore RS, Tani LY, et al: Revision of the Jones criteria for the diagnosis of acute rheumatic fever in the era of Doppler echocardiography: a scientific statement from the American Heart Association, *Circulation* 131:1806, 2015.

9. Texas Heart Institute Heart Information Center: Rheumatic fever. Retrieved from *www.texasheart.org/HIC/Topics/Cond/rheufev.cfm*.
10. Woods CJ, Levy CS: Medscape: Streptococcus Group B infections treatment & management. Retrieved from *http://emedicine.medscape.com/article/229091-treatment*.

*11. Nishimura RA, Otto CM, Bonow RO, et al: 2014 AHA/ACC Guideline for the management of patients with valvular heart disease: executive summary: a report of the American College of Cardiology/American Heart Association Task Force on Practice Guidelines, *Circulation* 129:2440, 2014.

*12. Meziani F, Debbal S, Atbi A: Analysis of the pathological severity degree of aortic stenosis (AS) and mitral stenosis (MS) using the discrete wavelet transform (DTW), *J Med Eng Tech* 37(1):61, 2013.

13. Mitral Valve Repair Center at the Mount Sinai Hospital: Mitral repair, 2015. Retrieved from *www.mitralvalverepair.org/content/view/64*.
14. Teehan S, McKee G, Dempsey O: Management of severe aortic stenosis, *WIN* 22(10):61, 2014/2015.
15. Mitral Valve Repair Center at the Mount Sinai Hospital: Minimally invasive heart surgery center, 2015. Retrieved from *www.mitralvalverepair.org/content/view/16*
16. Zhang P, Melander S: Transcatheter aortic valve replacement for severe aortic stenosis, *Crit Care Nurs Q* 37(4):346, 2014.
17. Medtronic: An advanced TAVR Design. CoreValve® Transcatheter Aortic Valve Implantation (TAVI) platform. Retrieved from *www.corevalve.com/intl/product/index.htm*.
18. Malaisrie SC, McDonald E, Kruse J, et al: Mortality while waiting for aortic valve replacement, *Ann Thorac Surg* 98(5):1564, 2014.
19. Padilla H, Paltoo B, Edsall R, et al: Recognizing and treating Takotsubo cardiomyopathy, *Nursing* 44(8):50, 2014.
20. Frustaci A, Petrosillo N, Farancone M, et al: Biopsy-proven autoimmune myocarditis in HIV-associated dilated cardiomyopathy, *BMC Infect Dis* 14:729, 2014.
21. Nicholson C: Chronic heart failure: pathophysiology, diagnosis and treatment, *Nurs Older People* 26(7):29, 2014.

*22. Al-Zaiti SS, Fallavollita JA, Cantry JM, et al: Electrocardiographic predictors of sudden and non-sudden cardiac death in patients with ischemic cardiomyopathy, *Heart Lung* 43:527, 2014.

23. American Heart Association: Prevention and treatment of cardiomyopathy. Retrieved from *www.heart.org/HEARTORG/Conditions/More/Cardiomyopathy/Prevention-and-Treatment-of-Cardiomyopathy_UCM_444176_Article.jsp*.
24. Hensley N, Deitrich J, Nyhan D, et al: Hypertrophic cardiomyopathy: a review, *Anesth Analg* 120(3):554, 2015.
25. Caselli S, Maron MS, Pandian NG, et al: Differentiating left ventricular hypertrophy in athletes from that in patients with hypertrophic cardiomyopathy, *Am J Cardiol* 114(9):1383, 2013.

*26. Chen YZ, Qiao SB, Hu FH, et al: Biventricular reverse remodeling after successful alcohol septal ablation for obstructive hypertrophic cardiomyopathy, *Am J Cardiol* 115(4):493, 2015.

*Evidence-based information for clinical practice.

37

Vascular Disorders

Deidre D. Wipke-Tevis, Kathleen A. Rich

Hardening of the heart ages people more quickly than hardening of the arteries.

Unknown

http://evolve.elsevier.com/Lewis/medsurg/

LEARNING OUTCOMES

1. Relate the major risk factors to the etiology and pathophysiology of peripheral artery disease (PAD).
2. Describe the clinical manifestations, interprofessional care, and nursing management of the patient with PAD of the lower extremities.
3. Plan appropriate nursing and interprofessional management for the patient with acute arterial ischemic disorders of the lower extremities.
4. Differentiate the pathophysiology, clinical manifestations, and nursing and interprofessional management of the patient with thromboangiitis obliterans (Buerger's disease) and Raynaud's phenomenon.
5. Differentiate the pathophysiology, clinical manifestations, interprofessional care, and nursing management of patients with different types of aortic aneurysms.
6. Select appropriate nursing interventions for a patient undergoing an aortic aneurysm repair.
7. Describe the pathophysiology, clinical manifestations, interprofessional care, and nursing management of the patient with aortic dissection.
8. Evaluate the risk factors predisposing patients to the development of superficial vein thrombosis and venous thromboembolism (VTE).
9. Differentiate between the clinical characteristics of superficial vein thrombosis and VTE.
10. Compare and contrast the interprofessional care and nursing management of patients with superficial vein thrombosis and VTE.
11. Prioritize the key aspects of nursing management of the patient receiving anticoagulant therapy.
12. Relate the pathophysiology and clinical manifestations to the interprofessional care, drug therapy, and interventional/surgical therapies of patients with varicose veins, chronic venous insufficiency, and venous leg ulcers.

KEY TERMS

acute arterial ischemia, p. 808
aneurysm, p. 810
aortic dissection, p. 814
chronic venous insufficiency (CVI), p. 826
critical limb ischemia, p. 804
deep vein thrombosis (DVT), p. 816
intermittent claudication, p. 803
peripheral artery disease (PAD), p. 802
post-thrombotic syndrome (PTS), p. 818
Raynaud's phenomenon, p. 809
superficial vein thrombosis, p. 816
thromboangiitis obliterans (Buerger's disease), p. 809
varicose veins, p. 825
venous thromboembolism (VTE), p. 816
venous thrombosis, p. 816
Virchow's triad, p. 816

Problems of the vascular system include disorders of the arteries, veins, and lymphatic vessels. Arterial disorders are classified as atherosclerotic, aneurysmal, and nonatherosclerotic vascular diseases. Atherosclerotic vascular disease is divided into coronary, cerebral, peripheral, mesenteric, and renal artery disease.[1] This chapter discusses peripheral artery disease, aortic aneurysm and dissection, and venous diseases.

PERIPHERAL ARTERY DISEASE

Peripheral artery disease (PAD) involves thickening of artery walls. This results in a progressive narrowing of the arteries of the upper and lower extremities. PAD prevalence increases with age. It typically becomes symptomatic in the sixth to eighth decades of life. In people with diabetes mellitus, PAD occurs earlier. In the United States, PAD prevalence is higher in those of lower socioeconomic status, women, and African Americans.[2]

PAD is strongly related to other types of cardiovascular disease (CVD) and their risk factors. Patients with PAD have a significantly higher risk of mortality (in general), CVD mortality, major coronary events, and stroke.[3] PAD is a marker of advanced systemic atherosclerosis. Patients with PAD are more likely to have coronary artery disease (CAD) and/or cerebral artery disease.

Unfortunately, low levels of public awareness of PAD and its risk factors exist in the United States. In general, PAD remains underdiagnosed and undertreated.

Etiology and Pathophysiology

The leading cause of PAD is *atherosclerosis,* a gradual thickening of the *intima* (the innermost layer of the arterial wall) and *media*

Reviewed by Rebecca Personett, RN, PhD, NEA-BC, Professor of Nursing, North Central Texas College, Gainesville, Texas and Brookhaven College, Dallas, Texas; Tara McMillan-Queen, RN, MSN, ANP, GNP, Faculty II, Mercy School of Nursing, Charlotte, North Carolina; and Janet M. Riggs, RN, MSN, DrNP, Clinical Research Coordinator, University of Pennsylvania, Philadelphia, Pennsylvania.

(middle layer of the arterial wall). This results from the deposit of cholesterol and lipids within the vessel walls and leads to progressive narrowing of the artery (see Fig. 33-1). Although the exact cause of atherosclerosis is unknown, inflammation and endothelial injury play a major role (see Chapter 33).

Risk factors for PAD are similar, but not identical, to coronary artery disease. Important risk factors for PAD are tobacco use (most important), chronic kidney disease, diabetes, hypertension, and hypercholesterolemia.[2] The additive presence of risk factors dramatically increases the risk of PAD, especially in women and African Americans.[2] Other risk factors include elevated C-reactive protein, family history, hypertriglyceridemia, increasing age, hyperhomocysteinemia, hyperuricemia, obesity, sedentary lifestyle, and stress.[4]

Atherosclerosis more commonly affects certain segments of the arterial tree. These include the coronary (see Chapter 33), carotid (see Chapter 57), and lower extremity arteries. Clinical symptoms occur when vessels are 60% to 75% blocked.

PERIPHERAL ARTERY DISEASE OF THE LOWER EXTREMITIES

Lower extremity PAD may affect the iliac, femoral, popliteal, tibial, or peroneal arteries, or any combination of these arteries (Fig. 37-1). The femoral popliteal area is the most common site in nondiabetic patients. Patients with diabetes tend to develop PAD in the arteries below the knee. In advanced PAD, multiple levels of occlusions are found.

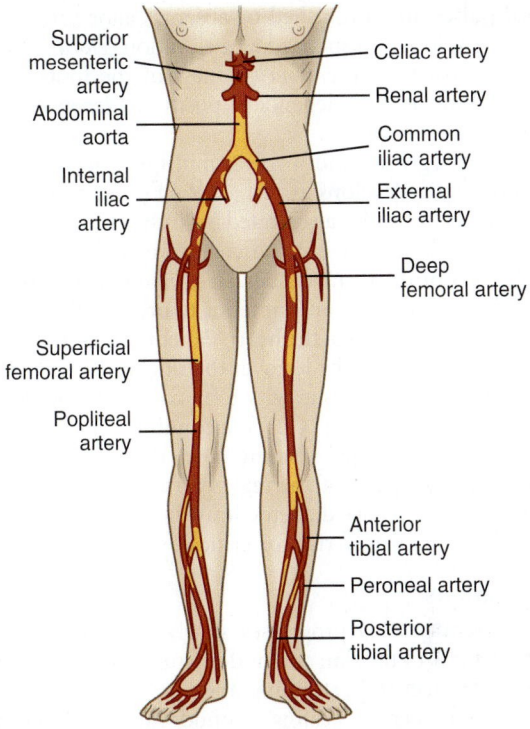

FIG. 37-1 Common anatomic locations of atherosclerotic lesions (shown in *yellow*) of the abdominal aorta and lower extremities.

GENDER DIFFERENCES

Vascular Disorders

Men

- Thromboangiitis obliterans (Buerger's disease) occurs predominantly in men <40 yr of age.
- Abdominal aortic aneurysms (AAAs) are more common in men than women.
- Men with AAAs are more likely to undergo endovascular aneurysm repair or open aneurysm repair than women.
- Sexual dysfunction in male patients is common after aortic surgery.
- Aortic dissection affects men more often than women.

Women

- Peripheral artery disease (PAD) prevalence is higher in women.
- Women with low lifetime recreational activity are at greater risk for PAD than similar men.
- Older women experience the classic signs of intermittent claudication less often than men.
- Women with PAD experience faster functional decline and greater mobility loss than men with PAD.
- Raynaud's phenomenon occurs primarily in women between 15 and 40 yr of age.
- Risk for venous thromboembolism (VTE) is greater in women over age 35 who use tobacco and oral contraceptives or oral hormone therapy, are pregnant or postpartum, or have a family history of VTE.
- Primary varicose veins are more common and more symptomatic in women than men.
- Risk for varicose veins is greater in multiparous women.
- Women with AAAs are at higher risk for rupture.
- In-hospital mortality is higher in women undergoing revascularization than men, regardless of disease severity or procedure performed.
- Women develop surgical site infections more often than men.
- Women, particularly African American and Hispanic women, experience more graft thrombosis and amputation after lower extremity bypass surgery than men.

Clinical Manifestations

Generally, the severity of the clinical manifestations depends on the site and extent of the blockage and the amount of collateral circulation. The classic symptom of lower extremity PAD is **intermittent claudication**. This ischemic muscle pain is caused by exercise, resolves within 10 minutes or less with rest, and is reproducible. The ischemic pain is a result of the buildup of lactic acid from anaerobic metabolism. Once the patient stops exercising, the lactic acid is cleared and the pain subsides. PAD of the iliac arteries produces claudication in the buttocks and thighs. Calf claudication indicates femoral or popliteal artery involvement.

As many as one third of patients with PAD report classic claudication symptoms. The remaining either have no symptoms or present with atypical leg symptoms (e.g., burning, heaviness, pressure, soreness, tightness, weakness) in atypical locations (e.g., ankle, foot, hamstring, hip, knee, shin). Older women experience classic claudication less often than men.[5] If PAD involves the internal iliac arteries, erectile dysfunction may result.

Paresthesia, or numbness or tingling, in the toes or feet may result from nerve tissue ischemia. True peripheral neuropathy occurs more often in patients with diabetes (see Chapter 48) and in those with long-standing ischemia. Neuropathy produces severe shooting or burning pain in the extremity. It does not follow particular nerve roots and may be present near ulcerated areas. Gradual, reduced blood flow to neurons produces loss of both pressure and deep pain sensations. Thus patients may not notice lower extremity injuries.

The limb's physical appearance provides important information about blood flow. The skin becomes thin, shiny, and taut, and hair loss occurs on the lower legs. Pedal, popliteal, or femoral pulses are diminished or absent. Pallor (blanching of the foot) develops in response to leg elevation *(elevation pallor)*. Conversely, *reactive hyperemia* (redness of the foot) develops when the limb is in a dependent position *(dependent rubor)* (Table 37-1).

As PAD progresses and involves multiple arterial segments, continuous pain develops at rest. *Rest pain* most often occurs in the foot or toes and is aggravated by limb elevation. Rest pain occurs when blood flow is insufficient to meet basic metabolic requirements of the distal tissues. Rest pain occurs more often at night because cardiac output tends to drop during sleep and the limbs are at the level of the heart. Patients often try to achieve pain relief by dangling the leg over the side of the bed or sleeping in a chair. This allows gravity to maximize blood flow.

Critical limb ischemia (CLI) is a condition characterized by chronic ischemic rest pain lasting more than 2 weeks, arterial leg ulcers, or gangrene of the leg as a result of PAD. Patients with PAD who also have diabetes, heart failure, and a history of a stroke are at increased risk for critical limb ischemia.[6]

Complications

Lower extremity PAD progresses slowly. Prolonged ischemia leads to atrophy of the skin and underlying muscles. Even minor trauma to the feet (e.g., stubbing one's toe, blister from shoes) can result in delayed healing, wound infection, and tissue necrosis, especially in the patient with diabetes. Arterial (ischemic) ulcers most often occur over bony prominences on the toes, feet, and lower legs (Table 37-1). Nonhealing arterial ulcers and gangrene are the most serious complications. If PAD is present for an extended period, collateral circulation may prevent gangrene of the extremity.

Amputation may be needed if adequate blood flow is not restored or if severe infection occurs. Uncontrolled pain and severe, spreading infection are indicators that an amputation is needed in people who are not candidates for revascularization.

Diagnostic Studies

Various tests can assess blood flow and the vascular system (Table 37-2). Doppler ultrasound with duplex imaging maps blood flow throughout the entire region of an artery. When palpation of a peripheral pulse is difficult because of severe PAD, the Doppler ultrasound can determine the degree of blood flow. A palpable pulse and a Doppler pulse are not equivalent, and the terms are not interchangeable.

Segmental blood pressures (BPs) are obtained (using Doppler ultrasound and a sphygmomanometer) at the thigh, below the knee, and at ankle level while the patient is supine. A drop in

TABLE 37-1 Comparison of Peripheral Artery and Venous Disease

Characteristic	Peripheral Artery Disease	Venous Disease
Peripheral pulses	Decreased or absent	Present, may be difficult to palpate with edema
Capillary refill	>3 sec	<3 sec
Ankle-brachial index	≤0.90	>0.90
Edema	Absent unless leg constantly in dependent position	Lower leg edema
Hair	Loss of hair on legs, feet, toes	Hair may be present or absent
Ulcer		
• Location	Tips of toes, foot, or lateral malleolus	Near medial malleolus
• Margin	Rounded, smooth, looks "punched out"	Irregularly shaped
• Drainage	Minimal	Moderate to large amount
• Tissue	Black eschar or pale pink granulation	Yellow slough or dark red, "ruddy" granulation
Pain	Intermittent claudication or rest pain in foot	Dull ache or heaviness in calf or thigh
	Ulcer may or may not be painful	Ulcer often painful
Nails	Thickened; brittle	Normal or thickened
Skin color	Dependent rubor, elevation pallor	Bronze-brown pigmentation
		Varicose veins may be visible
Skin texture	Thin, shiny, taut	Skin thick, hardened, and indurated
Skin temperature	Cool, temperature gradient down the leg	Warm, no temperature gradient
Dermatitis	Rarely occurs	Frequently occurs
Pruritus	Rarely occurs	Frequently occurs

TABLE 37-2 Interprofessional Care

Peripheral Artery Disease

Diagnostic Assessment

- Health history and physical examination, including palpation of peripheral pulses
- Doppler ultrasound studies
- Segmental blood pressures
- Ankle-brachial index (Table 37-3)
- Duplex imaging
- Angiography
- Magnetic resonance angiography

Management

- Cardiovascular disease risk factor modification
  - Tobacco cessation
  - Regular physical exercise
  - Achieve or maintain ideal body weight
  - Follow Dietary Approaches to Stop Hypertension (DASH) diet
  - Tight glucose control in diabetics including A1C monitoring
  - Tight BP control
  - Treatment of hyperlipidemia and hypertriglyceridemia (see Table 33-5)
  - Antiplatelet agent (aspirin or clopidogrel [Plavix])
  - Angiotensin-converting enzyme inhibitors (see Table 32-7)
- Treatment of claudication symptoms
  - Structured walking or exercise program
  - Cilostazol (Pletal) or pentoxifylline
- Nutritional therapy
- Physical/occupational therapy
- Proper foot care (see Table 48-21)

Surgical Therapy

- Percutaneous transluminal balloon angioplasty with or without stent
- Percutaneous transluminal atherectomy
- Percutaneous transluminal cryoplasty
- Peripheral artery bypass surgery
- Patch graft angioplasty, often in conjunction with bypass surgery
- Endarterectomy (for localized stenosis but rarely done as a stand-alone procedure)
- Thrombolytic therapy or mechanical clot extraction therapy (for acute ischemia only)
- Sympathectomy (for pain management only)
- Amputation

TABLE 37-3 Interpreting Ankle-Brachial Index Results

Ankle-Brachial Index (ABI)	Clinical Significance
>1.30	Noncompressible arteries
1.00-1.30	Normal ABI
0.91-0.99	Borderline ABI
≤0.90	Abnormal ABI
Classification of PAD Severity	
0.90-0.71	Mild PAD
0.70-0.41	Moderate PAD
≤0.40	Severe PAD

PAD, Peripheral artery disease.

segmental BP of greater than 30 mm Hg suggests PAD. Angiography and magnetic resonance angiography delineate the location and extent of PAD (see Table 31-6).

The *ankle-brachial index* (ABI) is a PAD screening tool. It is performed using a hand-held Doppler. The ABI is calculated by dividing the ankle systolic BPs by the higher of the left and right brachial systolic BPs. PAD guidelines recommend uniform reporting of ABI results[6] (Table 37-3). In older patients and those with diabetes, the arteries often are calcified and noncompressible. This results in a falsely elevated ABI.

Interprofessional Care

Table 37-2 summarizes the interprofessional care for a patient with PAD.

Risk Factor Modification. The first treatment goal in treating PAD is to reduce CVD risk factors in all patients with PAD regardless of the severity of symptoms. Risk factors must be modified with both drug therapy and lifestyle changes (see Tables 33-1 to 33-4).

Tobacco cessation is essential to reduce the risk of CVD events, PAD progression, and death. This is a complex and difficult process with a high incidence of relapse. Comprehensive tobacco cessation strategies are recommended (see Tables 10-4 to 10-6).

Diabetes is a major risk factor for PAD and increases the risk of amputation in these patients. It is recommended that patients with diabetes maintain a glycosylated hemoglobin (A1C) below 7.0% and, optimally, as near as possible to 6.0%.[7] (Chapter 48 discusses diabetes mellitus.)

Aggressive lipid management is essential for all patients with PAD. Both dietary interventions and drug therapy are needed. Statins (e.g., simvastatin [Zocor]) and a fibric acid derivative (gemfibrozil [Lopid]) may be used (see Table 33-5).

Hypertension is a well-known risk factor for PAD progression, as well as other CVD events (e.g., stroke, myocardial infarction [MI], heart failure). Current guidelines for the management of hypertension in people with PAD include BP less than 140/90 mm Hg.[6] In PAD patients with diabetes or renal insufficiency, BP less than 130/80 mm Hg is recommended.

Angiotensin-converting enzyme (ACE) inhibitors (e.g., ramipril [Altace]) are used for symptomatic patients with PAD. Lifestyle changes are encouraged and include reducing dietary sodium and following the Dietary Approaches to Stop Hypertension (DASH) diet. (Chapter 32 discusses hypertension.)

Drug Therapy. Antiplatelet agents are critical for reducing the risks of CVD events and death in PAD patients. Oral antiplatelet therapy should include 75 to 325 mg/day of aspirin. Aspirin-intolerant patients may take 75 mg of clopidogrel (Plavix) daily.

Combination antiplatelet therapy with aspirin and clopidogrel is not typically recommended. However, it may be used in select high-risk PAD patients. Anticoagulants (e.g., warfarin [Coumadin]) are not recommended for prevention of CVD events in PAD patients.

DRUG ALERT Clopidogrel (Plavix) and Omeprazole (Prilosec)

- Antiplatelet effect of clopidogrel is reduced by about half when given with omeprazole.
- This increases the risk of MI and stroke.

Two drugs are available to treat intermittent claudication: cilostazol (Pletal) and pentoxifylline. Cilostazol, a phosphodiesterase inhibitor, inhibits platelet aggregation and increases vasodilation. Pentoxifylline, a xanthine derivative, improves the deformability of RBCs and WBCs and decreases fibrinogen concentration, platelet adhesiveness, and blood viscosity.

DRUG ALERT Cilostazol (Pletal)

- Contraindicated in patients with heart failure of any severity.

Exercise Therapy. A supervised exercise program is recommended as an initial treatment for all patients with intermittent claudication. Exercise should be performed for 30 to 45 minutes/day, at least 3 times/week, for a minimum of 3 months. Although walking is the most commonly prescribed exercise for PAD patients, alternative modes of exercise (e.g., cycling) also improve walking ability and quality of life in patients with PAD.[8]

Encouragement of participation in exercise is particularly important for women with PAD, since women experience faster functional decline and greater mobility loss than men with PAD. Overall, patients with PAD who have higher levels of daily physical activity also have better survival rates.[6]

Nutritional Therapy. Teach patients with PAD to maintain a body mass index (BMI) less than 25 kg/m^2 and a waist circumference less than 40 inches for men and less than 35 inches for women. Even modest, sustained weight loss of 3% to 5% yields important reductions in triglycerides, glucose, A1C, and the risk of developing type 2 diabetes. Greater weight loss produces greater benefits.[9] Recommend a diet reduced in calories and salt for obese or overweight individuals with PAD.[10]

Complementary and Alternative Therapies. Patients taking antiplatelet agents, nonsteroidal antiinflammatory drugs (NSAIDs) (e.g., ibuprofen), and anticoagulants (e.g., warfarin) should consult with their HCP before taking any dietary or herbal supplements because of potential interactions and bleeding risks[11] (see the Complementary & Alternative Therapies box on p. 820).

Care of the Leg With Critical Limb Ischemia. Optimal therapy for the patient with critical limb ischemia is revascularization via bypass surgery using an *autogenous* (native) vein. If this is not feasible, percutaneous transluminal angioplasty (PTA) is recommended.[6] Patients with CLI who are not candidates for surgery or PTA may be treated with IV prostanoids (e.g., iloprost [Ventavis]). These drugs may decrease rest pain and improve ulcer healing. Patients with CLI should continue optimal drug therapy (e.g., statin, antiplatelet, ACE inhibitor, β-blocker) to reduce the risk of a CVD event.

Conservative management of critical limb ischemia includes protecting the extremity from trauma, decreasing ischemic pain, preventing and controlling infection, and improving perfusion. Carefully inspect, cleanse, and lubricate feet to prevent cracking of the skin and infection. Avoid lubrication between the toes and soaking the patient's feet to prevent skin *maceration* (or breakdown). If ulceration is present, keep the affected foot clean and dry. Cover any ulcers with a dry, sterile dressing to maintain cleanliness. Deep ulcers can be treated with a variety of wound care products, but healing is unlikely without increased blood flow. Systemic antibiotics are used in patients with CLI, skin ulcerations, and limb infection.[6]

Encourage the patient to select soft, roomy, and protective footwear and avoid extremes of heat and cold. Keep the patient's heels free of pressure. You can do this by placing a pillow under the calves so that the heels are off the mattress. Commercially available devices can also provide heel protection. Giving opioid analgesics and placing the bed in the reverse Trendelenburg position may control pain and increase perfusion to the lower extremities.

Spinal cord stimulation may be helpful in managing pain and preventing amputation in patients with CLI. Other promising strategies include growth factors and gene and stem cell therapy to stimulate blood vessel growth *(angiogenesis)*. Unfortunately, almost half of the patients with CLI will die within 5 years.[12]

Interventional Radiology Catheter-Based Procedures. Interventional radiology catheter-based procedures are alternatives to open surgical approaches for treatment of lower extremity PAD. These procedures take place in a catheterization laboratory rather than in an operating room. Determining which intervention to use depends on blockage location and lesion type and severity.

All these procedures are similar to angiography in that they involve the insertion of a specialized catheter into the femoral artery. The *percutaneous transluminal angioplasty* (PTA) procedure uses a catheter that contains a balloon at the tip. The end of the catheter is moved to the narrowed (stenotic) area of the artery. The balloon is then inflated, compressing the atherosclerotic intimal lining.[13]

Stents, expandable metallic devices, are placed within the artery immediately after the balloon angioplasty is done. The stent acts as a scaffold to keep the artery open. Both angioplasty balloons and peripheral stents may be coated with a drug-eluting agent (e.g., paclitaxel) to reduce restenosis. These drugs work by limiting the growth of new tissue in the treated stenotic area and improve long-term patency rates.[14]

Atherectomy is the removal of the obstructing plaque. A directional atherectomy device uses a high-speed cutting disk that cuts long strips of the atheroma. Laser atherectomy uses ultraviolet energy to break up the atheroma. Other types of atherectomy catheters have a diamond-coated tip that rotates at a high speed (similar to a dentist drill). These crush the calcium within the atheroma into particles smaller than a blood cell.[15]

Cryoplasty combines two procedures: PTA and cold therapy. A specialized balloon is filled with liquid nitrous oxide, which changes from liquid to gas as it enters the balloon. Expansion of the gas results in cooling to 14° F (−10° C). The cold temperature limits restenosis by reducing smooth muscle cell activity.[16]

Pre- and postprocedure nursing care is the same as for a diagnostic angiography (see Table 31-6). Antiplatelet agents are needed postprocedure to reduce the risk of restenosis. Long-term, low-dose aspirin therapy or clopidogrel is recommended.

Surgical Therapy. Various surgical approaches can be used to improve blood flow beyond a blocked artery. When possible, peripheral artery bypass surgery should be done with an autogenous vein to bypass (carry blood around) the lesion (Fig. 37-2).

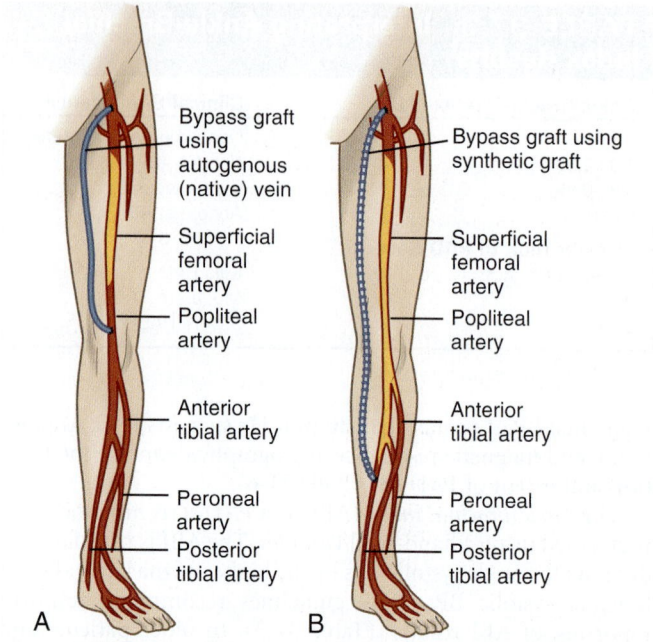

FIG. 37-2 **A,** Femoral-popliteal bypass graft around an occluded superficial femoral artery. **B,** Femoral–posterior tibial bypass graft around occluded superficial femoral, popliteal, and proximal tibial arteries.

Synthetic grafts typically are used for long bypasses such as an axillary-femoral bypass. When a person's own vein is not available, human umbilical vein or a composite sequential bypass graft (native vein plus synthetic graft) is an alternative.[6] PTA with stenting may also be used in combination with bypass surgery.

Other surgical options include *endarterectomy* (opening the artery and removing the obstructing plaque) and *patch graft angioplasty* (opening the artery, removing plaque, and sewing a patch to the opening to widen the lumen). In-hospital mortality is higher in women undergoing revascularization than men, regardless of disease severity or procedure performed.[17]

Amputation may be required if tissue necrosis is extensive, gangrene or osteomyelitis develops, or all major arteries in the limb are blocked, precluding the possibility of successful surgery. Every effort is made to preserve as much of the limb as possible to improve the potential for rehabilitation. (Amputation is discussed in Chapter 62.)

❖ NURSING MANAGEMENT: LOWER EXTREMITY PERIPHERAL ARTERY DISEASE

◆ Nursing Assessment

Table 37-4 presents subjective and objective data that you should obtain from a patient with PAD.

◆ Nursing Diagnoses

Nursing diagnoses for the patient with PAD may include, but are not limited to, the following:

- Ineffective peripheral tissue perfusion *related to* deficient knowledge of contributing factors
- Activity intolerance *related to* imbalance between O_2 supply and demand
- Chronic pain *related to* ischemia, inflammation, and swelling
- Ineffective health management *related to* lack of knowledge of disease and self-care measures

TABLE 37-4 Nursing Assessment

Peripheral Artery Disease

Subjective Data

Important Health Information

Past health history: Tobacco use, diabetes mellitus, hypertension, hyperlipidemia, hypertriglyceridemia, hyperuricemia, impaired renal function, obesity. ↑ high-sensitivity C-reactive protein, homocysteine, or lipoprotein (a) [Lp(a)] levels. Positive family history, sedentary lifestyle, stress

Functional Health Patterns

Health perception–health management: Family history of cardiovascular disease. Tobacco use, including exposure to environmental smoke

Nutritional-metabolic: High sodium, saturated fat, and cholesterol intake. Elevated A1C

Activity-exercise: Exercise intolerance

Cognitive-perceptual: Buttock, thigh, or calf pain that is precipitated by exercise and that subsides with rest (intermittent claudication) or progresses to pain at rest. Burning pain in feet and toes at rest. Numbness, tingling, sensation of cold in legs or feet. Progressive loss of sensation and deep pain in extremities

Sexuality-reproductive: Erectile dysfunction

Objective Data

Integumentary

Loss of hair on legs and feet. Thick toenails. Pallor with elevation. Dependent rubor. Thin, cool, shiny skin with muscle atrophy. Skin breakdown and arterial ulcers, especially over bony areas. Gangrene

Cardiovascular

Decreased or absent peripheral pulses. Feet cool to touch. Capillary refill >3 sec. Bruits may be present at pulse sites.

Neurologic

Mobility or sensation impairment

Possible Diagnostic Findings

Arterial stenosis evident with duplex imaging, ↓ Doppler pressures, ↓ ankle-brachial index, angiography indicative of peripheral atherosclerosis

Additional information on nursing diagnoses for the patient with PAD of the lower extremities is presented in eNursing Care Plan 37-1 on the website for this chapter.

◆ Planning

The overall goals for the patient who has lower extremity PAD include (1) adequate tissue perfusion; (2) relief of pain; (3) increased exercise tolerance; (4) intact, healthy skin on the extremities; and (5) increased knowledge of disease and treatment plan.

◆ Nursing Implementation

◆ **Health Promotion.** Assess the patient for CVD risk factors and provide instructions on how to control them (see Tables 33-1 to 33-2). Also teach diet modification to reduce the intake of cholesterol, saturated fat, and refined sugars (see Tables 33-3 to 33-4); proper care of the feet; and avoidance of injury to the extremities. Encourage patients with positive family histories of cardiac, diabetic, or vascular disease to obtain regular follow-up care.

◆ **Acute Care.** After surgical or radiologic intervention, the patient is moved to a recovery area for observation. Check the operative extremity every 15 minutes initially and then hourly for color, temperature, capillary refill, presence of peripheral pulses, and sensation and movement. Loss of palpable pulses or a change in the Doppler sound over a pulse requires immediate notification of the HCP and prompt intervention. Postoperative ABI measurements are not recommended as they place the patient at risk for graft thrombosis. Compare all assessment findings with the patient's baseline and with findings in the opposite limb.

Many PAD patients have a history of chronic ischemic rest pain and may have developed a tolerance to opioids. Thus aggressive pain management may be needed postoperatively.

After the patient leaves the recovery area, continue to monitor perfusion to the extremities. Assess for potential complications such as bleeding, hematoma, thrombosis, embolization, and compartment syndrome. A dramatic increase in pain, loss of previously palpable pulses, extremity pallor or cyanosis, numbness or tingling, or a cold extremity suggests blockage of the graft or stent. Report these findings to the HCP immediately.

Avoid placing the patient in a knee-flexed position except for exercise. Turn the patient and position frequently with pillows to support the incision. On postoperative day 1, assist the patient out of bed several times daily. Discourage prolonged sitting with leg dependency, since it may cause pain and edema, increase the risk of venous thrombosis, and place stress on the suture lines. If edema develops, position the patient supine and elevate the leg above heart level.

CHECK YOUR PRACTICE

You are caring for a 74-yr-old male patient who is recovering from left femoral-popliteal bypass graft surgery. When responding to the patient's call bell, the patient reports severe pain in the operative leg. On assessment, you note that the dorsalis pedis and posterior tibial pulses are no longer palpable and the foot is cold to touch.

- What are your next actions?

Graduated compression stockings may be used to help control leg edema. Walking even short distances is desirable. The use of a walker may be helpful, especially in frail, older patients.

Surgical site infection (SSI) occurs in about 5% of cases. Women develop SSIs more often than men.[18] Careful postoperative assessment and wound care are important. SSIs are associated with early graft loss, longer hospitalizations, reoperation, and sepsis. If no complications occur, discharge can be anticipated 3 to 5 days after surgery.

◆ **Ambulatory Care.** Assess for CVD risk factors and be alert for opportunities to teach health promotion strategies to patients and their caregivers (see Chapters 4 and 33). Continued tobacco use dramatically decreases the long-term patency rates of grafts and stents and increases the risk of an MI or stroke. Long-term antiplatelet therapy with aspirin or clopidogrel is recommended for patients after surgery. Patients having distal peripheral bypass surgery (i.e., below the knee) using synthetic graft materials are given dual antiplatelet therapy (clopidogrel plus aspirin) for 1 year, followed by lifelong single antiplatelet therapy.[19]

Encourage supervised exercise training after a successful revascularization. Explain that exercise decreases CVD risk

TABLE 37-5 Patient & Caregiver Teaching

Peripheral Artery Bypass Surgery

Include the following information in the teaching plan for a patient undergoing peripheral artery bypass surgery and the patient's caregiver.

1. Reduce risk factors by stopping the use of all tobacco products, controlling blood glucose levels (if diabetic) and blood pressure, lowering cholesterol and triglyceride levels, achieving or maintaining ideal body weight, and exercising regularly.
2. Provide teaching about the basic mechanism of action and side effects of drugs such as antiplatelets, antihypertensives, lipid-lowering therapy, and pain medication.
3. Eat healthy—it is essential to recovery. Drink plenty of fluids, eat a well-balanced diet (e.g., foods high in protein, vitamins C and A, and zinc; high-fiber foods; fresh fruits and vegetables), eat fewer high-fat foods, and reduce salt intake.
4. Participate in a supervised exercise program or take a daily walk. In the beginning, take several short walks a day and rest between activities. Gradually increase your walking to 30 to 40 min/day, 3 to 5 days/wk.
5. Care for feet and legs. Inspect feet and wash them daily. Wear clean cotton or wool socks and well-fitting shoes. File toenails straight across. Avoid sitting with legs crossed, extreme hot and cold temperatures, and prolonged standing.
6. Follow routine postoperative wound care that includes keeping incision clean and dry; do not disturb Steri-Strips (if present).
7. Monitor for signs and symptoms of impaired healing or infection of the leg incision, and notify HCP if any of the following occur:
   - Prolonged drainage or pus from the incision
   - Increased redness, warmth, pain, or hardness along incision
   - Separation of wound edges
   - Temperature >100°F (37.8°C)
8. Keep all follow-up appointments with HCP.
9. Notify HCP immediately of increased leg or foot pain or a change in the color or temperature of leg or foot.

factors, including hypertension, hyperlipidemia, obesity, and glucose levels. Teach foot care to all patients with PAD. Meticulous foot care is especially important in the patient with diabetes and PAD (see Table 48-21). Diabetic neuropathy increases the patient's risk for injury and results in delay in seeking treatment. Tell patients to inspect their legs and feet daily for mottling, changes in skin color or texture, and reduction in hair growth. Show patients how to check skin temperature and capillary refill and to palpate pulses. Stress that they must report any changes in these findings or the development of ulceration or inflammation to their HCP.

Thick or overgrown toenails and calluses are potentially serious and require regular attention by an HCP (e.g., podiatrist). Patients who have poor eyesight, back problems, obesity, or arthritis may need help with foot care. Encourage patients to wear clean, all-cotton or all-wool socks and comfortable shoes with rounded (not pointed) toes and soft insoles. Tell patients to lace shoes loosely and to break in new shoes gradually (Table 37-5).

◆ Evaluation

The expected outcomes are that a patient with PAD of the lower extremities will have:

- Adequate peripheral tissue perfusion
- Increased activity tolerance
- Effective pain management
- Knowledge of disease and treatment plan

Additional information on the expected outcomes for the patient with PAD of the lower extremities is presented in eNursing Care Plan 37-1 (available on the website for this chapter).

ACUTE ARTERIAL ISCHEMIC DISORDERS

Etiology and Pathophysiology

Acute arterial ischemia is a sudden interruption in the arterial blood supply to a tissue, an organ, or an extremity that, if left untreated, can result in tissue death. It is caused by embolism, thrombosis of a preexisting atherosclerotic artery, or trauma. *Embolization* of a thrombus from the heart is the most frequent cause of acute arterial occlusion. Heart conditions in which thrombi can develop include infective endocarditis, mitral valve disease, atrial fibrillation, cardiomyopathies, and prosthetic heart valves. Noncardiac sources of emboli include aneurysms, ulcerated atherosclerotic plaque, recent endovascular procedures, and venous thrombi.

The thrombi become dislodged and may travel anywhere in the systemic circulation if they originate in the left side of the heart. Most emboli block an artery of the lower extremity in areas where vessels branch (e.g., iliofemoral, popliteal, tibial) or there is atherosclerotic narrowing. Sudden local thrombosis may occur at the site of an atherosclerotic plaque. Hypovolemia (e.g., shock), hyperviscosity (e.g., polycythemia), and hypercoagulability (e.g., chemotherapy) predispose an individual to thrombotic arterial occlusion.

Traumatic injury to the extremity itself may cause partial or total blockage. Acute arterial occlusion may also develop as a result of arterial dissection in the carotid artery or aorta or as a result of a procedure-related arterial injury (e.g., after angiography).

Clinical Manifestations

Clinical manifestations of acute arterial ischemia include the *six Ps: pain, pallor, pulselessness, paresthesia, paralysis,* and *poikilothermia* (adaptation of the limb to the environmental temperature, most often cool). Without immediate intervention, ischemia may progress to tissue necrosis and gangrene within a few hours. If you detect these signs, immediately notify the HCP.

Paralysis is a late sign of acute arterial ischemia and signals the death of nerves supplying the extremity. Foot drop occurs as a result of nerve damage. Because nerve tissue is extremely sensitive to hypoxia, limb paralysis or ischemic neuropathy may persist even after revascularization.

Interprofessional Care

Early diagnosis and treatment are essential to keep the affected limb viable during acute arterial ischemia. Anticoagulant therapy with IV unfractionated heparin (UH) is started to prevent thrombus growth and inhibit further embolization. In patients undergoing embolectomy, UH should be followed by long-term anticoagulation with warfarin (see discussion of other anticoagulant options later in this chapter).

To restore blood flow, the thrombus is removed as soon as possible. Options consist of surgical thrombectomy (recommended procedure), percutaneous catheter-directed thrombolytic therapy, percutaneous mechanical thrombectomy with or without thrombolytic therapy, or surgical bypass. A mechanical catheter that is used with a thrombolytic is known as a *pharmacomechanical device.*[20]

Percutaneous catheter-directed thrombolytic therapy using tissue plasminogen activator (tPA [alteplase]) or urokinase

(Kinlytic) is recommended for acute arterial ischemia of duration less than 14 days.[6] A catheter is inserted into the femoral artery and moved to the site of the clot, and the thrombolytic drug is continuously infused. Thrombolytic agents work by directly dissolving the clot over a period of 24 to 48 hours. (Chapter 33 discusses thrombolytic therapy.)

The mechanical thrombectomy device is designed to extract or fragment the thrombus. Surgical revascularization may be used in a patient with trauma (e.g., laceration of the artery) or with significant arterial blockage. Amputation is reserved for patients with ischemic rest pain and tissue loss in whom limb salvage is not possible. If the patient remains at risk for further embolization from a persistent source (e.g., chronic atrial fibrillation), long-term anticoagulation is recommended to prevent further acute arterial ischemic episodes[21] (see Table 37-10 on p. 820).

THROMBOANGIITIS OBLITERANS

Thromboangiitis obliterans (Buerger's disease) is a nonatherosclerotic, segmental, recurrent inflammatory disorder of the small and medium arteries and veins of the upper and lower extremities. Rarely, systemic manifestations of the disease may involve cerebral, coronary, mesenteric, pulmonary, and/or renal arteries. The disease occurs mostly in young men (younger than 45 years of age) with a long history of tobacco and/or marijuana use and chronic periodontal infection but without other CVD risk factors (e.g., hypertension, hyperlipidemia, diabetes).[22]

In the acute phase of Buerger's disease, an inflammatory thrombus forms and blocks the vessel. Over time, the thrombus becomes more organized and the inflammation in the vessel wall subsides.[22]

During the chronic phase, thrombosis and fibrosis occur in the vessel, causing tissue ischemia. The symptoms of Buerger's disease often are confused with PAD and other autoimmune diseases (e.g., scleroderma). Patients may have intermittent claudication of the feet, hands, or arms. As the disease progresses, rest pain and ischemic ulcerations develop. Other signs and symptoms may include color and temperature changes of the limbs, paresthesia, superficial vein thrombosis, and cold sensitivity.

There are no laboratory or diagnostic tests specific to Buerger's disease. Diagnosis is made based on age of onset; history; clinical symptoms; involvement of distal vessels; presence of ischemic ulcerations; and exclusion of autoimmune disease, diabetes, thrombophilia (inherited tendency to clot), and other sources of emboli, such as atherosclerosis and aneurysm.[22]

The primary treatment for Buerger's disease is the complete cessation of tobacco and marijuana use in any form. Use of nicotine replacement products is contraindicated. Patients must choose between their tobacco or marijuana and their affected limb, but not both.

Conservative management includes avoiding limb exposure to cold temperatures, a supervised walking program, antibiotics to treat any infected ulcers, and analgesics to manage the ischemic pain. Teach patients to avoid trauma to the extremities.

A variety of drugs have been tried to treat Buerger's disease (e.g., calcium channel blockers, cilostazol, sildenafil [Viagra]). Although these drugs do not stop disease progression, they can be used to decrease pain.

One promising drug used to manage pain has been IV iloprost (Ventavis), a prostaglandin analog that promotes vasodilation. This drug improves rest pain, promotes healing of ischemic ulcers, and decreases the need for amputation.[22]

Surgical options include *sympathectomy* (transection of a nerve, ganglion, and/or plexus of the sympathetic nervous system), implantation of a spinal cord stimulator, and bypass surgery. Sympathectomy and implantation of a spinal cord stimulator can improve distal blood flow, reduce pain, and decrease the rate of amputation but neither alters the inflammatory process. Bypass surgery typically is not an option because of the involvement of smaller, distal vessels but may be used in selected patients with severe ischemia.

Painful ulcerations may require finger or toe amputations. Amputation below the knee may be needed in severe cases. The rate of amputation in patients who continue tobacco or marijuana use after diagnosis is much higher than in those who stop.[22]

RAYNAUD'S PHENOMENON

Raynaud's phenomenon is an episodic vasospastic disorder of small cutaneous arteries, most often involving the fingers and toes. It occurs primarily in young women (typically between 15 and 40 years of age), and it is more common in women than men. The pathogenesis of Raynaud's phenomenon is due to abnormalities in the vascular, intravascular, and neuronal mechanisms that cause an imbalance between vasodilation and vasoconstriction.[23]

Raynaud's phenomenon may occur in isolation *(primary Raynaud's phenomenon)* or in association with an underlying disease (e.g., rheumatoid arthritis, scleroderma, systemic lupus erythematosus) *(secondary Raynaud's phenomenon)*. Other contributing factors include occupation-related conditions, such as the use of vibrating machinery or work in cold environments, exposure to heavy metals (e.g., lead), and hyperhomocysteinemia.

Diagnosis is based on persistent symptoms for at least 2 years. Patients with Raynaud's phenomenon should have routine follow-up to monitor for development of connective tissue or autoimmune diseases.

Raynaud's phenomenon is characterized by vasospasm-induced color changes of fingers, toes, ears, and nose (white, blue, and red). Decreased perfusion results in pallor (white). The digits then appear cyanotic (bluish purple) (Fig. 37-3). These changes are followed by rubor (red), caused by the hyperemic response that occurs when blood flow is restored. The patient usually describes coldness and numbness in the vasoconstrictive phase. This is followed by throbbing, aching pain,

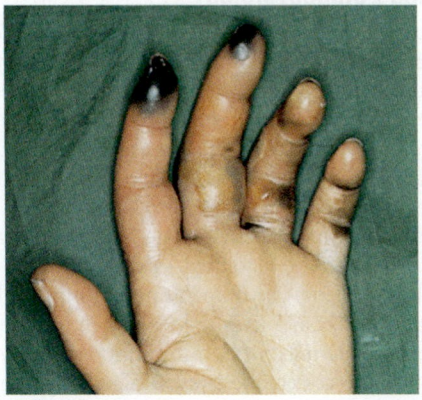

FIG. 37-3 Raynaud's phenomenon. (From Kamal A, Brockelhurst JC: *Colour atlas of geriatric medicine*, ed 2, 1991, Mosby-Year Book-Europe.)

tingling, and swelling in the hyperemic phase. An episode usually lasts only minutes but in severe cases may persist for several hours. Exposure to cold, emotional upsets, tobacco use, and caffeine often bring on symptoms.

After frequent, prolonged attacks the skin may become thickened and the nails brittle. Occasionally, complications include *punctate* (small hole) lesions of the fingertips and superficial gangrenous ulcers in advanced stages.

The primary focus of nursing management of Raynaud's phenomenon is patient teaching. Focus your instructions on preventing recurrent episodes. Tell patients to wear loose, warm clothing as protection from the cold, including gloves when handling cold objects. At all times, patients should avoid temperature extremes. Immersing hands in warm water often decreases the vasospasm. The patient should stop using all tobacco products and avoid caffeine and other drugs that have vasoconstrictive effects (e.g., cocaine, amphetamines, ergotamine, pseudoephedrine). Finally, provide patients with stress management strategies as appropriate.

When conservative management is ineffective, drug therapy is considered. Sustained-release calcium channel blockers (e.g., nifedipine [Procardia]) are the first-line drug therapy. Calcium channel blockers relax smooth muscles of the arterioles by blocking the influx of calcium into the cells. This reduces the frequency and severity of vasospastic attacks. If calcium channel blockers are not sufficient treatment, other vasodilators (e.g., transdermal glyceryl trinitrate [Nitro-Dur]) may be used.[24]

Prompt intervention is needed for patients with digital ulceration and/or critical ischemia. Treatment options include prostacyclin infusion therapy (e.g., iloprost), antibiotics, analgesics, and possibly an endothelin receptor antagonist (e.g., bosentan [Tracleer]) and surgical debridement of necrotic tissue. Statins may also lessen the severity of Raynaud's phenomenon.[24] Sympathectomy is considered only in advanced cases.

AORTIC ANEURYSMS

The aorta is the largest artery and supplies O_2, nutrients, and blood to all vital organs. One of the most common problems affecting the aorta is an **aneurysm**, which is a permanent, localized outpouching or dilation of the vessel wall. Aneurysms occur in men more often than in women and in whites more often than African Americans. The incidence increases with age.[25] Aneurysms may occur in more than one location. Peripheral artery aneurysms can also develop but are not common.

Etiology and Pathophysiology

Aortic aneurysms may involve the aortic arch and thoracic and/or abdominal aorta. Three fourths of aortic aneurysms occur in the abdominal aorta (Fig. 37-4) and one fourth in the thoracic aorta. Most abdominal aortic aneurysms (AAAs) occur below the renal arteries. Growth rates are higher in patients who smoke tobacco.[25] The larger the aneurysm, the greater the risk of rupture.

A variety of disorders are associated with aortic aneurysms. The primary causes are classified as degenerative, congenital, mechanical (e.g., penetrating or blunt trauma), inflammatory (e.g., aortitis [Takayasu's arteritis]), or infectious (e.g., aortitis [*Chlamydia pneumoniae,* human immunodeficiency virus]).

Risk factors for aortic aneurysms include age, male gender, hypertension, CAD, family history, tobacco use, high cholesterol, lower extremity PAD, carotid artery disease, previous stroke, and excess weight or obesity. Tobacco use is the most important modifiable risk factor.[25]

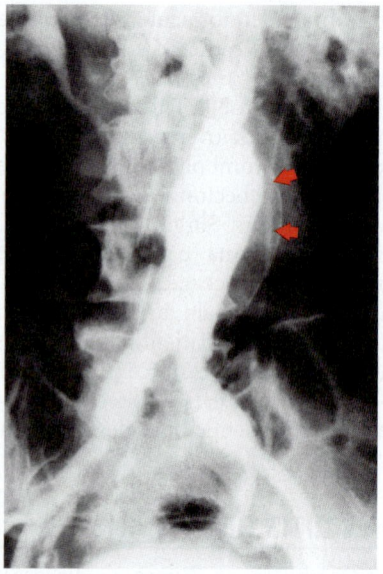

FIG. 37-4 Angiography demonstrating fusiform abdominal aortic aneurysm. Note calcification of the aortic wall *(arrows)* and extension of the aneurysm into the common iliac arteries. (Courtesy Jo Menzoian, Boston, Mass.)

Genetic Link

The development of both aortic aneurysm and aortic dissection has a strong genetic component. The familial tendency is related to a number of congenital anomalies. Examples include bicuspid aortic valve, coarctation of the aorta, Turner syndrome, autosomal dominant polycystic kidney disease, specific collagen defects (e.g., Ehlers-Danlos syndrome), and premature breakdown of vascular elastic tissue (e.g., Marfan's syndrome).[26]

Classification

Aneurysms are classified as true or false aneurysms (Fig. 37-5, *A* to *C*). A *true aneurysm* is one in which the wall of the artery forms the aneurysm, with at least one vessel layer still intact. True aneurysms are further subdivided into fusiform and saccular types. A *fusiform aneurysm* is circumferential and relatively uniform in shape. A *saccular aneurysm* is pouchlike with a narrow neck connecting the bulge to one side of the arterial wall.

A *false aneurysm,* or *pseudoaneurysm,* is not an aneurysm but a disruption of all arterial wall layers with bleeding that is contained by surrounding anatomic structures. False aneurysms may result from trauma, infection, peripheral artery bypass graft surgery (at the site of the graft-to-artery anastomosis), or arterial leakage after removal of cannulae (e.g., femoral artery catheters, intraaortic balloon pump devices).

Clinical Manifestations

Thoracic aortic aneurysms (TAAs) are often asymptomatic. When present, symptoms include deep, diffuse chest pain that may extend to the interscapular area. Ascending aorta and aortic arch aneurysms can cause (1) angina from decreased blood flow to the coronary arteries; (2) transient ischemic attacks from decreased blood flow to the carotid arteries; and (3) coughing, shortness of breath, hoarseness, and/or dysphagia

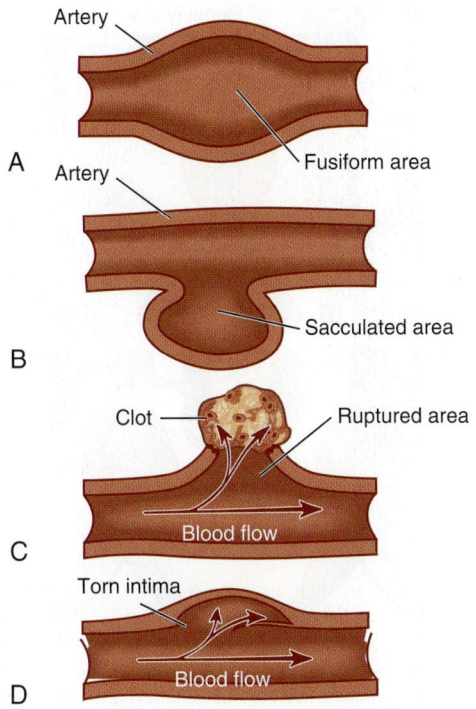

FIG. 37-5 **A,** True fusiform abdominal aortic aneurysm. **B,** True saccular aortic aneurysm. **C,** False aneurysm, or pseudoaneurysm. **D,** Aortic dissection.

(difficulty swallowing) from pressure on the laryngeal nerve. If the aneurysm presses on the superior vena cava, decreased venous return can result in jugular venous distention (distended neck veins) and edema of the face and arms.

AAAs are often asymptomatic and frequently found during routine physical examinations or evaluations for an unrelated problem (e.g., abdominal x-ray, CT scan). A pulsatile mass in the periumbilical area slightly to the left of the midline may be present. Bruits may be auscultated over the aneurysm. Physical findings may be more difficult to detect in obese individuals.

AAA symptoms may mimic pain associated with abdominal or back disorders. Compression of nearby anatomic structures and nerves may cause symptoms such as back pain, epigastric discomfort, altered bowel elimination, and intermittent claudication. Occasionally, aneurysms spontaneously embolize plaque, causing *"blue toe syndrome"* (patchy mottling of the feet and toes in the presence of palpable pedal pulses).

Complications

Rupture of an aneurysm is the most serious complication. It is more likely to occur in people who smoke tobacco.[3,25] If rupture occurs into the retroperitoneal space, bleeding may be controlled by surrounding anatomic structures, preventing exsanguination and death. In this case the patient often has severe back pain and may or may not have back or flank ecchymosis *(Grey Turner's sign)*.

If rupture occurs into the thoracic or abdominal cavity, patients can die from massive hemorrhage. The patient who reaches the hospital will be in hypovolemic shock with tachycardia, hypotension, pale clammy skin, decreased urine output, altered level of consciousness, and abdominal tenderness. (Shock is discussed in Chapter 66.) In this situation, simultaneous resuscitation and immediate surgical repair are necessary. For patients admitted to the hospital with a ruptured AAA, in-hospital mortality is high at 53%.[3,26]

Diagnostic Studies

Chest x-rays are done to reveal abnormal widening of the thoracic aorta. An abdominal x-ray may show calcification within the aortic wall. An electrocardiogram (ECG) may rule out MI, since thoracic aneurysm or dissection symptoms can mimic angina. Echocardiography assesses the function of the aortic valve. Ultrasound is useful for aneurysm screening and to monitor aneurysm size. A CT scan is the most accurate test to determine the length and cross-sectional diameter and the presence of thrombus in the aneurysm. MRI may also be used to diagnose and assess the location and severity of aneurysms. Angiography provides helpful information by using contrast imaging to map the entire aortic system. (Chapter 31 and Table 31-6 discuss angiography.)

Interprofessional Care

The primary goal of interprofessional care is to prevent the rupture of an aneurysm. Early detection and prompt treatment are essential. Conservative medical therapy of small, asymptomatic AAAs (4.0 to 5.4 cm) is the best practice.[6] This consists of risk factor modification (ceasing tobacco use, decreasing BP, optimizing lipid profile, gradually increasing physical activity) and monitoring of aneurysm size using ultrasound or CT every 6 to 12 months. Growth rates may be lowered with β-blockers (e.g., propranolol [Inderal]), ACE inhibitors (e.g., captopril [Capoten]), and angiotensin II receptor blockers (e.g., losartan [Cozaar]), statins (e.g., simvastatin [Zocor]), and antibiotics (e.g., doxycycline [Acticlate]).[26] Monitoring by ultrasound every 2 to 3 years is recommended for patients with AAAs smaller than 4.0 cm in diameter.[6]

Surgical repair is recommended in patients with asymptomatic aneurysms 5.5 cm in diameter or larger. Surgical intervention may occur sooner if the patient has a genetic disorder (e.g., Marfan's, Ehlers-Danlos syndrome), the aneurysm expands rapidly, it becomes symptomatic, or the risk of rupture is high.[6] A careful review of body systems is necessary to identify any co-morbidities, especially of the lungs, heart, or kidneys, because they affect the patient's surgical risk. Correction of existing carotid or coronary artery blockages may be needed before the aneurysm is repaired.

Surgical Therapy. For elective surgery, the patient needs to be well hydrated, and any electrolyte, coagulation, and hematocrit abnormalities are corrected preoperatively. If the aneurysm has ruptured, emergent surgical intervention is required.

The open aneurysm repair (OAR) involves a large abdominal incision through which the surgeon (1) cuts into the diseased aortic segment, (2) removes any thrombus or plaque, (3) sutures a synthetic graft to the aorta proximal and distal to the aneurysm, and (4) sutures the native aortic wall around the graft to act as a protective cover (Fig. 37-6). If the iliac arteries are also aneurysmal, a bifurcated graft replaces the entire diseased segment. With saccular aneurysms, it may be possible to excise only the bulbous lesion, repairing the artery by primary closure (suturing the artery together) or by application of an autogenous or synthetic patch graft.

All OARs require aortic cross-clamping proximal and distal to the aneurysm. Most resections are done in 30 to 45 minutes, after which the clamps are removed and blood flow is restored. If the cross clamp must be applied above the renal arteries,

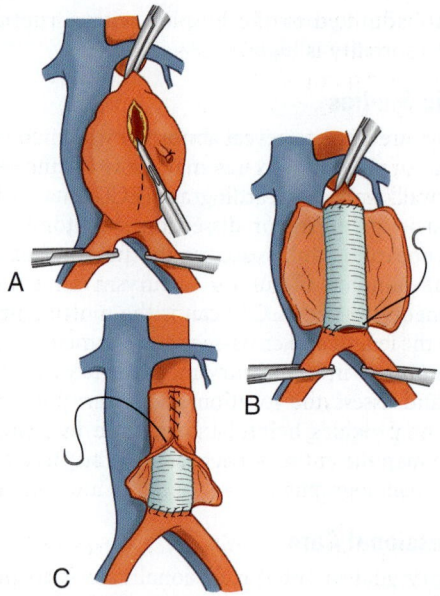

FIG. 37-6 Surgical repair of an abdominal aortic aneurysm. **A,** Incising the aneurysmal sac. **B,** Insertion of synthetic graft. **C,** Suturing native aortic wall over synthetic graft.

adequate renal blood flow after clamp removal should be determined before closure of the abdominal incision. The risk of postoperative renal complications such as acute kidney injury increases in patients who have OAR of AAAs above the level of the renal arteries.

Endovascular Graft Procedure. Minimally invasive endovascular aneurysm repair (EVAR) is an alternative to OAR for select patients. Eligibility criteria include iliofemoral vessels that allow for safe graft insertion and vessels of sufficient length and width to support the graft.[26]

EVAR involves the placement of a sutureless aortic graft into the abdominal aorta inside the aneurysm via the femoral artery. The grafts are made of various materials, such as a Dacron cylinder consisting of several sections, and are supported with multiple rings of flexible wire (Fig. 37-7).

The main section of the graft is bifurcated and delivered through a femoral artery catheter. The second part of the graft is inserted through the opposite femoral artery. When all graft components are in place, they are released (deployed) against the vessel wall by balloon inflation. The blood then flows through the endovascular graft, thus preventing further expansion of the aneurysm.

Postprocedure angiography is done to check for any leaks and to confirm patency of all stent-graft components. The aneurysmal wall will shrink over time because the blood is being diverted through the endograft.

Complications. EVAR is less invasive than OAR. EVAR also has fewer complications, such as paraplegia and death. In addition, hospital stays are shorter with EVAR.[27] Women have a higher rate of complications after EVAR compared to men. However, there are no gender differences in mortality rates.[28]

The most common complication of AAA repair is *endoleak,* the seepage of blood back into the old aneurysm. This may be the result of an inadequate seal at either graft end, a tear through the graft fabric, or leakage between overlapping graft segments. Repair may require coil embolization (insertion of beads) for hemostasis.

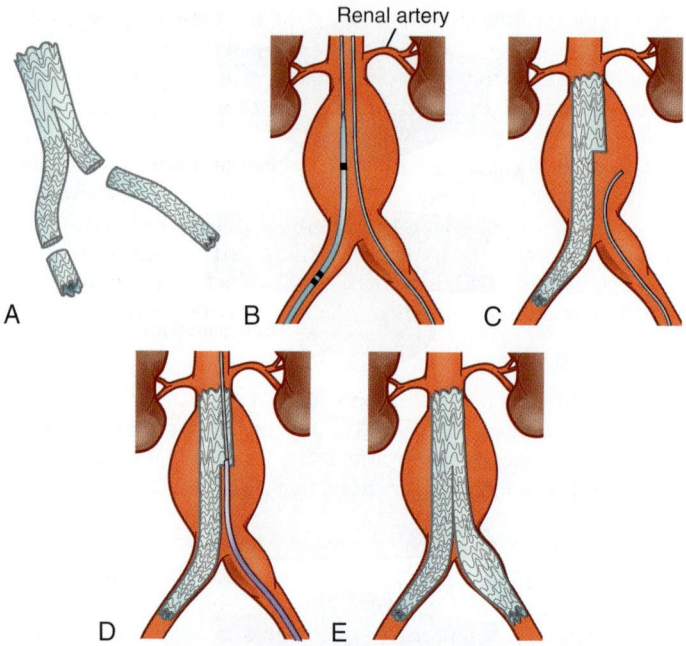

FIG. 37-7 Bifurcated (two-branched) endovascular stent grafting of an aneurysm. **A,** Insertion of a woven polyester tube (graft) covered by a tubular metal web (stent). **B,** The stent graft is inserted through a large blood vessel (e.g., femoral artery) using a delivery catheter. The catheter is positioned below the renal arteries in the area of the aneurysm. **C,** The stent graft is slowly released (deployed) into the blood vessel. When the stent comes in contact with the blood vessel, it expands to a preset size. **D,** A second stent graft can be inserted in the contralateral (opposite) vessel if necessary. **E,** Fully deployed bifurcated stent graft.

Other potential complications include aneurysm growth above or below the graft, aneurysm rupture, aortic dissection, bleeding, renal artery occlusion caused by stent migration, graft thrombosis, incisional site hematoma, and incisional infection. Patients undergoing EVAR require periodic imaging for the rest of their lives to monitor for an endoleak, document stability of the aneurysm sac, and determine the need for surgical intervention.

A potentially lethal complication in an emergency repair of a ruptured AAA is the development of *intraabdominal hypertension* (IAH) with associated *abdominal compartment syndrome* (ACS). Persistent IAH reduces blood flow to the viscera. ACS refers to the impaired organ perfusion caused by IAH and resulting multisystem organ failure.[29] IAH is confirmed by measuring the patient's intraabdominal pressure indirectly through a catheter and transducer system, typically by using an indwelling urinary catheter.

Treatment goals include control of situations that lead to IAH. Interventions include open (surgical) decompression, percutaneous drainage, and percutaneous drainage combined with tPA infusion. Conservative measures such as intubation, ventilation, patient positioning, gastric decompression, cautious fluid resuscitation, pain management, and temporary hemofiltration are also used.

❖ NURSING MANAGEMENT: AORTIC ANEURYSMS

◆ Nursing Assessment

Begin by performing a thorough history and physical assessment. Because atherosclerosis is a systemic disease, look for signs of coexisting cardiac, pulmonary, cerebral, and lower extremity vascular problems. Monitor the patient for signs of aneurysm rupture, such as diaphoresis; pallor; weakness; tachycardia; hypotension; abdominal, back, groin, or periumbilical pain; changes in level of consciousness; or a pulsating abdominal mass.

Establishing baseline data is critical for comparison with later postoperative assessments. Pay special attention to the character and quality of the patient's peripheral pulses, and renal and neurologic status. Before surgery, mark pedal pulse sites (dorsalis pedis and posterior tibial) with a single-use marker and document any skin lesions on the lower extremities.

Planning

The overall goals for a patient undergoing aortic surgery include (1) normal tissue perfusion; (2) intact motor and sensory function; and (3) no complications related to surgical repair, such as thrombosis, infection, or rupture.

Nursing Implementation

Health Promotion. To promote overall health, encourage the patient to reduce CVD risk factors (see Table 33-2), including controlling BP, ceasing tobacco use (see Chapter 10), increasing physical activity, and maintaining normal body weight and serum lipid levels. These measures also help ensure continued graft patency after surgical repair.

Acute Care. During the preoperative period, provide emotional support and teaching to the patient and caregiver. Preoperative teaching includes a brief explanation of the disease process, the planned surgical procedure(s), preoperative routines, what to expect immediately after surgery (e.g., recovery room, tubes and drains), and usual postoperative timelines. Specific preoperative routines vary by agency and surgeon. In general, aortic surgery patients have a bowel preparation (e.g., laxatives, enemas) and skin cleansing with an antimicrobial agent the day before surgery, have nothing by mouth (NPO) after midnight the day of surgery, and receive IV antibiotics immediately before the incision is made. If appropriate, a preoperative visit to the intensive care unit (ICU) may be helpful to the patient and caregiver. Patients with a history of CVD should receive a β-blocker (e.g., metoprolol [Lopressor]) preoperatively.

Postoperatively, aortic surgery patients typically go to an ICU for 24 to 48 hours for close monitoring. When the patient arrives in the ICU, various devices are in place. These include an endotracheal tube for mechanical ventilation, an arterial line, a central venous pressure (CVP) or pulmonary artery (PA) catheter, peripheral IV lines, an indwelling urinary catheter, and a nasogastric (NG) tube. The patient needs continuous ECG and pulse oximetry monitoring. If the thorax is opened during surgery, chest tubes will be in place. Pain medication is given via epidural catheter or patient-controlled analgesia (PCA).

In addition to the usual goals of care for a postoperative patient (e.g., maintaining adequate respiratory function, fluid and electrolyte balance, and pain control [see Chapter 19]), check for graft patency and renal perfusion. Also watch for and intervene to limit or treat cardiac ischemia, dysrhythmias, infections, VTE, and neurologic complications. eNursing Care Plan 37-2 for the patient with an aneurysm repair or other aortic surgery is available on the website for this chapter.

Graft Patency. An adequate BP is important to maintain graft patency. Prolonged low BP may result in graft thrombosis. Give IV fluids and blood components as ordered to maintain adequate blood flow. Monitor CVP or PA pressures and urine output hourly in the immediate postoperative period to assess the patient's hydration and perfusion status.

Avoid severe hypertension, since it may cause undue stress on the arterial anastomoses, resulting in leakage of blood or rupture at the suture lines. Drug therapy with IV diuretics (e.g., furosemide [Lasix]) or IV antihypertensive agents (e.g., labetalol [Normodyne], metoprolol, hydralazine [Apresoline], sodium nitroprusside [Nipride]) may be indicated.

Cardiovascular Status. Myocardial ischemia or infarction may occur in the perioperative period because of decreased myocardial O_2 supply or increased myocardial O_2 demands. Cardiac dysrhythmias may occur because of electrolyte imbalances, hypoxemia, hypothermia, or myocardial ischemia. Nursing interventions include continuous ECG monitoring; frequent electrolyte and arterial blood gas determinations; administration of O_2, IV antidysrhythmic and antihypertensive drugs, and electrolytes as needed; adequate pain control; and resumption of cardiac drugs.

Infection. A prosthetic vascular graft infection is a relatively rare but potentially life-threatening complication. Nursing interventions to prevent infection include giving a broad-spectrum antibiotic as prescribed. Assess temperature regularly, and promptly report elevations. Monitor laboratory data for an elevated white blood cell (WBC) count, which may be the first indication of an infection. Ensure adequate nutrition and assess the surgical incision for signs of infection (e.g., redness, swelling, drainage). Keep surgical incisions clean and dry and perform wound care as ordered.

Use strict aseptic technique in the care of all peripheral, arterial, and CVP or PA catheter insertion sites, since these are ports of entry for bacteria. Meticulous perineal care for the patient with an indwelling urinary catheter and early catheter removal are essential to minimize the risk of urinary tract infection.

Gastrointestinal Status. After OAR, postoperative ileus may develop as a result of anesthesia and the handling of the bowel during surgery. The intestines may become swollen and bruised, and peristalsis ceases for variable intervals. A retroperitoneal surgical approach can be used to decrease the risk of bowel complications.

An NG tube may be placed during surgery and connected to low, intermittent suction to decompress the stomach, prevent aspiration of stomach contents, and decrease pressure on suture lines. Record the amount and character of the NG output. While the patient is NPO, provide oral care frequently. Ice chips or lozenges can help soothe a dry or irritated throat. Assess for bowel sounds every 4 hours. The passing of flatus signals returning bowel function and should be noted. Encourage early ambulation, since this can help the return of bowel function. A postoperative ileus rarely lasts beyond the fourth postoperative day.

If the blood supply to the bowel is disrupted during surgery, temporary ischemia or infarction (death) of intestinal tissue may result. Clinical manifestations of this rare but serious complication include absent bowel sounds, fever, abdominal distention and pain, diarrhea, and bloody stools. If bowel infarction occurs, immediate reoperation is necessary to restore blood flow, with likely resection of the infarcted bowel.

Neurologic Status. Neurologic complications can occur after aortic surgery. When the ascending aorta and aortic arch are involved, assess the patient's level of consciousness, pupil size and response to light, facial symmetry, tongue position, speech, upper extremity movement, and quality of hand grasps (see

Chapter 55). When the descending aorta is involved, perform a neurovascular assessment of the lower extremities. Record all assessments and report changes from baseline to the HCP immediately.

◆ ***Peripheral Perfusion Status.*** The location of the aneurysm determines what type of peripheral perfusion assessment is done. Check and record all peripheral pulses hourly for several hours and then routinely (based on agency policy). When the ascending aorta and aortic arch are involved, assess the carotid, radial, and temporal artery pulses. For surgery of the descending aorta, assess the femoral, popliteal, posterior tibial, and dorsalis pedis pulses (see Fig. 31-6). You may need a Doppler to assess peripheral pulses. Check skin temperature and color, capillary refill time, and sensation and movement of the extremities (see Chapter 31).

Occasionally, lower extremity pulses may be absent for a short time after surgery because of vasospasm and hypothermia. A decreased or absent pulse together with a cool, pale, mottled, or painful extremity may indicate embolization or graft occlusion. Report these findings to the HCP immediately. Graft occlusion requires reoperation if identified early. Thrombolytic therapy may also be considered. In some patients, pulses may have been absent before surgery because of coexistent PAD. It is essential to compare your findings with the preoperative status to determine the cause of a decreased or absent pulse and the proper treatment.

◆ ***Renal Perfusion Status.*** The patient will have an indwelling urinary catheter after surgery. In the immediate postoperative period, record hourly urine output. Further evaluate renal function by monitoring daily blood urea nitrogen (BUN) and serum creatinine levels. CVP and PA pressures also provide important information about hydration status. Maintain accurate fluid intake and output and record daily weights until the patient resumes a regular diet.

Decreased renal perfusion can occur from embolization of the aortic thrombus or plaque to one or both of the renal arteries. This causes ischemia of one or both kidneys. Hypotension, dehydration, prolonged aortic clamping during surgery, or blood loss can also lead to decreased renal perfusion. Irreversible renal failure may occur after surgery, particularly in high-risk people (e.g., patients with diabetes). (Acute kidney injury is discussed in Chapter 46.)

◆ **Ambulatory Care.** Instruct the patient and caregiver to gradually increase activities once home. Fatigue, poor appetite, and irregular bowel habits are common. Teach the patient to avoid heavy lifting for 6 weeks after surgery. Any redness, swelling, increased pain, drainage from incisions, or fever greater than 100° F (37.8° C) should be reported to an HCP.

Teach the patient and caregiver to look for changes in color or warmth of the extremities. Patients and caregivers can learn to palpate peripheral pulses to assess changes in their quality.

Sexual dysfunction in male patients is common after aortic surgery. Preoperatively, document baseline sexual function and recommend counseling as appropriate. A referral to a urologist may be useful if erectile dysfunction occurs.

◆ Evaluation

Expected outcomes are that the patient who undergoes aortic surgery will have:

- Patent arterial graft with adequate distal perfusion
- Adequate urine output
- No signs of infection

AORTIC DISSECTION

Aortic dissection, often misnamed *"dissecting aneurysm,"* is not a type of aneurysm. Rather, dissection results from the creation of a false lumen between the intima (inner lining) and the media (middle layer) of arterial wall (Figs. 37-5, *D* and 37-8). Aortic dissection is classified based on the location of the dissection and duration of onset. *Type A dissection* affects the ascending aorta and arch. *Type B dissection* begins in the descending aorta. Dissections are also classified as acute (first 14 days), subacute (14 to 90 days), or chronic (greater than 90 days) based on symptom onset.[26] Approximately two thirds of dissections involve the ascending aorta and are acute in onset.[30] Chronic dissections are almost always Type B.

Etiology and Pathophysiology

Nontraumatic aortic dissection is caused by degenerated elastic fibers in the arterial wall. Chronic hypertension hastens this process. In aortic dissection a tear develops in the inner layer of the aorta. Blood surges through this tear into the middle layer of the aorta, causing the inner and middle layers to separate (dissect). If the blood-filled channel ruptures through the outside aortic wall, aortic dissection is often fatal.

As the heart contracts, each pulsation increases the pressure on the damaged area, which further increases the dissection. Extension of the dissection may cut off blood supply to critical areas such as the brain, kidneys, spinal cord, and extremities. The false lumen may remain patent, become thrombosed (clotted), rejoin the true lumen by way of a distal tear, or rupture.

Aortic dissection affects men 2 to 5 times more often than women and occurs most frequently in the sixth and seventh decades of life.[30] Predisposing factors include age, aortic diseases (e.g., aortitis, coarctation, arch hypoplasia), atherosclerosis, blunt or iatrogenic trauma, tobacco use, cocaine or methamphetamine use, congenital heart disease (e.g., bicuspid aortic valve), connective tissue disorders (e.g., Marfan's or Ehlers-Danlos syndrome), family history, history of heart surgery, male gender, pregnancy, and poorly controlled hypertension.[26] Nearly half of all acute aortic dissections in patients younger than 40 years of age occur in patients with Marfan's syndrome.[30]

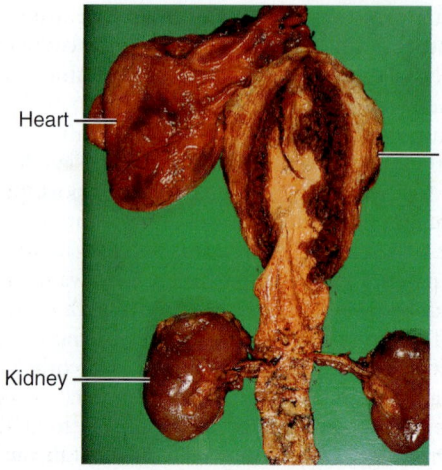

FIG. 37-8 Aortic dissection of the thoracic aorta. (From Damjanov I, Linder J, editors: *Anderson's pathology,* ed 10, St Louis, 1996, Mosby.)

Clinical Manifestations

About 80% of patients with an acute Type A aortic dissection report an abrupt onset of excruciating anterior chest pain. Patients with acute Type B aortic dissection are more likely to report pain located in their back, abdomen, or legs. Pain location may overlap between Type A and B dissections. The pain is frequently described as "sharp" and "worst ever," or as "tearing," "ripping," or "stabbing."

Dissection pain can be differentiated from MI pain, which is more gradual in onset and has increasing intensity. As the dissection progresses, pain may migrate and follow the path of the dissection. Older patients are less likely to have abrupt onset of chest or back pain and more likely to have hypotension and vague symptoms. Some patients have a painless aortic dissection, emphasizing the importance of the physical examination.

If the aortic arch is involved, the patient may exhibit neurologic deficits. These include altered level of consciousness, weakened or absent carotid and temporal pulses, and dizziness or syncope. Type A aortic dissection usually produces some degree of disruption in blood flow in the coronary arteries and aortic valve insufficiency. The patient may develop angina; MI; and a new, high-pitched heart murmur. In severe cases, these complications can result in left heart failure (e.g., dyspnea, orthopnea, pulmonary edema), cardiogenic shock, and death.[26] When either subclavian artery is involved, radial, ulnar, and brachial pulse quality and BP readings may be different between the left and right arms. As the dissection progresses down the aorta, the abdominal organs and lower extremities demonstrate evidence of decreased tissue perfusion.

Complications

A severe and life-threatening complication of an acute ascending aortic dissection is *cardiac tamponade.* This occurs when blood from the dissection leaks into the pericardial sac. Clinical manifestations of tamponade include hypotension, narrowed pulse pressure, jugular venous distention, muffled heart sounds, and pulsus paradoxus (see Chapter 36).

The aorta may rupture because it is weakened by the dissection. Hemorrhage may occur into the mediastinal, pleural, or abdominal cavities. Aortic rupture typically results in exsanguination and death. Dissection can lead to occlusion of the blood supply to vital organs. Spinal cord ischemia leads to weakness and decreased sensation and rarely to complete lower extremity paralysis. Renal ischemia can lead to renal failure. Abdominal (mesenteric) ischemia can occur and cause abdominal pain, decreased bowel sounds, altered bowel function, and bowel necrosis.

Diagnostic Studies

Diagnostic studies to detect aortic dissection are similar to those for suspected aneurysms (Table 37-6). An ECG can help rule out cardiac ischemia. A chest x-ray may show a widening of the mediastinum and pleural effusion. Three-dimensional (3-D) CT scanning, MRI, and transesophageal echocardiography (TEE) are equally reliable for the diagnosis of acute aortic dissection. A CT scan or MRI can provide more detailed information on the severity of the dissection and related complications (e.g., pericardial effusions, carotid dissection). TEE is preferred in very unstable patients or those with contraindications to CT or MRI (e.g., those with metal implants, allergies to contrast material).[26]

TABLE 37-6 Interprofessional Care

Aortic Dissection

Diagnostic Assessment	Management
• Health history and physical examination • ECG • Chest x-ray • CT scan • Transesophageal echocardiogram • MRI	• Bed rest • Pain relief with opioids • Blood transfusion (if needed) ***Drug Therapy*** *(see Table 32-7)* • IV β-blockers • IV calcium channel blockers • Angiotensin-converting enzyme inhibitors ***Surgical Therapy*** • Endovascular aortic dissection repair • Open surgical repair

Interprofessional Care

Patients with acute aortic dissection are managed in the ICU. The initial goals of therapy for acute aortic dissection without complications are heart rate (HR) and BP control and pain management. HR and BP control reduces aortic wall stress by decreasing systolic BP and myocardial contractility (Table 37-6). An IV β-blocker (e.g., esmolol [Brevibloc]) is titrated to a target HR of 60 beats/minute or less or to a systolic BP between 100 and 110 mm Hg.

A calcium channel blocker (e.g., diltiazem [Cardizem]) can be used to lower HR if a β-blocker is contraindicated. Reducing the HR, BP, and myocardial contractility limits extension of the dissection. Morphine is the preferred analgesic. It decreases sympathetic nervous system stimulation and relieves pain. Supportive treatment for an acute aortic dissection serves as a bridge to surgery.

Conservative Therapy. The patient with an acute or chronic Type B aortic dissection without complications can be treated conservatively. Conservative treatment includes pain relief, HR and BP control, and CVD risk factor modification along with close surveillance imaging with CT or MRI.

Endovascular Dissection Repair. Endovascular repair of acute Type B aortic dissections with complications (e.g., hemodynamic instability) and chronic Type B aortic dissection with complications (e.g., peripheral ischemia) is a treatment option. Thoracic endovascular aortic repair (TEVAR) is similar to EVAR. However, a temporary lumbar drain may be inserted for cerebrospinal fluid removal to reduce spinal cord edema and help prevent paralysis.[31] If a lumbar drain is used, strict aseptic techniques are essential to avoid introducing infection.

Surgical Therapy. An acute Type A aortic dissection is a surgical emergency. Mortality rate is 50% within 48 hours of symptom onset. Otherwise, surgery is indicated when conservative therapy is ineffective or when complications (e.g., heart failure) occur. Open surgical repair is recommended for patients with a chronic dissection who have a connective tissue disorder and a descending thoracic aortic diameter greater than 5.5 cm.[26]

The aorta is fragile after dissection. Thus surgery is delayed for as long as possible to allow time for edema to decrease and to permit clotting of the blood in the false lumen. Surgery involves resection of the aortic segment containing the intimal tear and replacement with a synthetic graft. Even with prompt surgical intervention, the in-hospital mortality and neurologic complications are high.[26] Causes of death include aortic rupture, mesenteric ischemia, MI, sepsis, stroke, and multiorgan failure.

❖ NURSING MANAGEMENT: AORTIC DISSECTION

Preoperatively, nursing management includes keeping the patient in bed in a semi-Fowler's position and maintaining a quiet environment. These measures help to keep the HR and systolic BP at the lowest possible level that maintains vital organ perfusion (typically HR less than 60 beats/minute; systolic BP between 110 and 120 mm Hg). Give opioids and sedatives as ordered. To prevent extension of the dissection, manage pain and anxiety because they can cause elevations in the HR and systolic BP.

Titrating IV antihypertensive agents requires careful supervision, including continuous ECG and arterial BP monitoring (see Chapters 32 and 65). Monitor vital signs frequently, sometimes as often as every 2 to 3 minutes, until target HR and BP are reached. Look for any changes in peripheral pulses and signs of increasing pain, restlessness, and anxiety. If the arteries branching off the aortic arch are involved, monitor the patient's level of consciousness, cranial nerve functions, and limb movement, sensation, and strength.[31] Postoperative care is similar to that after OAR (see earlier section on nursing management of aortic aneurysms on p. 813).

In preparation for discharge, focus on patient and caregiver teaching. All patients with a history of aortic dissection, regardless of location or treatment approach, require long-term health care to control HR and BP. Patients must understand that they need to take antihypertensive drugs daily for the rest of their lives. β-Blockers are used to control HR and BP and decrease myocardial contractility. It is important that patients understand the drug regimen and potential side effects (e.g., dizziness, depression, fatigue, erectile dysfunction). Tell the patient to discuss any side effects with the HCP before stopping the drug.

Follow-up with regularly scheduled MRIs or CTs is essential. The most common cause of death in long-term survivors is aortic rupture from redissection or aneurysm formation. Tell patients that if the pain or other symptoms return, they should activate emergency response system (ERS) for immediate care.

ACUTE AND CHRONIC VENOUS DISORDERS

PHLEBITIS

Generally, every hospitalized patient has an IV catheter inserted for giving fluids and/or drugs. *Phlebitis* is an acute inflammation of the walls of small cannulated veins of the hand or arm. Clinical manifestations include pain, tenderness, warmth, erythema, swelling, and a palpable cord. Phlebitis risk factors are mechanical irritation from the catheter, infusion of irritating drugs, and catheter location. Severe phlebitis is more likely to occur in the antecubital area, and IV catheter insertion in this area should be avoided when possible.[32]

Phlebitis is rarely infectious and usually resolves quickly after catheter removal. If edema is present, elevate the extremity to promote reabsorption of fluid into the vasculature. Apply warm, moist heat and give oral NSAIDs (e.g., diclofenac [Voltaren]) or topical NSAIDs (e.g., diclofenac gel [Solaraze]) to relieve pain and inflammation. In rare cases, surgical intervention may be needed.[32]

VENOUS THROMBOSIS

Venous thrombosis involves the formation of a *thrombus* (blood clot) in association with inflammation of the vein. It is the most common disorder of the veins and is classified as either superficial vein thrombosis or deep vein thrombosis. **Superficial vein thrombosis** is the formation of a thrombus in a superficial vein, usually the greater or lesser saphenous vein. **Deep vein thrombosis (DVT)** involves a thrombus in a deep vein, most commonly the iliac and/or femoral veins. **Venous thromboembolism (VTE)** is the preferred terminology and represents the spectrum of pathology from DVT to pulmonary embolism (PE) (Table 37-7). (Chapter 27 discusses PE.)

Superficial vein thrombosis has been considered a benign disorder. However, superficial vein thrombosis is serious. Nearly 25% of patients with superficial vein thrombosis may also have a DVT or PE at the time of diagnosis. Further, between 5% and 10% of these patients are at risk for developing recurrent VTE with the greatest risk being in the first 3 months after having the superficial vein thrombosis.[33]

Etiology

Three important factors (called **Virchow's triad**) in the etiology of venous thrombosis are (1) venous stasis, (2) damage of the endothelium (inner lining of the vein), and (3) hypercoagulability of the blood (Fig. 37-9). The patient at risk for the development of VTE usually has predisposing conditions to these three disorders (Table 37-8).

TABLE 37-7 Comparison of Superficial Vein Thrombosis and Venous Thromboembolism

	Superficial Vein Thrombosis	Venous Thromboembolism (VTE)
Usual location	Typically, superficial leg veins (e.g., varicosities). Occasionally superficial arm veins.	Deep veins of arms (e.g., axillary, subclavian), legs (e.g., femoral), pelvis (e.g., iliac), vena cava, and pulmonary system.
Clinical findings	Tenderness, itchiness, redness, warmth, pain, inflammation, and induration along the course of superficial vein. Vein appears as a palpable cord. Edema rarely occurs.	Tenderness to pressure over involved vein, induration of overlying muscle, venous distention. Edema. May have mild to moderate pain, deep reddish color to area caused by venous congestion. NOTE: Some patients may have no obvious physical changes in the affected extremity.
Sequelae	If untreated, clot may extend to deeper veins and VTE may occur.	Embolization to lungs (pulmonary embolism) may occur and may result in death.* Pulmonary hypertension and post-thrombotic syndrome with or without venous leg ulceration may develop.

*See Chapter 27 for clinical findings related to pulmonary embolism.

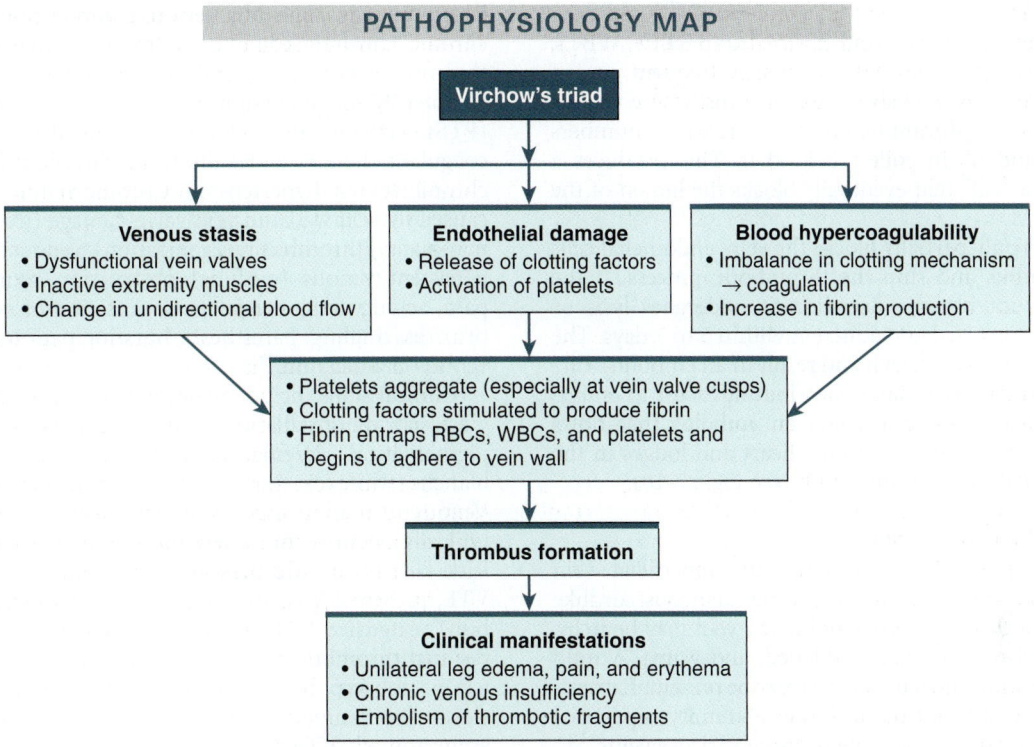

FIG. 37-9 Pathophysiology of venous thromboembolism.

TABLE 37-8 Risk Factors for Venous Thromboembolism

Venous Stasis
- Advanced age
- Atrial fibrillation
- Bed rest
- Chronic heart failure
- Fractured leg or hip
- Long trips without adequate exercise
- Obesity
- Orthopedic surgery (especially hip or lower extremity)
- Pregnancy and postpartum period
- Prolonged immobility
- Spinal cord injury or limb paralysis
- Stroke
- Varicose veins

Endothelial Damage
- Abdominal and pelvic surgery (e.g., gynecologic or urologic surgery)
- Caustic or hypertonic IV drugs
- Fractures of the pelvis, hip, or leg
- History of previous venous thromboembolism
- Indwelling, peripherally inserted central vein catheter
- IV drug abuse
- Trauma

Hypercoagulability of Blood
- Antiphospholipid antibody syndrome
- Antithrombin III deficiency
- Dehydration or malnutrition
- Elevated (clotting) factor VIII or lipoprotein (a)
- Erythropoiesis-stimulating drugs (e.g., epoetin alfa [Procrit])
- High altitudes
- Hormone therapy
- Hyperhomocysteinemia
- Cancer (especially breast, brain, hepatic, pancreatic, and gastrointestinal)
- Nephrotic syndrome
- Oral contraceptives, especially in women >35 yr who use tobacco
- Polycythemia vera
- Pregnancy and postpartum period
- Protein C deficiency
- Protein S deficiency
- Sepsis
- Severe anemias
- Tobacco use

Venous Stasis. Normal venous blood flow depends on the action of muscles in the extremities and the functional adequacy of venous valves, which allow flow in one direction. *Venous stasis* occurs when the valves are dysfunctional or the muscles of the extremities are inactive. Venous stasis occurs more frequently in people who are obese or pregnant, have chronic heart failure or atrial fibrillation, have been traveling on long trips without regular exercise, have a prolonged surgical procedure, or are immobile for long periods (e.g., spinal cord injury, fractured hip, limb paralysis).[34]

Endothelial Damage. Damage to the endothelium of the vein may be caused by direct (e.g., surgery, intravascular catheterization, trauma, burns, prior VTE) or indirect (chemotherapy, diabetes, sepsis) injury to the vessel. Damaged endothelium stimulates platelet activation and starts the coagulation cascade. This predisposes the patient to thrombus development.

Hypercoagulability of Blood. Hypercoagulability of blood occurs in many disorders. These include severe anemias; polycythemia; malignancies (e.g., cancers of the breast, brain, pancreas, and gastrointestinal tract); nephrotic syndrome; hyperhomocysteinemia; protein C, protein S, and antithrombin deficiency.[34] A patient with sepsis is predisposed to hypercoagulability because of endotoxins that are released. Some drugs (e.g., corticosteroids, estrogens) predispose a patient to thrombus formation.

Women of childbearing age who take estrogen-based oral contraceptives or postmenopausal women on oral hormone therapy are at increased risk for VTE. Women who use oral contraceptives and tobacco double their risk. Smoking causes hypercoagulability by increasing plasma fibrinogen and homocysteine levels and activating the intrinsic coagulation pathway. Women who use tobacco and oral contraceptives, are over 35 years old, and have a family history of VTE are at an extremely high risk for VTE.[34]

Pathophysiology

Localized platelet aggregation and fibrin entrap RBCs, WBCs, and more platelets to form a thrombus. A frequent site of thrombus formation is the valve cusps of veins, where venous stasis occurs. As the thrombus enlarges, increased numbers of blood cells and fibrin collect behind it. This produces a larger clot with a "tail" that eventually blocks the lumen of the vein.

If a thrombus only partially blocks the vein, endothelial cells cover the thrombus and stop the thrombotic process. If the thrombus does not become detached, it undergoes lysis or becomes firmly organized and adherent within 5 to 7 days. The organized thrombus may detach and result in an embolus. Turbulence of blood flow is a major contributing factor to embolization. The thrombus can become an embolus that flows through the venous circulation to the heart and lodges in the pulmonary circulation, becoming a PE (see Fig. 27-10).

Superficial Vein Thrombosis

Clinical Manifestations. The patient with superficial vein thrombosis may have a palpable, firm, subcutaneous cordlike vein (Table 37-7). The area surrounding the vein may be itchy, tender or painful to the touch, reddened, and warm. A mild temperature elevation and leukocytosis may be present. Extremity edema may or may not occur. Lower extremity superficial vein thrombosis often involves one or more varicose veins.

Risk factors for superficial vein thrombosis include increased age, pregnancy, obesity, malignancy, recent fracture(s), and thrombophilia; estrogen therapy; recent sclerotherapy (e.g., treatment for varicose veins); recent surgery or long-distance travel; and a history of chronic venous insufficiency (CVI), superficial vein thrombosis, or VTE.[33] It also can occur in people with endothelial alterations (e.g., Buerger's disease), or it may be unprovoked.

Interprofessional Care. Duplex ultrasound is used to confirm the diagnosis (clot 5 cm or larger) and to rule out clot extension to a deep vein.[34] For patients with a lower leg superficial vein thrombosis, subcutaneous fondaparinux (Arixtra) reduces symptomatic VTE, and superficial vein thrombosis extension and recurrence without causing major bleeding problems.[35]

If the superficial vein thrombosis affects a very short vein segment (less than 5 cm) and is not near the saphenofemoral junction, anticoagulants may not be necessary and oral NSAIDs can ease symptoms. Additional interventions to relieve symptoms include telling the patient to wear graduated compression stockings or bandages, elevate the affected limb above level of heart, apply topical NSAIDS, and perform mild exercise such as walking.

Venous Thromboembolism

Clinical Manifestations. The patient with lower extremity VTE may or may not have unilateral leg edema, pain, tenderness with palpation, dilated superficial veins, a sense of fullness in the thigh or the calf, paresthesias, warm skin, erythema, or a systemic temperature greater than 100.4° F (38° C) (Table 37-7). If the inferior vena cava is involved, both legs may be edematous and cyanotic. About 5% to 10% of VTEs involve the upper extremity veins and may extend into the internal jugular vein or superior vena cava. If the superior vena cava is involved, similar symptoms may occur in the arms, neck, back, and face. Diagnosis of an initial VTE is based on clinical assessment combined with D-dimer testing and/or duplex ultrasound.

Complications. The most serious complications of VTE are PE, chronic thromboembolic pulmonary hypertension, post-thrombotic syndrome, and phlegmasia cerulea dolens. (See Chapter 27 for discussion of PE.) **Post-thrombotic syndrome (PTS)** occurs in 20% to 50% of patients despite adequate anticoagulant therapy. It results from chronic inflammation and chronic venous hypertension. Chronic venous hypertension is caused by vein wall and vein valve damage (from acute inflammation and thrombus reorganization), venous valve reflux, and persistent venous (outflow) obstruction. Symptoms include pain, aching, fatigue, heaviness, sensation of swelling, cramps, pruritus, tingling, paresthesia, bursting pain with exercise, and venous claudication.[36]

Clinical signs include persistent edema, spider veins (telangiectasia), venous dilation (ectasia), redness, cyanosis, increased pigmentation, eczema, pain during compression, atrophie blanche (white scar tissue), and *lipodermatosclerosis* (Fig. 37-10). Venous ulceration can occur with severe PTS. Signs of PTS typically begin within a few months to a few years of a VTE. Risk factors include persistent leg symptoms 1 month after VTE, proximal VTE location (e.g., near the iliofemoral junction), extensive VTE, recurrent ipsilateral (same side) VTE, residual thrombus, obesity, older age, poor INR control, daily use of tobacco before pregnancy, increased D-dimer levels, elevated inflammatory markers, varicose veins, and possibly asymptomatic VTE.[36]

Phlegmasia cerulea dolens (swollen, blue, painful leg), a rare complication, may develop in a patient in the advanced stages of cancer. It results from severe lower extremity VTE(s) that involve(s) the major leg veins, causing near-total occlusion of venous outflow. Patients typically experience sudden, massive swelling; deep pain; and intense cyanosis of the extremity. If untreated, the venous obstruction causes arterial occlusion and gangrene and requires amputation.

Diagnostic Studies. Table 37-9 presents the various diagnostic studies used to determine the site or location and extent of a VTE.

Interprofessional Care

Prevention and Prophylaxis. VTE prophylaxis is a core measure of high-quality health care in high-risk hospitalized patients developed by the Joint Commission and the National Quality

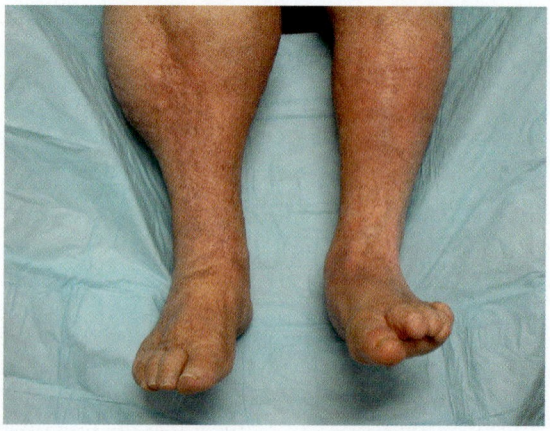

FIG. 37-10 Lipodermatosclerosis. Skin on lower leg becomes scarred, and the leg becomes tapered like an "inverted bottle." Hallmark signs of lipodermatosclerosis are leathery skin, brown discoloration, hyperpigmentation and hypopigmentation, and circumferential or near circumferential scarring and shrinking of the extremity. (From Etufugh CN, Phillips TJ: Venous ulcers, *Clin Dermatol* 25[1]:125, 2007.)

TABLE 37-9 Diagnostic Studies

Venous Thromboembolism*

Study	Description and Abnormal Findings
Blood Laboratory Studies	
ACT, aPTT, INR, bleeding time, Hgb, Hct, platelet count	Alterations if patient has underlying blood dyscrasia (e.g., increased Hgb and Hct in patient with polycythemia).
D-dimer	Fragment of fibrin formed as result of fibrin degradation and clot lysis. Elevated results suggest venous thromboembolism (VTE). *Normal results:* <250 ng/mL (<250 mcg/L)
Fibrin monomer complex	Forms when concentration of thrombin exceeds that of antithrombin. Presence is evidence of thrombus formation and suggests VTE. *Normal results:* <6.1 mg/L
Noninvasive Venous Studies	
Venous compression ultrasound	Evaluation of deep femoral, popliteal, and posterior tibial veins. *Normal finding:* Veins collapse with application of external pressure. *Abnormal finding:* Veins fail to collapse with application of external pressure. Failure to collapse suggests a thrombus.
Duplex ultrasound	Combination of compression ultrasound with spectral and color flow Doppler. Veins examined for compressibility and intraluminal filling defects to help determine location and extent of thrombus (most widely used test to diagnose VTE).
Invasive Venous Studies	
Computed tomography venography (CTV)	Uses spiral CT to evaluate veins in the pelvis, thighs, and calves after injection of contrast material. May be performed simultaneously with CT angiography of pulmonary vessels for patients being evaluated for VTE.
Magnetic resonance venography	Uses MRI with specialized software to evaluate blood flow through veins. Can be done with or without contrast. Highly accurate for pelvic and proximal veins. Less accurate for calf veins. Can distinguish acute and chronic thrombus.
Contrast venography (phlebogram)	X-ray determination of location and extent of clot using contrast media to outline filling defects. Identifies the presence of collateral circulation. Once the gold standard, but currently rarely performed.

ACT, Activated clotting time; *aPTT,* activated partial thromboplastin time; *INR,* international normalized ratio.
*See Table 27-26 for diagnostic studies for pulmonary embolism.

Forum. There are six VTE measures. These can be found at *www.jointcommission.org/venous_thromboembolism/default.aspx.* In addition, it is recommended that hospitals have a thromboprophylaxis policy that addresses VTE prevention on admission of all adult patients. As many as 80% of medically ill patients at risk for VTE do not receive appropriate thromboprophylaxis.[37]

In patients at risk for VTE, a variety of interventions are used. These are based on such factors as bleeding and thrombosis risk, past medical history, current drugs, medical diagnoses, scheduled procedures, and patient preferences.

Early and aggressive mobilization based on the patient's condition is the easiest and most cost-effective method to decrease VTE risk. Patients on bed rest should change position at least every 2 hours. Unless contraindicated, teach patients to flex and extend their feet, knees, and hips at least every 2 to 4 hours while awake. Patients who can get out of bed need to be in a chair for meals and walk at least four to six times per day as able. Tell the patient and caregiver about the importance of these measures. Early and frequent ambulation is sufficient prophylaxis for very low VTE–risk patients undergoing minor surgical procedures.[38] Anticoagulation and mechanical prophylaxis are not recommended for acutely ill medical patients at low risk for VTE.

Graduated compression stockings (e.g., thromboembolic deterrent [TED] hose) are a part of VTE prevention in hospitalized patients. When fitted correctly (both size and length) and worn properly and consistently from admission until discharge or full mobility, these stockings decrease VTE risk in surgical patients.[39] Proper use means the toe hole is under the toes, the heel patch is over the heel, the thigh gusset is on the inner thigh (thigh length only), and there are no wrinkles. The stockings are not to be rolled down, cut, or otherwise altered.

Knee-length stockings seem to be as effective as thigh-length stockings in the prevention of VTE in surgical patients. However, additional research is needed.[40] If the stockings are not fitted and worn correctly, venous return is impeded. This may promote the development of arterial ischemia, edema, skin breakdown, and VTE. VTE prevention is enhanced if graduated compression stockings are used along with anticoagulation.

Intermittent pneumatic compression devices (IPCs) use inflatable sleeves or boots to compress the calf and thigh and/or foot and ankle to improve venous return. The sleeves apply external pressure by means of an electric pump. IPCs may or may not be used with graduated compression stockings. Like graduated compression stockings, ensure correct fit by accurately measuring the extremities. IPCs will not be effective if they are not applied correctly, if the fit is incorrect, or if the patient does not wear the device continuously. Exceptions include during bathing, skin assessment, and ambulation. IPCs are not worn when a patient has an active VTE because of the risk of PE.[41]

Drug Therapy. Anticoagulants are used routinely for VTE prevention and treatment. The regimen depends on the patient's VTE risk. The goal of anticoagulant therapy for VTE prophylaxis is to prevent clot formation. The goals for treatment of a confirmed VTE are to prevent new clot development, spread of the clot, and embolization.[42]

Three major classes of anticoagulants are available: (1) vitamin K antagonists (VKA), (2) thrombin inhibitors (both indirect and direct), and (3) factor Xa inhibitors[43] (Table 37-10). Anticoagulant therapy does not dissolve the clot. Clot lysis begins naturally through the body's intrinsic fibrinolytic system (see Chapter 29).

Vitamin K antagonists. The oral anticoagulant for long-term or extended anticoagulation is warfarin, a VKA. Warfarin

TABLE 37-10 Drug Therapy

Anticoagulant Therapy

Drug	Route of Administration	Comments
Vitamin K Antagonists (VKA)		
warfarin (Coumadin)	PO	INR is used for monitoring therapeutic levels. Administer at the same time each day. Variations of certain genes (e.g., *CYP2CP, VKORC1*) may influence response to drug. *Antidote:* Vitamin K. For major VKA-related bleeding, treatment with four-factor prothrombin complex concentrate and IV vitamin K is recommended over fresh frozen plasma.
Thrombin Inhibitors: Indirect		
Unfractionated Heparin (UH)	Continuous IV Intermittent IV	Therapeutic effects measured at regular intervals by the aPTT or ACT. Monitor CBC counts at regular intervals and titrate according to parameters.
heparin sodium	Subcutaneous	If administering subcutaneously, inject deep into subcutaneous tissue (preferably into the abdominal fatty tissue or above the iliac crest), inserting the entire length of the needle. Hold skinfold during injection but release before removing needle. Do not aspirate. Do not inject IM. Do not rub site after injection. Rotate sites. *Antidote:* Protamine neutralizes the effect of UH.
Low-Molecular-Weight Heparin (LMWH)	Subcutaneous	Routine coagulation tests typically not required. Monitor CBC count at regular intervals. Do not expel air bubble before administering subcutaneously. Follow remaining administration guidelines as described above for UH. Reduced dosage needed in patients with renal impairment. Use extreme caution in patients with a history of HIT. *Antidote:* Protamine neutralizes the effects of LMWH.
enoxaparin (Lovenox) dalteparin (Fragmin)		
Thrombin Inhibitors: Direct		
Hirudin Derivatives		
bivalirudin (Angiomax)	IV	Therapeutic effect measured by ACT or aPTT. Used in patients with HIT when anticoagulation is still required. *Antidote:* None.
desirudin (Iprivask)	Subcutaneous	
Synthetic Thrombin Inhibitors		
argatroban	IV	Therapeutic effect measured by aPTT. Used in patients at risk for or with HIT. Used for VTE prevention in joint replacement surgery. VTE treatment option and for stroke prevention in nonvalvular atrial fibrillation. *Antidote:* idarucizumab (Praxbind) neutralizes the effect of dabigatran only.
dabigatran (Pradaxa)	PO	
Factor Xa Inhibitors		
fondaparinux (Arixtra)	Subcutaneous	Routine coagulation tests not required. Monitor complete blood count and creatinine at regular intervals. Do not expel air bubble before administering. Follow remaining administration guidelines as described for UH. All are approved for VTE prophylaxis and treatment. For surgical patients, initial dose should be given no earlier than 6 hr postoperatively. Use with caution in older patients. Assess creatinine level before giving fondaparinux. May cause thrombocytopenia. If uncontrollable bleeding occurs, treatment with recombinant factor VIIa may be effective. *Antidote:* Andexanet alfa is currently under FDA priority review. Andexanet alfa has been shown to reverse the effects of Factor Xa inhibitors.
rivaroxaban (Xarelto)	PO	
apixaban (Eliquis)	PO	
edoxaban (Savaysa)	PO	

ACT, Activated clotting time; *aPTT,* activated partial thromboplastin time; *HIT,* heparin-induced thrombocytopenia; *INR,* international normalized ratio; *VTE,* venous thromboembolism.

inhibits activation of the vitamin K–dependent coagulation factors II, VII, IX, and X, as well as the anticoagulant proteins C and S. (Fig. 29-4 displays the clotting pathways, and clotting factors are listed in Table 29-2.) Warfarin begins to take effect in 48 to 72 hours. It then takes several more days to achieve a maximum effect. Thus an overlap of a parenteral anticoagulant (e.g., UH or LMWH) and warfarin typically is required for 5 days. The level of anticoagulation is monitored daily using the international normalized ratio (INR). The INR is a standardized system of reporting prothrombin time (PT) (Table 37-11). The antidote for warfarin-related bleeding is vitamin K or Kcentra (Prothrombin Complex Concentrate [Human]).

Take a careful history before starting warfarin. Do not give antiplatelets or NSAIDs with warfarin, since these drugs increase bleeding risk.[43] Many other drugs, vitamins, minerals, and dietary and herbal supplements also interact with warfarin (see the Complementary & Alternative Therapies box on this page). A diet that frequently varies in vitamin K intake (e.g., green leafy vegetables) can make it hard to achieve and maintain a target INR level.

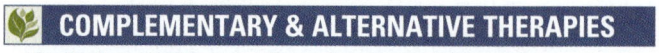

COMPLEMENTARY & ALTERNATIVE THERAPIES

Herbal and Dietary Supplements That May Affect Clotting

Scientific Evidence

The following herbs and dietary supplements may affect blood clotting: bilberry, black cohosh, chamomile, chondroitin sulfate, DHEA, feverfew, garlic, ginger, ginkgo biloba, ginseng, goldenseal, grapeseed extract, green tea, horse chestnut seed extract, melatonin, niacin, omega-3 fatty acids, psyllium, red yeast rice extract, saw palmetto, soy, turmeric.

Nursing Implications

- Inform patients that taking these herbs or dietary supplements may increase their risk of bleeding.
- Caution patients with bleeding disorders about the use of these herbs and dietary supplements. Advise them that they should consult with their HCP before using these substances.

DHEA, Dehydroepiandrosterone.

TABLE 37-11 Blood Coagulation Tests

Test and Drugs Monitored	Normal Value	Therapeutic Value
International normalized ratio (INR)	0.75-1.25	2-3
• Vitamin K antagonists (e.g., warfarin [Coumadin])		
Activated partial thromboplastin time (aPTT)	25-35 sec	46-70 sec
• Unfractionated heparin (e.g., heparin [Hep-Lock])		
• Hirudin derivatives (e.g., bivalirudin [Angiomax])		
• Synthetic thrombin inhibitors (e.g., argatroban [Acova], dabigatran [Pradaxa])		
Activated clotting time (ACT)	70-120 sec*	>300 sec
• Unfractionated heparin		
• Hirudin derivatives		
• Synthetic thrombin inhibitors		
Anti–factor Xa		
• Low-molecular-weight heparin (e.g., enoxaparin [Lovenox])	0 U/mL	0.6-1.0 U/mL
• Factor Xa inhibitors (e.g., fondaparinux [Arixtra], rivaroxaban [Xarelto])	0 U/mL	0.2-1.5 U/mL

*Varies based on type of system and test reagent or activator used.

Genetic variants in the genes *VKORC1* and cytochrome P450 2C9 *(CYP2C9)* may influence how some people respond to warfarin (see Table 12-5). Although genetic testing is available, pharmacogenetic-based dosing is not recommended in clinical practice at this time.[44]

Thrombin inhibitors. *Indirect thrombin inhibitors* are divided into two major classes: UH and LMWHs. UH (e.g., heparin) affects both the intrinsic and common pathways of blood coagulation by way of the plasma antithrombin. Antithrombin inhibits thrombin-mediated conversion of fibrinogen to fibrin by affecting factors II (prothrombin), IX, X, XI, and XII (see Fig. 29-4).

Heparin can be given subcutaneously for VTE prophylaxis or by continuous IV infusion for VTE treatment. When given IV, heparin requires frequent monitoring of clotting status as measured by activated partial thromboplastin time (aPTT) (Table 37-11). Protamine sulfate reverses the effect of heparin.

One serious side effect of heparin is *heparin-induced thrombocytopenia* (HIT). HIT is an immune reaction to heparin. It causes a severe, sudden reduction in the platelet count along with a paradoxical increase in venous or arterial thrombosis. HIT is diagnosed by measuring the presence of heparin antibodies in the blood. Treatment requires immediately stopping heparin therapy and, if further anticoagulation is required, using a non-heparin anticoagulant (e.g., fondaparinux).[45] Another side effect of long-term heparin therapy is osteoporosis.

LMWHs (e.g., enoxaparin [Lovenox]) are derived from UH. They have more bioavailability, more predictable dose response, longer half-life, and fewer bleeding complications than UH. LMWHs are less likely to cause HIT and osteoporosis. LMWHs typically do not require ongoing anticoagulant monitoring and dose adjustment and their antiinflammatory properties may help prevent PTS and venous ulcer development.[36] Protamine neutralizes the effect of LMWH.

Direct thrombin inhibitors are classified as hirudin derivatives or synthetic thrombin inhibitors. Hirudin is made using recombinant deoxyribonucleic acid (DNA) technology. It binds specifically with thrombin and directly inhibits its function without causing plasma protein and platelet interactions. Hirudin derivatives (e.g., bivalirudin [Angiomax]) are given by continuous IV infusion. Bivalirudin is approved for patients with or at risk for HIT having a percutaneous coronary intervention. Anticoagulant activity is monitored using aPTT or activated clotting time (ACT) (Table 37-11). If bleeding occurs, there is no antidote for hirudin derivatives.

Argatroban, a synthetic direct thrombin inhibitor, inhibits thrombin. Like bivalirudin, it is used as an alternative to heparin for the prevention and treatment of HIT and for patients with or at risk for HIT needing percutaneous coronary interventions. Dabigatran (Pradaxa), an oral direct thrombin inhibitor, is used for VTE prevention after elective joint replacement, for stroke prevention in nonvalvular atrial fibrillation, and as a treatment option in VTE. The effect of argatroban is not reversible. Anticoagulant effect is monitored for both drugs using aPTT or ACT. Idarucizumab (Praxbind) neutralizes the effect of dabigatran. There are no similar drugs for any other synthetic direct thrombin inhibitor.

Factor Xa inhibitors. *Factor Xa inhibitors* inhibit factor Xa directly or indirectly, producing rapid anticoagulation. These include fondaparinux (Arixtra), rivaroxaban (Xarelto), apixaban (Eliquis), and edoxaban (Savaysa). All are used for both VTE treatment and prophylaxis. Fondaparinux is given subcutaneously. Rivaroxaban, apixaban, and edoxaban are oral drugs. Although coagulation monitoring or dose adjustment is not needed, the drug's anticoagulant activity can be measured using anti-Xa assays (Table 37-11). If uncontrollable bleeding occurs, recombinant factor VIIa may be useful. Fondaparinux is contraindicated in patients with severe renal disease.

Anticoagulant therapy for VTE prophylaxis. For VTE prophylaxis in the hospitalized medical patient at risk for thrombosis who is not bleeding, low-dose UH, LMWH, or fondaparinux is used. If the patient is at low VTE risk, drug prophylaxis is not needed. Patients with moderate VTE risk (e.g., general, gynecologic, urologic surgery) should receive either UH or LMWH. Patients with high VTE risk (e.g., trauma) should receive UH or LMWH until discharge. Patients having abdominal or pelvic surgery for cancer or major orthopedic surgery (e.g., total knee or hip replacement) should be prescribed VTE prophylaxis.[44]

Anticoagulant therapy for VTE treatment. Patients with confirmed VTE should receive initial treatment with either LMWH, UH, or an oral Factor Xa drug. Oral VKA therapy may be considered. A therapeutic INR is maintained between 2.0 and 3.0 if VKA therapy is used. Subtherapeutic INR, especially in the first few months of therapy, is linked with PTS development.[36] Active treatment of VTE should continue for at least 3 months and may continue longer in some patients.[46]

Patients with multiple co-morbidities, complex medical issues, or a very large VTE usually are hospitalized for treatment. Parenteral administration of UH is the typical initial treatment. Depending on the clinical presentation and home situation, patients may be safely and effectively managed as outpatients.

Thrombolytic therapy for VTE treatment. Another treatment option for patients with a thrombus is catheter-directed administration of a thrombolytic drug (e.g., urokinase, tPA). It dissolves the clot(s), reduces the acute symptoms, improves deep venous flow, reduces valvular reflux, and may help to decrease the incidence of PTS. Catheter-directed thrombolysis is recommended for select patients who are at a low bleeding risk and present with an acute, extensive, symptomatic, proximal VTE. Systemic anticoagulation is recommended before, during, and after catheter-directed thrombolysis. (Chapter 33 discusses thrombolytic therapy.)

CHECK YOUR PRACTICE

Your 55-yr-old female patient is admitted with an extensive VTE in her right leg. She is receiving weight-based IV heparin per agency protocol: 18 U/kg/hr. You receive the following critical laboratory result: aPTT 122 seconds.

- Describe your next actions.

Surgical and Interventional Radiology Therapies. Although most VTE patients are managed medically, a small number of patients with extensive, acute, proximal VTE who are not candidates for catheter-directed thrombolysis and/or interventional radiology therapies (due to bleeding risk) may undergo surgery.[36] Surgical options include open venous thrombectomy and inferior vena cava interruption. *Venous thrombectomy* involves the removal of a thrombus through an incision in the vein. Anticoagulant therapy is recommended after venous thrombectomy.

Vena cava interruption devices (e.g., Greenfield, Vena Tech, TrapEase filters) can be placed percutaneously through the right femoral or right internal jugular veins. The filter device is opened, and the spokes penetrate the vessel walls (Fig. 37-11). The filters act as a "sieve-type" device, permitting filtration of clots without interruption of blood flow. Complications after the insertion are rare but include air embolism, improper placement, migration of the filter, and perforation of the vena cava with retroperitoneal bleeding. Over time, clots can clog the filter and completely block the vena cava, requiring filter removal and replacement. A filter device is recommended with acute PE or proximal VTE of the leg in patients with active bleeding or if anticoagulant therapy is contraindicated or ineffective. Patients with a filter device alone are at increased risk of developing a VTE. If the active bleeding or anticoagulation contraindication resolves, a course of anticoagulant therapy is suggested.[47]

Percutaneous endovascular interventional radiology procedures can be used along with catheter-directed thrombolytic therapy, especially for severely symptomatic patients with iliocaval or iliofemoral obstruction.[36] The interventional radiology procedures are similar to those used in the treatment of lower-extremity PAD. The difference is accessing an occluded vein instead of an artery. They include mechanical thrombectomy, pharmacomechanical devices, and post-thrombus extraction, angioplasty, and/or stenting.[47] Anticoagulation therapy is recommended after an iliofemoral interventional radiology procedure. Postprocedure nursing care focuses on (1) maintenance of catheter systems (if continuous infusions); (2) monitoring for bleeding, embolization, and impaired perfusion; and (3) VTE prevention teaching.[48]

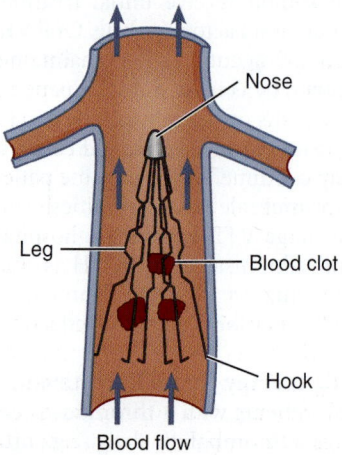

FIG. 37-11 Inferior vena caval interruption technique using Greenfield stainless steel filter to prevent pulmonary embolism. As blood travels up the vena cava, clots are trapped in the filter.

❖ NURSING MANAGEMENT: VENOUS THROMBOEMBOLISM

◆ Nursing Assessment

Table 37-12 presents the subjective and objective data to obtain from a patient with VTE.

TABLE 37-12 Nursing Assessment

Venous Thromboembolism

Subjective Data

Important Health Information *(Table 37-8)*

Past health history: Trauma to vein, intravascular catheter (e.g., peripherally inserted central catheter), varicose veins, pregnancy or recent childbirth, bacteremia, obesity, prolonged bed rest, irregular heartbeat (e.g., atrial fibrillation), COPD, HF, cancer, coagulation disorders and hypercoagulable states, systemic lupus erythematosus, MI, spinal cord injury, stroke, prolonged travel, recent bone fracture, dehydration

Medications: Use of estrogens (including oral contraceptives, hormone therapy), tamoxifen, raloxifene (Evista), corticosteroids, excessive amounts of vitamin E, erythropoiesis-stimulating drugs

Surgery or other treatments: Any recent surgery, especially orthopedic, gynecologic, gastric, or urologic. Previous surgery involving veins. Central venous catheter

Functional Health Patterns

Health perception–health management: IV drug abuse, tobacco use, obesity

Activity-exercise: Inactivity

Cognitive-perceptual: Pain in area on palpation or ambulation

Objective Data

General

Fever, anxiety, pain

Integumentary

Increased size of extremity when compared with other side. Taut, shiny, warm skin, erythematous, tender to palpation. No physical changes in the affected extremity in some patients

Cardiovascular

Distention and warmth of superficial veins in affected area. Edema and cyanosis of extremities, neck, back, and face (if superior vena cava involvement)

Possible Diagnostic Findings

Leukocytosis, abnormal coagulation, anemia or ↑ hematocrit and RBC count, ↑ D-dimer level, positive venous compression on duplex ultrasound study; positive CTV, magnetic resonance venogram, or contrast venogram study

COPD, Chronic obstructive pulmonary disease; *CTV,* computed tomography venogram; *HF,* heart failure; *MI,* myocardial infarction.

Nursing Diagnoses

Nursing diagnoses and collaborative problems for the patient with VTE include, but are not limited to, the following:

- Acute pain *related to* venous congestion, impaired venous return, and inflammation
- Ineffective health management *related to* lack of knowledge about disorder and its treatment
- Risk for impaired skin integrity *related to* altered peripheral tissue perfusion
- Potential complication: bleeding *related to* anticoagulant therapy
- Potential complication: PE *related to* embolization of thrombus, dehydration, and immobility

Planning

The overall goals for the patient with VTE include (1) pain relief, (2) decreased edema, (3) increased knowledge of disorder and treatment plan, (4) no skin ulceration, (5) no bleeding complications, and (6) no evidence of PE.

Nursing Implementation

Acute Care. Focus your nursing care for the patient with VTE on prevention of emboli formation and reduction of inflammation. Review with the patient any drugs, vitamins, minerals, and dietary and herbal supplements being taken that may interfere with anticoagulant therapy (see the Complementary & Alternative Therapies box on p. 820). Depending on the anticoagulant ordered, monitor INR, aPTT, ACT, anti–factor Xa levels, complete blood count (CBC), creatinine, factor X levels, hemoglobin, hematocrit, platelet levels, and/or liver enzymes.[49] Monitor platelet counts for patients getting UH or LMWH to assess for HIT. Titrate doses of UH, warfarin, and direct thrombin inhibitors based on results of blood studies and agency protocols. Direct thrombin inhibitors may need adjustment for patients with renal or liver disease. Always check the results of appropriate tests before starting, giving, or changing anticoagulant therapy.

Monitor for and reduce the risk of bleeding that may occur with anticoagulant therapy (Table 37-13). Be aware that the risk of bleeding is greater in people receiving LMWH or UH with an active gastroduodenal ulcer, prior bleeding history, low platelet count, hepatic or renal failure, rheumatic disease, cancer, or age greater than 85 years.[50] Patients receiving warfarin with an INR of 5.0 or more are also at increased risk for bleeding. In the event of anticoagulation above target goals, give reversal agents (e.g., protamine, vitamin K) or make dosage adjustments as ordered. In the event of major VKA-related bleeding, rapid treatment with four-factor prothrombin complex concentrate and IV vitamin K is recommended over fresh frozen plasma.

DRUG ALERT Anticoagulant Therapy

- Avoid IM injections.
- Observe closely for any signs of bleeding: hypotension, tachycardia, hematuria, melena, hematemesis, petechiae, ecchymosis, oozing or visible bleeding from trauma site or surgical incision.
- Tell patients to report any signs of bleeding: black or bloody stools, bleeding gums, bloody urine or sputum, coffee-ground or bloody vomit, excessive bruising, nosebleeds, excessive menstrual bleeding.
- Assess for mental status changes, especially in the older patient, since this may indicate cerebral bleeding.
- Tell patients to avoid taking aspirin, NSAIDs, fish oil supplements, garlic supplements, ginkgo biloba, and certain antibiotics (e.g., sulfamethoxazole and trimethoprim [Bactrim]).

TABLE 37-13 Nursing Interventions for Patients Taking Anticoagulants

Assessment

- Monitor vital signs as indicated.
- Examine urine and stool for overt and occult signs of blood.
- Inspect skin frequently, especially under any splinting devices.
- Evaluate platelet count for signs of heparin-induced thrombocytopenia.
- Evaluate appropriate laboratory coagulation tests for target therapeutic levels.
- Evaluate lower extremity for ecchymosis or hematoma development if intermittent pneumatic compression device used.
- Perform assessments frequently to observe for signs and symptoms of bleeding (e.g., hypotension, tachycardia) or clotting.
- Notify the HCP of any abnormalities in assessments, vital signs, or laboratory values.

Injections

- Avoid IM injections.
- Minimize venipunctures.
- Use small-gauge needles for venipunctures unless therapy requires a larger gauge.
- Apply manual pressure for at least 10 min (or longer if needed) on venipuncture sites.

Patient Care

- Avoid restrictive clothing.
- Apply moisturizing lotion to skin.
- Use electric razors, not straight razors.
- Perform physical care in a gentle manner.
- Tell patient not to forcefully blow nose.
- Avoid removing or disrupting established clots.
- Humidify O_2 source if supplemental O_2 is ordered.
- Use soft toothbrushes or foam swabs for oral care.
- Reposition the patient carefully at regular intervals.
- Limit tape application. Use paper tape as appropriate.
- Give stool softeners to avoid hard stools and straining.
- Lubricate tubes (e.g., suction catheter) adequately before insertion.
- Avoid restraints if possible. Use only soft, padded restraints if needed.
- Use support pads, mattresses, bed cradles, and therapeutic beds as indicated.
- Apply graduated compression stockings or intermittent pneumatic compression devices (if ordered) and with attention to proper size, application, and use.
- Perform risk for fall and skin breakdown assessments per agency policy and implement safety and preventive measures as needed.

Early ambulation when compared with bed rest does not increase the short-term risk of a PE in patients with VTE. In addition, early ambulation after acute VTE results in a more rapid decrease in edema and limb pain, fewer PTS symptoms, and better quality of life. Teach the patient and caregiver the importance of physical activity and assist the patient to ambulate several times a day. For patients with acute VTE with severe edema and limb pain, bed rest with limb elevation may initially be prescribed.

Ambulatory Care. Focus discharge teaching on modification of VTE risk factors, importance of monitoring laboratory values, dietary and drug instructions, and guidelines for follow-up. If appropriate, tell the patient to stop smoking and avoid all nicotine products. Instruct the patient to avoid constrictive clothing. If appropriate, tell women with a history of VTE to stop oral contraceptives or HT. Teach patients to limit standing or sitting in a motionless, leg-dependent position.

TEAMWORK & COLLABORATION

Caring for the Patient With Venous Thromboembolism (VTE)

All members of the interprofessional team have important roles in VTE prevention and management of a patient with VTE..

Role of Nursing Personnel

Registered Nurse (RN)

- Assess patients for VTE risk and monitor for VTE in at-risk patients.
- Teach patients who are at risk for VTE about preventive measures such as increasing mobility, using graduated compression stockings and intermittent pneumatic compression devices, and taking anticoagulant drugs.
- Assess for the use of dietary supplements or herbs that may affect the coagulation status before the start of anticoagulant therapy.
- Evaluate the effect of anticoagulant drugs by monitoring appropriate laboratory results and side effects of therapy.
- Assess for complications of VTE, including pulmonary embolism (PE) and chronic venous insufficiency.
- Teach the patient and caregiver the clinical manifestations of PE and the need to contact the ERS if these occur.
- Provide discharge teaching about use of graduated compression stockings, anticoagulant drugs, diet, laboratory testing, and administration of subcutaneous anticoagulants (if needed).
- Teach safety precautions to prevent falls or other injuries that might result in bleeding.
- Provide instructions about the use of pressure to stop bleeding and that the ERS should be contacted for persistent bleeding.
- Teach the patient about lifestyle measures to prevent VTE, including leg exercises, ambulation, and avoidance of nicotine and oral contraceptives.

Licensed Practical/Vocational Nurse (LPN/LVN)

- Give prescribed oral, subcutaneous, and IV anticoagulants (consider state nurse practice act and agency policies regarding administration of high-alert medications and IV medications).
- Measure patients for graduated compression stockings and/or intermittent pneumatic compression devices.

Unlicensed Assistive Personnel (UAP)

- Reposition patients who are on bed rest at least every 2 hr.
- Remind patients about the need to flex and extend the legs and feet at least every 2 hr while in bed.
- Help ambulatory patients to walk at least 4 to 6 times daily.
- Help patients with putting on graduated compression stockings.
- Apply intermittent pneumatic compression devices.

Role of Other Team Members

Physical Therapist

- Assess patient's mobility status.
- Develop exercise/muscle strengthening program as needed.

Dietitian

- Assess patient's diet and nutritional status.
- Provide diet teaching as needed.

When traveling long distances, tell patients to frequently exercise the calf muscles, take short walks, and drink nonalcoholic, noncaffeinated beverages. For those at high risk for VTE who are planning a long trip, recommend properly fitted, knee-high graduated compression stockings during travel to decrease edema and VTE risk. Aspirin or anticoagulant use is not suggested for long-distance travelers. Teach the patient and caregiver about signs and symptoms of PE such as sudden onset of dyspnea, tachypnea, and pleuritic chest pain. (Chapter 27 discusses PE.) They should contact ERS if these symptoms occur.

TABLE 37-14 Patient & Caregiver Teaching

Anticoagulant Therapy

Include the following information in the teaching plan for a patient receiving anticoagulant therapy and the patient's caregiver.

1. Give reasons for and action of anticoagulant drug and how long therapy will last.
2. Take drug at the same time each day (preferably in afternoon or evening).
3. Depending on drug prescribed, obtain blood tests to assess therapeutic effect of the drug and whether change in dosage is needed.
4. Contact ERS immediately for any of the following adverse side effects of drug therapy:
   - Blood in urine or stool; or black, tarry stools
   - Vomiting blood, coffee-ground emesis
   - Unusual bleeding from gums, skin, or nose, or heavy menstrual bleeding
   - Severe headaches or stomach pain
   - Chest pain, shortness of breath, palpitations (heart racing)
   - Weakness, dizziness, mental status changes
   - Cold, blue, or painful feet
5. Avoid any trauma or injury that may cause bleeding (e.g., vigorous brushing of teeth, contact sports, rollerblading, use of straight razor).
6. Avoid all aspirin-containing drugs and nonsteroidal antiinflammatory drugs.
7. Limit alcohol intake to small to moderate amounts (12 oz beer, 4 oz wine, 1 oz hard liquor/day).
8. Wear a Medic Alert device indicating what anticoagulant drug is being taken.
9. If taking warfarin (Coumadin), avoid frequent or dramatic changes in eating foods high in vitamin K (e.g., broccoli, spinach, kale, greens). Do not take supplemental vitamin K.
10. Consult with HCP before beginning or discontinuing any drug, vitamin, mineral, or dietary or herbal supplement (see Complementary & Alternative Therapies box on p. 820).
11. Inform all HCPs, including dentist, of anticoagulant therapy.
12. Correct dosing is essential. Provide supervision if patient experiences confusion or cognitive impairment.

Teach the patient and caregiver about drug dosage, actions, and side effects; the need for routine blood tests; and what symptoms need immediate medical attention (Table 37-14). Devices are available for home monitoring of INR. Teach patients taking LMWH or fondaparinux and their caregivers how to give the drug subcutaneously. Active or young patients need to avoid contact sports and high-risk (for trauma) activities (e.g., skiing). Teach older patients about safety precautions to prevent falls (e.g., avoid use of throw rugs). Tell the patient and caregiver to apply pressure for 10 to 15 minutes if bleeding occurs (e.g., nosebleed).

A well-balanced diet is important. Teach patients taking warfarin to follow a consistent diet of foods containing vitamin K and to avoid any supplements containing vitamin K (e.g., vitamins, green tea). Tell the patient to avoid excessive amounts of vitamin E and alcohol. Encourage proper hydration to prevent additional hypercoagulability of the blood, which may occur with dehydration.

The overweight patient needs to limit carbohydrates and total caloric intake and increase physical activity to achieve and maintain desired weight. Exercise does not harm and may benefit patients with VTE and PTS.[36] Help the patient develop an exercise program with an emphasis on leg strength training and aerobic activity. An exercise program also improves the patient's quality of life.

Graduated compression stockings reduce symptomatic swelling in patients with a diagnosis of proximal VTE.[36] Alternatively, IPCs may be used for patients with significant edema and moderate to severe PTS. The long-term use of graduated compression stockings may not prevent PTS development.

◆ Evaluation

The expected outcomes are that the patient with VTE will have:

- Minimal to no pain
- Intact skin
- Increased knowledge of disorder and treatment plan
- No signs of hemorrhage or occult bleeding

VARICOSE VEINS

Varicose veins, or *varicosities,* are dilated (3 mm or larger in diameter), tortuous superficial veins commonly found in the saphenous vein system. Varicosities may be small and harmless or large and bulging. *Primary varicose veins* (idiopathic) are due to a weakness of the vein walls and are more common in women. *Secondary varicose veins* result from direct injury, a previous VTE, or excessive vein distension. Secondary varicose veins may also occur in the esophagus (esophageal varices), vulva, spermatic cords (varicoceles), and anorectal area (hemorrhoids), and as abnormal arteriovenous (AV) connections.

Congenital varicose veins result from chromosomal defects which cause abnormal development of the venous system.[51] *Reticular veins* are smaller varicose veins that appear flat, less tortuous, and blue-green in color. *Telangiectasias* (often referred to as spider veins), are small visible vessels (generally less than 1 mm in diameter) that appear bluish black, purple, or red.

Etiology and Pathophysiology

The etiology of varicose veins is multifactorial. Superficial veins in the lower extremities become dilated and tortuous in response to backward (retrograde) blood flow and increased venous pressure. Risk factors include family history of chronic venous disease, weakness of the vein structure, female gender, Hispanic ethnicity, tobacco use, increasing age, obesity, multiparity, history of VTE, venous obstruction resulting from extrinsic pressure by tumors, thrombophilia, phlebitis, previous leg injury, and occupations that require prolonged standing or sitting.[52]

In primary varicose veins, weak vein walls allow the vein valve ring to enlarge, so the leaflets no longer fit together properly (incompetent). Incompetent vein valves allow backward blood flow, particularly when the patient is standing. This results in increased venous pressure and further venous distention. High pressure in the superficial veins can also be caused by vein valve dysfunction in the deep veins or perforator veins (veins that perforate the deep fascia of muscles to connect the superficial veins to the deep veins).

Clinical Manifestations and Complications

Discomfort from varicose veins varies among people and tends to be worse after episodes of superficial vein thrombosis. Self-reported symptoms typically are worse in women.[52] The most common varicose vein symptoms include a heavy, achy feeling or pain after prolonged standing or sitting, which is relieved by walking or limb elevation. Some patients feel pressure or complain of an itchy, burning, tingling, throbbing, or cramplike leg sensation. Swelling, restless or tired legs, fatigue, and nocturnal leg cramps also may occur.

Superficial venous thrombosis is the most frequent complication of varicose veins. It may occur spontaneously or after trauma, surgical procedures, or pregnancy. Rare complications include rupture of the varicose veins resulting in external bleeding and skin ulcerations.

Diagnostic Studies and Interprofessional Care

Superficial varicose veins can often be diagnosed by careful physical examination. Duplex ultrasound imaging is the gold standard to evaluate venous anatomy, valvular competence, and venous obstruction.[52] Conservative treatment involves rest with limb elevation; graduated compression stockings; leg strengthening exercise, such as walking; and weight loss, if indicated.

Drug Therapy

Venoactive drugs, derived from plant extracts, are powerful antioxidants that work by stimulating release of chemicals within the vein walls to strengthen the circulation and reduce inflammation and edema. Several natural and synthetic venoactive agents have been used to treat varicose veins and advanced chronic venous disease. These include coumarins (α-benzopyrenes), defibrotide, flavonoids (e.g., diosmin, hesperidin, micronized purified flavonoid fraction [Daflon]), rutosides (e.g., horse chestnut seed extract *[Aesculus hippocastanum]*), and other plant extracts such as butcher's broom *[Ruscus aculeatus]*), Gotu kola, pine bark, and red vine leaf.[36,52]

Therapeutic benefits of venoactive drugs include pain relief, edema reduction, and decreased leg cramping and restless legs. These drugs have been widely used in Europe. They are not approved by the Federal Drug Administration (FDA) in the United States. However, many are available over-the-counter as dietary or herbal supplements.

DRUG ALERT Horse Chestnut Seed Extract
(Aesculus hippocastanum)

- May interact with lithium and antidiabetes, antiplatelet, and anticoagulant drugs.
- Should not be taken by individuals with liver or kidney disease or with a latex allergy.

Interventional and Surgical Therapies

Sclerotherapy involves the direct IV injection of a liquid or foam sclerosing substance (e.g., hypertonic saline, polidocanol, glycerin) that chemically ablates (destroys) the treated veins. Sclerotherapy can be used on telangiectasias, perforator veins, reticular veins, varicose veins 5 mm in diameter or smaller, and venous malformations (Fig. 37-12). This procedure is performed in an office setting and causes minimal discomfort.

The most common complications of sclerotherapy are residual pigmentation and matting (new telangiectasias develop in the area).[53] Less common complications include headaches, migraines, skin necrosis, sensory nerve injury, visual disturbances, and distal VTE. After injection, a graduated compression stocking or compression bandage is recommended. Patients should not travel long distances during the first week after sclerotherapy to minimize the risk of a VTE.[53]

Other noninvasive options include transcutaneous laser therapy for telangiectasias and high-intensity pulsed-light

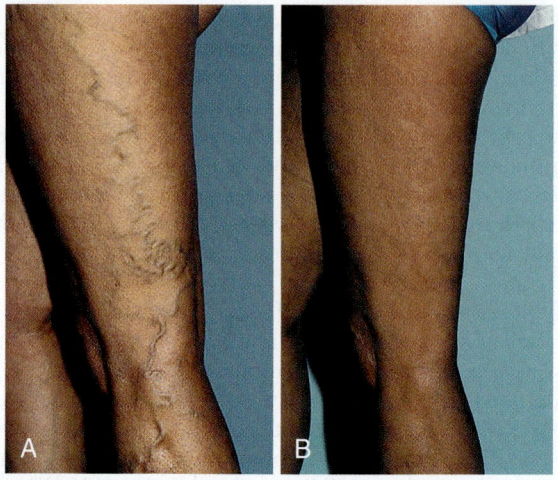

FIG. 37-12 **A,** Lateral aspect of varicose veins before treatment. **B,** Lateral aspect of varicose veins 2 years after initial treatment with sclerotherapy. (From Goldman MP, Guex JJ, Weiss RA: *Sclerotherapy: treatment of varicose and telangiectatic leg veins,* ed 5, Philadelphia, 2011, Mosby.)

therapy for reticular veins. Transcutaneous laser or light therapy is used for patients in whom sclerotherapy is contraindicated or has been ineffective.[52] Vascular lasers work by heating the hemoglobin in the vessels, resulting in vessel sclerosis. Potential complications of these therapies include pain, blistering, hyperpigmentation, and superficial erosions.

A minimally invasive treatment option for saphenous vein reflux is endovenous ablation using thermal energy from radiofrequency or laser therapy. A catheter is inserted into the vein to heat the vein wall, which then causes the vein to collapse. Potential complications include bruising, skin burns, hyperpigmentation, infection, paresthesia, superficial or deep vein thrombosis, and pulmonary embolism. Graduated compression stockings or bandages are recommended postprocedure. Endovenous thermal ablation may be done in combination with surgical ligation or phlebectomy.

Surgical intervention is indicated for recurrent superficial venous thrombosis or when symptoms cannot be controlled with medical or interventional therapy. The traditional surgical intervention involves ligation of the entire vein (usually the greater saphenous vein) and removal of its incompetent branches. An alternative but time-consuming technique is *ambulatory phlebectomy*. This involves pulling the varicosity through a "stab" incision followed by excision of the vein. *Transilluminated powered phlebectomy* involves the use of a tissue resector to destroy clusters of varicosities and removes the pieces via aspiration. Potential complications include bleeding, bruising, and infection. In up to 30% of patients, a new vein forms to replace the one removed.

❖ NURSING MANAGEMENT: VARICOSE VEINS

Prevention is a key factor related to varicose veins. Tell the patient to avoid sitting or standing for long periods, maintain ideal body weight, take precautions against injury to the extremities, avoid wearing constrictive clothing, and walk daily.

After vein ligation surgery, encourage the patient to deep breathe, which promotes venous return. Check the extremities regularly for color, movement, sensation, temperature, edema, and quality of pedal pulses. Some bruising and discoloration are normal. Elevate the legs 15 degrees to limit edema. Apply graduated compression stockings or bandages. Remove them every 8 hours for short periods and then reapply.

Long-term management of varicose veins is directed toward improving circulation and appearance, relieving discomfort, and avoiding complications and ulceration. Varicose veins can recur in other veins after surgery. Teach the patient the proper use and care of custom-fitted graduated compression stockings. The patient should apply stockings in bed before rising in the morning.

Emphasize the importance of periodic positioning of the legs above the heart. The overweight patient may need assistance with weight loss. The patient with a job that requires long periods of standing or sitting needs to frequently flex and extend her or his hips, legs, and ankles and change positions. Remind patients to consult with their HCP before taking any dietary or herbal supplements to avoid drug interactions.

CHRONIC VENOUS INSUFFICIENCY AND VENOUS LEG ULCERS

Chronic venous insufficiency (CVI), a common problem in older adults, describes long-standing functional abnormalities of the venous system that result in advanced venous signs and symptoms, such as edema, skin changes, and/or venous leg ulcers.[51] CVI can lead to *venous leg ulcers* (formerly called *venous stasis ulcers* or *varicose ulcers*). Although CVI and venous leg ulcers are not life-threatening diseases, they are painful, slow to heal, debilitating, and costly conditions that adversely affect patients' quality of life.

Etiology and Pathophysiology

Both long-standing primary varicose veins and PTS can progress to CVI. As a result of *ambulatory venous hypertension,* serous fluid and RBCs leak from the capillaries and venules into the tissue. This produces edema and chronic inflammatory changes. Enzymes in the tissue eventually break down RBCs, causing the release of *hemosiderin,* which causes a brownish skin discoloration. Over time, the skin and subcutaneous tissue around the ankle are replaced by fibrous tissue, resulting in thick, hardened, contracted skin. Although the causes of CVI are known, the exact pathophysiology of venous leg ulcers is unknown.

Clinical Manifestations and Complications

In individuals with CVI, the skin of the lower leg is leathery, with a characteristic brownish or "brawny" appearance from the hemosiderin deposition. Edema usually has been persistent for a prolonged period. Eczema is often present, and itching is a common complaint (Table 37-1).

Venous ulcers classically are located above the medial malleolus (Fig. 37-13). The ulcer is often quite painful, particularly when edema or infection is present. Pain may be worse when the leg is in a dependent position. If the venous ulcer is untreated, the wound becomes wider and deeper, increasing the likelihood of infection. Severe complications can include osteomyelitis and malignant changes.[54] On rare occasions, severe, long-standing CVI may result in the need for amputation.[52]

Interprofessional Care

Compression is essential for venous ulcer healing and prevention of venous ulcer recurrence.[36,55] A variety of options are available for compression therapy. These include custom-fitted

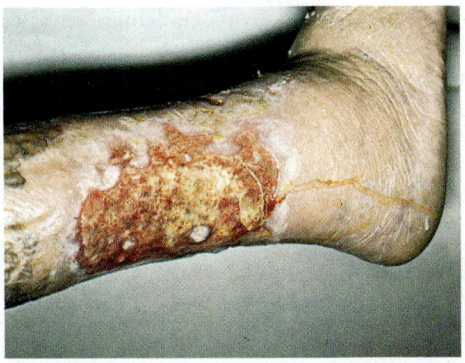

FIG. 37-13 Venous leg ulcer. (From Kamal A, Brockelhurst JC: *Colour atlas of geriatric medicine,* ed 2, 1991, Mosby-Year Book-Europe.)

graduated compression stockings, elastic tubular support bandages, a Velcro wrap (CircAid), IPCs, a paste bandage (Unna boot) with an elastic wrap, and multilayer (three or four) bandage systems (e.g., Profore).[52] There are benefits to each type of compression therapy. Evaluate patients individually when choosing a compression method. Before starting compression therapy, assess the arterial status to make sure that PAD is not also present. An ABI of 0.4 or less suggests severe PAD, and the patient should not have any type of compression therapy.[55]

Moist environment dressings are the basis of wound care.[50] A variety of these dressings are available, including transparent film dressings, hydrocolloids, hydrogels, foams, alginates, gauze, dextranomer, flax, and combination dressings. Dressing decisions should be based on wound characteristics, cost, best evidence, and clinician judgment. (Chapter 11 and Table 11-9 discuss dressings.)

Evaluate the nutritional status of a patient with a venous ulcer. A balanced diet with adequate protein, calories, and nutrients is essential. Foods high in protein (e.g., meat, beans, cheese, tofu), vitamin A (green leafy vegetables), vitamin C (citrus fruits, tomatoes, cantaloupe), and zinc (meat, seafood) are most important for healing. For patients with diabetes, maintaining normal blood glucose levels assists the healing process.

Venous leg ulcers are colonized by bacteria, but routine use of antibiotics is not indicated.[52] Clinical signs of infection include change in quantity, color, or odor of the drainage; pus; erythema of the wound edges; change in sensation around the wound; warmth around the wound; increased local pain, edema, or both; dark-colored granulation tissue; induration around the wound; delayed healing; and cellulitis. If signs of infection occur, obtain a wound culture. Antibiotic therapy should be guided by wound culture results. The usual treatment for infection is wound debridement, wound excision, and systemic antibiotics. Topical antibiotics are not recommended.

If the ulcer does not heal with conservative therapy, drug therapy should be considered. Pentoxifylline or micronized purified flavonoid fraction (Daflon) is recommended with compression therapy to improve healing.[36] Pentoxifylline minimizes WBC activation and adhesion to capillary endothelium and decreases oxidative stress. Micronized purified flavonoid fraction acts on WBCs to decrease inflammation and edema.[51]

Other treatments are recommended for large venous leg ulcers that do not respond to standard therapy after 4 to 6 weeks. These include coverage with a skin replacement or substitute such as split-thickness skin grafts, cultured keratinocyte grafts, artificial bioengineered skin, or porcine small intestinal submucosal tissue construct.[55] (Chapter 24 discusses skin grafting.) Although grafts may aid with healing, they do not replace the need for lifelong compression therapy. Neovalve reconstruction also may be considered in patients with long-standing, nonhealing ulcers.[36]

TEAMWORK & COLLABORATION

Caring for the Patient With Chronic Venous Insufficiency

Many patients with chronic venous insufficiency and venous ulcers are cared for in an outpatient setting. The registered nurse (RN) does an initial assessment of the wound, develops and implements the plan of care, and periodically evaluates the patient and venous ulcer. Much of the routine wound care is done by licensed practical/vocational nurses (LPN/LVNs) and unlicensed assistive personnel (UAP).

Role of Nursing Personnel

Registered Nurse (RN)

- Assess patients with chronic venous insufficiency for increases in edema, eczema, and venous leg ulcers.
- Assess patient's diet and nutritional status and make referrals as necessary.
- Assess for the use of venoactive dietary supplements or herbs that may adversely affect co-morbid conditions and/or prescription drugs.
- Choose appropriate options for compression therapy and wound care.
- Evaluate for the effectiveness of therapies and need for alternative approaches.
- Teach patient and caregiver about the clinical manifestations, complications, and treatment of venous insufficiency.

Licensed Practical/Vocational Nurse (LPN/LVN)

- Give prescribed analgesics, antibiotics, or other drugs.
- Apply compression therapy.
- Provide wound care for venous leg ulcers (consider state nurse practice act and agency policy).

Unlicensed Assistive Personnel (UAP)

- Assist patients in elevating legs to reduce edema and pain.
- Apply graduated compression stockings.
- Provide wound care for venous leg ulcers (consider state nurse practice act and agency policy).

Role of Other Team Members

Dietitian

- Assess patient's diet and nutritional status.
- Provide diet education as needed.

NURSING MANAGEMENT: CHRONIC VENOUS INSUFFICIENCY AND VENOUS LEG ULCERS

Long-term management of venous leg ulcers should focus on teaching the patient self-care measures. Demonstrate the correct application of graduated compression stockings and have the patient "show back" the skill. Prescription graduated compression stockings should be worn daily to prevent venous leg ulcer recurrence. Stress the importance of regular replacement every 4 to 6 months. Tell the patient and caregiver to avoid trauma to the limbs, and teach them proper foot and leg care to avoid additional skin trauma.

Patients with CVI have dry, flaky, itchy skin because of eczema. Daily moisturizing decreases itching and prevents cracking of the skin. Contact dermatitis may also result from contact with sensitizing products such as topical antimicrobial agents (e.g., gentamicin); additives in bandages or dressings (e.g., adhesives); ointments containing lanolin, alcohols, or benzocaine; and over-the-counter creams or lotions with fragrance or preservatives.[54] Assess the wound for signs of infection with each dressing change.

Be certain to discuss activity guidelines and proper limb positioning. Tell patients with CVI with or without a venous ulcer to avoid standing or sitting for long periods. Standing or sitting with the legs in a dependent position decreases blood flow to the lower extremities. Also tell patients to frequently elevate their legs above the level of the heart to reduce edema. Encourage patients to begin a daily walking program once an ulcer heals.

CASE STUDY

Peripheral Artery Disease

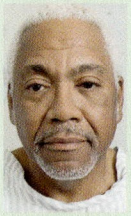

(©IPGGutenberg-UKLtd/iStock/Thinkstock)

Patient Profile

S.J., a 73-yr-old African American man, is admitted to the hospital with rest pain in both legs and a nonhealing ulcer of the big toe on the right foot.

Subjective Data

- History of a myocardial infarction, stroke, hypertension, heart failure, and type 1 diabetes mellitus
- Underwent a left femoral-popliteal bypass 5 yr ago
- Has a 45-pack-yr history of tobacco use
- Has been using insulin for 30 yr
- Complains of sudden, intense increase in right foot pain for past 2 hr
- Has slept in recliner with right leg in dependent position for several months

Current Medications

- Furosemide (Lasix) 40 mg/day PO
- Isosorbide dinitrate/hydralazine hydrochloride (BiDil) 1 tablet q8hr
- Aspart (NovoLog) insulin with meals
- Glargine insulin 50 U/day subcutaneously
- Diltiazem sustained release (Cardizem LA) 240 mg/day PO
- Aspirin 325 mg/day PO
- Fish oil daily (self-prescribed)

Objective Data

Physical Examination

- BP 148/92 mm Hg, irregular apical HR 90/min, respiratory rate 22/min, temperature 97.9°F (36.6°C)
- Alert and oriented but anxious, no apparent physical or mental deficits from previous stroke
- Has a diminished right femoral pulse, popliteal pulse by Doppler only, posterior tibial pulse by Doppler only, and dorsalis pedis pulse absent (not palpable or present by Doppler). Left leg pulses are weakly palpable
- Right leg ABI: 0.20. Left leg ABI: 0.68
- Has a 2-cm necrotic ulcer on tip of right big toe
- Has thickened toenails. Shiny, thin skin on legs. Hair absent on both lower legs
- Right foot is very cool, pale, and mottled in color with decreased sensation
- No peripheral edema present
- Bedside glucose measurement 298 mg/dL (last meal 4 hr before admission)

Discussion Questions

1. Assess S.J.'s risk factors for peripheral artery disease (PAD).
2. Differentiate S.J.'s signs and symptoms of chronic PAD and acute arterial ischemia.
3. Identify the possible cause(s) for the sudden, intense increase in right foot pain.
4. How would you interpret S.J.'s ABI findings?
5. What additional diagnostic tests can be performed to assess the extent of his PAD?
6. Given the physical examination data, what initial drug(s) would you expect the HCP to prescribe?
7. What treatment modalities are possible for S.J.?
8. ***Priority Decision:*** What are the priority nursing responsibilities in caring for S.J.?
9. ***Teamwork and Collaboration:*** Identify activities that can be delegated to unlicensed assistive personnel.
10. ***Priority Decision:*** Based on the assessment data presented, what are the priority nursing diagnoses? Are there any collaborative problems?
11. ***Evidence-Based Practice:*** When teaching S.J., what evidence-based advice would you give him regarding the use of dietary supplements such as fish oil?
12. ***Safety:*** To ensure S.J.'s safety, what nursing interventions are necessary to initiate?

Answers available at *http://evolve.elsevier.com/Lewis/medsurg.*

BRIDGE TO NCLEX EXAMINATION

The number of the question corresponds to the same-numbered outcome at the beginning of the chapter.

1. A 50-year-old woman weighs 95 kg and has a history of tobacco use, high blood pressure, high sodium intake, and sedentary lifestyle. When developing an individualized care plan for her, the nurse determines that the *most important* risk factors for peripheral artery disease (PAD) that must be modified are
   a. weight and diet.
   b. activity level and salt intake.
   c. tobacco use and high blood pressure.
   d. sedentary lifestyle and exercise training.
2. Rest pain is a manifestation of PAD that occurs due to a chronic
   a. vasospasm of small cutaneous arteries in the feet.
   b. increase in retrograde venous blood flow in the legs.
   c. decrease in arterial blood flow to the nerves of the feet.
   d. constriction in arterial blood flow to the leg muscles during exercise.
3. A patient with infective endocarditis develops sudden left leg pain with pallor, paresthesia, and a loss of peripheral pulses. The nurse's *initial* action should be to
   a. elevate the leg to promote venous return.
   b. start anticoagulant therapy with IV heparin.
   c. notify the HCP of the change in peripheral perfusion.
   d. place the bed in reverse Trendelenburg to promote perfusion.
4. Which clinical manifestations are seen in patients with either Buerger's disease or Raynaud's phenomenon *(select all that apply)*?
   a. Intermittent fevers
   b. Sensitivity to cold temperatures
   c. Gangrenous ulcers on fingertips
   d. Color changes of fingers and toes
   e. Episodes of superficial vein thrombosis

5. A patient is admitted to the hospital with a diagnosis of abdominal aortic aneurysm. Which signs and symptoms would suggest that his aneurysm has ruptured?
   a. Rapid onset of shortness of breath and hemoptysis
   b. Sudden, severe low back pain and bruising along his flank
   c. Gradually increasing substernal chest pain and diaphoresis
   d. Sudden, patchy blue mottling on feet and toes and rest pain
6. What are the *priority* nursing interventions after an abdominal aortic aneurysm repair?
   a. Assessment of cranial nerves and mental status
   b. Administration of IV heparin and monitoring of PT
   c. Administration of IV fluids and monitoring of kidney function
   d. Elevation of the legs and application of graduated compression stockings
7. The *first* priority of interprofessional care of a patient with a suspected acute aortic dissection is to
   a. reduce anxiety.
   b. monitor for chest pain.
   c. control blood pressure.
   d. increase myocardial contractility.
8. The patient at *highest* risk for venous thromboembolism (VTE) is
   a. a 62-year-old man with spider veins who is having arthroscopic knee surgery.
   b. a 32-year-old woman who smokes, takes oral contraceptives, and is planning a trip to Europe.
   c. a 26-year-old woman who is 3 days postpartum and received maintenance IV fluids for 12 hours during her labor.
   d. an active 72-year-old man at home recovering from transurethral resection of the prostate for benign prostatic hyperplasia.
9. Which are clinical findings in a person with an acute lower extremity VTE *(select all that apply)*?
   a. Pallor and coolness of foot and calf
   b. Mild to moderate calf pain and tenderness
   c. Grossly diminished or absent pedal pulses
   d. Unilateral edema and induration of the thigh
   e. Palpable cord along a superficial varicose vein
10. The recommended treatment for an initial VTE in an otherwise healthy person with no significant co-morbidities would include
   a. IV argatroban (Acova) as an inpatient.
   b. IV unfractionated heparin as an inpatient.
   c. subcutaneous unfractionated heparin as an outpatient.
   d. subcutaneous low-molecular-weight heparin as an outpatient.
11. A *key* aspect of teaching for the patient on anticoagulant therapy includes which instructions?
   a. Monitor for and report any signs of bleeding.
   b. Do not take acetaminophen (Tylenol) for a headache.
   c. Decrease your dietary intake of foods containing vitamin K.
   d. Arrange to have blood drawn twice a week to check drug effects.
12. In planning care and patient teaching for the patient with venous leg ulcers, the nurse recognizes that the *most* important intervention in healing and control of this condition is
   a. discussing activity guidelines.
   b. using moist environment dressings.
   c. taking horse chestnut seed extract daily.
   d. applying graduated compression stockings.

1. c, 2. c, 3. c, 4. b, c, d, 5. b, 6. c, 7. c, 8. b, 9. b, d, 10. d, 11. a, 12. d

For rationales to these answers and even more NCLEX review questions, visit *http://evolve.elsevier.com/Lewis/medsurg.*

EVOLVE WEBSITE

http://evolve.elsevier.com/Lewis/medsurg

Review Questions (Online Only)

Key Points

Answer Keys for Questions

- Rationales for Bridge to NCLEX Examination Questions
- Answer Guidelines for Case Study on p. 828
- Answer Guidelines for Managing Care of Multiple Patients Case Study (Section 7) on p. 831

Student Case Studies

- Patient With Abdominal Aortic Aneurysm
- Patient With Chronic Peripheral Artery Disease

Nursing Care Plans

- eNursing Care Plan 37-1: Patient With Peripheral Artery Disease of the Lower Extremities
- eNursing Care Plan 37-2: Patient After Surgical Repair of the Aorta

Conceptual Care Map Creator

Audio Glossary

Content Updates

REFERENCES

*1. Creager MA, Belkin B, Bluth EI, et al: 2012 ACCF/AHA/ACR/SCAI/SIR/STS/SVM/SVN/SVS key data elements and definitions for peripheral atherosclerotic vascular disease: a report of the American College of Cardiology Foundation/American Heart Association Task Force on Clinical Data Standards, *Circulation* 125:395, 2012. (Classic)

2. Eraso LH, Fukaya E, Mohler ER, et al: Peripheral arterial disease, prevalence, and cumulative risk factor profile analysis, *Eur Prevent Cardiol* 21:704, 2014.

3. Mozaffarian D, Benjamin EJ, Go AS, et al: Heart disease and stroke statistics—2015 update: a report from the American Heart Association, *Circulation* 131:29, 2015.

4. Rein P, Saely CH, Silbernagel G, et al: Systemic inflammation is higher in peripheral artery disease than in stable coronary artery disease, *Atherosclerosis* 239:299, 2015.

5. Schorr EN, Peden-McAlpine C, Treat-Jacobson D, et al: Characterization of the peripheral artery disease symptom experience, *Geriatric Nurs* 36(4):293, 2015.

*6. Anderson JL, Halperin JL, Albert NM, et al: Management of patients with peripheral artery disease (compilation of 2005 and 2011 ACCF/AHA guideline recommendations): a report of the American College of Cardiology Foundation/American Heart Association Task Force on Practice Guidelines, *J Am Coll Cardiol* 61:1555, 2013.

*7. American Diabetes Association: Standards of medical care in diabetes, *Diabetes Care* 38(Suppl):S1, 2015.

*8. Lauret GJ, Fakhry F, Fokkenrood HJP, et al: Modes of exercise training for intermittent claudication, *Cochrane Database Syst Rev* (7):CD009638, 2014.

*9. Jensen MD, Ryan DH, Apovian CM, et al: 2013 AHA/ACC/TOS guideline for the management of overweight and obesity in adults: a report of the American College of Cardiology/American Heart Association Task Force on Practice Guidelines and The Obesity Society, *J Am Coll Cardiol* 1:2985, 2014.

10. Nosova EV, Conte MS, Grenon SM: Advancing beyond the "heart-healthy diet" for peripheral artery disease, *J Vasc Surg* 61:265, 2015.

11. Kirk J, Dunker KS: Dietary counseling: the ingredient for successfully addressing the use of herbal supplements and probiotics in chronic kidney disease, *Adv Chronic Kidney Dis* 21:377, 2014.

*12. Rollins KE, Jackson D, Coughlin PA: Meta-analysis of contemporary short- and long-term mortality rates in patients diagnosed with critical limb ischaemia, *Br J Surg* 100:1002, 2013.

*13. Chowdhury MM, McLain AD, Twine CP: Angioplasty versus bare metal stenting for superficial femoral artery lesions, *Cochrane Database Syst Rev* (6):CD006767, 2014.

*14. Dake MD, Ansel GM, Jaff MR, et al: Sustained safety and effectiveness of paclitaxel-eluting stents for femoropopliteal lesions: 2-year follow-up from the Zilver PTX randomized and single-arm clinical studies, *J Am Coll Cardiol* 61:2417, 2013.

*15. Ambler GK, Radwan R, Hayes PD, et al: Atherectomy for peripheral arterial disease, *Cochrane Database Syst Rev* (3):CD006680, 2014.

*16. McCaslin JE, Andras A, Stansby G: Cryoplasty for peripheral arterial disease, *Cochrane Database Syst Rev* (8):CD005507, 2013.

17. Lo RC, Bensley RP, Dahlberg SE, et al: Presentation, treatment, and outcome differences between men and women undergoing revascularization or amputation for lower extremity peripheral arterial disease, *J Vasc Surg* 59:409, 2014.

18. Kalish JA, Farber A, Homa K, et al: Factors associated with surgical site infection after lower extremity bypass in the Society for Vascular Surgery (SVS) Vascular Quality Initiative (VQI), *J Vasc Surg* 60:1248, 2014.

*19. Alonso-Coello P, Bellmunt S, McGorrian C, et al: Antithrombotic therapy in peripheral artery disease: antithrombotic therapy and prevention of thrombosis, ed 9: American College of Chest Physicians evidence-based clinical practice guidelines, *Chest* 141:e669S, 2012. (Classic)

20. Byrne R, Taha A, Avgerinos E, et al: Contemporary outcomes of endovascular interventions for acute limb ischemia, *J Vasc Surg* 59:988, 2014.

*21. January C, Wann L, Alpert J, et al: 2014 AHA/ACC/HRS guideline for the management of patients with atrial fibrillation: executive summary, *J Am Coll Cardiol* 64:2246, 2014.

22. Vijayakumar A, Tiwari R, Prabhuswamy VK: Thromboangiitis obliterans (Buerger's disease)—current practices, *Int J Inflam* 2013:156905, 2013.

*23. Nietert PJ, Shaftman SR, Silver RM, et al: Raynaud phenomenon and mortality: 20+ years of follow-up of the Charleston Heart Study cohort, *Clin Epidemiol* 7:161, 2015.

24. Sinnathurai P, Schrieber L: Treatment of Raynaud phenomenon in systemic sclerosis, *Intern Med J* 43:476, 2013.

*25. Jahangir E, Lipworth L, Edwards TL, et al: Smoking, sex, risk factors and abdominal aortic aneurysms: a prospective study of 18782 persons aged above 65 years in the Southern Community Cohort Study, *J Epidemiol Community Health* 69:481, 2015.

*26. Erbel R, Aboyans V, Boileau C, et al: 2014 ESC guidelines on the diagnosis and treatment of aortic diseases, *Euro Heart J* 35:2873, 2014.

*27. Abraha I, Romagnoli C, Montedori A, et al: Thoracic stent graft versus surgery for thoracic aneurysm, *Cochrane Database Syst Rev* (9): CD006796, 2013.

28. Gloviczki P, Huang Y, Oderich GS, et al: Clinical presentation, comorbidities, and age, but not female gender predict survival after endovascular repair of abdominal aortic aneurysm, *J Vasc Surg* 61:853, 2015.

29. Rubenstein C, Bietz G, Davenport D, et al: Abdominal compartment syndrome associated with endovascular and open repair of ruptured abdominal aortic aneurysms, *J Vasc Surg* 61:648, 2015.

30. Conrad MF, Cambria RP: Aortic dissection. In Cronenwett JL, Johnston KW, editors: *Rutherford's vascular surgery*, ed 8, Philadelphia, 2014, Saunders.

31. Chen T, Crozier JA: Endovascular repair of thoracic aortic pathologies: postoperative nursing implications, *J Vasc Nurs* 32:63, 2014.

*32. Dunda SE, Demir E, Muffel OJ, et al: Management, clinical outcomes, and complications of acute cannula-related peripheral vein phlebitis of the upper extremity: a retrospective study, *Phlebology* 30:381, 2015.

*33. Cannegieter SC, Horváth-Puhó E, Schmidt M, et al: Risk of venous and arterial thrombotic events in patients diagnosed with superficial vein thrombosis: a nationwide cohort study, *Blood* 125:229, 2015.

34. Ver Hage A: Acute venous thromboembolism in critically ill patients, *Nursing Crit Care* 10:22, 2015.

*35. Di Nisio M, Wichers IM, Middledorp S: Treatment for superficial thrombophlebitis of the leg, *Cochrane Database Syst Rev* (4):CD004982, 2013.

*36. Kahn SR, Comerota AJ, Cushman M, et al: The postthrombotic syndrome: evidence-based prevention, diagnosis, and treatment strategies: a scientific statement from the American Heart Association, *Circulation* 130:1636, 2014.

37. Pendergraft T, Liu X, Edelsberg J, et al: Prophylaxis against venous thromboembolism in hospitalized medically ill patients, *Circ Cardiovasc Qual Outcomes* 6:75, 2013.

*38. Gould MK, Garcia DA, Wren SM, et al: Prevention of VTE in nonorthopedic surgical patients: antithrombotic therapy and prevention of thrombosis, ed 9: American College of Chest Physicians evidence-based clinical practice guidelines, *Chest* 141:e227S, 2012. (Classic)

*39. Sachdeva A, Dalton M, Amaragiri SV, et al: Graduated compression stockings for prevention of deep vein thrombosis, *Cochrane Database Syst Rev* (12):CD001484, 2014.

*40. Sajid MS, Desai M, Morris RW, et al: Knee length versus thigh length graduated compression stockings for prevention of deep vein thrombosis in postoperative surgical patients, *Cochrane Database Syst Rev* (5):CD007162, 2012. (Classic)

*41. Zhao JM, He ML, Xiao ZM, et al: Different types of intermittent pneumatic compression devices for preventing venous thromboembolism in patients after total hip replacement, *Cochrane Database Syst Rev* (12):CD009543, 2014.

*42. Garcia DA, Baglin TP, Weitz JI, et al: Parenteral anticoagulants: antithrombotic therapy and prevention of thrombosis, ed 9: American College of Chest Physicians evidence-based clinical practice guidelines, *Chest* 141:e24S, 2012. (Classic)

*43. Ageno W, Gallus AS, Wittkowsky A, et al: Oral anticoagulant therapy: antithrombotic therapy and prevention of thrombosis, ed 9: American College of Chest Physicians evidence-based clinical practice guidelines, *Chest* 141:e44S, 2012. (Classic)

*44. Guyatt GH, Akl EA, Crowther M, et al: Executive summary: antithrombotic therapy and prevention of thrombosis, ed 9: American College of Chest Physicians evidence-based clinical practice guidelines, *Chest* 141:7S, 2012. (Classic)

*45. Linkins LA, Dans AL, Moores LK, et al: Treatment and prevention of heparin-induced thrombocytopenia: antithrombotic therapy and prevention of thrombosis, ed 9: American College of Chest Physicians evidence-based clinical practice guidelines, *Chest* 141:e495S, 2012. (Classic)

46. Kearon C, Aki E: Duration of anticoagulation therapy for deep vein thrombosis and pulmonary embolism, *Blood* 123:1794, 2014.

47. Jenkins JS, Michael P: Deep venous thrombosis: an interventionalist's approach, *Ochsner J* 14:633, 2014.

48. Rich K: Iliofemoral deep vein thrombosis: percutaneous endovascular treatment options, *J Vasc Nurs* 23:47, 2015.

*49. Holbrook A, Schulman S, Witt DM, et al: Evidence-based management of anticoagulant therapy: antithrombotic therapy and prevention of thrombosis, ed 9: American College of Chest Physicians evidence-based clinical practice guidelines, *Chest* 141:e152S, 2012. (Classic)

50. Shoeb M, Fang M: Assessing bleeding risk in patients taking anticoagulants, *J Thromb Thrombolysis* 35:312, 2013.

51. Raffetto JD, Eberhardt RT: Chronic venous disorders. In Cronenwett JL, Johnston KW, editors: *Rutherford's vascular surgery*, ed 8, Philadelphia, 2014, Saunders.

*52. Wittens C, Davies AH, Baekgaard R, et al: Management of chronic venous disease: clinical practice guidelines of the European Society for Vascular Surgery (ESVS) 2015 European chronic venous disease guidelines, *Eur J Vasc Endovasc Surg* 49:678, 2015.

*53. Rabe E, Breu FX, Cavezzi A, et al: European guidelines for sclerotherapy in chronic venous disorders, *Phlebology* 29:338, 2014.

54. Vasudevan B: Venous leg ulcers: pathophysiology and classification, *Indian Dermatol Online J* 5:366, 2014.

*55. O'Donnell TF, Passman TA, Marston WA, et al: Management of venous leg ulcers: clinical practice guidelines of the Society for Vascular Surgery and the American Venous Forum, *J Vasc Surg* 60:3S, 2014.

*Evidence-based information for clinical practice.

CASE STUDY

Managing Care of Multiple Patients

You are working on the cardiovascular stepdown unit and have been assigned to care for the following six patients. You have one LPN and a UAP assigned to help you.

Patients

(©Jupiterimages/ Banana-Stock/ Thinkstock)

L.P. is a 63-yr-old man who was brought to the ED with complaints of chest pain, shortness of breath, palpitations, and dizziness. L.P.'s CK-MB and troponin levels are within normal limits. His ECG showed atrial fibrillation with a rapid ventricular response. He has been on IV diltiazem and IV heparin for 24 hr. Although his heart rate has decreased to 102 bpm, the atrial fibrillation persists.

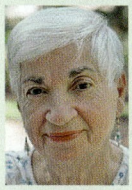

(©iStockphoto/ Thinkstock)

J.E. is a 70-yr-old woman admitted with complaints of increasing shortness of breath, fatigue, and weight gain. She has a systolic murmur and bilateral crackles. Her ejection fraction is 20%. She is currently receiving IV furosemide, oral potassium and enalapril (Vasotec), and a continuous infusion of nesiritide (Natrecor). She is receiving O_2 at 6 L via nasal cannula to keep her O_2 saturation >93%. Normal initial set of cardiac enzymes.

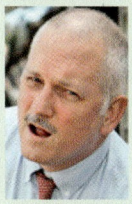

(©iStockphoto/ Thinkstock)

D.M. is a 51-yr-old man who was rushed to the hospital by ambulance after experiencing crushing substernal chest pain that radiated down his left arm. His ECG demonstrated marked ST segment elevation in the inferior leads. Cardiac catheterization showed a 90% blockage of his left anterior descending (LAD) artery. Coronary angioplasty was performed and a stent inserted. He is now 2 days post-PTCA, has had no recurrence of his chest pain, and is to be discharged today.

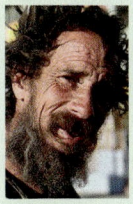

(©JennaDub/ iStock/ Thinkstock)

R.B. is a 50-yr-old man admitted for heart failure due to valvular heart disease. He has a history of IV drug and alcohol abuse. He complains of chest pain with minimal exertion. He has atrial fibrillation with a rapid ventricular response. His rhythm converted to normal sinus rhythm after receiving IV amiodarone. Transesophageal echocardiography shows left atrial and ventricular hypertrophy and mitral and aortic regurgitation.

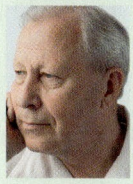

(©iStockphoto/ Thinkstock)

J.M. is a 68-yr-old man admitted 3 days ago with a diagnosis of acute decompensated HF. He had a cardiac arrest (pulseless VT) and was successfully defibrillated after one shock. He underwent electrophysiology studies and implantation of an implantable cardiodefibrillator (ICD). He now is being treated for his heart failure.

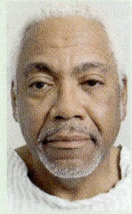

(©IPGGutenberg-UKLtd/iStock/ Thinkstock)

S.J. is a 73-yr-old man admitted with rest pain in both legs and a nonhealing ulcer of the big toe on the right foot. He has history of an MI, stroke, hypertension, heart failure, and type 1 diabetes mellitus. He underwent a left femoral-popliteal bypass 5 years ago. His right foot is cool, pale, and mottled in color with decreased sensation. He has a diminished right femoral pulse, right popliteal and posterior tibial pulses only obtained by Doppler, and his right dorsalis pedis pulse is absent (not palpable or present by Doppler). His left leg pulses are weak but palpable. His right leg ABI: 0.20; left leg ABI: 0.68.

Discussion Questions

1. ***Priority Decision:*** After receiving report, which patient should you see first? Second? Provide a rationale for your decision.
2. ***Teamwork and Collaboration:*** Which tasks could you delegate to the LPN *(select all that apply)*?
   a. Monitor L.P.'s heparin infusion.
   b. Report changes in pain or sensation of S.J.'s legs.
   c. Teach D.M. about activity restriction post-PTCA.
   d. Administer prescribed medications to R.B. and J.M.
   e. Hook up J.M. to 12-lead ECG and monitor for any dysrhythmias.
3. ***Priority Decision and Teamwork and Collaboration:*** As you are assessing L.P., the LPN informs you that S.J. is diaphoretic and complaining of chest pain. Which initial action would be *most* appropriate?
   a. Ask the LPN to notify S.J.'s HCP.
   b. Have the LPN administer prescribed nitroglycerin to S.J.
   c. Leave L.P.'s room to perform a focused assessment on S.J.
   d. Finish assessing L.P. while the UAP obtains a 12-lead ECG on S.J.

Case Study Progression

S.J. rates his chest pain as a 9/10. His blood pressure is 110/70, heart rate 110, respiratory rate 26, and O_2 saturation 93% on room air. You obtain a 12-lead ECG and administer 0.4 mg SL nitroglycerin with minimal pain relief after 5 minutes. The 12-lead ECG demonstrates new ST elevation in leads II, III, and aVF.

4. Which interventions would you expect the HCP to order for S.J. *(select all that apply)*?
   a. IV nitroglycerin
   b. IV morphine sulfate
   c. Emergent cardiac catheterization
   d. Furosemide 40 mg IV push stat
   e. Increase O_2 flow rate to 12 L/minute
5. Which statement would you include in patient teaching regarding ICDs with J.M. and his family?
   a. Avoid air travel.
   b. Avoid driving for 6 weeks.
   c. Avoid any sexual activity in case the ICD discharges.
   d. Avoid standing near antitheft devices in doorways of stores and public buildings.
6. Knowing the mechanism of action for nesiritide, you prioritize monitoring of J.E.'s
   a. blood pressure.
   b. respiratory rate.
   c. b-natriuretic peptide (BNP) level.
   d. troponin and CK-MB laboratory values.
7. ***Management Decision:*** You ask the UAP to take D.M.'s vital signs before and after having him walk 300 feet. When reviewing the patient's chart, you note documentation of the patient's walk but not his vital signs. What is your *best* initial action?
   a. Report the incident to the charge nurse for follow-up.
   b. Talk to the UAP to discuss why the vital signs were not documented.
   c. Walk D.M. yourself again and take his vital signs pre- and post-activity.
   d. Ask the LPN to ambulate D.M. and obtain his vital signs before and after.

Answers and rationales available at *http://evolve.elsevier.com/Lewis/medsurg.*

A

AB5000 Circulatory Support System, 754
Abacavir (Ziagen), 187*b*
Abandonment
elder mistreatment, 67*b*
fear of, at end of life, 139
Abatacept (Orencia), 1521*b*-1522*b*, 1529
ABCDE (Awakening and Breathing Trial Coordination, Daily Delirium Monitoring and Management, and Early Exercise and Mobility) bundle, 1582
ABCDE rule, 410, 410*f*
Abciximab (ReoPro), 715*b*-716*b*
Abdomen
abnormalities, 846*b*-847*b*
examination of, 843-844, 1112
auscultation, 843-844
inspection, 843
normal, 846*b*
palpation, 844, 844*f*
percussion, 844, 844*f*
secondary survey, 1633-1634
quadrants of, 843, 843*b*, 843*f*
Abdominal aortic aneurysms, 810, 810*f*-811*f*
clinical manifestations of, 811
interprofessional care for, 811
surgical repair of, 811, 812*f*
Abdominal breathing, 569
relaxation, **83-84**, 84*b*
Abdominal compartment syndrome, 812, 941, 1593
Abdominal distention, 597*b*-598*b*, 846*b*-847*b*
postoperative, 1063
Abdominal pain, 1197*b*
acute, **938-939**, 1013*b*
chronic, **940-941**
Abdominal paradox, 467*b*-468*b*
Abdominal thrusts, 1652*b*, 1652*f*
Abdominal trauma, **941**, 942*b*
Abdominal ultrasound, 603*t*, 847*t*-850*t*
focused abdominal sonography for trauma (FAST), 1633-1634
Abdominal wall, in older adults, 840*b*
Abdominal-perineal resection, 956
Abdominoplasty, 890*f*
Abducens nerve, 1305*b*, **1306**
Abduction, 1455*b*
Abiraterone (Zytiga), 1280*b*
Ablation surgery, 1391
ABO blood groups, 600, 601*b*
Abortion, 1243
induced, 1243, **1244**
methods for inducing, 1244*b*
spontaneous, 1243, 1243*b*, **1243-1244**
Abscesses
anorectal, **970**, 970*f*
brain, 1336*b*, **1338-1339**, 1339*b*
lactational breast, **1207**
lung, **512**
peritonsillar, **484**
Absence seizures, 1375-1376
Absent bowel sounds, 846*b*-847*b*
Absent breath sounds, 467*b*-468*b*
Absolute neutrophil count, 632
Absolute refractory phase or period, 761, 762*f*
Abuse
child sexual abuse, 1263
elder abuse, **66-67**, 67*b*, 1414*b*
ACA (Patient Protection and Affordable Care Act), 4
Acanthosis nigricans, 1151
Acapella airway clearance device, 570, 570*f*
Acarbose (Precose), 1131*b*
Accelerated idioventricular rhythm, 764*b*, 770
Acceptance, 728*b*, 1435*b*
Accessory nerve, 1305*b*
Accolate (zafirlukast), 479*b*-480*b*, 547, 548*b*-549*b*
Accountable care organizations (ACOs), 4
Acculturation, 22
AccuNeb (albuterol), 548*b*-549*b*
Accupril (quinapril), 691*b*-693*b*
Accutane (isotretinoin), 417*b*
Acebutolol (Sectral), 691*b*-693*b*
Aceon (perindopril), 691*b*-693*b*
Acetaminophen (Tylenol), 984*b*
for inflammation, 164, 164*b*
overdose, 1643*b*
for pain, 111-112, 111*b*
Acetazolamide, 381*b*, 1001*b*
Acetylsalicylic acid (aspirin), 1355
Achalasia, 905
Achilles tendon reflex, 1307
Achilles tendonitis, 1456*b*
Acid neutralizers, 903*b*
Acid-base imbalances, **286-297**, 288*b*, 289*f*
in chronic kidney disease, 1077
ROME memory device for, 291*b*
Acid-base regulation, **287-288**
Acid-fast bacteria smear and culture, 469*t*-471*t*
Acidosis, 287
diabetic ketoacidosis, **1142-1145**, 1154*b*
manifestations of, 290*b*
metabolic, 288*b*, **289**
in acute kidney injury, 1072
in chronic kidney disease, 1077
respiratory, 288*b*, **288**
Aciphex (rabeprazole), 903*b*
Aclidinium bromide (Tudorza, Pressair), 548*b*-549*b*
Acne, 403*b*
Acne vulgaris, 417, 417*f*, **419*b***
Acoustic neuroma, **387**, 1333*b*
Acquired immunodeficiency syndrome (AIDS), **221**. *See also* Human immunodeficiency virus (HIV) infection
diagnostic criteria for, 221, 221*b*
Acrochordons, 419*b*
Acromegaly, **1156-1157**
clinical manifestations of, 1157, 1157*f*
dermatologic manifestations of, 399*b*
Acromioplasty, 1466-1467
Acropachy, 1164, 1165*f*
ACS Cancer Survivors Network, 267*b*
Actemra (tocilizumab), 1521*b*-1522*b*, 1529
Actigraphy, **93**
Actinic keratosis, 397, **411**, 412*b*
Action potential, 659, 757-758, 758*b*
Activase (alteplase), 715*b*-716*b*
Activated clotting time, 601*t*, 821*b*
Activated partial thromboplastin time, 601*t*, 821*b*, 1659*b*
Active listening, 49
Active surveillance (watchful waiting), 1278
Active transport, 272
Activity-exercise pattern, 37*b*, 38. *See also* Physical activity
Actonel (risedronate), 1513
Actos (pioglitazone), 1131*b*
Acupressure, 1080*b*
Acupuncture, **121**, 1523*b*
Acute abdominal pain, **938-939**
emergency management of, 939*b*
etiology and pathophysiology of, 938, 938*f*
Acute abnormal uterine bleeding, 1246
Acute alcohol toxicity, **149**
Acute alcoholic hepatitis, 984
Acute angle-closure glaucoma, 380
Acute arterial ischemia, 808
Acute arterial ischemic disorders, **808-809**
Acute blood loss, **614-615**
clinical manifestations of, 615, 615*b*
laboratory results in, 610*b*
Acute bronchitis, **499-500**
Acute care
emergency nursing, 1634
for older adults, 71-74
Acute care nurse practitioners (ACNPs), 1555
Acute chest syndrome, 617
Acute cholecystitis, 1007*b*
Acute coronary syndrome, **718-734**, 718*f*
acute care for, 727-728
ambulatory care for, 730-732
diagnostic studies in, 721-722
drug therapy for, 715*b*-716*b*, 722, **725-726**
ECG changes in, 721, **775-777**, 776*b*
emotional and behavioral reactions to, 728
FITT activity guidelines for, 732, 732*b*
gender differences in, 705*b*
interprofessional care for, 714*f*, **722-726**
monitoring, 727
nursing assessment in, 726*b*
nursing diagnoses for, 726
nursing management of, **726-733**
nutritional therapy for, 726
patient & caregiver teaching for, 730-731, 731*b*
psychosocial responses to, 728*b*
rehabilitation after, 728*b*
sexual activity after, 732-733, 733*b*
Acute coryza, **478-480**
Acute decompensated heart failure
clinical manifestations of, 741-742
clinical mprofile, 742*b*
drug therapy for, 745-746, 745*b*
interprofessional care for, 744-746, 744*b*
Acute diarrhea, 929, 930*b*
Acute disease–related malnutrition, 857
Acute gastritis, 909-910
Acute gastroenteritis, 944
Acute gastrointestinal bleeding, 924, 924*b*
Acute glaucoma, 381*b*
Acute glomerulonephritis, 1041
Acute hemolytic reaction, 650*b*-651*b*
Acute hepatitis, 977-978
clinical manifestations of, 977, 977*b*
diagnostic findings in, 979, 979*b*
drug therapy for, 975
interprofessional care for, 980-981, 980*b*

NOTE: Disorder names and key terms are in **boldface**. Page numbers in **boldface** indicate main discussions. Page numbers followed by *f*, *t*, or *b* indicate figures, tables, or boxes, respectively.

Acute HIV infection, 219-220
Acute hypoparathyroidism, 1172*b*, 1173
Acute illness, 61*b*
Acute infectious diarrhea
causes and manifestations of, 930*b*
nursing assessment in, 932, 932*b*
nursing diagnoses for, 932
nursing management of, **932-933**
Acute inflammatory demyelinating polyneuropathy, 1440
Acute intracranial problems, 1314-1344
Acute kidney injury, 1069, **1069-1074**, 1070*b*
acute care for, 1075
ambulatory care for, 1075
causes of, 1069-1070, 1070*b*, 1070*f*
intrarenal, 1070-1071, 1070*b*, 1070*f*
postrenal, 1070*b*, 1070*f*, 1071
prerenal, 1070, 1070*b*, 1070*f*
clinical manifestations of, 1071-1072
diagnostic studies in, 1072-1073
diuretic phase, 1072
etiology and pathophysiology of, 1070-1071
health promotion for, 1074-1075
interprofessional care for, 1073-1074, 1073*b*
nursing diagnoses for, 1074
nursing management of, 1074-1075
nutritional therapy for, 1074
in older adults, 1075
oliguric phase, 1071-1072
recovery phase, 1072
RIFLE classification of, 1071, 1071*b*
Acute liver failure, 978, **996**
Acute low back pain, 1503-1504
Acute lung injury, 650*b*-651*b*
Acute lymphocytic leukemia, 636*b*, **636**, 639*b*
Acute marginal gingivitis, 846*b*-847*b*
Acute marijuana toxicity, 153
Acute myelogenous leukemia, 636*b*, **636**, 639*b*
Acute necrotizing ulcerative gingivitis, 897*b*
Acute osteomyelitis, 1497
Acute otitis media, 384
Acute pain, 103*b*, 107*b*, **107**
Acute pancreatitis, 999-1001, 999*f*
acute care for, 1002-1003
ambulatory care for, 1003
clinical manifestations of, 999-1000
complications of, 1000
conservative therapy for, 1000-1001
diagnostic findings in, 1000, 1000*b*
drug therapy for, 1001, 1001*b*
etiology and pathophysiology of, 999
health promotion for, 1002
interprofessional care for, 1000-1001, 1001*b*
nursing assessment in, 1002*b*
nursing diagnoses for, 1002
nursing management of, 1001-1003
nutritional therapy for, 1001
pathogenesis of, 999, 999*f*
respiratory distress in, 1002*b*
surgical therapy for, 1001
Acute pericarditis, 784-786, 785*f*
chest x-ray findings in, 785, 786*f*
interprofessional care for, 785-786, 786*b*
Acute pharyngitis, 484
Acute poststreptococcal glomerulonephritis, 1041-1042
Acute pulmonary embolism, 530*b*
Acute pyelonephritis, 1038-1039, 1038*f*
drug therapy for, 1039*b*
interprofessional care for, 1038, 1039*b*
Acute radiation syndrome, 1645
Acute rejection, 208
Acute respiratory distress syndrome, 1620-1623
case study, 1626*b*
chronic or late phase, 1622
clinical manifestations of, 1622-1623, 1622*f*
Acute respiratory distress syndrome *(Continued)*
clinical progression of, 1622
complications of, 1623, 1623*b*
diagnostic findings in, 1620*b*, 1622-1623
edema formation in, 1620, 1620*f*
etiology and pathophysiology of, 1620-1622, 1621*f*
fibrotic phase, 1622
injury or exudative phase, 1621-1622
interprofessional care for, 1624*b*
nursing and interprofessional management of, 1623-1625
nursing assessment in, 1624
nutritional support for, 1625
predisposing conditions, 1620*b*
reparative or proliferative phase, 1622
Acute Respiratory Distress Syndrome Clinical Network (ARDSNet) protocol, 1623
Acute respiratory failure, 503, **1609-1614**
clinical manifestations of, 1612-1614
diagnostic studies in, 1614
drug therapy for, 1618-1619
etiology and pathophysiology of, 1610-1612
interprofessional care for, 565, 1616*b*
medical supportive therapy for, 1619
nursing and interprofessional management of, 1614-1620
nursing assessment in, 1615*b*
nursing diagnoses related to, 1615
nutritional therapy for, 1619
oxygen therapy for, 1615-1616
prevention of, 1615
respiratory therapy for, 1615-1617
Acute sinusitis, 483, 483*b*
Acute soft tissue injury, 1464*b*
Acute stroke, 1359*b*
Acute subdural hematoma, 1329, 1329*b*
Acute thyroiditis, 1163
Acute thyrotoxicosis, 1167
Acute toxicity, 248
Acute transfusion reactions, 650*b*-651*b*, **652**
Acute tubular necrosis, 1071
Acute ulcers, 910, 910*f*
Acute urinary retention, 1059-1060, 1289*b*
Acute venous disorders, 816-828
Acute viral rhinitis, 478-480, 480
Adalat (nifedipine), 532*b*, 1059*b*
Adalimumab (Humira), 1521*b*-1522*b*, 1529
Adaptive grief, 133
Adcirca (tadalafil), 532*b*
Addiction, 123. *See also* Substance abuse
fear of, 124*b*
pseudoaddiction, 123
risk monitoring, 123
Addisonian crisis, 1178
Addison's disease, 1178
clinical manifestations of, 1175*b*, 1178, 1178*f*
dermatologic manifestations of, 399*b*
etiology and pathophysiology of, 1178
interprofessional care for, 1179*b*
nursing management of, 1179
patient & caregiver teaching for, 1179*b*
Adduction, 1455*b*
Adefovir (Hepsera), 980
Adenocarcinoma, 514*f*, 515*b*
Adenohypophysis (anterior pituitary gland), 1104*b*, **1105**
Adenomas
fibroadenoma, 1206*b*, **1207-1208**
mucous gland, **518**
Adenosine (Adenocard), 532*b*, 765*b*, 771*b*
Adenosine deaminase (ADA) deficiency, 188*f*
Adenoviruses, 214*b*
ADH stimulation (water deprivation) test, 1115*t*-1118*t*
Adhesions, 167*b*
Adipectomy, 890, 890*f*
Adjustable gastric banding, 885, 886*b*, 887*f*
Admission
nursing assessment on, 345*b*
to postanesthesia care unit (PACU), 330-332
same-day, 301
before surgery, 319
Admission, observation, and discharge (AOD) area, 316
Ado-trastuzumab emtansine (Kadcyla), 1217*b*, 1218
Adrenal androgens, 1104*b*, **1108**
Adrenal cortex, 275, **1107-1108**
disorders of, **1174-1181**
in older adults, 1108*b*
Adrenal glands, **1107-1108**, 1107*f*
Adrenal hormones, 1104*b*
Adrenal medulla, **1107**
disorders of, **1181-1182**
in older adults, 1108*b*
Adrenal studies, 1115*t*-1118*t*
Adrenalin (epinephrine), 202, 1599*b*
Adrenergic inhibitors, 690, 691*b*-693*b*
Adrenocortical insufficiency, 1178-1179
Adrenocorticotropic hormone (ACTH), 1104*b*, 1385*b*
measurement of, 1115*t*-1118*t*
Adrenocorticotropic hormone (ACTH) stimulation test, 1115*t*-1118*t*
Adrenocorticotropic hormone (ACTH) suppression test, 1115*t*-1118*t*
Adult day care, 68
Adult day health care, 68
Adult learners, 47-48, 55*b*
Adult learning, 47, 47*b*
Adult-onset diabetes, 1122
Advair Diskus or HFA (fluticasone/salmeterol), 548*b*-549*b*
Advance care planning, **135**
Advance directives, **135**, 136*b*, 575*b*
Advanced practice clinicians, 1274*b*
Advanced practice registered nurses (APRNs), 3, 1554-1555
Adventitious breath sounds, 466
Advocacy, 30
AeroChamber, 547*f*
Aesculus hippocastanum (horse chestnut seed extract), 825*b*
Affect
assessment of, 1304
in stroke, 1351
Afinitor (everolimus), 1217*b*, 1218
Afrezza (inhaled insulin), 1126*f*, 1130
African Americans, 19
arthritis and connective tissue disorders in, 1525*b*
chronic kidney disease in, 1076*b*
coronary artery disease in, 704, 704*b*
cultural characteristics of, 22*b*
cultural & ethnic health disparities in, 682*b*
culture-bound syndromes, 29*b*
in health care workplace, 24
integumentary problems in, 410*b*
lung cancer in, 514*b*
and medications, 28
obesity among, 875, 876*f*, 878*b*
older adults, 63
prostate cancer in, 1276
stroke in, 1347*b*
Afterdrop, **1639**
Afterload, 250, 661, **1560**
normal resting parameters, 1559*b*
Age spots, 398*b*
Ageism, 63
Agency for Healthcare Research and Quality (AHRQ)
clinical practice guidelines for treating tobacco use disorder, 146-147, 147*b*

Age-related changes, 64
in auditory system, 361
in breast, 1208
in cardiovascular system, 662-663
degeneration of the cornea, 353*b*, 353*f*
in drug metabolism, 72-73, 73*f*
in endocrine system, 1108
in gastrointestinal system, 839
health disparities, 20-21
in hematologic system, 593, 593*b*
in immune system, 196, 196*b*
in integumentary system, 396-397
in musculoskeletal system, 1450-1451
in nervous system, 1301
in reproductive systems, 1191
in respiratory system, 459
in sexual function, 1191*b*
in urinary system, 1019-1020
in visual system, 352
in wound healing, 168*b*
Age-related macular degeneration, 378-379
genetic risk alert, 355*b*
Agglutination, 199, 591
measurement of, 1198*t*-1201*t*
Aggrastat (tirofiban), 715*b*-716*b*
Aging
and Alzheimer's disease, 1402
attitudes toward, 63
biologic, 63, 64*f*
and COPD, 559
demographics of, 63
photoaging, 397, 397*f*
process of, 63, 64*f*
Agitation, 1618-1619, 1618*b*
Agranulocytes, 589
AIDS, 221. *See also* Human immunodeficiency virus (HIV) infection
diagnostic criteria for, 221, 221*b*
Air conduction, 360
Air pollutants, 539-540, 539*b*
Air pollution, 558
Air pouch/pneumatic technology, 1319
Airborne precautions, 218, 218*b*
Airway inflammation, 1618
Airway management
artificial airways, 1569-1570, **1570-1573**
in burns, 438-439
in cardiopulmonary resuscitation, 1651-1652
clearance devices, 570, 570*f*
clearance techniques, 569-570
primary survey, 1630, 1631*b*-1632*b*
stenting, 517
Airway obstruction, 484-485
etiology and relief of, 332, 335*f*
postoperative, 332, 333*b*, 1168*b*
Airway pressure release ventilation (APRV), 1576*b*, 1577
Airway suctioning, 1617
Akinesia
in Parkinson's disease, 1389
in stroke, 1350
Akynzeol (netupitant and palonosetron), 895*b*
Alanine aminotransferase
liver function test, 852*t*
reference values, 1655*b*-1658*b*
ALARA (as low as reasonably achievable) principle, 250
Alarm fatigue, 12, 1575*b*
Albiglutide (Tanzeum), 1131*b*, 1132
Albumin
blood component therapy, 648*b*
reference values, 1655*b*-1658*b*
serum, 859
Albustix (Dipstick) test, 1025*t*-1030*t*
Albuterol (Proventil HFA, Ventolin HFA, ProAir HFA, AccuNeb, VoSpire ER [oral only]), 548*b*-549*b*
Alcohol, **148-149**
binge drinking, 148
effects of chronic use of, 151*b*
effects of use and complications of, 148-149
moderation of intake of, 688-689
nontolerant drinkers, 148
recommendations for nutrient balance, 1133
risky drinking, 148
tolerant drinkers, 148
U.S. standard drink equivalents, 148, 148*f*
Alcohol toxicity, 149-150
acute, 149
Alcohol use disorder, 148, **149-150**
Alcohol Use Disorders Identification Test (AUDIT), 154, 154*b*
Alcohol withdrawal, 151*b*
Alcohol withdrawal delirium, 150, 338
Alcohol withdrawal syndrome, 150
Alcoholic hepatitis, 984
Alcoholism, 148
Aldactone. *See* Spironolactone
Aldesleukin (Proleukin), 195*b*
Aldolase, 1457*t*-1459*t*, 1655*b*-1658*b*
Aldosterone, 275, **1108**
factors affecting secretion of, 274-275, 275*f*
measurement of, 1115*t*-1118*t*
urine values, 1661*b*
Aldosterone antagonists
for heart failure, 748
for hypertension, 691*b*-693*b*
Alemtuzumab (Campath), 210, 211*b*
Alemtuzumab (Lemtrada), 1385*b*, 1386
Alendronate (Fosamax), 1513
Alertness, 1630, 1631*b*
Aleuts, 63
Aleve (naproxen), 111*b*
Alfentanil (Alfenta), 326*b*
Alfuzosin (Uroxatral), 1059*b*
Alginates, 169*b*
Alirocumab (Praluent), 711*b*
Aliskiren (Tekturna), 691*b*-693*b*
Alkaline phosphatase
in bone disease, 1457*t*-1459*t*
liver function test, 852*t*
reference values, 1655*b*-1658*b*
Alkalosis, 287
manifestations of, 290*b*
metabolic, 288*b*, **289**
respiratory, 288*b*, **288-289**
Alka-Seltzer (sodium bicarbonate), 903*b*
Alkylating agents, 247*b*
Allegra (fexofenadine), 479*b*-480*b*
Alleles, 178-179, 179*b*
dominant, 179, 179*b*
recessive, 179, 179*b*
Allen test, 1562
Allergens, 409, 539, 539*b*
patient & caregiver teaching for avoiding, 478*b*
recognition and control of, 201-202
Allergic disorders, 200-203. *See also* Hypersensitivity reactions
asthma, 540, 541*f*
chronic allergies, **201-202**
conjunctivitis, **371-372**
contact dermatitis, **200**, 203, 409, 418*b*
corticosteroid therapy for reactions, 1180*b*
dermatologic problems, 417, 418*b*
diagnostic studies in, 200-201
drug allergy check, 442*b*
drug therapy for, 202
Allergic disorders *(Continued)*
eye reactions, 357*b*
food allergies, 540
guidelines for preventing reactions, 204*b*
immunotherapy for, 202-203
insulin reactions, 1129
interprofessional care for, 201-203
latex allergies, **203-204**, 204
mediators of reactions, 197, 197*b*
mild transfusion reactions, 650*b*-651*b*
nursing assessment in, 200, 201*b*
nursing history, 36
patient & caregiver teaching for avoiding allergens, 478*b*
preoperative assessment of, 305, 305*b*
prevention of reactions, 1602*b*
rhinitis, 198, **477-478**, 478
severe transfusion reactions, 650*b*-651*b*
Allī (orlistat), 884*b*
AlloDerm, 445
Allodynia, 105, 1547
Allografts
bone grafts, 1506
skin grafts, 440
Allow Natural Death (AND) orders, 136, 136*b*
Alogliptin (Nesina), 1131*b*
Alopecia, 403*b*
in cancer, 251*b*-252*b*, 256
traction, 403-405, 404*f*
Alosetron (Lotronex), 941*b*
Aloxi (palonosetron), 895*b*
α-adrenergic agonists
for glaucoma, 381*b*
for pain, 116*b*, 117
for voiding dysfunction, 1059*b*
α-adrenergic antagonists
for BPH, 1271
for hypertension, 691*b*-693*b*
for voiding dysfunction, 1059*b*
α_1-antitrypsin, 1655*b*-1658*b*
α_1-antitrypsin deficiency, 558
genetics of, 558-559, 559*b*
α-fetoprotein, 240
liver function test, 852*t*
reference values, 1655*b*-1658*b*
α-interferon (Intron A), 195*b*
5α-reductase Inhibitors
for BPH, 1271
for voiding dysfunction, 1059*b*
Alport syndrome, 1052
Altace (ramipril), 691*b*-693*b*
Alteplase (Activase), 715*b*-716*b*
Aluminum and magnesium (Gelusil, Maalox, Mylanta, Aludrox), 903*b*
Aluminum and magnesium trisilicate (Gaviscon), 903*b*
Aluminum hydroxide, 903*b*
Alveolar edema, 741
Alveolar fractures, 1623
Alveolar hyperventilation, 1579
Alveolar hypoventilation, 1578-1579, **1612**
Alveolar macrophages, 459
Alveolar-capillary membrane, 455, 455*f*
Alveoli, 454-455, 455*f*
Alvesco (budesonide ciclesonide), 548*b*-549*b*
Alzheimer's disease, 1401-1409
acute care for, 1410
ambulatory care for, 1410-1414
cardiovascular factors, 1402-1403
case study, 1417*b*
clinical manifestations of, 1403-1404
cultural & ethnic health disparities, 1402*b*
diagnosis of, 1405, 1407*f*
diagnostic criteria for, 1404-1405, 1406*b*

Alzheimer's disease *(Continued)*
diagnostic studies for, 1405-1408
drug therapy for, 1408-1409, 1408*b*
early onset, 1402, 1402*b*
early warning signs, 1405*b*
etiology of, 1401-1402, 1404*f*
familial, 1402, 1402*b*
family & caregiver teaching in, 1414*b*
gender differences in, 1402*b*
genetics of, 1303*b*, 1402-1403, 1402*b*
health promotion for, 1409
impact of, 61*b*
infection prevention in, 1413
interprofessional care for, 1407*b*, 1408-1409
late onset, 1402*b*
memory loss in, 1406*b*
mild, 1414*b*
moderate, 1414*b*
nursing assessment in, 1409, 1409*b*
nursing diagnoses for, 1409
nursing management of, 1409-1414, 1412*b*
oral care in, 1412-1413
pathophysiology of, 1403, 1403*f*-1404*f*
preclinical, 1404-1405, 1406*b*
resources for, 1410
retrogenesis in, 1403-1404, 1407*f*
safety in, 1412
severe, 1414*b*
skin care in, 1413
sleep disturbances during, 92*b*
staff responsibilities in, 1412*b*
stages of, 1406*b*
support for caregivers in, 1413-1414, 1413*f*
Amantadine, 1390, 1391*b*
Amaryl (glimepiride), 1131*b*
Ambrisentan (Letairis), 532*b*
Ambu bag, 1570
Ambulation, after fracture, 1477
Ambulatory blood pressure monitoring, 687-688
Ambulatory peritoneal dialysis, continuous, 1086-1087
Ambulatory phlebectomy, 826
Ambulatory surgery, 302, **344-346**
discharge after, 344-345
discharge criteria, 344*b*
preoperative teaching, 309
Ambulatory venous hypertension, 826
Amenorrhea, 1190, 1246, 1246*b*
American Association of Critical-Care Nurses (AACN), 5
Certification Corporation, 1555
critical care certification (CCRN), 1555
critical care certification knowledge (CCRN-K), 1555
progressive care certification (PCCN), 1555
teleICU certification (CCRN-E), 1555
American Cancer Society, 256
American College of Cardiology (ACC), 681, 741, 741*b*
American College of Sports Medicine, 689
American Diabetes Association Act (ADA), 1141
American Geriatrics Society (AGS), 73
American Heart Association (AHA), 681
classification of heart failure, 741, 741*b*
Get With the Guidelines—Heart Failure program, 751
recommendations for physical activity, 689
American Indians or Alaska Natives, 19, 63
American Nurses Association (ANA), 2-3, 5
American Nurses Credentialing Center (ANCC), 5
American Parkinson Disease Association, 1392
American Red Cross, 1645, 1645*f*
American Society of Anesthesiologists, 307*b*, 322
American Spinal Injury Association (ASIA) Impairment Scale, 1421, 1422*f*
American Stroke Association (ASA), 1356, 1357*b*
American Urological Association (AUA), 1269, 1270*b*
Amidate (etomidate), 325*b*
Amikacin (Amikin), 509*b*
Amiloride (Midamor), 691*b*-693*b*
Amino acids, 610*b*
Aminoglycosides, 509*b*
Aminophylline, 548*b*-549*b*
5-Aminosalicylic acid, 947, 947*b*
Amiodarone (Cordarone), 771*b*
Amish, 26*b*
Amitriptyline, 116*b*, 1059*b*
Amlodipine (Norvasc), 691*b*-693*b*, 715*b*-716*b*
Ammonia, 852*t*
Ammonia salt encrustation, 1065, 1066*f*
Amputation, **1487**
acute care for, 1488-1490
ambulatory care for, 1490
bandaging, 1489, 1489*f*
diagnostic studies for, 1487
double amputee, 1489*f*
health promotion for, 1488
indications for, 1487
interprofessional care for, 1487, 1487*b*
lower extremity, 1490, 1490*b*
nursing management of, 1488-1490
in older adults, 1490
patient & caregiver teaching for, 1490, 1490*b*
postoperative care in, 1488-1490, 1489*f*
preoperative care in, 1488
sites of, 1488*f*
upper limb, 1490
Ampyra (dalfampridine), 1385*b*, 1386
Amsler grid test, 359*f*, 359*t*
Amylase
blood values, 847*t*-850*t*, 1655*b*-1658*b*
urine values, 1661*b*
Amylin, 1104*b*, 1136*f*
Amylin analogs, 1131*b*, 1132
Amyloid precursor protein, 1402
Amyloidosis, 1042*b*
Amyotrophic lateral sclerosis, **1395**
dementia in, 1401*b*
voice banking applications for, 1395*b*
Anakinra (Kineret), 195*b*, 1521*b*-1522*b*, 1529
Anal cancer, **970-971**
Anal fissures, **970**, 970*f*
Anal fistulas, **970**, 970*f*
Analgesia, 1308*b*-1309*b*
authorized agent controlled, 120
epidural, 340
via implantable pumps, 120
multimodal, 110
patient-controlled, **120**, 340, 340*b*
Analgesic ceiling, 111
Analgesics
adjuvant, 115-117, 116*b*
administration of, 117-120
buccal, 118
end-of-dose failure, 109
epidural, 119
equianalgesic dosing, 117-118, 117*b*
extended-release preparations, 118*b*
fear of hastening death by administering, 124-125
intranasal, 118
intraspinal, 119-120
intrathecal, 119
nonopioid, 111*b*, **111-112**
opioid, **112-115**, 113*b*-114*b*
oral, 118
parenteral, 119
rectal, 118
scheduling, 117
side effects of, 111, 111*b*
sustained-release preparations, 118*b*
titration of, 117
Analgesics *(Continued)*
transdermal, 118-119
transmucosal, 118
Anaphylactic shock, 1588*b*, 1590-1592
allergens causing, 197-198, 198*b*
clinical presentation of, 1591*b*
drug therapy for, 1599*b*
emergency management of, 202*b*
interprofessional care for, 1600*b*, 1601-1602
Anaphylaxis, **197-198**
clinical manifestations of, 197-198, 198*f*
interprofessional care for, 201
in operating room, 327
transfusion reactions, 650*b*-651*b*
Anasarca, 1594
Anastrozole (Arimidex), 1217*b*
Anatomic dead space, 454
Anatomic shunts, 1611
AND (Allow Natural Death) orders, 136, 136*b*
Andragogy, 47
Androgen deficiency, 399*b*
Androgen deprivation therapy, 1279-1280, 1280*b*
Androgen excess, 399*b*
Androgen receptor blockers, 259*b*, 1280, 1280*b*
Androgen synthesis inhibitors, 1279-1280, 1280*b*
Androgens, 1107
adrenal, 1104*b*, **1108**
Android obesity, 875, 876*b*
Anectine (succinylcholine), 326*b*
Anemia, **606-608**
acquired (extrinsic), 607*b*
acquired hemolytic, **619**
acute, 607*b*
from acute blood loss, **614-615**
aplastic, **614**
from blood loss, **614-615**
in cancer, 251*b*-252*b*, 253
cardiopulmonary manifestations of, 608
causes of, 606, 607*f*
chronic, 607*b*
of chronic disease, **613-614**
in chronic kidney disease, 1077-1078, 1081-1082
classification of, 606, 607*b*, 612, 612*b*
clinical manifestations of, 607-608, 608*b*
definition of, 606
dermatologic manifestations of, 399*b*
drug therapy for, 1081-1082
effects on wound healing, 168*b*
hemolytic, **615-619**
hereditary (intrinsic), 607*b*
integumentary manifestations of, 607-608, 608*b*
iron-deficiency, **609-611**
laboratory results in, 610*b*
megaloblastic, 612-613, 612*b*, **612-613**
nursing and interprofessional management of, 608
nursing assessment in, 609*b*
nursing diagnoses for, 608
in older adults, 608
pernicious, **612**
sickle cell, 610*b*, 616
Anesthesia, **322-329**, 1308*b*-1309*b*
balanced technique for, 323
dissociative, 323-324, 325*b*
epidural, **325-327**, 327*f*
fear of, 303
general, **322-324**, 323*b*, 325*b*
adjuncts to, 323, 326*b*
phases of, 324*b*
local, 323*b*, **324-327**, 340
monitored anesthesia care (MAC), **322**, 323*b*
regional, 120, 323*b*, **324-327**
spinal, **325-327**, 327*f*
techniques for, **322-327**, 323*b*
total intravenous anesthesia, 322

Anesthesia care provider (ACP), 318
  assisting, **320-321**
Anesthesiology, 318, 322
Anesthetics, 116*b*, 117
Aneuploidy, 1212-1213
Aneurysms
  aortic, **810-816**, 810*f*
  brain, 1336*b*
  cerebral, 1349
  clipping, 1356, 1356*f*
  coiling, 1356, 1356*f*
  dissecting, 814
  false, 810, 811*f*
  fusiform, 810, 811*f*
  left ventricular, 721
  pseudoaneurysms, 810, 811*f*
  saccular, 810, 811*f*
  true, 810, 811*f*
Anger
  in acute coronary syndrome, 728*b*
  of burn patients, 448*b*
  at end of life, 138
  in spinal cord injury, 1435*b*
Angina, 712
  chronic stable, **712-714**, 713*b*, 718*f*
    interprofessional care for, 714-718
    nursing management of, 726-733
  locations and patterns of pain during, 712*f*
  microvascular, 713*b*, **713-714**
  PQRST assessment of, 712, 712*b*
  precipitating factors, 713*b*
  Prinzmetal's, 713, 713*b*
  types of, 713*b*
  unstable, 713*b*, 714*f*, **719**
  variant, 713
Angina equivalent, 712
Angioedema, 199, 747
Angiogenesis, 703
Angiogenesis inhibitors, 257, 258*b*
Angiography
  cerebral, 1309*f*, 1310*t*-1312*t*
  cholangiography, 847*t*-850*t*
  computed tomography, 530, 1310*t*-1312*t*
  coronary, 673*t*-677*t*, 678, 678*f*, 722
  coronary CT, 673*t*-677*t*, 678
  fluorescein, 359*t*
  magnetic resonance, 673*t*-677*t*, 1025*t*-1030*t*, 1310*t*-1312*t*
  multigated acquisition (MUGA) radionuclide, 672, 673*t*-677*t*
  pulmonary, 469*t*-471*t*
  renal arteriogram, 1025*t*-1030*t*, 1027*f*
Angioma, 403*b*, 597*b*-598*b*
Angiomax (bivalirudin), 715*b*-716*b*, 820*b*
Angiopathy, **1147-1148**
Angioplasty
  balloon, 717
  patch graft, 806
  transluminal, 1353
Angiotensin-converting enzyme inhibitors
  for chronic stable angina and ACS, 715*b*-716*b*, 716-717
  for heart failure, 745*b*, 747
  for hypertension, 690, 691*b*-694*b*
Angiotensin-receptor blockers
  for chronic stable angina and ACS, 715*b*-716*b*, 716-717
  for heart failure, 745*b*, 747
  for hypertension, 690, 691*b*-694*b*
Angle of Louis, 453-454, 667
Animal bites, **1641-1642**, 1642
Animal-assisted therapy, 82*b*
Anions, 271, 272*b*, 272*f*
Anismus, 936
Anisocoria, 357*b*, 358, 1308*b*-1309*b*
Ankle arthroplasty, 1492
Ankle-brachial index, 805, 805*b*
Ankylosing spondylitis, 1536*b*, **1536-1537**, 1536*f*
Ankylosis, 1456*b*
Annuloplasty, 794
Annulus fibrosus, 1504-1505
Anorectal abscess, **970**, 970*f*
Anorectal problems, **968-971**
Anorexia
  in cancer, 251*b*-252*b*, 254-255
  at end of life, 140*b*-141*b*
  in nausea and vomiting, 894
Anorexia nervosa, **871-872**
Anorexins, 877*b*
Anoro Ellipta (umeclidinium/vilanterol), 548*b*-549*b*
Anosmia, 1306
Anosognosia, 1308*b*-1309*b*
Anovulation, 1189, 1246
Antacids
  for GERD, 902, 903*b*
  for pancreatitis, 1001*b*
  for peptic ulcers, 903*b*, 914
Antalgic gait, 1456*b*
Antegrade pyelography, 1025*t*-1030*t*
Anterior cord syndrome, 1422*b*
Anterior cruciate ligament tear, 1463*b*, **1467**, 1468, 1468*f*
Anterior pituitary gland, 1104*b*, **1105**
Anterior pituitary gland disorders, **1156-1159**
Anthrax Vaccine Adsorbed, 1645
Anthropometric measurements, 859
Antibiotic-resistant infection, 216, 217*b*
Antibiotics, 169*b*
  antitumor, 247*b*
  for arthritis, 1521*b*-1522*b*, 1529
  for burns, 441-442
  computer monitoring of, 1075*b*
  computer-based timing for administration of, 311*b*
  for dermatologic problems, 420-421
  empiric, 501
  for endocarditis, 783*b*
  for IBD, 947*b*
  nephrotoxic agents, 1020*b*
  for peptic ulcers, 913-914
  preoperative, 311, 311*b*
  resistant organisms, 216, 216*b*
  that cause photosensitivity, 408*b*
  for UTIs, 1036, 1036*b*
Antibodies
  HIV-antibody/antigen testing, 222*b*
  monoclonal, **209-210**, 211*b*
  panel of reactive antibodies (PRA), **208**
  polyclonal, **210**, 211*b*
Antibradycardia pacing, 772-773
Anticancer agents, 664*b*
Anticholinergics
  for asthma and COPD, 548*b*-549*b*, 551
  for multiple sclerosis, 1385*b*, 1386
  for nausea and vomiting, 895*b*
  for Parkinson's disease, 1390, 1391*b*
  preoperative, 311*b*
  for voiding dysfunction, 1059*b*
Anticipatory grief, 133
Anticoagulant therapy, 591
  for angina and ACS, 715*b*-716*b*
  for atrial fibrillation, 766*b*
  for burns, 441*b*
  drug alert, 823*b*
  for heart failure, 745*b*
  nursing interventions for patients on, 823*b*
  patient & caregiver teaching for, 824*b*
Anticoagulant therapy *(Continued)*
  safety alert, 1480*b*
  for VTE, 819, 820*b*, 821
Anticyclic-citrullinated peptide, 1457*t*-1459*t*
Antidepressants
  atypical, 1408*b*, 1409
  for burns, 441*b*
  for insomnia, 94
  for pain, 116*b*, 117
  that cause photosensitivity, 408*b*
Antidiabetics, preoperative, 311*b*
Antidiarrheal drugs, 931-932, 931*b*
Antidiuretic hormone, 1104*b*, 1105-1106, 1106*f*, 1159-1160
  regulation of water balance by, 274-275
  syndrome of inappropriate antidiuretic hormone, **1160**
Anti-DNA antibody, 1457*t*-1459*t*, 1659*b*
Antidysrhythmics, 771*b*
  for ACS, 725-726
  for heart failure, 745*b*
  that cause photosensitivity, 408*b*
Antiemetics
  for anesthesia, 326*b*
  preoperative, 311*b*
Anti-factor Xa, 821*b*
Antifungals, 408*b*
Antigens, **191**
  oncofetal, 239-240
  tumor-associated, 238-239, 239*f*
Antihemophilic factor, 592*b*
Antihistamines. *See also* Histamine (H_2)-receptor antagonists
  for allergic disorders, 202
  for dermatologic problems, 421
  drug alert, 478*b*
  for inflammation, 165
  for insomnia, 94-95, 94*b*
  for nausea and vomiting, 895*b*
  for Parkinson's disease, 1390, 1391*b*
  for rhinitis and sinusitis, 479*b*-480*b*
  that cause photosensitivity, 408*b*
Antihypertensive drugs, 689-693, 691*b*-693*b*
  combination therapy, 694*b*
  methods of action of, 690*f*
  patient and caregiver teaching related to, 690-693
  recommendations for, 689
  sites of action of, 690*f*
Anti-IgE, 548*b*-549*b*, 549
Anti-incontinence devices, 1057*b*
Antiinflammatory drugs
  for asthma, 546*b*, 547-549
  mechanism of action, 164, 164*b*
Anti-interleukin 5, 548*b*-549*b*, 549
Antimalarials, 1521*b*-1522*b*, 1528
Antimetabolites, 247*b*
Anti-mullerian hormone, 1198*t*-1201*t*
Antimuscarinics, 895*b*
Antinuclear antibody, 1457*t*-1459*t*, 1659*b*
Antiphospholipid syndrome, 1538
Antiplatelet therapy, **710**, 715*b*-716*b*, 805*b*
Antiproliferative drugs, 211*b*
Antipruritic drugs, 202
Antipsychotics
  for behavioral problems, 1408*b*, 1409
  cardiovascular effects of, 664*b*
  that cause photosensitivity, 408*b*
Antipyretic drugs, 164-165, 164*b*
Antireflux surgery, 902-903
Antiretroviral therapy, 219, 223
  drug interactions, 223*b*
  for HIV, 227-228
  patient & caregiver teaching for, 228*b*-229*b*
  side effects of, 230

Antiseizure drugs, **1377-1379**
drug alert, 1378*b*
for pain, 116*b*, 117
Antispasmodics, 1001*b*
Antitachycardia pacing, 772-773
Antithrombin, 601*t*
Antithrombotic therapy, 766*b*
Antithymocyte globulin
horse (Atgam), 209-210, 211*b*
rabbit (Thymoglobulin, ATG), 209-210, 211*b*
Antithyroid drugs, 1165-1166
Antitumor antibiotics, 247*b*
Antiulcer agents, 903*b*
Antivert (meclizine), 895*b*
Antiviral protein, 194, 195*f*
Antivirals, 981*b*
Anuria, 1025*b*, 1071
Anus
abnormalities, 846*b*-847*b*
normal, 846*b*, 1196*b*
in older adults, 840*b*
physical examination of, 845, 1195, 1196*b*
Anxiety
in acute coronary syndrome, 727-728, 728*b*
in burn patients, 448*b*
in critical care patients, 1556
at end of life, 138
preoperative, 302-303, 303*b*
in respiratory failure, 1618-1619
Anzemet (dolasetron), 326*b*, 895*b*
Aortic aneurysms, **810-816**, 810*f*
acute care for, 813-814
ambulatory care for, 814
classification of, 810
clinical manifestations of, 810-811
complications of, 811
diagnostic studies, 811
etiology and pathophysiology of, 810
genetics, 810
health promotion for, 813
interprofessional care for, 811-812
nursing management of, 812-814
surgical therapy for, 811-812, 812*f*
Aortic dissection, **814-816**, 814*f*
interprofessional care for, 815-816, 815*b*
nursing management of, **816**
Aortic valve regurgitation, 791*b*, **792-793**
Aortic valve stenosis, 791*b*, **792**
Aphasia, 1308*b*-1309*b*, 1345
expressive, 1351
global, 1351, 1351*b*
guidelines for communicating with patients with, 1361*b*
receptive, 1351
in stroke, 1351
types of, 1351*b*
Apheresis, **205**
Aphthous stomatitis, 897*b*
Apical pulse, 667, 668*b*
Apixaban (Eliquis), 820*b*
Aplastic anemia, **614**
causes of, 614*b*
laboratory data, 610*b*
Aplastic crisis, 617
Apneustic breathing, 1324*f*
Apocrine sweat glands, 396
Apolipoprotein E (ApoE), 1402
Apomorphine (Apokyn), 1391*b*
for Parkinson's disease, 1390-1391
Apoptosis, 235, 637
Appearance, general, 1304
Appendectomy, 840*b*
Appendicitis, **942**, 942*f*
Appetite, 834
Appetite-suppressing drugs, 884
Approach magnification, 369
Apps (applications)
patient teaching with, 1141*b*
translation apps, 31*b*
Apraclonidine (lopidine), 381*b*
Apraxia, 990, 1308*b*-1309*b*
Aprepitant (Emend), 895*b*
Aquapheresis, 744-745
Aqueous humor, 351
Arab Americans, 25
Arachidonic acid, 112*f*
Aranesp (darbepoetin alfa), 195*b*
Arava (leflunomide), 1521*b*-1522*b*, 1528
Arbovirus, 214*b*
Arcapta Neohaler (indacaterol), 548*b*-549*b*
Arcus senilis, 353*b*, 353*f*
ARDSNet (Acute Respiratory Distress Syndrome Clinical Network) protocol, 1623
Areola, 1187-1188
Arformoterol (Brovana), 548*b*-549*b*
Arginine vasopressin, 1106, 1159-1160
Argon laser trabeculoplasty, 380
Aricept (donepezil), 1390
Arimidex (anastrozole), 1217*b*
Arixtra (fondaparinux), 820*b*
Arm demi-span, 860-861
Arnuity Ellipta (fluticasone), 548*b*-549*b*
Aromasin (exemestane), 1217*b*
Aromatase inhibitors, 259*b*, 1217-1218, 1217*b*
Aromatherapy, 82*b*
Art therapy, 82*b*
Arterial blood gases, 289-290, **456**, 469*t*-471*t*
analysis of, 291*b*
normal exchange, 1609, 1610*f*
normal values, 290*b*, 457*b*
reference values, 1655*b*-1658*b*
in shock, 1590*t*
Arterial blood pressure, 662
Arterial blood pressure monitoring, **1561-1562**, 1562*f*
complications of, 1562
mean arterial pressure (MAP), 662
measurements, 662, 1561-1562
Arterial bruits, 667, 668*b*
Arterial oxygen saturation of hemoglobin (SpO_2), 457, 458*b*
noninvasive monitoring, 1565-1566
normal range, 1559*b*
Arterial pressure, 1562-1563
Arterial pressure-based cardiac output (APCO) monitoring, 1562-1563, 1562*f*
Arterial ulcers, 668*b*
Arteries and arterioles, **661**, 661*f*
of brain, 1299-1300, 1300*f*
cerebral, 1346*f*
palpation of, 666, 666*f*
Arteriography, peripheral, 673*t*-677*t*
Arteriovenous fistulas, 1087-1088, 1088*b*, 1088*f*
Arteriovenous grafts, 1088, 1088*b*, 1088*f*
Arteriovenous malformations, 1309*f*, 1336*b*
Arthralgia, 597*b*-598*b*, 783
Arthritis, **1517-1536**
cultural & ethnic health disparities, 1525*b*
drug therapy for, 1521*b*-1522*b*
impact of, 61*b*
in older adults, 1532
osteoarthritis, **1517-1523**, 1526*b*
psoriatic, **1537**
reactive, **1537-1538**
rheumatoid, **1525-1530**, 1526*b*
septic, **1535-1536**
sleep disturbances during, 92*b*
Arthritis Foundation, 1524
Arthritis mutilans, 1537
Arthrocentesis, 1457*t*-1459*t*, 1535
Arthrodesis, **1492**
Arthrofibrosis, 1466-1467
Arthropathy
seronegative, 1536
spondyloarthropathies, **1536-1549**
Arthroplasty, **1491-1492**
ankle, 1492
elbow and shoulder, 1491-1492
finger joint, 1491
hip, 1491, 1493*b*
knee, 1491
shoulder, 1491-1492
Arthroscopy, 1457*t*-1459*t*, 1460*f*
Artificial airways, **1569-1573**
Artificial discs, 1506, 1506*f*
Artificial heart, implantable, 1569
Artificial kidney, wearable, **1092**
Artificial skin, **445**
Aschoff's bodies, 788
Ascites, 846*b*-847*b*, 978, **988-990**, 989*f*
factors involved in, 988, 988*b*
interprofessional care for, 991
pathophysiology of, 988, 989*f*
Ascorbic acid. *See* Vitamin C
Asepsis, 316*f*, 320*b*, **320**, 320*f*
Ashworth scales, 1434
Asian Americans, 19
arthritis and connective tissue disorders in, 1525*b*
cross-cultural communication, 25-26
cultural characteristics of, 22*b*, 24
integumentary problems in, 410*b*
lung cancer in, 514*b*
older adults, 63
tuberculosis in, 28
Ask Me 3 (National Patient Safety Foundation), 50-51
Asmanex Twisthaler (budesonide mometasone), 548*b*-549*b*
Aspartate aminotransferase, 852*t*, 1655*b*-1658*b*
Aspergillus fumigatus, 215*b*
Asphyxiation, **430**
Aspiration
with ET tubes, 1573
postoperative, 333*b*, 334
in tube feedings, 866
Aspiration pneumonia, 500, **501-502**
Aspirin, 111-112, 111*b*
for arthritis, 1520-1523, 1521*b*-1522*b*, 1529
for atrial fibrillation, 766*b*
for inflammation, 164, 164*b*
for ischemic stroke, 1355
mechanism of action, 715*b*-716*b*
overdose, 1643*b*
for peripheral arterial disease, 805*b*
for stroke prevention, 1353
Assault
battery, 1644
sexual, **1263-1265**
Assessment, 5, 6*f*, 34
on admission to clinical unit, 345*b*
approaches for, 42-44
behavioral, 1304
comprehensive, 40, 44*b*
cultural, 29*b*, 30
culturally competent, 36
emergency, 40, 44*b*
focused, 40-42, 44*b*, 1455
head-to-toe, 1632-1634, 1633*b*
in older adults, 42*b*, 64*b*, 69-70
of pain, 107-110
pain assessment, 108*b*
in patient teaching, 51-53, 51*b*
secondary survey, 1632-1634, 1633*b*
SPICES tool, 70, 70*f*
spiritual, 134*b*
teamwork and collaboration in, 36*b*
types of, 40-44, 44*b*

Assignment, 11-12
Assist-control ventilation, 1575-1576, 1576*b*
Assisted mandatory ventilation, 1576*b*
Assisted reproductive technology (ART), 1243
Assisted suicide
  physician-assisted suicide, 136-137
  requests for, 125
Assistive devices
  for ambulation, 1477-1478
  for eating, 1361, 1361*f*
  for hearing loss and deafness, 389-391
  listening devices, 391
  for older adults, 72
Association of periOperative Registered Nurses (AORN), 5
Astelin (azelastine), 479*b*-480*b*
Astereognosis, 1308*b*-1309*b*
Asterixis, 990
Asthma, 198-199, 538, **539-553**
  acute care for, 554
  acute exacerbations, 544*b*, 545-547, 546*b*
  allergic, 540, 541*f*
  ambulatory care for, 554-557
  chest examination findings in, 468*b*
  classification of, 542-543, 542*b*
  clinical features of, 543*b*
  clinical manifestations of, 542
  complications of, 543
  control of, 544*b*
  and COPD, 559
  cough variant, 542
  cultural & ethnic health disparities in, 539*b*
  diagnostic studies in, 543-544, 543*b*
  drug therapy for, 545*f*, 546*b*, 547-553, 548*b*-549*b*
  early-phase response, 540
  exercise-induced, 539
  factors causing obstruction in, 540, 541*f*
  gender differences in, 539*b*
  genetics of, 539
  health promotion for, 554
  home monitoring, 551*b*
  images useful for, 85*b*
  immune response, 539
  intermittent, 544, 544*b*
  interprofessional care for, 544-547, 544*b*
  nursing assessment in, 553, 553*b*
  nursing diagnoses related to, 553
  nursing management of, **553-557**
  occupational, 540
  pathophysiology of, 540-542, 541*f*
  patient & caregiver teaching for, 552-553, 557*b*
  persistent, 544, 544*b*
  psychologic factors, 540
  risk factors for, 539-540
  sleep disturbances during, 92*b*
  triggers for attacks, 539-540, 539*b*
Asthma action plans, 554-555, 555*f*
Asthma Control Test (ACT), 544
Asthma exacerbation, 468*b*
Asthma triad, 540
Asthma-COPD overlap syndrome, 559
Astigmatism, 351, 368
Astrocytes, 1294-1295
Astrocytoma, 1333*b*
Asymmetric septal hypertrophy, 798
Asystole, 765, **770-771**
Atacand (candesartan), 691*b*-693*b*
Ataque de nervios, 29*b*
Ataxia, 597*b*-598*b*, 1308*b*-1309*b*
Ataxic gait, 1456*b*
Atelectasis, 455, 455*f*, 503, **528**, 1610
  chest examination findings in, 468*b*
  postoperative, 333*b*, 334, 335*f*
Atenolol (Tenormin), 691*b*-693*b*, 715*b*-716*b*
Atezolizumab (Tecentriq), 1037-1038
Atgam (horse antithymocyte globulin), 209-210, 211*b*
Atherectomy, 806
Atherosclerosis, 702-703, 703*f*
Athetosis, 1306, 1417
Ativan (lorazepam), 326*b*, 1378
Atopic dermatitis, 199, 199*f*, 418*b*
Atopic reactions, 198-199
Atopy, 539, 543
Atorvastatin (Lipitor), 711*b*
Atracurium, 326*b*
Atrial fibrillation, 764*b*, 766-767, 766*b*
Atrial flutter, 764*b*, 765-766, 765*f*
Atrial gallop, 669
Atrial natriuretic peptide, 275, 670
Atrioventricular block, 767*f*
  first-degree, 764*b*, **767-768**, 767*f*
  second-degree, 764*b*, 767*f*
    type I, **768**
    type II, **768**
  third-degree, 764*b*, 767*f*, 768
Atrium Medical Corporation, 523
Atrophy
  in insulin therapy, 1129
  muscle, 1456*b*, 1478*b*
  skin, 402*b*
Atrovent (ipratropium), 479*b*-480*b*, 548*b*-549*b*
Attitude(s), 21, 78
  toward aging, 63
Audiometry, **364**, 365*t*-366*t*
AUDIT (Alcohol Use Disorders Identification Test), 154, 154*b*
Auditory brainstem responses (ABRs), 365*t*-366*t*
Auditory evoked potentials (AEPs), 365*t*-366*t*
Auditory learning, 53
Auditory problems, 368*b*, **383-384**
Auditory system, **360-364**
  abnormalities, 365*b*
  assessment of, **361-364**, 364*b*
  diagnostic studies of, 364, 365*t*-366*t*
  health history, 362*b*
  normal, 364*b*
  in older adults, 361*b*, **361**
  physical examination of, 363-364
  structures and functions of, **360-361**
Augmentation mammoplasty, 1224
Augmented coughing, 1616, 1617*f*
Aura, 1370-1371
Auranofin (Ridaura), 1521*b*-1522*b*, 1529
Auricle (pinna), 360
Aurothioglucose, 1521*b*-1522*b*
Auscultation, **40**, 40*f*
  of chest, 466, 466*f*
  of pheripheral vascular system, 667
Auscultatory areas, 667, 667*f*
Auscultatory gap, 662
Auscultatory sounds, 466, 466*f*
Authorized agent controlled analgesia, 120
Autogenic drainage, 578
Autografts
  bone grafts, 1506
  for burns, 444
  cultured epithelial, **445**, 445*f*
  skin grafts, 427
Autoimmune diseases, 197, **205**
  examples, 205*b*
  genetic risks, 1453*b*
Autoimmune gastritis, 909
Autoimmune hepatitis, 985
Autoimmune liver diseases, 985
Autoimmune thyroiditis, 1163
Autoimmunity, 204-205
Autoinoculation, 1227
Autologous blood donation, 652
Autolytic debridement, 170*b*
Automated peritoneal dialysis, 1086, 1086*f*
Automatic external defibrillators (AEDs), 771-772, 772*f*, 1650, 1652*f*
  basic life support with, 1650-1651, 1651*b*
Automatic tube compensation (ATC), 1577
Automaticity, 760
Autonomic dysreflexia, 1431
Autonomic hyperreflexia, 1431, 1431*b*
Autonomic nervous system
  cardiovascular regulation by, 661
  structures and functions of, 1294, **1299**
Autonomic neuropathy, 1150
Auto-PEEP, 1577
Autoregulation, 687
Autosomal disorders, 181
Autosomal dominant disorders, 181, 181*b*
Autosomal recessive disorders, 181-182, 181*b*
Autosomes, 179*b*
Autosplenectomy, 617
Autotransfusion, 652, **652**
Avandia (rosiglitazone), 1131*b*
Avapro (irbesartan), 691*b*-693*b*
Avelox (moxifloxacin), 509*b*
Avodart (dutasteride), 1059*b*
Avonex (β-interferon), 195*b*
Avulsion, 1467, 1468*f*
Awakening and Breathing Trial Coordination, Daily Delirium Monitoring and Management, and Early Exercise and Mobility (ABCDE) bundle, 1582
Axid (nizatidine), 903*b*
Axillary lymph node dissection, 1212
Axillary lymph nodes, 1211-1212, 1212*f*, 1214
Axons, 1294
Azathioprine (Imuran)
  for arthritis, 1521*b*-1522*b*, 1529
  for immunosuppressive therapy, 209, 211*b*
Azelastine (Astelin), 479*b*-480*b*
Azilect (rasagiline), 1390, 1391*b*
Azilsartan (Edarbi), 691*b*-693*b*
Azopt (brinzolamide), 381*b*
Azotemia, 1069
Azulfidine (sulfasalazine), 947, 1521*b*-1522*b*, 1528

B

B cell depleting agents, 1521*b*-1522*b*
B cells, **192**, 193*f*, 239
Baby boomers, 55*b*
Bacille-Calmette-Guérin vaccine, 510
Back pain, 1502-1510
Baclofen, 116*b*, 1385*b*
Bacteremia, 503
Bacteria
  antibiotic-resistant organisms, 216, 216*b*
  disease-causing, 213-214, 214*b*
Bacterial food poisoning, 925, 925*b*
Bacterial infections
  conjunctivitis, 371
  infective endocarditis, **780-782**
  keratitis, 372
  skin infections, **413-415**, 414*b*
Bacterial meningitis, 1339-1340
  interprofessional care for, 1340, 1340*b*
  nursing diagnoses related to, 1340
  nursing management of, **1340-1341**
Bacterial peritonitis, 989-990
Bacterial vaginosis, 1250*b*
Bacteriuria, 1033
Bag-valve-mask, 1570
Balloon angioplasty, 717

Balloon kyphoplasty, 1485
Balloon tamponade, 991-992, 992*b*
Balloon valvuloplasty, **793-794**, 794*f*
Balloon-catheter systems, 1216
Balloons, intragastric, 885, 886*b*
Bandaging, residual limb, 1489, 1489*f*
Banding, 991
Baraclude (entecavir), 980
Barbiturates, 325*b*
Bariatric surgery, **885-887**
  ambulatory care considerations, 888-889
  home care considerations, 888-889
  postoperative care considerations, 888
  preoperative care considerations, 888
  procedures, 886*b*, 887*f*
  restrictive, 885
  for type 2 diabetes mellitus, 1137
Barium enema, 847*t*-850*t*
Barium swallow, 847*t*-850*t*
Baroreceptors, 661-662, 682, **683**
Barotrauma, 1578, 1623
Barrett's esophagus, 901
Basal body temperature assessment, 1198*t*-1201*t*
Basal cell carcinoma, **411**, 411*f*, 412*b*
Basal ganglia, 1297
Base deficit, 1590*t*
Basic life support, **1650-1652**, 1651*b*
Basiliximab (Simulect), 210
Basophils, 590, 1659*b*
Baths, 423
Battery (assault), 1644
Battle's sign, 1326, 1327*f*
B-cell lymphoma, 644*b*
Becker muscular dystrophy, 1501*b*-1502*b*, 1502
Beclomethasone (Beconase), 479*b*-480*b*
Beclomethasone (Qvar), 548*b*-549*b*
Bedaquiline (Sirturol), 509, 509*b*
Bedbugs, 416*b*
Bee stings, 416*b*
Beers Criteria (AGS), 73
Behavior modification
  for cardiovascular risk factors, 730*b*
  for weight loss, 883-884
Behavioral assessment, 1304
Behavioral changes
  in acute coronary syndrome, 728
  health behavior change, 47, 48*b*
  in heart failure, 743
Behavioral problems
  in Alzheimer's disease, 1411-1412
  drug therapy for, 1408*b*, 1409
Belatacept (Nulojix), 211*b*
Bell's palsy, **1439-1440**, 1439*f*
  clinical manifestations of, 1439*f*, 1440
  nursing management of, **1440**
Bell's phenomenon, 1440
Belviq (lorcaserin), 884*b*
Benazepril (Lotensin), 691*b*-693*b*, 745*b*
Bence-Jones protein, 603*t*, 645, 1661*b*
Benicar (olmesartan), 691*b*-693*b*
Benign paroxysmal positional vertigo, **386-387**
Benign prostatic hyperplasia, **1268-1273**, 1269*f*
  acute care for, 1274-1275
  ambulatory care for, 1275
  AUA symptom index, 1269, 1270*b*
  case study, 1289*b*
  clinical manifestations of, 1269
  complications of, 1269
  diagnostic studies for, 1269-1270
  drug therapy for, 1271
  etiology and pathophysiology of, 1268-1269
  health promotion for, 1273-1274
  herbal therapy for, 1271
  interprofessional care for, 1270-1273, 1270*b*
  invasive therapy (surgery) for, 1272-1273, 1272*b*
Benign prostatic hyperplasia *(Continued)*
  minimally invasive therapy for, 1271-1272, 1272*b*
  nursing assessment in, 1273*b*
  nursing diagnoses for, 1273
  nursing management of, **1273-1275**
  transurethral microwave thermotherapy for, 1271, 1272*b*
  treatment of, 1272*b*
Benzodiazepine-receptor–like agents, 94, 94*b*
Benzodiazepines
  for delirium, 1408*b*
  in general anesthesia, 326*b*
  for insomnia, 94, 94*b*
  overdose, **152**
  preoperative, 311*b*
Benztropine (Cogentin), 1391*b*
Bereavement, **133-134**
β-adrenergic agonists, for heart failure, 745*b*
β_2-adrenergic agonists
  for asthma, 548*b*-549*b*, 549-551
  long-acting, 548*b*-550*b*, 550
  for voiding dysfunction, 1059*b*
β-adrenergic antagonists (β-blockers), 771*b*
  for ACS, 715*b*-716*b*, 725
  for angina, 715*b*-716*b*, 717
  for glaucoma, 381*b*
  for heart failure, 745*b*, 748
  for hypertension, 691*b*-694*b*
  for hyperthyroidism, 1166
  preoperative, 311, 311*b*
β-amyloid, 1403
β-interferon, 1385*b*
Betapace (sotalol), 771*b*
Betaseron (β-interferon), 195*b*
Betaxolol (Betoptic), 381*b*, 691*b*-693*b*
Bethanechol (Urecholine), 903*b*, 1385*b*
Bias, 21
Bicalutamide (Casodex), 1280*b*
Bicarbonate, 1025*t*-1030*t*, 1655*b*-1658*b*
Biceps reflex, 1307, 1307*f*
Bicitra (sodium citrate), 903*b*
BiDil (isosorbide dinitrate/hydralazine), 745*b*, 748
Bigorexia, 871
Biguanides, 1130, 1131*b*, 1136*f*
Bile acid sequestrants, **710**, 711*b*
Bile reflux gastritis, 918
Bilevel positive airway pressure (BiPAP) ventilation, 97-98, 1577, 1617, 1618*f*
Biliary cirrhosis, **985**
Biliary colic, 1006
Biliary sludge, 999
Biliary tract, **838**
Biliary tract disorders, **1005-1010**
Biliary tract obstruction, 399*b*
Biliopancreatic diversion, 886*b*, 887*f*
Bilirubin, 837-838, 837*b*
  laboratory studies, 602*t*
  metabolism of, 837-838, 839*f*
  reference values, 1655*b*-1658*b*
  serum, 852*t*
  urinary, 852*t*, 1661*b*
Bilis or *colera*, 29*b*
Billroth I procedure, 917, 917*f*
Billroth II procedure, 917, 917*f*
Bimatoprost (Lumigan), 381*b*
Binge drinking, 148
Binge-eating disorder, 871
Biofeedback
  for fecal incontinence, 933
  for seizures, 1379
  for urinary incontinence, 1057*b*
Biologic aging, 63, 64*f*
Biologic response modifiers, 1521*b*-1522*b*, 1528-1529
Biologic therapy, 257, 1528
Biologic valves, 794-795
Biopsy, **243**
  core (core needle), 1206
  endoscopic, 243
  excisional, 243
  fine-needle aspiration (FNA), 1206
  hematologic, 602-604
  incisional, 243
  large-core, 243
  liver, 847*t*-850*t*, **851-852**
  lung, 469*t*-471*t*, **471-472**
  lymph node, 603*t*, 604
  neurologic pathology tests, 1310*t*-1312*t*
  percutaneous, 243
  punch, **422**, 422*f*
  renal, 1025*t*-1030*t*
  sentinel lymph node, 1212
  ultrasound-guided, 1198*t*-1201*t*
  vacuum-assisted, 1206
Bismuth subsalicylate (Pepto-Bismol), 931*b*
Bisoprolol (Zebeta), 691*b*-693*b*, 745*b*
Bisphosphonates, 1513, 1513*b*
Bites, **1640-1642**
  animal and human bites, 1641-1642, 1642*f*
  tick bites, 1641
Bivalirudin (Angiomax), 715*b*-716*b*, 820*b*
Biventricular assist device, 1568, 1568*f*
Biventricular failure, 738-739
Biventricular pacing, 774
Black cohosh, 1249*b*
Black light test (Wood's lamp), 405*t*
Black lung, 512-513
Blacks. *See* African Americans
Bladder
  neurogenic, 1423
    interprofessional care for, 1433*b*
    in spinal cord injury, **1432-1433**
    types of, 1432*b*
  orthotopic reconstruction of, 1065
  urinary, **1018-1019**
    cystoscopic examination of, 1025*t*-1030*t*, 1028*f*
    male, 1019*f*
    in older adults, 1020*b*
Bladder cancer, **1053-1054**, 1054*f*
  interprofessional care for, 1054, 1054*b*
  nursing and interprofessional management of, **1054-1055**
Bladder dysfunction, **1055-1060**, 1308*b*-1309*b*
Bladder irrigation, 1274, 1274*b*
Bladder management, 1430, 1433
Bladder neck support prostheses, 1057*b*
Bladder outlet obstruction, 1044, 1060
Bladder retraining, 1057*b*, 1360
Blastomyces dermatidis, 215*b*
Blebs, 444
Bleeding. *See also* Hemorrhage
  abnormal uterine bleeding, **1246-1247**
  in chronic kidney disease, 1078
  intermenstrual, 1246
  in peritoneal dialysis, 1087
  upper gastrointestinal, **921-923**
Bleeding varices, 994-995
Blepharitis, 357*b*, 370-371
Blindness, 358, 368
Blom-Singer voice prosthesis, 493, 493*f*
Blood, 587-590
  components of, 587-588, 589*f*
  contact with, 219
  functions of, 587, 588*b*
  hypercoagulability of, 817
  typing, **600**, 601*b*
  whole blood chemistries, 1655*b*-1658*b*
Blood bank personnel, 649*b*
Blood cells, 587-590, 588*f*
Blood coagulation tests, 821*b*

Blood component therapy, 647-652, 648*b*. *See also* Blood transfusions
administration procedure, 648-650
compatibilities for transfusions, 647, 649*b*
Blood cultures, 1590*t*
Blood flow, 658, 659*f*
Blood gases, **289-290**
arterial, 289-290, **456**, 469*t*-471*t*
analysis of, 291*b*
normal values, 457*b*
reference values, 1655*b*-1658*b*
in shock, 1590*t*
mixed venous, 456-457
normal values, 290*b*
reference values, 1655*b*-1658*b*
venous
normal values, 457*b*
reference values, 1655*b*-1658*b*
Blood glucose
drugs affecting, 1132
herbs and supplements that may affect, 1141*b*
Blood glucose monitoring, **1135-1137**, 1135*f*
instructions for patients & caregivers, 1136*b*, 1141*b*-1142*b*
self-monitoring, 1135
Blood groups, 600, 601*b*
Blood loss
acute, 610*b*, **614-615**
chronic, 610*b*, **615**
in hemodialysis, 1091
Blood pressure, **662**
alterations, 597*b*-598*b*
arterial, 662
classification of, 705-706
diastolic, 662
exercise for, 1142*b*
mean arterial pressure (MAP), 662, 699
regulation of, 681-683, 682*f*, 683*b*
segmental, 804-805
systolic, 662
Blood pressure monitoring
ambulatory, 687-688
home-based, 694*b*, **696-697**
informatics in, 697*b*
invasive
optimally damped system, 1561, 1561*f*
principles of, 1560-1561
steps for obtaining measurements, 1561*b*
system components, 1560, 1560*f*
types of, 1561-1565
zero reference stopcock positioning, 1561*b*
measurement, 662, **694-696**, 695*b*-696*b*
Blood products. *See also* Blood transfusions
for blood component therapy, 648*b*
contact with, 219
for shock, 1597*b*
Blood smear, 602*t*
Blood studies, 469*t*-471*t*, **601-602**, 602*t*
cardiovascular, 669-671, 673*t*-677*t*
communicating test results, 782*b*
gastrointestinal, 847*t*-850*t*
liver function studies, **852**, 852*t*
urinary, 1025*t*-1030*t*
Blood transfusion reactions, 650-652
acute, 650*b*-651*b*, **652**
delayed, 651*b*, 652
hemolytic, 199
massive, 650*b*-651*b*
Blood transfusions, 648. *See also* Blood component therapy
autotransfusion, 652
blood component compatibilities for, 647, 649*b*
safety alert, 648*b*
teamwork & collaboration for, 649*b*
Blood urea nitrogen (BUN), 1025*t*-1030*t*
reference values, 1655*b*-1658*b*
in shock, 1590*t*
Blood vessels, 661, **661**
Blood-brain barrier, 1294-1295, **1299-1300**
Blue toe syndrome, 811
Blunt trauma
abdominal, 941, 942*b*
chest, 519, 519*b*
renal, 1050
Blurred vision, 357*b*, 597*b*-598*b*
Board of Nursing, 1416*b*
Bobath method, 1364
Body fluid compartments, 271
Body image, 303
Body jacket brace, 1472
Body mass index (BMI), 861, **874**, 875*f*
Body shape, 875, 876*b*
Body water, 270, 271*f*. *See also* Fluid and electrolyte balance
Body weight. *See* Weight
Bone(s), **1446-1448**
cancellous, 1447
electrical stimulation of, **1474**
enlargement of, 1113*b*-1114*b*
flat, 1447-1448
functions of, 1446
irregular, 1447-1448
long, 1447
short, 1447
structure of, 1446-1447, 1447*f*
gross, 1447
microscopic, 1446-1447
types of, 1447-1448
Bone cancer
metastatic, **1501**
nursing management of, **1501**
Bone diseases
CKD mineral and bone disorder, **1078-1079**, 1079*f*, 1081
metabolic, **1510-1514**
Paget's disease of bone, 1514*b*, **1514**
Bone marrow, **587**
Bone marrow examination, 602-604, 603*t*, 604*f*
Bone marrow suppression, 250-253
Bone marrow transplantation, 259
Bone mineral density tests, 1457*t*-1459*t*
Bone pain, 597*b*-598*b*
Bone remodeling, 1447, 1470
Bone scans, 603*t*, 1457*t*-1459*t*
Bone tumors, 1500-1502
malignant, **1500-1501**
metastatic, 1514*b*-1515*b*
types of, 1500*b*
Boniva (ibandronate), 1513
Borborygmi, 843-844, 846*b*-847*b*, 917-918
Bosentan (Tracleer), 532*b*
Botox (botulinum toxin A), 1057, 1372
Botulism, 925*b*, **1442**
Bouchard's nodes, 1518
Boutonnière deformity, 1456*b*, 1527, 1527*f*
Bowel management
patterns at end of life, 140*b*-141*b*
in spinal cord injury, 1430, 1433*b*
Bowel obstruction, 950, 951*b*, 951*f*
Bowel sounds, absent, 846*b*-847*b*
Bowlegs, 1456*b*
Boxer's fracture, 1642
Brachioradialis reflex, 1307
Brachytherapy, **250**
balloon-catheter system, 1216
for breast cancer, 1216
high-dose, 1216, 1216*f*
Brachytherapy *(Continued)*
multicatheter method, 1216
for prostate cancer, 1279, 1279*f*
Braden Scale, 172
Bradycardia, 763, 763*f*
Bradykinesia, 1387, 1389
Brain. *See also under* Cerebral
components of, 1296, 1314, 1315*f*
functional areas of, 1333, 1334*f*
inflammatory conditions of, **1338-1342**
normal images of, 1309*f*
in older adults, 361*b*
structures and functions of, **1296-1298**
Brain abscesses, 1336*b*, **1338-1339**, 1339*b*
Brain aneurysms, 1336*b*
Brain attack, 1345
Brain death, 131, 1331*b*
Brain fag, 29*b*
Brain natriuretic peptide, 670, 673*t*-677*t*, 1655*b*-1658*b*
Brain stents, 1353-1354, 1354*f*
Brain tumors, 1333-1335
chemotherapy for, 1335
clinical manifestations of, 1333, 1334*b*
complications of, 1333
cultural & ethnic health disparities, 1333*b*
diagnostic studies for, 1334
interprofessional care for, 1334-1335
nursing diagnoses related to, 1335
nursing management of, **1335-1336**
radiation therapy for, 1335
surgical therapy for, 1334-1335, 1336*b*
targeted therapy for, 1335
types of, 1333, 1333*b*
Brainstem, 1297
Bravelle (urofollitropin), 1243*b*
BRCA genes, 1209-1210
Breakthrough pain, 108
Breast(s)
abnormalities, 1197*b*
age-related changes in, 1208
female, 1187-1188, 1196*b*
fibrocystic changes in, 1206*b*, **1207**, 1207*f*
lactating, 1187-1188, 1188*f*
lactational abscess in, **1207**
physical examination of, 1195-1196
Breast augmentation, **1224**
Breast cancer, 1208-1224
acute care for, 1219-1221
ambulatory care for, 1221-1222
brachytherapy for, 1216
case study, 1225*b*
chemotherapy for, 1216-1217
classification of, 1211*b*
clinical manifestations of, 1211
complications of, 1211
cultural & ethnic health disparities, 1218*b*
culturally competent care for, 1218
diagnostic studies for, 1211-1213
drug therapy for, 1216-1218, 1217*b*
etiology of, 1209
genetics of, 1192*b*, 1209-1210, 1210*b*
health promotion for, 1218-1219
hereditary breast and ovarian cancer (HBOC) syndrome, 1276
hormone therapy for, 1217-1218
immunotherapy for, 1217*b*, 1218
inflammatory, 1211
integrative therapies for, 1221*b*
interprofessional care for, 1213-1218, 1213*b*
metastasis of, 1211, 1212*b*
noninvasive, 1210
nursing assessment in, 1218, 1219*b*

Breast cancer *(Continued)*
nursing diagnoses related to, 1218
nursing management of, **1218-1222**
in older adults, 1222
palliative radiation therapy for, 1216
pathophysiology of, 1210
prophylactic oophorectomy and mastectomy for, 1210
psychosocial support for, 1220-1221
radiation therapy for, 1215-1216
recurrence of, 1211, 1212*b*
risk factors for, 1209, 1209*b*
risk factors for men, 1209-1210
screening guidelines, **1204-1205**
staging of, 1213, 1214*b*
surgery for, 1213-1215, 1214*f*, 1215*b*
targeted therapy for, 1217*b*, 1218
treatment of, 1220*b*
triple-negative, 1211
tumor size, 1212
types of, 1210-1211
Breast disorders, 1204-1226
assessment of, **1204-1206**
benign, 1206*b*, **1206-1208**
diagnostic studies of, **1205-1206**
in older adults, 1208
Breast implants and tissue expansion, 1215*b*, 1223, 1223*f*
Breast infections, 1206-1207
Breast pain
mastalgia, **1206**
phantom, 1215
Breast reconstruction, **1222-1224**, 1223*f*
indications for, 1223
tissue flap procedures, 1215*b*, 1223-1224
types of, 1223-1224
Breast reduction, **1224**
Breast self-examination, 1204-1205, 1205*f*
Breast-conserving surgery, 1213-1214, 1215*b*
Breath sounds
absent, 467*b*-468*b*
adventitious, 466
Breathing. *See also* Respiration
apneustic, 1324*f*
ataxic, 1324*f*
in cardiopulmonary resuscitation, 1651-1652
cluster, 1324*f*
in coma, 1324*f*
diaphragmatic (abdominal), 569
in increased ICP, 1324*b*
primary survey, 1630, 1631*b*-1632*b*
pursed-lip, 467*b*-468*b*, 554*b*, 569
relaxation, **83-84**
Breathing retraining or exercises, 568-569, 578
Breo Ellipta (fluticasone/vilanterol), 548*b*-549*b*
Breslow measurement, 412, 413*f*
Bretylium (Bretylol), 771*b*
Brevibloc (esmolol), 691*b*-693*b*, 771*b*
Brevital (methohexital), 325*b*
Brilinta (ticagrelor), 715*b*-716*b*
Brimonidine, 381*b*
Brinzolamide (Azopt), 381*b*
Bristol Stool Scale, 934
Broca's aphasia, 1351*b*
Broca's area, 1296
Bromocriptine (Cycloset), 1131*b*, 1390, 1390*b*-1391*b*
Brompheniramine, 479*b*-480*b*
Bronchial circulation, 455
Bronchial sounds, 466
Bronchiectasis, 538, 577, 577*f*, **580-581**
Bronchiolitis, 576-577
Bronchiolitis obliterans, 513, 534
Bronchitis
acute, **499-500**
chronic, 557
Bronchoalveolar lavage, 471
Bronchoconstriction, 454
Bronchoconstriction, reflex, 459
Bronchodilation, 454
Bronchodilators, 546*b*, 549-551
Bronchophony, 467*b*-468*b*
Bronchoscopes, fiberoptic, 467-471, 469*f*
Bronchoscopic laser therapy, 517
Bronchoscopic lung volume reduction surgery, 571
Bronchoscopy, **467-471**, 469*t*-471*t*, 526*b*
Bronchospasm
exercise-induced, 539
postoperative, 333*b*, 334-335
relief of, 1618
Bronchovesicualr sounds, 466
Brovana (arformoterol), 548*b*-549*b*
Brown-Séquard Syndrome, 1422*b*
Bruises easily, 1113*b*-1114*b*
Bruising. *See* Ecchymoses
Bruits, 667, 668*b*, 846*b*-847*b*
B-type natriuretic peptide, 275, 670, 673*t*-677*t*
Buck's traction, 1470, 1471*f*
Buddhism, 26*b*
Budesonide (Pulmicort Flexhaler), 547, 548*b*-549*b*
Budesonide (Rhinocort), 479*b*-480*b*
Budesonide ciclesonide (Alvesco), 548*b*-549*b*
Budesonide mometasone (Asmanex Twisthaler), 548*b*-549*b*
Budesonide/formoterol (Symbicort), 548*b*-549*b*
Buerger's disease (thromboangiitis obliterans), 399*b*, **809**
Buffalo hump, 1174
Buffers, **287**
Bulbourethral (Cowper's) glands, 1185
Bulimia nervosa, 872
Bullectomy, 571
Bull's eye rash, 1534, 1534*f*
Bullying, 730*b*
Bumetanide (Bumex), 691*b*-693*b*, 745*b*
BUN/creatinine ratio, 1025*t*-1030*t*
Bunion (hallux valgus), 1508, 1508*f*, 1509*b*, 1527*f*
Buprenorphine, 113*b*-114*b*, 114
Bupropion (Wellbutrin), 116*b*
Bupropion (Zyban), 147-148, 148*b*, 150*b*
Bupropion/naltrexone (Contrave), 884*b*
Burn centers, 432*b*
Burn shock, 434-436, 436*f*-437*f*
Burns, 429-451
airway management in, 438-439
burn center referral criteria for, 432*b*
care measures for, 441
case study, 449*b*
chemical, **429-430**
emergency management of, 436*b*
strategies to reduce injury, 430*b*
classification of injury, **431-433**, 432*b*
clinical manifestations of, 437, 442, 446
complications of, 437-438, 443, 446-447
definition of, 429
depth of, 431-432, 432*f*
drug therapy, 441-442, 441*b*
electrical, **431**, 431*f*
emergency management of, 435*b*
strategies to reduce injury, 430*b*
emergency care, **433-434**
emotional responses of patients, 448*b*
emotional/psychologic needs of patients and caregivers, **447-448**
excision and grafting, **444-445**
extent of, 432
fluid and electrolyte shifts in, 434-436, 436*f*-437*f*
fluid therapy for, 439
full-thickness, 432, 432*b*
Burns *(Continued)*
interprofessional care for, 438*b*
laboratory values, 442-443
location of, 433
Lund-Browder chart for, 432, 433*f*
lung injury associated with, 431*b*
management of, **434-448**
acute phase, **442-443**
emergent phase, **434-438**
rehabilitation phase, **446-447**
needs of nurses, **448**
nursing and interprofessional management of, **438-447**
nutritional therapy for, 441*b*, **442**, **446**
occupational therapy for, **446**
in older adults, 447
pain management in, 445-446
partial-thickness, 432, 432*b*
pathophysiology of, 434-437, 442, 446
physical therapy for, **446**
prehospital care for, **433-434**
risk factors for poor healing, 433
Rule of Nines for, 432, 433*f*
Sage Burn Diagram, 432
skin grafts for, 440, 440*b*, **444-445**, 444*f*
sources of injury, 430*b*
strategies to reduce injury, 430*b*
thermal, **429**
emergency management of, 434*b*
prehospital and emergency care for, 433
types of injury, 429-431, 430*f*
wound care, 439-440, 443-444
closed method, 440, 440*f*
open method, 440
Burr holes, 1337*b*
Bursae, 1450
Bursitis, 1468
Butorphanol (Stadol), 113*b*-114*b*, 114
Butterfly rash, 1538, 1539*f*
Butyrophenone, 895*b*
BVS 5000 Biventricular Support System, 754
Bydureon (exenatide extended-release), 1131*b*, 1132
Byetta (exenatide), 1131*b*-1132*b*, 1132
Bypass surgery
cardiopulmonary, 724-725
coronary artery, **724-725**, 724*f*
minimally invasive direct coronary artery bypass (MIDCAB), 725
off-pump coronary artery bypass graft (OPCAB), 725
peripheral artery, 806, 806*f*, 808*b*
robotic or totally endoscopic coronary artery bypass graft (TECAB), 725
Roux-en-Y gastric bypass, 885-887, 886*b*, 887*f*
Bystolic (nebivolol), 691*b*-693*b*

C

CAB, 433
Cachexia, cancer, 262
Caffeine, 96*b*, **153**
Calan (verapamil), 691*b*-693*b*, 715*b*-716*b*, 771*b*, 1059*b*
Calcaneus stress fracture, 1509*b*
Calcineurin inhibitors, **209**, 211*b*
Calcinosis cutis, 1545
Calcitonin, 1104*b*, **1107**
Calcium, 592*b*
blood values, 1025*t*-1030*t*, 1655*b*-1658*b*
in bone disease, 1457*t*-1459*t*
ionized, 1115*t*-1118*t*
measurement of, 1115*t*-1118*t*
sources of, 1513*b*
total, 1115*t*-1118*t*
urine values, 1661*b*
Calcium carbonate (Tums, Titralac), 903*b*

Calcium channel blockers, 771*b*
for chronic stable angina and ACS, 715*b*-716*b*, 717
for hypertension, 690, 691*b*-694*b*
for pulmonary hypertension, 532*b*
for voiding dysfunction, 1059*b*
Calcium gluconate, 1073*b*
Calcium glycerophosphate (Prelief), 1040
Calcium imbalances, **283-285**, 284*b*
Calcium oxalate stones, 1046*b*, 1047*f*
Calcium phosphate stones, 1046*b*
Calcium polyarbophil (Mitrolan), 931*b*
Calcium supplements
for menopausal symptoms, 1249
for osteoporosis, 1512
Calcium-scoring CT scans, 673*t*-677*t*, 678
Calculi, 1045
renal staghorn, 1045, 1046*f*
urinary tract, **1045-1048**
Callus, fracture, 1469
Calluses, 1509*b*
Calories (energy)
activities that affect expenditures, 1134*b*
estimation of requirements for, 854, 855*b*
high-calorie, high-protein diet, 863*b*
high-calorie diet, 1166
in parenteral nutrition, 869
Cambodian Americans, 29*b*
Campath (alemtuzumab), 210, 211*b*
***Campylobacter jejuni* infection**, 930*b*
Canagliflozin (Invokana), 1131*b*
Canal of Schlemm, 351
Canaliculi, 837
Cancer, 234-269
anal, **970-971**
associated with obesity, 879*f*, 880
biology of, 235-240
bladder, **1053-1054**, 1054*f*
bone
metastatic, **1501**
nursing management of, **1501**
breast, **1208-1224**
screening guidelines, **1204-1205**
cervical, **1256-1257**, 1256*f*
chemotherapy for, **245-248**
classification of, **240-241**, 240*b*-241*b*
cognitive effects of, 256
colorectal, 841*b*, **954-957**, 971*b*
combined modality therapy for, 243
complications of, **261-267**
control of, 244
coping with, 265*b*, **265-266**
cultural & ethnic health disparities, 267*b*
culturally competent care for, 267
cure of, 243-244
death rates, 234
development of, 236, 237*f*
diagnosis of, 242-243
diagnostic studies in, 242-243
early detection of, **241-243**, 242*b*
endometrial, **1257-1258**
esophageal, **905-906**
external ear malignancy, **384**
of female reproductive system, 1256*b*, **1256-1261**
nursing and interprofessional management of, **1259-1261**
radiation therapy for, 1261
gallbladder, 1010
gender differences in, 235*b*
gene therapy for, **261**
genetic links, 236-238
head and neck cancer, **491-493**
hematologic, 643*b*
Cancer *(Continued)*
hereditary breast and ovarian cancer (HBOC) syndrome, 1276
histologic grading of, 241
hormone therapy for, 259*b*, **259**
images useful for, 85*b*
immune system in, 238-240
immunotherapy for, **257-258**, 258*b*
impact of, 61*b*
incidence of, 234, 235*b*
infiltrative emergencies, 263*b*, 264
initiation of, 236
interprofessional care for, **243-261**
kidney, **1052-1053**
in kidney transplantation, 1096
laryngeal, 496*b*
latent, 238
liver, 986*b*, **996-997**
lung, **513-519**, 514*f*-515*f*, 535*b*
of male reproductive system, 1276*b*
management of symptoms, 248*b*
metabolic emergencies, 263*b*, 264
multimodality therapy for, 243
obstructive emergencies, 263*b*, 264
in older adults, 266
oral, **898-899**
ovarian, **1258-1259**
palliative care for, 244-245
pancreatic, 986*b*, **1004-1005**
of penis, **1284**
personalized medicine for, 244-245
prevention of, **241-243**, 242*b*, 245
progression of, 238
promotion of, 237-238
prostate, **1275-1281**
radiation therapy for, **248-250**
sleep disturbances during, 92*b*
staging of, 241
stomach, **919-920**
supportive care for, 245
surgery for, **245**, 245*f*
survivorship, **266-267**
testicular, 1284*f*, **1285**
thyroid, **1170-1171**
treatment goals, 243-244, 244*f*
vaginal, **1259**
vulvar, **1259**
warning signs of, 242*b*
Cancer cachexia, 262
Cancer pain, 264*b*, **264-265**
Cancer survivors, 267*b*
CancerCare, 267*b*
Cancer.Net, 267*b*
Candesartan (Atacand), 691*b*-693*b*
Candida albicans, 215*b*, 222*b*
Candidiasis, 222*b*, 418*b*
at end of life, 140*b*-141*b*
in mouth, 846*b*-847*b*
oral, 221, 221*f*, 897*b*
vulvovaginal, 1250, 1250*b*
Cangrelor (Kengreal), 715*b*-716*b*
Canker sores, 897*b*
Cannabinoids
for nausea and vomiting, 895*b*
for pain, 117-118
Cannabis use, **153**
Capillaries, **661**, 661*f*
fluid movement in, 273-274, 274*f*
Capillary fragility test, 601*t*
Capillary refill, 666-667
Capnography (end-tidal CO_2, $PetCO_2$) monitoring, 331, 469*t*-471*t*, 1571, 1614
Capreomycin (Capastat), 509*b*
Capsaicin
for arthritis, 1520-1523, 1521*b*-1522*b*
for pain, 116*b*, 118-119
Capsule endoscopy, 847*t*-850*t*, 851, 851*f*
Captopril, 691*b*-693*b*, 715*b*-716*b*, 745*b*, 747*b*
Carafate (sucralfate), 903*b*
Carbachol (Miostat, Isopto, Carbachol), 381*b*
Carbamazepine (Tegretol), 116*b*, 1377, 1378*b*
Carbapenem-resistant enterobacteriaceae (CRE), 216
Carbidopa, levodopa, and entacapone (Stalevo), 1390-1391
Carbidopa/levodopa, 1389-1390, 1390*b*-1391*b*
Carbohydrate counting, 1133-1134
Carbohydrates, 1133
Carbon dioxide (CO_2) monitoring, 457, 469*t*-471*t*, 1655*b*-1658*b*
Carbon dioxide (CO_2) narcosis, 565
Carbon monoxide poisoning, 1643*b*
Carbonic anhydrase inhibitors, 381*b*, 1001*b*
Carboxyhemoglobin, 430
Carbuncles, 414*b*
Carcinoembryonic antigen, 240, 1659*b*
Carcinogens, **237**, 238
chemical, 237
viral, 237
Carcinoma, 240-241
Carcinoma in situ, 241
Cardene (nicardipine), 715*b*-716*b*
Cardiac arrest, **1634-1635**, 1635*b*, 1650
Cardiac auscultatory areas, 667, 667*f*
Cardiac biomarkers, 669-670
in ACS, 721-722
after MI, 721-722, 722*f*
Cardiac blood pool scans, 672, 673*t*-677*t*
Cardiac catheterization, 673*t*-677*t*, **678-679**, 717-718, 729*b*
Cardiac cirrhosis, 986
Cardiac computed tomography, 673*t*-677*t*, **678**
Cardiac death, sudden, **733**, 771
Cardiac hypertrophy, 740, 741*f*
Cardiac index (CI), 660, **1559**
continuous CO (CCO)/continuous CI (CCI), 1562
normal, 1559*b*
Cardiac lesions, **788**
Cardiac muscle, 1448
Cardiac natriuretic peptide markers, **670**
Cardiac output (CO), 660, **1559**
in ARDS, 1625
arterial pressure-based, 1562-1563
continuous CO (CCO)/continuous CI (CCI), 1562
factors affecting, 660-661
normal, 1559*b*
in respiratory failure, 1619
Cardiac pacemakers, **773-775**
Cardiac parameters, 439
Cardiac rehabilitation, 707*b*, 730
Cardiac reserve, 661
Cardiac resynchronization therapy, 747*f*, **774**
Cardiac sinus node inhibitors, 745*b*, 748-749
Cardiac tamponade, 815
in cancer, 263*b*
emergency management of, 520*b*
in pericarditis, 785
Cardiac-specific troponin, 670, 673*t*-677*t*, 722
Cardiogenic shock, 1587-1589, 1588*b*
clinical presentation of, 1591*b*
drug therapy for, 1599*b*
interprofessional care for, 1598-1601, 1600*b*
after MI, 721
pathophysiology of, 1587, 1589*f*

Cardiomegaly, 797
Cardiomyocytes, 275
Cardiomyopathy, 796-799
causes of, 796, 796*b*
dilated, 796-797
genetic risk alert, 664*b*
hypertrophic, **798-799**
interprofessional care for, 797*b*
patient & caregiver teaching for, 800*b*
primary, 796
restrictive, **799**
secondary, 796
types of, 796, 797*b*
Cardiopulmonary bypass, 724-725
Cardiopulmonary resuscitation (CPR), 135-137, **1650-1652**, 1651*f*
hands-only, 1652
Cardiovascular disease
associated with obesity, 879, 879*f*
in chronic kidney disease, 1078
in kidney transplantation, 1096
monitoring for, 1148*b*
nursing diagnoses related to, 338
nursing management of, **337-338**
postoperative, **336-337**
risk factors for
behavioral interventions for, 730*b*
modification of, 696, 805
Cardiovascular magnetic resonance imaging (CMRI), **672-678**, 673*t*-677*t*
Cardiovascular system
abnormalities, 668*b*
aging and, 662-663
assessment of, **663-669**, 665*b*, 669*b*
physical examination, 666-669, 669*b*-670*b*
preoperative, 305, 307*b*
blood studies, 669-671, 673*t*-677*t*
case study, 663*b*, 666*b*, 669*b*, 679*b*
diagnostic studies, **669-679**, 673*t*-677*t*, 679*b*
at end of life, 132*b*
normal, 670*b*
nursing interventions for, 1359
in older adults, 662-663, 663*b*
regulation of, 661-662
structures and functions, **658-663**
Cardioversion
for atrial fibrillation, 772*b*
synchronized, 772
Carditis, 788
rheumatic, 789
Cardizem (diltiazem), 532*b*, 715*b*-716*b*, 771*b*, 1059*b*
Cardizem LA (diltiazem extended release), 691*b*-693*b*
Cardura (doxazosin), 691*b*-693*b*, 695*b*, 1059*b*
Care bundles, 1602
Caregiver stress, 50
Caregiver teaching, **46-59**. *See also* Patient and caregiver teaching
Caregivers, 49
in Alzheimer's disease, 1413-1414, 1413*f*
in burn care, 447-448
in critical care, 1557
family caregivers, **66**
needs assessment for, 49*b*
primary survey, 1631*b*, 1632
in shock, 1604
stressors on, 50*b*
support for, 49-50, 1413, 1413*f*
Caribbean and southern United States, 29*b*
Carina, 453-454
Carotene, 1655*b*-1658*b*
Carotenemia, 403*b*
Carotenosis, 403*b*
Carotid artery duplex scan, 1310*t*-1312*t*
Carotid artery rupture, 263*b*
Carpal tunnel syndrome, 1465-1466, 1466*f*
Carriers, 179*b*
Cartia XT (diltiazem), 532*b*
Cartilage, **1448**
elastic, 1448
enlargement of, 1113*b*-1114*b*
fibrous, 1448
hyaline, 1448
Carunculae myrtiformes, 1187
Carvedilol (Coreg)
for heart failure, 745*b*, 748, 748*b*
for hypertension, 691*b*-693*b*
mechanism of action, 715*b*-716*b*
Cascade disease pattern, 69
Case finding, 1238
Case management, 9
Casodex (bicalutamide), 1280*b*
Cast care, 1477, 1477*b*
Cast syndrome, 1472
Casts, 1471*b*, **1471-1473**, 1472*f*
hip spica, 1473
long arm, 1472, 1472*f*
for lower extremity injuries, 1472-1473
short arm, 1472, 1472*f*
for upper extremity injuries, 1472
for vertebral injuries, 1472
Cat bites, 1642
Cataflam (diclofenac K), 111*b*
Cataplexy, 98
Catapres (clonidine), 691*b*-693*b*, 699*b*
Cataract(s), 357*b*, **373-375**
acute care for, 375-376
ambulatory care for, 376
clinical manifestations of, 374
diagnostic studies in, 374
etiology and pathophysiology of, 374
interprofessional care for, 374-375, 374*b*
nonsurgical therapy for, 374
nursing diagnoses related to, 375
nursing management of, **375-376**
in older adults, 376
senile, 374
Cataract surgery, 374-375, 375*f*
nursing management of, 376
patient & caregiver teaching after, 376*b*
Catastrophic events, **327-329**
Catecholamines, 1102, 1107, 1661*b*
Catechol-*O*-methyltransferase inhibitors, 1391*b*
Cathartic colon syndrome, 934-935
Catheter ablation, **775**
Catheter site care, 870*b*
Catheter-associated urinary tract infections, 1034
prevention of, 1037, 1062*b*
Catheter-based procedures, 806
Catheterization
cardiac, 673*t*-677*t*, **678-679**, 717-718, 729*b*
intermittent, **1062-1063**
pulmonary artery, 1563*b*
suprapubic, 1062
urethral, **1061**, 1062*b*
urinary, **1060-1063**
Catheter-related infections, 870*b*
Catheters
central venous (CVCs), 294-295, 294*f*
centrally inserted, **294-295**, 294*f*
drainage from, 344*b*
fiberoptic, 1319
indwelling, 1061*b*-1062*b*
peripherally inserted central catheters (PICCs), **295**, 295*f*
placement for peritoneal dialysis, 1085-1086
pulmonary artery flow-directed, 1563-1564, 1563*f*
suprapubic, 1062
temporary vascular acess catheters for acute hemodialysis, 1088, 1089*f*
Catheters *(Continued)*
transhepatic biliary, 1008
ureteral, **1062**
urethral, **1061**, 1062*b*
urinary
construction of, **1061**
role of nursing personnel with, 1061*b*
types of, **1061-1063**, 1061*f*
Catholicism, 26*b*
Cations, 271, 272*b*, 272*f*
Cauda equina syndrome, 1422*b*, 1505
CD antigens (clusters of differentiation), 191
$CD4^+$ T cell (CD4 cells), 219
CD20 monoclonal antibody, 258*b*
Celecoxib (Celebrex), 111*b*, 1521*b*-1522*b*, 1523, 1529
Celiac disease, 966-967, 967*b*
Celiac Disease Foundation, 967
Celiac sprue, 966
Celiac Sprue Association, 967
Cell differentiation defects, 236
Cell phones, 889*b*
Cell proliferation, 235, 236*f*, 248, 248*b*
Cell proliferation defects, 235-236
CellCept (mycophenolate mofetil), 209, 211*b*, 1521*b*-1522*b*
Cell-mediated immunity, 196*b*, **196**
Cell-proliferative indices, 1213
Cellulitis, 172, 414*b*, 415*f*
Centers for Disease Control and Prevention (CDC), 878
Central cord syndrome, 1422*b*
Central cyanosis, 668*b*
Central herniation, 1318-1319
Central nervous system (CNS), 1294
divisions of, 1296, 1298*f*
structures and functions of, **1296-1298**
Central nervous system lymphoma, 222*b*, 1333*b*
Central neurogenic hyperventilation, 1324*f*
Central pain, 106*b*, 107
Central sensitization, 105, 105*f*
Central venous access devices (CVADs), 246, **294-296**
complications of, 296, 296*b*
indications for, 295*b*
nursing management of, **296-297**
removal of, 297
Central venous catheters (CVCs), 294-295, 294*f*
Central venous oxygen saturation ($ScvO_2$), 1564-1565, 1565*b*
Central venous pressure (CVP), 1564, 1565*f*
Centrally inserted catheters, **294-295**, 294*f*
Cerebellum, **1297-1298**
Cerebral aneurysms, 1336*b*
Cerebral angiography, 1309*f*, 1310*t*-1312*t*
Cerebral blood flow, 1315-1316
autoregulation of, 1315
factors affecting, 1316
regulation of, 1346
Cerebral circulation, **1299-1300**, 1300*f*, 1346, 1346*f*
Cerebral cortex
functional areas of, 1333, 1334*f*
stress response, 79
Cerebral edema, 1316-1317
causes of, 1317*b*
cytotoxic, 1317
interstitial, 1317
vasogenic, 1316
Cerebral herniation, 1316, 1317*f*
central, 1318-1319
tentorial, 1318-1319
uncal, 1318
Cerebral inflammatory conditions, 1338-1342, 1339*b*

Cerebral oxygenation monitoring, 1319-1322, 1321*f*
Cerebral perfusion pressure (CPP), 1315, 1315*b*
Cerebrospinal fluid, **1298**
analysis of, 1310*t*-1312*t*
drainage of, 1320-1321, 1321*f*
normal values, 1312*b*
reference values, 1662*b*
Cerebrovascular accident, 1345
Cerebrovascular disease, 686-687, 686*b*
Cerebrum, **1296-1297**, 1297*f*, 1298*b*
Certified perioperative nurse (CNOR), 317
Certolizumab (Cimzia), 1521*b*-1522*b*, 1529
Cerumen, impacted, 365*b*, **384**
Cervical cancer, **1256-1257**, 1256*f*
cultural & ethnic health disparities, 1256*b*
Pap test and, 1256*b*
staging and treatment of, 1257, 1257*b*
Cervical collars, 1630
Cervical cord injury, 1426*b*
Cervical disc disease, 1505
Cervical immobilization device, 1630
Cervical os, 1186*f*
Cervical polyps, **1255-1256**
Cervical spine injury, 1427*b*
Cervical spine stabilization, 1630, 1631*b*
Cervical traction, 1427, 1427*f*
Cervicitis, 1228, 1250, 1250*b*
Cervix, 1187
Cesamet (nabilone), 153, 895*b*
Cetirizine (Zyrtec), 479*b*-480*b*
Chalazion, 370
Chancres, 1235
Chantix (varenicline), 147-148, 148*b*, 150*b*
Charcot's foot, 1151
Charité artificial disc, 1506, 1506*f*
Chart review, 319
Cheilitis, 846*b*-847*b*
Cheilosis, 846*b*-847*b*
Chemical burns, **429-430**
emergency management of, 436*b*
prehospital and emergency care for, 433
strategies to reduce injury, 430*b*
Chemical carcinogens, 237
Chemical code, 136
Chemical hepatotoxicity, 984
Chemical pleurodesis, 528
Chemical pneumonitis, 513
Chemical restraints, 74
Chemical-induced liver diseases, **984**
Chemo brain, 251*b*-252*b*, 256
Chemobrain, 1217
Chemoreceptor trigger zone, 894
Chemoreceptors
in cardiovascular regulation, 662
in respiration, 458
Chemotaxis, 161
Chemotherapy, **245-248**, 247*b*
acute toxicity, 248
for breast cancer, 1216-1217
cardiotoxicity, 251*b*-252*b*
cell cycle phase–nonspecific drugs, 246, 247*b*
cell cycle phase–specific drugs, 246, 247*b*
chronic toxicity, 248
classification of drugs, 246
delayed effects of, 248
drugs that cause photosensitivity, 408*b*
effects on cells, 245-246
effects on normal tissues, 248
gastrointestinal effects of, 251*b*-252*b*, 253-255
genitourinary effects of, 251*b*-252*b*
goals of, 245, 246*f*
hematologic effects of, 251*b*-252*b*
induction stage, 638
Chemotherapy *(Continued)*
integumentary effects of, 251*b*-252*b*
intraarterial, 246-247
intraperitoneal, 247
intrathecal or intraventricular, 248
intravesical bladder, 248
late effects of, **256-257**
maintenance therapy, 638
methods of administration, 246, 248*b*
myeloablative, 260
nephrotoxicity, 251*b*-252*b*
nursing management of, **250-256**, 251*b*-252*b*
postinduction or postremission therapy, 638
preparation of, 246
pulmonary effects of, 256
regional administration of, 246-248
reproductive effects of, 256
skin changes in, 251*b*-252*b*, 255-256
stages of, 638
transarterial chemoembolization, 997
treatment plan, 248
Chest compression devices, 1634, 1635*f*
Chest compressions, 1650-1651, 1651*f*
Chest drainage, **524**, 525*b*
Chest drainage systems, 522-523, 523*b*, 523*f*, 525*b*
Chest examination, **463-466**
auscultation, 466, 466*f*
inspection, 463-464
palpation, 464-465
percussion, 465, 465*f*
in respiratory problems, 468*b*
secondary survey, 1633
sequence for, 464, 465*f*
Chest pain, 1113*b*-1114*b*
acute care for, 727
emergency management of, 723*b*
in heart failure, 743
in myocardial infarction, 720
Chest physiotherapy, 569-570, **1617**
Chest surgery, **524-527**
postoperative care, 527
preoperative care, 524
procedures, 524-526, 526*b*
Chest trauma, 519*b*, **519-527**
Chest tube dressings, 525*b*
Chest tubes, **522-523**, 525*b*
drainage from, 344*b*
insertion of, 522, 522*f*
removal of, 524
Chest wall
landmarks and structures of, 454, **454*f***
structures and functions of, **455-456**
Chest wounds, sucking, 521
Chest x-ray, 469*t*-471*t*, **671**, 671*f*, 673*t*-677*t*
in acute pericarditis, 785, 786*f*
in TB, 508
Chewing, 1546*b*
Cheyne-Stokes respiration, 132, 1324*f*
Child sexual abuse, 1263
Chinese Americans, 29*b*
Chlamydia trachomatis, 214*b*
Chlamydial infections, **1228-1230**
case study, 1240*b*
clinical manifestations of, 1228-1229, 1229*f*
conjunctivitis, 371
epididymitis, 1228-1229, 1229*f*
interprofessional care for, 1229-1230, 1229*b*
Chloride, 1655*b*-1658*b*, 1662*b*
Chloroma, 597*b*-598*b*, 637
Chlorothiazide (Diuril), 691*b*-693*b*
Chlorpheniramine (Chlor-Trimeton), 479*b*-480*b*
Chlorpromazine, 895*b*
Chlorthalidone, 691*b*-693*b*
Choking, 1652*b*
Cholangiography, 847*t*-850*t*
Cholangiopancreatography
endoscopic retrograde, 847*t*-850*t*, 851
magnetic resonance, 847*t*-850*t*
Cholangitis, 1006*b*, 1007
Choleclciferol (vitamin D_3), 409
Cholecystectomy, 840*b*
incisional (open), 1008-1009
laparoscopic, 1007-1009, 1010*b*
Cholecystitis, **1005-1008**
acute, 1007*b*
nursing assessment in, 1009*b*
Cholecystokinin, 836*b*, 877*b*, 877*f*
Choledochojejunostomy, 840*b*
Choledocholithiasis, 1007
Choledocholithotomy, 840*b*
Cholelithiasis, **1005-1008**, 1005*f*
conservative therapy for, 1007, 1007*b*
drug therapy for, 1007*b*, 1008
gender differences in, 1006*b*
interprofessional care for, 1007*b*
nursing assessment in, 1009*b*
surgical therapy for, 1007-1008, 1008*f*
Cholestasis, 985
Cholesterol, 673*t*-677*t*
reference values, 1655*b*-1658*b*
serum levels, 852*t*
Cholesterol absorption inhibitors, 710, 711*b*
Cholesterol gallstones, 1005
Cholestyramine (Prevalite), 711*b*
Choline magnesium trisalicylate (Trilisate), 111*b*
Cholinergic crisis, 1395*b*
Cholinergics
for GERD, 902, 903*b*
for glaucoma, 381*b*
for multiple sclerosis, 1385*b*
for peptic ulcers, 903*b*
Cholinesterase inhibitors, 1408*b*, 1409
Chondroitin, 1523*b*
Chondrosarcoma, 1500*b*, 1500*f*
Chordae tendineae, 658
Chordee, 1283
Chorea, 1306, 1395
Choroid, 352
Christmas disease, 626
Christmas factor, 592*b*
Chromosome disorders, 183
Chromosomes, **178-179**, 179*b*
Chronic abdominal pain, **940-941**
Chronic abnormal uterine bleeding, 1246
Chronic allergies, **201-202**
Chronic autoimmune thyroiditis, 1163
Chronic blood loss, 610*b*, **615**
Chronic bronchiolitis, 576-577
Chronic bronchitis, 557
Chronic constrictive pericarditis, **787**
Chronic dermatologic problems, 424-425
Chronic disease–related malnutrition, 857
Chronic fatigue syndrome, 1546, 1548
exercise therapy for, 1549*b*
sleep disturbances in, 92*b*
Chronic gastritis, 909-910
Chronic glaucoma, 381*b*
Chronic glomerulonephritis, 1041, **1043**
Chronic gout, 1533*f*
Chronic heart failure
clinical manifestations of, 742-743, 742*b*
drug therapy for, 747-749
interprofessional care for, 744*b*, 746-749
Chronic hepatitis, 978
clinical manifestations of, 977-978, 977*b*
interprofessional care for, 980*b*
Chronic hepatitis B, 980-981, 981*b*
Chronic hepatitis C, 981, 981*b*

Chronic hereditary nephritis, 1052
Chronic HIV infection, 220-221
Chronic illness, 60-63
anemia of chronic disease, 610*b*, **613-614**
characteristics of, 61*b*
impact of, 61*b*
nursing management of, **62-63**
in older adults, 64
tasks of, 62*b*
trajectory of, 60-61, 62*b*, 62*f*
Chronic inflammatory demyelinating polyradiculoneuropathy, 1441-1442
Chronic kidney disease, 1069, 1070*b*, **1075-1083**
acute care for, 1084
ambulatory care for, 1084
case study, 1097*b*
clinical manifestations of, 1076-1079, 1077*f*
cultural & ethnic health disparities, 1076*b*
dermatologic manifestations of, 399*b*
detection of, 1084*b*
diagnostic studies in, 1079
drug therapy for, 1080-1082
health promotion for, 1083-1084
interprofessional care for, 1079-1083, 1080*b*
nursing diagnoses for, 1083
nursing management of, **1083-1084**
nutritional therapy for, 1082-1083, 1082*b*-1083*b*
in older adults, 1096-1097
patient & caregiver teaching for, 1084*b*
prevention of, 1084*b*
risk factors for, 1081*b*
stages, 1076, 1076*b*
Chronic kidney disease mineral and bone disorder, 1078-1079, 1079*f*, 1081
Chronic liver disease, 92*b*
Chronic low back pain, 1504
Chronic lymphocytic leukemia, 636*b*, **636-637**, 639*b*
Chronic mechanical ventilation, 1582-1584
Chronic myelogenous leukemia, 636*b*, **636**, 639*b*
Chronic neurologic disorders, 1374-1383, 1386, 1386*f*
Chronic neurologic problems, 1368-1398
Chronic obstructive pulmonary disease (COPD), 538, **557-572**, 562*b*
activity considerations, 573-574, 574*b*
acute care for, 573
acute exacerbations, 564
ambulatory care for, 573-575
asthma-COPD overlap syndrome, 559
case study, 582*b*
chest examination findings in, 468*b*
classification of, 562
clinical features of, 543*b*
clinical manifestations of, 560-561
complications of, 561, 563-565
cultural & ethnic health disparities in, 539*b*
diagnostic studies in, 543*b*, 561-562
drug therapy for, 548*b*-549*b*, 562-563
end-of-life considerations, 575
etiology of, 558
gender differences in, 558*b*, 559
genetics of, 558
health promotion for, 572-573
impact of, 61*b*
interprofessional care for, 562-571, 562*b*
medication guidelines for, 563*b*
nursing assessment in, 572, 572*b*
nursing diagnoses for, 572
nursing management of, **572-576**
nutritional therapy for, 570-571, 571*b*
in older adults, 571-572
oxygen therapy for, 565-568
pathophysiology of, 559-560, 560*f*-561*f*
patient & caregiver teaching for, 573*b*
Chronic obstructive pulmonary disease (COPD) *(Continued)*
psychosocial considerations, 574
sleep disturbances during, 92*b*
stable, 562-563
surgical therapy for, 571
texting for, 573*b*
treatment of, 565-571
Chronic open-angle glaucoma, 380
Chronic osteomyelitis, 1497-1498, 1497*f*
Chronic otitis media, 385*b*, **385**
Chronic oxygen therapy, 568
Chronic pain, 107*b*, **107**
Chronic pancreatitis, 1003-1004
drug therapy for, 1001*b*
nursing management of, **1004**
Chronic pelvic pain, 1252-1253
Chronic peritoneal dialysis, 1087
Chronic prostatitis/chronic pelvic pain syndrome, 1282
Chronic pyelonephritis, 1039
Chronic rejection, 208-209
Chronic rheumatic carditis, 789
Chronic sensory polyneuropathy, 399*b*
Chronic sinusitis, 483, 483*b*
Chronic spinal cord injury, 1436*f*
Chronic stable angina, 712-714, 713*b*, 718*f*
drug therapy for, 714-717, 715*b*-716*b*
interprofessional care for, **714-718**, 714*f*
nursing management of, **726-733**
treatment of, 714, 714*b*
Chronic subdural hematoma, 1329, 1329*b*
Chronic toxicity, 248
Chronic ulcers, 910, 910*f*
Chronic urinary retention, 1059-1060
Chronic venous disorders, 816-828
Chronic venous insufficiency, 826-828, 827*b*
Church of Jesus Christ of Latter-Day Saints (Mormons), 26*b*
Chvostek's sign, 284, 284*f*
Chylomicrons, 670
Chylothorax, 521
Chyme, 836
Ciclesonide (Omnaris), 479*b*-480*b*
Cigarette smoking, 558
Cigarettes, electronic, 146
Cilostazol (Pletal), 805*b*
Cimetidine, 903*b*
Cimzia (certolizumab), 1521*b*-1522*b*, 1529
Cinquair (resilzumab), 548*b*-549*b*
for asthma and COPD, 549
Circadian rhythm disorders, 98
Circadian rhythms, **90**, 1105, 1105*f*
Circle of Willis, 1299, 1346, 1346*f*
Circulating nurse, 316-317
Circulation
bronchial, 455
cerebral, **1299-1300**, 1300*f*, 1346, 1346*f*
collateral, 703, 988
coronary, 658-659, 659*f*
primary survey, 1630, 1631*b*-1632*b*
return of spontaneous circulation, 1634
Circulatory assist devices, **1566-1569**
Circulatory overload reaction, 650*b*-651*b*
Circumduction, 1455*b*
Cirrhosis
biliary, **985**
cardiac, 986
of liver, **986-993**, 986*f*
acute care for, 994-995
ambulatory care for, 995
case study, 1010*b*
clinical manifestations of, 986-987, 987*f*-988*f*
compensated, 987-988
complications of, 987-990
cultural & ethnic health disparities, 986*b*
Cirrhosis *(Continued)*
diagnostic studies, 990
drug therapy for, 992, 993*b*
early manifestations of, 986
etiology and pathophysiology of, 986
health promotion for, 993-994
interprofessional care for, 991-993, 991*b*
late manifestations of, 986-987, 987*f*-988*f*
nursing assessment in, 993*b*
nursing diagnoses for, 993
nursing management of, **993-996**
nutritional therapy for, 992-993
pathophysiology of, 986, 987*f*
patient & caregiver teaching for, 995*b*
Cisatracurium (Nimbex), 326*b*
Clarinex (desloratadine), 479*b*-480*b*
Claritin (loratadine), 479*b*-480*b*
Clark level, 412
Classification systems, 6
Claudication, intermittent, 803
Clemastine, 479*b*-480*b*
Clevidipine (Cleviprex), 691*b*-693*b*
Clinical COPD Questionnaire (CCQ), 562
Clinical Institute Withdrawal Assessment of Alcohol Scale, Revised (CIWA-Ar), 150, 151*b*
Clinical manifestations, 35
Clinical pathways, **10-11**
Clinical questions, 15, 15*b*
Clinical reasoning, 9
Clipping aneurysms, 1356, 1356*f*
Clitoris, 1187
Clock drawing test, 1408, 1408*f*
Clomiphene (Clomid, Serophene), 1243*b*
Clonidine (Catapres), 691*b*-693*b*, 699*b*
Clonidine (Duraclon), 116*b*
Clonus, 1307
Clopatadine (Patanase), 479*b*-480*b*
Clopidogrel (Plavix), 187*b*
drug alert, 805*b*, 1353*b*
mechanism of action, 715*b*-716*b*
for peripheral arterial disease, 805*b*
Clostridia, 214*b*
Clostridial food poisoning, 925*b*
***Clostridium difficile* infection**, 929-931, 930*b*
interprofessional care for, **932**
Clostridium perfringens, 930*b*
Clotting
extrinsic pathway, 591, 591*f*
intrinsic pathway, 591, 591*f*
normal mechanisms, **590-592**, 591*f*
retraction and dissolution, 591-592
Clotting disorders, 399*b*
Clotting studies, 601*t*
Clubbing, 467*b*-468*b*, 598, 668*b*
Cluster breathing, 1324*f*
Cluster headache, 1370*f*, **1371**
drug therapy for, 1372
gender differences in, 1370*b*
interprofessional care for, 1369*b*
Clusters of differentiation (CD antigens), 191
Coaching, 581*b*
Coagulation. *See* Clotting
Coagulation factors, 592*b*, 628*b*
Cobalamin. *See* Vitamin B_{12}
Coccidioides immitis, 215*b*, 222*b*
Cochlear implants, 390-391, 391*f*
Codeine, 112, 113*b*-114*b*, 117*b*
Codominance, 179*b*
Cogentin (benztropine), 1391*b*
Cognitive changes
assessment of, 1304
in older adults, 64*b*
Cognitive impairment. *See also* Mild cognitive impairment
in cancer, 251*b*-252*b*, 256
drug therapy for, 1408*b*

Cognitive impairment *(Continued)*
in older adults, 64, 72*b*
postoperative, 338
Tai Chi for, 72*b*
tips to reduce risk of, 1410*b*
Cognitive-behavioral therapy
for insomnia, 93-94, 1080*b*
for pain, **122**
Cognitive-perceptual pattern, 37*b*, 38
Cogwheel rigidity, 1389
Coiling aneurysms, 1356, 1356*f*
Cold, common, 478-480
Cold extremities, 668*b*
Cold medications, 479*b*-480*b*
Cold sores, 897*b*, 1232
Cold therapy, **122**. *See also* Cryotherapy
patient & caregiver teaching for, 122*b*
RICE (Rest, ice, compression, and elevation), 165
Cold-related emergencies, 1637-1639
Colectomy, 840*b*
Colera, 29*b*
Colesevelam (WelChol), 711*b*
Colestipol (Colestid), 711*b*
Colic
biliary, 1006
renal, 1018, 1046
Collaboration, 4, 4*f*, 6*b*, **9-12**, 10*b*
Collaborative problems, 7-8
Collagen diseases, 1180*b*
Collateral circulation, 703, 988
Collecting bile duct, 1017*b*
Colles' fracture, 1480-1481, 1481*f*
Colloids, **293-294**, 1597*b*, 1598, 1600*b*
Colon cancer. *See* Colorectal cancer
Colonoscopy, 847*t*-850*t*
virtual, 847*t*-850*t*, 851
Colony-stimulating factors, 194, 195*b*
Color vision testing, 356*b*, 359
Colorectal cancer, 954-957
acute care for, 957-958
advanced disease, 955
ambulatory care for, 958
case study, 971*b*
chemotherapy for, 956-957
clinical manifestations of, 955, 955*f*
cultural & ethnic health disparities, 954*b*
diagnostic studies in, 955
early disease, 955
etiology and pathophysiology of, 954
genetic risks, 841*b*
health promotion for, 957
hereditary nonpolyposis colorectal cancer, 954*b*
interprofessional care for, 955-957, 955*b*
metastatic, 997*f*
nursing assessment in, 957*b*
nursing diagnoses for, 957
nursing management of, **957-958**
radiation therapy for, 957
risk factors for, 954*b*
signs and symptoms of, 955, 955*f*
staging, 954-955, 954*f*, 956*b*
surgical therapy for, 955-956
targeted therapy for, 956-957
TNM classification of, 955, 956*b*
Color-flow imaging (duplex), 671, 672*f*, 673*t*-677*t*
Colostomy, 840*b*, 958, 959*b*, 959*f*
loop, 959*f*
sigmoid, 959*f*
Colostomy care, 960-961
Colostomy irrigations, 961
Colposcopy, 1198*t*-1201*t*
Coma, 1317, 1324*f*
Combistix (Dipstick) test, 1025*t*-1030*t*
Combivent Respimat (ipratropium/albuterol), 548*b*-549*b*
Comedo, 403*b*
Comfort measures
in ED, 1632
in ET intubation, 1573
in shock, 1604
Commercial concentrates, 648*b*
Commissurotomy, 794
Common bile duct, 838*f*
Common bile duct obstruction, 1006, 1006*b*
Common cold, 478-480
Communication
for coordinating care, 10
with critical care patients, 1556
cross-cultural, **25-26**, 25*f*
cultural factors, 25*b*
culturally competent, 30-31
directives to physicians (DTPs), 135, 136*b*
at end of life, 139
with ET intubation, 1573
guidelines for communicating with patients with aphasia, 1361*b*
when no interpreter is available, 31*b*
with non-English-speaking patients, 52, 52*f*
nonverbal, 25, 25*f*, 49
nursing interventions for, 1361
for pain management, 122
for patient and caregiver teaching, 48-49, 49*f*
with patients with hearing impairment, 390*b*
postoperative SBAR hand-off, 345*b*
SBAR (Situation-Background-Assessment-Recommendation) technique, 10, 11*b*, 345*b*
after stroke, 1351
of test results, 782*b*
text messaging
for COPD, 573*b*
and diabetes, 1135*b*
verbal, 25, 25*f*
Communication devices, 494*b*
Community emergency response teams (CERTs), 1646
Community integration, 1365
Community-acquired pneumonia, 501*b*, **501**, 504*b*
Comparative genomic hybridization, 603*t*
Compartment syndrome, 1479
interprofessional care for, 1479, 1479*f*
secondary survey for, 1634
Competence, 754*b*
Complement, 1659*b*
total hemolytic (CH_{50}), 1457*t*-1459*t*
Complement system, **161-162**, 162*b*
Complementary & alternative therapies
assessment of use of herbs and dietary supplements, 38*b*
for insomnia, 95
for peripheral arterial disease, 805
Complete blood count, 599-600, 600*t*
Complex regional pain syndrome, 107
Compliance, 1315-1316
Complicated grief, 133-134
Compression
for inflammation, 165
RICE therapy, 165, 1464
for sprains and strains, 1464
Compression devices, 819
Compression stockings, 819
Computed tomography (CT)
abdominal, 603*t*, 1115*t*-1118*t*
of brain, 1309*f*, 1310*t*-1312*t*
calcium-scoring, 673*t*-677*t*, 678
Computed tomography (CT) *(Continued)*
cardiac, 673*t*-677*t*, 678
electron beam (EBCT), 673*t*-677*t*, 678, 678*f*
gastrointestinal, 847*t*-850*t*
multidetector (MDCT) scanning, 678
in musculoskeletal disorders, 1457*t*-1459*t*
of pelvis, 1198*t*-1201*t*
of respiratory system, 469*t*-471*t*
single-photon emission (SPECT), 603*t*, 672, 673*t*-677*t*, 1310*t*-1312*t*
spiral (helical) scan, 530
urogram, 1025*t*-1030*t*
Computed tomography angiography, 530, 1310*t*-1312*t*
coronary, 673*t*-677*t*, 678
Computer monitoring, 1075*b*
Computerized provider order entry (CPOE) systems, 14
Comtan (entacapone), 1390, 1391*b*
Concept maps, 8
Conceptual care maps, 8
Concussion, 1327
Condoms, 228*b*
Conductive hearing loss, 387
Confidentiality
and HIPAA, 1239*b*
protecting patient privacy, 1222*b*
Conflict resolution, 1159*b*
Confrontation visual field test, 356*b*
Confusion Assessment Method (CAM), 1415, 1416*b*, 1557
Congenital disorders, 179*b*
Conization, 1198*t*-1201*t*
Conjunctiva, 352
abnormalities, 357*b*
examination of, 358
in older adults, 353*b*
Conjunctivitis, 357*b*, **371-372**
allergic, 371-372
gonococcal, 1230
keratoconjunctivitis, 372
Connective tissue disease
cultural & ethnic health disparities, 1525*b*
drug therapy for, 1521*b*-1522*b*
mixed, **1545-1546**
Conn's syndrome, 1180
Consciousness
altered, 1308*b*-1309*b*, 1416*b*
in increased ICP, 1317-1318
unconsciousness, 1317-1318, 1652*b*
Consent
informed consent, 309, 310*b*
for surgery, 309-310
Constipation, 934-936, 1113*b*-1114*b*
in cancer, 251*b*-252*b*
causes of, 934, 935*b*
drug therapy for, 935-936, 936*b*
interprofessional care for, 935-936
nursing assessment in, 937*b*
nursing management of, 867*b*, **936-938**
nutritional therapy for, 936
opioid-induced, 114, 115*b*
patient & caregiver teaching for, 937*b*
postoperative, 341
probiotics and, 935
with tube feedings, 867*b*
Constraint-induced movement therapy, 1364
Constrictive pericarditis, 787
Consumerism, 4
Contact dermatitis, 200, 200*f*
allergic, 203, 409, 418*b*
irritant, 409
Contact lenses, 368

Contact precautions, 218, 218*b*
Contemplation, 47-48, 48*b*
Continence, 1019
Continent ileostomies, 958
Continent urinary diversion, 1065
Continuous ambulatory peritoneal dialysis, 1086-1087
Continuous bladder irrigation, 1274, 1274*b*
Continuous CO (CCO)/continuous CI (CCI), 1562
Continuous glucose monitoring (CGM) systems, 1135, 1136*f*
Continuous lateral rotation therapy, 1625, 1625*f*
Continuous positive airway pressure (CPAP), 97, 97*f*, 1576*b*, 1577
Continuous renal replacement therapy (CRRT), 1074, 1091*b*, **1091-1092**, 1092
Continuous subglottal suctioning, 1573, 1573*f*
Continuous venovenous hemodiafiltration, 1091, 1091*b*
Continuous venovenous hemodialysis, 1091, 1091*b*
Continuous venovenous hemofiltration, 1091, 1091*b*
Continuous venovenous therapy, 1091-1092, 1091*f*
Continuum of care, 8-9, 129, 130*f*
Contractility, 1560
Contractions
muscle, 1449
scar, 166, 166*b*
wound, 167*b*
Contractures
burn, 446, 447*f*
muscle or joint, 1456*b*, 1478*b*
Contrast echocardiography, 671, 673*t*-677*t*
Contrave (bupropion/naltrexone), 884*b*
Contrecoup injury, 1328
Contusions, 1328, 1469*b*
Conus medullaris syndrome, 1422*b*
Convulsive status epilepticus, 1376
Cooling methods, 1637
Coombs test, 602*t*
Coordinating care, **10-12**
Copaxone (glatiramer acetate), 1385*b*
COPD. *See* Chronic obstructive pulmonary disease
COPD Assessment Test (CAT), 562
Copeptin, 670, 673*t*-677*t*
Coping
with cancer, 265*b*, **265-266**
emotion-focused, 83*b*
problem-focused, 83*b*
strategies for, 82*b*, **82-83**
after stroke, 1362, 1364-1365
Coping–stress tolerance pattern, 37*b*, 39
Copper, 610*b*, 1655*b*-1658*b*
Cor pulmonale, 533
interprofessional care for, 533*b*, 563
nursing and interprofessional management of, **533**
pathophysiology of, 532*f*, 560, 563, 564*f*
Cordarone (amiodarone), 771*b*
Cordectomy, 491
Core (core needle) biopsy, 1206
Coreg (carvedilol), 691*b*-693*b*, 715*b*-716*b*, 745*b*, 748, 748*b*
CoreValve transcatheter aortic valve, 795, 795*f*
Corgard (nadolol), 691*b*-693*b*, 715*b*-716*b*, 993*b*
Corlanor (ivabradine), 745*b*
Corlopam (fenoldopam), 691*b*-693*b*
Cornea, 358
abnormalities, 357*b*
in older adults, 353*b*, 353*f*
Corneal abrasion, 357*b*
Corneal disorders, 373
Corneal scars, 373
Corneal transplant, 373, 373*f*
Corneal ulcers, 372, 372*f*
Corns, 1509*b*
Coronary angiography, 673*t*-677*t*, 678, 678*f*, 722
Coronary artery bypass graft surgery
minimally invasive direct, 725
off-pump, 725
robotic or totally endoscopic, 725
traditional, **724-725**, 724*f*
Coronary artery disease, 702-707, 718*f*
cultural & ethnic health disparities in, 704*b*
developmental stages, 703
etiology and pathophysiology of, 702-703
gender differences in, 704, 705*b*
genetics of, 664*b*, 704-707
health promotion for, 707-708
high-risk individuals, 707-708
hypertension and, 685
images useful for, 85*b*
impact of, 61*b*
lipid-lowering drug therapy for, 709-710
nursing and interprofessional management of, **707-712**
nutritional therapy for, 708-709
in older adults, 710-712
risk factors for, 703-704, 704*b*
modifiable, 703-707
nonmodifiable, 703-704
patient & caregiver teaching for reducing, 708*b*
psychologic, 706-707
Coronary artery stents, 717-718, 718*f*
Coronary circulation, 658-659, 659*f*
Coronary computed tomography angiography, 673*t*-677*t*, 678
Coronary microvascular disease, 713-714
Coronary revascularization, 717, 728-730
surgical, **724-725**
Coronavirus, 214*b*
Corrective glasses, 368, 392*b*
Cortical sensory functions, 1307
Corticosteroids
endogenous, 1104*b*, 1107
exogenous, **1179-1180**, 1180*b*
for allergic disorders, 202
for arthritis, 1521*b*-1522*b*, 1529
for asthma, 547-549, 548*b*-549*b*
for cancer, 259*b*
cardiovascular effects of, 664*b*
for dermatologic problems, **421**
drug alert, 1180*b*
effects on wound healing, 168*b*
for IBD, 947, 947*b*
for immunosuppressive therapy, 209, 211*b*
intravenous, 1618*b*
for multiple sclerosis, 1385*b*, 1386
for nausea and vomiting, 895*b*
for pain, 115, 116*b*
patient & caregiver teaching for, 1181*b*
for respiratory failure, 1618*b*
for rhinitis and sinusitis, 479*b*-480*b*
side effects of, 1096, 1180*b*
Cortisol, **1107**
circadian rhythm of, 1105, 1105*f*
free, 1115*t*-1118*t*
measurement of, 1115*t*-1118*t*
reference values, 1655*b*-1658*b*
regulation of water balance by, 275
Corvert (ibutilide), 771*b*
Corynebacterium, 214*b*
Coryza, acute, 478-480
Cosmetic procedures, 425-426, 426*b*
Cosmetic surgery, 301
nursing management of, **426**
for obesity, **890**
postoperative management of, 426
preoperative management of, 426
Costovertebral angle, 1023, 1024*f*
Cosyntropin, 1115*t*-1118*t*
Cough reflex, 458-459
Cough variant asthma, 542
Coughing
augmented (quad), 1616, 1617*f*
effective, 569-570, 1616-1617
huff, 569, 569*b*, 1616
staged, 1616
techniques for splinting incision when, 336, 336*f*
Coumadin. *See* Warfarin
Counseling
after fracture, 1478
sexual, 1288
Counterpulsation, 1567, 1567*b*
Counterregulatory mechanisms, 740
Coup-contrecoup injury, 1328, 1328*f*
Covera-HS (verapamil long-acting), 691*b*-693*b*
Cowper's (bulbourethral) glands, 1185
Coxsackievirus, 214*b*
Cozaar (losartan), 691*b*-693*b*, 715*b*-716*b*, 745*b*
Crackles, 466, 467*b*-468*b*
Cramps
heat cramps, **1637**
in hemodialysis, 1090-1091
Cranial nerve disorders, 1437-1440
Cranial nerves, **1299**, 1300*f*
abnormalities, 1308*b*-1309*b*
assessment of, 1304-1306, 1305*b*
normal, 1308*b*
Cranial radiation, prophylactic, 517
Cranial surgery, **1336-1337**
acute care for, 1337-1338
ambulatory care for, 1338
indications for, 1336*b*
nursing management of, **1337-1338**
types of, 1336-1337, 1337*b*
Craniectomy, 1337*b*
Cranioplasty, 1337*b*
Craniotomy, 1336, 1337*b*
C-reactive protein
in cardiac assessment, **670**, 673*t*-677*t*
in musculoskeletal disorders, 1457*t*-1459*t*
reference values, 1659*b*
Creatine
blood values, 1655*b*-1658*b*
urine values, 1661*b*
Creatine kinase, 670, 673*t*-677*t*, 722, 1457*t*-1459*t*
blood values, 1655*b*-1658*b*
in shock, 1590*t*
Creatinine, 1025*t*-1030*t*, 1031
in shock, 1590*t*
urine values, 1655*b*-1658*b*, 1661*b*
Creatinine clearance, 1025*t*-1030*t*, **1031**
Creon (pancrelipase), 1001*b*, 1004
Crepitation, 1456*b*, 1469*b*, 1518
CREST syndrome, 1542-1543
Crestor (rosuvastatin), 711*b*
Cretinism, 1168
Crisis management, 60-61
Critical appraisal, 15-16
Critical care nursing, 1554-1558, 1584*b*
case study, 1584*b*
culturally competent care, 1558
Critical care units (CCUs), 1554-1555
Critical incident stress management units, 1646
Critical limb ischemia, 804-806
Critical test results, 291*b*
Critical thinking, 9
Critically ill patients, 1555
Crizotinib (Xalkori), 187*b*
Crohn's disease, 944, 945*b*
clinical manifestations of, 945-946
genetics of, 944
pattern of inflammation in, 945, 945*f*
surgical therapy for, 948

Cromolyn spray, 479*b*-480*b*
Cross-cultural communication, **25-26**, 25*f*
Crossmatch, **208**
Cryoablation, 766-767
Cryopexy, **377**
Cryoplasty, 806
Cryoprecipitates
for blood component therapy, 648*b*
compatibilities for transfusions, 649*b*
Cryosurgery, **422**
Cryotherapy
for prostate cancer, 1279
for sprains and strains, 1464
Cryptococcus neoformans, 222*b*
Cryptorchidism, 1284
***Cryptosporidium* infection**, 930*b*
Cryptosporidium muris, 222*b*
Crystalloid solutions, 292, 293*b*, 1597*b*
Culdocentesis, 1198*t*-1201*t*
Culdoscopy, 1198*t*-1201*t*
Culdotomy, 1198*t*-1201*t*
Cullen's sign, 1000
Cultural assessment, 29*b*, 30
Cultural awareness, 23*b*
Cultural beliefs, 22, 25*b*
Cultural competence, **23-24**
development of, 23*b*
increasing, 29-31
National Standards for Culturally and Linguistically Appropriate Services in Health Care (CLAS standards), 30
patient assessment, 29-30
self-assessment, 29
Cultural conflict, 24
Cultural diversity, **24**, 24*f*
Cultural encounters, 23*b*
Cultural factors, **24-29**, 25*b*
Cultural groups, 22, 22*f*
Cultural imposition, 23
Cultural knowledge, 23*b*
Cultural safety, 23
Cultural skills, 23*b*
Cultural stereotyping, 856
Culturally competent care
in assessment, 36
for breast cancer, 1218
for critical care patients, 1558
for diabetes mellitus, 1137
for diabetic glycemic control and knowledge, 53*b*
end-of-life care, 134-135
for nutrition, 856
for older adults, 66
in patient teaching, 52
preoperative, 311-312
Culture, **21-31**, 22*b*
Culture-bound syndromes, 29, 29*b*
Cultured epithelial autografts, **445**, 445*f*
Cumulative trauma disorder, 1465
Cupped-hand position for percussion, 570, 570*f*
Cuprimine (penicillamine), 1521*b*-1522*b*, 1529
Curanderos (or *curanderas*), 24
CURB-65 scale, 501, 501*b*
Curettage, 422
Cushing syndrome, **1174-1176**
acute care for, 1177
ambulatory care for, 1177
clinical manifestations of, 1174, 1174*f*-1175*f*, 1175*b*
dermatologic manifestations of, 399*b*
health promotion for, 1177
interprofessional care for, 1175-1176, 1176*b*
nursing assessment in, 1176*b*
nursing diagnoses for, 1176-1177
nursing management of, **1176-1178**
Cushing syndrome *(Continued)*
postoperative care in, 1177
preoperative care in, 1177
Cushing's triad, 1316, 1318, 1324
Cutaneous lupus, subacute, 1538
Cutaneous melanoma, 411
Cutaneous T-cell lymphoma, 412*b*
Cyanide poisoning, 1643*b*
Cyanosis, 467*b*-468*b*, 597*b*-598*b*
central, 668*b*
in light- and dark-skinned persons, 404*b*
peripheral, 668*b*
Cyclic vomiting syndrome, 894
Cyclophosphamide (Cytosan)
for arthritis and connective tissue disorders, 1521*b*-1522*b*
for immunosuppressive therapy, 209, 211*b*
Cycloplegics, 374, 374*b*
Cycloset (bromocriptine), 1131*b*
Cyclosporine (Sandimmune, Neoral, Gengraf), 209, 209*b*, 211*b*
Cymbalta (duloxetine), 116*b*
Cyroprotective drug therapy, 903*b*, 914
Cyst(s), 403*b*
in breast, 1206*b*
ganglion, 1456*b*
medullary cystic disease, **1052**
ovarian, **1255**, 1255*f*
pancreatic pseudocysts, 1000
pilonidal, 846*b*-847*b*
polycystic kidney disease, **1051-1052**
polycystic ovary syndrome, **1255**, 1255*f*
sebaceous, 365*b*
Cystectomy
radical, 1054
segmental (partial), 1054
Cystic fibrosis, 538, **576-579**
clinical manifestations of, 577-578
complications of, 578
cultural & ethnic health disparities in, 539*b*
dermatologic manifestations of, 399*b*
diagnostic studies in, 578
etiology and pathophysiology of, 576-577
genetics of, 576-577, 576*b*, 576*f*
interprofessional care for, 578-579
nursing assessment in, 580*b*
nursing diagnoses for, 579
nursing management of, **579-580**
Cystic Fibrosis Foundation, 578
Cystic fibrosis transmembrane conductance regulator (CFTR) gene, 576, 576*f*
Cystine stones, 1046*b*
Cystitis, 1034
hemorrhagic, 251*b*-252*b*
interstitial, **1040-1041**
Cystocele, **1262**, 1262*f*
Cystography, 1025*t*-1030*t*
Cystolitholapaxy, 1047
Cystometrography, 1025*t*-1030*t*
Cystoscopic examination, 1025*t*-1030*t*, 1028*f*
Cystoscopic lithotripsy, 1047
Cystoscopy, 1025*t*-1030*t*
Cystotomy, 1048
Cytogenetics, molecular, 603*t*, 604
Cytokines, **194**, 195*b*
clinical uses, 194, 195*b*
immunotherapy, 258*b*
in inflammation, 162*b*, 163
Cytology, 469*t*-471*t*, 1025*t*-1030*t*
Cytolytic reactions, 199
Cytomegalovirus, 214*b*, 222*b*
Cytomegalovirus retinitis, 382
Cytoreductive procedures, 245
Cytotec (misoprostol), 903*b*, 1523
Cytotoxic cerebral edema, 1317
Cytotoxic drugs, 211*b*
Cytotoxic reactions, 197*b*, **199**
Cytotoxic T cells, 208, 209*f*, 239
Cytoxan, 614

D

da Vinci, Leonardo, 270
da Vinci system, 1278
Dabigatran (Pradaxa), 820*b*, 821
Daclizumab (Zenapax), 210, 211*b*
Daclizumab (Zinbryta), 1378*b*
Daily weights, **277**
Dalfampridine (Ampyra), 1385*b*, 1386
Daliresp (roflumilast), 548*b*-549*b*
Dalteparin (Fragmin), 715*b*-716*b*, 820*b*
Dancing, 1390*b*
Dantrolene (Dantrium), 1385*b*
Dapagliflozin (Farxiga), 1131*b*
Daranide (dichlorphenamide), 381*b*
Darbepoetin alfa (Aranesp), 195*b*
Darifenacin (Enablex), 1059*b*
Dark skin
assessment of, 174*b*, 402-405, 403*f*
pigmented nail beds in, 396, 396*f*
variations in, 404*b*
Dark-field microscopy, 1198*t*-1201*t*
DASH (Dietary Approaches to Stop Hypertension) diet, 688, 693-694, 749
DAST-10 (Drug Abuse Screening Test), 154, 155*b*
Data collection, **34-36**, 36*b*
types of data, 35
Data organization, 35-36
Databases, 34
Dawn phenomenon, 1130
Daypro (oxaprozin), 1521*b*-1522*b*
Daytime sleepiness, 90, 90*f*
D-dimer, 530, 601*t*, 1659*b*
Deafferentation pain, 106*b*, 107
Deafness, **387-388**. *See also* Hearing loss
Death, **131-132**
brain death, 131
in ED, 1635
fear of, 303
fear of hastening, 124-125
sudden cardiac death, **733**, 771
Death rattle, 132
Debridement, 439
enzymatic, 443-444
surgical, 439, 440*f*, **1491**
types of, 170*b*
Debulking procedures, 245
Decannulation, 490
Deceased donors, 1093-1094
Decerebrate posturing, 1318, 1318*f*
Decongestants, 202, 479*b*-480*b*
Decorticate posturing, 1318, 1318*f*
Decortication, 526*b*
Deep brain stimulation, 1391, 1391*f*
Deep inferior epigastric artery perforator (DIEP) flap, 1215*b*, 1223-1224
Deep pain, 106
Deep somatic pain, 106*b*
Deep tendon reflexes
abnormalities, 1308*b*-1309*b*
increased, 1113*b*-1114*b*
Deep vein thrombosis, 816
Defecation, 836
Defecography, 847*t*-850*t*
Defibrillation, **771-773**, 772*b*, 772*f*, 1651
Deformity, 1518-1519
Degarelix (Firmagon), 1280*b*
Degenerative disc disease, 1504-1505, 1505*f*
Degenerative neurologic disorders, **1383-1396**

Deglutition, 834
Dehiscence, 167*b*, 167*f*
Dehydration
at end of life, 140*b*-141*b*
nursing management of, 867*b*
with tube feedings, 867*b*
Delayed emergence, 338
Delayed hypersensitivity reactions, 197*b*, **199-200**
Delayed transfusion reactions, 651*b*, 652
Delegation, 11-12
Five Rights of Nursing Delegation, 11-12, 12*b*
safe, 868*b*
Delirium, 1399, 1400*b*, **1414-1417**
alcohol withdrawal, 150, 338
in critical care patients, 1557
drug therapy for, 1417
emergence, 338
at end of life, 140*b*-141*b*
etiology and pathophysiology of, 1415, 1415*b*
factors that precipitate, 1415*b*
mnemonic for causes of, 1415*b*
nursing and interprofessional management of, 1416-1417
postoperative, 338
Delivery of nursing care, 9
Delta virus, 976-977
Demadex (torsemide), 691*b*-693*b*
Demand pacemakers, 773
Dementia, **1399-1414**, 1400*b*
causes of, 1399, 1400*b*-1401*b*, 1400*f*
cultural & ethnic health disparities, 1402*b*
and depression, 1399
due to Alzheimer's disease, 1406*b*
gender differences in, 1402*b*
guidelines for dealing with patients, 1414*b*
with Lewy bodies, 1401*b*
mixed, 1400
modifying risk factors for, 1410*b*
multiinfarct, 1400
nursing and interprofessional management of, **1401**
tips to reduce risk of, 1410*b*
vascular, 1400
Demerol (meperidine), 114, 114*b*
Demographics
of aging, **63**
diverse population, **4**
Dendrites, 1294
Dendritic cells, 194
Dengue fever, 216*b*
Denial
in ACS, 728*b*
in spinal cord injury, 1435*b*
Denosumab (Prolia), 1513
Dentists, 10*b*
Deoxyribonucleic acid (DNA), **179-180**, 180*f*
Depen (penicillamine), 1521*b*-1522*b*
Dependence
in ACS, 728*b*
physical, 123
Dependent rubor, 803-804
Depigmentation, 1113*b*-1114*b*
Depolarization, 660-661
Depo-Medrol (methylprednisolone acetate), 1521*b*-1522*b*
Depressant toxicity, **152**, 152*b*
Depressant use, **152-153**
Depressant withdrawal, **152-153**
Depression, 1399, 1400*b*
in acute coronary syndrome, 728*b*
in burn patients, 448*b*
and dementia, 1399
drug therapy for, 1408*b*, 1409
at end of life, 138
images useful for, 85*b*
Depression *(Continued)*
in older adults, 73-74
in spinal cord injury, 1435, 1435*b*
Dermatitis
atopic, 199, 199*f*, 418*b*
contact, **200**, 200*f*
allergic, 203, 409, 418*b*
irritant, 409
incontinence-associated, 934
Dermatitis herpetiformis, 966
Dermatologic problems
allergic, 417, 418*b*
ambulatory care for, 422-425
benign conditions, **417-427**, 419*b*
chronic, 424-425
diabetes-related dermopathy, 1151
diagnostic studies of, 420
drug therapy for, **420-422**
interprofessional care for, **420-422**
nursing management of, **422-425**
psychologic effects of, 424-425
of scrotum, **1284**
self-treatment for, 410
in systemic lupus erythematosus, 1538
Dermatomes, 444, 1298, 1299*f*, 1421
Dermatomyositis, **1544-1545**
dermatologic manifestations of, 399*b*
nursing and interprofessional management of, **1545**
skin changes in, 1545, 1545*f*
Dermatosis papulosa nigra, 403-405
Dermis, **395**, 432
Desflurane (Suprane), 325*b*
Desipramine (Norpramin), 116*b*
Desirudin (Iprivask), 820*b*
Desloratadine (Clarinex), 479*b*-480*b*
Desquamation
dry, 255, 255*f*
wet, 255, 255*f*
Detrol (tolterodine), 1057*b*, 1059*b*
Deviated septum, **475**
Dexamethasone
for arthritis, 1521*b*-1522*b*
in general anesthesia, 326*b*
for nausea and vomiting, 895*b*
Dexamethasone suppression test, 1115*t*-1118*t*
Dexchlorpheniramine (Polaramine), 479*b*-480*b*
DexcomG4 Platinum, 1135
Dexlansoprazole (Dexilant), 903*b*
Dexmedetomidine (Precedex), 326*b*
Dextrose solutions, 293*b*
DiaBeta (glyburide), 1131*b*
Diabetes exchange lists, 1134
Diabetes Forecast, 1141
Diabetes insipidus, **1161**
central, 1161*b*
genetic risks, 1109*b*
nephrogenic, 1161*b*
neurogenic, 1109*b*
nursing and interprofessional management of, **1162**
pathophysiology of, 1161, 1161*f*
primary, 1161*b*
types of, 1161*b*
Diabetes mellitus, **1120-1137**
acute care for, 1139
acute complications of, **1142-1147**
adult-onset, 1122
ambulatory care for, 1139-1141
bariatric surgery for, 1137
and CAD, 706
CF-related, 577
chronic complications of, **1147-1153**
combination oral therapy for, 1131*b*, 1132
complications of, in feet and lower extremities, **1150-1151**, 1150*f*
Diabetes mellitus *(Continued)*
cultural & ethnic health disparities, 1137*b*
culturally appropriate education for, 53*b*
culturally competent care for, 1137
dermatologic manifestations of, 399*b*
diagnostic studies for, 1124
drug therapy for, 1125-1132, 1125*b*, 1131*b*
early detection of, 1138*b*
education text messaging and, 1135*b*
etiology and pathophysiology of, 1120-1122
exercise for, 1134-1135, 1134*b*, 1142*b*
genetics of, 1109*b*, 1122*b*
gestational, **1123-1124**
health promotion for, 708*b*, 1137-1138
idiopathic, 1122
impact of, 61*b*
infection in, **1151-1152**
insulin therapy for, 1125-1130, 1125*b*, 1139-1140
insulin-dependent, 1121-1122
integumentary complications of, **1151**
interprofessional care for, 1124-1125, 1125*b*
juvenile-onset, 1121-1122
latent autoimmune diabetes in adults, 1122
long-term complications of, 1147-1148, 1147*f*, 1148*b*
macrovascular complications of, 1148
management of, 1141*b*
maturity-onset, of the young, 1122*b*
medical identification and travel with, 1140
microvascular complications of, 1148
monitoring for long-term complications, 1148, 1148*b*
noninsulin injectable agents for, 1130-1132, 1131*b*, 1140
non–insulin-dependent, 1122
nursing assessment in, 1137, 1138*b*
nursing diagnoses related to, 1137
nursing management of, **1137-1141**, 1152*b*
nutritional therapy for, 1132-1134, 1133*b*
and obesity, 879
in older adults, 1152-1153
oral agents for, 1130-1132, 1131*b*, 1140
other types, 1124
pancreas transplantation for, 1137
patient & caregiver teaching for, 1134*b*, 1140-1141, 1141*b*-1142*b*
prediabetes, 1123
prevention and early detection of, 1138*b*
psychologic considerations, **1152-1153**
resources for patients, 1141
screening for, 1138, 1138*b*
sleep disturbances during, 92*b*
tight or intensive therapy for, 1147-1148
type 1, 1121*b*, **1121-1122**
clinical manifestations of, 1124
etiology and pathophysiology of, 1122, 1123*f*
genetics of, 1122, 1122*b*
nutritional therapy for, 1132-1133
onset of disease, 1122
type 2, 1121*b*, **1122**, 1124
clinical manifestations of, 1124
drug therapy for, 1136*f*
etiology and pathophysiology of, 1122, 1123*f*
genetics of, 1122-1124, 1122*b*
nutritional therapy for, 1133
onset of disease, 1123
Diabetic ketoacidosis, **1142-1145**, 1145*b*
case study, 1154*b*
emergency management of, 1144*b*
etiology and pathophysiology of, 1142-1143, 1143*f*
interprofessional care for, 1144-1145, 1144*b*
nursing management of, **1145-1146**
Diabetic nephropathy, 1042*b*, 1148*b*, **1149**
Diabetic neuropathy, 1148*b*, **1149-1150**, 1150*f*

Diabetic retinopathy, 376, 376*f*, **1148-1149**
case study, 392*b*
monitoring for, 1148*b*
Diagnostic studies. *See also specific tests*
communicating results, 782*b*
preoperative, 307*b*-308*b*, 308
Dialysate, 1089
Dialysis, **1084-1097**
general principles of, 1085, 1085*f*
hemodialysis, 1084, 1085*b*, **1087-1091**
complications of, 1096*b*
for elevated potassium levels, 1073, 1073*b*
nonpharmacologic interventions for sleep in patients on, 1080*b*
peritoneal, 1084, 1085*b*, **1085-1087**
complications of, 1096*b*
Dialyzers, 1089
Diaphragm, 456
Diaphragmatic (abdominal) breathing, 569
Diaphragmatic hernia, 904
Diaphysis, 1447
Diarrhea, **929-932**
acute, 929
acute infectious
causes and manifestations of, 930*b*
nursing management of, **932-933**
in cancer, 251*b*-252*b*, 254
drug therapy for, 931-932, 931*b*
interprofessional care for, 931-932
nursing assessment in, 932*b*
nursing management of, 867*b*
osmotic, 931
secretory, 930
with tube feedings, 867*b*
Diarthrodial (synovial) joints, 1448, 1448*f*-1449*f*
movements of, 1454, 1455*b*
Diastole, 658-660
Diastolic blood pressure, 662
Diastolic failure, 738
Diazepam (Valium), 326*b*, 1378, 1385*b*
Dichlorphenamide (Daranide), 381*b*
Diclofenac, 1521*b*-1522*b*, 1523
Diclofenac K (Cataflam), 111*b*, 118, 1521*b*-1522*b*
Diet(s)
for chronic kidney disease, 1082, 1082*b*
culturally competent, 856
for diabetes mellitus, 1133
for elevated potassium levels, 1073*b*
and gastritis, 909
gluten-free, 967, 967*b*
Halal practices, 856
health impact of well-balanced diet, 855*b*
heart-healthy food preparation, 749
high-calorie, high-protein, 863*b*
for hypertension, 688
for hyperthyroidism, 1166
incomplete, 857-858
ketogenic, 1379
Kosher practices, 856
low-sodium, 749*b*
for postmenopausal women, 1249
therapeutic lifestyle changes, 709*b*
tips for, 709*b*
vegetarian, **855-856**
for weight loss, 882*b*
Dietary Approaches to Stop Hypertension (DASH) diet, 688, 693-694, 749
Dietary Guidelines for Americans 2010, 861
Dietary Reference Intake (DRI) recommendations, 855, 858*b*
Dietary supplements
assessment of use of, 38*b*
iron, 610-611, 611*b*
for menopausal symptoms, 1249, 1249*b*
Dietary supplements *(Continued)*
for osteoporosis, 1512
that may affect blood glucose, 1141*b*
Dietitians, 10*b*
role in caring for chronic venous insufficiency and venous ulcers, 827*b*
role in caring for diabetic patients, 1152*b*
role in caring for the patient with hypertension, 696*b*
role in caring for VTE patients, 824*b*
role in nasogastric and gastric tubes and enteral feedings, 867*b*
role in wound care, 170*b*
Differential count, 599-600
Diffuse axonal injury, 1327
Diffuse parenchymal lung disease, 528
Diffusion, 271, 272*f*, 1085
facilitated, 272
Diffusion limitation, 1611-1612, 1611*f*
Digestion, 834, **835-836**
physiology of, 835-836
regulation of, 877, 877*f*
Digestive system, 833. *See also* Gastrointestinal system
Digital immigrants, 55*b*
Digital mammography, 1205
Digital natives, 55*b*
Digital photography, 175*b*
Digital technology, 53*f*, 55
Digitalis, 745*b*, 746, 748
Digitalis toxicity, 748
Digoxin
drug alerts, 748*b*, 787*b*
for dysrhythmia, 771*b*
for heart failure, 745*b*, 748
Dihydropyridines, 691*b*-693*b*
Dilantin (phenytoin), 116*b*, 771*b*
Dilated cardiomyopathy, **796-797**, 797*b*, 797*f*
etiology and pathophysiology of, 796-797, 796*b*
nursing and interprofessional management of, **798**
Dilated cardiomypathy, 738-739
Dilation and curettage (D&C), 1198*t*-1201*t*
Dilaudid (hydromorphone), 112, 113*b*-114*b*, 326*b*
Diltiazem (Cardizem, Cartia XT, Tiazac)
for dysrhythmia, 771*b*
mechanism of action, 715*b*-716*b*
for pulmonary hypertension, 532*b*
for voiding dysfunction, 1059*b*
Diltiazem extended release (Cardizem LA), 691*b*-693*b*
Dilutional hyponatremia, 442
Dimenhydrinate (Dramamine), 895*b*
Dimethyl fumarate (Tecfidera), 1385*b*, 1386
Diovan (valsartan), 691*b*-693*b*, 715*b*-716*b*, 745*b*
Dipeptidyl peptidase-4 (DPP-4) inhibitors, 1130, 1131*b*, 1136*f*
Diphenhydramine
in general anesthesia, 326*b*
for nausea and vomiting, 895*b*
for Parkinson's disease, 1391*b*
for rhinitis and sinusitis, 479*b*-480*b*
Diphenoxylate with atropine (Lomotil), 931*b*
Diphtheria, 216*b*
Dipivefrin (Propine), 381*b*
Diplopia, 357*b*, 597*b*-598*b*, 1308*b*-1309*b*
Diprivan (propofol), 325*b*
Dipstick (Albustix, Combistix) test, 1025*t*-1030*t*
Direct antihuman globulin test, 1659*b*
Direct Coombs test, 1659*b*
Direct thrombin inhibitors
for angina and ACS, 715*b*-716*b*
for VTE, 820*b*, 821
Directives to physicians (DTPs), 135, 136*b*
Dirty bombs, 1645
Disability survey, 1631*b*-1632*b*, 1632
Disaster medical assistance teams (DMATs), 1646
Disaster nursing, **1628-1648**
Disc herniation, 1504-1505, 1505*b*
Discectomy, 1506
Discharge
after ambulatory surgery, 344-345
from PACU, 344*b*, **344**
planning for, 345-346
Discharge, in ear canal, 365*b*
Discharge teaching, 345*b*
Disciplinary action, 1416*b*
Discomfort
fear of, 303
postoperative, **339**
Disconjugate gaze, 1306
Discrimination, 21
Disease-modifying antirheumatic drugs, 1521*b*-1522*b*, 1523, 1528
Diskography, 1457*t*-1459*t*
Dislocation, 1456*b*, **1464-1465**, 1465*f*
nursing and interprofessional management of, **1465**
Disopyramide (Norpace), 771*b*
Disorganization, 133, 133*f*
Disorganized thinking, 1416*b*
Dissecting aneurysm, 814
Disseminated gonococcal infections, 1230, 1231*f*
Disseminated intravascular coagulation, **629-631**
acute, 630*b*
bleeding manifestations of, 629*f*-630*f*, 630
interprofessional care for, 630-631
laboratory findings in, 623*b*, 630*b*
nursing diagnoses for, 631
nursing management of, **631**
risk factors for, 629*b*
screen for, 1590*t*
sites of action for therapies for, 630, 631*f*
thrombotic manifestations of, 630
Dissociative anesthesia, 323-324, 325*b*
Distraction, **122**
Distributive shock, 1588*b*, 1590-1593, 1591*b*
Ditropan (oxybutynin), 1059*b*
Ditropan XL (oxybutynin), 1385*b*
Diuretics
for cirrhosis, 993*b*
for heart failure, 745, 745*b*, 747
for hypertension, 690, 691*b*-694*b*
that cause photosensitivity, 408*b*
Diuril (chlorothiazide), 691*b*-693*b*
Diversity, **4**
cultural, **24**, 24*f*
Diverticula
esophageal, **907-908**, 907*f*
gastrointestinal, 963, 963*f*
urethral, **1040**
Diverticulitis, **963-964**, 963*f*
clinical manifestations of, 963
complications of, 963, 964*f*
diagnostic studies, 963-964
interprofessional care for, 964*b*
nursing and interprofessional management of, **933**
Diverticulosis, **963-964**
interprofessional care for, 964*b*
nursing and interprofessional management of, **933**
Dizziness, 361
DNA (deoxyribonucleic acid), **179-180**, 180*f*
DNA finger printing, 186
DNA microarrays (DNA chips), 186
DNP (doctor of nursing practice) degree, 3

DNR (do-not-resuscitate) orders, 135, 136*b*, 794*b*
out-of-hospital DNR, 136
Dobutamine
for heart failure, 745*b*, 746
for shock, 1599*b*
Doctor of nursing practice (DNP) degree, 3
Documentation
asthma action plans, 554-555, 555*f*
electronic health records (EHRs), **14-15**, 15*f*
for end-of-life care, 136*b*
PACU hand-off report, 331*b*
of pain assessment, 110
of physical examination, 40
postanesthesia hand-off report, 331
Dofetilide (Tikosyn), 771*b*
Dog bites, 1642
Dolasetron (Anzemet), 326*b*, 895*b*
Doll's eye reflex, 1324
Dolophine (methadone), 112*b*-114*b*, 326*b*
Donepezil (Aricept), 1390
Donnagel-PG, 931*b*
Donor nephrectomy
laparoscopic, 1094
open (conventional), 1094
Donor sources, 1093-1094
Do-not-resuscitate (DNR) orders, 135, 136*b*, 794*b*
out-of-hospital DNR, 136
Dopamine
endogenous, 1107
exogenous
for heart failure, 745*b*-746*b*, 746
for shock, 1599*b*
Dopamine receptor agonists
for diabetes mellitus, 1131*b*, 1132
for Parkinson's disease, 1391*b*
Dopaminergics, 1391*b*
Doppler ultrasound, 671, 672*f*
transcranial, 1310*t*-1312*t*
Dorsal horn processing, 105
Dorsiflexion, 1455*b*
Dorzolamide (Trusopt), 381*b*
Double amputee, 1489*f*
Double effect, 137
Double-barreled stomas, 959, 959*f*
Doubling time, 236
Dowager's hump, 1456*b*, 1485, 1511
Down syndrome, 1401*b*
Doxazosin (Cardura)
for hypertension, 691*b*-693*b*, 695*b*
for voiding dysfunction, 1059*b*
Doxepin, 116*b*
Doxorubicin, 1217*b*
Doxycycline (vibramycin)
for arthritis, 1521*b*-1522*b*
for chlamydial infections, 1229, 1229*b*
Drainage
autogenic, 578
chest systems, 525*b*
pleural, **522-524**, 525*b*
postural, 570
percussion for, 569, **570**, 570*f*
vibration for, 569, **570**
from surgical wounds, 343
from tubes, drains, and catheters, 343, 344*b*
water-seal, 525*b*
Dressings, 168
chest tube, 525*b*
types of, 169*b*
Dressler syndrome, 721, 784
Dronabinol (Marinol), 153
for nausea and vomiting, 894, 895*b*
Dronedarone (Multaq), 771*b*
Drop attacks, 1376
Droperidol, 895*b*
Droplet precautions, 218, 218*b*
Drowning, 1639
Drucker, Peter, 2
Drug Abuse Screening Test (DAST-10), 154, 155*b*
Drug allergy check, 442*b*
Drug metabolism, 72-73, 73*f*
Drug reactions
asthma, 540
skin reactions, 418*b*
Drug resistance
antimicrobial-resistant organisms, 216, 216*b*
patient & caregiver teaching to decrease risk for, 216, 217*b*
Drug therapy. *See also specific drugs*
adjuvant, 1216
cardiovascular effects of, 664*b*
drugs that cause photosensitivity, 408*b*
drugs that restrict lipoprotein production, 709-710
inhalation devices for, 551-552
lipid-lowering, 709-710
neoadjuvant, 1216
nephrotoxic agents, 1020*b*
nonprescription combination drugs, 553
nutrient interactions, 858
risk reduction, 225-226
topical medications, 423*b*, **423-424**
Drug tolerance, 122-123, 124*b*
Drug use. *See also* Addiction; Substance abuse
by older adults, 72-73, 74*b*
Drug-induced liver diseases, **984**
Drug-induced liver injury, 984
Drug-induced photosensitivity, 408-409, 409*f*
Drusen, 378
Dry desquamation, 255, 255*f*
Dry eye disorders, 357*b*, **373**
Dry powder inhalers, 551, 552*b*, 552*f*
Dual-energy X-ray absorptiometry, 1457*t*-1459*t*
Duchenne muscular dystrophy, 1501*b*-1502*b*, 1502
Duct system, 838*f*
Ductal carcinoma, 1210
invasive (infiltrating), 1210-1211
Ductal carcinoma in situ, 1210
Ductal ectasia, 1206*b*, 1208
Ductus (vas) deferens, 1184-1185, 1185*f*
Dulaglutide (Trulicity), 1131*b*-1132*b*, 1132
Dulera (mometasone furoate/formoterol fumarate), 548*b*-549*b*
Duloxetine (Cymbalta), 116*b*
Dumping syndrome, 886-887
postgastrectomy, 917-918, 918*b*
Duodenal ulcers, 910*f*, 911*b*, **912**, 912*f*
DuoNeb (ipratropium/albuterol), 548*b*-549*b*
Duplex (color-flow) imaging, 671, 672*f*, 673*t*-677*t*
venous Doppler thermography, 1457*t*-1459*t*
Dura mater, 1300
Durable power of attorney for health care, 135, 1153*b*
Duraclon (clonidine), 116*b*
Duragesic (fentanyl patch), 113*b*-114*b*, 118-119, 118*b*
Dust, occupational, 558
Dutasteride (Avodart), 1059*b*
Dyrenium (triamterene), 691*b*-693*b*
Dysarthria, 1308*b*-1309*b*
hypokinetic, 1388
after stroke, 1351
Dysgeusia, 254, 262
Dyskinesia, 1308*b*-1309*b*
Dyslipidemia, 1077, 1082. *See also* Hyperlipidemia
Dysmenorrhea, **1245-1246**
Dyspareunia, 1194, 1546
Dyspepsia, 846*b*-847*b*, 901
Dysphagia, 846*b*-847*b*, 898, 1308*b*-1309*b*
in cancer, 254
at end of life, 140*b*-141*b*
Dysphasia, 1308*b*-1309*b*, 1351
Dysplastic nevus, 412*b*, **413**, 413*f*, 427*b*
Dysplastic nevus syndrome, 413
Dyspnea, 456
at end of life, 140*b*-141*b*
in heart failure, 742
paroxysmal nocturnal, 742-743
Dysreflexia, autonomic, 1431
Dysrhythmias, **757-779**, 1113*b*-1114*b*
case study, 778*b*
causes of, 762*b*
characteristics of, 764*b*
electrophysiologic mechanisms of, 760-761
emergency management of, 763*b*
evaluation of, 761-762
in heart failure, 743
junctional, **767**
after myocardial infarction, 720
postoperative, 337
treatment of, **757-775**
types of, 763-771
Dystonia, 1306
Dysuria, 1025*b*

E

Ear protection, 388*b*
Eardrum. *See* Tympanic membrane
Eating
assistive devices for, 1361, 1361*f*
mindless, 878
regulation of, 877, 877*f*
in Sjögren's syndrome, 1546*b*
Eating disorders, **871-872**
in Alzheimer's disease, 1412
Internet-based interventions for, 871*b*
Ebola, 214*b*, 215
Ecchymoses (bruising), 403*b*, 597*b*-598*b*, 598, 623
in hemophilia, 626-627, 627*f*
in light- and dark-skinned persons, 404*b*
Eccrine sweat glands, 396
Echinacea, 480*b*
Echocardiography, **671-672**, 673*t*-677*t*
contrast, 671, 673*t*-677*t*
motion-mode (M-mode), 671, 673*t*-677*t*
pharmacologic, 673*t*-677*t*
stress, 671, 673*t*-677*t*
transesophageal, 671-672, 673*t*-677*t*
two-dimensional (2-D), 671, 672*f*, 673*t*-677*t*
Echovirus, 214*b*
Economic factors, 25*b*
Ectopic pregnancy, **1247**, 1247*f*
laparoscopic treatment of, 1248, 1248*f*
nursing and interprofessional management of, **1247-1248**
Ectropion, 357*b*
Edarbi (azilsartan), 691*b*-693*b*
Edema, 273-274, 1113*b*-1114*b*
in acute respiratory distress syndrome, 1620, 1620*f*
alveolar, 741
angioedema, 199, 747
cerebral, 1316-1317
in fracture healing, 1469*b*
in heart failure, 743
interstitial, 741
laryngeal, 333*b*
lymphedema, 592, 1214, 1215*f*
myxedema, 1113*b*-1114*b*, 1169, 1169*f*
papilledema, 376, 1308*b*-1309*b*
periorbital, 1042*b*
peripheral, 988-990
pitting, 668*b*
postoperative, 333*b*, 334
pulmonary, **529**, 741-742
chest examination findings in, 468*b*
postoperative, 333*b*, 334

Edematous pancreatitis, 999, 999*f*
Edoxaban (Savaysa), 820*b*
Education
culturally appropriate, 53*b*
health disparities, 20
pain, **123-124**
patient and caregiver teaching, **46-59**
STI-related programs, 1238-1239
text messaging and diabetes, 1135*b*
Effient (prasugrel), 715*b*-716*b*
Effusion
otitis media with, 384
pleural, **527-528**
Egophony, 467*b*-468*b*
ehealth literacy, 53
Ejaculate, 1185
Ejaculation, 1190
retrograde, 1274
Ejection fraction, 671, 737
Elastic recoil, 456
Elbow and shoulder arthroplasty, 1491-1492
Eldepril (selegiline), 1390, 1391*b*
Elder abuse, 1414*b*
Elder mistreatment, **66-67**
nursing assessment and intervention for, 67*b*
risk factors for, 66
types of, 67*b*
Elective phlebotomy, 652
Elective surgery, 301, 425-426
Electrical burns, **431**, 431*f*
emergency management of, 435*b*
strategies to reduce injury, 430*b*
Electrical stimulation
for bone growth, **1474**
for urinary incontinence, 1057*b*
Electrocardiography (ECG), **660**, 667*f*, **671**, 673*t*-677*t*, **757-760**
in acute coronary syndrome, 721, **775-777**, 776*b*, 776*f*-777*f*
ambulatory, 673*t*-677*t*
artifacts, 760*f*
continuous monitoring, 762
event monitoring, 671, 673*t*-677*t*
Holter monitoring, 762
HR estimation from, 759, 760*f*
lead placement, 758, 759*f*
loop recorder for, 671, 673*t*-677*t*
normal waveforms, 759*f*-761*f*
patient monitoring, 777
recording leads, 758*f*
signal-averaged, 673*t*-677*t*, 762
time and voltage on, 758-759, 759*f*
waveforms and values, 760, 761*b*
wireless monitoring, 760*b*
Electrocoagulation, **422**
Electrocochleography, 365*t*-366*t*
Electrodessication, **422**
Electroencephalography (EEG), 1310*t*-1312*t*
Electrohydraulic lithotripsy, 1048
Electrolarynx, 493, 493*f*
Electrolytes, **271**. *See also* Fluid and electrolyte balance; Fluid and electrolyte imbalance
in chronic kidney disease, 1077
composition of, 271
effects of stress on, 275*f*
in increased ICP, 1325
measurement of, 271
mechanisms controlling movement of, 271-273
in older adults, 276
in parenteral nutrition, 869
preoperative review of, 306
serum
normal values, 272*b*
in shock, 1590*t*
Electromagnetic radiation, 249
Electromyography (EMG), 1025*t*-1030*t*, 1310*t*-1312*t*
Electron beam computed tomography (EBCT), 673*t*-677*t*, 678, 678*f*
Electroneurography, 1310*t*-1312*t*
Electronic cigarettes, 146
Electronic health records (EHRs), **14-15**, 15*f*
Electronic ICU, 1554
Electronystagmography, 365*t*-366*t*
Electrophysiology study, 673*t*-677*t*, **679**, 762
Electrosurgery
loop electrosurgical excision procedure (LEEP), 1198*t*-1201*t*
safety considerations, 321, 321*f*
Electrothermoplasty, intradiscal (IDET), 1506
Electrovaporization, transurethral, of prostate (TUVP), 1272*b*
Elevation
for inflammation, 165
for sprains and strains, 1464
Elevation pallor, 803-804
Eligard (leuprolide), 1280*b*
Elimination, 834, **836-837**
assessment of, 37*b*, 38
Elimination problems
in Alzheimer's disease, 1413
in stroke, 1352
Eliquis (apixaban), 820*b*
EM, 1457*t*-1459*t*
Emancipated minors, 310
Emboli, 780-781
Embolic stroke, 1348*b*, 1348*f*, 1349
Embolism
fat embolism syndrome, **1480**
pulmonary, **529-531**, 529*f*
nursing management of, **531**
postoperative, 333*b*
venous. *See* Venous thromboembolism
Embolization, 808
Emend (aprepitant), 895*b*
Emergence delirium, 338
Emergency, 1645
Emergency assessment, 40, 44*b*
primary survey, 1630-1632, 1631*b*
secondary survey, 1632-1634, 1633*b*
Emergency care, 1628, **1628-1636**
acute care and evaluation, 1634
cold-related emergencies, **1637-1639**
comfort measures, 1632
environmental emergencies, **1636-1646**
heat-related emergencies, **1636-1637**
for older adults, 1635-1636
Emergency management tables, 1629*b*
Emergency Medical Treatment and Active Labor Act (EMTALA), 1482*b*
Emergency preparedness, 1645-1646
Emergency response plans, 1646
Emergency response system (ERS), 1650
Emergency Severity Index (ESI), 1629, 1629*b*
Emergency surgery, 301
Emotional reactions
in acute coronary syndrome, 728
atypical responses, 1364
in burns, 448*b*
Emotional support, 1604
Emotion-focused coping, 83*b*
Empacho, 29*b*
Empagliflozin (Jardiance), 1131*b*
Emphysema, 557
Empyema, 456, 503, 527
Enablex (darifenacin), 1059*b*
Enbrel (etanercept), 195*b*, 1529
Encephalitis, 1339*b*, **1341-1342**
Enchondroma, 1500*b*
End of life, 132
case study, 142*b*
palliative care for, **129-144**
physical manifestations of, 132, 132*b*
psychosocial manifestations of, 132-133, 132*b*
spiritual distress at, 142*b*
End stoma, 958
Endarterectomy, 806
Endemic fungal infections, 512, 512*b*
Endoanal (endorectal) ultrasound, 971
Endocarditis
infective, **780-782**, 1042*b*
risk factors for, 781*b*
Endocardium, 658, 780
Endocervical gonorrhea, 1230, 1230*f*
Endocervix, 1186
Endocrine diseases, **1156-1183**
in cirrhosis, 987
corticosteroid therapy for, 1180*b*
gender differences in, 1163*b*
in obesity, 879*f*
Endocrine glands, **1102**, 1103*f*, 1104*b*
Endocrine hormones, 1104*b*
Endocrine system
abnormalities, 1113*b*-1114*b*
assessment, **1108-1112**
assessment checklist, 1114*b*
blood pressure regulation by, 683
case study, 1109*b*, 1111*b*-1112*b*, 1118*b*
diagnostic studies of, **1114**, 1115*t*-1118*t*
health history, 1110*b*
in older adults, 1108*b*, **1108**
physical examination of, 1111-1112, 1112*b*
preoperative review of, 306
stress response, 79-80
structures and functions of, **1102-1108**
End-of-life care, **132-135**. *See also* Hospice care
for COPD patients, 575
culturally competent care, **134-135**
documents used in, 136*b*
ethical/legal dilemmas, 137*b*
for family caregivers, 142
for heart failure patients, 752-753
legal and ethical issues, **135-137**
for nurses, 142
nursing management, **137-139**, 138*b*
physical care, 139, 140*b*-141*b*
psychosocial care, 138-139, 138*b*, 139*f*
spiritual needs in, 134, 134*f*
Endoleaks, 812
Endometrial cancer, **1257-1258**
cultural & ethnic health disparities, 1256*b*
interprofessional care for, 1257-1258
Endometriosis, **1253-1254**
drug therapy for, 1253
interprofessional care for, 1253-1254, 253*b*
nursing management of, **1254**
sites of, 1253, 1253*f*
surgical therapy for, 1253-1254
Endometrium, 1186
Endomysium, 1448
Endophthalmitis, 382
Endorectal ultrasound, 971
Endoscopic biopsy, 243
Endoscopic carpal tunnel release, 1466
Endoscopic gastrostomy, percutaneous, 865-866
Endoscopic retrograde cholangiopancreatography, 847*t*-850*t*, 851
Endoscopic sleeve gastroplasty, 885
Endoscopic sphincterotomy, 1007, 1007*f*
Endoscopic ultrasound, 847*t*-850*t*

Endoscopy, **467-471**, 469*t*-471*t*, 1025*t*-1030*t*
capsule, 851, 851*f*
gastrointestinal, 847*t*-850*t*, 851, 851*f*
video capsule, 847*t*-850*t*, 851*f*
Endothelial damage, 817
Endothelial dysfunction, 685
Endothelin, 739
Endothelin receptor antagonists, 532*b*
Endotracheal intubation, 1569
complications of, 1573
fostering comfort and communication, 1573
maintaining correct placement, 1571
maintaining proper cuff inflation, 1571
maintaining skin integrity, 1572-1573
maintaining tube patency, 1571-1572
monitoring oxygenation and ventilation, 1571
nasal, 1569-1570
oral care, 1572-1573
procedure, 1570
tube placement, 1571*b*
unplanned extubation, 1573*b*
Endotracheal tubes, 1569-1570, 1569*f*
Endoureterotomy, 1050
Endourologic procedures, 1047
Endovascular therapy
aneurysm repair, 812, 812*f*
aortic dissection repair, 815
for ischemic stroke, 1355
for TIAs and stroke prevention, 1353-1354
End-stage kidney disease
RIFLE classification of, 1071*b*
sleep disturbances during, 92*b*
End-tidal CO_2 ($PetCO_2$) (capnography) monitoring, 331, 469*t*-471*t*
Energy conservation, 1524*b*
Energy costs, 731, 731*b*
Energy (calorie) requirements, 854, 855*b*
Energy source, 1449-1450
Enoxaparin (Lovenox), 715*b*-716*b*, 820*b*
ENROUTE device, 1355
Entacapone (Comtan), 1390, 1391*b*
***Entamoeba histolytica* infection**, 930*b*
Entecavir (Baraclude), 980
Enteral nutrition, 864*f*, **865-868**
feeding tube misconnections, 868
feeding tube placement locations, 865-866, 865*f*
nursing management of, 867*b*
for older adults, 868-869
tips to help decrease misconnections, 868*b*
Enterobacteriaceae, carbapenem-resistant, 216
Enterococci, vancomycin-resistant, 216, 216*b*
Entitlement to treatment, 1482*b*
Entresto (valsartan/sacubitril), 745*b*, 747-748
Entropion, 357*b*
Enucleation, **382-383**
Enuresis, 1025*b*
Environmental control, 1631*b*, 1632
Environmental emergencies, **1636-1646**
Environmental hazards, **407-409**
Environmental lung diseases, **513**
Environmental noise, 388, 389*f*
Environmental noise control, **388**
Enzalutamide (Xtandi), 1280*b*
Enzymatic debridement, 170*b*
Eosinophilic esophagitis, **907**
Eosinophils, 590, 1659*b*
Ependymal cells, 1295
Ependymoma, 1333*b*
Epicardial pacing, 775
Epicondylitis, lateral, 1456*b*
Epidemic keratoconjunctivitis, 372
Epidemics, 480-481
Epidermal growth factor receptor-2, 257, 258*b*
Epidermis, **394-395**, 395*f*, 431-432
Epidermophyton, 215*b*
Epididymis, 1184, 1185*f*
Epididymitis, **1284**, 1284*f*
chlamydial, 1228-1229, 1229*f*
Epidural analgesia, 340
Epidural anesthesia (epidural block), **325-327**, 327*f*
Epidural hematoma, 1328-1329, 1328*f*
Epigenetics, 183
Epiglottis, 453-454
Epilepsy, **1374-1379**
case study, 1396*b*
with headache, 1396*b*
idiopathic generalized, 1374
interprofessional care for, 1377-1379, 1377*b*
medically refractory, 1379
nursing assessment in, 1380*b*
nursing diagnoses related to, 1379
nursing management of, **1379-1382**
sudden unexplained or unexpected death in (SUDEP), 1376-1377
surgical therapy for, 1379
Epimysium, 1448
Epinephrine (Adrenalin)
for glaucoma, 381*b*
for hypersensitivity reactions, 202
for shock, 1599*b*
Epinephrine (adrenaline), 1104*b*, 1107, 1661*b*
Epiphyseal plate, 1447
Epiphysis, 1447
Epistaxis, **476**, 597*b*-598*b*, 1486*b*
nursing and interprofessional management of, **476-477**
Epistaxis balloon, 477, 477*f*
Epivir (lamivudine), 980
Eplerenone (Inspra)
for heart failure, 745*b*, 748
for hypertension, 691*b*-693*b*
Epoetin alfa (Epogen, Procrit), 195*b*
Epoprostenol (Flolan, Veletri), 532*b*
Eprosartan (Teveten), 691*b*-693*b*
Epstein-Barr virus, 214*b*
Eptifibatide (Integrilin), 715*b*-716*b*
Equianalgesic dosing, 117-118, 117*b*
Equipment, 40, 40*b*
Erb's point, 667
Erectile dysfunction, **1286-1288**
interprofessional care for, 1287-1288, 1287*b*
nursing management of, **1288**
risk factors for, 1287*b*
after spinal cord injury, 1434
Erectile mechanism problems, **1283-1284**
Erection
psychogenic, 1434
reflex erections, 1434
Erectogenic drugs, 1271, 1288
Erosions, penile, 1198*b*
Eructation, 846*b*-847*b*
Erysipelas, 414*b*
Erythema, 403*b*
in light- and dark-skinned persons, 404*b*
nonblanchable, 173*b*
palmar, 986
penile, 1198*b*
scrotal, 1198*b*
vulvar, 1197*b*
Erythema marginatum, 789
Erythema migrans, 1534, 1534*f*
Erythrocyte sedimentation rate, 602*t*, 1659*b*
Erythrocytes, 588-589, 1659*b*
Erythroleukemia, 612, 612*b*
Erythromelalgia, 621
Erythroplasia, 898
Erythropoiesis, 588-589, 609
nutrients for, 610*b*
Erythropoietin, 588-589, 602*t*
for cancer, 260*b*
clinical uses, 195*b*
Escharotomy, 437, 437*f*
Escherichia coli, 214*b*
***Escherichia coli* infection**
diarrhea in, 930*b*
urinary tract infection, 1033
***Escherichia coli* O157:H7 infection**
diarrhea in, 929-930, 930*b*
food poisoning, 925*b*, **925-926**
Eskimos, 63
Esmolol (Brevibloc)
for dysrhythmia, 771*b*
for hypertension, 691*b*-693*b*
Esomeprazole (Nexium), 903*b*
Esophageal achalasia, **908**, 908*f*
Esophageal cancer, **905-906**
acute care for, 906-907
ambulatory care for, 907
chemotherapy for, 906
cultural & ethnic health disparities, 898*b*
endoscopic therapy for, 906
health promotion for, 906
interprofessional care for, 905-906, 905*b*
nursing diagnoses, 906
nursing management of, **906-907**
nutritional therapy for, 906
postoperative care in, 907
preoperative care in, 906-907
radiation therapy for, 906
surgical therapy for, 905-906
targeted therapy for, 906
Esophageal disorders, **900-908**
Esophageal diverticula, **907-908**, 907*f*
Esophageal hernia, 904
Esophageal speech, 493
Esophageal strictures, **908**
Esophageal ulcerations, 901*f*
Esophageal varices, **908**, 988, 991-992
Esophagectomy, 905-906
Esophagitis, 901, 901*f*
in cancer, 251*b*-252*b*
eosinophilic, **907**
medication-induced, 905
Esophagoenterostomy, 840*b*, 905-906
Esophagogastroduodenoscopy, 847*t*-850*t*, 913, 913*f*
Esophagogastrostomy, 840*b*, 905-906
Esophagojejunostomy, 920, 920*f*
Esophagus, 835
abnormalities, 846*b*-847*b*
Barrett's, 901
in older adults, 840*b*
Esotropia, 373
Essential fatty acids deficiency, 399*b*
Estradiol, 1104*b*, 1198*t*-1201*t*
Estrogen
endogenous, 1104*b*
regulation of reproductive system by, 1188-1189
urine values, 1661*b*
exogenous, for cancer, 259*b*
Estrogen cream (Premarin), 1059*b*
Estrogen deficiency, 1248, 1248*b*
Estrogen receptor blockers, 259*b*, 1217, 1217*b*
Estrogen receptor modulators, 259*b*, 1217*b*, 1218
Estrogen receptors, 1212-1213
Estrogen replacement therapy, 1513
Estrogen vaginal ring (Estring), 1059*b*
Estrogen vaginal tablets (Vagifem), 1059*b*
Etanercept (Enbrel), 195*b*, 1521*b*-1522*b*, 1529
Ethambutol (Myambutol), 509*b*
Ethical/legal issues
advance directives, 575*b*
Board of Nursing disciplinary action, 1416*b*
brain death, 1331*b*
competence, 754*b*
confidentiality and HIPAA, 1239*b*

Ethical/legal issues *(Continued)*
do not resuscitate, 794*b*
durable power of attorney for health care, 1153*b*
in end-of-life care, **135-137**, 137*b*
entitlement to treatment, 1482*b*
family presence and visitation in the adult ICU, 1558*b*
in genetic testing, 185*b*
good samaritans, 1646*b*
health disparities, 19*b*
individual versus public health protection, 226*b*
informed consent, 310*b*
medical futility, 266*b*
for older adults, **69**
in pain management, **124-126**, 619*b*
patient adherence, 510*b*
preparation for surgery, 309-310
rationing, 995*b*
religious beliefs, 649*b*
resource allocation, 1093*b*
right to refuse treatment, 1424*b*
scope and standards of practice, 770*b*
in social networking, 5*b*
withdrawing treatment, 1097*b*
withholding treatment, 1338*b*
Ethnic groups, 22*b*
Ethnicity, **19-20**
Ethnocentrism, 23
Ethnogeriatrics, 66
Ethylene glycol poisoning, 1643*b*
Etomidate (Amidate), 325*b*
European Americans
cultural characteristics of, 22*b*
and medications, 28
older adults, 63
Euthanasia, 136
Evaluation
emergency nursing, 1634
nursing, 5, 6*f*
Everolimus (Afinitor), 1217*b*, 1218
Everolimus (Zortress), 211*b*
Eversion, 1455*b*
Evidence-based practice (EBP), 6*b*, **15-16**
culturally appropriate education, 53*b*
hierarchy of evidence for, 15, 15*f*
steps of, 15-16, 15*b*
Evil eye (or *mal ojo*), 27-28
Evisceration, 167*b*
Evista (raloxifene), 1217*b*, 1513
Evoked potentials, 1310*t*-1312*t*
Evolocumab (Repatha), 711*b*
Ewing's sarcoma, 1500*b*
Excess granulation tissue, 167*b*
Excision, **422**
Excitability, 761
Excoriations, 402*b*, 597*b*-598*b*
Exelon (rivastigmine), 1390
Exemestane (Aromasin), 1217*b*
Exenatide (Byetta), 1131*b*-1132*b*, 1132
Exenatide extended-release (Bydureon), 1131*b*, 1132
Exercise(s)
as coping strategy, 82*b*
for diabetes patients, 1134-1135, 1142*b*
instructions, 1142*b*
patient & caregiver teaching, 1134*b*
for fatigue in chronic fatigue syndrome, 1549*b*
and hematologic cancer, 643*b*
neck, 1508*b*
for osteoarthritis, 1519-1520
for pain, **121**
pelvic floor muscle (Kegel), 1037, 1057*b*-1058*b*
for peripheral arterial disease, 805
Exercise(s) *(Continued)*
postoperative, for masetctomy and lumpectomy patients, 1219, 1220*f*
for rheumatoid arthritis, 1531-1532
and skin, 409
for sleep in dialysis patients, 1080*b*
and sport injuries, 1476*b*
for stroke risk reduction, 1347
for weight loss, 883
Exercise stress perfusion imaging, 672, 673*t*-677*t*
Exercise testing, 469*t*-471*t*, **671**, 673*t*-677*t*, 762
Exercise-induced asthma, 539
Exercise-induced bronchospasm, 539
Exercise-induced headaches, 1370*b*
Exophthalmos, 357*b*, 1113*b*-1114*b*
Exostosis, 365*b*
Exotropia, 373
Expedited Partner Therapy (EPT), 1230
Expiratory reserve volume (ERV), 473*b*
Exploratory surgery, 301
Explosive devices, 1645
Exposure, 1631*b*, 1632
Extension, 1455*b*
Extensor plantar response, 1308*b*-1309*b*
External beam radiation therapy, 250, 1216, 1279
External counterpulsation (EECP), 718
External ear, **360**, 360*f*
abnormalities, 365*b*
malignancy of, **384**
in older adults, 361*b*
physical examination of, 364
External ear canal
cerumen in, **384**
foreign bodies in, **384**
physical examination of, 364
External ear problems, **383-384**
External fixation, **1473**
External fixators, 1473, 1473*f*
External genitalia
female, 1187, 1187*f*
male, 1185
normal, 1196*b*
physical examination of, 1196
External otitis, **383**
nursing and interprofessional management of, **383-384**
patient & caregiver teaching for prevention of, 384*b*
External rotation, 1455*b*
Extracapsular cataract extraction procedure, 375
Extracellular fluid, 271
Extracellular space, 271
Extracorporeal membrane oxygenation, 1578
Extracorporeal shock wave lithotripsy, 1048
Extraocular disorders, **370-373**
Extraocular movement, 1306*f*
Extraocular muscles, 352, 357*b*, 358
Extravasation injury, 246, 246*f*
Extremities
abnormalities in, 668*b*
physical examination of, 1112
secondary survey, 1634
Extubation, 1582
Exudate
formation of, 162
types of, 162*b*
Eye(s)
abnormalities, 1308*b*-1309*b*
external structures and functions of, 352, 352*f*
inflammation and infection of, **370-372**
internal structures and functions of, 352
Eye care, 370*b*
Eye injury, 371*b*
Eye surgery, 376*b*
Eye trauma, **370**, 371*b*
Eyeball, **350**, 351*f*
Eyebrows
assessment of, 358
in older adults, 353*b*
Eyeglasses, corrective, 368
Eyelashes
assessment of, 358
in older adults, 353*b*
Eyelids
abnormalities, 357*b*
assessment of, 358
in older adults, 353*b*
Ezetimibe (Zetia), 710, 711*b*

F

Face masks, 566*b*-567*b*, 566*f*
Face-lift, 425, 425*f*
FACES HF symptoms, 742
Facial assessment, 1633
Facial fractures, 1486*b*, **1486**
Facial nerve, 1305*b*
Factor VIII, 628*b*
Factor VIII deficiency, 626
Factor IX, 628*b*
Factor IX deficiency, 626
Factor 10a inhibitors, 820*b*, 821
Faith-based organizations, 889*b*
Falling out, 29*b*
Fallopian tubes, 1186
Falls
and osteoarthritis, 1520*b*
preventing, 1392*b*, 1412*b*
safety alert, 1462*b*
False aneurysms, 810, 811*f*
Falx cerebri, 1300, 1318
Familial adenomatous polyposis, 953, 953*b*
Familial Alzheimer's disease, 1402, 1402*b*
Familial disorders, 179*b*
Familial hypercholesterolemia, 704*b*
Familial prostate cancer, 1276
Family caregivers, **66**. *See also* Caregivers
in adult ICU, 1558*b*
end-of-life care for, 142
patient helpers, 1632
primary survey, 1631*b*, 1632
Family history, 189
Family members, **26-27**, 27*f*. *See also* Family caregivers
Family pedigrees, 181, 181*f*-182*f*, 188
Family presence, 1632
Family violence, 1644
Famotidine (Pepcid), 903*b*
Fareston (toremifene), 1217*b*
Farxiga (dapagliflozin), 1131*b*
Fascia, 1450
Fasciculi, 1448
Fascioscapulohumeral muscular dystrophy, 1501*b*
Fasciotomy, 1479, 1479*f*
Faslodex (fulvestrant), 1217*b*
FAST warning signs, 1346*b*
Fasting, preoperative, 309, 309*b*
Fasting blood glucose, 1115*t*-1118*t*
impaired, 1123
Fat embolism syndrome, **1480**
Fat mass and obesity-associated gene *(FTO)*, 877
Fat necrosis, 1206*b*
Fatalism, 22, 124*b*
Fatigue
alarm fatigue, 1575*b*
in cancer, 251*b*-252*b*, 253

Fatigue *(Continued)*
chronic fatigue syndrome, 1546, 1548
exercise therapy for, 1549*b*
sleep disturbances in, 92*b*
at end of life, 140*b*-141*b*
exercise therapy for, 1549*b*
in heart failure, 742
heat exhaustion, **1637**
Fats, 855
recommendations for nutrient balance, 1133
saturated, 855
Fat-soluble vitamins, 855
Fatty acids
essential, 399*b*
omega-3, 689*b*, 710*b*-711*b*
Fatty streaks, 703, 703*f*
Fear
in acute coronary syndrome, 728*b*
in burn patients, 448*b*
of disruption of life functioning, 303
at end of life, 139
preoperative, 303-304
Fecal analysis, 847*t*-850*t*, 1662*b*
Fecal incontinence, **933-934**
causes of, 933, 933*b*
interprofessional care for, 933-934
nursing management of, **934**
in spinal cord injury, 1423-1424
Fecal tests, 847*t*-850*t*
Federal Emergency Management Agency (FEMA), 1645
Feedback
negative, 1103-1104
positive, 1104
simple, 1103-1104, 1105*f*
Feeding
assistive devices for, 1361, 1361*f*
in Sjögren's syndrome, 1546*b*
after stroke, 1360*b*
Feeding tubes
enteral placement locations, 865-866, 865*f*
gastrostomy tubes, 865-866, 865*f*
jejunostomy tubes, 865-866, 865*f*
misconnection, 868
nasogastric, 865, 865*f*
nasointestinal, 865
orogastric, 865
patency of, 868
position of, 867-868
site care for, 868
teamwork & collaboration for, 867*b*
Feet. *See* Foot care
Feldene (piroxicam), 164*b*, 1521*b*-1522*b*
Felodipine, 691*b*-693*b*, 715*b*-716*b*
Felty syndrome, 1527
Female athlete triad, 871, 1194
Female breasts, 1187-1188
lactating, 1187-1188, 1188*f*
physical examination of, 1195-1196
Female external genitalia, 1187, 1187*f*
physical examination of, 1196
Female pelvis, 1187, 1202*f*
Female reproductive system
abnormalities, 1191*b*, 1197*b*
assessment of, **1191-1196**, 1196*b*
benign tumors of, **1254-1256**
cancers of, **1256-1261**
cultural & ethnic health disparities, 1256*b*
health promotion for, 1260
nursing and interprofessional management of, **1259-1261**
nursing diagnoses for, 1259-1260
radiation therapy for, 1261
case study, 1191*b*, 1195*b*-1196*b*, 1202*b*
diagnostic studies of, 1198*t*-1201*t*
lower genital tract infections, **1250-1251**
Female reproductive system *(Continued)*
normal, 1196*b*
in older adults, 1191*b*
physical examination of, 1195-1196, 1196*b*
problems of, **1242-1267**
structures and functions of, **1185-1188**, 1186*f*
surgical procedures involving, 1260-1261, 1260*b*
Female sexual response, 1190-1191
Femara (letrozole), 1217*b*
Femitus, 464
Femoral hernia, 965, 965*f*
Femoral shaft fracture, **1484-1485**
Fenofibrate (Tricor), 711*b*
Fenoldopam (Corlopam), 691*b*-693*b*
Fentanyl (Sublimaze), 113*b*-114*b*
equinanalgesic dosing, 117*b*
in general anesthesia, 326*b*
transdermal, 113*b*-114*b*, 118-119
transmucosal, 113*b*-114*b*, 118
Fentanyl patch (Duragesic), 113*b*-114*b*, 118-119, 118*b*
Ferritin, 602, 602*t*, 1655*b*-1658*b*
Fertility studies, 1198*t*-1201*t*
Fertinex (urofollitropin), 1243*b*
Fesoterodine (Toviaz), 1059*b*
Festinating gait, 1456*b*
Festination, 1389
Fetor hepaticus, 990
Fever, **163**
acute care for, 164
in myocardial infarction, 720
postoperative, 340-341, 340*b*
production of, 163, 163*f*
Fever blisters, 897*b*, 1232, 1232*f*
Fexofenadine (Allegra), 479*b*-480*b*
Fiber, dietary, 937*b*
Fiberoptic bronchoscopes, 467-471, 469*f*
Fiberoptic catheters, 1319
Fibric acid derivatives, **710**, 711*b*
Fibrin degradation products, 591-592, 601*t*, 1659*b*
Fibrin split products, 591-592, 601*t*, 630, 1659*b*
Fibrinogen, 592*b*, 601*t*, 1659*b*
Fibrinolysis, 591-592, 592*f*
Fibrin-stabilizing factor, 592*b*
Fibroadenoma, 1206*b*, **1207-1208**
Fibroblasts, 166, 395
Fibrocystic changes, 1206*b*, **1207**, 1207*f*
nursing and interprofessional management of, **1207**
Fibrocystic complex, 1207
Fibrocystic conditions, 1207
Fibrocystic disease, 1207
Fibroids, uterine, 1254
Fibromyalgia, 1546-1548
clinical features of, 1547, 1547*b*
diagnostic criteria for, 1547
interprofessional care for, 1547-1548
nursing management of, **1548**
sleep disturbances during, 92*b*
tender points, 1547*f*
Fibroscan (ultrasound elastography), 847*t*-850*t*
Fibrous or scar tissue, 166
Fibrous plaque, 703, 703*f*
Fight-or-flight response, 79, 80*f*, 1299
Filgrastim (Neupogen), 195*b*
Filtration of air, 458
Financial abuse, 67*b*
Financing, health care, 4
Finasteride (Proscar)
for BPH, 1271, 1271*b*
for voiding dysfunction, 1059*b*
Fine-needle aspiration (FNA), 243
Fine-needle aspiration biopsy, 1206
Finger joint arthroplasty, 1491
Fingernails, 396, 396*f*
Fingers: clubbing of, 467*b*-468*b*, 598, 668*b*
Fingolimod (Gilenya), 1385*b*
Firmagon (degarelix), 1280*b*
First spacing, 274
Fish oil, 689*b*
Fissures, 402*b*
anal, 846*b*-847*b*, **970**, 970*f*
Fistulas
anal, **970**, **970*f***
formation of, 167*b*
gastrointestinal, **962-963**
vaginal, **1263**, 1263*f*
FITT activity guidelines, 732, 732*b*
Fitzpatrick Classification of Skin Type, 410, 410*b*
Five *P*s of Sexual Health, 1194, 1195*b*
Five Rights of Nursing Delegation, 11-12, 12*b*
5 As, 146-147, 147*b*
5 Rs, 146-147, 147*b*
Fixation, intermaxillary, 1486, 1486*f*
Flail chest, 520*b*, **521-522**, 521*f*
Flanks, 1633-1634
Flatfoot, 1456*b*, 1509*b*
Flatulence, 836
Flatus, 836
Flavoxate (Urispas), 1059*b*
Flaxseed, 710*b*
Flecainide, 771*b*
Flexion, 1455*b*
Flolan (epoprostenol), 532*b*
Flomax (tamsulosin), 1059*b*
FloTrac sensor, 1562*f*
Flovent (fluticasone), 548*b*-549*b*
Flu (influenza), **480-481**
Fluid and electrolyte balance. *See also* Water balance
in ARDS, 1625
calculation of gain or loss, 271
in increased ICP, 1325
mechanisms controlling movement of, 271-273
movement in capillaries, 273-274, 274*f*
normal adult, 274, 274*b*
in older adults, 276
osmotic movement of, 273
preoperative review of, 306
in stress, 275*f*
Fluid and electrolyte imbalance(s)
abnormalities in, 291, 292*b*
assessment of, **290-291**
in burns, 434-436, 436*f*-437*f*
case study, 297*b*
Fluid and electrolyte replacement
IV, **292-294**
oral, **292**
Fluid compartments, 271
Fluid creep, 439
Fluid management, 1429-1430
Fluid overload, 1113*b*-1114*b*
Fluid responsiveness, 1598
Fluid restriction, 1082-1083, 1082*b*
Fluid resuscitation, 439*b*
Parkland (Baxter) formula for, 439, 439*b*
safety alert, 1598*b*
in shock, 1596-1598, 1600*b*, 1601
Fluid shifts, 273-274
Fluid spacing, **274**
Fluid therapy, **278**
in burns, 439
in shock, 1597*b*
Fluid volume deficit, **276**
causes and manifestations of, 276*b*
interprofessional care for, 276
laboratory findings, 277
nursing diagnoses, 276-277
patient safety in, 277
Fluid volume excess, **276**
causes and manifestations of, 276*b*
interprofessional care for, 276

Fluid volume excess *(Continued)*
laboratory findings, 277
nursing diagnoses, 277
Fluid volume imbalances, 276-278
cardiovascular care in, 277
fluid therapy, 278
nursing diagnoses, 276-277
nursing management of, **276-278**
patient safety in, 277
respiratory care in, 277
skin care in, 277-278
Flumazenil (Romazicon), 152
Flunisolide, 479*b*-480*b*
Fluorescein angiography, 359*t*
Fluorescent in situ hybridization, 603*t*, 604
Fluorescent treponemal antibody absorption (FTA-Abs) test, 1198*t*-1201*t*, 1236, 1659*b*
Fluoroquinolones, 509*b*
Fluorouracil, topical, 421
Flushing, 597*b*-598*b*
Flutamide, 1280*b*
Fluticasone (Arnuity Ellipta, Flonase, Flovent, Veramyst), 548*b*-549*b*
Fluticasone (Flonase, Veramyst), 479*b*-480*b*
Fluticasone/salmeterol (Advair Diskus or HFA), 548*b*-549*b*
Fluticasone/vilanterol (Breo Ellipta), 548*b*-549*b*
Flutter mucus clearance device, 570
Flutter valve, 522, 523*f*
Fluvastatin (Lescol), 711*b*
Foams, 169*b*
Focal segmental glomerulosclerosis, 1042*b*
Focused abdominal sonography for trauma (FAST), 1633-1634
Focused assessment, 40-42, 44*b*, 1307
Folic acid (folate), 602*t*, 610*b*
recommended daily intake, 858*b*
reference values, 1655*b*-1658*b*
Folic acid deficiency, 610*b*, 612*b*, **613**
Folk healers, 22, **24**
Folk medicine, 24
Follicle-stimulating hormone, 1104*b*
measurement of, 1115*t*-1118*t*, 1198*t*-1201*t*
regulation of reproductive system by, 1188
Follicle-stimulating hormone agonists, 1243*b*
Folliculitis, 414*b*
Follitropin (Gonal-f, Follistim), 1243*b*
Follow-up care, 345-346
Fondaparinux (Arixtra), 820*b*
Food(s)
absorption of, 834-835, **835-836**
caffeine content, 96*b*
guidelines for heart-healthy preparation, 749
high in iron, 856*b*
high in protein, 855*b*
high-calorie, 262*b*
high-fiber, 937*b*
high-potassium, 1083*b*
instructions for patients with diabetes, 1142*b*
maximizing intake, 571, 571*b*
portion sizes, 878, 878*b*, 883
protein foods with high biologic value, 262*b*
recommendations for nutrient balance, 1133
and stoma output, 961*b*
tips for choices and preparation, 709*b*
traditional, 856
Food additives, 539*b*, 540
Food allergies, 540
Food insecurity, 857
Food poisoning, 925-926
bacterial, 925, 925*b*
Escherichia coli O157:H7, 925*b*, **925-926**
prevention of, 926*b*
Foot care
acute care, 1508-1509
ambulatory care, 1509-1510
health promotion, 1508
nursing management, **1508-1510**
patient & caregiver teaching for, 1151*b*
postoperative care, 1508-1509, 1508*f*
Foot disorders, 1508, 1509*b*
diabetes-related complications, **1150-1151**, 1150*f*
in older adults, 1510
paresthesias, 597*b*-598*b*
Footdrop, 1478*b*
Foramen magnum, 1300
Forane (isoflurane), 325*b*
Forced expiratory volume in first second of expiration (FEV_1), 473*b*
Forced midexpiratory flow rate ($FEF_{25\%-75\%}$), 473*b*
Forced vital capacity (FVC), 473*b*
Foreign bodies
in external ear canal, **384**
in nose and sinuses, **484**
Forgetfulness, 1406*b*
Formoterol (Foradil Aerolizer, Perforomist), 548*b*-549*b*, 550
Forteo (teriparatide), 1513
Fosamax (alendronate), 1513
Fosinopril, 691*b*-693*b*
Fotamet (metformin), 1131*b*
Fourth heart sound (S_4), 668*b*, 669
Fovea centralis, 352
Fraction of inspired O_2 (FIO_2), 1575*b*
Fractional flow reserve, 679
Fracture(s), 1468-1480
acute care for, 1475-1477
ambulatory care for, 1477-1478
boxer's, 1642
classification of, 1468, 1468*f*
clinical manifestations of, 1468, 1469*b*
closed, 1468, 1468*f*
comminuted, 1468, 1469*f*
complete, 1468
complications of, **1478-1480**
counseling, 1478
displaced, 1468
drug therapy for, 1474
emergency management of, 1474*b*
facial, **1486**
greenstick, 1469*f*
health promotion for, 1475
hip, 1493*b*
immobilization, 1470*b*, 1471-1473
incomplete, 1468
interprofessional care for, 1470-1474, 1470*b*
nasal, **475-476**
nondisplaced, 1468
nursing assessment in, 1474-1475, 1475*b*
nursing diagnoses related to, 1475
nursing management of, **1474-1478**
nutritional therapy for, 1474
oblique, 1468, 1469*f*
open, 1468, 1468*f*, 1470*b*
pathologic, 1468, 1469*f*, 1514*b*-1515*b*
postoperative care for, 1476
preoperative care for, 1476
psychosocial problems with, 1477
reduction of, 1470-1471, 1470*b*
closed, 1470
open, 1470
referrals, 1478
refracture, 1470*b*
rib, **521**
skull, 1326-1327
spiral, 1469*f*
stress, 1469*f*
Fracture(s) *(Continued)*
transverse, 1469*f*
types of, 1468, 1469*f*, **1480-1490**
Fracture healing, **1469-1470**, 1470*b*
Fracture hematoma, 1464
Fracture Risk Assessment (FRAX) tool, 1512
Fragility fracture, 1480
Fragmin (dalteparin), 715*b*-716*b*, 820*b*
Frailty, 63, 65
Frank-Starling's law, 660-661, 740, 1560
Free thyroxine (T_4), 1115*t*-1118*t*
Free triiodothyronine (T_3), 1115*t*-1118*t*
Fresh frozen plasma, 648*b*-649*b*
Frontal bone fracture, 1486*b*
Frontotemporal lobar degeneration, 1401*b*
Frostbite, 1637-1638, 1638*f*
Frozen red blood cells, 648*b*
FTO (fat mass and obesity-associated gene), 877
Full code, 136
Full Outline of Unresponsiveness (FOUR) scale, 1323
Fulminant hepatic failure, 996
Fulvestrant (Faslodex), 1217*b*
Functional health patterns, 35-36
assessment of, 38-39
health history format, 37*b*
Functional residual capacity (FRC), 473*b*
Fungal infections, 214
disease-causing fungi, 215*b*
endemic, 512, 512*b*
opportunistic, 512, 512*b*
pulmonary, 512, 512*b*
skin, 417, 418*b*
Furadantin (nitrofurantoin), 1036*b*
Furosemide (Lasix)
for cirrhosis, 993*b*
for heart failure, 745*b*
for hypertension, 691*b*-693*b*
Furuncles, 414*b*
Furunculosis, 414*b*
Fusiform aneurysms, 810, 811*f*
Futility, medical, 266*b*
Future directions, 5*b*
The Future of Nursing: Leading Change, Advancing Health (IOM), 5

G

GABA receptor agonists, 116*b*, 117
Gabapentin (Neurontin), 116*b*
Gait abnormalities, 1456*b*
Galactorrhea, 1197*b*, 1208
Gallbladder, 835*b*, 838*f*
Gallbladder cancer, 1010
Gallbladder disease
acute care for, 1009
ambulatory care for, 1009-1010
cultural & ethnic health disparities, 986*b*
health promotion for, 1008-1009
nursing diagnoses for, 1008
nursing management of, **1008-1010**
nutritional therapy for, 1008
postoperative care in, 1009
Gallstones
cholesterol, 1005, 1005*f*
diagnosis of, 1007
interprofessional care for, 1007-1008
Gaming, 438*b*
Gamma knife radiosurgery, 250, 1438*b*
γ-glutamyltransferase, 852*t*, 1655*b*-1658*b*
Gandhi, Mahatma, 18
Ganglion cyst, 1456*b*
Ganglionic blockers, 691*b*-693*b*
Gangrene, 630*f*

Garlic, 710*b*
Gas exchange, normal, 1609, 1610*f*
Gastrectomy, 840*b*
postgastrectomy dumping, 917-918, 918*b*
total, 920, 920*f*
Gastric banding, adjustable, 885
Gastric bypass, Roux-en-Y, 885-887, 886*b*, 887*f*
Gastric cancer. *See* Stomach cancer
Gastric emptying studies, 847*t*-850*t*
Gastric feeding tubes, 867*b*
Gastric inhibitory peptide, 836*b*
Gastric lavage, 1642-1643
Gastric outlet obstruction, 913, 915-916
Gastric plication, 885, 886*b*
Gastric secretion, 836*b*
Gastric sleeve (sleeve gastrectomy), 885, 886*b*, 887*f*
Gastric ulcers, 911*b*, **912**
Gastric varices, 988, 991-992
Gastrin, 836*b*, 847*t*-850*t*
Gastritis, 909
acute, 909-910
autoimmune, 909
bile reflux, 918
causes of, 909*b*
chronic, 909-910
drug therapy for, 910*b*
drug-related, 909
nursing and interprofessional management of, **909-910**
risk factors for, 909
Gastroduodenostomy, 917, 917*f*
Gastroenteritis, 944
Gastroesophageal reflux disease, 900-904
with asthma, 540
drug therapy for, 902, 903*b*
endoscopic therapy for, 904
interprofessional care for, 901-904, 901*b*
lifestyle modifications for, 901
nursing management of, **904**
nutritional therapy for, 902
in older adults, 905
pathogenesis of, 900, 900*f*
patient & caregiver teaching for, 902*b*
sleep disturbances in, 92*b*
surgical therapy for, 902-904
Gastrointestinal bleeding
scintigraphy of, 847*t*-850*t*
upper gastrointestinal bleeding, **921-923**
Gastrointestinal motility, 836*b*
Gastrointestinal problems
associated with obesity, 879, 879*f*
in burns, 441*b*
corticosteroid therapy for, 1180*b*
fistulas, **962-963**
lower gastrointestinal problems, **929-973**
nursing management of, 342
postoperative, **341-342**
upper gastrointestinal problems, **893-928**
Gastrointestinal secretions, 835*b*-836*b*
Gastrointestinal stromal tumors, 968
Gastrointestinal system
abnormalities, 846*b*-847*b*
assessment of, **839-845**, 841*b*, 846*b*
preoperative, 307*b*
case study, 839*b*, 843*b*, 845*b*, 852*b*
diagnostic studies of, 845-852, 847*t*-850*t*, 852*b*
effects of chemotherapy and radiation on, 253
at end of life, 132*b*
normal, 846*b*
in older adults, 839, 840*b*
physical examination of, 842-845, 845*b*-846*b*
radiologic studies of, 845-851
regulation of water balance by, 275
structures and functions of, **833-839**, 834*f*
surgeries of, 840*b*
Gastrojejunostomy (G-J), 917, 917*f*
Gastrojejunostomy (G-J) tubes, 866
Gastropexy, 904-905
Gastrostomy, 840*b*
percutaneous endoscopic, 865-866, 866*f*
Gastrostomy tubes, 344*b*, 865-866, 865*f*
Gauze dressings, 169*b*
Gaviscon (aluminum/magnesium trisilicate), 903*b*
Gelusil (aluminum and magnesium), 903*b*
Gemfibrozil (Lopid), 710*b*-711*b*
Gender differences
health disparities, 20, 21*f*
of older adults, 63*b*
Gene therapy, **187**, 188*f*
for cancer, **261**
General anesthesia, **322-324**, 323*b*, 325*b*. *See also* Anesthesia
adjuncts to, 323, 326*b*
phases of, 324*b*
General survey, 39
General survey statements, 39
Generation X, 55*b*
Generation Y, 55*b*
Genes, **178-179**, 179*b*
Genetic analysis, 603*t*, 604
finger printing, 186
Genetic counselors, 185
Genetic disorders, 182-183, 183*b*
characteristics of, 181, 181*b*
liver diseases, **985**
multifactorial, **182-183**
single gene disorders, 182, 182*f*
Genetic Information Nondiscrimination Act (GINA), 184*b*
Genetic mutations, 180-181
Genetic risk factors, 179*b*
Genetic technology, 186
Genetic testing, **183-186**, 184*b*
direct-to-consumer tests, 185
ethical/legal dilemmas, 185*b*
interpreting results, 183-185
patient & family teaching for, 185*b*
Genetic variations, 28
Genetics, **178-182**, 179*b*
epigenetics, 183
nursing management of, **188-189**
pharmacogenetics, **186**
Gengraf (cyclosporine), 209, 211*b*
Genital herpes, 1232-1234
clinical manifestations of, 1232-1233, 1233*f*
drug therapy for, 1233-1234
interprofessional care for, 1233-1234, 1233*b*
primary episode, 1232-1233
recurrent, 1233
Genital lesions or ulcers, 1232-1240
Genital problems
female, **1242-1267**
male, **1268-1291**
Genital warts, 1234-1235, 1250
clinical manifestations of, 1234, 1234*f*
drug therapy for, 1235
interprofessional care for, 1234-1235, 1250-1251
Genitalia, external
female, 1187, 1187*f*
male, 1185
physical examination of, 1112
Genitourinary system
preoperative assessment of, 306, 307*b*
problems associated with obesity, 879*f*
Genitourinary tuberculosis, 1041
Genomes, 179*b*
Genome-wide association studies (GWAS), 179*b*, **186**
Genomic assay, 1213
Genomic tests, 1213
Genomics, **178-182**, 179*b*
nursing management of, **188-189**
pharmacogenomics, **186**
Genotypes, 179, 179*b*
Gentamicin, 1498*b*
Geographic tongue, 846*b*-847*b*
Geriatrics, 66
Gerontologic nursing, 69. *See also* Older adults
Gestational diabetes, 1123-1124
Get With the Guidelines—Heart Failure program, 751
Ghon lesion, 506
Ghost sickness, 29*b*
Ghrelin, 834, 877*b*, 877*f*, 878
Giant cell tumor, 1500*b*
Giardia lamblia, 929-931, 930*b*
Giardiasis, 216*b*
Gilenya (fingolimod), 1385*b*
GINA (Genetic Information Nondiscrimination Act), 184*b*
Ginger, 895*b*
Gingivitis, 846*b*-847*b*, 897*b*
Glans, 1185
Glasgow Coma Scale, 1323*b*, **1323**
Glatiramer acetate (Copaxone), 1385*b*
Glaucoma, 351, **379-380**, 380*f*
acute care for, 382
ambulatory care for, 382
angle-closure, 379-380
case study, 392*b*
drug therapy for, 381*b*
genetic risk alert, 355*b*
interprofessional care for, 379-380, 380*b*
nursing diagnoses related to, 380
nursing management of, **380-382**
in older adults, 382
open-angle, 379-380
Glial cells, **1294-1295**
Glimepiride (Amaryl), 1131*b*
Glioblastoma, 1333*b*, 1334*f*
Gliomas, 1333*b*
Gliosis, 1294-1295, 1374
Glipizide (Glucotrol, Glucotrol XL), 1131*b*
Gliptins, 1130-1132
Globe, 357*b*
Globus sensation, 901
Glomerular filtration rate (GFR), 1017, 1080*b*
Glomerulations, 1040
Glomerulonephritis, 1041-1042
acute, 1041
acute poststreptococcal, **1041-1043**
causes of, 1041, 1042*b*
chronic, 1041, **1043**
poststreptococcal, 1042*b*
rapidly progressive, **1043**
risk factors for, 1042*b*
Glomerulus, **1016-1017**, 1016*f*, 1017*b*
Glossectomy, 840*b*, 899
Glossitis, 846*b*-847*b*
Glossopharyngeal nerve, 1305*b*
Gloving, **320**
Glucagon, 1104*b*, **1108**
Glucagon-like peptide-1 (GLP-1), 877*b*, 1136*f*
Glucagon-like peptide-1 (GLP-1) receptor agonists, 1131*b*, 1132
Glucocorticoid excess, 399*b*
Glucocorticoids, 275, 1107
Gluconeogenesis, 1107
Glucophage (metformin), 1131*b*
Glucosamine, 1523*b*
Glucose
altered levels, 1113*b*-1114*b*
blood levels
drugs that affect, 1132
herbs and supplements that may affect, 1141*b*
estimated average (eAG), 1124

Glucose *(Continued)*
fasting, 1115*t*-1118*t*, 1123
normal metabolism of, 1120-1121, 1121*f*
reference values, 1655*b*-1658*b*, 1661*b*-1662*b*
in shock, 1590*t*
urinary, 1115*t*-1118*t*, 1661*b*
Glucose monitoring, **1135-1137**, 1135*f*
continuous glucose monitoring (CGM) systems, 1135, 1136*f*
instructions for patients & caregivers, 1136*b*, 1141*b*-1142*b*
self-monitoring, 1135
Glucose tolerance, impaired, 1123
Glucose-lowering agents, 1129*b*
α-Glucosidase inhibitors, 1130, 1131*b*, 1136*f*
Glucotrol (glipizide), 1131*b*
Glumetza (metformin), 1131*b*
Gluten-free diet, 967, 967*b*
Gluten-sensitive enteropathy, 966
Glyburide (DiaBeta, Glynase PresTab), 1131*b*
Glycerol rhizotomy, 1438*b*, 1439*f*
Glycoprotein IIb/IIIa inhibitors, 715*b*-716*b*
Glynase PresTab (glyburide), 1131*b*
Glyset (miglitol), 1131*b*
Goiter, 1112, 1113*b*-1114*b*, 1162, **1162**, 1162*f*
Goitrogens, 1162, 1162*b*
Gold compounds, 1521*b*-1522*b*, 1529
Gold sodium thiomalate (Myochrysine), 1521*b*-1522*b*, 1529
Golimumab (Simponi), 1521*b*-1522*b*, 1529
Gonadal feedback mechanisms, 1189, 1189*b*
Gonadotropic hormones, 1104*b*
Gonadotropin-releasing hormone (GnRH) agonists, 1253
Gonadotropin-releasing hormone (GnRH) antagonists, 1243*b*
Gonads, 1108*b*, 1184
Gonal-f (follitropin), 1243*b*
Goniometry, 1454, 1454*f*
Gonococcal infections, 1230-1231
case study, 1240*b*
clinical manifestations of, 1230, 1230*f*
disseminated, 1230, 1231*f*
drug therapy for, 1231
endocervical gonorrhea, 1230, 1230*f*
interprofessional care for, 1231, 1231*b*
Gonorrhea, 1230, 1230*f*. *See also* Gonococcal infections
endocervical, 1230, 1230*f*
Good lung down position, 1617
Good samaritans, 1646*b*
Goodpasture syndrome, 199, 1042*b*, **1043**
Goserelin (Zoladex), 1280*b*
Gottron's papules, 1545, 1545*f*
Gottron's sign, 1545
Gout, 1532-1534
chronic, 1533*f*
drug therapy for, 1533-1534
factors that may cause attacks, 1534
gender differences in, 1533*b*
interprofessional care for, 1533-1534, 1533*b*
nursing management of, **1534**
nutritional therapy for, 1534
Gowning, **320**
Graduated compression stockings, 819
Graft patency, 813
Grafts
arteriovenous, 1088, 1088*b*, 1088*f*
bone, 1506
for burns, 440, 440*b*, **444-445**, 444*f*
coronary artery bypass surgery, **724-725**, 724*f*
cultured epithelial autografts, **445**, 445*f*
Grafts *(Continued)*
HeRO (Hemodialysis Reliable Outflow), 1088, 1088*f*
patch angioplasty, 806
skin, **426-427**, 440
for burns, 440, 440*b*, **444-445**, 444*f*
vascular, 813
Graft-versus-host disease, 210
Gram stain, 469*t*-471*t*, 1198*t*-1201*t*
Granisetron, 326*b*, 895*b*
Granulation, 166, 166*b*
Granulation tissue, 1469
Granulocyte colony-stimulating factor, 260*b*
Granulocyte-macrophage colony-stimulating factor, 260*b*
Granulocytes, **589-590**
Granulocytopenia, 632
Granulomatous thyroiditis, 1163
Graphesthesia, 1307
Graves' disease, 1168. *See also* Hyperthyroidism
case study, **1182*b***
clinical manifestations of, 1162-1164, 1162*f*
etiology and pathophysiology of, 1163
laboratory findings in, 1165
Grey Turner's spots or sign, 811, 1000
Grief, 133-134
adaptive, 133
anticipatory, 133
complicated, 133-134
Kübler-Ross model of, 133*b*
prolonged, 133-134
in spinal cord injury, 1435, 1435*b*
Grief wheel, 133, 133*f*
Group A *Streptococcus* infection, 788*b*, 789
Growth hormone, 1104*b*, 1105, 1115*t*-1118*t*
Growth hormone stimulation test, 1115*t*-1118*t*
Guanabenz, 691*b*-693*b*
Guanfacine (Tenex), 691*b*-693*b*
Guglielmi detachable coil (GDC), 1356, 1356*f*
Guided imagery, 84
Guillain-Barré syndrome, 1440-1441
Guillotine amputation, 1487
Guilt, 448*b*
Gynecomastia
in men, 1208
senescent, 1208
Gynoid obesity, 875, 876*b*

H

Habit retraining, 1057*b*
Haemophilus, 214*b*
Hageman factor, 592*b*
Halal dietary practices, 856
Halitosis, 483, 908
Hallux rigidus, 1509*b*
Hallux valgus, 1508, 1508*f*, 1509*b*, 1527*f*
Halo sign, 1326-1327, 1327*f*
Halo vest, 1427-1428, 1428*b*, 1428*f*
Hamartomas, 518
Hammer toe, 1509*b*
Hands: paresthesias of, 597*b*-598*b*
Hands-only CPR, 1652
Haptoglobin, 1655*b*-1658*b*
Hardiness, 78
Hartford Institute for Geriatric Nursing, 70
Hartmann's pouch, 958
Hartmann's (lactated Ringer's) solution, 292, 293*b*
Harvest procedures, 260-261
Hashimoto's thyroiditis, 1163, 1168
Hawthorn, 749*b*
Head and neck arteries, 1300*f*
Head and neck assessment
physical examination, 1112
secondary survey, 1633
Head and neck cancer, 491-493
acute care for, 494-495
ambulatory care for, 495-496
chemotherapy for, 492
health promotion for, 494
interprofessional care for, 491-493, 491*b*
nursing assessment in, 494*b*
nursing diagnoses related to, 493-494
nursing management of, **493-496**
nutritional therapy for, 492-493
physical therapy for, 493
psychosocial needs in, 495
radiation therapy for, 249*f*, **492**, 495
staging of, 491
surgical therapy for, 491-492, 494-495
targeted therapy for, 492
Head and neck squamous cell carcinoma, 898
Head blocks, 1630
Head injury, 1326-1330
acute care for, 1330-1332
ambulatory care for, 1332-1333
emergency management of, 1330*b*
health promotion for, 1330
interprofessional care for, 1329-1330
nursing assessment in, 1331*b*
nursing diagnoses related to, 1330
nursing management of, **1330-1333**
patient & caregiver teaching for, 1332*b*
types of, 1326-1328
Head tilt–chin lift maneuver, 1650-1651, 1650*f*
Head trauma, 1327-1328, 1403
Headaches, 597*b*-598*b*, **1368-1374**
case study, 1396*b*
cluster, **1371**
diagnostic studies in, 1370*t*
drug therapy for, 1372-1373
epilepsy with, 1396*b*
exercise-induced, 1370*b*
gender differences in, 1370*b*
genetic risks, 1303*b*
in increased ICP, 1318
interprofessional care for, 1369*b*, **1371-1373**
location of pain, 1370*f*
migraine, **1370-1371**
nursing assessment in, 1373, 1373*b*
nursing diagnoses for, 1373
nursing management of, **1373-1374**
patient & caregiver teaching for, 1374*b*
primary, 1368
secondary, 1368
stress, **1370**
tension-type, **1370**
types of, **1371**
Head-to-toe assessment, 1632-1634, 1633*b*
Head-up tilt-test, 777
Healing. *See* Wound healing
Health
cultural factors, 24-29, 25*b*
determinants of, 18-19
dysfunctional patterns, 38
effects of stress on, 81*b*, **81-82**
Health assessment, 38
preoperative, 307*b*
Health behavior change, 47, 48*b*
Health care
cultural factors, 24-29, 25*b*
financing, 4
Health care environment, 3-4, 4*f*
cultural diversity in, 24, 24*f*
Health care providers
attitudes of, 21
cultural diversity among, 24
preventive measures for viral hepatitis, 983*b*

Health care systems, 4, 25*b*
Health care-associated infections, 217-218
Health disparities, 19*b*-20*b*, **19-21**
case study, 32*b*
factors and conditions leading to, 19-21, 19*b*
nursing interventions to reduce, 30*b*
nursing management of, **29-31**
Health equity, 19-21
Health history, 34-45. *See also* History taking
functional health pattern format, 37*b*
medical history, **34**
Health illiteracy, 52
Health Insurance Portability and Accountability Act (HIPAA), 14
confidentiality and, 1239*b*
violations, 5*b*
Health literacy, 20, 52
ehealth literacy, 53
Health maintenance organizations (HMOs), 4
Health perception–health management pattern, 37*b*, 38
Health policy, 4
Health promotion
models for, 47-48
for older adults, 70-71, 70*f*
skin-related, **407-410**
Health status, 18
Health-related beliefs and practices, 26*b*
Healthy People 2020, 4
lesbian, gay, bisexual, and transgender (LGBT) goals, 21*b*
overarching goals, 5*b*
Hearing aids, **389-390**, 390*b*, 392*b*
Hearing loss, 387-388
assistive devices and techniques for, **389-391**
causes of, 387*f*
central, 387-388
classification of, 388, 388*b*
communication with patients with, 390*b*
conductive, 360, 387
functional, 387-388
mixed, 387
nursing and interprofessional management of, **388-391**
in older adults, 391
sensorineural, 387
tinnitus and, 388
types of, 387-388
Heart, **658-661**
blood flow through, 658, 659*f*
conduction system of, 659-660, 660*f*, **757**
intrinsic rates of, 762*b*
dilation of, 740, 741*f*
effects of autonomic nervous system on, 661
implantable artificial, 1569
layers of, 780, 781*f*
mechanical system of, 660-661
nervous control of, **757**
orientation of, 667, 667*f*
structure of, 658, 659*f*
Heart block. *See also* Atrioventricular block
complete, 768
Heart cells, 757, 758*b*
Heart disease. *See also* Cardiovascular disease
hypertensive, 685-686, 686*b*
inflammatory disorders, **780-790**
rheumatic, **788-789**
valvular, 790-796
case study, 800*b*
diagnostic studies for, **793**
interprofessional care for, 793*b*, **793-795**
nursing assessment in, 795*b*
nursing diagnoses related to, 796
nursing management of, **795-796**
Heart failure, 737-749
acute care for, 751
acute decompensated
clinical manifestations of, 741-742
clinical profile, 742*b*
interprofessional care for, 744-746, 744*b*
ambulatory care for, 751-752
biventricular, 738-739
case study, 755*b*
causes of
precipitating, 737-738, 738*b*
primary, 737-738, 738*b*
chronic
clinical manifestations of, 742-743, 742*b*
interprofessional care for, 744*b*, 746-749
classification of, 741, 741*b*
clinical manifestations of, 741-743, 742*b*
compensatory mechanisms, 739-740
complications of, 743
counterregulatory mechanisms, 740
cultural & ethnic health disparities, 738*b*
diagnostic studies, 743-744
diastolic, 738
drug therapy for, 745-746, 745*b*
end-of-life care for, 752-753
etiology of, 737-738, 738*b*
gender differences in, 739*b*
genetics of, 738
health promotion for, 750-753
home care for, 752*b*
hypertension and, 686
impact of, 61*b*
interprofessional care for, 744*b*, 746-749
left-sided, 738-739, 742*b*
mixed systolic and diastolic, 738-739
after myocardial infarction, 720-721
neurohormonal response to, 739-740
nursing assessment in, 750, 750*b*
nursing care plan for, 8*b*
nursing diagnoses related to, 750
nursing management of, **750-753**
nutritional therapy for, 749
palliative care for, 752-753
pathophysiology of, 738-740, 739*f*-740*f*
patient & caregiver teaching for, 751*b*
with preserved EF, 737, **738**
with reduced EF, 737, **738**
right-sided, 739, 742*b*
signs of, 1113*b*-1114*b*
sleep disturbances during, 92*b*
systolic, 738
Heart murmurs, 668*b*, 669
Heart rate
estimation of, 759, 760*f*
normal range, 1559*b*
Heart rhythms
assessment of, 760, 762*b*
identification of, **757-775**
Heart sounds, 667, 667*f*
abnormal, 668*b*, 669
Heart surgery DVD/TV, 795*b*
Heart transplantation, 753-754
bridge to, 754
contraindications to, 753*b*
criteria for selection for, 753-754
indications for, 753*b*
posttransplantation, 754
surgical procedure, 754
Heart valves, 658, 659*f*
deformities of, **788**
prosthetic, 794-795, 795*f*
Heartburn (pyrosis), 900-901
Heart-healthy food preparation, 749
Heart-lung transplantation, 534
HeartWare LVAD, 754
Heat cramps, 1637
Heat exhaustion, 1637
Heat or eat phenomenon, 857
Heat therapy, **122**
active external or surface rewarming, 1639
active internal or core rewarming, 1639
for inflammation, 165
passive or spontaneous rewarming, 1639
patient & caregiver teaching for, 122*b*
Heat-related emergencies, 1636*b*, **1636-1637**
Heatstroke, 1637
cooling methods for, 1637
interprofessional care for, 1637
Heaves, 667
Heavy menstrual bleeding, 1246
Heberden's nodes, 1518, 1519*f*
Heel pain, 1509*b*
Heimlich maneuver, 1652*b*, 1652*f*
Heimlich valve, 522, 523*f*
Helicobacter pylori, 214*b*
***Helicobacter pylori* infection**
drug therapy for, 910*b*
gastritis and, 909
peptic ulcers and, 911
Heliotrope, 1545
Hemaglobin, 469*t*-471*t*
Hemangioblastoma, 1333*b*
Hemarthrosis, 626-627, 627*f*
Hematemesis, 460, 846*b*-847*b*
Hematocrit, 469*t*-471*t*, 599, 1659*b*
Hematologic problems, 606-655
in acute kidney injury, 1072
in cirrhosis, 986-987
cultural & ethnic health disparities in, 607*b*
exercise and, 643*b*
genetic risks, 594*b*
in systemic lupus erythematosus, 1539
Hematologic system
abnormalities, 597*b*-598*b*
assessment of, **593-598**, 595*b*, 599*b*
biopsies, 602-604
case study, 593*b*, 596*b*, 599*b*, 604*b*
diagnostic studies, 599-604, 602*t*-603*t*, 604*b*
effects of aging on, 593, 593*b*
effects of chemotherapy and radiation therapy on, 251*b*-252*b*
laboratory studies, 599-602
in older adults, 593, 593*b*
physical examination of, 596-598, 599*b*
reference values, 1659*b*
structures and functions of, **587-593**
Hematoma, 403*b*, 597*b*-598*b*
epidural, 1328-1329, 1328*f*
fracture, 1464
intracerebral, 1329
subdural, 1329, 1329*b*
Hematopoiesis, 587
Hematopoietic growth factors, **259**, 260*b*
Hematopoietic stem cell transplantation, **259-261**
allogeneic, 638-639
autologous, 638-639
complications of, 261
conditioning regimens, 261
harvest procedures, 260-261
indications for, 260*b*
for leukemia, 638-639
preparative regimens, 261
procedures, 260-261
syngeneic, 638-639
types of, 260
Hematuria, 1025*b*
Hemianopsia, homonymous, 1308*b*-1309*b*, 1362
Hemiglossectomy, 840*b*, 899
Hemiparesis, 1345

Hemiplegia, 1308*b*-1309*b*
Hemochromatosis, **619-620**, **985**
genetics of, 620, 620*b*
hereditary, **620**, 985
Hemodiafiltration, continuous venovenous, 1091, 1091*b*
Hemodialysis, 1084, 1085*b*, **1087-1091**, 1088*b*
complications of, 1090-1091, 1096*b*
continuous venovenous, 1091, 1091*b*
effectiveness of, 1091
for elevated potassium levels, 1073, 1073*b*
home, 1090, 1090*f*
procedure for, 1089-1090
settings and schedules, 1090
system components, 1089, 1090*f*
temporary vascular acess for, 1088-1089, 1089*f*
vascular access sites, 1087-1089
Hemodynamic monitoring, 673*t*-677*t*, **1558-1566**
noninvasive, 1566
nursing and interprofessional management of, **1566**
resting parameters, 1559*b*
terminology for, 1559-1560
Hemoglobin, 588, 599
arterial oxygen saturation (SpO_2), 457, 458*b*
noninvasive monitoring, 1565-1566
normal range, 1559*b*
glycosylated (hemoglobin A1C [A1C]), 1115*t*-1118*t*, 1659*b*
maintenance of, 1619
reference values, 1659*b*
urine values, 1661*b*
venous oxygen saturation (SvO_2), **456-457**, 1564-1565
central ($ScvO_2$), 1564-1565, 1565*b*
interpreting measurements, 1565*b*
invasive monitoring, 1564-1565
normal range, 1559*b*
Hemoglobin electrophoresis, 602*t*
Hemolysis, 589
extravascular, 615, 616*f*
Hemolytic anemia, **615-619**
acquired, 615, **619**
intrinsic, 615
laboratory data, 610*b*
Hemolytic transfusion reactions, 199
acute hemolytic reaction, 650*b*-651*b*
delayed, 651*b*
Hemolytic-uremic syndrome, 622
Hemophilia, **626-628**
acute care for, 628
ambulatory care for, 628
classic, 626
clinical manifestations of, 626-627, 627*f*
complications of, 626-627, 627*f*
diagnostic studies in, 627
drug therapy for, 628*b*
health promotion for, 628
interprofessional care for, 627-628
laboratory results, 627*b*
nursing management of, **628-629**
replacement factors for, 628*b*
types of, 626*b*
Hemophilia A, 626, 626*b*-627*b*
Hemophilia B, 626, 626*b*-627*b*
Hemopneumothorax, 520-521
Hemoptysis, 460
Hemorrhage, 167*b*, 1345
intracerebral, 1348*b*, 1349
in peptic ulcer disease, 912, 916
splinter hemorrhages, 668*b*
subarachnoid, 1348*b*, 1349-1350
subconjunctival, 357*b*
Hemorrhagic cystitis, 251*b*-252*b*
Hemorrhagic stroke, 1348*b*, 1348*f*, **1349-1350**
acute care for, 1355-1356
drug therapy for, 1355
surgical therapy for, 1355-1356
Hemorrhoids, 846*b*-847*b*, **968-969**, 969*f*
interprofessional care for, 969
nursing management of, **969-970**
Hemosiderin, 826
Hemostasis, 590
problems of, **622-640**
Hemothorax, 520-521, 520*b*
Heparin
for angina and ACS, 715*b*-716*b*
low-molecular-weight, 715*b*-716*b*, 820*b*, 821
unfractionated, 820*b*, 821
for VTE, 820*b*, 821
Heparin-induced thrombocytopenia, **622-623**, 821
interprofessional care for, 625*b*, **625**
Hepatic encephalopathy, **990**
acute care for, 995
factors precipitating, 990, 990*b*
grading scale, 990, 990*b*
interprofessional care for, 992
Hepatic failure. *See also* Liver failure
fulminant, 996
Hepatitis, **974-981**
acute, 977-978
clinical manifestations of, 977, 977*b*
diagnostic findings in, 979, 979*b*
interprofessional care for, 980*b*
acute alcoholic, 984
autoimmune, **985**
chronic, 978
clinical manifestations of, 977, 977*b*
interprofessional care for, 980*b*
cultural & ethnic health disparities, 986*b*
in hemodialysis, 1091
nursing assessment in, 982*b*
viral, **974-977**
acute care for, 983-984
ambulatory care for, 984
clinical manifestations of, 977-978, 977*b*
complications of, 977-978
diagnostic studies, 979-980, 979*t*
health promotion for, 982-983
interprofessional care for, 980-981, 980*b*
nursing assessment in, 982*b*
nursing diagnoses for, 982
nursing management of, **982-984**
nutritional therapy for, 981
pathophysiology of, 977
preventive measures for, 983*b*
systemic effects of, 977
Hepatitis A
course of infection, 975, 975*f*
health promotion against, 982-983
preventive measures against, 982-983, 983*b*
Hepatitis A virus, 214*b*, **974-975**, 975*b*
Hepatitis A virus vaccine, 982
Hepatitis B
chronic, 980-981
clinical manifestations of, 222*b*
course of infection, 976, 976*f*
delayed transfusion reaction, 651*b*
drug therapy for, 980-981, 981*b*
health promotion against, 983
preventive measures for, 983*b*
Hepatitis B immune globulin, 983
Hepatitis B virus, 214*b*, 975*b*, **975-976**
Hepatitis B virus vaccine, 983
Hepatitis C
chronic, 981
clinical manifestations of, 222*b*
delayed transfusion reaction, 651*b*
Hepatitis C *(Continued)*
drug therapy for, 981, 981*b*
health promotion against, 983
preventive measures for, 983*b*
screening and testing for, 977*b*
Hepatitis C virus, 214*b*, 975*b*, **976**
Hepatitis D virus, 975*b*, **976-977**
Hepatitis E virus, 975*b*, **977**
Hepatobiliary scintigraphy, 847*t*-850*t*
Hepatocytes, 837
Hepatomegaly, 597*b*-598*b*, 846*b*-847*b*
in heart failure, 743
Hepatopulmonary syndrome, 1611-1612
Hepatorenal syndrome, **990**
Hepatotoxicity
in cancer, 251*b*-252*b*
chemical, 984
Hepcidin, 592-593
Hepsera (adefovir), 980
Herbal products
assessment of use of, 38*b*
for menopausal symptoms, 1249*b*
and surgery, 304
that may affect blood glucose, 1141*b*
Herceptin. *See* Trastuzumab
Hereditary breast and ovarian cancer (HBOC) syndrome, 1276
Hereditary hemochromatosis, **620**, 985
Hereditary kidney diseases, **1051-1052**
Hereditary nephritis, chronic, 1052
Hereditary nonpolyposis colorectal cancer, 954*b*
Hereditary (inherited) prostate cancer, 1276
Hering-Breuer reflex, 458
Hernias, 846*b*-847*b*, **933-934**
cerebral herniation, 1316, 1317*f*
diaphragmatic, 904
esophageal, 904
femoral, 965, 965*f*
gender differences in, 965*b*
hiatal, **904**
interprofessional care for, 901*b*
rolling or paraesophageal, 904, 904*f*
sliding, 904, 904*f*
surgical repair of, 902-903, 903*f*
incarcerated, 964
incisional, 965
inguinal, 964-965, 965*f*
strangulated, 951*f*
irreducible, 964
nursing and interprofessional management of, **965**
in peritoneal dialysis, 1087
reducible, 964
types of, 964-965
umbilical, 965, 965*f*
ventral, 965
Herniated disc, 1504-1505
Herniorrhaphy, 840*b*, 904-905
Herniotomy, 904-905
HeRO (Hemodialysis Reliable Outflow) grafts, 1088, 1088*f*
Herpes simplex virus (HSV) infection, 214*b*
clinical manifestations of, 222*b*
genital herpes, **1232-1234**, 1233*f*
oral, 846*b*-847*b*, 897*b*
orolabial, 1232, 1232*f*
skin infection, 415*b*
Herpes zoster (shingles), 415, 415*b*, 416*f*
Herpesviruses, 214*b*
Hetlioz (tasimelteon), 370
Hiatal hernia, **904**
interprofessional care for, 901*b*
nursing and interprofessional management of, **904-905**

Hiatal hernia *(Continued)*
in older adults, 905
rolling or paraesophageal, 904, 904*f*
sliding, 904, 904*f*
surgical repair of, 902-903, 903*f*
Hiccups, postoperative, 341-342
High-density lipoproteins (HDLs), 670, 673*t*-677*t*, 1655*b*-1658*b*
High-frequency chest wall oscillation, 570
High-frequency oscillatory ventilation (HFOV), 1578
Hilus, 454
Hinduism, 26*b*
Hip: soft tissue injury of, 1464-1465, 1465*f*
Hip fracture, 1481-1482
ambulatory care for, 1484
case study, 1493*b*
interprofessional care for, 1482
nursing management of, **1482-1484**
in older adults, 1484
periprosthetic, 1493*b*
postoperative care in, 1483-1484
preoperative care in, 1482-1483
surgical repair of, 1482, 1482*f*
types of, 1481-1482, 1481*f*
Hip replacement
case study, 1493*b*
patient & caregiver teaching for, 1483, 1483*b*
postoperative care in, 1483, 1483*f*
revision arthroplasty, 1493*b*
total, 1482, 1482*f*
web-based community for, 1477*b*
Hip resurfacing arthroplasty, 1491
Hip spica cast, 1473
HIPAA. *See* Health Insurance Portability and Accountability Act
Hirsutism, 403*b*
Hispanics, 19
arthritis in, 1525*b*
chronic kidney disease in, 1076*b*
connective tissue disorders in, 1525*b*
coronary artery disease in, 704*b*
cross-cultural communication, 25
cultural traditions, 22, 22*b*, 24
culture-bound syndromes, 29*b*
in health care workplace, 24
integumentary problems in, 410*b*
lung cancer in, 514*b*
obesity among, 875, 876*f*, 878*b*
older adults, 63
tuberculosis in, 28
Histamine, 162*b*
Histamine (H_2)-receptor antagonists. *See also* Antihistamines
for GERD, 902, 903*b*
for peptic ulcers, 903*b*, 914
preoperative, 311*b*
Histamine (HT_3)-receptor antagonists, 895*b*
Histoplasma capsulatum, 222*b*
History taking. *See also* Health history
family history, 189
Five Ps of, 1194, 1195*b*
interview considerations, 35
nursing history, 34-35, 35*f*, **36-39**
obstetric history, 1194
SAMPLE mnemonic for, 1632-1633
secondary survey, 1632-1634, 1633*b*
sexual history, 1194, 1195*b*
HIV/AIDS. *See* Human immunodeficiency virus (HIV) infection
Hives, 199
HMG-CoA reductase inhibitors (statins), 709-710, 711*b*
HMOs (health maintenance organizations), 4
Hodgkin's disease, 640-641
Hodgkin's lymphoma, 640-641, 641*b*
B symptoms, 641
clinical manifestations of, 641, 641*f*
dermatologic manifestations of, 399*b*
exercise and, 643*b*
nursing and interprofessional management of, **641-642**
staging, 641, 642*f*
Holding area, 315-316
Holter monitoring, 673*t*-677*t*, 762
Home health care, 68. *See also specific disorders*
after bariatric surgery, 888-889
BP monitoring, 694*b*, **696-697**
for heart failure, 752*b*
hemodialysis, 1090, 1090*f*
nutritional support, 871
oxygen delivery systems, 568, 568*b*
oxygen therapy, 568, 569*b*
palliative care, 131*b*
in spinal cord injury, 1431-1435
STI testing, 1229*b*
telehealth monitoring, 752, 752*f*
Homeless older adults, 65
Homeostasis, 191, **270**
Homocysteine
and CAD, 707
cardiac assessment, **670**, 673*t*-677*t*
hematologic assessment, 602*t*
Homograft (allograft) skin, 440
Homonymous hemianopsia, 1308*b*-1309*b*, 1362
Hope, preoperative, 304
Hopefulness, 448*b*
Hopelessness, 138-139
Hordeolum (sty), 357*b*, 370, 370*f*
Hormone receptors, 1103
Hormone therapy
for breast cancer, 1217-1218
for cancer, 259*b*, **259**
cardiovascular effects of, 664*b*
corticosteroid therapy, 1180*b*
for menopausal symptoms, 1249
for voiding dysfunction, 1059*b*
Hormones, **1102-1105**
counterregulatory, 1121
endocrine, 1104*b*
of hypothalamus, 1105, 1105*b*, 1106*f*
lipid-soluble, **1103**, 1103*f*
regulation of, **1103-1105**
that control GI secretions and motility, 836*b*
tropic, 1105
water-soluble, **1103**, 1103*f*
Horse chestnut seed extract *(Aesculus hippocastanum)*, 825*b*
Hospice care, **130-131**, 130*f*
inpatient settings, 130, 131*f*
Hospital-acquired pneumonia, 501*b*, **501**
Hospitalization
of older adults, 71*b*
sleep disturbances during, **91**
Hostility, 728*b*
Hot flashes, 1248-1249
Huff coughing, 569, 569*b*, 1616
Human bites, 1641-1642, 1642*f*
Human chorionic gonadotropin
for infertility, 1243*b*
measurement of, 1198*t*-1201*t*
Human epidermal growth factor receptor-2 (HER-2), 1210, 1213
Human Genome Project (HGP), 182
Human immunodeficiency virus (HIV), 214*b*, 218-219, 219*f*-220*f*
Human immunodeficiency virus (HIV) infection, 218-231
acute, **219-220**
acute care for, 227-229
acute exacerbations, 229
Human immunodeficiency virus (HIV) infection *(Continued)*
ambulatory care for, 229-230
antiretroviral therapy for, 227-228
asymptomatic, 220-221
case study, 231*b*
chronic, **220-221**
clinical manifestations and complications, 219-221
condom use and, 227
delaying disease progression, 228-229
dermatologic manifestations of, 399*b*
diagnosis of, 221-222, 227
diagnostic studies in, 221-223
drug therapy for, 223, 224*b*
early detection of, 226*b*
early intervention for, 227-229
end-of-life care in, 230
health promotion in, 224-227
impact of, 61*b*
interprofessional care for, 223
laboratory studies in, 222-223
nursing assessment in, 223-224, 225*b*
nursing interventions for, 227*b*
nursing management of, **223-231**
with Internet and mobile devices, 229*b*
in older adults, 230
opportunistic diseases associated with, 221, 222*b*
pathophysiology of, 219, 220*f*
patient & caregiver teaching for, 229*b*
prevention of, 223-226, 226*b*
signs and symptoms patients need to report, 229*b*
sleep disturbances during, 92*b*
stigma of, 229-230
symptomatic, 221
testing for, 222*b*, 227
typical course, 219, 220*f*
window period, 221-222
Human leukocyte antigen (HLA), **206-207**
disease associations, 206-207
patterns of inheritance, 206, 207*f*
tissue typing, 208
Human leukocyte antigen (HLA)-B27, 1457*t*-1459*t*
Human papillomavirus (HPV) infection, 1192-1193
genital warts, **1234-1235**, 1234*f*
testing for, 1256-1257
vaccines against, 1234-1235, 1235*b*
Humanity, 3
Humeral shaft fracture, 1481
Humidification, 565, 1617
Humira (adalimumab), 1521*b*-1522*b*, 1529
Humor, 82*b*
Humoral immunity, **195-196**, 196*b*, 196*f*
Huntington's disease, 1395-1396, 1396*b*
dementia in, 1401*b*
genetic risks, 1303*b*
Hwa-byung, 29*b*
Hyaline cartilage, 1448
Hyaluronic acid, 1523
Hydralazine, 691*b*-693*b*, 745*b*
Hydration, 1617
Hydrocele, 1284*f*-1285*f*, **1285**
Hydrocephalus, 1298, 1317
indications for cranial surgery for, 1336*b*
normal pressure, 1400
Hydrochlorothiazide (HydroDIURIL), 691*b*-693*b*, 745*b*
Hydrocodone, 112, 113*b*-114*b*, 117*b*
Hydrocolloids, 169*b*
Hydrocortisone (Solu-Cortef)
for arthritis, 1521*b*-1522*b*
for asthma and COPD, 548*b*-549*b*
for shock, 1599*b*
Hydrogels, 169*b*

Hydrogen ion (H^+)concentration, **286-287**
Hydromorphone (Dilaudid), 112, 113*b*-114*b*
equinanalgesic dosing, 117*b*
in general anesthesia, 326*b*
Hydronephrosis, 1044, 1045*f*, 1071, 1269
Hydrostatic pressure, 273-274
Hydroureter, 1044
Hydroxychloroquine (Plaquenil), 1521*b*-1522*b*, 1528
Hydroxyzine (Vistaril), 895*b*
Hygiene, 1240
in diabetes mellitus, 1140
oral, 900*b*
in shock, 1603-1604
skin, 409. *See also* Skin care
Hygiene hypothesis, 539
Hymen, 1187
Hymenopteran stings, 1640*b*, **1640**
Hyoscyamine (Levsin, Levbid), 1059*b*
Hyperacute rejection, **208**
Hyperaldosteronism, **1180-1181**
primary, 1180, **1181**
secondary, 1180
Hyperalgesia, 105, 115
Hyperbaric oxygen therapy, **170**
Hypercalcemia, **283**
in cancer, 263*b*
causes and manifestations of, 284*b*
nursing and interprofessional management of, **283-284**
nursing diagnoses, 283
Hypercapnia, 96, 335, 1609
clinical manifestations of, 1613*b*
permissive, 1623
Hypercapnic respiratory failure, 1609-1610, 1610*b*, 1612
Hypercholesterolemia, familial, 704*b*
Hypercoagulability, 817
Hyperemia, reactive, 803-804
Hyperesthesia, 1440
Hyperextension, 1455*b*
Hyperglycemia, 1143*b*
hyperosmolar hyperglycemic syndrome, 1144*b*, **1145**
in parenteral nutrition, 870*b*
Hyperinsulinemia, 685
Hyperkalemia, **280-281**
in acute kidney injury, 1072
with burns, 443
causes of, 280-281, 281*b*
clinical manifestations of, 281, 281*b*, 281*f*
drug therapy for, 1080-1081
ECG changes in, 281, 281*f*
nursing diagnoses, 281-282
nursing management of, **281-282**
therapy for, 1073, 1073*b*
Hyperlipidemia. *See also* Dyslipidemia
in antiretroviral therapy, 230
drug therapy for, 711*b*
Hypermagnesemia, 286*b*, **286**
Hypermetabolic state, 442
Hypernatremia, **279**
with burns, 442
causes of, 279, 279*b*
clinical manifestations of, 279, 279*b*
nursing and interprofessional management of, **279-280**
nursing diagnoses, 279
Hyperopia, 351, 368
Hyperosmolar hyperglycemic syndrome, 1144*b*, **1145**
interprofessional care for, 1145
nursing management of, **1145-1146**
pathophysiology of, 1145, 1145*f*
Hyperparathyroidism, **1171-1173**
clinical manifestations of, 1172, 1172*b*
interprofessional care for, 1173
nonsurgical therapy for, 1173
nursing management of, **1173**
primary, 1172
secondary, 1172
surgical therapy for, 1173
tertiary, 1172
Hyperphosphatemia, 285*b*, **285**
Hyperpigmentation, 1113*b*-1114*b*
Hyperpituitarism, 399*b*
Hyperplasia, 876, 1208
Hyperreflexia
autonomic, 1431, 1431*b*
patient & caregiver teaching for, 1431*b*
in stroke, 1350
Hyperresonance, 467*b*-468*b*, 846*b*-847*b*
Hypersensitivity pneumonitis, 513
Hypersensitivity reactions, **197-200**
microbial, 200
type I (IgE-mediated), 197-199, 197*b*, 198*f*
type II (cytotoxic), 197*b*, 199
type III (immune-complex), 197*b*, 199
type IV (delayed), 197*b*, **199-200**
types of, 197, 197*b*
Hypersplenism, 647
Hypertension, 1113*b*-1114*b*
ambulatory care for, 696-698
ambulatory venous, 826
and CAD, 705-706
case study, 700*b*
in chronic kidney disease, 1078, 1081
classification of, 684, 684*b*
clinical manifestations of, 685
complications of, 685-687, 686*b*
cultural & ethnic health disparities in, 682*b*
definition of, 684
diagnostic studies in, 687-688
drug therapy for, 689-693, 691*b*-694*b*, 1081
etiology of, 684
gender differences, 682*b*
genetics of, 664*b*, 684-685
and glomerulonephritis, 1042*b*
health promotion for, 693-696, 708*b*
interprofessional care for, 687*b*, 688-693
intraabdominal, 812
lifestyle changes for, 688-689, 688*b*
nursing assessment in, 695*b*
nursing management of, **693-698**, 696*b*
in older adults, 698
pathophysiology of, 684
patient adherence to treatment plans, 697-698
patient & caregiver teaching for, 697*b*
patient evaluation, 694
portal, 988, 988*b*
postoperative, 337
prehypertension, 705-706
psychosocial risk factors for, 689
pulmonary, 529-530, **531-534**, 532*f*, 564*f*
resistant, 693, 695*b*
risk factors for, 685*b*, 689
screening for, 694*b*, 696
secondary, 684, 684*b*
sleep disturbances during, 92*b*
systolic, isolated, 684
target organ diseases, 685, 686*b*
white coat, 687
Hypertensive crisis, **698-699**
causes of, 698*b*
nursing and interprofessional management of, 699-700
Hypertensive emergency, 698
Hypertensive encephalopathy, 698
Hypertensive retinopathy, 698, 699*f*
Hypertensive urgency, 698
Hyperthermia
emergency management of, 1636*b*
malignant
in operating room, 327-329
postoperative, 341
Hyperthyroidism, **1163-1166**
acute care for, 1167-1168
ambulatory care for, 1168
clinical manifestations of, 1163-1164, 1164*b*-1165*b*
dermatologic manifestations of, 399*b*
drug therapy for, 1165-1166
interprofessional care for, 1165-1166, 1165*b*
laboratory findings in, 1164*b*
nursing assessment in, 1167*b*
nursing diagnoses for, 1166
nursing management of, **1166-1168**
nutritional therapy for, 1166
in older adults, 1165*b*
radioactive iodine therapy for, 1166
surgical therapy for, 1166
in younger adults, 1165*b*
Hypertonia, 1306
Hypertonic solutions, 273, 273*f*, 292-293, 293*b*, 1597*b*
Hypertrophic cardiomyopathy, 797*b*, **798-799**, 798*f*
causes of, 796*b*
nursing and interprofessional management of, **799**
Hypertrophic obstructive cardiomyopathy, 798
Hypertrophic scars, 167*b*, 167*f*
Hypertrophy, 876, 1129
Hypertropia, 373
Hyperuricemia, 1532
in cancer, 251*b*-252*b*
causes of, 1532*b*
Hyperventilation
alveolar, 1579
central neurogenic, 1324*f*
Hyperviscosity, **620**
Hyperviscosity syndrome, 645
Hypervolemia, **620**
Hypnosis, **122**
Hypnotics
for anesthesia, 325*b*
benzodiazepine, 94
for burns, 441*b*
for insomnia, 94
non-benzodiazepine, 94, 94*b*
Hypocalcemia, **284**
causes and manifestations of, 284*b*
nursing and interprofessional management of, **284-285**
nursing diagnoses, 284
tests for, 284, 287*f*
Hypochromia, 611
Hypocretin, 90
Hypoglossal nerve, 1305*b*
Hypoglycemia, 1143*b*, **1146**
interprofessional care for, 1146*b*
nursing and interprofessional management of, **1146-1147**
in parenteral nutrition, 870*b*
postprandial, 918
Rule of 15 for, 1146-1147
Hypoglycemia unawareness, 1146
Hypoglycemics, 408*b*
Hypogonadism, **1288-1289**
Hypokalemia, **282**
with burns, 443
causes of, 281*b*
clinical manifestations of, 281*b*, 282

Hypokalemia *(Continued)*
nursing and interprofessional management of, **282-283**
nursing diagnoses, 282
postoperative, 337
prevention of, 283*b*
Hypokinetic dysarthria, 1388
Hypomagnesemia, 286*b*, **286**
Hyponatremia, **280**
with burns, 442
dilutional, 442
nursing and interprofessional management of, **280**
nursing diagnoses, 280
Hypoparathyroidism, **1173**, 1174*b*
acute, 1172*b*, 1173
clinical manifestations of, 399*b*, 1172*b*, 1173
nursing and interprofessional management of, **1173-1174**
Hypophosphatemia, 285*b*, **285-286**
Hypophysectomy, 1158
Hypophysis, **1105-1106**
Hypopigmentation, 403*b*
Hypopituitarism, **1158**
clinical manifestations of, 1158, 1158*b*
nursing and interprofessional management of, **1158**
Hypopnea, 96
Hyporeflexia, 1350
Hypospadias, 1283
Hypotension
in hemodialysis, 1090
orthostatic, 695
postoperative, 337
postprandial, 663
Hypothalamic-pituitary-adrenal axis, 79, 79*f*, 274-275
Hypothalamic-pituitary-gonadal axis, 1188, 1188*f*
Hypothalamus, **1105**, 1297
hormones of, 1105, 1105*b*, 1106*f*
stress response, 79
Hypothalamus-hypophyseal portal system, 1105
Hypothermia, **1638-1639**
emergency management of, 1639*b*
interprofessional care for, 1639
postoperative, 340, 340*b*
prevention of, 322
therapeutic, **1634-1635**, 1635*b*
Hypothyroidism, **1168-1169**
acute care for, 1170
ambulatory care for, 1170
clinical manifestations of, 1164*b*, 1168-1169
dermatologic manifestations of, 399*b*
health promotion for, 1170
interprofessional care for, 1169, 1169*b*
laboratory findings in, 1164*b*
nursing diagnoses for, 1170
nursing management of, **1169-1170**
patient & caregiver teaching for, 1170*b*
primary, 1168
secondary, 1168
subclinical, 1168
Hypotonia, 1306
Hypotonic solutions, 273, 273*f*, **292**, 293*b*
Hypotropia, 373
Hypoventilation
alveolar, 1578-1579, **1612**
postoperative, 333*b*, 335
Hypovolemia
absolute, 1588*b*
in acute kidney injury, 1072
relative, 1588*b*
Hypovolemic shock, 1588*b*, 1589
in burns, 434
clinical presentation of, 1591*b*
emergency management of, 939*b*
Hypovolemic shock *(Continued)*
interprofessional care for, 1600*b*, 1601
pathophysiology of, 1589, 1589*f*
Hypoxemia, 96, 1609
clinical manifestations of, 1613, 1613*b*
postoperative, 332-334, 333*b*
refractory, 1621
Hypoxemic respiratory failure, 1609-1612, 1610*b*
Hypoxia, 1613
Hysterectomy, 1254, 1257, 1258*f*
acute intervention for, 1260-1261
surgical procedures, 1260*b*
Hysterosalpingography, 1198*t*-1201*t*
Hysteroscopy, 1198*t*-1201*t*

I

Ibandronate (Boniva), 1513
Ibrance (palbociclib), 1217*b*, 1218
Ibuprofen (Nuprin), 111*b*
for arthritis, 1521*b*-1522*b*, 1523
for inflammation, 164, 164*b*
Ibutilide (Corvert), 771*b*
Icosapent ethyl (Vascepa), 711*b*
ICU psychosis, 1557
Idiopathic generalized epilepsy, 1374-1375
Idiopathic pulmonary arterial hypertension, 531, **531-532**
Idiopathic pulmonary fibrosis, **528**
Idiopathic thrombocytopenic purpura, 622
I/E ratio, 1575*b*, 1577
Ileal conduit (ileal loop), 1064-1065, 1064*b*, 1064*f*
Ileal conduit appliances, 1066*b*
Ileal pouch/anal anastomosis, 948, 948*f*
Ileoanal pouch, 948, 948*f*
Ileostomy, 840*b*, 958, 959*b*, 959*f*
continent, 958
permanent, 948
Ileostomy care, 961-962
postoperative, 948-949
Ileus, postoperative, 341
Illegal drug use. *See* Substance abuse
Iloprost (Ventavis), 532*b*
Image-guided radiation therapy, 249
Imagery
digital photography, 175*b*
for pain management, 1221*b*
for stress management, **84**, 85*b*, 85*f*
Imipramine (Tofranil), 116*b*, 1059*b*
Immigrants, **28**, 28*f*
Immigration, **28**
Immobilization
cervical spine, 1630, 1631*b*
fracture, 1470*b*, 1471-1473
for inflammation, 165
spinal cord, 1427-1428, 1427*f*-1428*f*
Immobilization devices, 249, 249*f*
Immune response(s)
altered, **196-200**
in asthma, 539
in burns, 437
in cancer, 238-240
cells involved in, 192-194, 193*f*
functions of, 191
normal, 191-196
in older adults, 196, 196*b*
primary, 196, 196*f*
secondary, 196, 196*f*
stress response, 80-81, 80*f*
Immune system
inhibition of, 80, 80*f*
organs of, 192*f*
preoperative assessment of, 306, 307*b*
Immune thrombocytopenic purpura, 622
clinical manifestations of, 623, 623*f*
interprofessional care for, **624**, 625*b*
Immune-complex reactions, 197*b*, **199**
Immunity, 191
acquired, 192
active, 192, 192*b*
passive, 192, 192*b*
autoimmunity, **204-205**
cell-mediated, 196*b*, **196**
humoral, **195-196**, 196*b*, 196*f*
innate, 191
types of, 191-192
Immunizations, 389. *See also* Vaccines
Immunocompetence, 196-197
Immunodeficiency disorders, **205-206**
primary, 206, 206*b*
secondary, 206, 206*b*
Immunofluorescent skin studies, 405*t*
Immunoglobulin A, 194*b*
Immunoglobulin A nephropathy, 1042*b*
Immunoglobulin D, 194*b*
Immunoglobulin E, 194*b*
Immunoglobulin E-mediated reactions, 197*b*, **197-199**, 198*f*
Immunoglobulin G, 194*b*
Immunoglobulin M, 194*b*
Immunoglobulins, 192
characteristics of, 194*b*
intravenous
drug alert, 1545*b*
for polymyositis and dermatomyositis, 1545
rabies immune globulin (RIG), 1642
tetanus immune globulin (TIG), 1634*b*
for viral hepatitis, 983*b*
Immunologic escape, 239, 240*f*
Immunologic surveillance, 238-239
Immunology, 1660*b*
Immunomodulators, 258*b*. *See also* Targeted therapy
for dermatologic problems, 421-422
for hepatitis, 981*b*
for IBD, 947, 947*b*
for multiple sclerosis, 1385*b*
Immunosenescence, 196
Immunosuppressants
for arthritis, 1529
for IBD, 947, 947*b*
for multiple sclerosis, 1385*b*
Immunosuppressive therapy, **209-210**
drug therapy, 209, 211*b*
images useful for, 85*b*
for kidney transplantation, 1095
sites of action, 209, 210*f*
Immunotherapy
administration of, 203
for allergic disorders, 202-203
for arthritis, 1521*b*-1522*b*, 1528
for breast cancer, 1217*b*, 1218
for cancer, **257-258**, 258*b*. *See also specific cancers*
nursing management of, **258-259**
mechanism of action, 203
nursing management of, **203-204**
side effects of, 257-258
subcutaneous, 203
sublingual, 203
Imodium A-D (loperamide), 931*b*
Impacted cerumen, **384**
Impaired fasting glucose, 1123
Impaired glucose tolerance, 1123
Impaired nurses, 125*b*
Impedance cardiography, 1566
Impetigo, 414*b*
Impingement syndrome, 1463*b*
Implantable artificial heart, 1569
Implantable cardioverter-defibrillators (ICDs), **772-773**, 773*f*
patient & caregiver teaching for, 773*b*
Implantable contact lenses, 368

Implantable gastric stimulation, 886*b*, 887
Implantable hearing devices, 390
Implanted gastric stimulation devices, 886*b*
Implanted infusion ports, **295**, 295*f*
Implants
breast, 1215*b*, 1223
cochlear, 390-391, 391*f*
penile, 1288
for visual problems, 367
Implementation, 5, 6*f*
Imuran. *See* Azathioprine
Inagliptin (Tradjenta), 1131*b*
Inattention, 1416*b*
Incentive spirometers, 336, 336*f*
Incest, 1263
Incident Command System (ICS), 1646
Incisional hernias, 965
Income disparities, 20
Incontinence. *See* Fecal incontinence; Urinary incontinence
Incontinence clamps, 1057*b*
Incontinence-associated dermatitis, 934
Incontinent urinary diversion, 1064-1065
Incruse Ellipta (umeclidinium), 548*b*-549*b*
Incus, 361
Indacaterol (Arcapta Neohaler), 548*b*-549*b*
Indapamide, 691*b*-693*b*
Inderal (propranolol), 691*b*-693*b*, 771*b*, 993*b*
Indomethacin, 1521*b*-1522*b*
Indwelling catheters, 1061*b*
Infection(s), 213-218
antibiotic-resistant, 216, 217*b*
in breast, 1206-1207
in cancer, 262
case study, 176*b*
catheter-related, 870*b*
chlamydial, 1228-1230
in chronic kidney disease, 1078
and COPD, 558
in diabetes, 1151-1152
disseminated, 213
emerging, 215-216, 215*b*
exit site, 1087
in eye, 370-373
in fracture, 1478-1479
fungal, 214, 512
disease-causing fungi, 215*b*
pulmonary, 512, 512*b*
skin, 417, 418*b*
genital herpes, 1232-1234
gonococcal, 1230-1231
health care-associated, 217-218
images useful for, 85*b*
intraocular, 382
in kidney transplantation, 1095-1096
localized, 213
lower genital tract, 1250-1251
lower respiratory tract, 499-513
in older adults, 217-218
oral, 897, 897*b*
in oxygen therapy, 565
precautions against, 218
prevention and control, 218, 1606-1607
in Alzheimer's disease, 1413
for wound healing, 171
pulmonary, 1618
pulmonary fungal, 512
reemerging, 215-216, 216*b*
respiratory tract, 540
scrotum and testes, 1284
sexually transmitted, 1227-1241
skin, 413-417
surgical site, 343
systemic, 213
Infection(s) *(Continued)*
in systemic lupus erythematosus, 1539-1540
urinary system, **1033-1041**
urinary tract, 1033-1036
vascular graft, 813
wound, 167*b*-168*b*, 171
yeast, 1250
Infectious diarrhea, acute, 930*b*, **932-933**
Infective endocarditis, 780-782, 781*f*
acute, 780
ambulatory care for, 784
drug therapy for, 782
etiology and pathophysiology of, 780-781, 781*f*
and glomerulonephritis, 1042*b*
health promotion for, 783-784
interprofessional care for, 782
nursing assessment in, 783, 783*b*
nursing diagnoses related to, 783
nursing management of, **783-784**
pathogenesis of, 781, 782*f*
prophylactic treatment of, 782, 783*b*
subacute, 780
Inferior vena cava, 661
Inferior vena cava interruption, 822, 822*f*
Infertility
female, **1242-1243**
drug therapy for, 1243*b*
interprofessional care for, 1243*b*
nursing and interprofessional management of, **1243**
male, **1289**
posttesticular, 1289
pretesticular, 1289
Infestations, 415-417, 416*b*
Infiltrative emergencies, 263*b*, 264
Inflammation, 160-177
acute, 163
acute care for, 164-165
airway, 1618
in burns, 436-437
case study, 176*b*
cerebral, 1338-1342, 1339*b*
chronic, 163
clinical manifestations of, 162-163
drug therapy for, 164-165, 164*b*
in eye, **370-373**
health promotion in, 163-165
heart disorders, **780-790**
intraocular, **382**
local, 162-163, 163*b*, 163*f*
lower gastrointestinal disorders, **942-965**
nursing and interprofessional management of, **163-165**
and nutritional status, 858-859
oral, 897*b*, **897**
pelvic inflammatory disease, **1251-1252**
of scrotum and testes, **1284**
subacute, 163
systemic, 162-163
types of, 163
urinary system, **1033-1041**
Inflammatory bowel disease, 944-949
complications of, 946, 946*b*
dermatologic manifestations of, 399*b*
drug therapy for, 946-948, 947*b*
genetics, 841*b*, 944-945
interprofessional care for, 946-949, 946*b*
nursing assessment in, 949*b*
nursing diagnoses related to, 949
nursing management of, **949-950**
nutritional therapy for, 949
in older adults, 950
postoperative care in, 948-949
surgical therapy for, 948-949, 948*b*
Inflammatory breast cancer, 1211
Inflammatory exudate, 162, 162*b*
Inflammatory prostatitis, asymptomatic, 1282
Inflammatory response, 160-163, 161*f*, 162*b*
Infliximab (Remicade), 1521*b*-1522*b*, 1529
Influenza, 480-481
Influenza A virus, 214*b*
Influenza B virus, 214*b*
Influenza vaccination, 482*b*
Informatics, 6*b*, **13-15**
blood pressure monitoring, 697*b*
cell phones, 889*b*
computer monitoring, 1075*b*
heart surgery DVD/TV, 795*b*
importing monitor and ventilator data, 1578*b*
social media, 1371*b*
video games, 1363*b*
voice banking applications, 1395*b*
web-based knee and hip replacement community, 1477*b*
wireless ECG monitoring, 760*b*
Information access, 53*f*, 55, 65*f*
Internet use, 635*b*
Informed consent, 309, 310*b*
Infusion ports, implanted, **295**, 295*f*
Infusion pumps, 746*b*
smart, 1556*b*
Ingestion, **834-835**
Inguinal hernia, 964, 965*f*
strangulated, 951*f*
Inguinal masses, 1198*b*
Inhalant use, 153
Inhalation agents, 323, 325*b*
Inhalation devices, 551-552
Inhalation injury, 430-431, 435*b*
Inhalers, **551**
Inheritance patterns, 181-182, 181*f*-182*f*, 189*f*
HLA, 206, 207*f*
Injection therapy
fear of injections, 124*b*
intracavernosal injections, 1288
Injury. *See also* Trauma
acute soft tissue, 1464*b*
anterior cruciate ligament, **1467**, 1468*f*
head, **1326-1330**
lower extremity, 1472-1473
meniscus, 1463*b*, **1467**, 1467*f*
repetitive strain, 1465
rotator cuff, **1466-1467**
soft tissue, **1462-1468**, 1464*b*
spinal cord, **1419-1426**
sports-related, 1463*b*
submersion, **1639-1640**
thoracic, **519-527**, 520*b*
traumatic brain, 1326, 1342*b*
upper extremity, 1472
vertebral, 1472
Injury-related malnutrition, 857
Inner ear, 360*f*, 361*b*, **361**
Inner ear problems, 386-391
Inotropic therapy
for heart failure, 746, 748
negative inotropes, 1560
positive inotropes, 1560
Inoue technique, 793, 794*f*
Insect bites, 415-417, 416*b*
Insect stings, 1640, 1640*b*
Insomnia, 91-95
acute, 91-92
case study, 100*b*
chronic, 91-92
drug therapy for, 93*b*-94*b*, **94-95**
interprofessional care for, 93-95, 93*b*

Insomnia *(Continued)*
nursing assessment in, 95, 95*b*
nursing diagnoses related to, 95
nursing interventions for, 95-96
nursing management of, **95-96**
pathophysiology of, 92-93
Inspection, **39**
Inspiratory capacity (IC), 473*b*
Inspiratory reserve volume (IRV), 473*b*
Inspra (eplerenone), 691*b*-693*b*, 745*b*, 748
Insulet Corporation, 1128-1129, 1129*f*
Insulin, 877*b*, 877*f*, 1104*b*, **1108**
endogenous
metabolism of, 1120-1121, 1121*f*
reference values, 1655*b*-1658*b*
exogenous, 1122
administration of, 1127-1129
allergic reactions to, 1129
combination therapy, 1126
commercially available preparations, 1125*b*, 1126*f*
continuous, 1126
for diabetes mellitus, **1125-1130**, 1126*b*, 1139-1140
for elevated potassium levels, 1073*b*
inhaled, 1126*f*, 1130
injection, 1127-1128
injection sites, 1127-1128, 1128*f*
intensive, 1125
long- or intermediate-acting (basal) background, 1126, 1126*f*
mealtime (bolus), 1125-1126
for pancreatitis, 1001*b*
patient & caregiver teaching for, 1128*b*
physiologic, 1125
problems with, 1129-1130
regimens, 1125, 1127*b*
regular insulin IV, 1073*b*, 1126*f*
storage of, 1127
types of, 1125, 1125*b*
Insulin pens, 1128, 1128*f*
Insulin pumps, 1128-1129, 1129*f*
Insulin resistance, 685, 1123
Insulin-dependent diabetes, 1121-1122
Insulin-like growth factor-1, 1115*t*-1118*t*
Intake and output, **277**
Integrase inhibitors, 224*b*
Integrative therapies, 1221*b*
Integrilin (eptifibatide), 715*b*-716*b*
Integument
abnormalities, 1113*b*-1114*b*
physical examination of, 1111-1112
Integumentary problems, 407-428
cultural & ethnic health disparities in, 410*b*
diabetes-related complications, **1151**
postoperative, **343**
Integumentary system, 394
abnormalities, 403*b*
assessment of, **397-405**, 398*b*, 400*b*, 402*b*, 404*b*, 406*b*
normal, 397*b*
preoperative, 306, 307*b*
case study, 398*b*, 400*b*, 404*b*, 406*b*
diagnostic studies of, **405-406**, 405*t*, 406*b*
at end of life, 132*b*
functions of, **396**
in older adults, 396-397, 397*b*
Intellectual impairments, 1351. *See also* Cognitive impairment
Intensity-modulated radiation therapy, 249
Intensive Care Delirium Screening Checklist, 1557
Intensive care units (ICUs), 1554-1555, 1556*f*
electronic ICU, 1554
family presence and visitation in, 1558*b*
teleICU, 1554
Interferon(s)
clinical uses, 194, 195*b*
functions of, 194, 195*b*, 195*f*
for hepatitis, 981
Interferon β-1a, 1385*b*
Interferon β-1b, 1385*b*
Interferon-γ (IFN-gamma) release assays (IGRAs), **508**
Interleukin-1 receptor antagonist, 195*b*, 1521*b*-1522*b*, 1529
Interleukin-6 receptor antagonist, 1521*b*-1522*b*, 1529
Interleukin-11, 260*b*
Interleukins
clinical uses, 194, 195*b*
functions of, 194, 195*b*
Intermaxillary fixation, 1486*f*
Intermediate care units, 1555
Intermenstrual bleeding, 1246
Intermittent catheterization, **1062-1063**
Intermittent claudication, 803
Intermittent mandatory ventilation, 1576*b*
Intermittent pneumatic compression devices, 819
Internal fixation, **1473**, 1473*f*
Internal fixation devices, 1473, 1473*f*
Internal rotation, 1455*b*
International Association of Laryngectomees, 493
International normalized ratio (INR), 601*t*, 821*b*, 852*t*
International Prognostic Index (IPI), 644
International Standards for Neurologic Classification of Spinal Cord Injury, 1425
Internet access, 55
for eating disorders, 871*b*
HIV management, 229*b*
information access, 635*b*
for older adults, 65*b*, 65*f*
web-based knee and hip replacement community, 1477*b*
Interpreters, 31, 31*b*
Interprofessional teams, **9-10**, 10*b*, 15*f*, 24*f*
Interspinous process decompression system, 1506
Interstitial cells of Cajal, 968
Interstitial cell–stimulating hormone (ICSH), 1105, 1188
Interstitial cerebral edema, 1317
Interstitial cystitis/painful bladder syndrome, 1040-1041
Interstitial edema, 741
Interstitial fluid, 271, 273-274
Interstitial laser coagulation (ILC), 1272
Interstitial lung diseases, 528-529
Interstitial oncotic pressure, 274
Interstitial pancreatitis, 999
Intertriginous areas, 399
Intertrigo, 401, 401*f*, 403*b*, 1208
Interventional radiology
catheter-based procedures, 806
for peripheral arterial disease, 806
for varicose veins, 825-826
for VTE treatment, 822
Intervertebral disc disease, 1504-1506
interprofessional care for, 1505-1506, 1506*b*
surgical therapy for, 1506
Intervertebral foramen, 1505
Interviews
considerations for patient interviews, 35
motivational interviewing, 47, 48*b*
preoperative, **302**
Intestinal infarction, 951
Intestinal obstruction, 950-952
clinical manifestations of, 951-952, 951*b*
interprofessional care for, 952
nursing diagnoses for, 952
nursing management of, **952-953**
pseudo-obstruction, 951
types of, 950-951
Intestinal secretagogues, 936, 936*b*
Intestinal strangulation, 951, 951*f*
Intestinal transplantation, 968
Intima, 802-803
Intimate partner violence, 1263, 1644
Intoxication. *See also specific intoxicants*
alcohol toxicity, **149-150**
paradoxic, 1390
poisonings, **1642-1644**, 1643*b*
water, 442
Intraabdominal hypertension, 812
Intraaortic balloon pump, 1566-1568, 1567*f*
complications of, 1567-1568, 1568*b*
indications and contraindications to, 1566*b*
Intraaortic balloon pump machine, 1567, 1567*f*
Intracavernosal injections, 1288
Intracellular fluid, 271
Intracellular space, 271
Intracerebral hematoma, 1329
Intracerebral hemorrhage, 1348*b*, **1349**
hypertensive, 1349, 1349*f*
Intracranial bleeding, 1336*b*
Intracranial pressure, **1314-1316**
changes in, 1315-1316, 1316*f*
increased, **1316-1323**
acute care for, 1324-1326
clinical manifestations of, 1317-1318
complications of, 1318-1319
diagnostic studies for, 1319
drug therapy for, 1322
interprofessional care for, 1319*b*, 1322-1323
mechanisms of, 1316
nursing assessment in, 1323-1324
nursing diagnoses related to, 1324
nursing management of, **1323-1326**
nutritional therapy for, 1322-1323
ocular signs of, 1318
progression of, 1316, 1317*f*
psychologic considerations, 1326
monitoring, 1319-1322, 1320*f*
acute care, 1325
indications for, 1319
methods for, 1319-1320
sites for placement of devices, 1319, 1319*f*
normal, 1314-1315
normal compensatory adaptations, 1315
normal waveforms, 1320*b*
radiation effects on, 251*b*-252*b*
regulation and maintenance of, 1314-1315
Intracranial pressure-volume curve, 1315-1316, 1316*f*
Intracranial problems, acute, **1314-1344**
Intradermal tests, 201
Intradiscal electrothermoplasty, 1506
Intraductal papilloma, 1208
Intragastric balloons, 885, 886*b*
Intraocular disorders, 373-383
Intraocular pressure testing, 356*b*, 358
Intraoperative care, 315-329
case study, 328*b*
nursing activities, 317*b*
nursing management after surgery, **322**
nursing management before surgery, **318-319**
nursing management during surgery, **319-322**
Intraosseous access, 1596, 1596*b*
Intraperitoneal chemotherapy, 247
Intrapleural space, 455-456
Intrapulmonary shunts, 1611
Intrathecal or intraventricular chemotherapy, 248
Intraurethral devices, 1288
Intravascular ultrasound, 673*t*-677*t*, 678-679
Intravascular volume depletion, 434
Intravenous immunoglobulin (IVIG), 1545, 1545*b*
Intravenous pyelography (IVP), 1025*t*-1030*t*
Intravenous (IV) therapy, **292-294**, 294*b*
additives, 293
agents for anesthesia, 323, 325*b*

Intraventricular chemotherapy, 248
Intravesical bladder chemotherapy, 248
Intrinsic factor, 612
Intron A (α-interferon), 195*b*
Intubation
  endotracheal, 1569
  nasal ET, 1569-1570
  oral, 1569-1570
  rapid-sequence, 1570
Invasive blood pressure monitoring
  arterial blood pressure, 1561-1562
  arterial pressure-based cardiac output (APCO) monitoring, 1562-1563, 1562*f*
  central venous or right atrial pressure measurement, 1564
  optimally damped system, 1561, 1561*f*
  principles of, 1560-1561
  steps for obtaining measurements, 1561*b*
  system components, 1560, 1560*f*
  types of, 1561-1565
  venous oxygen saturation monitoring, 1564-1565
  zero reference stopcock positioning, 1561*b*
Invasive ductal carcinoma, 1210-1211
Invasive lobular carcinoma, 1211
Inversion, 1455*b*
Invokana (canagliflozin), 1131*b*
Involucrum, 1496-1497
Iodine, 1166
  radioactive, 1166
Ionizing radiation, 1645
Ipratropium (Atrovent HFA), 548*b*-549*b*
Ipratropium bromide (Atrovent), 479*b*-480*b*
Ipratropium/albuterol (Combivent Respimat, DuoNeb), 548*b*-549*b*
Iprivask (desirudin), 820*b*
Irbesartan (Avapro), 691*b*-693*b*
Iris, 353*b*, 358
Iron
  blood studies, 601-602, 602*t*
  food sources, 610*b*, 856*b*
  metabolism of, **590**, 590*f*, 601-602
  overdose, 1643*b*
  reference values, 1655*b*-1658*b*
  supplemental, 610-611, 611*b*
Iron overload, 651*b*
Iron-binding capacity, 1655*b*-1658*b*
Iron-deficiency anemia, **609-611**
  drug therapy for, 610-611
  interprofessional care for, 610-611, 611*b*
  laboratory studies, 610, 610*b*
  nursing management of, **611**
Irritable bowel syndrome, 940*b*, **940-941**
Irritant contact dermatitis, 409
Irritants, 409
Ischemia, 703, 1345
  acute arterial ischemic disorders, **808-809**
  critical limb ischemia, 804-806
  myocardial, 712, 776, 776*f*
  silent, 713
  transient ischemic attacks, **1347-1348**
Ischemic stroke, 1348-1349, 1348*b*
  acute care for, 1354-1355
  drug therapy for, 1355
  endovascular therapy for, 1355
Ishihara test, 356*b*
Islam, 26*b*
Islamic Food and Nutrition Council of America, 856
Isoflurane (Forane), 325*b*
Isografts, 427
Isolated systolic hypertension, 684
Isolation precautions, 218*b*
Isometric activities, 732
Isoniazid (INH), 509*b*
Isoptin (verapamil), 1059*b*
Isopto (carbachol), 381*b*
Isopto Carpine (pilocarpine), 381*b*
Isosorbide dinitrate (Isordil), 715*b*-716*b*, 716
Isosorbide dinitrate/hydralazine (BiDil), 745*b*, 748
Isosorbide mononitrate, 715*b*-716*b*, 716
Isotonic solutions, 273, 273*f*, 292, 293*b*, 1597*b*
Isotretinoin (Accutane), 417*b*
Isradipine, 691*b*-693*b*
Istalol (timolol maleate), 381*b*
Itching. *See* Pruritus
Ivabradine (Corlanor), 745*b*
Ivacaftor (Kalydeco), 579
Ivacaftor/lumicaftor (Orkambi), 579

J

J reflex, 1622
Jaeger chart, 356*b*
Jakson-Pratt drainage devices, 168, 169*f*
Janus kinase (JAK) inhibitors, 1521*b*-1522*b*, 1528
Janus kinase-2 (JAK2) gene, 620
Januvia (sitagliptin), 1131*b*
Jardiance (empagliflozin), 1131*b*
Jaundice, 403*b*, 597*b*-598*b*, 975, 975*f*, **986**
  classification of, 978*b*
  in hepatitis, 977-978
  in light- and dark-skinned persons, 404*b*
  obstructive, 1006*b*
Jaw-thrust maneuver, 1630, 1630*f*, 1651
JC papovavirus, 222*b*
Jehovah's Witness, 26*b*
Jejunostomy tubes (J-tubes), 865-866, 865*f*
Jet lag disorder, 98
The Joint Commission (TJC), 12, 124
  Speak Up initiative, 50-51, 51*b*
  venous thromboembolism measures, 818-819
Joint surgery, 1490
  complications of, 1492
  interprofessional care in, 1492
  nursing management of, **1492-1493**
  postoperative management in, 1492
  preoperative management in, 1492
  procedures, **1490-1493**
  types of, 1490-1492
Joint swelling, 597*b*-598*b*
Joints, **1448**
  classification of, 1448*f*
  diarthrodial, 1448, 1448*f*-1449*f*
  mobility assessment, 1454
  osteoarthritis in, 1518
  patient & caregiver teaching for protection of, 1524*b*, 1531*b*
  protection of, 1519, **1531**
  rheumatoid arthritis in, 1526-1527
  in scleroderma, 1543
Journaling, 82*b*
Judaism, 26*b*
Jugular venous bulb oximetry, 1322
Jugular venous distention, 666, 668*b*
Junctional dysrhythmias, 764*b*, **767**, 767*f*
Juvenile-onset diabetes, 1121-1122

K

Kadcyla (ado-trastuzumab emtansine), 1217*b*, 1218
Kalydeco (ivacaftor), 579
Kaposi sarcoma, 221, 221*f*, 222*b*
Katz Index, 859
Kayexalate (sodium polystyrene sulfonate), 1073, 1073*b*
Kegel (pelvic floor muscle) exercises, 933, 1057*b*-1058*b*
Keloid scarring, 167*b*, 167*f*
Keloids, 403-405, 403*b*, 403*f*
Kengreal (cangrelor), 715*b*-716*b*
Keratinocytes, 394
Keratitis, 371, **372**
Keratoconjunctivitis, 372
Keratoconjunctivitis sicca, 373
Keratoconus, **373**
Keratometry, 356*b*
Ketamine (Ketalar), 325*b*
Ketogenic diet, 1379
Ketones, urinary, 1115*t*-1118*t*, 1661*b*
Ketoprofen, 1521*b*-1522*b*
Ketorolac, 111*b*
17-Ketosteroids, 1115*t*-1118*t*
Kidney(s). *See also under* Renal
  acid-base regulation by, 288
  blood supply, 1016
  functions of, **1015-1018**
    indicators of, 1080*b*
    regulation of blood pressure, 683
    regulation of water balance, 275
  macrostructure of, 1015-1016, 1016*f*
  microstructure of, 1016, 1016*f*
  in older adults, 1020*b*
  palpation of, 1023, 1023*f*
  structures of, **1015-1018**, 1018*f*
  wearable artificial, **1092**
Kidney cancer, **1052-1053**, 1053*b*
Kidney disease
  hereditary, **1051-1052**
  hypertension and, 686*b*, 687
  immunologic disorders, **1041-1044**
  recurrence after kidney transplantation, 1096
  in systemic lupus erythematosus, 1538-1539
Kidney Disease Improving Global Outcomes (KDIGO) Clinical Practice Guidelines, 1076
Kidney failure, 1069. *See also* Renal failure
Kidney punch, 1023
Kidney stone dance, 1046
Kidney stones, **1045**, 1048*b*
Kidney transplantation, **1092-1095**
  complications of, 1095-1096, 1096*b*
  corticosteroid-related complications of, 1096
  histocompatibility studies for, 1093
  immunosuppressive therapy for, 1095
  live donor, 1094-1095
  nursing management of transplant recipients, **1095-1097**
  postoperative care in, 1095
  preoperative care in, 1095
  selection of recipients, 1092-1093
  sources of donors for, 1093-1094
  surgical placement, 1094-1095, 1094*f*
  surgical procedure, 1094-1095
Kidneys, ureters, bladder (KUB) x-ray, 1025*t*-1030*t*
Kineret (anakinra), 195*b*, 1521*b*-1522*b*, 1529
Kinetic therapy, 1625
Kinins, 162*b*
Kit chroeun, 29*b*
Klebsiella pneumoniae, 216*b*
Klebsiella-Enterobacter, 214*b*
Knee arthroplasty, 1491
Knee arthroscopy, 1460*f*
Knee immobilizer, 1473, 1473*f*
Knee replacement, 1477*b*
Knock-knees, 1456*b*
Knowledge
  advances in, 3-4
  cultural, 23*b*
  need for, 47*b*, 53
Knowles, Malcolm, 47
Kock pouch, 1065, 1065*f*
Korean Americans, 29*b*

Korotkoff sounds, 664
Kosher dietary practices, 856
Kosher Quest, 856
Koucharang or *kit chroeun*, 29*b*
KUB (kidneys, ureters, bladder) x-ray, 1025*t*-1030*t*
Kübler-Ross model of grief, 133*b*
Kupffer cells, 837
Kussmaul respirations, 467*b*-468*b*
Kwashiorkor, 856
Kyphoplasty, 646, 1513
Kyphosis, 663*b*, 1456*b*, 1511, 1512*f*

L

Labetalol, 691*b*-693*b*, 699*b*
Labile factor, 592*b*
Laboratory reference values, **1655**
Lacerations, scalp, 1326-1328
Lachman's test, 1467
Lacrimal apparatus, 352*f*, 353*b*
Lactase deficiency, 967
Lactate, 1590*t*
Lactated Ringer's (Hartmann's) solution, 292, 293*b*
Lactating female breasts, 1187-1188, 1188*f*
Lactational breast abscess, 1207
Lactational mastitis, 1206, 1206*b*
Lactic dehydrogenase, 602*t*, 1655*b*-1658*b*
Lactulose, 993*b*
Laminectomy, 1506
Lamivudine (Epivir), 980
Lamotrigine (Lamictal), 116*b*
Langerhans' cells, 194, 395
Language differences, 25*b*
Lansoprazole (Prevacid), 903*b*
Lanugo, 871
Laparoscopic cholecystectomy, 1007-1009, 1010*b*
Laparoscopic nephrectomy, 1063, 1094
Laparoscopy, 847*t*-850*t*
Lapatinib (Tykerb), 257, 1217*b*, 1218
Large cell carcinoma, 515*b*
Large intestine, **836-837**
  anatomic locations, 836, 837*f*
  obstruction of, 951*b*
  in older adults, 840*b*
  polyps of, **953**, 953*f*
Laryngeal cancer, 496*b*
Laryngeal edema, postoperative, 333*b*
Laryngeal polyps, 490
Laryngeal problems, 484-496
Laryngeal stridor, 1168
Laryngectomy, 491, 492*f*, 494*b*
Laryngopharynx, 453
Laryngospasm, postoperative, 333*b*
Laser ablation
  bronchoscopic therapy, 517
  contact laser techniques, 1272
  cosmetic procedures, 425
  for dermatologic problems, 420, 420*b*
  for head and neck cancer, 491
  interstitial coagulation (ILC), 1272
  photocoagulation, 377
  prostatectomy, 1271-1272, 1272*b*
  transmyocardial revascularization, 725
  visual, of the prostate (VLAP), 1272
Laser-assisted in situ keratomileusis (LASIK), 368
Laser-assisted subepithelial keratomileusis (LASEK), 368
Lasix (furosemide)
  for cirrhosis, 993*b*
  for heart failure, 745*b*
  for hypertension, 691*b*-693*b*
Latanoprost (Xalatan), 381*b*
Late potentials, 762
Latent autoimmune diabetes in adults, 1122
Lateral epicondylitis, 1456*b*
Latex allergy, 203-204, 327
  guidelines for preventing, 204*b*
  nursing and interprofessional management of, **204**
  types of, 203
Latex-food syndrome, 203-204
Latinos, 19
  cultural characteristics of, 22*b*
  culture-bound syndromes, 29*b*
  in health care workplace, 24
  older adults, 63
Latissimus dorsi flap, 1223-1224
Lawton Scale, 859
Laxatives, 935-936, 936*b*
Leadership, 646*b*, 1090*b*
  in changing environments, 1365*b*
  conflict resolution, 1159*b*
  development of, 86*b*, 125*b*
  safe delegation, 868*b*
Learning
  adult learning principles, 47, 47*b*
  auditory, 53
  factors affecting teaching, 51*b*, 53
  motivation for, 47*b*
  orientation to, 47*b*
  physical, 53
  process of, 46-51
  readiness for, 47*b*, 53
  setting goals for, 54
  visual, 53
  writing goals for, 54*b*
Learning materials, 54-55, 54*f*
Learning needs, 53
Learning styles, 53
Leflunomide (Arava), 1521*b*-1522*b*, 1528
Left atrial appendage occlusion, 767, 1353
Left ventricular aneurysm, 721
Left ventricular assist devices, 747*f*
Left ventricular end-diastolic pressure, 1559-1560
Left ventricular free wall rupture, 721
Left ventricular hypertrophy, 685-686, 686*f*
Left ventricular thrombus, 743
Left-sided heart failure, 738-739, 742*b*
Leg ulcers, 597*b*-598*b*
  venous, **826-827**, 827*b*, 827*f*
Legal blindness, 358, 368
Legal issues. *See also* Ethical/legal issues
  in end-of-life care, **135-137**, 137*b*
  for older adults, **69**
  preparation for surgery, 309-310
Legionella pneumophila, 214*b*
Leininger, Madeleine, 23
Leiomyomas, 1254-1255, 1254*f*
Lemtrada (alemtuzumab), 1385*b*, 1386
Lens, of eye, 352
  abnormalities, 357*b*
  contact lenses, 368
  intraocular
    phakic, 368
    refractive, 368
  Morgan, 370
  in older adults, 353*b*
Lentigo, 419*b*
Leptin, 834, 877, 877*b*, 877*f*
Lesbian, gay, bisexual, and transgender (LGBT) individuals, 21*b*, **21**
Lescol (fluvastatin), 711*b*
Lesions. *See also* Skin lesions
  cardiac, **788**
  ear, 365*b*
  genital, **1232-1240**
  Ghon, 506
  punctate, 810
  skip, 945
Letairis (ambrisentan), 532*b*
Lethargy, 1113*b*-1114*b*
Letrozole (Femara), 1217*b*
Leukemia, 635-639
  acute care for, 640
  acute lymphocytic leukemia, 636*b*, **636**, 639*b*
  acute myelogenous leukemia, 636*b*, **636**, 639*b*
  ambulatory care for, 640
  case study, 652*b*
  chronic lymphocytic leukemia, 636*b*, **636-637**, 639*b*
  chronic myelogenous leukemia, 636*b*, **636**, 639*b*
  classification of, 240-241, 635-637
  clinical manifestations of, 637
  diagnostic studies in, 637-638
  drug therapy for, 638, 639*b*
  etiology of, 635
  genetics of, 636
  interprofessional care for, 638-639
  lymphoma overlap, 637
  minimal residual disease, 638
  nursing assessment in, 639*b*
  nursing management of, **639-640**
  pathophysiology of, 637, 637*f*
  remission of, 638
  treatment of, 638
  types of, 636*b*
Leukine (sargramostim), 195*b*
Leukocytes. *See* White blood cells
Leukopenia, 599, 632
  in cancer, 251*b*-252*b*
Leukoplakia, 846*b*-847*b*, 898
Leukotriene modifiers, 547-549, 548*b*-549*b*
Leukotriene receptor antagonists, **202**
  for asthma, 547, 548*b*-549*b*
  for rhinitis and sinusitis, 479*b*-480*b*
Leukotrienes, 162, **162**, 162*f*
Leuprolide (Lupron, Eligard)
  for endometriosis, 1243*b*, 1253*b*
  for prostate cancer, 1280*b*
Levalbuterol (Xopenex), 548*b*-549*b*
Levbid (hyoscyamine), 1059*b*
Level of consciousness
  altered consciousness, 1308*b*-1309*b*
  in increased ICP, 1317-1318
  unconsciousness, 1317-1318, 1652*b*
Levobunolol (Betagan), 381*b*
Levocetirizine (Xyzal), 479*b*-480*b*
Levodopa (L-dopa), 1391*b*
Levofloxacin (Levaquin), 509*b*
Levophed (norepinephrine), 1599*b*
Levorphanol (Levo-Dromoran), 112, 113*b*-114*b*, 117*b*
Levothyroxine (Synthroid), 1169, 1169*b*
Levsin (hyoscyamine), 1059*b*
Lewy bodies, 1387-1388
Lewy body dementia, 1401*b*
Lhermitte's sign, 1384
Lice, 416*b*
Licensed practical/vocational nurses (LPN/LVNs), 11
  intraoperative activities, **317**
  role in assessment and data collection, 36*b*
  role in bladder irrigation, 1274*b*
  role in blood transfusions, 649*b*
  role in cardiac catheterization and PCI, 729*b*
  role in caring for acute stroke patients, 1359*b*
  role in caring for Alzheimer's patients, 1412*b*
  role in caring for arthritis patients, 1529*b*
  role in caring for chronic venous insufficiency and venous ulcers, 827*b*
  role in caring for diabetic patients, 1152*b*
  role in caring for incontinent patients, 1059*b*
  role in caring for neutropenia patients, 632*b*
  role in caring for osteomyelitis patients, 1498*b*
  role in caring for patients with casts or in traction, 1471*b*
  role in caring for seizure patients, 1380*b*

Licensed practical/vocational nurses (LPN/LVNs) *(Continued)*
role in caring for the patient with hypertension, 696*b*
role in caring for VTE patients, 824*b*
role in IV therapy, 294*b*
role in nasogastric and gastric tubes and enteral feedings, 867*b*
role in ostomy care, 960*b*
role in oxygen administration, 568*b*
role in pain management, 123*b*
role in postoperative care, 334*b*
role in skin care, 425*b*
role in suctioning and tracheostomy care, 490*b*
role in wound care, 170*b*
role with corrective lenses and hearing aids, 392*b*
role with urinary catheters, 1061*b*
Lichen sclerosis, 1250
Lichenification, 403*b*, 424
LICOX brain tissue O_2 system, 1321-1322, 1321*f*, 1352-1353
Lidocaine (Lidoderm), 116*b*
for pain, 118-119
LifePak defibrillator, 771-772, 772*f*
Lifestyle modifications
MyPlate tips for health, 862*b*
therapeutic, 708-709
therapeutic diet for, 709*b*
tips for, 709*b*
for urinary incontinence, 1057*b*
Ligament injury, 1463*b*
Ligaments, 1450
Light skin, 404*b*
Limb-girdle muscular dystrophy, 1501*b*
Limbic system, 79, 1297
Linear accelerators, 250, 250*f*
LINX Reflux Management System, 903-904
Liotrix, 1169
Lip cancer, 898*b*
Lip reading, 390
Lipase, 847*t*-850*t*
Lipectomy, 890, 890*f*
Lipid-lowering agents, 709-710, 710*b*
for ACS, 715*b*-716*b*, 725-726
for angina, 715*b*-716*b*, 717
mechanism of action, 715*b*-716*b*
Lipids, serum, **670**, 673*t*-677*t*
elevated, 704-706
Lipitor (atorvastatin), 711*b*
Lipodermatosclerosis, 818, 818*f*
Lipodystrophy
in antiretroviral therapy, 230
clinical manifestations of, 230, 230*f*
in insulin therapy, 1129
Lipoma, **419*b***
Lipoprotein (a), 670, 673*t*-677*t*
Lipoprotein-associated phospholipase A_2, **671**, 673*t*-677*t*
Lipoproteins, 670, 673*t*-677*t*
drugs that increase removal of, 710, 711*b*
drugs that restrict production of, 709-710, 711*b*
Liposuction, 426, 890
Liquid oxygen (O_2), 565*f*, 568, 568*f*
Liraglutide (Saxenda), 884*b*
Liraglutide (Victoza), 1131*b*-1132*b*, 1132
Lisinopril (Zestril), 691*b*-693*b*, 715*b*-716*b*
Listening, active, 49
Literacy, 52
ehealth literacy, 53
health literacy, 20, 52
Lithiasis, 1045
choledocholithiasis, 1007
cholelithiasis, **1005-1008**, 1005*f*
Lithiasis *(Continued)*
microlithiasis, 999
nephrolithiasis, 1045
Lithotripsy, **1047-1048**
cystoscopic, 1047
electrohydraulic, 1048
extracorporeal shock wave lithotripsy, 1048
laser, 1047
percutaneous ultrasonic, 1048
Lithotrites, 1047
Live donor kidney transplantation
postoperative care in, 1095
surgical procedure, 1094
Live donors, 1093
Liver, **592-593**. *See also under* Hepatic
assessment of
palpation, 598, 844, 845*f*
preoperative, 306, 307*b*
functions of, 837*b*, **837-838**
nodular, 846*b*-847*b*
in older adults, 840*b*
secretions of, 835*b*
structure of, **837-838**, 838*f*
Liver biopsy, 847*t*-850*t*, **851-852**
Liver cancer, **996-997**
cultural & ethnic health disparities, 986*b*
metastatic carcinoma, 996, 997*f*
nursing and interprofessional management of, **997**
Liver disorders, **974-999**
associated with obesity, 879
autoimmune diseases, **985**
chemical-induced diseases, **984**
corticosteroid therapy for, 1180*b*
cultural & ethnic health disparities, 986*b*
dermatologic manifestations of, 399*b*
drug-induced diseases, **984**
drug-induced liver injury, 984
genetic diseases, **985**
metabolic diseases, **985**
in older adults, **998-999**
Liver dullness, 846*b*-847*b*
Liver enzymes, 1590*t*
Liver failure
acute, 978, **996**
fulminant, 996
Liver function studies, **852**, 852*t*
Liver transplantation, **998-999**
Liver ultrasound, 603*t*
Living will, 135, 136*b*
LMNOP mnemonic for resuscitation aids, 1632
Lobectomy, 526*b*
Lobular carcinoma, 1210
invasive (infiltrating), 1211
Lobular carcinoma in situ, 1210
Local anesthesia, 323*b*, **324-327**
methods of administration, 324-327
perineural, 340
Lockjaw, 1442
Lomotil (diphenoxylate with atropine), 931*b*
Loneliness, 139
Long-term care, 8
Long-term care facilities, **68-69**, 69*f*
Loop colostomy, 959*f*
Loop diuretics
for heart failure, 745*b*, 747
for hypertension, 691*b*-693*b*
Loop electrosurgical excision procedure (LEEP), 1198*t*-1201*t*
Loop of Henle, 1017, 1017*b*
Loop stoma, 958
Loopography, 1025*t*-1030*t*
Looser's transformation zones, 1510
Loperamide (Imodium A-D, Pepto Diarrhea Control), 931*b*
Lopid (gemfibrozil), 710*b*-711*b*
Lopressor (metoprolol), 691*b*-693*b*, 715*b*-716*b*, 771*b*
Loratadine (Claritin), 479*b*-480*b*
Lorazepam (Ativan), 326*b*, 1378
Lorcaserin (Belviq), 884*b*
Lordosis, 1456*b*, 1485
Losartan (Cozaar)
for heart failure, 745*b*
for hypertension, 691*b*-693*b*
mechanism of action, 715*b*-716*b*
Loss of protective sensation, 1151
Lotensin (benazepril), 691*b*-693*b*, 745*b*
Lotronex (alosetron), 941*b*
Lou Gehrig's disease, 1395
Lovastatin, 711*b*
Lovecraft, H.P., 301
Lovenox (enoxaparin), 715*b*-716*b*, 820*b*
Low back pain, **1502-1510**
acute, **1503-1504**
chronic, **1504**
nursing assessment in, 1503*b*
patient & caregiver teaching for, 1504*b*
in peritoneal dialysis, 1087
Low vision, 368
Low-density lipoprotein cholesterol, 1148
Low-density lipoproteins (LDLs), 670, 673*t*-677*t*, 1655*b*-1658*b*
Lower airway injury, **431**, 437
Lower esophageal sphincter, 835
Lower esophageal sphincter pressure, 900, 900*b*
Lower extremities
casts for, 1472-1473
diabetes-related complications, **1150-1151**, 1150*f*
peripheral arterial disease of, **803-808**, 803*f*
Lower extremity amputation, 1490, 1490*b*
Lower gastrointestinal problems, **929-973**
Lower gastrointestinal series, 845-851, 847*t*-850*t*, 851*f*
Lower genital tract infections, 1250*b*, **1250-1251**
Lower motor neurons, 1296
Lower respiratory tract
problems of, **499-537**
structures and functions of, **454-455**, **454*f***, 455*f*
Lower respiratory tract infections, **499-513**
Lower urinary tract symptoms, 1034, 1035*b*
Low-molecular-weight heparins
for angina and ACS, 715*b*-716*b*
for VTE, 820*b*, 821
LUCAS 2 Mechanical Chest Compression Device, 1634, 1635*f*
Lumbar disc disease, 1505
Lumbar disc herniation, 1505*b*
Lumbar puncture, 603*t*, 1310*t*-1312*t*
Lumigan (bimatoprost), 381*b*
Lumpectomy, 1213-1214, 1214*f*
postoperative exercises, 1219, 1220*f*
with radiation therapy, 1215*b*
Lund-Browder chart, 432, 433*f*
Lung(s)
blood supply, 455
compliance of, 456
normal gas exchange, 1609, 1610*f*
normal regional V/Q differences, 1610, 1611*f*
physical examination of, **463-466**
white, 1622-1623, 1622*f*
Lung abscess, 503, **512-513**
Lung biopsy, 469*t*-471*t*, **471-472**, 472*f*

Lung cancer, **513-519**, 514*f*-515*f*
acute care for, 517-518
ambulatory care for, 518
bronchoscopic laser therapy for, 517
case study, 535*b*
chemotherapy for, 516
clinical manifestations of, 515
cultural & ethnic health disparities in, 514*b*
diagnostic studies in, 515-516
etiology of, 514
gender differences in, 514*b*
health promotion for, 517
immunotherapy for, 517
interprofessional care for, 516-517, 516*b*
nursing assessment in, 517, 518*b*
nursing diagnoses related to, 517
nursing management of, **517-518**
pathophysiology of, 514-515
photodynamic therapy for, 517
prophylactic cranial radiation for, 517
radiation therapy for, 516
screening for, 516
surgical therapy for, 516
targeted therapy for, 516-517
types of, 501*b*
Lung diseases
diffuse parenchymal, 528
environmental, **513**
interstitial, **528-529**
obstructive, **538-584**
restrictive disorders, **527-528**
extrapulmonary conditions, 527, 527*b*
intrapulmonary conditions, 527, 527*b*
vascular disorders, **529-531**
Lung injury
acute transfusion-related reaction, 650*b*-651*b*
associated with burns, 431*b*
Lung resection, 526*b*
Lung transplantation, **533-534**, 571
bilateral, 534
heart-lung, 534
indications for, 533*b*
postoperative care for, 534
preoperative care for, 533-534
single-lung, 534
surgical procedure, 534
Lung tumors, 518-519
Lung volume reduction surgery, 526*b*, 571
Lung volumes and capacities, 473*b*
Lupron (leuprolide), 1243*b*, 1280*b*
Lupus. *See* Systemic lupus erythematosus
Luteinizing hormone, 1104*b*
measurement of, 1115*t*-1118*t*, 1198*t*-1201*t*
regulation of reproductive system by, 1188
Lyme disease, **1534-1535**, 1534*f*, 1535*b*
Lymph node biopsy, 603*t*, 604
Lymph node removal, 492
Lymph nodes, 592
assessment of, 596-598
axillary, 1211, 1212*f*
analysis of, 1212, 1214
dissection of, 1212
functions of, 192
sentinel, 238
Lymph system, **592**
Lymphadenopathy, 597*b*-598*b*
Lymphedema, 592, 1214, 1215*f*
Lymphocytes, 161, **192-194**, **590**, 1659*b*
Lymphoid organs, 192, 192*f*
Lymphoma, **640-652**
classification of, 240-241
CNS, 1333*b*
cutaneous T-cell, 412*b*
Hodgkin's, **640-641**, 641*b*, 641*f*
leukemia overlap, 637
non-Hodgkin's, 639, 641*b*, **642-644**
Lynch syndrome, 954*b*
Lyrica (pregabalin), 116*b*

M

M proteins, 645
Maalox (aluminum and magnesium), 903*b*
Macitentan (Opsumit), 532*b*
Macrobid (nitrofurantoin), 1036
Macrodantin (nitrofurantoin), 1036, 1036*b*
Macroglial cells, 1294-1295
Macrophage colony-stimulating factor, 260*b*
Macrophages, 193*f*, 239, 459
Macula, 352
Macules, 401*b*
Maestro Rechargeable System, 886*b*, 887, 887*f*
Magnesium, 771*b*, 1655*b*-1658*b*
Magnesium imbalances, 286*b*, **286**
in chronic kidney disease, 1077
hypermagnesemia, 286*b*, **286**
hypomagnesemia, 286*b*, **286**
Magnesium oxide (MagOx), 903*b*
Magnesium sulfate, 993*b*
Magnet Recognition Program (ANCC), 5
Magnetic resonance angiography, 673*t*-677*t*, 1025*t*-1030*t*, 1310*t*-1312*t*
Magnetic resonance cholangiopancreatography, 847*t*-850*t*
Magnetic resonance imaging
abdominal, 1115*t*-1118*t*
of brain, 1309*f*, 1310*t*-1312*t*
of breast, 1198*t*-1201*t*
cardiovascular, 672-678, 673*t*-677*t*
in endocrine disorders, 1115*t*-1118*t*
functional (fMRI), 1310*t*-1312*t*
gastrointestinal, 847*t*-850*t*
in hematologic disorders, 603*t*
in musculoskeletal disorders, 1457*t*-1459*t*
of reproductive system, 1198*t*-1201*t*
of respiratory system, 469*t*-471*t*
of urinary system, 1025*t*-1030*t*
Magnetic resonance spectroscopy, 1310*t*-1312*t*
Magnetoencephalography (MEG), 1310*t*-1312*t*
Major histocompatibility antigens, 199
Malabsorption syndrome, 857, **965-968**
causes of, 965, 965*b*
clinical manifestations of, 965, 966*b*
dermatologic manifestations of, 399*b*
Malabsorptive surgery, 885-887, 886*b*
Male external genitalia, 1185
Male reproductive system
abnormalities, 1191*b*, 1198*b*
areas in which problems are likely to develop, 1268, 1269*f*
assessment of, **1191-1196**, 1196*b*
diagnostic studies of, 1198*t*-1201*t*
normal, 1196*b*
in older adults, 1191*b*
physical examination of, 1195, 1196*b*
problems of, **1268-1291**
structures and functions of, **1184-1185**, 1185*f*
Male sexual function, **1286-1289**
Male sexual response, 1190
Malignancy. *See also* Cancer
of external ear, **384**
in kidney transplantation, 1096
Malignant bone tumors, **1500-1501**
Malignant external otitis, 383
Malignant hyperthermia
in operating room, 327-329
postoperative, 341
Malignant melanoma, **411-413**, 412*b*
Breslow measurement, 412, 413*f*
case study, 427*b*
Clark level, 412
interprofessional care for, 411-413
Malignant neoplasms, **240**
Malignant nephrosclerosis, 1050
Malleus, 361
Mallory-Weiss tears, 894
Malnutrition, **856-859**, 857*f*, 859*f*
acute care for, 862-863
acute disease–related, 857
ambulatory care for, 863
in cancer, 261-262
chronic disease–related, 857
clinical manifestations of, 859, 859*f*
conditions that increase risk for, 857*b*
contributing factors, 857-858
diagnostic studies in, 859
etiology of, 856-857
gerontologic considerations, **863-864**
health promotion for, 861
injury-related, 857
laboratory studies, 859
nursing and interprofessional management of, **859-864**
nursing assessment in, 859-861, 860*b*
nursing diagnoses for, 861
protein-calorie, 856
starvation-related, 857
Malocclusion, 1486
Malunion, 1470*b*
Mammalian target of rapamycin (mTOR), 1053
MammaPrint, 1213
Mammography, 1198*t*-1201*t*
digital, 1205
screening, 1205, 1205*f*
stereotactic, 1206
three-dimensional (3D), 1205
Mammoplasty, **1222-1224**
augmentation, 1224
MammoSite system, 1216
Mammostrat, 1213
Management, 1090*b*
Mandibular fracture, 1486*b*, **1486-1487**
Mandibulectomy, 840*b*, 899
Mantoux test, 508
Marasmus, 856
Marijuana, **153**
Marinol (dronabinol), 153, 894, 895*b*
Mass casualty incident (MCI), 1645
Mass casualty incident preparedness, 1645-1646
Massage, **85**, **121**
Masses
abdominal, 846*b*-847*b*
inguinal, 1198*b*
penile, 1198*b*
in rectum and anus, 846*b*-847*b*
scrotal, 1198*b*, 1284*f*
Mast cell stabilizers, 202, 479*b*-480*b*
Mast cells, 590
Mastalgia, **1206**
Mastectomy, 1214, 1214*f*
modified radical, 1214, 1214*f*, 1215*b*
nipple-sparing, 1214
postoperative exercises, 1219, 1220*f*
prophylactic, 1210
surgical procedures, 1215*b*
total or simple, 1214, 1214*f*, 1215*b*
Mastication, 834
Mastitis, **1206**
lactational, 1206, 1206*b*
Mastoid problems, **384-386**
Mastoidectomy, 385
Mastoiditis, **384-385**
Maturity-onset diabetes, of the young, 1122*b*
Mavik (trandolapril), 691*b*-693*b*
Maxillary fracture, 1486*b*
Maximal voluntary ventilation (MVV), 473*b*
Meals, 878, 878*b*, 883
Mean arterial pressure (MAP), 662, 699
Meaninglessness, 139

Measles, 215-216, 216*b*
Mechanical chest compression devices, 1634, 1635*f*
Mechanical debridement, 170*b*
Mechanical overventilation, 1579
Mechanical receptors, 458
Mechanical valves, 794-795
Mechanical ventilation, **1574-1584**, 1574*f*
alarms, 1575*b*
case study, 1584*b*
chronic, 1582-1584
importing monitor and ventilator data, 1578*b*
indications for weaning from, 1583*b*
malfunction, 1581
modes, 1576*b*
nursing management of patients receiving, 1584
nursing management of patients requiring, 1581*b*
oral care for patients on, 1572*b*
psychosocial needs during, 1580-1581
settings of, 1574-1575, 1575*b*
suctioning procedures for patients on, 1572*b*
types of, 1574
Meclizine (Antivert), 895*b*
Meclofenamate, 1521*b*-1522*b*
Media, 802-803
Mediastinal chest tubes, 344*b*
Mediastinoscopy, 469*t*-471*t*
Mediastinum, 455
Medic Alert bracelets or necklaces, 1140, 1140*f*
Medicaid, **68**
Medical doctors (physicians), 10*b*
Medical futility, 266*b*
Medical history, **34**
Medical identification, 1140, 1140*f*
Medical interpreters, 31, 31*b*, 52
Medical Order for Life-Sustaining Treatment (MOLST), 135, 136*b*
Medical power of attorney, 135, 136*b*
Medically underserved, 20
Medicare, **68**
Medicare Advantage Plans, 68
Medication errors, 73, 73*b*
Medication overuse headache, 1372-1373
Medication use. *See also* Substance abuse
by older adults, 72-73, 74*b*
Medications
cultural factors, 28-29
ineffective, 124*b*
nursing history, 36
preoperative, 311, 311*b*
preoperative assessment of, 304-305
Meditation, 84*b*, **84**
Medrol (methylprednisolone), 548*b*-549*b*
Medullary cystic disease, **1052**
Medulloblastoma, 1333*b*
Megakaryocytes, 590, 624
Megaloblastic anemia, **612-613**
classification of, 612, 612*b*
nursing management of, **613**
Meglitinides, 1130, 1131*b*, 1136*f*
Meiosis, 180
Melanocytes, 395
Melanocyte-stimulating hormone, 1104*b*
Melanoma
ABCDEs of, 410, 410*f*
cutaneous, 411
genetic risk alert, 399*b*
malignant, **411-413**, 412*b*, 427*b*
uveal, 382, 383*f*
Melanonychia striata, 396
Melatonin, 90, 95*b*
Melatonin-receptor agonists, 94, 94*b*
Melena, 846*b*-847*b*
Meloxicam (Mobic), 1521*b*-1522*b*
Memory loss
in Alzheimer's disease, 1406*b*
drug therapy for, 1408*b*
in mild cognitive impairment, 1406*b*
in stroke, 1351
Men. *See also* Gender differences
acute coronary syndrome in, 705*b*
coronary artery disease in, 704, 705*b*
gynecomastia in, 1208
heart failure in, 739*b*
HPV vaccine and young men, 1235*b*
risk factors for breast cancer, 1209-1210
vascular disorders in, 803*b*
Men who have sex with men (MSM), 1238*b*
Menarche, 1189, 1190*b*, 1244
Ménière's disease, 386*b*, **386**
Meninges, **1300**, 1301*f*
Meningioma, 1333*b*, 1334*f*
Meningitis, 503, 1339, 1339*b*
bacterial, **1339-1340**
viral, **1341**
Meningococcal vaccines, 1340
Meniscectomy, 1467
Meniscus injury, 1463*b*, **1467**, 1467*f*
Menopause, 1190, 1248
induced, 1248
perimenopause, **1248-1249**
postmenopause, **1248-1249**
sleep disturbances associated with, 1249*b*
Menorrhagia, 1246
Menotropins, 1243*b*
Menstrual cycle, 1189-1190, 1189*f*
Menstruation
patient teaching about, 1190*b*
problems related to, **1244-1254**
Mental status
assessment of, 1304
normal, 1308*b*
Mental status abnormalities, 1308*b*-1309*b*. *See also* Cognitive impairment; Mild cognitive impairment
Meperidine (Demerol), 114, 114*b*, 117*b*
Mepolizumab (Nucala), 548*b*-549*b*, 549
Merkel cells, 395
Mesotheliomas, **518**
Metabolic acidosis, 288*b*, **289**, 290*b*
in acute kidney injury, 1072
in chronic kidney disease, 1077
Metabolic alkalosis, 288*b*, **289**, 290*b*
Metabolic asphyxiation, **430**
Metabolic bone diseases, **1510-1514**, 1514
Metabolic emergencies, 263*b*, 264
Metabolic equivalents (METs), 731, 731*b*
Metabolic liver diseases, **985**
Metabolic problems
associated with obesity, 879*f*
in chronic kidney disease, 1076-1077
in SIRS or MODS, 1607
Metabolic syndrome, 880, **890-891**, 985
and CAD, 706
diagnostic criteria for, 890*b*
nursing and interprofessional management of, **891-892**
pathophysiology of, 890, 891*f*
Metabolism
drug metabolism, 72-73, 73*f*
regulation of, 877, 877*f*
Metamorphopsia, 378
Metanephrine, 1115*t*-1118*t*, 1661*b*
Metaphysis, 1447
Metaplasia, esophageal, 901
Metastasis, 238
bone cancer, **1501**, 1514*b*-1515*b*
brain tumors, 1333*b*
Metastasis *(Continued)*
hematogenous, 238
liver cancer, 996, 997*f*
main sites, 238, 238*f*
pathogenesis of, 238, 239*f*
prostate cancer, 1276*f*
skip, 238
Metered-dose inhalers, 547, 547*f*, 550*f*, 551, 551*b*-552*b*
Metformin (Glucophage, Glucophage XR, Riomet, Fotamet, Glumetza)
for diabetes, 1130, 1131*b*
drug alert, 1130*b*
Methadone (Dolophine), 112, 113*b*-114*b*
drug alert, 112*b*
equinanalgesic dosing, 117*b*
in general anesthesia, 326*b*
Methazolamide, 381*b*
Methicillin-resistant *Staphylococus aureus*, 216, 216*b*
Methohexital (Brevital), 325*b*
Methotrexate (Trexall), 1521*b*-1522*b*, 1528
N-Methyl-D-aspartate receptor antagonists, 1408*b*, 1409
Methyldopa, 691*b*-693*b*
Methylmalonic acid, 602*t*
Methylprednisolone (Medrol, Depo-Medrol, Solu-Medrol)
for arthritis, 1521*b*-1522*b*
for asthma, 548*b*-549*b*, 551
for immunosuppressive therapy, 209, 211*b*
for multiple sclerosis, 1385*b*
Methylxanthines, 548*b*-549*b*
Metoclopramide (Reglan)
in general anesthesia, 326*b*
for GERD, 894*b*, 903*b*
for nausea and vomiting, 895*b*
Metolazone (Zaroxolyn)
for heart failure, 745*b*
for hypertension, 691*b*-693*b*
Metoprolol (Lopressor, Toprol XL), 715*b*-716*b*
for dysrhythmia, 771*b*
for heart failure, 745*b*
for hypertension, 691*b*-693*b*
Metrorrhagia, 1246
Mexican Americans, 28, 682*b*
Mexiletine (Mexitil), 116*b*, 771*b*
Micardis (telmisartan), 691*b*-693*b*
Microagression, 26
Microbial hypersensitivity reactions, 200
Microcytosis, 611
Microglia, 1294
Microglobulin, 602*t*
Microlithiasis, 999
Microscopy, dark-field, 1198*t*-1201*t*
Microsporum, 215*b*
Microsurgery, reconstructive, 427
Microvascular angina, 713*b*, **713-714**
Microwave thermotherapy, transurethral (TUMT), 1271, 1272*b*
Micturition, 1019
Midamor (amiloride), 691*b*-693*b*
Midazolam, 326*b*
Middle ear, **360-361**, 360*f*
in older adults, 361*b*
problems of, **384-386**
Midwives *(parteras)*, 24
Mifflin–St. Jeor equation, 854, 855*b*
Miglitol (Glyset), 1131*b*
Migraine headache, **1370-1371**, 1370*f*
drug therapy for, 1372
gender differences in, 1370*b*
interprofessional care for, 1369*b*
social media for patients with, 1371*b*

Migraine with aura, 1370
Migraine without aura, 1370
Mild cognitive impairment
due to Alzheimer's disease, 1405, 1406*b*
memory loss in, 1406*b*
Miliary tuberculosis, 508
Milk thistle (silymarin), 980*b*
Millennials, 55*b*
Milnacipran (Savella), 116*b*
Milrinone (Primacor), 745*b*, 746
Mind-body-spirit connection, **81**, 81*f*
Mineral oil slides, 405*t*
Mineral salts, 855
Mineralocorticoids, 1104*b*, 1107. *See also* Corticosteroids
regulation of water balance by, 275
Minerals, 855, 856*b*
Mini Nutritional Assessment (MNA), 860
Mini-Cog, 1408, 1408*b*
Minimal leak technique (MLT), 1571
Minimal occluding volume (MOV) technique, 1571
Minimally invasive direct coronary artery bypass graft (MIDCAB), 725
Minimally invasive surgery (MIS), 315
Minimally invasive valvuloplasty, 794
MiniMed® 530/730G with Enlite and Guardian REAL-Time, 1135, 1136*f*
Mini-Mental State Examination (MMSE), 1408, 1408*b*
Minimum Data Set (MDS), 860
Minipress (prazosin), 691*b*-693*b*
Minocycline (Minocin), 1521*b*-1522*b*, 1529
Minoxidil, 691*b*-693*b*
Miostat (carbachol), 381*b*
Miotics, 381*b*
Mirabegron (Myrbetriq), 1059*b*
Mirapex (pramipexole), 1391*b*
Mirror therapy, 1489, 1489*f*
Miscarriage, 1243
Misoprostol (Cytotec)
for arthritis, 1523
for peptic ulcers, 903*b*, 914
Mitomycin, 1055
Mitosis, 180
Mitotic inhibitors, 247*b*
Mitoxantrone, 1385*b*, 1386
Mitral valve endocarditis, 781*f*
Mitral valve prolapse, **791-792**, 792*f*
clinical manifestations of, 791*b*, 792
patient & caregiver teaching for, 792*b*
Mitral valve regurgitation, 791*b*, **791**
Mitral valve stenosis, 791*b*, **791**
Mitral valvuloplasty, 794*f*
Mitrolan (calcium polyarbophil), 931*b*
Mixed acid-base disorders, **289**
Mixed connective tissue disease, **1545-1546**
Mixed dementia, 1400
Mixed venous oxygen saturation (SvO_2), **456-457**, 1564-1565
central ($ScvO_2$), 1564-1565, 1565*b*
interpreting measurements, 1565*b*
invasive monitoring, 1564-1565
normal range, 1559*b*
Mobi-C disc, 1506
Mobile devices, 229*b*
Mobitz I heart block, **768**
Mobitz II heart block, **768**
Moexipril (Univasc), 691*b*-693*b*
Mohs surgery, 422, 423*f*
Molecular cytogenetics, 603*t*, 604
Moles, 403*b*
Mometasone (Nasonex), 479*b*-480*b*
Mometasone furoate/formoterol fumarate (Dulera), 548*b*-549*b*
Moniliasis, 897*b*
Monitored anesthesia care (MAC), **322**, 323*b*
Monoamine oxidase inhibitors, 1390, 1391*b*
Monoarthritis, 788-789
Monoclonal antibodies, **209-210**
for asthma and COPD, 548*b*-549*b*, 549
for immunosuppressive therapy, 211*b*
for multiple sclerosis, 1385*b*
Monocytes, **590**
in cancer, 239
inflammatory response, **161**
reference values, 1659*b*
Monofilament testing, 1151
Mononuclear cells, 589
Mononuclear phagocytes, 192
Monro-Kellie doctrine, 1315
Mons pubis, 1187
Montelukast (Singulair), 479*b*-480*b*, 547, 548*b*-549*b*
Mood, 1304
Moon face, 1113*b*-1114*b*, 1174
Morgan lens, 370
Mormons (Church of Jesus Christ of Latter-Day Saints), 26*b*
Morphine (Roxanol, MSIR, MS Contin, Avinza, Kadian, Epimorph, Oramorph SR), 112, 113*b*-114*b*
for ACS, 715*b*-716*b*, 725
drug alert, 112*b*
epidural, 119
equinanalgesic dosing, 117*b*
in general anesthesia, 326*b*
for heart failure, 745*b*, 746
intrathecal, 119
for pancreatitis, 1001*b*
Morton's neuroma, 1508, 1509*b*
Motion-mode (M-mode) echocardiography, 671, 673*t*-677*t*
Motivational interviewing, 47, 48*b*
Motor deficits
in increased ICP, 1318
in stroke, 1350-1351
Motor system
abnormalities, 1308*b*-1309*b*
assessment of, 1306
normal, 1308*b*
Mouth, **834**
abnormalities, 846*b*-847*b*
assessment of
inspection, 842
palpation, 842-843
physical examination, **463**, 842-843
infections and inflammation of, 897*b*, **897**
normal, 846*b*
in older adults, 840*b*
Movement therapy, constraint-induced, 1364
Moxifloxacin (Avelox, Vigamox), 509*b*
Mucociliary clearance system, 458
Mucociliary escalator, 458
Mucositis, 251*b*-252*b*, 254
Mucous gland adenoma, **518**
Mucus clearance devices, 570
Multaq (dronedarone), 771*b*
Multidetector CT (MDCT) scanning, 678
Multidrug-resistant tuberculosis, 506
Multigated acquisition (MUGA) radionuclide angiography, 672, 673*t*-677*t*
Multiinfarct dementia, 1400
Multimodality therapy, 243
Multinucleated giant cells, 161
Multiple chemical sensitivity, **204**
Multiple dressing change, 440, 440*f*
Multiple endocrine neoplasia, 1109*b*, **1171**
Multiple myeloma, **645-647**
Multiple organ dysfunction syndrome (MODS), 1587, 1588*f*, **1604-1605**
clinical manifestations of, 1605, 1606*b*
nursing and interprofessional management of, **1606-1608**
Multiple sclerosis, **1383-1386**, 1384*f*
drug therapy for, 1385-1386, 1385*b*
etiology and pathophysiology of, 1383-1384, 1384*f*
genetic risks, 1303*b*
interprofessional care for, 1385-1386, 1385*b*
nursing assessment in, 1386*b*
nursing diagnoses related to, 1387
nursing management of, **1386-1387**
pathogenesis of, 1383-1384, 1383*f*
patterns of, 1384*b*
Multiple sleep latency tests, 99
Mumps, surgical, 897*b*
Mumps virus, 214*b*
Murmurs, 662, 668*b*, 669
Muromonab-CD3 (Orthoclone OKT3), 209, 211*b*
Muscarinic receptor blockers, 1059*b*
Muscle(s), **1448-1450**
structure of, 1448-1449, 1450*f*
types of, 1448
Muscle atrophy, 1456*b*, 1478*b*
Muscle contractions, 1449
isometric, 1449
isotonic, 1449
Muscle cramps, 1090-1091
Muscle fibers, 1449
Muscle relaxants, 1385*b*, 1386
Muscle spasms, 1469*b*, 1478*b*
Muscle spasticity, 1456*b*
Muscle stretch reflex, 1307, 1307*f*
Muscle-strength scale, 1455*b*
Muscle-strength testing, 1454
Muscular dystrophy, **1501-1502**
safety alert, 1502*b*
types of, 1501*b*
Muscular Dystrophy Association, 1502
Musculoskeletal system
abnormalities, 1456*b*
assessment of, **1451-1455**
checklist for, 1457*b*
palpation, 1453-1454
preoperative, 306, 307*b*
case study, 1451*b*, 1454*b*, 1457*b*, 1460*b*
diagnostic studies of, **1455-1457**, 1457*t*-1459*t*
at end of life, 132*b*
health history, 1452, 1452*b*
interventions to optimize function, 1359-1360
measurement of, 1454-1455
nontraumatic problems, 1465
normal, 1455*b*
in older adults, 1450-1451, 1451*b*
physical examination, 1453-1455
problems associated with obesity, 879*f*, 880
problems in systemic lupus erythematosus, 1538
problems unrelated to trauma, **1496-1516**
stroke rehabilitation interventions, 1363-1364
structures and functions of, **1446-1451**
Musculoskeletal trauma, **1462-1495**
in older adults, 1463*b*
patient & caregiver teaching for prevention of, 1463*b*
problems associated with, 1478*b*
regional disorders, 1465
work-related disorders, 1465
Music, **85**
Music therapy, 303*b*, 319*b*
Muslims, 25
Mustard gas, 1645
Mutations, 179*b*, 180-181, 180*f*
acquired (somatic), 181
germline, 181
types of, 181
Mutilation, 303
Myalgia, 1456*b*
Myambutol (ethambutol), 509*b*

Myasthenia gravis, **1393-1394**
clinical manifestations of, 1393, 1393*f*
drug therapy for, 1394
interprofessional care for, 1394, 1394*b*
nursing diagnoses for, 1394
nursing management of, **1394**
surgical therapy for, 1394
Myasthenic crisis, 1393, 1395*b*
Mycobacteria, 214*b*
atypical, **511-512**
Mycobacterium avium complex (MAC), 222*b*, 512
Mycobacterium tuberculosis, 222*b*, 506
Mycophenolate mofetil (CellCept, Myfortic), **209**
for arthritis and connective tissue disorders, 1521*b*-1522*b*
drug alert, 209*b*
for immunosuppressive therapy, 209, 211*b*
Mycosis,, 214
Mydriatics, 374, 374*b*
Myectomy, 799
Myelin sheath, 1294
Myelodysplastic syndrome, **634-635**
Myelography, 1310*t*-1312*t*, 1457*t*-1459*t*
Myeloma, multiple, **645-646**
Mylanta (aluminum and magnesium), 903*b*
Myocardial infarction, 719, 719*f*
case study, 734*b*
ECG changes in, 776-777, 777*f*
healing process, 720
non–ST-segment-elevation (NSTEMI), 718, **719-721**
ST-segment-elevation (STEMI), 714*f*, 718, **719-721**
Myocardial ischemia, 712
ECG changes in, 776, 776*f*
Myocarditis, **787-788**
in cancer, 251*b*-252*b*
interprofessional care for, 787-788
nursing management of, **788**
Myocardium
blood supply, 658-659
oxygen needs, 712, 712*b*
Myochrysine (gold sodium thiomalate), 1529
Myoclonic seizures, 1376
Myoclonus, 140*b*-141*b*, 1306
Myofascial pain syndrome, **1546**
Myoglobin, 670, 673*t*-677*t*, 722, 1661*b*
Myometrium, 1186
Myopia, 351, 367
Myositis ossificans, 1470*b*
Myotomes, 1298
MyPlate, 861, 861*f*, 862*b*, 1134
Myringoplasty, 385
Myringotomy, 384
Myxedema, 1113*b*-1114*b*, 1169, 1169*f*

N

Nabilone (Cesamet), 153, 895*b*
Nabumetone, 1521*b*-1522*b*
Nadolol (Corgard), 691*b*-693*b*, 715*b*-716*b*, 993*b*
Nafarelin (Synarel), 1243*b*
Nail(s), 396, 396*f*
Nail beds
clubbing of, 467*b*-468*b*, 598, 668*b*
pigmented, 396, 396*f*
Nalbuphine (Nubain), 114
Naloxone (Narcan), 152
NANDA, NOC, and NIC (NNN) linkages, 7*b*, **7**
NANDA International (NANDA-I), 7, **7**
Naproxen (Naprosyn, Aleve), 111*b*, 1521*b*-1522*b*
Narcolepsy, 90, **98-99**
Nasal bone fracture, 1486*b*
Nasal cannulas, 566*b*-567*b*, 566*f*, 568
high-flow, 566*b*-567*b*, 567*f*
Nasal endotracheal intubation, 1569-1570
Nasal fracture, **475-476**
Nasal packing, 477, 477*f*
Nasal polyps, **483-484**
Nasal sprays, 479*b*-480*b*
Nasal surgery, **476**
Nasogastric feeding tubes, 865, 865*f*
drainage from, 344*b*
nursing management of, 867*b*
Nasointestinal feeding tubes, 865
Nasopharynx, 453
Natalizumab (Tysabri), 1385*b*, 1386
Nateglinide (Starlix), 1131*b*
National Academy of Medicine, 5
National Association of Anorexia Nervosa and Associated Disorders (ANAD), 872
National Cancer Institute (NCI), 267*b*
National Coalition for Cancer Survivoship, 267*b*
National Database of Nursing Quality Indicators (NDNQI), **13**, 14*b*
National Disaster Medical System (NDMS), 1646
National Heart, Lung, and Blood Institute (NHLBI)
educational materials, 694
guidelines for heart-healthy food preparation, 749
National Incident Management System (NIMS), 1646
National Institute for Occupational Safety and Health (NIOSH), 204*b*
National Institute on Alcohol Abuse and Alcoholism, 148, 148*f*
National Institutes of Health Stroke Scale (NIHSS), 1358*b*, 1359
National Osteoporosis Foundation, 1512
National Patient Safety Foundation, 50-51
National Patient Safety Goals (NPSGs), **12**, 13*b*, 316
National Quality Forum (NQF), 12
National Standards for Culturally and Linguistically Appropriate Services in Health Care (CLAS standards), 30
Native Americans and Native Alaskans, 19
arthritis and connective tissue disorders in, 1525*b*
chronic kidney disease in, 1076*b*
coronary artery disease in, 704*b*
cross-cultural communication, 25-26
cultural traditions, 22*b*, 24
culture-bound syndromes, 29*b*
in health care workplace, 24
Native Hawaiians and other Pacific Islanders, 19
Natrecor (nesiritide), 745*b*
Natural death acts, 135
Natural killer (NK)-cell lymphoma, 644*b*
Natural killer (NK) cells, 193*f*, **194**, 239, 590
Nausea and vomiting, 846*b*-847*b*, **893-895**
acute care for, 896
ambulatory care for, 896
anticipatory, 254
in cancer, 251*b*-252*b*, 253-254
cultural & ethnic health disparities, 898*b*
cyclic vomiting syndrome, 894
definition of, 893
delayed, 254
drug therapy for, 895*b*, 907*f*
at end of life, 140*b*-141*b*
interprofessional care for, 894-895
in myocardial infarction, 720
nondrug therapy for, 895
nursing assessment in, 895-896, 896*b*
nursing diagnoses related to, 342, 896
nursing management of, **895-897**
nutritional therapy for, 894-895
in older adults, 897
opioid-induced nausea, 114-115
Nausea and vomiting
pathophysiology of, 893-894, 894*f*
postoperative, 341
projectile vomiting, 894
Nebivolol (Bystolic), 691*b*-693*b*
Nebulization, 565
Nebulizers, **551-552**
Neck assessment
physical examination, **463**, 1112
secondary survey, 1633
Neck dissection
modified radical, 492
radical, 492
selective, 492
Neck exercises, 1508*b*
Neck pain, 1507*b*, **1507-1508**
Necrobiosis lipoidica diabeticorum, 1151, 1152*f*
Necrotizing pancreatitis, 999
Necrotizing pneumonia, 502
Necrotizing ulcerative gingivitis, 897*b*
Need to know, 47*b*, 53
Needle ablation, transurethral (TUNA), 1271, 1272*b*
Needs assessment, 49*b*
Negative feedback, 1103-1104, 1189, 1189*b*
Negative-pressure ventilation, 1574, 1574*f*
Negative-pressure wound therapy, 169-170, 171*f*
Neglect, 67*b*
Neisseria gonorrhea, 216*b*
Neisseriae, 214*b*
Neointimal hyperplasia, 718
Neomycin sulfate, 993*b*
Neoplasms
benign, **240**
malignant, **240**
Neoral (cyclosporine), 209, 211*b*
Neostigmine, 1385*b*
Neovascularization, 1149
Nephrectomy
indications for, 1063
laparoscopic, 1063, 1094
open (conventional), 1094
postoperative management in, 1063
preoperative management in, 1063
surgical procedure, 1063
Nephritis. *See also* Glomerulonephritis; Pyelonephritis
chronic hereditary, 1052
Nephrolithiasis, 1045
Nephrolithotomy, 1047-1048
Nephrons, 1016-1017, 1017*b*
Nephropathy, diabetic, 1148*b*, **1149**
Nephrosclerosis, 687, **1050**
accelerated (malignant), 1050
benign, 1050
Nephrostography, 1025*t*-1030*t*
Nephrostomy, 1064*b*, 1064*f*
Nephrostomy tubes, 1062
Nephrotic syndrome, **1043-1044**
Nephrotoxic agents, 1020*b*
Nerve agent poisoning, 1645
Nerve blocks, 120
Nerve conduction enhancers, 1385*b*
Nerve conduction studies, 1310*t*-1312*t*
Nerve impulses, **1295-1296**, 1296*f*
Nerve regeneration, **1295**
Nervous system
abnormalities, 1308*b*-1309*b*
assessment of, **1301-1307**
focused, 1307, 1308*b*
health history, 1303*b*
physical examination, 1304-1307
case study, 1302*b*, 1304*b*, 1307*b*, 1312*b*
cells of, 1294-1295

Nervous system *(Continued)*
diagnostic studies of, **1307**, 1310*t*-1312*t*
normal, 1308*b*
in older adults, 1301, 1302*b*
primary afferent fibers, 104
stress response, 79
structures and functions of, **1294-1301**
in systemic lupus erythematosus, 1539
Nesina (alogliptin), 1131*b*
Nesiritide (Natrecor), 745-746, 745*b*
Netupitant and palonosetron (Akynzeol), 895*b*
Neulasta (pegfilgrastim), 195*b*
Neumega (oprelvekin), 195*b*
Neupogen (filgrastim), 195*b*
Neupro (rotigotine), 1391*b*
Neurectomy, 120
Neuroablative interventions, 120
Neurofibrillary tangles, 1403
Neurogenic bladder, 1423
interprofessional care for, 1433*b*
in spinal cord injury, **1432-1433**
types of, 1432*b*
Neurogenic bowel, 1423-1424, 1430, 1433-1434
Neurogenic hyperventilation, central, 1324*f*
Neurogenic shock, 1420, 1588*b*, 1590
clinical presentation of, 1591*b*
drug therapy for, 1599*b*
interprofessional care for, 1600*b*, 1601
pathophysiology of, 1590, 1592*f*
Neurohypophysis (posterior pituitary gland), 1104*b*, **1105-1106**
Neurokinin-1 receptor antagonists, 895*b*
Neurologic assessment, **1301-1307**
in increased ICP, 1323-1324
pathology tests, 1310*t*-1312*t*
preoperative, 305-306, 307*b*
Neurologic disorders
in acute kidney injury, 1072
chronic, **1374-1383**
corticosteroid therapy for, 1180*b*
degenerative, **1383-1396**
Neurologic problems
chronic, **1368-1398**
nursing diagnoses related to, 339
nursing management of, **339**
postoperative, **338**
Neuromuscular blocking agents
in general anesthesia, 326*b*
safety alert, 1619*b*
Neuromuscular conditions, 1612
Neuromuscular junction, 1449, 1450*f*
Neurons, **1294**, 1295*f*
second-order, 105
third-order, 105-106
Neurontin (gabapentin), 116*b*
Neuroohypophysis (posterior piruitary gland), 1104*b*
Neuropathic pain, 106*b*, **106-107**
chronic, 119
in spinal cord injury, 1424
Neuropathy
acute inflammatory demyelinating polyneuropathy, 1440
autonomic, 1150
chronic inflammatory demyelinating polyradiculoneuropathy, **1441-1442**
diabetic, 1148*b*, **1149-1150**, 1150*f*
diabetic sensory, 1150-1151
peripheral, 106*b*
acute care for, 1541
in cancer, 251*b*-252*b*
in chronic kidney disease, 1078
in cirrhosis, 987
polyneuropathies, **1440-1442**
stocking-glove, 1150
Neuropeptide Y, 877, 877*b*
Neuroplasticity, 105
Neurosurgery, 120, 121*f*
Neurotransmitters, **1295-1296**
Neurotrophic ulcerations, 1150, 1150*f*
Neurovent catheters, 1321-1322
Neutropenia, 600, **632-633**
causes of, 632, 633*b*
in chemotherapy, 253
definition of, 632
nursing and interprofessional management of, 632*b*-633*b*, **633-634**
patient & caregiver teaching for, 634*b*
safety alert, 632*b*
severe, 632
Neutrophils, **161**, 589
absolute neutrophil count, 632
polymorphonuclear segmented (segs), 599-600
segmented, 161, 589-590
Never events, 12
Nevus, 403*b*, **419*b***
atypical or dysplastic, 412*b*, **413**, 413*f*, 427*b*
spider nevus, 597*b*-598*b*, 598
Nevus of Ota, 403-405, 404*f*
New York Heart Association (NYHA), 741, 741*b*
Nexium (esomeprazole), 903*b*
Niacin (Niaspan), 610*b*, 710, 710*b*-711*b*
Niacin (nicotinic acid) deficiency, 399*b*
Nicardipine (Cardene), 691*b*-693*b*, 715*b*-716*b*
Nicotine, **145-146**
Nicotine replacement therapy, 147, 150*b*
Nicotinic acid (niacin) deficiency, 399*b*
Nifedipine (Adalat CC, Nifedical XL, Procardia), 532*b*, 715*b*-716*b*, 1059*b*
Nifedipine long acting (Procardia XL), 691*b*-693*b*
Night terrors, 99
Nightingale, Florence, 86
Nightmares, 99
NIH Stroke Scale, 1323
Nilutamide (Nilandron), 1280*b*
Nimbex (cisatracurium), 326*b*
Nimodipine, 1356, 1356*b*
Nipple discharge, 1197*b*, **1208**
Nipple discharge test, 1198*t*-1201*t*
Nipple-areolar reconstruction, 1223*f*, 1224
Nipples, 1197*b*
Nipple-sparing mastectomy, 1214
Nipress (sodium nitroprusside)
for heart failure, 745
for hypertension, 691*b*-693*b*
for shock, 1599*b*
Nisoldipine (Sular), 691*b*-693*b*
Nissen fundoplication, 902-903, 903*f*
Nitrates, 716*b*
for chronic stable angina and ACS, 715*b*-716*b*
for heart failure, 745*b*, 748
long-acting, 716
short-acting, 714-716
transdermal controlled-release, 716
Nitric oxide, 1578
Nitrofurantoin (Furadantin, Macrodantin), 1036, 1036*b*
Nitroglycerin (Nitro-Bid)
for ACS, 715*b*-716*b*, 725
drug alert, 792*b*
for hypertension, 691*b*-693*b*
mechanism of action, 715*b*-716*b*
for shock, 1599*b*
sublingual, 715*b*-716*b*, 716
transdermal, 715*b*-716*b*, 716
Nitroglycerin ointment, 715*b*-716*b*, 716
Nitroprusside (Nipride), 745*b*
Nitrosoureas, 247*b*
Nitrous oxide, 325*b*
Nizatidine (Axid), 903*b*
Nociception, 103, 104*f*
Nociceptive pain, 104, 104*f*, 106*b*, **106**
in spinal cord injury, 1424
Nocturia, 743, 1025*b*
Nocturnal dyspnea, paroxysmal, 742-743
Nodes of Ranvier, 1295
Nodular goiters, 1162
Nodular liver, 846*b*-847*b*
Nodules
subcutaneous, 789
thyroid, **1170-1171**
Noise control, **388**
Nomenclatures, 6
Non–24-hour sleep-wake disorder, 369
Nonalcoholic fatty liver disease, **985**
Nonalcoholic steatohepatitis, **985**
Non-English-speaking patients, 52, 52*f*
Nongonococcal urethritis, 1228
Non-Hodgkin's lymphoma, 639, 641*b*, **642-644**
classification of, 643, 644*b*
clinical manifestations of, 643, 643*f*
dermatologic manifestations of, 399*b*
nursing and interprofessional management of, **644-645**
staging, 642*f*, 643-644
treatment of, 644*b*
Non–insulin-dependent diabetes mellitus, 1122
Nonnucleoside reverse transcriptase inhibitors (NNRTIs), 224*b*
Non–rapid eye movement (NREM) sleep, 90-91, **91**
Nonsalicylates, 111*b*
Non-small cell lung cancer, 514, 515*b*
staging of, 516, 516*b*
Nonsteroidal antiinflammatory drugs
for arthritis, 1521*b*-1522*b*, 1523, 1529
cardiovascular effects of, 664*b*
drug alert, 112*b*
for inflammation, 164, 164*b*
mechanism of action, 112, 112*f*
overdose, 1643*b*
for pain, 111*b*, 112
that cause photosensitivity, 408*b*
Nonstructural protein 5A (NS5A) inhibitors, 981*b*
Nonverbal patients, 126*b*
Norepinephrine (Levophed), 1599*b*
Norepinephrine (noradrenaline), 1104*b*, 1107, 1661*b*
Norovirus, 216, 930*b*, 944
Norpramin (desipramine), 116*b*
Nortriptyline (Pamelor), 116*b*
Norvasc (amlodipine), 691*b*-693*b*, 715*b*-716*b*
Norwalk-like virus infection, 930*b*
Nose. *See also under* Nasal
obstruction of, **483-484**
physical examination of, **463**
Nose problems, **475-484**, 540
Nosebleed (epistaxis), **476**
NPSGs (National Patient Safety Goals), **12**, 13*b*, 316
NQF (National Quality Forum), 12
NT-Pro-BNP, 673*t*-677*t*
Nubain (nalbuphine), 114
Nucala (mepolizumab), 548*b*-549*b*, 549
Nuchal rigidity, 597*b*-598*b*, 1339
Nuclear cardiology, **672**, 673*t*-677*t*
Nuclear imaging
gastrointestinal scans, 847*t*-850*t*
pharmacologic, 673*t*-677*t*
Nucleic acid amplification test (NAAT), 1198*t*-1201*t*
Nucleoside and nucleotide analogs, 980-981, 981*b*
Nucleoside reverse transcriptase inhibitors (NRTIs), 224*b*
Nucleotide reverse transcriptase inhibitors (NtRTIs), 224*b*
Nucleotides, 179-180

Nucynta (tapentadol), 113*b*-114*b*, 114
Nulojix (belatacept), 211*b*
Nuprin (ibuprofen), 111*b*
Nurse(s), 2, 3*f*
advanced practice registered nurses (APRNs), 3
cultural diversity among, 24
end-of-life care for, 142
impaired, 125*b*
self-assessment, 29
sleep needs, **100-101**
special needs, **448**
as teachers, 48-49
Nurse anesthetists, 318
Nurse practitioners
acute care nurse practitioners (ACNPs), 1555
role in bladder irrigation, 1274*b*
Nursing
coaching in, 581*b*
continuum of care, 8-9, 129, 130*f*
critical care, **1554-1558**
definitions of, 2-3
delivery of care, 9
focus of, 34-35
gerontologic, 69-70
intraoperative activities, 317*b*
key messages, 5*b*
perioperative activities, 318*b*
planning, 70
professional practice, **2-3**
self-care in, 86*b*
telehealth, 9, 9*f*
transcultural, 23, 30*f*
view of humanity, 3
Nursing: A Social Policy Statement (ANA), 3
Nursing care plans, **7-8**, 8*b*
Nursing diagnoses, 5, 6*f*, **1653-1654**
development of, 44
NANDA-I list, 7
Nursing history, 34-35, 35*f*, **36-39**
Nursing Interventions Classification (NIC), 7, 7*b*, **7**
Nursing Outcomes Classification (NOC), 7, 7*b*, **7**
Nursing practice, **2-3**
domain of, 2
scope of, 3
Nursing process, **5**, 6*f*
Nursing-sensitive patient outcomes, 7
Nutrient-drug interactions, 858
Nutrition Facts food labels, 861, 862*f*
Nutrition labels, 749, 750*f*
Nutritional assessment, 37*b*, 38
components of, 860, 861*b*
in older adults, 65, 66*b*
preoperative review, 306-307
SCALES, 66*b*
Nutritional deficiency, **854**
in cancer, 261-262
in critical care, 1557
and wound healing, 168*b*
Nutritional support, 854
algorithm for, 864*f*
for ARDS, 1625
for celiac disease, 967, 967*b*
for critical care patients, 1557
cultural factors, 28
culturally competent care, 856
enteral nutrition, **865-868**
foods high in iron, 856*b*
foods high in protein, 855*b*
high-calorie foods, 262*b*
high-fiber foods, 937*b*
home support, 871
low-sodium diets, 749*b*
maximizing food intake, 571, 571*b*
Nutritional support *(Continued)*
in multiple organ dysfunction syndrome, 1607
MyPlate tips, 862*b*
normal, **854-855**
oral feeding, **865**
parenteral nutrition, **869-870**
patient teaching related to, 1133-1134
protein foods with high biologic value, 262*b*
recommendations for nutrient balance, 1133
for respiratory failure, 1619
in shock, 1598
in SIRS or MODS, 1607
skin, 409
specialized, **865-870**
in spinal cord injury, 1429-1430
therapeutic lifestyle changes diet, 709*b*
tips for diet and lifestyle changes, 709*b*
transitioning to oral feeding, 870*b*
for weight loss, 881-883, 882*b*
Nystagmus, 361, 1306, 1308*b*-1309*b*

O

Obesity, **874-878**, 875*f*
android, 875, 876*b*
and CAD, 706
case study, 891*b*
centripetal, 1174
classification of, 874-875, 875*b*
cultural & ethnic health disparities, 878*b*
drug therapy for, 884-885, 884*b*
effects of, 61*b*
environmental factors, 878
epidemiology of, 875, 876*f*
etiology and pathophysiology of, 875-876
extreme, 874, 875*b*
faith-based interventions for, 889*b*
genetic links, 877-878
gynoid, 875, 876*b*
health risks associated with, 878-880, 879*f*
health-promoting behaviors for, 708*b*
hormones and peptides in, 877, 877*b*, 877*f*
interprofessional care for, 882*b*
morbid, 874
nursing and interprofessional management of, **880-885**
nursing assessment in, 880-881, 880*b*-881*b*
nutritional therapy for, 881-883, 882*b*
in older adults, 889-890
perioperative care in, **887-890**
physiologic regulatory mechanisms in, 877-878, 877*f*
postoperative care in, 888
preoperative care in, 888
psychosocial factors, 878
severe, 874
skin problems in, 409
sleep disturbances with, 92*b*
surgical therapy for, 886*b*
bariatric, **885-887**
cosmetic, **890**
wound healing in, 168*b*
Obstetric history, 1194
Obstipation, 930
Obstructive cardiomyopathy, hypertrophic, 798
Obstructive emergencies, 263*b*, 264
Obstructive jaundice, 1006*b*
Obstructive pulmonary diseases, **538-584**, 539*b*
Obstructive shock, 1588*b*, 1593-1594, 1593*f*
clinical presentation of, 1591*b*
interprofessional care for, 1600*b*, 1602
pathophysiology of, 1593
Obstructive sleep apnea, 92*b*, **96-97**, 96*f*
Obstructive sleep apnea–hypopnea syndrome, 96
Obstructive uropathies, **1044-1050**
Ocaliva (oeticholic acid), 985
Occupational asthma, 540
Occupational chemicals and dusts, 558
Occupational disparities, 20
Occupational Safety and Health Administration (OSHA), 217*b*, 218
Occupational therapists, 10*b*
role in caring for arthritis patients, 1529*b*
role in caring for osteomyelitis patients, 1498*b*
role in caring for patients with casts or in traction, 1471*b*
role in caring for seizure patients, 1380*b*
Octreotide acetate (Sandostatin), 931*b*, 993*b*
Ocular tumors, **382**
Oculomotor nerve, 1305*b*, **1306**
Odynophagia, 254, 846*b*-847*b*
Oeticholic acid (Ocaliva), 985
Off-pump coronary artery bypass graft (OPCAB), 725
Older adults, **63-74**
acute care for, 71-74
acute kidney injury in, 1075
ambulatory care for, 71-74
amputation in, 1490
anemia in, 608
arthritis in, 1532
assessment of, 42*b*, 64*b*
assistive devices for, 72
breast cancer in, 1222
burns in, 447
cardiovascular system in, 662-663
care alternatives for, 68-69
care transitions for, 71
case study, 75*b*
cataracts in, 376
chronic kidney disease in, 1096-1097
chronically ill, 64
cognitive function in, 64*b*
cognitively impaired, 64
COPD in, 571-572
coronary artery disease in, 710-712
culturally competent care for, 66
daily requirements for maintaining weight, 863-864
depression in, 73-74
enteral nutrition for, 868-869
evaluation of nursing care for, 74*b*
fluids and electrolytes, 276
foot problems in, 1510
frail, 63, 65
gastrointestinal system in, 839
gender differences, 63*b*
GERD in, 905
glaucoma in, 382
health promotion for, 70-71, 70*f*
hearing loss in, 391
hiatal hernia in, 905
hip fracture in, 1484
homeless, 65
hospitalized, 71*b*
hypertension in, 698
hyperthyroidism in, 1165*b*
IBD in, 950
infections in, 217-218
informaton access, 53*f*
integumentary system in, 396-397
legal and ethical issues, 69
liver disease in, 998-999
malnutrition in, 863-864
medication errors, 73, 73*b*
medication use, 72-73, 74*b*
metabolic bone diseases in, 1514
musculoskeletal system in, 1450-1451, 1451*b*
nausea and vomiting in, 897

Older adults *(Continued)*
nursing assessment in, 69-70
nursing evaluation of, 74
nursing implementation for, 70-74
nursing management of, 69-74
nursing planning with, 70
nutritional assessment of, 65, 66*b*
obesity in, 889-890
old-old adults, 63
pain in, 125-126
peptic ulcer disease in, 919
physical examination adaptations for, 40
postoperative care for, 346
preoperative care for, 312-313
prevention of musculoskeletal problems in, 1463*b*
rehabilitation for, 71-72, 71*f*
reproductive system in, 1191
respiratory failure in, 1619-1620
respiratory system in, 459, 459*b*
rural, 64, 65*f*
safety with, 72
seizures in, 1379
sleep disturbances, 99-100, 99*f*
social services for, 67
social support for, 66-67
special populations, 64-66
spinal cord injury in, 1435-1436, 1436*f*
stroke in, 1365-1367
surgery for, 327
visual impairment in, 370
visual system in, 353*b*
wound healing in, 168*b*
young-old adults, 63
Old-old adults, 63
Olfactory nerve, 1305*b*, **1306**
Oligodendrocytes, 1295
Oligodendroglioma, 1333*b*
Oliguria, 1025*b*, 1071
postoperative, 342
Olmesartan (Benicar), 691*b*-693*b*
Olodaterol (Striverdi Respimat), 548*b*-549*b*
Omalizumab (Xolair), 548*b*-549*b*, 549
Omega-3 fatty acids, 689*b*, 710*b*-711*b*
Omeprazole (Prilosec), 805*b*, 903*b*
Omeprazole and sodium bicarbonate (Zegerid), 903*b*
Omnaris (ciclesonide), 479*b*-480*b*
OmniPod Insulin Management System, 1129*f*
Onabotulinumtoxin A (Botox), 1057
Oncogenes, 179*b*, 236
Oncologic emergencies, 262-264, 263*b*
Oncology Nursing Society (ONS), 5
Oncotic pressure, 273
interstitial, 274
plasma, 274
Oncotype DX test, 1213
Ondansetron (Zofran), 326*b*, 895*b*
Onglyza (saxagliptin), 1131*b*
ONS (Oncology Nursing Society), 5
Onychomycosis, 417, 417*f*, 418*b*
Oophorectomy
acute intervention for, 1261
prophylactic, 1210
Opana (oxymorphone), 112, 113*b*-114*b*
Open aneurysm repair, 811-813
Open release surgery, 1466
Operating room, **316**, 316*f*
catastrophic events, **327-329**
physical environment of, **315-316**
principles of aseptic technique for, 320*b*
room preparation, **319**
transportation to, 311
Ophthalmia neonatorum, 1230
Ophthalmopathy, 1163-1164
Ophthalmoplegia, 1308*b*-1309*b*
Ophthalmoscopy, 356*b*, 358
Opioid Risk Tool, 123
Opioid withdrawal, **152-153**
Opioid withdrawal syndrome, 124*b*
Opioid-induced hyperalgesia, 115
Opioids, **112-115**, 113*b*-114*b*
abuse of, **152**
to avoid, 114
for chronic stable angina and ACS, 715*b*-716*b*
equianalgesic dosing, 117*b*
in general anesthesia, 326*b*
mechanism of action, 715*b*-716*b*
overdose, **152**
preoperative, 311*b*
risk monitoring, 123
side effects of, 114-115
types of, 112-114
Opioid-sparing effect, 111
Opisthotonos, 1442
Opportunistic diseases, 219
associated with HIV infection, 221, 222*b*
drug therapy for, 223
fungal infections, 512, 512*b*
Opportunistic pneumonia, 502
Opposition, 1455*b*
Oprelvekin (Neumega), 195*b*
Opsumit (macitentan), 532*b*
Optic disc cupping, 379
Optic nerve, 358-359, 1305*b*, **1306**
Optical devices for vision enhancement, 369
Oral cancer, **898-899**
characteristics of, 898*b*
interprofessional care for, 898*b*, 899
nonsurgical therapy for, 899
nursing assessment in, 899*b*
nursing diagnoses for, 899
nursing management of, **899-900**
nutritional therapy for, 899
surgical therapy for, 899
types of, 898*b*
Oral candidiasis, 897*b*
Oral care
for intubated patients, 1572-1573
for patients on mechanical ventilators, 1572*b*
Oral cavity cancer, 898*b*, **898**
Oral contraceptives, 664*b*
Oral feeding, **865**
after stroke, 1360*b*
transitioning to, 870*b*
Oral fluid and electrolyte replacement, **292**
Oral glucose tolerance test, 1115*t*-1118*t*
Oral hairy leukoplakia, 221, 221*f*
Oral hygiene, 900*b*
Oral inflammation and infections, 897*b*, **897**
Oral intubation, 1569-1570
Oral thrush, 221, 221*f*
Orchiectomy, 1280
Orchitis, **1284**
Orencia (abatacept), 1521*b*-1522*b*, 1529
Orexin-receptor antagonists, 94, 94*b*
Orexins, 90, 877*b*
Organ donation, **135**
deceased donors, 1093-1094
live donors, 1093
paired, 1093
sources of donors, 1093-1094
Organ transplantation, **207-210**, 207*f*
Orgasm, 1190
Orientation to learning, 47*b*
Orkambi (ivacaftor/lumicaftor), 579
Orlistat (Xenical, Allī), 884*b*
Orogastric feeding tubes, 865
Oropharyngeal cancer, 898*b*, **898**
Oropharynx, 453
Orthoclone OKT3 (muromonab-CD3), 209, 211*b*
Orthopnea, 742
Orthotopic bladder reconstruction, 1065
Osmolality, 272-273
measurement of, 273
plasma, 273, 1106, 1106*f*
reference values, 1655*b*-1658*b*, 1661*b*
Osmolarity, 272-273
Osmoreceptors, 1106
Osmosis, 272-273, 273*f*, 1085
Osmotic diarrhea, 931
Osmotic pressure, 272-273
Ossification, 1447, 1469-1470
Osteitis deformans, 1514
Osteitis fibrosa, 1079
Osteoarthritis, **1517-1523**, 1526*b*
acute care for, 1524
ambulatory care for, 1524
causes of, 1518, 1518*b*
cold therapy for, 1519
complementary & alternative therapies for, 1520
drug therapy for, 1520-1523, 1521*b*-1522*b*
falls and, 1520*b*
gender differences in, 1518*b*
health promotion for, 1524
heat therapy for, 1519
interprofessional care for, 1519-1523, 1520*b*
joints most frequently involved in, 1518, 1520*f*
nursing diagnoses, 1524
nursing management of, **1523-1524**
nutritional therapy for, 1519-1520
pathologic changes in, 1518, 1519*f*
patient & caregiver teaching for, 1524*b*
prevention of, 1523*b*
surgical therapy for, 1523
Osteoblasts, 1447
Osteochondroma, 1500*b*, **1500**
Osteoclastoma, 1500*b*
Osteocytes, 1447
Osteomalacia, 1079, **1510**
Osteomyelitis, **1496-1498**, 1497*f*
acute, 1497
acute care for, 1499
ambulatory care for, 1499
chronic, 1497, 1497*f*
direct entry, 1496
etiology and pathophysiology of, 1496-1497, 1497*b*, 1497*f*
health promotion for, 1499
indirect entry, 1496
interprofessional care for, 1497-1498, 1498*b*
nursing assessment in, 1499*b*
nursing diagnoses for, 1498
nursing management of, **1498-1500**
Osteons, 1446-1447
Osteopenia, 1511
Osteophytes, 1517-1518
Osteoporosis, **1510-1512**, 1510*f*
clinical manifestations of, 1511, 1512*f*
cultural & ethnic health disparities, 1511*b*
drug therapy for, 1513-1514
gender differences in, 1511*b*
interprofessional care for, 1512*b*
nursing and interprofessional management of, **1512-1514**
risk factors for, 1511*b*
Osteosarcoma, 1500*b*, **1500-1501**, 1500*f*
Osteotomy, **1490-1491**
Ostomy
psychologic adaptation to, 962
types of, 958, 959*f*
Ostomy care, 960*b*-961*b*
Ostomy surgery, **958-959**
nursing management of, **959-962**
postoperative care in, 960
preoperative care in, 960
sexual function after, 962
types of, 958-959

Otalgia, 383
Otitis media, **384-385**
acute, 384
chronic, 385*b*, **385**
with effusion, 384
Otorrhea, 1326, 1327*f*
Otosclerosis, 385*b*, **385-386**
Ototoxic substances, 389
Outcome and Assessment Information Set (OASIS), 860
Out-of-hospital DNR, 136
Out-patient surgery, 302
Ovarian cancer, **1258-1259**
cultural & ethnic health disparities, 1256*b*
genetics of, 1192*b*, 1258, 1258*b*
hereditary breast and ovarian cancer (HBOC) syndrome, 1276
interprofessional care for, 1259, 1259*b*
Ovarian cysts, **1255**, 1255*f*
Ovaries, 1185-1186
Overdrive pacing, 772-773
Overflow incontinence, 1056*b*, 1059-1060
Overnutrition, 856
Overuse syndrome, 1465
Overweight, 874, 875*b*
Oxaprozin (Daypro), 1521*b*-1522*b*
Oximetry, **457**, 469*t*-471*t*, 1322
Oxybutynin (Ditropan IR, Ditropan XL, Oxytrol Transdermal System)
for multiple sclerosis, 1385*b*
for voiding dysfunction, 1059*b*
Oxycodone (OxyContin, Roxicodone), 112, 113*b*-114*b*, 117*b*
OxyContin (oxycodone), 113*b*-114*b*
Oxygen masks
partial and non-rebreather masks, 566*b*-567*b*, 566*f*
simple face masks, 566*b*-567*b*, 566*f*
Venturi mask, 566*b*-567*b*, 567*f*
Oxygen saturation of hemoglobin
arterial (SpO_2), 457, 458*b*
noninvasive monitoring, 1565-1566
normal range, 1559*b*
low, 597*b*-598*b*
monitoring, 1564-1565
reference values, 1655*b*-1658*b*
venous
central ($ScvO_2$), 1564-1565, 1565*b*
mixed (SvO_2), **456-457**, 1559*b*, 1564-1565
monitoring, 1564-1565
normal range, 1559*b*
Oxygen therapy, **565-568**
for acute respiratory failure, 1615-1616
administration, 568*b*
for ARDS, 1624
chronic, 568
complications of, 565
drug alert, 1579*b*
at home, 568, 569*b*
home delivery systems, 568, 568*b*
methods of administration, 565, 565*f*, 566*b*-567*b*
patient & caregiver teaching for, 569*b*
portable systems, 565*f*, 568, 568*f*
for shock, 1596
Oxygen toxicity, **565**, 1616
Oxygenation
cerebral: monitoring, 1319-1322, 1321*f*
inadequate: signs of, 331*b*, 457*b*
monitoring, 469*t*-471*t*, 1571
myocardial needs, 712, 712*b*
physiology of, **456**
tissue needs, 1612
Oxygenation failure, 1609-1610
Oxygen-conserving cannula, 566*b*-567*b*, 566*f*
Oxyhemoglobin, 588
Oxymetazoline, 479*b*-480*b*
Oxymorphone (Opana), 112, 113*b*-114*b*, 117*b*
Oxytocin, 1104*b*, 1159-1160

P

Pacemakers, **773-775**, 773*f*-774*f*
failure to capture, 775
failure to sense, 775
monitoring patients with, 775
patient & caregiver teaching for, 776*b*
permanent, 774*b*, **774**
temporary, 774-775, 774*b*, 774*f*
transcutaneous, 775, 775*f*
Pacific Islander Americans, 19, 22*b*, 63, 514*b*
Pacing leads, 747*f*
Packed red blood cells, 648*b*-649*b*
Paget's disease of bone, 1514*b*, **1514**
Paget's disease of breast, 399*b*, 1211
Pain, **102-128**
abdominal, 1197*b*
acute, **938-939**
chronic, **940-941**
acute, 107*b*, **107**
anginal, 712*f*. *See also* Angina
associated symptoms, 109
bone, 597*b*-598*b*
breakthrough, 108
breast (mastalgia), **1206**
cancer, **264-265**
case study, 127*b*
central, 106*b*, 107
chest
acute care for, 727
emergency management of, 723*b*
in heart failure, 743
in myocardial infarction, 720
chronic, 107*b*, **107**
chronic pelvic, **1252-1253**
chronic prostatitis/chronic pelvic pain syndrome, 1282
classification of, **106-107**
in compartment syndrome, 1479
complex regional pain syndrome, 107
continuous, background, 445
in critical care patients, 1556
deafferentation, 106*b*, 107
deep, 106
deep somatic, 106*b*
definitions of, 102-106
diffuse, 1502
dimensions of, 102-106, 103*b*
dorsal horn processing, 105
in ear, 365*b*
in eye, 357*b*
fear of
at end of life, 139
preoperative, 303
in fracture healing, 1469*b*
gender differences, 102-106
headache, **1368-1374**
localized, 1502
low back pain, **1502-1510**
magnitude of the problem, 102
mechanisms of, 103-106, 105*f*
modulation of, 104*f*, 106
with musculoskeletal injuries, 1478*b*
neck, **1507-1508**
neuropathic, 106*b*, **106-107**
chronic, 119
in spinal cord injury, 1424
nociceptive, 104, 104*f*, 106*b*, **106**, 1424
Pain *(Continued)*
nursing and interprofessional management of, **122-123**
nursing diagnoses, 339
nursing management of, **339-340**
in older adults, 125-126
pelvic, chronic, **1252-1253**
perception of, 104*f*, 106
persistent, 107
phantom breast pain, 1215
post-breast therapy syndrome, 1214-1215
postoperative, 333*b*, **339**
radicular, 1502
referred, 105, 105*f*, 1502
rest pain, 804
sleep disturbances during, 92*b*
somatic, 106
after spinal cord injury, 1424
superficial, 106, 106*b*
sympathetically maintained, 106*b*, 107
transmission of, 104-106, 104*f*
transmission to spinal cord, 104-105
transmission to thalamus and cortex, 105-106
treatment-induced, 445
on urination, 1025*b*
visceral, 106, 106*b*
Pain assessment, **107-110**, 108*b*, 1306
in cancer, 264, 264*b*
documentation of, 110
elements of, 107-110
in nonverbal patients, 126*b*
with placebos, 125
principles of, 108*b*
reassessment, 110
Pain education, **123-124**
Pain management, **110-122**. *See also* Analgesics
in Alzheimer's disease, 1412
basic principles of, 110-111
in burns, 445-446
in cancer, 264-265
communication for, 122
complementary & alternative therapies for, 1221*b*
in critical care patients, 1556
drug therapy, 110, 111*b*, **111-120**
at end of life, 140*b*-141*b*
ethical issues in, **124-126**
ethical/legal dilemmas, 619*b*
holistic approach to, 110
images useful for, 85*b*
institutionalization of, **123-124**
interprofessional approach to, 110
interventional therapy, 120-121
multimodal approach to, 110
neuroablative techniques, 120
neurosurgical procedures for, 120, 121*f*
nondrug therapies, 121*b*, **121-122**
patient & caregiver teaching for, 111, 123*b*
for patients unable to self-report pain, 126
with placebos, 125
in respiratory failure, 1618-1619
safety alert, 1618*b*
in special populations, **126**
after spinal cord injury, 1430, 1434
strategies for, 109, 1632
in substance abuse, 126
teamwork & collaboration for, 123*b*
Pain pattern, 108-109
Pain thermometer sclae, 109*f*
Pain treatment plans, 110-111
Painful bladder syndrome, **1040-1041**, 1067*b*
Painful heels, 1509*b*
Paired organ donation, 1093
Palbociclib (Ibrance), 1217*b*, 1218

Palliative care, **129-130**, 130*f*
in cancer, 244
at end of life, **129-144**
goals of, 129*b*, 130*f*
in heart failure, 752-753
home, 131*b*
radiation therapy, 1216
sedation, 136-137
surgical, 301
Pallidotomy, 1391
Pallor, 597*b*-598*b*
in compartment syndrome, 1479
elevation, 803-804
in light- and dark-skinned persons, 404*b*
Palmar erythema, 986
PALM-COIEN classification system, 1246*f*
Palonosetron (Aloxi), 895*b*
Palpation, **39**, 39*f*
Palpitations, 597*b*-598*b*
Pamelor (nortriptyline), 116*b*
Pancarditis, rheumatic, 788
Pancreas, **1108**
functions of, **838-839**, 1108
in older adults, 840*b*, 1108*b*
secretions, 835*b*
structure of, **838-839**, 838*f*
Pancreatic cancer, **1004-1005**
cultural & ethnic health disparities, 986*b*
interprofessional care for, 1004-1005
nursing management of, **1005**
Pancreatic disorders, 986*b*, **999-1005**
Pancreatic enzyme products, 1001*b*, 1004
Pancreatic hormones, 1104*b*, **1108**
Pancreatic polypeptide, 1104*b*
Pancreatic pseudocysts, 1000
Pancreatic studies, 1115*t*-1118*t*
Pancreatic transplantation, 1137
Pancreaticoduodenectomy, 1004-1005, 1005*f*
Pancreatitis
acute, **999-1001**, 999*f*
diagnostic findings in, 1000, 1000*b*
drug therapy for, 1001*b*
interprofessional care for, 1000-1001, 1001*b*
nursing management of, **1001-1003**
pathogenesis of, 999, 999*f*
chronic, **1003-1004**
drug therapy for, 1001*b*
nursing management of, **1004**
edematous, 999, 999*f*
interstitial, 999
mild, 999
necrotizing, 999
severe, 999
Pancrelipase (Pancrease, Zenpep, Creon, Viokace), 1001*b*, 1004
Pancuronium, 326*b*
Pancytopenia, 599
Panel of reactive antibodies (PRA), **208**
Pannus, 1536
Pantoprazole (Protonix), 903*b*
Pantothenic acid (vitamin B_5), 610*b*
Papanicolaou (Pap) test, 1198*t*-1201*t*, 1256-1257, 1256*b*
Papillary muscle dysfunction or rupture, 721
Papillary transitional cell carcinoma, 1053, 1054*f*
Papilledema, 376, 1308*b*-1309*b*, 1318
Papilloma, intraductal, 1208
Papillomavirus, 214*b*
Papules, 401*b*
Paracentesis, 991
Paracrine action, 1102
Paradoxic breathing, 1614
Paradoxic intoxication, 1390
Paraesophageal hiatal hernia, 904, 904*f*
Parainfluenza virus, 214*b*
Paralysis, 1479
Paralytic ileus, 950-951
Paranasal sinus problems, **475-484**
Paraneoplastic syndrome, 514-515
Paraphimosis, 1283, 1283*f*
Paraplegia, 1308*b*-1309*b*, 1420, 1423*b*
Parasomnias, **99-100**
Parasympathetic nervous system, 1299
Parathormone, 1104*b*, 1107
Parathyroid disorders, **1171-1174**
Parathyroid glands, **1107**, 1107*f*
in older adults, 1108*b*
scan of, 1115*t*-1118*t*
Parathyroid hormone, 1104*b*, **1107**, 1115*t*-1118*t*
Parathyroid studies, 1115*t*-1118*t*
Paregoric, 931*b*
Parenteral nutrition, 864*f*, **869-870**
assessment of, 870*b*
catheter site care, 870*b*
central, 869
complications of, 870-871, 871*b*
home support, 871
indications for, 869*b*
management of infusions, 870*b*
methods of administration, 869-870
nursing management of, **870-871**
peripheral, 870
preparation of solutions, 870*b*
transitioning to oral nutrition, 870*b*
Paresthesias, 803, 1308*b*-1309*b*, 1456*b*
in compartment syndrome, 1479
of feet and hands, 597*b*-598*b*
Parietal pleura, 455
Parkinsonism, 1387, 1388*f*
atypical, 1387
Parkinson's disease, **1387-1391**
clinical manifestations of, 1388-1389, 1389*f*
complications of, 1389
dancing and, 1390*b*
dementia in, 1401*b*
diagnostic studies for, 1389
drug therapy for, 1389-1391, 1391*b*
etiology and pathophysiology of, 1387-1388, 1388*f*
familial cases, 1387
genetics of, 1303*b*, 1388
interprofessional care for, 1389-1391, 1389*b*
nursing assessment in, 1392*b*
nursing diagnoses for, 1391
nursing management of, **1391-1393**
nutritional therapy for, 1391
off episodes, 1390-1391
sleep disturbances during, 92*b*
surgical therapy for, 1391
TRAP mnemonic for, 1388
Parkland (Baxter) formula, 439, 439*b*
Parotitis, 897*b*
Paroxysmal nocturnal dyspnea, 742-743
Paroxysmal supraventricular tachycardia, 764*b*, **765**, 765*f*
Parteras (midwives), 24
Partial pressure of CO_2 in arterial blood ($PaCO_2$), 1655*b*-1658*b*
Partial pressure of CO_2 in venous blood ($PvCO_2$), 1655*b*-1658*b*
Partial pressure of O_2 in arterial blood (PaO_2), 457*b*-458*b*, 1655*b*-1658*b*
Partial pressure of O_2 in venous blood (PvO_2), 1655*b*-1658*b*
Partial thromboplastin time, activated (aPTT), 821*b*
Parturition, 1187
Parvovirus, 214*b*
Pasero Opioid-Induced Sedation Scale (POSS), 115*b*
Passive leg raise challenge, 1601
Passive warming measures, 341
Passy-Muir speaking tracheostomy valve, 490, 490*f*
Past health history, 36. *See also* Health history
Pastoral care, 10*b*
Patanase (clopatadine), 479*b*-480*b*
Patch graft angioplasty, 806
Patch tests, 201, 405*f*, 405*t*
Patellar reflex, 1307, 1307*f*
Pathogens, 213-215
Pathologic fracture, 1514*b*-1515*b*
Patient adherence to treatment, 510*b*
Patient and caregiver teaching, **46-59**. *See also specific disorders and procedures*
assessment of factors affecting, 51-53, 51*b*
case study, 57*b*
challenges in, 49
communication for, 48-49, 49*f*
cultural considerations, 52
discharge teaching, 345*b*
evaluation of, 56-57, 57*b*
learner factors, 51*b*, 52-53
materials for, 54-55, 54*f*
physical factors, 51, 51*b*
planning, 54-55
preoperative, 308-309, 309*b*
process of, 51-57
psychologic factors, 51-52, 51*b*
regulatory mandates for, 50-51
required competencies for, 48-49
role of, 46
with smart phone apps, 1141*b*
sociocultural factors, 51*b*, 52-53
socioeconomic considerations, 52-53
teaching strategies for, 54-55, 54*f*, 55*b*-56*b*, 56*f*
text messaging, 1135*b*
Patient and visitor violence/abuse, 1644*b*
Patient interviews
considerations for, 35
motivational interviewing, 47, 48*b*
preoperative, **302**
Patient positioning
grounding, 321, 321*f*
postoperative, 332-334, 336, 336*f*
during surgery, **321**
for tube feedings, 866
Patient privacy, 1222*b*
Patient Protection and Affordable Care Act (ACA), 4
Patient rights, 1482*b*
Patient-centered care, **5-9**, 6*b*
Patient-controlled analgesia, **120**, 340, 340*b*
Patient-controlled epidural analgesia, 120
PBS. *See* Painful bladder syndrome
PCV13 (pneumococcal conjugate vaccine), 504*b*
Peak expiratory flow rate (PEFR), 473*b*
Peak flow meters, 556*b*
Peale, Norman Vincent, 82
Pectoriloquy, 467*b*-468*b*
Pedicles, 427
Pediculosis, 416*b*
Pedigree, 179*b*
Peek sign, 1393*f*
Pegfilgrastim (Neulasta), 195*b*
Pelvic examination
internal, 1196
secondary survey, 1634
Pelvic exenteration, 1261, 1261*f*
Pelvic floor muscle exercises (Kegel), 1037, 1057*b*-1058*b*
Pelvic floor muscle rehabilitation, 1057*b*
Pelvic fracture, **1481**
Pelvic inflammatory disease, **1251-1252**, 1251*f*
interprofessional care for, 1251-1252
nursing assessment in, 1252*b*
nursing management of, **1252**
Pelvic organ prolapse, **1261-1265**

Pelvic organs, 1185-1187
Pelvic pain, chronic, **1252-1253**
Pelvis, female, 1187, 1198*t*-1201*t*
Pencil in cup deformity, 1537
Penetrating injuries
abdominal trauma, 941, 942*b*
chest trauma, 519, 519*b*
renal, 1050
Penicillamine (Cuprimine, Depen), 1521*b*-1522*b*, 1529
Penicillin-resistant *Streptococcus pneumoniae*, 216, 216*b*
Penile discharge, 1198*b*
Penile erythema, 1198*b*
Penile growths or masses, 1198*b*
Penile implants, 1288
Penis
cancer of, **1284**
congenital problems of, **1283**
physical examination of, 1195
problems of, **1283-1284**
Pentazocine (Talwin), 113*b*-114*b*, 114
Pepcid (famotidine), 903*b*
Peptic ulcers, 910-915
acute, 910, 910*f*
acute care for, 915-916
acute exacerbation, 915
ambulatory care for, 916-917
case study, 926*b*
chronic, 910, 910*f*
clinical manifestations of, 912
complications of, 912-913, 915, 917-918
conservative therapy for, 913-915
cyroprotective drug therapy for, 914
diagnostic studies in, 913
drug therapy for, 903*b*, 913-915
etiology of, 910-912
health promotion for, 915
interprofessional care for, 913-915, 914*b*, 917-918
lifestyle factors, 912
medication-induced, 911-912
nursing assessment in, 915*b*
nursing diagnoses related to, 915
nursing management of, **915-918**
nutritional therapy for, 915
in older adults, 919
pathophysiology of, 910-912, 911*f*
patient & caregiver teaching for, 916*b*
postoperative care for, 918-919
postoperative complications of, 917-918
preoperative care for, 918
surgical therapy for, 917-918
nursing management of, **918-919**
nutritional therapy after, 918
types of, 910, 910*f*
Peptide YY, 877*b*, 877*f*
Pepto Diarrhea Control (loperamide), 931*b*
Pepto-Bismol (bismuth subsalicylate), 931*b*
Perceptual deficits, 1362, 1362*f*
Percussion, **39-40**, 40*f*
of chest, 465, 465*f*
cupped-hand position for, 570, 570*f*
for postural drainage, 569, **570**, 570*f*
Percussion sounds, 465*b*, 465*f*
Percutaneous biopsy, 243
Percutaneous coronary intervention (PCI), 717
emergent, 722-723
nursing management of, 729*b*
Percutaneous discectomy, 1506
Percutaneous endoscopic gastrostomy, 865-866, 866*f*
Percutaneous nephrolithotomy, 1047
Percutaneous tracheostomy, 485
Percutaneous transhepatic cholangiography, 847*t*-850*t*
Percutaneous transluminal angioplasty, 806
Percutaneous transluminal balloon valvuloplasty, **793-794**, 794*f*
Percutaneous transluminal septal myocardial ablation, 799
Percutaneous ultrasonic lithotripsy, 1048
Perennial rhinitis, 477
Perforomist (formoterol), 548*b*-549*b*
Perfusion
peripheral, 814
renal, 814
Perfusion imaging, 672
Perfusion scanning, 530
Pericardial effusion, 785
Pericardial friction rubs, 668*b*, 669, 785
Pericardial space, 658
Pericardiocentesis, 786, 786*f*
Pericarditis, 784
acute, 721, **784-786**, 785*f*
in cancer, 251*b*-252*b*
causes of, 784, 784*b*
chronic constrictive, **787**
after myocardial infarction, 721
Pericardium, 658, 781*f*
Perimenopause, **1248-1249**
clinical manifestations of, 1248-1249, 1248*b*
interprofessional care for, 1249
nursing management of, **1249-1250**
Perimetrium, 1186
Perimetry (visual field) testing, 359*t*
Perimysium, 1448
Perinatal transmission, 219, 226
Perindopril (Aceon), 691*b*-693*b*
Perineum, 1634
Perineural local anesthesia, 340
Periodic limb movement disorder, 98
Periodic limb movements in sleep, 98
Perioperative nurses, 316-317
Perioperative nursing, 318*b*
care for obese patients, **887-890**
Perioperative Nursing Data Set (PNDS), 322
Periorbital bone fracture, 1486*b*
Periorbital edema, 1042*b*
Periosteum, 1447
Peripheral adenocarcinoma, 514*f*
Peripheral arteriography, 673*t*-677*t*
Peripheral artery bypass surgery, 806, 806*f*, 808*b*
Peripheral artery disease, 802-810, 804*b*
ambulatory care for, 807-808
case study, 828*b*
clinical manifestations of, 803-804
complementary & alternative therapies for, 805
complications of, 804
dermatologic manifestations of, 399*b*
diagnostic studies in, 804-805
drug therapy for, 805
etiology and pathophysiology of, 802-803
exercise therapy for, 805
hypertension and, 686*b*, 687
interprofessional care for, 804*b*, 805-806
of lower extremities, **803-806**, 803*f*
acute care for, 807
health promotion for, 807
nursing management of, **806-808**
nursing assessment in, 807*b*
nursing diagnoses for, 806
nutritional therapy for, 805
in obesity, 1151
after spinal cord injury, 1424
surgical therapy for, 806, 806*f*
Peripheral blood smear, 602*t*
Peripheral cyanosis, 668*b*
Peripheral edema, 988-990
Peripheral nervous system, 1294, **1298-1299**
Peripheral neuropathy, 106*b*
acute care for, 1541
in cancer, 251*b*-252*b*
in chronic kidney disease, 1078
in cirrhosis, 987
Peripheral perfusion, 814
Peripheral sensitization, 104, 105*f*
Peripheral stem cell transplantation, 259
Peripheral vascular disease. *See* Peripheral artery disease
Peripheral vascular system, 666-667
Peripherally inserted central catheters (PICCs), **295**, 295*f*
Periprosthetic hip fracture, 1493*b*
Peristalsis, 835
Peritoneal dialysis, 1084, 1085*b*, **1085-1087**
automated, 1086, 1086*f*
catheter exit site, 1085-1086, 1086*f*
catheter placement for, 1085-1086
chronic, 1087
complications of, 1087, 1096*b*
continuous ambulatory, 1086-1087
exit site infection, 1087
solutions and cycles, 1086
systems, 1086-1087
Peritoneoscopy, 847*t*-850*t*
Peritoneum, 938
Peritonitis, 943
causes of, 943, 943*b*
interprofessional care for, 943, 943*b*
nursing diagnoses for, 944
nursing management of, **943-944**
in peritoneal dialysis, 1087
spontaneous bacterial, 989-990
Peritonsillar abscess, 484
Permissive hypercapnia, 1623
Pernicious anemia, 612
Perphenazine, 895*b*
PERRL (Pupils are Equal [in size], Round, and Reactive to Light), 1306
PERRLA (Pupils are Equal, Round, and Reactive to Light and Accommodation), 358, 1306
Persistent pain, 107
Personal Diabetes Manager (PDM), 1129*f*
Personal hygiene. *See* Hygiene
Personal protective equipment (PPE), 217*b*, 218, 1643
Personal space, 27, 27*f*
Personalized cancer medicine, 244-245
Personhood, 1632
Perspiration, sensible, 274
Pertussis, 216*b*, **500**
Pertuzumab (Perjeta), 1217*b*
Pes cavus, 1509*b*
Pes planus, 1456*b*, 1509*b*
Pessaries, 1057*b*
Pet therapy, 82*b*, 83*f*
Petechiae, 403*b*-404*b*, 597*b*-598*b*, 598, 623, 623*f*
Pethidine, 114
Peyronie's disease, 1283-1284
pH, **286-287**
normal range, 287, 287*f*
reference values, 1655*b*-1658*b*, 1661*b*
Phacoemulsification, 374-375
Phagocytes, 192
Phagocytosis, 589
Phakic intraocular lens, 368
Phantom breast pain, 1215
Phantom limb sensation, 1488
Pharmacists, 10*b*, 294*b*
Pharmacogenetics, 179*b*, **186**, 187*b*, 244
Pharmacogenomics, 179*b*, **186**, 244
Pharmacologic echocardiography, 673*t*-677*t*
Pharmacologic nuclear imaging, 673*t*-677*t*

Pharmacomechanical devices, 808
Pharyngectomy, 491
Pharyngitis, acute, **484**
Pharynx, **834**
physical examination of, **463**
problems of, **484**
Phenothiazines, 895*b*
Phenotypes, 179*b*
Phenteramine/topiramate (Qsymia), 884*b*
Phentolamine (Regitine), 691*b*-693*b*
Phenylalanine, 1655*b*-1658*b*
Phenylephrine, 479*b*-480*b*, 1599*b*
Phenylpropanolamine, 1059*b*
Phenytoin (Dilantin), 116*b*, 771*b*
Pheochromocytoma, **1181-1182**
Philadelphia chromocome, 183, 636
Phimosis, 1283, 1283*f*
Phlebectomy, 826
Phlebitis, **816**
Phlebostatic axis, 1560, 1561*f*
Phlebotomy, elective, 652
Phlegmasia cerulea dolens, 818
Phoenix Society, 448
Phonophobia, 1370
Phosgene, 1645
Phosphate, 1115*t*-1118*t*, 1655*b*-1658*b*
Phosphate imbalances, 285*b*, **285-286**
Phosphate restriction, 1082*b*, 1083
Phosphodiesterase inhibitors, 745*b*
Phosphodiesterase type 5 (PDE5) inhibitors, 532*b*, 1288*b*
Phospholipase A_2, lipoprotein-associated, **671**, 673*t*-677*t*
Phosphorus
blood values, 1025*t*-1030*t*
in bone disease, 1457*t*-1459*t*
reference values, 1655*b*-1658*b*
Photoaging, 397, 397*f*
Photodynamic therapy, 379, 517
Photography, digital, 175*b*
Photophobia, 357*b*, 1370
Photorefractive keratectomy, 368
Photosensitivity
drug-induced, 408-409, 408*b*, 409*f*
in systemic lupus erythematosus, 1538
Phototherapy, 420
Photovaporization of the prostate (PVP), 1272
Phyllodes tumor, 1211
Physical abuse
child sexual abuse, 1263
elder abuse, **66-67**, 67*b*, 1414*b*
Physical activity
activity-exercise pattern, 37*b*, 38
for acute coronary syndrome, 731-732
for CAD, 706, 708
caloric expenditures, 1134*b*
in COPD, 573-574, 574*b*
energy costs of, 731, 731*b*
guidelines for, 689, 732, 732*b*
health impact of, 1464*b*
health-promoting behaviors for, 708*b*
high-energy activities, 731*b*
for hypertension, 689
isometric activities, 732
low-energy activities, 731*b*
moderate-energy activities, 731*b*
and sport injuries, 1476*b*
very-high-energy activities, 731*b*
Physical Classification System (ASA), 307*b*, 322
Physical dependence, 123
Physical examination, 35*f*, **39-40**
equipment for, 40, 40*b*
example findings, 43*b*-44*b*
general survey, 39
internal pelvic examination, 1196
negative findings, 39
Physical examination *(Continued)*
in older adults, 40
organization of, 40, 41*b*-42*b*
positive findings, 39
preoperative, 307-308, 307*b*
recording, 40
before surgery, 318
techniques for, 39-40
Physical learning, 53
Physical restraints, 74
Physical therapists, 10*b*
role in caring for acute stroke patients, 1359*b*
role in caring for arthritis patients, 1529*b*
role in caring for hypertensive patients, 696*b*
role in caring for patients with casts or in traction, 1471*b*
role in caring for seizure patients, 1380*b*
role in caring for VTE patients, 824*b*
role in postoperative care, 334*b*
role in stroke rehabilitation, 1364, 1364*f*
Physical therapy
for burns, **446**
chest physiotherapy, **1617**
for head and neck cancer, 493
Physician assistants, 10*b*, 1274*b*
Physician Order for Life-Sustaining Treatment (POLST), 135, 136*b*
Physician-assisted suicide, 136-137
Physicians (medical doctors), 10*b*, 1274*b*
Physiologic stress ulcers, **922**
Pia mater, 1300
PICOT format, 2, 15
Pilocarpine (Isopto Carpine, Pilocar, Pilopine-HS, Piloptic, Pilostat), 381*b*
Pilonidal cysts, 846*b*-847*b*
Pilonidal sinus, **971**
Pindolol, 691*b*-693*b*
Pineal gland, **1106**
Pinna (auricle), 360
Pioglitazone (Actos), 1131*b*
Piroxicam (Feldene), 164*b*, 1521*b*-1522*b*
Pitressin (vasopressin), 993*b*, 1599*b*
Pitting edema, 668*b*
Pituitary adenoma, 1333*b*
Pituitary gland, **1105-1106**, 1106*f*
anterior, 1104*b*, **1105**, **1156-1159**
disorders of, **1156-1162**
genetic risks, 1109*b*
hypofunction of, **1158**
posterior, 1104*b*, **1105-1106**, **1159-1162**
studies of, 1115*t*-1118*t*
Pituitary surgery, **1158**
nursing management of, **1158-1159**
transsphenoidal approach to, 1158, 1159*f*
Place disparities, 20
Placebos, 125
Planning
for discharge and follow-up care, 345-346
in nursing process, 5, 6*f*
Plant sterols, 710*b*
Plantar fasciitis, 1456*b*
Plantar flexion, 1455*b*
Plantar warts, 415*b*, 416*f*, 1509*b*
Plaque
characteristics of, 401*b*
fibrous, 703, 703*f*
on lips or in mouth, 846*b*-847*b*
Plaquenil (hydroxychloroquine), 1528
Plasma, 271, 587-588
reference values, 1655*b*-1658*b*
shifts of interstitial fluid to, 274
shifts to interstitial fluid, 273-274
Plasma cell myeloma, 645
Plasma cells, 192
Plasma oncotic pressure, 274
Plasma osmolality, 273, 1106, 1106*f*
Plasma thromboplastin antecedent, 592*b*
Plasmacytoma, 597*b*-598*b*
Plasmapheresis, **205**
Plasminogen, 601*t*
Plasticity, 105
Platelet adhesions, 591
Platelet count, 600, 601*t*
Platelet growth factor, 195*b*, 260*b*
Platelets, 590
activation of, 591
aggregation of, 591
for blood component therapy, 648*b*
plug formation, 591
reference values, 1659*b*
for transfusions, 649*b*
Platinum drugs, 247*b*
Plavix (clopidogrel), 187*b*, 715*b*-716*b*, 805*b*
Pletal (cilostazol), 805*b*
Plethysmography, 1457*t*-1459*t*
Pleura, 455
Pleural chest tubes, 344*b*
Pleural drainage, **522-524**
Pleural effusion, 456, 503, **527-528**
chest examination findings in, 468*b*
exudative, 527
in heart failure, 743
interprofessional care for, 528
transudative, 527
Pleural friction rub, 467*b*-468*b*
Pleural space, 519
Pleural tuberculosis, 508
Pleurisy, 503, **528**
Pleuritis (pleurisy), **528**
Pneumatic compression devices, 819
Pneumatic retinopexy, 377
Pneumatic technology, 1319
Pneumaturia, 1025*b*
Pneumococcal conjugate vaccine (PCV13, Prevnar 13), 504*b*
Pneumococcal polysaccharide vaccine (PPSV23, Pneumovax 23), 504*b*
Pneumoconioses, 512-513
Pneumocystis jiroveci, 215*b*
***Pneumocystis jiroveci* pneumonia (PJP)**, 222*b*, 502
Pneumomediastinum, 1578
Pneumonectomy, 526*b*
Pneumonia, **500-505**
acute care for, 506
ambulatory care for, 506
aspiration, 500, **501-502**
assessment of, 501, 501*b*
case study, 535*b*
chest examination findings in, 468*b*
clinical manifestations of, 502-503
community-acquired, 501*b*, **501**, 504*b*
complications of, 503
diagnostic studies in, 503
drug therapy for, 504, 504*b*
empiric antibiotic therapy for, 501
etiology of, 500
health promotion for, 505-506
hospital-acquired, 501*b*, **501**
interprofessional care for, 503-505, 503*b*
necrotizing, 502
nosocomial, 501
nursing assessment in, 505*b*
nursing diagnoses related to, 505
nursing management of, **505-506**
nutritional therapy for, 504-505
opportunistic, 502
organisms that cause, 500, 501*b*
pathophysiology of, 502, 502*f*
risk factors for, 501*b*
types of, 501-502
ventilator-associated, 501, **1579**, 1623

Pneumonitis
in cancer, 251*b*-252*b*, 256
chemical, 513
hypersensitivity, 513
Pneumothorax, 503, **519-521**
closed, 521
emergency management of, 520*b*
iatrogenic, 520
interprofessional care for, 521
open, 519*f*, 521
spontaneous, 519-520
tension, 520, 520*f*
types of, 519-521
Pneumovax 23 (pneumococcal polysaccharide vaccine), 504*b*
Podagra, 1532-1533
Poikiloderma, 1545
Poikilothermia, 808
Poikilothermism, 1424
Point of maximal impulse (PMI), 667
Poison control centers, 1642
Poisonings, **1642-1644**, 1643*b*
Poliovirus, 214*b*
Pollution, air, 558
Polyarteritis, 1042*b*
Polyarthralgia, 1538
Polyarthritis, 788-789
Polyclonal antibodies, **210**, 211*b*
Polycystic kidney disease, **1051-1052**, 1051*f*
genetics of, 1021*b*, 1051-1052, 1051*b*
nursing and interprofessional management of, **1052**
Polycystic ovary syndrome, 1255, **1255**, 1255*f*
Polycythemia, **620-621**
interprofessional care for, 621
primary, 620, 621*f*
secondary, 620-621, 621*f*
Polycythemia vera, 620
clinical manifestations of, 621
diagnostic studies in, 621
genetics, 620
nursing management of, **621-622**
Polydipsia, 1113*b*-1114*b*
in acromegaly, 1157
in diabetes mellitus, 1122, 1124
Polymerase chain reaction (PCR), 186
Polymerase inhibitors, 981*b*
Polymorphisms, 180
Polymorphonuclear leukocytes, 589
Polymorphonuclear segmented neutrophils (segs), 599-600
Polymyositis, **1544-1545**
Polyneuropathy, **1440-1442**
acute inflammatory demyelinating, 1440
chronic inflammatory demyelinating polyradiculoneuropathy, **1441-1442**
chronic sensory polyneuropathy, 399*b*
Polyphagia, 1122, 1124
Polypharmacy, 73
Polyps
adenomatous, 953
cervical, **1255-1256**
hyperplastic, 953
of large intestine, 953, **953**, 953*f*
laryngeal, **490**
nasal, **483-484**
pedunculated, 953, 953*f*
types of, 953
Polysomnography, 90-91, **93**
Polysubstance use, 154
Polyuria, 1025*b*, 1113*b*-1114*b*
in acromegaly, 1157
in diabetes mellitus, 1122, 1124
Populations, 4
Portal hypertension, 988, 988*b*
Portion sizes, 878, 878*b*, 883
Portosystemic shunts, 992, 992*f*
Position sense, 1307
Positional therapy, 97
Positioning
acute care in increased ICP, 1325
for ARDS, 1624-1625
for mobilization of secretions, 1616-1617
prone, 1578
for sleep apnea, 97
Positive end-expiratory pressure (PEEP), 1575*b*-1576*b*, 1577
Positive expiratory pressure (PEP), 570
Positive feedback, 1104, 1189*b*
Positive inotropes, 746, 748
Positive reinforcement, 53
Positive-pressure ventilation (PPV), 1574
for ARDS, 1624-1625
bilevel positive airway pressure (BiPAP), 97-98, 1577, 1617, 1618*f*
complications of, 1578-1581
continuous positive airway pressure (CPAP), 97, 97*f*
indications for weaning from, 1583*b*
nutritional support, 1581-1582
in respiratory failure, 1617
weaning from, 1582, 1583*b*
Positron emission tomography (PET)
in Alzheimer's disease, 1405, 1407*f*
of brain, 1310*t*-1312*t*
in cancer, 243, 243*f*
cardiac, 672, 673*t*-677*t*
hematologic assessment, 603*t*
of respiratory system, 469*t*-471*t*
Postanesthesia care, 330-331, 330*b*
Postanesthesia care unit (PACU), 330
admission to, 330-332
cardiovascular problems in, 336-338
discharge from, 344*b*, **344**
initial assessment in, 331-332, 331*b*
neurologic and psychologic problems in, 338-339
progression through, 330-331
respiratory problems in, 332-335
Postanesthesia hand-off report, 331, 331*b*
Post-breast therapy pain syndrome, 1214-1215
Postconcussion syndrome, 1327
Posterior chest inspection, 464
Posterior forchette, 1187
Posterior pituitary gland, 1104*b*, **1105-1106**
Posterior pituitary gland disorders, **1159-1162**
Posterior surfaces, 1633*b*
Postexposure prophylaxis (PEP), 226
Postherpetic neuralgia, 107
Postmenopause, **1248-1249**
clinical manifestations of, 1248-1249, 1248*b*
interprofessional care for, 1249
nursing management of, **1249-1250**
nutritional therapy for, 1249
Postmortem care, 139
Postoperative care, **330-348**, 334*b*
in bariatric surgery, 888
case study, 346*b*
in chest surgery, 527
in joint surgery, 1492
after lung transplantation, 534
nursing assessment on admission to clinical unit, 345*b*
for obese patients, 888
for older adults, 346
Postoperative care *(Continued)*
in ostomy surgery, 960
patient positioning, 332-334, 336, 336*f*
potential problems, 331, 332*f*
SBAR hand-off communication, 345*b*
in thyroid surgery, 1167-1168
Postoperative cognitive dysfunction, 338
Postoperative ileus, 341
Postoperative nausea and vomiting, 341
Postprandial hypoglycemia, 918
Post-thrombotic syndrome, 818
Post-transplant lymphoproliferative disorder
classification of, 644*b*
after kidney transplantation, 1096
Postural drainage, 570
percussion for, 569, **570**, 570*f*
vibration for, 569, **570**
Postural instability
in Parkinson's disease, 1389
after stroke, 1363, 1363*f*
Posturography, 365*t*-366*t*
Potassium
in burns, 443
high-potassium foods, 1083*b*
in musculoskeletal disorders, 1457*t*-1459*t*
reference values, 1655*b*-1658*b*
in shock, 1590*t*
sodium-potassium pump, 272*f*
in urinary assessment, 1025*t*-1030*t*
Potassium channel blockers, 771*b*
Potassium chloride (KCl), 282, 282*b*
Potassium excess. *See also* Hyperkalemia
in acute kidney injury, 1072
therapy for, 1073, 1073*b*
Potassium hydroxide (KOH), 405*t*
Potassium imbalances, **280-283**
causes and manifestations of, 281*b*
in chronic kidney disease, 1077
Potassium restriction, 1082*b*, 1083
Potassium-sparing diuretics, 691*b*-693*b*, 745*b*
Power of attorney for health care, 135, 136*b*
Powered phlebectomy, trans-illuminated, 826
Powerlessness, 138-139
Pox virus, 214*b*
PPSV23 (pneumococcal polysaccharide vaccine), 504*b*
PQRST assessment, 35, 712, 712*b*
Pradaxa (dabigatran), 820*b*, 821
Praluent (alirocumab), 711*b*
Pramipexole (Mirapex), 1391*b*
Pramlintide (Symlin), 1131*b*-1132*b*, 1132
Prandin (repaglinide), 1131*b*
Prasugrel (Effient), 715*b*-716*b*
Pravastatin (Pravachol), 711*b*
Prayer, 84
Prazosin (Minipress), 691*b*-693*b*
Prealbumin, 859
Precautions
standard, 218
transmission-based, 218
Precedex (dexmedetomidine), 326*b*
Precontemplation, 47, 48*b*
Precose (acarbose), 1131*b*
Prediabetes, 1123
Prednisone
for arthritis, 1521*b*-1522*b*
for asthma and COPD, 548*b*-549*b*
for immunosuppressive therapy, 209, 211*b*
for multiple sclerosis, 1385*b*
Preferred provider organizations (PPOs), 4
Pregabalin (Lyrica), 116*b*, 1378
Pregnancy
early loss of, **1243-1244**

Pregnancy *(Continued)*
ectopic, **1247**, 1247*f*
laparoscopic treatment of, 1248, 1248*f*
nursing and interprofessional management of, **1247-1248**
lupus and, 1542
Prehypertension, 684, 705-706
Prelief (calcium glycerophosphate), 1040
Preload, 660-661, 1559*b*, **1559-1560**
Preload responsiveness, 1562
Premarin (estrogen cream), 1059*b*
Premature atrial contractions, 764*b*, **764-765**, 764*f*
Premature ventricular contractions, 764*b*, 768, **768-769**, 769*f*
Premenstrual dysphoric disorder, 1244
Premenstrual syndrome, **1244-1245**
interprofessional care for, 1244-1245, 1245*b*
nursing management of, **1245**
Preoperative care, **301-314**
in bariatric surgery, 888
case study, 292*b*
in chest surgery, 524
culturally competent, 311-312
day-of-surgery preparation, 310-311, 310*f*
fasting recommendations, 309, 309*b*
in joint surgery, 1492
in lung transplantation, 533-534
medications, 311, 311*b*
nursing assessment in, **302-308**
nursing management, **308-313**
for obese patients, 888
for older adults, 312-313
in ostomy surgery, 960
patient interview, **302**
patient teaching, 308-309, 309*b*
psychosocial assessment in, 302-304, 303*b*
in thyroid surgery, 1167
Preoperative checklist, 311*b*-312*b*
Preoperative holding area, 315-316
Prepuce problems, **1283**
Presbycusis, 361, 391, 391*b*
Presbyopia, 351, 368
Presenilin-1, 1402
Presenilin-2, 1402
Pressair (aclidinium bromide), 548*b*-549*b*
Pressoreceptors, 682
Pressure support ventilation (PSV), 1576, 1576*b*
Pressure ulcers, **172**
acute care for, 174-175
ambulatory care for, 175-176
assessment of patients with dark skin, 174*b*
in compartment syndrome, 1479
health promotion in, 174
nursing and interprofessional management of, **172-177**
nursing assessment for, 172, 172*b*, 174*b*
nursing diagnoses, 172
patient & caregiver teaching for, 175*b*
prevention of, 174*b*
repositioning and, 174*b*
risk factors for, 172, 172*b*
safety alerts, 172*b*, 174*b*
stages/categories of, 172, 173*b*
Pressure ventilation, 1574, 1576-1577
Pressure-control inverse ratio ventilation (PC-IRV), 1576-1577, 1576*b*
Pressure-control ventilation (PCV), 1576-1577
Prestige cervical disc, 1506
Prevacid (lansoprazole), 903*b*
Prevalite (cholestyramine), 711*b*
Prevention
in cancer, 301
in chronic illness, 61-62
infection prevention and control, 171, **218**
primary, 61-62
secondary, 61-62
Prevnar 13 (pneumococcal conjugate vaccine), 504*b*
Priapism, 1283, 1434
Priftin (rifapentiine), 509*b*
Prilosec (omeprazole), 805*b*, 903*b*
Primary afferent fibers, 104
Primary biliary cirrhosis, **985**
Primary sclerosing cholangitis, **985**
Primary survey, 1630-1632, 1631*b*-1632*b*
Principle of double effect, 137
Prinzmetal's angina, 713, 713*b*
Prions, 214-215
Prior experiences, 47*b*
Privacy, patient, 1222*b*
ProAir HFA (albuterol), 548*b*-549*b*
Probiotics, 935
Problem identification, 44
Problem-focused coping, 83*b*
Procainamide, 771*b*
Procardia (nifedipine), 532*b*, 715*b*-716*b*
Procardia XL (nifedipine long acting), 691*b*-693*b*
Prochlorperazine, 326*b*, 895*b*
Procoagulants, 591
Proconvertin, 592*b*
Procrit (epoetin alfa), 195*b*
Proctocolectomy, total
with ileal pouch/anal anastomosis, 948, 948*f*
with permanent ileostomy, 948
ProDisc-L, 1506
Prodysrhythmia, **771**
Professional nursing organizations, 5
Professional nursing practice, **2-3**
Progesterone, 1104*b*, 1188-1189
measurement of, 1198*t*-1201*t*
reference values, 1655*b*-1658*b*
Progesterone receptor status, 1212-1213
Prograf (tacrolimus), 209, 211*b*
Programmed death receptor (PD)-1, 258*b*
Programs for All-Inclusive Care for the Elderly (PACE), **69**
Progressive care units (PCUs), 1555
Projectile vomiting, 894
Prokinetic agents
for GERD, 903*b*
for nausea and vomiting, 895*b*
for peptic ulcers, 903*b*
Prolactin, 1104*b*, 1188, 1198*t*-1201*t*
Prolactinoma, 1157
Prolamines, 966
Prolapse
pelvic organ, **1261-1265**
uterine, **1261-1262**, 1262*f*
Proleukin (aldesleukin), 195*b*
Prolia (denosumab), 1513
Prolonged grief disorder, 133-134
Promethazine
in general anesthesia, 326*b*
injection alert, 894*b*
for nausea and vomiting, 895*b*
Prompted voiding, 1057*b*
Pronation, 1455*b*
Pronator drift, 1306
Prone positioning, 1578
Propafenone (Rytmol), 771*b*
Propantheline (Pro-Banthine), 1059*b*, 1385*b*
Propine (dipivefrin), 381*b*
Propofol (Diprivan), 325*b*
Propranolol (Inderal), 691*b*-693*b*, 771*b*, 993*b*
Proprioception, 1307
Proprotein convertase subtilisin/kexin 9 (PCSK9) inhibitors, **710**, 711*b*
Proscar (finasteride), 1059*b*, 1271*b*
Prosigna, 1213
Prostaglandins, 162*b*, **162**, 162*f*
synthetic, 903*b*
Prostate, 1185, 1269*f*
photovaporization of (PVP), 1272
problems of, **1268-1283**
transurethral incision of (TUIP), 1272*b*, 1273
transurethral resection of (TURP), 1272-1273, 1272*b*, 1273*f*
visual laser ablation of (VLAP), 1272
Prostate cancer, **1275-1281**
acute care for, 1281
ambulatory care for, 1281-1282
androgen deprivation therapy for, 1279-1280, 1280*b*
brachytherapy for, 1279, 1279*f*
chemotherapy for, 1280
clinical manifestations of, 1276
complications of, 1276
cryotherapy for, 1279
cultural & ethnic health disparities, 1276*b*
culturally competent care for, 1280-1281
diagnostic studies for, 1276-1277
drug therapy for, 1279-1280
etiology and pathophysiology of, 1275-1276
familial, 1276
genetics of, 1192*b*, 1276
health promotion for, 1281-1282
hereditary (inherited), 1276
hormone-refractory, 1279
interprofessional care for, 1277-1280, 1278*b*
metastasis, 1276*f*
nursing assessment in, 1281*b*
nursing diagnoses for, 1281
nursing management of, **1281-1282**
radiation therapy for, 1279-1280
sporadic, 1276
staging of, 1277, 1277*b*
surgical therapy for, 1278-1279
Prostate surgery, 1278-1279
ambulatory care after, 1275
bladder irrigation after, 1274, 1274*b*
postoperative care in, 1274-1275
preoperative care in, 1274
Prostatectomy
approaches to, 1278, 1278*f*
laser, 1271-1272, 1272*b*
nerve-sparing proceure, 1279
open, 1272*b*
perineal, 1278, 1278*f*
radical, 1278
retropubic, 1278, 1278*f*
robotic-assisted, 1278
Prostate-specific antigen (PSA)
measurement of, 1198*t*-1201*t*
reference values, 1655*b*-1658*b*
Prostatitis, **1282**
asymptomatic inflammatory, 1282
chronic, 1282
nursing and interprofessional management of, **1282-1283**
Prostheses
for amputations, 1488, 1489*f*
bladder neck support, 1057*b*
periprosthetic hip fracture, 1493*b*
Prosthetic heart valves, 794-795, 795*f*
Protease inhibitors (PIs), 224*b*, 981*b*
Proteasome inhibitors, 258*b*
Proteasomes, 257
Protected health information (PHI), 14
Protein(s), 855
complete, 855
dietary, 409
foods high in, 855*b*
high-calorie, high-protein diet, 863*b*
incomplete, 855
negative acute phase, 859
in parenteral nutrition, 869

Protein(s) *(Continued)*
positive acute phase, 859
recommendations for nutrient balance, 1133
reference values, 1655*b*-1658*b*, 1661*b*-1662*b*
serum levels, 852*t*
synthesis of, 180
Protein deficiency, 168*b*
Protein foods with high biologic value, 262*b*
Protein restriction, 1082, 1082*b*
Protein-calorie malnutrition, 856
Protest, 133, 133*f*
Proteus, 214*b*
Prothrombin, 592*b*
Prothrombin time, 601*t*, 852*t*, 1659*b*
Protonix (pantoprazole), 903*b*
Proton-pump inhibitors (PPIs), 902*b*
for cirrhosis, 993*b*
for GERD, 902, 903*b*
for pancreatitis, 1001*b*
for peptic ulcers, 903*b*, 914
Protooncogenes, 179*b*, 236
Protozoa, 214
Proud flesh (excess granulation tissue), 167*b*
Proventil HFA (albuterol), 548*b*-549*b*
Pruritus, 399, 597*b*-598*b*, 1006*b*
control of, **424**
with jaundice, 978
opioid-induced, 115
Pseudoaddiction, 123
Pseudoaneurysms, 810, 811*f*
Pseudoarthrosis, 1470*b*
Pseudocysts, pancreatic, 1000
Pseudoephedrine (Sudafed)
for rhinitis and sinusitis, 478*b*-480*b*
for voiding dysfunction, 1059*b*
Pseudofolliculitis, 403-405
Pseudogout, 1533
Pseudohypoparathyroidism, **1173**
Pseudomonas aeruginosa, 214*b*
Pseudo-obstruction, intestinal, 951
Psoriasis, 417, 417*f*, **419*b***
Psoriatic arthritis, **1537**
Psoriatic spondylitis, 1537
Psychogenic erection, 1434
Psychogenic seizures, 1376
Psychologic abuse, 67*b*
Psychologic factors, 29, 706-707
Psychologic problems
nursing diagnoses related to, 339
nursing management of, **339**
postoperative, **338**
Psychologic support
for rheumatoid arthritis patients, 1532
for STI patients, 1239
Psychoneuroimmunology, 80
Psychosocial care
attempting to normalize social interactions, 61
for breast cancer patients, 1220-1221
for COPD patients, 574
at end of life, 138-139, 138*b*, 139*f*
during mechanical ventilation, 1580-1581
preoperative assessment, 302-304, 303*b*, 318
in systemic lupus erythematosus, 1542
Psychosocial problems
with fractures, 1477
management of risk factors, 689
with obesity, 879*f*, 880
Psychostimulants, 664*b*
Psyllium, 710*b*
Ptosis, 357*b*, 1306
Pubis, 1195
Public health, 226*b*
Pull test, 1389
Pulmicort Flexhaler (budesonide), 547, 548*b*-549*b*
Pulmonary angiography, 469*t*-471*t*
Pulmonary artery (PA) catheter, 457, **1563-1564**, 1563*f*
indications and contraindications to catheterization, 1563*b*
insertion, 1564, 1564*f*
Pulmonary artery occlusive pressure, 1558-1559
Pulmonary artery wedge pressure, 678
Pulmonary congestion, 1618
Pulmonary diseases
corticosteroid therapy for, 1180*b*
obstructive, **538-584**
Pulmonary edema, **529**, 741-742
causes of, 529*b*
chest examination findings in, 468*b*
postoperative, 333*b*, 334
Pulmonary embolism, **529-531**, 529*f*
acute, 530*b*
drug therapy for, 530-531
interprofessional care for, 530-531, 530*b*
nursing management of, **531**
postoperative, 333*b*
surgical therapy for, 531
Pulmonary fibrosis, 512-513
chest examination findings in, 468*b*
idiopathic, **528**
Pulmonary function tests, 469*t*-471*t*, **472**, 473*b*
Pulmonary hypertension, 529-530, **531-534**
drug therapy for, 532, 532*b*
idiopathic, 531, **531-532**
nursing and interprofessional management of, **532-533**
pathophysiology of, 532*f*, 564*f*
primary, 531
secondary, 531, **533**
Pulmonary infections
fungal, 512*b*, **512**
treatment of, 1618
Pulmonary rehabilitation, 573
Pulmonary vascular resistance (PVR), 1559-1560
Pulmonic stenosis, 791*b*, **793**
Pulse abnormalities, 668*b*
Pulse deficits, 667-669, 668*b*
Pulse oximetry, 439*b*, 457, 1565-1566
Pulse pressure, 662
Pulseless electrical activity, **771**
Pulselessness, 1479
Pulsus alternans, 668*b*
Pulsus paradoxus, 785, 785*b*
Punch biopsy, 405*t*, 422, 422*f*
Punctate lesions, 810
Punnett squares, 188, 189*f*
Pupil(s), 352
abnormalities, 357*b*
assessment of, 356*b*, 358
Pupillary check, 1323, 1324*f*
Pupillometers, 1323
Purkinje fibers, 659-660
Purpura, 597*b*-598*b*, 623
Pursed-lip breathing, 467*b*-468*b*, 554*b*, 569
Pus, 161, 162*b*
Pustules, 401*b*
Pyelography
antegrade, 1025*t*-1030*t*
intravenous, 1025*t*-1030*t*
retrograde, 1025*t*-1030*t*
Pyelolithotomy, 1048
Pyelonephritis, 1034, 1038
acute, **1038**, 1038*f*
chronic, **1039**
Pyloroplasty, 840*b*, 917
Pyorrhea, 846*b*-847*b*
Pyramid effects, 236
Pyramidal tract, 1296
Pyrazinamide (PZA), 509*b*
Pyridoxine (vitamin B_6), 610*b*, 858*b*
Pyrosis, 846*b*-847*b*, 900-901

Q

Qsymia (phenteramine/topiramate), 884*b*
Quad coughing, 1616
Quadriplegia, 1308*b*-1309*b*, 1420
Quality and Safety Education for Nurses (QSEN) Institute, 5, 6*b*
Quality improvement, 6*b*, **12-13**
Quality improvement (QI) programs, 13, 13*f*
Quantitative protein test, 1025*t*-1030*t*
Quantitative ultrasound, 1457*t*-1459*t*
Questions, open-ended, 57*b*
Quinapril (Accupril), 691*b*-693*b*
Quinidine (Quinora), 771*b*
Qvar (beclomethasone), 548*b*-549*b*

R

Rabeprazole (Aciphex), 903*b*
Rabies, 1642, 1642*b*
Rabies immun globulin (RIG), 1642
Raccoon eyes, 1326, 1327*f*
Race, **19-20**
Racism, 26
Radiation, 237, 249
acute radiation syndrome, 1645
electromagnetic, 249
external, 250
internal, 250
ionizing, 1645
late effects of, **256-257**
particulate, 249
skin hazards, 409
Radiation skin changes, 251*b*-252*b*, 255, 255*b*
Radiation therapy, **248-250**
acute intervention for, 1261
for cancer. *See specific cancers*
cardiovascular effects of, 256
cranial, 517
for dermatologic problems, 420
external beam, 250, 1216, 1279
gastrointestinal effects of, 251*b*-252*b*, 253-255
genitourinary effects of, 251*b*-252*b*
hematologic effects of, 251*b*-252*b*
image-guided, 249
immobilization devices for, 249, 249*f*
integumentary effects of, 251*b*-252*b*
intensity-modulated, 249
nursing management of, **250-256**, 251*b*-252*b*
palliative, 1216
pulmonary effects of, 256
reproductive effects of, 256
safety principles, 250
simulation and treatment planning, 249
stereotactic body radiotherapy, 516
transarterial radioembolization, 997
treatment, 249-250
Radical cystectomy, 1054
Radical neck dissection, 492
modified, 492
reconstructive surgery after, 492*f*
Radiculopathy, 1505
Radioactive iodine therapy, 1166
Radioactive iodine uptake (RAIU) test, 1115*t*-1118*t*
Radiobiology, 249
Radiofrequency ablation
catheter ablation therapy, **775**
for lung cancer, 517
Radiofrequency discal nucleoplasty, 1506
Radiography. *See* X-rays

Radioisotope studies, 603*t*, 1457*t*-1459*t*
Radiologic dispersal devices (RDDs), 1645
Radiologic studies. *See also specific techniques*
of breast, 1205
hematologic, 603*t*
lower gastrointestinal series, 845-851, 847*t*-850*t*, 851*f*
small bowel series, 847*t*-850*t*
upper gastrointestinal series, 845, 847*t*-850*t*
Radionuclide cystography, 1025*t*-1030*t*
Radiosensitivity, tumor, 249, 249*b*
Radiosurgery, stereotactic, 1335, 1337*b*, **1337**, 1337*f*
Raloxifene (Evista), 1217*b*, 1513
Ramipril (Altace), 691*b*-693*b*
Range of motion
assessment of, 1454, 1454*f*
limited, 1456*b*
Ranitidine (Zantac), 903*b*
Rapamune (sirolimus), 209, 211*b*
Rape, statutory, 1263
Rapid eye movement (REM) sleep, **90-91**
Rapid HIV-antibody testing, 222*b*
Rapid plasma reagin (RPR), 1198*t*-1201*t*, 1659*b*
Rapid postanesthesia care unit progression, 330-331
Rapid response teams (RRTs), 1554
Rapidly progressive glomerulonephritis, **1043**
Rapid-sequence intubation, 1570, 1630
Rasagiline (Azilect), 1390, 1391*b*
Rash
bull's eye, 1534, 1534*f*
butterfly, 1538, 1539*f*
in light- and dark-skinned persons, 404*b*
Rationing, 995*b*
Raynaud's phenomenon, **809-810**, 809*f*, **1543**
Reactive hyperemia, 803-804
Readiness to learn, 47*b*, 53
Real-time three-dimensional (3-D) ultrasound, 671, 673*t*-677*t*
Rebif (β-interferon), 195*b*
Rebound tenderness, abdominal, 846*b*-847*b*
Reclast (zoledronic acid), 1513
Recording the physical examination, 40
Recruitment, 365*b*
Rectocele, **1262**, 1262*f*
Rectum
abnormalities, 846*b*-847*b*
in older adults, 840*b*
physical examination of, 845
Red blood cells
disorders of, **619-622**
indices, 599
laboratory studies, 599
in shock, 1590*t*
Red yeast rice, 710*b*
Reed-Sternberg cells, 640-641
Reese, Della, 1120
Refeeding symdrome, 870-871
Referred pain, 105
areas of, 105*f*
low back pain, 1502
Reflex arcs, 1296, 1297*f*
Reflex bronchoconstriction, 459
Reflex erections, 1434
Reflex incontinence, 1056*b*
Reflexes, 1296
abnormalities, 1308*b*-1309*b*
assessment of, 1307, 1307*f*
normal, 1308*b*
in spinal cord injury, 1431
Reflux, gastroesophageal, **900-904**
Refraction, 351
Refractive errors, 351, **367-368**
Refractive intraocular lens, 368
Refractive media, 350-351
Refractometry, 359*t*
Refractory epilepsy, 1379
Refractory hypoxemia, 1621
Refractory phase or period, 761, 762*f*
Refusal of treatment, 1424*b*
Regional anesthesia, 323*b*, 324-327, **324-327**
Registered nurse(s). *See also* Nurse(s)
intraoperative activities, **316-317**, 317*b*
role in assessment and data collection, 36*b*
role in bladder irrigation, 1274*b*
role in blood transfusions, 649*b*
role in cardiac catheterization and PCI, 729*b*
role in caring for acute stroke patients, 1359*b*
role in caring for Alzheimer's patients, 1412*b*
role in caring for arthritis patients, 1529*b*
role in caring for diabetic patients, 1152*b*
role in caring for incontinent patients, 1059*b*
role in caring for neutropenia patients, 632*b*
role in caring for osteomyelitis patients, 1498*b*
role in caring for patients with casts or in traction, 1471*b*
role in caring for patients with chronic venous insufficiency and venous ulcers, 827*b*
role in caring for patients with hypertension, 696*b*
role in caring for seizure patients, 1380*b*
role in caring for VTE patients, 824*b*
role in IV therapy, 294*b*
role in nasogastric and gastric tubes and enteral feedings, 867*b*
role in ostomy care, 960*b*
role in oxygen administration, 568*b*
role in pain management, 123*b*
role in postoperative care, 334*b*
role in skin care, 425*b*
role in suctioning and tracheostomy care, 490*b*
role in wound care, 170*b*
role with corrective lenses and hearing aids, 392*b*
role with urinary catheters, 1061*b*
Registered nurse first assistant (RNFA), 317
Regitine (phentolamine), 691*b*-693*b*
Reglan (metoclopramide)
drug alert, 894*b*
in general anesthesia, 326*b*
for GERD, 903*b*
for nausea and vomiting, 895*b*
Regurgitation, 894
aortic valve, 791*b*, **792-793**
mitral valve, 791*b*, **791**
valvular, 790-791, 790*f*
Rehabilitation
cardiac, 707*b*, 730
for older adults, 71-72, 71*f*
pelvic floor muscle, 1057*b*
pulmonary, 573
respiratory, 1432
after spinal cord injury, 1421, 1422*f*, 1423*b*, 1431-1435, 1432*f*
stroke, 1363
Reiter's syndrome, 1537
Rejection
acute, **208**
chronic, **208-209**
hyperacute, **208**
kidney transplant, 1095
transplant, **208-209**
Relative refractory period, 761, 762*f*
Relaxation breathing, **83-84**, 84*b*
Relaxation response, 83
Relaxation strategies, 83*b*, **83-85**
for pain management, **122**
Religion, **24-25**
Religious beliefs, 649*b*
Religious groups, 26*b*
Relocation stress syndrome, 69
Remicade (infliximab), 1521*b*-1522*b*, 1529
Remifentanil (Ultiva), 326*b*
Remodeling, bone, 1470
Remodulin (treprostinil), 532*b*
Renal arteriography, 1025*t*-1030*t*, 1027*f*
Renal artery stenosis, **1050-1051**
Renal biopsy, 1025*t*-1030*t*
Renal cell carcinoma, 1052-1053, 1052*f*, 1053*b*
Renal colic, 1018, 1046
Renal failure, 1017, 1069
in ARDS, 1623
in heart failure, 743
Renal perfusion, 814
Renal problems, **1033-1068**
Renal replacement therapy, 1074
continuous (CRRT), 1074, 1091*b*, **1091-1092**
Renal scans, 1025*t*-1030*t*
Renal staghorn calculus, 1045, 1046*f*
Renal surgery, **1063**
Renal trauma, **1050**
blunt, 1050
penetrating injuries, 1050
Renal tubules, 1017, 1017*b*
Renal ultrasound, 1025*t*-1030*t*
Renal vascular problems, **1050-1051**
Renal vein thrombosis, **1051**
Renin inhibitors, 691*b*-693*b*
Renin-angiotensin-aldosterone system, 1017-1018, 1018*f*
in heart failure, 739
in hypertension, 684-685
Renin-angiotensin-aldosterone system inhibitors, 745*b*, 747-748
Renova (tretinoin), 426*b*
ReoPro (abciximab), 715*b*-716*b*
Reorganization, 133, 133*f*
Reovirus, 214*b*
Repaglinide (Prandin), 1131*b*
Repatha (evolocumab), 711*b*
Reperfusion therapy, 722
Repetitive strain injury, **1465**
Repetitive trauma disorder, 1465
Reproductive system
abnormalities, 1191*b*
assessment of, **1191-1196**
focused, 1196, 1196*b*
health history, 1193*b*
in cancer, 251*b*-252*b*, 256
diagnostic studies of, **1196**
female, **1185-1188**, 1186*f*
female problems, **1242-1267**
male, **1184-1185**, 1185*f*
male problems, **1268-1291**
neuroendocrine regulation of, 1188-1189
in older adults, 1191*b*, **1191**
problems associated with obesity, 879*f*
structures and functions of, **1184-1191**
Requip (ropinirole), 1391*b*
Reserpine, 691*b*-693*b*
Residual limb bandaging, 1489, 1489*f*
Residual volume (RV), 473*b*
Resilience, 78
Resilzumab (Cinquair), 548*b*-549*b*, 549
Resource allocation, 1093*b*
Respect, 27-28
Respiration. *See also* Breathing
abnormal patterns associated with coma, 1324*f*
control of, 458
defense mechanisms, 458-459
in increased ICP, 1324-1325
Kussmaul respirations, 467*b*-468*b*
monitoring, 336*b*
in older adults, 459
physiology of, **456-457**
Respiratory acidosis, 288*b*, **288**, 290*b*
Respiratory alkalosis, 288*b*, **288-289**, 290*b*
Respiratory depression, opioid-induced, 115

Respiratory diseases
chest examination findings in, 468*b*
dermatologic manifestations of, 399*b*
genetic risk alert, 461*b*
lower respiratory problems, **499-537**
postoperative problems, **332-335**
nursing diagnoses related to, 335-336
nursing management of, **335-336**
prevention of, **500*b***
problems associated with obesity, 879*f*, 880
restrictive disorders, **527-528**
upper respiratory problems, **475-498**
Respiratory distress, 1002*b*
Respiratory failure
acute, **1609-1614**
classification of, 1609-1610, 1610*f*
hypercapnic, 1609-1610
hypoxemic, 1609-1610
in older adults, 1619-1620
Respiratory gases, 455, 455*f*
Respiratory rate, 1575*b*
Respiratory rehabilitation, 1432
Respiratory syncytial virus, 214*b*
Respiratory system. *See also under* Pulmonary
abnormalities, 467*b*-468*b*
acid-base regulation by, 287-288
assessment of, **459-466**, 461*b*, 466*b*
preoperative, 305, 307*b*
case study, 460*b*, 463*b*-464*b*, 473*b*
diagnostic studies of, **467-472**, 469*t*-471*t*, 473*b*
at end of life, 132*b*
health history, 461*b*
normal, 467*b*
in older adults, 459, 459*b*
physical examination of, **463-466**
structures and functions of, **453-459**, **454*f***
Respiratory therapists, 10*b*
role in cardiac catheterization and PCI, 729*b*
role in caring for seizure patients, 1380*b*
role in oxygen administration, 568*b*
role in postoperative care, 334*b*
role in suctioning and tracheostomy care, 490*b*
Respiratory therapy, **1615-1617**, 1624*b*
Respiratory tract infections, 540
Rest, ice, compression, and elevation (RICE), 165, 1464
Rest pain, 804
Resting hemodynamic parameters, 1559*b*
Restless legs syndrome, **1382**
diagnostic criteria for, 1382
nursing management of, **1382-1383**
Restraints
chemical, 74
physical, 74
use of, 74
Restrictive cardiomyopathy, 797*b*, **799**
causes of, 796*b*
nursing and interprofessional management of, **799**
Restrictive respiratory disorders, **527-528**
extrapulmonary conditions, 527, 527*b*
intrapulmonary conditions, 527, 527*b*
Resuscitation, **135-137**
Resuscitation adjuncts, 1631*b*, 1632
Reteplase (Retavase), 715*b*-716*b*
Reticular activating system, 79, 90, 1297
Reticular formation, 79, 1297
Reticular veins, 825
Reticulocyte count, 602*t*, 1659*b*
Reticulocytes, 589, 1659*b*
Retina, 352
assessment of, 358-359, 359*f*
in older adults, 353*b*
Retin-A (tretinoin), 426*b*
Retinal breaks, 377
Retinal detachment, **376-378**
interprofessional care for, 377-378, 377*b*
postoperative considerations, 378
risk factors for, 377*b*
surgical therapy for, 377-378
Retinal holes, 377
Retinal tears, 377
Retinitis, cytomegalovirus, 382
Retinol. *See* Vitamin A
Retinopathy, **376**
diabetic, 376, 376*f*, **1148-1149**
case study, 392*b*
monitoring for, 1148*b*
hypertension and, 686*b*, 687
hypertensive, 376, 698, 699*f*
nonproliferative, 376, 1149
proliferative, 376, 1149
Retracted eardrum, 365*b*
Retrogenesis, 1403-1404, 1407*f*
Retrograde ejaculation, 1274
Retrograde pyelography, 1025*t*-1030*t*
Retroviruses, 219
Return of spontaneous circulation, 1634
Revatio (sildenafil), 532*b*
Reverse transcriptase, 219
Reverse transcriptase inhibitors, 224*b*
Rewarming
active external or surface, 1639
active internal or core, 1639
passive or spontaneous, 1639
Rezira oral solution (hydrocodone and pseudoephedrine), 479*b*-480*b*
Rh blood groups, 600, 601*b*
Rh factor, 600
Rhabdomyolysis, 1478, 1637
Rhabdovirus, 214*b*
Rheumatic carditis, chronic, 789
Rheumatic diseases, 1517
Rheumatic fever, **788-789**
acute care for, 790
ambulatory care for, 790
diagnostic criteria for, 788-789, 788*b*
extracardiac lesions of, 788
health promotion for, 790
interprofessional care for, 789, 789*b*
nursing assessment in, 789, 789*b*
nursing diagnoses related to, 790
nursing management of, **789-790**
Rheumatic heart disease, **788-789**
dermatologic manifestations of, 399*b*
nursing assessment in, 789, 789*b*
nursing diagnoses related to, 790
nursing management of, **789-790**
Rheumatic pancarditis, 788
Rheumatoid arthritis, **1525-1530**, 1526*b*
acute care for, 1530-1531
ambulatory care for, 1531-1532
case study, 1549*b*
clinical manifestations of, 1526-1527, 1527*f*
cold therapy for, 1531-1532
diagnostic criteria for, 1528*b*
drug therapy for, 1528-1529
etiology and pathophysiology of, 1525-1526, 1525*f*
extraarticular manifestations, 1527, 1527*f*
genetic links, 1526
health promotion for, 1530
heat therapy for, 1531-1532
interprofessional care for, 1528-1530, 1528*b*-1529*b*
nursing assessment in, 1530*b*
nursing diagnoses for, 1530
nursing management of, **1530-1532**
Rheumatoid arthritis *(Continued)*
nutritional therapy for, 1529-1530
stages, 1526*b*
surgical therapy for, 1530
Rheumatoid factor, 1457*t*-1459*t*, 1525
Rheumatoid nodules, 1527
Rhinitis
acute viral, **478-480**
allergic, **477-478**
drug therapy for, 479*b*-480*b*
perennial, 477
seasonal, 477
Rhinocort (budesonide), 479*b*-480*b*
Rhinoplasty, **476**
Rhinorrhea, 1326, 1327*f*
Rhinosinusitis, 482
Rhinovirus, 214*b*
Rhizotomy, 120
glycerol, 1438*b*, 1439*f*
percutaneous radiofrequency, 1438*b*
Rhytidectomy, 425
Rib fractures, **521**
Ribavirin (Rebetol, Copegus, Ribasphere), 981*b*
Riboflavin (vitamin B_2), 610*b*
Riboflavin (vitamin B_2) deficiency, 399*b*
Ribonucleic acid (RNA), **180**
RICE (rest, ice, compression, and elevation), 165, 1464
Ridaura (auranofin), 1521*b*-1522*b*, 1529
Rifampin (Rifadin), 509*b*
Rifapentiine (Priftin), 509*b*
Rifaximin (Xifaxan), 993*b*
RIFLE classification, 1071, 1071*b*
Right atrial pressure measurement, 1564
Right to refuse treatment, 1424*b*
Right ventricular ejection fraction (RVEF), 1559*b*
Rights
of delegation, 11-12, 12*b*
personal, 67*b*
Right-sided heart failure, 739, 742*b*
Rigidity
cogwheel, 1389
nuchal, 597*b*-598*b*
in Parkinson's disease, 1389
Ring sign, 1326-1327, 1327*f*
Ringer's solution, 293*b*
Rinne test, 365*t*-366*t*
Riomet (metformin), 1131*b*
Risedronate (Actonel), 1513
Risk monitoring, 123
Risky drinking, 148
Rituals, 24-25
Rituximab (Rituxan)
for arthritis, 1521*b*-1522*b*, 1529
for non-Hodgkin's lymphoma, 644, 644*b*
Rivaroxaban (Xarelto), 820*b*
Rivastigmine (Exelon), 1390
RNA (ribonucleic acid), **180**
Robert Wood Johnson Foundation, 5
Robotic or totally endoscopic coronary artery bypass graft, 725
Robotic-assisted prostatectomy, 1278
Rocky Mountain spotted fever, 1641
Rocuronium, 326*b*
Roflumilast (Daliresp), 548*b*-549*b*
Role-relationship pattern, 37*b*, 38-39
Rolling or paraesophageal hiatal hernia, 904, 904*f*
Romberg test, 1307
ROME (memory device for acid-base imbalances), 291*b*
R-on-T phenomenon, 768-769
Ropinirole (Requip), 1391*b*
Rosiglitazone (Avandia), 1131*b*
Rosuvastatin (Crestor), 711*b*

Rotary chair testing, 365*t*-366*t*
Rotator cuff tear, 1463*b*, **1466-1467**, 1467*f*
Rotavirus, 214*b*, 216, 930*b*
Rotigotine (Neupro), 1391*b*
RotoProne bed (ArjoHuntleigh), 1625*f*
RotoRest Therapy System, 1428, 1428*f*
Roux-en-Y gastric bypass, 885-887, 886*b*, 887*f*
Roxicodone (oxycodone), 113*b*-114*b*
Rubella virus, 214*b*
Rubeola virus, 214*b*
Rubor, dependent, 803-804
Rugae, 1187
Rule of 15, 1146-1147
Rule of Nines, 432, 433*f*
Rumpel-Leede test, 601*t*
Rural older adults, 64, 65*f*
Rytmol (propafenone), 771*b*

S

Saccular aneurysms, 810, 811*f*
Sacroiliitis, 1536
Saddle embolus, 529
Safe Practices (NQF), 12
Safety, 6*b*, **12**
in Alzheimer's disease, 1412
antibiotic, 1075*b*
cultural, 23
in delegation, 868*b*
National Patient Safety Goals (NPSGs), **12**, 13*b*
with older adults, 72
in parenteral nutrition, 870*b*
sexual activities, 225
during surgery, **321**
Safety net programs, 857
Sage Burn Diagram, 432
Salicylates (aspirin), 111-112, 111*b*
for arthritis, 1520-1523, 1521*b*-1522*b*
for inflammation, 164, 164*b*
Saline solutions, 292, 293*b*
Salivary glands, 835*b*
Salmeterol (Serevent Diskus), 548*b*-549*b*, 550
Salmonella, 214*b*, 930-931, 930*b*
***Salmonella* food poisoning**, 925*b*
Salpingectomy, 1261
Salt intake. *See also* Sodium
dietary reduction of, 688
and hypertension, 684, 686*f*
Salt resistance, 684
Salt sensitivity, 684
Same-day admission, 301
Same-day surgery, 302
SAMPLE history taking, 1632-1633
Sanctura (trospium chloride), 1059*b*
Sandimmune (cyclosporine), 209, 211*b*
Sandostatin (octreotide acetate), 931*b*, 993*b*
Sarcoidosis, **528-529**
Sarcoma, 240-241, 1500
Sarcomeres, 1448-1449
Sargramostim (Leukine), 195*b*
Satiety, early, 919
Savaysa (edoxaban), 820*b*
Savella (milnacipran), 116*b*
Saw palmetto *(Serenoa repens)*, 1271
Saxagliptin (Onglyza), 1131*b*
Saxenda (liraglutide), 884*b*
SBAR (Situation-Background-Assessment-Recommendation) communication, 10, 11*b*, 345*b*
SBIRT (Screening, Brief Intervention, and Referral to Treatment) approach, 153-154, 153*f*
Scabies, 416*b*
Scales, 365*b*, 402*b*
SCALES nutritional assessment, 66*b*
Scalp lacerations, 1326-1328
Scar contraction, 166, 166*b*
Scar tissue, 166
Scars
characteristics of, 402*b*
corneal, **373**
hypertrophic, 167*b*, 167*f*
keloid, 167*b*, 167*f*
in light- and dark-skinned persons, 404*b*
Scheduled voiding regimens, 1057*b*
Schwann cells, 1295
Schwannoma, 1333*b*
Schwartz's sign, 385
Sciatica, 1502
Scintigraphy, 847*t*-850*t*
Sclera, 352
examination of, 358
in older adults, 353*b*
Scleral buckling, **377**
Sclerodactyly, 1543, 1543*f*
Scleroderma, 1042*b*, **1542-1544**
clinical manifestations of, 1542-1543, 1543*f*
dermatologic manifestations of, 399*b*
drug therapy for, 1543-1544
interprofessional care for, 1543-1544, 1544*b*
localized, 1542
nursing management of, **1544**
Sclerotherapy
for esophageal or gastric varices, 991
for varicosities, 825, 826*f*
Scoliosis, 1455, 1455*f*, 1456*b*
Scope and standards of practice, 770*b*
Scopolamine (Transderm-Scōp), 326*b*, 895*b*
Scotomas, 378
Screener and Opioid Assessment for Patient Pain, 123
Screening, Brief Intervention, and Referral to Treatment (SBIRT) approach, 153-154, 153*f*
Screening mammography, 1205, 1205*f*
Scrotal erythema, 1198*b*
Scrotal masses, 1198*b*, 1284*f*
Scrotum
physical examination of, 1195
problems of, **1284-1286**
Scrub nurse, 316
Scrubbing, **320**
Seasonal rhinitis, **477**
Sebaceous cysts, 365*b*
Sebaceous glands, 396
Seborrheic keratoses, **419*b***
Sebum, 396
Second spacing, 274
Secondary cardiomyopathy, 796
Secondary intention, 166
Secondary polycythemia, 620-621, 621*f*
Secondary prevention, 61-62
Secondary pulmonary arterial hypertension, 531, **533**
Secondary skin infections, 424
Secondary skin lesions, 401, 402*b*
Secondary spinal cord injury, 1420, 1420*f*
Secondary survey, 1632-1634, 1633*b*
Secondary syphilis, 1236*b*, 1236*f*
Second-order neurons, 105
Secretin, 836*b*
Secretions: mobilization of, 1616-1617
positioning for, 1616-1617
Secretory diarrhea, 930
Sectral (acebutolol), 691*b*-693*b*
Secure-C artificial cervical disc, 1506
Sedation
moderate to deep, **322**, 323*b*
opioid-induced, 115, 115*b*
palliative, 136-137
Pasero Opioid-Induced Sedation Scale (POSS), 115*b*
safety alert, 1618*b*
Sedation holidays, 1618
Sedation scales, 115, 115*b*
Sedative-hypnotics
abuse of, **152**
for burns, 441, 441*b*
toxicity of, **152**
withdrawal from, **152**
Sedimentation, 458
Segmental (partial) cystectomy, 1054
Seizure disorders, **1374-1379**
acute care for, 1380
ambulatory care for, 1381-1382
diagnostic studies in, 1377
drug therapy for, 1377-1379
health promotion for, 1380
interprofessional care for, 1377-1379, 1377*b*
nursing assessment in, 1380*b*
nursing diagnoses related to, 1379
nursing management of, **1379-1382**
in older adults, 1379
patient & caregiver teaching for, 1381*b*
Seizures, 1113*b*-1114*b*, 1374
absence
atypical, 1376
typical, 1375-1376
akinetic, 1376
atonic, 1376
classification of, 1375, 1375*b*, 1375*f*
clinical manifestations of, 1375-1376
clonic, 1376
complications of, 1376-1377
focal, 1375-1376, 1375*b*
complex, 1376
patient & caregiver teaching for, 1381*b*
simple, 1376
generalized, 1375-1376, 1375*b*
myoclonic, 1376
nursing management of, 1380*b*
partial, 1376
partial focal, 1376
psychogenic, 1376
safety alert, 1380*b*
subclinical, 1376
surgical therapy for, 1379
tonic, 1376
tonic-clonic, 1375
emergency management of, 1378*b*
patient & caregiver teaching for, 1381*b*
Selective estrogen receptor modulators, 1243*b*
Selective serotonin-reuptake inhibitors, 1408*b*, 1409
Selegiline (Eldepril), 1390, 1391*b*
Self-assessment, 29
Self-care, 86*b*
Self-concept, 47*b*
Self-efficacy, 48, 52
Self-management, 62
Self-monitoring of blood glucose, 1135, 1136*b*
Self-neglect, 67
Self-perception–self-concept pattern, 37*b*, 38
Self-report, 126
Self-treatment, 410
Semen, 1185
Semen analysis, 1198*t*-1201*t*
Semilunar valves, 658
Seminal vesicles, 1185
Seminiferous tubules, 1185*f*
Senescent gynecomastia, 1208
Senior centers, 68, 68*f*
Sensible perspiration, 274
Sensitivity testing, 1035-1036
Sensorineural hearing loss, 387
Sensory deprivation, 1430
Sensory neuropathy, diabetic, 1150-1151
Sensory polyneuropathy, chronic, 399*b*

Sensory system
abnormalities, 1308*b*-1309*b*
assessment of, 1306-1307
at end of life, 132*b*
normal, 1308*b*
Sensory-perceptual alterations
in critical care patients, 1557
in stroke, 1361-1362
Sentinel events, 12, 652
Sentinel lymph node biopsy, 1212
Sentinel lymph nodes, 238
Sepsis, 503, 1592, 1604-1605
diagnostic criteria for, 1592*b*
severe, 1592
transfusion reaction, 650*b*-651*b*
Septal hypertrophy, asymmetric, 798
Septal myocardial ablation, percutaneous transluminal, 799
Septic arthritis, **1535-1536**
Septic shock, 503, 1588*b*, **1592-1593**
clinical presentation of, 1591*b*
drug therapy for, 1599*b*
interprofessional care for, 1600*b*, 1601
pathophysiology of, 1592-1593, 1593*f*
Septum, deviated, **475**
Sequestra, 1496-1497
Serevent Diskus (salmeterol), 548*b*-549*b*, 550
Serious reportable events (SREs), 4, **12**, 652
Serology, 1660*b*
Serophene (clomiphene), 1243*b*
Serotonin norepinephrine reuptake inhhibitor antidepressants, 162*b*
for pain, 116*b*, 117
Serotonin (5-HT_3) receptor antagonists. *See* Histamine (HT_3)-receptor antagonists
Serum, 587-588, 1655*b*-1658*b*
Serum cardiac biomarkers, 721-722
Serum electrolytes, 1590*t*
Serum lipids, **670**, 673*t*-677*t*
elevated, 704-706, 708*b*
Serum protein electrophoresis, 602*t*
Seventh-Day Adventism, 26*b*
Sevoflurane (Ultane), 325*b*
Sexual abuse
child, 1263
elder mistreatment, 67*b*
Sexual activity, 1240
after ACS, 732-733, 733*b*
and COPD, 575
decreasing risks related to sexual intercourse, 225
nursing interventions for, 1365
risk-reducing activities, 225
safe sexual activities, 225
after spinal cord injury, 1434-1435
Sexual assault, **1263-1265**
Sexual assault nurse examiners (SANEs), 1644
Sexual counseling, 1288
Sexual function
female response, 1190-1191
gender differences in, 1191*b*
male, **1286-1289**
male response, 1190
in older adults, 1191*b*
after ostomy surgery, 962
response phases of, 1190-1191
after stroke, 1365
Sexual history, 1194
Five Ps of taking, 1194, 1195*b*
Sexual orientation, 21
Sexual transmission, 219
Sexuality, 21
Sexuality-reproductive pattern, 37*b*, 39
Sexually transmitted infections, **1227-1241**
acute care for, 1239-1240
ambulatory care for, 1240
case finding, 1238
causes of, 1227, 1228*b*
cultural & ethnic health disparities, 1228*b*
drug therapy for, 1229-1230
educational and research programs, 1238-1239
follow-up, 1239-1240
gender differences in, 1231*b*
health promotion for, 1238-1239
home-based testing for, 1229*b*
incidence factors, **1227-1228**
measures to prevent, 1238
nursing assessment in, 1237, 1237*b*
nursing diagnoses for, 1237-1238
nursing management of, **1237-1240**
patient teaching for, 1239*b*
psychologic support for patients with, 1239
risk factors for, 1228*b*
risk in special populations, 1238*b*
screening for, 1238
Shamans, 24
Shenjing shuairuo, 29*b*
Shielding, 250
Shift work sleep disorder, 100
Shigella, 214*b*
***Shigella* infection**, 930*b*
Shin splints, 1463*b*
Shingles (herpes zoster), 415, 415*b*, 416*f*
Shock, **1587-1602**, 1588*f*
acute care for, 1602-1604
ambulatory care for, 1604
anaphylactic, 1588*b*, 1590-1592
allergens causing anaphylactic shock, 197-198, 198*b*
emergency management of, 202*b*
cardiogenic, 1587-1589, 1588*b*
interprofessional care for, 1598-1601
after myocardial infarction, 721
case study, 1607*b*
classification of, 1587-1594, 1588*b*
clinical presentations of, 1591*b*
diagnostic studies in, 1590*t*, 1596
distributive, 1588*b*, 1590-1593
drug therapy for, 1598, 1599*b*
emergency management of, 1597*b*
fluid therapy in, 1597*b*
general measures for, 1596-1598
in grief, 133, 133*f*
health promotion for, 1602
hypovolemic, 1588*b*, 1589
in burns, 434
emergency management of, 939*b*
interprofessional care for, 1596-1602, 1600*b*
neurogenic, 1420, 1588*b*, 1590
nursing assessment in, 1602
nursing diagnoses related to, 1602
nursing management of, **1602-1604**
nutritional therapy for, 1598
obstructive, 1588*b*, 1593-1594
septic, 503, 1588*b*, 1592-1593
spinal, 1420
in spinal cord injury, 1435*b*
stages of, 1594-1596, 1595*b*
Short bowel syndrome, 948, **967-968**
Short Michigan Alcoholism Screening Test–Geriatric version (SMAST-G), 156
Short-leg gait, 1456*b*
Shortness of breath, 139
Shoulder arthroplasty, 1491-1492
Shower cart, 440*f*
Showing back, 56, 56*b*
Shunts
anatomic, 1611
cranial, 1337*b*
intrapulmonary, 1611
portosystemic, 992, 992*f*
for varices, 992, 992*f*
ventricular, 1335
V/Q mismatch, 1611, 1611*f*
Sickle cell anemia, 610*b*, 616
Sickle cell crisis, 617
Sickle cell disease, **616-617**
clinical manifestations of, 617, 618*f*
complications of, 617, 618*f*
etiology and pathophysiology of, 616-617, 616*f*
genetics of, 180*f*, 616, 616*b*
nursing and interprofessional management of, **617-619**
Sickle cell Hgb C, 616
Sickle cell trait, 616
Sickle cell–thalassemia, 616
Sickling, 616-617
Sigmoid colostomy, 959*f*
Sigmoidoscopy, 847*t*-850*t*
Sign language, 390
Signs, 35
Sildenafil (Revatio), 532*b*
Silence, 25
Silent, painless thyroiditis, 1163
Silent chest, 546, 546*b*
Silent ischemia, 713
Silymarin (milk thistle), 980*b*
Simponi (golimumab), 1521*b*-1522*b*, 1529
Simulect (basiliximab), 210
Simvastatin (Zocor), 710*b*-711*b*
Single-Item Literacy Screener (SILS), 52*f*
Single-photon emission computed tomography (SPECT), 603*t*, 672, 673*t*-677*t*, 1310*t*-1312*t*
Singulair (montelukast), 479*b*-480*b*, 547, 548*b*-549*b*
Singultus, postoperative, 341-342
Sinus bradycardia, **763**, 763*f*, 764*b*
Sinus problems, 540
Sinus rhythm, normal, 760, 760*f*
Sinus tachycardia, **763-764**, 763*f*, 764*b*
Sinuses
location of, 482*f*
obstruction of, **483-484**
Sinusitis, **482-483**
acute, 483, 483*b*
chronic, 483, 483*b*
drug therapy for, 479*b*-480*b*
nursing and interprofessional management of, **483**
patient & caregiver teaching for, 483*b*
subacute, 483
Sinusoids, 837
Sirolimus (Rapamune), 209, 211*b*
Sirturol (bedaquiline), 509, 509*b*
Sitagliptin (Januvia), 1131*b*
Situation-Background-Assessment-Recommendation (SBAR) communication, 10, 11*b*, 345*b*
6-min walk test, 469*t*-471*t*, 673*t*-677*t*
Sjögren's syndrome, 1527, 1546*b*
Skeletal muscle, 1448
Skeletal traction, 1470-1471, 1471*f*
Skeletal x-ray, 603*t*
Skene's glands, 1187
Skin
artificial, **445**
assessment of, 598
case study, 404*b*
effects of sun on, 407, 408*b*

Skin *(Continued)*
Fitzpatrick classification of, 410, 410*b*
health promotion related to, **407-410**
physical examination of, 400-402, 404*b*
structures of, **394-396**, 395*f*
Skin appendages, **395-396**
Skin biopsy, 405*t*
Skin breakdown
at end of life, 140*b*-141*b*
prevention of, 1360
Skin cancer, 410-413
genetic risk alert, 399*b*
nonmelanoma, **410-411**
tanning booths and, 408*b*
Skin care, 424, 425*b*
feeding tube site, 868
for intubated patients, 1572-1573
patient & caregiver teaching for, 1434*b*
after spinal cord injury, 1430-1431, 1434, 1434*b*
Skin changes
in chemotherapy, 251*b*-252*b*, 255-256
in heart failure, 743
radiation, 251*b*-252*b*, 255, 255*b*
in scleroderma, 1543, 1543*f*
in shock, 1603
Skin culture, 405*t*
Skin grafts, **426-427**
allograft (homograft), 440
for burns, 440, 440*b*, **444-445**, 444*f*
types of, 427
Skin infections, 413-417
bacterial, 413-415, 414*b*
fungal, 417, 418*b*
prevention of secondary infections, 424
prevention of spread, 424
secondary, 424
viral, 415, 415*b*
Skin lesions
characteristics of, 401, 401*b*-402*b*
in cirrhosis, 986
disseminated gonococcal infections, 1230, 1231*f*
distribution terminology, 402*b*
primary, 401, 401*b*
secondary, 401, 402*b*
Skin nutrition, 409
Skin scraping, **422**
Skin tags, 419*b*
Skin tears, 166
Skin tests, **467**
for allergies, 200-201
diagnostic studies, 405*t*
Skin traction, 1470
Skin ulceration, 1113*b*-1114*b*
Skip lesions, 945
Skip metastasis, 238
Skull, **1300**
Skull fractures, 1326-1327
clinical manifestations of, 1327*b*
indications for cranial surgery, 1336*b*
types of, 1326*b*
Skull x-rays, 1310*t*-1312*t*
Sleep, **89-91**
and COPD, 575
insufficient, **91**
non–rapid eye movement (NREM), **90-91**
nurse's needs for, **100-101**
in older adults, 99-100
physiologic mechanisms of, **90-91**
rapid eye movement (REM), **90-91**
and skin, 409
Sleep apnea
conservative treatment of, 97-98
diagnosis and monitoring of, 97*b*
mild, 97
Sleep apnea *(Continued)*
nursing and interprofessional management of, **97-98**
obstructive sleep apnea, 92*b*, **96-97**
obstructive sleep apnea–hypopnea syndrome, 96
positive airway pressure devices for, 97, 97*f*
surgical treatment of, 98
Sleep architecture, 90-91
Sleep behavior, 90
Sleep deprivation, 91, 91*f*
Sleep disorders, 89, 90*f*-91*f*, **91-101**
Sleep disturbances, 89, **91**, 92*b*
associated with menopause, 1249*b*
associated with obesity, 880
in critical care patients, 1556
in dialysis patients, 1080*b*
drug therapy for, 1408*b*
in hospital, **91**
nonpharmacologic interventions for, 1080*b*
in older adults, **99-100**, 99*f*
Sleep hygiene, 93, 93*b*
Sleep terrors, 99
Sleep-disordered breathing, 96-97
Sleepiness
daytime, 90, 90*f*
postprandial, 90
Sleep-rest pattern
assessment of, 37*b*, 38
in older adults, 74
Sleep-wake cycle, 90
Sleepwalking, 99
Sleeve gastrectomy (gastric sleeve), 885, 886*b*, 887*f*
Sliding hiatal hernia, 904, 904*f*
Slipped disc, 1504-1505
Sludge, biliary, 999
Small bowel series, 847*t*-850*t*
Small cell carcinoma, 515*b*
Small cell lung cancer, 514, 515*b*
Small intestine, **835**
obstruction of, 951*b*
in older adults, 840*b*
secretions, 835*b*
Small joints: protection of, 1531*b*
Smart infusion pumps, 1556*b*
Smart phone apps, 1141*b*
SmartVest, 570
SMAST-G (Short Michigan Alcoholism Screening Test–Geriatric version), 156
Smoke and inhalation injury, 430-431
Smoker's patch, 898
Smoking cessation. *See also* Tobacco cessation
for COPD, 562
drug therapy for, 147, 150*b*
nicotine replacement therapy for, 147
patient teaching guide for, 149*b*
Smoking cigarettes, 168*b*, **558**
Smooth muscle, 1448
Smooth tongue, 597*b*-598*b*, 846*b*-847*b*
Snellen eye chart, 356*b*, 358
Social interactions, 61. *See also* Psychosocial care
Social isolation, 61
Social networking
ethical/legal dilemmas, 5*b*
for migraine headache patients, 1371*b*
Social services, 67
Social support, 82*b*
for older adults, **66-67**
Social workers, 10*b*, 1529*b*
Sodium
blood levels, 1025*t*-1030*t*
in burns, 442
reference values, 1655*b*-1658*b*, 1661*b*
serum levels, 1590*t*
in shock, 1590*t*
Sodium bicarbonate (Alka-Seltzer), 903*b*, 1073*b*
Sodium channel blockers, 771*b*
Sodium citrate (Bicitra), 903*b*
Sodium imbalances, 278-280, 278*f*, 1077
Sodium nitroprusside (Nipress)
for heart failure, 745, 745*b*
for hypertension, 691*b*-693*b*
for shock, 1599*b*
Sodium polystyrene sulfonate (Kayexalate), 1073, 1073*b*
Sodium restriction
for chronic kidney disease, 1082*b*, 1083
for hypertension, 684, 686*f*, 688
Sodium retention, 684
Sodium-glucose co-transporter 2 (SGLT2) inhibitors, 1131*b*, 1132, 1136*f*
Sodium-potassium pump, 272*f*
Soft corns, 1509*b*
Soft tissue expansion, 427
Soft tissue injuries, 1462-1468
emergency management of, 1464*b*
of hip, 1464-1465, 1465*f*
Solar keratosis, 411
Solifenacin (VESIcare), 1059*b*
Solu-Cortef (hydrocortisone)
for arthritis, 1521*b*-1522*b*
for asthma, 548*b*-549*b*
for shock, 1599*b*
Solu-Medrol (methylprednisolone)
for arthritis, 1521*b*-1522*b*
for asthma and COPD, 548*b*-549*b*
for immunosuppressive therapy, 209, 211*b*
Somatic (acquired) mutations, 181
Somatic pain, 106
deep, 106*b*
superficial, 106*b*
Somatomedin C, 1115*t*-1118*t*
Somatosensory evoked potentials, 1457*t*-1459*t*
Somatostatin, 1104*b*
Somatotropin, 1104*b*, 1115*t*-1118*t*
Somogyi effect, 1129-1130
Sotalol (Betapace), 771*b*
Sound: transmission of, 361
Soy, 710*b*, 1249*b*
Space, personal, 27, 27*f*
Spastic gait, 1456*b*
Spasticity
muscle, 1456*b*
after spinal cord injury, 1434
Spatial-perceptual deficits, 1351-1352, 1362, 1362*f*
Speak Up initiative (TJC), 50-51, 51*b*
Speaking tracheostomy tube, 486*b*, 489
Spectral karyotyping, 603*t*, 604
Speech
abnormalities of, 1308*b*-1309*b*
esophageal, 493
with tracheostomy tube, **489-490**
Speech pathologists, 10*b*
Speech reading, 390
Speech therapists, 1359*b*
Spermatocele, 1284*f*, **1285**
Spermatogenesis, 1184
Spermatozoa, 1184
Sphincter electromyography (EMG), 1025*t*-1030*t*
Sphincterotomy, 1001, 1007, 1007*f*
Sphingosine 1-phosphate modulators, 1385*b*
SPICES assessment, 70, 70*f*
Spider angiomas, 986
Spider nevi, 597*b*-598*b*, 598, 986
Spinal adjustment, 1435, 1435*b*
Spinal anatomy, 119, 119*f*
Spinal anesthesia, **325-327**, 327*f*
Spinal cord
abnormalities, 1308*b*-1309*b*
ascending tracts, 1296
descending tracts, 1296
pain transmission to, 104-105
structures and functions of, **1296**

Spinal cord compression, 263*b*
Spinal cord injury, 1419-1437
acute care for, 1425-1431
bladder management in, 1430, 1433
bowel management in, 1430, 1433*b*
case study, 1443*b*
cervical cord injury, 1426*b*
cervical spine injury, 1427*b*
chronic, 1436*f*
classification of, 1420-1421
clinical manifestations of, 1421-1424
complete, 1420-1421
degree of, 1420-1421
dermatologic manifestations of, 399*b*
diagnostic studies in, 1424
drug therapy for, 1426
emergency management of, 1425*b*
fluid management in, 1429-1430
grief response in, 1435, 1435*b*
health promotion for, 1426-1435
home care for, 1431-1435
immobilization of, 1427-1428, 1427*f*-1428*f*
incomplete, 1420-1421, 1422*b*
interprofessional care for, 1424-1426, 1426*b*
mechanisms of, 1420, 1421*f*
metabolic needs in, 1424
motor effects of, 1421
nursing assessment in, 1427*b*
nursing diagnoses related to, 1426
nursing interventions for, 1426-1427
nursing management of, **1426-1436**
nutritional management in, 1429-1430
in older adults, 1435-1436, 1436*f*
pain management in, 1430
pathophysiology of, 1420-1421, 1420*f*
prehospital care in, 1424-1425
primary, 1420
rehabilitation in, 1421, 1422*f*, 1423*b*, 1431-1435, 1432*f*
respiratory complications of, 1421-1422, 1429
respiratory rehabilitation in, 1432
secondary, 1420, 1420*f*
sensory effects of, 1421
skeletal level, 1420, 1422*f*, 1423*b*
skin care in, 1430-1431, 1434, 1434*b*
stabilization of, 1425
surgical therapy for, 1425-1426
temperature control in, 1430
types of, 1420
Spinal cord tumors, 1436-1437, 1436*f*
classification of, 1436*b*
extradural, 1436, 1436*f*
intradural-extramedullary, 1436, 1436*f*
intradural-intramedullary, 1436*f*
intramedullary, 1436
nursing and interprofessional management of, **1437**
types of, 1436*f*
Spinal fusion, 1506
Spinal nerves, **1298**, 1299*f*
Spinal shock, 1420
Spinal stenosis, 1504
Spine x-rays, 1310*t*-1312*t*
Spinocerebellar tracts, 1296
Spinothalamic tracts, 1296
Spiral (helical) CT scan, 530
Spiritual assessment, 134*b*
Spiritual distress, 142*b*
Spirituality, **24-25**, 134
end-of-life care for, 134, 134*f*
mind-body-spirit connection, **81**, 81*f*
Spiriva HandiHaler (tiotropium), 548*b*-549*b*
Spironolactone (Aldactone)
for cirrhosis, 993*b*
for heart failure, 745*b*, 748, 748*b*
for hypertension, 691*b*-693*b*
Spleen, **592**
disorders of, **647**
palpation of, 598
ultrasound of, 603*t*
Splenomegaly, 597*b*-598*b*, 647, 647*b*, 846*b*-847*b*
Splinter hemorrhages, 668*b*
Splinting, respiratory, 467*b*-468*b*
Splints, sugar-tong, 1472
Spondyloarthropathies, 1536-1549
Spontaneous awakening trial (SAT), 1582
Spontaneous bacterial peritonitis, 989-990
Spontaneous breathing trial (SBT), 1582
Spontaneous circulation: return of, 1634
Sporothrix schenckii, 215*b*
Sports-related injuries, 1463*b*, 1476*b*
Sprains and strains, 1463
acute care for, 1464
ambulatory care for, 1464
health promotion for, 1463-1464
nursing management of, **1463-1464**
Sputum induction, 467
Sputum studies, **467**, 469*t*-471*t*
Squamocolumnar junction, 1186-1187, 1186*f*
Squamous cell carcinoma, 411, 412*b*, 515*b*
SREs. *See* Serious reportable events
St. John's wort, 28
Stable factor, 592*b*
Stadol (butorphanol), 113*b*-114*b*, 114
Staff helpers, 1632
Staff training, 438*b*
Staged cough, 1616
Staghorn calculus, 1045, 1046*f*
Stalevo (carbidopa, levodopa, and entacapone), 1390-1391
Standard precautions, 218, 218*b*
Standardized guidelines, 30
Standardized nursing terminologies, 5-7
Standards of practice, 770*b*
Stapedotomy, 385
Stapes, 361
Staphylococcus aureus, 214*b*
***Staphylococcus aureus* infection**, 930*b*
food poisoning, 925*b*
methicillin-resistant, 216, 216*b*
vancomycin-resistant, 216
Staphylococcus epidermidis, 216*b*
Starlix (nateglinide), 1131*b*
Starvation, 858-859
Starvation-related malnutrition, 857
State Board of Nursing, 1416*b*
Statins (HMG-CoA reductase inhibitors), 709-710, 711*b*
Status epilepticus, 1376, 1378
Statutory rape, 1263
Steal syndrome, 1088
Steatorrhea, 846*b*-847*b*, 859, 965, 1006*b*
Stem cell therapy, **187-188**
autologous transplantation, 260, 260*f*
infusions, 261
syngeneic transplantation, 260
Stem cells, 188
adult, 188
embryonic, 188
hematopoietic, 587
Stenosis, valvular, 790-791, 790*f*
Stents
airway, 517
brain, 1353-1354, 1354*f*
coronary artery, 717-718, 718*f*
for peripheral arterial disease, 806
Step-down units, 1555
Steppage gait, 1456*b*
Stereognosis, 1307
Stereopsis, 359
Stereotactic body radiotherapy, 516
Stereotactic mammography, 1206
Stereotactic radiosurgery, 1335, 1337*b*, **1337**, 1337*f*
Stereotyping, 23, 856
Sternal tenderness, 597*b*-598*b*
Sternal-occipital-mandibular immobilizer brace, 1427, 1428*f*
Stimulant toxicity, 151, 151*b*, **151**
Stimulant use, 150, **151**
Stimulant withdrawal, 151
Stings and bites, 1640-1642
Stocking-glove neuropathy, 1150
Stoma(s), 958
characteristics of, 960*b*
double-barreled, 959, 959*f*
effects of food on output, 961*b*
end, 958
loop, 958
urinary, 1064-1065, 1064*f*, 1066*f*
Stoma care, 495, 1066*f*
Stomach, **835**
abnormalities, 846*b*-847*b*
in older adults, 840*b*
secretions, 835*b*
Stomach cancer, 919-920, 919*f*
acute care for, 921
ambulatory care for, 921
chemotherapy for, 920
cultural & ethnic health disparities, 898*b*
health promotion for, 921
interprofessional care for, 919-920, 920*b*
nursing assessment in, 920
nursing diagnoses for, 920-921
nursing management of, **920-921**
postoperative care in, 921
PPIs and, 902*b*
preoperative care in, 921
radiation therapy for, 920
surgical therapy for, 920, 920*f*
targeted therapy for, 920
Stomach disorders, 909-926
Stomatitis, 897*b*
aphthous, 897*b*
in cancer, 251*b*-252*b*
Stool culture, 847*t*-850*t*
Stool softeners, 726, 936*b*
Strabismus, 357*b*, **373**
Straight-leg-raising test, 1455
Strains, 1463-1464
Streptococcus, 214*b*
Streptococcus pneumoniae, penicillin-resistant, 216, 216*b*
Streptomycin, 509*b*
Stress, 77-88
caregiver stress, 50
case study, 87*b*
definition of, **77-78**
examples, 77
and fluid and electrolyte balance, 275, 275*f*
and health, 81-82, 81*b*
and hypertension, 685
nursing management of, **86-88**, 86*f*
relocation stress syndrome, 69
Stress echocardiography, 671, 673*t*-677*t*
Stress headache, 1370
Stress incontinence, 1025*b*, 1056*b*
Stress management, **77-88**
implementation in practice, 87*b*
personal tips for, 87*b*

Stress perfusion imaging, 672, 673*t*-677*t*
Stress response
factors affecting, 78, 78*b*, 78*f*
physiologic, **78-81**, 79*f*
summary, 80
Stress testing, **671**, 673*t*-677*t*
Stress ulcers
in ARDS, 1623
physiologic, **922**
in spinal cord injury, 1430
Stressors, 50*b*, 77, 78*f*
Stress-related mucosal disease, 912, **922**
Stretch reflex, 1307, 1307*f*
Striae, 1113*b*-1114*b*
Strictures, **1049-1050**
ureteral, **1049-1050**
urethral, **1050**
Stridor, 467*b*-468*b*
laryngeal, 1168
Striverdi Respimat (olodaterol), 548*b*-549*b*
Stroke, **1345-1367**
acute, 1359*b*
acute care for, 1358-1362
ambulatory care for, 1362-1365
case study, 1366*b*
clinical manifestations of, 1350*b*, **1350-1352**, 1350*f*
core measures for, 1356, 1357*b*
cultural & ethnic health disparities, 1347*b*
definition of, 1345
diagnostic studies for, **1352-1353**, 1352*t*
embolic, 1348*b*, 1348*f*, 1349
emergency management of, 1354*b*
FAST warning signs of, 1346*b*
gerontologic considerations, **1365-1367**
health promotion for, 1358
heatstroke, **1637**
hemorrhagic, 1348*b*, 1348*f*, 1349-1350, 1355-1356
impact of, 61*b*
interprofessional care for, 1353*b*, **1353-1356**
ischemic, 1348-1349, 1348*b*
acute care for, 1354-1355
drug therapy for, 1355
endovascular therapy for, 1355
nursing assessment in, 1356-1357, 1357*b*
nursing diagnoses for, 1357
nursing management of, **1356-1367**, 1359*b*
oral feeding after, 1360*b*
pathophysiology of, **1346**
prevention of, 1353-1354, 1353*b*
rehabilitation care after, 1356
risk factors for, **1346-1348**
spatial-perceptual deficits in, 1351-1352, 1362, 1362*f*
thrombotic, 1348-1349, 1348*b*, 1348*f*
types of, 1348-1350, 1348*b*
Stroke rehabilitation, 1363, 1364*f*
Bobath method, 1364
constraint-induced movement therapy, 1364
exercise, 1347
musculoskeletal interventions, 1363-1364
video games, 1363*b*
virtual reality for, 1363*b*
walking, 1364*b*
Stroke survivorship, 1364-1365
Stroke volume (SV), 1559, 1559*b*
Stroke volume index (SVI), 1559, 1559*b*
Stroke volume variation (SVV), 1559*b*, 1562
Struvite stones, 1046*b*
Stuart-Prower factor, 592*b*
Sty (hordeolum), 357*b*
Subacute cutaneous lupus, 1538
Subacute sinusitis, 483
Subacute subdural hematoma, 1329, 1329*b*
Subarachnoid hemorrhage, 1348*b*, **1349-1350**
Subarachnoid space, 1300
Subconjunctival hemorrhage, 357*b*
Subcutaneous immunotherapy, 203
Subcutaneous nodules, 789
Subcutaneous tissue, 395, 432
Subdural hematoma, 1329
acute, 1329, 1329*b*
chronic, 1329, 1329*b*
subacute, 1329, 1329*b*
types of, 1329*b*
Subglottal suctioning, continuous, 1573, 1573*f*
Sublimaze (fentanyl), 326*b*
Sublingual immunotherapy, 203
Subluxation, 1456*b*, **1464-1465**, 1465*f*
in rheumatoid arthritis, 1527
Submersion injuries, **1639-1640**
emergency management of, 1641*b*
interprofessional care for, 1640
pathophysiology of, 1639-1640, 1640*f*
Substance abuse
acute intervention for, 155
brief screening tools for, 154, 154*b*
and CAD, 707
case study, 156*b*
and glomerulonephritis, 1042*b*
health problems related to, 145, 146*b*
health promotion in, 155
manifestations suggesting, 155*b*
medication use, 72-73, 74*b*
nursing management of, **153-156**
in older adults, 72-73, 74*b*, 155-156, 156*f*
pain management in, 126
polysubstance use, 154
Substance use disorders, **145-157**
criteria for, 145, 146*b*
drugs associated with, **145-146**
nursing diagnoses for, 154-155
Subthalamic nucleotomy, 1391
Succinylcholine (Anectine), 326*b*
Sucking chest wound, 521
Sucralfate (Carafate), 903*b*, 914
Suctioning
airway, 1617
complications of, 1571-1572
indications for, 1571
procedures for patients on mechanical ventilators, 1572*b*
subglottal continuous, 1573, 1573*f*
tracheal, 487, 487*f*, 488*b*, 490*b*
closed system, 1570, 1570*f*
closed-suction technique, 1571, 1572*b*
open-suction technique, 1571, 1572*b*
Sudafed (pseudoephedrine), 478*b*-480*b*
Sudden cardiac death, **704**, **733**, 771
Sudden unexplained or unexpected death in epilepsy (SUDEP), 1376-1377
Sufentanil (Sufenta), 326*b*
Sugar-tong splints, 1472
Suicide. *See also* Assisted suicide
physician-assisted, 136-137
Sular (nisoldipine), 691*b*-693*b*
Sulfasalazine (Azulfidine)
for arthritis, 1521*b*-1522*b*, 1528
for inflammatory bowel disease, 947, 947*b*
Sulfonylureas, 1130, 1131*b*, 1136*f*
Sumatriptan (Imitrex), 1372, 1372*b*
Sumatriptan transdermal system (Zecuity), 1372
Sun exposure, **407-409**, 408*b*
Sun protection factor (SPF), 408
Sundowning, 1411-1412
Sunscreens, 408
Superficial pain, 106
Superficial somatic pain, 106*b*
Superficial vein thrombosis, 816, 816*b*, **818**
Superior vena cava, 661
Superior vena cava syndrome, 263*b*, 264*f*
Superoptic nuclei cells, 1017
Supination, 1455*b*
Supplemental Nutrition Assistance Program (SNAP), 863
Supplements. *See* Dietary supplements
Support groups, 773
for caregivers, 1413, 1413*f*
for weight loss, 884
Suprane (desflurane), 325*b*
Suprapubic catheterization, 1062
Suprapubic catheters, 1062
Surface rewarming, 1639
Surfactant, **455**
Surgeons, **317**
Surgeon's assistant, 317
Surgery
site preparation, **322**
Surgery, 301
ablation, 1391
ambulatory, 302, **344-346**
antireflux, 902-903
bariatric, **885-887**
procedures, 886*b*, 887*f*
special considerations, 888
for type 2 diabetes mellitus, 1137
breast augmentation, **1224**
breast cancer, 1213-1215, 1214*f*, 1215*b*
breast reconstruction, **1222-1224**, 1223*f*
breast reduction, **1224**
breast-conserving, 1213-1214, 1215*b*
for cancer, **245**, 245*f*. *See also specific cancers*
cataract, 374-375, 375*f*
chest, **524-527**, 526*b*
consent for, 309-310
coronary revascularization, **724-725**
cosmetic, 301
nursing management of, **426**
for obesity, **890**
procedures, 425-426
cranial, **1336-1337**
cryosurgery, **422**
curative, 301
diagnostic, 301
discharge criteria, 344*b*
elective, 301, 425-426
emergency, 301
exploratory, 301
female reproductive system procedures, 1260-1261, 1260*b*
of gastrointestinal system, 840*b*
heart surgery DVD/TV, 795*b*
heart transplantation, 754
herbal products and, 304
incontinence after, 1056*b*
intraoperative care, **315-329**
joint procedures, **1490-1493**
kidney transplantation, 1094-1095
laser, 425
legal preparation for, 309-310
loop electrosurgical excision procedure (LEEP), 1198*t*-1201*t*
lung volume reduction, 526*b*
malabsorptive, 885-887, 886*b*
minimally invasive surgery (MIS), 315
Mohs surgery, 422, 423*f*
nasal, **476**
neurosurgical procedures for pain relief, 120, 121*f*
nipple-areolar reconstruction, 1223*f*, 1224
nursing history, 36
nursing management after surgery, **322**
nursing management before surgery, **318-319**
nursing management during surgery, **319-322**
in older adults, 327

Surgery *(Continued)*
ostomy, **958-959**
out-patient, 302
palliative, 301
pituitary, **1158**
postoperative care, **330-348**
preoperative care, **301-314**
preventive, 301
reconstructive microsurgery, 427
renal, **1063**
safety considerations, **321**
same-day, 302
settings for, **301-302**
shunting procedures, 992, 992*f*
stereotactic radiosurgery, 1335
suffixes describing procedures, 302*b*
thyroid, 1167-1168
ureteral, **1063**
urinary diversion, **1063-1065**, 1433
urinary tract, **1063-1066**
vertebral disc, 1506, **1507**
video-assisted thoracoscopic surgery, 526*b*, **526**
Surgical attire, 320*f*
Surgical biopsy, 243
Surgical Care Improvement Project (SCIP), 315-316
Surgical cholangiography, 847*t*-850*t*
Surgical debridement, 170*b*, 439, 440*f*
Surgical site infection, 343
Surgical suite, 315
Surgical team, **316-318**
Surgical technologist, **317**
Surgical time-out, 321*b*
Surgical tracheostomy, 485
Surgical wounds
nursing diagnoses related to, 343
nursing management of, **343**
Surveillance, immunologic, 238-239
Suspensory ligament, 351
Sustained maximal inspiration, 336
Susto, 29*b*
Swallowing
in Sjögren's syndrome, 1546*b*
with tracheostomy, **489**
Swallowing difficulties, 1412. *See also* Dysphagia
Swan neck deformity, 1456*b*, 1527, 1527*f*
Swayback, 1456*b*
Sweat glands
apocrine, 396
eccrine, 396
Swelling, 1456*b*
in fracture healing, 1469*b*
joint, 597*b*-598*b*
of pinna, 365*b*
Swine flu, 215
Sydenham's chorea, 789
Symbicort (budesonide/formoterol), 548*b*-549*b*
Syme's amputation, 1487, 1488*f*
Symlin (pramlintide), 1131*b*-1132*b*, 1132
Sympathectomy, 120, 809
Sympathetic nervous system, 1299
blood pressure regulation by, 682-683, 683*b*, 685
in heart failure, 739-740
in myocardial infarction, 720
Sympathetic overdrive, 151
Sympathoadrenal response, 79
Sympathomimetic drugs
for allergic disorders, 202
for shock, 1598
Symptoms, 35
controlling, 61
investigation of, 35, 36*b*
Synapses, **1295**, 1296*f*
Synaptic transmission, 1294-1295
Synarel (nafarelin), 1243*b*
Synchronized cardioversion, 772
Synchronized intermittent mandatory ventilation, 1576, 1576*b*
Syncope, **777-778**
postoperative, 337
Syndrome of inappropriate antidiuretic hormone, 1159-1160, **1160**
in cancer, 263*b*
causes of, 1160, 1160*b*
nursing and interprofessional management of, **1160-1161**
pathophysiology of, 1160, 1160*f*
Syndrome X, 713-714
Synovectomy, **1490**
Synovial joints, 1448, 1448*f*-1449*f*
movements of, 1454, 1455*b*
Synthroid (levothyroxine), 1169, 1169*b*
Syphilis, **1235-1237**
chancres of, 1235, 1236*f*
dermatologic manifestations of, 399*b*
interprofessional care for, 1237, 1237*b*
secondary, 1236*b*, 1236*f*
stages of, 1235, 1236*b*
tertiary, 1236*b*, 1236*f*
Systemic exertion intolerance disease, **1548**
clinical features of, 1546, 1547*b*, 1548
nursing and interprofessional management of, **1548-1549**
Systemic inflammatory response syndrome (SIRS), 1587, 1588*f*, **1604-1605**
clinical manifestations of, 1605, 1606*b*
nursing and interprofessional management of, **1606-1608**
Systemic lupus erythematosus, 1042*b*, **1538-1540**
acute care for, 1541
ambulatory care for, 1542
clinical manifestations of, 1538-1540, 1539*f*
complications of, 1538-1540, 1539*f*
dermatologic manifestations of, 399*b*
diagnostic criteria for, 1540*b*
health promotion for, 1541
interprofessional care for, 1540, 1540*b*
nursing assessment in, 1541*b*
nursing diagnoses related to, 1541
nursing management of, **1541-1542**
patient & caregiver teaching for, 1542*b*
and pregnancy, 1542
Systemic sclerosis, **1542-1544**
Systemic vascular resistance (SVR), 662, 681-682, 1559-1560
Systole, 660
Systolic blood pressure, 662
Systolic dysfunction, 1587
Systolic failure, 738

T

T cell activation inhibitors, 1521*b*-1522*b*
T cells, **192-194**, 193*f*
cytotoxic, 193*f*, **194**, 208, 209*f*, 239
dendritic, **194**
helper, 193*f*, **194**
T tubes
placement of, 1008, 1008*f*
postoperative care for, 1009
Tachycardia, 597*b*-598*b*, **743**
sinus, **763-764**, 763*f*
Tachypnea, 467*b*-468*b*
Tacrolimus (Prograf), 209, 209*b*, 211*b*
Tadalafil (Adcirca), 532*b*
Tai Chi, 72*b*
Tail of Spence, 1187-1188, 1188*f*
Takedown, 958
Takotsubo cardiomyopathy, 796
Talwin (pentazocine), 113*b*-114*b*, 114
Tamoxifen, 1217, 1217*b*
Tamsulosin (Flomax), 1059*b*
Tanning booths, 408*b*
Tanzeum (albiglutide), 1131*b*
Tapentadol (Nucynta), 113*b*-114*b*, 114
Tardive dyskinesia, 1417
Target cell concept, 1103*f*
Targeted therapy, **257-258**
for breast cancer, 1217*b*, 1218
for IBD, 947-948, 947*b*
nursing management of, **258-259**
side effects of, 257-258
sites of action, 257, 259*f*
Tasimelteon (Hetlioz), 370
Tasmar (tolcapone), 1390
Taste alterations, 262
tau, 1403
Taxanes, 247*b*
Taxonomies, 6
T-cell lymphoma
classification of, 644*b*
cutaneous, 412*b*
Teachable moments, 46
Teachable plans, 46
Teaching
nurses as teachers, 48-49
patient and caregiver, **46-59**
process of, 46-51
resources for, 56*b*
Teaching back, 56, 56*b*-57*b*
Teaching materials, 54-55, 54*f*
Teaching strategies, 54-55, 54*f*, 55*b*-56*b*, 56*f*
Teamwork, 6*b*, **9-12**, 10*b*
interprofessional teams, **9-10**
Tecentriq (atezolizumab), 1037-1038
Tecfidera (dimethyl fumarate), 1385*b*, 1386
Technology
advances in, 3-4
genetic, 186
patient teaching with, 53*f*, 55
Tegretol (carbamazepine), 116*b*
Tekturna (aliskiren), 691*b*-693*b*
Telangiectasias, 403*b*, 422, 597*b*-598*b*, 598, 825
in cirrhosis, 986
Telbivudine (Tyzeka), 980
Telehealth, 9, 9*f*, 55, 752, 752*f*
Tele-intensive care unit (tele-ICU), 1554, 1555*f*
Telemedicine, 55
Telemetry monitoring, 760
Teletherapy, **250**
Television, 795*b*
Telmisartan (Micardis), 691*b*-693*b*
Temozolomide (Temodar), 1335, 1335*b*
Temperature
assessment of, 1306
in spinal cord injury, 1430
Temperature alterations
nursing diagnoses related to, 341
nursing management of, **341**
postoperative, 340*b*
Temporary vascular acess, 1088-1089, 1089*f*
Tenderness, sternal, 597*b*-598*b*
Tendonitis, 1463*b*
Tendons, 1450
Tenecteplase (TNKase), 715*b*-716*b*
Tenesmus, 846*b*-847*b*
Tenex (guanfacine), 691*b*-693*b*
Tennis elbow, 1456*b*
Tenofovir (Viread), 980
Tenormin (atenolol), 691*b*-693*b*, 715*b*-716*b*
Tenosynovitis, 1456*b*

Tension pneumothorax, 520, 520*b*, 520*f*
Tension-type headache, **1370**, 1370*f*
drug therapy for, 1372-1373
gender differences in, 1370*b*
interprofessional care for, 1369*b*
Tenting, 277, 403*b*
Tentorial herniation, 1318-1319
Tentorium cerebelli, 1318
Terazosin, 691*b*-693*b*, 1059*b*
Teriflunomide (Aubagio), 1385-1386, 1385*b*
Teriparatide (Forteo), 1513
Terminology
genetic and genomic, 179*b*
hemodynamic, 1559-1560
lesion distribution, 402*b*
NANDA, NOC, and NIC (NNN) linkages, 7*b*, **7**
standardized nursing terminologies, 5-7
suffixes describing surgical procedures, 302*b*
Terrorism, **1645**
Testes, **1184**, 1185*f*
Testicular cancer, 1284*f*, **1285**
cultural & ethnic health disparities, 1276*b*
nursing and interprofessional management of, **1285-1286**
Testicular problems, **1284-1286**, 1289
Testicular torsion, 1284*f*, **1285**
Testosterone, 1104*b*
measurement of, 1198*t*-1201*t*
plasma levels, 1288, 1288*f*
reference values, 1655*b*-1658*b*
regulation of reproductive system by, 1189
Tetanus, **1442**
Tetanus immune globulin (TIG), 1634*b*
Tetanus immunization, 441
Tetanus vaccines, 1634*b*
Tetany, 284, 1113*b*-1114*b*
Tetraplegia, 1308*b*-1309*b*, 1420, 1423*b*
Teveten (eprosartan), 691*b*-693*b*
Text messaging
for COPD, 573*b*
and diabetes, 1135*b*
Thalamotomy, 1391
Thalamus, 105-106, 1297
Thalassemia, **611-612**, 612
Thalassemia major, 610*b*, 611
Thalassemia minor, 611
Theophylline, 548*b*-549*b*, 551*b*
TheraPEP Therapy System, 570
Therapeutic hypothermia, **1634-1635**, 1635*b*
Thermal burns, **429**, 433, 434*b*
Thermoregulation, 1113*b*-1114*b*
Thermotherapy, transurethral microwave (TUMT), 1271, 1272*b*
Thiamine (vitamin B_1), 858*b*
Thiamine (vitamin B_1) deficiency, 399*b*
Thiazide diuretics, 691*b*-693*b*, 745*b*, 747
Thiazolidinediones, 1130, 1131*b*, 1136*f*
Thin blood, 29*b*
Third heart sound (S_3), 668*b*, 669
Third space syndrome, 263*b*
Third spacing, 274, 434
Thoracentesis, 469*t*-471*t*, **472**, 472*f*, 527-528
Thoracic aortic aneurysms, 810-811
Thoracic aortic dissection, 814, 814*f*
Thoracic cage, 455
Thoracic expansion, 464, 464*f*
Thoracic injury, **519-527**, 520*b*
Thoracoscopic surgery, video-assisted, 526*b*, **526**
Thoracotomy, **524-526**, 526*b*
Thoratec HeartMate II, 754
Thorax
assessment of, 667-669
physical examination of, **463-466**, 1112
Three-dimensional (3D) mammography, 1205
Three-dimensional (3D) ultrasound, real-time, 671, 673*t*-677*t*
Thrills, 666, 668*b*
Thrombin inhibitors
for angina and ACS, 715*b*-716*b*
for VTE, 820*b*, 821
Thrombin time, 601*t*
Thromboangiitis obliterans, 399*b*, **809**
Thrombocytes, 590, 1659*b*
Thrombocytopenia, 600, **622-625**
acquired, 622, 622*b*
acute care for, 625-626
ambulatory care for, 626
in cancer, 251*b*-252*b*, 253
clinical manifestations of, 623, 623*f*
from decreased platelet production, 625*b*, **625**
diagnostic studies in, 623-624
etiology of, 622-623, 622*b*
health promotion for, 625
heparin-induced, **622-623**, 625*b*, **625**, 821
interprofessional care for, 624-625, 625*b*, **625**
laboratory results, 623*b*
nursing assessment in, 624*b*
nursing diagnoses for, 625
nursing management of, **625-626**
patient & caregiver teaching for, 626*b*
Thrombocytosis, 600
Thromboembolism. *See* Venous thromboembolism
Thrombolytic therapy
for acute coronary syndrome, 715*b*-716*b*, 723-724
for angina, 715*b*-716*b*
contraindications to, 723-724, 724*b*
indications for, 723-724
procedure for, 724
safety alert, 724*b*
for VTE treatment, 821-822
Thrombopoietin, 590
Thrombotic stroke, 1348-1349, 1348*b*, 1348*f*
Thrombotic thrombocytopenic purpura, **622**, **624-625**, 625*b*
Thromboxane, 162, 162*f*
Thrombus, 816
Thrush, 221, 897*b*
Thymoglobulin (rabbit antithymocyte globulin), 210, 211*b*
Thyroglobulin, 1115*t*-1118*t*
Thyroid acropachy, 1164, 1165*f*
Thyroid antibodies, 1115*t*-1118*t*
Thyroid cancer, **1170-1171**
anaplastic, 1171
follicular, 1171
nursing and interprofessional management of, **1171**
papillary, 1171
Thyroid gland, **1106-1107**, 1107*f*
disorders of, 1109*b*, **1162-1171**, 1162*f*
in older adults, 1108*b*
palpation of, 1112, 1112*f*
physical examination of, 1112
studies of, 1115*t*-1118*t*
Thyroid hormones, 1104*b*, 1106
Thyroid nodules, 1113*b*-1114*b*, **1170-1171**
Thyroid scan, 1115*t*-1118*t*
Thyroid surgery
nursing management of, 1167
postoperative care in, 1167-1168
preoperative care in, 1167
Thyroidectomy
nursing interventions for, 1168
subtotal, 1166, 1166*f*
Thyroiditis, 1162, **1163**
acute, 1163
chronic autoimmune, 1163
Hashimoto's, 1163
silent, painless, 1163
subacute granulomatous, 1163
Thyroid-stimulating hormone, 1104*b*, 1115*t*-1118*t*, 1655*b*-1658*b*
Thyrotoxic crisis, 1164-1165
Thyrotoxic storm, 1164-1165
Thyrotoxicosis
acute, 1164-1165, 1167
drug therapy for, 1166
Thyrotropin, 1104*b*, 1115*t*-1118*t*
Thyroxine (T_4), 1104*b*, **1107**
measurement of, 1115*t*-1118*t*
reference values, 1655*b*-1658*b*
Tiazac (diltiazem), 532*b*
Tibial fracture, **1485**
Tic douloureux, 1437-1438
Ticagrelor (Brilinta), 715*b*-716*b*
Tick bites, **1641**
Tick removal, 1641, 1641*f*
Ticks, 416*b*
Ticlopidine, 1353*b*
Tidal volume (V_T), 454, 473*b*, 1575*b*
Tidaling, 523
Tigan (trimethobenzamide), 895*b*
Tikosyn (dofetilide), 771*b*
Time management
for patient and caregiver teaching, 49
reordering time, 61
Time orientation, 25*b*
Timed voiding, 1057*b*
Timolol maleate (Timoptic, Istalol), 381*b*
Tinea corporis, 418*b*
Tinea cruris, 418*b*
Tinea pedis, 418*b*
Tinea unguium, 417, 417*f*, 418*b*
Tinnitus, 361, 388
Tiotropium (Spiriva HandiHaler), 548*b*-549*b*
Tirofiban (Aggrastat), 715*b*-716*b*
Tissue(s)
oxygen needs, 1612
subcutaneous, 395, 432
Tissue donation, **135**
Tissue expansion, 1215*b*, 1223, 1223*f*
Tissue factor, 592*b*
Tissue oxygenation, 1607
Tissue perfusion, 1625
Tissue regeneration, 165, 165*b*
Tissue thromboplastin, 592*b*
Tissue typing, **208**
Titin, 738
Titralac (calcium carbonate), 903*b*
Tizanidine (Zanaflex)
for multiple sclerosis, 1385*b*
for pain, 116*b*
TNKase (tenecteplase), 715*b*-716*b*
Tobacco cessation, **146-148**, 148*b*
5 As for users, 146-147, 147*b*
5 Rs to motivate, 146-147, 147*b*
health-promoting behaviors for, 708*b*
for hypertension, 689
inpatient interventions, 147*b*
patient teaching guide for, 149*b*
Tobacco smoke, 558, 558*b*
Tobacco use disorder, **145-146**. *See also* Smoking
and CAD, 706
clinical practice guidelines for treating, 146-147, 147*b*
nursing and interprofessional management of, **146-150**
Tocilizumab (Actemra), 1521*b*-1522*b*, 1529
Toenails, 396, 396*f*
Tofacitinib (Xeljanz), 1521*b*-1522*b*, 1528
Tofranil (imipramine), 116*b*, 1059*b*
Tolcapone (Tasmar), 1390, 1391*b*
Tolerant drinkers, 148
Tolmetin, 1521*b*-1522*b*
Tolterodine (Detrol), 1057*b*, 1059*b*
Tomosynthesis mammography, 1205

Tongue
  geographic, 846*b*-847*b*
  smooth, 597*b*-598*b*, 846*b*-847*b*
Tongue cancer, 898*b*
Tonometry, 356*b*
Tophi, 365*b*, 1533, 1533*f*
Topical medications, 423*b*, **423-424**
Topiramate (Topamax), 1372*b*
Topoisomerase inhibitors, 247*b*
Toprol XL (metoprolol), 745*b*
Toremifene (Fareston), 1217*b*
Torsades de pointes, 769
Torsemide (Demadex), 691*b*-693*b*
Torticollis, 1456*b*
Total ankle arthroplasty, 1492
Total hip arthroplasty, 1491
Total intravenous anesthesia, 322
Total lung capacity (TLC), 473*b*
Total proctocolectomy
  with ileal pouch/anal anastomosis, 948, 948*f*
  with permanent ileostomy, 948
TotalCare SpO_2RT Bed System, 1625*f*
Totally endoscopic coronary artery bypass graft (TECAB), 725
Touch, 27-28, 1306
Tourniquet test, 601*t*
Toviaz (fesoterodine), 1059*b*
Toxic nodular goiters, 1162
Toxoplasma gondii, 222*b*
Trace elements, 856*b*, 869
Tracheal deviation, 467*b*-468*b*
Tracheal problems, **484-496**
Tracheal suction
  closed system, 1570, 1570*f*
  closed-suction technique, 1571
  open-suction technique, 1571
Tracheostomy, **485-486**, 491, 1486, 1569
  complications of, 487, 487*b*
  decannulation, 490
  nursing management of, 486*b*, **486-490**, 487*f*
  percutaneous, 485
  surgical, 485
  swallowing dysfunction with, 489
Tracheostomy care, 488*b*, 489*f*, 490*b*
  acute care, 486-489, 487*f*
  changing tapes, 488*b*, 489*f*
  chronic care, 489
  suctioning, 487, 487*f*, 488*b*, 490*b*
Tracheostomy collars, 566*b*-567*b*, 567*f*
Tracheostomy T bar, 566*b*-567*b*, 567*f*
Tracheostomy tubes, 485, 485*f*
  nursing management of, 486*b*
  speaking tracheostomy tube, 486*b*, 489
  speech with, **489-490**
Tracheotomy, 1569
Trachoma, 371
Tracleer (bosentan), 532*b*
Traction, **1470-1471**
  cervical, 1427, 1427*f*
  nursing implementation, 1476-1477
  nursing management of patients in, 1471*b*
  skeletal, 1470-1471, 1471*f*
Traction alopecia, 403-405, 404*f*
Traditional foods, 856
Traditional healers, 24
Traditionalists, 55*b*
Traditions, **24**
Tradjenta (inagliptin), 1131*b*
Training, 438*b*
Train-of-four (TOF) assessment, 1580, 1580*f*
Traits, 179*b*
Tramadol (Ultram), 113*b*-114*b*, 114
Trandolapril (Mavik), 691*b*-693*b*
Trans fat, 855
Transarterial chemoembolization, 997
Transarterial radioembolization, 997
Transbronchial lung biopsy, 471
Transcellular fluids, 271
Transcranial Doppler ultrasound, 1310*t*-1312*t*
Transcultural nursing, 23, 30*f*
Transcutaneous carbon dioxide ($PtcCO_2$), 331
Transcutaneous electrical nerve stimulation, **121**, 121*f*
Transcutaneous pacemakers, 775, 775*f*
Transderm-Scōp (scopolamine), 326*b*, 895*b*
Transduction, 103-104, 104*f*
Transesophageal echocardiography, 671-672, 673*t*-677*t*
Transesophageal puncture (TEP), 493
Transferrin, 602*t*, 1655*b*-1658*b*
Transferrin saturation, 601, 602*t*
Transferring the patient, **319-320**
Transformation zone, 1186-1187, 1186*f*
Transfusion-related acute lung injury (TRALI) reaction, 650*b*-651*b*
Transgender individuals, 1238*b*
Transhepatic biliary catheter, 1008
Transhepatic cholangiography, percutaneous, 847*t*-850*t*
Transient ischemic attacks, **1347-1348**, 1353-1354
Trans-illuminated powered phlebectomy, 826
Transitional care, 8
Transitional Care Model (TCM), 71
Transitional cell carcinoma, papillary, 1053, 1054*f*
Transitions of care, 8-9
Transjugular intrahepatic portosystemic shunt, 992
Translation applications, 31*b*
Translation services, 52, 52*f*
Transluminal angioplasty, 1353
Transluminal balloon valvuloplasty, percutaneous, **793-794**, 794*f*
Transluminal septal myocardial ablation, percutaneous, 799
Transmissible spongiform encephalopathies (TSEs), 214-215
Transmission-based precautions, 218, 218*b*
Transmyocardial laser revascularization, 725
Transparent films, 169*b*
Transplant rejection, **208-209**
Transplantation
  bone marrow, 259
  corneal, 373, 373*f*
  heart, **753-754**
  hematopoietic stem cell, **259-261**, 260*b*, 638-639
  kidney, **1092-1095**
  liver, **998-999**
  lung, **533-534**, 571
  organ, **207-210**, 207*f*
  pancreas, 1137
  for Parkinson's disease, 1391
Transportation
  to operating room, 311
  transferring the patient, **319-320**
Transrectal ultrasound (TRUS), 1270
Transtheoretical model of health behavior change, 47, 48*b*
Transurethral electrovaporization of prostate (TUVP), 1272*b*
Transurethral incision of prostate (TUIP), 1272*b*, 1273
Transurethral microwave thermotherapy (TUMT), 1271, 1272*b*
Transurethral needle ablation (TUNA), 1271, 1272*b*
Transurethral resection of the bladder tumor (TURBT), 1054
Transurethral resection of the prostate (TURP), 1272-1273, 1272*b*, 1273*f*
  postoperative care in, 1274-1275
  preoperative care in, 1274
Transurethral resection syndrome, 1273
Transvenous pacemakers, 774-775, 774*f*
Transverse rectus abdominis musculocutaneous (TRAM) flap, 1215*b*, 1223, 1224*f*
Trastuzumab (Herceptin), 187*b*, 257, 1217*b*-1218*b*
Trauma, 808
  abdominal, **941**
  case study, 1647*b*
  chest, 519*b*, **519-527**
  cumulative disorder, 1465
  to external ear, **383**
  eye, **370**, 371*b*
  focused abdominal sonography for (FAST), 1633-1634
  head, 1327-1328, 1403
  incontinence after, 1056*b*
  musculoskeletal, **1462-1495**
  renal, **1050**
  repetitive disorder, 1465
  spinal cord, 399*b*
Traumatic brain injury, 1326, 1342*b*
Travel, 1140
Travoprost (Travatan), 381*b*
Treatments
  carrying out regimens, 61
  nursing history, 36
  refusal of, 1424*b*
  withdrawing, 1097*b*
  withholding, 1338*b*
Trelstar (triptorelin), 1280*b*
Tremor, 1388-1389
Trench mouth, 897*b*
Treponema pallidum, 214*b*
Treponema pallidum particle agglutination (TP-PA) test, 1236
Treprostinil (Remodulin), 532*b*
Treprostinil (Tyvaso), 532*b*
Tretinoin (Retin-A, Renova), 426*b*
Trexall (methotrexate), 1521*b*-1522*b*
Triage, **1628-1630**
Triamcinolone (Aristospan), 479*b*-480*b*, 1521*b*-1522*b*
Triamterene (Dyrenium), 691*b*-693*b*
Triceps reflex, 1307
Trichomonas vaginalis, 1231
***Trichomonas* vaginitis**, 1250*b*
Trichomoniasis, **1231-1232**
  drug therapy for, 1232
  interprofessional care for, 1232
Trichophyton, 215*b*
Tricor (fenofibrate), 711*b*
Tricuspid stenosis, 791*b*, **793**
Tricyclic antidepressants
  cardiovascular effects of, 664*b*
  overdose, 1643*b*
  for pain, 116*b*, 117
  for voiding dysfunction, 1059*b*
Trifluoperazine, 895*b*
Trigeminal nerve, 1305*b*, 1437, 1437*f*
Trigeminal neuralgia, **1437-1438**
  drug therapy for, 1438
  interprofessional care for, 1438, 1438*b*
  nursing management of, **1438-1439**
  surgical therapy for, 1438, 1438*b*, 1439*f*
Trigger points, 121
Triggered beats, 760-761
Triglycerides, 670, 673*t*-677*t*
  in chronic kidney disease, 1077
  reference values, 1655*b*-1658*b*
Trihexyphenidyl, 1391*b*

Triiodothyronine (T_3), 1104*b*, **1107**
measurement of, 1115*t*-1118*t*
reference values, 1655*b*-1658*b*
uptake test, 1115*t*-1118*t*
Trilisate (choline magnesium trisalicylate), 111*b*
Trimethobenzamide (Tigan), 895*b*
Tripod position, 1613-1614, 1614*f*
Tripod position, 467*b*-468*b*
Triptorelin (Trelstar), 1280*b*
Trismus, 1442
Trochlear nerve, 1305*b*, **1306**
Trolamine salicylate, 118
Trophic feeding, 1598
Tropic hormones, 1105
excess of, **1157-1158**
Troponins
cardiac-specific, 670, 673*t*-677*t*, 722
reference values, 1655*b*-1658*b*
in shock, 1590*t*
Trospium chloride (Sanctura), 1059*b*
Trousseau's sign, 284, 284*f*
Trulicity (dulaglutide), 1131*b*-1132*b*
Trusopt (dorzolamide), 381*b*
Try This Series (Hartford Institute for Geriatric Nursing), 70
T-tubes, 344*b*
Tube feeding, 865
aspiration risk, 866
nursing management of, 866*b*-867*b*
patient position for, 866
safety, 866-868
Tuberculin skin test, 472*b*, **508**
Tuberculosis, 28, 216*b*, **506-510**
active disease, 507, 509
acute care for, 511
ambulatory care for, 511
bacteriologic studies in, 508
classification of, 507, 507*b*
clinical manifestations of, 507-508
complications of, 508
cultural & ethnic health disparities in, 506*b*
diagnostic studies in, 508
directly observed therapy for, 509
drug therapy for, 509-510, 509*b*-510*b*
directly observed therapy, 509
patient adherence to, 510*b*
etiology and pathophysiology of, 506-507
genitourinary, **1041**
health promotion for, 511
interprofessional care for, 508-510, 508*b*
latent infection, 507, 507*b*, 509-510, 510*b*
miliary, 508
multidrug-resistant, 506
nursing diagnoses related to, 511
nursing management of, **510-511**
pleural, 508
primary, 507
pulmonary, 508*b*
reactivation, 507
Tudorza (aclidinium bromide), 548*b*-549*b*
Tumor angiogenesis, 238
Tumor lysis syndrome, 263*b*
Tumor markers, 239-240
Tumor necrosis factor, 195*b*
Tumor necrosis factor inhibitors
for arthritis, 1521*b*-1522*b*, 1529
drug alert, 1529*b*
Tumor necrosis factor receptors, 195*b*
Tumor suppressor genes, 236
Tumor treatment fields, 1335
Tumor-associated antigens, 238-239, 239*f*
Tumors
benign, **1254-1256**
bone, **1500-1502**
brain, 1333-1335
Tumors *(Continued)*
of female reproductive system, **1254-1256**
gastrointestinal stromal tumors, **968**
lung, 518-519
malignant. *See* Cancer
ocular, **382**
phyllodes, 1211
radiosensitivity of, 249, 249*b*
spinal cord, **1436-1437**, 1436*f*
urinary tract, 1052-1055
Tums (calcium carbonate), 903*b*
Tuning fork tests, 365*t*-366*t*
Turbinates, 453
Turgor, 401
Twain, Mark, 1156
Twinrix, 982
Two-dimensional (2-D) echocardiography, 671, 672*f*, 673*t*-677*t*
Two-point discrimination, 1307
Tykerb (lapatinib), 257, 1217*b*, 1218
Tylenol. *See* Acetaminophen
Tympanic membrane (eardrum), 360
abnormalities, 365*b*
normal, 364*f*
perforation of, 385*f*
physical examination of, 364
retracted, 365*b*
Tympanometry, 365*t*-366*t*
Tympanoplasty, 385
Tympanum, 364
Tympany, 844
Tyrosine kinase inhibitors, 257, 258*b*
Tysabri (natalizumab), 1385*b*, 1386
Tyvaso (treprostinil), 532*b*
Tyzeka (telbivudine), 980
Tzanck test (Wright's and Giemsa's stain), 405*t*

U

Ulcerative colitis, 944, 945*b*
clinical manifestations of, 946
pattern of inflammation in, 945, 945*f*
surgical therapy for, 948
Ulcerative gingivitis, acute necrotizing, 897*b*
Ulcers
arterial, 668*b*
corneal, **372**, 372*f*
duodenal, 910*f*, 911*b*, **912**, 912*f*
esophageal, 901*f*
gastric, 911*b*, **912**
genital, **1232-1240**
leg ulcers, 597*b*-598*b*
in mouth, 846*b*-847*b*
neurotrophic, 1150, 1150*f*
penile, 1198*b*
peptic, **910-915**, 910*f*, 926*b*
pressure, **172**
skin, 402*b*, 1113*b*-1114*b*
STIs characterized by, **1232-1240**
stress
in ARDS, 1623
physiologic, **922**
in spinal cord injury, 1430
venous, 399*b*, 668*b*, **826-827**, 827*b*, 827*f*
Ulnar deviation, 1456*b*
Ulnar drift, 1456*b*, 1527, 1527*f*
Ultane (sevoflurane), 325*b*
Ultiva (remifentanil), 326*b*
Ultradian rhythms, 1105
Ultrafiltration, 744-745, 1085
Ultram (tramadol), 113*b*-114*b*, 114
Ultrasound
abdominal, 603*t*, 847*t*-850*t*
of breast, 1206
endoanal (endorectal), 971
endorectal, 971
endoscopic, 847*t*-850*t*
Ultrasound *(Continued)*
focused abdominal sonography for trauma (FAST), 1633-1634
gastrointestinal, 847*t*-850*t*
intravascular, 673*t*-677*t*, 678-679
liver, 603*t*
of nervous system, 1310*t*-1312*t*
quantitative, 1457*t*-1459*t*
real-time three-dimensional (3-D), 671, 673*t*-677*t*
renal, 1025*t*-1030*t*
of reproductive system, 1198*t*-1201*t*
spleen, 603*t*
thyroid, 1115*t*-1118*t*
transrectal (TRUS), 1270
of visual system, 359*t*
Ultrasound elastography, 847*t*-850*t*
Ultrasound-guided biopsy, 1198*t*-1201*t*
Ultraviolet light, 407, 408*b*
Umbilical hernia, 965, 965*f*
Umeclidinium (Incruse Ellipta), 548*b*-549*b*
Umeclidinium/vilanterol (Anoro Ellipta), 548*b*-549*b*
Uncal herniation, 1318
Unconsciousness, 1317-1318, 1652*b*
Undernutrition, 856, 872*b*
Underweight, 875*b*
Uniform Anatomical Gift Act, 208
United Network for Organ Sharing (UNOS), 207-208, 1094
United Ostomy Associations of America, 962
Univasc (moexipril), 691*b*-693*b*
Universal Protocol, 321
Unlicensed assistive personnel (UAP), 11
role in assessment and data collection, 36*b*
role in bladder irrigation, 1274*b*
role in blood transfusions, 649*b*
role in cardiac catheterization and PCI, 729*b*
role in caring for acute stroke patients, 1359*b*
role in caring for Alzheimer's patients, 1412*b*
role in caring for arthritis patients, 1529*b*
role in caring for chronic venous insufficiency and venous ulcers, 827*b*
role in caring for diabetic patients, 1152*b*
role in caring for incontinent patients, 1059*b*
role in caring for neutropenia patients, 632*b*
role in caring for osteomyelitis patients, 1498*b*
role in caring for patients with casts or in traction, 1471*b*
role in caring for seizure patients, 1380*b*
role in caring for the patient with hypertension, 696*b*
role in IV therapy, 294*b*
role in nasogastric and gastric tubes and enteral feedings, 867*b*
role in ostomy care, 960*b*
role in oxygen administration, 568*b*
role in pain management, 123*b*
role in postoperative care, 334*b*
role in skin care, 425*b*
role in suctioning and tracheostomy care, 490*b*
role in wound care, 170*b*
role with corrective lenses and hearing aids, 392*b*
role with urinary catheters, 1061*b*
Upper airway burns, **430-431**, 437
Upper esophageal sphincter, 835
Upper extremity injuries, 1472
Upper gastrointestinal bleeding, **921-923**
acute, 924, 924*b*
acute care for, 924-925
ambulatory care for, 925
causes of, 922, 922*b*
drug therapy for, 923
emergency assessment and management of, 922-923
emergency management of, 924, 924*b*
endoscopic therapy for, 923
health promotion for, 924

Upper gastrointestinal bleeding *(Continued)*
interprofessional care for, 922-923
nursing assessment in, 923-924, 923*b*
nursing diagnoses related to, 924
nursing management of, **923-925**
surgical therapy, 923
types of, 922, 922*b*
Upper gastrointestinal problems, 893-928
Upper gastrointestinal series, 845, 847*t*-850*t*
Upper limb amputation, 1490
Upper motor neurons, 1296
Upper respiratory tract
problems of, **475-498**
structures and functions of, **453-454**
Upper small intestine disorders, 909-926
Urecholine (bethanechol), 903*b*, 1385*b*
Uremia, 1076
Uremic fetor, 1078
Ureteral catheters, **1062**
Ureteral strictures, 1049-1050
Ureteral surgery, **1063**
Ureteroileosigmoidostomy, 1064*f*
Ureterolithotomy, 1048
Ureteroneocystostomy, 1050
Ureteropelvic junction, 1018
Ureteroscopes, 1047
Ureterostomy, 1064*b*, 1064*f*
Ureteroureterostomy, 1050
Ureterovesical junctions, 1018
Ureters, 1016*f*, **1018**, 1020*b*
Urethra, **1019**
female, 1016*f*, 1019
male, 1016*f*, 1019
in older adults, 1020*b*
Urethral catheterization, **1061**, 1062*b*
Urethral diverticula, 1040
Urethral plugs, 1057*b*
Urethral strictures, 1050
Urethritis, 1034, **1039-1040**, 1228
nongonococcal, 1228
Urethrography, 1025*t*-1030*t*
Urethroplasty, 1050
Urethrovesical unit, **1019**
Urge incontinence, 1056*b*
Urge-suppression strategies, 1057*b*
Uric acid
blood levels, 1025*t*-1030*t*
in bone disease, 1457*t*-1459*t*
reference values, 1655*b*-1658*b*, 1661*b*
Uric acid stones, 1046*b*
Urinalysis, **1024-1031**, 1025*t*-1030*t*
Urinary bladder, **1018-1019**, 1019*f*
Urinary catheterization, **1060-1063**
complications of, **1060-1061**
indications for, **1060-1061**, 1061*b*
Urinary catheters, 1061*b*
construction of, **1061**
types of, **1061-1063**, 1061*f*
Urinary diversion, 1054, **1063-1065**, 1064*b*
continent, 1065
incontinent, 1064-1065
methods of, 1064*f*
nursing management of, **1065-1066**
postoperative management in, 1065-1066
preoperative management in, 1065
in spinal cord injury, 1433
Urinary frequency, 1025*b*, 1067*b*
Urinary hesitancy, 1025*b*
Urinary incontinence, 1025*b*, **1055-1058**
diagnostic studies in, 1055
drug therapy for, 1057, 1059*b*
at end of life, 140*b*-141*b*
functional, 1056*b*
gender differences in, 1055*b*
Urinary incontinence *(Continued)*
interprofessional care for, 1055-1058, 1059*b*
interventions for, 1055-1057, 1057*b*
nursing management of, **1058-1059**
in spinal cord injury, 1423
surgical therapy for, 1057-1058
after trauma or surgery, 1056*b*
types of, 1056*b*
Urinary obstruction, 1044, 1044*f*
Urinary retention, 1025*b*, **1059-1060**
acute, 1059-1060, 1289*b*
case study, 1289*b*
chronic, 1059-1060
drug therapy, 1060
interprofessional care for, 1060
nursing management of, **1060**
surgical therapy for, 1060
Urinary stoma, 1064-1065, 1064*f*, 1066*f*
Urinary system
abnormalities, 1025*b*
assessment of, **1020-1023**
checklist for, 1024*b*
health history, 1021*b*
physical examination, 1023
case study, 1020*b*, 1023*b*-1024*b*, 1031*b*
diagnostic studies of, **1024-1031**, 1025*t*-1030*t*, 1031*b*
at end of life, 132*b*
lower, 1015
normal, 1023*b*
in older adults, 1019-1020, 1020*b*
organs of, 1015, 1016*f*
structures and functions of, **1015-1020**
surgery of, **1063-1066**
upper, 1015, 1016*f*
Urinary tract calculi, 1045-1048, 1047*f*
clinical manifestations of, 1046
diagnostic studies in, 1046-1047
etiology and pathophysiology of, 1045
gender differences in, 1045*b*
interprofessional care for, 1047-1048
nursing assessment in, 1049*b*
nursing management of, **1048-1049**
nutritional therapy for, 1048, 1049*b*
risk factors for, 1045*b*
surgical therapy for, 1048
types of, 1045, 1046*b*
Urinary tract infections, 1033-1036
acute care for, 1037
ambulatory care for, 1037-1038
catheter-associated, 1034
prevention of, 1037, 1062*b*
causes of, 1033, 1034*b*
clinical manifestations of, 1034-1035
complicated, 1033
diagnostic studies in, 1035-1036
drug therapy for, 1036, 1036*b*
etiology of, 1034
health promotion for, 1036-1038
interprofessional care for, 1036, 1036*b*
nursing assessment in, 1037*b*
nursing management of, 1036-1038
pathophysiology of, 1034
patient & caregiver teaching for, 1037*b*
recurrent, 1036*b*
risk factors for, 1035*b*
sites of, 1034, 1034*f*
uncomplicated, 1033, 1036*b*
Urinary tract tumors, 1052-1055
Urination, 1019, 1025*b*
Urine, 1016-1017
Urine culture, 1025*t*-1030*t*, 1035
Urine output, 439
postoperative, 1063
Urine studies, 603*t*, **1024-1031**, 1025*t*-1030*t*, 1661*b*
Urispas (flavoxate), 1059*b*
Urodynamic studies, 1025*t*-1030*t*, **1031**
Urofollitropin (Fertinex, Bravelle), 1243*b*
Urogram, CT, 1025*t*-1030*t*
Urologic disorders
clinical manifestations of, 1022*b*
cultural & ethnic health disparities, 1034*b*
genetic risks, 1021*b*
infectious, **1033-1041**
inflammatory, **1033-1041**
nursing diagnoses related to, 342-343
nursing management of, **342-343**
postoperative, **342**
Urosepsis, 1034, 1038
Uroxatral (alfuzosin), 1059*b*
Urticaria, 199, 418*b*
U.S. Department of Health and Human Services, 1646
U.S. Department of Homeland Security (DHS), 1646
Uterine bleeding, abnormal, **1246-1247**
classification of, 1246, 1246*f*
interprofessional care for, 1246-1247, 1246*b*
nursing management of, 1247
Uterine cancer, 1192*b*
Uterine fibroids, 1254
Uterine prolapse, 1261-1262, 1262*f*
Uterus, 1186-1187
Uveal melanoma, 382, 383*f*
Uveitis, 382, 1536

V

Vaccines
bacille-Calmette-Guérin, 510
HPV, 1234-1235, 1235*b*
immunotherapy, 258*b*
influenza, 482*b*
meningococcal, 1340
pneumococcal, 504*b*
tetanus, 441, 1634*b*
Vacuum erection devices, 1288
Vacuum-assisted biopsy, 1206
Vagal nerve stimulation, 1379
Vagifem (estrogen vaginal tablets), 1059*b*
Vagina, 1187
fistulas involving, **1263**, 1263*f*
Vaginal cancer, 1259
Vaginal weight training, 1057*b*
Vaginitis, 1250*b*
Vaginosis, 1250*b*
Vagotomy, 840*b*, 917
Vagus nerve, 1305*b*
Valgus deformity, 1456*b*, 1519
Valium (diazepam), 326*b*, 1378, 1385*b*
Valsalva maneuver, 726, 836-837
Valsartan (Diovan)
for heart failure, 745*b*
for hypertension, 691*b*-693*b*
mechanism of action, 715*b*-716*b*
Valsartan/sacubitril (Entresto), 745*b*, 747-748
Value-belief pattern, 37*b*, 39
Values, 21-22
Valve repair, 794
Valve replacement, 794-795
Valvular heart disease, 790-796
acute care for, 796
ambulatory care for, 796
case study, 800*b*
clinical manifestations of, 791*b*
conservative therapy for, 793-794
diagnostic studies for, **793**

Valvular heart disease *(Continued)*
health promotion for, 796
interprofessional care for, 793*b*, **793-795**
nursing assessment in, 795*b*
nursing diagnoses related to, 796
nursing management of, **795-796**
surgical therapy for, 794-795
Valvular regurgitation, 790-791, 790*f*
Valvular stenosis, 790-791, 790*f*
Valvuloplasty, 794, 794*f*
balloon, **793-794**, 794*f*
minimally invasive, 794
Valvulotomy, 794
Vancomycin-resistant enterococci (VRE), 216, 216*b*
Vancomycin-resistant *Staphylococus aureus*, 216
Vanillylmandelic acid, 1115*t*-1118*t*, 1661*b*
Varenicline (Chantix), 147-148, 148*b*, 150*b*
Variant angina, 713
Varicella-zoster virus, 214*b*, 222*b*
Varices
acute care for, 994-995
bleeding, 994-995
esophageal, **908**, 988, 991-992
gastric, 988, 991-992
interprofessional care for, 991-992
Varicocele, 1284*f*, **1285**
Varicose veins, 668*b*, **825-826**, 826*f*
drug therapy for, 825
interprofessional care for, 825
interventional and surgical therapy for, 825-826, 826*f*
nursing management of, **826**
Varicosities, 403*b*, 825-826
Varus deformity, 1456*b*, 1519
Vas (ductus) deferens, 1184-1185, 1185*f*
Vascepa (icosapent ethyl), 711*b*
Vascular access, for hemodialysis
sites for, 1087-1089, 1088*f*
temporary, 1088-1089, 1089*f*
Vascular dementia, 1400
Vascular disorders, **802-830**
gender differences in, 803*b*
lung disorders, **529-531**
renal problems, **1050-1051**
Vascular endothelium, 683
Vascular graft infection, 813
Vascular injury, 590-591
Vascular resistance, 1560
Vascular system, **661**. *See also* Cardiovascular system
inflammatory response, 160, 161*f*
Vasectomy, **1286**, 1286*f*
reversals, 1286
Vasodilators
for heart failure, 745-746, 745*b*, 748
for hypertension, 690, 691*b*-693*b*
for pulmonary hypertension, 532*b*
for shock, 1598
Vasoepididymostomy, 1286
Vasogenic cerebral edema, 1316
Vasomotor instability, 1248-1249
Vasopressin (Pitressin)
for shock, 1599*b*, 1601
for upper gastrointestinal bleeding, 993*b*, 1104*b*
Vasopressors, 1598, 1601
Vasovotomy, 1286
Vegetarian diet, **855-856**
Vegetations, 780-781, 781*f*
Veins and venules, **661**, 661*f*
Veletri (epoprostenol), 532*b*
Vemurafenib (Zelboraf), 187*b*
Vena cava interruption, 822
Vena cava interruption devices, 822, 822*f*
Venereal Disease Research Laboratory (VDRL) test, 1236, 1659*b*
Venlafaxine, 116*b*
Venography, 673*t*-677*t*
Venous blood gases
mixed, 456-457
normal values, 457*b*
reference values, 1655*b*-1658*b*
Venous disorders
acute, **816-828**
chronic, **816-828**
Venous hydrostatic pressure, 274
Venous hypertension, ambulatory, 826
Venous insufficiency, chronic, **826-827**
Venous leg ulcers, **826-828**, 827*b*, 827*f*
Venous oxygen saturation of hemoglobin
central ($ScvO_2$), 1564-1565, 1565*b*
mixed (SvO_2), **456-457**, 1559*b*, 1564-1565
monitoring, 1564-1565
normal range, 1559*b*
Venous stasis, 817
Venous thrombectomy, 822
Venous thromboembolism, 529, 816, 816*b*, **818-822**, 1479-1480
acute care for, 823
ambulatory care for, 823-825
anticoagulant therapy for, 821
clinical manifestations of, 818
complications of, 818
diagnostic studies, 819*t*
drug therapy for, 819-822, 820*b*
interprofessional care for, 818-822
nursing assessment in, 822*b*
nursing diagnoses for, 823
nursing management of, **822-825**, 824*b*
pathophysiology of, 816, 817*f*
postoperative, 337
prevention and prophylaxis of, 442, 818-819
risk factors for, 817*b*
surgical and interventional radiology therapy for, 822
thrombolytic therapy for, 821-822
Venous thrombosis, **816-822**
deep vein thrombosis, 816
renal vein thrombosis, **1051**
Venous ulcers, 399*b*, 668*b*
Venovenous hemodiafiltration, continuous, 1091, 1091*b*
Venovenous hemodialysis, continuous, 1091, 1091*b*
Venovenous hemofiltration, continuous, 1091, 1091*b*
Venovenous therapy, continuous, 1091*f*
Ventavis (iloprost), 532*b*
Ventilation
mechanical. *See* Mechanical ventilation
monitoring, 1571
physiology of, **456**
for shock, 1596
Ventilation scanning, 530
Ventilation-perfusion (V/Q) mismatch, 1610-1611, 1611*f*
range of relationships, 1611, 1611*f*
regional differences, 1610, 1611*f*
shunts, 1611, 1611*f*
Ventilation-perfusion (V/Q) scan, 469*t*-471*t*, 530
Ventilator bundle protocols, 1623, 1623*b*
Ventilator-associated pneumonia, 501, **1579**, 1623
Ventilators. *See also* Mechanical ventilation
disconnection or malfunction, 1581
importing monitor and ventilator data, 1578*b*
settings of, 1574-1575, 1575*b*
Ventolin HFA (albuterol), 548*b*-549*b*
Ventral hernias, 965
Ventricles, **1298**
Ventricular assist devices, 747*f*, 1568-1569
biventricular assist device, 1568, 1568*f*
contraindications to, 1568-1569
Ventricular bigeminy, 768
Ventricular fibrillation, 764*b*, **770**, 770*f*
Ventricular gallop, 669
Ventricular hypertrophy, 661
Ventricular remodeling, 740
Ventricular septal wall rupture, 721
Ventricular shunts, 1335
Ventricular tachycardia, 764*b*, **768-769**, 769*f*
monomorphic, 769
polymorphic, 769
Ventricular trigeminy, 768
Ventriculomyotomy and myectomy, 799
Ventriculostomy, 1319, 1320*f*-1321*f*
Venturi mask, 566*b*-567*b*, 567*f*
Verapamil (Calan, Isoptin), 715*b*-716*b*
for dysrhythmia, 771*b*
for hypertension, 691*b*-693*b*
for voiding dysfunction, 1059*b*
Verapamil long-acting (Covera-HS), 691*b*-693*b*
Verapamil timed-release (Verelan PM), 691*b*-693*b*
Verbal communication, 25, 25*f*
Verruca vulgaris, 415*b*
Vertebral column, 1300-1301, 1301*f*
Vertebral disc surgery, 1506, **1507**
Vertebral injuries
casts for, 1472
fractures, **1485-1486**
Vertebroplasty, 1485, 1513
Vertigo, 361
benign paroxysmal positional vertigo, **386-387**
Very-low-density lipoproteins (VLDLs), 670
Vesicants, 246
VESIcare (solifenacin), 1059*b*
Vesicles, 401*b*
penile, 1198*b*
Vesicular sounds, 466
Vest Airway system, 570
Vestibular tests, 365*t*-366*t*
Vestibule, 1187
Vestibulocochlear nerve, 1305*b*
Veterans, 55*b*
Vibramycin (doxycycline), 1229*b*, 1521*b*-1522*b*
Vibration, 569, **570**
Vibration sense, 1307
Victoza (liraglutide), 1131*b*-1132*b*, 1132
Video capsule endoscopy, 847*t*-850*t*, 851*f*
Video games, 1363*b*
Video-assisted thoracoscopic surgery, 526*b*, **526**
Videourodynamics, 1025*t*-1030*t*
Vigamox (moxifloxacin), 509*b*
Vigileo monitor, 1562*f*
Vinca alkaloids, 247*b*
Vincent's infection, 897*b*
Viokace (pancrelipase), 1001*b*, 1004
Violence, **1644-1645**. *See also* Physical abuse; Trauma
family, 1644
intimate partner violence, 1263, 1644
patient and visitor violence/abuse, 1644*b*
rape, 1263
workplace, 1644, 1644*b*
Viral carcinogens, 237
Viral infections
conjunctivitis, 371
and glomerulonephritis, 1042*b*
hepatitis, **974-977**
keratitis, 372
meningitis, **1341**
rhinitis, **478-480**
skin, 415*b*, **415**
Virchow's triad, 816
Viread (tenofovir), 980
Virtual colonoscopy, 847*t*-850*t*, 851
Virtual reality, 1363*b*
Viruses, 214*b*
disease-causing, 214, 214*b*
hepatitis, 975*b*

Visceral pain, 106, 106*b*
Visceral pleura, 455
Viscosupplementation, 1523
Vision, **350-352**
Visitation, 1558*b*
Visitor violence/abuse, 1644*b*
Vistaril (hydroxyzine), 895*b*
Visual acuity testing, 356*b*, 358
Visual field cuts, 597*b*-598*b*
Visual field defects, 357*b*
Visual field (perimetry) testing, 359*t*
Visual fields, 1306*f*
Visual impairment, 368-369
acute care for, 369
ambulatory care for, 369-370
cultural & ethnic health disparities in, 368*b*
nonoptical methods for vision enhancement, 369
nonsurgical corrections, 368
nursing management of, **369-370**
in older adults, 370
optical devices for vision enhancement, 369-370
severe, 368
surgical therapy for, 368
Visual laser ablation of the prostate (VLAP), 1272
Visual learning, 53
Visual pathways, 351-352, 351*f*
Visual problems, 367-370
Visual system, **350-359**
abnormalities, 357*b*
assessment of, **352-359**, 353*b*, 356*b*, 359*b*-360*b*
physical examination, 355-359
techniques for, 356*b*, 359
case study, 353*b*, 356*b*, 359*b*-360*b*
diagnostic studies of, 359, 359*t*
health history, 354*b*
normal, 356*b*
in older adults, 352, 353*b*
structures and functions of, **350-352**
Vital capacity (VC), 473*b*
Vital signs
assessment of, 666-669
in increased ICP, 1318
in inflammation, 164
Vitamin A, 409
recommended daily intake, 858*b*
reference values, 1655*b*-1658*b*
Vitamin A deficiency, 858*b*
Vitamin B complex, 409
Vitamin B_1, 858*b*
Vitamin B_1 deficiency, 399*b*, 858*b*
Vitamin B_2, 610*b*
Vitamin B_2 deficiency, 399*b*
Vitamin B_6, 610*b*, 858*b*
Vitamin B_6 deficiency, 858*b*
Vitamin B_{12}, 602*t*, 610*b*
recommended daily intake, 858*b*
reference values, 1655*b*-1658*b*
Vitamin B_{12} deficiency, 612
classification of, 612*b*
clinical manifestations of, 858*b*
interprofessional care for, 613
laboratory data, 610*b*
Vitamin C, 409, 610*b*
recommended daily intake, 858*b*
reference values, 1655*b*-1658*b*
Vitamin C deficiency
clinical manifestations of, 858*b*
dermatologic manifestations of, 399*b*
and wound healing, 168*b*
Vitamin D, 858*b*
Vitamin D deficiency, 858*b*
Vitamin D supplements, 1512
Vitamin D_3 (choleclciferol), 409
Vitamin E, 610*b*, 858*b*
Vitamin E deficiency, 858*b*
Vitamin K, 409, 993*b*
liver function test, 852*t*
recommended daily intake, 858*b*
Vitamin K antagonists, 715*b*-716*b*, 819-821, 820*b*
Vitamin K deficiency, 858*b*
Vitamins, 855
fat-soluble, 855
for inflammation, 164*b*
in parenteral nutrition, 869
recommended daily intakes, 858*b*
water-soluble, 855
Vitiligo, 403-405, 403*b*, 404*f*, 1113*b*-1114*b*
Vitrectomy, 377-378
Vitreous humor, 351, 353*b*
Vocal cord stripping, 491
Voice banking applications, 1395*b*
Voiding, 1019
drug therapy for dysfunction of, 1059*b*
prompted, 1057*b*
scheduled regimens, 1057*b*
timed, 1057*b*
Voiding cystourethrography, 1025*t*-1030*t*
Voiding pressure flow tudy, 1025*t*-1030*t*
Volatile liquids, 325*b*
Volume ventilation, 1574-1576
Volutrauma, 1578, 1623
Volvulus, 950, 951*f*
Vomiting
cyclic vomiting syndrome, 894
definition of, 893
at end of life, 140*b*-141*b*
in increased ICP, 1318
nausea and vomiting, **893-895**
nursing management of, 867*b*
projectile, 894
with tube feedings, 867*b*
Von Willebrand disease, 626*b*, **626-628**
Von Willebrand factor, 628*b*
Vorapaxar (Zontivity), 715*b*-716*b*
VoSpire ER (albuterol), 548*b*-549*b*
Vulva, 1187
Vulvar cancer, 1259
Vulvar discharge, 1197*b*
Vulvar erythema, 1197*b*
Vulvar growths, 1197*b*
Vulvar intraepithelial neoplasia, 1259
Vulvectomy, 1261
Vulvovaginal candidiasis, 1250, 1250*b*

W

Waist circumference, 874-875
Waist-to-hip ratio (WHR), **875**
Wake behavior, 90
Walking, 1364*b*
Warfarin (Coumadin)
for atrial fibrillation, 766*b*
mechanism of action, 715*b*-716*b*
pharmacogenetics of, 186, 187*b*, 187*f*
for VTE, 819-821
Warm extremities, 668*b*
Warming
active measures, 341
passive measures, 341
Warts, 415, 415*b*, 416*f*
genital, **1234-1235**, 1234*f*, 1250-1251
Wasp stings, 416*b*
Watchful waiting, 1255, 1270
Water balance. *See also* Fluid and electrolyte balance
regulation of, 274-276
adrenal cortical, 275
cardiac, 275
Water balance *(Continued)*
gastrointestinal, 275
hypothalamic-pituitary, 274-275
renal, 275
Water content, 270, 271*f*
Water deficit, 273
Water deprivation (restriction) (ADH stimulation) test, 1115*t*-1118*t*
Water intoxication, 442
Water loss, insensible, 274
Water retention, 684
Water therapy, 1386, 1386*f*
Waterhouse-Friderichsen syndrome, 1340
Water-seal drainage, 525*b*
Water-soluble vitamins, 855
Weakness, 140*b*-141*b*, 597*b*-598*b*
Wearable artificial kidney, **1092**
Web-based health information, 53*f*, 55
Web-based knee and hip replacement community, 1477*b*
Weber test, 365*t*-366*t*
Wedge resection, 526*b*
Wegener's granulomatosis, 1042*b*
Weight
changes in, 743, 1113*b*-1114*b*
classification of, 874-875
daily, **277**
healthy, 878*b*
in heart failure, 743
Weight loss
1200-calorie–restricted weight-reduction diet for, 882*b*
diet programs for, 882*b*
for hypertension, 688
Weight training, vaginal, 1057*b*
WelChol (colesevelam), 711*b*
Wellbutrin (bupropion), 116*b*
Wenckebach heart block, **768**
Wernicke-Korsakoff syndrome, 149
Wernicke's aphasia, 1351*b*
Wernicke's receptive speech area, 1296
West Nile virus, 214*b*
Wet compresses, 422-423
Wet desquamation, 255, 255*f*
Wet mouonts, 1198*t*-1201*t*
What Happens Next?, 1410
Wheal-and-flare reaction, 197
Wheals, 401*b*
Wheezes, 466, 467*b*-468*b*
Whipple procedure, 1004-1005, 1005*f*
Whitaker study, 1025*t*-1030*t*
White blood cells
laboratory studies, 599-600
leukocytes, 589
reference values, 1659*b*
in shock, 1590*t*
White coat hypertension, 687
White lung, 1622-1623, 1622*f*
Whiteout, 1622-1623, 1622*f*
Whites, 19, 514*b*, 704*b*
Wilson's disease, 985
Windup, 105
Withdrawal
alcohol, **150**, 151*b*
opioid, 124*b*
stimulant, 151
Withdrawing treatment, 1097*b*
Withholding treatment, 1338*b*
Women. *See also* Gender differences
acute coronary syndrome in, 705*b*
coronary artery disease in, 704, 705*b*
heart failure in, 739*b*
lesbian, 21
osteoarthritis in, 1518*b*

Women *(Continued)*
risk factors for breast cancer, 1209
vascular disorders in, 803*b*
Women who have sex with women (WSW), 1238*b*
Wood's lamp (black light), 405*t*
Workplace bullying, 730*b*
Workplace conflict resolution, 1159*b*
Workplace infection, 226
Workplace violence, 1644, 1644*b*
Work-related musculoskeletal disorder, 1465
Wound care, 170*b*
for burns, 439-440
closed method, 440, 440*f*
dressings, 168, 169*b*
open method, 440
for surgical wounds, **343**
tetanus vaccines and TIG for, 1634*b*
Wound dehiscence, 343
Wound healing, 720
in burns, 436-437
complications of, 166, 167*b*
drug therapy for, 170
factors delaying, 167, 168*b*
in fractures, **1469-1470**
granulation phase, 166, 166*b*
hyperbaric oxygen therapy for, 170
initial phase, 166, 166*b*
maturation phase, 166, 166*b*
nursing and interprofessional management of, **166-172**
nutritional therapy for, 170-171
patient teaching for, 171-172
primary intention, 165-166, 165*f*, 166*b*
process of, **165-166**
secondary intention, 166
tertiary intention, 166
types of, 165, 165*f*
Wound Ostomy Continence Nurses Society, 962
Wounds
chronic, 167
classification of, 166
clean, 168
contaminated, 168-169
full-thickness, 166
Wounds *(Continued)*
measurements, 166, 168*f*
partial-thickness, 166
postoperative infection in, 343
psychologic implications of, 171
superficial, 166
Wright's and Giemsa's stain (Tzanck test), 405*t*
Wryneck, 1456*b*

X

Xalatan (latanoprost), 381*b*
Xalkori (crizotinib), 187*b*
Xarelto (rivaroxaban), 820*b*
Xeljanz (tofacitinib), 1521*b*-1522*b*, 1528
Xenical (orlistat), 884*b*
Xerostomia, 254, 495
Xifaxan (rifaximin), 993*b*
X-linked disorders, 181
X-linked dominant disorders, 182
X-linked genes, 179*b*
X-linked recessive disorders, 181*b*, 182
Xolair (omalizumab), 548*b*-549*b*, 549
Xopenex (levalbuterol), 548*b*-549*b*
Xpert EV test, 1341
X-rays, 1455-1457
chest, 469*t*-471*t*, **671**, 671*f*, 673*t*-677*t*
in acute pericarditis, 785, 786*f*
in TB, 508
kidneys, ureters, bladder (KUB), 1025*t*-1030*t*
lower gastrointestinal series, 845-851, 847*t*-850*t*, 851*f*
skeletal, 603*t*
skull, 1310*t*-1312*t*
small bowel series, 847*t*-850*t*
spine, 1310*t*-1312*t*
standard, 1457*t*-1459*t*
upper gastrointestinal series, 845, 847*t*-850*t*
Xtandi (enzalutamide), 1280*b*
Xyzal (levocetirizine), 479*b*-480*b*

Y

Yeast infections, 1250
Yoga, 83*b*
Young men, 1235*b*
Young-old adults, 63

Z

Zafirlukast (Accolate), 479*b*-480*b*, 547, 548*b*-549*b*
Zanaflex (tizanidine), 116*b*, 1385*b*
Zantac (ranitidine), 903*b*
Zaroxolyn (metolazone), 691*b*-693*b*, 745*b*
Zebeta (bisoprolol), 691*b*-693*b*, 745*b*
Zecuity (sumatriptan transdermal system), 1372
Zegerid (omeprazole and sodium bicarbonate), 903*b*
Zenapax (daclizumab), 210, 211*b*
Zenker's diverticulum, 907
Zenpep (pancrelipase), 1001*b*, 1004
Zestril (lisinopril), 691*b*-693*b*, 715*b*-716*b*
Zetia (ezetimibe), 711*b*
Ziagen (abacavir), 187*b*
Zig-zag deformity, 1527
Zileuton (Zyflo), 479*b*-480*b*, 547, 548*b*-549*b*
Zinbryta (daclizumab), 1378*b*
Zinc, 482*b*, 1655*b*-1658*b*
Zinc deficiency, 168*b*
Zocor (simvastatin), 710*b*-711*b*
Zofran (ondansetron), 326*b*, 895*b*
Zoladex (goserelin), 1280*b*
Zoledronic acid (Reclast), 1513
Zoledronic acid (Zometa), 646, 646*b*
Zollinger-Ellison syndrome, 912
Zontivity (vorapaxar), 715*b*-716*b*
Zonule, 351
Zoonosis, 215
Zortress (everolimus), 211*b*
Zutripro oral solution (hydrocodone, chlorpheniramine, and pseudoephedrine), 479*b*-480*b*
Zyban (bupropion), 147-148, 148*b*, 150*b*
Zyflo (zileuton), 479*b*-480*b*, 547, 548*b*-549*b*
Zygomatic arch fracture, 1486*b*
Zyrtec (cetirizine), 479*b*-480*b*
Zytiga (abiraterone), 1280*b*

ABBREVIATIONS

ABG	arterial blood gas
ACE	angiotensin-converting enzyme
ACLS	advanced cardiac life support
ACS	acute coronary syndrome
ACTH	adrenocorticotropic hormone
ADH	antidiuretic hormone
AED	automatic external defibrillator
AIDS	acquired immunodeficiency syndrome
AKA	above-knee amputation
AKI	acute kidney injury
ALI	acute lung injury
ALL	acute lymphocytic leukemia
ALS	amyotrophic lateral sclerosis
AMI	acute myocardial infarction
ANA	antinuclear antibody
ANS	autonomic nervous system
AORN	Association of periOperative Room Nurses
APD	automated peritoneal dialysis
aPTT	activated partial thromboplastin time
ARDS	acute respiratory distress syndrome
ATN	acute tubular necrosis
BCLS	basic cardiac life support
BKA	below-knee amputation
BMI	body mass index
BMR	basal metabolic rate
BMT	bone marrow transplantation
BPH	benign prostatic hyperplasia
BSE	breast self-examination
BUN	blood urea nitrogen
CABG	coronary artery bypass graft
CAD	coronary artery disease; circulatory assist device
CAPD	continuous ambulatory peritoneal dialysis
CAVH	continuous arteriovenous hemofiltration
CBC	complete blood count
CCU	coronary care unit; critical care unit
CDC	Centers for Disease Control and Prevention
CIS	carcinoma in situ
CKD	chronic kidney disease
CLL	chronic lymphocytic leukemia
CML	chronic myelocytic leukemia
CMP	cardiomyopathy
CN	cranial nerve
CNS	central nervous system
CO	cardiac output
COPD	chronic obstructive pulmonary disease
CPAP	continuous positive airway pressure
CPR	cardiopulmonary resuscitation
CRRT	continuous renal replacement therapy
CRNA	certified registered nurse anesthetist
CSF	cerebrospinal fluid
CT	computed tomography
CVA	cerebrovascular accident; costovertebral angle
CVAD	central venous access device
CVI	chronic venous insufficiency
CVP	central venous pressure
D&C	dilation and curettage
DDD	degenerative disk disease
DI	diabetes insipidus
DIC	disseminated intravascular coagulation
DJD	degenerative joint disease
DKA	diabetic ketoacidosis
DM	diabetes mellitus; diastolic murmur
DRE	digital rectal examination
DVT	deep vein thrombosis
ECF	extracellular fluid
ECG	electrocardiogram
ED	emergency department; erectile dysfunction
EEG	electroencephalogram
EMG	electromyogram
EMS	emergency medical services
ENT	ear, nose, and throat
ERCP	endoscopic retrograde cholangiopancreatography
ERT	estrogen replacement therapy
ESKD	end-stage kidney disease
ESR	erythrocyte sedimentation rate
ET	endotracheal
FEV	forced expiratory volume
FRC	functional residual capacity
FUO	fever of unknown origin
GCS	Glasgow Coma Scale
GERD	gastroesophageal reflux disease
GFR	glomerular filtration rate
GH	growth hormone
GI	glycemic index
GTT	glucose tolerance test
GU	genitourinary
GYN, Gyn	gynecologic
HAI	health care–associated infection
HAV	hepatitis A virus
Hb, Hgb	hemoglobin
HBV	hepatitis B virus
Hct	hematocrit
HCV	hepatitis C virus
HD	hemodialysis, Huntington's disease
HDL	high-density lipoprotein
HF	heart failure
HIV	human immunodeficiency virus
H&P	history and physical examination
HPV	human papillomavirus
HSCT	hematopoietic stem cell transplantation
IABP	intraaortic balloon pump
IBS	irritable bowel syndrome
ICP	intracranial pressure
I&D	incision and drainage
IE	infective endocarditis
IFG	impaired fasting glucose
IGT	impaired glucose tolerance
INR	international normalized ratio
IOP	intraocular pressure
IPPB	intermittent positive-pressure breathing
ITP	idiopathic thrombocytopenic purpura
IUD	intrauterine device
IV	intravenous
IVP	intravenous push; intravenous pyelogram
JVD	jugular venous distention
KS	Kaposi sarcoma
KUB	kidney, ureters, and bladder (x-ray)
KVO	keep vein open
LAD	left anterior descending
LDL	low-density lipoprotein